PRODUCT ALERT

Ingenix has you covered!

April ICD-9-CM Updates

CMS has proposed semi-annual ICD-9-CM changes effective April 1 and October 1 to comply with the provision of the Medicare Prescription Drug, Improvement, and Modernization Act of 2003 (MMA). That means now, more than ever in order to be compliant with HIPAA regulations, it's important to be ready with up-to-date ICD-9-CM coding information.

Ingenix is committed to providing you and your staff with the ICD-9-CM code update information you need to code accurately and efficiently. We are offering several ways to make sure you are always up-to-date.

- **Updateable Edition of ICD-9-CM Expert.** With three updates a year, you never have to worry about your codes being out of date. Whether you already own an *ICD-9-CM Expert Updateable* edition or you are thinking about purchasing one, you can be confident that you will have code changes in your mailbox before their effective dates.

- **IngenixExpert.com.** Access the same features of *ICD-9-CM Expert* right through your Internet connection. The same trusted information you already use—is now online for even greater speed and convenience. You'll never have to worry about outdated codes again with up-to-the-minute updates every time you log on.

- **ICD-9-CM Expert and Professional coding books.** For customers who own or are thinking about buying *ICD-9-CM Expert* or *ICD-9-CM Professional,* Ingenix will help you prepare for the additional ICD-9-CM code changes in April

by providing the code changes to you online at no additional cost. Just visit IngenixOnline often and look for the ICD-9-CM update icon to review the latest available updates.

No extra charges for code changes. No additional cost for updated books. No hassle for you or your staff.

Revised Coding Guidelines

Under HIPAA regulations failure to comply with the official coding guidelines may result in denied and delayed claims. Ingenix includes the complete official coding guidelines in every ICD-9-CM code book.

Due to the extensive changes to the ICD-9-CM code set effective October 1, 2004, the ICD-9-CM Coordination and Maintenance Committee is in the process of revising the coding guidelines.

The ICD-9-CM Coordination and Maintenance Committee had not released the revised official coding guidelines in time to be included in the 2005 editions. The guidelines are expected to be released in October and will be included in the February update for the *ICD-9-CM Expert Updateable* editions.

For all our customers, the revised guidelines will be available on our web site. Please visit www.ingenixonline.com and look for the ICD-9-CM update icon to review the latest available information.

Look for this icon:

ICD-9-CM Special Notice:
Ingenix has you covered ⚠

2005 Web Products

Up-to-Date. Affordable. Accurate. Fast. The IngenixExpert.com Product Suite

ICD-9-CM Expert.com for Physicians

Item No.: 1402   Available: Now
$79.95

ICD-9-CM Expert.com for Hospitals

Item No.: 1403   Available: Now
$89.95

HCPCS Expert.com

Item No.: 1401   Available: Now
$69.95

CPT® Expert.com

Item No.: 1400   Available: Now
$74.95

FREE 30 Day Trial!

You can access the same features of our best-selling *ICD-9-CM Expert, HCPCS Level II Expert,* and *CPT® Expert* code books, in real-time, right through your Internet connection! It's the same trusted information you already use—now online for even greater speed and convenience.

- **Bypass the index!** Our powerful search engine takes you to the codes you need. Enter a term, abbreviation, or acronym to get clinical code results instantly.

- **Get continuously updated content.** Know you are coding efficiently from the latest codes, descriptions, and guidelines, including revisions and errata.

- **Code more confidently with robust clinical information and color-coded edits.** Extensive appendices, commonly miscoded procedures, Medicare requirements, and glossaries are on-screen, right at your fingertips.

- **Improve your understanding of procedures and anatomy.** Anatomical illustrations are included to help you make the best possible coding selection.

If it's in the book, it's better online!

Discover the speed, precision, and value that only **IngenixExpert.com** products can provide…FREE for 30 days! Visit www.ingenixexpert.com to sign up for your trial today!

100% Money Back Guarantee:
If our merchandise* ever fails to meet your expectations, please contact our Customer Service Department toll-free at 1.800.INGENIX (464.3649), option 1, for an immediate response.
*Software: Credit will be granted for unopened packages only.

CPT® Expert is not a replacement for the American Medical Association's CPT® Standard and Professional code books. CPT is a registered trademark of the American Medical Association.

SAVE 5% when you order at www.ingenixonline.com (reference source code FOBW5)

or call toll-free 1.800.INGENIX (464.3649), option 1.

Also available from your medical bookstore or distributor.   FOBA5

ingenix

Instantly Access Current, Code-specific Information ONLINE.

EncoderPro.com

Standard	Item No.: 1137	**$249.95***
Professional	Item No.: 1221	**$499.95***
Expert	Item No.: 1127	**$899.95***

*Call for multi-user pricing.

Available: Now
High speed Internet connection recommended.

Rely on real-time information to make the right code selections—don't wait for updates! Count on our market-leading customer support team to assist you with any *EncoderPro.com* questions.

EncoderPro.com

- **Easily search all three code sets simultaneously.** Powerful Code Lookup across CPT®, HCPCS, and ICD-9-CM code sets with Ingenix Code Logic™ Search Engine.

- **Enhance your understanding of procedures.** Ingenix lay descriptions help you identify the differences between and among procedures with easy-to-understand explanations.

- **Expand your understanding of anatomy.** Illustrations detailing body parts and procedures can help you make the best possible coding selection.

- **Quickly reference important coding guidelines.** HCPCS annotations and ICD-9-CM section notes help even beginner coders select the correct codes quickly.

EncoderPro.com/Professional offers all of the features from *EncoderPro.com*, plus:

- **Access medically necessary diagnoses for your selected procedures by using LMRP medical necessity edits.**

- **Minimize billing errors by referencing Medicare NCCI edits.** Receive quarterly NCCI unbundling edits.

EncoderPro.com/Expert offers even more value:

- **Stay in compliance and increase accurate reimbursement.** Use the compliance edit module to check for medical necessity verification, unbundled codes, and ICD-9-CM specificity.

- **Quickly reference charges for procedures in the Medicare physician fee schedule.** Includes calculated fees by locality.

CPT is a registered trademark of the American Medical Association.

SAVE 5% when you order at www.ingenixonline.com (reference source code FOBW5)

or call toll-free 1.800.INGENIX (464.3649), option 1.

Also available from your medical bookstore or distributor.

FOBA5

2005 Publications

Expedite claim submission with an enhanced CPT® coding resource

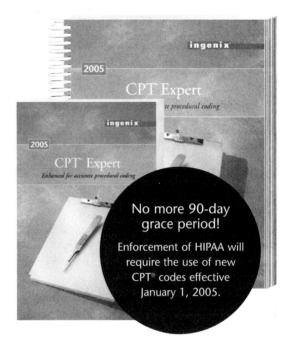

No more 90-day grace period!

Enforcement of HIPAA will require the use of new CPT® codes effective January 1, 2005.

2005 CPT® Expert (Spiral)

Item No.: 4566   **$94.95**
Available: December 2004   ISBN: 1-56337-562-1

2005 CPT® Expert (Compact)

Item No.: 4565   **$79.95**
Available: December 2004   ISBN: 1-56337-563-X

Interpret annual CPT® code changes, understand their implications, and apply them appropriately to expedite claim submission with the *CPT® Expert*. A one-of-a-kind resource, the *CPT® Expert* provides not only 2005 CPT® codes, but guidance on how to improve your coding precision and increase coding efficiency. Stop searching through more complicated code books and software for answers to easily solvable coding questions— reach for the *CPT® Expert.*

- **NEW! Find out how to best apply a CPT® code.** *CPT® Assistant* references are included to help provide guidance and practical advice.

- **EXCLUSIVE! Improve the precision of CPT® coding selection.** Information from the AMA, CMS, the *Medicare Coverage Manual,* the *Coverage Issues Manual* and Ingenix experts helps you better understand the rules, regulations, and guidelines that affect your CPT® code selection.

- **Access a complete, comprehensive listing of CPT® codes.** All 2005 CPT® codes are included, along with their official, full descriptions.

- **Determine which codes are payable under OPPS and how.** APC status indicators are included.

- **Know which codes can be billed using ASC groupings.** ASC designation symbols are provided.

- **Complete unfinished claims requiring deleted 2004 CPT® codes.** Deleted codes from 2004 and their complete descriptions are included, but denoted with strike-outs.

- **Easily identify commonly miscoded codes, unlisted codes, and codes not covered by Medicare.** Color keys mark the CPT® codes that can affect your Medicare reimbursement.

- **Know how to best report particular codes.** Icons identify the codes that are affected by Medicare rules.

- **Increase claim submission speed.** Short, simple introductions to each chapter provide tips and instruction.

- **Save time locating the information you need.** An extensive index helps you code with increased speed and proficiency.

- **Keep current with corrections to CPT® codes and other late-breaking news.** Alerts are sent via e-mail to provide valuable code change information.

100% Money Back Guarantee:

If our merchandise* ever fails to meet your expectations, please contact our Customer Service Department toll-free at 1.800.INGENIX (464.3649), option 1, for an immediate response.
*Software: Credit will be granted for unopened packages only.

The *CPT® Expert* is not a replacement for the American Medical Association's *CPT® Standard* and *Professional* code books. CPT is a registered trademark of the American Medical Association.

SAVE 5% when you order at www.ingenixonline.com (reference source code FOBW5)

or call toll-free 1.800.INGENIX (464.3649), option 1.

Also available from your medical bookstore or distributor.

The official source for procedural codes and guidelines—the 2005 AMA CPT® books

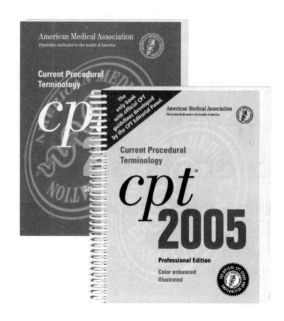

2005 CPT® Standard (Perfect Bound)

Item No.: 4474   **$62.95**

Available: October 2004   ISBN: 1-57947-578-7

2005 CPT® Professional (Spiral)

Item No.: 4457   **$86.95**

Available: October 2004   ISBN: 1-57947-579-5

The American Medical Association (AMA) makes hundreds of CPT® code changes each year. Coders need the official, comprehensive resource to help them avoid using the wrong codes and prevent potential delays in reimbursement.

The *CPT® Standard* and the *CPT® Professional*, published by the AMA, are the official sources of this information. Easy-to-use and easy-to-understand, each reference provides over 7,000 official CPT® codes and the rules you need to know to use them efficiently for optimal reimbursement.

- **EXCLUSIVE to the 2005 CPT® Professional book! Access the latest official codes.** Use of the official codes is required by CMS to be in compliance with HIPAA regulations.

- **EXCLUSIVE to the 2005 CPT® Professional book! Improve efficiency when searching for specific CPT® codes.** Each page includes color-coding, icons, and bars—all designed to help you code with increased speed and proficiency.

- **EXCLUSIVE to the 2005 CPT® Professional book! Locate descriptions, tips, and rulings regarding specific CPT® codes with ease.** *CPT® Assistant* references are included to help provide guidance and practical advice.

- **Stay up-to-date on hundreds of code changes.** All of the CPT® codes, their descriptions, and the official rules and guidelines are included.

- **Quickly find the CPT® code you need.** A comprehensive index—by procedure, service, organ, condition, eponym, synonym, and abbreviation—makes searching fast.

- **Better understand rules and procedures.** Refer to the visual references for help with coding selection.

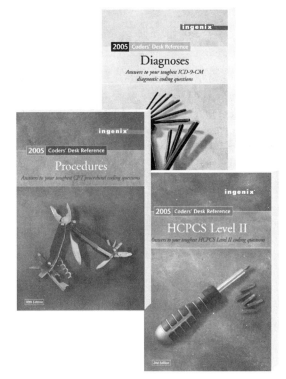

Answers to the toughest coding questions

2005 Coders' Desk References

Coders' Desk Reference for Procedures
Item No.: 5764   Available: December 2004
ISBN: 1-56337-598-2   **$119.95**

Coders' Desk Reference for Diagnoses
Item No.: 5766   Available: September 2004
ISBN: 1-56337-599-0   **$119.95**

Coders' Desk Reference for HCPCS Level II
Item No.: 4975   Available: December 2004
ISBN: 1-56337-600-8   **$119.95**

With the nationwide shortage of coders continuing, new coders are expected to be proficient right away...while experienced coders are under pressure to be more productive than ever before. That's why Ingenix has created a comprehensive *Coders' Desk Reference* suite for all three code sets, creating an essential power suite for every health care professional.

- **Decrease coding time with comprehensive lay descriptions.** Clinical explanations clarify procedures in *Coders' Desk Reference for Procedures,* indicate the disease processes and causes of conditions in *Coders' Desk Reference for Diagnoses* and simplify HCPCS Level II codes by describing supplies and services in *Coders' Desk Reference for HCPCS.*

- **Reduce costly claim delays and denials by always using the latest code sets.** All *Coders' Desk References* conform to standard code book organization and use updated codes for 2005.

- **New coders: Master the intricacies of coding, documentation, and billing. Veteran health care professionals: Code faster and more efficiently.** The suite offers advice to avoid common coding errors and includes anatomical charts, eponyms, acronyms and medical abbreviations.

100% Money Back Guarantee:
If our merchandise* ever fails to meet your expectations, please contact our Customer Service Department toll-free at 1.800.INGENIX (464.3649), option 1, for an immediate response.
*Software: Credit will be granted for unopened packages only.

CPT is a registered trademark of the American Medical Association.

Four simple ways to place an order.

Call
1.800.ingenix (464.3649), **option 1.** Mention source code FOBA5 when ordering.

Mail
PO Box 27116
Salt Lake City, UT 84127-0116
With payment and/or purchase order.

Fax
801.982.4033
With credit card information and/or purchase order.

Click
www.ingenixonline.com
Save 5% when you order online today—use source code FOBW5.

ingenix *e*smart
ingenix online frequent buyer program

GET REWARDS FOR SHOPPING ONLINE!
To find out more, visit IngenixOnline.com

E-Smart program available only to Ingenix customers who are not part of Medallion, Gold Medallion or Partner Accounts programs. You must be registered at Ingenix Online to have your online purchases tracked for rewards purposes. Shipping charges and taxes still apply and cannot be used for rewards. Offer valid online only.

100% Money Back Guarantee
If our merchandise* ever fails to meet your expectations, please contact our Customer Service Department toll-free at 1.800.ingenix (464.3649), option 1 for an immediate response.

*Software: Credit will be granted for unopened packages only.

Customer Service Hours
7:00 am - 5:00 pm Mountain Time
9:00 am - 7:00 pm Eastern Time

Shipping and Handling

no. of items	fee
1	$10.95
2-4	$12.95
5-7	$14.95
8-10	$19.95
11+	Call

---

ingenix

Order Form

Information

Customer No. _____ Contact No. _____

Purchase Order No. _____ Source Code _____
ATTACH COPY OF PURCHASE ORDER

Contact Name _____

Title _____ Specialty _____

Company _____

Street Address _____
NO PO BOXES, PLEASE

City _____ State _____ Zip _____

Telephone ( ) _____ Fax ( ) _____
IN CASE WE HAVE QUESTIONS ABOUT YOUR ORDER

E-mail _____ @ _____
REQUIRED FOR ORDER CONFIRMATION AND SELECT PRODUCT DELIVERY.

Ingenix respects your right to privacy. We will not sell or rent your e-mail address or fax number to anyone outside Ingenix and its business partners. If you would like to remove your name from Ingenix promotion, please call 1.800.ingenix (464.3649), option 1.

Product

Item No.	Qty	Description	Price	Total

Subtotal _____

UT, OH, & VA residents, please add applicable Sales tax _____

(See chart on the left) Shipping & handling charges _____
All foreign orders, please call for shipping costs

Total _____

Payment

○ Please bill my credit card ○ MasterCard ○ VISA ○ Amex ○ Discover

Card No. | | | | | | | | | | | | | | | | | Expires |
MONTH   YEAR

Signature _____

○ Check enclosed, made payable to: Ingenix, Inc. ○ Please bill my office

Purchase Order No. _____

© 2004 Ingenix, Inc. All prices subject to change without notice.

FOBA5

2005

ingenix®

ICD-9-CM
Expert

for Physicians
Volumes 1 & 2

International Classification of Diseases
9th Revision
Clinical Modification

Sixth Edition

Edited by:
Anita C. Hart, RHIA, CCS, CCS-P
Catherine A. Hopkins, CPC

Ingenix is committed to providing you with the ICD-9-CM code update information you need to code accurately and to be in compliance with HIPAA regulations. In the case of adoption of additional ICD-9-CM code changes effective April 1, 2005, Ingenix will provide these code changes to you at no additional cost! Just check back at http://www.IngenixOnline.com and look for the ICD-9-CM Update icon to review the latest information concerning any new code changes.

Codes Valid October 1, 2004, through September 30, 2005

Additional copies may be ordered from:

Your local bookstore
or
1-800-INGENIX (464-3649)

IPES ISBN 1-56337-584-2

PUBLISHER'S NOTICE

All the codes, indexes and other material in the ICD-9-CM are compiled from official ICD-9-CM codes and instructions as well as the Medicare regulations and manuals issued or authorized by the Centers for Medicare and Medicaid Services (formerly know as Health Care Financing Administration). The code book is designed to provide accurate and authoritative information in regard to the subject covered, and every reasonable effort has been made to ensure the accuracy of the information within these pages. However, the ultimate responsibility for correct coding lies with the provider of services.

Ingenix, Inc., its employees, agents and staff make no representation, warranty or guarantee that this compilation of codes and narratives is error-free or that the use of this code book will prevent differences of opinion or disputes with Medicare or other third-party payers as to the codes that are accepted or the amounts that will be paid to providers of services, and will bear no responsibility or liability for the results or consequences of the use of this code book.

CONTINUING EDUCATION UNITS FOR AAPC CERTIFIED MEMBERS

This publication has prior approval by the American Academy of Professional Coders for continuing education units. Granting of prior approval in no way constitutes endorsement by AAPC of the publication content nor the publisher. Instructions to submit CEUs are available at www.aapc.com/education/ceus.htm.

SPECIAL REPORTS AND ANNOUNCEMENTS

Purchase of this publication entitles you to Special Reports and announcements via e-mail. Please call customer service at 800 INGENIX (464-3649) or contact your bookstore to take advantage of this exciting new free service that will keep you abreast of important code changes and regulatory developments.

Review, download, and print the Special Reports in .pdf format. Log on to http://www.ingenixonline.com/content/2005I9Expert

Preface

ICD-9-CM for Physicians has been designed with the physician office coder in mind. The most recent official government versions of volumes 1 and 2 have been combined to provide physicians and their office staff with an ICD-9-CM book that is easy to use.

In addition, our technical experts have drawn upon their extensive hands-on experience to enhance the government's official version with valuable features essential to correct coding and reimbursement. With these enhancements, physician office health information professionals will increase the efficiency and timeliness of claim submission for both Medicare and other third-party payers.

As you review the content, you'll find the following:

- All the official ICD-9-CM codes, indexes, notes, footnotes and symbols
- Complete official coding guidelines
- Our exclusive color coding, symbols, and footnotes that alert coders to coding and reimbursement issues. Medicare outpatient code edits, such as invalid fourth or fifth digit for diagnosis codes and circumstances under which Medicare may be secondary payer (MSP), are identified.
- Illustrations and clinically oriented definitions to aid in correct code assignment
- Symbols identifying new codes and text revisions; pages are dated to indicate when the changes were made
- Exclusive QuickFlip Color Tabs for quick, easy location of terms and codes in the index and tabular list

USE OF OFFICIAL SOURCES

This *ICD-9-CM for Physicians* contains the official U.S. Department of Health and Human Services, ICD-9-CM codes, effective for the current year.

The color coding, footnotes and symbols, which identify coding and reimbursement issues, are derived from official federal government sources, including the Medicare Outpatient Code Editor as well as the knowledge of our technical experts.

The American Hospital Association's (AHA) *Coding Clinic for ICD-9-CM* references are used with permission of the AHA.

IMPORTANT INFORMATION ABOUT YOUR SUBSCRIPTION SERVICE

If you have purchased the updateable *ICD-9-CM for Physicians*, your subscription includes an updating service throughout the year to keep the code book current and accurate. Whenever CMS issues changes or corrections to the ICD-9-CM codes, We will issue an update to the book. In July you will receive a list of all new, revised, and invalid codes for the upcoming year.

TECHNICAL EDITORS

Anita C. Hart, RHIA, CCS, CCS-P
Product Manager, Ingenix, Inc.

Ms. Hart's experience includes 15 years conducting and publishing research in clinical medicine and human genetics for Yale University, Massachusetts General Hospital, and Massachusetts Institute of Technology. In addition, Ms. Hart has supervised medical records management, health information management, coding and reimbursement, and worker's compensation issues as the office manager for a physical therapy rehabilitation clinic. Ms. Hart is an expert in physician and facility coding, reimbursement systems, and compliance issues. Ms. Hart developed the *Complete Coding Tutor, ICD-9-CM Changes: An Insider View,* and has served as technical consultant for numerous other publications for hospital and physician practices. Currrently, Ms. Hart is the Product Manager and Technical Editor for the ICD-9-CM, ICD-10-CM/PCS and DRG product lines.

Catherine A. Hopkins, CPC
Clinical/Technical Editor, Ingenix, Inc.

Ms. Hopkins has 17 years of experience in the health care field. Her experience includes six years as office manager and senior coding specialist for a large multi-specialty practice. Ms. Hopkins has written several coding manuals and newsletters and has taught seminars on CPT, HCPCS, and ICD-9-CM coding. She also serves as technical support for various software products.

In addition to the editors, the following people have contributed to this book:

Sheri Bernard, *Senior Product Director*
Lynn Speirs, *Senior Director, Publishing Services*
Stacy Perry, *Desktop Publishing Manager*
Kerrie Hornsby, *Desktop Publishing Manager*
Tracy Betzler, *Desktop Publishing Specialist*
Irene Day, *Desktop Publishing Specialist*
Gregory Kemp, *Desktop Publishing Specialist*
Paul Driscoll, *Illustrator*

WHAT TO DO IF YOU HAVE QUESTIONS

If you have any questions call our customer service department toll-free at 800-INGENIX (464-3649), option 1.

If you have comments on the content of this book, please e-mail them to customerservice@ingenix.com or fax to 801-982-4033.

ADDITIONAL COPIES

Contact the customer service order department toll-free at 800-INGENIX (464-3649), option 1.

Introduction

HISTORY AND FUTURE OF ICD-9

The *International Classification of Diseases, Ninth Revision, Clinical Modification* (ICD-9-CM) is based on the official version of the World Health Organization's Ninth Revision, International Classification of Diseases (ICD-9). ICD-9-CM classifies morbidity and mortality information for statistical purposes, indexing of hospital records by disease and operations, data storage, and retrieval.

This modification of ICD-9 supplants the Eighth Revision International Classification of Diseases, Adapted for Use in the United States (ICDA-8) and the Hospital Adaptation of ICDA (H-ICDA).

The concept of extending the *International Classification of Diseases* for use in hospital indexing was originally developed in response to a need for a more efficient basis for storage and retrieval of diagnostic data. In 1950, the U.S. Public Health Service and the Veterans Administration began independent tests of the International Classification of Diseases for hospital indexing purposes. The following year, the Columbia Presbyterian Medical Center in New York City adopted the International Classification of Diseases, Sixth Revision, with some modifications for use in its medical record department. A few years later, the Commission on Professional and Hospital Activities (CPHA) in Ann Arbor, Mich., adopted the International Classification of Diseases with similar modifications for use in hospitals participating in the Professional Activity Study.

The problem of adapting ICD for indexing hospital records was addressed by the U.S. National Committee on Vital and Health Statistics through its subcommittee on hospital statistics. The subcommittee reviewed the modifications made by the various users of ICD and proposed that uniform changes be made. This was done by a small working party.

In view of the growing interest in the use of the International Classification of Diseases for hospital indexing, a study was undertaken in 1956 by the American Hospital Association and the American Medical Record Association (then the American Association of Medical Record Librarians) of the relative efficiencies of coding systems for diagnostic indexing. This study indicated the International Classification of Diseases provided a suitable and efficient framework for indexing hospital records. The major users of the International Classification of Diseases for hospital indexing purposes then consolidated their experiences, and an adaptation was first published in December 1959. A revision was issued in 1962 and the first "Classification of Operations and Treatments" was included.

In 1966, the international conference for revising the International Classification of Diseases noted the eighth revision of ICD had been constructed with hospital indexing in mind and considered the revised classification suitable, in itself, for hospital use in some countries. However, it was recognized that the basic classification might provide inadequate detail for diagnostic indexing in other countries. A group of consultants was asked to study the eighth revision of ICD (ICD-8) for applicability to various users in the United States. This group recommended that further detail be provided for coding of hospital and morbidity data. The American Hospital Association was requested to develop the needed adaptation proposals. This was done by an advisory committee (the Advisory Committee to the Central Office on ICDA). In 1968 the United States Public Health Service published the product, Eighth Revision International Classification of Diseases, Adapted for Use in the United States. This became commonly known as ICDA-8, and beginning in 1968 it served as the basis for coding diagnostic data for both official morbidity and mortality statistics in the United States.

In 1968, the CPHA published the Hospital Adaptation of ICDA (H-ICDA) based on both the original ICD-8 and ICDA-8. In 1973, CPHA published a revision of H-ICDA, referred to as H-ICDA-2. Hospitals throughout the United States were divided in their use of these classifications until January 1979, when ICD-9-CM was made the single classification intended primarily for use in the United States, replacing these earlier related, but somewhat dissimilar, classifications.

Physicians have been required by law to submit diagnosis codes for Medicare reimbursement since the passage of the Medicare Catastrophic Coverage Act of 1988. This act requires physician offices to include the appropriate diagnosis codes when billing for services provided to Medicare beneficiaries on or after April 1, 1989. The Centers for Medicare and Medicaid Services (CMS) designated ICD-9-CM as the coding system physicians must use.

In 1993 the World Health Organization published the newest version of International Classification of Diseases, Tenth Revision, ICD-10. This version contains the greatest number of changes in the history of ICD. There are more codes (5,500 more than ICD-9) to allow more specific reporting of diseases and newly recognized conditions. ICD-10 consists of three volumes; tabular list (volume I), instructions (volume 2) and the alphabetic index (volume 3). It contains 21 chapters including two supplementary ones. The codes are alphanumeric (A00–T98, V01–Y98 and Z00–Z99). Currently ICD-10 is being used in some European countries with implementation expected after the year 2007 in the United States.

ICD-9-CM BACKGROUND

In February 1977, a steering committee was convened by the National Center for Health Statistics to provide advice and counsel in developing a clinical modification of ICD-9. The organizations represented on the steering committee included the following:

- American Association of Health Data Systems
- American Hospital Association
- American Medical Record Association
- Association for Health Records
- Council on Clinical Classifications
- Centers for Medicare and Medicaid Services (formerly known as Health Care Financing Administration), Department of Health and Human Services
- WHO Center for Classification of Diseases for North America, sponsored by the National Center for Health Statistics, Department of Health and Human Services

The Council on Clinical Classifications was sponsored by the following:

- American Academy of Pediatrics
- American College of Obstetricians and Gynecologists
- American College of Physicians
- American College of Surgeons
- American Psychiatric Association
- Commission on Professional and Hospital Activities

The steering committee met periodically in 1977. Clinical guidance and technical input were provided by task forces on classification from the Council on Clinical Classification's sponsoring organizations.

ICD-9-CM is a clinical modification of the World Health Organization's ICD-9. The term "clinical" is used to emphasize the modification's intent: to serve as a useful tool to classify morbidity data for indexing medical records, medical care review, and ambulatory and other medical care programs, as well as for basic health statistics. To describe the clinical picture of the patient, the codes must be more precise than those needed only for statistical groupings and trend analysis.

CHARACTERISTICS OF ICD-9-CM

ICD-9-CM far exceeds its predecessors in the number of codes provided. The disease classification has been expanded to include health-related conditions and to provide greater specificity at the fifth-digit level of detail. These fifth digits are not optional; they are intended for use in recording the information substantiated in the clinical record.

Volume I (tabular list) of ICD-9-CM contains four appendices:

Appendix A:	Morphology of Neoplasms
Appendix B:	Deleted effective October 1, 2004
Appendix C:	Classification of Drugs by American Hospital Formulary Service List Number and Their ICD-9-CM Equivalents

These appendices are included as a reference to provide further information about the patient's clinical picture, to further define a diagnostic statement, to aid in classifying new drugs or to reference three-digit categories.

Volume 2 (alphabetic index) of ICD-9-CM contains many diagnostic terms that do not appear in volume I since the index includes most diagnostic terms currently in use.

THE DISEASE CLASSIFICATION

ICD-9-CM is totally compatible with its parent system, ICD-9, thus meeting the need for comparability of morbidity and mortality statistics at the international level. A few fourth-digit codes were created in existing three-digit rubrics only when the necessary detail could not be accommodated by the use of a fifth-digit subclassification. To ensure that each rubric of ICD-9-CM collapses back to its ICD-9 counterpart the following specifications governed the ICD-9-CM disease classification:

Specifications for the tabular list:

1. Three-digit rubrics and their contents are unchanged from ICD-9.

2. The sequence of three-digit rubrics is unchanged from ICD-9.

3. Three-digit rubrics are not added to the main body of the classification.

4. Unsubdivided three-digit rubrics are subdivided where necessary to
    *   add clinical detail
    *   isolate terms for clinical accuracy

5. The modification in ICD-9-CM is accomplished by adding a fifth digit to existing ICD-9 rubrics, except as noted under #7 below.

6. The optional dual classification in ICD-9 is modified.
    *   Duplicate rubrics are deleted:
        –   four-digit manifestation categories duplicating etiology entries
        –   manifestation inclusion terms duplicating etiology entries

    *   Manifestations of disease are identified, to the extent possible, by creating five-digit codes in the etiology rubrics.
    *   When the manifestation of a disease cannot be included in the etiology rubrics, provision for its identification is made by retaining the ICD-9 rubrics used for classifying manifestations of disease.

7. The format of ICD-9-CM is revised from that used in ICD-9.
    *   American spelling of medical terms is used.
    *   Inclusion terms are indented beneath the titles of codes.
    *   Codes not to be used for primary tabulation of disease are printed in italics with the notation, "*code first underlying disease.*"

Specifications for the alphabetic index:

1. The format of the alphabetic index follows that of ICD-9.

2. When two codes are required to indicate etiology and manifestation, the manifestation code appears in brackets (e.g., diabetic cataract 250.5 *[366.41]*).

THE ICD-9-CM COORDINATION AND MAINTENANCE COMMITTEE

The four cooperating parties involved in maintaining the ICD-9-CM classification system include representatives of the American Hospital Association (AHA), the Centers for Medicare and Medicaid Services (CMS), the National Center for Health Statistics (NCHS), and the American Health Information Management Association (AHIMA).

Proposals for changes to the ICD-9-CM classification system are submitted and discussed in two open forum meetings held in April and October of each year at the Headquarters of the Centers for Medicare and Medicaid Services, Baltimore, Maryland. Comments received during and after the meetings are then discussed by the Committee. A notice of the new codes and code revisions approved by the Committee are published in the Federal Register as part of the proposed and final rule for the changes to the inpatient prospective payment system. The complete official document of changes to the classification system is released as the Addenda for the *International Classification of Diseases, Ninth Revision, Clinical Modification, Sixth Edition, Volumes 1, 2 and 3.*

How to Use the ICD-9-CM for Physicians (Volumes 1 & 2)

This *ICD-9-CM for Physicians* is based on the official version of the International Classification of Diseases, Ninth Revision, Clinical Modification, Sixth Edition, issued by the U.S. Department of Health and Human Services. Annual code changes are implemented by the government and are effective Oct. 1 and valid through Sept. 30 of the following year.

To accommodate the coder's approach to coding, the alphabetic index (Volume 2) has been placed before the tabular list (Volume 1). This allows the user to locate the term in the index, then confirm the accuracy of the code in the tabular list.

10 STEPS TO CORRECT CODING

To code accurately, it is necessary to have a working knowledge of medical terminology and to understand the characteristics, terminology and conventions of ICD-9-CM. Transforming descriptions of diseases, injuries, conditions and procedures into numerical designations (coding) is a complex activity and should not be undertaken without proper training.

Originally, coding allowed retrieval of medical information by diagnoses and operations for medical research, education and administration. Coding today is used to describe the medical necessity of a procedure which then facilitates payment of health services, to evaluate utilization patterns and to study the appropriateness of health care costs. Coding provides the basis for epidemiological studies and research into the quality of health care. Incorrect or inaccurate coding can lead to investigations of fraud and abuse. Therefore, coding must be performed correctly and consistently to produce meaningful statistics to aid in planning for the health needs of the nation.

Follow the steps below to code correctly:

Step 1: Identify the reason for the visit (e.g., sign, symptom, diagnosis, condition to be coded).

Physicians describe the patient's condition using terminology that includes specific diagnoses as well as symptoms, problems or reasons for the encounter. If symptoms are present but a definitive diagnosis has not yet been determined, code the symptoms. Do not code conditions that are referred to as "rule out," "suspected," "probable" or "questionable."

Step 2: Always consult the Alphabetic Index, Volume 2, before turning to the tabular list.

The most critical rule is to begin a code search in the index. Never turn first to the Tabular List (Volume 1), as this will lead to coding errors and less specificity in code assignments. To prevent coding errors, use both the alphabetic index and the tabular list when locating and assigning a code.

Step 3: Locate the main entry term.

The Alphabetic Index is arranged by condition. Conditions may be expressed as nouns, adjectives and eponyms. Some conditions have multiple entries under their synonyms. Main terms are identified using boldface type.

Step 4: Read and interpret any notes listed with the main term

Notes are identified using italicized type.

Step 5: Review entries for modifiers

Nonessential modifiers are in parentheses. These parenthetical terms are supplementary words or explanatory information that may either be present or absent in the diagnostic statement and do not affect code assignment.

Step 6: Interpret abbreviations, cross-references, symbols and brackets

Cross-references used are "*see*," "*see* category" or "*see also*." The abbreviation NEC may follow main terms or subterms. NEC (not elsewhere classified) indicates that there is no specific code for the condition even though the medical documentation may be very specific. The ☑ box

indicates the code requires an additional digit. If the appropriate digits are not found in the index, in a box beneath the main term, you MUST refer to the tabular list. Italicized brackets *[ ]*, are used to enclose a second code number that must be used with the code immediately preceding it and in that sequence.

Step 7: Choose a tentative code and locate it in the tabular list.

Be guided by any inclusion or exclusion terms, notes or other instructions, such as "*code first*" and "use additional code," that would direct the use of a different or additional code from that selected in the index for a particular diagnosis, condition or disease.

Step 8: Determine whether the code is at the highest level of specificity.

Assign three-digit codes (category codes) if there are no four-digit codes within the code category. Assign four-digit codes (subcategory codes) if there are no five-digit codes for that category. Assign five-digit codes (fifth-digit subclassification codes) for those categories where they are available.

Step 9: Consult the color coding and reimbursement prompts, including the age, sex and Medicare as secondary payer edits.

Consult the official ICD-9-CM guidelines for coding and reporting, and refer to the AHA's *Coding Clinic for ICD-9-CM* for coding guidelines governing the use of specific codes.

Step 10: Assign the code.

ORGANIZATION

Introduction

The introductory material in this book includes the history and future of ICD-9-CM as well as an overview of the classification system

Official ICD-9-CM Conventions

This section provides a full explanation of all the official footnotes, symbols, instructional notes, and conventions found in the official government version

Additional Conventions

Exclusive color-coding, symbols, and notations have been included in the *ICD-9-CM for Physicians, Volumes 1 and 2* to alert coders to important coding and reimbursement issues. This section provides a full explanation of the additional conventions used throughout this book.

Synopsis of Code Changes

This section includes a complete listing of all code changes for the current year.

Summary of AHA's Coding Clinic for ICD-9-CM Topics

This is a brief summary of the official advice concerning coding topics covered in the latest issues of *AHA's ICD-9-CM Coding Clinic for ICD-9-CM* and is found only in the *ICD-9-CM Expert for Physicians* updateable edition.

Coding Guidelines

Included in this book are the official ICD-9-CM coding guidelines as approved by the four cooperating parties of the ICD-9-CM Coordination and Maintenance Committee. Failure to comply with these official coding guidelines may result in denied or delayed claims.

NOTE: Due to the extensive nature of the revisions, the ICD-9-CM Coordination and Maintenance Committee had not released the revised official coding guidelines in time to be included in this edition. The new guidelines are expected to be released in October and will be available on our web site. Please visit www.IngenixOnline.com and look for the ICD-9-CM update icon to review the latest available information.

Disease Classification: Alphabetic Index to Diseases

The Alphabetic Index to Diseases is separated by tabs labeled with the letters of the alphabet, contains diagnostic terms for illnesses, injuries and reasons for encounters with health care professionals. Both the Table of Drugs and Chemicals and the Alphabetic Index to External Causes of Injury and Poisoning are easily located with the tabs in this section.

Disease Classification: Tabular List of Diseases

The Tabular List of Diseases arranges the ICD-9-CM codes and descriptors numerically. Tabs divide this section into chapters, identified by the code range on the tab.

The tabular list includes two supplementary classifications:

- V Codes—Supplementary Classification of Factors Influencing Health Status and Contact with Health Services (V01–V84)
- E Codes—Supplementary Classification of External Causes of Injury and Poisoning (E800–E999)

ICD-9-CM includes four official appendixes.

- Appendix A   Morphology of Neoplasms
- Appendix B   Deleted effective October 1, 2004
- Appendix C   Classification of Drugs by AHFS List
- Appendix D   Classification of Industrial Accidents According to Agency
- Appendix E   List of Three-digit Categories

These appendices are included as a reference to provide further information about the patient's circumstances, help further define a diagnostic statement, maintain a tumor registry and aid in classifying new drugs.

Resources

Listed below are the exclusive resources found ONLY in the *ICD-9-CM Expert for Physicians, Volumes 1 & 2*.

Valid Three-digit Code Table

ICD-9-CM is composed of codes with either 3, 4, or 5 digits. A code is invalid if it has not been coded to the full number of digits required for that code. There are a certain number codes that are valid for reporting as three digit codes. A list of these valid three-digit code is included as a convenient reference when auditing claims.

Code Tables

Exclusive coding tables covering abortion, burns, complications, diabetes, hernia, pregnancy, and others are provided to simplify those complex coding issues.

ICD-9-CM Official Conventions

ICD-9-CM FOOTNOTES, SYMBOLS, INSTRUCTIONAL NOTES AND CONVENTIONS

This *ICD-9-CM for Physicians* preserves all the footnotes, symbols, instructional notes and conventions found in the government's official version. Accurate coding depends upon understanding the meaning of these elements.

The following appear in the disease tabular list, unless otherwise noted.

OFFICIAL GOVERNMENT SYMBOLS

§ The section mark preceding a code denotes a footnote on the page. This symbol is used only in the Tabular List of Diseases.

ICD-9-CM CONVENTIONS USED IN THE TABULAR LIST

In addition to the symbols and footnotes above, the ICD-9-CM disease tabular has certain abbreviations, punctuation, symbols and other conventions. Our *ICD-9-CM for Physicians* preserves these conventions. Proper use of the conventions will lead to efficient and accurate coding.

Abbreviations

NEC Not elsewhere classifiable

This abbreviation is used when the ICD-9-CM system does not provide a code specific for the patient's condition.

NOS Not otherwise specified

This abbreviation is the equivalent of 'unspecified' and is used only when the coder lacks the information necessary to code to a more specific four-digit subcategory.

[ ] Brackets enclose synonyms, alternative terminology or explanatory phrases:

482.2 Pneumonia due to Hemophilus influenzae [H. influenzae]

Brackets that appear beneath a code indicate the fifth digits that are considered valid fifth digits for the code. This convention is applied for those instances in ICD-9-CM where not all common fifth digits are considered valid for each subcategory within a category.

715.0 Osteoarthrosis, generalized
[0,4,9]

Generalized arthrosis can only be assigned in cases for which the degenerative joint disease involves multiple joints. Therefore, this code is considered for arthrosis in the sites described as unspecified, hand (which consists of multiple joints), or multiple sites. Therefore, only fifth digits 0, 4, and 9 are valid with subcategory 715.0.

[ ] Slanted brackets that appear in the Alphabetic Index indicates mandatory multiple coding. Both codes must be assigned to fully describe the condition and are sequenced in the order listed.

Tachycardia
ventricular (paroxysmal)
psychogenic 316 *[427.1]*

Psychogenic paroxysmal tachycardia is reported using both 316, Psychogenic factors associated with diseases classified elsewhere, and 427.1, Paroxysmal ventricular tachycardia.

( ) Parentheses enclose supplementary words, called nonessential modifiers, that may be present in the narrative description of a disease without affecting the code assignment:

198.4 Other parts of nervous system
Meninges (cerebral) (spinal)

: Colons are used in the tabular list after an incomplete term that needs one or more of the modifiers that follow in order to make it assignable to a given category:

021.1 Enteric tularemia
Tularemia:
cryptogenic
intestinal
typhoidal

} Braces enclose a series of terms, each of which is modified by the statement appearing to the right of the brace:

560.2 Volvulus
Knotting
Strangulation
Torsion
Twist
} of intestine, bowel, or colon

OTHER CONVENTIONS

Boldface Boldface type is used for all codes and titles in the tabular list.

Italicized Italicized type is used for all exclusion notes and to identify codes that should not be used for describing the primary diagnosis.

INSTRUCTIONAL NOTES

These notes appear only in the Tabular List of Diseases

Includes An includes note further defines or clarifies the content of the chapter, subchapter, category, subcategory or subclassification. The includes note in the example below applies only to category 461.

Excludes Terms following the word "*Excludes*" are not classified to the chapter, subchapter, category, subcategory or specific subclassification code under which it is found. The note also may provide the location of the excluded diagnosis. Excludes notes are italicized.

461 Acute sinusitis

INCLUDES
abscess
empyema
infection
inflammation
suppuration
} acute, of sinus
(accessory)
(nasal)

EXCLUDES *chronic or unspecified sinusitis (473.0-473.9)*

Use additional code:

This instruction signals the coder that an additional code should be used if the information is available to provide a more complete picture of that diagnosis.

362.13 Changes in vascular appearance
Vascular sheathing of retina
Use additional code for any associated atherosclerosis (440.8)

There are coding circumstances outside of the etiology/ manifestation convention when multiple coding for a single condition is required. The 'Use additional code' note will be found under the associated condition code in the tabular. In the index, the multiple coding requirement is indicated by the use of the slanted bracket. The two codes are to be sequenced as listed in the index. For example, retinal arteriosclerosis must be coded using two codes sequenced as listed in the index.

Arteriosclerosis, arteriosclerotic
retinal (vascular) 440.8 *[362.13]*

Code first underlying disease:

The *Code first underlying disease* instructional note found under certain codes is a sequencing rule. Most often this sequencing rule applies to the etiology/manifestation convention and is found under the manifestation code. The manifestation code may never be used alone or as a primary diagnosis (i.e., sequenced first). The instructional note, the code and its descriptor appear in italics in the tabular list.

590.81   *Pyelitis or pyelonephritis in diseases classified elsewhere*

> *Code first underlying disease as:*
> tuberculosis (016.0)

Not all codes with a 'Code first underlying disease' instructional note are part of the etiology/manifestation convention. The 'Code first' note will appear, but the title of the code and the instructional note are not in italics. These codes may be reported alone or as the secondary diagnosis. For example, disseminated chorioretinitis may be reported as a principal diagnosis. However, if the underlying condition that caused disseminated chorioretinitis is known, such as tuberculous disseminated chorioretinitis, two codes are required and sequenced as listed in the index.

363.13   Disseminated choroiditis and chorioretinitis, generalized

> Code first underlying disease as:
> tuberculosis (017.3)

Code, if applicable, any causal condition first:

A code with this note indicates that this code may be assigned as a principal diagnosis when the causal condition is unknown or not applicable. If a causal condition is known, then the code for that condition should be sequenced as the principal or first-listed diagnosis.

590.0   Chronic pyelonephritis

> Chronic pyelitis
> Chronic pyonephrosis
> Code, if applicable, any causal condition first

Omit code:

"*Omit code*" is used to instruct the coder that no code is to be assigned. When this instruction is found in the Alphabetic Index to Diseases the medical term should not be coded as a diagnosis.

> **Metaplasia**
> cervix—*omit code*

See Condition:

The "*see condition*' note found in the Alphabetic Index to Disease instructs the coder to refer to a main term for the condition. This note will follow index terms that are nouns for anatomical sites or adjectival forms of disease term. In the example below, the index terms 'Cervix' and 'Diffuse' are followed by the — see condition. Coders should search the index using a condition term such as atrophy or prolapse.

> **Cervix** — *see* condition
> **Diffuse**— *see* condition

Morphology Codes:

For each neoplastic disease listed in the index, a morphology code is provided that identifies histological type and behavior.

> **Myelolipoma** (M8870/0)—*see* Neoplasm, by site, benign

The histology is identified by the first four digits and the behavior is identified by the digit following the slash. Appendix A of Volume 1 contains a listing of morphology codes. This appendix is helpful when the pathology report identifies the neoplasm by using an M code. The coder may refer to Appendix A to determine the nomenclature of the neoplasm that will be the main term to search in the Index. The behavior classification is as follows:

0	Benign
1	Uncertain behavior
2	Carcinoma in situ
3	Malignant, primary site
6	Malignant, secondary site.

Additional Conventions

SYMBOLS AND NOTATIONS

New and Revised Text Symbols

●   A bullet at a code or line of text indicates that that the entry is new.

▲   A triangle in the Tabular List indicates that the code title is revised. In the Alphabetic Index the triangle indicates that a code has changed.

►◄   These symbols appear at the beginning and at the end of a section of new or revised text.

When these symbols appear on a page there will be a date on the lower outside corner of the page indicating the date of the change, (e.g., October 2004).

Additional Digits Required

☑4ᵗʰ   This symbol indicates that the code requires a fourth digit.

☑5ᵗʰ   This symbol indicates that a code requires a fifth digit.

☑   This symbol found only in the alphabetic index sections and the Table of Drugs and Chemicals indicates that an additional digit is required. Referring to the tabular section is essential to locate the appropriate additional digit.

AHA's Coding Clinic for ICD-9-CM References

The four cooperating parties have designated the AHA's *Coding Clinic for ICD-9-CM* as the official publication for coding guidelines. The references are identified by the notation AHA: followed by the issue, year and page number.

In the example below, AHA's *Coding Clinic for ICD-9-CM*, third quarter 1991, page 15, contains a discussion on code assignment for vitreous hemorrhage:

379.23   **Vitreous hemorrhage**
         AHA: 3Q, '91, 15

The table below explains the abbreviations in the Coding Clinic references:

J-F	January/February
M-A	March/April
M-J	May/June
J-A	July/August
S-O	September/October
N-D	November/December
1Q	First quarter
2Q	Second quarter
3Q	Third quarter
4Q	Fourth quarter

Age and Sex Edit Symbols

The age edits below address OCE edits and are used to detect inconsistencies between the patient's age and diagnosis. They appear in the Tabular List of Diseases to the right of the code description.

Newborn Age: 0

These diagnoses are intended for newborns and neonates and the patient's age must be 0 years

Pediatric Age: 0-17

These diagnoses are intended for children and the patient's age must between 0 and 17 years

Maternity Age: 12-55

These diagnoses are intended for the patients between the age of 12 and 55 years

Adult Age 15-124

These diagnoses are intended for the patients between the age of 15 and 124 years.

The sex symbols below address OCE edits and are used to detect inconsistencies between the patient's sex and diagnosis. They appear in the Tabular List of Diseases to the right of the code description:

♂   **Male diagnosis only**

This symbol appears to the right of the code description. This reference appears in the disease tabular list.

♀   **Female diagnosis only**

This symbol appears to the right of the code description. This reference appears in the disease tabular list.

COLOR CODING

To alert the coder to Medicare outpatient code edits and other important reimbursement issues, color bars have been added over the code descriptors in the tabular list. Some codes carry more than one color.

Carriers use the Medicare Outpatient Code Editor (OCE) to examine claims for coding and billing accuracy and completeness. Color codes in this book signify Medicare code edits for E codes and manifestation codes as a primary diagnosis, Medicare secondary payer alerts and when a more specific diagnosis or code should be used.

Manifestation Code

These codes will appear in italic type as well as with a blue color bar over the code title. A manifestation code is not allowed to be reported as a primary diagnosis because each describes a manifestation of some other underlying disease, not the disease itself. This is referred to as mandatory multiple coding of etiology and manifestation. Code the underlying disease first. A *Code first underlying disease* instructional note will appear with underlying disease codes identified. In the Alphabetic Index these codes are listed as the secondary code in slanted brackets with the code for the underlying disease listed first.

Other Specified Code

These codes will appear with a gray color bar over the code title. Use these codes when the documentation indicates a specified diagnosis, but the ICD-9-CM system does not have a specific code that describes the diagnosis. These codes are may be stated as "Other" or "Not elsewhere classified (NEC)."

Unspecified Code

These codes will have a yellow color bar over the code title. Use these codes when the neither the diagnostic statement nor the documentation provides enough information to assign a more specified diagnosis code. These codes may be stated as "Unspecified" or "Not otherwise specified (NOS)." Note: Do not assign these codes when a more specific diagnosis has been determined.

OTHER NOTATIONS

DEF: This symbol indicates a definition of disease or procedure term. The definition will appear in blue type in the Disease Tabular Lists.

MSP   This identifies specific trauma codes that alert the carrier that another carrier should be billed first and Medicare billed second if payment from the first payer does not equal or exceed the amount Medicare would pay.

PDx   This symbol identifies a V code that can only be used as a primary diagnosis

SDx   This symbol identifies a V code that can only be used as a secondary diagnosis

      Note: A V code without a symbol may be used as either a primary or secondary diagnosis

Summary of Code Changes

DISEASE TABULAR LIST (VOLUME 1)

Special note: Effective October 1, 2004 the Glossary of Mental Disorders, Appendix B, has been removed from ICD-9-CM.

▲ 041.82 ~~Bacillus~~ ▶Bacteroides◀ fragilis

041.84 Includes term deleted

042 Excludes term revised

062.8 Excludes term revised

066.4 Includes terms deleted

● 066.40 West Nile fever, unspecified
Includes terms added

● 066.41 West Nile fever with encephalitis
Includes terms added

● 066.42 West Nile fever with other neurologic manifestation
Use additional code note added

● 066.49 West Nile fever with other complications
Use additional code note added

▲ 070.41 Acute ~~or unspecified~~ hepatitis C with hepatic coma

▲ 070.51 Acute ~~or unspecified~~ hepatitis C without mention of hepatic coma

070.6 Excludes note added

● 070.7 Unspecified viral hepatitis C

● 070.70 Unspecified viral hepatitis C without hepatic coma
Includes term added

● 070.71 Unspecified viral hepatitis C with hepatic coma

070.9 Excludes note added

176.1 Includes terms revised

176.8 Includes term revised

233.1 Cervix uteri
Includes terms added
Excludes note added

▲ 250.00 Diabetes mellitus without mention of complication, type II ~~[non-insulin dependent type] [NIDDM type] [adult-onset type]~~ or unspecified type, not stated as uncontrolled
Instructional note revised
Use additional code note added

▲ 250.01 Diabetes mellitus without mention of complication, type I ~~[insulin dependent type] [IDDM]~~ [juvenile type], not stated as uncontrolled

▲ 250.02 Diabetes mellitus without mention of complication, type II ~~[non-insulin dependent type] [NIDDM type] [adult-onset type]~~ or unspecified type, uncontrolled
Instructional note revised
Use additional code note added

▲ 250.03 Diabetes mellitus without mention of complication, type I ~~[insulin dependent type] [IDDM]~~ [juvenile type], uncontrolled

▲ 250.10 Diabetes with ketoacidosis, type II ~~[non-insulin dependent type] [NIDDM type] [adult-onset type]~~ or unspecified type, not stated as uncontrolled
Instructional note revised
Use additional code note added

▲ 250.11 Diabetes with ketoacidosis, type I ~~[insulin dependent type] [IDDM]~~ [juvenile type], not stated as uncontrolled

▲ 250.12 Diabetes with ketoacidosis, type II ~~[non-insulin dependent type] [NIDDM type] [adult-onset type]~~ or unspecified type, uncontrolled
Instructional note revised
Use additional code note added

▲ 250.13 Diabetes with ketoacidosis, type I ~~[insulin dependent type] [IDDM]~~ [juvenile type], uncontrolled

▲ 250.20 Diabetes with hyperosmolarity, type II ~~[non-insulin dependent type] [NIDDM type] [adult-onset type]~~ or unspecified type, not stated as uncontrolled
Instructional note revised
Use additional code note added

▲ 250.21 Diabetes with hyperosmolarity, type I ~~[insulin dependent type] [IDDM]~~ [juvenile type], not stated as uncontrolled

▲ 250.22 Diabetes with hyperosmolarity, type II ~~[non-insulin dependent type] [NIDDM type] [adult-onset type]~~ or unspecified type, uncontrolled
Instructional note revised
Use additional code note added

▲ 250.23 Diabetes with hyperosmolarity, type I ~~[insulin dependent type] [IDDM]~~ [juvenile type], uncontrolled

▲ 250.30 Diabetes with other coma, type II ~~[non-insulin dependent type] [NIDDM type] [adult-onset type]~~ or unspecified type, not stated as uncontrolled
Instructional note revised
Use additional code note added

▲ 250.31 Diabetes with other coma, type I ~~[insulin dependent type] [IDDM]~~ [juvenile type], not stated as uncontrolled

▲ 250.32 Diabetes with other coma, type II ~~[non-insulin dependent type] [NIDDM type] [adult-onset type]~~ or unspecified type, uncontrolled
Instructional note revised
Use additional code note added

▲ 250.33 Diabetes with other coma, type I ~~[insulin dependent type] [IDDM]~~ [juvenile type], uncontrolled

▲ 250.40 Diabetes with renal manifestations, type II ~~[non-insulin dependent type] [NIDDM type] [adult-onset type]~~ or unspecified type, not stated as uncontrolled
Instructional note revised
Use additional code note added

▲ 250.41 Diabetes with renal manifestations, type I ~~[insulin dependent type] [IDDM]~~ [juvenile type], not stated as uncontrolled

▲ 250.42 Diabetes with renal manifestations, type II ~~[non-insulin dependent type] [NIDDM type] [adult-onset type]~~ or unspecified type, uncontrolled
Instructional note revised
Use additional code note added

▲ 250.43 Diabetes with renal manifestations, type I ~~[insulin dependent type] [IDDM]~~ [juvenile type], uncontrolled

▲ 250.50 Diabetes with ophthalmic manifestations, type II ~~[non-insulin dependent type] [NIDDM type] [adult-onset type]~~ or unspecified type, not stated as uncontrolled
Instructional note revised
Use additional code note added

▲ 250.51 Diabetes with ophthalmic manifestations, type I ~~[insulin dependent type] [IDDM]~~ [juvenile type], not stated as uncontrolled

▲ 250.52 Diabetes with ophthalmic manifestations, type II ~~[non-insulin dependent type] [NIDDM type] [adult-onset type]~~ or unspecified type, uncontrolled
Instructional note revised
Use additional code note added

▲ 250.53 Diabetes with ophthalmic manifest-ions, type I ~~[insulin dependent type] [IDDM]~~ [juvenile type], uncontrolled

▲ 250.60 Diabetes with neurological manifestations, type II ~~[non-insulin dependent type] [NIDDM type] [adult-onset type]~~ or unspecified type, not stated as uncontrolled
Instructional note revised
Use additional code note added
Use additional code terms added

▲ 250.61 Diabetes with neurological manifestations, type I ~~[insulin dependent type] [IDDM]~~ [juvenile type], not stated as uncontrolled
Use additional code terms added

▲ 250.62 Diabetes with neurological manifestations, type II ~~[non-insulin dependent type] [NIDDM type] [adult-onset type]~~ or unspecified type, uncontrolled
Instructional note revised
Use additional code note added
Use additional code terms added

▲ 250.63 Diabetes with neurological manifestations, type I ~~[insulin dependent type] [IDDM]~~ [juvenile type], uncontrolled
Use additional code terms added

▲ 250.70 Diabetes with peripheral circulatory disorders, type II ~~[non-insulin dependent type] [NIDDM type] [adult-onset type]~~ or unspecified type, not stated as uncontrolled
Instructional note revised
Use additional code note added

▲ 250.71 Diabetes with peripheral circulatory disorders, type I ~~[insulin dependent type] [IDDM]~~ [juvenile type], not stated as uncontrolled

▲ 250.72 Diabetes with peripheral circulatory disorders, type II ~~[non-insulin dependent type] [NIDDM type] [adult-onset type]~~ or unspecified type, uncontrolled
Instructional note revised
Use additional code note added

▲ 250.73 Diabetes with peripheral circulatory disorders, type I ~~[insulin dependent type] [IDDM]~~ [juvenile type], uncontrolled

▲ 250.80 Diabetes with other specified manifestations, type II ~~[non-insulin dependent type] [NIDDM type] [adult-onset type]~~ or unspecified type, not stated as uncontrolled
Instructional note revised
Use additional code note added

▲ 250.81 Diabetes with other specified manifestations, type I ~~[insulin dependent type] [IDDM]~~ [juvenile type], not stated as uncontrolled

▲ 250.82 Diabetes with other specified manifestations, type II ~~[non-insulin dependent type] [NIDDM type] [adult-onset type]~~ or unspecified type, uncontrolled
Instructional note revised
Use additional code note added

▲ 250.83 Diabetes with other specified manifestations, type I ~~[insulin dependent type] [IDDM]~~ [juvenile type], uncontrolled

▲ 250.90 Diabetes with unspecified complication, type II ~~[non-insulin dependent type] [NIDDM type] [adult-onset type]~~ or unspecified type, not stated as uncontrolled
Instructional note revised
Use additional code note added

▲ 250.91 Diabetes with other unspecified complication, type I ~~[insulin dependent type] [IDDM]~~ [juvenile type], not stated as uncontrolled

▲ 250.92 Diabetes with other unspecified complication, type II ~~[non-insulin dependent type] [NIDDM type] [adult-onset type]~~ or unspecified type, uncontrolled
Instructional note revised
Use additional code note added

▲ 250.93 Diabetes with other unspecified complication, type I ~~[insulin dependent type] [IDDM]~~ [juvenile type], uncontrolled

252.0 Includes terms deleted
Excludes term deleted

● 252.00 Hyperparathyroidism, unspecified

● 252.01 Primary hyperparathyroidism
Includes term revised

● 252.02 Secondary hyperparathyroidism, non-renal
Excludes note added

▶◀ Revised Text ● New Code ▲ Revised Code Title

● 252.08 Other hyperparathyroidism
Includes term added
255.10 Excludes note added
255.11 Excludes note added
● 273.4 Alpha-1-antitrypsin deficiency
Includes term added
275.4 Excludes term revised
277.6 Includes term deleted
● 277.85 Disorders of fatty acid oxidation
Includes terms added
Excludes note added
● 277.86 Peroxisomal disorders
Includes terms added
Excludes note added
● 277.87 Disorders of mitochondrial metabolism
Includes terms added
Use additional code note added
Excludes note added
286.5 Includes term added
Use additional code note deleted
▲ 290 ~~Senile and presenile organic psychotic conditions~~ ▶Dementias◀
Excludes terms added
▲ 290.4 ~~Arteriosclerotic~~ ▶Vascular◀ dementia
▲ 290.40 ~~Arteriosclerotic~~ ▶Vascular◀ dementia, uncomplicated
▲ 290.41 ~~Arteriosclerotic~~ ▶Vascular◀ dementia, with delirium
▲ 290.42 ~~Arteriosclerotic~~ ▶Vascular◀ dementia, with ~~delusional features~~ delusions
▲ 290.43 ~~Arteriosclerotic~~ ▶Vascular◀ dementia, with ~~depressive features~~ depressed mood
▲ 291 ~~Alcoholic psychoses~~ ▶Alcohol-induced mental disorders◀
▲ 291.1 Alcohol ▶-induced persisting◀ amnestic ~~syndrome~~ disorder
▲ 291.2 ~~Other alcoholic~~ ▶Alcohol-induced persisting◀ dementia
▲ 291.3 Alcohol ~~withdrawal hallucinosis~~ ▶-induced psychotic disorder with hallucinations◀
▲ 291.5 Alcoholic ~~jealousy~~ ▶-induced psychotic disorder with delusions◀
▲ 291.8 Other specified ~~alcoholic psychosis~~ ▶alcohol-induced mental disorders◀
291.89 Includes terms added
▲ 291.9 Unspecified ~~alcoholic psychosis~~ ▶alcohol-induced mental disorders◀
Includes term added
▲ 292 ~~Drug psychoses~~ ▶Drug-induced mental disorders◀
Includes term deleted
▲ 292.0 Drug withdrawal ~~syndrome~~
▲ 292.1 ~~Paranoid and/or hallucinatory states induced by drugs~~ ▶Drug-induced psychotic disorders◀
▲ 292.11 Drug-induced ~~organic delusional syndrome~~ ▶psychotic disorder with delusions◀
▲ 292.12 Drug-induced ~~hallucinosis~~ ▶psychotic disorder with hallucinations◀
▲ 292.82 Drug-induced ▶persisting◀ dementia
▲ 292.83 Drug-induced ▶persisting◀ amnestic ~~syndrome~~ disorder
▲ 292.84 Drug-induced ~~organic affective syndrome~~ ▶mood disorder◀
292.89 Includes terms added
292.9 Includes term added
▲ 293 Transient ~~organic psychotic conditions~~ ▶mental disorders due to conditions classified elsewhere◀
▲ 293.0 ~~Acute delirium~~ ▶Delirium due to conditions classified elsewhere◀
▲ 293.8 Other specified transient ~~organic~~ ▶mental disorders due to conditions classified elsewhere◀
▲ 293.81 ~~Organic delusional syndrome~~ ▶Psychotic disorder with delusions in conditions classified elsewhere◀
▲ 293.82 ~~Organic hallucinosis syndrome~~ ▶Psychotic disorder with hallucinations in conditions classified elsewhere◀
▲ 293.83 ~~Organic affective syndrome~~ ▶Mood disorder in conditions classified elsewhere◀
▲ 293.84 ~~Organic anxiety syndrome~~ ▶Anxiety disorder in conditions classified elsewhere◀
293.89 Includes term added

▲ 293.9 Unspecified transient ~~organic~~ mental disorder ▶in conditions classified elsewhere◀
▲ 294 ~~Other organic psychotic conditions (chronic)~~ ▶Persistent mental disorders due to conditions classified elsewhere◀
▲ 294.0 Amnestic ~~syndrome~~ ▶disorder in conditions classified elsewhere◀
Code first note added
294.1 Includes term added
▲ 294.8 Other ~~specified organic brain syndromes (chronic)~~ ▶persistent mental disorders due to conditions classified elsewhere◀
Includes terms added
▲ 294.9 Unspecified ~~organic brain syndrome (chronic)~~ ▶persistent mental disorders due to conditions classified elsewhere◀
Includes terms added
▲ 295.4 ~~Acute schizophrenic episode~~ ▶Schizophreniform disorder◀
Includes term deleted
▲ 295.6 Residual ▶type◀ ~~schizophrenia~~
▲ 295.7 ~~Schizo-affective type~~ ▶Schizoaffective disorder◀
295.9 Includes term added
▲ 296 ~~Affective psychoses~~ ▶Episodic mood disorders◀
▲ 296.0 ▶Bipolar I disorder, single manic◀ ~~disorder, single~~ episode
▲ 296.4 Bipolar ~~affective~~ ▶I◀ disorder, ▶most recent episode (or current)◀ manic
▲ 296.5 Bipolar ~~affective~~ ▶I◀ disorder, ▶most recent episode (or current)◀ depressed
▲ 296.6 Bipolar ~~affective~~ ▶I◀ disorder, ▶most recent episode (or current)◀ mixed
▲ 296.7 Bipolar ~~affective~~ ▶I◀ disorder, ▶most recent episode (or current)◀ unspecified
▲ 296.8 ~~Manic-depressive psychosis,~~ ▶Other and unspecified bipolar disorders◀
▲ 296.80 ~~Manic-depressive psychosis,~~ ▶Bipolar disorder,◀ unspecified
Includes term added
296.89 Includes term added
▲ 296.9 Other and unspecified ~~affective psychoses~~ ▶episodic mood disorder◀
▲ 296.90 Unspecified ~~affective psychosis~~ ▶episodic mood disorder◀
Includes term added
▲ 296.99 Other specified ~~affective psychoses~~ ▶episodic mood disorder◀
▲ 297 ~~Paranoid states~~ ▶Delusional disorders◀
▲ 297.1 ~~Paranoia~~ ▶Delusional disorder◀
▲ 297.3 Shared ~~paranoid~~ ▶psychotic◀ disorder
298.8 Includes term added
298.9 Includes term added
▲ 299 ~~Psychoses with origin specific to childhood~~ ▶Pervasive developmental disorders◀
Includes note deleted
▲ 299.0 ~~Infantile autism~~ ▶Autistic disorder◀
▲ 299.1 ~~Disintegrative psychosis~~ ▶Childhood disintegrative disorder◀
▲ 299.8 Other specified ~~early childhood psychoses~~ ▶pervasive developmental disorders◀
Includes term added
▲ 299.9 Unspecified ▶pervasive developmental disorder◀
Includes term added
▲ 300 ~~Neurotic disorders~~ ▶Anxiety, dissociative and somatoform disorders◀
▲ 300.01 Panic disorder ▶without agoraphobia◀
Excludes note added
▲ 300.1 ~~Hysteria~~ Dissociative, conversion and factitious disorders
▲ 300.12 ~~Psychogenic~~ ▶Dissociative◀ amnesia
▲ 300.13 ~~Psychogenic~~ ▶Dissociative◀ fugue
▲ 300.14 ~~Multiple personality~~ ▶Dissociative identity disorder◀
Includes term deleted
▲ 300.16 Factitious ~~illness~~ ▶disorder◀ with ▶predominantly◀ psychological ▶signs and◀ symptoms
300.19 Includes term revised
▲ 300.21 Agoraphobia with panic ~~attacks~~ ▶disorder◀
Includes term added
Excludes note added
▲ 300.29 Other isolated or ~~simple~~ ▶specific◀ phobias

▲ 300.4 ~~Neurotic depression~~ ▶Dysthymic disorder◀
Includes term deleted
▲ 300.6 Depersonalization ~~syndrome~~ ▶disorder◀
Includes term added
▲ 300.8 ~~Other neurotic disorders~~ ▶Somatoform disorders◀
▲ 300.89 Other ▶somatoform disorders◀
▲ 300.9 ~~Unspecified neurotic disorder~~ ▶Unspecified nonpsychotic mental disorder◀
Includes term deleted
▲ 301.22 Schizotypal personality ▶disorder◀
▲ 301.4 ▶Obsessive-◀ compulsive personality disorder
▲ 301.81 Narcissistic personality ▶disorder◀
▲ 301.82 Avoidant personality ▶disorder◀
▲ 301.83 Borderline personality ▶disorder◀
▲ 302 Sexual ~~deviations~~ and ▶gender identity◀ disorders
▲ 302.0 Ego-dystonic ~~homosexuality~~ ▶sexual orientation◀
Includes term revised
▲ 302.3 ~~Transvestism~~ ▶Transvestic fetishism◀
▲ 302.6 ~~Disorders of psychosexual identity~~ ▶Gender identity disorder in children◀
Includes term deleted
Includes term added
Excludes term deleted
302.70 Includes term added
▲ 302.71 ~~With inhibited~~ ▶Hypoactive◀ sexual desire ▶disorder◀
302.72 Includes terms added
▲ 302.73 ~~With inhibited~~ Female orgasmic ▶disorder◀
▲ 302.74 ~~With inhibited~~ Male orgasmic ▶disorder◀
▲ 302.75 ~~With~~ Premature ejaculation
▲ 302.76 ~~With functional~~ Dyspareunia, ▶psychogenic◀
Includes term deleted
302.79 Includes term added
▲ 302.85 Gender identity disorder ~~of adolescent or adult life~~ ▶in adolescents or adults◀
Excludes note added
302.89 Includes terms added
302.9 Includes terms added
▲ 304.1 ~~Barbiturate and similarly acting~~ Sedative, ~~or~~ hypnotic ▶or anxiolytic◀ dependence
304.6 Includes terms added
▲ 305.4 ~~Barbiturate and similarly acting~~ Sedative, ~~or~~ hypnotic or ▶anxiolytic◀ abuse
305.9 Includes term added
▲ 307.0 ~~Stammering and~~ Stuttering
307.20 Includes term added
▲ 307.21 Transient tic disorder ~~of childhood~~
▲ 307.22 Chronic motor ▶or vocal◀ tic disorder
▲ 307.23 ~~Gilles de la~~ Tourette's disorder
▲ 307.3 ~~Stereotyped repetitive movements~~ ▶Stereotypic movement disorder◀
307.4 Excludes term revised
▲ 307.45 ~~Phase-shift disruption of 24-hour sleep-wake cycle~~ ▶Circadian rhythm sleep disorder◀
▲ 307.46 ~~Somnambulism or night terrors~~ ▶Sleep arousal disorder◀
Includes terms added
307.47 Includes terms added
307.50 Includes term added
▲ 307.51 Bulimia ▶nervosa◀
▲ 307.53 ~~Psychogenic~~ Rumination ▶disorder◀
307.59 Includes term added
▲ 307.8 ~~Psychalgia~~ ▶Pain disorders related to psychological factors◀
307.89 Includes term deleted
Code first note added
Excludes note revised
307.9 Includes term added
308.3 Includes term added
Includes term added
▲ 309.0 ~~Brief depressive reaction~~ ▶Adjustment disorder with depressed mood◀
Includes term deleted
▲ 309.24 Adjustment ~~reaction~~ ▶disorder◀ with ~~anxious mood~~ ▶anxiety◀
▲ 309.28 Adjustment ~~reaction~~ ▶disorder◀ with mixed ~~emotional features~~ ▶anxiety and depressed mood◀
▲ 309.3 ▶Adjustment disorder◀ with ~~predominant~~ disturbance of conduct

▶◀ Revised Text   ● New Code   ▲ Revised Code Title

▲ 309.4 ▶Adjustment disorder◀ with mixed disturbance of emotions and conduct
▲ 309.81 Prolonged Posttraumatic stress disorder
Includes term added
Excludes term added
▲ 310 Specific nonpsychotic mental disorders due to organic brain damage
▲ 310.1 Organic Personality change syndrome ▶due to conditions classified elsewhere◀
Includes term deleted
310.8 Includes term added
312.39 Includes term added
312.89 Includes term added
312.9 Includes term added
▲ 313.23 Elective ▶Selective◀ mutism
▲ 313.81 Oppositional ▶defiant◀ disorder
313.82 Includes term added
313.89 Includes term added
▲ 313.9 Unspecified emotional disturbance of childhood ▶or adolescence◀
Includes term added
▲ 315.1 Specific arithmetical ▶Mathematics◀ disorder
315.2 Includes term added
▲ 315.31 Developmental ▶Expressive◀ language disorder
Includes term deleted
▲ 315.32 ▶Mixed◀ receptive▶-expressive◀ language disorder (mixed)
Includes term deleted
315.39 Includes term added
▲ 315.4 ▶Developmental◀ coordination disorder
315.9 Includes term added
337.3 Use additional code note revised
● 347.0 Narcolepsy
● 347.00 Narcolepsy, Without cataplexy
Includes term added
● 347.01 Narcolepsy, With cataplexy
● 347.1 Narcolepsy in conditions classified elsewhere
Code first note added
● 347.10 Narcolepsy in conditions classified elsewhere, Without cataplexy
● 347.11 Narcolepsy in conditions classified elsewhere, With cataplexy
▲ 380.0 Perichondritis ▶and chondritis◀ of pinna
Includes term added
● 380.03 Chondritis of pinna
402 Includes note revised
436 Includes terms deleted
Excludes terms added
● 453.4 Venous embolism and thrombosis of deep vessels of lower extremity
● 453.40 Venous embolism and thrombosis of unspecified deep vessels of lower extremity
Includes terms added
● 453.41 Venous embolism and thrombosis of deep vessels of proximal lower extremity
Includes terms added
● 453.42 Venous embolism and thrombosis of deep vessels of distal lower extremity
Includes terms added
466.0 Excludes note added
● 477.2 Due to animal (cat) (dog) hair and dander
491.21 Includes terms deleted
● 491.22 Obstructive chronic bronchitis, With acute bronchitis
492.8 Excludes term revised
493.2 Excludes term revised
496 Excludes terms revised
520.6 Excludes term deleted
521.05 Excludes term revised
● 521.06 Dental caries pit and fissure
● 521.07 Dental caries of smooth surface
● 521.08 Dental caries of root surface
▲ 521.1 Diseases of hard tissues of teeth, Excessive attrition ▶(approximal wear) (occlusal wear)◀
Includes terms deleted
● 521.10 Diseases of hard tissues of teeth, Excessive attrition, unspecified
● 521.11 Diseases of hard tissues of teeth, Excessive attrition, limited to enamel
● 521.12 Diseases of hard tissues of teeth, Excessive attrition, extending into dentine
● 521.13 Diseases of hard tissues of teeth, Excessive attrition, extending into pulp

● 521.14 Diseases of hard tissues of teeth, Excessive attrition, localized
● 521.15 Diseases of hard tissues of teeth, Excessive attrition, generalized
● 521.20 Diseases of hard tissues of teeth, Abrasion, unspecified
● 521.21 Diseases of hard tissues of teeth, Abrasion, limited to enamel
● 521.22 Diseases of hard tissues of teeth, Abrasion, extending into dentine
● 521.23 Diseases of hard tissues of teeth, Abrasion, extending into pulp
● 521.24 Diseases of hard tissues of teeth, Abrasion, localized
● 521.25 Diseases of hard tissues of teeth, Abrasion, generalized
● 521.30 Diseases of hard tissues of teeth, Erosion, unspecified
● 521.31 Diseases of hard tissues of teeth, Erosion, limited to enamel
● 521.32 Diseases of hard tissues of teeth, Erosion, extending into dentine
● 521.33 Diseases of hard tissues of teeth, Erosion, extending into pulp
● 521.34 Diseases of hard tissues of teeth, Erosion, localized
● 521.35 Diseases of hard tissues of teeth, Erosion, generalized
521.4 Includes terms deleted
● 521.40 Diseases of hard tissues of teeth, Pathological resorption, unspecified
● 521.41 Diseases of hard tissues of teeth, Pathological resorption, internal
● 521.42 Diseases of hard tissues of teeth, Pathological resorption, external
● 521.49 Diseases of hard tissues of teeth, Other pathological resorption
Includes term added
▲ 521.7 ▶Intrinsic◀ posteruptive color changes
Excludes term added
523.2 Includes term revised
● 523.20 Gingival recession, unspecified
● 523.21 Gingival recession, minimal
● 523.22 Gingival recession, moderate
● 523.23 Gingival recession, severe
● 523.24 Gingival recession, localized
● 523.25 Gingival recession, generalized
523.6 Includes term added
Excludes note added
● 524.07 Excessive tuberosity of jaw
524.2 Includes terms deleted
Excludes note added
● 524.20 Unspecified anomaly of dental arch relationship
● 524.21 Anomaly of dental arch relationship, Angle's class I
Includes term added
● 524.22 Anomaly of dental arch relationship, Angle's class II
Includes terms added
● 524.23 Anomaly of dental arch relationship, Angle's class III
Includes term added
● 524.24 Anomaly of dental arch relationship, Open anterior occlusal relationship
● 524.25 Anomaly of dental arch relationship, Open posterior occlusal relationship
● 524.26 Anomaly of dental arch relationship, Excessive horizontal overlap
● 524.27 Anomaly of dental arch relationship, Reverse articulation
Includes term added
● 524.28 Anomalies of interarch distance
Includes term added
● 524.29 Other anomalies of dental arch relationship
▲ 524.3 Anomalies of tooth position ▶of fully erupted teeth◀
Includes terms deleted
Excludes note added
● 524.30 Unspecified anomaly of tooth position
Includes terms added
● 524.31 Crowding of teeth
● 524.32 Excessive spacing of teeth
● 524.33 Horizontal displacement of teeth
Includes term added
● 524.34 Vertical displacement of teeth
Includes terms added
● 524.35 Rotation of teeth

● 524.36 Insufficient interocclusal distance of teeth (ridge)
● 524.37 Excessive interocclusal distance of teeth
Includes term added
● 524.39 Other anomalies of tooth position
524.5 Includes terms deleted
● 524.50 Dentofacial functional abnormality, unspecified
● 524.51 Dentofacial functional abnormality, Abnormal jaw closure
Includes term added
● 524.52 Dentofacial functional abnormality, Limited mandibular range of motion
● 524.53 Dentofacial functional abnormality, Deviation in opening and closing of the mandible
● 524.54 Dentofacial functional abnormality, Insufficient anterior guidance
● 524.55 Dentofacial functional abnormality, Centric occlusion maximum intercuspation discrepancy
● 524.56 Dentofacial functional abnormality, Non-working side interference
● 524.57 Dentofacial functional abnormality, Lack of posterior occlusal support
● 524.59 Other dentofacial functional abnormalities
Includes terms added
● 524.64 Temporomandibular joint sounds on opening and/or closing the jaw
● 524.75 Vertical displacement of alveolus and teeth
Includes term added
● 524.76 Occlusal plane deviation
● 524.81 Other specified dentofacial anomalies, Anterior soft tissue impingement
● 524.82 Other specified dentofacial anomalies, Posterior soft tissue impingement
● 524.89 Other specified dentofacial anomalies
● 525.20 Unspecified atrophy of edentulous alveolar ridge
Includes terms added
● 525.21 Minimal atrophy of the mandible
● 525.22 Moderate atrophy of the mandible
● 525.23 Severe atrophy of the mandible
● 525.24 Minimal atrophy of the maxilla
● 525.25 Moderate atrophy of the maxilla
● 525.26 Severe atrophy of the maxilla
528.6 Excludes term revised
528.7 Includes terms deleted
● 528.71 Minimal keratinized residual ridge mucosa
● 528.72 Excessive keratinized residual ridge mucosa
● 528.79 Other disturbances of oral epithelium, including tongue
Includes terms added
529.8 Excludes term revised
● 530.86 Infection of esophagostomy
Use additional code note added
● 530.87 Mechanical complication of esophagostomy
Includes term added
536.3 Includes term added
560.89 Includes term added
588.8 Includes terms deleted
● 588.81 Secondary hyperparathyroidism (of renal origin)
Includes term added
● 588.89 Other specified disorders resulting from impaired renal function
Includes term added
596.8 Excludes terms revised
599.5 Excludes term revised
615 Excludes term revised
618.0 Includes terms deleted
● 618.00 Prolapse of vaginal walls without mention of uterine prolapse, Unspecified prolapse of vaginal walls
Includes term added
● 618.01 Prolapse of vaginal walls without mention of uterine prolapse, Cystocele, midline
Includes term added
● 618.02 Prolapse of vaginal walls without mention of uterine prolapse, Cystocele, lateral
Includes term added
● 618.03 Prolapse of vaginal walls without mention of uterine prolapse, Urethrocele

▶◀ Revised Text ● New Code ▲ Revised Code Title

- 618.04 Prolapse of vaginal walls without mention of uterine prolapse, Rectocele
  Includes term added
- 618.05 Prolapse of vaginal walls without mention of uterine prolapse, Perineocele
- 618.09 Other prolapse of vaginal walls without mention of uterine prolapse
  Includes term added
  618.8 Includes terms deleted
- 618.81 Incompetence or weakening of pubocervical tissue
- 618.82 Incompetence or weakening of rectovaginal tissue
- 618.83 Pelvic muscle wasting
  Includes term added
- 618.89 Other specified genital prolapse
- ▲ 621.3 Endometrial ~~cystic~~ hyperplasia
- 621.30 Endometrial hyperplasia, unspecified
  Includes term added
- 621.31 Simple endometrial hyperplasia without atypia
- 621.32 Complex endometrial hyperplasia without atypia
- 621.33 Endometrial hyperplasia with atypia
  622.1 Includes terms deleted
  Excludes term added
- 622.10 Dysplasia of cervix, unspecified
  Includes term added
- 622.11 Mild dysplasia of cervix
  Includes term added
- 622.12 Moderate dysplasia of cervix
  Includes term added
  Excludes note added
- 629.2 Female genital mutilation status
  Includes term added
- 629.20 Female genital mutilation status, unspecified
  Includes term added
- 629.21 Female genital mutilation Type I status
  Includes term added
- 629.22 Female genital mutilation Type II status
  Includes term added
- 629.23 Female genital mutilation Type III status
  Includes term added
  648.6 Other cardiovascular diseases
  Excludes term added
- 692.84 Contact dermatitis and other eczema, Due to animal (cat) (dog) dander
  Includes term added
  692.89 Includes term deleted
  Excludes term deleted
  Excludes terms added
- 705.2 Focal hyperhidrosis
  Excludes note added
- 705.21 Primary focal hyperhidrosis
  Includes terms added
- 705.22 Secondary focal hyperhidrosis
  Includes term added
  705.89 Excludes term revised
- 707.00 Decubitus ulcer, Unspecified site
- 707.01 Decubitus ulcer, Elbow
- 707.02 Decubitus ulcer, Upper back
  Includes term added
- 707.03 Decubitus ulcer, Lower back
  Includes term added
- 707.04 Decubitus ulcer, Hip
- 707.05 Decubitus ulcer, Buttock
- 707.06 Decubitus ulcer, Ankle
- 707.07 Decubitus ulcer, Heel
- 707.09 Decubitus ulcer, Other site
  Includes term added
  713.0 Code first note revised
  718 Excludes term revised
  719 Excludes term revised
  719.8 Excludes term revised
  728.2 Excludes term added
  733 Excludes term revised
  733.29 Excludes term revised
  737.4 Code first note revised
  758 Use additional code note added
  758.3 Includes terms deleted
- 758.31 Cri-du-chat syndrome
  Includes term added
- 758.32 Velo-cardio-facial syndrome
  Includes term added
- 758.33 Other microdeletions
  Includes terms added
- 758.39 Other autosomal deletions

- ▲ 760.7 Noxious influences affecting fetus ▶or newborn◀ via placenta or breast milk
  771.8 Use additional code note revised
- 780.58 Sleep related movement disorder
  Includes term added
  Excludes note added
- ▲ 780.8 ▶Generalized◀ hyperhidrosis
  Includes term added
  Excludes term added
  785.52 Includes terms added
  Code first term added
  785.59 Includes terms deleted
- ▲ 788.3 ▶Urinary incontinence◀
  Code, if applicable note revised
- 788.38 Overflow incontinence
- 790.95 Elevated C-reactive protein (CRP)
- ▲ 795 ▶Other and◀ nonspecific abnormal ▶cytological,◀ histological, ~~and~~ immunological ▶and DNA test findings◀
- ▲ 795.0 ~~Nonspecific~~ Abnormal Papanicolaou smear of cervix ▶and cervical HPV◀
  Includes terms added
  Excludes terms revised
  Excludes terms deleted
  Excludes terms added
- ▲ 795.00 ~~Nonspecific~~ Abnormal ▶glandular◀ Papanicolaou smear of cervix ~~unspecified~~
  Includes terms added
- ▲ 795.01 ~~Atypical squamous cell changes of undetermined significance favor benign (ASCUS favor benign)~~ ▶Papanicolaou smear of cervix with atypical squamous cells of undetermined significance (ASC-US)◀
  Includes term deleted
- ▲ 795.02 ~~Atypical squamous cell changes of undetermined significance favor dysplasia (ASCUS favor dysplasia)~~ ▶Papanicolaou smear of cervix with atypical squamous cells cannot exclude high grade squamous intraepithelial lesion (ASC-H)◀
  Includes term deleted
- 795.03 Papanicolaou smear of cervix with low grade squamous intraepithelial lesion (LGSIL)
- 795.04 Papanicolaou smear of cervix with high grade squamous intraepithelial lesion (HGSIL)
  Includes term added
- 795.05 Cervical high risk human papillomavirus (HPV) DNA test positive
- 795.08 Unsatisfactory smear
  Includes term added
- ▲ 795.09 Other ~~nonspecific~~ abnormal Papanicolaou smear of cervix ▶and cervical HPV◀
  Includes terms deleted
  Includes term added
  Use additional code note added
  Excludes note added
- 796.6 Abnormal findings on neonatal screening
  Excludes note added
  995.9 Code first note revised
  995.92 Use additional code term deleted
  995.94 Use additional code term deleted
  996.4 Excludes term revised
  997.4 Excludes terms added
  SUPPLEMENTARY CLASSIFICATION OF FACTORS INFLUENCING HEALTH STATUS AND CONTACT WITH HEALTH SERVICES ▶(V01-V84)◀
- V01.71 Contact with or exposure to, Varicella
- V01.79 Contact with or exposure to, Other viral diseases
- V01.83 Contact with or exposure to, Escherichia coli (E. coli)
- V01.84 Contact with or exposure to, Meningococcus
- ▲ V07.4 ~~Postmenopausal~~ Hormone replacement therapy ▶(postmenopausal)◀
  V08 Excludes term revised
  V09.0 Includes term added
  V09.8 Includes terms added
  V22 Excludes term revised
  V45.77 Excludes note added
- V46.11 Dependence on respirator, status
- V46.12 Encounter for respirator dependence during power failure
- V49.83 Awaiting organ transplant status

- V58.44 Aftercare following organ transplant
  Use additional code note added
  V58.6 Excludes term added
  V58.61 Excludes note added
  V58.63 Excludes note added
  V58.64 Excludes note added
- V58.66 Long-term (current) use of aspirin
- V58.67 Long-term (current) use of insulin
  V58.7 Excludes note added
- V69.4 Lack of adequate sleep
  Includes term added
  Excludes note added
  PERSONS WITHOUT REPORTED DIAGNOSIS ENCOUNTERED DURING EXAMINATION AND INVESTIGATION OF INDIVIDUALS AND POPULATIONS ▶(V70-V84)◀
  V72.3 Includes terms deleted
  Use additional code note deleted
- V72.31 Routine gynecological examination
  Includes terms added
  Use additional code note added
- V72.32 Encounter for Papanicolaou cervical smear to confirm findings of recent normal smear following initial abnormal smear
- ▲ V72.4 Pregnancy examination or test, ~~pregnancy unconfirmed~~
  Includes term deleted
- V72.40 Pregnancy examination or test, pregnancy unconfirmed
  Includes term added
- V72.41 Pregnancy examination or test, negative result
  V76.2 Excludes term revised
  V82.81 Use additional code term revised
- V84 Genetic susceptibility to disease
  Includes note added
  Use additional code note added
- V84.0 Genetic susceptibility to malignant neoplasm
  Code first, if applicable note added
  Use additional code, if applicable note added
- V84.01 Genetic susceptibility to malignant neoplasm of breast
- V84.02 Genetic susceptibility to malignant neoplasm of ovary
- V84.03 Genetic susceptibility to malignant neoplasm of prostate
- V84.04 Genetic susceptibility to malignant neoplasm of endometrium
- V84.09 Genetic susceptibility to other malignant neoplasm
- V84.8 Genetic susceptibility to other disease

▶◀ Revised Text   ● New Code   ▲ Revised Code Title

Coding Guidelines

ICD-9-CM OFFICIAL GUIDELINES FOR CODING AND REPORTING

Effective October 1, 2003
Revised December 15, 2003

The Centers for Medicare and Medicaid Services (CMS) formerly the Health Care Financing Administration (HCFA) and the National Center for Health Statistics (NCHS), two departments within the Department of Health and Human Services (DHHS) present the following guidelines for coding and reporting using the International Classification of Diseases, 9th Revision, Clinical Modification (ICD-9-CM). These guidelines should be used as a companion document to the official version of the ICD-9-CM as published on CD-ROM.

These guidelines for coding and reporting have been developed and approved by the Cooperating Parties for ICD-9-CM: the American Hospital Association, the American Health Information Management Association, CMS, and the NCHS. These guidelines, published by the Department of Health and Human Services have also appeared in the *Coding Clinic for ICD-9-CM*, published by the American Hospital Association.

These guidelines have been developed to assist the user in coding and reporting in situations where the ICD-9-CM does not provide direction. Coding and sequencing instructions in volumes I, II, and III of ICD-9-CM take precedence over any guidelines. The conventions, general guidelines and chapter-specific guidelines apply to the proper use of ICD-9-CM, regardless of the health care setting. A joint effort between the attending physician and coder is essential to achieve complete and accurate documentation, code assignment, and reporting of diagnoses and procedures. These guidelines have been developed and approved by the Cooperating Parties to assist both the physician and the coder in identifying those diagnoses that are to be reported. The importance of consistent, complete documentation in the medical record cannot be overemphasized. Without such documentation the application of all coding guidelines is a difficult, if not impossible, task.

These guidelines are not exhaustive. The cooperating parties are continuing to conduct reviews of these guidelines and develop new guidelines as needed. Users of the ICD-9-CM should be aware that only guidelines approved by the cooperating parties are official. Revision of these guidelines and new guidelines will be published by the U.S. Department of Health and Human Services when they are approved by the cooperating parties. The term "admitted" is used generally to mean a health care encounter in any setting.

The guidelines have been reorganized into several new sections including an enhanced introduction that provides more detail about the structure and conventions of the classification usually found in the classification itself. The other new section, General Guidelines, brings together overarching guidelines that were previously found throughout the various sections of the guidelines. The new format of the guidelines also includes a resequencing of the disease-specific guidelines. They are sequenced in the same order as they appear in the tabular list chapters (Infectious and Parasitic diseases, Neoplasms, etc.)

These changes will make it easier for coders, experienced and beginners, to more easily find the specific portion of the coding guideline information they seek.

TABLE OF CONTENTS

Section I Conventions, General Coding Guidelines and Chapter-Specific Guidelines

The conventions, general guidelines and chapter-specific guidelines are applicable to all health care settings unless otherwise indicated.

A. Conventions for the ICD-9-CM

The conventions for the ICD-9-CM are the general rules for use of the classification independent of the guidelines. These conventions are incorporated within the index and tabular of the ICD-9-CM as instructional notes. The conventions are as follows:

1. Format: The ICD-9-CM uses an indented format for ease in reference

2. Abbreviations

    a. Index Abbreviations

    NEC "Not elsewhere classifiable" This abbreviation in the index represents "other specified" When a specific code is not available for a condition the index directs the coder to the "other specified" code in the tabular.

    b. Tabular Abbreviations

    NEC "Not elsewhere classifiable" This abbreviation in the tabular represents "other specified" When a specific code is not available for a condition the tabular includes an NEC entry under a code to identify the code as the "other specified" code. (see "Other" codes)

    NOS "Not otherwise specified" This abbreviation is the equivalent of unspecified. (see "Unspecified" codes)

3. Punctuation

    [ ] Brackets are used in the tabular list to enclose synonyms, alternative wording or explanatory phrases. Brackets are used in the index to identify manifestation codes. (see etiology/manifestations).

    ( ) Parentheses are used in both the index and tabular to enclose supplementary words which may be present or absent in the statement of a disease or procedure without affecting the code number to which it is assigned. The terms within the parentheses are referred to as nonessential modifiers.

    : Colons are used in the Tabular list after an incomplete term which needs one or more of the modifiers following the colon to make it assignable to a given category.

4. Includes and Excludes Notes and Inclusion terms

    Includes:

    This note appears immediately under a three-digit code title to further define, or give examples of, the content of the category.

    Excludes:

    An excludes note under a code indicate that the terms excluded from the code are to be coded elsewhere. In some cases the codes for the excluded terms should not be used in conjunction with the code from which it is excluded. An example of this is a congenital condition excluded from an acquired form of the same condition. The congenital and acquired codes should not be used together. In other cases, the excluded terms may be used together with an excluded code. An example of this is when fractures of different bones are coded to different codes. Both codes may be used together if both types of fractures are present.

    Inclusion terms:

    List of terms are included under certain four and five digit codes. These terms are the conditions for which that code number is to be used. The terms may be synonyms of the code title, or, in the case of "other specified" codes, the terms are a list of the various conditions assigned to that code. The inclusion terms are not necessarily exhaustive. Additional terms found only in the index may also be assigned to a code.

5. Other and Unspecified codes

    a. "Other" codes

    Codes titled "other" or "other specified" (usually a code with a 4th digit 8 or fifth-digit 9 for diagnosis codes) are for use when the information in the medical record provides detail for which a specific code does not exist. Index entries with NEC in the line designate "other" codes in the tabular. These index entries represent specific disease entities for which no specific code exists so the term is included within an "other" code.

b. "Unspecified" codes
Codes (usually a code with a 4th digit 9 or 5th digit 0 for diagnosis codes) titled "unspecified" are for use when the information in the medical record is insufficient to assign a more specific code.

6. Etiology/manifestation convention ("code first", "use additional code" and "in diseases classified elsewhere" notes)

Certain conditions have both an underlying etiology and multiple body system manifestations due to the underlying etiology. For such conditions the ICD-9-CM has a coding convention that requires the underlying condition be sequenced first followed by the manifestation. Where ever such a combination exists there is a "use additional code" note at the etiology code, and a "code first" note at the manifestation code. These instructional notes indicate the proper sequencing order of the codes, etiology followed by manifestation.

In most cases the manifestation codes will have in the code title, "in diseases classified elsewhere." Codes with this title are a component of the etiology/ manifestation convention. The code title indicates that it is a manifestation code. "In diseases classified elsewhere" codes are never permitted to be used as first listed or principal diagnosis codes. They must be used in conjunction with an underlying condition code and they must be listed following the underlying condition.

There are manifestation codes that do not have "in diseases classified elsewhere" in the title. For such codes a "use additional code" note will still be present and the rules for sequencing apply.

In addition to the notes in the tabular, these conditions also have a specific index entry structure. In the index both conditions are listed together with the etiology code first followed by the manifestation codes in brackets. The code in brackets is always to be sequenced second.

The most commonly used etiology/manifestation combinations are the codes for Diabetes mellitus, category 250. For each code under category 250 there is a use additional code note for the manifestation that is specific for that particular diabetic manifestation. Should a patient have more than one manifestation of diabetes more than one code from category 250 may be used with as many manifestation codes as are needed to fully describe the patient's complete diabetic condition. The 250 diabetes codes should be sequenced first, followed by the manifestation codes.

"Code first" and "Use additional code" notes are also used as sequencing rules in the classification for certain codes that are not part of an etiology/ manifestation combination. See - Other multiple coding for a single condition in the General Guidelines section.

B. General Coding Guidelines

1. Use of Both Alphabetic Index and Tabular List
Use both the Alphabetic Index and the Tabular List when locating and assigning a code. Reliance on only the Alphabetic Index or the Tabular List leads to errors in code assignments and less specificity in code selection.

2. Locate each term in the Alphabetic Index and verify the code selected in the Tabular List. Read and be guided by instructional notations that appear in both the Alphabetic Index and the Tabular List.

3. Level of Detail in Coding
Diagnosis and procedure codes are to be used at their highest number of digits available.

ICD-9-CM diagnosis codes are composed of codes with either 3, 4, or 5 digits. Codes with three digits are included in ICD-9-CM as the heading of a category of codes that may be further subdivided by the use of fourth and/or fifth digits, which provide greater detail.

A three-digit code is to be used only if it is not further subdivided. Where fourth-digit subcategories and/or fifth-digit subclassifications are provided, they must be assigned. A code is invalid if it has not been coded to the full number of digits required for that code. For example, Acute myocardial infarction, code 410, has fourth digits that describe the location of the infarction (e.g., 410.2, Of inferolateral wall), and fifth digits that identify the episode of care. It would be incorrect to report a code in category 410 without a fourth and fifth digit.

ICD-9-CM Volume 3 procedure codes are composed of codes with either 3 or 4 digits. Codes with two digits are included in ICD-9-CM as the heading of a category of codes that may be further subdivided by the use of third and/or fourth digits, which provide greater detail.

4. The appropriate code or codes from 001.0 through V83.89 must be used to identify diagnoses, symptoms, conditions, problems, complaints or other reason(s) for the encounter/visit.

5. The selection of codes 001.0 through 999.9 will frequently be used to describe the reason for the admission/encounter. These codes are from the section of ICD-9-CM for the classification of diseases and injuries (e.g., infectious and parasitic diseases; neoplasms; symptoms, signs, and ill-defined conditions, etc.).

6. Codes that describe symptoms and signs, as opposed to diagnoses, are acceptable for reporting purposes when a related definitive diagnosis has not been established (confirmed) by the physician. Chapter 16 of ICD-9-CM, Symptoms, Signs, and Ill-defined conditions (codes 780.0 -799.9) contain many, but not all codes for symptoms.

7. Conditions that are an integral part of a disease process
Signs and symptoms that are integral to the disease process should not be assigned as additional codes.

8. Conditions that are not an integral part of a disease process
Additional signs and symptoms that may not be associated routinely with a disease process should be coded when present.

9. Multiple coding for a single condition
In addition to the etiology/manifestation convention that requires two codes to fully describe a single condition that affects multiple body systems, there are other single conditions that also require more than one code. "Use additional code" notes are found in the tabular at codes that are not part of an etiology/manifestation pair where a secondary code is useful to fully describe a condition. The sequencing rule is the same, "use additional code" indicates that a secondary code should be added.

For example, for infections that are not included in chapter 1, a secondary code from category 041, Bacterial infection in conditions classified elsewhere and of unspecified site, may be required to identify the bacterial organism causing the infection. A "use additional code" note will normally be found at the infection code indicates a need for the organism code to be added as a secondary code.

"Code first" notes are also under certain codes that are not specifically manifestation codes but may be due to an underlying cause. When a "code first" note is present and an underlying condition is present the underlying condition should be sequenced first.

"Code, if applicable, any causal condition first", notes indicate that this code may be assigned as a principal diagnosis when the causal condition is unknown or not applicable. If a causal condition is known, then the code for that condition should be sequenced as the principal or first-listed diagnosis.

Multiple codes may be needed for late effects, complication codes and obstetric codes to more fully describe a condition. See the specific guidelines for these conditions for further instruction.

10. Acute and Chronic Conditions
If the same condition is described as both acute (subacute) and chronic, and separate subentries exist in the Alphabetic Index at the same indentation level, code both and sequence the acute (subacute) code first.

11. Combination Code
A combination code is a single code used to classify: two diagnoses, or
A diagnosis with an associated secondary process (manifestation)
A diagnosis with an associated complication

Combination codes are identified by referring to subterm entries in the Alphabetic Index and by reading the inclusion and exclusion notes in the Tabular List.

Assign only the combination code when that code fully identifies the diagnostic conditions involved or when the Alphabetic Index so directs. Multiple coding should not be used when the classification provides a combination code that clearly identifies all of the elements documented in the diagnosis. When the combination code lacks necessary specificity in describing the manifestation or complication, an additional code may be used as a secondary code.

12. Late Effects

A late effect is the residual effect (condition produced) after the acute phase of an illness or injury has terminated. There is no time limit on when a late effect code can be used. The residual may be apparent early, such as in cerebrovascular accident cases, or it may occur months or years later, such as that due to a previous injury. Coding of late effects generally requires two codes sequenced in the following order: The condition or nature of the late effect is sequenced first. The late effect code is sequenced second.

An exception to the above guidelines are those instances where the code for late effect is followed by a manifestation code identified in the Tabular List and title, or the late effect code has been expanded (at the fourth and fifth-digit levels) to include the manifestation(s). The code for the acute phase of an illness or injury that led to the late effect is never used with a code for the late effect.

13. Impending or Threatened Condition

Code any condition described at the time of discharge as "impending" or "threatened" as follows: If it did occur, code as confirmed diagnosis. If it did not occur, reference the Alphabetic Index to determine if the condition has a subentry term for "impending" or "threatened" and also reference main term entries for "Impending" and for "Threatened." If the subterms are listed, assign the given code. If the subterms are not listed, code the existing underlying condition(s) and not the condition described as impending or threatened.

C. Chapter-Specific Coding Guidelines

In addition to general coding guidelines, there are guidelines for specific diagnoses and/or conditions in the classification. Unless otherwise indicated, these guidelines apply to all health care settings.

C1. Infectious and Parasitic Diseases

A. Human Immunodeficiency Virus (HIV) Infections

1. Code only confirmed cases of HIV infection/illness. This is an exception to the hospital inpatient guideline Section II, H.

In this context, "confirmation" does not require documentation of positive serology or culture for HIV; the physician's diagnostic statement that the patient is HIV positive, or has an HIV-related illness is sufficient.

2. Selection and sequencing

a. If a patient is admitted for an HIV-related condition, the principal diagnosis should be 042, followed by additional diagnosis codes for all reported HIV-related conditions.

b. If a patient with HIV disease is admitted for an unrelated condition (such as a traumatic injury), the code for the unrelated condition (e.g., the nature of injury code) should be the principal diagnosis. Other diagnoses would be 042 followed by additional diagnosis codes for all reported HIV-related conditions.

c. Whether the patient is newly diagnosed or has had previous admissions/encounters for HIV conditions is irrelevant to the sequencing decision.

d. V08 Asymptomatic human immunodeficiency virus [HIV] infection, is to be applied when the patient without any documentation of symptoms is listed as being "HIV positive," "known HIV," "HIV test positive," or similar terminology. Do not use this code if the term "AIDS" is used or if the patient is treated for any HIV-related illness or is described as having any condition(s) resulting from his/her HIV positive status; use 042 in these cases.

e. Patients with inconclusive HIV serology, but no definitive diagnosis or manifestations of the illness, may be assigned code 795.71, Inconclusive serologic test for Human Immunodeficiency Virus [HIV]

f. Previously diagnosed HIV-related illness

Patients with any known prior diagnosis of an HIV-related illness should be coded to 042. Once a patient had developed an HIV-related illness, the patient should always be assigned code 042 on every subsequent admission/encounter. Patients previously diagnosed with any HIV illness (042) should never be assigned to 795.71 or V08.

g. HIV Infection in Pregnancy, Childbirth and the Puerperium

During pregnancy, childbirth or the puerperium, a patient admitted (or presenting for a health care encounter) because of an HIV-related illness should receive a principal diagnosis of 647.6X, Other specified infectious and parasitic diseases in the mother classifiable elsewhere, but complicating the pregnancy, childbirth or the puerperium, followed by 042 and the code(s) for the HIV-related illness(es). Codes from Chapter 15 always take sequencing priority.

Patients with asymptomatic HIV infection status admitted (or presenting for a health care encounter) during pregnancy, childbirth, or the puerperium should receive codes of 647.6X and V08.

h. Encounters for Testing for HIV

If a patient is being seen to determine his/her HIV status, use code V73.89, Screening for other specified viral disease. Use code V69.8, Other problems related to lifestyle, as a secondary code if an asymptomatic patient is in a known high risk group for HIV. Should a patient with signs or symptoms or illness, or a confirmed HIV related diagnosis be tested for HIV, code the signs and symptoms or the diagnosis. An additional counseling code V65.44 may be used if counseling is provided during the encounter for the test.

When a patient returns to be informed of his/her HIV test results use code V65.44, HIV counseling, if the results of the test are negative.

If the results are positive but the patient is asymptomatic use code V08, Asymptomatic HIV infection. If the results are positive and the patient is symptomatic use code 042, HIV infection, with codes for the HIV related symptoms or diagnosis. The HIV counseling code may also be used if counseling is provided for patients with positive test results.

B. ► Septicemia, Systemic Inflammatory Response Syndrome (SIRS), Sepsis, Severe Sepsis, and Septic Shock ◄

1. ► In most cases, it will be a code from category 038, Septicemia, that will be used in conjunction with a code from subcategory 995.9.

a. If the documentation in the record states streptococcal sepsis, codes 038.0 and code 995.91 should be used, in that sequence.

b. If the documentation states streptococcal septicemia, only code 038.0 should be assigned, however, the physician should be queried whether the patient has sepsis, an infection with SIRS.

c. Either the term sepsis or SIRS must be documented, to assign a code from subcategory 995.9. ◄

2. ► If the terms sepsis, severe sepsis, or SIRS are used with an underlying infection other than septicemia, such as pneumonia, cellulitis or a nonspecified urinary tract infection, code 038.9 should be assigned first, then code 995.91, followed by the code for the initial infection. The use of the terms sepsis or SIRS indicates that the patient's infection has advanced to the point of a systemic infection so the systemic infection should be sequenced before the localized infection. The instructional note under subcategory 995.9 instructs to assign the underlying condition first.

Note: The term urosepsis is a nonspecific term. If that is the only term documented then only code 599.0 should be assigned based on the default for the term in the ICD-9-CM index, in addition to the code for the causal organism if known. ◄

3. ►For patients with severe sepsis, the code for the systemic infection (038.x) or trauma should be sequenced first, followed by either code 995.92, Systemic inflammatory response syndrome due to infectious process with organ dysfunction, or code 995.94, Systemic inflammatory response syndrome due to noninfectious process with organ dysfunction. Codes for the specific organ dysfunctions should also be assigned.◄

4. ►If septic shock is documented, it is necessary to code first the initiating systemic infection or trauma, then either code 995.92 or 995.94, followed by code 785.52, Septic shock.◄

5. Sepsis and septic shock associated with abortion, ectopic pregnancy, and molar pregnancy are classified to category codes in Chapter 11 (630-639).

6. Negative or inconclusive blood cultures do not preclude a diagnosis of septicemia ►or sepsis◄ in patients with clinical evidence of the condition, ►however, the physician should be queried.◄

C2. Neoplasms

Chapter 2 of the ICD-9-CM contains the code for most benign and all malignant neoplasms. Certain benign neoplasms, such as prostatic adenomas, may be found in the specific body system chapters. To properly code a neoplasm it is necessary to determine from the record if the neoplasm is benign, in-situ, malignant, or of uncertain histologic behavior. If malignant, any secondary (metastatic) sites should also be determined.

The neoplasm table in the Alphabetic Index should be referenced first. If the histological term is documented, that term should be referenced first, rather than going immediately to the Neoplasm Table, in order to determine which column in the Neoplasm Table is appropriate. For example, if the documentation indicates "adenoma," refer to the term in the Alphabetic Index to review the entries under this term and the instructional note to "see also neoplasm, by site, benign." The table provides the proper code based on the type of neoplasm and the site. It is important to select the proper column in the table that corresponds to the type of neoplasm. The tabular should then be referenced to verify that the correct code has been selected from the table and that a more specific site code does not exist.

A. If the treatment is directed at the malignancy, designate the malignancy as the principal diagnosis.

B. When a patient is admitted because of a primary neoplasm with metastasis and treatment is directed toward the secondary site only, the secondary neoplasm is designated as the principal diagnosis even though the primary malignancy is still present.

C. Coding and sequencing of complications associated with the malignant neoplasm or with the therapy thereof are subject to the following guidelines:

1. When admission/encounter is for management of an anemia associated with the malignancy, and the treatment is only for anemia, the anemia is designated at the principal diagnosis and is followed by the appropriate code(s) for the malignancy.

2. When the admission/encounter is for management of an anemia associated with chemotherapy or radiotherapy and the only treatment is for the anemia, the anemia is sequenced first followed by the appropriate code(s) for the malignancy.

3. When the admission/encounter is for management of dehydration due to the malignancy or the therapy, or a combination of both, and only the dehydration is being treated (intravenous rehydration), the dehydration is sequenced first, followed by the code(s) for the malignancy.

4. When the admission/encounter is for treatment of a complication resulting from a surgical procedure performed for the treatment of an intestinal malignancy, designate the complication as the principal or first-listed diagnosis if treatment is directed at resolving the complication.

D. When a primary malignancy has been previously excised or eradicated from its site and there is no further treatment directed to that site and there is no evidence of any existing primary malignancy, a code from category V10, Personal history of malignant neoplasm, should be used to indicate the former site of the malignancy. Any mention of extension, invasion, or metastasis to another site is coded as a secondary malignant neoplasm to that site. The secondary site may be the principal or first-listed with the V10 code used as a secondary code.

E. Admissions/Encounters involving chemotherapy and radiation therapy

1. When an episode of care involves the surgical removal of a neoplasm, primary or secondary site, followed by chemotherapy or radiation treatment, the neoplasm code should be assigned as principal or first-listed diagnosis. When an episode of inpatient care involves surgical removal of a primary site or secondary site malignancy followed by adjunct chemotherapy or radiotherapy, code the malignancy as the principal or first-listed diagnosis, using codes in the 140-198 series or where appropriate in the 200-203 series.

2. If a patient admission/encounter is solely for the administration of chemotherapy or radiation therapy code V58.0, Encounter for radiation therapy, or V58.1, Encounter for chemotherapy, should be the first-listed or principal diagnosis. If a patient receives both chemotherapy and radiation therapy both codes should be listed, in either order of sequence.

3. When a patient is admitted for the purpose of radiotherapy or chemotherapy and develops complications such as uncontrolled nausea and vomiting or dehydration, the principal or first-listed diagnosis is V58.0, Encounter for radiotherapy, or V58.1, Encounter for chemotherapy.

F. When the reason for admission/encounter is to determine the extent of the malignancy, or for a procedure such as paracentesis or thoracentesis, the primary malignancy or appropriate metastatic site is designated as the principal or first-listed diagnosis, even though chemotherapy or radiotherapy is administered.

G. Symptoms, signs, and ill-defined conditions listed in Chapter 16 characteristic of, or associated with, an existing primary or secondary site malignancy cannot be used to replace the malignancy as principal or first-listed diagnosis, regardless of the number of admissions or encounters for treatment and care of the neoplasm.

C3. Endocrine, Nutritional, and Metabolic Diseases and Immunity Disorders

Reserved for future guideline expansion

C4. Diseases of Blood and Blood Forming Organs

Reserved for future guideline expansion

C5. Mental Disorders

Reserved for future guideline expansion

C6. Diseases of Nervous System and Sense Organs

Reserved for future guideline expansion

C7. Diseases of Circulatory System

A. Hypertension

The Hypertension Table, found under the main term, "Hypertension", in the Alphabetic Index, contains a complete listing of all conditions due to or associated with hypertension and classifies them according to malignant, benign, and unspecified.

1. Hypertension, Essential, or NOS Assign hypertension (arterial) (essential) (primary) (systemic) (NOS) to category code 401 with the appropriate fourth digit to indicate malignant (.0), benign (.1), or unspecified (.9). Do not use either .0 malignant or .1 benign unless medical record documentation supports such a designation.

2. Hypertension with Heart Disease

Heart conditions (425.8, 429.0-429.3, 429.8, 429.9) are assigned to a code from category 402 when a causal relationship is stated (due to hypertension) or implied (hypertensive). Use an additional code from category 428 to identify the type of heart failure in those patients with heart failure. More than one code from category 428 may be assigned if the patient has systolic or diastolic failure and congestive heart failure.

The same heart conditions (425.8, 428, 429.0-429.3, 429.8, 429.9) with hypertension, but without a stated casual relationship, are coded separately. Sequence according to the circumstances of the admission/encounter.

3. Hypertensive Renal Disease with Chronic Renal Failure

Assign codes from category 403, Hypertensive renal disease, when conditions classified to categories 585-587 are present.

Unlike hypertension with heart disease, ICD-9-CM presumes a cause-and-effect relationship and classifies renal failure with hypertension as hypertensive renal disease.

4. Hypertensive Heart and Renal Disease

Assign codes from combination category 404, Hypertensive heart and renal disease, when both hypertensive renal disease and hypertensive heart disease are stated in the diagnosis. Assume a relationship between the hypertension and the renal disease, whether or not the condition is so designated. Assign an additional code from category 428, to identify the type of heart failure. More than one code from category 428 may be assigned if the patient has systolic or diastolic failure and congestive heart failure.

5. Hypertensive Cerebrovascular Disease

First assign codes from 430-438, Cerebrovascular disease, then the appropriate hypertension code from categories 401-405.

6. Hypertensive Retinopathy

Two codes are necessary to identify the condition. First assign the code from subcategory 362.11, Hypertensive retinopathy, then the appropriate code from categories 401-405 to indicate the type of hypertension.

7. Hypertension, Secondary

Two codes are required: one to identify the underlying etiology and one from category 405 to identify the hypertension. Sequencing of codes is determined by the reason for admission/encounter.

8. Hypertension, Transient

Assign code 796.2, Elevated blood pressure reading without diagnosis of hypertension, unless patient has an established diagnosis of hypertension. Assign code 642.3x for transient hypertension of pregnancy.

9. Hypertension, Controlled

Assign appropriate code from categories 401-405. This diagnostic statement usually refers to an existing state of hypertension under control by therapy.

10. Hypertension, Uncontrolled

Uncontrolled hypertension may refer to untreated hypertension or hypertension not responding to current therapeutic regimen. In either case, assign the appropriate code from categories 401-405 to designate the stage and type of hypertension. Code to the type of hypertension.

11. Elevated Blood Pressure

For a statement of elevated blood pressure without further specificity, assign code 796.2, Elevated blood pressure reading without diagnosis of hypertension, rather than a code from category 401.

B. Late Effects of Cerebrovascular Disease

Category 438 is used to indicate conditions classifiable to categories 430-437 as the causes of late effects (neurologic deficits), themselves classified elsewhere. These "late effects" include neurologic deficits that persist after initial onset of conditions classifiable to 430-437. The neurologic deficits caused by cerebrovascular disease may be present from the onset or may arise at any time after the onset of the condition classifiable to 430-437.

Codes from category 438 may be assigned on a health care record with codes from 430-437, if the patient has a current cerebrovascular accident (CVA) and deficits from an old CVA. Assign code V12.59 (and not a code from category 438) as an additional code for history of cerebrovascular disease when no neurologic deficits are present.

C8. Diseases of Respiratory System

Reserved for future guideline expansion

C9. Diseases of Digestive System

Reserved for future guideline expansion

C10. Diseases of Genitourinary System

Reserved for future guideline expansion

C11. Complications of Pregnancy, Childbirth, and the Puerperium

A. General Rules for Obstetric Cases

1. Obstetric cases require codes from chapter 11, codes in the range 630-677, Complications of Pregnancy, Childbirth, and the Puerperium. Should the physician document that the pregnancy is incidental to the encounter, then code V22.2 should be used in place of any chapter 11 codes. It is the physician's responsibility to state that the condition being treated is not affecting the pregnancy.

2. Chapter 11 codes have sequencing priority over codes from other chapters. Additional codes from other chapters may be used in conjunction with chapter 11 codes to further specify conditions. For example, sepsis and septic shock associated with abortion, ectopic pregnancy, and molar pregnancy are classified to category codes in Chapter 11 (630-639).

3. Chapter 11 codes are to be used only on the maternal record, never on the record of the newborn.

4. Categories 640-648, 651-676 have required fifth-digits, which indicate whether the encounter is antepartum, postpartum and whether a delivery has also occurred.

5. The fifth-digits, which are appropriate for each code number, are listed in brackets under each code. The fifth-digits on each code should all be consistent with each other. That is, should a delivery occur all of the fifth-digits should indicate the delivery.

6. For prenatal outpatient visits for patients with high-risk pregnancies, a code from category V23, Supervision of high-risk pregnancy, should be used as the principal or first-listed diagnosis. Secondary chapter 11 codes may be used in conjunction with these codes if appropriate. A thorough review of any pertinent excludes note is necessary to be certain that these V codes are being used properly.

7. An outcome of delivery code, V27.0-V27.9, should be included on every maternal record when a delivery has occurred. These codes are not to be used on subsequent records or on the newborn record.

8. For routine outpatient prenatal visits when no complications are present codes V22.0, Supervision of normal first pregnancy, and V22.1, Supervision of other normal pregnancy, should be used as the first-listed diagnoses. These codes should not be used in conjunction with chapter 11 codes.

B. Selection of OB Principal or First-listed Diagnosis

1. In episodes when no delivery occurs, the principal diagnosis should correspond to the principal complication of the pregnancy, which necessitated the encounter. Should more than one complication exist, all of which are treated or monitored, any of the complications codes may be sequenced first.

2. When a delivery occurs, the principal diagnosis should correspond to the main circumstances or complication of the delivery.

In cases of cesarean delivery, the selection of the principal diagnosis should correspond to the reason the cesarean delivery was performed unless the reason for admission/encounter was unrelated to the condition resulting in the cesarean delivery.

C. Fetal Conditions Affecting the Management of the Mother

Codes from category 655, Known or suspected fetal abnormality affecting management of the mother, and category 656, Other fetal and placental problems affecting the management of the mother, are assigned only when the fetal condition is actually responsible for modifying the management of the mother, i.e., by requiring diagnostic studies, additional observation, special care, or termination of pregnancy. The fact that the fetal condition exists does not justify assigning a code from this series to the mother's record.

D. HIV Infection in Pregnancy, Childbirth and the Puerperium

During pregnancy, childbirth or the puerperium, a patient admitted because of an HIV-related illness should receive a principal diagnosis of 647.6X, Other specified infectious and parasitic diseases in the mother classifiable elsewhere, but complicating the pregnancy, childbirth or the puerperium, followed by 042 and the code(s) for the HIV-related illness(es). This is an exception to the sequencing rule found in above.

Patients with asymptomatic HIV infection status admitted during pregnancy, childbirth, or the puerperium should receive codes of 647.6X and V08.

E. Normal Delivery, 650

1. Code 650 is for use in cases when a woman is admitted for a full-term normal delivery and delivers a single, healthy infant without any complications antepartum, during the delivery, or postpartum during the delivery episode.

2. Code 650 may be used if the patient had a complication at some point during her pregnancy but the complication is not present at the time of the admission for delivery.

3. Code 650 is always a principal diagnosis. It is not to be used if any other code from chapter 11 is needed to describe a current complication of the antenatal, delivery, or perinatal period. Additional codes from other chapters may be used with code 650 if they are not related to or are in any way complicating the pregnancy.

4. V27.0, Single liveborn, is the only outcome of delivery code appropriate for use with 650.

F. The Postpartum Period

1. The postpartum period begins immediately after delivery and continues for six weeks following delivery.

2. A postpartum complication is any complication occurring within the six-week period.

3. Chapter 11 codes may also be used to describe pregnancy-related complications after the six-week period should the physician document that a condition is pregnancy related.

4. Postpartum complications that occur during the same admission as the delivery are identified with a fifth digit of "2." Subsequent admissions/encounters for postpartum complications should identified with a fifth digit of "4."

5. When the mother delivers outside the hospital prior to admission and is admitted for routine postpartum care and no complications are noted, code V24.0, Postpartum care and examination immediately after delivery, should be assigned as the principal diagnosis.

6. A delivery diagnosis code should not be used for a woman who has delivered prior to admission to the hospital. Any postpartum procedures should be coded.

G. Code 677, Late effect of complication of pregnancy, childbirth, and the puerperium

1. Code 677, Late effect of complication of pregnancy, childbirth, and the puerperium is for use in those cases when an initial complication of a pregnancy develops a sequelae requiring care or treatment at a future date.

2. This code may be used at any time after the initial postpartum period.

3. This code, like all late effect codes, is to be sequenced following the code describing the sequelae of the complication.

H. Abortions

1. Fifth-digits are required for abortion categories 634-637. Fifth-digit 1, incomplete, indicates that all of the products of conception have not been expelled from the uterus. Fifth-digit 2, complete, indicates that all products of conception have been expelled from the uterus prior to the episode of care.

2. A code from categories 640-648 and 651-657 may be used as additional codes with an abortion code to indicate the complication leading to the abortion.

   Fifth digit 3 is assigned with codes from these categories when used with an abortion code because the other fifth digits will not apply. Codes from the 660-669 series are not to be used for complications of abortion.

3. Code 639 is to be used for all complications following abortion. Code 639 cannot be assigned with codes from categories 634-638.

4. Abortion with Liveborn Fetus.

   When an attempted termination of pregnancy results in a liveborn fetus assign code 644.21, Early onset of delivery, with an appropriate code from category V27, Outcome of Delivery. The procedure code for the attempted termination of pregnancy should also be assigned.

5. Retained Products of Conception following an abortion.

Subsequent admissions for retained products of conception following a spontaneous or legally induced abortion are assigned the appropriate code from category 634, Spontaneous abortion, or legally induced abortion, with a fifth digit of "1" (incomplete). This advice is appropriate even when the patient was discharged previously with a discharge diagnosis of complete abortion.

C12. Diseases Skin and Subcutaneous Tissue

Reserved for future guideline expansion

C13. Diseases of Musculoskeletal and Connective Tissue

Reserved for future guideline expansion

C14. Congenital Anomalies

Reserved for future guideline expansion

C15. Newborn (Perinatal) Guidelines

For coding and reporting purposes the perinatal period is defined as birth through the 28th day following birth. The following guidelines are provided for reporting purposes. Hospitals may record other diagnoses as needed for internal data use.

A. General Perinatal Rule

All clinically significant conditions noted on routine newborn examination should be coded. A condition is clinically significant if it requires: clinical evaluation; or therapeutic treatment; or diagnostic procedures; or extended length of hospital stay; or increased nursing care and/or monitoring; or has implications for future health care needs.

Note: The perinatal guidelines listed above are the same as the general coding guidelines for "additional diagnoses," except for the final point regarding implications for future health care needs. Whether or not a condition is clinically significant can only be determined by the physician.

B. Use of Codes V30-V39

When coding the birth of an infant, assign a code from categories V30-V39, according to the type of birth. A code from this series is assigned as a principal diagnosis, and assigned only once to a newborn at the time of birth.

C. Newborn Transfers

If the newborn is transferred to another institution, the V30 series is not used at the receiving hospital.

D. Use of Category V29

1. Assign a code from category V29, Observation and evaluation of newborns and infants for suspected conditions not found, to identify those instances when a healthy newborn is evaluated for a suspected condition that is determined after study not to be present. Do not use a code from category V29 when the patient has identified signs or symptoms of a suspected problem; in such cases, code the sign or symptom.

2. A V29 code is to be used as a secondary code after the V30, Outcome of delivery, code. It may also be assigned as a principal code for readmissions or encounters when the V30 code no longer applies. It is for use only for healthy newborns and infants for which no condition after study is found to be present.

E. Maternal Causes of Perinatal Morbidity

Codes from categories 760-763, Maternal causes of perinatal morbidity and mortality, are assigned only when the maternal condition has actually affected the fetus or newborn. The fact that the mother has an associated medical condition or experiences some complication of pregnancy, labor or delivery does not justify the routine assignment of codes from these categories to the newborn record.

F. Congenital Anomalies

Assign an appropriate code from categories 740-759, Congenital Anomalies, as an additional diagnosis when a specific abnormality is diagnosed for an infant. Congenital anomalies may also be the principal or first listed diagnosis for admissions/encounters subsequent to the newborn admission. Such abnormalities may occur as a set of symptoms or multiple malformations. A code should be assigned for each presenting manifestation of the syndrome if the syndrome is not specifically indexed in ICD-9-CM.

G. Coding of Additional Perinatal Diagnoses

1. Assign codes for conditions that require treatment or further investigation, prolong the length of stay, or require resource utilization.

2. Assign codes for conditions that have been specified by the physician as having implications for future health care needs.

   Note: This guideline should not be used for adult patients.

3. Assign a code for Newborn conditions originating in the perinatal period (categories 760-779), as well as complications arising during the current episode of care classified in other chapters, only if the diagnoses have been documented by the responsible physician at the time of transfer or discharge as having affected the fetus or newborn.

H. Prematurity and Fetal Growth Retardation

Codes from category 764 and subcategories 765.0 and 765.1 should not be assigned based solely on recorded birthweight or estimated gestational age, but on the attending physician's clinical assessment of maturity of the infant. NOTE: Since physicians may utilize different criteria in determining prematurity, do not code the diagnosis of prematurity unless the physician documents this condition.

A code from subcategory 765.2, Weeks of gestation, should be assigned as an additional code with category 764 and codes from 765.0 and 765.1 to specify weeks of gestation as documented by the physician.

C16. Signs, Symptoms and Ill-Defined Conditions

Reserved for future guideline expansion

C17. Injury and Poisoning

A. Coding of Injuries

When coding injuries, assign separate codes for each injury unless a combination code is provided, in which case the combination code is assigned. Multiple injury codes are provided in ICD-9-CM, but should not be assigned unless information for a more specific code is not available. These codes are not to be used for normal, healing surgical wounds or to identify complications of surgical wounds.

The code for the most serious injury, as determined by the physician, is sequenced first.

1. Superficial injuries such as abrasions or contusions are not coded when associated with more severe injuries of the same site.

2. When a primary injury results in minor damage to peripheral nerves or blood vessels, the primary injury is sequenced first with additional code(s) from categories 950-957, Injury to nerves and spinal cord, and/or 900-904, Injury to blood vessels. When the primary injury is to the blood vessels or nerves, that injury should be sequenced first.

B. Coding of Fractures

The principles of multiple coding of injuries should be followed in coding fractures. Fractures of specified sites are coded individually by site in accordance with both the provisions within categories 800-829 and the level of detail furnished by medical record content. Combination categories for multiple fractures are provided for use when there is insufficient detail in the medical record (such as trauma cases transferred to another hospital), when the reporting form limits the number of codes that can be used in reporting pertinent clinical data, or when there is insufficient specificity at the fourth-digit or fifth-digit level. More specific guidelines are as follows:

1. Multiple fractures of same limb classifiable to the same three-digit or four-digit category are coded to that category.

2. Multiple unilateral or bilateral fractures of same bone(s) but classified to different fourth-digit subdivisions (bone part) within the same three-digit category are coded individually by site.

3. Multiple fracture categories 819 and 828 classify bilateral fractures of both upper limbs (819) and both lower limbs (828), but without any detail at the fourth-digit level other than open and closed type of fractures.

4. Multiple fractures are sequenced in accordance with the severity of the fracture and the physician should be asked to list the fracture diagnoses in the order of severity.

C. Coding of Burns

Current burns (940-948) are classified by depth, extent and by agent (E code). Burns are classified by depth as first degree (erythema), second degree (blistering), and third degree (full-thickness involvement).

1. Sequence first the code that reflects the highest degree of burn when more than one burn is present.

2. Classify burns of the same local site (three-digit category level, (940-947) but of different degrees to the subcategory identifying the highest degree recorded in the diagnosis.

3. Non-healing burns are coded as acute burns.

   Necrosis of burned skin should be coded as a non-healed burn.

4. Assign code 958.3, Posttraumatic wound infection, not elsewhere classified, as an additional code for any documented infected burn site.

5. When coding burns, assign separate codes for each burn site. Category 946 Burns of Multiple specified sites, should only be used if the location of the burns are not documented.

   Category 949, Burn, unspecified, is extremely vague and should rarely be used.

6. Assign codes from category 948, Burns classified according to extent of body surface involved, when the site of the burn is not specified or when there is a need for additional data. It is advisable to use category 948 as additional coding when needed to provide data for evaluating burn mortality, such as that needed by burn units. It is also advisable to use category 948 as an additional code for reporting purposes when there is mention of a third-degree burn involving 20 percent or more of the body surface.

   In assigning a code from category 948: Fourth-digit codes are used to identify the percentage of total body surface involved in a burn (all degree).

   Fifth-digits are assigned to identify the percentage of body surface involved in third-degree burn.

   Fifth-digit zero (0) is assigned when less than 10 percent or when no body surface is involved in a third-degree burn.

   Category 948 is based on the classic "rule of nines" in estimating body surface involved: head and neck are assigned nine percent, each arm nine percent, each leg 18 percent, the anterior trunk 18 percent, posterior trunk 18 percent, and genitalia one percent. Physicians may change these percentage assignments where necessary to accommodate infants and children who have proportionately larger heads than adults and patients who have large buttocks, thighs, or abdomen that involve burns.

7. Encounters for the treatment of the late effects of burns (i.e., scars or joint contractures) should be coded to the residual condition (sequelae) followed by the appropriate late effect code (906.5-906.9). A late effect E code may also be used, if desired.

8. When appropriate, both a sequelae with a late effect code, and a current burn code may be assigned on the same record.

D. Coding of Debridement of Wound, Infection, or Burn

Excisional debridement may be performed by a physician and/or other health care provider and involves an excisional, as opposed to a mechanical (brushing, scrubbing, washing) debridement.

For coding purposes, excisional debridement, 86.22.

Nonexcisional debridement is assigned to 86.28.

Modified based on Coding Clinic, 2nd Quarter 2000, p. 9.

E. Adverse Effects, Poisoning and Toxic Effects

The properties of certain drugs, medicinal and biological substances or combinations of such substances, may cause toxic reactions. The occurrence of drug toxicity is classified in ICD-9-CM as follows:

1. Adverse Effect

   When the drug was correctly prescribed and properly administered, code the reaction plus the appropriate code from the E930-E949 series. Codes from the E930-E949 series must be used to identify the causative substance for an adverse effect of drug, medicinal and biological substances, correctly prescribed and properly administered. The effect, such as tachycardia, delirium, gastrointestinal hemorrhaging, vomiting, hypokalemia, hepatitis, renal failure, or respiratory failure, is coded and followed by the appropriate code from the E930-E949 series.

Adverse effects of therapeutic substances correctly prescribed and properly administered (toxicity, synergistic reaction, side effect, and idiosyncratic reaction) may be due to (1) differences among patients, such as age, sex, disease, and genetic factors, and (2) drug-related factors, such as type of drug, route of administration, duration of therapy, dosage, and bioavailability.

2. Poisoning

a. When an error was made in drug prescription or in the administration of the drug by physician, nurse, patient, or other person, use the appropriate poisoning code from the 960-979 series.

b. If an overdose of a drug was intentionally taken or administered and resulted in drug toxicity, it would be coded as a poisoning (960-979 series).

c. If a nonprescribed drug or medicinal agent was taken in combination with a correctly prescribed and properly administered drug, any drug toxicity or other reaction resulting from the interaction of the two drugs would be classified as a poisoning.

d. When coding a poisoning or reaction to the improper use of a medication (e.g., wrong dose, wrong substance, wrong route of administration) the poisoning code is sequenced first, followed by a code for the manifestation. If there is also a diagnosis of drug abuse or dependence to the substance, the abuse or dependence is coded as an additional code.

C18. Classification of Factors Influencing Health Status and Contact with Health Service

A. ICD-9-CM provides codes to deal with encounters for circumstances other than a disease or injury. The Supplementary Classification of Factors Influencing Health Status and Contact with Health Services (V01.0 - V83.89) is provided to deal with occasions when circumstances other than a disease or injury (codes 001-999) are recorded as a diagnosis or problem.

There are four primary circumstances for the use of V codes:

1. When a person who is not currently sick encounters the health services for some specific reason, such as to act as an organ donor, to receive prophylactic care, such as inoculations or health screenings, or to receive counseling on health related issue.

2. When a person with a resolving disease or injury, or a chronic, long-term condition requiring continuous care, encounters the health care system for specific aftercare of that disease or injury (e.g.,dialysis for renal disease; chemotherapy for malignancy; cast change). A diagnosis/symptom code should be used whenever a current, acute, diagnosis is being treated or a sign or symptom is being studied.

3. When circumstances or problems influence a person's health status but are not in themselves a current illness or injury.

4. For newborns, to indicate birth status.

B. V codes are for use in both the inpatient and outpatient setting but are generally more applicable to the outpatient setting. V codes may be used as either a first listed (principal diagnosis code in the inpatient setting) or secondary code depending on the circumstances of the encounter. Certain V codes may only be used as first listed, others only as secondary codes.

C. V Codes indicate a reason for an encounter. They are not procedure codes. A corresponding procedure code must accompany a V code to describe the procedure performed.

D. Categories of V Codes

1. Contact/Exposure

Category V01 indicates contact with or exposure to communicable diseases. These codes are for patients who do not show any sign or symptom of a disease but have been exposed to it by close personal contact with an infected individual or are in an area where a disease is epidemic. These codes may be used as a first listed code to explain an encounter for testing, or, more commonly, as a secondary code to identify a potential risk.

2. Inoculations and vaccinations

Categories V03-V06 are for encounters for inoculations and vaccinations. They indicate that a patient is being seen to receive a prophylactic inoculation against a disease. The injection itself must be represented by the appropriate procedure code. A code from V03-V06 may be used as a secondary code if the inoculation is given as a routine part of preventive health care, such as a well-baby visit.

3. Status

Status codes indicate that a patient is either a carrier of a disease or has the sequelae or residual of a past disease or condition. This includes such things as the presence of prosthetic or mechanical devices resulting from past treatment. A status code is informative because the status may affect the course of treatment and its outcome. A status code is distinct from a history code. The history code indicates that the patient no longer has the condition.

The status V codes/categories are:

V02	Carrier or suspected carrier of infectious diseases Carrier status, indicates that a person harbors the specific organisms of a disease without manifest symptoms and is capable of transmitting the infection.
V08	Asymptomatic HIV infection status This code indicates that a patient has tested positive for HIV but has manifested no signs or symptoms of the disease.
V09	Infection with drug-resistant microorganisms This category indicates that a patient has an infection which is resistant to drug treatment. Sequence the infection code first.
V21	Constitutional states in development
V22.2	Pregnant state, incidental This code is a secondary code only for use when the pregnancy is in no way complicating the reason for visit. Otherwise, a code from the obstetric chapter is required.
V26.5x	Sterilization status
V42	Organ or tissue replaced by transplant
V43	Organ or tissue replaced by other means
V44	Artificial opening status
V45	Other postsurgical states
V46	Other dependence on machines
V49.6	Upper limb amputation status
V49.7	Lower limb amputation status
V48.81	Postmenopausal status
V49.82	Dental sealant status
V58.6	Long-term (current) drug use This subcategory indicates a patient's continuous use of a prescribed drug (including such things as aspirin therapy) for the long-term treatment of a condition or for prophylactic use. It is not for use for patients who have addictions to drugs.
V83	Genetic carrier status Categories V42-V46, and subcategories V49.6, V49.7 are for use only if there are no complications or malfunctions of the organ or tissue replaced, the amputation site or the equipment on which the patient is dependent. These are always secondary codes.

4. History (of)

There are two types of history V codes, personal and family. Personal history codes explain a patient's past medical condition that no longer exists and is not receiving any treatment but that has the potential for recurrence, and, therefore, may require continued monitoring. The exceptions to this general rule are category V14, Personal history of allergy to medicinal agents and subcategory V15.0, Allergy, other than to medicinal agents. A person who has had an allergic episode to a substance or food in the past should always be considered allergic to the substance.

Family history codes are for use when a patient has a family member(s) who has had a particular disease that causes the patient to be at higher risk of also contracting the disease.

Personal history codes may be used in conjunction with follow-up codes and family history codes may be use in conjunction with screening codes to explain the need for a test or procedure. History codes are also acceptable on any medical record regardless of the reason for visit. A history of an illness, even if no longer present, is important information that may alter the type of treatment ordered.

The history V code categories are:

V10	Personal history of malignant neoplasm
V12	Personal history of certain other diseases
V13	Personal history of other diseases Except: V13.4, Personal history of arthritis, and V13.6, Personal history of congenital malformations. These conditions are life-long so are not true history codes.
V14	Personal history of allergy to medicinal agents
V15	Other personal history presenting hazards to health Except: V15.7, Personal history of contraception.
V16	Family history of malignant neoplasm
V17	Family history of certain chronic disabling diseases
V18	Family history of certain other specific diseases
V19	Family history of other conditions

5. Screening

Screening is the testing for disease or disease precursors in seemingly well individuals so that early detection and treatment can be provided for those who test positive for the disease. Screenings that are recommended for many subgroups in a population include: routine mammograms for women over 40, a fecal occult blood test for everyone over 50, an amniocentesis to rule out a fetal anomaly for pregnant women over 35, because the incidence of breast cancer and colon cancer in these subgroups is higher than in the general population, as is the incidence of Down's syndrome in older mothers.

The testing of a person to rule out or confirm a suspected diagnosis because the patient has some sign or symptom is a diagnostic examination, not a screening. In these cases, the sign or symptom is used to explain the reason for the test.

A screening code may be a first listed code if the reason for the visit is specifically the screening exam. It may also be used as an additional code if the screening is done during an office visit for other health problems. A screening code is not necessary if the screening is inherent to a routine examination, such as a pap smear done during a routine pelvic examination.

Should a condition be discovered during the screening then the code for the condition may be assigned as an additional diagnosis.

The V code indicates that a screening exam is planned. A procedure code is required to confirm that the screening was performed.

The screening V code categories:

V28	Antenatal screening
V73-V82	Special screening examinations

6. Observation

There are two observation V code categories. They are for use in very limited circumstances when a person is being observed for a suspected condition that is ruled out. The observation codes are not for use if an injury or illness or any signs or symptoms related to the suspected condition are present. In such cases the diagnosis/symptom code is used with the corresponding E code to identify any external cause.

The observation codes are to be used as principal diagnosis only. The only exception to this is when the principal diagnosis is required to be a code from the V30, Live born infant, category. Then the V29 observation code is sequenced after the V30 code. Additional codes may be used in addition to the observation code but only if they are unrelated to the suspected condition being observed.

The observation V code categories:

V29	Observation and evaluation of newborns for suspected condition not found A code from category V30 should be sequenced before the V29 code.
V71	Observation and evaluation for suspected condition not found

7. Aftercare

Aftercare visit codes cover situations when the initial treatment of a disease or injury has been performed and the patient requires continued care during the healing or recovery phase, or for the long-term consequences of the disease. The aftercare V code should not be used if treatment is directed at a current, acute disease or injury, the diagnosis code is to be used in these cases. Exceptions to this rule are codes V58.0, Radiotherapy, and V58.1, Chemotherapy. These codes are to be first listed, followed by the diagnosis code when a patient's encounter is solely to receive radiation therapy or chemotherapy for the treatment of a neoplasm. Should a patient receive both chemotherapy and radiation therapy during the same encounter code V58.0 and V58.1 may be used together on a record with either one being sequenced first.

The aftercare codes are generally first listed to explain the specific reason for the encounter. An aftercare code may be used as an additional code when some type of aftercare is provided in addition to the reason for admission and no diagnosis code is applicable. An example of this would be the closure of a colostomy during an encounter for treatment of another condition.

Certain aftercare V code categories need a secondary diagnosis code to describe the resolving condition or sequelae, for others, the condition is inherent in the code title.

Additional V code aftercare category terms include, fitting and adjustment, and attention to artificial openings.

The aftercare V category/codes:

V52	Fitting and adjustment of prosthetic device and implant
V53	Fitting and adjustment of other device
V54	Other orthopedic aftercare
V55	Attention to artificial openings
V56	Encounter for dialysis and dialysis catheter care
V57	Care involving the use of rehabilitation procedures
V58.0	Radiotherapy
V58.1	Chemotherapy
V58.3	Attention to surgical dressings and sutures
V58.41	Encounter for planned post-operative wound closure
V58.42	Aftercare, surgery, neoplasm
V58.43	Aftercare, surgery, trauma
V58.49	Other specified aftercare following surgery
V58.71–V58.78	Aftercare following surgery
V58.81	Fitting and adjustment of vascular catheter
V58.82	Fitting and adjustment of non-vascular catheter
V58.83	Monitoring therapeutic drug
V58.89	Other specified aftercare

8. Follow-up

The follow-up codes are for use to explain continuing surveillance following completed treatment of a disease, condition, or injury. They infer that the condition has been fully treated and no longer exists. They should not be confused with aftercare codes which explain current treatment for a healing condition or its sequelae. Follow-up codes may be used in conjunction with history codes to provide the full picture of the healed condition and its treatment. The follow-up code is sequenced first, followed by the history code.

A follow-up code may be used to explain repeated visits. Should a condition be found to have recurred on the follow-up visit, then the diagnosis code should be used in place of the follow-up code.

The follow-up V code categories:

| V24 | Postpartum care and evaluation |
| V67 | Follow-up examination |

9. Donor

Category V59 is the donor codes. They are for use for living individuals who are donating blood or other body tissue. These codes are only for individuals donating for others, not for self donations. They are not for use to identify cadaveric donations.

10. Counseling

Counseling V codes are for use for when a patient or family member receives assistance in the aftermath of an illness or injury, or when support is required in coping with family or social problems. They are not necessary for use in conjunction with a diagnosis code when the counseling component of care is considered integral to standard treatment.

The counseling V categories/codes:

V25.0	General counseling and advice for contraceptive management
V26.3	Genetic counseling
V26.4	General counseling and advice for procreative management
V61	Other family circumstances
V65.1	Person consulted on behalf of another person
V65.3	Dietary surveillance and counseling
V65.4	Other counseling, not elsewhere classified

11. Obstetrics and related conditions

See the Obstetrics guidelines for further instruction on the use of these codes.

V codes for pregnancy are for use in those circumstances when none of the problems or complications included in the codes from the Obstetrics chapter exist (a routine prenatal visit or postpartum care) V22.0, Supervision of normal first pregnancy, and V22.1, Supervision of other normal pregnancy, are always first listed and are not to be used with any other code from the OB chapter.

The outcome of delivery, category V27, should be included on all maternal delivery records. It is always a secondary code.

V codes for family planning (contraceptive) or procreative management and counseling should be included on an obstetric record either during the pregnancy or the postpartum stage, if applicable.

Obstetrics and related conditions V code categories:

V22	Normal pregnancy
V23	Supervision of high-risk pregnancy Except: V23.2, Pregnancy with history of abortion. Code 646.3, Habitual aborter, from the OB chapter is required to indicate a history of abortion during a pregnancy.
V24	Postpartum care and evaluation
V25	Encounter for contraceptive management Except V25.0x (See counseling above)
V26	Procreative management Except V26.5x, Sterilization status, V26.3 and V26.4 (Counseling)
V27	Outcome of delivery
V28	Antenatal screening See Screening - see section 5 of this article

12. Newborn, infant and child

See the newborn guidelines for further instruction on the use of these codes.

Newborn V code categories:

| V20 | Health supervision of infant or child |
| V29 | Observation and evaluation of newborns for suspected condition not found-see Observation, section 6 of this article. |

V30-V39 Liveborn infant according to type of birth

13. Routine and administrative examinations

The V codes allow for the description of encounters for routine examinations, such as, a general check-up, or, examinations for administrative purposes, such as, a pre-employment physical. The codes are for use as first listed codes only and are not to be used if the examination is for diagnosis of a suspected condition or for treatment purposes. In such cases the diagnosis code is used. During a routine exam, should a diagnosis or condition be discovered, it should be coded as an additional code. Pre-existing and chronic conditions, and history codes may also be included as additional codes as long as the examination is for administrative purposes and not focused on any particular condition.

Pre-operative examination V codes are for use only in those situations when a patient is being cleared for surgery and no treatment is given.

The V codes categories/code for routine and administrative examinations:

V20.2	Routine infant or child health check Any injections given should have a corresponding procedure code.
V70	General medical examination
V72	Special investigations and examinations Except V72.5 and V72.6

14. Miscellaneous V codes

The miscellaneous V codes capture a number of other health care encounters that do not fall into one of the other categories. Certain of these codes identify the reason for the encounter, others are for use as additional codes which provide useful information on circumstances which may affect a patient's care and treatment.

Miscellaneous V code categories/codes:

V07	Need for isolation and other prophylactic measures
V50	Elective surgery for purposes other than remedying health states
V58.5	Orthodontics
V60	Housing, household, and economic circumstances
V62	Other psychosocial circumstances
V63	Unavailability of other medical facilities for care
V64	Persons encountering health services for specific procedures, not carried out
V66	Convalescence and Palliative Care
V68	Encounters for administrative purposes
V69	Problems related to lifestyle

15. Nonspecific V codes

Certain V codes are so non-specific, or potentially redundant with other codes in the classification that there can be little justification for their use in the inpatient setting. Their use in the outpatient setting should be limited to those instances when there is no further documentation to permit more precise coding. Otherwise, any sign or symptom or any other reason for visit which is captured in another code should be used.

Nonspecific V code categories/codes:

V11	Personal history of mental disorder A code from the mental disorders chapter, with an in remission fifth-digit, should be used.
V13.4	Personal history of arthritis
V13.6	Personal history of congenital malformations
V15.7	Personal history of contraception
V23.2	Pregnancy with history of abortion
V40	Mental and behavioral problems
V41	Problems with special senses and other special functions
V47	Other problems with internal organs
V48	Problems with head, neck, and trunk
V49	Problems with limbs and other problems Exceptions: V49.6 Upper limb amputation status, V49.7 Lower limb amputation status,

V49.81 Postmenopausal status, V49.82 Dental sealant status

V51   Aftercare involving the use of plastic surgery

V58.2   Blood transfusion, without reported diagnosis

V58.9   Unspecified aftercare

V72.5   Radiological examination, NEC

V72.6   Laboratory examination
Codes V72.5 and V72.6 are not to be used if any sign or symptoms, or reason for a test is documented. See section K and L of the outpatient guidelines.

C19. Supplemental Classification of External Causes of Injury and Poisoning (E-codes)

Introduction: These guidelines are provided for those who are currently collecting E codes in order that there will be standardization in the process. If your institution plans to begin collecting E codes, these guidelines are to be applied. The use of E codes is supplemental to the application of ICD-9-CM diagnosis codes. E codes are never to be recorded as principal diagnosis (first-listed in noninpatient setting) and are not required for reporting to CMS.

External causes of injury and poisoning codes (E codes) are intended to provide data for injury research and evaluation of injury prevention strategies. E codes capture how the injury or poisoning happened (cause), the intent (unintentional or accidental; or intentional, such as suicide or assault), and the place where the event occurred. Some major categories of E codes include:

- transport accidents
- poisoning and adverse effects of drugs, medicinal substances and biologicals
- accidental falls
- accidents caused by fire and flames
- accidents due to natural and environmental factors
- late effects of accidents, assaults or self injury
- assaults or purposely inflicted injury
- suicide or self inflicted injury

These guidelines apply for the coding and collection of E codes from records in hospitals, outpatient clinics, emergency departments, other ambulatory care settings and physician offices, and nonacute care settings, except when other specific guidelines apply. (See Section III, Reporting Diagnostic Guidelines for Hospital-based Outpatient Services/Reporting Requirements for Physician Billing.)

A.   General E Code Coding Guidelines

1.   An E code may be used with any code in the range of 001-V83.89, which indicates an injury, poisoning, or adverse effect due to an external cause.

2.   Assign the appropriate E code for all initial treatments of an injury, poisoning, or adverse effect of drugs.

3.   Use a late effect E code for subsequent visits when a late effect of the initial injury or poisoning is being treated. There is no late effect E code for adverse effects of drugs.

4.   Use the full range of E codes to completely describe the cause, the intent and the place of occurrence, if applicable, for all injuries, poisonings, and adverse effects of drugs.

5.   Assign as many E codes as necessary to fully explain each cause. If only one E code can be recorded, assign the E code most related to the principal diagnosis.

6.   The selection of the appropriate E code is guided by the Index to External Causes, which is located after the alphabetical index to diseases and by Inclusion and Exclusion notes in the Tabular List.

7.   An E code can never be a principal (first listed) diagnosis.

B.   Place of Occurrence Guidelines
Use an additional code from category E849 to indicate the Place of Occurrence for injuries and poisonings. The Place of Occurrence describes the place where the event occurred and not the patient's activity at the time of the event.

Do not use E849.9 if the place of occurrence is not stated.

C.   Adverse Effects of Drugs, Medicinal and Biological Substances Guidelines

1.   Do not code directly from the Table of Drugs and Chemicals. Always refer back to the Tabular List.

2.   Use as many codes as necessary to describe completely all drugs, medicinal or biological substances.

3.   If the same E code would describe the causative agent for more than one adverse reaction, assign the code only once.

4.   If two or more drugs, medicinal or biological substances are reported, code each individually unless the combination code is listed in the Table of Drugs and Chemicals. In that case, assign the E code for the combination.

5.   When a reaction results from the interaction of a drug(s) and alcohol, use poisoning codes and E codes for both.

6.   If the reporting format limits the number of E codes that can be used in reporting clinical data, code the one most related to the principal diagnosis. Include at least one from each category (cause, intent, place) if possible.

If there are different fourth digit codes in the same three digit category, use the code for "Other specified" of that category. If there is no "Other specified" code in that category, use the appropriate "Unspecified" code in that category.

If the codes are in different three digit categories, assign the appropriate E code for other multiple drugs and medicinal substances.

7.   Codes from the E930-E949 series must be used to identify the causative substance for an adverse effect of drug, medicinal and biological substances, correctly prescribed and properly administered. The effect, such as tachycardia, delirium, gastrointestinal hemorrhaging, vomiting, hypokalemia, hepatitis, renal failure, or respiratory failure, is coded and followed by the appropriate code from the E930-E949 series.

D.   Multiple Cause E Code Coding Guidelines

If two or more events cause separate injuries, an E code should be assigned for each cause. The first listed E code will be selected in the following order:

E codes for child and adult abuse take priority over all other E codes - see Child and Adult abuse guidelines.

E codes for terrorism events take priority over all other E codes except child and adult abuse.

E codes for cataclysmic events take priority over all other E codes except child and adult abuse and terrorism.

E codes for transport accidents take priority over all other E codes except cataclysmic events and child and adult abuse and terrorism.

The first-listed E code should correspond to the cause of the most serious diagnosis due to an assault, accident, or self-harm, following the order of hierarchy listed above.

E.   Child and Adult Abuse Guidelines

1.   When the cause of an injury or neglect is intentional child or adult abuse, the first listed E code should be assigned from categories E960-E968, Homicide and injury purposely inflicted by other persons, (except category E967). An E code from category E967, Child and adult battering and other maltreatment, should be added as an additional code to identify the perpetrator, if known.

2.   In cases of neglect when the intent is determined to be accidental E code E904.0, Abandonment or neglect of infant and helpless person, should be the first listed E code.

F.   Unknown or Suspected Intent Guidelines

1.   If the intent (accident, self-harm, assault) of the cause of an injury or poisoning is unknown or unspecified, code the intent as undetermined E980-E989.

2.   If the intent (accident, self-harm, assault) of the cause of an injury or poisoning is questionable, probable or suspected, code the intent as undetermined E980-E989.

G.   Undetermined Cause Guidelines

When the intent of an injury or poisoning is known, but the cause is unknown, use codes: E928.9, Unspecified accident, E958.9, Suicide and self-inflicted injury by unspecified means, and E968.9, Assault by unspecified means.

These E codes should rarely be used, as the documentation in the medical record, in both the inpatient outpatient and other settings, should normally provide sufficient detail to determine the cause of the injury.

H.   Late Effects of External Cause Guidelines

1. Late effect E codes exist for injuries and poisonings but not for adverse effects of drugs, misadventures and surgical complications.
2. A late effect E code (E929, E959, E969, E977, E989, or E999.1) should be used with any report of a late effect or sequela resulting from a previous injury or poisoning (905-909).
3. A late effect E code should never be used with a related current nature of injury code.

I. Misadventures and Complications of Care Guidelines

1. Assign a code in the range of E870-E876 if misadventures are stated by the physician.
2. Assign a code in the range of E878-E879 if the physician attributes an abnormal reaction or later complication to a surgical or medical procedure, but does not mention misadventure at the time of the procedure as the cause of the reaction.

J. Terrorism Guidelines

1. When the cause of an injury is identified by the Federal Government (FBI) as terrorism, the first-listed E-code should be a code from category E979, Terrorism. The definition of terrorism employed by the FBI is found at the inclusion note at E979. The terrorism E-code is the only E-code that should be assigned. Additional E codes from the assault categories should not be assigned.
2. When the cause of an injury is suspected to be the result of terrorism a code from category E979 should not be assigned. Assign a code in the range of E codes based circumstances on the documentation of intent and mechanism.
3. Assign code E979.9, Terrorism, secondary effects, for conditions occurring subsequent to the terrorist event. This code should not be assigned for conditions that are due to the initial terrorist act.
4. For statistical purposes these codes will be tabulated within the category for assault, expanding the current category from E960-E969 to include E979 and E999.1.

Section II Selection of Principal Diagnosis(es) for Inpatient, Short-term, Acute Care, ▶and Long Term Care◀ Hospital Records

The circumstances of inpatient admission always govern the selection of principal diagnosis. The principal diagnosis is defined in the Uniform Hospital Discharge Data Set (UHDDS) as "that condition established after study to be chiefly responsible for occasioning the admission of the patient to the hospital for care."

The UHDDS definitions are used by acute care short-term hospitals to report inpatient data elements in a standardized manner. These data elements and their definitions can be found in the July 31, 1985, *Federal Register* (Vol. 50, No, 147), pp. 31038-40.

In determining principal diagnosis the coding conventions in the ICD-9-CM, Volumes I and II take precedence over these official coding guidelines. (See Section IA).

The importance of consistent, complete documentation in the medical record cannot be overemphasized. Without such documentation the application of all coding guidelines is a difficult, if not impossible, task.

A. Codes for symptoms, signs, and ill-defined conditions

Codes for symptoms, signs, and ill-defined conditions from Chapter 16 are not to be used as principal diagnosis when a related definitive diagnosis has been established.

B. Two or more interrelated conditions, each potentially meeting the definition for principal diagnosis

When there are two or more interrelated conditions (such as diseases in the same ICD-9-CM chapter or manifestations characteristically associated with a certain disease) potentially meeting the definition of principal diagnosis, either condition may be sequenced first, unless the circumstances of the admission, the therapy provided, the Tabular List, or the Alphabetic Index indicate otherwise.

C. Two or more diagnoses that equally meet the definition for principal diagnosis

In the unusual instance when two or more diagnoses equally meet the criteria for principal diagnosis as determined by the circumstances of admission, diagnostic workup and/or therapy provided, and the Alphabetic Index, Tabular List, or another coding guidelines does not provide sequencing direction, any one of the diagnoses may be sequenced first.

D. Two or more comparative or contrasting conditions

In those rare instances when two or more contrasting or comparative diagnoses are documented as "either/or" (or similar terminology), they are coded as if the diagnoses were confirmed and the diagnoses are sequenced according to the circumstances of the admission. If no further determination can be made as to which diagnosis should be principal, either diagnosis may be sequenced first.

E. A symptom(s) followed by contrasting/comparative diagnoses

When a symptom(s) is followed by contrasting/comparative diagnoses, the symptom code is sequenced first. All the contrasting/comparative diagnoses should be coded as additional diagnoses.

F. Original treatment plan not carried out

Sequence as the principal diagnosis the condition, which after study occasioned the admission to the hospital, even though treatment may not have been carried out due to unforeseen circumstances.

G. Complications of surgery and other medical care

When the admission is for treatment of a complication resulting from surgery or other medical care, the complication code is sequenced as the principal diagnosis. If the complication is classified to the 996-999 series, an additional code for the specific complication may be assigned.

H. Uncertain Diagnosis

If the diagnosis documented at the time of discharge is qualified as "probable", "suspected", "likely", "questionable", "possible", or "still to be ruled out", code the condition as if it existed or was established. The bases for these guidelines are the diagnostic workup, arrangements for further workup or observation, and initial therapeutic approach that correspond most closely with the established diagnosis.

Section III Reporting Additional Diagnoses for Inpatient, Short-term, Acute Care, ▶and Long Term Care◀ Hospital Records

General Rules for Other (Additional) Diagnoses

For reporting purposes the definition for "other diagnoses" is interpreted as additional conditions that affect patient care in terms of requiring: clinical evaluation; or therapeutic treatment; or diagnostic procedures; or extended length of hospital stay; or increased nursing care and/or monitoring.

The UHDDS item #11-b defines Other Diagnoses as "all conditions that coexist at the time of admission, that develop subsequently, or that affect the treatment received and/or the length of stay. Diagnoses that relate to an earlier episode which have no bearing on the current hospital stay are to be excluded." UHDDS definitions apply to inpatients in acute care, short-term, hospital setting The UHDDS definitions are used by acute care short-term hospitals to report inpatient data elements in a standardized manner. These data elements and their definitions can be found in the July 31, 1985, *Federal Register* (Vol. 50, No, 147), pp. 31038-40.

The following guidelines are to be applied in designating "other diagnoses" when neither the Alphabetic Index nor the Tabular List in ICD-9-CM provide direction. The listing of the diagnoses in the patient record is the responsibility of the attending physician.

A. Previous conditions

If the physician has included a diagnosis in the final diagnostic statement, such as the discharge summary or the face sheet, it should ordinarily be coded. Some physicians include in the diagnostic statement resolved conditions or diagnoses and status-post procedures from previous admission that have no bearing on the current stay. Such conditions are not to be reported and are coded only if required by hospital policy.

However, history codes (V10-V19) may be used as secondary codes if the historical condition or family history has an impact on current care or influences treatment.

B.   Abnormal findings

Abnormal findings (laboratory, x-ray, pathologic, and other diagnostic results) are not coded and reported unless the physician indicates their clinical significance. If the findings are outside the normal range and the attending physician has ordered other tests to evaluate the condition or prescribed treatment, it is appropriate to ask the physician whether the abnormal finding should be added.

Please note: This differs from the coding practices in the outpatient setting for coding encounters for diagnostic tests that have been interpreted by a physician.

C.   Uncertain Diagnosis

If the diagnosis documented at the time of discharge is qualified as "probable", "suspected", "likely", "questionable", "possible", or "still to be ruled out", code the condition as if it existed or was established. The bases for these guidelines are the diagnostic workup, arrangements for further workup or observation, and initial therapeutic approach that correspond most closely with the established diagnosis.

Section IV Diagnostic Coding and Reporting Guidelines for Outpatient Services

These coding guidelines for outpatient diagnoses have been approved for use by hospitals/physicians in coding and reporting hospital-based outpatient services and physician office visits.

Information about the use of certain abbreviations, punctuation, symbols, and other conventions used in the ICD-9-CM Tabular List (code numbers and titles), can be found in Section IA of these guidelines, under "Conventions Used in the Tabular List." Information about the correct sequence to use in finding a code is also described in Section I.

The terms encounter and visit are often used interchangeably in describing outpatient service contacts and, therefore, appear together in these guidelines without distinguishing one from the other.

Though the conventions and general guidelines apply to all settings, coding guidelines for outpatient and physician reporting of diagnoses will vary in a number of instances from those for inpatient diagnoses, recognizing that:

The Uniform Hospital Discharge Data Set (UHDDS) definition of principal diagnosis applies only to inpatients in acute, short-term, general, ▶and long term care◀ hospitals.

Coding guidelines for inconclusive diagnoses (probable, suspected, rule out, etc.) were developed for inpatient reporting and do not apply to outpatients.

A.   Selection of first-listed condition

In the outpatient setting, the term first-listed diagnosis is used in lieu of principal diagnosis.

In determining the first-listed diagnosis the coding conventions of ICD-9-CM, as well as the general and disease specific guidelines take precedence over the outpatient guidelines.

Diagnoses often are not established at the time of the initial encounter/visit. It may take two or more visits before the diagnosis is confirmed.

The most critical rule involves beginning the search for the correct code assignment through the Alphabetic Index. Never begin searching initially in the Tabular List as this will lead to coding errors.

B.   The appropriate code or codes from 001.0 through V83.89 must be used to identify diagnoses, symptoms, conditions, problems, complaints, or other reason(s) for the encounter/visit.

C.   For accurate reporting of ICD-9-CM diagnosis codes, the documentation should describe the patient's condition, using terminology which includes specific diagnoses as well as symptoms, problems, or reasons for the encounter. There are ICD-9-CM codes to describe all of these.

D.   The selection of codes 001.0 through 999.9 will frequently be used to describe the reason for the encounter. These codes are from the section of ICD-9-CM for the classification of diseases and injuries (e.g. infectious and parasitic diseases; neoplasms; symptoms, signs, and ill-defined conditions, etc.).

E.   Codes that describe symptoms and signs, as opposed to diagnoses, are acceptable for reporting purposes when a diagnosis has not been established (confirmed) by the physician. Chapter 16 of ICD-9-CM, Symptoms, Signs, and Ill-defined conditions (codes 780.0 - 799.9) contain many, but not all codes for symptoms.

F.   ICD-9-CM provides codes to deal with encounters for circumstances other than a disease or injury. The Supplementary Classification of

factors Influencing Health Status and Contact with Health Services (V01.0- V83.89) is provided to deal with occasions when circumstances other than a disease or injury are recorded as diagnosis or problems.

G.   Level of Detail in Coding

1.   ICD-9-CM is composed of codes with either 3, 4, or 5 digits. Codes with three digits are included in ICD-9-CM as the heading of a category of codes that may be further subdivided by the use of fourth and/or fifth digits, which provide greater specificity.

2.   A three-digit code is to be used only if it is not further subdivided. Where fourth-digit subcategories and/or fifth-digit subclassifications are provided, they must be assigned. A code is invalid if it has not been coded to the full number of digits required for that code. See also discussion under Section I, General Coding Guidelines, Level of Detail.

H.   List first the ICD-9-CM code for the diagnosis, condition, problem, or other reason for encounter/visit shown in the medical record to be chiefly responsible for the services provided. List additional codes that describe any coexisting conditions.

I.   Do not code diagnoses documented as "probable", "suspected," "questionable," "rule out," or "working diagnosis". Rather, code the condition(s) to the highest degree of certainty for that encounter/visit, such as symptoms, signs, abnormal test results, or other reason for the visit.

Please note: This differs from the coding practices used by hospital medical record departments for coding the diagnosis of acute care, short-term hospital inpatients.

J.   Chronic diseases treated on an ongoing basis may be coded and reported as many times as the patient receives treatment and care for the condition(s).

K.   Code all documented conditions that coexist at the time of the encounter/visit, and require or affect patient care treatment or management. Do not code conditions that were previously treated and no longer exist. However, history codes (V10-V19) may be used as secondary codes if the historical condition or family history has an impact on current care or influences treatment.

L.   For patients receiving diagnostic services only during an encounter/visit, sequence first the diagnosis, condition, problem, or other reason for encounter/visit shown in the medical record to be chiefly responsible for the outpatient services provided during the encounter/visit. Codes for other diagnoses (e.g., chronic conditions) may be sequenced as additional diagnoses.

For outpatient encounters for diagnostic tests that have been interpreted by a physician, and the final report is available at the time of coding, code any confirmed or definitive diagnosis(es) documented in the interpretation. Do not code related signs and symptoms as additional diagnoses.

Please note: This differs from the coding practice in the hospital inpatient setting regarding abnormal findings on test results.

M.   For patients receiving therapeutic services only during an encounter/visit, sequence first the diagnosis, condition, problem, or other reason for encounter/visit shown in the medical record to be chiefly responsible for the outpatient services provided during the encounter/visit. Codes for other diagnoses (e.g., chronic conditions) may be sequenced as additional diagnoses.

The only exception to this rule is that when the primary reason for the admission/encounter is chemotherapy, radiation therapy, or rehabilitation, the appropriate V code for the service is listed first, and the diagnosis or problem for which the service is being performed listed second.

N.   For patient's receiving preoperative evaluations only, sequence a code from category V72.8, Other specified examinations, to describe the pre-op consultations. Assign a code for the condition to describe the reason for the surgery as an additional diagnosis. Code also any findings related to the pre-op evaluation.

O.   For ambulatory surgery, code the diagnosis for which the surgery was performed. If the postoperative diagnosis is known to be different from the preoperative diagnosis at the time the diagnosis is confirmed, select the postoperative diagnosis for coding, since it is the most definitive.

P.   For routine outpatient prenatal visits when no complications are present codes V22.0, Supervision of normal first pregnancy, and V22.1, Supervision of other normal pregnancy, should be used as principal diagnoses. These codes should not be used in conjunction with chapter 11 codes.

A

AAT (alpha-1 antitrypsin) deficiency 273.4 ●

AAV (disease) (illness) (infection) — *see* Human immunodeficiency virus (disease) (illness) (infection)

Abactio — *see* Abortion, induced

Abactus venter — *see* Abortion, induced

Abarognosis 781.99

Abasia (-astasia) 307.9
  atactica 781.3
  choreic 781.3
  hysterical 300.11
  paroxysmal trepidant 781.3
  spastic 781.3
  trembling 781.3
  trepidans 781.3

Abderhalden-Kaufmann-Lignac syndrome (cystinosis) 270.0

Abdomen, abdominal — *see also* condition
  accordion 306.4
  acute 789.0 ☑
  angina 557.1
  burst 868.00
  convulsive equivalent (*see also* Epilepsy) 345.5 ☑
  heart 746.87
  muscle deficiency syndrome 756.79
  obstipum 756.79

Abdominalgia 789.0 ☑
  periodic 277.3

Abduction contracture, hip or other joint — *see* Contraction, joint

Abercrombie's syndrome (amyloid degeneration) 277.3

Aberrant (congenital) — *see also* Malposition, congenital
  adrenal gland 759.1
  blood vessel NEC 747.60
    arteriovenous NEC 747.60
    cerebrovascular 747.81
    gastrointestinal 747.61
    lower limb 747.64
    renal 747.62
    spinal 747.82
    upper limb 747.63
  breast 757.6
  endocrine gland NEC 759.2
  gastrointestinal vessel (peripheral) 747.61
  hepatic duct 751.69
  lower limb vessel (peripheral) 747.64
  pancreas 751.7
  parathyroid gland 759.2
  peripheral vascular vessel NEC 747.60
  pituitary gland (pharyngeal) 759.2
  renal blood vessel 747.62
  sebaceous glands, mucous membrane, mouth 750.26
  spinal vessel 747.82
  spleen 759.0
  testis (descent) 752.51
  thymus gland 759.2
  thyroid gland 759.2
  upper limb vessel (perpipheral) 747.63

Aberratio
  lactis 757.6
  testis 752.51

Aberration — *see also* Anomaly
  chromosome — *see* Anomaly, chromosome(s)
  distantal 368.9
  mental (*see also* Disorder, mental, nonpsychotic) 300.9

Abetalipoproteinemia 272.5

Abionarce 780.79

Abiotrophy 799.89

Ablatio
  placentae — *see* Placenta, ablatio
  retinae (*see also* Detachment, retina) 361.9

Ablation
  pituitary (gland) (with hypofunction) 253.7
  placenta — *see* Placenta, ablatio
  uterus 621.8

Ablepharia, ablepharon, ablephary 743.62

Ablepsia — *see* Blindness

Ablepsy — *see* Blindness

Ablutomania 300.3

Abnormal, abnormality, abnormalities — *see also* Anomaly
  acid-base balance 276.4
    fetus or newborn — *see* Distress, fetal
  adaptation curve, dark 368.63
  alveolar ridge 525.9
  amnion 658.9 ☑
    affecting fetus or newborn 762.9
  anatomical relationship NEC 759.9
  apertures, congenital, diaphragm 756.6
  auditory perception NEC 388.40
  autosomes NEC 758.5
    13 758.1
    18 758.2
    21 or 22 758.0
    D_1 758.1
    E_3 758.2
    G 758.0
  ballistocardiogram 794.39
  basal metabolic rate (BMR) 794.7
  biosynthesis, testicular androgen 257.2
  blood level (of)
    cobalt 790.6
    copper 790.6
    iron 790.6
    lithium 790.6
    magnesium 790.6
    mineral 790.6
    zinc 790.6
  blood pressure
    elevated (without diagnosis of hypertension) 796.2
    low (*see also* Hypotension) 458.9
      reading (incidental) (isolated) (nonspecific) 796.3
  bowel sounds 787.5
  breathing behavior — *see* Respiration
  caloric test 794.19
  cervix (acquired) NEC 622.9
    congenital 752.40
    in pregnancy or childbirth 654.6 ☑
      causing obstructed labor 660.2 ☑
        affecting fetus or newborn 763.1
  chemistry, blood NEC 790.6
  chest sounds 786.7
  chorion 658.9 ☑
    affecting fetus or newborn 762.9
  chromosomal NEC 758.89
    analysis, nonspecific result 795.2
    autosomes (*see also* Abnormal, autosomes NEC) 758.5
    fetal, (suspected) affecting management of pregnancy 655.1 ☑
    sex 758.81
  clinical findings NEC 796.4
  communication — *see* Fistula
  configuration of pupils 379.49
  coronary
    artery 746.85
    vein 746.9
  cortisol-binding globulin 255.8
  course, Eustachian tube 744.24
  dentofacial NEC 524.9
    functional 524.50 ▲
    specified type NEC 524.89 ▲
  development, developmental NEC 759.9
    bone 756.9
    central nervous system 742.9
  direction, teeth 524.30 ▲
  Dynia (*see also* Defect, coagulation) 286.9
  Ebstein 746.2
  echocardiogram 793.2
  echoencephalogram 794.01
  echogram NEC — *see* Findings, abnormal, structure
  electrocardiogram (ECG) (EKG) 794.31
  electroencephalogram (EEG) 794.02
  electromyogram (EMG) 794.17
    ocular 794.14
  electro-oculogram (EOG) 794.12
  electroretinogram (ERG) 794.11
  erythrocytes 289.9
    congenital, with perinatal jaundice 282.9 [774.0]

Abnormal, abnormality, abnormalities — *see also* Anomaly — *continued*
  Eustachian valve 746.9
  excitability under minor stress 301.9
  fat distribution 782.9
  feces 787.7
  fetal heart rate — *see* Distress, fetal
  fetus NEC
    affecting management of pregnancy — *see* Pregnancy, management affected by, fetal
    causing disproportion 653.7 ☑
      affecting fetus or newborn 763.1
      causing obstructed labor 660.1 ☑
        affecting fetus or newborn 763.1
  findings without manifest disease — *see* Findings, abnormal
  fluid
    amniotic 792.3
    cerebrospinal 792.0
    peritoneal 792.9
    pleural 792.9
    synovial 792.9
    vaginal 792.9
  forces of labor NEC 661.9 ☑
    affecting fetus or newborn 763.7
  form, teeth 520.2
  function studies
    auditory 794.15
    bladder 794.9
    brain 794.00
    cardiovascular 794.30
    endocrine NEC 794.6
    kidney 794.4
    liver 794.8
    nervous system
      central 794.00
      peripheral 794.19
    oculomotor 794.14
    pancreas 794.9
    placenta 794.9
    pulmonary 794.2
    retina 794.11
    special senses 794.19
    spleen 794.9
    thyroid 794.5
    vestibular 794.16
  gait 781.2
    hysterical 300.11
  gastrin secretion 251.5
  globulin
    cortisol-binding 255.8
    thyroid-binding 246.8
  glucagon secretion 251.4
  glucose 790.29
    in pregnancy, childbirth, or puerperium 648.8 ☑
      fetus or newborn 775.0
    non-fasting 790.29
  gravitational (G) forces or states 994.9
  hair NEC 704.2
  hard tissue formation in pulp 522.3
  head movement 781.0
  heart
    rate
      fetus, affecting liveborn infant
        before the onset of labor 763.81
        during labor 763.82
        unspecified as to time of onset 763.83
      intrauterine
        before the onset of labor 763.81
        during labor 763.82
        unspecified as to time of onset 763.83
      newborn
        before the onset of labor 763.81
        during labor 763.82
        unspecified as to time of onset 763.83
    shadow 793.2
    sounds NEC 785.3
  hemoglobin (*see also* Disease, hemoglobin) 282.7
    trait — *see* Trait, hemoglobin, abnormal
  hemorrhage, uterus — *see* Hemorrhage, uterus
  histology NEC 795.4

Abnormal, abnormality, abnormalities — *see
also* Anomaly — *continued*
  increase
    in
      appetite 783.6
      development 783.9
  involuntary movement 781.0
  jaw closure 524.51   ▲
  karyotype 795.2
  knee jerk 796.1
  labor NEC 661.9 ☑
    affecting fetus or newborn 763.7
  laboratory findings — *see* Findings, abnormal
  length, organ or site, congenital — *see*
    Distortion
  loss of height 781.91
  loss of weight 783.21
  lung shadow 793.1
  mammogram 793.80
    microcalcification 793.81
  Mantoux test 795.5
  membranes (fetal)
    affecting fetus or newborn 762.9
    complicating pregnancy 658.8 ☑
  menstruation — *see* Menstruation
  metabolism (*see also* condition) 783.9
  movement 781.0
    disorder NEC 333.90
      sleep related 780.58   ●
      specified NEC 333.99
    head 781.0
    involuntary 781.0
    specified type NEC 333.99
  muscle contraction, localized 728.85
  myoglobin (Aberdeen) (Annapolis) 289.9
  narrowness, eyelid 743.62
  optokinetic response 379.57
  organs or tissues of pelvis NEC
    in pregnancy or childbirth 654.9 ☑
      affecting fetus or newborn 763.89
      causing obstructed labor 660.2 ☑
        affecting fetus or newborn 763.1
  origin — *see* Malposition, congenital
  palmar creases 757.2
  Papanicolaou (smear)
    cervix 795.00   ●
      with
        ►atypical squamous cells◄   ●
          cannot exclude high grade   ●
            squamous intraepithelial   ●
            lesion (ASC-H) 795.02   ●
          of undetermined significance   ●
            (ASC-US) 795.01   ●
          high grade squamous   ●
            intraepithelial lesion   ●
            (HGSIL) 795.04   ●
          low grade squamous   ●
            intraepithelial lesion   ●
            (LGSIL) 795.03   ●
        nonspecific finding NEC 795.09
    other site 795.1
  parturition
    affecting fetus or newborn 763.9
    mother — *see* Delivery, complicated
  pelvis (bony) — *see* Deformity, pelvis
  percussion, chest 786.7
  periods (grossly) (*see also* Menstruation) 626.9
  phonocardiogram 794.39
  placenta — *see* Placenta, abnormal
  plantar reflex 796.1
  plasma protein — *see* Deficiency, plasma,
    protein
  pleural folds 748.8
  position — *see also* Malposition
    gravid uterus 654.4 ☑
      causing obstructed labor 660.2 ☑
        affecting fetus or newborn 763.1
  posture NEC 781.92
  presentation (fetus) — *see* Presentation, fetus,
    abnormal
  product of conception NEC 631
  puberty — *see* Puberty
  pulmonary
    artery 747.3
    function, newborn 770.89

Abnormal, abnormality, abnormalities — *see
also* Anomaly — *continued*
  pulmonary — *continued*
    test results 794.2
    ventilation, newborn 770.89
      hyperventilation 786.01
  pulsations in neck 785.1
  pupil reflexes 379.40
  quality of milk 676.8 ☑
  radiological examination 793.9
    abdomen NEC 793.6
    biliary tract 793.3
    breast 793.89
      mammogram NOS 793.80
      mammographic microcalcification 793.81
    gastrointestinal tract 793.4
    genitourinary organs 793.5
    head 793.0
    intrathoracic organ NEC 793.2
    lung (field) 793.1
    musculoskeletal system 793.7
    retroperitoneum 793.6
    skin and subcutaneous tissue 793.9
    skull 793.0
  red blood cells 790.09
    morphology 790.09
    volume 790.09
  reflex NEC 796.1
  renal function test 794.4
  respiration signs — *see* Respiration
  response to nerve stimulation 794.10
  retinal correspondence 368.34
  rhythm, heart — *see also* Arrhythmia
    fetus — *see* Distress, fetal
  saliva 792.4
  scan
    brain 794.09
    kidney 794.4
    liver 794.8
    lung 794.2
    thyroid 794.5
  secretion
    gastrin 251.5
    glucagon 251.4
  semen 792.2
  serum level (of)
    acid phosphatase 790.5
    alkaline phosphatase 790.5
    amylase 790.5
    enzymes NEC 790.5
    lipase 790.5
  shape
    cornea 743.41
    gallbladder 751.69
    gravid uterus 654.4 ☑
      affecting fetus or newborn 763.89
      causing obstructed labor 660.2 ☑
        affecting fetus or newborn 763.1
    head (*see also* Anomaly, skull) 756.0
    organ or site, congenital NEC — *see*
      Distortion
  sinus venosus 747.40
  size
    fetus, complicating delivery 653.5 ☑
      causing obstructed labor 660.1 ☑
    gallbladder 751.69
    head (*see also* Anomaly, skull) 756.0
    organ or site, congenital NEC — *see*
      Distortion
    teeth 520.2
  skin and appendages, congenital NEC 757.9
  soft parts of pelvis — *see* Abnormal, organs or
    tissues of pelvis
  spermatozoa 792.2
  sputum (amount) (color) (excessive) (odor)
    (purulent) 786.4
  stool NEC 787.7
    bloody 578.1
      occult 792.1
    bulky 787.7
    color (dark) (light) 792.1
    content (fat) (mucus) (pus) 792.1
    occult blood 792.1
  synchondrosis 756.9
  test results without manifest disease — *see*
    Findings, abnormal

Abnormal, abnormality, abnormalities — *see
also* Anomaly — *continued*
  thebesian valve 746.9
  thermography — *see* Findings, abnormal,
    structure
  threshold, cones or rods (eye) 368.63
  thyroid-binding globulin 246.8
  thyroid product 246.8
  toxicology (findings) NEC 796.0
  tracheal cartilage (congenital) 748.3
  transport protein 273.8
  ultrasound results — *see* Findings, abnormal,
    structure
  umbilical cord
    affecting fetus or newborn 762.6
    complicating delivery 663.9 ☑
    specified NEC 663.8 ☑
  union
    cricoid cartilage and thyroid cartilage 748.3
    larynx and trachea 748.3
    thyroid cartilage and hyoid bone 748.3
  urination NEC 788.69
    psychogenic 306.53
    stream
      intermittent 788.61
      slowing 788.62
      splitting 788.61
      weak 788.62
    urgency 788.63
  urine (constituents) NEC 791.9
  uterine hemorrhage (*see also* Hemorrhage,
    uterus) 626.9
    climacteric 627.0
    postmenopausal 627.1
  vagina (acquired) (congenital)
    in pregnancy or childbirth 654.7 ☑
      affecting fetus or newborn 763.89
      causing obstructed labor 660.2 ☑
        affecting fetus or newborn 763.1
  vascular sounds 785.9
  vectorcardiogram 794.39
  visually evoked potential (VEP) 794.13
  vulva (acquired) (congenital)
    in pregnancy or childbirth 654.8 ☑
      affecting fetus or newborn 763.89
      causing obstructed labor 660.2 ☑
        affecting fetus or newborn 763.1
  weight
    gain 783.1
      of pregnancy 646.1 ☑
        with hypertension — *see* Toxemia, of
          pregnancy
    loss 783.21
  x-ray examination — *see* Abnormal,
    radiological examination

Abnormally formed uterus — *see* Anomaly,
  uterus

Abnormity (any organ or part) — *see* Anomaly

ABO
  hemolytic disease 773.1
  incompatibility reaction 999.6

Abocclusion 524.20   ▲

Abolition, language 784.69

Aborter, habitual or recurrent NEC
  without current pregnancy 629.9
  current abortion (*see also* Abortion,
    spontaneous) 634.9 ☑
    affecting fetus or newborn 761.8
  observation in current pregnancy 646.3 ☑

Abortion (complete) (incomplete) (inevitable) (with
  retained products of conception) 637.9 ☑

*Note — Use the following fifth-digit
subclassification with categories 634–637:*

  0   unspecified
  1   incomplete
  2   complete

  with
    complication(s) (any) following previous
      abortion — *see* category 639 ☑
    damage to pelvic organ (laceration) (rupture)
      (tear) 637.2 ☑

Abortion — *continued*
  with — *continued*
    embolism (air) (amniotic fluid) (blood clot)
      (pulmonary) (pyemic) (septic) (soap)
      637.6 ☑
    genital tract and pelvic infection 637.0 ☑
    hemorrhage, delayed or excessive 637.1 ☑
    metabolic disorder 637.4 ☑
    renal failure (acute) 637.3 ☑
    sepsis (genital tract) (pelvic organ) 637.0 ☑
      urinary tract 637.7 ☑
    shock (postoperative) (septic) 637.5 ☑
    specified complication NEC 637.7 ☑
    toxemia 637.3 ☑
    unspecified complication(s) 637.8 ☑
    urinary tract infection 637.7 ☑
  accidental — *see* Abortion, spontaneous
  artificial — *see* Abortion, induced
  attempted (failed) — *see* Abortion, failed
  criminal — *see* Abortion, illegal
  early — *see* Abortion, spontaneous
  elective — *see* Abortion, legal
  failed (legal) 638.9
    with
      damage to pelvic organ (laceration)
        (rupture) (tear) 638.2
      embolism (air) (amniotic fluid) (blood clot)
        (pulmonary) (pyemic) (septic) (soap)
        638.6
      genital tract and pelvic infection 638.0
      hemorrhage, delayed or excessive 638.1
      metabolic disorder 638.4
      renal failure (acute) 638.3
      sepsis (genital tract) (pelvic organ) 638.0
        urinary tract 638.7
      shock (postoperative) (septic) 638.5
      specified complication NEC 638.7
      toxemia 638.3
      unspecified complication(s) 638.8
      urinary tract infection 638.7
  fetal indication — *see* Abortion, legal
  fetus 779.6
  following threatened abortion — *see* Abortion,
    by type
  habitual or recurrent (care during pregnancy)
    646.3 ☑
    with current abortion (*see also* Abortion,
      spontaneous) 634.9 ☑
    affecting fetus or newborn 761.8
    without current pregnancy 629.9
  homicidal — *see* Abortion, illegal
  illegal 636.9 ☑
    with
      damage to pelvic organ (laceration)
        (rupture) (tear) 636.2 ☑
      embolism (air) (amniotic fluid) (blood clot)
        (pulmonary) (pyemic) (septic) (soap)
        636.6 ☑
      genital tract and pelvic infection 636.0 ☑
      hemorrhage, delayed or excessive
        636.1 ☑
      metabolic disorder 636.4 ☑
      renal failure 636.3 ☑
      sepsis (genital tract) (pelvic organ)
        636.0 ☑
        urinary tract 636.7 ☑
      shock (postoperative) (septic) 636.5 ☑
      specified complication NEC 636.7 ☑
      toxemia 636.3 ☑
      unspecified complication(s) 636.8 ☑
      urinary tract infection 636.7 ☑
    fetus 779.6
  induced 637.9 ☑
    illegal — *see* Abortion, illegal
    legal indications — *see* Abortion, legal
    medical indications — *see* Abortion, legal
    therapeutic — *see* Abortion, legal
  late — *see* Abortion, spontaneous
  legal (legal indication) (medical indication)
    (under medical supervision) 635.9 ☑
    with
      damage to pelvic organ (laceration)
        (rupture) (tear) 635.2 ☑
      embolism (air) (amniotic fluid) (blood clot)
        (pulmonary) (pyemic) (septic) (soap)
        635.6 ☑
      genital tract and pelvic infection 635.0 ☑

Abortion — *continued*
  legal — *continued*
    with — *continued*
      hemorrhage, delayed or excessive
        635.1 ☑
      metabolic disorder 635.4 ☑
      renal failure (acute) 635.3 ☑
      sepsis (genital tract) (pelvic organ)
        635.0 ☑
        urinary tract 635.7 ☑
      shock (postoperative) (septic) 635.5 ☑
      specified complication NEC 635.7 ☑
      toxemia 635.3 ☑
      unspecified complication(s) 635.8 ☑
      urinary tract infection 635.7 ☑
    fetus 779.6
  medical indication — *see* Abortion, legal
  mental hygiene problem — *see* Abortion, legal
  missed 632
  operative — *see* Abortion, legal
  psychiatric indication — *see* Abortion, legal
  recurrent — *see* Abortion, spontaneous
  self-induced — *see* Abortion, illegal
  septic — *see* Abortion, by type, with sepsis
  spontaneous 634.9 ☑
    with
      damage to pelvic organ (laceration)
        (rupture) (tear) 634.2 ☑
      embolism (air) (amniotic fluid) (blood clot)
        (pulmonary) (pyemic) (septic) (soap)
        634.6 ☑
      genital tract and pelvic infection 634.0 ☑
      hemorrhage, delayed or excessive
        634.1 ☑
      metabolic disorder 634.4 ☑
      renal failure 634.3 ☑
      sepsis (genital tract) (pelvic organ)
        634.0 ☑
        urinary tract 634.7 ☑
      shock (postoperative) (septic) 634.5 ☑
      specified complication NEC 634.7 ☑
      toxemia 634.3 ☑
      unspecified complication(s) 634.8 ☑
      urinary tract infection 634.7 ☑
    fetus 761.8
    threatened 640.0 ☑
      affecting fetus or newborn 762.1
  surgical — *see* Abortion, legal
  therapeutic — *see* Abortion, legal
  threatened 640.0 ☑
    affecting fetus or newborn 762.1
  tubal — *see* Pregnancy, tubal
  voluntary — *see* Abortion, legal

Abortus fever 023.9

Aboulomania 301.6

Abrachia 755.20

Abrachiatism 755.20

Abrachiocephalia 759.89

Abrachiocephalus 759.89

Abrami's disease (acquired hemolytic jaundice)
  283.9

Abramov-Fiedler myocarditis (acute isolated
  myocarditis) 422.91

Abrasion — *see also* Injury, superficial, by site
  cornea 918.1
  dental 521.20 ▲
    extending into ●
      dentine 521.22 ●
      pulp 521.23 ●
    generalized 521.25 ●
    limited to enamel 521.21 ●
    localized 521.24 ●
  teeth, tooth (dentifrice) (habitual) (hard tissues)
    (occupational) (ritual) (traditional) (wedge
    defect) ▶(*see also* Abrasion, dental)◀
    521.20 ▲

Abrikossov's tumor (M9580/0) — *see also*
  Neoplasm, connective tissue, benign
  malignant (M9580/3) — *see* Neoplasm,
    connective tissue, malignant

Abrism 988.8

Abruption, placenta — *see* Placenta, abruptio

Abruptio placentae — *see* Placenta, abruptio

Abscess (acute) (chronic) (infectional)
  (lymphangitic) (metastatic) (multiple)
  (pyogenic) (septic) (with lymphangitis) (*see
  also* Cellulitis) 682.9
  abdomen, abdominal
    cavity — *see* Abscess, peritoneum
    wall 682.2
  abdominopelvic — *see* Abscess, peritoneum
  accessory sinus (chronic) (*see also* Sinusitis)
    473.9
  adrenal (capsule) (gland) 255.8
  alveolar 522.5
    with sinus 522.7
  amebic 006.3
    bladder 006.8
    brain (with liver or lung abscess) 006.5
    liver (without mention of brain or lung
      abscess) 006.3
      with
        brain abscess (and lung abscess)
          006.5
        lung abscess 006.4
    lung (with liver abscess) 006.4
      with brain abscess 006.5
    seminal vesicle 006.8
    specified site NEC 006.8
    spleen 006.8
  anaerobic 040.0
  ankle 682.6
  anorectal 566
  antecubital space 682.3
  antrum (chronic) (Highmore) (*see also* Sinusitis,
    maxillary) 473.0
  anus 566
  apical (tooth) 522.5
    with sinus (alveolar) 522.7
  appendix 540.1
  areola (acute) (chronic) (nonpuerperal) 611.0
    puerperal, postpartum 675.1 ☑
  arm (any part, above wrist) 682.3
  artery (wall) 447.2
  atheromatous 447.2
  auditory canal (external) 380.10
  auricle (ear) (staphylococcal) (streptococcal)
    380.10
  axilla, axillary (region) 682.3
    lymph gland or node 683
  back (any part) 682.2
  Bartholin's gland 616.3
    with
      abortion — *see* Abortion, by type, with
        sepsis
      ectopic pregnancy (*see also* categories
        633.0-633.9) 639.0
      molar pregnancy (*see also* categories 630-
        632) 639.0
    complicating pregnancy or puerperium
      646.6 ☑
    following
      abortion 639.0
      ectopic or molar pregnancy 639.0
  bartholinian 616.3
  Bezold's 383.01
  bile, biliary, duct or tract (*see also*
    Cholecystitis) 576.8
  bilharziasis 120.1
  bladder (wall) 595.89
    amebic 006.8
  bone (subperiosteal) (*see also* Osteomyelitis)
    730.0 ☑
    accessory sinus (chronic) (*see also* Sinusitis)
      473.9
    acute 730.0 ☑
    chronic or old 730.1 ☑
    jaw (lower) (upper) 526.4
    mastoid — *see* Mastoiditis, acute
    petrous (*see also* Petrositis) 383.20
    spinal (tuberculous) (*see also* Tuberculosis)
      015.0 ☑ *[730.88]*
      nontuberculous 730.08
  bowel 569.5
  brain (any part) 324.0
    amebic (with liver or lung abscess) 006.5
    cystic 324.0
    late effect — *see* category 326
    otogenic 324.0
    tuberculous (*see also* Tuberculosis) 013.3 ☑

Abscess (see also Cellulitis) — continued
- breast (acute) (chronic) (nonpuerperal) 611.0
  - newborn 771.5
  - puerperal, postpartum 675.1 ☑
  - tuberculous (see also Tuberculosis) 017.9 ☑
- broad ligament (chronic) (see also Disease, pelvis, inflammatory) 614.4
  - acute 614.3
- Brodie's (chronic) (localized) (see also Osteomyelitis) 730.1 ☑
- bronchus 519.1
- buccal cavity 528.3
- bulbourethral gland 597.0
- bursa 727.89
  - pharyngeal 478.29
- buttock 682.5
- canaliculus, breast 611.0
- canthus 372.20
- cartilage 733.99
- cecum 569.5
  - with appendicitis 540.1
- cerebellum, cerebellar 324.0
  - late effect — see category 326
- cerebral (embolic) 324.0
  - late effect — see category 326
- cervical (neck region) 682.1
  - lymph gland or node 683
  - stump (see also Cervicitis) 616.0
- cervix (stump) (uteri) (see also Cervicitis) 616.0
- cheek, external 682.0
  - inner 528.3
- chest 510.9
  - with fistula 510.0
  - wall 682.2
- chin 682.0
- choroid 363.00
- ciliary body 364.3
- circumtonsillar 475
- cold (tuberculous) — see also Tuberculosis, abscess
  - articular — see Tuberculosis, joint
- colon (wall) 569.5
- colostomy or enterostomy 569.61
- conjunctiva 372.00
- connective tissue NEC 682.9
- cornea 370.55
  - with ulcer 370.00
- corpus
  - cavernosum 607.2
  - luteum (see also Salpingo-oophoritis) 614.2
- Cowper's gland 597.0
- cranium 324.0
- cul-de-sac (Douglas') (posterior) (see also Disease, pelvis, inflammatory) 614.4
  - acute 614.3
- dental 522.5
  - with sinus (alveolar) 522.7
- dentoalveolar 522.5
  - with sinus (alveolar) 522.7
- diaphragm, diaphragmatic — see Abscess, peritoneum
- digit NEC 681.9
- Douglas' cul-de-sac or pouch (see also Disease, pelvis, inflammatory) 614.4
  - acute 614.3
- Dubois' 090.5
- ductless gland 259.8
- ear
  - acute 382.00
  - external 380.10
  - inner 386.30
  - middle — see Otitis media
- elbow 682.3
- endamebic — see Abscess, amebic
- entamebic — see Abscess, amebic
- enterostomy 569.61
- epididymis 604.0
- epidural 324.9
  - brain 324.0
  - late effect — see category 326
  - spinal cord 324.1
- epiglottis 478.79
- epiploon, epiploic — see Abscess, peritoneum
- erysipelatous (see also Erysipelas) 035
- esophagostomy 530.86 ●
- esophagus 530.19

Abscess (see also Cellulitis) — continued
- ethmoid (bone) (chronic) (sinus) (see also Sinusitis, ethmoidal) 473.2
- external auditory canal 380.10
- extradural 324.9
  - brain 324.0
  - late effect — see category 326
  - spinal cord 324.1
- extraperitoneal — see Abscess, peritoneum
- eye 360.00
- eyelid 373.13
- face (any part, except eye) 682.0
- fallopian tube (see also Salpingo-oophoritis) 614.2
- fascia 728.89
- fauces 478.29
- fecal 569.5
- femoral (region) 682.6
- filaria, filarial (see also Infestation, filarial) 125.9
- finger (any) (intrathecal) (periosteal) (subcutaneous) (subcuticular) 681.00
- fistulous NEC 682.9
- flank 682.2
- foot (except toe) 682.7
- forearm 682.3
- forehead 682.0
- frontal (sinus) (chronic) (see also Sinusitis, frontal) 473.1
- gallbladder (see also Cholecystitis, acute) 575.0
- gastric 535.0 ☑
- genital organ or tract NEC
  - female 616.9
    - with
      - abortion — see Abortion, by type, with sepsis
      - ectopic pregnancy (see also categories 633.0-633.9) 639.0
      - molar pregnancy (see also categories 630-632) 639.0
    - following
      - abortion 639.0
      - ectopic or molar pregnancy 639.0
    - puerperal, postpartum, childbirth 670.0 ☑
  - male 608.4
- genitourinary system, tuberculous (see also Tuberculosis) 016.9 ☑
- gingival 523.3
- gland, glandular (lymph) (acute) NEC 683
- glottis 478.79
- gluteal (region) 682.5
- gonorrheal NEC (see also Gonococcus) 098.0
- groin 682.2
- gum 523.3
- hand (except finger or thumb) 682.4
- head (except face) 682.8
- heart 429.89
- heel 682.7
- helminthic (see also Infestation, by specific parasite) 128.9
- hepatic 572.0
  - amebic (see also Abscess, liver, amebic) 006.3
  - duct 576.8
- hip 682.6
  - tuberculous (active) (see also Tuberculosis) 015.1 ☑
- ileocecal 540.1
- ileostomy (bud) 569.61
- iliac (region) 682.2
  - fossa 540.1
- iliopsoas (tuberculous) (see also Tuberculosis) 015.0 ☑ [730.88]
  - nontuberculous 728.89
- infraclavicular (fossa) 682.3
- inguinal (region) 682.2
  - lymph gland or node 683
- intersphincteric (anus) 566
- intestine, intestinal 569.5
  - rectal 566
- intra-abdominal (see also Abscess, peritoneum) 567.2
  - postoperative 998.59
- intracranial 324.0
  - late effect — see category 326
- intramammary — see Abscess, breast
- intramastoid (see also Mastoiditis, acute) 383.00

Abscess (see also Cellulitis) — continued
- intraorbital 376.01
- intraperitoneal — see Abscess, peritoneum
- intraspinal 324.1
  - late effect — see category 326
- intratonsillar 475
- iris 364.3
- ischiorectal 566
- jaw (bone) (lower) (upper) 526.4
  - skin 682.0
- joint (see also Arthritis, pyogenic) 711.0 ☑
  - vertebral (tuberculous) (see also Tuberculosis) 015.0 ☑ [730.88]
    - nontuberculous 724.8
- kidney 590.2
  - with
    - abortion — see Abortion, by type, with urinary tract infection
    - calculus 592.0
    - ectopic pregnancy (see also categories 633.0-633.9) 639.8
    - molar pregnancy (see also categories 630-632) 639.8
    - complicating pregnancy or puerperium 646.6 ☑
      - affecting fetus or newborn 760.1
    - following
      - abortion 639.8
      - ectopic or molar pregnancy 639.8
- knee 682.6
  - joint 711.06
  - tuberculous (active) (see also Tuberculosis) 015.2 ☑
- labium (majus) (minus) 616.4
  - complicating pregnancy, childbirth, or puerperium 646.6 ☑
- lacrimal (passages) (sac) (see also Dacryocystitis) 375.30
  - caruncle 375.30
  - gland (see also Dacryoadenitis) 375.00
- lacunar 597.0
- larynx 478.79
- lateral (alveolar) 522.5
  - with sinus 522.7
- leg, except foot 682.6
- lens 360.00
- lid 373.13
- lingual 529.0
  - tonsil 475
- lip 528.5
- Littre's gland 597.0
- liver 572.0
  - amebic 006.3
    - with
      - brain abscess (and lung abscess) 006.5
      - lung abscess 006.4
    - due to Entamoeba histolytica 006.3
    - dysenteric (see also Abscess, liver, amebic) 006.3
  - pyogenic 572.0
  - tropical (see also Abscess, liver, amebic) 006.3
- loin (region) 682.2
- lumbar (tuberculous) (see also Tuberculosis) 015.0 ☑ [730.88]
  - nontuberculous 682.2
- lung (miliary) (putrid) 513.0
  - amebic (with liver abscess) 006.4
    - with brain abscess 006.5
- lymph, lymphatic, gland or node (acute) 683
  - any site, except mesenteric 683
  - mesentery 289.2
- lymphangitic, acute — see Cellulitis
- malar 526.4
- mammary gland — see Abscess, breast
- marginal (anus) 566
- mastoid (process) (see also Mastoiditis, acute) 383.00
  - subperiosteal 383.01
- maxilla, maxillary 526.4
  - molar (tooth) 522.5
    - with sinus 522.7
  - premolar 522.5
  - sinus (chronic) (see also Sinusitis, maxillary) 473.0
- mediastinum 513.1

☑ Additional Digit Required   ►◄ Revised Text   ● New Line   ▲ Revised Code

Abscess (*see also* Cellulitis) — *continued*
meibomian gland 373.12
meninges (*see also* Meningitis) 320.9
mesentery, mesenteric — *see* Abscess,
   peritoneum
mesosalpinx (*see also* Salpingo-oophoritis)
   614.2
milk 675.1 ☑
Monro's (psoriasis) 696.1
mons pubis 682.2
mouth (floor) 528.3
multiple sites NEC 682.9
mural 682.2
muscle 728.89
myocardium 422.92
nabothian (follicle) (*see also* Cervicitis) 616.0
nail (chronic) (with lymphangitis) 681.9
   finger 681.02
   toe 681.11
nasal (fossa) (septum) 478.1
   sinus (chronic) (*see also* Sinusitis) 473.9
nasopharyngeal 478.29
nates 682.5
navel 682.2
   newborn NEC 771.4
neck (region) 682.1
   lymph gland or node 683
nephritic (*see also* Abscess, kidney) 590.2
nipple 611.0
   puerperal, postpartum 675.0 ☑
nose (septum) 478.1
   external 682.0
omentum — *see* Abscess, peritoneum
operative wound 998.59
orbit, orbital 376.01
ossifluent — *see* Abscess, bone
ovary, ovarian (corpus luteum) (*see also*
   Salpingo-oophoritis) 614.2
oviduct (*see also* Salpingo-oophoritis) 614.2
palate (soft) 528.3
   hard 526.4
palmar (space) 682.4
pancreas (duct) 577.0
paradontal 523.3
parafrenal 607.2
parametric, parametrium (chronic) (*see also*
   Disease, pelvis, inflammatory) 614.4
   acute 614.3
paranephric 590.2
parapancreatic 577.0
parapharyngeal 478.22
pararectal 566
parasinus (*see also* Sinusitis) 473.9
parauterine (*see also* Disease, pelvis,
   inflammatory) 614.4
   acute 614.3
paravaginal (*see also* Vaginitis) 616.10
parietal region 682.8
parodontal 523.3
parotid (duct) (gland) 527.3
   region 528.3
parumbilical 682.2
   newborn 771.4
pectoral (region) 682.2
pelvirectal — *see* Abscess, peritoneum
pelvis, pelvic
   female (chronic) (*see also* Disease, pelvis,
      inflammatory) 614.4
      acute 614.3
   male, peritoneal (cellular tissue) — *see*
      Abscess, peritoneum
   tuberculous (*see also* Tuberculosis) 016.9 ☑
penis 607.2
   gonococcal (acute) 098.0
      chronic or duration of 2 months or over
         098.2
perianal 566
periapical 522.5
   with sinus (alveolar) 522.7
periappendiceal 540.1
pericardial 420.99
pericecal 540.1
pericemental 523.3
pericholecystic (*see also* Cholecystitis, acute)
   575.0
pericoronal 523.3
peridental 523.3

Abscess (*see also* Cellulitis) — *continued*
perigastric 535.0 ☑
perimetric (*see also* Disease, pelvis,
   inflammatory) 614.4
   acute 614.3
perinephric, perinephritic (*see also* Abscess,
   kidney) 590.2
perineum, perineal (superficial) 682.2
   deep (with urethral involvement) 597.0
   urethra 597.0
periodontal (parietal) 523.3
   apical 522.5
periosteum, periosteal (*see also* Periostitis)
   730.3 ☑
   with osteomyelitis (*see also* Osteomyelitis)
      730.2 ☑
      acute or subacute 730.0 ☑
      chronic or old 730.1 ☑
peripleuritic 510.9
   with fistula 510.0
periproctic 566
periprostatic 601.2
perirectal (staphylococcal) 566
perirenal (tissue) (*see also* Abscess, kidney)
   590.2
perisinuous (nose) (*see also* Sinusitis) 473.9
peritoneum, peritoneal (perforated) (ruptured)
   567.2
   with
      abortion — *see* Abortion, by type, with
         sepsis
      appendicitis 540.1
      ectopic pregnancy (*see also* categories
         633.0-633.9) 639.0
      molar pregnancy (*see also* categories 630-
         632) 639.0
   following
      abortion 639.0
      ectopic or molar pregnancy 639.0
   pelvic, female (*see also* Disease, pelvis,
      inflammatory) 614.4
      acute 614.3
   postoperative 998.59
   puerperal, postpartum, childbirth 670.0 ☑
   tuberculous (*see also* Tuberculosis) 014.0 ☑
peritonsillar 475
perityphlic 540.1
periureteral 593.89
periurethral 597.0
   gonococcal (acute) 098.0
      chronic or duration of 2 months or over
         098.2
periuterine (*see also* Disease, pelvis,
   inflammatory) 614.4
   acute 614.3
perivesical 595.89
pernicious NEC 682.9
petrous bone — *see* Petrositis
phagedenic NEC 682.9
   chancroid 099.0
pharynx, pharyngeal (lateral) 478.29
phlegmonous NEC 682.9
pilonidal 685.0
pituitary (gland) 253.8
pleura 510.9
   with fistula 510.0
popliteal 682.6
postanal 566
postcecal 540.1
postlaryngeal 478.79
postnasal 478.1
postpharyngeal 478.24
posttonsillar 475
posttyphoid 002.0
Pott's (*see also* Tuberculosis) 015.0 ☑ [730.88]
pouch of Douglas (chronic) (*see also* Disease,
   pelvis, inflammatory) 614.4
premammary — *see* Abscess, breast
prepatellar 682.6
prostate (*see also* Prostatitis) 601.2
   gonococcal (acute) 098.12
      chronic or duration of 2 months or over
         098.32
psoas (tuberculous) (*see also* Tuberculosis)
   015.0 ☑ [730.88]
   nontuberculous 728.89
pterygopalatine fossa 682.8

Abscess (*see also* Cellulitis) — *continued*
pubis 682.2
puerperal — Puerperal, abscess, by site
pulmonary — *see* Abscess, lung
pulp, pulpal (dental) 522.0
   finger 681.01
   toe 681.10
pyemic — *see* Septicemia
pyloric valve 535.0 ☑
rectovaginal septum 569.5
rectovesical 595.89
rectum 566
regional NEC 682.9
renal (*see also* Abscess, kidney) 590.2
retina 363.00
retrobulbar 376.01
retrocecal — *see* Abscess, peritoneum
retrolaryngeal 478.79
retromammary — *see* Abscess, breast
retroperineal 682.2
retroperitoneal — *see* Abscess, peritoneum
retropharyngeal 478.24
   tuberculous (*see also* Tuberculosis) 012.8 ☑
retrorectal 566
retrouterine (*see also* Disease, pelvis,
   inflammatory) 614.4
   acute 614.3
retrovesical 595.89
root, tooth 522.5
   with sinus (alveolar) 522.7
round ligament (*see also* Disease, pelvis,
   inflammatory) 614.4
   acute 614.3
rupture (spontaneous) NEC 682.9
sacrum (tuberculous) (*see also* Tuberculosis)
   015.0 ☑ [730.88]
   nontuberculous 730.08
salivary duct or gland 527.3
scalp (any part) 682.8
scapular 730.01
sclera 379.09
scrofulous (*see also* Tuberculosis) 017.2 ☑
scrotum 608.4
seminal vesicle 608.0
   amebic 006.8
septal, dental 522.5
   with sinus (alveolar) 522.7
septum (nasal) 478.1
serous (*see also* Periostitis) 730.3 ☑
shoulder 682.3
side 682.2
sigmoid 569.5
sinus (accessory) (chronic) (nasal) (*see also*
   Sinusitis) 473.9
   intracranial venous (any) 324.0
      late effect — *see* category 326
Skene's duct or gland 597.0
skin NEC 682.9
   tuberculous (primary) (*see also*
      Tuberculosis) 017.0 ☑
sloughing NEC 682.9
specified site NEC 682.8
   amebic 006.8
spermatic cord 608.4
sphenoidal (sinus) (*see also* Sinusitis,
   sphenoidal) 473.3
spinal
   cord (any part) (staphylococcal) 324.1
      tuberculous (*see also* Tuberculosis)
         013.5 ☑
   epidural 324.1
spine (column) (tuberculous) (*see also*
   Tuberculosis) 015.0 ☑ [730.88]
   nontuberculous 730.08
spleen 289.59
   amebic 006.8
staphylococcal NEC 682.9
stitch 998.59
stomach (wall) 535.0 ☑
strumous (tuberculous) (*see also* Tuberculosis)
   017.2 ☑
subarachnoid 324.9
   brain 324.0
   cerebral 324.0
   late effect — *see* category 326
   spinal cord 324.1

Abscess

☑ Additional Digit Required   ►◄ Revised Text   ● New Line   ▲ Revised Code

Abscess (*see also* Cellulitis) — *continued*
  subareolar — *see also* Abscess, breast
      puerperal, postpartum 675.1 ☑
  subcecal 540.1
  subcutaneous NEC 682.9
  subdiaphragmatic — *see* Abscess, peritoneum
  subdorsal 682.2
  subdural 324.9
    brain 324.0
    late effect — *see* category 326
    spinal cord 324.1
  subgaleal 682.8
  subhepatic — *see* Abscess, peritoneum
  sublingual 528.3
    gland 527.3
  submammary — *see* Abscess, breast
  submandibular (region) (space) (triangle) 682.0
    gland 527.3
  submaxillary (region) 682.0
    gland 527.3
  submental (pyogenic) 682.0
    gland 527.3
  subpectoral 682.2
  subperiosteal — *see* Abscess, bone
  subperitoneal — *see* Abscess, peritoneum
  subphrenic — *see also* Abscess, peritoneum
    postoperative 998.59
  subscapular 682.2
  subungual 681.9
  suburethral 597.0
  sudoriparous 705.89
  suppurative NEC 682.9
  supraclavicular (fossa) 682.3
  suprahepatic — *see* Abscess, peritoneum
  suprapelvic (*see also* Disease, pelvis,
      inflammatory) 614.4
    acute 614.3
  suprapubic 682.2
  suprarenal (capsule) (gland) 255.8
  sweat gland 705.89
  syphilitic 095.8
  teeth, tooth (root) 522.5
    with sinus (alveolar) 522.7
    supporting structures NEC 523.3
  temple 682.0
  temporal region 682.0
  temporosphenoidal 324.0
    late effect — *see* category 326
  tendon (sheath) 727.89
  testicle — *see* Orchitis
  thecal 728.89
  thigh (acquired) 682.6
  thorax 510.9
    with fistula 510.0
  throat 478.29
  thumb (intrathecal) (periosteal) (subcutaneous)
      (subcuticular) 681.00
  thymus (gland) 254.1
  thyroid (gland) 245.0
  toe (any) (intrathecal) (periosteal)
      (subcutaneous) (subcuticular) 681.10
  tongue (staphylococcal) 529.0
  tonsil(s) (lingual) 475
  tonsillopharyngeal 475
  tooth, teeth (root) 522.5
    with sinus (alveolar) 522.7
    supporting structure NEC 523.3
  trachea 478.9
  trunk 682.2
  tubal (*see also* Salpingo-oophoritis) 614.2
  tuberculous — *see* Tuberculosis, abscess
  tubo-ovarian (*see also* Salpingo-oophoritis)
      614.2
  tunica vaginalis 608.4
  umbilicus NEC 682.2
    newborn 771.4
  upper arm 682.3
  upper respiratory 478.9
  urachus 682.2
  urethra (gland) 597.0
  urinary 597.0
  uterus, uterine (wall) (*see also* Endometritis)
      615.9
    ligament (*see also* Disease, pelvis,
        inflammatory) 614.4
      acute 614.3
    neck (*see also* Cervicitis) 616.0

Abscess (*see also* Cellulitis) — *continued*
  uvula 528.3
  vagina (wall) (*see also* Vaginitis) 616.10
  vaginorectal (*see also* Vaginitis) 616.10
  vas deferens 608.4
  vermiform appendix 540.1
  vertebra (column) (tuberculous) (*see also*
      Tuberculosis) 015.0 ☑ *[730.88]*
    nontuberculous 730.0 ☑
  vesical 595.89
  vesicouterine pouch (*see also* Disease, pelvis,
      inflammatory) 614.4
  vitreous (humor) (pneumococcal) 360.04
  vocal cord 478.5
  von Bezold's 383.01
  vulva 616.4
    complicating pregnancy, childbirth, or
        puerperium 646.6 ☑
  vulvovaginal gland (*see also* Vaginitis) 616.3
  web-space 682.4
  wrist 682.4
Absence (organ or part) (complete or partial)
  acoustic nerve 742.8
  adrenal (gland) (congenital) 759.1
    acquired V45.79
  albumin (blood) 273.8
  alimentary tract (complete) (congenital) (partial)
      751.8
    lower 751.5
    upper 750.8
  alpha-fucosidase 271.8
  alveolar process (acquired) 525.8
    congenital 750.26
  anus, anal (canal) (congenital) 751.2
  aorta (congenital) 747.22
  aortic valve (congenital) 746.89
  appendix, congenital 751.2
  arm (acquired) V49.60
    above elbow V49.66
    below elbow V49.65
    congenital (*see also* Deformity, reduction,
        upper limb) 755.20
      lower — *see* Absence, forearm, congenital
      upper (complete) (partial) (with absence of
          distal elements, incomplete) 755.24
        with
          complete absence of distal elements
              755.21
          forearm (incomplete) 755.23
  artery (congenital) (peripheral) NEC (*see also*
      Anomaly, peripheral vascular system)
      747.60
    brain 747.81
    cerebral 747.81
    coronary 746.85
    pulmonary 747.3
    umbilical 747.5
  atrial septum 745.69
  auditory canal (congenital) (external) 744.01
  auricle (ear) (with stenosis or atresia of
      auditory canal), congenital 744.01
  bile, biliary duct (common) or passage
      (congenital) 751.61
  bladder (acquired) V45.74
    congenital 753.8
  bone (congenital) NEC 756.9
    marrow 284.9
      acquired (secondary) 284.8
      congenital 284.0
      hereditary 284.0
      idiopathic 284.9
    skull 756.0
  bowel sounds 787.5
  brain 740.0
    specified part 742.2
  breast(s) (acquired) V45.71
    congenital 757.6
  broad ligament (congenital) 752.19
  bronchus (congenital) 748.3
  calvarium, calvaria (skull) 756.0
  canaliculus lacrimalis, congenital 743.65
  carpal(s) (congenital) (complete) (partial) (with
      absence of distal elements, incomplete)
      (*see also* Deformity, reduction, upper
      limb) 755.28
    with complete absence of distal elements
        755.21

Absence — *continued*
  cartilage 756.9
  caudal spine 756.13
  cecum (acquired) (postoperative)
      (posttraumatic) V45.72
    congenital 751.2
  cementum 520.4
  cerebellum (congenital) (vermis) 742.2
  cervix (acquired) (uteri) V45.77
    congenital 752.49
  chin, congenital 744.89
  cilia (congenital) 743.63
    acquired 374.89
  circulatory system, part NEC 747.89
  clavicle 755.51
  clitoris (congenital) 752.49
  coccyx, congenital 756.13
  cold sense (*see also* Disturbance, sensation)
      782.0
  colon (acquired) (postoperative) V45.72
    congenital 751.2
  congenital
    lumen — *see* Atresia
    organ or site NEC — *see* Agenesis
    septum — *see* Imperfect, closure
  corpus callosum (congenital) 742.2
  cricoid cartilage 748.3
  diaphragm (congenital) (with hernia) 756.6
    with obstruction 756.6
  digestive organ(s) or tract, congenital (complete)
      (partial) 751.8
    acquired V45.79
    lower 751.5
    upper 750.8
  ductus arteriosus 747.89
  duodenum (acquired) (postoperative) V45.72
    congenital 751.1
  ear, congenital 744.09
    acquired V45.79
    auricle 744.01
    external 744.01
    inner 744.05
    lobe, lobule 744.21
    middle, except ossicles 744.03
      ossicles 744.04
    ossicles 744.04
  ejaculatory duct (congenital) 752.89
  endocrine gland NEC (congenital) 759.2
  epididymis (congenital) 752.89
    acquired V45.77
  epiglottis, congenital 748.3
  epileptic (atonic) (typical) (*see also* Epilepsy)
      345.0 ☑
  erythrocyte 284.9
  erythropoiesis 284.9
    congenital 284.0
  esophagus (congenital) 750.3
  Eustachian tube (congenital) 744.24
  extremity (acquired)
    congenital (*see also* Deformity, reduction)
        755.4
    lower V49.70
    upper V49.60
  extrinsic muscle, eye 743.69
  eye (acquired) V45.78
    adnexa (congenital) 743.69
    congenital 743.00
    muscle (congenital) 743.69
  eyelid (fold), congenital 743.62
    acquired 374.89
  face
    bones NEC 756.0
    specified part NEC 744.89
  fallopian tube(s) (acquired) V45.77
    congenital 752.19
  femur, congenital (complete) (partial) (with
      absence of distal elements, incomplete)
      (*see also* Deformity, reduction, lower
      limb) 755.34
    with
      complete absence of distal elements
          755.31
      tibia and fibula (incomplete) 755.33
  fibrin 790.92
  fibrinogen (congenital) 286.3
    acquired 286.6

Absence — *continued*
    fibula, congenital (complete) (partial) (with
        absence of distal elements, incomplete)
        (*see also* Deformity, reduction, lower
        limb) 755.37
        with
            complete absence of distal elements
                755.31
            tibia 755.35
                with
                    complete absence of distal elements
                        755.31
                    femur (incomplete) 755.33
                        with complete absence of distal
                            elements 755.31
    finger (acquired) V49.62
        congenital (complete) (partial) (*see also*
            Deformity, reduction, upper limb)
            755.29
            meaning all fingers (complete) (partial)
                755.21
            transverse 755.21
    fissures of lungs (congenital) 748.5
    foot (acquired) V49.73
        congenital (complete) 755.31
    forearm (acquired) V49.65
        congenital (complete) (partial) (with absence
            of distal elements, incomplete) (*see
            also* Deformity, reduction, upper limb)
            755.25
            with
                complete absence of distal elements
                    (hand and fingers) 755.21
                humerus (incomplete) 755.23
    fovea centralis 743.55
    fucosidase 271.8
    gallbladder (acquired) V45.79
        congenital 751.69
    gamma globulin (blood) 279.00
    genital organs
        acquired V45.77
        congenital
            female 752.89
                external 752.49
                internal NEC 752.89
            male 752.89
                penis 752.69
    genitourinary organs, congenital NEC
        752.89
    glottis 748.3
    gonadal, congenital NEC 758.6
    hair (congenital) 757.4
        acquired — *see* Alopecia
    hand (acquired) V49.63
        congenital (complete) (*see also* Deformity,
            reduction, upper limb) 755.21
    heart (congenital) 759.89
        acquired — *see* Status, organ replacement
    heat sense (*see also* Disturbance, sensation)
        782.0
    humerus, congenital (complete) (partial) (with
        absence of distal elements, incomplete)
        (*see also* Deformity, reduction, upper
        limb) 755.24
        with
            complete absence of distal elements
                755.21
            radius and ulna (incomplete) 755.23
    hymen (congenital) 752.49
    ileum (acquired) (postoperative) (posttraumatic)
        V45.72
        congenital 751.1
    immunoglobulin, isolated NEC 279.03
        IgA 279.01
        IgG 279.03
        IgM 279.02
    incus (acquired) 385.24
        congenital 744.04
    internal ear (congenital) 744.05
    intestine (acquired) (small) V45.72
        congenital 751.1
            large 751.2
        large V45.72
            congenital 751.2
    iris (congenital) 743.45
    jaw — *see* Absence, mandible

Absence — *continued*
    jejunum (acquired) V45.72
        congenital 751.1
    joint, congenital NEC 755.8
    kidney(s) (acquired) V45.73
        congenital 753.0
    labium (congenital) (majus) (minus) 752.49
    labyrinth, membranous 744.05
    lacrimal apparatus (congenital) 743.65
    larynx (congenital) 748.3
    leg (acquired) V49.70
        above knee V49.76
        below knee V49.75
        congenital (partial) (unilateral) (*see also*
            Deformity, reduction, lower limb)
            755.31
            lower (complete) (partial) (with absence of
                distal elements, incomplete) 755.35
                with
                    complete absence of distal elements
                        (foot and toes) 755.31
                    thigh (incomplete) 755.33
                        with complete absence of distal
                            elements 755.31
            upper — *see* Absence, femur
    lens (congenital) 743.35
        acquired 379.31
    ligament, broad (congenital) 752.19
    limb (acquired)
        congenital (complete) (partial) (*see also*
            Deformity, reduction) 755.4
            lower 755.30
                complete 755.31
                incomplete 755.32
                longitudinal — *see* Deficiency, lower
                    limb, longitudinal
                transverse 755.31
            upper 755.20
                complete 755.21
                incomplete 755.22
                longitudinal — *see* Deficiency, upper
                    limb, longitudinal
                transverse 755.21
        lower NEC V49.70
        upper NEC V49.60
    lip 750.26
    liver (congenital) (lobe) 751.69
    lumbar (congenital) (vertebra) 756.13
        isthmus 756.11
        pars articularis 756.11
    lumen — *see* Atresia
    lung (bilateral) (congenital) (fissure) (lobe)
        (unilateral) 748.5
        acquired (any part) V45.76
    mandible (congenital) 524.09
    maxilla (congenital) 524.09
    menstruation 626.0
    metacarpal(s), congenital (complete) (partial)
        (with absence of distal elements,
        incomplete) (*see also* Deformity,
        reduction, upper limb) 755.28
        with all fingers, complete 755.21
    metatarsal(s), congenital (complete) (partial)
        (with absence of distal elements,
        incomplete) (*see also* Deformity,
        reduction, lower limb) 755.38
        with complete absence of distal elements
            755.31
    muscle (congenital) (pectoral) 756.81
        ocular 743.69
    musculoskeletal system (congenital) NEC 756.9
    nail(s) (congenital) 757.5
    neck, part 744.89
    nerve 742.8
    nervous system, part NEC 742.8
    neutrophil 288.0
    nipple (congenital) 757.6
    nose (congenital) 748.1
        acquired 738.0
    nuclear 742.8
    ocular muscle (congenital) 743.69
    organ
        of Corti (congenital) 744.05
        or site
            acquired V45.79
            congenital NEC 759.89

Absence — *continued*
    osseous meatus (ear) 744.03
    ovary (acquired) V45.77
        congenital 752.0
    oviduct (acquired) V45.77
        congenital 752.19
    pancreas (congenital) 751.7
        acquired (postoperative) (posttraumatic)
            V45.79
    parathyroid gland (congenital) 759.2
    parotid gland(s) (congenital) 750.21
    patella, congenital 755.64
    pelvic girdle (congenital) 755.69
    penis (congenital) 752.69
        acquired V45.77
    pericardium (congenital) 746.89
    perineal body (congenital) 756.81
    phalange(s), congenital 755.4
        lower limb (complete) (intercalary) (partial)
            (terminal) (*see also* Deformity,
            reduction, lower limb) 755.39
            meaning all toes (complete) (partial)
                755.31
            transverse 755.31
        upper limb (complete) (intercalary) (partial)
            (terminal) (*see also* Deformity,
            reduction, upper limb) 755.29
            meaning all digits (complete) (partial)
                755.21
            transverse 755.21
    pituitary gland (congenital) 759.2
    postoperative — *see* Absence, by site, acquired
    prostate (congenital) 752.89
        acquired V45.77
    pulmonary
        artery 747.3
        trunk 747.3
        valve (congenital) 746.01
        vein 747.49
    punctum lacrimale (congenital) 743.65
    radius, congenital (complete) (partial) (with
        absence of distal elements, incomplete)
        755.26
        with
            complete absence of distal elements
                755.21
            ulna 755.25
                with
                    complete absence of distal elements
                        755.21
                    humerus (incomplete) 755.23
    ray, congenital 755.4
        lower limb (complete) (partial) (*see also*
            Deformity, reduction, lower limb)
            755.38
            meaning all rays 755.31
            transverse 755.31
        upper limb (complete) (partial) (*see also*
            Deformity, reduction, upper limb)
            755.28
            meaning all rays 755.21
            transverse 755.21
    rectum (congenital) 751.2
        acquired V45.79
    red cell 284.9
        acquired (secondary) 284.8
        congenital 284.0
        hereditary 284.0
        idiopathic 284.9
    respiratory organ (congenital) NEC 748.9
    rib (acquired) 738.3
        congenital 756.3
    roof of orbit (congenital) 742.0
    round ligament (congenital) 752.89
    sacrum, congenital 756.13
    salivary gland(s) (congenital) 750.21
    scapula 755.59
    scrotum, congenital 752.89
    seminal tract or duct (congenital) 752.89
        acquired V45.77
    septum (congenital) — *see also* Imperfect,
        closure, septum
        atrial 745.69
            and ventricular 745.7
        between aorta and pulmonary artery 745.0
        ventricular 745.3
            and atrial 745.7

Absence

Absence — Acalcicosis

Absence — *continued*
  sex chromosomes 758.81
  shoulder girdle, congenital (complete) (partial) 755.59
  skin (congenital) 757.39
  skull bone 756.0
    with
      anencephalus 740.0
      encephalocele 742.0
      hydrocephalus 742.3
        with spina bifida (*see also* Spina bifida) 741.0 ☑
      microcephalus 742.1
  spermatic cord (congenital) 752.89
  spinal cord 742.59
  spine, congenital 756.13
  spleen (congenital) 759.0
    acquired V45.79
  sternum, congenital 756.3
  stomach (acquired) (partial) (postoperative) V45.75
    with postgastric surgery syndrome 564.2
    congenital 750.7
  submaxillary gland(s) (congenital) 750.21
  superior vena cava (congenital) 747.49
  tarsal(s), congenital (complete) (partial) (with absence of distal elements, incomplete) (*see also* Deformity, reduction, lower limb) 755.38
  teeth, tooth (congenital) 520.0
    with abnormal spacing 524.30 ▲
    acquired 525.10
      with malocclusion 524.30 ▲
      due to
        caries 525.13
        extraction 525.10
        periodontal disease 525.12
        trauma 525.11
  tendon (congenital) 756.81
  testis (congenital) 752.89
    acquired V45.77
  thigh (acquired) 736.89
  thumb (acquired) V49.61
    congenital 755.29
  thymus gland (congenital) 759.2
  thyroid (gland) (surgical) 246.8
    with hypothyroidism 244.0
    cartilage, congenital 748.3
    congenital 243
  tibia, congenital (complete) (partial) (with absence of distal elements, incomplete) (*see also* Deformity, reduction, lower limb) 755.36
    with
      complete absence of distal elements 755.31
      fibula 755.35
        with
          complete absence of distal elements 755.31
        femur (incomplete) 755.33
          with complete absence of distal elements 755.31
  toe (acquired) V49.72
    congenital (complete) (partial) 755.39
      meaning all toes 755.31
      transverse 755.31
    great V49.71
  tongue (congenital) 750.11
  tooth, teeth, (congenital) 520.0
    with abnormal spacing 524.30 ▲
    acquired 525.10
      with malocclusion 524.30 ▲
      due to
        caries 525.13
        extraction 525.10
        periodontal disease 525.12
        trauma 525.11
  trachea (cartilage) (congenital) (rings) 748.3
  transverse aortic arch (congenital) 747.21
  tricuspid valve 746.1
  ulna, congenital (complete) (partial) (with absence of distal elements, incomplete) (*see also* Deformity, reduction, upper limb) 755.27

Absence — *continued*
  ulna, congenital — *continued*
    with
      complete absence of distal elements 755.21
      radius 755.25
        with
          complete absence of distal elements 755.21
          humerus (incomplete) 755.23
  umbilical artery (congenital) 747.5
  ureter (congenital) 753.4
    acquired V45.74
  urethra, congenital 753.8
    acquired V45.74
  urinary system, part NEC, congenital 753.8
    acquired V45.74
  uterus (acquired) V45.77
    congenital 752.3
  uvula (congenital) 750.26
  vagina, congenital 752.49
    acquired V45.77
  vas deferens (congenital) 752.89
    acquired V45.77
  vein (congenital) (peripheral) NEC (*see also* Anomaly, peripheral vascular system) 747.60
    brain 747.81
    great 747.49
    portal 747.49
    pulmonary 747.49
  vena cava (congenital) (inferior) (superior) 747.49
  ventral horn cell 742.59
  ventricular septum 745.3
  vermis of cerebellum 742.2
  vertebra, congenital 756.13
  vulva, congenital 752.49

Absentia epileptica (*see also* Epilepsy) 345.0 ☑
Absinthemia (*see also* Dependence) 304.6 ☑
Absinthism (*see also* Dependence) 304.6 ☑
Absorbent system disease 459.89
Absorption
  alcohol, through placenta or breast milk 760.71
  antibiotics, through placenta or breast milk 760.74
  anti-infective, through placenta or breast milk 760.74
  chemical NEC 989.9
    specified chemical or substance — *see* Table of Drugs and Chemicals
    through placenta or breast milk (fetus or newborn) 760.70
      alcohol 760.71
      anti-infective agents 760.74
      cocaine 760.75
      "crack" 760.75
      diethylstilbestrol [DES] 760.76
      hallucinogenic agents 760.73
      medicinal agents NEC 760.79
      narcotics 760.72
      obstetric anesthetic or analgesic drug 763.5
      specified agent NEC 760.79
      suspected, affecting management of pregnancy 655.5 ☑
  cocaine, through placenta or breast milk 760.75
  drug NEC (*see also* Reaction, drug)
    through placenta or breast milk (fetus or newborn) 760.70
      alcohol 760.71
      anti-infective agents 760.74
      cocaine 760.75
      "crack" 760.75
      diethylstilbestrol [DES] 760.76
      hallucinogenic agents 760.73
      medicinal agents NEC 760.79
      narcotics 760.72
      obstetric anesthetic or analgesic drug 763.5
      specified agent NEC 760.79

Absorption — *continued*
  drug NEC (*see also* Reaction, drug) — *continued*
    through placenta or breast milk — *continued*
      suspected, affecting management of pregnancy 655.5 ☑
  fat, disturbance 579.8
  hallucinogenic agents, through placenta or breast milk 760.73
  immune sera, through placenta or breast milk 760.79
  lactose defect 271.3
  medicinal agents NEC, through placenta or breast milk 760.79
  narcotics, through placenta or breast milk 760.72
  noxious substance, — *see* Absorption, chemical
  protein, disturbance 579.8
  pus or septic, general — *see* Septicemia
  quinine, through placenta or breast milk 760.74
  toxic substance, — *see* Absorption, chemical
  uremic — *see* Uremia
Abstinence symptoms or syndrome
  alcohol 291.81
  drug 292.0
Abt-Letterer-Siwe syndrome (acute histiocytosis X) (M9722/3) 202.5 ☑
Abulia 799.89
Abulomania 301.6
Abuse
  adult 995.80
    emotional 995.82
    multiple forms 995.85
    neglect (nutritional) 995.84
    physical 995.81
    psychological 995.82
    sexual 995.83
  alcohol (*see also* Alcoholism) 305.0 ☑
    dependent 303.9 ☑
    non-dependent 305.0 ☑
  child 995.50
    counseling
      perpetrator
        non-parent V62.83
        parent V61.22
      victim V61.21
    emotional 995.51
    multiple forms 995.59
    neglect (nutritional) 995.52
    psychological 995.51
    physical 995.54
      shaken infant syndrome 995.55
    sexual 995.53
  drugs, nondependent 305.9 ☑

> *Note — Use the following fifth-digit subclassification with the following codes: 305.0, 305.2-305.9:*
>
> | 0 | unspecified | 2 | episodic |
> |---|---|---|---|
> | 1 | continuous | 3 | in remission |

    amphetamine type 305.7 ☑
    antidepressants 305.8 ☑
    anxiolytic 305.4 ☑ ●
    barbiturates 305.4 ☑
    caffeine 305.9 ☑
    cannabis 305.2 ☑
    cocaine type 305.6 ☑
    hallucinogens 305.3 ☑
    hashish 305.2 ☑
    hypnotic 305.4 ☑ ●
    inhalant 305.9 ☑ ●
    LSD 305.3 ☑
    marijuana 305.2 ☑
    mixed 305.9 ☑
    morphine type 305.5 ☑
    opioid type 305.5 ☑
    phencyclidine (PCP) 305.9 ☑
    sedative 305.4 ☑ ●
    specified NEC 305.9 ☑
    tranquilizers 305.4 ☑
  spouse 995.80
  tobacco 305.1
Acalcerosis 275.40
Acalcicosis 275.40

☑ Additional Digit Required   ►◄ Revised Text   ● New Line   ▲ Revised Code

Acalculia 784.69
 developmental 315.1
Acanthocheilonemiasis 125.4
Acanthocytosis 272.5
Acanthokeratodermia 701.1
Acantholysis 701.8
 bullosa 757.39
Acanthoma (benign) (M8070/0) — *see also*
  Neoplasm, by site, benign
 malignant (M8070/3) — *see* Neoplasm, by site,
  malignant
Acanthosis (acquired) (nigricans) 701.2
 adult 701.2
 benign (congenital) 757.39
 congenital 757.39
 glycogenic
  esophagus 530.89
 juvenile 701.2
 tongue 529.8
Acanthrocytosis 272.5
Acapnia 276.3
Acarbia 276.2
Acardia 759.89
Acardiacus amorphus 759.89
Acardiotrophia 429.1
Acardius 759.89
Acariasis 133.9
 sarcoptic 133.0
Acaridiasis 133.9
Acarinosis 133.9
Acariosis 133.9
Acarodermatitis 133.9
 urticarioides 133.9
Acarophobia 300.29
Acatalasemia 277.89
Acatalasia 277.89
Acatamathesia 784.69
Acataphasia 784.5
Acathisia 781.0
 due to drugs 333.99
Acceleration, accelerated
 atrioventricular conduction 426.7
 idioventricular rhythm 427.89
Accessory (congenital)
 adrenal gland 759.1
 anus 751.5
 appendix 751.5
 atrioventricular conduction 426.7
 auditory ossicles 744.04
 auricle (ear) 744.1
 autosome(s) NEC 758.5
  21 or 22 758.0
 biliary duct or passage 751.69
 bladder 753.8
 blood vessels (peripheral) (congenital) NEC (*see
  also* Anomaly, peripheral vascular
  system) 747.60
  cerebral 747.81
  coronary 746.85
 bone NEC 756.9
  foot 755.67
 breast tissue, axilla 757.6
 carpal bones 755.56
 cecum 751.5
 cervix 752.49
 chromosome(s) NEC 758.5
  13-15 758.1
  16-18 758.2
  21 or 22 758.0
  autosome(s) NEC 758.5
  D$_1$ 758.1
  E$_3$ 758.2
  G 758.0
  sex 758.81
 coronary artery 746.85
 cusp(s), heart valve NEC 746.89
  pulmonary 746.09
 cystic duct 751.69
 digits 755.00
 ear (auricle) (lobe) 744.1
 endocrine gland NEC 759.2
 external os 752.49

Accessory — *continued*
 eyelid 743.62
 eye muscle 743.69
 face bone(s) 756.0
 fallopian tube (fimbria) (ostium) 752.19
 fingers 755.01
 foreskin 605
 frontonasal process 756.0
 gallbladder 751.69
 genital organ(s)
  female 752.89
   external 752.49
   internal NEC 752.89
  male NEC 752.89
   penis 752.69
 genitourinary organs NEC 752.89
 heart 746.89
  valve NEC 746.89
   pulmonary 746.09
 hepatic ducts 751.69
 hymen 752.49
 intestine (large) (small) 751.5
 kidney 753.3
 lacrimal canal 743.65
 leaflet, heart valve NEC 746.89
  pulmonary 746.09
 ligament, broad 752.19
 liver (duct) 751.69
 lobule (ear) 744.1
 lung (lobe) 748.69
 muscle 756.82
 navicular of carpus 755.56
 nervous system, part NEC 742.8
 nipple 757.6
 nose 748.1
 organ or site NEC — *see* Anomaly, specified
  type NEC
 ovary 752.0
 oviduct 752.19
 pancreas 751.7
 parathyroid gland 759.2
 parotid gland (and duct) 750.22
 pituitary gland 759.2
 placental lobe — *see* Placenta, abnormal
 preauricular appendage 744.1
 prepuce 605
 renal arteries (multiple) 747.62
 rib 756.3
  cervical 756.2
 roots (teeth) 520.2
 salivary gland 750.22
 sesamoids 755.8
 sinus — *see* condition
 skin tags 757.39
 spleen 759.0
 sternum 756.3
 submaxillary gland 750.22
 tarsal bones 755.67
 teeth, tooth 520.1
  causing crowding 524.31   ▲
 tendon 756.89
 thumb 755.01
 thymus gland 759.2
 thyroid gland 759.2
 toes 755.02
 tongue 750.13
 tragus 744.1
 ureter 753.4
 urethra 753.8
 urinary organ or tract NEC 753.8
 uterus 752.2
 vagina 752.49
 valve, heart NEC 746.89
  pulmonary 746.09
 vertebra 756.19
 vocal cords 748.3
 vulva 752.49
Accident, accidental — *see also* condition
 birth NEC 767.9
 cardiovascular (*see also* Disease,
  cardiovascular) 429.2
 cerebral (*see also* Disease, cerebrovascular,
  acute) 434.91   ▲
 cerebrovascular (current) (CVA) (*see also*
  Disease, cerebrovascular, acute)
  434.91   ▲

Accident, accidental — *see also* condition —
  continued
 cerebrovascular (*see also* Disease,
   cerebrovascular, acute) — *continued*
   embolic 434.11   ●
   healed or old V12.59
   impending 435.9
   ischemic 434.91   ●
   late effect — *see* Late effect(s) (of)
    cerebrovascular disease
   postoperative 997.02
   thrombotic 434.01   ●
  coronary (*see also* Infarct, myocardium)
   410.9 ☑
  craniovascular (*see also* Disease,
   cerebrovascular, acute) 436
  during pregnancy, to mother
   affecting fetus or newborn 760.5
  heart, cardiac (*see also* Infarct, myocardium)
   410.9 ☑
  intrauterine 779.89
  vascular — *see* Disease, cerebrovascular, acute
Accommodation
 disorder of 367.51
  drug-induced 367.89
  toxic 367.89
 insufficiency of 367.4
 paralysis of 367.51
  hysterical 300.11
 spasm of 367.53
Accouchement — *see* Delivery
Accreta placenta (without hemorrhage) 667.0 ☑
 with hemorrhage 666.0 ☑
Accretio cordis (nonrheumatic) 423.1
Accretions on teeth 523.6
Accumulation secretion, prostate 602.8
Acephalia, acephalism, acephaly 740.0
Acephalic 740.0
Acephalobrachia 759.89
Acephalocardia 759.89
Acephalocardius 759.89
Acephalochiria 759.89
Acephalochirus 759.89
Acephalogaster 759.89
Acephalostomus 759.89
Acephalothorax 759.89
Acephalus 740.0
Acetonemia 790.6
 diabetic 250.1 ☑
Acetonglycosuria 982.8
Acetonuria 791.6
Achalasia 530.0
 cardia 530.0
 digestive organs congenital NEC 751.8
 esophagus 530.0
 pelvirectal 751.3
 psychogenic 306.4
 pylorus 750.5
 sphincteral NEC 564.89
Achard-Thiers syndrome (adrenogenital) 255.2
Ache(s) — *see* Pain
Acheilia 750.26
Acheiria 755.21
Achillobursitis 726.71
Achillodynia 726.71
Achlorhydria, achlorhydric 536.0
 anemia 280.9
 diarrhea 536.0
 neurogenic 536.0
 postvagotomy 564.2
 psychogenic 306.4
 secondary to vagotomy 564.2
Achloroblepsia 368.52
Achloropsia 368.52
Acholia 575.8
Acholuric jaundice (familial) (splenomegalic) (*see
  also* Spherocytosis) 282.0
 acquired 283.9
Achondroplasia 756.4
Achrestic anemia 281.8

Achroacytosis, lacrimal gland 375.00
  tuberculous (*see also* Tuberculosis) 017.3 ☑
Achroma, cutis 709.00
Achromate (congenital) 368.54
Achromatopia 368.54
Achromatopsia (congenital) 368.54
Achromia
  congenital 270.2
  parasitica 111.0
  unguium 703.8
Achylia
  gastrica 536.8
    neurogenic 536.3
    psychogenic 306.4
  pancreatica 577.1
Achylosis 536.8
Acid
  burn — *see also* Burn, by site
    from swallowing acid — *see* Burn, internal
      organs
  deficiency
    amide nicotinic 265.2
    amino 270.9
    ascorbic 267
    folic 266.2
    nicotinic (amide) 265.2
    pantothenic 266.2
  intoxication 276.2
  peptic disease 536.8
  stomach 536.8
    psychogenic 306.4
Acidemia 276.2
  arginosuccinic 270.6
  fetal
    affecting management of pregnancy 656.3 ☑
    before onset of labor, in liveborn infant
      768.2
    during labor, in liveborn infant 768.3
    intrauterine — *see* Distress, fetal 656.3 ☑
    unspecified as to time of onset, in liveborn
      infant 768.4
  pipecolic 270.7
Acidity, gastric (high) (low) 536.8
  psychogenic 306.4
Acidocytopenia 288.0
Acidocytosis 288.3
Acidopenia 288.0
Acidosis 276.2
  diabetic 250.1 ☑
  fetal, affecting management of pregnancy
    756.8 ☑
  fetal, affecting newborn 768.9
  kidney tubular 588.89 ▲
  lactic 276.2
  metabolic NEC 276.2
    with respiratory acidosis 276.4
    late, of newborn 775.7
  renal
    hyperchloremic 588.89 ▲
    tubular (distal) (proximal) 588.89 ▲
  respiratory 276.2
    complicated by
      metabolic acidosis 276.4
      metabolic alkalosis 276.4
Aciduria 791.9
  arginosuccinic 270.6
  beta-aminoisobutyric (BAIB) 277.2
  glutaric ●
    type I 270.7 ●
    type II (type IIA, IIB, IIC) 277.85 ●
    type III 277.86 ●
  glycolic 271.8
  methylmalonic 270.3
    with glycinemia 270.7
  organic 270.9
  orotic (congenital) (hereditary) (pyrimidine
    deficiency) 281.4
Acladiosis 111.8
  skin 111.8
Aclasis
  diaphyseal 756.4
  tarsoepiphyseal 756.59
Acleistocardia 745.5
Aclusion 524.4

Acmesthesia 782.0
Acne (pustular) (vulgaris) 706.1
  agminata (*see also* Tuberculosis) 017.0 ☑
  artificialis 706.1
  atrophica 706.0
  cachecticorum (Hebra) 706.1
  conglobata 706.1
  conjunctiva 706.1
  cystic 706.1
  decalvans 704.09
  erythematosa 695.3
  eyelid 706.1
  frontalis 706.0
  indurata 706.1
  keloid 706.1
  lupoid 706.0
  necrotic, necrotica 706.0
    miliaris 704.8
  nodular 706.1
  occupational 706.1
  papulosa 706.1
  rodens 706.0
  rosacea 695.3
  scorbutica 267
  scrofulosorum (Bazin) (*see also* Tuberculosis)
    017.0 ☑
  summer 692.72
  tropical 706.1
  varioliformis 706.0
Acneiform drug eruptions 692.3
Acnitis (primary) (*see also* Tuberculosis) 017.0 ☑
Acomia 704.00
Acontractile bladder 344.61
Aconuresis (*see also* Incontinence) 788.30
Acosta's disease 993.2
Acousma 780.1
Acoustic — *see* condition
Acousticophobia 300.29
Acquired — *see* condition
Acquired immune deficiency syndrome — *see*
    Human immunodeficiency virus (disease)
    (illness) (infection)
Acquired immunodeficiency syndrome — *see*
    Human immunodeficiency virus (disease)
    (illness) (infection)
Acragnosis 781.99
Acrania 740.0
Acroagnosis 781.99
Acroasphyxia, chronic 443.89
Acrobrachycephaly 756.0
Acrobystiolith 608.89
Acrobystitis 607.2
Acrocephalopolysyndactyly 755.55
Acrocephalosyndactyly 755.55
Acrocephaly 756.0
Acrochondrohyperplasia 759.82
Acrocyanosis 443.89
  newborn 770.83
Acrodermatitis 686.8
  atrophicans (chronica) 701.8
  continua (Hallopeau) 696.1
  enteropathica 686.8
  Hallopeau's 696.1
  perstans 696.1
  pustulosa continua 696.1
  recalcitrant pustular 696.1
Acrodynia 985.0
Acrodysplasia 755.55
Acrohyperhidrosis ▶(*see also* Hyperhidrosis)◀
    780.8
Acrokeratosis verruciformis 757.39
Acromastitis 611.0
Acromegaly, acromegalia (skin) 253.0
Acromelalgia 443.89
Acromicria acromikria 756.59
Acronyx 703.0
Acropachy, thyroid (*see also* Thyrotoxicosis)
    242.9 ☑
Acropachyderma 757.39
Acroparesthesia 443.89
  simple (Schultz's type) 443.89

Acroparesthesia — *continued*
  vasomotor (Nothnagel's type) 443.89
Acropathy thyroid (*see also* Thyrotoxicosis)
    242.9 ☑
Acrophobia 300.29
Acroposthitis 607.2
Acroscleriasis (*see also* Scleroderma) 710.1
Acroscleroderma (*see also* Scleroderma) 710.1
Acrosclerosis (*see also* Scleroderma) 710.1
Acrosphacelus 785.4
Acrosphenosyndactylia 755.55
Acrospiroma, eccrine (M8402/0) — *see*
    Neoplasm, skin, benign
Acrostealgia 732.9
Acrosyndactyly (*see also* Syndactylism) 755.10
Acrotrophodynia 991.4
Actinic — *see also* condition
  cheilitis (due to sun) 692.72
    chronic NEC 692.74
    due to radiation, except from sun 692.82
  conjunctivitis 370.24
  dermatitis (due to sun) (*see also* Dermatitis,
    actinic 692.70
    due to
      roentgen rays or radioactive substance
        692.82
      ultraviolet radiation, except from sun
        692.82
      sun NEC 692.70
  elastosis solare 692.74
  granuloma 692.73
  keratitis 370.24
  ophthalmia 370.24
  reticuloid 692.73
Actinobacillosis, general 027.8
Actinobacillus
  lignieresii 027.8
  mallei 024
  muris 026.1
Actinocutitis NEC (*see also* Dermatitis, actinic)
    692.70
Actinodermatitis NEC (*see also* Dermatitis,
    actinic) 692.70
Actinomyces
  israelii (infection) — *see* Actinomycosis
  muris-ratti (infection) 026.1
Actinomycosis, actinomycotic 039.9
  with
    pneumonia 039.1
  abdominal 039.2
  cervicofacial 039.3
  cutaneous 039.0
  pulmonary 039.1
  specified site NEC 039.8
  thoracic 039.1
Actinoneuritis 357.89
Action, heart
  disorder 427.9
    postoperative 997.1
  irregular 427.9
    postoperative 997.1
    psychogenic 306.2
Active — *see* condition
Activity decrease, functional 780.99
Acute — *see also* condition
  abdomen NEC 789.0 ☑
  gallbladder (*see also* Cholecystitis, acute) 575.0
Acyanoblepsia 368.53
Acyanopsia 368.53
Acystia 753.8
Acystinervia — *see* Neurogenic, bladder
Acystineuria — *see* Neurogenic, bladder
Adactylia, adactyly (congenital) 755.4
  lower limb (complete) (intercalary) (partial)
    (terminal) (*see also* Deformity, reduction,
    lower limb) 755.39
    meaning all digits (complete) (partial) 755.31
    transverse (complete) (partial) 755.31
  upper limb (complete) (intercalary) (partial)
    (terminal) (*see also* Deformity, reduction,
    upper limb) 755.29

☑ Additional Digit Required   ▶◀ Revised Text   ● New Line   ▲ Revised Code

Adactylia, adactyly — *continued*
  upper limb (*see also* Deformity, reduction,
      upper limb) — *continued*
    meaning all digits (complete) (partial) 755.21
    transverse (complete) (partial) 755.21
Adair-Dighton syndrome (brittle bones and blue
    sclera, deafness) 756.51
Adamantinoblastoma (M9310/0) — *see*
    Ameloblastoma
Adamantinoma (M9310/0) — *see* Ameloblastoma
Adamantoblastoma (M9310/0) — *see*
    Ameloblastoma
Adams-Stokes (-Morgagni) disease or syndrome
    (syncope with heart block) 426.9
Adaptation reaction (*see also* Reaction,
    adjustment) 309.9
Addiction — *see also* Dependence
  absinthe 304.6 ✅
  alcoholic (ethyl) (methyl) (wood) 303.9 ✅
    complicating pregnancy, childbirth, or
        puerperium 648.4 ✅
      affecting fetus or newborn 760.71
      suspected damage to fetus affecting
          management of pregnancy 655.4 ✅
  drug (*see also* Dependence) 304.9 ✅
  ethyl alcohol 303.9 ✅
  heroin 304.0 ✅
  hospital 301.51
  methyl alcohol 303.9 ✅
  methylated spirit 303.9 ✅
  morphine (-like substances) 304.0 ✅
  nicotine 305.1
  opium 304.0 ✅
  tobacco 305.1
  wine 303.9 ✅
Addison's
  anemia (pernicious) 281.0
  disease (bronze) (primary adrenal insufficiency)
      255.4
    tuberculous (*see also* Tuberculosis) 017.6 ✅
  keloid (morphea) 701.0
  melanoderma (adrenal cortical hypofunction)
      255.4
Addison-Biermer anemia (pernicious) 281.0
Addison-Gull disease — *see* Xanthoma
Addisonian crisis or melanosis (acute
    adrenocortical insufficiency) 255.4
Additional — *see also* Accessory
  chromosome(s) 758.5
    13-15 758.1
    16-18 758.2
    21 758.0
    autosome(s) NEC 758.5
    sex 758.81
Adduction contracture, hip or other joint — *see*
    Contraction, joint
Adenasthenia gastrica 536.0
Aden fever 061
Adenitis (*see also* Lymphadenitis) 289.3
  acute, unspecified site 683
    epidemic infectious 075
  axillary 289.3
    acute 683
    chronic or subacute 289.1
  Bartholin's gland 616.8
  bulbourethral gland (*see also* Urethritis) 597.89
  cervical 289.3
    acute 683
    chronic or subacute 289.1
  chancroid (Ducrey's bacillus) 099.0
  chronic (any lymph node, except mesenteric)
      289.1
    mesenteric 289.2
  Cowper's gland (*see also* Urethritis) 597.89
  epidemic, acute 075
  gangrenous 683
  gonorrheal NEC 098.89
  groin 289.3
    acute 683
    chronic or subacute 289.1
  infectious 075
  inguinal (region) 289.3
    acute 683
    chronic or subacute 289.1

Adenitis (*see also* Lymphadenitis) — *continued*
  lymph gland or node, except mesenteric 289.3
    acute 683
    chronic or subacute 289.1
    mesenteric (acute) (chronic) (nonspecific)
        (subacute) 289.2
  mesenteric (acute) (chronic) (nonspecific)
      (subacute) 289.2
    due to Pasteurella multocida (P. septica)
        027.2
  parotid gland (suppurative) 527.2
  phlegmonous 683
  salivary duct or gland (any) (recurring)
      (suppurative) 527.2
  scrofulous (*see also* Tuberculosis) 017.2 ✅
  septic 289.3
  Skene's duct or gland (*see also* Urethritis)
      597.89
  strumous, tuberculous (*see also* Tuberculosis)
      017.2 ✅
  subacute, unspecified site 289.1
  sublingual gland (suppurative) 527.2
  submandibular gland (suppurative) 527.2
  submaxillary gland (suppurative) 527.2
  suppurative 683
  tuberculous — *see* Tuberculosis, lymph gland
  urethral gland (*see also* Urethritis) 597.89
  venereal NEC 099.8
  Wharton's duct (suppurative) 527.2
Adenoacanthoma (M8570/3) — *see* Neoplasm, by
    site, malignant
Adenoameloblastoma (M9300/0) 213.1
  upper jaw (bone) 213.0
Adenocarcinoma (M8140/3) — *see also*
    Neoplasm, by site, malignant

> *Note* — *The following list of adjectival modifiers
> is not exhaustive. A description of
> adenocarcinoma that does not appear in this list
> should be coded in the same manner as
> carcinoma with that description. Thus, "mixed
> acidophil-basophil adenocarcinoma," should be
> coded in the same manner as "mixed acidophil-
> basophil carcinoma," which appears in the list
> under "Carcinoma."*
>
> *Except where otherwise indicated, the
> morphological varieties of adenocarcinoma in the
> list should be coded by site as for "Neoplasm,
> malignant."*

  with
    apocrine metaplasia (M8573/3)
    cartilaginous (and osseous) metaplasia
        (M8571/3)
    osseous (and cartilaginous) metaplasia
        (M8571/3)
    spindle cell metaplasia (M8572/3)
    squamous metaplasia (M8570/3)
  acidophil (M8280/3)
    specified site — *see* Neoplasm, by site,
        malignant
    unspecified site 194.3
  acinar (M8550/3)
  acinic cell (M8550/3)
  adrenal cortical (M8370/3) 194.0
  alveolar (M8251/3)
    and
      epidermoid carcinoma, mixed (M8560/3)
      squamous cell carcinoma, mixed
          (M8560/3)
  apocrine (M8401/3)
    breast — *see* Neoplasm, breast, malignant
    specified site NEC — *see* Neoplasm, skin,
        malignant
    unspecified site 173.9
  basophil (M8300/3)
    specified site — *see* Neoplasm, by site,
        malignant
    unspecified site 194.3
  bile duct type (M8160/3)
    liver 155.1
    specified site NEC — *see* Neoplasm, by site,
        malignant
    unspecified site 155.1
  bronchiolar (M8250/3) — *see* Neoplasm, lung,
      malignant
  ceruminous (M8420/3) 173.2

Adenocarcinoma (M8140/3) — *see also*
    Neoplasm, by site, malignant — *continued*
  chromophobe (M8270/3)
    specified site — *see* Neoplasm, by site,
        malignant
    unspecified site 194.3
  clear cell (mesonephroid type) (M8310/3)
  colloid (M8480/3)
  cylindroid type (M8200/3)
  diffuse type (M8145/3)
    specified site — *see* Neoplasm, by site,
        malignant
    unspecified site 151.9
  duct (infiltrating) (M8500/3)
    with Paget's disease (M8541/3) — *see*
        Neoplasm, breast, malignant
    specified site — *see* Neoplasm, by site,
        malignant
    unspecified site 174.9
  embryonal (M9070/3)
  endometrioid (M8380/3) — *see* Neoplasm, by
      site, malignant
  eosinophil (M8280/3)
    specified site — *see* Neoplasm, by site
        malignant
    unspecified site 194.3
  follicular (M8330/3)
    and papillary (M8340/3) 193
    moderately differentiated type (M8332/3) 193
    pure follicle type (M8331/3) 193
    specified site — *see* Neoplasm, by site,
        malignant
    trabecular type (M8332/3) 193
    unspecified type 193
    well differentiated type (M8331/3) 193
  gelatinous (M8480/3)
  granular cell (M8320/3)
  Hürthle cell (M8290/3) 193
  in
    adenomatous
        polyp (M8210/3)
        polyposis coli (M8220/3) 153.9
    polypoid adenoma (M8210/3)
    tubular adenoma (M8210/3)
    villous adenoma (M8261/3)
  infiltrating duct (M8500/3)
    with Paget's disease (M8541/3) — *see*
        Neoplasm, breast, malignant
    specified site — *see* Neoplasm, by site,
        malignant
    unspecified site 174.9
  inflammatory (M8530/3)
    specified site — *see* Neoplasm, by site,
        malignant
    unspecified site 174.9
  in situ (M8140/2) — *see* Neoplasm, by site, in
      situ
  intestinal type (M8144/3)
    specified site — *see* Neoplasm, by site,
        malignant
    unspecified site 151.9
  intraductal (noninfiltrating) (M8500/2)
    papillary (M8503/2)
      specified site — *see* Neoplasm, by site, in
          situ
      unspecified site 233.0
    specified site — *see* Neoplasm, by site, in
        situ
    unspecified site 233.0
  islet cell (M8150/3)
    and exocrine, mixed (M8154/3)
      specified site — *see* Neoplasm, by site,
          malignant
      unspecified site 157.9
    pancreas 157.4
    specified site NEC — *see* Neoplasm, by site,
        malignant
    unspecified site 157.4
  lobular (M8520/3)
    specified site — *see* Neoplasm, by site,
        malignant
    unspecified site 174.9
  medullary (M8510/3)
  mesonephric (M9110/3)
  mixed cell (M8323/3)
  mucinous (M8480/3)
  mucin-producing (M8481/3)

✅ Additional Digit Required   ▶◀ Revised Text   ● New Line   ▲ Revised Code

Adenocarcinoma (M8140/3) — *see also*
  Neoplasm, by site, malignant — *continued*
  mucoid (M8480/3) — *see also* Neoplasm, by
    site, malignant
    cell (M8300/3)
      specified site — *see* Neoplasm, by site,
        malignant
      unspecified site 194.3
  nonencapsulated sclerosing (M8350/3) 193
  oncocytic (M8290/3)
  oxyphilic (M8290/3)
  papillary (M8260/3)
    and follicular (M8340/3) 193
    intraductal (noninfiltrating) (M8503/2)
      specified site — *see* Neoplasm, by site, in
        situ
      unspecified site 233.0
    serous (M8460/3)
      specified site — *see* Neoplasm, by site,
        malignant
      unspecified site 183.0
  papillocystic (M8450/3)
    specified site — *see* Neoplasm, by site,
      malignant
    unspecified site 183.0
  pseudomucinous (M8470/3)
    specified site — *see* Neoplasm, by site,
      malignant
    unspecified site 183.0
  renal cell (M8312/3) 189.0
  sebaceous (M8410/3)
  serous (M8441/3) — *see also* Neoplasm, by
    site, malignant
    papillary
      specified site — *see* Neoplasm, by site
        malignant
      unspecified site 183.0
  signet ring cell (M8490/3)
  superficial spreading (M8143/3)
  sweat gland (M8400/3) — *see* Neoplasm, skin,
    malignant
  trabecular (M8190/3)
  tubular (M8211/3)
  villous (M8262/3)
  water-clear cell (M8322/3) 194.1
Adenofibroma (M9013/0)
  clear cell (M8313/0) — *see* Neoplasm, by site,
    benign
  endometrioid (M8381/0) 220
    borderline malignancy (M8381/1) 236.2
    malignant (M8381/3) 183.0
  mucinous (M9015/0)
    specified site — *see* Neoplasm, by site,
      benign
    unspecified site 220
  prostate 600.20
    with urinary retention 600.21
  serous (M9014/0)
    specified site — *see* Neoplasm, by site,
      benign
    unspecified site 220
  specified site — *see* Neoplasm, by site, benign
  unspecified site 220
Adenofibrosis
  breast 610.2
  endometrioid 617.0
Adenoiditis 474.01
  acute 463
  chronic 474.01
    with chronic tonsillitis 474.02
Adenoids (congenital) (of nasal fossa) 474.9
  hypertrophy 474.12
  vegetations 474.2
Adenolipomatosis (symmetrical) 272.8
Adenolymphoma (M8561/0)
  specified site — *see* Neoplasm, by site, benign
  unspecified 210.2
Adenoma (sessile) (M8140/0) — *see also*
  Neoplasm, by site, benign

Note — Except where otherwise indicated, the morphological varieties of adenoma in the list below should be coded by site as for "Neoplasm, benign."

Adenoma (M8140/0) — *see also* Neoplasm, by
  site, benign — *continued*
  acidophil (M8280/0)
    specified site — *see* Neoplasm, by site,
      benign
    unspecified site 227.3
  acinar (cell) (M8550/0)
  acinic cell (M8550/0)
  adrenal (cortex) (cortical) (functioning)
    (M8370/0) 227.0
    clear cell type (M8373/0) 227.0
    compact cell type (M8371/0) 227.0
    glomerulosa cell type (M8374/0) 227.0
    heavily pigmented variant (M8372/0) 227.0
    mixed cell type (M8375/0) 227.0
  alpha cell (M8152/0)
    pancreas 211.7
    specified site NEC — *see* Neoplasm, by site,
      benign
    unspecified site 211.7
  alveolar (M8251/0)
  apocrine (M8401/0)
    breast 217
    specified site NEC — *see* Neoplasm, skin,
      benign
    unspecified site 216.9
  basal cell (M8147/0)
  basophil (M8300/0)
    specified site — *see* Neoplasm, by site,
      benign
    unspecified site 227.3
  beta cell (M8151/0)
    pancreas 211.7
    specified site NEC — *see* Neoplasm, by site,
      benign
    unspecified site 211.7
  bile duct (M8160/0) 211.5
  black (M8372/0) 227.0
  bronchial (M8140/1) 235.7
    carcinoid type (M8240/3) — *see* Neoplasm,
      lung, malignant
    cylindroid type (M8200/3) — *see* Neoplasm,
      lung, malignant
  ceruminous (M8420/0) 216.2
  chief cell (M8321/0) 227.1
  chromophobe (M8270/0)
    specified site — *see* Neoplasm, by site,
      benign
    unspecified site 227.3
  clear cell (M8310/0)
  colloid (M8334/0)
    specified site — *see* Neoplasm, by site,
      benign
    unspecifted site 226
  cylindroid type, bronchus (M8200/3) — *see*
    Neoplasm, lung, malignant
  duct (M8503/0)
  embryonal (M8191/0)
  endocrine, multiple (M8360/1)
    single specified site — *see* Neoplasm, by site,
      uncertain behavior
    two or more specified sites 237.4
    unspecified site 237.4
  endometrioid (M8380/0) — *see also* Neoplasm,
    by site, benign
    borderline malignancy (M8380/1) — *see*
      Neoplasm, by site, uncertain behavior
  eosinophil (M8280/0)
    specified site — *see* Neoplasm, by site,
      benign
    unspecified site 227.3
  fetal (M8333/0)
    specified site — *see* Neoplasm, by site,
      benign
    unspecified site 226
  follicular (M8330/0)
    specified site — *see* Neoplasm, by site,
      benign
    unspecified site 226
  hepatocellular (M8170/0) 211.5
  Hürthle cell (M8290/0) 226
  intracystic papillary (M8504/0)
  islet cell (functioning) (M8150/0)
    pancreas 211.7
    specified site NEC — *see* Neoplasm, by site,
      benign
    unspecified site 211.7

Adenoma (M8140/0) — *see also* Neoplasm, by
  site, benign — *continued*
  liver cell (M8170/0) 211.5
  macrofollicular (M8334/0)
    specified site NEC — *see* Neoplasm, by site,
      benign
    unspecified site 226
  malignant, malignum (M8140/3) — *see*
    Neoplasm, by site, malignant
  mesonephric (M9110/0)
  microfollicular (M8333/0)
    specified site — *see* Neoplasm, by site,
      benign
    unspecified site 226
  mixed cell (M8323/0)
  monomorphic (M8146/0)
  mucinous (M8480/0)
  mucoid cell (M8300/0)
    specified site — *see* Neoplasm, by site,
      benign
    unspecified site 227.3
  multiple endocrine (M8360/1)
    single specified site — *see* Neoplasm, by site,
      uncertain behavior
    two or more specified sites 237.4
    unspecified site 237.4
  nipple (M8506/0) 217
  oncocytic (M8290/0)
  oxyphilic (M8290/0)
  papillary (M8260/0) — *see also* Neoplasm, by
    intracystic (M8504/0)
  papillotubular (M8263/0)
  Pick's tubular (M8640/0)
    specified site — *see* Neoplasm, by site,
      benign
    unspecified site
      female 220
      male 222.0
  pleomorphic (M8940/0)
  polypoid (M8210/0)
  prostate (benign) 600.20
    with urinary retention 600.21
  rete cell 222.0
  sebaceous, sebaceum (gland) (senile) (M8410/0)
    — *see also* Neoplasm, skin, benign
    disseminata 759.5
  Sertoli cell (M8640/0)
    specified site — *see* Neoplasm, by site,
      benign
    unspecified site
      female 220
      male 222.0
  skin appendage (M8390/0) — *see* Neoplasm,
    skin, benign
  sudoriferous gland (M8400/0) — *see* Neoplasm,
    skin, benign
  sweat gland or duct (M8400/0) — *see*
    Neoplasm, skin, benign
  testicular (M8640/0)
    specified site — *see* Neoplasm, by site, benign
    unspecified site
      female 220
      male 222.0
  thyroid 226
  trabecular (M8190/0)
  tubular (M8211/0) — *see also* Neoplasm, by
    site, benign
    papillary (M8460/3)
    Pick's (M8640/0)
      specified site — *see* Neoplasm, by site,
        benign
      unspecified site
        female 220
        male 222.0
  tubulovillous (M8263/0)
  villoglandular (M8263/0)
  villous (M8261/1) — *see* Neoplasm, by site,
    uncertain behavior
  water-clear cell (M8322/0) 227.1
  wolffian duct (M9110/0)
Adenomatosis (M8220/0)
  endocrine (multiple) (M8360/1)
    single specified site — *see* Neoplasm, by site,
      uncertain behavior
    two or more specified sites 237.4
    unspecified site 237.4

Adenomatosis (M8220/0) — *continued*
  erosive of nipple (M8506/0) 217
  pluriendocrine — *see* Adenomatosis, endocrine
  pulmonary (M8250/1) 235.7
    malignant (M8250/3) — *see* Neoplasm, lung,
      malignant
    specified site — *see* Neoplasm, by site, benign
    unspecified site 211.3
Adenomatous
  cyst, thyroid (gland) — *see* Goiter, nodular
  goiter (nontoxic) (*see also* Goiter, nodular)
    241.9
    toxic or with hyperthyroidism 242.3 ☑
Adenomyoma (M8932/0) — *see also* Neoplasm,
    by site, benign
  prostate 600.20
    with urinary retention 600.21
Adenomyometritis 617.0
Adenomyosis (uterus) (internal) 617.0
Adenopathy (lymph gland) 785.6
  inguinal 785.6
  mediastinal 785.6
  mesentery 785.6
  syphilitic (secondary) 091.4
  tracheobronchial 785.6
    tuberculous (*see also* Tuberculosis) 012.1 ☑
      primary, progressive 010.8 ☑
  tuberculous (*see also* Tuberculosis, lymph
    gland) 017.2 ☑
    tracheobronchial 012.1 ☑
      primary, progressive 010.8 ☑
Adenopharyngitis 462
Adenophlegmon 683
Adenosalpingitis 614.1
Adenosarcoma (M8960/3) 189.0
Adenosclerosis 289.3
Adenosis
  breast (sclerosing) 610.2
  vagina, congenital 752.49
Adentia (complete) (partial) (*see also* Absence,
    teeth) 520.0
Adherent
  labium (minus) 624.4
  pericardium (nonrheumatic) 423.1
    rheumatic 393
  placenta 667.0 ☑
    with hemorrhage 666.0 ☑
  prepuce 605
  scar (skin) NEC 709.2
  tendon in scar 709.2
Adhesion(s), adhesive (postinfectional)
    (postoperative)
  abdominal (wall) (*see also* Adhesions,
    peritoneum) 568.0
  amnion to fetus 658.8 ☑
    affecting fetus or newborn 762.8
  appendix 543.9
  arachnoiditis — *see* Meningitis
  auditory tube (Eustachian) 381.89
  bands — *see also* Adhesions, peritoneum
    cervix 622.3
    uterus 621.5
  bile duct (any) 576.8
  bladder (sphincter) 596.8
  bowel (*see also* Adhesions, peritoneum) 568.0
  cardiac 423.1
    rheumatic 398.99
  cecum (*see also* Adhesions, peritoneum) 568.0
  cervicovaginal 622.3
    congenital 752.49
    postpartal 674.8 ☑
      old 622.3
  cervix 622.3
  clitoris 624.4
  colon (*see also* Adhesions, peritoneum) 568.0
  common duct 576.8
  congenital — *see also* Anomaly, specified type
    NEC
    fingers (*see also* Syndactylism, fingers)
      755.11
    labium (majus) (minus) 752.49
    omental, anomalous 751.4
    ovary 752.0
    peritoneal 751.4

Adhesion(s), adhesive — *continued*
  congenital — *see also* Anomaly, specified type
    NEC — *continued*
    toes (*see also* Syndactylism, toes) 755.13
    tongue (to gum or roof of mouth) 750.12
  conjunctiva (acquired) (localized) 372.62
    congenital 743.63
    extensive 372.63
  cornea — *see* Opacity, cornea
  cystic duct 575.8
  diaphragm (*see also* Adhesions, peritoneum)
    568.0
  due to foreign body — *see* Foreign body
  duodenum (*see also* Adhesions, peritoneum)
    568.0
    with obstruction 537.3
  ear, middle — *see* Adhesions, middle ear
  epididymis 608.89
  epidural — *see* Adhesions, meninges
  epiglottis 478.79
  Eustachian tube 381.89
  eyelid 374.46
    postoperative 997.99
      surgically created V45.69
  gallbladder (*see also* Disease, gallbladder)
    575.8
  globe 360.89
  heart 423.1
    rheumatic 398.99
  ileocecal (coil) (*see also* Adhesions, peritoneum)
    568.0
  ileum (*see also* Adhesions, peritoneum) 568.0
  intestine (postoperative) (*see also* Adhesions,
    peritoneum) 568.0
    with obstruction 560.81
      with hernia — *see also* Hernia, by site,
        with obstruction
        gangrenous — *see* Hernia, by site,
          with gangrene
  intra-abdominal (*see also* Adhesions,
    peritoneum) 568.0
  iris 364.70
    to corneal graft 996.79
  joint (*see also* Ankylosis) 718.5 ☑
  kidney 593.89
  labium (majus) (minus), congenital 752.49
  liver 572.8
  lung 511.0
  mediastinum 519.3
  meninges 349.2
    cerebral (any) 349.2
      congenital 742.4
    congenital 742.8
    spinal (any) 349.2
      congenital 742.59
    tuberculous (cerebral) (spinal) (*see also*
      Tuberculosis, meninges) 013.0 ☑
  mesenteric (*see also* Adhesions, peritoneum)
    568.0
  middle ear (fibrous) 385.10
    drum head 385.19
      to
        incus 385.11
        promontorium 385.13
        stapes 385.12
    specified NEC 385.19
  nasal (septum) (to turbinates) 478.1
  nerve NEC 355.9
    spinal 355.9
      root 724.9
        cervical NEC 723.4
        lumbar NEC 724.4
        lumbosacral 724.4
        thoracic 724.4
  ocular muscle 378.60
  omentum (*see also* Adhesions, peritoneum)
    568.0
  organ or site, congenital NEC — *see* Anomaly,
    specified type NEC
  ovary 614.6
    congenital (to cecum, kidney, or omentum)
      752.0
  parauterine 614.6
  parovarian 614.6
  pelvic (peritoneal)
    female (postoperative) (postinfection) 614.6

Adhesion(s), adhesive — *continued*
  pelvic — *continued*
    male (postoperative) (postinfection) (*see also*
      Adhesions, peritoneum) 568.0
    postpartal (old) 614.6
    tuberculous (*see also* Tuberculosis) 016.9 ☑
  penis to scrotum (congenital) 752.69
  periappendiceal (*see also* Adhesions,
    peritoneum) 568.0
  pericardium (nonrheumatic) 423.1
    rheumatic 393
    tuberculous (*see also* Tuberculosis) 017.9 ☑
      [420.0]
  pericholecystic 575.8
  perigastric (*see also* Adhesions, peritoneum)
    568.0
  periovarian 614.6
  periprostatic 602.8
  perirectal (*see also* Adhesions, peritoneum)
    568.0
  perirenal 593.89
  peritoneum, peritoneal (fibrous) (postoperative)
    568.0
    with obstruction (intestinal) 560.81
      with hernia — *see also* Hernia, by site,
        with obstruction
        gangrenous — *see* Hernia, by site,
          with gangrene
      duodenum 537.3
    congenital 751.4
    female (postoperative) (postinfective) 614.6
    pelvic, female 614.6
    pelvic, male 568.0
    postpartal, pelvic 614.6
    to uterus 614.6
  peritubal 614.6
  periureteral 593.89
  periuterine 621.5
  perivesical 596.8
  perivesicular (seminal vesicle) 608.89
  pleura, pleuritic 511.0
    tuberculous (*see also* Tuberculosis, pleura)
      012.0 ☑
  pleuropericardial 511.0
  postoperative (gastrointestinal tract) (*see also*
    Adhesions, peritoneum) 568.0
    eyelid 997.99
      surgically created V45.69
    pelvic female 614.9
    pelvic male 568.0
    urethra 598.2
  postpartal, old 624.4
  preputial, prepuce 605
  pulmonary 511.0
  pylorus (*see also* Adhesions, peritoneum) 568.0
  Rosenmüller's fossa 478.29
  sciatic nerve 355.0
  seminal vesicle 608.89
  shoulder (joint) 726.0
  sigmoid flexure (*see also* Adhesions,
    peritoneum) 568.0
  spermatic cord (acquired) 608.89
    congenital 752.89
  spinal canal 349.2
    nerve 355.9
      root 724.9
        cervical NEC 723.4
        lumbar NEC 724.4
        lumbosacral 724.4
        thoracic 724.4
  stomach (*see also* Adhesions, peritoneum)
    568.0
  subscapular 726.2
  tendonitis 726.90
    shoulder 726.0
  testicle 608.89
  tongue (congenital) (to gum or roof of mouth)
    750.12
    acquired 529.8
  trachea 519.1
  tubo-ovarian 614.6
  tunica vaginalis 608.89
  ureter 593.89
  uterus 621.5
    to abdominal wall 614.6
      in pregnancy or childbirth 654.4 ☑
        affecting fetus or newborn 763.89

☑ Additional Digit Required   ▶◀ Revised Text   ● New Line   ▲ Revised Code

Adhesion(s), adhesive — continued
  vagina (chronic) (postoperative) (postradiation)
      623.2
  vaginitis (congenital) 752.49
  vesical 596.8
  vitreous 379.29
Adie (-Holmes) syndrome (tonic pupillary
      reaction) 379.46
Adiponecrosis neonatorum 778.1
Adiposa dolorosa 272.8
Adiposalgia 272.8
Adiposis
  cerebralis 253.8
  dolorosa 272.8
  tuberosa simplex 272.8
Adiposity 278.00
  heart (see also Degeneration, myocardial) 429.1
  localized 278.1
Adiposogenital dystrophy 253.8
Adjustment
  prosthesis or other device — see Fitting of
  reaction — see Reaction, adjustment
Administration, prophylactic
  antibiotics V07.39
  antitoxin, any V07.2
  antivenin V07.2
  chemotherapeutic agent NEC V07.39
  chemotherapy V07.39
  diphtheria antitoxin V07.2
  fluoride V07.31
  gamma globulin V07.2
  immune sera (gamma globulin) V07.2
  passive immunization agent V07.2
  RhoGAM V07.2
Admission (encounter)
  as organ donor — see Donor
  by mistake V68.9
  for
      adequacy testing (for)
          hemodialysis V56.31
          peritoneal dialysis V56.32
      adjustment (of)
          artificial
              arm (complete) (partial) V52.0
              eye V52.2
              leg (complete) (partial) V52.1
          brain neuropacemaker V53.02
          breast
              implant V52.4
              prosthesis V52.4
          cardiac device V53.39
              defibrillator, automatic implantable
                  V53.32
              pacemaker V53.31
                  carotid sinus V53.39
          catheter
              non-vascular V58.82
              vascular V58.81
          cerebral ventricle (communicating) shunt
              V53.01
          colostomy belt V55.3
          contact lenses V53.1
          cystostomy device V53.6
          dental prosthesis V52.3
          device, unspecified type V53.90
              abdominal V53.5
              cardiac V53.39
                  defibrillator, automatic implantable
                      V53.32
                  pacemaker V53.31
              carotid sinus V53.39
              cerebral ventricle (communicating)
                  shunt V53.01
              insulin pump V53.91
              intrauterine contraceptive V25.1
              nervous system V53.09
              orthodontic V53.4
              other device V53.99
              prosthetic V52.9
                  breast V52.4
                  dental V52.3
                  eye V52.2
                  specified type NEC V52.8
              special senses V53.09

Admission — continued
  for — continued
      adjustment (of) — continued
          device, unspecified type — continued
              substitution
                  auditory V53.09
                  nervous system V53.09
                  visual V53.09
              urinary V53.6
          dialysis catheter
              extracorporeal V56.1
              peritoneal V56.2
          diaphragm (contraceptive) V25.02
          growth rod V54.02
          hearing aid V53.2
          ileostomy device V55.2
          intestinal appliance or device NEC V53.5
          intrauterine contraceptive device V25.1
          neuropacemaker (brain) (peripheral nerve)
              (spinal cord) V53.02
          orthodontic device V53.4
          orthopedic (device) V53.7
              brace V53.7
              cast V53.7
              shoes V53.7
          pacemaker
              brain V53.02
              cardiac V53.31
              carotid sinus V53.39
              peripheral nerve V53.02
              spinal cord V53.02
          prosthesis V52.9
              arm (complete) (partial) V52.0
              breast V52.4
              dental V52.3
              eye V52.2
              leg (complete) (partial) V52.1
              specified type NEC V52.8
          spectacles V53.1
          wheelchair V53.8
      adoption referral or proceedings V68.89
      aftercare (see also Aftercare) V58.9
          cardiac pacemaker V53.31
          chemotherapy V58.1
          dialysis
              extracorporeal (renal) V56.0
              peritoneal V56.8
              renal V56.0
          fracture (see also Aftercare, fracture)
              V54.9
          medical NEC V58.89
          organ transplant V58.44   •
          orthopedic V54.9
              specified care NEC V54.89
          pacemaker device
              brain V53.02
              cardiac V53.31
              carotid sinus V53.39
              nervous system V53.02
              spinal cord V53.02
          postoperative NEC V58.49
              wound closure, planned V58.41
          postpartum
              immediately after delivery V24.0
              routine follow-up V24.2
          postradiation V58.0
          radiation therapy V58.0
          removal of
              non-vascular catheter V58.82
              vascular catheter V58.81
          specified NEC V58.89
          surgical NEC V58.49
              wound closure, planned V58.41
      artificial insemination V26.1
      attention to artificial opening (of) V55.9
          artificial vagina V55.7
          colostomy V55.3
          cystostomy V55.5
          enterostomy V55.4
          gastrostomy V55.1
          ileostomy V55.2
          jejunostomy V55.4
          nephrostomy V55.6
          specified site NEC V55.8
              intestinal tract V55.4
              urinary tract V55.6
          tracheostomy V55.0

Admission — continued
  for — continued
      attention to artificial opening — continued
          ureterostomy V55.6
          urethrostomy V55.6
      battery replacement
          cardiac pacemaker V53.31
      boarding V65.0
      breast
          augmentation or reduction V50.1
          removal, prophylactic V50.41
      change of
          cardiac pacemaker (battery) V53.31
          carotid sinus pacemaker V53.39
          catheter in artificial opening — see
              Attention to, artificial, opening
          dressing V58.3
          fixation device
              external V54.89
              internal V54.01
          Kirschner wire V54.89
          neuropacemaker device (brain)
              (peripheral nerve) (spinal cord)
              V53.02
          pacemaker device
              brain V53.02
              cardiac V53.31
              carotid sinus V53.39
              nervous system V53.02
          plaster cast V54.89
          splint, external V54.89
          Steinmann pin V54.89
          surgical dressing V58.3
          traction device V54.89
      checkup only V70.0
      chemotherapy V58.1
      circumcision, ritual or routine (in absence of
          medical indication) V50.2
      clinical research investigation (control)
          (normal comparison) (participant)
          V70.7
      closure of artificial opening — see Attention
          to, artificial, opening
      contraceptive
          counseling V25.09
              emergency V25.03
              postcoital V25.03
          management V25.9
              specified type NEC V25.8
      convalescence following V66.9
          chemotherapy V66.2
          psychotherapy V66.3
          radiotherapy V66.1
          surgery V66.0
          treatment (for) V66.5
              combined V66.6
              fracture V66.4
              mental disorder NEC V66.3
              specified condition NEC V66.5
      cosmetic surgery NEC V50.1
          following healed injury or operation V51
      counseling (see also Counseling) V65.40
          without complaint or sickness V65.49
          contraceptive management V25.09
              emergency V25.03
              postcoital V25.03
          dietary V65.3
          exercise V65.41
          for
              nonattending third party V65.19
              pediatric pre-birth visit for
                  expectant mother V65.11
              victim of abuse
                  child V61.21
                  partner or spouse V61.11
          genetic V26.3
          gonorrhea V65.45
          HIV V65.44
          human immunodeficiency virus V65.44
          injury prevention V65.43
          insulin pump training V65.46
          procreative management V26.4
          sexually transmitted disease NEC V65.45
              HIV V65.44
          specified reason NEC V65.49
          substance use and abuse V65.42
          syphilis V65.45

Admission — *continued*
  for — *continued*
    counseling (*see also* Counseling) — *continued*
      victim of abuse
        child V61.21
        partner or spouse V61.11
    desensitization to allergens V07.1
    dialysis V56.0
      catheter
        fitting and adjustment
          extracorporeal V56.1
          peritoneal V56.2
        removal or replacement
          extracorporeal V56.1
          peritoneal V56.2
      extracorporeal (renal) V56.0
      peritoneal V56.8
      renal V56.0
    dietary surveillance and counseling V65.3
    drug monitoring, therapeutic V58.83
    ear piercing V50.3
    elective surgery V50.9
      breast
        augmentation or reduction V50.1
        removal, prophylactic V50.41
      circumcision, ritual or routine (in absence of medical indication) V50.2
      cosmetic NEC V50.1
        following healed injury or operation V51
      ear piercing V50.3
      face-lift V50.1
      hair transplant V50.0
      plastic
        cosmetic NEC V50.1
        following healed injury or operation V51
      prophylactic organ removal V50.49
        breast V50.41
        ovary V50.42
      repair of scarred tissue (following healed injury or operation) V51
      specified type NEC V50.8
    end-of-life care V66.7
    examination (*see also* Examination) V70.9
      administrative purpose NEC V70.3
      adoption V70.3
      allergy V72.7
      at health care facility V70.0
      athletic team V70.3
      camp V70.3
      cardiovascular, preoperative V72.81
      clinical research investigation (control) (participant) V70.7
      dental V72.2
      developmental testing (child) (infant) V20.2
      donor (potential) V70.8
      driver's license V70.3
      ear V72.1
      employment V70.5
      eye V72.0
      follow-up (routine) — *see* Examination, follow-up
      for admission to
        old age home V70.3
        school V70.3
      general V70.9
        specified reason NEC V70.8
      gynecological V72.31 ▲
      health supervision (child) (infant) V20.2
      hearing V72.1
      immigration V70.3
      insurance certification V70.3
      laboratory V72.6
      marriage license V70.3
      medical (general) (*see also* Examination, medical) V70.9
      medicolegal reasons V70.4
      naturalization V70.3
      pelvic (annual) (periodic) V72.31 ▲
      postpartum checkup V24.2
      pregnancy (possible) (unconfirmed) V72.40 ▲
        negative result V72.41 ●

Admission — *continued*
  for — *continued*
    examination (*see also* Examination) — *continued*
      preoperative V72.84
        cardiovascular V72.81
        respiratory V72.82
        specified NEC V72.83
      prison V70.3
      psychiatric (general) V70.2
        requested by authority V70.1
      radiological NEC V72.5
      respiratory, preoperative V72.82
      school V70.3
      screening — *see* Screening
      skin hypersensitivity V72.7
      specified type NEC V72.85
      sport competition V70.3
      vision V72.0
      well baby and child care V20.2
    exercise therapy V57.1
    face-lift, cosmetic reason V50.1
    fitting (of)
      artificial
        arm (complete) (partial) V52.0
        eye V52.2
        leg (complete) (partial) V52.1
      biliary drainage tube V58.82
      brain neuropacemaker V53.02
      breast V52.4
        implant V52.4
        prosthesis V52.4
      cardiac pacemaker V53.31
      catheter
        non-vascular V58.82
        vascular V58.81
      cerebral ventricle (communicating) shunt V53.01
      chest tube V58.82
      colostomy belt V55.2
      contact lenses V53.1
      cystostomy device V53.6
      dental prosthesis V52.3
      device, unspecified type V53.90
        abdominal V53.5
        cerebral ventricle (communicating) shunt V53.01
        insulin pump V53.91
        intrauterine contraceptive V25.1
        nervous system V53.09
        orthodontic V53.4
        other device V53.99
        prosthetic V52.9
          breast V52.4
          dental V52.3
          eye V52.2
        special senses V53.09
        substitution
          auditory V53.09
          nervous system V53.09
          visual V53.09
      diaphragm (contraceptive) V25.02
      fistula (sinus tract) drainage tube V58.82
      growth rod V54.02
      hearing aid V53.2
      ileostomy device V55.2
      insulin pump titration V53.91
      insulin pump training V65.46
      intestinal appliance or device NEC V53.5
      intrauterine contraceptive device V25.1
      neuropacemaker (brain) (peripheral nerve) (spinal cord) V53.02
      orthodontic device V53.4
      orthopedic (device) V53.7
        brace V53.7
        cast V53.7
        shoes V53.7
      pacemaker
        brain V53.02
        cardiac V53.31
        carotid sinus V53.39
        spinal cord V53.02
      pleural drainage tube V58.82
      prosthesis V52.9
        arm (complete) (partial) V52.0
        breast V52.4
        dental V52.3

Admission — *continued*
  for — *continued*
    examination (*see also* Examination) — *continued*
      prosthesis — *continued*
        eye V52.2
        leg (complete) (partial) V52.1
        specified type NEC V52.8
      spectacles V53.1
      wheelchair V53.8
    follow-up examination (routine) (following) V67.9
      cancer chemotherapy V67.2
      chemotherapy V67.2
      high-risk medication NEC V67.51
      injury NEC V67.59
      psychiatric V67.3
      psychotherapy V67.3
      radiotherapy V67.1
      specified surgery NEC V67.09
      surgery V67.00
        vaginal pap smear V67.01
      treatment (for) V67.9
        combined V67.6
        fracture V67.4
        involving high-risk medication NEC V67.51
        mental disorder V67.3
        specified NEC V67.59
    hair transplant, for cosmetic reason V50.0
    health advice, education, or instruction V65.4 ☑
    hormone replacement therapy (postmenopausal) V07.4 ●
    hospice care V66.7
    insertion (of)
      subdermal implantable contraceptive V25.5
    intrauterine device
      insertion V25.1
      management V25.42
    investigation to determine further disposition V63.8
    isolation V07.0
    issue of
      medical certificate NEC V68.0
      repeat prescription NEC V68.1
        contraceptive device NEC V25.49
    kidney dialysis V56.0
    lengthening of growth rod V54.02
    mental health evaluation V70.2
      requested by authority V70.1
    nonmedical reason NEC V68.89
    nursing care evaluation V63.8
    observation (without need for further medical care) (*see also* Observation) V71.9
      accident V71.4
      alleged rape or seduction V71.5
      criminal assault V71.6
      following accident V71.4
        at work V71.3
      foreign body ingestion V71.89
      growth and development variations, childhood V21.0
      inflicted injury NEC V71.6
      ingestion of deleterious agent or foreign body V71.89
      injury V71.6
      malignant neoplasm V71.1
      mental disorder V71.09
      newborn — *see* Observation, suspected, condition, newborn
      rape V71.5
      specified NEC V71.89
      suspected disorder V71.9
        abuse V71.81
        accident V71.4
          at work V71.3
        benign neoplasm V71.89
        cardiovascular V71.7
        exposure
          anthrax V71.82
          biological agent NEC V71.83
          SARS V71.83
        heart V71.7
        inflicted injury NEC V71.6
        malignant neoplasm V71.1

Admission (vertical text, right margin)

Admission — *continued*
  for — *continued*
    observation (*see also* Observation) —
      continued
      suspected disorder — *continued*
        mental NEC V71.09
        neglect V71.81
        specified condition NEC V71.89
        tuberculosis V71.2
      tuberculosis V71.2
    occupational therapy V57.21
    organ transplant, donor — *see* Donor
    ovary, ovarian removal, prophylactic V50.42
    palliative care V66.7
    Papanicolaou smear
      cervix V76.2
        for suspected malignant neoplasm V76.2
          no disease found V71.1
        routine, as part of gynecological examination V72.31 ▲
        to confirm findings of recent ●
          normal smear following initial ●
          abnormal smear V72.32 ●
      vaginal V76.47
        following hysterectomy for malignant condition V67.01
    passage of sounds or bougie in artificial opening — *see* Attention to, artificial, opening
    paternity testing V70.4
    peritoneal dialysis V56.32
    physical therapy NEC V57.1
    plastic surgery
      cosmetic NEC V50.1
      following healed injury or operation V51
    postmenopausal hormone replacement therapy V07.4
    postpartum observation
      immediately after delivery V24.0
      routine follow-up V24.2
    poststerilization (for restoration) V26.0
    procreative management V26.9
      specified type NEC V26.8
    prophylactic
      administration of
        antibiotics V07.39
        antitoxin, any V07.2
        antivenin V07.2
        chemotherapeutic agent NEC V07.39
        chemotherapy NEC V07.39
        diphtheria antitoxin V07.2
        fluoride V07.31
        gamma globulin V07.2
        immune sera (gamma globulin) V07.2
        RhoGAM V07.2
        tetanus antitoxin V07.2
      breathing exercises V57.0
      chemotherapy NEC V07.39
        fluoride V07.31
      measure V07.9
        specified type NEC V07.8
      organ removal V50.49
        breast V50.41
        ovary V50.42
    psychiatric examination (general) V70.2
      requested by authority V70.1
    radiation management V58.0
    radiotherapy V58.0
    reforming of artificial opening — *see* Attention to, artificial, opening
    rehabilitation V57.9
      multiple types V57.89
      occupational V57.21
      orthoptic V57.4
      orthotic V57.81
      physical NEC V57.1
      specified type NEC V57.89
      speech V57.3
      vocational V57.22
    removal of
      cardiac pacemaker V53.31
      cast (plaster) V54.89
      catheter from artificial opening — *see* Attention to, artificial, opening
      cerebral ventricle (communicating) shunt V53.01

Admission — *continued*
  for — *continued*
    removal of — *continued*
      cystostomy catheter V55.5
      device
        cerebral ventricle (communicating) shunt V53.01
        fixation
          external V54.89
          internal V54.01
        intrauterine contraceptive V25.42
        traction, external V54.89
      dressing V58.3
      fixation device
        external V54.89
        internal V54.01
      intrauterine contraceptive device V25.42
      Kirschner wire V54.89
      neuropacemaker (brain) (peripheral nerve) (spinal cord) V53.02
      orthopedic fixation device
        external V54.89
        internal V54.01
      pacemaker device
        brain V53.02
        cardiac V53.31
        carotid sinus V53.39
        nervous system V53.02
      plaster cast V54.89
      plate (fracture) V54.01
      rod V54.01
      screw (fracture) V54.01
      splint, traction V54.89
      Steinmann pin V54.89
      subdermal implantable contraceptive V25.43
      surgical dressing V58.3
      sutures V58.3
      traction device, external V54.89
      ureteral stent V53.6
    repair of scarred tissue (following healed injury or operation) V51
    reprogramming of cardiac pacemaker V53.31
    respirator dependence, during power failure V46.12 ●●
    restoration of organ continuity (poststerilization) (tuboplasty) (vasoplasty) V26.0
    sensitivity test — *see also* Test, skin
      allergy NEC V72.7
      bacterial disease NEC V74.9
      Dick V74.8
      Kveim V82.89
      Mantoux V74.1
      mycotic infection NEC V75.4
      parasitic disease NEC V75.8
      Schick V74.3
      Schultz-Charlton V74.8
    social service (agency) referral or evaluation V63.8
    speech therapy V57.3
    sterilization V25.2
    suspected disorder (ruled out) (without need for further care) — *see* Observation
    terminal care V66.7
    tests only — *see* Test
    therapeutic drug monitoring V58.83
    therapy
      blood transfusion, without reported diagnosis V58.2
      breathing exercises V57.0
      chemotherapy V58.1
        prophylactic NEC V07.39
        fluoride V07.31
      dialysis (intermittent) (treatment)
        extracorporeal V56.0
        peritoneal V56.8
        renal V56.0
        specified type NEC V56.8
      exercise (remedial) NEC V57.1
        breathing V57.0
      long-term (current) drug use NEC V58.69
        antibiotics V58.62
        ►anticoagulants◄ V58.61
        anti-inflammatories, non-steroidal (NSAID) V58.64

Admission — *continued*
  for — *continued*
    therapy — *continued*
      long-term drug use NEC — *continued*
        ►antiplatelets◄ V58.63
        ►antithrombotics◄ V58.63
        aspirin V58.66 ●
        insulin V58.67 ●
        steroids V58.65
      occupational V57.21
      orthoptic V57.4
      physical NEC V57.1
      radiation V58.0
      speech V57.3
      vocational V57.22
    toilet or cleaning
      of artificial opening — *see* Attention to, artificial, opening
      of non-vascular catheter V58.82
      of vascular catheter V58.81
    tubal ligation V25.2
    tuboplasty for previous sterilization V26.0
    vaccination, prophylactic (against)
      arthropod-borne virus, viral NEC V05.1
        disease NEC V05.1
        encephalitis V05.0
      Bacille Calmette Guérin (BCG) V03.2
      BCG V03.2
      chickenpox V05.4
      cholera alone V03.0
        with typhoid-paratyphoid (cholera + TAB) V06.0
      common cold V04.7
      dengue V05.1
      diphtheria alone V03.5
      diphtheria-tetanus-pertussis (DTP) (DTaP) V06.1
        with
          poliomyelitis (DTP + polio) V06.3
          typhoid-paratyphoid (DTP + TAB) V06.2
      diphtheria-tetanus [Td] [DT] without pertussis V06.5
      disease (single) NEC V05.9
        bacterial NEC V03.9
          specified type NEC V03.89
        combinations NEC V06.9
          specified type NEC V06.8
        specified type NEC V05.8
        viral NEC V04.89
      encephalitis, viral, arthropod-borne V05.0
      Hemophilus infuenzae, type B [Hib] V03.81
      hepatitis, viral V05.3
      immune sera (gamma globulin) V07.2
      influenza V04.81
        with
          Streptococcus pneumoniae [pneumococcus] V06.6
      Leishmaniasis V05.2
      measles alone V04.2
      measles-mumps-rubella (MMR) V06.4
      mumps alone V04.6
        with measles and rubella (MMR) V06.4
      not done because of contraindication V64.0
      pertussis alone V03.6
      plague V03.3
      pneumonia V03.82
      poliomyelitis V04.0
        with diphtheria-tetanus-pertussis (DTP+ polio) V06.3
      rabies V04.5
      respiratory syncytial virus (RSV) V04.82
      rubella alone V04.3
        with measles and mumps (MMR) V06.4
      smallpox V04.1
      specified type NEC V05.8
      Streptococcus pneumoniae [pneumococcus] V03.82
        with
          influenza V06.6
      tetanus toxoid alone V03.7
        with diphtheria [Td] [DT] V06.5
          and pertussis (DTP) (DTaP) V06.1

☑ Additional Digit Required   ►◄ Revised Text   ● New Line   ▲ Revised Code

Admission — *continued*
  for — *continued*
    vaccination, prophylactic — *continued*
      tuberculosis (BCG) V03.2
      tularemia V03.4
      typhoid alone V03.1
        with diphtheria-tetanus-pertussis (TAB + DTP) V06.2
      typhoid-paratyphoid alone (TAB) V03.1
      typhus V05.8
      varicella (chicken pox) V05.4
      viral encephalitis, arthropod-borne V05.0
      viral hepatitis V05.3
      yellow fever V04.4
    vasectomy V25.2
    vasoplasty for previous sterilization V26.0
    vision examination V72.0
    vocational therapy V57.22
    waiting period for admission to other facility V63.2
      undergoing social agency investigation V63.8
    well baby and child care V20.2
    x-ray of chest
      for suspected tuberculosis V71.2
      routine V72.5

Adnexitis (suppurative) (*see also* Salpingo-oophoritis) 614.2

Adolescence NEC V21.2

Adoption
  agency referral V68.89
  examination V70.3
  held for V68.89

Adrenal gland — *see* condition

Adrenalism 255.9
  tuberculous (*see also* Tuberculosis) 017.6 ☑

Adrenalitis, adrenitis 255.8
  meningococcal hemorrhagic 036.3

Adrenarche, precocious 259.1

Adrenocortical syndrome 255.2

Adrenogenital syndrome (acquired) (congenital) 255.2
  iatrogenic, fetus or newborn 760.79

Adrenoleukodystrophy 277.86   ●
  neonatal 277.86   ●
  x-linked 277.86   ●

Adrenomyeloneuropathy 277.86   ●

Adventitious bursa — *see* Bursitis

Adynamia (episodica) (hereditary) (periodic) 359.3

Adynamic
  ileus or intestine (*see also* Ileus) 560.1
  ureter 753.22

Aeration lung, imperfect, newborn 770.5

Aerobullosis 993.3

Aerocele — *see* Embolism, air

Aerodermectasia
  subcutaneous (traumatic) 958.7
    surgical 998.81
  surgical 998.81

Aerodontalgia 993.2

Aeroembolism 993.3

Aerogenes capsulatus infection (*see also* Gangrene, gas) 040.0

Aero-otitis media 993.0

Aerophagy, aerophagia 306.4
  psychogenic 306.4

Aerosinusitis 993.1

Aerotitis 993.0

Affection, affections — *see also* Disease
  sacroiliac (joint), old 724.6
  shoulder region NEC 726.2

Afibrinogenemia 286.3
  acquired 286.6
  congenital 286.3
  postpartum 666.3 ☑

African
  sleeping sickness 086.5
  tick fever 087.1
  trypanosomiasis 086.5
    Gambian 086.3
    Rhodesian 086.4

Aftercare V58.9
  artificial openings — *see* Attention to, artificial, opening
  blood transfusion without reported diagnosis V58.2
  breathing exercise V57.0
  cardiac device V53.39
    defibrillator, automatic implantable V53.32
    pacemaker V53.31
      carotid sinus V53.39
  carotid sinus pacemaker V53.39
  cerebral ventricle (communicating) shunt V53.01
  chemotherapy session (adjunctive) (maintenance) V58.1
  defibrillator, automatic implantable cardiac V53.32
  exercise (remedial) (therapeutic) V57.1
    breathing V57.0
  extracorporeal dialysis (intermittent) (treatment) V56.0
  following surgery NEC V58.49
    for
      injury V58.43
      neoplasm V58.42
      organ transplant V58.44   ●
      trauma V58.43
    joint replacement V54.81
    of
      circulatory system V58.73
      digestive system V58.75
      genital organs V58.76
      genitourinary system V58.76
      musculoskeletal system V58.78
      nervous system V58.72
      oral cavity V58.75
      respiratory system V58.74
      sense organs V58.71
      skin V58.77
      subcutaneous tissue V58.77
      teeth V58.75
      urinary system V58.76
    wound closure, planned V58.41
  fracture V54.9
    healing V54.89
      pathologic
        ankle V54.29
        arm V54.20
          lower V54.22
          upper V54.21
        finger V54.29
        foot V54.29
        hand V54.29
        hip V54.23
        leg V54.24
          lower V54.26
          upper V54.25
        pelvis V54.29
        specified site NEC V54.29
        toe(s) V54.29
        vertebrae V54.27
        wrist V54.29
      traumatic
        ankle V54.19
        arm V54.10
          lower V54.12
          upper V54.11
        finger V54.19
        foot V54.19
        hand V54.19
        hip V54.13
        leg V54.14
          lower V54.16
          upper V54.15
        pelvis V54.19
        specified site NEC V54.19
        toe(s) V54.19
        vertebrae V54.17
        wrist V54.19
    removal of
      external fixation device V54.89
      internal fixation device V54.01
      specified care NEC V54.89
  gait training V57.1
    for use of artificial limb(s) V57.81
  internal fixation device V54.09

Aftercare — *continued*
  involving
    dialysis (intermittent) (treatment)
      extracorporeal V56.0
      peritoneal V56.8
      renal V56.0
    gait training V57.1
      for use of artificial limb(s) V57.81
    growth rod
      adjustment V54.02
      lengthening V54.02
    internal fixation device V54.09
    orthoptic training V57.4
    orthotic training V57.81
    radiotherapy session V58.0
    removal of
      dressings V58.3
      fixation device
        external V54.89
        internal V54.01
      fracture plate V54.01
      pins V54.01
      plaster cast V54.89
      rods V54.01
      screws V54.01
      surgical dressings V58.3
      sutures V58.3
      traction device, external V54.89
    neuropacemaker (brain) (peripheral nerve) (spinal cord) V53.02
    occupational therapy V57.21
    orthodontic V58.5
    orthopedic V54.9
      change of external fixation or traction device V54.89
      following joint replacement V54.81
      internal fixation device V54.09
      removal of fixation device
        external V54.89
        internal V54.01
      specified care NEC V54.89
    orthoptic training V57.4
    orthotic training V57.81
    pacemaker
      brain V53.02
      cardiac V53.31
      carotid sinus V53.39
      peripheral nerve V53.02
      spinal cord V53.02
    peritoneal dialysis (intermittent) (treatment) V56.8
    physical therapy NEC V57.1
      breathing exercises V57.0
    radiotherapy session V58.0
    rehabilitation procedure V57.9
      breathing exercises V57.0
      multiple types V57.89
      occupational V57.21
      orthoptic V57.4
      orthotic V57.81
      physical therapy NEC V57.1
      remedial exercises V57.1
      specified type NEC V57.89
      speech V57.3
      therapeutic exercises V57.1
      vocational V57.22
    renal dialysis (intermittent) (treatment) V56.0
    specified type NEC V58.89
      removal of non-vascular catheter V58.82
      removal of vascular catheter V58.81
    speech therapy V57.3
    vocational rehabilitation V57.22

After-cataract 366.50
  obscuring vision 366.53
  specified type, not obscuring vision 366.52

Agalactia 676.4 ☑

Agammaglobulinemia 279.00
  with lymphopenia 279.2
  acquired (primary) (secondary) 279.06
  Bruton's X-linked 279.04
  infantile sex-linked (Bruton's) (congenital) 279.04
  Swiss-type 279.2

Aganglionosis (bowel) (colon) 751.3

Age (old) (*see also* Senile) 797

Agenesis — *see also* Absence, by site, congenital
  acoustic nerve 742.8
  adrenal (gland) 759.1
  alimentary tract (complete) (partial) NEC 751.8
    lower 751.2
    upper 750.8
  anus, anal (canal) 751.2
  aorta 747.22
  appendix 751.2
  arm (complete) (partial) (*see also* Deformity, reduction, upper limb) 755.20
  artery (peripheral) NEC (*see also* Anomaly, peripheral vascular system) 747.60
    brain 747.81
    coronary 746.85
    pulmonary 747.3
    umbilical 747.5
  auditory (canal) (external) 744.01
  auricle (ear) 744.01
  bile, biliary duct or passage 751.61
  bone NEC 756.9
  brain 740.0
    specified part 742.2
  breast 757.6
  bronchus 748.3
  canaliculus lacrimalis 743.65
  carpus NEC (*see also* Deformity, reduction, upper limb) 755.28
  cartilage 756.9
  cecum 751.2
  cerebellum 742.2
  cervix 752.49
  chin 744.89
  cilia 743.63
  circulatory system, part NEC 747.89
  clavicle 755.51
  clitoris 752.49
  coccyx 756.13
  colon 751.2
  corpus callosum 742.2
  cricoid cartilage 748.3
  diaphragm (with hernia) 756.6
  digestive organ(s), or tract (complete) (partial) NEC 751.8
    lower 751.2
    upper 750.8
  ductus arteriosus 747.89
  duodenum 751.1
  ear NEC 744.09
    auricle 744.01
    lobe 744.21
  ejaculatory duct 752.89
  endocrine (gland) NEC 759.2
  epiglottis 748.3
  esophagus 750.3
  Eustachian tube 744.24
  extrinsic muscle, eye 743.69
  eye 743.00
    adnexa 743.69
  eyelid (fold) 743.62
  face
    bones NEC 756.0
    specified part NEC 744.89
  fallopian tube 752.19
  femur NEC (*see also* Absence, femur, congenital) 755.34
  fibula NEC (*see also* Absence, fibula, congenital) 755.37
  finger NEC (*see also* Absence, finger, congenital) 755.29
  foot (complete) (*see also* Deformity, reduction, lower limb) 755.31
  gallbladder 751.69
  gastric 750.8
  genitalia, genital (organ)
    female 752.89
      external 752.49
      internal NEC 752.89
    male 752.89
      penis 752.69
  glottis 748.3
  gonadal 758.6
  hair 757.4
  hand (complete) (*see also* Deformity, reduction, upper limb) 755.21

Agenesis — *see also* Absence, by site, congenital — *continued*
  heart 746.89
    valve NEC 746.89
      aortic 746.89
      mitral 746.89
      pulmonary 746.01
  hepatic 751.69
  humerus NEC (*see also* Absence, humerus, congenital) 755.24
  hymen 752.49
  ileum 751.1
  incus 744.04
  intestine (small) 751.1
    large 751.2
  iris (dilator fibers) 743.45
  jaw 524.09
  jejunum 751.1
  kidney(s) (partial) (unilateral) 753.0
  labium (majus) (minus) 752.49
  labyrinth, membranous 744.05
  lacrimal apparatus (congenital) 743.65
  larynx 748.3
  leg NEC (*see also* Deformity, reduction, lower limb) 755.30
  lens 743.35
  limb (complete) (partial) (*see also* Deformity, reduction) 755.4
    lower NEC 755.30
    upper 755.20
  lip 750.26
  liver 751.69
  lung (bilateral) (fissures) (lobe) (unilateral) 748.5
  mandible 524.09
  maxilla 524.09
  metacarpus NEC 755.28
  metatarsus NEC 755.38
  muscle (any) 756.81
  musculoskeletal system NEC 756.9
  nail(s) 757.5
  neck, part 744.89
  nerve 742.8
  nervous system, part NEC 742.8
  nipple 757.6
  nose 748.1
  nuclear 742.8
  organ
    of Corti 744.05
    or site not listed — *see* Anomaly, specified type NEC
  osseous meatus (ear) 744.03
  ovary 752.0
  oviduct 752.19
  pancreas 751.7
  parathyroid (gland) 759.2
  patella 755.64
  pelvic girdle (complete) (partial) 755.69
  penis 752.69
  pericardium 746.89
  perineal body 756.81
  pituitary (gland) 759.2
  prostate 752.89
  pulmonary
    artery 747.3
    trunk 747.3
    vein 747.49
  punctum lacrimale 743.65
  radioulnar NEC (*see also* Absence, forearm, congenital) 755.25
  radius NEC (*see also* Absence, radius, congenital) 755.26
  rectum 751.2
  renal 753.0
  respiratory organ NEC 748.9
  rib 756.3
  roof of orbit 742.0
  round ligament 752.89
  sacrum 756.13
  salivary gland 750.21
  scapula 755.59
  scrotum 752.89
  seminal duct or tract 752.89
  septum
    atrial 745.69
    between aorta and pulmonary artery 745.0
    ventricular 745.3

Agenesis — *see also* Absence, by site, congenital — *continued*
  shoulder girdle (complete) (partial) 755.59
  skull (bone) 756.0
    with
      anencephalus 740.0
      encephalocele 742.0
      hydrocephalus 742.3
        with spina bifida (*see also* Spina bifida) 741.0 ☑
      microcephalus 742.1
  spermatic cord 752.89
  spinal cord 742.59
  spine 756.13
    lumbar 756.13
      isthmus 756.11
      pars articularis 756.11
  spleen 759.0
  sternum 756.3
  stomach 750.7
  tarsus NEC 755.38
  tendon 756.81
  testicular 752.89
  testis 752.89
  thymus (gland) 759.2
  thyroid (gland) 243
    cartilage 748.3
  tibia NEC (*see also* Absence, tibia, congenital) 755.36
  tibiofibular NEC 755.35
  toe (complete) (partial) (*see also* Absence, toe, congenital) 755.39
  tongue 750.11
  trachea (cartilage) 748.3
  ulna NEC (*see also* Absence, ulna, congenital) 755.27
  ureter 753.4
  urethra 753.8
  urinary tract NEC 753.8
  uterus 752.3
  uvula 750.26
  vagina 752.49
  vas deferens 752.89
  vein(s) (peripheral) NEC (*see also* Anomaly, peripheral vascular system) 747.60
    brain 747.81
    great 747.49
    portal 747.49
    pulmonary 747.49
  vena cava (inferior) (superior) 747.49
  vermis of cerebellum 742.2
  vertebra 756.13
    lumbar 756.13
      isthmus 756.11
      pars articularis 756.11
  vulva 752.49

Ageusia (*see also* Disturbance, sensation) 781.1

Aggressiveness 301.3

Aggressive outburst (*see also* Disturbance, conduct) 312.0 ☑
  in children ►or◄ adolescents 313.9

Aging skin 701.8

Agitated — *see* condition

Agitation 307.9
  catatonic (*see also* Schizophrenia) 295.2 ☑

Aglossia (congenital) 750.11

Aglycogenosis 271.0

Agnail (finger) (with lymphangitis) 681.02

Agnosia (body image) (tactile) 784.69
  verbal 784.69
    auditory 784.69
      secondary to organic lesion 784.69
    developmental 315.8
    secondary to organic lesion 784.69
    visual 784.69
      developmental 315.8
      secondary to organic lesion 784.69
  visual 368.16
    developmental 315.31

Agoraphobia 300.22
  with panic ►disorder◄ 300.21

Agrammatism 784.69

Agranulocytopenia 288.0

☑ Additional Digit Required   ►◄ Revised Text   ● New Line   ▲ Revised Code

Agranulocytosis (angina) (chronic) (cyclical) (genetic) (infantile) (periodic) (pernicious) 288.0

Agraphia (absolute) 784.69
  with alexia 784.61
  developmental 315.39

Agrypnia (*see also* Insomnia) 780.52

Ague (*see also* Malaria) 084.6
  brass-founders' 985.8
  dumb 084.6
  tertian 084.1

Agyria 742.2

Ahumada-del Castillo syndrome (nonpuerperal galactorrhea and amenorrhea) 253.1

AIDS 042

AIDS-associated retrovirus (disease) (illness) 042
  infection — *see* Human immunodeficiency virus, infection

AIDS-associated virus (disease) (illness) 042
  infection — *see* Human immunodeficiency virus, infection

AIDS-like disease (illness) (syndrome) 042

AIDS-related complex 042

AIDS-related conditions 042

AIDS-related virus (disease) (illness) 042
  infection — *see* Human immunodeficiency virus, infection

AIDS virus (disease) (illness) 042
  infection — *see* Human immunodeficiency virus, infection

Ailment, heart — *see* Disease, heart

Ailurophobia 300.29

Ainhum (disease) 136.0

Air
  anterior mediastinum 518.1
  compressed, disease 993.3
  embolism (any site) (artery) (cerebral) 958.0
    with
      abortion — *see* Abortion, by type, with embolism
      ectopic pregnancy (*see also* categories 633.0-633.9) 639.6
      molar pregnancy (*see also* categories 630-632) 639.6
    due to implanted device — *see* Complications, due to (presence of) any device, implant, or graft classified to 996.0-996.5 NEC
    following
      abortion 639.6
      ectopic or molar pregnancy 639.6
    infusion, perfusion, or transfusion 999.1
    in pregnancy, childbirth, or puerperium 673.0 ☑
    traumatic 958.0
  hunger 786.09
    psychogenic 306.1
  leak (lung) (pulmonary) (thorax) 512.8
    iatrogenic 512.1
    postoperative 512.1
  rarefied, effects of — *see* Effect, adverse, high altitude
  sickness 994.6

Airplane sickness 994.6

Akathisia, acathisia 781.0
  due to drugs 333.99

Akinesia algeria 352.6

Akiyami 100.89

Akureyri disease (epidemic neuromyasthenia) 049.8

Alacrima (congenital) 743.65

Alactasia (hereditary) 271.3

Alalia 784.3
  developmental 315.31
    receptive-expressive 315.32
  secondary to organic lesion 784.3

Alaninemia 270.8

Alastrim 050.1

Albarrán's disease (colibacilluria) 791.9

Albers-Schönberg's disease (marble bones) 756.52

Albert's disease 726.71

Albinism, albino (choroid) (cutaneous) (eye) (generalized) (isolated) (ocular) (oculocutaneous) (partial) 270.2

Albinismus 270.2

Albright (-Martin) (-Bantam) disease (pseudohypoparathyroidism) 275.49

Albright (-McCune) (-Sternberg) syndrome (osteitis fibrosa disseminata) 756.59

Albuminous — *see* condition

Albuminuria, albuminuric (acute) (chronic) (subacute) 791.0
  Bence-Jones 791.0
  cardiac 785.9
  complicating pregnancy, childbirth, or puerperium 646.2 ☑
    with hypertension — *see* Toxemia, of pregnancy
    affecting fetus or newborn 760.1
  cyclic 593.6
  gestational 646.2 ☑
  gravidarum 646.2 ☑
    with hypertension — *see* Toxemia, of pregnancy
    affecting fetus or newborn 760.1
  heart 785.9
  idiopathic 593.6
  orthostatic 593.6
  postural 593.6
  pre-eclamptic (mild) 642.4 ☑
    affecting fetus or newborn 760.0
    severe 642.5 ☑
      affecting fetus or newborn 760.0
  recurrent physiologic 593.6
  scarlatinal 034.1

Albumosuria 791.0
  Bence-Jones 791.0
  myelopathic (M9730/3) 203.0 ☑

Alcaptonuria 270.2

Alcohol, alcoholic
  abstinence 291.81
  acute intoxication 305.0 ☑
    with dependence 303.0 ☑
  addiction (*see also* Alcoholism) 303.9 ☑
    maternal
      with suspected fetal damage affecting management of pregnancy 655.4 ☑
      affecting fetus or newborn 760.71
  amnestic disorder, persisting 291.1
  anxiety 291.89
  brain syndrome, chronic 291.2
  cardiopathy 425.5
  chronic (*see also* Alcoholism) 303.9 ☑
  cirrhosis (liver) 571.2
  delirium 291.0
    acute 291.0
    chronic 291.1
    tremens 291.0
    withdrawal 291.0
  dementia NEC 291.2
  deterioration 291.2
  drunkenness (simple) 305.0 ☑
  hallucinosis (acute) 291.3
  induced ●
    mental disorder 291.9 ●
      anxiety 291.89 ●
      mood 291.89 ●
      sexual 291.89 ●
      sleep 291.89 ●
      specified type 291.89 ●
    persisting ●
      amnestic disorder 291.1 ●
      dementia 291.2 ●
    psychotic disorder ●
      with ●
        delusions 291.5 ●
        hallucinations 291.3 ●
  insanity 291.9
  intoxication (acute) 305.0 ☑
    with dependence 303.0 ☑
    pathological 291.4
  jealousy 291.5
  Korsakoff's, Korsakov's, Korsakow's 291.1
  liver NEC 571.3
    acute 571.1

Alcohol, alcoholic — *continued*
  liver NEC — *continued*
    chronic 571.2
  mania (acute) (chronic) 291.9
  mood 291.89
  paranoia 291.5
  paranoid (type) psychosis 291.5
  pellagra 265.2
  poisoning, accidental (acute) NEC 980.9
    specified type of alcohol — *see* Table of Drugs and Chemicals
  psychosis (*see also* Psychosis, alcoholic) 291.9
    Korsakoff's, Korsakov's, Korsakow's 291.1
    polyneuritic 291.1
    with
      delusions 291.5
      hallucinations 291.3
  related disorder 291.9 ●
  withdrawal symptoms, syndrome NEC 291.81
    delirium 291.0
    hallucinosis 291.3

Alcoholism 303.9 ☑

> *Note* — Use the following fifth-digit subclassification with category 303:
>
> 0   unspecified
> 1   continuous
> 2   episodic
> 3   in remission

  with psychosis (*see also* Psychosis, alcoholic) 291.9
  acute 303.0 ☑
  chronic 303.9 ☑
    with psychosis 291.9
  complicating pregnancy, childbirth, or puerperium 648.4 ☑
    affecting fetus or newborn 760.71
  history V11.3
  Korsakoff's, Korsakov's, Korsakow's 291.1
  suspected damage to fetus affecting management of pregnancy 655.4 ☑

Alder's anomaly or syndrome (leukocyte granulation anomaly) 288.2

Alder-Reilly anomaly (leukocyte granulation) 288.2

Aldosteronism (primary) 255.10
  congenital 255.10
  familial type I 255.11
  glucocorticoid-remediable 255.11
  secondary 255.14

Aldosteronoma (M8370/1) 237.2

Aldrich (-Wiskott) syndrome (eczema-thrombocytopenia) 279.12

Aleppo boil 085.1

Aleukemic — *see* condition

Aleukia
  congenital 288.0
  hemorrhagica 284.9
    acquired (secondary) 284.8
    congenital 284.0
    idiopathic 284.9
  splenica 289.4

Alexia (congenital) (developmental) 315.01
  secondary to organic lesion 784.61

Algoneurodystrophy 733.7

Algophobia 300.29

Alibert's disease (mycosis fungoides) (M9700/3) 202.1 ☑

Alibert-Bazin disease (M9700/3) 202.1 ☑

Alice in Wonderland syndrome 293.89

Alienation, mental (*see also* Psychosis) 298.9

Alkalemia 276.3

Alkalosis 276.3
  metabolic 276.3
    with respiratory acidosis 276.4
  respiratory 276.3

Alkaptonuria 270.2

Allen-Masters syndrome 620.6

Allergic bronchopulmonary aspergillosis 518.6

Allergy, allergic (reaction) 995.3
air-borne substance (*see also* Fever, hay) 477.9
specified allergen NEC 477.8
alveolitis (extrinsic) 495.9
due to
Aspergillus clavatus 495.4
cryptostroma corticale 495.6
organisms (fungal, thermophilic
actinomycete, other) growing in
ventilation (air conditioning
systems) 495.7
specified type NEC 495.8
anaphylactic shock 999.4
due to food — *see* Anaphylactic shock, due
to, food
angioneurotic edema 995.1
animal ▶(cat) (dog)◀ (epidermal) 477.8
dander 477.2 ●
hair 477.2 ●
arthritis (*see also* Arthritis, allergic) 716.2 ☑
asthma — *see* Asthma
bee sting (anaphylactic shock) 989.5
biological — *see* Allergy, drug
bronchial asthma — *see* Asthma
conjunctivitis (eczematous) 372.14
dander, ▶animal (cat) (dog)◀ 477.2 ▲
dandruff 477.8
dermatitis (venenata) — *see* Dermatitis
diathesis V15.09
drug, medicinal substance, and biological (any)
(correct medicinal substance properly
administered) (external) (internal) 995.2
wrong substance given or taken NEC 977.9
specified drug or substance — *see* Table
of Drugs and Chemicals
dust (house) (stock) 477.8
eczema — *see* Eczema
endophthalmitis 360.19
epidermal (animal) 477.8
feathers 477.8
food (any) (ingested) 693.1
atopic 691.8
in contact with skin 692.5
gastritis 535.4 ☑
gastroenteritis 558.3
gastrointestinal 558.3
grain 477.0
grass (pollen) 477.0
asthma (*see also* Asthma) 493.0 ☑
hay fever 477.0
hair, ▶animal (cat) (dog)◀ 477.2
hay fever (grass) (pollen) (ragweed) (tree) (*see
also* Fever, hay) 477.9
history (of) V15.09
to
eggs V15.03
food additives V15.05
insect bite V15.06
latex V15.07
milk products V15.02
nuts V15.05
peanuts V15.01
radiographic dye V15.08
seafood V15.04
specified food NEC V15.05
spider bite V15.06
horse serum — see Allergy, serum
inhalant 477.9
dust 477.8
pollen 477.0
specified allergen other than pollen 477.8
kapok 477.8
medicine — *see* Allergy, drug
migraine 346.2 ☑
milk protein 558.3
pannus 370.62
pneumonia 518.3
pollen (any) (hay fever) 477.0
asthma (*see also* Asthma) 493.0 ☑
primrose 477.0
primula 477.0
purpura 287.0
ragweed (pollen) (Senecio jacobae) 477.0
asthma (*see also* Asthma) 493.0 ☑
hay fever 477.0

Allergy, allergic — *continued*
respiratory (*see also* Allergy, inhalant) 477.9
due to
drug — *see* Allergy, drug
food — *see* Allergy, food
rhinitis (*see also* Fever, hay) 477.9
due to food 477.1
rose 477.0
Senecio jacobae 477.0
serum (prophylactic) (therapeutic) 999.5
anaphylactic shock 999.4
shock (anaphylactic) (due to adverse effect of
correct medicinal substance properly
administered) 995.0
food — *see* Anaphylactic shock, due to, food
from serum or immunization 999.5
anaphylactic 999.4
sinusitis (*see also* Fever, hay) 477.9
skin reaction 692.9
specified substance — *see* Dermatitis, due
to
tree (any) (hay fever) (pollen) 477.0
asthma (*see also* Asthma) 493.0 ☑
upper respiratory (*see also* Fever, hay) 477.9
urethritis 597.89
urticaria 708.0
vaccine — *see* Allergy, serum
Allescheriosis 117.6
Alligator skin disease (ichthyosis congenita)
757.1
acquired 701.1
Allocheiria, allochiria (*see also* Disturbance,
sensation) 782.0
Almeida's disease (Brazilian blastomycosis) 116.1
Alopecia (atrophicans) (pregnancy) (premature)
(senile) 704.00
adnata 757.4
areata 704.01
celsi 704.01
cicatrisata 704.09
circumscripta 704.01
congenital, congenitalis 757.4
disseminata 704.01
effluvium (telogen) 704.02
febrile 704.09
generalisata 704.09
hereditaria 704.09
marginalis 704.01
mucinosa 704.09
postinfectional 704.09
seborrheica 704.09
specific 091.82
syphilitic (secondary) 091.82
telogen effluvium 704.02
totalis 704.09
toxica 704.09
universalis 704.09
x-ray 704.09
Alpers' disease 330.8
Alpha-lipoproteinemia 272.4
Alpha thalassemia 282.49
Alphos 696.1
Alpine sickness 993.2
Alport's syndrome (hereditary
hematurianephropathy-deafness) 759.89
Alteration (of), **altered**
awareness 780.09
transient 780.02
consciousness 780.09
persistent vegetative state 780.03
transient 780.02
mental status 780.99
amnesia (retrograde) 780.93
memory loss 780.93
Alternaria (infection) 118
Alternating — *see* condition
Altitude, high (effects) — *see* Effect, adverse, high
altitude
Aluminosis (of lung) 503
Alvarez syndrome (transient cerebral ischemia)
435.9
Alveolar capillary block syndrome 516.3

Alveolitis
allergic (extrinsic) 495.9
due to organisms (fungal, thermophilic
actinomycete, other) growing in
ventilation (air conditioning systems)
495.7
specified type NEC 495.8
due to
Aspergillus clavatus 495.4
Cryptostroma corticale 495.6
fibrosing (chronic) (cryptogenic) (lung) 516.3
idiopathic 516.3
rheumatoid 714.81
jaw 526.5
sicca dolorosa 526.5
Alveolus, alveolar — *see* condition
Alymphocytosis (pure) 279.2
Alymphoplasia, thymic 279.2
Alzheimer's
dementia (senile)
with behavioral disturbance 331.0 *[294.11]*
without behavioral disturbance 331.0
[294.10]
disease or sclerosis 331.0
with dementia — *see* Alzheimer's, dementia
Amastia (*see also* Absence, breast) 611.8
Amaurosis (acquired) (congenital) (*see also*
Blindness) 369.00
fugax 362.34
hysterical 300.11
Leber's (congenital) 362.76
tobacco 377.34
uremic — *see* Uremia
Amaurotic familial idiocy (infantile) (juvenile)
(late) 330.1
Ambisexual 752.7
Amblyopia (acquired) (congenital) (partial) 368.00
color 368.59
acquired 368.55
deprivation 368.02
ex anopsia 368.00
hysterical 300.11
nocturnal 368.60
vitamin A deficiency 264.5
refractive 368.03
strabismic 368.01
suppression 368.01
tobacco 377.34
toxic NEC 377.34
uremic — *see* Uremia
Ameba, amebic (histolytica) — *see also* Amebiasis
abscess 006.3
bladder 006.8
brain (with liver and lung abscess) 006.5
liver 006.3
with
brain abscess (and lung abscess)
006.5
lung abscess 006.4
lung (with liver abscess) 006.4
with brain abscess 006.5
seminal vesicle 006.8
spleen 006.8
carrier (suspected of) V02.2
meningoencephalitis
due to Naegleria (gruberi) 136.2
primary 136.2
Amebiasis NEC 006.9
with
brain abscess (with liver or lung abscess)
006.5
liver abscess (without mention of brain or
lung abscess) 006.3
lung abscess (with liver abscess) 006.4
with brain abscess 006.5
acute 006.0
bladder 006.8
chronic 006.1
cutaneous 006.6
cutis 006.6
due to organism other than Entamoeba
histolytica 007.8
hepatic (*see also* Abscess, liver, amebic) 006.3
nondysenteric 006.2
seminal vesicle 006.8

☑ Additional Digit Required   ▶◀ Revised Text   ● New Line   ▲ Revised Code

Amebiasis NEC — *continued*
  specified
    organism NEC 007.8
    site NEC 006.8
Ameboma 006.8
Amelia 755.4
  lower limb 755.31
  upper limb 755.21
Ameloblastoma (M9310/0) 213.1
  jaw (bone) (lower) 213.1
    upper 213.0
  long bones (M9261/3) — *see* Neoplasm, bone,
    malignant
  malignant (M9310/3) 170.1
    jaw (bone) (lower) 170.1
      upper 170.0
  mandible 213.1
  tibial (M9261/3) 170.7
Amelogenesis imperfecta 520.5
  nonhereditaria (segmentalis) 520.4
Amenorrhea (primary) (secondary) 626.0
  due to ovarian dysfunction 256.8
  hyperhormonal 256.8
Amentia (*see also* Retardation, mental) 319
  Meynert's (nonalcoholic) 294.0
    alcoholic 291.1
  nevoid 759.6
American
  leishmaniasis 085.5
  mountain tick fever 066.1
  trypanosomiasis — *see* Trypanosomiasis,
    American
Ametropia (*see also* Disorder, accommodation)
  367.9
Amianthosis 501
Amimia 784.69
Amino acid
  deficiency 270.9
    anemia 281.4
  metabolic disorder (*see also* Disorder, amino
    acid) 270.9
Aminoaciduria 270.9
  imidazole 270.5
Amnesia (retrograde) 780.93
  auditory 784.69
    developmental 315.31
    secondary to organic lesion 784.69
  dissociative 300.12
  hysterical or dissociative type 300.12
  psychogenic 300.12
  transient global 437.7
Amnestic (confabulatory) **syndrome** 294.0
  alcohol-induced ▶persisting◀ 291.1
  drug-induced ▶persisting◀ 292.83
  posttraumatic 294.0
Amniocentesis screening (for) V28.2
  alphafetoprotein level, raised V28.1
  chromosomal anomalies V28.0
Amnion, amniotic — *see also* condition
  nodosum 658.8 ☑
Amnionitis (complicating pregnancy) 658.4 ☑
  affecting fetus or newborn 762.7
Amoral trends 301.7
Amotio retinae (*see also* Detachment, retina)
  361.9
Ampulla
  lower esophagus 530.89
  phrenic 530.89
Amputation
  any part of fetus, to facilitate delivery 763.89
  cervix (supravaginal) (uteri) 622.8
    in pregnancy or childbirth 654.6 ☑
      affecting fetus or newborn 763.89
  clitoris — *see* Wound, open, clitoris
  congenital
    lower limb 755.31
    upper limb 755.21
  neuroma (traumatic) — *see also* Injury, nerve,
    by site
    surgical complication (late) 997.61
  penis — *see* Amputation, traumatic, penis
  status (without complication) — *see* Absence,
    by site, acquired

Amputation — *continued*
  stump (surgical) (posttraumatic)
    abnormal, painful, or with complication
      (late) 997.60
    healed or old NEC — *see also* Absence, by
      site, acquired
      lower V49.70
      upper V49.60
  traumatic (complete) (partial)

> *Note* — "Complicated" includes traumatic
> amputation with delayed healing, delayed
> treatment, foreign body, or infection.

    arm 887.4
      at or above elbow 887.2
        complicated 887.3
      below elbow 887.0
        complicated 887.1
      both (bilateral) (any level(s)) 887.6
        complicated 887.7
      complicated 887.5
    finger(s) (one or both hands) 886.0
      with thumb(s) 885.0
        complicated 885.1
      complicated 886.1
    foot (except toe(s) only) 896.0
      and other leg 897.6
        complicated 897.7
      both (bilateral) 896.2
        complicated 896.3
      complicated 896.1
      toe(s) only (one or both feet) 895.0
        complicated 895.1
    genital organ(s) (external) NEC 878.8
      complicated 878.9
    hand (except finger(s) only) 887.0
      and other arm 887.6
        complicated 887.7
      both (bilateral) 887.6
        complicated 887.7
      complicated 887.1
      finger(s) (one or both hands) 886.0
        with thumb(s) 885.0
          complicated 885.1
        complicated 886.1
      thumb(s) (with fingers of either hand)
        885.0
        complicated 885.1
    head 874.9
    late effect — *see* Late, effects (of),
      amputation
    leg 897.4
      and other foot 897.6
        complicated 897.7
      at or above knee 897.2
        complicated 897.3
      below knee 897.0
        complicated 897.1
      both (bilateral) 897.6
        complicated 897.7
      complicated 897.5
    lower limb(s) except toe(s) — *see*
      Amputation, traumatic, leg
    nose — *see* Wound, open, nose
    penis 878.0
      complicated 878.1
    sites other than limbs — *see* Wound, open,
      by site
    thumb(s) (with finger(s) of either hand) 885.0
      complicated 885.1
    toe(s) (one or both feet) 895.0
      complicated 895.1
    upper limb(s) — *see* Amputation, traumatic,
      arm
Amputee (bilateral) (old) — *see also* Absence, by
  site, acquired V49.70
Amusia 784.69
  developmental 315.39
  secondary to organic lesion 784.69
Amyelencephalus 740.0
Amyelia 742.59
Amygdalitis — *see* Tonsillitis
Amygdalolith 474.8
Amyloid disease or degeneration 277.3
  heart 277.3 *[425.7]*

Amyloidosis (familial) (general) (generalized)
  (genetic) (primary) (secondary) 277.3
  with lung involvement 277.3 *[517.8]*
  heart 277.3 *[425.7]*
  nephropathic 277.3 *[583.81]*
  neuropathic (Portuguese) (Swiss) 277.3 *[357.4]*
  pulmonary 277.3 *[517.8]*
  systemic, inherited 277.3
Amylopectinosis (brancher enzyme deficiency)
  271.0
Amylophagia 307.52
Amyoplasia, congenita 756.89
Amyotonia 728.2
  congenita 358.8
Amyotrophia, amyotrophy, amyotrophic 728.2
  congenita 756.89
  diabetic 250.6 ☑ *[358.1]*
  lateral sclerosis (syndrome) 335.20
  neuralgic 353.5
  sclerosis (lateral) 335.20
  spinal progressive 335.21
Anacidity, gastric 536.0
  psychogenic 306.4
Anaerosis of newborn 768.9
Analbuminemia 273.8
Analgesia (*see also* Anesthesia) 782.0
Analphalipoproteinemia 272.5
Anaphylactic shock or reaction (correct
  substance properly administered) 995.0
  due to
    food 995.60
      additives 995.66
      crustaceans 995.62
      eggs 995.68
      fish 995.65
      fruits 995.63
      milk products 995.67
      nuts (tree) 995.64
      peanuts 995.61
      seeds 995.64
      specified NEC 995.69
      tree nuts 995.64
      vegetables 995.63
    immunization 999.4
    overdose or wrong substance given or taken
      977.9
      specified drug — *see* Table of Drugs and
        Chemicals
    serum 999.4
  following sting(s) 989.5
  purpura 287.0
  serum 999.4
Anaphylactoid shock or reaction — *see*
  Anaphylactic shock
Anaphylaxis — *see* Anaphylactic shock
Anaplasia, cervix 622.10   ▲
Anarthria 784.5
Anarthritic rheumatoid disease 446.5
Anasarca 782.3
  cardiac (*see also* Failure, heart) 428.0
  fetus or newborn 778.0
  lung 514
  nutritional 262
  pulmonary 514
  renal (*see also* Nephrosis) 581.9
Anaspadias 752.62
Anastomosis
  aneurysmal — *see* Aneurysm
  arteriovenous, congenital NEC (*see also*
    Anomaly, arteriovenous) 747.60
    ruptured, of brain (*see also* Hemorrhage,
      subarachnoid) 430
  intestinal 569.89
    complicated NEC 997.4
      involving urinary tract 997.5
  retinal and choroidal vessels 743.58
    acquired 362.17
Anatomical narrow angle (glaucoma) 365.02
Ancylostoma (infection) (infestation) 126.9
  americanus 126.1
  braziliense 126.2
  caninum 126.8
  ceylanicum 126.3

Ancylostoma — *continued*
  duodenale 126.0
  Necator americanus 126.1

Ancylostomiasis (intestinal) 126.9
  Ancylostoma
    americanus 126.1
    caninum 126.8
    ceylanicum 126.3
    duodenale 126.0
  braziliense 126.2
  Necator americanus 126.1

Anders' disease or syndrome (adiposis tuberosa simplex) 272.8

Andersen's glycogen storage disease 271.0

Anderson's disease 272.7

Andes disease 993.2

Andrews' disease (bacterid) 686.8

Androblastoma (M8630/1)
  benign (M8630/0)
    specified site — *see* Neoplasm, by site, benign
    unspecified site
      female 220
      male 222.0
  malignant (M8630/3)
    specified site — *see* Neoplasm, by site, malignant
    unspecified site
      female 183.0
      male 186.9
  specified site — *see* Neoplasm, by site, uncertain behavior
  tubular (M8640/0)
    with lipid storage (M8641/0)
      specified site — *see* Neoplasm, by site, benign
      unspecified site
        female 220
        male 222.0
    specified site — *see* Neoplasm, by site, benign
    unspecified site
      female 220
      male 222.0
  unspecified site
    female 236.2
    male 236.4

Android pelvis 755.69
  with disproportion (fetopelvic) 653.3 ☑
    affecting fetus or newborn 763.1
    causing obstructed labor 660.1 ☑
      affecting fetus or newborn 763.1

Anectasis, pulmonary (newborn or fetus) 770.5

Anemia 285.9
  with
    disorder of
      anaerobic glycolysis 282.3
      pentose phosphate pathway 282.2
    koilonychia 280.9
  6-phosphogluconic dehydrogenase deficiency 282.2
  achlorhydric 280.9
  achrestic 281.8
  Addison's (pernicious) 281.0
  Addison-Biermer (pernicious) 281.0
  agranulocytic 288.0
  amino acid deficiency 281.4
  aplastic 284.9
    acquired (secondary) 284.8
    congenital 284.0
    constitutional 284.0
    due to
      chronic systemic disease 284.8
      drugs 284.8
      infection 284.8
      radiation 284.8
    idiopathic 284.9
    myxedema 244.9
    of or complicating pregnancy 648.2 ☑
    red cell (acquired) (pure) (with thymoma) 284.8
      congenital 284.0
    specified type NEC 284.8
    toxic (paralytic) 284.8
  aregenerative 284.9
    congenital 284.0

Anemia — *continued*
  asiderotic 280.9
  atypical (primary) 285.9
  autohemolysis of Selwyn and Dacie (type I) 282.2
  autoimmune hemolytic 283.0
  Baghdad Spring 282.2
  Balantidium coli 007.0
  Biermer's (pernicious) 281.0
  blood loss (chronic) 280.0
    acute 285.1
  bothriocephalus 123.4
  brickmakers' (*see also* Ancylostomiasis) 126.9
  cerebral 437.8
  childhood 282.9   ▲
  chlorotic 280.9
  chronica congenita aregenerativa 284.0
  chronic simple 281.9
  combined system disease NEC 281.0 *[336.2]*
    due to dietary deficiency 281.1 *[336.2]*
  complicating pregnancy or childbirth 648.2 ☑
  congenital (following fetal blood loss) 776.5
    aplastic 284.0
    due to isoimmunization NEC 773.2
    Heinz-body 282.7
    hereditary hemolytic NEC 282.9
    nonspherocytic
      Type I 282.2
      Type II 282.3
    pernicious 281.0
    spherocytic (*see also* Spherocytosis) 282.0
  Cooley's (erythroblastic) 282.49
  crescent — *see* Disease, sickle-cell
  cytogenic 281.0
  Dacie's (nonspherocytic)
    type I 282.2
    type II 282.3
  Davidson's (refractory) 284.9
  deficiency 281.9
    2, 3 diphosphoglycurate mutase 282.3
    2, 3 PG 282.3
    6-PGD 282.2
    6-phosphogluronic dehydrogenase 282.2
    amino acid 281.4
    combined B_{12} and folate 281.3
    enzyme, drug-induced (hemolytic) 282.2
    erythrocytic glutathione 282.2
    folate 281.2
      dietary 281.2
      drug-induced 281.2
    folic acid 281.2
      dietary 281.2
      drug-induced 281.2
    G-6-PD 282.2
    GGS-R 282.2
    glucose-6-phosphate dehydrogenase (G-6-PD) 282.2
    glucose-phosphate isomerase 282.3
    glutathione peroxidase 282.2
    glutathione reductase 282.2
    glyceraldehyde phosphate dehydrogenase 282.3
    GPI 282.3
    G SH 282.2
    hexokinase 282.3
    iron (Fe) 280.9
      specified NEC 280.8
    nutritional 281.9
      with
        poor iron absorption 280.9
        specified deficiency NEC 281.8
      due to inadequate dietary iron intake 280.1
      specified type NEC 281.8
    of or complicating pregnancy 648.2 ☑
    pentose phosphate pathway 282.2
    PFK 282.3
    phosphofructo-aldolase 282.3
    phosphofructokinase 282.3
    phosphoglycerate kinase 282.3
    PK 282.3
    protein 281.4
    pyruvate kinase (PK) 282.3
    TPI 282.3
    triosephosphate isomerase 282.3
    vitamin B_{12} NEC 281.1
      dietary 281.1

Anemia — *continued*
  deficiency — *continued*
    vitamin B_{12} NEC — *continued*
      pernicious 281.0
  Diamond-Blackfan (congenital hypoplastic) 284.0
  dibothriocephalus 123.4
  dimorphic 281.9
  diphasic 281.8
  diphtheritic 032.89
  Diphyllobothrium 123.4
  drepanocytic (*see also* Disease, sickle-cell) 282.60
  due to
    blood loss (chronic) 280.0
      acute 285.1
    defect of Embden-Meyerhof pathway glycolysis 282.3
    disorder of glutathione metabolism 282.2
    fetal blood loss 776.5
    fish tapeworm (D. latum) infestation 123.4
    glutathione metabolism disorder 282.2
    hemorrhage (chronic) 280.0
      acute 285.1
    hexose monophosphate (HMP) shunt deficiency 282.2
    impaired absorption 280.9
    loss of blood (chronic) 280.0
      acute 285.1
    myxedema 244.9
    Necator americanus 126.1
    prematurity 776.6
    selective vitamin B_{12} malabsorption with proteinuria 281.1
  Dyke-Young type (secondary) (symptomatic) 283.9
  dyserythropoietic (congenital) (types I, II, III) 285.8
  dyshemopoietic (congenital) 285.8
  Egypt (*see also* Ancylostomiasis) 126.9
  elliptocytosis (*see also* Elliptocytosis) 282.1
  enzyme deficiency, drug-induced 282.2
  epidemic (*see also* Ancylostomiasis) 126.9
  EPO resistant 285.21
  erythroblastic
    familial 282.49
    fetus or newborn (*see also* Disease, hemolytic) 773.2
    late 773.5
  erythrocytic glutathione deficiency 282.2
  erythropoietin-resistant (EPO resistant anemia) 285.21
  essential 285.9
  Faber's (achlorhydric anemia) 280.9
  factitious (self-induced blood letting) 280.0
  familial erythroblastic (microcytic) 282.49
  Fanconi's (congenital pancytopenia) 284.0
  favism 282.2
  fetal, following blood loss 776.5
  fetus or newborn
    due to
      ABO
        antibodies 773.1
        incompatibility, maternal/fetal 773.1
        isoimmunization 773.1
      Rh
        antibodies 773.0
        incompatibility, maternal/fetal 773.0
        isoimmunization 773.0
    following fetal blood loss 776.5
  fish tapeworm (D. latum) infestation 123.4
  folate (folic acid) deficiency 281.2
    dietary 281.2
    drug-induced 281.2
  folate malabsorption, congenital 281.2
  folic acid deficiency 281.2
    dietary 281.2
    drug-induced 281.2
  G-6-PD 282.2
  general 285.9
  glucose-6-phosphate dehydrogenase deficiency 282.2
  glutathione-reductase deficiency 282.2
  goat's milk 281.2
  granulocytic 288.0
  Heinz-body, congenital 282.7
  hemoglobin deficiency 285.9

Anemia — *continued*
  hemolytic 283.9
    acquired 283.9
      with hemoglobinuria NEC 283.2
      autoimmune (cold type) (idiopathic)
          (primary) (secondary) (symptomatic)
          (warm type) 283.0
      due to
        cold reactive antibodies 283.0
        drug exposure 283.0
        warm reactive antibodies 283.0
      fragmentation 283.19
      idiopathic (chronic) 283.9
      infectious 283.19
        autoimmune 283.0
      non-autoimmune NEC 283.10
      toxic 283.19
      traumatic cardiac 283.19
    acute 283.9
      due to enzyme deficiency NEC 282.3
      fetus or newborn (*see also* Disease,
          hemolytic) 773.2
        late 773.5
      Lederer's (acquired infectious hemolytic
          anemia) 283.19
    autoimmune (acquired) 283.0
    chronic 282.9
      idiopathic 283.9
    cold type (secondary) (symptomatic) 283.0
    congenital (spherocytic) (*see also*
        Spherocytosis) 282.0
      nonspherocytic — *see* Anemia, hemolytic,
          nonspherocytic, congenital
    drug-induced 283.0
      enzyme deficiency 282.2
    due to
      cardiac conditions 283.19
      drugs 283.0
      enzyme deficiency NEC 282.3
        drug-induced 282.2
      presence of shunt or other internal
          prosthetic device 283.19
      thrombotic thrombocytopenic purpura
          446.6
    elliptocytotic (*see also* Elliptocytosis) 282.1
    familial 282.9
    hereditary 282.9
      due to enzyme deficiency NEC 282.3
        specified NEC 282.8
    idiopathic (chronic) 283.9
    infectious (acquired) 283.19
    mechanical 283.19
    microangiopathic 283.19
    non-autoimmune NEC 283.10
    nonspherocytic
      congenital or hereditary NEC 282.3
        glucose-6-phosphate dehydrogenase
            deficiency 282.2
        pyruvate kinase (PK) deficiency 282.3
        type I 282.2
        type II 282.3
      type I 282.2
      type II 282.3
    of or complicating pregnancy 648.2 ☑
    resulting from presence of shunt or other
        internal prosthetic device 283.19
    secondary 283.19
      autoimmune 283.0
    sickle-cell — *see* Disease, sickle-cell
    Stransky-Regala type (Hb-E) (*see also*
        Disease, hemoglobin) 282.7
    symptomatic 283.19
      autoimmune 283.0
    toxic (acquired) 283.19
    uremic (adult) (child) 283.11
    warm type (secondary) (symptomatic) 283.0
  hemorrhagic (chronic) 280.0
    acute 285.1
  HEMPAS 285.8
  hereditary erythroblast multinuclearity-positive
      acidified serum test 285.8
  Herrick's (hemoglobin S disease) 282.61
  hexokinase deficiency 282.3
  high A₂ 282.49
  hookworm (*see also* Ancylostomiasis) 126.9
  hypochromic (idiopathic) (microcytic)
      (normoblastic) 280.9

Anemia — *continued*
  hypochromic — *continued*
    with iron loading 285.0
    due to blood loss (chronic) 280.0
      acute 285.1
    familial sex linked 285.0
    pyridoxine-responsive 285.0
  hypoplasia, red blood cells 284.8
    congenital or familial 284.0
  hypoplastic (idiopathic) 284.9
    congenital 284.0
    familial 284.0
    of childhood 284.0
  idiopathic 285.9
    hemolytic, chronic 283.9
  in
    chronic illness NEC 285.29
    end-stage renal disease 285.21
    neoplastic disease 285.22
  infantile 285.9
  infective, infectional 285.9
  intertropical (*see also* Ancylostomiasis) 126.9
  iron (Fe) deficiency 280.9
    due to blood loss (chronic) 280.0
      acute 285.1
    of or complicating pregnancy 648.2 ☑
    specified NEC 280.8
  Jaksch's (pseudoleukemia infantum) 285.8
  Joseph-Diamond-Blackfan (congenital
      hypoplastic) 284.0
  labyrinth 386.50
  Lederer's (acquired infectious hemolytic
      anemia) 283.19
  leptocytosis (hereditary) 282.49
  leukoerythroblastic 285.8
  macrocytic 281.9
    nutritional 281.2
    of or complicating pregnancy 648.2 ☑
    tropical 281.2
  malabsorption (familial), selective B₁₂ with
      proteinuria 281.1
  malarial (*see also* Malaria) 084.6
  malignant (progressive) 281.0
  malnutrition 281.9
  marsh (*see also* Malaria) 084.6
  Mediterranean (with hemoglobinopathy)
      282.49
  megaloblastic 281.9
    combined B₁₂ and folate deficiency 281.3
    nutritional (of infancy) 281.2
    of infancy 281.2
    of or complicating pregnancy 648.2 ☑
    refractory 281.3
    specified NEC 281.3
  megalocytic 281.9
  microangiopathic hemolytic 283.19
  microcytic (hypochromic) 280.9
    due to blood loss (chronic) 280.0
      acute 285.1
    familial 282.49
    hypochromic 280.9
  microdrepanocytosis 282.49
  miners' (*see also* Ancylostomiasis) 126.9
  myelopathic 285.8
  myelophthisic (normocytic) 285.8
  newborn (*see also* Disease, hemolytic) 773.2
    due to isoimmunization (*see also* Disease,
        hemolytic) 773.2
    late, due to isoimmunization 773.5
    posthemorrhagic 776.5
  nonregenerative 284.9
  nonspherocytic hemolytic — *see* Anemia,
      hemolytic, nonspherocytic
  normocytic (infectional) (not due to blood loss)
      285.9
    due to blood loss (chronic) 280.0
      acute 285.1
    myelophthisic 284.8
  nutritional (deficiency) 281.9
    with
      poor iron absorption 280.9
      specified deficiency NEC 281.8
    due to inadequate dietary iron intake 280.1
    megaloblastic (of infancy) 281.2
  of childhood 282.9   ▲
  of chronic illness NEC 285.29

Anemia — *continued*
  of or complicating pregnancy 648.2 ☑
    affecting fetus or newborn 760.8
  of prematurity 776.6
  orotic aciduric (congenital) (hereditary) 281.4
  osteosclerotic 289.89
  ovalocytosis (hereditary) (*see also* Elliptocytosis)
      282.1
  paludal (*see also* Malaria) 084.6
  pentose phosphate pathway deficiency 282.2
  pernicious (combined system disease)
      (congenital) (dorsolateral spinal
      degeneration) (juvenile) (myelopathy)
      (neuropathy) (posterior sclerosis)
      (primary) (progressive) (spleen) 281.0
    of or complicating pregnancy 648.2 ☑
  pleochromic 285.9
    of sprue 281.8
  portal 285.8
  posthemorrhagic (chronic) 280.0
    acute 285.1
    newborn 776.5
  postoperative   ●
    due to blood loss 285.1   ●
    other 285.9   ●
  postpartum 648.2 ☑
  pressure 285.9
  primary 285.9
  profound 285.9
  progressive 285.9
    malignant 281.0
    pernicious 281.0
  protein-deficiency 281.4
  pseudoleukemica infantum 285.8
  puerperal 648.2 ☑
  pure red cell 284.8
    congenital 284.0
  pyridoxine-responsive (hypochromic) 285.0
  pyruvate kinase (PK) deficiency 282.3
  refractoria sideroblastica 285.0
  refractory (primary) 284.9
    with hemochromatosis 285.0
    megaloblastic 281.3
    sideroblastic 285.0
    sideropenic 280.9
  Rietti-Greppi-Micheli (thalassemia minor)
      282.49
  scorbutic 281.8
  secondary (to) 285.9
    blood loss (chronic) 280.0
      acute 285.1
    hemorrhage 280.0
      acute 285.1
    inadequate dietary iron intake 280.1
  semiplastic 284.9
  septic 285.9
  sickle-cell (*see also* Disease, sickle-cell) 282.60
  sideroachrestic 285.0
  sideroblastic (acquired) (any type) (congenital)
      (drug-induced) (due to disease)
      (hereditary) (primary) (refractory)
      (secondary) (sex-linked hypochromic)
      (vitamin B₆ responsive) 285.0
  sideropenic (refractory) 280.9
    due to blood loss (chronic) 280.0
      acute 285.1
  simple chronic 281.9
  specified type NEC 285.8
  spherocytic (hereditary) (*see also* Spherocytosis)
      282.0
  splenic 285.8
    familial (Gaucher's) 272.7
  splenomegalic 285.8
  stomatocytosis 282.8
  syphilitic 095.8
  target cell (oval) 282.49
  thalassemia 282.49
  thrombocytopenic (*see also* Thrombocytopenia)
      287.5
  toxic 284.8
  triosephosphate isomerase deficiency 282.3
  tropical, macrocytic 281.2
  tuberculous (*see also* Tuberculosis) 017.9 ☑
  vegan's 281.1
  vitamin
    B₆-responsive 285.0

Anemia — *continued*
  vitamin — *continued*
    B_{12} deficiency (dietary) 281.1
      pernicious 281.0
  von Jaksch's (pseudoleukemia infantum) 285.8
  Witts' (achlorhydric anemia) 280.9
  Zuelzer (-Ogden) (nutritional megaloblastic
    anemia) 281.2

Anencephalus, anencephaly 740.0
  fetal, affecting management of pregnancy
    655.0 ☑

Anergasia (*see also* Psychosis, organic) 294.9
  senile 290.0

Anesthesia, anesthetic 782.0
  complication or reaction NEC 995.2
    due to
      correct substance properly administered
        995.2
      overdose or wrong substance given 968.4
        specified anesthetic — *see* Table of
          Drugs and Chemicals
  cornea 371.81
  death from
    correct substance properly administered
      995.4
    during delivery 668.9 ☑
    overdose or wrong substance given 968.4
    specified anesthetic — *see* Table of Drugs
      and Chemicals
  eye 371.81
  functional 300.11
  hyperesthetic, thalamic 348.8
  hysterical 300.11
  local skin lesion 782.0
  olfactory 781.1
  sexual (psychogenic) 302.72
  shock
    due to
      correct substance properly administered
        995.4
      overdose or wrong substance given 968.4
      specified anesthetic — *see* Table of Drugs
        and Chemicals
  skin 782.0
  tactile 782.0
  testicular 608.9
  thermal 782.0

Anetoderma (maculosum) 701.3

Aneuploidy NEC 758.5

Aneurin deficiency 265.1

Aneurysm (anastomotic) (artery) (cirsoid) (diffuse)
  (false) (fusiform) (multiple) (ruptured)
  (saccular) (varicose) 442.9
  abdominal (aorta) 441.4
    ruptured 441.3
    syphilitic 093.0
  aorta, aortic (nonsyphilitic) 441.9
    abdominal 441.4
      dissecting 441.02
      ruptured 441.3
      syphilitic 093.0
    arch 441.2
      ruptured 441.1
    arteriosclerotic NEC 441.9
      ruptured 441.5
    ascending 441.2
      ruptured 441.1
    congenital 747.29
    descending 441.9
      abdominal 441.4
        ruptured 441.3
      ruptured 441.5
      thoracic 441.2
        ruptured 441.1
    dissecting 441.00
      abdominal 441.02
      thoracic 441.01
      thoracoabdominal 441.03
    due to coarctation (aorta) 747.10
    ruptured 441.5
    sinus, right 747.29
    syphilitic 093.0
    thoracoabdominal 441.7
      ruptured 441.6

Aneurysm — *continued*
  aorta, aortic — *continued*
    thorax, thoracic (arch) (nonsyphilitic) 441.2
      dissecting 441.01
      ruptured 441.1
      syphilitic 093.0
    transverse 441.2
      ruptured 441.1
    valve (heart) (*see also* Endocarditis, aortic)
      424.1
  arteriosclerotic NEC 442.9
    cerebral 437.3
      ruptured (*see also* Hemorrhage,
        subarachnoid) 430
  arteriovenous (congenital) (peripheral) NEC (*see
    also* Anomaly, arteriovenous) 747.60
    acquired NEC 447.0
      brain 437.3
        ruptured (*see also* Hemorrhage
          subarachnoid) 430
      coronary 414.11
      pulmonary 417.0
    brain (cerebral) 747.81
      ruptured (*see also* Hemorrhage,
        subarachnoid) 430
    coronary 746.85
    pulmonary 747.3
    retina 743.58
    specified site NEC 747.89
      acquired 447.0
    traumatic (*see also* Injury, blood vessel, by
      site) 904.9
  basal — *see* Aneurysm, brain
  berry (congenital) (ruptured) (*see also*
    Hemorrhage, subarachnoid) 430
  brain 437.3
    arteriosclerotic 437.3
      ruptured (*see also* Hemorrhage,
        subarachnoid) 430
    arteriovenous 747.81
      acquired 437.3
        ruptured (*see also* Hemorrhage,
          subarachnoid) 430
      ruptured (*see also* Hemorrhage,
        subarachnoid) 430
    berry (congenital) (ruptured) (*see also*
      Hemorrhage, subarachnoid) 430
    congenital 747.81
      ruptured (*see also* Hemorrhage,
        subarachnoid) 430
    meninges 437.3
      ruptured (*see also* Hemorrhage,
        subarachnoid) 430
    miliary (congenital) (ruptured) (*see also*
      Hemorrhage, subarachnoid) 430
    mycotic 421.0
      ruptured (*see also* Hemorrhage,
        subarachnoid) 430
    nonruptured 437.3
    ruptured (*See also* Hemorrhage,
      subarachnoid) 430
    syphilitic 094.87
    syphilitic (hemorrhage) 094.87
    traumatic — *see* Injury, intracranial
  cardiac (false) (*see also* Aneurysm, heart)
    414.10
  carotid artery (common) (external) 442.81
    internal (intracranial portion) 437.3
      extracranial portion 442.81
      ruptured into brain (*see also*
        Hemorrhage, subarachnoid) 430
    syphilitic 093.89
      intracranial 094.87
  cavernous sinus (*see also* Aneurysm, brain)
    437.3
    arteriovenous 747.81
      ruptured (*see also* Hemorrhage,
        subarachnoid) 430
    congenital 747.81
      ruptured (*see also* Hemorrhage,
        subarachnoid) 430
  celiac 442.84
  central nervous system, syphilitic 094.89
  cerebral — *see* Aneurysm, brain
  chest — *see* Aneurysm, thorax

Aneurysm — *continued*
  circle of Willis (*see also* Aneurysm, brain) 437.3
    congenital 747.81
      ruptured (*see also* Hemorrhage,
        subarachnoid) 430
    ruptured (*see also* Hemorrhage,
      subarachnoid) 430
  common iliac artery 442.2
  congenital (peripheral) NEC 747.60
    brain 747.81
      ruptured (*see also* Hemorrhage,
        subarachnoid) 430
    cerebral — *see* Aneurysm, brain, congenital
    coronary 746.85
    gastrointestinal 747.61
    lower limb 747.64
    pulmonary 747.3
    renal 747.62
    retina 743.58
    specified site NEC 747.89
    spinal 747.82
    upper limb 747.63
  conjunctiva 372.74
  conus arteriosus (*see also* Aneurysm, heart)
    414.10
  coronary (arteriosclerotic) (artery) (vein) (*see
    also* Aneurysm, heart) 414.11
    arteriovenous 746.85
    congenital 746.85
    syphilitic 093.89
  cylindrical 441.9
    ruptured 441.5
    syphilitic 093.9
  dissecting 442.9
    aorta (any part) 441.00
      abdominal 441.02
      thoracic 441.01
      thoracoabdominal 441.03
    syphilitic 093.9
  ductus arteriosus 747.0
  embolic — *see* Embolism, artery
  endocardial, infective (any valve) 421.0
  femoral 442.3
  gastroduodenal 442.84
  gastroepiploic 442.84
  heart (chronic or with a stated duration of over
    8 weeks) (infectional) (wall) 414.10
    acute or with a stated duration of 8 weeks
      or less (*see also* Infarct, myocardium)
      410.9 ☑
    congenital 746.89
    valve — *see* Endocarditis
  hepatic 442.84
  iliac (common) 442.2
  infective (any valve) 421.0
  innominate (nonsyphilitic) 442.89
    syphilitic 093.89
  interauricular septum (*see also* Aneurysm,
    heart) 414.10
  interventricular septum (*see also* Aneurysm,
    heart) 414.10
  intracranial — *see* Aneurysm, brain
  intrathoracic (nonsyphilitic) 441.2
    ruptured 441.1
    syphilitic 093.0
  jugular vein 453.8
  lower extremity 442.3
  lung (pulmonary artery) 417.1
  malignant 093.9
  mediastinal (nonsyphilitic) 442.89
    syphilitic 093.89
  miliary (congenital) (ruptured) (*see also*
    Hemorrhage, subarachnoid) 430
  mitral (heart) (valve) 424.0
  mural (arteriovenous) (heart) (*see also*
    Aneurysm, heart) 414.10
  mycotic, any site 421.0
    ruptured, brain (*see also* Hemorrhage,
      subarachnoid) 430
  myocardium (*see also* Aneurysm, heart) 414.10
  neck 442.81
  pancreaticoduodenal 442.84
  patent ductus arteriosus 747.0
  peripheral NEC 442.89
    congenital NEC (*see also* Aneurysm,
      congenital) 747.60
  popliteal 442.3

☑ Additional Digit Required   ▶◀ Revised Text   ● New Line   ▲ Revised Code

Aneurysm — *continued*
pulmonary 417.1
  arteriovenous 747.3
    acquired 417.0
  syphilitic 093.89
  valve (heart) (*see also* Endocarditis,
    pulmonary) 424.3
racemose 442.9
  congenital (peripheral) NEC 747.60
radial 442.0
Rasmussen's (*see also* Tuberculosis) 011.2 ☑
renal 442.1
retinal (acquired) 362.17
  congenital 743.58
  diabetic 250.5 ☑ *[362.01]*
sinus, aortic (of Valsalva) 747.29
specified site NEC 442.89
spinal (cord) 442.89
  congenital 747.82
  syphilitic (hemorrhage) 094.89
spleen, splenic 442.83
subclavian 442.82
  syphilitic 093.89
superior mesenteric 442.84
syphilitic 093.9
  aorta 093.0
  central nervous system 094.89
  congenital 090.5
  spine, spinal 094.89
thoracoabdominal 441.7
  ruptured 441.6
thorax, thoracic (arch) (nonsyphilitic) 441.2
  dissecting 441.0 ☑
  ruptured 441.1
  syphilitic 093.0
traumatic (complication) (early) — *see* Injury,
  blood vessel, by site
tricuspid (heart) (valve) — *see* Endocarditis,
  tricuspid
ulnar 442.0
upper extremity 442.0
valve, valvular — *see* Endocarditis
venous 456.8
  congenital NEC (*see also* Aneurysm,
    congenital) 747.60
ventricle (arteriovenous) (*see also* Aneurysm,
  heart) 414.10
visceral artery NEC 442.84
Angiectasis 459.89
Angiectopia 459.9
Angiitis 447.6
allergic granulomatous 446.4
hypersensitivity 446.20
  Goodpasture's syndrome 446.21
  specified NEC 446.29
necrotizing 446.0
Wegener's (necrotizing respiratory
  granulomatosis) 446.4
Angina (attack) (cardiac) (chest) (effort) (heart)
  (pectoris) (syndrome) (vasomotor) 413.9
abdominal 557.1
accelerated 411.1
agranulocytic 288.0
aphthous 074.0
catarrhal 462
crescendo 411.1
croupous 464.4
cruris 443.9
  due to atherosclerosis NEC (*see also*
    Arteriosclerosis, extremities) 440.20
decubitus 413.0
diphtheritic (membranous) 032.0
erysipelatous 034.0
erythematous 462
exudative, chronic 476.0
faucium 478.29
gangrenous 462
  diphtheritic 032.0
infectious 462
initial 411.1
intestinal 557.1
ludovici 528.3
Ludwig's 528.3
malignant 462
  diphtheritic 032.0

Angina — *continued*
membranous 464.4
  diphtheritic 032.0
mesenteric 557.1
monocytic 075
nocturnal 413.0
phlegmonous 475
  diphtheritic 032.0
preinfarctional 411.1
Prinzmetal's 413.1
progressive 411.1
pseudomembranous 101
psychogenic 306.2
pultaceous, diphtheritic 032.0
scarlatinal 034.1
septic 034.0
simple 462
stable NEC 413.9
staphylococcal 462
streptococcal 034.0
stridulous, diphtheritic 032.3
syphilitic 093.9
  congenital 090.5
tonsil 475
trachealis 464.4
unstable 411.1
variant 413.1
Vincent's 101
Angioblastoma (M9161/1) — *see* Neoplasm,
  connective tissue, uncertain behavior
Angiocholecystitis (*see also* Cholecystitis, acute)
  575.0
Angiocholitis (*see also* Cholecystitis, acute) 576.1
Angiodysgensis spinalis 336.1
Angiodysplasia (intestinalis) (intestine) 569.84
with hemorrhage 569.85
duodenum 537.82
  with hemorrhage 537.83
stomach 537.82
  with hemorrhage 537.83
Angioedema (allergic) (any site) (with urticaria)
  995.1
hereditary 277.6
Angioendothelioma (M9130/1) — *see also*
  Neoplasm, by site, uncertain behavior
benign (M9130/0) (*see also* Hemangioma, by
  site) 228.00
bone (M9260/3) — *see* Neoplasm, bone,
  malignant
Ewing's (M9260/3) — *see* Neoplasm, bone,
  malignant
nervous system (M9130/0) 228.09
Angiofibroma (M9160/0) — *see also* Neoplasm,
  by site, benign
juvenile (M9160/0) 210.7
  specified site — *see* Neoplasm, by site,
    benign
  unspecified site 210.7
Angiohemophilia (A) (B) 286.4
Angioid streaks (choroid) (retina) 363.43
Angiokeratoma (M9141/0) — *see also* Neoplasm,
  skin, benign
corporis diffusum 272.7
Angiokeratosis
diffuse 272.7
Angioleiomyoma (M8894/0) — *see* Neoplasm,
  connective tissue, benign
Angioleucitis 683
Angiolipoma (M8861/0) (*see also* Lipoma, by site)
  214.9
infiltrating (M8861/1) — *see* Neoplasm,
  connective tissue, uncertain behavior
Angioma (M9120/0) (*see also* Hemangioma, by
  site) 228.00
capillary 448.1
hemorrhagicum hereditaria 448.0
malignant (M9120/3) — *see* Neoplasm,
  connective tissue, malignant
pigmentosum et atrophicum 757.33
placenta — *see* Placenta, abnormal
plexiform (M9131/0) — *see* Hemangioma, by
  site
senile 448.1
serpiginosum 709.1

Angioma (M9120/0) (*see also* Hemangioma, by
  site) — *continued*
spider 448.1
stellate 448.1
Angiomatosis 757.32
bacillary 083.8
corporis diffusum universale 272.7
cutaneocerebral 759.6
encephalocutaneous 759.6
encephalofacial 759.6
encephalotrigeminal 759.6
hemorrhagic familial 448.0
hereditary familial 448.0
heredofamilial 448.0
meningo-oculofacial 759.6
multiple sites 228.09
neuro-oculocutaneous 759.6
retina (Hippel's disease) 759.6
retinocerebellosa 759.6
retinocerebral 759.6
systemic 228.09
Angiomyolipoma (M8860/0)
specified site — *see* Neoplasm, connective
  tissue, benign
unspecified site 223.0
Angiomyoliposarcoma (M8860/3) — *see*
  Neoplasm, connective tissue, malignant
Angiomyoma (M8894/0) — *see* Neoplasm,
  connective tissue, benign
Angiomyosarcoma (M8894/3) — *see* Neoplasm,
  connective tissue, malignant
Angioneurosis 306.2
Angioneurotic edema (allergic) (any site) (with
  urticaria) 995.1
hereditary 277.6
Angiopathia, angiopathy 459.9
diabetic (peripheral) 250.7 ☑ *[443.81]*
peripheral 443.9
  diabetic 250.7 ☑ *[443.81]*
  specified type NEC 443.89
retinae syphilitica 093.89
retinalis (juvenilis) 362.18
  background 362.10
  diabetic 250.5 ☑ *[362.01]*
  proliferative 362.29
  tuberculous (*see also* Tuberculosis) 017.3 ☑
    [362.18]
Angiosarcoma (M9120/3) — *see* Neoplasm,
  connective tissue, malignant
Angiosclerosis — *see* Arteriosclerosis
Angioscotoma, enlarged 368.42
Angiospasm 443.9
brachial plexus 353.0
cerebral 435.9
cervical plexus 353.2
nerve
  arm 354.9
    axillary 353.0
    median 354.1
    ulnar 354.2
  autonomic (*see also* Neuropathy, peripheral,
    autonomic) 337.9
  axillary 353.0
  leg 355.8
    plantar 355.6
  lower extremity — *see* Angiospasm, nerve,
    leg
  median 354.1
  peripheral NEC 355.9
  spinal NEC 355.9
  sympathetic (*see also* Neuropathy,
    peripheral, autonomic) 337.9
  ulnar 354.2
  upper extremity — *see* Angiospasm, nerve,
    arm
peripheral NEC 443.9
traumatic 443.9
  foot 443.9
  leg 443.9
vessel 443.9
Angiospastic disease or edema 443.9
Angle's   ●
class I 524.21   ●
class II 524.22   ●

Aneurysm — Angle's

☑ Additional Digit Required   ►◄ Revised Text   ● New Line   ▲ Revised Code

Angle's — continued
    class III 524.23   ●
Anguillulosis 127.2
Angulation
    cecum (see also Obstruction, intestine) 560.9
    coccyx (acquired) 738.6
        congenital 756.19
    femur (acquired) 736.39
        congenital 755.69
    intestine (large) (small) (see also Obstruction,
        intestine) 560.9
    sacrum (acquired) 738.5
        congenital 756.19
    sigmoid (flexure) (see also Obstruction,
        intestine) 560.9
    spine (see also Curvature, spine) 737.9
    tibia (acquired) 736.89
        congenital 755.69
    ureter 593.3
    wrist (acquired) 736.09
        congenital 755.59
Angulus infectiosus 686.8
Anhedonia 302.72
Anhidrosis (lid) (neurogenic) (thermogenic) 705.0
Anhydration 276.5
    with
        hypernatremia 276.0
        hyponatremia 276.1
Anhydremia 276.5
    with
        hypernatremia 276.0
        hyponatremia 276.1
Anidrosis 705.0
Aniridia (congenital) 743.45
Anisakiasis (infection) (infestation) 127.1
Anisakis larva infestation 127.1
Aniseikonia 367.32
Anisocoria (pupil) 379.41
    congenital 743.46
Anisocytosis 790.09
Anisometropia (congenital) 367.31
Ankle — see condition
Ankyloblepharon (acquired) (eyelid) 374.46
    filiforme (adnatum) (congenital) 743.62
    total 743.62
Ankylodactly (see also Syndactylism) 755.10
Ankyloglossia 750.0
Ankylosis (fibrous) (osseous) 718.50
    ankle 718.57
    any joint, produced by surgical fusion V45.4
    cricoarytenoid (cartilage) (joint) (larynx) 478.79
    dental 521.6
    ear ossicle NEC 385.22
        malleus 385.21
    elbow 718.52
    finger 718.54
    hip 718.55
    incostapedial joint (infectional) 385.22
    joint, produced by surgical fusion NEC V45.4
    knee 718.56
    lumbosacral (joint) 724.6
    malleus 385.21
    multiple sites 718.59
    postoperative (status) V45.4
    sacroiliac (joint) 724.6
    shoulder 718.51
    specified site NEC 718.58
    spine NEC 724.9
    surgical V45.4
    teeth, tooth (hard tissues) 521.6
    temporomandibular joint 524.61
    wrist 718.53
Ankylostoma — see Ancylostoma
Ankylostomiasis (intestinal) — see
    Ancylostomiasis
Ankylurethria (see also Stricture, urethra) 598.9
Annular — see also condition
    detachment, cervix 622.8
    organ or site, congenital NEC — see Distortion
    pancreas (congenital) 751.7
Anodontia (complete) (partial) (vera) 520.0
    with abnormal spacing 524.30   ▲

Anodontia — continued
    acquired 525.10
        causing malocclusion 524.30   ▲
        due to
            caries 525.13
            extraction 525.10
            periodontal disease 525.12
            trauma 525.11
Anomaly, anomalous (congenital) (unspecified
    type) 759.9
    abdomen 759.9
    abdominal wall 756.70
    acoustic nerve 742.9
    adrenal (gland) 759.1
    Alder (-Reilly) (leukocyte granulation) 288.2
    alimentary tract 751.9
        lower 751.5
        specified type NEC 751.8
        upper (any part, except tongue) 750.9
            tongue 750.10
                specified type NEC 750.19
    alveolar 524.70   ▲
        ridge (process) 525.8   ●
        specified NEC 524.79   ●
    ankle (joint) 755.69
    anus, anal (canal) 751.5
    aorta, aortic 747.20
        arch 747.21
        coarctation (postductal) (preductal) 747.10
        cusp or valve NEC 746.9
        septum 745.0
        specified type NEC 747.29
    aorticopulmonary septum 745.0
    apertures, diaphragm 756.6
    appendix 751.5
    aqueduct of Sylvius 742.3
        with spina bifida (see also Spina bifida)
            741.0 ☑
    arm 755.50
        reduction (see also Deformity, reduction,
            upper limb) 755.20
    arteriovenous (congenital) (peripheral) NEC
        747.60
        brain 747.81
        cerebral 747.81
        coronary 746.85
        gastrointestinal 747.61
        lower limb 747.64
        renal 747.62
        specified site NEC 747.69
        spinal 747.82
        upper limb 747.63
    artery (see also Anomaly, peripheral vascular
        system) NEC 747.60
        brain 747.81
        cerebral 747.81
        coronary 746.85
        eye 743.9
        pulmonary 747.3
        renal 747.62
        retina 743.9
        umbilical 747.5
    arytenoepiglottic folds 748.3
    atrial
        bands 746.9
        folds 746.9
        septa 745.5
    atrioventricular
        canal 745.69
        common 745.69
        conduction 426.7
        excitation 426.7
        septum 745.4
    atrium — see Anomaly, atrial
    auditory canal 744.3
        specified type NEC 744.29
            with hearing impairment 744.02
    auricle
        ear 744.3
            causing impairment of hearing 744.02
        heart 746.9
            septum 745.5
    autosomes, autosomal NEC 758.5
    Axenfeld's 743.44
    back 759.9

Anomaly, anomalous — continued
    band
        atrial 746.9
        heart 746.9
        ventricular 746.9
    Bartholin's duct 750.9
    biliary duct or passage 751.60
        atresia 751.61
    bladder (neck) (sphincter) (trigone) 753.9
        specified type NEC 753.8
    blood vessel 747.9
        artery — see Anomaly, artery
        peripheral vascular — see Anomaly,
            peripheral vascular system
        vein — see Anomaly, vein
    bone NEC 756.9
        ankle 755.69
        arm 755.50
        chest 756.3
        cranium 756.0
        face 756.0
        finger 755.50
        foot 755.67
        forearm 755.50
        frontal 756.0
        head 756.0
        hip 755.63
        leg 755.60
        lumbosacral 756.10
        nose 748.1
        pelvic girdle 755.60
        rachitic 756.4
        rib 756.3
        shoulder girdle 755.50
        skull 756.0
            with
                anencephalus 740.0
                encephalocele 742.0
                hydrocephalus 742.3
                    with spina bifida (see also Spina
                        bifida) 741.0 ☑
                microcephalus 742.1
        toe 755.66
    brain 742.9
        multiple 742.4
        reduction 742.2
        specified type NEC 742.4
        vessel 747.81
    branchial cleft NEC 744.49
        cyst 744.42
        fistula 744.41
        persistent 744.41
        sinus (external) (internal) 744.41
    breast 757.9
    broad ligament 752.10
        specified type NEC 752.19
    bronchus 748.3
    bulbar septum 745.0
    bulbus cordis 745.9
        persistent (in left ventricle) 745.8
    bursa 756.9
    canal of Nuck 752.9
    canthus 743.9
    capillary NEC (see also Anomaly, peripheral
        vascular system) 747.60
    cardiac 746.9
        septal closure 745.9
            acquired 429.71
        valve NEC 746.9
            pulmonary 746.00
            specified type NEC 746.89
    cardiovascular system 746.9
        complicating pregnancy, childbirth, or
            puerperium 648.5 ☑
    carpus 755.50
    cartilage, trachea 748.3
    cartilaginous 756.9
    caruncle, lacrimal, lachrymal 743.9
    cascade stomach 750.7
    cauda equina 742.59
    cecum 751.5
    cerebral — see also Anomaly, brain vessels
        747.81
    cerebrovascular system 747.81
    cervix (uterus) 752.40
        with doubling of vagina and uterus 752.2

☑ Additional Digit Required   ►◄ Revised Text   ● New Line   ▲ Revised Code

Anomaly, anomalous — *continued*
cervix — *continued*
in pregnancy or childbirth 654.6 ☑
affecting fetus or newborn 763.89
causing obstructed labor 660.2 ☑
affecting fetus or newborn 763.1
Chédiak-Higashi (-Steinbrinck) (congenital
gigantism of peroxidase granules) 288.2
cheek 744.9
chest (wall) 756.3
chin 744.9
specified type NEC 744.89
chordae tendineae 746.9
choroid 743.9
plexus 742.9
chromosomes, chromosomal 758.9
13 (13-15) 758.1
18 (16-18) 758.2
21 or 22 758.0
autosomes NEC (*see also* Abnormality,
autosomes) 758.5
deletion 758.39 ▲
Christchurch 758.39 ▲
D₁ 758.1
E₃ 758.2
G 758.0
mitochondrial 758.9
mosaics 758.89
sex 758.81
complement, XO 758.6
complement, XXX 758.81
complement, XXY 758.7
complement, XYY 758.81
gonadal dysgenesis 758.6
Klinefelter's 758.7
Turner's 758.6
trisomy 21 758.0
cilia 743.9
circulatory system 747.9
specified type NEC 747.89
clavicle 755.51
clitoris 752.40
coccyx 756.10
colon 751.5
common duct 751.60
communication
coronary artery 746.85
left ventricle with right atrium 745.4
concha (ear) 744.3
connection
renal vessels with kidney 747.62
total pulmonary venous 747.41
connective tissue 756.9
specified type NEC 756.89
cornea 743.9
shape 743.41
size 743.41
specified type NEC 743.49
coronary
artery 746.85
vein 746.89
cranium — *see* Anomaly, skull
cricoid cartilage 748.3
cushion, endocardial 745.60
specified type NEC 745.69
cystic duct 751.60
dental arch relationship 524.20 ▲
angle's class I 524.21 ●
angle's class II 524.22 ●
angle's class III 524.23 ●
articulation ●
anterior 524.27 ●
posterior 524.27 ●
reverse 524.27 ●
disto-occlusion 524.22 ●
division I 524.22 ●
division II 524.22 ●
excessive horizontal overlap 524.26 ●
interarch distance (excessive)
(inadequate) 524.28 ●
mesio-occlusion 524.23 ●
neutro-occlusion 524.21 ●
open ●
anterior occlusal relationship 524.24 ●
posterior occlusal relationship 524.25 ●
specified NEC 524.29 ●
dentition 520.6

Anomaly, anomalous — *continued*
dentofacial NEC 524.9
functional 524.50 ▲
specified type NEC 524.89 ▲
dermatoglyphic 757.2
Descemet's membrane 743.9
specified type NEC 743.49
development
cervix 752.40
vagina 752.40
vulva 752.40
diaphragm, diaphragmatic (apertures) NEC
756.6
digestive organ(s) or system 751.9
lower 751.5
specified type NEC 751.8
upper 750.9
distribution, coronary artery 746.85
ductus
arteriosus 747.0
Botalli 747.0
duodenum 751.5
dura 742.9
brain 742.4
spinal cord 742.59
ear 744.3
causing impairment of hearing 744.00
specified type NEC 744.09
external 744.3
causing impairment of hearing 744.02
specified type NEC 744.29
inner (causing impairment of hearing)
744.05
middle, except ossicles (causing impairment
of hearing) 744.03
ossicles 744.04
ossicles 744.04
prominent auricle 744.29
specified type NEC 744.29
with hearing impairment 744.09
Ebstein's (heart) 746.2
tricuspid valve 746.2
ectodermal 757.9
Eisenmenger's (ventricular septal defect) 745.4
ejaculatory duct 752.9
specified type NEC 752.89
elbow (joint) 755.50
endocardial cushion 745.60
specified type NEC 745.69
endocrine gland NEC 759.2
epididymis 752.9
epiglottis 748.3
esophagus 750.9
specified type NEC 750.4
Eustachian tube 744.3
specified type NEC 744.24
eye (any part) 743.9
adnexa 743.9
specified type NEC 743.69
anophthalmos 743.00
anterior
chamber and related structures 743.9
angle 743.9
specified type NEC 743.44
specified type NEC 743.44
segment 743.9
combined 743.48
multiple 743.48
specified type NEC 743.49
cataract (*see also* Cataract) 743.30
glaucoma (*see also* Buphthalmia) 743.20
lid 743.9
specified type NEC 743.63
microphthalmos (*see also* Microphthalmos)
743.10
posterior segment 743.9
specified type NEC 743.59
vascular 743.58
vitreous 743.9
specified type NEC 743.51
ptosis (eyelid) 743.61
retina 743.9
specified type NEC 743.59
sclera 743.9
specified type NEC 743.47
specified type NEC 743.8
eyebrow 744.89

Anomaly, anomalous — *continued*
eyelid 743.9
specified type NEC 743.63
face (any part) 744.9
bone(s) 756.0
specified type NEC 744.89
fallopian tube 752.10
specified type NEC 752.19
fascia 756.9
specified type NEC 756.89
femur 755.60
fibula 755.60
finger 755.50
supernumerary 755.01
webbed (*see also* Syndactylism, fingers)
755.11
fixation, intestine 751.4
flexion (joint) 755.9
hip or thigh (*see also* Dislocation, hip,
congenital) 754.30
folds, heart 746.9
foot 755.67
foramen
Botalli 745.5
ovale 745.5
forearm 755.50
forehead (*see also* Anomaly, skull) 756.0
form, teeth 520.2
fovea centralis 743.9
frontal bone (*see also* Anomaly, skull) 756.0
gallbladder 751.60
Gartner's duct 752.11
gastrointestinal tract 751.9
specified type NEC 751.8
vessel 747.61
genitalia, genital organ(s) or system
female 752.9
external 752.40
specified type NEC 752.49
internal NEC 752.9
male (external and internal) 752.9
epispadias 752.62
hidden penis 752.65
hydrocele, congenital 778.6
hypospadias 752.61
micropenis 752.64
testis, undescended 752.51
retractile 752.52
specified type NEC 752.89
genitourinary NEC 752.9
Gerbode 745.4
globe (eye) 743.9
glottis 748.3
granulation or granulocyte, genetic 288.2
constitutional 288.2
leukocyte 288.2
gum 750.9
gyri 742.9
hair 757.9
specified type NEC 757.4
hand 755.50
hard tissue formation in pulp 522.3
head (*see also* Anomaly, skull) 756.0
heart 746.9
auricle 746.9
bands 746.9
fibroelastosis cordis 425.3
folds 746.9
malposition 746.87
maternal, affecting fetus or newborn 760.3
obstructive NEC 746.84
patent ductus arteriosus (Botalli) 747.0
septum 745.9
acquired 429.71
aortic 745.0
aorticopulmonary 745.0
atrial 745.5
auricular 745.5
between aorta and pulmonary artery
745.0
endocardial cushion type 745.60
specified type NEC 745.69
interatrial 745.5

☑ Additional Digit Required ▶◀ Revised Text ● New Line ▲ Revised Code

Anomaly, anomalous — *continued*
  heart — *continued*
    septum — *continued*
      interventricular 745.4
        with pulmonary stenosis or atresia,
          dextraposition of aorta, and
          hypertrophy of right ventricle
          745.2
        acquired 429.71
      specified type NEC 745.8
      ventricular 745.4
        with pulmonary stenosis or atresia,
          dextraposition of aorta, and
          hypertrophy of right ventricle
          745.2
        acquired 429.71
    specified type NEC 746.89
    tetralogy of Fallot 745.2
    valve NEC 746.9
      aortic 746.9
        atresia 746.89
        bicuspid valve 746.4
        insufficiency 746.4
        specified type NEC 746.89
        stenosis 746.3
          subaortic 746.81
          supravalvular 747.22
      mitral 746.9
        atresia 746.89
        insufficiency 746.6
        specified type NEC 746.89
        stenosis 746.5
      pulmonary 746.00
        atresia 746.01
        insufficiency 746.09
        stenosis 746.02
          infundibular 746.83
          subvalvular 746.83
      tricuspid 746.9
        atresia 746.1
        stenosis 746.1
    ventricle 746.9
  heel 755.67
  Hegglin's 288.2
  hemianencephaly 740.0
  hemicephaly 740.0
  hemicrania 740.0
  hepatic duct 751.60
  hip (joint) 755.63
  hourglass
    bladder 753.8
    gallbladder 751.69
    stomach 750.7
  humerus 755.50
  hymen 752.40
  hypersegmentation of neutrophils, hereditary
    288.2
  hypophyseal 759.2
  ileocecal (coil) (valve) 751.5
  ileum (intestine) 751.5
  ilium 755.60
  integument 757.9
    specified type NEC 757.8
  interarch distance (excessive) (inadequate) ●
    524.28 ●
  intervertebral cartilage or disc 756.10
  intestine (large) (small) 751.5
    fixational type 751.4
  iris 743.9
    specified type NEC 743.46
  ischium 755.60
  jaw NEC 524.9
    closure 524.51 ▲
    size (major) NEC 524.00
    specified type NEC 524.89 ▲
  jaw-cranial base relationship 524.10
    specified NEC 524.19
  jejunum 751.5
  joint 755.9
    hip
      dislocation (*see also* Dislocation, hip,
        congenital) 754.30
      predislocation (*see also* Subluxation,
        congenital, hip) 754.32
      preluxation (*see also* Subluxation,
        congenital, hip) 754.32

Anomaly, anomalous — *continued*
  joint — *continued*
    hip — *continued*
      subluxation (*see also* Subluxation,
        congenital, hip) 754.32
    lumbosacral 756.10
      spondylolisthesis 756.12
      spondylosis 756.11
    multiple arthrogryposis 754.89
    sacroiliac 755.69
  Jordan's 288.2
  kidney(s) (calyx) (pelvis) 753.9
    vessel 747.62
  Klippel-Feil (brevicollis) 756.16
  knee (joint) 755.64
  labium (majus) (minus) 752.40
  labyrinth, membranous (causing impairment of
    hearing) 744.05
  lacrimal
    apparatus, duct or passage 743.9
      specified type NEC 743.65
    gland 743.9
      specified type NEC 743.64
  Langdon Down (mongolism) 758.0
  larynx, laryngeal (muscle) 748.3
    web, webbed 748.2
  leg (lower) (upper) 755.60
    reduction NEC (*see also* Deformity,
      reduction, lower limb) 755.30
  lens 743.9
    shape 743.36
    specified type NEC 743.39
  leukocytes, genetic 288.2
    granulation (constitutional) 288.2
  lid (fold) 743.9
  ligament 756.9
    broad 752.10
    round 752.9
  limb, except reduction deformity 755.9
    lower 755.60
      reduction deformity (*see also* Deformity,
        reduction, lower limb) 755.30
      specified type NEC 755.69
    upper 755.50
      reduction deformity (*see also* Deformity,
        reduction, upper limb) 755.20
      specified type NEC 755.59
  lip 750.9
    harelip (*see also* Cleft, lip) 749.10
    specified type NEC 750.26
  liver (duct) 751.60
    atresia 751.69
  lower extremity 755.60
    vessel 747.64
  lumbosacral (joint) (region) 756.10
  lung (fissure) (lobe) NEC 748.60
    agenesis 748.5
    specified type NEC 748.69
  lymphatic system 759.9
  Madelung's (radius) 755.54
  mandible 524.9
    size NEC 524.00
  maxilla 524.9
    size NEC 524.00
  May (-Hegglin) 288.2
  meatus urinarius 753.9
    specified type NEC 753.8
  meningeal bands or folds, constriction of 742.8
  meninges 742.9
    brain 742.4
    spinal 742.59
  meningocele (*see also* Spina bifida) 741.9 ☑
  mesentery 751.9
  metacarpus 755.50
  metatarsus 755.67
  middle ear, except ossicles (causing impairment
    of hearing) 744.03
    ossicles 744.04
  mitral (leaflets) (valve) 746.9
    atresia 746.89
    insufficiency 746.6
    specified type NEC 746.89
    stenosis 746.5
  mouth 750.9
    specified type NEC 750.26
  multiple NEC 759.7
    specified type NEC 759.89

Anomaly, anomalous — *continued*
  muscle 756.9
    eye 743.9
      specified type NEC 743.69
    specified type NEC 756.89
  musculoskeletal system, except limbs 756.9
    specified type NEC 756.9
  nail 757.9
    specified type NEC 757.5
  narrowness, eyelid 743.62
  nasal sinus or septum 748.1
  neck (any part) 744.9
    specified type NEC 744.89
  nerve 742.9
    acoustic 742.9
      specified type NEC 742.8
    optic 742.9
      specified type NEC 742.8
    specified type NEC 742.8
  nervous system NEC 742.9
    brain 742.9
      specified type NEC 742.4
    specified type NEC 742.8
  neurological 742.9
  nipple 757.6 ▲
  nonteratogenic NEC 754.89
  nose, nasal (bone) (cartilage) (septum) (sinus)
    748.1
  ocular muscle 743.9
  omphalomesenteric duct 751.0
  opening, pulmonary veins 747.49
  optic
    disc 743.9
      specified type NEC 743.57
    nerve 742.9
  opticociliary vessels 743.9
  orbit (eye) 743.9
    specified type NEC 743.66
  organ
    of Corti (causing impairment of hearing)
      744.05
    or site 759.9
      specified type NEC 759.89
  origin
    both great arteries from same ventricle
      745.11
    coronary artery 746.85
    innominate artery 747.69
    left coronary artery from pulmonary artery
      746.85
    pulmonary artery 747.3
    renal vessels 747.62
    subclavian artery (left) (right) 747.21
  osseous meatus (ear) 744.03
  ovary 752.0
  oviduct 752.10
  palate (hard) (soft) 750.9
    cleft (*see also* Cleft, palate) 749.00
  pancreas (duct) 751.7
  papillary muscles 746.9
  parathyroid gland 759.2
  paraurethral ducts 753.9
  parotid (gland) 750.9
  patella 755.64
  Pelger-Huët (hereditary hyposegmentation)
    288.2
  pelvic girdle 755.60
    specified type NEC 755.69
  pelvis (bony) 755.60
    complicating delivery 653.0 ☑
    rachitic 268.1
      fetal 756.4
  penis (glans) 752.69
  pericardium 746.89
  peripheral vascular system NEC 747.60
    gastrointestinal 747.61
    lower limb 747.64
    renal 747.62
    specified site NEC 747.69
    spinal 747.82
    upper limb 747.63
  Peter's 743.44
  pharynx 750.9
    branchial cleft 744.41
    specified type NEC 750.29
  Pierre Robin 756.0

Anomaly, anomalous

Anomaly, anomalous — *continued*
  pigmentation NEC 709.00
    congenital 757.33
  pituitary (gland) 759.2
  pleural folds 748.8
  portal vein 747.40
  position tooth, teeth 524.30 ▲
    crowding 524.31 ●
    displacement 524.30 ●
      horizontal 524.33 ●
      vertical 524.34 ●
    distance ●
      interocclusal ●
        excessive 524.37 ●
        insufficient 524.36 ●
    excessive spacing 524.32 ●
    rotation 524.35 ●
    specified NEC 524.39 ●
  preauricular sinus 744.46
  prepuce 752.9
  prostate 752.9
  pulmonary 748.60
    artery 747.3
    circulation 747.3
    specified type NEC 748.69
    valve 746.00
      atresia 746.01
      insufficiency 746.09
      specified type NEC 746.09
      stenosis 746.02
        infundibular 746.83
        subvalvular 746.83
    vein 747.40
    venous
      connection 747.49
        partial 747.42
        total 747.41
      return 747.49
        partial 747.42
        total (TAPVR) (complete)
          (subdiaphragmatic)
          (supradiaphrag-matic) 747.41
  pupil 743.9
  pylorus 750.9
    hypertrophy 750.5
    stenosis 750.5
  rachitic, fetal 756.4
  radius 755.50
  rectovaginal (septum) 752.40
  rectum 751.5
  refraction 367.9
  renal 753.9
    vessel 747.62
  respiratory system 748.9
    specified type NEC 748.8
  rib 756.3
    cervical 756.2
  Rieger's 743.44
  rings, trachea 748.3
  rotation — *see also* Malrotation
    hip or thigh (*see also* Subluxation,
      congenital, hip) 754.32
  round ligament 752.9
  sacroiliac (joint) 755.69
  sacrum 756.10
  saddle
    back 754.2
    nose 754.0
      syphilitic 090.5
  salivary gland or duct 750.9
    specified type NEC 750.26
  scapula 755.50
  sclera 743.9
    specified type NEC 743.47
  scrotum 752.9
  sebaceous gland 757.9
  seminal duct or tract 752.9
  sense organs 742.9
    specified type NEC 742.8
  septum
    heart — *see* Anomaly, heart, septum
    nasal 748.1
  sex chromosomes NEC (*see also* Anomaly,
    chromosomes) 758.81
  shoulder (girdle) (joint) 755.50
    specified type NEC 755.59
  sigmoid (flexure) 751.5

Anomaly, anomalous — *continued*
  sinus of Valsalva 747.29
  site NEC 759.9
  skeleton generalized NEC 756.50
  skin (appendage) 757.9
    specified type NEC 757.39
  skull (bone) 756.0
    with
      anencephalus 740.0
      encephalocele 742.0
      hydrocephalus 742.3
        with spina bifida (*see also* Spina
          bifida) 741.0 ☑
      microcephalus 742.1
  specified type NEC
    adrenal (gland) 759.1
    alimentary tract (complete) (partial) 751.8
      lower 751.5
      upper 750.8
    ankle 755.69
    anus, anal (canal) 751.5
    aorta, aortic 747.29
      arch 747.21
    appendix 751.5
    arm 755.59
    artery (peripheral) NEC (*see also* Anomaly,
      peripheral vascular system) 747.60
      brain 747.81
      coronary 746.85
      eye 743.58
      pulmonary 747.3
      retinal 743.58
      umbilical 747.5
    auditory canal 744.29
      causing impairment of hearing 744.02
    bile duct or passage 751.69
    bladder 753.8
      neck 753.8
    bone(s) 756.9
      arm 755.59
      face 756.0
      leg 755.69
      pelvic girdle 755.69
      shoulder girdle 755.59
      skull 756.0
        with
          anencephalus 740.0
          encephalocele 742.0
          hydrocephalus 742.3
            with spina bifida (*see also* Spina
              bifida) 741.0 ☑
          microcephalus 742.1
    brain 742.4
    breast 757.6
    broad ligament 752.19
    bronchus 748.3
    canal of Nuck 752.89
    cardiac septal closure 745.8
    carpus 755.59
    cartilaginous 756.9
    cecum 751.5
    cervix 752.49
    chest (wall) 756.3
    chin 744.89
    ciliary body 743.46
    circulatory system 747.89
    clavicle 755.51
    clitoris 752.49
    coccyx 756.19
    colon 751.5
    common duct 751.69
    connective tissue 756.89
    cricoid cartilage 748.3
    cystic duct 751.69
    diaphragm 756.6
    digestive organ(s) or tract 751.8
      lower 751.5
      upper 750.8
    duodenum 751.5
    ear 744.29
      auricle 744.29
        causing impairment of hearing 744.02
      causing impairment of hearing 744.09
      inner (causing impairment of hearing)
        744.05
      middle, except ossicles 744.03
        ossicles 744.04

Anomaly, anomalous — *continued*
  specified type — *continued*
    ejaculatory duct 752.89
    endocrine 759.2
    epiglottis 748.3
    esophagus 750.4
    Eustachian tube 744.24
    eye 743.8
      lid 743.63
      muscle 743.69
    face 744.89
      bone(s) 756.0
    fallopian tube 752.19
    fascia 756.89
    femur 755.69
    fibula 755.69
    finger 755.59
    foot 755.67
    fovea centralis 743.55
    gallbladder 751.69
    Gartner's duct 752.89
    gastrointestinal tract 751.8
    genitalia, genital organ(s)
      female 752.89
        external 752.49
        internal NEC 752.89
      male 752.89
        penis 752.69
        scrotal transposition 752.81
    genitourinary tract NEC 752.89
    glottis 748.3
    hair 757.4
    hand 755.59
    heart 746.89
      valve NEC 746.89
        pulmonary 746.09
    hepatic duct 751.69
    hydatid of Morgagni 752.89
    hymen 752.49
    integument 757.8
    intestine (large) (small) 751.5
      fixational type 751.4
    iris 743.46
    jejunum 751.5
    joint 755.8
    kidney 753.3
    knee 755.64
    labium (majus) (minus) 752.49
    labyrinth, membranous 744.05
    larynx 748.3
    leg 755.69
    lens 743.39
    limb, except reduction deformity 755.8
      lower 755.69
        reduction deformity (*see also*
          Deformity, reduction, lower limb)
          755.30
      upper 755.59
        reduction deformity (*see also*
          Deformity, reduction, upper
          limb) 755.20
    lip 750.26
    liver 751.69
    lung (fissure) (lobe) 748.69
    meatus urinarius 753.8
    metacarpus 755.59
    mouth 750.26
    muscle 756.89
      eye 743.69
    musculoskeletal system, except limbs 756.9
    nail 757.5
    neck 744.89
    nerve 742.8
      acoustic 742.8
      optic 742.8
    nervous system 742.8
    nipple 757.6
    nose 748.1
    organ NEC 759.89
      of Corti 744.05
    osseous meatus (ear) 744.03
    ovary 752.0
    oviduct 752.19
    pancreas 751.7
    parathyroid 759.2
    patella 755.64
    pelvic girdle 755.69

☑ Additional Digit Required   ▶◀ Revised Text   ● New Line   ▲ Revised Code

Anomaly, anomalous — *continued*
  specified type — *continued*
    penis 752.69
    pericardium 746.89
    peripheral vascular system NEC (*see also*
        Anomaly, peripheral vascular system)
        747.60
    pharynx 750.29
    pituitary 759.2
    prostate 752.89
    radius 755.59
    rectum 751.5
    respiratory system 748.8
    rib 756.3
    round ligament 752.89
    sacrum 756.19
    salivary duct or gland 750.26
    scapula 755.59
    sclera 743.47
    scrotum 752.89
      transposition 752.81
    seminal duct or tract 752.89
    shoulder girdle 755.59
    site NEC 759.89
    skin 757.39
    skull (bone(s)) 756.0
      with
        anencephalus 740.0
        encephalocele 742.0
        hydrocephalus 742.3
          with spina bifida (*see also* Spina
            bifida) 741.0 ☑
        microcephalus 742.1
  specified organ or site NEC 759.89
  spermatic cord 752.89
  spinal cord 742.59
  spine 756.19
  spleen 759.0
  sternum 756.3
  stomach 750.7
  tarsus 755.67
  tendon 756.89
  testis 752.89
  thorax (wall) 756.3
  thymus 759.2
  thyroid (gland) 759.2
    cartilage 748.3
  tibia 755.69
  toe 755.66
  tongue 750.19
  trachea (cartilage) 748.3
  ulna 755.59
  urachus 753.7
  ureter 753.4
    obstructive 753.29
  urethra 753.8
    obstructive 753.6
  urinary tract 753.8
  uterus 752.3
  uvula 750.26
  vagina 752.49
  vascular NEC (*see also* Anomaly, peripheral
    vascular system) 747.60
    brain 747.81
  vas deferens 752.89
  vein(s) (peripheral) NEC (*see also* Anomaly,
    peripheral vascular system) 747.60
    brain 747.81
    great 747.49
    portal 747.49
    pulmonary 747.49
    vena cava (inferior) (superior) 747.49
  vertebra 756.19
  vulva 752.49
  spermatic cord 752.9
  spine, spinal 756.10
    column 756.10
    cord 742.9
      meningocele (*see also* Spina bifida)
        741.9 ☑
      specified type NEC 742.59
      spina bifida (*see also* Spina bifida)
        741.9 ☑
      vessel 747.82
    meninges 742.59
    nerve root 742.9
  spleen 759.0

Anomaly, anomalous — *continued*
  Sprengel's 755.52
  sternum 756.3
  stomach 750.9
    specified type NEC 750.7
  submaxillary gland 750.9
  superior vena cava 747.40
  talipes — *see* Talipes
  tarsus 755.67
    with complete absence of distal elements
      755.31
  teeth, tooth NEC 520.9
    position 524.30   ▲
      crowding 524.31   ●
      displacement 524.30   ●
        horizontal 524.33   ●
        vertical 524.34   ●
      distance
        interocclusal
          excessive 524.37   ●
          insufficient 524.36   ●
      excessive spacing 524.32   ●
      rotation 524.35   ●
      specified NEC 524.39   ●
    spacing 524.30   ▲
  tendon 756.9
    specified type NEC 756.89
  termination
    coronary artery 746.85
  testis 752.9
  thebesian valve 746.9
  thigh 755.60
    flexion (*see also* Subluxation, congenital,
      hip) 754.32
  thorax (wall) 756.3
  throat 750.9
  thumb 755.50
    supernumerary 755.01
  thymus gland 759.2
  thyroid (gland) 759.2
    cartilage 748.3
  tibia 755.60
    saber 090.5
  toe 755.66
    supernumerary 755.02
    webbed (*see also* Syndactylism, toes) 755.13
  tongue 750.10
    specified type NEC 750.19
  trachea, tracheal 748.3
    cartilage 748.3
    rings 748.3
  tragus 744.3
  transverse aortic arch 747.21
  trichromata 368.59
  trichromatopsia 368.59
  tricuspid (leaflet) (valve) 746.9
    atresia 746.1
    Ebstein's 746.2
    specified type NEC 746.89
    stenosis 746.1
  trunk 759.9
  Uhl's (hypoplasia of myocardium, right
    ventricle) 746.84
  ulna 755.50
  umbilicus 759.9
    artery 747.5
  union, trachea with larynx 748.3
  unspecified site 759.9
  upper extremity 755.50
    vessel 747.63
  urachus 753.7
    specified type NEC 753.7
  ureter 753.9
    obstructive 753.20
    specified type NEC 753.4
      obstructive 753.29
  urethra (valve) 753.9
    obstructive 753.6
    specified type NEC 753.8
  urinary tract or system (any part, except
    urachus) 753.9
    specified type NEC 753.8
    urachus 753.7
  uterus 752.3
    with only one functioning horn 752.3

Anomaly, anomalous — *continued*
  uterus — *continued*
    in pregnancy or childbirth 654.0 ☑
      affecting fetus or newborn 763.89
      causing obstructed labor 660.2 ☑
        affecting fetus or newborn 763.1
  uvula 750.9
  vagina 752.40
  valleculae 748.3
  valve (heart) NEC 746.9
    formation, ureter 753.29
    pulmonary 746.00
    specified type NEC 746.89
  vascular NEC (*see also* Anomaly, peripheral
    vascular system) 747.60
    ring 747.21
  vas deferens 752.9
  vein(s) (peripheral) NEC (*see also* Anomaly,
    peripheral vascular system) 747.60
    brain 747.81
    cerebral 747.81
    coronary 746.89
    great 747.40
      specified type NEC 747.49
    portal 747.40
    pulmonary 747.40
    retina 743.9
  vena cava (inferior) (superior) 747.40
  venous return (pulmonary) 747.49
    partial 747.42
    total 747.41
  ventricle, ventricular (heart) 746.9
    bands 746.9
    folds 746.9
    septa 745.4
  vertebra 756.10
  vesicourethral orifice 753.9
  vessels NEC (*see also* Anomaly, peripheral
    vascular system) 747.60
    optic papilla 743.9
  vitelline duct 751.0
  vitreous humor 743.9
    specified type NEC 743.51
  vulva 752.49
  wrist (joint) 755.50

Anomia 784.69

Anonychia 757.5
  acquired 703.8

Anophthalmos, anophthalmus (clinical)
  (congenital) (globe) 743.00
  acquired V45.78

Anopsia (altitudinal) (quadrant) 368.46

Anorchia 752.89

Anorchism, anorchidism 752.89

Anorexia 783.0
  hysterical 300.11
  nervosa 307.1

Anosmia (*see also* Disturbance, sensation) 781.1
  hysterical 300.11
  postinfectional 478.9
  psychogenic 306.7
  traumatic 951.8

Anosognosia 780.99

Anosphrasia 781.1

Anosteoplasia 756.50

Anotia 744.09

Anovulatory cycle 628.0

Anoxemia 799.0
  newborn 768.9

Anoxia 799.0
  altitude 993.2
  cerebral 348.1
    with
      abortion — *see* Abortion, by type, with
        specified complication NEC
      ectopic pregnancy (*see also* categories
        633.0-633.9) 639.8
      molar pregnancy (*see also* categories 630-
        632) 639.8
    complicating
      delivery (cesarean) (instrumental)
        669.4 ☑
      ectopic or molar pregnancy 639.8

☑ Additional Digit Required   ◄► Revised Text   ● New Line   ▲ Revised Code

Anoxia — *continued*
cerebral — *continued*
complicating — *continued*
obstetric anesthesia or sedation 668.2 ☑
during or resulting from a procedure 997.01
following
abortion 639.8
ectopic or molar pregnancy 639.8
newborn (*see also* Distress, fetal, liveborn
infant) 768.9
due to drowning 994.1
fetal, affecting newborn 768.9
heart — *see* Insufficiency, coronary
high altitude 993.2
intrauterine
fetal death (before onset of labor) 768.0
during labor 768.1
liveborn infant — *see* Distress, fetal,
liveborn infant
myocardial — *see* Insufficiency, coronary
newborn 768.9
mild or moderate 768.6
severe 768.5
pathological 799.0
Anteflexion — *see* Anteversion
Antenatal
care, normal pregnancy V22.1
first V22.0
screening (for) V28.9
based on amniocentesis NEC V28.2
chromosomal anomalies V28.0
raised alphafetoprotein levels V28.1
chromosomal anomalies V28.0
fetal growth retardation using ultrasonics
V28.4
isoimmunization V28.5
malformations using ultrasonics V28.3
raised alphafetoprotein levels in amniotic
fluid V28.1
specified condition NEC V28.8
Streptococcus B V28.6
Antepartum — *see* condition
Anterior — *see also* condition
spinal artery compression syndrome 721.1
Antero-occlusion 524.24   ▲
Anteversion
cervix (*see also* Anteversion, uterus) 621.6
femur (neck), congenital 755.63
uterus, uterine (cervix) (postinfectional)
(postpartal, old) 621.6
congenital 752.3
in pregnancy or childbirth 654.4 ☑
affecting fetus or newborn 763.89
causing obstructed labor 660.2 ☑
affecting fetus or newborn 763.1
Anthracosilicosis (occupational) 500
Anthracosis (lung) (occupational) 500
lingua 529.3
Anthrax 022.9
with pneumonia 022.1 *[484.5]*
colitis 022.2
cutaneous 022.0
gastrointestinal 022.2
intestinal 022.2
pulmonary 022.1
respiratory 022.1
septicemia 022.3
specified manifestation NEC 022.8
Anthropoid pelvis 755.69
with disproportion (fetopelvic) 653.2 ☑
affecting fetus or newborn 763.1
causing obstructed labor 660.1 ☑
affecting fetus or newborn 763.1
Anthropophobia 300.29
Antibioma, breast 611.0
Antibodies
maternal (blood group) (*see also*
Incompatibility) 656.2 ☑
anti-D, cord blood 656.1 ☑
fetus or newborn 773.0
Antibody deficiency syndrome
agammaglobulinemic 279.00
congenital 279.04

Antibody deficiency syndrome — *continued*
hypogammaglobulinemic 279.00
Anticoagulant, circulating (*see also* Circulating
anticoagulants) 286.5
Antimongolism syndrome 758.39   ▲
Antimonial cholera 985.4
Antisocial personality 301.7
Antithrombinemia (*see also* Circulating
anticoagulants) 286.5
Antithromboplastinemia (*see also* Circulating
anticoagulants) 286.5
Antithromboplastinogenemia (*see also*
Circulating anticoagulants) 286.5
Antitoxin complication or reaction — *see*
Complications, vaccination
Anton (-Babinski) syndrome
(hemiasomatognosia) 307.9
Antritis (chronic) 473.0
acute 461.0
Antrum, antral — *see* condition
Anuria 788.5
with
abortion — *see* Abortion, by type, with renal
failure
ectopic pregnancy (*see also* categories
633.0-633.9) 639.3
molar pregnancy (*see also* categories 630-
632) 639.3
calculus (impacted) (recurrent) 592.9
kidney 592.0
ureter 592.1
congenital 753.3
due to a procedure 997.5
following
abortion 639.3
ectopic or molar pregnancy 639.3
newborn 753.3
postrenal 593.4
puerperal, postpartum, childbirth 669.3 ☑
specified as due to a procedure 997.5
sulfonamide
correct substance properly administered
788.5
overdose or wrong substance given or taken
961.0
traumatic (following crushing) 958.5
Anus, anal — *see* condition
Anusitis 569.49
Anxiety (neurosis) (reaction) (state) 300.00
alcohol-induced 291.89
depression 300.4
drug-induced 292.89
due to or associated with physical condition
293.84
generalized 300.02
hysteria 300.20
in
acute stress reaction 308.0
transient adjustment reaction 309.24
panic type 300.01
separation, abnormal 309.21
syndrome (organic) (transient) 293.84
Aorta, aortic — *see* condition
Aortectasia 441.9
Aortitis (nonsyphilitic) 447.6
arteriosclerotic 440.0
calcific 447.6
Döhle-Heller 093.1
luetic 093.1
rheumatic (*see also* Endocarditis, acute,
rheumatic) 391.1
rheumatoid — *see* Arthritis, rheumatoid
specific 093.1
syphilitic 093.1
congenital 090.5
Apethetic thyroid storm (*see also* Thyrotoxicosis)
242.9 ☑
Apepsia 536.8
achlorhydric 536.0
psychogenic 306.4
Aperistalsis, esophagus 530.0
Apert's syndrome (acrocephalosyndactyly) 755.55

Apert-Gallais syndrome (adrenogenital) 255.2
Apertognathia 524.20   ▲
Aphagia 787.2
psychogenic 307.1
Aphakia (acquired) (bilateral) (postoperative)
(unilateral) 379.31
congenital 743.35
Aphalangia (congenital) 755.4
lower limb (complete) (intercalary) (partial)
(terminal) 755.39
meaning all digits (complete) (partial) 755.31
transverse 755.31
upper limb (complete) (intercalary) (partial)
(terminal) 755.29
meaning all digits (complete) (partial) 755.21
transverse 755.21
Aphasia (amnestic) (ataxic) (auditory) (Broca's)
(choreatic) (classic) (expressive) (global)
(ideational) (ideokinetic) (ideomotor) (jargon)
(motor) (nominal) (receptive) (semantic)
(sensory) (syntactic) (verbal) (visual)
(Wernicke's) 784.3
developmental 315.31
syphilis, tertiary 094.89
uremic — *see* Uremia
Aphemia 784.3
uremic — *see* Uremia
Aphonia 784.41
clericorum 784.49
hysterical 300.11
organic 784.41
psychogenic 306.1
Aphthae, aphthous — *see also* condition
Bednar's 528.2
cachectic 529.0
epizootic 078.4
fever 078.4
oral 528.2
stomatitis 528.2
thrush 112.0
ulcer (oral) (recurrent) 528.2
genital organ(s) NEC
female 629.8
male 608.89
larynx 478.79
Apical — *see* condition
Aplasia — *see also* Agenesis
alveolar process (acquired) 525.8
congenital 750.26
aorta (congenital) 747.22
aortic valve (congenital) 746.89
axialis extracorticalis (congenital) 330.0
bone marrow (myeloid) 284.9
acquired (secondary) 284.8
congenital 284.0
idiopathic 284.9
brain 740.0
specified part 742.2
breast 757.6
bronchus 748.3
cementum 520.4
cerebellar 742.2
congenital pure red cell 284.0
corpus callosum 742.2
erythrocyte 284.8
congenital 284.0
extracortical axial 330.0
eye (congenital) 743.00
fovea centralis (congenital) 743.55
germinal (cell) 606.0
iris 743.45
labyrinth, membranous 744.05
limb (congenital) 755.4
lower NEC 755.30
upper NEC 755.20
lung (bilateral) (congenital) (unilateral) 748.5
nervous system NEC 742.8
nuclear 742.8
ovary 752.0
Pelizaeus-Merzbacher 330.0
prostate (congenital) 752.89
red cell (pure) (with thymoma) 284.8
acquired (secondary) 284.8
congenital 284.0
hereditary 284.0

Aplasia — *see also* Agenesis — *continued*
    red cell — *continued*
        of infants 284.0
        primary 284.0
    round ligament (congenital) 752.89
    salivary gland 750.21
    skin (congenital) 757.39
    spinal cord 742.59
    spleen 759.0
    testis (congenital) 752.89
    thymic, with immunodeficiency 279.2
    thyroid 243
    uterus 752.3
    ventral horn cell 742.59
Apleuria 756.3
Apnea, apneic (spells) 786.03
    newborn, neonatorum 770.81
        essential 770.81
        obstructive 770.82
        primary 770.81
        sleep 770.81
        specified NEC 770.82
    psychogenic 306.1
    sleep NEC 780.57
        with
            hypersomnia 780.53
            hyposomnia 780.51
            insomnia 780.51
            sleep disturbance NEC 780.57
Apneumatosis newborn 770.4
Apodia 755.31
Apophysitis (bone) (*see also* Osteochondrosis)
    732.9
    calcaneus 732.5
    juvenile 732.6
Apoplectiform convulsions (*see also* Disease,
    cerebrovascular, acute) 436
Apoplexia, apoplexy, apoplectic (*see also*
    Disease, cerebrovascular, acute) 436
    abdominal 569.89
    adrenal 036.3
    attack 436
    basilar (*see also* Disease, cerebrovascular,
        acute) 436
    brain (*see also* Disease, cerebrovascular, acute)
        436
    bulbar (*see also* Disease, cerebrovascular,
        acute) 436
    capillary (*see also* Disease, cerebrovascular,
        acute) 436
    cardiac (*see also* Infarct, myocardium) 410.9 ☑
    cerebral (*see also* Disease, cerebrovascular
        acute) 436
    chorea (*see also* Disease, cerebrovascular,
        acute) 436
    congestive (*see also* Disease, cerebrovascular,
        acute) 436
        newborn 767.4
    embolic (*see also* Embolism, brain) 434.1 ☑
    fetus 767.0
    fit (*see also* Disease, cerebrovascular, acute)
        436
    healed or old V12.59
    heart (auricle) (ventricle) (*see also* Infarct,
        myocardium) 410.9 ☑
    heat 992.0
    hemiplegia (*see also* Disease, cerebrovascular,
        acute) 436
    hemorrhagic (stroke) (*see also* Hemorrhage,
        brain) 432.9
    ingravescent (*see also* Disease, cerebrovascular,
        acute) 436
    late effect — *see* Late effect(s) (of)
        cerebrovascular disease
    lung — *see* Embolism, pulmonary
    meninges, hemorrhagic (*see also* Hemorrhage
        subarachnoid) 430
    neonatorum 767.0
    newborn 767.0
    pancreatitis 577.0
    placenta 641.2 ☑
    progressive (*see also* Disease, cerebrovascular,
        acute) 436

Apoplexia, apoplexy, apoplectic (*see also*
    Disease, cerebrovascular, acute) — *continued*
    pulmonary (artery) (vein) — *see* Embolism,
        pulmonary
    sanguineous (*see also* Disease,
        cerebrovascular, acute) 436
    seizure (*see also* Disease, cerebrovascular,
        acute) 436
    serous (*see also* Disease, cerebrovascular,
        acute) 436
    spleen 289.59
    stroke (*see also* Disease, cerebrovascular,
        acute) 436
    thrombotic (*see also* Thrombosis, brain)
        434.0 ☑
    uremic — *see* Uremia
    uteroplacental 641.2 ☑
Appendage
    fallopian tube (cyst of Morgagni) 752.11
    intestine (epiploic) 751.5
    preauricular 744.1
    testicular (organ of Morgagni) 752.89
Appendicitis 541
    with
        perforation, peritonitis (generalized), or
            rupture 540.0
            with peritoneal abscess 540.1
        peritoneal abscess 540.1
    acute (catarrhal) (fulminating) (gangrenous)
        (inflammatory) (obstructive) (retrocecal)
        (suppurative) 540.9
        with
            perforation, peritonitis, or rupture 540.0
                with peritoneal abscess 540.1
            peritoneal abscess 540.1
    amebic 006.8
    chronic (recurrent) 542
    exacerbation — *see* Appendicitis, acute
    fulminating — *see* Appendicitis, acute
    gangrenous — *see* Appendicitis, acute
    healed (obliterative) 542
    interval 542
    neurogenic 542
    obstructive 542
    pneumococcal 541
    recurrent 542
    relapsing 542
    retrocecal 541
    subacute (adhesive) 542
    subsiding 542
    suppurative — *see* Appendicitis, acute
    tuberculous (*see also* Tuberculosis) 014.8 ☑
Appendiclausis 543.9
Appendicolithiasis 543.9
Appendicopathia oxyurica 127.4
Appendix, appendicular — *see also* condition
    Morgagni (male) 752.89
        fallopian tube 752.11
Appetite
    depraved 307.52
    excessive 783.6
        psychogenic 307.51
    lack or loss (*see also* Anorexia) 783.0
        nonorganic origin 307.59
    perverted 307.52
        hysterical 300.11
Apprehension, apprehensiveness (abnormal)
    (state) 300.00
    specified type NEC 300.09
Approximal wear 521.10 ▲
Apraxia (classic) (ideational) (ideokinetic)
    (ideomotor) (motor) 784.69
    oculomotor, congenital 379.51
    verbal 784.69
Aptyalism 527.7
Aqueous misdirection 365.83
Arabicum elephantiasis (*see also* Infestation,
    filarial) 125.9
Arachnidism 989.5
Arachnitis — *see* Meningitis
Arachnodactyly 759.82
Arachnoidism 989.5

Arachnoiditis (acute) (adhesive) (basic) (brain)
    (cerebrospinal) (chiasmal) (chronic) (spinal)
    (*see also* Meningitis) 322.9
    meningococcal (chronic) 036.0
    syphilitic 094.2
    tuberculous (*see also* Tuberculosis meninges)
        013.0 ☑
Araneism 989.5
Arboencephalitis, Australian 062.4
Arborization block (heart) 426.6
Arbor virus, arbovirus (infection) NEC 066.9
ARC 042
Arches — *see* condition
Arcuatus uterus 752.3
Arcus (cornea)
    juvenilis 743.43
        interfering with vision 743.42
    senilis 371.41
Arc-welders' lung 503
Arc-welders' syndrome (photokeratitis) 370.24
Areflexia 796.1
Areola — *see* condition
Argentaffinoma (M8241/1) — *see also* Neoplasm,
    by site, uncertain behavior
    benign (M8241/0) — *see* Neoplasm, by site,
        benign
    malignant (M8241/3) — *see* Neoplasm, by site,
        malignant
    syndrome 259.2
Argentinian hemorrhagic fever 078.7
Arginosuccinicaciduria 270.6
Argonz-Del Castillo syndrome (nonpuerperal
    galactorrhea and amenorrhea) 253.1
**Argyll-Robertson phenomenon, pupil, or
    syndrome** (syphilitic) 094.89
    atypical 379.45
    nonluetic 379.45
    nonsyphilitic 379.45
    reversed 379.45
Argyria, argyriasis NEC 985.8
    conjunctiva 372.55
    cornea 371.16
    from drug or medicinal agent
        correct substance properly administered
            709.09
        overdose or wrong substance given or taken
            961.2
Arhinencephaly 742.2
Arias-Stella phenomenon 621.30 ▲
Ariboflavinosis 266.0
Arizona enteritis 008.1
Arm — *see* condition
Armenian disease 277.3
Arnold-Chiari obstruction or syndrome (*see also*
    Spina bifida) 741.0 ☑
    type I 348.4
    type II (*see also* Spina bifida) 741.0 ☑
    type III 742.0
    type IV 742.2
Arrest, arrested
    active phase of labor 661.1 ☑
        affecting fetus or newborn 763.7
    any plane in pelvis
        complicating delivery 660.1 ☑
            affecting fetus or newborn 763.1
    bone marrow (*see also* Anemia, aplastic) 284.9
    cardiac 427.5
        with
            abortion — *see* Abortion, by type, with
                specified complication NEC
            ectopic pregnancy (*see also* categories
                633.0-633.9) 639.8
            molar pregnancy (*see also* categories 630-
                632) 639.8
        complicating
            anesthesia
                correct substance properly
                    administered 427.5
                obstetric 668.1 ☑
                overdose or wrong substance given 968.4
                    specified anesthetic — *see* Table of
                        Drugs and Chemicals

Aplasia — Arrest, arrested

Arrest, arrested — *continued*
  cardiac — *continued*
    complicating — *continued*
      delivery (cesarean) (instrumental) 669.4 ☑
      ectopic or molar pregnancy 639.8
      surgery (nontherapeutic) (therapeutic) 997.1
    fetus or newborn 779.89
    following
      abortion 639.8
      ectopic or molar pregnancy 639.8
    postoperative (immediate) 997.1
    long-term effect of cardiac surgery 429.4
  cardiorespiratory (*see also* Arrest, cardiac) 427.5
  deep transverse 660.3 ☑
    affecting fetus or newborn 763.1
  development or growth
    bone 733.91
    child 783.40
    fetus 764.9 ☑
      affecting management of pregnancy 656.5 ☑
    tracheal rings 748.3
  epiphyseal 733.91
  granulopoiesis 288.0
  heart — *see* Arrest, cardiac
  respiratory 799.1
    newborn 770.89
  sinus 426.6
  transverse (deep) 660.3 ☑
    affecting fetus or newborn 763.1
Arrhenoblastoma (M8630/1)
  benign (M8630/0)
    specified site — *see* Neoplasm, by site, benign
    unspecified site
      female 220
      male 222.0
  malignant (M8630/3)
    specified site — *see* Neoplasm, by site, malignant
    unspecified site
      female 183.0
      male 186.9
  specified site — *see* Neoplasm, by site, uncertain behavior
  unspecified site
    female 236.2
    male 236.4
Arrhinencephaly 742.2
  due to
    trisomy 13 (13-15) 758.1
    trisomy 18 (16-18) 758.2
Arrhythmia (auricle) (cardiac) (cordis) (gallop rhythm) (juvenile) (nodal) (reflex) (sinus) (supraventricular) (transitory) (ventricle) 427.9
  bigeminal rhythm 427.89
  block 426.9
  bradycardia 427.89
  contractions, premature 427.60
  coronary sinus 427.89
  ectopic 427.89
  extrasystolic 427.60
  postoperative 997.1
  psychogenic 306.2
  vagal 780.2
Arrillaga-Ayerza syndrome (pulmonary artery sclerosis with pulmonary hypertension) 416.0
Arsenical
  dermatitis 692.4
  keratosis 692.4
  pigmentation 985.1
  from drug or medicinal agent
    correct substance properly administered 709.09
    overdose or wrong substance given or taken 961.1
Arsenism 985.1
  from drug or medicinal agent
    correct substance properly administered 692.4

Arsenism — *continued*
  from drug or medicinal agent — *continued*
    overdose or wrong substance given or taken 961.1
Arterial — *see* condition
Arteriectasis 447.8
Arteriofibrosis — *see* Arteriosclerosis
Arteriolar sclerosis — *see* Arteriosclerosis
Arteriolith — *see* Arteriosclerosis
Arteriolitis 447.6
  necrotizing, kidney 447.5
  renal — *see* Hypertension, kidney
Arteriolosclerosis — *see* Arteriosclerosis
Arterionephrosclerosis (*see also* Hypertension, kidney) 403.90
Arteriopathy 447.9
Arteriosclerosis, arteriosclerotic (artery) (deformans) (diffuse) (disease) (endarteritis) (general) (obliterans) (obliterative) (occlusive) (senile) (with calcification) 440.9
  with
    gangrene 440.24
    psychosis (*see also* Psychosis, arteriosclerotic) 290.40
    ulceration 440.23
  aorta 440.0
  arteries of extremities — *see* Arteriosclerosis, extremities
  basilar (artery) (*see also* Occlusion, artery, basilar) 433.0 ☑
  brain 437.0
  bypass graft
    coronary artery 414.05
      autologous artery (gastroepiploic) (internal mammary) 414.04
      autologous vein 414.02
      nonautologous biological 414.03
      of transplanted heart 414.07
    extremity 440.30
      autologous vein 440.31
      nonautologous biological 440.32
  cardiac — *see* Arteriosclerosis, coronary
  cardiopathy — *see* Arteriosclerosis, coronary
  cardiorenal (*see also* Hypertension, cardiorenal) 404.90
  cardiovascular (*see also* Disease, cardiovascular) 429.2
  carotid (artery) (common) (internal) (*see also* Occlusion, artery, carotid) 433.1 ☑
  central nervous system 437.0
  cerebral 437.0
    late effect — *see* Late effect(s) (of) cerebrovascular disease
  cerebrospinal 437.0
  cerebrovascular 437.0
  coronary (artery) 414.00
    graft — *see* Arteriosclerosis, bypass graft
    native artery 414.01
      of transplanted heart 414.06
  extremities (native artery) NEC 440.20
    bypass graft 440.30
      autologous vein 440.31
      nonautologous biological 440.32
    claudication (intermittent) 440.21
    and
      gangrene 440.24
      rest pain 440.22
      and
        gangrene 440.24
        ulceration 440.23
          and gangrene 440.24
      ulceration 440.23
        and gangrene 440.24
    gangrene 440.24
    rest pain 440.22
    and
      gangrene 440.24
      ulceration 440.23
        and gangrene 440.24
    specified site NEC 440.29
    ulceration 440.23
      and gangrene 440.24

Arteriosclerosis, arteriosclerotic — *continued*
  heart (disease) — *see also* Arteriosclerosis, coronary
  valve 424.99
    aortic 424.1
    mitral 424.0
    pulmonary 424.3
    tricuspid 424.2
  kidney (*see also* Hypertension, kidney) 403.90
  labyrinth, labyrinthine 388.00
  medial NEC 440.20
  mesentery (artery) 557.1
  Mönckeberg's 440.20
  myocarditis 429.0
  nephrosclerosis (*see also* Hypertension, kidney) 403.90
  peripheral (of extremities) — *see* Arteriosclerosis, extremities
  precerebral 433.9 ☑
    specified artery NEC 433.8 ☑
  pulmonary (idiopathic) 416.0
  renal (*see also* Hypertension, kidney) 403.90
    arterioles (*see also* Hypertension, kidney) 403.90
    artery 440.1
  retinal (vascular) 440.8 *[362.13]*
  specified artery NEC 440.8
    with gangrene 440.8 *[785.4]*
  spinal (cord) 437.0
  vertebral (artery) (*see also* Occlusion, artery, vertebral) 433.2 ☑
Arteriospasm 443.9
Arteriovenous — *see* condition
Arteritis 447.6
  allergic (*see also* Angiitis, hypersensitivity) 446.20
  aorta (nonsyphilitic) 447.6
    syphilitic 093.1
  aortic arch 446.7
  brachiocephalica 446.7
  brain 437.4
    syphilitic 094.89
  branchial 446.7
  cerebral 437.4
    late effect — *see* Late effect(s) (of) cerebrovascular disease
    syphilitic 094.89
  coronary (artery) — *see also* Arteriosclerosis, coronary
    rheumatic 391.9
      chronic 398.99
    syphilitic 093.89
  cranial (left) (right) 446.5
  deformans — *see* Arteriosclerosis
  giant cell 446.5
  necrosing or necrotizing 446.0
  nodosa 446.0
  obliterans — *see also* Arteriosclerosis
    subclaviocarotica 446.7
  pulmonary 417.8
  retina 362.18
  rheumatic — *see* Fever, rheumatic
  senile — *see* Arteriosclerosis
  suppurative 447.2
  syphilitic (general) 093.89
    brain 094.89
    coronary 093.89
    spinal 094.89
  temporal 446.5
  young female, syndrome 446.7
Artery, arterial — *see* condition
Arthralgia (*see also* Pain, joint) 719.4 ☑
  allergic (*see also* Pain, joint) 719.4 ☑
  in caisson disease 993.3
  psychogenic 307.89
  rubella 056.71
  Salmonella 003.23
  temporomandibular joint 524.62
Arthritis, arthritic (acute) (chronic) (subacute) 716.9 ☑
  meaning Osteoarthritis — *see* Osteoarthrosis

Arthritis, arthritic — *continued*

Note — *Use the following fifth-digit subclassification with categories 711-712, 715-716:*

0	*site unspecified*
1	*shoulder region*
2	*upper arm*
3	*forearm*
4	*hand*
5	*pelvic region and thigh*
6	*lower leg*
7	*ankle and foot*
8	*other specified sites*
9	*multiple sites*

allergic 716.2 ☑
ankylosing (crippling) (spine) 720.0
   sites other than spine 716.9 ☑
atrophic 714.0
   spine 720.9
back (*see also* Arthritis, spine) 721.90
Bechterew's (ankylosing spondylitis) 720.0
blennorrhagic 098.50
cervical, cervicodorsal (*see also* Spondylosis, cervical) 721.0
Charcôt's 094.0 *[713.5]*
   diabetic 250.6 ☑ *[713.5]*
   syringomyelic 336.0 *[713.5]*
   tabetic 094.0 *[713.5]*
chylous (*see also* Filariasis) 125.9 *[711.7]* ☑
climacteric NEC 716.3 ☑
coccyx 721.8
cricoarytenoid 478.79
crystal (-induced) — *see* Arthritis, due to crystals
deformans (*see also* Osteoarthrosis) 715.9 ☑
   spine 721.90
      with myelopathy 721.91
degenerative (*see also* Osteoarthrosis) 715.9 ☑
   idiopathic 715.09
   polyarticular 715.09
   spine 721.90
      with myelopathy 721.91
dermatoarthritis, lipoid 272.8 *[713.0]*
due to or associated with
   acromegaly 253.0 *[713.0]*
   actinomycosis 039.8 *[711.4]* ☑
   amyloidosis 277.3 *[713.7]*
   bacterial disease NEC 040.89 *[711.4]* ☑
   Behçet's syndrome 136.1 *[711.2]* ☑
   blastomycosis 116.0 *[711.6]* ☑
   brucellosis (*see also* Brucellosis) 023.9 *[711.4]* ☑
   caisson disease 993.3
   coccidioidomycosis 114.3 *[711.6]* ☑
   coliform (Escherichia coli) 711.0 ☑
   colitis, ulcerative (*see also* Colitis, ulcerative) 556.9 *[713.1]*
   cowpox 051.0 *[711.5]* ☑
   crystals — *see also* Gout
      dicalcium phosphate 275.49 *[712.1]* ☑
      pyrophosphate 275.49 *[712.2]* ☑
      specified NEC 275.49 *[712.8]* ☑
   dermatoarthritis, lipoid 272.8 *[713.0]*
   dermatological disorder NEC 709.9 *[713.3]*
   diabetes 250.6 ☑ *[713.5]*
   diphtheria 032.89 *[711.4]* ☑
   dracontiasis 125.7 *[711.7]* ☑
   dysentery 009.0 *[711.3]* ☑
   endocrine disorder NEC 259.9 *[713.0]*
   enteritis NEC 009.1 *[711.3]* ☑
      infectious (*see also* Enteritis, infectious) 009.0 *[711.3]* ☑
         specified organism NEC 008.8 *[711.3]* ☑
      regional (*see also* Enteritis, regional) 555.9 *[713.1]*
         specified organism NEC 008.8 *[711.3]* ☑
   epiphyseal slip, nontraumatic (old) 716.8 ☑
   erysipelas 035 *[711.4]* ☑

Arthritis, arthritic — *continued*
due to or associated with — *continued*
   erythema
      epidemic 026.1
         multiforme 695.1 *[713.3]*
         nodosum 695.2 *[713.3]*
   Escherichia coli 711.0 ☑
   filariasis NEC 125.9 *[711.7]* ☑
   gastrointestinal condition NEC 569.9 *[713.1]*
   glanders 024 *[711.4]* ☑
   Gonococcus 098.50
   gout 274.0
   H. influenzae 711.0 ☑
   helminthiasis NEC 128.9 *[711.7]* ☑
   hematological disorder NEC 289.9 *[713.2]*
   hemochromatosis 275.0 *[713.0]*
   hemoglobinopathy NEC (*see also* Disease, hemoglobin) 282.7 *[713.2]*
   hemophilia (*see also* Hemophilia) 286.0 *[713.2]*
   Hemophilus influenzae (H. influenzae) 711.0 ☑
   Henoch (-Schönlein) purpura 287.0 *[713.6]*
   histoplasmosis NEC (*see also* Histoplasmosis) 115.99 *[711.6]* ☑
   hyperparathyroidism 252.00 *[713.0]*   ▲
   hypersensitivity reaction NEC 995.3 *[713.6]*
   hypogammaglobulinemia (*see also* Hypogamma-globulinemia) 279.00 *[713.0]*
   hypothyroidism NEC 244.9 *[713.0]*
   infection (*see also* Arthritis, infectious) 711.9 ☑
   infectious disease NEC 136.9 *[711.8]* ☑
   leprosy (*see also* Leprosy) 030.9 *[711.4]* ☑
   leukemia NEC (M9800/3) 208.9 ☑ *[713.2]*
   lipoid dermatoarthritis 272.8 *[713.0]*
   Lyme disease 088.81 *[711.8]* ☑
   Mediterranean fever, familial 277.3 *[713.7]*
   meningococcal infection 036.82
   metabolic disorder NEC 277.9 *[713.0]*
   multiple myelomatosis (M9730/3) 203.0 ☑ *[713.2]*
   mumps 072.79 *[711.5]* ☑
   mycobacteria 031.8 *[711.4]* ☑
   mycosis NEC 117.9 *[711.6]* ☑
   neurological disorder NEC 349.9 *[713.5]*
   ochronosis 270.2 *[713.0]*
   O'Nyong Nyong 066.3 *[711.5]* ☑
   parasitic disease NEC 136.9 *[711.8]* ☑
   paratyphoid fever (*see also* Fever, paratyphoid) 002.9 *[711.3]* ☑
   Pneumococcus 711.0 ☑
   poliomyelitis (*see also* Poliomyelitis) 045.9 ☑ *[711.5]* ☑
   Pseudomonas 711.0 ☑
   psoriasis 696.0
   pyogenic organism (E. coli) (H. influenzae) (Pseudomonas) (Streptococcus) 711.0 ☑
   rat-bite fever 026.1 *[711.4]* ☑
   regional enteritis (*see also* Enteritis, regional) 555.9 *[713.1]*
   Reiter's disease 099.3 *[711.1]* ☑
   respiratory disorder NEC 519.9 *[713.4]*
   reticulosis, malignant (M9720/3) 202.3 *[713.2]*
   rubella 056.71
   salmonellosis 003.23
   sarcoidosis 135 *[713.7]*
   serum sickness 999.5 *[713.6]*
   Staphylococcus 711.0 ☑
   Streptococcus 711.0 ☑
   syphilis (*see also* Syphilis) 094.0 *[711.4]* ☑
   syringomyelia 336.0 *[713.5]*
   thalassemia 282.49 *[713.2]*
   tuberculosis (*see also* Tuberculosis, arthritis) 015.9 ☑ *[711.4]* ☑
   typhoid fever 002.0 *[711.3]* ☑
   ulcerative colitis (*see also* Colitis, ulcerative) 556.9 *[713.1]*
   urethritis
      nongonococcal (*see also* Urethritis, nongonococcal) 099.40 *[711.1]* ☑
      nonspecific (*see also* Urethritis, nongonococcal) 099.40 *[711.1]* ☑
      Reiter's 099.3 *[711.1]* ☑

Arthritis, arthritic — *continued*
due to or associated with — *continued*
   viral disease NEC 079.99 *[711.5]* ☑
erythema epidemic 026.1
gonococcal 098.50
gouty (acute) 274.0
hypertrophic (*see also* Osteoarthrosis) 715.9 ☑
   spine 721.90
      with myelopathy 721.91
idiopathic, blennorrheal 099.3
in caisson disease 993.3 *[713.8]*
infectious or infective (acute) (chronic) (subacute) NEC 711.9 ☑
   nonpyogenic 711.9 ☑
   spine 720.9
inflammatory NEC 714.9
juvenile rheumatoid (chronic) (polyarticular) 714.30
   acute 714.31
   monoarticular 714.33
   pauciarticular 714.32
lumbar (*see also* Spondylosis, lumbar) 721.3
meningococcal 036.82
menopausal NEC 716.3 ☑
migratory — *see* Fever, rheumatic
neuropathic (Charcôt's) 094.0 *[713.5]*
   diabetic 250.6 ☑ *[713.5]*
   nonsyphilitic NEC 349.9 *[713.5]*
   syringomyelic 336.0 *[713.5]*
   tabetic 094.0 *[713.5]*
nodosa (*see also* Osteoarthrosis) 715.9 ☑
   spine 721.90
      with myelopathy 721.91
nonpyogenic NEC 716.9 ☑
   spine 721.90
      with myelopathy 721.91
ochronotic 270.2 *[713.0]*
palindromic (*see also* Rheumatism, palindromic) 719.3 ☑
pneumococcal 711.0 ☑
postdysenteric 009.0 *[711.3]* ☑
postrheumatic, chronic (Jaccoud's) 714.4
primary progressive 714.0
   spine 720.9
proliferative 714.0
   spine 720.0
psoriatic 696.0
purulent 711.0 ☑
pyogenic or pyemic 711.0 ☑
rheumatic 714.0
   acute or subacute — *see* Fever, rheumatic
   chronic 714.0
   spine 720.9
rheumatoid (nodular) 714.0
   with
      splenoadenomegaly and leukopenia 714.1
      visceral or systemic involvement 714.2
   aortitis 714.89
   carditis 714.2
   heart disease 714.2
   juvenile (chronic) (polyarticular) 714.30
      acute 714.31
      monoarticular 714.33
      pauciarticular 714.32
   spine 720.0
rubella 056.71
sacral, sacroiliac, sacrococcygeal (*see also* Spondylosis, sacral) 721.3
scorbutic 267
senile or senescent (*see also* Osteoarthrosis) 715.9 ☑
   spine 721.90
      with myelopathy 721.91
septic 711.0 ☑
serum (nontherapeutic) (therapeutic) 999.5 *[713.6]*
specified form NEC 716.8 ☑
spine 721.90
   with myelopathy 721.91
   atrophic 720.9
   degenerative 721.90
      with myelopathy 721.91
   hypertrophic (with deformity) 721.90
      with myelopathy 721.91
   infectious or infective NEC 720.9
   Marie-Strümpell 720.0

☑ Additional Digit Required   ▶◀ Revised Text   ● New Line   ▲ Revised Code

Arthritis, arthritic — *continued*
  spine — *continued*
    nonpyogenic 721.90
      with myelopathy 721.91
    pyogenic 720.9
    rheumatoid 720.0
    traumatic (old) 721.7
    tuberculous (*see also* Tuberculosis) 015.0 ☑
      [720.81]
  staphylococcal 711.0 ☑
  streptococcal 711.0 ☑
  suppurative 711.0 ☑
  syphilitic 094.0 *[713.5]*
    congenital 090.49 *[713.5]*
  syphilitica deformans (Charcôt) 094.0 *[713.5]*
  temporomandibular joint 524.69
  thoracic (*see also* Spondylosis, thoracic) 721.2
  toxic of menopause 716.3 ☑
  transient 716.4 ☑
  traumatic (chronic) (old) (post) 716.1 ☑
    current injury — *see* nature of injury
  tuberculous (*see also* Tuberculosis, arthritis)
    015.9 *[711.4]* ☑
  urethritica 099.3 *[711.1]* ☑
  urica, uratic 274.0
  venereal 099.3 *[711.1]* ☑
  vertebral (*see also* Arthritis, spine) 721.90
  villous 716.8 ☑
  von Bechterew's 720.0
Arthrocele (*see also* Effusion, joint) 719.0 ☑
Arthrochondritis — *see* Arthritis
Arthrodesis status V45.4
Arthrodynia (*see also* Pain, joint) 719.4 ☑
  psychogenic 307.89
Arthrodysplasia 755.9
Arthrofibrosis, joint (*see also* Ankylosis) 718.5 ☑
Arthrogryposis 728.3
  multiplex, congenita 754.89
Arthrokatadysis 715.35
Arthrolithiasis 274.0
Arthro-onychodysplasia 756.89
Arthro-osteo-onychodysplasia 756.89
Arthropathy (*see also* Arthritis) 716.9 ☑

> *Note* — Use the following fifth-digit
> *subclassification with categories 711-712, 716:*
>
> 0   *site unspecified*
> 1   *shoulder region*
> 2   *upper arm*
> 3   *forearm*
> 4   *hand*
> 5   *pelvic region and thigh*
> 6   *lower leg*
> 7   *ankle and foot*
> 8   *other specified sites*
> 9   *multiple sites*

  Behçets 136.1 *[711.2]* ☑
  Charcôt's 094.0 *[713.5]*
    diabetic 250.6 ☑ *[713.5]*
    syringomyelic 336.0 *[713.5]*
    tabetic 094.0 *[713.5]*
  crystal (-induced) — *see* Arthritis, due to
    crystals
  gouty 274.0
  neurogenic, neuropathic (Charcôt's) (tabetic)
    094.0 *[713.5]*
    diabetic 250.6 ☑ *[713.5]*
    nonsyphilitic NEC 349.9 *[713.5]*
    syringomyelic 336.0 *[713.5]*
  postdysenteric NEC 009.0 *[711.3]* ☑
  postrheumatic, chronic (Jaccoud's) 714.4
  psoriatic 696.0
  pulmonary 731.2
  specified NEC 716.8 ☑
  syringomyelia 336.0 *[713.5]*
  tabes dorsalis 094.0 *[713.5]*
  tabetic 094.0 *[713.5]*
  transient 716.4 ☑
  traumatic 716.1 ☑
  uric acid 274.0

Arthophyte (*see also* Loose, body, joint) 718.1 ☑
Arthrophytis 719.80
  ankle 719.87
  elbow 719.82
  foot 719.87
  hand 719.84
  hip 719.85
  knee 719.86
  multiple sites 719.89
  pelvic region 719.85
  shoulder (region) 719.81
  specified site NEC 719.88
  wrist 719.83
Arthropyosis (*see also* Arthritis, pyogenic)
  711.0 ☑
**Arthroscopic surgical procedure converted
to open procedure** V64.43
Arthrosis (deformans) (degenerative) (*see also*
  Osteoarthrosis) 715.9 ☑
  Charcôt's 094.0 *[713.5]*
  polyarticular 715.09
  spine (*see also* Spondylosis) 721.90
Arthus' phenomenon 995.2
  due to
    correct substance properly administered
      995.2
    overdose or wrong substance given or taken
      977.9
      specified drug — *see* Table of Drugs and
        Chemicals
    serum 999.5
Articular — *see also* condition
  disc disorder (reducing or non-reducing)
    524.63
  spondylolisthesis 756.12
Articulation   ●
  anterior 524.27   ●
  posterior 524.27   ●
  reverse 524.27   ●
Artificial
  device (prosthetic) — *see* Fitting, device
  insemination V26.1
  menopause (states) (symptoms) (syndrome)
    627.4
  opening status (functioning) (without
    complication) V44.9
    anus (colostomy) V44.3
    colostomy V44.3
    cystostomy V44.50
      appendico-vesicostomy V44.52
      cutaneous-vesicostomy V44.51
      specified type NEC V44.59
    enterostomy V44.4
    gastrostomy V44.1
    ileostomy V44.2
    intestinal tract NEC V44.4
    jejunostomy V44.4
    nephrostomy V44.6
    specified site NEC V44.8
    tracheostomy V44.0
    ureterostomy V44.6
    urethrostomy V44.6
    urinary tract NEC V44.6
    vagina V44.7
  vagina status V44.7
ARV (disease) (illness) (infection) — *see* Human
  immunodeficiency virus (disease) (illness)
  (infection)
Arytenoid — *see* condition
Asbestosis (occupational) 501
Asboe-Hansen's disease (incontinentia
  pigmenti) 757.33
Ascariasis (intestinal) (lung) 127.0
Ascaridiasis 127.0
Ascaris 127.0
  lumbricoides (infestation) 127.0
  pneumonia 127.0
Ascending — *see* condition
Aschoff's bodies (*see also* Myocarditis,
  rheumatic) 398.0
Ascites 789.5
  abdominal NEC 789.5
  cancerous (M80000/6) 197.6

Ascites — *continued*
  cardiac 428.0
  chylous (nonfilarial) 457.8
    filarial (*see also* Infestation, filarial) 125.9
  congenital 778.0
  due to S. japonicum 120.2
  fetal, causing fetopelvic disproportion 653.7 ☑
  heart 428.0
  joint (*see also* Effusion, joint) 719.0 ☑
  malignant (M8000/6) 197.6
  pseudochylous 789.5
  syphilitic 095.2
  tuberculous (*see also* Tuberculosis) 014.0 ☑
Ascorbic acid (vitamin C) **deficiency** (scurvy) 267
▶**ASC-US**◀ (atypical squamous ▶cells◀ of
  undetermined significance) 795.01   ▲
ASC-H (atypical squamous cells cannot   ●
  exclude high grade squamous   ●
  intraepithelial lesion) 795.02   ●
ASCVD (arteriosclerotic cardiovascular disease)
  429.2
Aseptic — *see* condition
Asherman's syndrome 621.5
Asialia 527.7
Asiatic cholera (*see also* Cholera) 001.9
Asocial personality or trends 301.7
Asomatognosia 781.8
Aspergillosis 117.3
  with pneumonia 117.3 *[484.6]*
  allergic bronchopulmonary 518.6
  nonsyphilitic NEC 117.3
Aspergillus (flavus) (fumigatus) (infection)
  (terreus) 117.3
Aspermatogenesis 606.0
Aspermia (testis) 606.0
Asphyxia, asphyxiation (by) 799.0
  antenatal — *see* Distress, fetal
  bedclothes 994.7
  birth (*see also* Ashpyxia, newborn) 768.9
  bunny bag 994.7
  carbon monoxide 986
  caul (*see also* Asphyxia, newborn)
  cave-in 994.7
    crushing — *see* Injury, internal,
      intrathoracic organs
  constriction 994.7
  crushing — *see* Injury, internal, intrathoracic
    organs
  drowning 994.1
  fetal, affecting newborn 768.9
  food or foreign body (in larynx) 933.1
    bronchioles 934.8
    bronchus (main) 934.1
    lung 934.8
    nasopharynx 933.0
    nose, nasal passages 932
    pharynx 933.0
    respiratory tract 934.9
      specified part NEC 934.8
    throat 933.0
    trachea 934.0
  gas, fumes, or vapor NEC 987.9
    specified — *see* Table of Drugs and
      Chemicals
  gravitational changes 994.7
  hanging 994.7
  inhalation — *see* Inhalation
  intrauterine
    fetal death (before onset of labor) 768.0
      during labor 768.1
    liveborn infant — *see* Distress, fetal,
      liveborn infant
  local 443.0
  mechanical 994.7
    during birth (*see also* Distress, fetal)
      768.9
  mucus 933.1
    bronchus (main) 934.1
    larynx 933.1
    lung 934.8
    nasal passages 932
    newborn 770.1
    pharynx 933.0

Asphyxia, asphyxiation — *continued*
 mucus — *continued*
  respiratory tract 934.9
   specfied part NEC 934.8
  throat 933.0
  trachea 934.0
  vaginal (fetus or newborn) 770.1
 newborn 768.9
  blue 768.6
  livida 768.6
  mild or moderate 768.6
  pallida 768.5
  severe 768.5
  white 768.5
 pathological 799.0
 plastic bag 994.7
 postnatal (*see also* Asphyxia, newborn) 768.9
  mechanical 994.7
 pressure 994.7
 reticularis 782.61
 strangulation 994.7
 submersion 994.1
 traumatic NEC — *see* Injury, internal,
   intrathoracic organs
 vomiting, vomitus — *see* Asphyxia, food or
   foreign body
Aspiration
 acid pulmonary (syndrome) 997.3
  obstetric 668.0 ☑
 amniotic fluid 770.1
 bronchitis 507.0
 contents of birth canal 770.1
 fetal pneumonitis 770.1
 food, foreign body, or gasoline (with asphyxiation)
   — *see* Asphyxia, food or foreign body
 meconium 770.1
 mucus 933.1
  into
   bronchus (main) 934.1
   lung 934.8
   respiratory tract 934.9
    specified part NEC 934.8
   trachea 934.0
  newborn 770.1
  vaginal (fetus or newborn) 770.1
 newborn 770.1
 pneumonia 507.0
 pneumonitis 507.0
  fetus or newborn 770.1
  obstetric 668.0 ☑
 syndrome of newborn (massive) (meconium)
   770.1
 vernix caseosa 770.1
Asplenia 759.0
 with mesocardia 746.87
Assam fever 085.0
Assimilation, pelvis
 with disproportion 653.2 ☑
  affecting fetus or newborn 763.1
  causing obstructed labor 660.1 ☑
   affecting fetus or newborn 763.1
Assmann's focus (*see also* Tuberculosis) 011.0 ☑
Astasia (-asbasia) 307.9
 hysterical 300.11
Asteatosis 706.8
 cutis 706.8
Astereognosis 780.99
Asterixis 781.3
 in liver disease 572.8
Asteroid hyalitis 379.22
Asthenia, asthenic 780.79
 cardiac (*see also* Failure, heart) 428.9
  psychogenic 306.2
 cardiovascular (*see also* Failure, heart) 428.9
  psychogenic 306.2
 heart (*see also* Failure, heart) 428.9
  psychogenic 306.2
 hysterical 300.11
 myocardial (*see also* Failure, heart) 428.9
  psychogenic 306.2
 nervous 300.5
 neurocirculatory 306.2
 neurotic 300.5
 psychogenic 300.5
 psychoneurotic 300.5

Asthenia, asthenic — *continued*
 psychophysiologic 300.5
 reaction, psychoneurotic 300.5
 senile 797
 Stiller's 780.79
 tropical anhidrotic 705.1
Asthenopia 368.13
 accommodative 367.4
 hysterical (muscular) 300.11
 psychogenic 306.7
Asthenospermia 792.2
Asthma, asthmatic (bronchial) (catarrh)
  (spasmodic) 493.9 ☑

> Note — *The following fifth-digit subclassification
> is for use with codes 493.0-493.2, 493.9:*
>
> 0 *unspecified*
> 1 *with status asthmaticus*
> 2 *with (acute) exacerbation*

 with
  chronic obstructive pulmonary disease
   (COPD) 493.2 ☑
  hay fever 493.0 ☑
  rhinitis, allergic 493.0 ☑
 allergic 493.9 ☑
  stated cause (external allergen) 493.0 ☑
 atopic 493.0 ☑
 cardiac (*see also* Failure, ventricular, left) 428.1
 cardiobronchial (*see also* Failure, ventricular,
   left) 428.1
 cardiorenal (*see also* Hypertension, cardiorenal)
   404.90
 childhood 493.0 ☑
 colliers' 500
 cough variant 493.82
 croup 493.9 ☑
 detergent 507.8
 due to
  detergent 507.8
  inhalation of fumes 506.3
  internal immunological process 493.0 ☑
 endogenous (intrinsic) 493.1 ☑
 eosinophilic 518.3
 exercise induced bronchospasm 493.81
 exogenous (cosmetics) (dander or dust) (drugs)
   (dust) (feathers) (food) (hay) (platinum)
   (pollen) 493.0 ☑
 extrinsic 493.0 ☑
 grinders' 502
 hay 493.0 ☑
 heart (*see also* Failure, ventricular, left) 428.1
 IgE 493.0 ☑
 infective 493.1 ☑
 intrinsic 493.1 ☑
 Kopp's 254.8
 late-onset 493.1 ☑
 meat-wrappers' 506.9
 Millar's (laryngismus stridulus) 478.75
 millstone makers' 502
 miners' 500
 Monday morning 504
 New Orleans (epidemic) 493.0 ☑
 platinum 493.0 ☑
 pneumoconiotic (occupational) NEC 505
 potters' 502
 psychogenic 316 [493.9] ☑
 pulmonary eosinophilic 518.3
 red cedar 495.8
 Rostan's (*see also* Failure, ventricular, left)
   428.1
 sandblasters' 502
 sequoiosis 495.8
 stonemasons' 502
 thymic 254.8
 tuberculous (*see also* Tuberculosis, pulmonary)
   011.9 ☑
 Wichmann's (laryngismus stridulus) 478.75
 wood 495.8
Astigmatism (compound) (congenital) 367.20
 irregular 367.22
 regular 367.21
Astroblastoma (M9430/3)
 nose 748.1
 specified site — *see* Neoplasm, by site,
   malignant
 unspecified site 191.9

Astrocytoma (cystic) (M9400/3)
 anaplastic type (M9401/3)
  specified site — *see* Neoplasm, by site,
    malignant
  unspecified site 191.9
 fibrillary (M9420/3)
  specified site — *see* Neoplasm, by site,
    malignant
  unspecified site 191.9
 fibrous (M9420/3)
  specified site — *see* Neoplasm, by site,
    malignant
  unspecified site 191.9
 gemistocytic (M9411/3)
  specified site — *see* Neoplasm, by site,
    malignant
  unspecified site 191.9
 juvenile (M9421/3)
  specified site — *see* Neoplasm, by site,
    malignant
  unspecified site 191.9
 nose 748.1
 pilocytic (M9421/3)
  specified site — *see* Neoplasm, by site,
    malignant
  unspecified site 191.9
 piloid (M9421/3)
  specified site — *see* Neoplasm, by site,
    malignant
  unspecified site 191.9
 protoplasmic (M9410/3)
  specified site — *see* Neoplasm, by site,
    malignant
  unspecified site 191.9
 specified site — *see* Neoplasm, by site,
   malignant
 subependymal (M9383/1) 237.5
  giant cell (M9384/1) 237.5
 unspecified site 191.9
Astroglioma (M9400/3)
 nose 748.1
 specified site — *see* Neoplasm, by site,
   malignant
 unspecified site 191.9
Asymbolia 784.60
Asymmetrical breathing 786.09
Asymmetry — *see also* Distortion
 chest 786.9
 face 754.0
 jaw NEC 524.12
  maxillary 524.11
 pelvis with disproportion 653.0 ☑
  affecting fetus or newborn 763.1
  causing obstructed labor 660.1 ☑
   affecting fetus or newborn 763.1
Asynergia 781.3
Asynergy 781.3
 ventricular 429.89
Asystole (heart) (*see also* Arrest, cardiac) 427.5
Ataxia, ataxy, ataxic 781.3
 acute 781.3
 brain 331.89
 cerebellar 334.3
  hereditary (Marie's) 334.2
  in
   alcoholism 303.9 ☑ [334.4]
   myxedema (*see also* Myxedema) 244.9
     [334.4]
   neoplastic disease NEC 239.9 [334.4]
 cerebral 331.89
 family, familial 334.2
  cerebral (Marie's) 334.2
  spinal (Friedreich's) 334.0
 Friedreich's (heredofamilial) (spinal) 334.0
 frontal lobe 781.3
 gait 781.2
  hysterical 300.11
 general 781.3
 hereditary NEC 334.2
  cerebellar 334.2
  spastic 334.1
  spinal 334.0
 heredofamilial (Marie's) 334.2
 hysterical 300.11

☑ Additional Digit Required   ▶◀ Revised Text   ● New Line   ▲ Revised Code

Ataxia, ataxy, ataxic — *continued*
  locomotor (progressive) 094.0
    diabetic 250.6 ☑ *[337.1]*
    Marie's (cerebellar) (heredofamilial) 334.2
    nonorganic origin 307.9
    partial 094.0
    postchickenpox 052.7
    progressive locomotor 094.0
    psychogenic 307.9
    Sanger-Brown's 334.2
    spastic 094.0
      hereditary 334.1
      syphilitic 094.0
    spinal
      hereditary 334.0
      progressive locomotor 094.0
    telangiectasia 334.8
Ataxia-telangiectasia 334.8
Atelectasis (absorption collapse) (complete)
    (compression) (massive) (partial)
    (postinfective) (pressure collapse)
    (pulmonary) (relaxation) 518.0
  newborn (congenital) (partial) 770.5
    primary 770.4
  primary 770.4
  tuberculous (*see also* Tuberculosis, pulmonary)
    011.9 ☑
Ateleiosis, ateliosis 253.3
Atelia — *see* Distortion
Ateliosis 253.3
Atelocardia 746.9
Atelomyelia 742.59
Athelia 757.6
Atheroembolism
  extremity
    lower 445.02
    upper 445.01
  kidney 445.81
  specified site NEC 445.89
Atheroma, atheromatous (*see also*
    Arteriosclerosis) 440.9
  aorta, aortic 440.0
    valve (*see also* Endocarditis, aortic) 424.1
  artery — *see* Arteriosclerosis
  basilar (artery) (*see also* Occlusion, artery,
    basilar) 433.0 ☑
  carotid (artery) (common) (internal) (*see also*
    Occlusion, artery, carotid) 433.1 ☑
  cerebral (arteries) 437.0
  coronary (artery) — *see* Arteriosclerosis,
    coronary
  degeneration — *see* Arteriosclerosis
  heart, cardiac — *see* Arteriosclerosis, coronary
  mitral (valve) 424.0
  myocardium, myocardial — *see*
    Arteriosclerosis, coronary
  pulmonary valve (heart) (*see also* Endocarditis,
    pulmonary) 424.3
  skin 706.2
  tricuspid (heart) (valve) 424.2
  valve, valvular — *see* Endocarditis
  vertebral (artery) (*see also* Occlusion, artery,
    vertebral) 433.2 ☑
Atheromatosis — *see also* Arteriosclerosis
  arterial, congenital 272.8
Atherosclerosis — *see* Arteriosclerosis
Athetosis (acquired) 781.0
  bilateral 333.7
  congenital (bilateral) 333.7
  double 333.7
  unilateral 781.0
Athlete's
  foot 110.4
  heart 429.3
Athletic team examination V70.3
Athrepsia 261
Athyrea (acquired) (*see also* Hypothyroidism)
    244.9
  congenital 243
Athyreosis (congenital) 243
  acquired — *see* Hypothyroidism

Athyroidism (acquired) (*see also* Hypothyroidism)
    244.9
  congenital 243
Atmospheric pyrexia 992.0
Atonia, atony, atonic
  abdominal wall 728.2
  bladder (sphincter) 596.4
    neurogenic NEC 596.54
      with cauda equina syndrome 344.61
  capillary 448.9
  cecum 564.89
    psychogenic 306.4
  colon 564.89
    psychogenic 306.4
    congenital 779.89
  dyspepsia 536.3
    psychogenic 306.4
  intestine 564.89
    psychogenic 306.4
  stomach 536.3
    neurotic or psychogenic 306.4
    psychogenic 306.4
  uterus 666.1 ☑
    affecting fetus or newborn 763.7
  vesical 596.4
Atopy NEC V15.09
Atransferrinemia, congenital 273.8
Atresia, atretic (congenital) 759.89
  alimentary organ or tract NEC 751.8
    lower 751.2
    upper 750.8
  ani, anus, anal (canal) 751.2
  aorta 747.22
    with hypoplasia of ascending aorta and
      defective development of left ventricle
      (with mitral valve atresia) 746.7
    arch 747.11
    ring 747.21
  aortic (orifice) (valve) 746.89
    arch 747.11
  aqueduct of Sylvius 742.3
    with spina bifida (*see also* Spina bifida)
      741.0 ☑
  artery NEC (*see also* Atresia, blood vessel)
    747.60
    cerebral 747.81
    coronary 746.85
    eye 743.58
    pulmonary 747.3
    umbilical 747.5
  auditory canal (external) 744.02
  bile, biliary duct (common) or passage 751.61
    acquired (*see also* Obstruction, biliary)
      576.2
  bladder (neck) 753.6
  blood vessel (peripheral) NEC 747.60
    cerebral 747.81
    gastrointestinal 747.61
    lower limb 747.64
    pulmonary artery 747.3
    renal 747.62
    spinal 747.82
    upper limb 747.63
  bronchus 748.3
  canal, ear 744.02
  cardiac
    valve 746.89
      aortic 746.89
      mitral 746.89
      pulmonary 746.01
      tricuspid 746.1
  cecum 751.2
  cervix (acquired) 622.4
    congenital 752.49
    in pregnancy or childbirth 654.6 ☑
      affecting fetus or newborn 763.89
      causing obstructed labor 660.2 ☑
        affecting fetus or newborn 763.1
  choana 748.0
  colon 751.2
  cystic duct 751.61
    acquired 575.8
      with obstruction (*see also* Obstruction,
        gallbladder) 575.2
  digestive organs NEC 751.8
  duodenum 751.1

Atresia, atretic — *continued*
  ear canal 744.02
  ejaculatory duct 752.89
  epiglottis 748.3
  esophagus 750.3
  Eustachian tube 744.24
  fallopian tube (acquired) 628.2
    congenital 752.19
  follicular cyst 620.0
  foramen of
    Luschka 742.3
      with spina bifida (*see also* Spina bifida)
        741.0 ☑
    Magendie 742.3
      with spina bifida (*see also* Spina bifida)
        741.0 ☑
  gallbladder 751.69
  genital organ
    external
      female 752.49
      male NEC 752.89
        penis 752.69
    internal
      female 752.89
      male 752.89
  glottis 748.3
  gullet 750.3
  heart
    valve NEC 746.89
      aortic 746.89
      mitral 746.89
      pulmonary 746.01
      tricuspid 746.1
  hymen 752.42
    acquired 623.3
    postinfective 623.3
  ileum 751.1
  intestine (small) 751.1
    large 751.2
  iris, filtration angle (*see also* Buphthalmia)
    743.20
  jejunum 751.1
  kidney 753.3
  lacrimal, apparatus 743.65
    acquired — *see* Stenosis, lacrimal
  larynx 748.3
  ligament, broad 752.19
  lung 748.5
  meatus urinarius 753.6
  mitral valve 746.89
    with atresia or hypoplasia of aortic orifice or
      valve, with hypoplasia of ascending
      aorta and defective development of left
      ventricle 746.7
  nares (anterior) (posterior) 748.0
  nasolacrimal duct 743.65
  nasopharynx 748.8
  nose, nostril 748.0
    acquired 738.0
  organ or site NEC — *see* Anomaly, specified
    type NEC
  osseous meatus (ear) 744.03
  oviduct (acquired) 628.2
    congenital 752.19
  parotid duct 750.23
    acquired 527.8
  pulmonary (artery) 747.3
    valve 746.01
    vein 747.49
  pulmonic 746.01
  pupil 743.46
  rectum 751.2
  salivary duct or gland 750.23
    acquired 527.8
  sublingual duct 750.23
    acquired 527.8
  submaxillary duct or gland 750.23
    acquired 527.8
  trachea 748.3
  tricuspid valve 746.1
  ureter 753.29
  ureteropelvic junction 753.21
  ureterovesical orifice 753.22
  urethra (valvular) 753.6
  urinary tract NEC 753.29
  uterus 752.3
    acquired 621.8

Ataxia, ataxy, ataxic — Atresia, atretic

Atresia, atretic — *continued*
  vagina (acquired) 623.2
    congenital 752.49
    postgonococcal (old) 098.2
    postinfectional 623.2
    senile 623.2
  vascular NEC (*see also* Atresia, blood vessel)
    747.60
    cerebral 747.81
  vas deferens 752.89
  vein NEC (*see also* Atresia, blood vessel) 747.60
    cardiac 746.89
    great 747.49
    portal 747.49
    pulmonary 747.49
  vena cava (inferior) (superior) 747.49
  vesicourethral orifice 753.6
  vulva 752.49
    acquired 624.8

Atrichia, atrichosis 704.00
  congenital (universal) 757.4

Atrioventricularis commune 745.69

Atrophia — *see also* Atrophy
  alba 709.09
  cutis 701.8
    idiopathica progressiva 701.8
    senilis 701.8
  dermatological, diffuse (idiopathic) 701.8
  flava hepatis (acuta) (subacuta) (*see also*
    Necrosis, liver) 570
  gyrata of choroid and retina (central) 363.54
    generalized 363.57
  senilis 797
    dermatological 701.8
  unguium 703.8
    congenita 757.5

Atrophoderma, atrophodermia 701.9
  diffusum (idiopathic) 701.8
  maculatum 701.3
    et striatum 701.3
      due to syphilis 095.8
    syphilitic 091.3
  neuriticum 701.8
  pigmentosum 757.33
  reticulatum symmetricum faciei 701.8
  senile 701.8
  symmetrical 701.8
  vermiculata 701.8

Atrophy, atrophic
  adrenal (autoimmune) (capsule) (cortex) (gland)
    255.4
    with hypofunction 255.4
  alveolar process or ridge (edentulous)
    525.20 ▲
    mandible 525.20 ●
      minimal 525.21 ●
      moderate 525.22 ●
      severe 525.23 ●
    maxilla 525.20 ●
      minimal 525.24 ●
      moderate 525.25 ●
      severe 525.26 ●
  appendix 543.9
  Aran-Duchenne muscular 335.21
  arm 728.2
  arteriosclerotic — *see* Arteriosclerosis
  arthritis 714.0
    spine 720.9
  bile duct (any) 576.8
  bladder 596.8
  blanche (of Milian) 701.3
  bone (senile) 733.99
    due to
      disuse 733.7
      infection 733.99
      tabes dorsalis (neurogenic) 094.0
    posttraumatic 733.99
  brain (cortex) (progressive) 331.9
    with dementia 290.10
    Alzheimer's 331.0
      with dementia — *see* Alzheimer's,
        dementia
    circumscribed (Pick's) 331.11
      with dementia
        with behavioral disturbance
          331.11 *[294.11]*

Atrophy, atrophic — *continued*
  brain — *continued*
    circumscribed — *continued*
      with dementia — *continued*
        without behavioral disturbance
          331.11 *[294.10]*
    congenital 742.4
    hereditary 331.9
    senile 331.2
  breast 611.4
    puerperal, postpartum 676.3 ☑
  buccal cavity 528.9
  cardiac (brown) (senile) (*see also* Degeneration,
    myocardial) 429.1
  cartilage (infectional) (joint) 733.99
  cast, plaster of Paris 728.2
  cerebellar — *see* Atrophy, brain
  cerebral — *see* Atrophy, brain
  cervix (endometrium) (mucosa) (myometrium)
    (senile) (uteri) 622.8
    menopausal 627.8
  Charcôt-Marie-Tooth 356.1
  choroid 363.40
    diffuse secondary 363.42
    hereditary (*see also* Dystrophy, choroid)
      363.50
      gyrate
        central 363.54
        diffuse 363.57
        generalized 363.57
    senile 363.41
  ciliary body 364.57
  colloid, degenerative 701.3
  conjunctiva (senile) 372.89
  corpus cavernosum 607.89
  cortical (*see also* Atrophy, brain) 331.9
  Cruveilhier's 335.21
  cystic duct 576.8
  dacryosialadenopathy 710.2
  degenerative
    colloid 701.3
    senile 701.3
  Déjérine-Thomas 333.0
  diffuse idiopathic, dermatological 701.8
  disuse
    bone 733.7
    muscle 728.2
    pelvic muscles and anal spincter 618.83 ●
  Duchenne-Aran 335.21
  ear 388.9
  edentulous alveolar ridge 525.20 ▲
    mandible 525.20 ●
      minimal 525.21 ●
      moderate 525.22 ●
      severe 525.23 ●
    maxilla 525.20 ●
      minimal 525.24 ●
      moderate 525.25 ●
      severe 525.26 ●
  emphysema, lung 492.8
  endometrium (senile) 621.8
    cervix 622.8
  enteric 569.89
  epididymis 608.3
  eyeball, cause unknown 360.41
  eyelid (senile) 374.50
  facial (skin) 701.9
  facioscapulohumeral (Landouzy-Déjérine) 359.1
  fallopian tube (senile), acquired 620.3
  fatty, thymus (gland) 254.8
  gallbladder 575.8
  gastric 537.89
  gastritis (chronic) 535.1 ☑
  gastrointestinal 569.89
  genital organ, male 608.89
  glandular 289.3
  globe (phthisis bulbi) 360.41
  gum ►(*see also* Recession, gingival)◄
    523.20 ▲
  hair 704.2
  heart (brown) (senile) (*see also* Degeneration,
    myocardial) 429.1
  hemifacial 754.0
    Romberg 349.89
  hydronephrosis 591

Atrophy, atrophic — *continued*
  infantile 261
    paralysis, acute (*see also* Poliomyelits, with
      paralysis) 045.1 ☑
  intestine 569.89
  iris (generalized) (postinfectional) (sector
    shaped) 364.59
    essential 364.51
    progressive 364.51
    sphincter 364.54
  kidney (senile) (*see also* Sclerosis, renal) 587
    with hypertension (*see also* Hypertension,
      kidney) 403.90
    congenital 753.0
    hydronephrotic 591
    infantile 753.0
  lacrimal apparatus (primary) 375.13
    secondary 375.14
  Landouzy-Déjérine 359.1
  laryngitis, infection 476.0
  larynx 478.79
  Leber's optic 377.16
  lip 528.5
  liver (acute) (subacute) (*see also* Necrosis, liver)
    570
    chronic (yellow) 571.8
    yellow (congenital) 570
      with
        abortion — *see* Abortion, by type, with
          specified complication NEC
        ectopic pregnancy (*see also* categories
          633.0-633.9) 639.8
        molar pregnancy (*see also* categories
          630-632) 639.8
      chronic 571.8
      complicating pregnancy 646.7 ☑
      following
        abortion 639.8
        ectopic or molar pregnancy 639.8
      from injection, inoculation or transfusion
        (onset within 8 months after
        administration) — *see* Hepatitis,
        viral
      healed 571.5
      obstetric 646.7 ☑
      postabortal 639.8
      postimmunization — *see* Hepatitis, viral
      posttransfusion — *see* Hepatitis, viral
      puerperal, postpartum 674.8 ☑
  lung (senile) 518.89
    congenital 748.69
  macular (dermatological) 701.3
    syphilitic, skin 091.3
      striated 095.8
  muscle, muscular 728.2
    disuse 728.2
    Duchenne-Aran 335.21
    extremity (lower) (upper) 728.2
    familial spinal 335.11
    general 728.2
    idiopathic 728.2
    infantile spinal 335.0
    myelopathic (progressive) 335.10
    myotonic 359.2
    neuritic 356.1
    neuropathic (peroneal) (progressive) 356.1
    peroneal 356.1
    primary (idiopathic) 728.2
    progressive (familial) (hereditary) (pure)
      335.21
      adult (spinal) 335.19
      infantile (spinal) 335.0
      juvenile (spinal) 335.11
      spinal 335.10
        adult 335.19
          Aran-Duchenne 335.10
          hereditary or familial 335.11
          infantile 335.0
    pseudohypertrophic 359.1
    spinal (progressive) 335.10
      adult 335.19
      Aran-Duchenne 335.21
      familial 335.11
      hereditary 335.11
      infantile 335.0
      juvenile 335.11
    syphilitic 095.6

☑ Additional Digit Required   ►◄ Revised Text   ● New Line   ▲ Revised Code

Atrophy, atrophic — *continued*
  myocardium (*see also* Degeneration,
      myocardial) 429.1
  myometrium (senile) 621.8
      cervix 622.8
  myotatic 728.2
  myotonia 359.2
  nail 703.8
      congenital 757.5
  nasopharynx 472.2
  nerve — *see also* Disorder, nerve
      abducens 378.54
      accessory 352.4
      acoustic or auditory 388.5
      cranial 352.9
          first (olfactory) 352.0
          second (optic) (*see also* Atrophy, optic
              nerve) 377.10
          third (oculomotor)(partial) 378.51
              total 378.52
          fourth (trochlear) 378.53
          fifth (trigeminal) 350.8
          sixth (abducens) 378.54
          seventh (facial) 351.8
          eighth (auditory) 388.5
          ninth (glossopharyngeal) 352.2
          tenth (pneumogastric) (vagus) 352.3
          eleventh (accessory) 352.4
          twelfth (hypoglossal) 352.5
      facial 351.8
      glossopharyngeal 352.2
      hypoglossal 352.5
      oculomotor (partial) 378.51
      total 378.52
      olfactory 352.0
      peripheral 355.9
      pneumogastric 352.3
      trigeminal 350.8
      trochlear 378.53
      vagus (pneumogastric) 352.3
  nervous system, congenital 742.8
  neuritic (*see also* Disorder, nerve) 355.9
  neurogenic NEC 355.9
      bone
          tabetic 094.0
  nutritional 261
  old age 797
  olivopontocerebellar 333.0
  optic nerve (ascending) (descending)
      (infectional) (nonfamilial) (papillomacular
      bundle) (postretinal) (secondary NEC)
      (simple) 377.10
      associated with retinal dystrophy 377.13
      dominant hereditary 377.16
      glaucomatous 377.14
      hereditary (dominant) (Leber's) 377.16
      Leber's (hereditary) 377.16
      partial 377.15
      postinflammatory 377.12
      primary 377.11
      syphilitic 094.84
          congenital 090.49
          tabes dorsalis 094.0
  orbit 376.45
  ovary (senile), acquired 620.3
  oviduct (senile), acquired 620.3
  palsy, diffuse 335.20
  pancreas (duct) (senile) 577.8
  papillary muscle 429.81
  paralysis 355.9
  parotid gland 527.0
  patches skin 701.3
      senile 701.8
  penis 607.89
  pharyngitis 472.1
  pharynx 478.29
  pluriglandular 258.8
  polyarthritis 714.0
  prostate 602.2
  pseudohypertrophic 359.1
  renal (*see also* Sclerosis, renal) 587
  reticulata 701.8
  retina (*see also* Degeneration, retina) 362.60
      hereditary (*see also* Dystrophy, retina)
          362.70
  rhinitis 472.0
  salivary duct or gland 527.0

Atrophy, atrophic — *continued*
  scar NEC 709.2
  sclerosis, lobar (of brain) 331.0
      with dementia
          with behavioral disturbance
              331.0 *[294.11]*
          without behavioral disturbance
              331.0 *[294.10]*
  scrotum 608.89
  seminal vesicle 608.89
  senile 797
      degenerative, of skin 701.3
  skin (patches) (senile) 701.8
  spermatic cord 608.89
  spinal (cord) 336.8
      acute 336.8
      muscular (chronic) 335.10
          adult 335.19
          familial 335.11
          juvenile 335.10
      paralysis 335.10
          acute (*see also* Poliomyelitis, with
              paralysis) 045.1 ☑
  spine (column) 733.99
  spleen (senile) 289.59
  spots (skin) 701.3
      senile 701.8
  stomach 537.89
  striate and macular 701.3
      syphilitic 095.8
  subcutaneous 701.9
      due to injection 999.9
  sublingual gland 527.0
  submaxillary gland 527.0
  Sudeck's 733.7
  suprarenal (autoimmune) (capsule) (gland)
      255.4
      with hypofunction 255.4
  tarso-orbital fascia, congenital 743.66
  testis 608.3
  thenar, partial 354.0
  throat 478.29
  thymus (fat) 254.8
  thyroid (gland) 246.8
      with
          cretinism 243
          myxedema 244.9
      congenital 243
  tongue (senile) 529.8
      papillae 529.4
      smooth 529.4
  trachea 519.1
  tunica vaginalis 608.89
  turbinate 733.99
  tympanic membrane (nonflaccid) 384.82
      flaccid 384.81
  ulcer (*see also* Ulcer, skin) 707.9
  upper respiratory tract 478.9
  uterus, uterine (acquired) (senile) 621.8
      cervix 622.8
      due to radiation (intended effect) 621.8
  vagina (senile) 627.3
  vascular 459.89
  vas deferens 608.89
  vertebra (senile) 733.99
  vulva (primary) (senile) 624.1
  Werdnig-Hoffmann 335.0
  yellow (acute) (congenital) (liver) (subacute) (*see
      also* Necrosis, liver) 570
      chronic 571.8
      resulting from administration of blood,
          plasma, serum, or other biological
          substance (within 8 months of
          administration) — *see* Hepatitis, viral

Attack
  akinetic (*see also* Epilepsy) 345.0 ☑
  angina — *see* Angina
  apoplectic (*see also* Disease, cerebrovascular,
      acute) 436
  benign shuddering 333.93
  bilious — *see* Vomiting
  cataleptic 300.11
  cerebral (*see also* Disease, cerebrovascular,
      acute) 436
  coronary (*see also* Infarct, myocardium)
      410.9 ☑

Attack — *continued*
  cyanotic, newborn 770.83
  epileptic (*see also* Epilepsy) 345.9 ☑
  epileptiform 780.39
  heart (*see also* Infarct, myocardium) 410.9 ☑
  hemiplegia (*see also* Disease, cerebrovascular,
      acute) 436
  hysterical 300.11
  jacksonian (*see also* Epilepsy) 345.5 ☑
  myocardium, myocardial (*see also* Infarct,
      myocardium) 410.9 ☑
  myoclonic (*see also* Epilepsy) 345.1 ☑
  panic 300.01
  paralysis (*see also* Disease, cerebrovascular,
      acute) 436
  paroxysmal 780.39
  psychomotor (*see also* Epilepsy) 345.4 ☑
  salaam (*see also* Epilepsy) 345.6 ☑
  schizophreniform (*see also* Schizophrenia)
      295.4 ☑
  sensory and motor 780.39
  syncope 780.2
  toxic, cerebral 780.39
  transient ischemic (TIA) 435.9
  unconsciousness 780.2
      hysterical 300.11
  vasomotor 780.2
  vasovagal (idiopathic) (paroxysmal) 780.2

Attention to
  artificial opening (of) V55.9
      digestive tract NEC V55.4
      specified site NEC V55.8
      urinary tract NEC V55.6
      vagina V55.7
  colostomy V55.3
  cystostomy V55.5
  gastrostomy V55.1
  ileostomy V55.2
  jejunostomy V55.4
  nephrostomy V55.6
  surgical dressings V58.3
  sutures V58.3
  tracheostomy V55.0
  ureterostomy V55.6
  urethrostomy V55.6

Attrition
  gum ►(*see also* Recession, gingival)◄
      523.20   ▲
  teeth (hard tissues) 521.10   ▲
      excessive 521.10   ●
          extending into   ●
              dentine 521.12   ●
              pulp 521.13   ●
          generalized 521.15   ●
          limited to enamel 521.11   ●
          localized 521.14   ●

Atypical — *see also* condition
  cells
      endocervical 795.00   ●
      endometrial 795.00   ●
      glandular 795.00   ●
  distribution, vessel (congenital) (peripheral)
      NEC 747.60
  endometrium 621.9
  kidney 593.89

Atypism, cervix 622.10   ▲

Audible tinnitus (*see also* Tinnitus) 388.30

Auditory — *see* condition

Audry's syndrome (acropachyderma) 757.39

Aujeszky's disease 078.89

Aura, jacksonian (*see also* Epilepsy) 345.5 ☑

Aurantiasis, cutis 278.3

Auricle, auricular — *see* condition

Auriculotemporal syndrome 350.8

Australian
  Q fever 083.0
  X disease 062.4

Autism, autistic (child) (infantile) 299.0 ☑

Autodigestion 799.89

Autoerythrocyte sensitization 287.2

Autographism 708.3

Autoimmune
  cold sensitivity 283.0

☑ Additional Digit Required   ►◄ Revised Text   ● New Line   ▲ Revised Code

Autoimmune — *continued*
disease NEC 279.4
hemolytic anemia 283.0
thyroiditis 245.2
Autoinfection, septic — *see* Septicemia
Autointoxication 799.89
Automatism 348.8
epileptic (*see also* Epilepsy) 345.4 ☑
paroxysmal, idiopathic (*see also* Epilepsy) 345.4 ☑
Autonomic, autonomous
bladder 596.54
neurogenic NEC 596.54
with cauda equina 344.61
dysreflexia 337.3
faciocephalalgia (*see also* Neuropathy, peripheral, autonomic) 337.9
hysterical seizure 300.11
imbalance (*see also* Neuropathy, peripheral, autonomic) 337.9
Autophony 388.40
Autosensitivity, erythrocyte 287.2
Autotopagnosia 780.99
Autotoxemia 799.89
Autumn — *see* condition
Avellis' syndrome 344.89
Aviators
disease or sickness (*see also* Effect, adverse, high altitude) 993.2
ear 993.0
effort syndrome 306.2
Avitaminosis (multiple NEC) (*see also* Deficiency, vitamin) 269.2
A 264.9
B 266.9
with
beriberi 265.0
pellagra 265.2
B_1 265.1
B_2 266.0
B_6 266.1
B_{12} 266.2
C (with scurvy) 267
D 268.9
with
osteomalacia 268.2
rickets 268.0
E 269.1
G 266.0
H 269.1
K 269.0
multiple 269.2
nicotinic acid 265.2
P 269.1
Avulsion (traumatic) 879.8
blood vessel — *see* Injury, blood vessel, by site
cartilage — *see* Dislocation, by site
knee, current (*see also* Tear, meniscus) 836.2
symphyseal (inner), complicating delivery 665.6 ☑
complicated 879.9
diaphragm — *see* Injury, internal, diaphragm
ear — *see* Wound, open, ear
epiphysis of bone — *see* Fracture, by site
external site other than limb — *see* Wound, open, by site
eye 871.3
fingernail — *see* Wound, open, finger
fracture — *see* Fracture, by site
genital organs, external — *see* Wound, open, genital organs
head (intracranial) NEC — *see also* Injury, intracranial, with open intracranial wound
complete 874.9
external site NEC 873.8
complicated 873.9
internal organ or site — *see* Injury, internal, by site
joint — *see also* Dislocation, by site
capsule — *see* Sprain, by site
ligament — *see* Sprain, by site

Avulsion — *continued*
limb — *see also* Amputation, traumatic, by site
skin and subcutaneous tissue — *see* Wound, open, by site
muscle — *see* Sprain, by site
nerve (root) — *see* Injury, nerve, by site
scalp — *see* Wound, open, scalp
skin and subcutaneous tissue — *see* Wound, open, by site
symphyseal cartilage (inner), complicating delivery 665.6 ☑
tendon — *see also* Sprain, by site
with open wound — *see* Wound, open, by site
toenail — *see* Wound, open, toe(s)
tooth 873.63
complicated 873.73
Awaiting organ transplant status V49.83 ●
Awareness of heart beat 785.1
Axe grinders' disease 502
Axenfeld's anomaly or syndrome 743.44
Axilla, axillary — *see also* condition
breast 757.6
Axonotmesis — *see* Injury, nerve, by site
Ayala's disease 756.89
Ayerza's disease or syndrome (pulmonary artery sclerosis with pulmonary hypertension) 416.0
Azoospermia 606.0
Azotemia 790.6
meaning uremia (*see also* Uremia) 586
Aztec ear 744.29
Azorean disease (of the nervous system) 334.8
Azygos lobe, lung (fissure) 748.69

B

Baader's syndrome (erythema multiforme exudativum) 695.1
Baastrup's syndrome 721.5
Babesiasis 088.82
Babesiosis 088.82
Babington's disease (familial hemorrhagic telangiectasia) 448.0
Babinski's syndrome (cardiovascular syphilis) 093.89
Babinski-Fröhlich syndrome (adiposogenital dystrophy) 253.8
Babinski-Nageotte syndrome 344.89
Bacillary — *see* condition
Bacilluria 791.9
asymptomatic, in pregnancy or puerperium 646.5 ☑
tuberculous (*see also* Tuberculosis) 016.9 ☑
Bacillus — *see also* Infection, bacillus
abortus infection 023.1
anthracis infection 022.9
coli
infection 041.4
generalized 038.42
intestinal 008.00
pyemia 038.42
septicemia 038.42
Flexner's 004.1
fusiformis infestation 101
mallei infection 024
Shiga's 004.0
suipestifer infection (*see also* Infection, Salmonella) 003.9
Back — *see* condition
Backache (postural) 724.5
psychogenic 307.89
sacroiliac 724.6
Backflow (pyelovenous) (*see also* Disease, renal) 593.9
Backknee (*see also* Genu, recurvatum) 736.5
Bacteremia 790.7
newborn 771.83
Bacteria
in blood (*see also* Bacteremia) 790.7
in urine (*see also* Bacteriuria) 599.0

Bacterial — *see* condition
Bactericholia (*see also* Cholecystitis, acute) 575.0
Bacterid, bacteride (Andrews' pustular) 686.8
Bacteriuria, bacteruria 791.9
with
urinary tract infection 599.0
asymptomatic 791.9
in pregnancy or puerperium 646.5 ☑
affecting fetus or newborn 760.1
Bad
breath 784.9
heart — *see* Disease, heart
trip (*see also* Abuse, drugs, nondependent) 305.3 ☑
Baehr-Schiffrin disease (thrombotic thrombocytopenic purpura) 446.6
Baelz's disease (cheilitis glandularis apostematosa) 528.5
Baerensprung's disease (eczema marginatum) 110.3
Bagassosis (occupational) 495.1
Baghdad boil 085.1
Bagratuni's syndrome (temporal arteritis) 446.5
Baker's
cyst (knee) 727.51
tuberculous (*see also* Tuberculosis) 015.2 ☑
itch 692.82
Bakwin-Krida syndrome (craniometaphyseal dysplasia) 756.89
Balanitis (circinata) (gangraenosa) (infectious) (vulgaris) 607.1
amebic 006.8
candidal 112.2
chlamydial 099.53
due to Ducrey's bacillus 099.0
erosiva circinata et gangraenosa 607.1
gangrenous 607.1
gonococcal (acute) 098.0
chronic or duration of 2 months or over 098.2
nongonococcal 607.1
phagedenic 607.1
venereal NEC 099.8
xerotica obliterans 607.81
Balanoposthitis 607.1
chlamydial 099.53
gonococcal (acute) 098.0
chronic or duration of 2 months or over 098.2
ulcerative NEC 099.8
Balanorrhagia — *see* Balanitis
Balantidiasis 007.0
Balantidiosis 007.0
Balbuties, balbutio 307.0
Bald
patches on scalp 704.00
tongue 529.4
Baldness (*see also* Alopecia) 704.00
Balfour's disease (chloroma) 205.3 ☑
Balint's syndrome (psychic paralysis of visual fixation) 368.16
Balkan grippe 083.0
Ball
food 938
hair 938
Ballantyne (-Runge) syndrome (postmaturity) 766.22
Balloon disease (*see also* Effect, adverse, high altitude) 993.2
Ballooning posterior leaflet syndrome 424.0
Baló's disease or concentric sclerosis 341.1
Bamberger's disease (hypertrophic pulmonary osteoarthropathy) 731.2
Bamberger-Marie disease (hypertrophic pulmonary osteoarthropathy) 731.2
Bamboo spine 720.0
Bancroft's filariasis 125.0
Band(s)
adhesive (*see also* Adhesions, peritoneum) 568.0

☑ Additional Digit Required   ▶◀ Revised Text   ● New Line   ▲ Revised Code

Band(s) — *continued*
  amniotic 658.8 ☑
    affecting fetus or newborn 762.8
  anomalous or congenital — *see also* Anomaly,
      specified type NEC
    atrial 746.9
    heart 746.9
    intestine 751.4
    omentum 751.4
    ventricular 746.9
  cervix 622.3
  gallbladder (congenital) 751.69
  intestinal (adhesive) (*see also* Adhesions,
      peritoneum) 568.0
    congenital 751.4
  obstructive (*see also* Obstruction, intestine)
      560.81
  periappendiceal (congenital) 751.4
  peritoneal (adhesive) (*see also* Adhesions,
      peritoneum) 568.0
    with intestinal obstruction 560.81
    congenital 751.4
  uterus 621.5
  vagina 623.2
Bandl's ring (contraction)
  complicating delivery 661.4 ☑
    affecting fetus or newborn 763.7
Bang's disease (Brucella abortus) 023.1
Bangkok hemorrhagic fever 065.4
Bannister's disease 995.1
Bantam-Albright-Martin disease
    (pseudohypoparathyroidism) 275.49
Banti's disease or syndrome (with cirrhosis)
    (with portal hypertension) — *see* Cirrhosis,
    liver
Bar
  calcaneocuboid 755.67
  calcaneonavicular 755.67
  cubonavicular 755.67
  prostate 600.90
    with urinary retention 600.91
  talocalcaneal 755.67
Baragnosis 780.99
Barasheh, barashek 266.2
Barcoo disease or rot (*see also* Ulcer, skin) 707.9
Bard-Pic syndrome (carcinoma, head of pancreas)
    157.0
Bärensprung's disease (eczema marginatum)
    110.3
Baritosis 503
Barium lung disease 503
Barlow's syndrome (meaning mitral valve
    prolapse) 424.0
Barlow (-Möller) disease or syndrome (meaning
    infantile scurvy) 267
Barodontalgia 993.2
Baron Münchausen syndrome 301.51
Barosinusitis 993.1
Barotitis 993.0
Barotrauma 993.2
  odontalgia 993.2
  otitic 993.0
  sinus 993.1
Barraquer's disease or syndrome (progressive
    lipodystrophy) 272.6
Barré-Guillain syndrome 357.0
Barré-Liéou syndrome (posterior cervical
    sympathetic) 723.2
Barrel chest 738.3
Barrett's esophagus 530.85 ●
Barrett's syndrome or ulcer (chronic peptic ulcer
    of esophagus) 530.85
Bársony-Polgár syndrome (corkscrew esophagus)
    530.5
Bársony-Teschendorf syndrome (corkscrew
    esophagus) 530.5
Bartholin's
  adenitis (*see also* Bartholinitis) 616.8
  gland — *see* condition

Bartholinitis (suppurating) 616.8
  gonococcal (acute) 098.0
    chronic or duration of 2 months or over
      098.2
Bartonellosis 088.0
Bartter's syndrome (secondary
    hyperaldosteronism with juxtaglomerular
    hyperplasia) 255.13
Basal — *see* condition
Basan's (hidrotic) **ectodermal dysplasia** 757.31
Baseball finger 842.13
Basedow's disease or syndrome (exophthalmic
    goiter) 242.0 ☑
Basic — *see* condition
Basilar — *see* condition
Bason's (hidrotic) **ectodermal dysplasia** 757.31
Basopenia 288.0
Basophilia 288.8
Basophilism (corticoadrenal) (Cushing's)
    (pituitary) (thymic) 255.0
Bassen-Kornzweig syndrome
    (abetalipoproteinemia) 272.5
Bat ear 744.29
Bateman's
  disease 078.0
  purpura (senile) 287.2
Bathing cramp 994.1
Bathophobia 300.23
Batten's disease, retina 330.1 [362.71]
Batten-Mayou disease 330.1 [362.71]
Batten-Steinert syndrome 359.2
Battered
  adult (syndrome) 995.81
  baby or child (syndrome) 995.54
  spouse (syndrome) 995.81
Battey mycobacterium infection 031.0
Battledore placenta — *see* Placenta, abnormal
Battle exhaustion (*see also* Reaction, stress,
    acute) 308.9
Baumgarten-Cruveilhier (cirrhosis) **disease, or
    syndrome** 571.5
Bauxite
  fibrosis (of lung) 503
  workers' disease 503
Bayle's disease (dementia paralytica) 094.1
Bazin's disease (primary) (*see also* Tuberculosis)
    017.1 ☑
Beach ear 380.12
Beaded hair (congenital) 757.4
Beals syndrome 759.82 ●
Beard's disease (neurasthenia) 300.5
Bearn-Kunkel (-Slater) syndrome (lupoid
    hepatitis) 571.49
Beat
  elbow 727.2
  hand 727.2
  knee 727.2
Beats
  ectopic 427.60
  escaped, heart 427.60
    postoperative 997.1
  premature (nodal) 427.60
    atrial 427.61
    auricular 427.61
    postoperative 997.1
    specified type NEC 427.69
    supraventricular 427.61
    ventricular 427.69
Beau's
  disease or syndrome (*see also* Degeneration,
    myocardial) 429.1
  lines (transverse furrows on fingernails) 703.8
Bechterew's disease (ankylosing spondylitis)
    720.0
Bechterew-Strümpell-Marie syndrome
    (ankylosing spondylitis) 720.0
Beck's syndrome (anterior spinal artery
    occlusion) 433.8 ☑

Becker's
  disease (idiopathic mural endomyocardial
    disease) 425.2
  dystrophy 359.1
Beckwith (-Wiedemann) syndrome 759.89
Bedclothes, asphyxiation or suffocation by
    994.7
Bednar's aphthae 528.2
Bedsore 707.00 ▲
  with gangrene 707.00 [785.4] ▲
Bedwetting (*see also* Enuresis) 788.36
Beer-drinkers' heart (disease) 425.5
Bee sting (with allergic or anaphylactic shock)
    989.5
Begbie's disease (exophthalmic goiter) 242.0 ☑
Behavior disorder, disturbance — *see also*
    Disturbance, conduct
  antisocial, without manifest psychiatric
      disorder
    adolescent V71.02
    adult V71.01
    child V71.02
  dyssocial, without manifest psychiatric disorder
    adolescent V71.02
    adult V71.01
    child V71.02
  high risk — *see* Problem
Behçet's syndrome 136.1
Behr's disease 362.50
Beigel's disease or morbus (white piedra) 111.2
Bejel 104.0
Bekhterev's disease (ankylosing spondylitis)
    720.0
Bekhterev-Strümpell-Marie syndrome
    (ankylosing spondylitis) 720.0
Belching (*see also* Eructation) 787.3
Bell's
  disease (*see also* Psychosis, affective) 296.0 ☑
  mania (*see also* Psychosis, affective) 296.0 ☑
  palsy, paralysis 351.0
    infant 767.5
    newborn 767.5
    syphilitic 094.89
  spasm 351.0
**Bence-Jones albuminuria, albuminosuria, or
    proteinuria** 791.0
Bends 993.3
Benedikt's syndrome (paralysis) 344.89
Benign — *see also* condition
  cellular changes, cervix 795.09
  prostate
    hyperplasia 600.20 ▲
      with urinary retention 600.21 ▲
    neoplasm 222.2
Bennett's
  disease (leukemia) 208.9 ☑
  fracture (closed) 815.01
    open 815.11
Benson's disease 379.22
Bent
  back (hysterical) 300.11
  nose 738.0
    congenital 754.0
Bereavement V62.82
  as adjustment reaction 309.0
Berger's paresthesia (lower limb) 782.0
Bergeron's disease (hysteroepilepsy) 300.11
Beriberi (acute) (atrophic) (chronic) (dry)
    (subacute) (wet) 265.0
  with polyneuropathy 265.0 [357.4]
  heart (disease) 265.0 [425.7]
  leprosy 030.1
  neuritis 265.0 [357.4]
Berlin's disease or edema (traumatic) 921.3
Berloque dermatitis 692.72
Bernard-Horner syndrome (*see also* Neuropathy,
    peripheral, autonomic) 337.9
Bernard-Sergent syndrome (acute adrenocortical
    insufficiency) 255.4
Bernard-Soulier disease or thrombopathy 287.1

Bernhardt's disease or paresthesia 355.1
Bernhardt-Roth disease or syndrome
(paresthesia) 355.1
Bernheim's syndrome (*see also* Failure, heart)
428.0
Bertielliasis 123.8
Bertolotti's syndrome (sacralization of fifth
lumbar vertebra) 756.15
Berylliosis (acute) (chronic) (lung) (occupational)
503
Besnier's
lupus pernio 135
prurigo (atopic dermatitis) (infantile eczema)
691.8
Besnier-Boeck disease or sarcoid 135
Besnier-Boeck-Schaumann disease (sarcoidosis)
135
Best's disease 362.76
Bestiality 302.1
**Beta-adrenergic hyperdynamic circulatory
state** 429.82
Beta-aminoisobutyric aciduria 277.2
Beta-mercaptolactate-cysteine disulfiduria
270.0
Beta thalassemia (major) (minor) (mixed) 282.49
Beurmann's disease (sporotrichosis) 117.1
Bezoar 938
intestine 936
stomach 935.2
Bezold's abscess (*see also* Mastoiditis) 383.01
Bianchi's syndrome (aphasia-apraxia-alexia)
784.69
Bicornuate or bicornis uterus 752.3
in pregnancy or childbirth 654.0 ☑
with obstructed labor 660.2 ☑
affecting fetus or newborn 763.1
affecting fetus or newborn 763.89
Bicuspid aortic valve 746.4
Biedl-Bardet syndrome 759.89
Bielschowsky's disease 330.1
Bielschowsky-Jansky
amaurotic familial idiocy 330.1
disease 330.1
Biemond's syndrome (obesity, polydactyly, and
mental retardation) 759.89
Biermer's anemia or disease (pernicious anemia)
281.0
Biett's disease 695.4
Bifid (congenital) — *see also* Imperfect, closure
apex, heart 746.89
clitoris 752.49
epiglottis 748.3
kidney 753.3
nose 748.1
patella 755.64
scrotum 752.89
toe 755.66
tongue 750.13
ureter 753.4
uterus 752.3
uvula 749.02
with cleft lip (*see also* Cleft, palate, with cleft
lip) 749.20
Biforis uterus (suprasimplex) 752.3
Bifurcation (congenital) — *see also* Imperfect,
closure
gallbladder 751.69
kidney pelvis 753.3
renal pelvis 753.3
rib 756.3
tongue 750.13
trachea 748.3
ureter 753.4
urethra 753.8
uvula 749.02
with cleft lip (*see also* Cleft, palate, with cleft
lip) 749.20
vertebra 756.19
Bigeminal pulse 427.89
Bigeminy 427.89
Big spleen syndrome 289.4

Bilateral — *see* condition
Bile duct — *see* condition
Bile pigments in urine 791.4
Bilharziasis (*see also* Schistosomiasis) 120.9
chyluria 120.0
cutaneous 120.3
galacturia 120.0
hematochyluria 120.0
intestinal 120.1
lipemia 120.9
lipuria 120.0
Oriental 120.2
piarhemia 120.9
pulmonary 120.2
tropical hematuria 120.0
vesical 120.0
Biliary — *see* condition
Bilious (attack) — *see also* Vomiting
fever, hemoglobinuric 084.8
Bilirubinuria 791.4
Biliuria 791.4
Billroth's disease
meningocele (*see also* Spina bifida) 741.9 ☑
Bilobate placenta — *see* Placenta, abnormal
Bilocular
heart 745.7
stomach 536.8
Bing-Horton syndrome (histamine cephalgia)
346.2 ☑
Binswanger's disease or dementia 290.12
Biörck (-Thorson) syndrome (malignant
carcinoid) 259.2
Biparta, bipartite — *see also* Imperfect, closure
carpal scaphoid 755.59
patella 755.64
placenta — *see* Placenta, abnormal
vagina 752.49
Bird
face 756.0
fanciers' lung or disease 495.2
Bird's disease (oxaluria) 271.8
Birth
abnormal fetus or newborn 763.9
accident, fetus or newborn — *see* Birth, injury
complications in mother — *see* Delivery,
complicated
compression during NEC 767.9
defect — *see* Anomaly
delayed, fetus 763.9
difficult NEC, affecting fetus or newborn 763.9
dry, affecting fetus or newborn 761.1
forced, NEC, affecting fetus or newborn 763.89
forceps, affecting fetus or newborn 763.2
hematoma of sternomastoid 767.8
immature 765.1 ☑
extremely 765.0 ☑
inattention, after or at 995.52
induced, affecting fetus or newborn 763.89
infant — *see* Newborn
injury NEC 767.9
adrenal gland 767.8
basal ganglia 767.0
brachial plexus (paralysis) 767.6
brain (compression) (pressure) 767.0
cerebellum 767.0
cerebral hemorrhage 767.0
conjunctiva 767.8
eye 767.8
fracture
bone, any except clavicle or spine 767.3
clavicle 767.2
femur 767.3
humerus 767.3
long bone 767.3
radius and ulna 767.3
skeleton NEC 767.3
skull 767.3
spine 767.4
tibia and fibula 767.3
hematoma 767.8
liver (subcapsular) 767.8
mastoid 767.8
skull 767.19
sternomastoid 767.8

Birth — *continued*
injury NEC — *continued*
hematoma — *continued*
testes 767.8
vulva 767.8
intracranial (edema) 767.0
laceration
brain 767.0
by scalpel 767.8
peripheral nerve 767.7
liver 767.8
meninges
brain 767.0
spinal cord 767.4
nerves (cranial, peripheral) 767.7
brachial plexus 767.6
facial 767.5
paralysis 767.7
brachial plexus 767.6
Erb (-Duchenne) 767.6
facial nerve 767.5
Klumpke (-Déjérine) 767.6
radial nerve 767.6
spinal (cord) (hemorrhage) (laceration)
(rupture) 767.4
rupture
intracranial 767.0
liver 767.8
spinal cord 767.4
spleen 767.8
viscera 767.8
scalp 767.19
scalpel wound 767.8
skeleton NEC 767.3
specified NEC 767.8
spinal cord 767.4
spleen 767.8
subdural hemorrhage 767.0
tentorial, tear 767.0
testes 767.8
vulva 767.8
instrumental, NEC, affecting fetus or newborn
763.2
lack of care, after or at 995.52
multiple
affected by maternal complications of
pregnancy 761.5
healthy liveborn — *see* Newborn, multiple
neglect, after or at 995.52
newborn — *see* Newborn
palsy or paralysis NEC 767.7
precipitate, fetus or newborn 763.6
premature (infant) 765.1 ☑
prolonged, affecting fetus or newborn 763.9
retarded, fetus or newborn 763.9
shock, newborn 779.89
strangulation or suffocation
due to aspiration of amniotic fluid 770.1
mechanical 767.8
trauma NEC 767.9
triplet
affected by maternal complications of
pregnancy 761.5
healthy liveborn — *see* Newborn, multiple
twin
affected by maternal complications of
pregnancy 761.5
healthy liveborn — *see* Newborn, twin
ventouse, affecting fetus or newborn 763.3
Birthmark 757.32
Bisalbuminemia 273.8
Biskra button 085.1
Bite(s)
with intact skin surface — *see* Contusion
animal — *see* Wound, open, by site
intact skin surface — *see* Contusion
centipede 989.5
chigger 133.8
fire ant 989.5
flea — *see* Injury, superficial, by site
human (open wound) — *see also* Wound, open,
by site
intact skin surface — *see* Contusion

Bite(s) — *continued*
　insect
　　nonvenomous — *see* Injury, superficial, by
　　　site
　　venomous 989.5
　mad dog (death from) 071
　poisonous 989.5
　red bug 133.8
　reptile 989.5
　　nonvenomous — *see* Wound, open, by site
　snake 989.5
　　nonvenomous — *see* Wound, open, by site
　spider (venomous) 989.5
　　nonvenomous — *see* Injury, superficial, by
　　　site
　venomous 989.5
Biting
　cheek or lip 528.9
　nail 307.9
Black
　death 020.9
　eye NEC 921.0
　hairy tongue 529.3
　lung disease 500
Blackfan-Diamond anemia or syndrome
　(congenital hypoplastic anemia) 284.0
Blackhead 706.1
Blackout 780.2
Blackwater fever 084.8
Bladder — *see* condition
Blast
　blindness 921.3
　concussion — *see* Blast, injury
　injury 869.0
　　with open wound into cavity 869.1
　　abdomen or thorax — *see* Injury, internal,
　　　by site
　　brain (*see also* Concussion, brain) 850.9
　　　with skull fracture — *see* Fracture, skull
　　ear (acoustic nerve trauma) 951.5
　　　with perforation, tympanic membrane —
　　　　see Wound, open, ear, drum
　　lung (*see also* Injury, internal, lung) 861.20
　　otitic (explosive) 388.11
Blastomycosis, blastomycotic (chronic)
　(cutaneous) (disseminated) (lung)
　(pulmonary) (systemic) 116.0
　Brazilian 116.1
　European 117.5
　keloidal 116.2
　North American 116.0
　primary pulmonary 116.0
　South American 116.1
Bleb(s) 709.8
　emphysematous (bullous) (diffuse) (lung)
　　(ruptured) (solitary) 492.0
　filtering, eye (postglaucoma) (status) V45.69
　　with complication 997.99
　　postcataract extraction (complication)
　　　997.99
　lung (ruptured) 492.0
　　congenital 770.5
　subpleural (emphysematous) 492.0
Bleeder (familial) (hereditary) (*see also* Defect,
　coagulation) 286.9
　nonfamilial 286.9
Bleeding (*see also* Hemorrhage) 459.0
　anal 569.3
　anovulatory 628.0
　atonic, following delivery 666.1 ☑
　capillary 448.9
　due to subinvolution 621.1
　　puerperal 666.2 ☑
　ear 388.69
　excessive, associated with menopausal onset
　　627.0
　familial (*see also* Defect, coagulation) 286.9
　following intercourse 626.7
　gastrointestinal 578.9
　gums 523.8
　hemorrhoids — *see* Hemorrhoids, bleeding
　intermenstrual
　　irregular 626.6
　　regular 626.5

Bleeding (*see also* Hemorrhage) — *continued*
　intraoperative 998.11
　irregular NEC 626.4
　menopausal 627.0
　mouth 528.9
　nipple 611.79
　nose 784.7
　ovulation 626.5
　postclimacteric 627.1
　postcoital 626.7
　postmenopausal 627.1
　　following induced menopause 627.4
　postoperative 998.11
　preclimacteric 627.0
　puberty 626.3
　　excessive, with onset of menstrual periods
　　　626.3
　rectum, rectal 569.3
　tendencies (*see also* Defect, coagulation) 286.9
　throat 784.8
　umbilical stump 772.3
　umbilicus 789.9
　unrelated to menstrual cycle 626.6
　uterus, uterine 626.9
　　climacteric 627.0
　　dysfunctional 626.8
　　functional 626.8
　　unrelated to menstrual cycle 626.6
　vagina, vaginal 623.8
　　functional 626.8
　vicarious 625.8
Blennorrhagia, blennorrhagic — *see* Blennorrhea
Blennorrhea (acute) 098.0
　adultorum 098.40
　alveolaris 523.4
　chronic or duration of 2 months or over 098.2
　gonococcal (neonatorum) 098.40
　inclusion (neonatal) (newborn) 771.6
　neonatorum 098.40
Blepharelosis (*see also* Entropion) 374.00
Blepharitis (eyelid) 373.00
　angularis 373.01
　ciliaris 373.00
　　with ulcer 373.01
　marginal 373.00
　　with ulcer 373.01
　scrofulous (*see also* Tuberculosis) 017.3 ☑
　　[373.00]
　squamous 373.02
　ulcerative 373.01
Blepharochalasis 374.34
　congenital 743.62
Blepharoclonus 333.81
Blepharoconjunctivitis (*see also* Conjunctivitis)
　372.20
　angular 372.21
　contact 372.22
Blepharophimosis (eyelid) 374.46
　congenital 743.62
Blepharoplegia 374.89
Blepharoptosis 374.30
　congenital 743.61
Blepharopyorrhea 098.49
Blepharospasm 333.81
Blessig's cyst 362.62
Blighted ovum 631
Blind
　bronchus (congenital) 748.3
　eye — *see also* Blindness
　　hypertensive 360.42
　　hypotensive 360.41
　loop syndrome (postoperative) 579.2
　sac, fallopian tube (congenital) 752.19
　spot, enlarged 368.42
　tract or tube (congenital) NEC — *see* Atresia
Blindness (acquired) (congenital) (both eyes)
　369.00
　blast 921.3
　　with nerve injury — *see* Injury, nerve, optic
　Bright's — *see* Uremia
　color (congenital) 368.59
　　acquired 368.55
　　blue 368.53
　　green 368.52

Blindness — *continued*
　color — *continued*
　　red 368.51
　　total 368.54
　concussion 950.9
　cortical 377.75
　day 368.10
　　acquired 368.10
　　congenital 368.10
　　hereditary 368.10
　　specified type NEC 368.10
　due to
　　injury NEC 950.9
　　refractive error — *see* Error, refractive
　eclipse (total) 363.31
　emotional 300.11
　hysterical 300.11
　legal (both eyes) (USA definition) 369.4
　　with impairment of better (less impaired) eye
　　　near-total 369.02
　　　　with
　　　　　lesser eye impairment 369.02
　　　　　　near-total 369.04
　　　　　　total 369.03
　　　profound 369.05
　　　　with
　　　　　lesser eye impairment 369.05
　　　　　　near-total 369.07
　　　　　　profound 369.08
　　　　　　total 369.06
　　　severe 369.21
　　　　with
　　　　　lesser eye impairment 369.21
　　　　　　blind 369.11
　　　　　　near-total 369.13
　　　　　　profound 369.14
　　　　　　severe 369.22
　　　　　　total 369.12
　　　total
　　　　with lesser eye impairment
　　　　　total 369.01
　mind 784.69
　moderate
　　both eyes 369.25
　　　with impairment of lesser eye (specified
　　　　as)
　　　　blind, not further specified 369.15
　　　　low vision, not further specified 369.23
　　　　near-total 369.17
　　　　profound 369.18
　　　　severe 369.24
　　　　total 369.16
　　one eye 369.74
　　　with vision of other eye (specified as)
　　　　near-normal 369.75
　　　　normal 369.76
　near-total
　　both eyes 369.04
　　　with impairment of lesser eye (specified
　　　　as)
　　　　blind, not further specified 369.02
　　　　total 369.03
　　one eye 369.64
　　　with vision of other eye (specified as)
　　　　near-normal 369.65
　　　　normal 369.66
　night 368.60
　　acquired 368.62
　　congenital (Japanese) 368.61
　　hereditary 368.61
　　specified type NEC 368.69
　　vitamin A deficiency 264.5
　nocturnal — *see* Blindness, night
　one eye 369.60
　　with low vision of other eye 369.10
　profound
　　both eyes 369.08
　　　with impairment of lesser eye (specified
　　　　as)
　　　　blind, not further specified 369.05
　　　　near-total 369.07
　　　　total 369.06
　　one eye 369.67
　　　with vision of other eye (specified as)
　　　　near-normal 369.68
　　　　normal 369.69
　psychic 784.69

☑ Additional Digit Required　　　　　▶◀ Revised Text　　　　　● New Line　　　　　▲ Revised Code

Blindness — *continued*

severe

both eyes 369.22

with impairment of lesser eye (specified as)

blind, not further specified 369.11

low vision, not further specified 369.21

near-total 369.13

profound 369.14

total 369.12

one eye 369.71

with vision of other eye (specified as)

near-normal 369.72

normal 369.73

snow 370.24

sun 363.31

temporary 368.12

total

both eyes 369.01

one eye 369.61

with vision of other eye (specified as)

near-normal 369.62

normal 369.63

transient 368.12

traumatic NEC 950.9

word (developmental) 315.01

acquired 784.61

secondary to organic lesion 784.61

Blister — *see also* Injury, superficial, by site

beetle dermatitis 692.89

due to burn — *see* Burn, by site, second degree

fever 054.9

multiple, skin, nontraumatic 709.8

Bloating 787.3

Bloch-Siemens syndrome (incontinentia pigmenti) 757.33

Bloch-Stauffer dyshormonal dermatosis 757.33

Bloch-Sulzberger disease or syndrome (incontinentia pigmenti) (melanoblastosis) 757.33

Block

alveolar capillary 516.3

arborization (heart) 426.6

arrhythmic 426.9

atrioventricular (AV) (incomplete) (partial) 426.10

with

2:1 atrioventricular response block 426.13

atrioventricular dissociation 426.0

first degree (incomplete) 426.11

second degree (Mobitz type I) 426.13

Mobitz (type) II 426.12

third degree 426.0

complete 426.0

congenital 746.86

congenital 746.86

Mobitz (incomplete)

type I (Wenckebach's) 426.13

type II 426.12

partial 426.13

auriculoventricular (*see also* Block, atrioventricular) 426.10

complete 426.0

congenital 746.86

congenital 746.86

bifascicular (cardiac) 426.53

bundle branch (complete) (false) (incomplete) 426.50

bilateral 426.53

left (complete) (main stem) 426.3

with right bundle branch block 426.53

anterior fascicular 426.2

with

posterior fascicular block 426.3

right bundle branch block 426.52

hemiblock 426.2

incomplete 426.2

with right bundle branch block 426.53

posterior fascicular 426.2

with

anterior fascicular block 426.3

right bundle branch block 426.51

Block — *continued*

bundle branch — *continued*

right 426.4

with

left bundle branch block (incomplete) (main stem) 426.53

left fascicular block 426.53

anterior 426.52

posterior 426.51

Wilson's type 426.4

cardiac 426.9

conduction 426.9

complete 426.0

Eustachian tube (*see also* Obstruction, Eustachian tube) 381.60

fascicular (left anterior) (left posterior) 426.2

foramen Magendie (acquired) 331.3

congenital 742.3

with spina bifida (*see also* Spina bifida) 741.0 ☑

heart 426.9

first degree (atrioventricular) 426.11

second degree (atrioventricular) 426.13

third degree (atrioventricular) 426.0

bundle branch (complete) (false) (incomplete) 426.50

bilateral 426.53

left (*see also* Block, bundle branch, left) 426.3

right (*see also* Block, bundle branch, right) 426.4

complete (atrioventricular) 426.0

congenital 746.86

incomplete 426.13

intra-atrial 426.6

intraventricular NEC 426.6

sinoatrial 426.6

specified type NEC 426.6

hepatic vein 453.0

intraventricular (diffuse) (myofibrillar) 426.6

bundle branch (complete) (false) (incomplete) 426.50

bilateral 426.53

left (*see also* Block, bundle branch, left) 426.3

right (*see also* Block, bundle branch, right) 426.4

kidney (*see also* Disease, renal) 593.9

postcystoscopic 997.5

myocardial (*see also* Block, heart) 426.9

nodal 426.10

optic nerve 377.49

organ or site (congenital) NEC — *see* Atresia

parietal 426.6

peri-infarction 426.6

portal (vein) 452

sinoatrial 426.6

sinoauricular 426.6

spinal cord 336.9

trifascicular 426.54

tubal 628.2

vein NEC 453.9

Blocq's disease or syndrome (astasia-abasia) 307.9

Blood

constituents, abnormal NEC 790.6

disease 289.9

specified NEC 289.89

donor V59.01

other blood components V59.09

stem cells V59.02

whole blood V59.01

dyscrasia 289.9

with

abortion — *see* Abortion, by type, with hemorrhage, delayed or excessive

ectopic pregnancy (*see also* categories 633.0-633.9) 639.1

molar pregnancy (*see also* categories 630-632) 639.1

fetus or newborn NEC 776.9

following

abortion 639.1

ectopic or molar pregnancy 639.1

puerperal, postpartum 666.3 ☑

Blood — *continued*

flukes NEC (*see also* Infestation, Schistosoma) 120.9

in

feces (*see also* Melena) 578.1

occult 792.1

urine (*see also* Hematuria) 599.7

mole 631

occult 792.1

poisoning (*see also* Septicemia) 038.9

pressure

decreased, due to shock following injury 958.4

fluctuating 796.4

high (*see also* Hypertension) 401.9

incidental reading (isolated) (nonspecific), without diagnosis of hypertension 796.2

low (*see also* Hypotension) 458.9

incidental reading (isolated) (nonspecific), without diagnosis of hypotension 796.3

spitting (*see also* Hemoptysis) 786.3

staining cornea 371.12

transfusion

without reported diagnosis V58.2

donor V59.01

stem cells V59.02

reaction or complication — *see* Complications, transfusion

tumor — *see* Hematoma

vessel rupture — *see* Hemorrhage

vomiting (*see also* Hematemesis) 578.0

Blood-forming organ disease 289.9

Bloodgood's disease 610.1

Bloodshot eye 379.93

Bloom (-Machacek) (-Torre) syndrome 757.39

Blotch, palpebral 372.55

Blount's disease (tibia vara) 732.4

Blount-Barber syndrome (tibia vara) 732.4

Blue

baby 746.9

bloater 491.20

with

acute bronchitis 491.22 ●

exacerbation (acute) 491.21 ●

diaper syndrome 270.0

disease 746.9

dome cyst 610.0

drum syndrome 381.02

sclera 743.47

with fragility of bone and deafness 756.51

toe syndrome 445.02

Blueness (*see also* Cyanosis) 782.5

Blurring, visual 368.8

Blushing (abnormal) (excessive) 782.62

Boarder, hospital V65.0

infant V65.0

Bockhart's impetigo (superficial folliculitis) 704.8

Bodechtel-Guttmann disease (subacute sclerosing panencephalitis) 046.2

Boder-Sedgwick syndrome (ataxia-telangiectasia) 334.8

Body, bodies

Aschoff (*see also* Myocarditis, rheumatic) 398.0

asteroid, vitreous 379.22

choroid, colloid (degenerative) 362.57

hereditary 362.77

cytoid (retina) 362.82

drusen (retina) (*see also* Drusen) 362.57

optic disc 377.21

fibrin, pleura 511.0

foreign — *see* Foreign body

Hassall-Henle 371.41

loose

joint (*see also* Loose, body, joint) 718.1 ☑

knee 717.6

knee 717.6

sheath, tendon 727.82

Mallory's 034.1

Mooser 081.0

Negri 071

rice (joint) (*see also* Loose, body, joint) 718.1 ☑

knee 717.6

☑ Additional Digit Required   ▶◀ Revised Text   ● New Line   ▲ Revised Code

Body, bodies — *continued*
  rocking 307.3
Boeck's
  disease (sarcoidosis) 135
  lupoid (miliary) 135
  sarcoid 135
Boerhaave's syndrome (spontaneous esophageal
    rupture) 530.4
Boggy
  cervix 622.8
  uterus 621.8
Boil (*see also* Carbuncle) 680.9
  abdominal wall 680.2
  Aleppo 085.1
  ankle 680.6
  anus 680.5
  arm (any part, above wrist) 680.3
  auditory canal, external 680.0
  axilla 680.3
  back (any part) 680.2
  Baghdad 085.1
  breast 680.2
  buttock 680.5
  chest wall 680.2
  corpus cavernosum 607.2
  Delhi 085.1
  ear (any part) 680.0
  eyelid 373.13
  face (any part, except eye) 680.0
  finger (any) 680.4
  flank 680.2
  foot (any part) 680.7
  forearm 680.3
  Gafsa 085.1
  genital organ, male 608.4
  gluteal (region) 680.5
  groin 680.2
  hand (any part) 680.4
  head (any part, except face) 680.8
  heel 680.7
  hip 680.6
  knee 680.6
  labia 616.4
  lacrimal (*see also* Dacryocystitis) 375.30
    gland (*see also* Dacryoadenitis) 375.00
    passages (duct) (sac) (*see also*
      Dacryocystitis) 375.30
  leg, any part except foot 680.6
  multiple sites 680.9
  natal 085.1
  neck 680.1
  nose (external) (septum) 680.0
  orbit, orbital 376.01
  partes posteriores 680.5
  pectoral region 680.2
  penis 607.2
  perineum 680.2
  pinna 680.0
  scalp (any part) 680.8
  scrotum 608.4
  seminal vesicle 608.0
  shoulder 680.3
  skin NEC 680.9
  specified site NEC 680.8
  spermatic cord 608.4
  temple (region) 680.0
  testis 608.4
  thigh 680.6
  thumb 680.4
  toe (any) 680.7
  tropical 085.1
  trunk 680.2
  tunica vaginalis 608.4
  umbilicus 680.2
  upper arm 680.3
  vas deferens 608.4
  vulva 616.4
  wrist 680.4
Bold hives (*see also* Urticaria) 708.9
Bolivian hemorrhagic fever 078.7
Bombé, iris 364.74
Bomford-Rhoads anemia (refractory) 284.9
Bone — *see* condition
Bonnevie-Ullrich syndrome 758.6
Bonnier's syndrome 386.19

Bonvale Dam fever 780.79
Bony block of joint 718.80
  ankle 718.87
  elbow 718.82
  foot 718.87
  hand 718.84
  hip 718.85
  knee 718.86
  multiple sites 718.89
  pelvic region 718.85
  shoulder (region) 718.81
  specified site NEC 718.88
  wrist 718.83
Borderline
  intellectual functioning V62.89
  pelvis 653.1 ☑
    with obstruction during labor 660.1 ☑
      affecting fetus or newborn 763.1
  psychosis (*see also* Schizophrenia) 295.5 ☑
    of childhood (*see also* Psychosis, childhood)
      299.8 ☑
  schizophrenia (*see also* Schizophrenia) 295.5 ☑
Borna disease 062.9
Bornholm disease (epidemic pleurodynia) 074.1
Borrelia vincentii (mouth) (pharynx) (tonsils) 101
Bostock's catarrh (*see also* Fever, hay) 477.9
Boston exanthem 048
Botalli, ductus (patent) (persistent) 747.0
Bothriocephalus latus infestation 123.4
Botulism 005.1
Bouba (*see also* Yaws) 102.9
Bouffée délirante 298.3
Bouillaud's disease or syndrome (rheumatic
    heart disease) 391.9
Bourneville's disease (tuberous sclerosis) 759.5
Boutonneuse fever 082.1
Boutonniere
  deformity (finger) 736.21
  hand (intrinsic) 736.21
Bouveret (-Hoffmann) disease or syndrome
    (paroxysmal tachycardia) 427.2
Bovine heart — *see* Hypertrophy, cardiac
Bowel — *see* condition
Bowen's
  dermatosis (precancerous) (M8081/2) — *see*
    Neoplasm, skin, in situ
  disease (M8081/2) — *see* Neoplasm, skin, in
    situ
  epithelioma (M8081/2) — *see* Neoplasm, skin,
    in situ
  type
    epidermoid carcinoma in situ (M8081/2) —
      see Neoplasm, skin, in situ
    intraepidermal squamous cell carcinoma
      (M8081/2) — *see* Neoplasm, skin, in
      situ
Bowing
  femur 736.89
    congenital 754.42
  fibula 736.89
    congenital 754.43
  forearm 736.09
    away from midline (cubitus valgus) 736.01
    toward midline (cubitus varus) 736.02
  leg(s), long bones, congenital 754.44
  radius 736.09
    away from midline (cubitus valgus) 736.01
    toward midline (cubitus varus) 736.02
  tibia 736.89
    congenital 754.43
Bowleg(s) 736.42
  congenital 754.44
  rachitic 268.1
Boyd's dysentery 004.2
Brachial — *see* condition
Brachman-de Lange syndrome (Amsterdam
    dwarf, mental retardation, and
    brachycephaly) 759.89
Brachycardia 427.89
Brachycephaly 756.0
Brachymorphism and ectopia lentis 759.89

Bradley's disease (epidemic vomiting) 078.82
Bradycardia 427.89
  chronic (sinus) 427.81
  newborn 779.81
  nodal 427.89
  postoperative 997.1
  reflex 337.0
  sinoatrial 427.89
    with paroxysmal tachyarrhythmia or
      tachycardia 427.81
    chronic 427.81
  sinus 427.89
    with paroxysmal tachyarrhythmia or
      tachycardia 427.81
    chronic 427.81
    persistent 427.81
    severe 427.81
  tachycardia syndrome 427.81
  vagal 427.89
Bradypnea 786.09
Brailsford's disease 732.3
  radial head 732.3
  tarsal scaphoid 732.5
Brailsford-Morquio disease or syndrome
    (mucopolysac-charidosis IV) 277.5
Brain — *see also* condition
  death 348.8
  syndrome (acute) (chronic) (nonpsychotic)
    (organic) (with neurotic reaction) (with
    behavioral reaction) (*see also* Syndrome,
    brain) 310.9
    with
      presenile brain disease 290.10
      psychosis, psychotic reaction (*see also*
        Psychosis, organic) 294.9
    congenital (*see also* Retardation, mental)
      319
Branched-chain amino-acid disease 270.3
Branchial — *see* condition
Branchopulmonitis — *see* Pneumonia, broncho-
Brandt's syndrome (acrodermatitis enteropathica)
    686.8
Brash (water) 787.1
Brass-founders', ague 985.8
Bravais-Jacksonian epilepsy (*see also* Epilepsy)
    345.5 ☑
Braxton Hicks contractions 644.1 ☑
Braziers' disease 985.8
Brazilian
  blastomycosis 116.1
  leishmaniasis 085.5
BRBPR (bright red blood per rectum) 569.3   ●
Break
  cardiorenal — *see* Hypertension, cardiorenal
  retina (*see also* Defect, retina) 361.30
Breakbone fever 061
Breakdown
  device, implant, or graft — *see* Complications,
    mechanical
  nervous (*see also* Disorder, mental,
    nonpsychotic) 300.9
  perineum 674.2 ☑
Breast — *see* condition
Breast feeding difficulties 676.8 ☑
Breath
  foul 784.9
  holder, child 312.81
  holding spells 786.9
  shortness 786.05
Breathing
  asymmetrical 786.09
  bronchial 786.09
  exercises V57.0
  labored 786.09
  mouth 784.9
  periodic 786.09
  tic 307.20
Breathlessness 786.09
Breda's disease (*see also* Yaws) 102.9
Breech
  delivery, affecting fetus or newborn 763.0

Breech — *continued*
  extraction, affecting fetus or newborn 763.0
  presentation (buttocks) (complete) (frank)
      652.2 ☑
    with successful version 652.1 ☑
      before labor, affecting fetus or newborn
          761.7
      during labor, affecting fetus or newborn
          763.0
Breisky's disease (kraurosis vulvae) 624.0
Brennemann's syndrome (acute mesenteric
      lymphadenitis) 289.2
Brenner's
  tumor (benign) (M9000/0) 220
    borderline malignancy (M9000/1) 236.2
    malignant (M9000/3) 183.0
    proliferating (M9000/1) 236.2
Bretonneau's disease (diphtheritic malignant
      angina) 032.0
Breus' mole 631
Brevicollis 756.16
Bricklayers' itch 692.89
Brickmakers' anemia 126.9
Bridge
  myocardial 746.85
Bright red blood per rectum (BRBPR) 569.3 ●
Bright's
  blindness — *see* Uremia
  disease (*see also* Nephritis) 583.9
    arteriosclerotic (*see also* Hypertension,
        kidney) 403.90
Brill's disease (recrudescent typhus) 081.1
  flea-borne 081.0
  louse-borne 081.1
Brill-Symmers disease (follicular lymphoma)
      (M9690/3) 202.0 ☑
Brill-Zinsser disease (recrudescent typhus) 081.1
Brinton's disease (linitis plastica) (M8142/3)
      151.9
Brion-Kayser disease (*see also* Fever,
      paratyphoid) 002.9
Briquet's disorder or syndrome 300.81
Brissaud's
  infantilism (infantile myxedema) 244.9
  motor-verbal tic 307.23
Brissaud-Meige syndrome (infantile myxedema)
      244.9
Brittle
  bones (congenital) 756.51
  nails 703.8
    congenital 757.5
Broad — *see also* condition
  beta disease 272.2
  ligament laceration syndrome 620.6
Brock's syndrome (atelectasis due to enlarged
      lymph nodes) 518.0
Brocq's disease 691.8
  atopic (diffuse) neurodermatitis 691.8
  lichen simplex chronicus 698.3
  parakeratosis psoriasiformis 696.2
  parapsoriasis 696.2
Brocq-Duhring disease (dermatitis herpetiformis)
      694.0
Brodie's
  abscess (localized) (chronic) (*see also*
      Osteomyelitis) 730.1 ☑
  disease (joint) (*see also* Osteomyelitis) 730.1 ☑
Broken
  arches 734
    congenital 755.67
  back — *see* Fracture, vertebra, by site
  bone — *see* Fracture, by site
  compensation — *see* Disease, heart
  implant or internal device — *see* listing under
      Complications, mechanical
  neck — *see* Fracture, vertebra, cervical
  nose 802.0
    open 802.1
  tooth, teeth 873.63
    complicated 873.73
Bromhidrosis 705.89

Bromidism, bromism
  acute 967.3
    correct substance properly administered
        349.82
    overdose or wrong substance given or taken
        967.3
  chronic (*see also* Dependence) 304.1 ☑
Bromidrosiphobia 300.23
Bromidrosis 705.89
Bronchi, bronchial — *see* condition
Bronchiectasis (cylindrical) (diffuse) (fusiform)
      (localized) (moniliform) (postinfectious)
      (recurrent) (saccular) 494.0
  with acute exacerbation 494.1
  congenital 748.61
  tuberculosis (*see also* Tuberculosis) 011.5 ☑
Bronchiolectasis — *see* Bronchiectasis
Bronchiolitis (acute) (infectious) (subacute)
      466.19
  with
    bronchospasm or obstruction 466.19
    influenza, flu, or grippe 487.1
  catarrhal (acute) (subacute) 466.19
  chemical 506.0
    chronic 506.4
  chronic (obliterative) 491.8
  due to external agent — *see* Bronchitis, acute,
      due to
  fibrosa obliterans 491.8
  influenzal 487.1
  obliterans 491.8
    with organizing pneumonia (B.O.O.P.) 516.8
    status post lung transplant 996.84
  obliterative (chronic) (diffuse) (subacute) 491.8
    due to fumes or vapors 506.4
  respiratory syncytial virus 466.11
  vesicular — *see* Pneumonia, broncho-
Bronchitis (diffuse) (hypostatic) (infectious)
      (inflammatory) (simple) 490
  with
    emphysema — *see* Emphysema
    influenza, flu, or grippe 487.1
    obstruction airway, chronic 491.20
      with
        acute bronchitis 491.22   ●
        exacerbation (acute) 491.21   ●
    tracheitis 490
      acute or subacute 466.0
        with bronchospasm or obstruction
            466.0
      chronic 491.8
  acute or subacute 466.0
    with
      bronchospasm 466.0
      obstruction 466.0
      tracheitis 466.0
    chemical (due to fumes or vapors) 506.0
    due to
      fumes or vapors 506.0
      radiation 508.8
  allergic (acute) (*see also* Asthma) 493.9 ☑
  arachidic 934.1
  aspiration 507.0
    due to fumes or vapors 506.0
  asthmatic (acute) 493.90
    with
      acute exacerbation 493.92
      status asthmaticus 493.91
    chronic 493.2 ☑
  capillary 466.19
    with bronchospasm or obstruction 466.19
    chronic 491.8
  caseous (*see also* Tuberculosis) 011.3 ☑
  Castellani's 104.8
  catarrhal 490
    acute — *see* Bronchitis, acute
    chronic 491.0
  chemical (acute) (subacute) 506.0
    chronic 506.4
    due to fumes or vapors (acute) (subacute)
        506.0
      chronic 506.4
  chronic 491.9
    with
      tracheitis (chronic) 491.8

Bronchitis — *continued*
  chronic — *continued*
    asthmatic 493.2 ☑
    catarrhal 491.0
    chemical (due to fumes and vapors) 506.4
    due to
      fumes or vapors (chemical) (inhalation)
          506.4
      radiation 508.8
      tobacco smoking 491.0
    mucopurulent 491.1
    obstructive 491.20
      with
        acute bronchitis 491.22   ●
        exacerbation (acute) 491.21   ●
    purulent 491.1
    simple 491.0
    specified type NEC 491.8
  croupous 466.0
    with bronchospasm or obstruction 466.0
    due to fumes or vapors 506.0
  emphysematous 491.20
    with
      acute bronchitis 491.22   ●
      exacerbation (acute) 491.21   ●
  exudative 466.0
  fetid (chronic) (recurrent) 491.1
  fibrinous, acute or subacute 466.0
    with bronchospasm or obstruction 466.0
  grippal 487.1
  influenzal 487.1
  membranous, acute or subacute 466.0
    with bronchospasm or obstruction 466.0
  moulders' 502
  mucopurulent (chronic) (recurrent) 491.1
    acute or subacute 466.0
  non-obstructive 491.0
  obliterans 491.8
  obstructive (chronic) 491.20
    with
      acute bronchitis 491.22   ●
      exacerbation (acute) 491.21   ●
  pituitous 491.1
  plastic (inflammatory) 466.0
  pneumococcal, acute or subacute 466.0
    with bronchospasm or obstruction 466.0
  pseudomembranous 466.0
  purulent (chronic) (recurrent) 491.1
    acute or subacute 466.0
      with bronchospasm or obstruction 466.0
  putrid 491.1
  scrofulous (*see also* Tuberculosis) 011.3 ☑
  senile 491.9
  septic, acute or subacute 466.0
    with bronchospasm or obstruction 466.0
  smokers' 491.0
  spirochetal 104.8
  suffocative, acute or subacute 466.0
  summer (*see also* Asthma) 493.9 ☑
  suppurative (chronic) 491.1
    acute or subacute 466.0
  tuberculous (*see also* Tuberculosis) 011.3 ☑
  ulcerative 491.8
    Vincent's 101
  Vincent's 101
  viral, acute or subacute 466.0
Bronchoalveolitis 485
Bronchoaspergillosis 117.3
Bronchocele
  meaning
    dilatation of bronchus 519.1
    goiter 240.9
Bronchogenic carcinoma 162.9
Bronchohemisporosis 117.9
Broncholithiasis 518.89
  tuberculous (*see also* Tuberculosis) 011.3 ☑
Bronchomalacia 748.3
Bronchomoniliasis 112.89
Bronchomycosis 112.89
Bronchonocardiosis 039.1
Bronchopleuropneumonia — *see* Pneumonia,
      broncho-
Bronchopneumonia — *see* Pneumonia, broncho-

☑ Additional Digit Required   ►◄ Revised Text   ● New Line   ▲ Revised Code

Bronchopneumonitis — *see* Pneumonia, broncho-
Bronchopulmonary — *see* condition
Bronchorrhagia 786.3
    newborn 770.3
    tuberculous (*see also* Tuberculosis) 011.3 ☑
Bronchorrhea (chronic) (purulent) 491.0
    acute 466.0
Bronchospasm 519.1
    with
        asthma — *see* Asthma
        bronchiolitis
            due to respiratory syncytial virus 466.11
        bronchitis — *see* Bronchitis
        chronic obstructive pulmonary disease (COPD) 496
        emphysema — *see* Emphysema
        due to external agent — *see* Condition, respiratory, acute, due to
    exercise induced 493.81
Bronchospirochetosis 104.8
Bronchostenosis 519.1
Bronchus — *see* condition
Bronze, bronzed
    diabetes 275.0
    disease (Addison's) (skin) 255.4
        tuberculous (*see also* Tuberculosis) 017.6 ☑
Brooke's disease or tumor (M8100/0) — *see* Neoplasm, skin, benign
Brown's tendon sheath syndrome 378.61
Brown enamel of teeth (hereditary) 520.5
Brown-Séquard's paralysis (syndrome) 344.89
Brow presentation complicating delivery 652.4 ☑
Brucella, brucellosis (infection) 023.9
    abortus 023.1
    canis 023.3
    dermatitis, skin 023.9
    melitensis 023.0
    mixed 023.8
    suis 023.2
Bruck's disease 733.99
Bruck-de Lange disease or syndrome (Amsterdam dwarf, mental retardation, and brachycephaly) 759.89
Brugada syndrome 746.89
Brugsch's syndrome (acropachyderma) 757.39
Brug's filariasis 125.1
Bruhl's disease (splenic anemia with fever) 285.8
Bruise (skin surface intact) — *see also* Contusion
    with
        fracture — *see* Fracture, by site
        open wound — *see* Wound, open, by site
    internal organ (abdomen, chest, or pelvis) — *see* Injury, internal, by site
    umbilical cord 663.6 ☑
        affecting fetus or newborn 762.6
Bruit 785.9
    arterial (abdominal) (carotid) 785.9
    supraclavicular 785.9
Brushburn — *see* Injury, superficial, by site
Bruton's X-linked agammaglobulinemia 279.04
Bruxism 306.8
Bubbly lung syndrome 770.7
Bubo 289.3
    blennorrhagic 098.89
    chancroidal 099.0
    climatic 099.1
    due to Hemophilus ducreyi 099.0
    gonococcal 098.89
    indolent NEC 099.8
    inguinal NEC 099.8
        chancroidal 099.0
        climatic 099.1
        due to H. ducreyi 099.0
    scrofulous (*see also* Tuberculosis) 017.2 ☑
    soft chancre 099.0
    suppurating 683
    syphilitic 091.0
        congenital 090.0
    tropical 099.1

Bubo — *continued*
    venereal NEC 099.8
    virulent 099.0
Bubonic plague 020.0
Bubonocele — *see* Hernia, inguinal
Buccal — *see* condition
Buchanan's disease (juvenile osteochondrosis of iliac crest) 732.1
Buchem's syndrome (hyperostosis corticalis) 733.3
Buchman's disease (osteochondrosis, juvenile) 732.1
Bucket handle fracture (semilunar cartilage) (*see also* Tear, meniscus) 836.2
Budd-Chiari syndrome (hepatic vein thrombosis) 453.0
Budgerigar-fanciers' disease or lung 495.2
Büdinger-Ludloff-Läwen disease 717.89
Buerger's disease (thromboangiitis obliterans) 443.1
Bulbar — *see* condition
Bulbus cordis 745.9
    persistent (in left ventricle) 745.8
Bulging fontanels (congenital) 756.0
Bulimia 783.6
    nervosa 307.51   ●
    nonorganic origin 307.51
Bulky uterus 621.2
Bulla(e) 709.8
    lung (emphysematous) (solitary) 492.0
Bullet wound — *see also* Wound, open, by site
    fracture — *see* Fracture, by site, open
    internal organ (abdomen, chest, or pelvis) — *see* Injury, internal, by site, with open wound
    intracranial — *see* Laceration, brain, with open wound
Bullis fever 082.8
Bullying (*see also* Disturbance, conduct) 312.0 ☑
Bundle
    branch block (complete) (false) (incomplete) 426.50
        bilateral 426.53
        left (*see also* Block, bundle branch, left) 426.3
            hemiblock 426.2
        right (*see also* Block, bundle branch, right) 426.4
    of His — *see* condition
    of Kent syndrome (anomalous atrioventricular excitation) 426.7
Bungpagga 040.81
Bunion 727.1
Bunionette 727.1
Bunyamwera fever 066.3
Buphthalmia, buphthalmos (congenital) 743.20
    associated with
        keratoglobus, congenital 743.22
        megalocornea 743.22
        ocular anomalies NEC 743.22
    isolated 743.21
    simple 743.21
Bürger-Grütz disease or syndrome (essential familial hyperlipemia) 272.3
Buried roots 525.3
Burke's syndrome 577.8
Burkitt's
    tumor (M9750/3) 200.2 ☑
    type malignant, lymphoma, lymphoblastic, or undifferentiated (M9750/3) 200.2 ☑

Burn (acid) (cathode ray) (caustic) (chemical) (electric heating appliance) (electricity) (fire) (flame) (hot liquid or object) (irradiation) (lime) (radiation) (steam) (thermal) (x-ray) 949.0

> *Note* — *Use the following fifth-digit subclassification with category 948 to indicate the percent of body surface with third degree burn:*
>
> 0   *Less than 10% or unspecified*
> 1   *10–19%*
> 2   *20–29%*
> 3   *30–39%*
> 4   *40–49%*
> 5   *50–59%*
> 6   *60–69%*
> 7   *70–79%*
> 8   *80–89%*
> 9   *90% or more of body surface*

    with
        blisters — *see* Burn, by site, second degree
        erythema — *see* Burn, by site, first degree
        skin loss (epidermal) — *see also* Burn, by site, second degree
            full thickness — *see also* Burn, by site, third degree
                with necrosis of underlying tissues — *see* Burn, by site, third degree, deep
    first degree — *see* Burn, by site, first degree
    second degree — *see* Burn, by site, second degree
    third degree — *see* Burn, by site, third degree
        deep — *see* Burn, by site, third degree, deep
    abdomen, abdominal (muscle) (wall) 942.03
        with
            trunk — *see* Burn, trunk, multiple sites
        first degree 942.13
        second degree 942.23
        third degree 942.33
            deep 942.43
                with loss of body part 942.53
    ankle 945.03
        with
            lower limb(s) — *see* Burn, leg, multiple sites
        first degree 945.13
        second degree 945.23
        third degree 945.33
            deep 945.43
                with loss of body part 945.53
    anus — *see* Burn, trunk, specified site NEC
    arm(s) 943.00
        first degree 943.10
        second degree 943.20
        third degree 943.30
            deep 943.40
                with loss of body part 943.50
        lower — *see* Burn, forearm(s)
        multiple sites, except hand(s) or wrist(s) 943.09
            first degree 943.19
            second degree 943.29
            third degree 943.39
                deep 943.49
                    with loss of body part 943.59
        upper 943.03
            first degree 943.13
            second degree 943.23
            third degree 943.33
                deep 943.43
                    with loss of body part 943.53
    auditory canal (external) — *see* Burn, ear
    auricle (ear) — *see* Burn, ear
    axilla 943.04
        with
            upper limb(s) except hand(s) or wrist(s) — *see* Burn, arm(s), multiple sites
        first degree 943.14
        second degree 943.24
        third degree 943.34
            deep 943.44
                with loss of body part 943.54

Burn — *continued*
  back 942.04
    with
      trunk — *see* Burn, trunk, multiple sites
    first degree 942.14
    second degree 942.24
    third degree 942.34
      deep 942.44
        with loss of body part 942.54
  biceps
    brachii — *see* Burn, arm(s), upper
    femoris — *see* Burn, thigh
  breast(s) 942.01
    with
      trunk — *see* Burn, trunk, multiple sites
    first degree 942.11
    second degree 942.21
    third degree 942.31
      deep 942.41
        with loss of body part 942.51
  brow — *see* Burn, forehead
  buttock(s) — *see* Burn, back
  canthus (eye) 940.1
    chemical 940.0
  cervix (uteri) 947.4
  cheek (cutaneous) 941.07
    with
      face or head — *see* Burn, head, multiple sites
    first degree 941.17
    second degree 941.27
    third degree 941.37
      deep 941.47
        with loss of body part 941.57
  chest wall (anterior) 942.02
    with
      trunk — *see* Burn, trunk, multiple sites
    first degree 942.12
    second degree 942.22
    third degree 942.32
      deep 942.42
        with loss of body part 942.52
  chin 941.04
    with
      face or head — *see* Burn, head, multiple sites
    first degree 941.14
    second degree 941.24
    third degree 941.34
      deep 941.44
        with loss of body part 941.54
  clitoris — *see* Burn, genitourinary organs, external
  colon 947.3
  conjunctiva (and cornea) 940.4
    chemical
      acid 940.3
      alkaline 940.2
  cornea (and conjunctiva) 940.4
    chemical
      acid 940.3
      alkaline 940.2
  costal region — *see* Burn, chest wall
  due to ingested chemical agent — *see* Burn, internal organs
  ear (auricle) (canal) (drum) (external) 941.01
    with
      face or head — *see* Burn, head, multiple sites
    first degree 941.11
    second degree 941.21
    third degree 941.31
      deep 941.41
        with loss of a body part 941.51
  elbow 943.02
    with
      hand(s) and wrist(s) — *see* Burn, multiple specified sites
      upper limb(s) except hand(s) or wrist(s) — *see also* Burn, arm(s), multiple sites
    first degree 943.12
    second degree 943.22
    third degree 943.32
      deep 943.42
        with loss of body part 943.52
  electricity, electric current — *See* Burn, by site

Burn — *continued*
  entire body — *see* Burn, multiple, specified sites
  epididymis — *see* Burn, genitourinary organs, external
  epigastric region — *see* Burn, abdomen
  epiglottis 947.1
  esophagus 947.2
  extent (percent of body surface)
    less than 10 percent 948.0 ☑
    10-19 percent 948.1 ☑
    20-29 percent 948.2 ☑
    30-39 percent 948.3 ☑
    40-49 percent 948.4 ☑
    50-59 percent 948.5 ☑
    60-69 percent 948.6 ☑
    70-79 percent 948.7 ☑
    80-89 percent 948.8 ☑
    90 percent or more 948.9 ☑
  extremity
    lower — *see* Burn, leg
    upper — *see* Burn, arm(s)
  eye(s) (and adnexa) (only) 940.9
    with
      face, head, or neck 941.02
        first degree 941.12
        second degree 941.22
        third degree 941.32
          deep 941.42
            with loss of body part 941.52
      other sites (classifiable to more than one category in 940-945) — *see* Burn, multiple, specified sites
      resulting rupture and destruction of eyeball 940.5
      specified part — *see* Burn, by site
  eyeball — *see also* Burn, eye
    with resulting rupture and destruction of eyeball 940.5
  eyelid(s) 940.1
    chemical 940.0
  face — *see* Burn, head
  finger (nail) (subungual) 944.01
    with
      hand(s) — *see* Burn, hand(s), multiple sites
      other sites — *see* Burn, multiple, specified sites
      thumb 944.04
        first degree 944.14
        second degree 944.24
        third degree 944.34
          deep 944.44
            with loss of body part 944.54
    first degree 944.11
    second degree 944.21
    third degree 944.31
      deep 944.41
        with loss of body part 944.51
    multiple (digits) 944.03
      with thumb — *see* Burn, finger, with thumb
      first degree 944.13
      second degree 944.23
      third degree 944.33
        deep 944.43
          with loss of body part 944.53
  flank — *see* Burn, abdomen
  foot 945.02
    with
      lower limb(s) — *see* Burn, leg, multiple sites
    first degree 945.12
    second degree 945.22
    third degree 945.32
      deep 945.42
        with loss of body part 945.52
  forearm(s) 943.01
    with
      upper limb(s) except hand(s) or wrist(s) — *see* Burn, arm(s), multiple sites
    first degree 943.11
    second degree 943.21
    third degree 943.31
      deep 943.41
        with loss of body part 943.51

Burn — *continued*
  forehead 941.07
    with
      face or head — *see* Burn, head, multiple sites
    first degree 941.17
    second degree 941.27
    third degree 941.37
      deep 941.47
        with loss of body part 941.57
  fourth degree — *see* Burn, by site, third degree, deep
  friction — *see* Injury, superficial, by site
  from swallowing caustic or corrosive substance NEC — *see* Burn, internal organs
  full thickness — *see* Burn, by site, third degree
  gastrointestinal tract 947.3
  genitourinary organs
    external 942.05
      with
        trunk — *see* Burn, trunk, multiple sites
      first degree 942.15
      second degree 942.25
      third degree 942.35
        deep 942.45
          with loss of body part 942.55
    internal 947.8
  globe (eye) — *see* Burn, eyeball
  groin — *see* Burn, abdomen
  gum 947.0
  hand(s) (phalanges) (and wrist) 944.00
    first degree 944.10
    second degree 944.20
    third degree 944.30
      deep 944.40
        with loss of body part 944.50
    back (dorsal surface) 944.06
      first degree 944.16
      second degree 944.26
      third degree 944.36
        deep 944.46
          with loss of body part 944.56
    multiple sites 944.08
      first degree 944.18
      second degree 944.28
      third degree 944.38
        deep 944.48
          with loss of body part 944.58
  head (and face) 941.00
    eye(s) only 940.9
      specified part — *see* Burn, by site
    first degree 941.10
    second degree 941.20
    third degree 941.30
      deep 941.40
        with loss of body part 941.50
    multiple sites 941.09
      with eyes — *see* Burn, eyes, with face, head, or neck
      first degree 941.19
      second degree 941.29
      third degree 941.39
        deep 941.49
          with loss of body part 941.59
  heel — *see* Burn, foot
  hip — *see* Burn, trunk, specified site NEC
  iliac region — *see* Burn, trunk, specified site NEC
  infected 958.3
  inhalation (*see also* Burn, internal organs) 947.9
  internal organs 947.9
    from caustic or corrosive substance (swallowing) NEC 947.9
    specified NEC (*see also* Burn, by site) 947.8
  interscapular region — *see* Burn, back
  intestine (large) (small) 947.3
  iris — *see* Burn, eyeball
  knee 945.05
    with
      lower limb(s) — *see* Burn, leg, multiple sites
    first degree 945.15
    second degree 945.25

☑ Additional Digit Required   ▶◀ Revised Text   ● New Line   ▲ Revised Code

Burn — *continued*
  knee — *continued*
    third degree 945.35
      deep 945.45
        with loss of body part 945.55
  labium (majorus) (minus) — *see* Burn,
    genitourinary organs, external
  lacrimal apparatus, duct, gland, or sac 940.1
    chemical 940.0
  larynx 947.1
  late effect — *see* Late, effects (of), burn
  leg 945.00
    first degree 945.10
    second degree 945.20
    third degree 945.30
      deep 945.40
        with loss of body part 945.50
    lower 945.04
      with other part(s) of lower limb(s) — *see*
        Burn, leg, multiple sites
      first degree 945.14
      second degree 945.24
      third degree 945.34
        deep 945.44
          with loss of body part 945.54
    multiple sites 945.09
      first degree 945.19
      second degree 945.29
      third degree 945.39
        deep 945.49
          with loss of body part 945.59
    upper — *see* Burn, thigh
  lightning — *see* Burn, by site
  limb(s)
    lower (including foot or toe(s)) — *see* Burn,
      leg
    upper (except wrist and hand) — *see* Burn,
      arm(s)
  lip(s) 941.03
    with
      face or head — *see* Burn, head, multiple
        sites
    first degree 941.13
    second degree 941.23
    third degree 941.33
      deep 941.43
        with loss of body part 941.53
  lumbar region — *see* Burn, back
  lung 947.1
  malar region — *see* Burn, cheek
  mastoid region — *see* Burn, scalp
  membrane, tympanic — *see* Burn, ear
  midthoracic region — *see* Burn, chest wall
  mouth 947.0
  multiple (*see also* Burn, unspecified) 949.0
    specified sites classifiable to more than one
      category in 940-945 946.0
      first degree 946.1
      second degree 946.2
      third degree 946.3
        deep 946.4
          with loss of body part 946.5
  muscle, abdominal — *see* Burn, abdomen
  nasal (septum) — *see* Burn, nose
  neck 941.08
    with
      face or head — *see* Burn, head, multiple
        sites
    first degree 941.18
    second degree 941.28
    third degree 941.38
      deep 941.48
        with loss of body part 941.58
  nose (septum) 941.05
    with
      face or head — *see* Burn, head, multiple
        sites
    first degree 941.15
    second degree 941.25
    third degree 941.35
      deep 941.45
        with loss of body part 941.55
  occipital region — *see* Burn, scalp
  orbit region 940.1
    chemical 940.0
  oronasopharynx 947.0
  palate 947.0

Burn — *continued*
  palm(s) 944.05
    with
      hand(s) and wrist(s) — *see* Burn, hand(s),
        multiple sites
    first degree 944.15
    second degree 944.25
    third degree 944.35
      deep 944.45
        with loss of a body part 944.55
  parietal region — *see* Burn, scalp
  penis — *see* Burn, genitourinary organs,
    external
  perineum — *see* Burn, genitourinary organs,
    external
  periocular area 940.1
    chemical 940.0
  pharynx 947.0
  pleura 947.1
  popliteal space — *see* Burn, knee
  prepuce — *see* Burn, genitourinary organs,
    external
  pubic region — *see* Burn, genitourinary organs,
    external
  pudenda — *see* Burn, genitourinary organs,
    external
  rectum 947.3
  sac, lacrimal 940.1
    chemical 940.0
  sacral region — *see* Burn, back
  salivary (ducts) (glands) 947.0
  scalp 941.06
    with
      face or neck — *see* Burn, head, multiple
        sites
    first degree 941.16
    second degree 941.26
    third degree 941.36
      deep 941.46
        with loss of body part 941.56
  scapular region 943.06
    with
      upper limb(s), except hand(s) or wrist(s)
        — *see* Burn, arm(s), multiple sites
    first degree 943.16
    second degree 943.26
    third degree 943.36
      deep 943.46
        with loss of body part 943.56
  sclera — *see* Burn, eyeball
  scrotum — *see* Burn, genitourinary organs,
    external
  septum, nasal — *see* Burn, nose
  shoulder(s) 943.05
    with
      hand(s) and wrist(s) — *see* Burn,
        multiple, specified sites
      upper limb(s), except hand(s) or wrist(s)
        — *see* Burn, arm(s), multiple sites
    first degree 943.15
    second degree 943.25
    third degree 943.35
      deep 943.45
        with loss of body part 943.55
  skin NEC (*see also* Burn, unspecified) 949.0
  skull — *see* Burn, head
  small intestine 947.3
  sternal region — *see* Burn, chest wall
  stomach 947.3
  subconjunctival — *see* Burn, conjunctiva
  subcutaneous — *see* Burn, by site, third
    degree
  submaxillary region — *see* Burn, head
  submental region — *see* Burn, chin
  sun — *see* Sunburn
  supraclavicular fossa — *see* Burn, neck
  supraorbital — *see* Burn, forehead
  temple — *see* Burn, scalp
  temporal region — *see* Burn, scalp
  testicle — *see* Burn, genitourinary organs,
    external
  testis — *see* Burn, genitourinary organs,
    external
  thigh 945.06
    with
      lower limb(s) — *see* Burn, leg, multiple
        sites

Burn — *continued*
  thigh — *continued*
    first degree 945.16
    second degree 945.26
    third degree 945.36
      deep 945.46
        with loss of body part 945.56
  thorax (external) — *see* Burn, chest wall
  throat 947.0
  thumb(s) (nail) (subungual) 944.02
    with
      finger(s) — *see* Burn, finger, with other
        sites, thumb
      hand(s) and wrist(s) — *see* Burn, hand(s),
        multiple sites
    first degree 944.12
    second degree 944.22
    third degree 944.32
      deep 944.42
        with loss of body part 944.52
  toe (nail) (subungual) 945.01
    with
      lower limb(s) — *see* Burn, leg, multiple
        sites
    first degree 945.11
    second degree 945.21
    third degree 945.31
      deep 945.41
        with loss of body part 945.51
  tongue 947.0
  tonsil 947.0
  trachea 947.1
  trunk 942.00
    first degree 942.10
    second degree 942.20
    third degree 942.30
      deep 942.40
        with loss of body part 942.50
    multiple sites 942.09
      first degree 942.19
      second degree 942.29
      third degree 942.39
        deep 942.49
          with loss of body part 942.59
    specified site NEC 942.09
      first degree 942.19
      second degree 942.29
      third degree 942.39
        deep 942.49
          with loss of body part 942.59
  tunica vaginalis — *see* Burn, genitourinary
    organs, external
  tympanic membrane — *see* Burn, ear
  tympanum — *see* Burn, ear
  ultraviolet 692.82
  unspecified site (multiple) 949.0
    with extent of body surface involved
      specified
      less than 10 percent 948.0 ☑
      10-19 percent 948.1 ☑
      20-29 percent 948.2 ☑
      30-39 percent 948.3 ☑
      40-49 percent 948.4 ☑
      50-59 percent 948.5 ☑
      60-69 percent 948.6 ☑
      70-79 percent 948.7 ☑
      80-89 percent 948.8 ☑
      90 percent or more 948.9 ☑
    first degree 949.1
    second degree 949.2
    third degree 949.3
      deep 949.4
        with loss of body part 949.5
  uterus 947.4
  uvula 947.0
  vagina 947.4
  vulva — *see* Burn, genitourinary organs,
    external
  wrist(s) 944.07
    with
      hand(s) — *see* Burn, hand(s), multiple
        sites
    first degree 944.17
    second degree 944.27
    third degree 944.37
      deep 944.47
        with loss of body part 944.57

Burn

☑ Additional Digit Required   ▶◀ Revised Text   ● New Line   ▲ Revised Code

Calcium — *continued*
  deposits — *see also* Calcification, by site —
    continued
      in tendon (sheath) 727.82
        with bursitis, synovitis or tenosynovitis
          727.82
  salts or soaps in vitreous 379.22
Calciuria 791.9
Calculi — *see* Calculus
Calculosis, intrahepatic — *see*
  Choledocholithiasis
Calculus, calculi, calculous 592.9
  ampulla of Vater — *see* Choledocholithiasis
  anuria (impacted) (recurrent) 592.0
  appendix 543.9
  bile duct (any) — *see* Choledocholithiasis
  biliary — *see* Cholelithiasis
  bilirubin, multiple — *see* Cholelithiasis
  bladder (encysted) (impacted) (urinary) 594.1
    diverticulum 594.0
  bronchus 518.89
  calyx (kidney) (renal) 592.0
    congenital 753.3
  cholesterol (pure) (solitary) — *see* Cholelithiasis
  common duct (bile) — *see* Choledocholithiasis
  conjunctiva 372.54
  cystic 594.1
    duct — *see* Cholelithiasis
  dental 523.6
    subgingival 523.6
    supragingival 523.6
  epididymis 608.89
  gallbladder — *see also* Cholelithiasis
    congenital 751.69
  hepatic (duct) — *see* Choledocholithiasis
  intestine (impaction) (obstruction) 560.39
  kidney (impacted) (multiple) (pelvis) (recurrent)
    (staghorn) 592.0
    congenital 753.3
  lacrimal (passages) 375.57
  liver (impacted) — *see* Choledocholithiasis
  lung 518.89
  nephritic (impacted) (recurrent) 592.0
  nose 478.1
  pancreas (duct) 577.8
  parotid gland 527.5
  pelvis, encysted 592.0
  prostate 602.0
  pulmonary 518.89
  renal (impacted) (recurrent) 592.0
    congenital 753.3
  salivary (duct) (gland) 527.5
  seminal vesicle 608.89
  staghorn 592.0
  Stensen's duct 527.5
  sublingual duct or gland 527.5
    congenital 750.26
  submaxillary duct, gland, or region 527.5
  suburethral 594.8
  tonsil 474.8
  tooth, teeth 523.6
  tunica vaginalis 608.89
  ureter (impacted) (recurrent) 592.1
  urethra (impacted) 594.2
  urinary (duct) (impacted) (passage) (tract) 592.9
    lower tract NEC 594.9
      specified site 594.8
  vagina 623.8
  vesical (impacted) 594.1
  Wharton's duct 527.5
Caliectasis 593.89
California
  disease 114.0
  encephalitis 062.5
Caligo cornea 371.03
Callositas, callosity (infected) 700
Callus (infected) 700
  bone 726.91
  excessive, following fracture — *see also* Late,
    effect (of), fracture
Calvé (-Perthes) disease (osteochondrosis,
  femoral capital) 732.1
Calvities (*see also* Alopecia) 704.00
Cameroon fever (*see also* Malaria) 084.6

Camptocormia 300.11
Camptodactyly (congenital) 755.59
Camurati-Engelmann disease (diaphyseal
  sclerosis) 756.59
Canal — *see* condition
Canaliculitis (lacrimal) (acute) 375.31
  Actinomyces 039.8
  chronic 375.41
Canavan's disease 330.0
Cancer (M8000/3) — *see also* Neoplasm, by site,
  malignant

> *Note* — *The term "cancer" when modified by an
> adjective or adjectival phrase indicating a
> morphological type should be coded in the same
> manner as "carcinoma" with that adjective or
> phrase. Thus, "squamous-cell cancer" should be
> coded in the same manner as "squamous-cell
> carcinoma," which appears in the list under
> "Carcinoma."*

  bile duct type (M8160/3), liver 155.1
  hepatocellular (M8170/3) 155.0
Cancerous (M8000/3) — *see* Neoplasm, by site,
  malignant
Cancerphobia 300.29
Cancrum oris 528.1
Candidiasis, candidal 112.9
  with pneumonia 112.4
  balanitis 112.2
  congenital 771.7
  disseminated 112.5
  endocarditis 112.81
  esophagus 112.84
  intertrigo 112.3
  intestine 112.85
  lung 112.4
  meningitis 112.83
  mouth 112.0
  nails 112.3
  neonatal 771.7
  onychia 112.3
  otitis externa 112.82
  otomycosis 112.82
  paronychia 112.3
  perionyxis 112.3
  pneumonia 112.4
  pneumonitis 112.4
  skin 112.3
  specified site NEC 112.89
  systemic 112.5
  urogenital site NEC 112.2
  vagina 112.1
  vulva 112.1
  vulvovaginitis 112.1
Candidiosis — *see* Candidiasis
Candiru infection or infestation 136.8
Canities (premature) 704.3
  congenital 757.4
Canker (mouth) (sore) 528.2
  rash 034.1
Cannabinosis 504
Canton fever 081.9
Cap
  cradle 690.11
Capillariasis 127.5
Capillary — *see* condition
Caplan's syndrome 714.81
Caplan-Colinet syndrome 714.81
Capsule — *see* condition
Capsulitis (joint) 726.90
  adhesive (shoulder) 726.0
  hip 726.5
  knee 726.60
  labyrinthine 387.8
  thyroid 245.9
  wrist 726.4
Caput
  crepitus 756.0
  medusae 456.8
  succedaneum 767.19
Carapata disease 087.1

Carate — *see* Pinta
Carboxyhemoglobinemia 986
Carbuncle 680.9
  abdominal wall 680.2
  ankle 680.6
  anus 680.5
  arm (any part, above wrist) 680.3
  auditory canal, external 680.0
  axilla 680.3
  back (any part) 680.2
  breast 680.2
  buttock 680.5
  chest wall 680.2
  corpus cavernosum 607.2
  ear (any part) (external) 680.0
  eyelid 373.13
  face (any part except eye) 680.0
  finger (any) 680.4
  flank 680.2
  foot (any part) 680.7
  forearm 680.3
  genital organ (male) 608.4
  gluteal (region) 680.5
  groin 680.2
  hand (any part) 680.4
  head (any part except face) 680.8
  heel 680.7
  hip 680.6
  kidney (*see also* Abscess, kidney) 590.2
  knee 680.6
  labia 616.4
  lacrimal
    gland (*see also* Dacryoadenitis) 375.00
    passages (duct) (sac) (*see also*
      Dacryocystitis) 375.30
  leg, any part except foot 680.6
  lower extremity, any part except foot 680.6
  malignant 022.0
  multiple sites 680.9
  neck 680.1
  nose (external) (septum) 680.0
  orbit, orbital 376.01
  partes posteriores 680.5
  pectoral region 680.2
  penis 607.2
  perineum 680.2
  pinna 680.0
  scalp (any part) 680.8
  scrotum 608.4
  seminal vesicle 608.0
  shoulder 680.3
  skin NEC 680.9
  specified site NEC 680.8
  spermatic cord 608.4
  temple (region) 680.0
  testis 608.4
  thigh 680.6
  thumb 680.4
  toe (any) 680.7
  trunk 680.2
  tunica vaginalis 608.4
  umbilicus 680.2
  upper arm 680.3
  urethra 597.0
  vas deferens 608.4
  vulva 616.4
  wrist 680.4
Carbunculus (*see also* Carbuncle) 680.9
Carcinoid (tumor) (M8240/1) — *see also*
  Neoplasm, by site, uncertain behavior
  and struma ovarii (M9091/1) 236.2
  argentaffin (M8241/1) — *see* Neoplasm, by site,
    uncertain behavior
    malignant (M8241/3) — *see* Neoplasm, by
      site, malignant
  benign (M9091/0) 220
  composite (M8244/3) — *see* Neoplasm, by site,
    malignant
  goblet cell (M8243/3) — *see* Neoplasm, by site,
    malignant
  malignant (M8240/3) — *see* Neoplasm, by site,
    malignant
  nonargentaffin (M8242/1) — *see also*
    Neoplasm, by site, uncertain behavior
    malignant (M8242/3) — *see* Neoplasm, by
      site, malignant

☑ Additional Digit Required   ▶◀ Revised Text   ● New Line   ▲ Revised Code

Carcinoid (tumor) (M8240/1) — *see also*
    Neoplasm, by site, uncertain behavior —
    continued
      strumal (M9091/1) 236.2
      syndrome (intestinal) (metastatic) 259.2
      type bronchial adenoma (M8240/3) — *see*
        Neoplasm, lung, malignant
Carcinoidosis 259.2
Carcinoma (M8010/3) — *see also* Neoplasm, by
    site, malignant

> *Note* — *Except where otherwise indicated, the*
> *morphological varieties of carcinoma in the list*
> *below should be coded by site as for "Neoplasm,*
> *malignant."*

    with
      apocrine metaplasia (M8573/3)
      cartilaginous (and osseous) metaplasia
        (M8571/3)
      osseous (and cartilaginous) metaplasia
        (M8571/3)
      productive fibrosis (M8141/3)
      spindle cell metaplasia (M8572/3)
      squamous metaplasia (M8570/3)
    acidophil (M8280/3)
      specified site — *see* Neoplasm, by site,
        malignant
      unspecified site 194.3
    acidophil-basophil, mixed (M8281/3)
      specified site — *see* Neoplasm, by site,
        malignant
      unspecified site 194.3
    acinar (cell) (M8550/3)
    acinic cell (M8550/3)
    adenocystic (M8200/3)
    adenoid
      cystic (M8200/3)
      squamous cell (M8075/3)
    adenosquamous (M8560/3)
    adnexal (skin) (M8390/3) — *see* Neoplasm,
      skin, malignant
    adrenal cortical (M8370/3) 194.0
    alveolar (M8251/3)
      cell (M8250/3) — *see* Neoplasm, lung,
        malignant
    anaplastic type (M8021/3)
    apocrine (M8401/3)
      breast — *see* Neoplasm, breast, malignant
      specified site NEC — *see* Neoplasm, skin,
        malignant
      unspecified site 173.9
    basal cell (pigmented) (M8090/3) — *see also*
      Neoplasm, skin, malignant
      fibro-epithelial type (M8093/3) — *see*
        Neoplasm, skin, malignant
      morphea type (M8092/3) — *see* Neoplasm,
        skin, malignant
      multicentric (M8091/3) — *see* Neoplasm,
        skin, malignant
    basaloid (M8123/3)
    basal-squamous cell, mixed (M8094/3) — *see*
      Neoplasm, skin, malignant
    basophil (M8300/3)
      specified site — *see* Neoplasm, by site,
        malignant
      unspecified site 194.3
    basophil-acidophil, mixed (M8281/3)
      specified site — *see* Neoplasm, by site,
        malignant
      unspecified site 194.3
    basosquamous (M8094/3) — *see* Neoplasm,
      skin, malignant
    bile duct type (M8160/3)
      and hepatocellular, mixed (M8180/3) 155.0
      liver 155.1
      specified site NEC — *see* Neoplasm, by site,
        malignant
      unspecified site 155.1
    branchial or branchiogenic 146.8
    bronchial or bronchogenic — *see* Neoplasm,
      lung, malignant
    bronchiolar (terminal) (M8250/3) — *see*
      Neoplasm, lung, malignant
    bronchiolo-alveolar (M8250/3) — *see*
      Neoplasm, lung, malignant
    bronchogenic (epidermoid) 162.9

Carcinoma — *see also* Neoplasm, by site,
    malignant — *continued*
    C cell (M8510/3)
      specified site — *see* Neoplasm, by site,
        malignant
      unspecified site 193
    ceruminous (M8420/3) 173.2
    chorionic (M9100/3)
      specified site — *see* Neoplasm, by site,
        malignant
      unspecified site
        female 181
        male 186.9
    chromophobe (M8270/3)
      specified site — *see* Neoplasm, by site,
        malignant
      unspecified site 194.3
    clear cell (mesonephroid type) (M8310/3)
    cloacogenic (M8124/3)
      specified site — *see* Neoplasm, by site,
        malignant
      unspecified site 154.8
    colloid (M8480/3)
    cribriform (M8201/3)
    cylindroid type (M8200/3)
    diffuse type (M8145/3)
      specified site — *see* Neoplasm, by site,
        malignant
      unspecified site 151.9
    duct (cell) (M8500/3)
      with Paget's disease (M8541/3) — *see*
        Neoplasm, breast, malignant
      infiltrating (M8500/3)
        specified site — *see* Neoplasm, by site,
          malignant
        unspecified site 174.9
    ductal (M8500/3)
    ductular, infiltrating (M8521/3)
    embryonal (M9070/3)
      and teratoma, mixed (M9081/3)
      combined with choriocarcinoma (M9101/3)
        — *see* Neoplasm, by site, malignant
      infantile type (M9071/3)
      liver 155.0
      polyembryonal type (M9072/3)
    endometrioid (M8380/3)
    eosinophil (M8280/3)
      specified site — *see* Neoplasm, by site,
        malignant
      unspecified site 194.3
    epidermoid (M8070/3) — *see also* Carcinoma,
      squamous cell
      and adenocarcinoma, mixed (M8560/3)
      in situ, Bowen's type (M8081/2) — *see*
        Neoplasm, skin, in situ
      intradermal — *see* Neoplasm, skin, in situ
    fibroepithelial type basal cell (M8093/3) — *see*
      Neoplasm, skin, malignant
    follicular (M8330/3)
      and papillary (mixed) (M8340/3) 193
      moderately differentiated type (M8332/3)
        193
      pure follicle type (M8331/3) 193
      specified site — *see* Neoplasm, by site,
        malignant
      trabecular type (M8332/3) 193
      unspecified site 193
      well differentiated type (M8331/3) 193
    gelatinous (M8480/3)
    giant cell (M8031/3)
      and spindle cell (M8030/3)
    granular cell (M8320/3)
    granulosa cell (M8620/3) 183.0
    hepatic cell (M8170/3) 155.0
    hepatocellular (M8170/3) 155.0
      and bile duct, mixed (M8180/3) 155.0
    hepatocholangiolitic (M8180/3) 155.0
    Hürthle cell (thyroid) 193
    hypernephroid (M8311/3)
    in
      adenomatous
        polyp (M82l0/3)
        polyposis coli (M8220/3) 153.9
      pleomorphic adenoma (M8940/3)
      polypoid adenoma (M8210/3)
      situ (M8010/3) — *see* Carcinoma, in situ
      tubular adenoma (M8210/3)

Carcinoma — *see also* Neoplasm, by site,
    malignant — *continued*
  in — *continued*
      villous adenoma (M8261/3)
    infiltrating duct (M8500/3)
      with Paget's disease (M8541/3) — *see*
        Neoplasm, breast, malignant
      specified site — *see* Neoplasm, by site,
        malignant
      unspecified site 174.9
    inflammatory (M8530/3)
      specified site — *see* Neoplasm, by site,
        malignant
      unspecified site 174.9
    in situ (M8010/2) — *see also* Neoplasm, by
      site, in situ
      epidermoid (M8070/2) — *see also* Neoplasm,
        by site, in situ
        with questionable stromal invasion
          (M8076/2)
          specified site — *see* Neoplasm, by site,
            in situ
          unspecified site 233.1
        Bowen's type (M8081/2) — *see*
          Neoplasm, skin, in situ
      intraductal (M8500/2)
        specified site — *see* Neoplasm, by site, in
          situ
        unspecified site 233.0
      lobular (M8520/2)
        specified site — *see* Neoplasm, by site, in
          situ
        unspecified site 233.0
      papillary (M8050/2) — *see* Neoplasm, by
        site, in situ
      squamous cell (M8070/2) — *see also*
        Neoplasm, by site, in situ
        with questionable stromal invasion
          (M8076/2)
          specified site — *see* Neoplasm, by site,
            in situ
          unspecified site 233.1
      transitional cell (M8120/2) — *see* Neoplasm,
        by site, in situ
    intestinal type (M8144/3)
      specified site — *see* Neoplasm, by site,
        malignant
      unspecified site 151.9
    intraductal (noninfiltrating) (M8500/2)
      papillary (M8503/2)
        specified site — *see* Neoplasm, by site, in
          situ
        unspecified site 233.0
      specified site — *see* Neoplasm, by site, in
        situ
      unspecified site 233.0
    intraepidermal (M8070/2) — *see also*
      Neoplasm, skin, in situ
      squamous cell, Bowen's type (M8081/2) —
        see Neoplasm, skin, in situ
    intraepithelial (M8010/2) — *see also* Neoplasm,
      by site, in situ
      squamous cell (M8072/2) — *see* Neoplasm,
        by site, in situ
    intraosseous (M9270/3) 170.1
      upper jaw (bone) 170.0
    islet cell (M8150/3)
      and exocrine, mixed (M8154/3)
        specified site — *see* Neoplasm, by site,
          malignant
        unspecified site 157.9
      pancreas 157.4
      specified site NEC — *see* Neoplasm, by site,
        malignant
      unspecified site 157.4
    juvenile, breast (M8502/3) — *see* Neoplasm,
      breast, malignant
    Kulchitsky's cell (carcinoid tumor of intestine)
      259.2
    large cell (M8012/3)
      squamous cell, nonkeratinizing type
        (M8072/3)
    Leydig cell (testis) (M8650/3)
      specified site — *see* Neoplasm, by site,
        malignant

Carcinoma — *see also* Neoplasm, by site, malignant — *continued*
 Leydig cell (testis) (M8650/3) — *continued*
  unspecified site 186.9
   female 183.0
   male 186.9
 liver cell (M8170/3) 155.0
 lobular (infiltrating) (M8520/3)
  non-infiltrating (M8520/3)
   specified site — *see* Neoplasm, by site, in situ
   unspecified site 233.0
  specified site — *see* Neoplasm, by site, malignant
  unspecified site 174.9
 lymphoepithelial (M8082/3)
 medullary (M8510/3)
  with
   amyloid stroma (M8511/3)
    specified site — *see* Neoplasm, by site, malignant
    unspecified site 193
   lymphoid stroma (M8512/3)
    specified site — *see* Neoplasm, by site, malignant
    unspecified site 174.9
 mesometanephric (M9110/3)
 mesonephric (M9110/3)
 metastatic (M8010/6) — *see* Metastasis, cancer
 metatypical (M8095/3) — *see* Neoplasm, skin, malignant
 morphea type basal cell (M8092/3) — *see* Neoplasm, skin, malignant
 mucinous (M8480/3)
 mucin-producing (M8481/3)
 mucin-secreting (M8481/3)
 mucoepidermoid (M8430/3)
 mucoid (M8480/3)
  cell (M8300/3)
   specified site — *see* Neoplasm, by site, malignant
   unspecified site 194.3
 mucous (M8480/3)
 nonencapsulated sclerosing (M8350/3) 193
 noninfiltrating
  intracystic (M8504/2) — *see* Neoplasm, by site, in situ
  intraductal (M8500/2)
   papillary (M8503/2)
    specified site — *see* Neoplasm, by site, in situ
    unspecified site 233.0
   specified site — *see* Neoplasm, by site, in situ
   unspecified site 233.0
  lobular (M8520/2)
   specified site — *see* Neoplasm, by site, in situ
   unspecified site 233.0
 oat cell (M8042/3)
  specified site — *see* Neoplasm, by site, malignant
  unspecified site 162.9
 odontogenic (M9270/3) 170.1
  upper jaw (bone) 170.0
 onocytic (M8290/3)
 oxyphilic (M8290/3)
 papillary (M8050/3)
  and follicular (mixed) (M8340/3) 193
  epidermoid (M8052/3)
  intraductal (noninfiltrating) (M8503/2)
   specified site — *see* Neoplasm, by site, in situ
   unspecified site 233.0
  serous (M8460/3)
   specified site — *see* Neoplasm, by site, malignant
  surface (M8461/3)
   specified site — *see* Neoplasm, by site, malignant
   unspecified site 183.0
  unspecified site 183.0
  squamous cell (M8052/3)
  transitional cell (M8130/3)
 papillocystic (M8450/3)
  specified site — *see* Neoplasm, by site, malignant

Carcinoma — *see also* Neoplasm, by site, malignant — *continued*
 papillocystic (M8450/3) — *continued*
  unspecified site 183.0
 parafollicular cell (M8510/3)
  specified site — *see* Neoplasm, by site, malignant
  unspecified site 193
 pleomorphic (M8022/3)
 polygonal cell (M8034/3)
 prickle cell (M8070/3)
 pseudoglandular, squamous cell (M8075/3)
 pseudomucinous (M8470/3)
  specified site — *see* Neoplasm, by site, malignant
  unspecified site 183.0
 pseudosarcomatous (M8033/3)
 regaud type (M8082/3) — *see* Neoplasm, nasopharynx, malignant
 renal cell (M8312/3) 189.0
 reserve cell (M8041/3)
 round cell (M8041/3)
 Schmincke (M8082/3) — *see* Neoplasm, nasopharynx, malignant
 Schneiderian (M8121/3)
  specified site — *see* Neoplasm, by site, malignant
  unspecified site 160.0
 scirrhous (M8141/3)
 sebaceous (M8410/3) — *see* Neoplasm, skin, malignant
 secondary (M8010/6) — *see* Neoplasm, by site, malignant, secondary
 secretory, breast (M8502/3) — *see* Neoplasm, breast, malignant
 serous (M8441/3)
  papillary (M8460/3)
   specified site — *see* Neoplasm, by site, malignant
   unspecified site 183.0
  surface, papillary (M8461/3)
   specified site — *see* Neoplasm, by site, malignant
   unspecified site 183.0
 Sertoli cell (M8640/3)
  specified site — *see* Neoplasm, by site, malignant
  unspecified site 186.9
 signet ring cell (M8490/3)
  metastatic (M8490/6) — *see* Neoplasm, by site, secondary
 simplex (M8231/3)
 skin appendage (M8390/3) — *see* Neoplasm, skin, malignant
 small cell (M8041/3)
  fusiform cell type (M8043/3)
  squamous cell, non-keratinizing type (M8073/3)
 solid (M8230/3)
  with amyloid stroma (M8511/3)
   specified site — *see* Neoplasm, by site, malignant
   unspecified site 193
 spheroidal cell (M8035/3)
 spindle cell (M8032/3)
  and giant cell (M8030/3)
 spinous cell (M8070/3)
 squamous (cell) (M8070/3)
  adenoid type (M8075/3)
  and adenocarcinoma, mixed (M8560/3)
  intraepidermal, Bowen's type — *see* Neoplasm, skin, in situ
  keratinizing type (large cell) (M8071/3)
  large cell, non-keratinizing type (M8072/3)
  microinvasive (M8076/3)
   specified site — *see* Neoplasm, by site, malignant
   unspecified site 180.9
  non-keratinizing type (M8072/3)
  papillary (M8052/3)
  pseudoglandular (M8075/3)
  small cell, non-keratinizing type (M8073/3)
  spindle cell type (M8074/3)
  verrucous (M805l/3)
 superficial spreading (M8143/3)
 sweat gland (M8400/3) — *see* Neoplasm, skin, malignant

Carcinoma — *see also* Neoplasm, by site, malignant — *continued*
 theca cell (M8600/3) 183.0
 thymic (M8580/3) 164.0
 trabecular (M8190/3)
 transitional (cell) (M8120/3)
  papillary (M8130/3)
  spindle cell type (M8122/3)
 tubular (M8211/3)
 undifferentiated type (M8020/3)
 urothelial (M8120/3)
 ventriculi 151.9
 verrucous (epidermoid) (squamous cell) (M8051/3)
 villous (M8262/3)
 water-clear cell (M8322/3) 194.1
 wolffian duct (M9110/3)

Carcinomaphobia 300.29

Carcinomatosis
 peritonei (M8010/6) 197.6
 specified site NEC (M8010/3) — *see* Neoplasm, by site, malignant
 unspecified site (M8010/6) 199.0

Carcinosarcoma (M8980/3) — *see also* Neoplasm, by site, malignant
 embryonal type (M8981/3) — *see* Neoplasm, by site, malignant

Cardia, cardial — *see* condition

Cardiac — *see also* condition
 death — *see* Disease, heart
 device
  defibrillator, automatic implantable V45.02
  in situ NEC V45.00
  pacemaker
   cardiac
    fitting or adjustment V53.31
    in situ V45.01
   carotid sinus
    fitting or adjustment V53.39
    in situ V45.09
 pacemaker — *see* Cardiac, device, pacemaker
 tamponade 423.9

Cardialgia (*see also* Pain, precordial) 786.51

Cardiectasis — *see* Hypertrophy, cardiac

Cardiochalasia 530.81

Cardiomalacia (*see also* Degeneration, myocardial) 429.1

Cardiomegalia glycogenica diffusa 271.0

Cardiomegaly (*see also* Hypertrophy, cardiac) 429.3
 congenital 746.89
 glycogen 271.0
 hypertensive (*see also* Hypertension, heart) 402.90
 idiopathic 429.3

Cardiomyoliposis (*see also* Degeneration, myocardial) 429.1

Cardiomyopathy (congestive) (constrictive) (familial) (infiltrative) (obstructive) (restrictive) (sporadic) 425.4
 alcoholic 425.5
 amyloid 277.3 [425.7]
 beriberi 265.0 [425.7]
 cobalt-beer 425.5
 congenital 425.3
 due to
  amyloidosis 277.3 [425.7]
  beriberi 265.0 [425.7]
  cardiac glycogenosis 271.0 [425.7]
  Chagas' disease 086.0
  Friedreich's ataxia 334.0 [425.8]
  hypertension —*see* Hypertension, with, heart involvement
  mucopolysaccharidosis 277.5 [425.7]
  myotonia atrophica 359.2 [425.8]
  progressive muscular dystrophy 359.1 [425.8]
  sarcoidosis 135 [425.8]
 glycogen storage 271.0 [425.7]
 hypertensive — *see* Hypertension, with, heart involvement
 hypertrophic
  nonobstructive 425.4

Cardiomyopathy — continued
  hypertrophic — continued
    obstructive 425.1
      congenital 746.84
  idiopathic (concentric) 425.4
  in
    Chagas' disease 086.0
    sarcoidosis 135 *[425.8]*
  ischemic 414.8
  metabolic NEC 277.9 *[425.7]*
    amyloid 277.3 *[425.7]*
    thyrotoxic (*see also* Thyrotoxicosis) 242.9 ☑
      [425.7]
    thyrotoxicosis (*see also* Thyrotoxicosis)
      242.9 ☑ *[425.7]*
    nutritional 269.9 *[425.7]*
    beriberi 265.0 *[425.7]*
  obscure of Africa 425.2
  peripartum 674.5 ☑
  postpartum 674.5 ☑
  primary 425.4
  secondary 425.9
  thyrotoxic (*see also* Thyrotoxicosis) 242.9 ☑
    [425.7]
  toxic NEC 425.9
  tuberculous (*see also* Tuberculosis) 017.9 ☑
    [425.8]
Cardionephritis — *see* Hypertension, cardiorenal
Cardionephropathy — *see* Hypertension, cardiorenal
Cardionephrosis — *see* Hypertension, cardiorenal
Cardioneurosis 306.2
Cardiopathia nigra 416.0
Cardiopathy (*see also* Disease, heart) 429.9
  hypertensive (*see also* Hypertension, heart) 402.90
  idiopathic 425.4
  mucopolysaccharidosis 277.5 *[425.7]*
Cardiopericarditis (*see also* Pericarditis) 423.9
Cardiophobia 300.29
Cardioptosis 746.87
Cardiorenal — *see* condition
Cardiorrhexis (*see also* Infarct, myocardium) 410.9 ☑
Cardiosclerosis — *see* Arteriosclerosis, coronary
Cardiosis — *see* Disease, heart
Cardiospasm (esophagus) (reflex) (stomach) 530.0
  congenital 750.7
Cardiostenosis — *see* Disease, heart
Cardiosymphysis 423.1
Cardiothyrotoxicosis — *see* Hyperthyroidism
Cardiovascular — *see* condition
Carditis (acute) (bacterial) (chronic) (subacute) 429.89
  Coxsackie 074.20
  hypertensive (*see also* Hypertension, heart) 402.90
  meningococcal 036.40
  rheumatic — *see* Disease, heart, rheumatic
  rheumatoid 714.2
Care (of)
  child (routine) V20.1
  convalescent following V66.9
    chemotherapy V66.2
    medical NEC V66.5
    psychotherapy V66.3
    radiotherapy V66.1
    surgery V66.0
    surgical NEC V66.0
    treatment (for) V66.5
      combined V66.6
      fracture V66.4
      mental disorder NEC V66.3
      specified type NEC V66.5
  end-of-life V66.7
  family member (handicapped) (sick)
    creating problem for family V61.49
    provided away from home for holiday relief V60.5
    unavailable, due to
      absence (person rendering care) (sufferer) V60.4

Care (of) — continued
  family member — continued
    unavailable, due to — continued
      inability (any reason) of person rendering care V60.4
  holiday relief V60.5
  hospice V66.7
  lack of (at or after birth) (infant) (child) 995.52
    adult 995.84
  lactation of mother V24.1
  palliative V66.7
  postpartum
    immediately after delivery V24.0
    routine follow-up V24.2
  prenatal V22.1
    first pregnancy V22.0
    high risk pregnancy V23.9
      specified problem NEC V23.89
  terminal V66.7
  unavailable, due to
    absence of person rendering care V60.4
    inability (any reason) of person rendering care V60.4
  well baby V20.1
Caries (bone) (*see also* Tuberculosis, bone) 015.9 ☑ *[730.8]*
  arrested 521.04
  cementum 521.03
  cerebrospinal (tuberculous) 015.0 ☑ *[730.88]*
  dental (acute) (chronic) (incipient) (infected) 521.00 ▲
    with pulp exposure 521.03
    extending to
      dentine 521.02
      pulp 521.03
    other specified NEC 521.09
    pit and fissure 521.06 ●
    root surface 521.08 ●
    smooth surface 521.07 ●
  dentin (acute) (chronic) 521.02
  enamel (acute) (chronic) (incipient) 521.01
  external meatus 380.89
  hip (*see also* Tuberculosis) 015.1 ☑ *[730.85]*
  initial 521.01 ●
  knee 015.2 ☑ *[730.86]*
  labyrinth 386.8
  limb NEC 015.7 ☑ *[730.88]*
  mastoid (chronic) (process) 383.1
  middle ear 385.89
  nose 015.7 ☑ *[730.88]*
  orbit 015.7 ☑ *[730.88]*
  ossicle 385.24
  petrous bone 383.20
  sacrum (tuberculous) 015.0 ☑ *[730.88]*
  spine, spinal (column) (tuberculous) 015.0 ☑ *[730.88]*
  syphilitic 095.5
    congenital 090.0 *[730.8]* ☑
  teeth (internal) 521.00
    initial 521.01
  vertebra (column) (tuberculous) 015.0 ☑ *[730.88]*
Carini's syndrome (ichthyosis congenita) 757.1
Carious teeth 521.00
Carneous mole 631
Carnosinemia 270.5
Carotid body or sinus syndrome 337.0
Carotidynia 337.0
Carotinemia (dietary) 278.3
Carotinosis (cutis) (skin) 278.3
Carpal tunnel syndrome 354.0
Carpenter's syndrome 759.89
Carpopedal spasm (*see also* Tetany) 781.7
Carpoptosis 736.05
Carrier (suspected) of
  amebiasis V02.2
  bacterial disease (meningococcal, staphylococcal, streptococcal) NEC V02.59
  cholera V02.0
  cystic fibrosis gene V83.81
  defective gene V83.89
  diphtheria V02.4

Carrier (suspected) of — continued
  dysentery (bacillary) V02.3
    amebic V02.2
  Endamoeba histolytica V02.2
  gastrointestinal pathogens NEC V02.3
  genetic defect V83.89
  gonorrhea V02.7
  group B streptococcus V02.51
  HAA (hepatitis Australian-antigen) V02.61
  hemophilia A (asymptomatic) V83.01
    symptomatic V83.02
  hepatitis V02.60
    Australian-antigen (HAA) V02.61
    B V02.61
    C V02.62
    serum V02.61
    specified type NEC V02.69
    viral V02.60
  infective organism NEC V02.9
  malaria V02.9
  paratyphoid V02.3
  Salmonella V02.3
    typhosa V02.1
  serum hepatitis V02.61
  Shigella V02.3
  Staphylococcus NEC V02.59
  Streptococcus NEC V02.52
    group B V02.51
  typhoid V02.1
  venereal disease NEC V02.8
Carrión's disease (Bartonellosis) 088.0
Car sickness 994.6
Carter's
  relapsing fever (Asiatic) 087.0
Cartilage — *see* condition
Caruncle (inflamed)
  abscess, lacrimal (*see also* Dacryocystitis) 375.30
  conjunctiva 372.00
    acute 372.00
  eyelid 373.00
  labium (majus) (minus) 616.8
  lacrimal 375.30
  urethra (benign) 599.3
  vagina (wall) 616.8
Cascade stomach 537.6
Caseation lymphatic gland (*see also* Tuberculosis) 017.2 ☑
Caseous
  bronchitis — *see* Tuberculosis, pulmonary
  meningitis 013.0 ☑
  pneumonia — *see* Tuberculosis, pulmonary
Cassidy (-Scholte) syndrome (malignant carcinoid) 259.2
Castellani's bronchitis 104.8
Castleman's tumor or lymphoma (mediastinal lymph node hyperplasia) 785.6
Castration, traumatic 878.2
  complicated 878.3
Casts in urine 791.7
Cat's ear 744.29
Catalepsy 300.11
  catatonic (acute) (*see also* Schizophrenia) 295.2 ☑
  hysterical 300.11
  schizophrenic (*see also* Schizophrenia) 295.2 ☑
Cataphasia 307.0
Cataplexy (idiopathic) ►— *see* Narcolepsy◄
Cataract (anterior cortical) (anterior polar) (black) (capsular) (central) (cortical) (hypermature) (immature) (incipient) (mature) 366.9
  anterior
    and posterior axial embryonal 743.33
    pyramidal 743.31
    subcapsular polar
      infantile, juvenile, or presenile 366.01
      senile 366.13
  associated with
    calcinosis 275.40 *[366.42]*
    craniofacial dysostosis 756.0 *[366.44]*
    galactosemia 271.1 *[366.44]*
    hypoparathyroidism 252.1 *[366.42]*
    myotonic disorders 359.2 *[366.43]*

☑ Additional Digit Required   ►◄ Revised Text   ● New Line   ▲ Revised Code

Cataract — *continued*
  associated with — *continued*
    neovascularization 366.33
  blue dot 743.39
  cerulean 743.39
  complicated NEC 366.30
  congenital 743.30
    capsular or subcapsular 743.31
    cortical 743.32
    nuclear 743.33
    specified type NEC 743.39
    total or subtotal 743.34
    zonular 743.32
  coronary (congenital) 743.39
    acquired 366.12
  cupuliform 366.14
  diabetic 250.5 ☑ *[366.41]*
  drug-induced 366.45
  due to
    chalcosis 360.24 *[366.34]*
    chronic choroiditis (*see also* Choroiditis)
      363.20 *[366.32]*
    degenerative myopia 360.21 *[366.34]*
    glaucoma (*see also* Glaucoma) 365.9
      [366.31]
    infection, intraocular NEC 366.32
    inflammatory ocular disorder NEC 366.32
    iridocyclitis, chronic 364.10 *[366.33]*
    pigmentary retinal dystrophy 362.74
      [366.34]
    radiation 366.46
  electric 366.46
  glassblowers' 366.46
  heat ray 366.46
  heterochromic 366.33
  in eye disease NEC 366.30
  infantile (*see also* Cataract, juvenile) 366.00
  intumescent 366.12
  irradiational 366.46
  juvenile 366.00
    anterior subcapsular polar 366.01
    combined forms 366.09
    cortical 366.03
    lamellar 366.03
    nuclear 366.04
    posterior subcapsular polar 366.02
    specified NEC 366.09
    zonular 366.03
  lamellar 743.32
    infantile, juvenile, or presenile 366.03
  morgagnian 366.18
  myotonic 359.2 *[366.43]*
  myxedema 244.9 *[366.44]*
  nuclear 366.16
  posterior, polar (capsular) 743.31
    infantile, juvenile, or presenile 366.02
    senile 366.14
  presenile (*see also* Cataract, juvenile) 366.00
  punctate
    acquired 366.12
    congenital 743.39
  secondary (membrane) 366.50
    obscuring vision 366.53
    specified type, not obscuring vision 366.52
  senile 366.10
    anterior subcapsular polar 366.13
    combined forms 366.19
    cortical 366.15
    hypermature 366.18
    immature 366.12
    incipient 366.12
    mature 366.17
    nuclear 366.16
    posterior subcapsular polar 366.14
    specified NEC 366.19
    total or subtotal 366.17
  snowflake 250.5 ☑ *[366.41]*
  specified NEC 366.8
  subtotal (senile) 366.17
    congenital 743.34
  sunflower 360.24 *[366.34]*
  tetanic NEC 252.1 *[366.42]*
  total (mature) (senile) 366.17
    congenital 743.34
    localized 366.21
    traumatic 366.22
  toxic 366.45

Cataract — *continued*
  traumatic 366.20
    partially resolved 366.23
    total 366.22
  zonular (perinuclear) 743.32
    infantile, juvenile, or presenile 366.03
Cataracta 366.10
  brunescens 366.16
  cerulea 743.39
  complicata 366.30
  congenita 743.30
  coralliformis 743.39
  coronaria (congenital) 743.39
    acquired 366.12
  diabetic 250.5 ☑ *[366.41]*
  floriformis 360.24 *[366.34]*
  membranacea
    accreta 366.50
    congenita 743.39
  nigra 366.16
Catarrh, catarrhal (inflammation) (*see also*
    condition) 460
  acute 460
  asthma, asthmatic (*see also* Asthma) 493.9 ☑
  Bostock's (*see also* Fever, hay) 477.9
  bowel — *see* Enteritis
  bronchial 490
    acute 466.0
    chronic 491.0
    subacute 466.0
  cervix, cervical (canal) (uteri) — *see* Cervicitis
  chest (*see also* Bronchitis) 490
  chronic 472.0
  congestion 472.0
  conjunctivitis 372.03
  due to syphilis 095.9
    congenital 090.0
  enteric — *see* Enteritis
  epidemic 487.1
  Eustachian 381.50
  eye (acute) (vernal) 372.03
  fauces (*see also* Pharyngitis) 462
  febrile 460
  fibrinous acute 466.0
  gastroenteric — *see* Enteritis
  gastrointestinal — *see* Enteritis
  gingivitis 523.0
  hay (*see also* Fever, hay) 477.9
  infectious 460
  intestinal — *see* Enteritis
  larynx (*see also* Laryngitis, chronic) 476.0
  liver 070.1
    with hepatic coma 070.0
  lung (*see also* Bronchitis) 490
    acute 466.0
    chronic 491.0
  middle ear (chronic) — *see* Otitis media,
    chronic
  mouth 528.0
  nasal (chronic) (*see also* Rhinitis) 472.0
    acute 460
  nasobronchial 472.2
  nasopharyngeal (chronic) 472.2
    acute 460
  nose — *see* Catarrh, nasal
  ophthalmia 372.03
  pneumococcal, acute 466.0
  pulmonary (*see also* Bronchitis) 490
    acute 466.0
    chronic 491.0
  spring (eye) 372.13
  suffocating (*see also* Asthma) 493.9 ☑
  summer (hay) (*see also* Fever, hay) 477.9
  throat 472.1
  tracheitis 464.10
    with obstruction 464.11
  tubotympanal 381.4
    acute (*see also* Otitis media, acute,
      nonsuppurative) 381.00
    chronic 381.10
  vasomotor (*see also* Fever, hay) 477.9
  vesical (bladder) — *see* Cystitis
Catarrhus aestivus (*see also* Fever, hay) 477.9
Catastrophe, cerebral (*see also* Disease,
    cerebrovascular, acute) 436

Catatonia, catatonic (acute) 781.99
  with
    affective psychosis — *see* Psychosis,
      affective
  agitation 295.2 ☑
  Churg-Strauss syndrome 446.4
  dementia (praecox) 295.2 ☑
  due to or associated with physical condition
    293.89
  excitation 295.2 ☑
  excited type 295.2 ☑
  in conditions classified elsewhere 293.89   ●
  schizophrenia 295.2 ☑
  stupor 295.2 ☑
Cat-scratch — *see also* Injury, superficial disease
    or fever 078.3
Cauda equina — *see also* condition
  syndrome 344.60
Cauliflower ear 738.7
Caul over face 768.9
Causalgia 355.9
  lower limb 355.71
  upper limb 354.4
Cause
  external, general effects NEC 994.9
  not stated 799.9
  unknown 799.9
Caustic burn — *see also* Burn, by site
  from swallowing caustic or corrosive substance
    — *see* Burn, internal organs
Cavare's disease (familial periodic paralysis)
    359.3
Cave-in, injury
  crushing (severe) (*see also* Crush, by site)
    869.1
  suffocation 994.7
Cavernitis (penis) 607.2
  lymph vessel — *see* Lymphangioma
Cavernositis 607.2
Cavernous — *see* condition
Cavitation of lung (*see also* Tuberculosis)
    011.2 ☑
  nontuberculous 518.89
  primary, progressive 010.8 ☑
Cavity
  lung — *see* Cavitation of lung
  optic papilla 743.57
  pulmonary — *see* Cavitation of lung
  teeth 521.00
  vitreous (humor) 379.21
Cavovarus foot, congenital 754.59
Cavus foot (congenital) 754.71
  acquired 736.73
Cazenave's
  disease (pemphigus) NEC 694.4
  lupus (erythematosus) 695.4
Cecitis — *see* Appendicitis
Cecocele — *see* Hernia
Cecum — *see* condition
Celiac
  artery compression syndrome 447.4
  disease 579.0
  infantilism 579.0
Cell, cellular — *see also* condition
  anterior chamber (eye) (positive aqueous ray)
    364.04
Cellulitis (diffuse) (with lymphangitis) (*see also*
    Abscess) 682.9
  abdominal wall 682.2
  anaerobic (*see also* Gas gangrene) 040.0
  ankle 682.6
  anus 566
  areola 611.0
  arm (any part, above wrist) 682.3
  auditory canal (external) 380.10
  axilla 682.3
  back (any part) 682.2
  breast 611.0
    postpartum 675.1 ☑
  broad ligament (*see also* Disease, pelvis,
    inflammatory) 614.4
    acute 614.3

Cataract — Cellulitis

Cellulitis (see also Abscess) — continued
buttock 682.5
cervical (neck region) 682.1
cervix (uteri) (see also Cervicitis) 616.0
cheek, external 682.0
   internal 528.3
chest wall 682.2
chronic NEC 682.9
corpus cavernosum 607.2
digit 681.9
Douglas' cul-de-sac or pouch (chronic) (see also Disease, pelvis, inflammatory) 614.4
   acute 614.3
drainage site (following operation) 998.59
ear, external 380.10
enterostomy 569.61
erysipelar (see also Erysipelas) 035
esophagostomy 530.86   ●
eyelid 373.13
face (any part, except eye) 682.0
finger (intrathecal) (periosteal) (subcutaneous) (subcuticular) 681.00
flank 682.2
foot (except toe) 682.7
forearm 682.3
gangrenous (see also Gangrene) 785.4
genital organ NEC
   female — see Abscess, genital organ, female
   male 608.4
glottis 478.71
gluteal (region) 682.5
gonococcal NEC 098.0
groin 682.2
hand (except finger or thumb) 682.4
head (except face) NEC 682.8
heel 682.7
hip 682.6
jaw (region) 682.0
knee 682.6
labium (majus) (minus) (see also Vulvitis) 616.10
larynx 478.71
leg, except foot 682.6
lip 528.5
mammary gland 611.0
mouth (floor) 528.3
multiple sites NEC 682.9
nasopharynx 478.21
navel 682.2
   newborn NEC 771.4
neck (region) 682.1
nipple 611.0
nose 478.1
   external 682.0
orbit, orbital 376.01
palate (soft) 528.3
pectoral (region) 682.2
pelvis, pelvic
   with
      abortion — see Abortion, by type, with sepsis
      ectopic pregnancy (see also categories 633.0— 633.9) 639.0
      molar pregnancy (see also categories 630— 632) 639.0
   female (see also Disease, pelvis, inflammatory) 614.4
      acute 614.3
   following
      abortion 639.0
      ectopic or molar pregnancy 639.0
   male (see also Abscess, peritoneum) 567.2
   puerperal, postpartum, childbirth 670.0 ☑
penis 607.2
perineal, perineum 682.2
perirectal 566
peritonsillar 475
periurethral 597.0
periuterine (see also Disease, pelvis, inflammatory) 614.4
   acute 614.3
pharynx 478.21
phlegmonous NEC 682.9
rectum 566
retromammary 611.0
retroperitoneal (see also Peritonitis) 567.2

Cellulitis (see also Abscess) — continued
round ligament (see also Disease, pelvis, inflammatory) 614.4
   acute 614.3
scalp (any part) 682.8
   dissecting 704.8
scrotum 608.4
seminal vesicle 608.0
septic NEC 682.9
shoulder 682.3
specified sites NEC 682.8
spermatic cord 608.4
submandibular (region) (space) (triangle) 682.0
   gland 527.3
submaxillary 528.3
   gland 527.3
submental (pyogenic) 682.0
   gland 527.3
suppurative NEC 682.9
testis 608.4
thigh 682.6
thumb (intrathecal) (periosteal) (subcutaneous) (subcuticular) 681.00
toe (intrathecal) (periosteal) (subcutaneous) (subcuticular) 681.10
tonsil 475
trunk 682.2
tuberculous (primary) (see also Tuberculosis) 017.0 ☑
tunica vaginalis 608.4
umbilical 682.2
   newborn NEC 771.4
vaccinal 999.3
vagina — see Vaginitis
vas deferens 608.4
vocal cords 478.5
vulva (see also Vulvitis) 616.10
wrist 682.4

Cementoblastoma, benign (M9273/0) 213.1
   upper jaw (bone) 213.0
Cementoma (M9273/0) 213.1
   gigantiform (M9276/0) 213.1
      upper jaw (bone) 213.0
   upper jaw (bone) 213.0
Cementoperiostitis 523.4
Cephalgia, cephalalgia (see also Headache) 784.0
   histamine 346.2 ☑
   nonorganic origin 307.81
   psychogenic 307.81
   tension 307.81
Cephalhematocele, cephalematocele
   due to birth injury 767.19
   fetus or newborn 767.19
   traumatic (see also Contusion, head) 920
Cephalhematoma, cephalematoma (calcified)
   due to birth injury 767.19
   fetus or newborn 767.19
   traumatic (see also Contusion, head) 920
Cephalic — see condition
Cephalitis — see Encephalitis
Cephalocele 742.0
Cephaloma — see Neoplasm, by site, malignant
Cephalomenia 625.8
Cephalopelvic — see condition
Cercomoniasis 007.3
Cerebellitis — see Encephalitis
Cerebellum (cerebellar) — see condition
Cerebral — see condition
Cerebritis — see Encephalitis
Cerebrohepatorenal syndrome 759.89
Cerebromacular degeneration 330.1
Cerebromalacia (see also Softening, brain) 434.9 ☑
Cerebrosidosis 272.7
Cerebrospasticity — see Palsy, cerebral
Cerebrospinal — see condition
Cerebrum — see condition
Ceroid storage disease 272.7
Cerumen (accumulation) (impacted) 380.4
Cervical — see also condition
   auricle 744.43

Cervical — see also condition — continued
   high risk human papillomavirus (HPV) DNA test positive 795.05   ●
   low risk human papillomavirus (HPV) DNA test positive 795.09   ●
   rib 756.2
Cervicalgia 723.1
Cervicitis (acute) (chronic) (nonvenereal) (subacute) (with erosion or ectropion) 616.0
   with
      abortion — see Abortion, by type, with sepsis
      ectopic pregnancy (see also categories 633.0-633.9) 639.0
      molar pregnancy (see also categories 630-632) 639.0
      ulceration 616.0
   chlamydial 099.53
   complicating pregnancy or puerperium 646.6 ☑
      affecting fetus or newborn 760.8
   following
      abortion 639.0
      ectopic or molar pregnancy 639.0
   gonococcal (acute) 098.15
      chronic or duration of 2 months or more 098.35
   senile (atrophic) 616.0
   syphilitic 095.8
   trichomonal 131.09
   tuberculous (see also Tuberculosis) 016.7 ☑
Cervicoaural fistula 744.49
Cervicocolpitis (emphysematosa) (see also Cervicitis) 616.0
Cervix — see condition
Cesarean delivery, operation or section NEC 669.7 ☑
   affecting fetus or newborn 763.4
   post mortem, affecting fetus or newborn 761.6
   previous, affecting management of pregnancy 654.2 ☑
Céstan's syndrome 344.89
Céstan-Chenais paralysis 344.89
Céstan-Raymond syndrome 433.8 ☑
Cestode infestation NEC 123.9
   specified type NEC 123.8
Cestodiasis 123.9
Chabert's disease 022.9
Chacaleh 266.2
Chafing 709.8
Chagas' disease (see also Trypanosomiasis, American) 086.2
   with heart involvement 086.0
Chagres fever 084.0
Chalasia (cardiac sphincter) 530.81
Chalazion 373.2
Chalazoderma 757.39
Chalcosis 360.24
   cornea 371.15
   crystalline lens 360.24 [366.34]
   retina 360.24
Chalicosis (occupational) (pulmonum) 502
Chancre (any genital site) (hard) (indurated) (infecting) (primary) (recurrent) 091.0
   congenital 090.0
   conjunctiva 091.2
   Ducrey's 099.0
   extragenital 091.2
   eyelid 091.2
   Hunterian 091.0
   lip (syphilis) 091.2
   mixed 099.8
   nipple 091.2
   Nisbet's 099.0
   of
      carate 103.0
      pinta 103.0
      yaws 102.0
   palate, soft 091.2
   phagedenic 099.0
   Ricord's 091.0
   Rollet's (syphilitic) 091.0

Cellulitis — Chancre

☑ Additional Digit Required   ►◄ Revised Text   ● New Line   ▲ Revised Code

Childhood, period of rapid growth V21.0

Chill(s) 780.99
  with fever 780.6
  congestive 780.99
    in malarial regions 084.6
  septic — see Septicemia
  urethral 599.84

Chilomastigiasis 007.8

Chin — see condition

Chinese dysentery 004.9

Chiropractic dislocation (see also Lesion, nonallopathic, by site) 739.9

Chitral fever 066.0

Chlamydia, chlamydial — see condition

Chloasma 709.09
  cachecticorum 709.09
  eyelid 374.52
    congenital 757.33
    hyperthyroid 242.0 ☑
  gravidarum 646.8 ☑
  idiopathic 709.09
  skin 709.09
  symptomatic 709.09

Chloroma (M9930/3) 205.3 ☑

Chlorosis 280.9
  Egyptian (see also Ancylostomiasis) 126.9
  miners' (see also Ancylostomiasis) 126.9

Chlorotic anemia 280.9

Chocolate cyst (ovary) 617.1

Choked
  disk or disc — see Papilledema
  on food, phlegm, or vomitus NEC (see also Asphyxia, food) 933.1
  phlegm 933.1
  while vomiting NEC (see also Asphyxia, food) 933.1

Chokes (resulting from bends) 993.3

Choking sensation 784.9

Cholangiectasis (see also Disease, gallbladder) 575.8

Cholangiocarcinoma (M8160/3)
  and hepatocellular carcinoma, combined (M8180/3) 155.0
  liver 155.1
  specified site NEC — see Neoplasm, by site, malignant
  unspecified site 155.1

Cholangiohepatitis 575.8
  due to fluke infestation 121.1

Cholangiohepatoma (M8180/3) 155.0

Cholangiolitis (acute) (chronic) (extrahepatic) (gangrenous) 576.1
  intrahepatic 575.8
  paratyphoidal (see also Fever, paratyphoid) 002.9
  typhoidal 002.0

Cholangioma (M8160/0) 211.5
  malignant — see Cholangiocarcinoma

Cholangitis (acute) (ascending) (catarrhal) (chronic) (infective) (malignant) (primary) (recurrent) (sclerosing) (secondary) (stenosing) (suppurative) 576.1
  chronic nonsuppurative destructive 571.6
  nonsuppurative destructive (chronic) 571.6

Cholecystdocholithiasis — see Choledocholithiasis

Cholecystitis 575.10
  with
    calculus, stones in
      bile duct (common) (hepatic) — see Choledocholithiasis
      gallbladder — see Cholelithiasis
  acute 575.0
  acute and chronic 575.12
  chronic 575.11
  emphysematous (acute) (see also Cholecystitis, acute) 575.0
  gangrenous (see also Cholecystitis, acute) 575.0
  paratyphoidal, current (see also Fever, paratyphoid) 002.9

Cholecystitis — continued
  suppurative (see also Cholecystitis, acute) 575.0
  typhoidal 002.0

Choledochitis (suppurative) 576.1

Choledocholith — see Choledocholithiasis

Choledocholithiasis 574.5 ☑

> Note — Use the following fifth-digit subclassification with category 574:
>
> 0   without mention of obstruction
> 1   with obstruction

  with
    cholecystitis 574.4 ☑
      acute 574.3 ☑
      chronic 574.4 ☑
    cholelithiasis 574.9 ☑
      with
        cholecystitis 574.7 ☑
          acute 574.6 ☑
            and chronic 574.8 ☑
          chronic 574.7 ☑

Cholelithiasis (impacted) (multiple) 574.2 ☑

> Note — Use the following fifth-digit subclassification with category 574:
>
> 0   without mention of obstruction
> 1   with obstruction

  with
    cholecystitis 574.1 ☑
      acute 574.0 ☑
      chronic 574.1 ☑
    choledocholithiasis 574.9 ☑
      with
        cholecystitis 574.7 ☑
          acute 574.6 ☑
            and chronic 574.8 ☑
          chronic cholecystitis 574.7 ☑

Cholemia (see also Jaundice) 782.4
  familial 277.4
  Gilbert's (familial nonhemolytic) 277.4

Cholemic gallstone — see Cholelithiasis

Choleperitoneum, choleperitonitis (see also Disease, gallbladder) 567.8

Cholera (algid) (Asiatic) (asphyctic) (epidemic) (gravis) (Indian) (malignant) (morbus) (pestilential) (spasmodic) 001.9
  antimonial 985.4
  carrier (suspected) of V02.0
  classical 001.0
  contact V01.0
  due to
    Vibrio
      cholerae (Inaba, Ogawa, Hikojima serotypes) 001.0
      El Tor 001.1
  El Tor 001.1
  exposure to V01.0
  vaccination, prophylactic (against) V03.0

Cholerine (see also Cholera) 001.9

Cholestasis 576.8

Cholesteatoma (ear) 385.30
  attic (primary) 385.31
  diffuse 385.35
  external ear (canal) 380.21
  marginal (middle ear) 385.32
    with involvement of mastoid cavity 385.33
    secondary (with middle ear involvement) 385.33
  mastoid cavity 385.30
  middle ear (secondary) 385.32
    with involvement of mastoid cavity 385.33
  postmastoidectomy cavity (recurrent) 383.32
  primary 385.31
  recurrent, postmastoidectomy cavity 383.32
  secondary (middle ear) 385.32
    with involvement of mastoid cavity 385.33

Cholesteatosis (middle ear) (see also Cholesteatoma) 385.30
  diffuse 385.35

Cholesteremia 272.0

Cholesterin
  granuloma, middle ear 385.82
  in vitreous 379.22

Cholesterol
  deposit
    retina 362.82
    vitreous 379.22
  imbibition of gallbladder (see also Disease, gallbladder) 575.6

Cholesterolemia 272.0
  essential 272.0
  familial 272.0
  hereditary 272.0

Cholesterosis, cholesterolosis (gallbladder) 575.6
  with
    cholecystitis — see Cholecystitis
    cholelithiasis — see Cholelithiasis
  middle ear (see also Cholesteatoma) 385.30

Cholocolic fistula (see also Fistula, gallbladder) 575.5

Choluria 791.4

Chondritis (purulent) 733.99
  auricle 380.03 ●
  costal 733.6
    Tietze's 733.6
  patella, posttraumatic 717.7
  pinna 380.03 ●
  posttraumatica patellae 717.7
  tuberculous (active) (see also Tuberculosis) 015.9 ☑
    intervertebral 015.0 ☑ [730.88]

Chondroangiopathia calcarea seu punctate 756.59

Chondroblastoma (M9230/0) — see also Neoplasm, bone, benign
  malignant (M9230/3) — see Neoplasm, bone, malignant

Chondrocalcinosis (articular) (crystal deposition) (dihydrate) (see also Arthritis, due to, crystals) 275.49 [712.3] ☑
  due to
    calcium pyrophosphate 275.49 [712.2] ☑
    dicalcium phosphate crystals 275.49 [712.1] ☑
    pyrophosphate crystals 275.49 [712.2] ☑

Chondrodermatitis nodularis helicis 380.00

Chondrodysplasia 756.4
  angiomatose 756.4
  calcificans congenita 756.59
  epiphysialis punctata 756.59
  hereditary deforming 756.4
  rhizomelic punctata 277.86 ●

Chondrodystrophia (fetalis) 756.4
  calcarea 756.4
  calcificans congenita 756.59
  fetalis hypoplastica 756.59
  hypoplastica calcinosa 756.59
  punctata 756.59
  tarda 277.5

Chondrodystrophy (familial) (hypoplastic) 756.4

Chondroectodermal dysplasia 756.55

Chondrolysis 733.99

Chondroma (M9220/0) — see also Neoplasm cartilage, benign
  juxtacortical (M9221/0) — see Neoplasm, bone, benign
  periosteal (M9221/0) — see Neoplasm, bone, benign

Chondromalacia 733.92
  epiglottis (congenital) 748.3
  generalized 733.92
  knee 717.7
  larynx (congenital) 748.3
  localized, except patella 733.92
  patella, patellae 717.7
  systemic 733.92
  tibial plateau 733.92
  trachea (congenital) 748.3

Chondromatosis (M9220/1) — see Neoplasm, cartilage, uncertain behavior

Chondromyxosarcoma (M9220/3) — see Neoplasm, cartilage, malignant

☑ Additional Digit Required   ▶◀ Revised Text   ● New Line   ▲ Revised Code

Chondro-osteodysplasia (Morquio- Brailsford type) 277.5

Chondro-osteodystrophy 277.5

Chondro-osteoma (M9210/0) — *see* Neoplasm, bone, benign

Chondropathia tuberosa 733.6

Chondrosarcoma (M9220/3) — *see also* Neoplasm, cartilage, malignant
  juxtacortical (M9221/3) — *see* Neoplasm, bone, malignant
  mesenchymal (M9240/3) — *see* Neoplasm, connective tissue, malignant

Chordae tendineae rupture (chronic) 429.5

Chordee (nonvenereal) 607.89
  congenital 752.63
  gonococcal 098.2

Chorditis (fibrinous) (nodosa) (tuberosa) 478.5

Chordoma (M9370/3) — *see* Neoplasm, by site, malignant

Chorea (gravis) (minor) (spasmodic) 333.5
  with
    heart involvement — *see* Chorea with rheumatic heart disease
    rheumatic heart disease (chronic, inactive, or quiescent) (conditions classifiable to 393-398) — *see also* Rheumatic heart condition involved
      active or acute (conditions classifiable to 391) 392.0
  acute — *see* Chorea, Sydenham's
  apoplectic (*see also* Disease, cerebrovascular, acute) 436
  chronic 333.4
  electric 049.8
  gravidarum — *see* Eclampsia, pregnancy
  habit 307.22
  hereditary 333.4
  Huntington's 333.4
  posthemiplegic 344.89
  pregnancy — *see* Eclampsia, pregnancy
  progressive 333.4
    chronic 333.4
    hereditary 333.4
  rheumatic (chronic) 392.9
    with heart disease or involvement — *see* Chorea, with rheumatic heart disease
  senile 333.5
  Sydenham's 392.9
    with heart involvement — *see* Chorea, with rheumatic heart disease
      nonrheumatic 333.5
  variabilis 307.23

Choreoathetosis (paroxysmal) 333.5

Chorioadenoma (destruens) (M9100/1) 236.1

Chorioamnionitis 658.4 ☑
  affecting fetus or newborn 762.7

Chorioangioma (M9120/0) 219.8

Choriocarcinoma (M9100/3)
  combined with
    embryonal carcinoma (M9101/3) — *see* Neoplasm, by site, malignant
    teratoma (M9101/3) — *see* Neoplasm, by site, malignant
  specified site — *see* Neoplasm, by site, malignant
  unspecified site
    female 181
    male 186.9

Chorioencephalitis, lymphocytic (acute) (serous) 049.0

Chorioepithelioma (M9100/3) — *see* Choriocarcinoma

Choriomeningitis (acute) (benign) (lymphocytic) (serous) 049.0

Chorionepithelioma (M9100/3) — *see* Choriocarcinoma

Chorionitis (*see also* Scleroderma) 710.1

Chorioretinitis 363.20
  disseminated 363.10
    generalized 363.13
    in
      neurosyphilis 094.83
      secondary syphilis 091.51

Chorioretinitis — *continued*
  disseminated — *continued*
    peripheral 363.12
    posterior pole 363.11
    tuberculous (*see also* Tuberculosis) 017.3 ☑ [363.13]
  due to
    histoplasmosis (*see also* Histoplasmosis) 115.92
    toxoplasmosis (acquired) 130.2
      congenital (active) 771.2
  focal 363.00
    juxtapapillary 363.01
    peripheral 363.04
    posterior pole NEC 363.03
  juxtapapillaris, juxtapapillary 363.01
  progressive myopia (degeneration) 360.21
  syphilitic (secondary) 091.51
    congenital (early) 090.0 [363.13]
      late 090.5 [363.13]
    late 095.8 [363.13]
  tuberculous (*see also* Tuberculosis) 017.3 ☑ [363.13]

Choristoma — *see* Neoplasm, by site, benign

Choroid — *see* condition

Choroideremia, choroidermia (initial stage) (late stage) (partial or total atrophy) 363.55

Choroiditis (*see also* Chorioretinitis) 363.20
  leprous 030.9 [363.13]
  senile guttate 363.41
  sympathetic 360.11
  syphilitic (secondary) 091.51
    congenital (early) 090.0 [363.13]
      late 090.5 [363.13]
    late 095.8 [363.13]
  Tay's 363.41
  tuberculous (*see also* Tuberculosis) 017.3 ☑ [363.13]

Choroidopathy NEC 363.9
  degenerative (*see also* Degeneration, choroid) 363.40
  hereditary (*see also* Dystrophy, choroid) 363.50
  specified type NEC 363.8

Choroidoretinitis — *see* Chorioretinitis

Choroidosis, central serous 362.41

Choroidretinopathy, serous 362.41

Christian's syndrome (chronic histiocytosis X) 277.89

Christian-Weber disease (nodular nonsuppurative panniculitis) 729.30

Christmas disease 286.1

Chromaffinoma (M8700/0) — *see also* Neoplasm, by site, benign
  malignant (M8700/3) — *see* Neoplasm, by site, malignant

Chromatopsia 368.59

Chromhidrosis, chromidrosis 705.89

Chromoblastomycosis 117.2

Chromomycosis 117.2

Chromophytosis 111.0

Chromotrichomycosis 111.8

Chronic — *see* condition

Churg-Strauss syndrome 446.4

Chyle cyst, mesentery 457.8

Chylocele (nonfilarial) 457.8
  filarial (*see also* Infestation, filarial) 125.9
  tunica vaginalis (nonfilarial) 608.84
    filarial (*see also* Infestation, filarial) 125.9

Chylomicronemia (fasting) (with hyperprebetalipoproteinemia) 272.3

Chylopericardium (acute) 420.90

Chylothorax (nonfilarial) 457.8
  filarial (*see also* Infestation, filarial) 125.9

Chylous
  ascites 457.8
  cyst of peritoneum 457.8
  hydrocele 603.9
  hydrothorax (nonfilarial) 457.8
    filarial (*see also* Infestation, filarial) 125.9

Chyluria 791.1
  bilharziasis 120.0

Chyluria — *continued*
  due to
    Brugia (malayi) 125.1
    Wuchereria (bancrofti) 125.0
      malayi 125.1
  filarial (*see also* Infestation, filarial) 125.9
  filariasis (*see also* Infestation, filarial) 125.9
  nonfilarial 791.1

Cicatricial (deformity) — *see* Cicatrix

Cicatrix (adherent) (contracted) (painful) (vicious) 709.2
  adenoid 474.8
  alveolar process 525.8
  anus 569.49
  auricle 380.89
  bile duct (*see also* Disease, biliary) 576.8
  bladder 596.8
  bone 733.99
  brain 348.8
  cervix (postoperative) (postpartal) 622.3
    in pregnancy or childbirth 654.6 ☑
      causing obstructed labor 660.2 ☑
  chorioretinal 363.30
    disseminated 363.35
    macular 363.32
    peripheral 363.34
    posterior pole NEC 363.33
  choroid — *see* Cicatrix, chorioretinal
  common duct (*see also* Disease, biliary) 576.8
  congenital 757.39
  conjunctiva 372.64
  cornea 371.00
    tuberculous (*see also* Tuberculosis) 017.3 ☑ [371.05]
  duodenum (bulb) 537.3
  esophagus 530.3
  eyelid 374.46
    with
      ectropion — *see* Ectropion
      entropion — *see* Entropion
  hypopharynx 478.29
  knee, semilunar cartilage 717.5
  lacrimal
    canaliculi 375.53
    duct
      acquired 375.56
      neonatal 375.55
    punctum 375.52
    sac 375.54
  larynx 478.79
  limbus (cystoid) 372.64
  lung 518.89
  macular 363.32
    disseminated 363.35
    peripheral 363.34
  middle ear 385.89
  mouth 528.9
  muscle 728.89
  nasolacrimal duct
    acquired 375.56
    neonatal 375.55
  nasopharynx 478.29
  palate (soft) 528.9
  penis 607.89
  prostate 602.8
  rectum 569.49
  retina 363.30
    disseminated 363.35
    macular 363.32
    peripheral 363.34
    posterior pole NEC 363.33
  semilunar cartilage — *see* Derangement, meniscus
  seminal vesicle 608.89
  skin 709.2
    infected 686.8
    postinfectional 709.2
    tuberculous (*see also* Tuberculosis) 017.0 ☑
  specified site NEC 709.2
  throat 478.29
  tongue 529.8
  tonsil (and adenoid) 474.8
  trachea 478.9
  tuberculous NEC (*see also* Tuberculosis) 011.9 ☑
  ureter 593.89

Cicatrix — continued
urethra 599.84
uterus 621.8
vagina 623.4
in pregnancy or childbirth 654.7 ☑
causing obstructed labor 660.2 ☑
vocal cord 478.5
wrist, constricting (annular) 709.2
CIN I [cervical intraepithelial neoplasia I]
622.11 ▲
CIN II [cervical intraepithelial neoplasia II]
622.12 ▲
CIN III [cervical intraepithelial neoplasia III] 233.1
Cinchonism
correct substance properly administered 386.9
overdose or wrong substance given or taken
961.4
Circine herpes 110.5
Circle of Willis — see condition
Circular — see also condition
hymen 752.49
Circulating anticoagulants 286.5
following childbirth 666.3 ☑
postpartum 666.3 ☑
Circulation
collateral (venous), any site 459.89
defective 459.9
congenital 747.9
lower extremity 459.89
embryonic 747.9
failure 799.89
fetus or newborn 779.89
peripheral 785.59
fetal, persistent 747.83
heart, incomplete 747.9
Circulatory system — see condition
Circulus senilis 371.41
Circumcision
in absence of medical indication V50.2
ritual V50.2
routine V50.2
Circumscribed — see condition
Circumvallata placenta — see Placenta,
abnormal
Cirrhosis, cirrhotic 571.5
with alcoholism 571.2
alcoholic (liver) 571.2
atrophic (of liver) — see Cirrhosis, portal
Baumgarten-Cruveilhier 571.5
biliary (cholangiolitic) (cholangitic) (cholestatic)
(extrahepatic) (hypertrophic)
(intrahepatic) (nonobstructive)
(obstructive) (pericholangiolitic)
(posthepatic) (primary) (secondary)
(xanthomatous) 571.6
due to
clonorchiasis 121.1
flukes 121.3
brain 331.9
capsular — see Cirrhosis, portal
cardiac 571.5
alcoholic 571.2
central (liver) — see Cirrhosis, liver
Charcôt's 571.6
cholangiolitic — see Cirrhosis, biliary
cholangitic — see Cirrhosis, biliary
cholestatic — see Cirrhosis, biliary
clitoris (hypertrophic) 624.2
coarsely nodular 571.5
congestive (liver) — see Cirrhosis, cardiac
Cruveilhier-Baumgarten 571.5
cryptogenic (of liver) 571.5
alcoholic 571.2
dietary (see also Cirrhosis, portal) 571.5
due to
bronzed diabetes 275.0
congestive hepatomegaly — see Cirrhosis,
cardiac
cystic fibrosis 277.00
hemochromatosis 275.0
hepatolenticular degeneration 275.1
passive congestion (chronic) — see
Cirrhosis, cardiac
Wilson's disease 275.1

Cirrhosis, cirrhotic — continued
due to — continued
xanthomatosis 272.2
extrahepatic (obstructive) — see Cirrhosis,
biliary
fatty 571.8
alcoholic 571.0
florid 571.2
Glisson's — see Cirrhosis, portal
Hanot's (hypertrophic) — see Cirrhosis, biliary
hepatic — see Cirrhosis, liver
hepatolienal — see Cirrhosis, liver
hobnail — see Cirrhosis, portal
hypertrophic — see also Cirrhosis, liver
biliary — see Cirrhosis, biliary
Hanot's — see Cirrhosis, biliary
infectious NEC — see Cirrhosis, portal
insular — see Cirrhosis, portal
intrahepatic (obstructive) (primary) (secondary)
— see Cirrhosis, biliary
juvenile (see also Cirrhosis, portal) 571.5
kidney (see also Sclerosis, renal) 587
Laennec's (of liver) 571.2
nonalcoholic 571.5
liver (chronic) (hepatolienal) (hypertrophic)
(nodular) (splenomegalic) (unilobar) 571.5
with alcoholism 571.2
alcoholic 571.2
congenital (due to failure of obliteration of
umbilical vein) 777.8
cryptogenic 571.5
alcoholic 571.2
fatty 571.8
alcoholic 571.0
macronodular 571.5
alcoholic 571.2
micronodular 571.5
alcoholic 571.2
nodular, diffuse 571.5
alcoholic 571.2
pigmentary 275.0
portal 571.5
alcoholic 571.2
postnecrotic 571.5
alcoholic 571.2
syphilitic 095.3
lung (chronic) (see also Fibrosis, lung) 515
macronodular (of liver) 571.5
alcoholic 571.2
malarial 084.9
metabolic NEC 571.5
micronodular (of liver) 571.5
alcoholic 571.2
monolobular — see Cirrhosis, portal
multilobular — see Cirrhosis, portal
nephritis (see also Sclerosis, renal) 587
nodular — see Cirrhosis, liver
nutritional (fatty) 571.5
obstructive (biliary) (extrahepatic) (intrahepatic)
— see Cirrhosis, biliary
ovarian 620.8
paludal 084.9
pancreas (duct) 577.8
pericholangiolitic — see Cirrhosis, biliary
periportal — see Cirrhosis, portal
pigment, pigmentary (of liver) 275.0
portal (of liver) 571.5
alcoholic 571.2
posthepatitic (see also Cirrhosis, postnecrotic)
571.5
postnecrotic (of liver) 571.5
alcoholic 571.2
primary (intrahepatic) — see Cirrhosis, biliary
pulmonary (see also Fibrosis, lung) 515
renal (see also Sclerosis, renal) 587
septal (see also Cirrhosis, postnecrotic) 571.5
spleen 289.51
splenomegalic (of liver) — see Cirrhosis, liver
stasis (liver) — see Cirrhosis, liver
stomach 535.4 ☑
Todd's (see also Cirrhosis, biliary) 571.6
toxic (nodular) — see Cirrhosis, postnecrotic
trabecular — see Cirrhosis, postnecrotic
unilobar — see Cirrhosis, liver
vascular (of liver) — see Cirrhosis, liver

Cirrhosis, cirrhotic — continued
xanthomatous (biliary) (see also Cirrhosis,
biliary) 571.6
due to xanthomatosis (familial) (metabolic)
(primary) 272.2
Cistern, subarachnoid 793.0
Citrullinemia 270.6
Citrullinuria 270.6
Ciuffini-Pancoast tumor (M8010/3) (carcinoma,
pulmonary apex) 162.3
Civatte's disease or poikiloderma 709.09
Clam diggers' itch 120.3
Clap — see Gonorrhea
Clark's paralysis 343.9
Clarke-Hadfield syndrome (pancreatic
infantilism) 577.8
Clastothrix 704.2
Claude's syndrome 352.6
Claude Bernard-Horner syndrome (see also
Neuropathy, peripheral, autonomic) 337.9
Claudication, intermittent 443.9
cerebral (artery) (see also Ischemia, cerebral,
transient) 435.9
due to atherosclerosis 440.21
spinal cord (arteriosclerotic) 435.1
syphilitic 094.89
spinalis 435.1
venous (axillary) 453.8
Claudicatio venosa intermittens 453.8
Claustrophobia 300.29
Clavus (infected) 700
Clawfoot (congenital) 754.71
acquired 736.74
Clawhand (acquired) 736.06
congenital 755.59
Clawtoe (congenital) 754.71
acquired 735.5
Clay eating 307.52
Clay shovelers' fracture — see Fracture,
vertebra, cervical
Cleansing of artificial opening (see also
Attention to artificial opening) V55.9
Cleft (congenital) — see also Imperfect, closure
alveolar process 525.8
branchial (persistent) 744.41
cyst 744.42
clitoris 752.49
cricoid cartilage, posterior 748.3
facial (see also Cleft, lip) 749.10
lip 749.10
with cleft palate 749.20
bilateral (lip and palate) 749.24
with unilateral lip or palate 749.25
complete 749.23
incomplete 749.24
unilateral (lip and palate) 749.22
with bilateral lip or palate 749.25
complete 749.21
incomplete 749.22
bilateral 749.14
with cleft palate, unilateral 749.25
complete 749.13
incomplete 749.14
unilateral 749.12
with cleft palate, bilateral 749.25
complete 749.11
incomplete 749.12
nose 748.1
palate 749.00
with cleft lip 749.20
bilateral (lip and palate) 749.24
with unilateral lip or palate 749.25
complete 749.23
incomplete 749.24
unilateral (lip and palate) 749.22
with bilateral lip or palate 749.25
complete 749.21
incomplete 749.22
bilateral 749.04
with cleft lip, unilateral 749.25
complete 749.03
incomplete 749.04

☑ Additional Digit Required   ▶◀ Revised Text   ● New Line   ▲ Revised Code

Cleft — *see also* Imperfect, closure — *continued*
  palate — *continued*
    unilateral 749.02
      with cleft lip, bilateral 749.25
      complete 749.01
      incomplete 749.02
    penis 752.69
    posterior, cricoid cartilage 748.3
    scrotum 752.89
    sternum (congenital) 756.3
    thyroid cartilage (congenital) 748.3
    tongue 750.13
    uvula 749.02
      with cleft lip (*see also* Cleft, lip, with cleft
        palate) 749.20
    water 366.12
Cleft hand (congenital) 755.58
Cleidocranial dysostosis 755.59
Cleidotomy, fetal 763.89
Cleptomania 312.32
Clérambault's syndrome 297.8
    erotomania 302.89
Clergyman's sore throat 784.49
Click, clicking
    systolic syndrome 785.2
Clifford's syndrome (postmaturity) 766.22
Climacteric (*see also* Menopause) 627.2
    arthritis NEC (*see also* Arthritis, climacteric)
      716.3 ☑
    depression (*see also* Psychosis, affective)
      296.2 ☑
    disease 627.2
      recurrent episode 296.3 ☑
      single episode 296.2 ☑
    female (symptoms) 627.2
    male (symptoms) (syndrome) 608.89
    melancholia (*see also* Psychosis, affective)
      296.2 ☑
      recurrent episode 296.3 ☑
      single episode 296.2 ☑
    paranoid state 297.2
    paraphrenia 297.2
    polyarthritis NEC 716.39
      male 608.89
    symptoms (female) 627.2
Clinical research investigation (control)
      (participant) V70.7
Clinodactyly 755.59
Clitoris — *see* condition
Cloaca, persistent 751.5
Clonorchiasis 121.1
Clonorchiosis 121.1
Clonorchis infection, liver 121.1
Clonus 781.0
Closed bite 524.20   ▲
**Closed surgical procedure converted to
    open procedure**
    arthroscopic V64.43
    laparoscopic V64.41
    thoracoscopic V64.42
Closure
    artificial opening (*see also* Attention to artificial
      opening) V55.9
    congenital, nose 748.0
    cranial sutures, premature 756.0
    defective or imperfect NEC — *see* Imperfect,
      closure
    fistula, delayed — *see* Fistula
    fontanelle, delayed 756.0
    foramen ovale, imperfect 745.5
    hymen 623.3
    interauricular septum, defective 745.5
    interventricular septum, defective 745.4
    lacrimal duct 375.56
      congenital 743.65
      neonatal 375.55
    nose (congenital) 748.0
      acquired 738.0
    vagina 623.2
    valve — *see* Endocarditis
    vulva 624.8

Clot (blood)
    artery (obstruction) (occlusion) (*see also*
      Embolism) 444.9
    bladder 596.7
    brain (extradural or intradural) (*see also*
      Thrombosis, brain) 434.0 ☑
      late effects — *see* Late effect(s) (of)
        cerebrovascular disease
    circulation 444.9
    heart (*see also* Infarct, myocardium) 410.9 ☑
    vein (*see also* Thrombosis) 453.9
Clotting defect NEC (*see also* Defect, coagulation)
      286.9
Clouded state 780.09
    epileptic (*see also* Epilepsy) 345.9 ☑
    paroxysmal (idiopathic) (*see also* Epilepsy)
      345.9 ☑
Clouding
    corneal graft 996.51
Cloudy
    antrum, antra 473.0
    dialysis effluent 792.5
Clouston's (hidrotic) ectodermal dysplasia
      757.31
Clubbing of fingers 781.5
Clubfinger 736.29
    acquired 736.29
    congenital 754.89
Clubfoot (congenital) 754.70
    acquired 736.71
    equinovarus 754.51
    paralytic 736.71
Club hand (congenital) 754.89
    acquired 736.07
Clubnail (acquired) 703.8
    congenital 757.5
Clump kidney 753.3
Clumsiness 781.3
    syndrome 315.4
Cluttering 307.0
Clutton's joints 090.5
Coagulation, intravascular (diffuse)
      (disseminated) (*see also* Fibrinolysis) 286.6
    newborn 776.2
Coagulopathy (*see also* Defect, coagulation) 286.9
    consumption 286.6
    intravascular (disseminated) NEC 286.6
      newborn 776.2
Coalition
    calcaneoscaphoid 755.67
    calcaneus 755.67
    tarsal 755.67
Coal miners'
    elbow 727.2
    lung 500
Coal workers' lung or pneumoconiosis 500
Coarctation
    aorta (postductal) (preductal) 747.10
    pulmonary artery 747.3
Coated tongue 529.3
Coats' disease 362.12
Cocainism (*see also* Dependence) 304.2 ☑
Coccidioidal granuloma 114.3
Coccidioidomycosis 114.9
    with pneumonia 114.0
    cutaneous (primary) 114.1
    disseminated 114.3
    extrapulmonary (primary) 114.1
    lung 114.5
      acute 114.0
      chronic 114.4
      primary 114.0
    meninges 114.2
    primary (pulmonary) 114.0
      acute 114.0
    prostate 114.3
    pulmonary 114.5
      acute 114.0
      chronic 114.4
      primary 114.0
    specified site NEC 114.3

Coccidioidosis 114.9
    lung 114.5
      acute 114.0
      chronic 114.4
      primary 114.0
    meninges 114.2
Coccidiosis (colitis) (diarrhea) (dysentery) 007.2
Cocciuria 791.9
Coccus in urine 791.9
Coccydynia 724.79
Coccygodynia 724.79
Coccyx — *see* condition
Cochin-China
    diarrhea 579.1
      anguilluliasis 127.2
    ulcer 085.1
Cock's peculiar tumor 706.2
Cockayne's disease or syndrome (microcephaly
      and dwarfism) 759.89
Cockayne-Weber syndrome (epidermolysis
      bullosa) 757.39
Cocked-up toe 735.2
Codman's tumor (benign chondroblastoma)
      (M9230/0) — *see* Neoplasm, bone, benign
Coenurosis 123.8
Coffee workers' lung 495.8
Cogan's syndrome 370.52
    congenital oculomotor apraxia 379.51
    nonsyphilitic interstitial keratitis 370.52
Coiling, umbilical cord — *see* Complications,
      umbilical cord
Coitus, painful (female) 625.0
    male 608.89
    psychogenic 302.76
Cold 460
    with influenza, flu, or grippe 487.1
    abscess — *see also* Tuberculosis, abscess
      articular — *see* Tuberculosis, joint
    agglutinin
      disease (chronic) or syndrome 283.0
        hemoglobinuria 283.0
          paroxysmal (cold) (nocturnal) 283.2
    allergic (*see also* Fever, hay) 477.9
    bronchus or chest — *see* Bronchitis
      with grippe or influenza 487.1
    common (head) 460
      vaccination, prophylactic (against) V04.7
    deep 464.10
    effects of 991.9
      specified effect NEC 991.8
    excessive 991.9
      specified effect NEC 991.8
    exhaustion from 991.8
    exposure to 991.9
      specified effect NEC 991.8
    grippy 487.1
    head 460
    injury syndrome (newborn) 778.2
    intolerance 780.99
    on lung — *see* Bronchitis
    rose 477.0
    sensitivity, autoimmune 283.0
    virus 460
Coldsore (*see also* Herpes, simplex) 054.9
Colibacillosis 041.4
    generalized 038.42
Colibacilluria 791.9
Colic (recurrent) 789.0 ☑
    abdomen 789.0 ☑
      psychogenic 307.89
    appendicular 543.9
    appendix 543.9
    bile duct — *see* Choledocholithiasis
    biliary — *see* Cholelithiasis
    bilious — *see* Cholelithiasis
    common duct — *see* Choledocholithiasis
    Devonshire NEC 984.9
      specified type of lead — *see* Table of Drugs
        and Chemicals
    flatulent 787.3
    gallbladder or gallstone — *see* Cholelithiasis
    gastric 536.8
    hepatic (duct) — *see* Choledocholithiasis

Colic — *continued*
  hysterical 300.11
  infantile 789.0 ☑
  intestinal 789.0 ☑
  kidney 788.0
  lead NEC 984.9
    specified type of lead — *see* Table of Drugs and Chemicals
  liver (duct) — *see* Choledocholithiasis
  mucous 564.9
    psychogenic 316 *[564.9]*
  nephritic 788.0
  painter's NEC 984.9
  pancreas 577.8
  psychogenic 306.4
  renal 788.0
  saturnine NEC 984.9
    specified type of lead — *see* Table of Drugs and Chemicals
  spasmodic 789.0 ☑
  ureter 788.0
  urethral 599.84
    due to calculus 594.2
  uterus 625.8
    menstrual 625.3
  vermicular 543.9
  virus 460
  worm NEC 128.9
Colicystitis (*see also* Cystitis) 595.9
Colitis (acute) (catarrhal) (croupous) (cystica superficialis) (exudative) (hemorrhagic) (noninfectious) (phlegmonous) (presumed noninfectious) 558.9
  adaptive 564.9
  allergic 558.3
  amebic (*see also* Amebiasis) 006.9
    nondysenteric 006.2
  anthrax 022.2
  bacillary (*see also* Infection, Shigella) 004.9
  balantidial 007.0
  chronic 558.9
    ulcerative (*see also* Colitis, ulcerative) 556.9
  coccidial 007.2
  dietetic 558.9
  due to radiation 558.1
  functional 558.9
  gangrenous 009.0
  giardial 007.1
  granulomatous 555.1
  gravis (*see also* Colitis, ulcerative) 556.9
  infectious (*see also* Enteritis, due to, specific organism) 009.0
    presumed 009.1
  ischemic 557.9
    acute 557.0
    chronic 557.1
    due to mesenteric artery insufficiency 557.1
  membranous 564.9
    psychogenic 316 *[564.9]*
  mucous 564.9
    psychogenic 316 *[564.9]*
  necrotic 009.0
  polyposa (*see also* Colitis, ulcerative) 556.9
  protozoal NEC 007.9
  pseudomembranous 008.45
  pseudomucinous 564.9
  regional 555.1
  segmental 555.1
  septic (*see also* Enteritis, due to, specific organism) 009.0
  spastic 564.9
    psychogenic 316 *[564.9]*
  staphylococcus 008.41
    food 005.0
  thromboulcerative 557.0
  toxic 558.2
  transmural 555.1
  trichomonal 007.3
  tuberculous (ulcerative) 014.8 ☑
  ulcerative (chronic) (idiopathic) (nonspecific) 556.9
    entero- 556.0
    fulminant 557.0
    ileo- 556.1
    left-sided 556.5
    procto- 556.2

Colitis — *continued*
  ulcerative — *continued*
    proctosigmoid 556.3
    psychogenic 316 *[556]* ☑
    specified NEC 556.8
    universal 556.6
Collagen disease NEC 710.9
  nonvascular 710.9
  vascular (allergic) (*see also* Angiitis, hypersensitivity) 446.20
Collagenosis (*see also* Collagen disease) 710.9
  cardiovascular 425.4
  mediastinal 519.3
Collapse 780.2
  adrenal 255.8
  cardiorenal (*see also* Hypertension, cardiorenal) 404.90
  cardiorespiratory 785.51
    fetus or newborn 779.89
  cardiovascular (*see also* Disease, heart) 785.51
    fetus or newborn 779.89
  circulatory (peripheral) 785.59
    with
      abortion — *see* Abortion, by type, with shock
      ectopic pregnancy (*see also* categories 633.0-633.9) 639.5
      molar pregnancy (*see also* categories 630-632) 639.5
    during or after labor and delivery 669.1 ☑
    fetus or newborn 779.89
    following
      abortion 639.5
      ectopic or molar pregnancy 639.5
  during or after labor and delivery 669.1 ☑
    fetus or newborn 779.89
  external ear canal 380.50
    secondary to
      inflammation 380.53
      surgery 380.52
      trauma 380.51
  general 780.2
  heart — *see* Disease, heart
  heat 992.1
  hysterical 300.11
  labyrinth, membranous (congenital) 744.05
  lung (massive) (*see also* Atelectasis) 518.0
    pressure, during labor 668.0 ☑
  myocardial — *see* Disease, heart
  nervous (*see also* Disorder, mental, nonpsychotic) 300.9
  neurocirculatory 306.2
  nose 738.0
  postoperative (cardiovascular) 998.0
  pulmonary (see also Atelectasis) 518.0
    fetus or newborn 770.5
      partial 770.5
      primary 770.4
  thorax 512.8
    iatrogenic 512.1
    postoperative 512.1
  trachea 519.1
  valvular — *see* Endocarditis
  vascular (peripheral) 785.59
    with
      abortion — *see* Abortion, by type, with shock
      ectopic pregnancy (*see also* categories 633.0-633.9) 639.5
      molar pregnancy (*see also* categories 630-632) 639.5
    cerebral (*see also* Disease, cerebrovascular, acute) 436
    during or after labor and delivery 669.1 ☑
    fetus or newborn 779.89
    following
      abortion 639.5
      ectopic or molar pregnancy 639.5
  vasomotor 785.59
  vertebra 733.13
Collateral — *see also* condition
  circulation (venous) 459.89
  dilation, veins 459.89
Colles' fracture (closed) (reversed) (separation) 813.41
  open 813.51

Collet's syndrome 352.6
Collet-Sicard syndrome 352.6
Colliculitis urethralis (*see also* Urethritis) 597.89
Colliers'
  asthma 500
  lung 500
  phthisis (*see also* Tuberculosis) 011.4 ☑
Collodion baby (ichthyosis congenita) 757.1
Colloid milium 709.3
Coloboma NEC 743.49
  choroid 743.59
  fundus 743.52
  iris 743.46
  lens 743.36
  lids 743.62
  optic disc (congenital) 743.57
    acquired 377.23
  retina 743.56
  sclera 743.47
Coloenteritis — *see* Enteritis
Colon — *see* condition
Coloptosis 569.89
Color
  amblyopia NEC 368.59
    acquired 368.55
  blindness NEC (congenital) 368.59
    acquired 368.55
Colostomy
  attention to V55.3
  fitting or adjustment V53.5
  malfunctioning 569.62
  status V44.3
Colpitis (*see also* Vaginitis) 616.10
Colpocele 618.6
Colpocystitis (*see also* Vaginitis) 616.10
Colporrhexis 665.4 ☑
Colpospasm 625.1
Column, spinal, vertebral — *see* condition
Coma 780.01
  apoplectic (*see also* Disease, cerebrovascular, acute) 436
  diabetic (with ketoacidosis) 250.3 ☑
    hyperosmolar 250.2 ☑
  eclamptic (*see also* Eclampsia) 780.39
  epileptic 345.3
  hepatic 572.2
  hyperglycemic 250.2 ☑
  hyperosmolar (diabetic) (nonketotic) 250.2 ☑
  hypoglycemic 251.0
    diabetic 250.3 ☑
  insulin 250.3 ☑
    hypersmolar 250.2 ☑
    non-diabetic 251.0
    organic hyperinsulinism 251.0
  Kussmaul's (diabetic) 250.3 ☑
  liver 572.2
  newborn 779.2
  prediabetic 250.2 ☑
  uremic — *see* Uremia
Combat fatigue (*see also* Reaction, stress, acute) 308.9
Combined — *see* condition
Comedo 706.1
Comedocarcinoma (M8501/3) — *see also* Neoplasm, breast, malignant
  noninfiltrating (M8501/2)
    specified site — *see* Neoplasm, by site, in situ
    unspecified site 233.0
Comedomastitis 610.4
Comedones 706.1
  lanugo 757.4
Comma bacillus, carrier (suspected) of V02.3
Comminuted fracture — *see* Fracture, by site
Common
  aortopulmonary trunk 745.0
  atrioventricular canal (defect) 745.69
  atrium 745.69
  cold (head) 460
    vaccination, prophylactic (against) V04.7
  truncus (arteriosus) 745.0
  ventricle 745.3

☑ Additional Digit Required   ▶◀ Revised Text   ● New Line   ▲ Revised Code

Commotio (current)
    cerebri (*see also* Concussion, brain) 850.9
        with skull fracture — *see* Fracture, skull, by
            site
    retinae 921.3
    spinalis — *see* Injury, spinal, by site
Commotion (current)
    brain (without skull fracture) (*see also*
        Concussion, brain) 850.9
        with skull fracture — *see* Fracture, skull, by
            site
    spinal cord — *see* Injury, spinal, by site
Communication
    abnormal — *see also* Fistula
        between
            base of aorta and pulmonary artery 745.0
            left ventricle and right atrium 745.4
            pericardial sac and pleural sac 748.8
            pulmonary artery and pulmonary vein
                747.3
        congenital, between uterus and anterior
            abdominal wall 752.3
            bladder 752.3
            intestine 752.3
            rectum 752.3
        left ventricular— right atrial 745.4
        pulmonary artery— pulmonary vein 747.3
Compensation
    broken — *see* Failure, heart
    failure — *see* Failure, heart
    neurosis, psychoneurosis 300.11
Complaint — *see also* Disease
    bowel, functional 564.9
        psychogenic 306.4
    intestine, functional 564.9
        psychogenic 306.4
    kidney (*see also* Disease, renal) 593.9
    liver 573.9
    miners' 500
Complete — *see* condition
Complex
    cardiorenal (*see also* Hypertension, cardiorenal)
        404.90
    castration 300.9
    Costen's 524.60
    ego-dystonic homosexuality 302.0
    Eisenmenger's (ventricular septal defect) 745.4
    homosexual, ego-dystonic 302.0
    hypersexual 302.89
    inferiority 301.9
    jumped process
        spine — *see* Dislocation, vertebra
    primary, tuberculosis (*see also* Tuberculosis)
        010.0 ☑
    Taussig-Bing (transposition, aorta and
        overriding pulmonary artery) 745.11
Complications
    abortion NEC — *see* categories 634-639
    accidental puncture or laceration during a
        procedure 998.2
    amputation stump (late) (surgical) 997.60
        traumatic — *see* Amputation, traumatic
    anastomosis (and bypass) NEC — *see also*
        Complications, due to (presence of) any
        device, implant, or graft classified to
        996.0-996.5 NEC
        hemorrhage NEC 998.11
        intestinal (internal) NEC 997.4
            involving urinary tract 997.5
        mechanical — *see* Complications,
            mechanical, graft
        urinary tract (involving intestinal tract)
            997.5
    anesthesia, anesthetic NEC (*see also*
        Anesthesia, complication) 995.2
        in labor and delivery 668.9 ☑
            affecting fetus or newborn 763.5
            cardiac 668.1 ☑
            central nervous system 668.2 ☑
            pulmonary 668.0 ☑
            specified type NEC 668.8 ☑
    aortocoronary (bypass) graft 996.03
        atherosclerosis — *see* Arteriosclerosis,
            coronary
        embolism 996.72

Complications — *continued*
    aortocoronary graft — *continued*
        occlusion NEC 996.72
        thrombus 996.72
    arthroplasty 996.4
    artificial opening
        cecostomy 569.60
        colostomy 569.60
        cystostomy 997.5
        enterostomy 569.60
        esophagostomy   ●
            infection 530.86   ●
            mechanical 530.87   ●
        gastrostomy 536.40
        ileostomy 569.60
        jejunostomy 569.60
        nephrostomy 997.5
        tracheostomy 519.00
        ureterostomy 997.5
        urethrostomy 997.5
    bariatric surgery 997.4   ●
    bile duct implant (prosthetic) NEC 996.79
        infection or inflammation 996.69
        mechanical 996.59
    bleeding (intraoperative) (postoperative) 998.11
    blood vessel graft 996.1
        aortocoronary 996.03
            atherosclerosis — *see* Arteriosclerosis,
                coronary
            embolism 996.72
            occlusion NEC 996.72
            thrombus 996.72
        atherosclerosis — *see* Arteriosclerosis,
            extremities
        embolism 996.74
        occlusion NEC 996.74
        thrombus 996.74
    bone growth stimulator 996.78
        infection or inflammation 996.67
    bone marrow transplant 996.85
    breast implant (prosthetic) NEC 996.79
        infection or inflammation 996.69
        mechanical 996.54
    bypass — *see also* Complications, anastomosis
        aortocoronary 996.03
            atherosclerosis — *see* Arteriosclerosis,
                coronary
            embolism 996.72
            occlusion NEC 996.72
            thrombus 996.72
        carotid artery 996.1
            atherosclerosis — *see* Arteriosclerosis,
                extremities
            embolism 996.74
            occlusion NEC 996.74
            thrombus 996.74
    cardiac (*see also* Disease, heart) 429.9
        device, implant, or graft NEC 996.72
            infection or inflammation 996.61
            long-term effect 429.4
            mechanical (*see also* Complications,
                mechanical, by type) 996.00
            valve prosthesis 996.71
                infection or inflammation 996.61
        postoperative NEC 997.1
            long-term effect 429.4
    cardiorenal (*see also* Hypertension, cardiorenal)
        404.90
    carotid artery bypass graft 996.1
        atherosclerosis — *see* Arteriosclerosis,
            extremities
        embolism 996.74
        occlusion NEC 996.74
        thrombus 996.74
    cataract fragments in eye 998.82
    catheter device NEC — *see also* Complications,
        due to (presence of) any device, implant,
        or graft classified to 996.0-996.5 NEC
        mechanical — *see* Complications,
            mechanical, catheter
    cecostomy 569.60
    cesarean section wound 674.3 ☑
    chin implant (prosthetic) NEC 996.79
        infection or inflammation 996.69
        mechanical 996.59
    colostomy (enterostomy) 569.60
        specified type NEC 569.69

Complications — *continued*
    contraceptive device, intrauterine NEC 996.76
        infection 996.65
        inflammation 996.65
        mechanical 996.32
    cord (umbilical) — *see* Complications, umbilical
        cord
    cornea
        due to
            contact lens 371.82
    coronary (artery) bypass (graft) NEC 996.03
        atherosclerosis — *see* Arterio-sclerosis,
            coronary
        embolism 996.72
        infection or inflammation 996.61
        mechanical 996.03
        occlusion NEC 996.72
        specified type NEC 996.72
        thrombus 996.72
    cystostomy 997.5
    delivery 669.9 ☑
        procedure (instrumental) (manual) (surgical)
            669.4 ☑
        specified type NEC 669.8 ☑
    dialysis (hemodialysis) (peritoneal) (renal) NEC
        999.9
        catheter NEC — *see also* Complications, due
            to (presence of) any device, implant or
            graft classified to 996.0-996.5 NEC
        infection or inflammation 996.62
            peritoneal 996.68
        mechanical 996.1
            peritoneal 996.56
    due to (presence of) any device, implant, or
        graft classified to 996.0-996.5 NEC
        996.70
        with infection or inflammation — *see*
            Complications, infection or
            inflammation, due to (presence of) any
            device, implant, or graft classified to
            996.0-996.5 NEC
        arterial NEC 996.74
            coronary NEC 996.03
                atherosclerosis — *see* Arteriosclerosis,
                    coronary
                embolism 996.72
                occlusion NEC 996.72
                specified type NEC 996.72
                thrombus 996.72
            renal dialysis 996.73
        arteriovenous fistula or shunt NEC 996.74
        bone growth stimulator 996.78
        breast 996.70
        cardiac NEC 996.72
            defibrillator 996.72
            pacemaker 996.72
            valve prosthesis 996.71
        catheter NEC 996.79
            spinal 996.75
            urinary, indwelling 996.76
            vascular NEC 996.74
                renal dialysis 996.73
            ventricular shunt 996.75
        coronary (artery) bypass (graft) NEC 996.03
            atherosclerosis — *see* Arteriosclerosis,
                coronary
            embolism 996.72
            occlusion NEC 996.72
            thrombus 996.72
        electrodes
            brain 996.75
            heart 996.72
        gastrointestinal NEC 996.79
        genitourinary NEC 996.76
        heart valve prosthesis NEC 996.71
        infusion pump 996.74
        insulin pump 996.57
        internal
            joint prosthesis 996.77
            orthopedic NEC 996.78
            specified type NEC 996.79
        intrauterine contraceptive device NEC
            996.76
        joint prosthesis, internal NEC 996.77
        mechanical — *see* Complications,
            mechanical
        nervous system NEC 996.75

Commotio — Complications

☑ Additional Digit Required   ▶◀ Revised Text   ● New Line   ▲ Revised Code

Complications — *continued*
due to (presence of) any device, implant, or
graft classified to 996.0-996.5 —
continued
  ocular lens NEC 996.79
  orbital NEC 996.79
  orthopedic NEC 996.78
    joint, internal 996.77
  renal dialysis 996.73
  specified type NEC 996.79
  urinary catheter, indwelling 996.76
  vascular NEC 996.74
  ventricular shunt 996.75
during dialysis NEC 999.9
ectopic or molar pregnancy NEC 639.9
electroshock therapy NEC 999.9
enterostomy 569.60
  specified type NEC 569.69
esophagostomy
  infection 530.86   ●
  mechanical 530.87   ●
external (fixation) device with internal
component(s) NEC 996.78
  infection or inflammation 996.67
  mechanical 996.4
extracorporeal circulation NEC 999.9
eye implant (prosthetic) NEC 996.79
  infection or inflammation 996.69
  mechanical
    ocular lens 996.53
    orbital globe 996.59
gastrointestinal, postoperative NEC (*see also*
Complications, surgical procedures)
997.4
gastrostomy 536.40
  specified type NEC 536.49
genitourinary device, implant or graft NEC
996.76
  infection or inflammation 996.65
    urinary catheter, indwelling 996.64
  mechanical (*see also* Complications,
    mechanical, by type) 996.30
  specified NEC 996.39
graft (bypass) (patch) NEC — *see also*
Complications, due to (presence of) any
device, implant, or graft classified to
996.0-996.5 NEC
  bone marrow 996.85
  corneal NEC 996.79
    infection or inflammation 996.69
    rejection or reaction 996.51
  mechanical — *see* Complications,
    mechanical, graft
  organ (immune or nonimmune cause)
    (partial) (total) 996.80
    bone marrow 996.85
    heart 996.83
    intestines 996.87
    kidney 996.81
    liver 996.82
    lung 996.84
    pancreas 996.86
    specified NEC 996.89
  skin NEC 996.79
    infection or inflammation 996.69
    rejection 996.52
      artificial 996.55
      decellularized allodermis 996.55
heart — *see also* Disease, heart transplant
(immune or nonimmune cause) 996.83
hematoma (intraoperative) (postoperative)
998.12
hemorrhage (intraoperative) (postoperative)
998.11
hyperalimentation therapy NEC 999.9
immunization (procedure) — *see*
Complications, vaccination
implant — *see also* Complications, due to
(presence of) any device, implant, or graft
classified to 996.0-996.5 NEC
  mechanical — *see* Complications,
    mechanical, implant

Complications — *continued*
infection and inflammation
  due to (presence of) any device, implant or
graft classified to 996.0-996.5 NEC
996.60
  arterial NEC 996.62
    coronary 996.61
    renal dialysis 996.62
  arteriovenous fistula or shunt 996.62
  artificial heart 996.61
  bone growth stimulator 996.67
  breast 996.69
  cardiac 996.61
  catheter NEC 996.69
    peritoneal 996.68
    spinal 996.63
    urinary, indwelling 996.64
    vascular NEC 996.62
    ventricular shunt 996.63
  coronary artery bypass 996.61
  electrodes
    brain 996.63
    heart 996.61
  gastrointestinal NEC 996.69
  genitourinary NEC 996.65
    indwelling urinary catheter 996.64
  heart assist device 996.61
  heart valve 996.61
  infusion pump 996.62
  insulin pump 996.69
  intrauterine contraceptive device 996.65
  joint prosthesis, internal 996.66
  ocular lens 996.69
  orbital (implant) 996.69
  orthopedic NEC 996.67
    joint, internal 996.66
  specified type NEC 996.69
  urinary catheter, indwelling 996.64
  ventricular shunt 996.63
infusion (procedure) 999.9
  blood — *see* Complications, transfusion
  infection NEC 999.3
  sepsis NEC 999.3
inhalation therapy NEC 999.9
injection (procedure) 999.9
  drug reaction (*see also* Reaction, drug) 995.2
  infection NEC 999.3
  sepsis NEC 999.3
  serum (prophylactic) (therapeutic) — *see*
    Complications, vaccination
  vaccine (any) — *see* Complications,
    vaccination
inoculation (any) — *see* Complications,
vaccination
insulin pump 996.57
internal device (catheter) (electronic) (fixation)
(prosthetic) NEC — *see also*
Complications, due to (presence of) any
device, implant, or graft classified to
996.0-996.5 NEC
  mechanical — *see* Complications,
    mechanical
intestinal transplant (immune or nonimmune
cause) 996.87
intraoperative bleeding or hemorrhage 998.11
intrauterine contraceptive device 996.76 — *see*
also Complications, contraceptive device
  with fetal damage affecting management of
    pregnancy 655.8 ☑
  infection or inflammation 996.65
jejunostomy 569.60
kidney transplant (immune or nonimmune
cause) 996.81
labor 669.9 ☑
  specified condition NEC 669.8 ☑
liver transplant (immune or nonimmune cause)
996.82
lumbar puncture 349.0
mechanical
  anastomosis — *see* Complications,
    mechanical, graft
  artificial heart 996.09   ▲
  bypass — *see* Complications, mechanical,
    graft
  catheter NEC 996.59
    cardiac 996.09
    cystostomy 996.39

Complications — *continued*
mechanical — *continued*
  catheter NEC — *continued*
    dialysis (hemodialysis) 996.1
      peritoneal 996.56
    during a procedure 998.2
    urethral, indwelling 996.31
  colostomy 569.62
  device NEC 996.59
    balloon (counterpulsation), intra-aortic
      996.1
    cardiac 996.00
      automatic implantable defibrillator
        996.04
      long-term effect 429.4
      specified NEC 996.09
    contraceptive, intrauterine 996.32
    counterpulsation, intra-aortic 996.1
    fixation, external, with internal
      components 996.4
    fixation, internal (nail, rod, plate) 996.4
    genitourinary 996.30
      specified NEC 996.39
    insulin pump 996.57
    nervous system 996.2
    orthopedic, internal 996.4
    prosthetic NEC 996.59
    umbrella, vena cava 996.1
    vascular 996.1
  dorsal column stimulator 996.2
  electrode NEC 996.59
    brain 996.2
    cardiac 996.01
    spinal column 996.2
  enterostomy 569.62
  esophagostomy 530.87   ▲
  fistula, arteriovenous, surgically created
    996.1
  gastrostomy 536.42
  graft NEC 996.52
    aortic (bifurcation) 996.1
    aortocoronary bypass 996.03
    blood vessel NEC 996.1
    bone 996.4
    cardiac 996.00
    carotid artery bypass 996.1
    cartilage 996.4
    corneal 996.51
    coronary bypass 996.03
    decellularized allodermis 996.55
    genitourinary 996.30
      specified NEC 996.39
    muscle 996.4
    nervous system 996.2
    organ (immune or nonimmune cause)
      996.80
      heart 996.83
      intestines 996.87
      kidney 996.81
      liver 996.82
      lung 996.84
      pancreas 996.86
      specified NEC 996.89
    orthopedic, internal 996.4
    peripheral nerve 996.2
    prosthetic NEC 996.59
    skin 996.52
      artificial 996.55
    specified NEC 996.59
    tendon 996.4
    tissue NEC 996.52
    tooth 996.59
    ureter, without mention of resection
      996.39
    vascular 996.1
  heart valve prosthesis 996.02
    long-term effect 429.4
  implant NEC 996.59
    cardiac 996.00
      automatic implantable defibrillator
        996.04
      long-term effect 429.4
      specified NEC 996.09
    electrode NEC 996.59
      brain 996.2
      cardiac 996.01
      spinal column 996.2

Complications — *continued*
  mechanical — *continued*
    implant NEC — *continued*
      genitourinary 996.30
      nervous system 996.2
      orthopedic, internal 996.4
      prosthetic NEC 996.59
        in
          bile duct 996.59
          breast 996.54
          chin 996.59
          eye
            ocular lens 996.53
            orbital globe 996.59
        vascular 996.1
      insulin pump 996.57
      nonabsorbable surgical material 996.59
      pacemaker NEC 996.59
        brain 996.2
        cardiac 996.01
        nerve (phrenic) 996.2
      patch — *see* Complications, mechanical,
        graft
      prosthesis NEC 996.59
        bile duct 996.59
        breast 996.54
        chin 996.59
        ocular lens 996.53
        reconstruction, vas deferens 996.39
      reimplant NEC 996.59
        extremity (*see also* Complications,
          reattached, extremity) 996.90
        organ (*see also* Complications,
          transplant, organ, by site) 996.80
      repair — *see* Complications, mechanical,
        graft
      shunt NEC 996.59
        arteriovenous, surgically created 996.1
        ventricular (communicating) 996.2
      stent NEC 996.59
      tracheostomy 519.02
      vas deferens reconstruction 996.39
  medical care NEC 999.9
    cardiac NEC 997.1
    gastrointestinal NEC 997.4
    nervous system NEC 997.00
    peripheral vascular NEC 997.2
    respiratory NEC 997.3
    urinary NEC 997.5
    vascular
      mesenteric artery 997.71
      other vessels 997.79
      peripheral vessels 997.2
      renal artery 997.72
  nephrostomy 997.5
  nervous system
    device, implant, or graft NEC 349.1
      mechanical 996.2
    postoperative NEC 997.00
  obstetric 669.9 ☑
    procedure (instrumental) (manual) (surgical)
      669.4 ☑
    specified NEC 669.8 ☑
    surgical wound 674.3 ☑
  ocular lens implant NEC 996.79
    infection or inflammation 996.69
    mechanical 996.53
  organ transplant — *see* Complications,
    transplant, organ, by site
  orthopedic device, implant, or graft
    internal (fixation) (nail) (plate) (rod) NEC
      996.78
      infection or inflammation 996.67
      joint prosthesis 996.77
        infection or inflammation 996.66
      mechanical 996.4
  pacemaker (cardiac) 996.72
    infection or inflammation 996.61
    mechanical 996.01
  pancreas transplant (immune or nonimmune
    cause) 996.86
  perfusion NEC 999.9
  perineal repair (obstetrical) 674.3 ☑
    disruption 674.2 ☑
  pessary (uterus) (vagina) — *see* Complications,
    contraceptive device
  phototherapy 990

Complications — *continued*
  postcystoscopic 997.5
  postmastoidectomy NEC 383.30
  postoperative — *see* Complications, surgical
    procedures
  pregnancy NEC 646.9 ☑
    affecting fetus or newborn 761.9
  prosthetic device, internal NEC — *see also*
    Complications, due to (presence of) any
    device, implant or graft classified to
    996.0-996.5 NEC
    mechanical NEC (*see also* Complications,
      mechanical) 996.59
  puerperium NEC (*see also* Puerperal) 674.9 ☑
  puncture, spinal 349.0
  pyelogram 997.5
  radiation 990
  radiotherapy 990
  reattached
    body part, except extremity 996.99
    extremity (infection) (rejection) 996.90
      arm(s) 996.94
      digit(s) (hand) 996.93
        foot 996.95
      finger(s) 996.93
      foot 996.95
      forearm 996.91
      hand 996.92
      leg 996.96
      lower NEC 996.96
      toe(s) 996.95
      upper NEC 996.94
  reimplant NEC — *see also* Complications, to
    (presence of) any device, implant, or graft
    classified to 996.0-996.5 NEC
    bone marrow 996.85
    extremity (*see also* Complications,
      reattached, extremity) 996.90
      due to infection 996.90
    mechanical — *see* Complications,
      mechanical, reimplant
    organ (immune or nonimmune cause)
      (partial) (total) (*see also* Complications,
      transplant, organ, by site) 996.80
  renal allograft 996.81
  renal dialysis — *see* Complications, dialysis
  respiratory 519.9
    device, implant or graft NEC 996.79
      infection or inflammation 996.69
      mechanical 996.59
    distress syndrome, adult, following trauma
      or surgery 518.5
    insufficiency, acute, postoperative 518.5
    postoperative NEC 997.3
    therapy NEC 999.9
  sedation during labor and delivery 668.9 ☑
    affecting fetus or newborn 763.5
    cardiac 668.1 ☑
    central nervous system 668.2 ☑
    pulmonary 668.0 ☑
    specified type NEC 668.8 ☑
  seroma (intraoperative) (postoperative)
    (noninfected) 998.13
    infected 998.51
  shunt NEC — *see also* Complications, due to
    (presence of) any device, implant, or graft
    classified to 996.0-996.5 NEC
    mechanical — *see* Complications,
      mechanical, shunt
  specified body system NEC
    device, implant, or graft NEC — *see*
      Complications, due to (presence of)
      any device, implant, or graft classified
      to 996.0-996.5 NEC
    postoperative NEC 997.99
  spinal puncture or tap 349.0
  stoma, external
    gastrointestinal tract
      colostomy 569.60
      enterostomy 569.60
      esophagostomy   ●
        infection 530.86   ●
        mechanical 530.87   ●
      gastrostomy 536.40
    urinary tract 997.5
  stomach banding 997.4   ●
  stomach stapling 997.4   ●

Complications — *continued*
  surgical procedures 998.9
    accidental puncture or laceration 998.2
    amputation stump (late) 997.60
    anastomosis — *see* Complications,
      anastomosis
    burst stitches or sutures (external) 998.32
      internal 998.31
    cardiac 997.1
      long-term effect following cardiac surgery
        429.4
    cataract fragments in eye 998.82
    catheter device — *see* Complications,
      catheter device
    cecostomy malfunction 569.62
    colostomy malfunction 569.62
    cystostomy malfunction 997.5
    dehiscence (of incision) (external) 998.32
      internal 998.31
    dialysis NEC (*see also* Complications,
      dialysis) 999.9
    disruption
      anastomosis (internal) — *see*
        Complications, mechanical, graft
      internal suture (line) 998.31
      wound (external) 998.32
        internal 998.31
    dumping syndrome (postgastrectomy) 564.2
    elephantiasis or lymphedema 997.99
      postmastectomy 457.0
    emphysema (surgical) 998.81
    enterostomy malfunction 569.62
    esophagostomy malfunction 530.87   ●
    evisceration 998.32
    fistula (persistent postoperative) 998.6
    foreign body inadvertently left in wound
      (sponge) (suture) (swab) 998.4
    from nonabsorbable surgical material
      (Dacron) (mesh) (permanent suture)
      (reinforcing) (Teflon) — *see*
      Complications, due to (presence of)
      any device, implant, or graft classified
      to 996.0-996.5 NEC
    gastrointestinal NEC 997.4
    gastrostomy malfunction 536.42
    hematoma 998.12
    hemorrhage 998.11
    ileostomy malfunction 569.62
    internal prosthetic device NEC (*see also*
      Complications, internal device) 996.70
      hemolytic anemia 283.19
      infection or inflammation 996.60
      malfunction — *see* Complications,
        mechanical
      mechanical complication — *see*
        Complications, mechanical
      thrombus 996.70
    jejunostomy malfunction 569.62
    nervous system NEC 997.00
    obstruction, internal anastomosis — *see*
      Complications, mechanical, graft
    other body system NEC 997.99
    peripheral vascular NEC 997.2
    postcardiotomy syndrome 429.4
    postcholecystectomy syndrome 576.0
    postcommissurotomy syndrome 429.4
    postgastrectomy dumping syndrome 564.2
    postmastectomy lymphedema syndrome
      457.0
    postmastoidectomy 383.30
      cholesteatoma, recurrent 383.32
      cyst, mucosal 383.31
      granulation 383.33
      inflammation, chronic 383.33
    postvagotomy syndrome 564.2
    postvalvulotomy syndrome 429.4
    reattached extremity (infection) (rejection)
      (*see also* Complications, reattached,
      extremity) 996.90
    respiratory NEC 997.3
    seroma 998.13
    shock (endotoxic) (hypovolemic) (septic)
      998.0

Complications — *continued*
  surgical procedures — *continued*
    shunt, prosthetic (thrombus) — *see also*
        Complications, due to (presence of)
        any device, implant, or graft classified
        to 996.0-996.5 NEC
      hemolytic anemia 283.19
    specified complication NEC 998.89
    stitch abscess 998.59
    transplant — *see* Complications, graft
    ureterostomy malfunction 997.5
    urethrostomy malfunction 997.5
    urinary NEC 997.5
    vascular
      mesenteric artery 997.71
      other vessels 997.79
      peripheral vessels 997.2
      renal artery 997.72
    wound infection 998.59
  therapeutic misadventure NEC 999.9
    surgical treatment 998.9
  tracheostomy 519.00
  transfusion (blood) (lymphocytes) (plasma) NEC
      999.8
    atrophy, liver, yellow, subacute (within 8
        months of administration) — *see*
        Hepatitis, viral
    bone marrow 996.85
    embolism
      air 999.1
      thrombus 999.2
    hemolysis NEC 999.8
      bone marrow 996.85
    hepatitis (serum) (type B) (within 8 months
        after administration) — *see* Hepatitis,
        viral
    incompatibility reaction (ABO) (blood group)
        999.6
      Rh (factor) 999.7
    infection 999.3
    jaundice (serum) (within 8 months after
        administration) — *see* Hepatitis, viral
    sepsis 999.3
    shock or reaction NEC 999.8
      bone marrow 996.85
    subacute yellow atrophy of liver (within 8
        months after administration) — *see*
        Hepatitis, viral
    thromboembolism 999.2
  transplant NEC — *see also* Complications, due
      to (presence of) any device, implant, or
      graft classified to 996.0-996.5 NEC
    bone marrow 996.85
    organ (immune or nonimmune cause)
        (partial) (total) 996.80
      bone marrow 996.85
      heart 996.83
      intestines 996.87
      kidney 996.81
      liver 996.82
      lung 996.84
      pancreas 996.86
      specified NEC 996.89
  trauma NEC (early) 958.8
  ultrasound therapy NEC 999.9
  umbilical cord
    affecting fetus or newborn 762.6
    complicating delivery 663.9 ☑
      affecting fetus or newborn 762.6
      specified type NEC 663.8 ☑
  urethral catheter NEC 996.76
    infection or inflammation 996.64
    mechanical 996.31
  urinary, postoperative NEC 997.5
  vaccination 999.9
    anaphylaxis NEC 999.4
    cellulitis 999.3
    encephalitis or encephalomyelitis 323.5
    hepatitis (serum) (type B) (within 8 months
        after administration) — *see* Hepatitis,
        viral
    infection (general) (local) NEC 999.3
    jaundice (serum) (within 8 months after
        administration) — *see* Hepatitis, viral
    meningitis 997.09 *[321.8]*
    myelitis 323.5
    protein sickness 999.5

Complications — *continued*
  vaccination — *continued*
    reaction (allergic) 999.5
      Herxheimer's 995.0
      serum 999.5
    sepsis 999.3
    serum intoxication, sickness, rash, or other
        serum reaction NEC 999.5
    shock (allergic) (anaphylactic) 999.4
    subacute yellow atrophy of liver (within 8
        months after administration) — *see*
        Hepatitis, viral
    vaccinia (generalized) 999.0
      localized 999.3
  vascular
    device, implant, or graft NEC 996.74
      infection or inflammation 996.62
      mechanical NEC 996.1
        cardiac (*see also* Complications,
            mechanical, by type) 996.00
    following infusion, perfusion, or transfusion
        999.2
    postoperative NEC 997.2
      mesenteric artery 997.71
      other vessels 997.79
      peripheral vessels 997.2
      renal artery 997.72
  ventilation therapy NEC 999.9

Compound presentation, complicating delivery
    652.8 ☑
  causing obstructed labor 660.0 ☑

Compressed air disease 993.3

Compression
  with injury — *see* specific injury
  arm NEC 354.9
  artery 447.1
    celiac, syndrome 447.4
  brachial plexus 353.0
  brain (stem) 348.4
    due to
      contusion, brain — *see* Contusion, brain
      injury NEC — *see also* Hemorrhage,
          brain, traumatic
        birth — *see* Birth, injury, brain
      laceration, brain — *see* Laceration, brain
    osteopathic 739.0
  bronchus 519.1
  by cicatrix — *see* Cicatrix
  cardiac 423.9
  cauda equina 344.60
    with neurogenic bladder 344.61
  celiac (artery) (axis) 447.4
  cerebral — *see* Compression, brain
  cervical plexus 353.2
  cord (umbilical) — *see* Compression, umbilical
      cord
  cranial nerve 352.9
    second 377.49
    third (partial) 378.51
      total 378.52
    fourth 378.53
    fifth 350.8
    sixth 378.54
    seventh 351.8
  divers' squeeze 993.3
  duodenum (external) (*see also* Obstruction,
      duodenum) 537.3
  during birth 767.9
  esophagus 530.3
    congenital, external 750.3
  Eustachian tube 381.63
  facies (congenital) 754.0
  fracture — *see* Fracture, by site
  heart — *see* Disease, heart
  intestine (*see also* Obstruction, intestine) 560.9
    with hernia — *see* Hernia, by site, with
        obstruction
  laryngeal nerve, recurrent 478.79
  leg NEC 355.8
  lower extremity NEC 355.8
  lumbosacral plexus 353.1
  lung 518.89
  lymphatic vessel 457.1
  medulla — *see* Compression, brain
  nerve NEC — *see also* Disorder, nerve
    arm NEC 354.9

Compression — *continued*
  nerve NEC — *see also* Disorder, nerve —
      continued
    autonomic nervous system (*see also*
        Neuropathy, peripheral, autonomic)
        337.9
    axillary 353.0
    cranial NEC 352.9
    due to displacement of intervertebral disc
        722.2
      with myelopathy 722.70
      cervical 722.0
        with myelopathy 722.71
      lumbar, lumbosacral 722.10
        with myelopathy 722.73
      thoracic, thoracolumbar 722.11
        with myelopathy 722.72
    iliohypogastric 355.79
    ilioinguinal 355.79
    leg NEC 355.8
    lower extremity NEC 355.8
    median (in carpal tunnel) 354.0
    obturator 355.79
    optic 377.49
    plantar 355.6
    posterior tibial (in tarsal tunnel) 355.5
    root (by scar tissue) NEC 724.9
      cervical NEC 723.4
      lumbar NEC 724.4
      lumbosacral 724.4
      thoracic 724.4
    saphenous 355.79
    sciatic (acute) 355.0
    sympathetic 337.9
    traumatic — *see* Injury, nerve
    ulnar 354.2
    upper extremity NEC 354.9
  peripheral — *see* Compression, nerve
  spinal (cord) (old or nontraumatic) 336.9
    by displacement of intervertebral disc — *see*
        Displacement, intervertebral disc
    nerve
      root NEC 724.9
        postoperative 722.80
          cervical region 722.81
          lumbar region 722.83
          thoracic region 722.82
        traumatic — *see* Injury, nerve, spinal
      traumatic — *see* Injury, nerve, spinal
    spondylogenic 721.91
      cervical 721.1
      lumbar, lumbosacral 721.42
      thoracic 721.41
    traumatic — *see also* Injury, spinal, by site
      with fracture, vertebra — *see* Fracture,
          vertebra, by site, with spinal cord
          injury
  spondylogenic — *see* Compression, spinal cord,
      spondylogenic
  subcostal nerve (syndrome) 354.8
  sympathetic nerve NEC 337.9
  syndrome 958.5
  thorax 512.8
    iatrogenic 512.1
    postoperative 512.1
  trachea 519.1
    congenital 748.3
  ulnar nerve (by scar tissue) 354.2
  umbilical cord
    affecting fetus or newborn 762.5
      cord prolapsed 762.4
    complicating delivery 663.2 ☑
      cord around neck 663.1 ☑
      cord prolapsed 663.0 ☑
  upper extremity NEC 354.9
  ureter 593.3
  urethra — *see* Stricture, urethra
  vein 459.2
  vena cava (inferior) (superior) 459.2
  vertebral NEC — *see* Compression, spinal
      (cord)

Compulsion, compulsive
  eating 307.51
  neurosis (obsessive) 300.3

☑ Additional Digit Required   ▶◀ Revised Text   ● New Line   ▲ Revised Code

Compulsion, compulsive — *continued*
  personality 301.4
  states (mixed) 300.3
  swearing 300.3
    in Gilles de la Tourette's syndrome 307.23
  tics and spasms 307.22
  water drinking NEC (syndrome) 307.9
Concato's disease (pericardial polyserositis) 423.2
  peritoneal 568.82
  pleural — *see* Pleurisy
Concavity, chest wall 738.3
Concealed
  hemorrhage NEC 459.0
  penis 752.65
Concentric fading 368.12
Concern (normal) **about sick person in family**
  V61.49
Concrescence (teeth) 520.2
Concretio cordis 423.1
  rheumatic 393
Concretion — *see also* Calculus
  appendicular 543.9
  canaliculus 375.57
  clitoris 624.8
  conjunctiva 372.54
  eyelid 374.56
  intestine (impaction) (obstruction) 560.39
  lacrimal (passages) 375.57
  prepuce (male) 605
    female (clitoris) 624.8
  salivary gland (any) 527.5
  seminal vesicle 608.89
  stomach 537.89
  tonsil 474.8
Concussion (current) 850.9
  with
    loss of consciousness 850.5
      brief (less than one hour)
        30 minutes or less 850.11
        31-59 minutes 850.12
      moderate (1-24 hours) 850.2
      prolonged (more than 24 hours) (with
        complete recovery) (with return to
        pre-existing conscious level) 850.3
        without return to pre-existing
          conscious level 850.4
    mental confusion or disorientation (without
      loss of consciousness) 850.0
    with loss of consciousness — *see*
      Concussion, with, loss of
      consciousness
  without loss of consciousness 850.0
  blast (air) (hydraulic) (immersion) (underwater)
    869.0
    with open wound into cavity 869.1
    abdomen or thorax — *see* Injury, internal,
      by site
    brain — *see* Concussion, brain
    ear (acoustic nerve trauma) 951.5
      with perforation, tympanic membrane —
        see Wound, open, ear drum
    thorax — *see* Injury, internal, intrathoracic
      organs NEC
  brain or cerebral (without skull fracture) 850.9
    with
      loss of consciousness 850.5
        brief (less than one hour)
          30 minutes or less 850.11
          31-59 minutes 850.12
        moderate (1-24 hours) 850.2
        prolonged (more than 24 hours) (with
          complete recovery) (with return
          to pre-existing conscious level)
          850.3
          without return to pre-existing
            conscious level 850.4
      mental confusion or disorientation
        (without loss of consciousness)
        850.0
      with loss of consciousness — *see*
        Concussion, brain, with, loss of
        consciousness
    skull fracture — *see* Fracture, skull, by
      site

Concussion — *continued*
  brain or cerebral — *continued*
    without loss of consciousness 850.0
  cauda equina 952.4
  cerebral — *see* Concussion, brain
  conus medullaris (spine) 952.4
  hydraulic — *see* Concussion, blast
  internal organs — *see* Injury, internal, by site
  labyrinth — *see* Injury, intracranial
  ocular 921.3
  osseous labyrinth — *see* Injury, intracranial
  spinal (cord) — *see also* Injury, spinal, by site
    due to
      broken
        back — *see* Fracture, vertebra, by site,
          with spinal cord injury
        neck — *see* Fracture, vertebra,
          cervical, with spinal cord injury
      fracture, fracture dislocation, or
        compression fracture of spine or
        vertebra — *see* Fracture, vertebra,
        by site, with spinal cord injury
  syndrome 310.2
  underwater blast — *see* Concussion, blast
Condition — *see also* Disease
  psychiatric 298.9
  respiratory NEC 519.9
    acute or subacute NEC 519.9
      due to
        external agent 508.9
          specified type NEC 508.8
          fumes or vapors (chemical) (inhalation)
          506.3
          radiation 508.0
    chronic NEC 519.9
      due to
        external agent 508.9
          specified type NEC 508.8
          fumes or vapors (chemical) (inhalation)
          506.4
          radiation 508.1
    due to
      external agent 508.9
        specified type NEC 508.8
      fumes or vapors (chemical) (inhalation)
        506.9
Conduct disturbance (*see also* Disturbance,
  conduct) 312.9
  adjustment reaction 309.3
  hyperkinetic 314.2
Condyloma NEC 078.10
  acuminatum 078.11
  gonorrheal 098.0
  latum 091.3
  syphilitic 091.3
    congenital 090.0
  venereal, syphilitic 091.3
Confinement — *see* Delivery
Conflagration — *see also* Burn, by site
  asphyxia (by inhalation of smoke, gases, fumes,
    or vapors) 987.9
    specified agent — *see* Table of Drugs and
      Chemicals
Conflict
  family V61.9
    specified circumstance NEC V61.8
  interpersonal NEC V62.81
  marital V61.10
    involving divorce or estrangement V61.0
  parent-child V61.20
  partner V61.10
Confluent — *see* condition
Confusion, confused (mental) (state) (*see also*
  State, confusional) 298.9
  acute 293.0
  epileptic 293.0
  postoperative 293.9
  psychogenic 298.2
  reactive (from emotional stress, psychological
    trauma) 298.2
  subacute 293.1
Congelation 991.9
Congenital — *see also* condition
  aortic septum 747.29
  intrinsic factor deficiency 281.0

Congenital — *see also* condition — *continued*
  malformation — *see* Anomaly
Congestion, congestive (chronic) (passive)
  asphyxia, newborn 768.9
  bladder 596.8
  bowel 569.89
  brain (*see also* Disease, cerebrovascular NEC)
    437.8
    malarial 084.9
  breast 611.79
  bronchi 519.1
  bronchial tube 519.1
  catarrhal 472.0
  cerebral — *see* Congestion, brain
  cerebrospinal — *see* Congestion, brain
  chest 514
  chill 780.99
    malarial (*see also* Malaria) 084.6
  circulatory NEC 459.9
  conjunctiva 372.71
  due to disturbance of circulation 459.9
  duodenum 537.3
  enteritis — *see* Enteritis
  eye 372.71
  fibrosis syndrome (pelvic) 625.5
  gastroenteritis — *see* Enteritis
  general 799.89
  glottis 476.0
  heart (*see also* Failure, heart) 428.0
  hepatic 573.0
  hypostatic (lung) 514
  intestine 569.89
  intracranial — *see* Congestion, brain
  kidney 593.89
  labyrinth 386.50
  larynx 476.0
  liver 573.0
  lung 514
    active or acute (*see also* Pneumonia) 486
      congenital 770.0
    chronic 514
    hypostatic 514
    idiopathic, acute 518.5
    passive 514
  malaria, malarial (brain) (fever) (*see also*
    Malaria) 084.6
  medulla — *see* Congestion, brain
  nasal 478.1
  orbit, orbital 376.33
    inflammatory (chronic) 376.10
      acute 376.00
  ovary 620.8
  pancreas 577.8
  pelvic, female 625.5
  pleural 511.0
  prostate (active) 602.1
  pulmonary — *see* Congestion, lung
  renal 593.89
  retina 362.89
  seminal vesicle 608.89
  spinal cord 336.1
  spleen 289.51
    chronic 289.51
  stomach 537.89
  trachea 464.11
  urethra 599.84
  uterus 625.5
    with subinvolution 621.1
  viscera 799.89
Congestive — *see* Congestion
Conical
  cervix 622.6
  cornea 371.60
  teeth 520.2
Conjoined twins 759.4
  causing disproportion (fetopelvic) 653.7 ☑
Conjugal maladjustment V61.10
  involving divorce or estrangement V61.0
Conjunctiva — *see* condition
Conjunctivitis (exposure) (infectious)
  (nondiphtheritic) (pneumococcal) (pustular)
  (staphylococcal) (streptococcal) NEC 372.30
  actinic 370.24
  acute 372.00
    atopic 372.05

Conjunctivitis — *continued*
  acute — *continued*
    contagious 372.03
    follicular 372.02
    hemorrhagic (viral) 077.4
  adenoviral (acute) 077.3
  allergic (chronic) 372.14
    with hay fever 372.05
  anaphylactic 372.05
  angular 372.03
  Apollo (viral) 077.4
  atopic 372.05
  blennorrhagic (neonatorum) 098.40
  catarrhal 372.03
  chemical 372.05
  chlamydial 077.98
    due to
      Chlamydia trachomatis — *see* Trachoma
      paratrachoma 077.0
  chronic 372.10
    allergic 372.14
    follicular 372.12
    simple 372.11
    specified type NEC 372.14
    vernal 372.13
  diphtheritic 032.81
  due to
    dust 372.05
    enterovirus type 70 077.4
    erythema multiforme 695.1 *[372.33]*
    filiariasis (*see also* Filiariasis) 125.9 *[372.15]*
    mucocutaneous
      disease NEC 372.33
      leishmaniasis 085.5 *[372.15]*
    Reiter's disease 099.3 *[372.33]*
    syphilis 095.8 *[372.10]*
    toxoplasmosis (acquired) 130.1
      congenital (active) 771.2
    trachoma — *see* Trachoma
  dust 372.05
  eczematous 370.31
  epidemic 077.1
    hemorrhagic 077.4
  follicular (acute) 372.02
    adenoviral (acute) 077.3
    chronic 372.12
  glare 370.24
  gonococcal (neonatorum) 098.40
  granular (trachomatous) 076.1
    late effect 139.1
  hemorrhagic (acute) (epidemic) 077.4
  herpetic (simplex) 054.43
    zoster 053.21
  inclusion 077.0
  infantile 771.6
  influenzal 372.03
  Koch-Weeks 372.03
  light 372.05
  medicamentosa 372.05
  membranous 372.04
  meningococcic 036.89
  Morax-Axenfeld 372.02
  mucopurulent NEC 372.03
  neonatal 771.6
    gonococcal 098.40
  Newcastle's 077.8
  nodosa 360.14
  of Beal 077.3
  parasitic 372.15
    filiariasis (*see also* Filiariasis) 125.9 *[372.15]*
    mucocutaneous leishmaniasis 085.5
      [372.15]
  Parinaud's 372.02
  petrificans 372.39
  phlyctenular 370.31
  pseudomembranous 372.04
    diphtheritic 032.81
  purulent 372.03
  Reiter's 099.3 *[372.33]*
  rosacea 695.3 *[372.31]*
  serous 372.01
    viral 077.99
  simple chronic 372.11
  specified NEC 372.39
  sunlamp 372.04
  swimming pool 077.0

Conjunctivitis — *continued*
  trachomatous (follicular) 076.1
    acute 076.0
    late effect 139.1
  traumatic NEC 372.39
  tuberculous (*see also* Tuberculosis) 017.3 ☑
    [370.31]
  tularemic 021.3
  tularensis 021.3
  vernal 372.13
    limbar 372.13 *[370.32]*
  viral 077.99
    acute hemorrhagic 077.4
    specified NEC 077.8
Conjunctivochalasis 372.81
Conjunctoblepharitis — *see* Conjunctivitis
Conn (-Louis) syndrome (primary aldosteronism)
  255.12
Connective tissue — *see* condition
Conradi (-Hünermann) syndrome or disease
  (chondrodysplasia calcificans congenita)
  756.59
Consanguinity V19.7
Consecutive — *see* condition
Consolidated lung (base) — *see* Pneumonia, lobar
Constipation 564.00
  atonic 564.09
  drug induced
    correct substance properly administered
      564.09
    overdose or wrong substance given or taken
      977.9
      specified drug — *see* Table of Drugs and
        Chemicals
  neurogenic 564.09
  other specified NEC 564.09
  outlet dysfunction 564.02
  psychogenic 306.4
  simple 564.00
  slow transit 564.01
  spastic 564.09
Constitutional — *see also* condition
  arterial hypotension (*see also* Hypotension)
    458.9
  obesity 278.00
    morbid 278.01
  psychopathic state 301.9
  short stature in childhood 783.43
  state, developmental V21.9
    specified development NEC V21.8
  substandard 301.6
Constitutionally substandard 301.6
Constriction
  anomalous, meningeal bands or folds 742.8
  aortic arch (congenital) 747.10
  asphyxiation or suffocation by 994.7
  bronchus 519.1
  canal, ear (*see also* Stricture, ear canal,
    acquired) 380.50
  duodenum 537.3
  gallbladder (*see also* Obstruction, gallbladder)
    575.2
    congenital 751.69
  intestine (*see also* Obstruction, intestine) 560.9
  larynx 478.74
    congenital 748.3
  meningeal bands or folds, anomalous 742.8
  organ or site, congenital NEC — *see* Atresia
  prepuce (congenital) 605
  pylorus 537.0
    adult hypertrophic 537.0
    congenital or infantile 750.5
    newborn 750.5
  ring (uterus) 661.4 ☑
    affecting fetus or newborn 763.7
  spastic — *see also* Spasm
    ureter 593.3
    urethra — *see* Stricture, urethra
  stomach 537.89
  ureter 593.3
  urethra — *see* Stricture, urethra
  visual field (functional) (peripheral) 368.45
Constrictive — *see* condition

Consultation
  medical — *see also* Counseling, medical
  specified reason NEC V65.8
  without complaint or sickness V65.9
    feared complaint unfounded V65.5
    specified reason NEC V65.8
Consumption — *see* Tuberculosis
Contact
  with
    AIDS virus V01.79 ▲
    anthrax V01.81
    cholera V01.0
    communicable disease V01.9
      specified type NEC V01.89
      viral NEC V01.79 ▲
    Escherichia coli (E. coli) V01.83 ●
    German measles V01.4
    gonorrhea V01.6
    HIV V01.79 ▲
    human immunodeficiency virus V01.79 ▲
    meningococcus V01.84 ●
    parasitic disease NEC V01.89
    poliomyelitis V01.2
    rabies V01.5
    rubella V01.4
    SARS-associated coronavirus V01.82
    smallpox V01.3
    syphilis V01.6
    tuberculosis V01.1
    varicella V01.71 ●
    venereal disease V01.6
    viral disease NEC V01.79 ▲
  dermatitis — *see* Dermatitis
Contamination, food (*see also* Poisoning, food)
  005.9
Contraception, contraceptive
  advice NEC V25.09
    family planning V25.09
    fitting of diaphragm V25.02
    prescribing or use of
      oral contraceptive agent V25.01
      specified agent NEC V25.02
  counseling NEC V25.09
    emergency V25.03
    family planning V25.09
    fitting of diaphragm V25.02
    prescribing or use of
      oral contraceptive agent V25.01
        emergency V25.03
        postcoital V25.03
      specified agent NEC V25.02
  device (in situ) V45.59
    causing menorrhagia 996.76
    checking V25.42
    complications 996.32
    insertion V25.1
    intrauterine V45.51
    reinsertion V25.42
    removal V25.42
    subdermal V45.52
  fitting of diaphragm V25.02
  insertion
    intrauterine contraceptive device V25.1
    subdermal implantable V25.5
  maintenance V25.40
    examination V25.40
      subdermal implantable V25.43
        intrauterine device V25.42
      oral contraceptive V25.41
      specified method NEC V25.49
    intrauterine device V25.42
    oral contraceptive V25.41
    specified method NEC V25.49
    subdermal implantable V25.43
  management NEC V25.49
  prescription
    oral contraceptive agent V25.01
      emergency V25.03
      postcoital V25.03
      repeat V25.41
    specified agent NEC V25.02
      repeat V25.49
  sterilization V25.2
  surveillance V25.40
    intrauterine device V25.42

(side tab) Conjunctivitis — Contraception, contraceptive

Contraception, contraceptive — *continued*
  surveillance — *continued*
    oral contraceptive agent V25.41
      subdermal implantable V25.43
    specified method NEC V25.49
Contraction, contracture, contracted
  Achilles tendon (*see also* Short, tendon,
    Achilles) 727.81
  anus 564.89
  axilla 729.9
  bile duct (*see also* Disease, biliary) 576.8
  bladder 596.8
    neck or sphincter 596.0
  bowel (*see also* Obstruction, intestine) 560.9
  Braxton Hicks 644.1 ☑
  bronchus 519.1
  burn (old) — *see* Cicatrix
  cecum (*see also* Obstruction, intestine) 560.9
  cervix (*see also* Stricture, cervix) 622.4
    congenital 752.49
  cicatricial — *see* Cicatrix
  colon (*see also* Obstruction, intestine) 560.9
  conjunctiva trachomatous, active 076.1
    late effect 139.1
  Dupuytren's 728.6
  eyelid 374.41
  eye socket (after enucleation) 372.64
  face 729.9
  fascia (lata) (postural) 728.89
    Dupuytren's 728.6
    palmar 728.6
    plantar 728.71
  finger NEC 736.29
    congenital 755.59
    joint (*see also* Contraction, joint) 718.44
  flaccid, paralytic
    joint (*see also* Contraction, joint) 718.4 ☑
    muscle 728.85
      ocular 378.50
  gallbladder (*see also* Obstruction, gallbladder)
    575.2
  hamstring 728.89
    tendon 727.81
  heart valve — *see* Endocarditis
  Hicks' 644.1 ☑
  hip (*see also* Contraction, joint) 718.4 ☑
  hourglass
    bladder 596.8
      congenital 753.8
    gallbladder (*see also* Obstruction,
      gallbladder) 575.2
      congenital 751.69
    stomach 536.8
      congenital 750.7
      psychogenic 306.4
    uterus 661.4 ☑
      affecting fetus or newborn 763.7
  hysterical 300.11
  infantile (*see also* Epilepsy) 345.6 ☑
  internal os (*see also* Stricture, cervix) 622.4
  intestine (*see also* Obstruction, intestine) 560.9
  joint (abduction) (acquired) (adduction) (flexion)
    (rotation) 718.40
    ankle 718.47
    congenital NEC 755.8
      generalized or multiple 754.89
        lower limb joints 754.89
      hip (*see also* Subluxation, congenital, hip)
        754.32
      lower limb (including pelvic girdle) not
        involving hip 754.89
      upper limb (including shoulder girdle)
        755.59
    elbow 718.42
    foot 718.47
    hand 718.44
    hip 718.45
    hysterical 300.11
    knee 718.46
    multiple sites 718.49
    pelvic region 718.45
    shoulder (region) 718.41
    specified site NEC 718.48
    wrist 718.43
  kidney (granular) (secondary) (*see also*
    Sclerosis, renal) 587

Contraction, contracture, contracted —
  continued
  kidney (*see also* Sclerosis, renal) — *continued*
    congenital 753.3
    hydronephritic 591
    pyelonephritic (*see also* Pyelitis, chronic)
      590.00
    tuberculous (*see also* Tuberculosis) 016.0 ☑
  ligament 728.89
    congenital 756.89
  liver — *see* Cirrhosis, liver
  muscle (postinfectional) (postural) NEC 728.85
    congenital 756.89
      sternocleidomastoid 754.1
    extraocular 378.60
    eye (extrinsic) (*see also* Strabismus) 378.9
      paralytic (*see also* Strabismus, paralytic)
        378.50
    flaccid 728.85
    hysterical 300.11
    ischemic (Volkmann's) 958.6
    paralytic 728.85
    posttraumatic 958.6
    psychogenic 306.0
      specified as conversion reaction 300.11
  myotonic 728.85
  neck (*see also* Torticollis) 723.5
    congenital 754.1
    psychogenic 306.0
  ocular muscle (*see also* Strabismus) 378.9
    paralytic (*see also* Strabismus, paralytic)
      378.50
  organ or site, congenital NEC — *see* Atresia
  outlet (pelvis) — *see* Contraction, pelvis
  palmar fascia 728.6
  paralytic
    joint (*see also* Contraction, joint) 718.4 ☑
    muscle 728.85
      ocular (*see also* Strabismus, paralytic)
        378.50
  pelvis (acquired) (general) 738.6
    affecting fetus or newborn 763.1
    complicating delivery 653.1 ☑
      causing obstructed labor 660.1 ☑
      generally contracted 653.1 ☑
        causing obstructed labor 660.1 ☑
      inlet 653.2 ☑
        causing obstructed labor 660.1 ☑
      midpelvic 653.8 ☑
        causing obstructed labor 660.1 ☑
      midplane 653.8 ☑
        causing obstructed labor 660.1 ☑
      outlet 653.3 ☑
        causing obstructed labor 660.1 ☑
  plantar fascia 728.71
  premature
    atrial 427.61
    auricular 427.61
    auriculoventricular 427.61
    heart (junctional) (nodal) 427.60
    supraventricular 427.61
    ventricular 427.69
  prostate 602.8
  pylorus (*see also* Pylorospasm) 537.81
  rectosigmoid (*see also* Obstruction, intestine)
    560.9
  rectum, rectal (sphincter) 564.89
    psychogenic 306.4
  ring (Bandl's) 661.4 ☑
    affecting fetus or newborn 763.7
  scar — *see* Cicatrix
  sigmoid (*see also* Obstruction, intestine) 560.9
  socket, eye 372.64
  spine (*see also* Curvature, spine) 737.9
  stomach 536.8
    hourglass 536.8
      congenital 750.7
    psychogenic 306.4
  tendon (sheath) (*see also* Short, tendon) 727.81
  toe 735.8
  ureterovesical orifice (postinfectional) 593.3
  urethra 599.84
  uterus 621.8
    abnormal 661.9 ☑
      affecting fetus or newborn 763.7
    clonic, hourglass or tetanic 661.4 ☑
      affecting fetus or newborn 763.7

Contraction, contracture, contracted —
  continued
  uterus — *continued*
    dyscoordinate 661.4 ☑
      affecting fetus or newborn 763.7
    hourglass 661.4 ☑
      affecting fetus or newborn 763.7
    hypotonic NEC 661.2 ☑
      affecting fetus or newborn 763.7
    incoordinate 661.4 ☑
      affecting fetus or newborn 763.7
    inefficient or poor 661.2 ☑
      affecting fetus or newborn 763.7
    irregular 661.2 ☑
      affecting fetus or newborn 763.7
    tetanic 661.4 ☑
      affecting fetus or newborn 763.7
  vagina (outlet) 623.2
  vesical 596.8
    neck or urethral orifice 596.0
  visual field, generalized 368.45
  Volkmann's (ischemic) 958.6
Contusion (skin surface intact) 924.9
  with
    crush injury — *see* Crush
    dislocation — *see* Dislocation, by site
    fracture — *see* Fracture, by site
    internal injury — *see also* Injury, internal,
      by site
      heart — *see* Contusion, cardiac
      kidney — *see* Contusion, kidney
      liver — *see* Contusion, liver
      lung — *see* Contusion, lung
      spleen — *see* Contusion, spleen
    intracranial injury — *see* Injury, intracranial
    nerve injury — *see* Injury, nerve
    open wound — *see* Wound, open, by site
  abdomen, abdominal (muscle) (wall) 922.2
    organ(s) NEC 868.00
  adnexa, eye NEC 921.9
  ankle 924.21
    with other parts of foot 924.20
  arm 923.9
    lower (with elbow) 923.10
    upper 923.03
      with shoulder or axillary region 923.09
  auditory canal (external) (meatus) (and other
    part(s) of neck, scalp, or face, except eye)
    920
  auricle, ear (and other part(s) of neck, scalp, or
    face except eye) 920
  axilla 923.02
    with shoulder or upper am 923.09
  back 922.31
  bone NEC 924.9
  brain (cerebral) (membrane) (with hemorrhage)
    851.8 ☑

Note — Use the following fifth-digit
subclassification with categories 851-854:

  0 unspecified state of consciousness
  1 with no loss of consciousness
  2 with brief [less than one hour] loss of
    consciousness
  3 with moderate [1-24 hours] loss of
    consciousness
  4 with prolonged [more than 24 hours] loss
    of consciousness and return to pre-
    existing conscious level
  5 with prolonged [more than 24 hours] loss
    of consciousness, without return to pre-
    existing conscious level
  Use fifth-digit 5 to designate when a patient
    is unconscious and dies before regaining
    consciousness, regardless of the duration
    of the loss of consciousness
  6 with loss of consciousness of unspecified
    duration
  9 with concussion, unspecified

  with
    open intracranial wound 851.9 ☑
    skull fracture — *see* Fracture, skull, by
      site
  cerebellum 851.4 ☑
    with open intracranial wound 851.5 ☑

Contusion — *continued*
  brain — *continued*
    cortex 851.0 ☑
      with open intracranial wound 851.1 ☑
    occipital lobe 851.4 ☑
      with open intracranial wound 851.5 ☑
    stem 851.4 ☑
      with open intracranial wound 851.5 ☑
  breast 922.0
  brow (and other part(s) of neck, scalp, or face, except eye) 920
  buttock 922.32
  canthus 921.1
  cardiac 861.01
    with open wound into thorax 861.11
  cauda equina (spine) 952.4
  cerebellum — *see* Contusion, brain, cerebellum
  cerebral — *see* Contusion, brain
  cheek(s) (and other part(s) of neck, scalp, or face, except eye) 920
  chest (wall) 922.1
  chin (and other part(s) of neck, scalp, or face, except eye) 920
  clitoris 922.4
  conjunctiva 921.1
  conus medullaris (spine) 952.4
  cornea 921.3
  corpus cavernosum 922.4
  cortex (brain) (cerebral) — *see* Contusion, brain, cortex
  costal region 922.1
  ear (and other part(s) of neck, scalp, or face except eye) 920
  elbow 923.11
    with forearm 923.10
  epididymis 922.4
  epigastric region 922.2
  eye NEC 921.9
  eyeball 921.3
  eyelid(s) (and periocular area) 921.1
  face (and neck, or scalp, any part except eye) 920
  femoral triangle 922.2
  fetus or newborn 772.6
  finger(s) (nail) (subungual) 923.3
  flank 922.2
  foot (with ankle) (excluding toe(s)) 924.20
  forearm (and elbow) 923.10
  forehead (and other part(s) of neck, scalp, or face, except eye) 920
  genital organs, external 922.4
  globe (eye) 921.3
  groin 922.2
  gum(s) (and other part(s) of neck, scalp, or face, except eye) 920
  hand(s) (except fingers alone) 923.20
  head (any part, except eye) (and face) (and neck) 920
  heart — *see* Contusion, cardiac
  heel 924.20
  hip 924.01
    with thigh 924.00
  iliac region 922.2
  inguinal region 922.2
  internal organs (abdomen, chest, or pelvis) NEC — *see* Injury, internal, by site
  interscapular region 922.33
  iris (eye) 921.3
  kidney 866.01
    with open wound into cavity 866.11
  knee 924.11
    with lower leg 924.10
  labium (majus) (minus) 922.4
  lacrimal apparatus, gland, or sac 921.1
  larynx (and other part(s) of neck, scalp, or face, except eye) 920
  late effect — *see* Late, effects (of), contusion
  leg 924.5
    lower (with knee) 924.10
  lens 921.3
  lingual (and other part(s) of neck, scalp, or face, except eye) 920
  lip(s) (and other part(s) of neck, scalp, or face, except eye) 920

Contusion — *continued*
  liver 864.01
    with
      laceration — *see* Laceration, liver
      open wound into cavity 864.11
  lower extremity 924.5
    multiple sites 924.4
  lumbar region 922.31
  lung 861.21
    with open wound into thorax 861.31
  malar region (and other part(s) of neck, scalp, or face, except eye) 920
  mandibular joint (and other part(s) of neck, scalp, or face, except eye) 920
  mastoid region (and other part(s) of neck, scalp. or face, except eye) 920
  membrane, brain — *see* Contusion, brain
  midthoracic region 922.1
  mouth (and other part(s) of neck, scalp, or face, except eye) 920
  multiple sites (not classifiable to same three-digit category) 924.8
    lower limb 924.4
    trunk 922.8
    upper limb 923.8
  muscle NEC 924.9
  myocardium — *see* Contusion, cardiac
  nasal (septum) (and other part(s) of neck, scalp, or face, except eye) 920
  neck (and scalp, or face any part, except eye) 920
  nerve — *see* Injury, nerve, by site
  nose (and other part(s) of neck, scalp, or face, except eye) 920
  occipital region (scalp) (and neck or face, except eye) 920
    lobe — *see* Contusion, brain, occipital lobe
  orbit (region) (tissues) 921.2
  palate (soft) (and other part(s) of neck, scalp, or face, except eye) 920
  parietal region (scalp) (and neck, or face, except eye) 920
    lobe — *see* Contusion, brain
  penis 922.4
  pericardium — *see* Contusion, cardiac
  perineum 922.4
  periocular area 921.1
  pharynx (and other part(s) of neck, scalp, or face, except eye) 920
  popliteal space (*see also* Contusion, knee) 924.11
  prepuce 922.4
  pubic region 922.4
  pudenda 922.4
  pulmonary — *see* Contusion, lung
  quadriceps femoralis 924.00
  rib cage 922.1
  sacral region 922.32
  salivary ducts or glands (and other part(s) of neck, scalp, or face, except eye) 920
  scalp (and neck, or face any part, except eye) 920
  scapular region 923.01
    with shoulder or upper arm 923.09
  sclera (eye) 921.3
  scrotum 922.4
  shoulder 923.00
    with upper arm or axillar regions 923.09
  skin NEC 924.9
  skull 920
  spermatic cord 922.4
  spinal cord — *see also* Injury, spinal, by site
    cauda equina 952.4
    conus medullaris 952.4
  spleen 865.01
    with open wound into cavity 865.11
  sternal region 922.1
  stomach — *see* Injury, internal, stomach
  subconjunctival 921.1
  subcutaneous NEC 924.9
  submaxillary region (and other part(s) of neck, scalp, or face, except eye) 920
  submental region (and other part(s) of neck, scalp, or face, except eye) 920
  subperiosteal NEC 924.9
  supraclavicular fossa (and other part(s) of neck, scalp, or face, except eye) 920

Contusion — *continued*
  supraorbital (and other part(s) of neck, scalp, or face, except eye) 920
  temple (region) (and other part(s) of neck, scalp, or face, except eye) 920
  testis 922.4
  thigh (and hip) 924.00
  thorax 922.1
    organ — *see* Injury, internal, intrathoracic
  throat (and other part(s) of neck, scalp, or face, except eye) 920
  thumb(s) (nail) (subungual) 923.3
  toe(s) (nail) (subungual) 924.3
  tongue (and other part(s) of neck, scalp, or face, except eye) 920
  trunk 922.9
    multiple sites 922.8
    specified site — *see* Contusion, by site
  tunica vaginalis 922.4
  tympanum (membrane) (and other part(s) of neck, scalp, or face, except eye) 920
  upper extremity 923.9
    multiple sites 923.8
  uvula (and other part(s) of neck, scalp, or face, except eye) 920
  vagina 922.4
  vocal cord(s) (and other part(s) of neck, scalp, or face, except eye) 920
  vulva 922.4
  wrist 923.21
    with hand(s), except finger(s) alone 923.20
Conus (any type) (congenital) 743.57
  acquired 371.60
  medullaris syndrome 336.8
Convalescence (following) V66.9
  chemotherapy V66.2
  medical NEC V66.5
  psychotherapy V66.3
  radiotherapy V66.1
  surgery NEC V66.0
  treatment (for) NEC V66.5
    combined V66.6
    fracture V66.4
    mental disorder NEC V66.3
    specified disorder NEC V66.5
Conversion
  closed surgical procedure to open procedure
    arthroscopic V64.43
    laparoscopic V64.41
    thoracoscopic V64.42
  hysteria, hysterical, any type 300.11
  neurosis, any 300.11
  reaction, any 300.11
Converter, tuberculosis (test reaction) 795.5
Convulsions (idiopathic) 780.39
  apoplectiform (*see also* Disease, cerebrovascular, acute) 436
  brain 780.39
  cerebral 780.39
  cerebrospinal 780.39
  due to trauma NEC — *see* Injury, intracranial
  eclamptic (*see also* Eclampsia) 780.39
  epileptic (*see also* Epilepsy) 345.9 ☑
  epileptiform (*see also* Seizure, epileptiform) 780.39
  epileptoid (*see also* Seizure, epileptiform) 780.39
  ether
    anesthetic
      correct substance properly administered 780.39
      overdose or wrong substance given 968.2
    other specified type — *see* Table of Drugs and Chemicals
  febrile 780.31
  generalized 780.39
  hysterical 300.11
  infantile 780.39
    epilepsy — *see* Epilepsy
  internal 780.39
  jacksonian (*see also* Epilepsy) 345.5 ☑
  myoclonic 333.2
  newborn 779.0
  paretic 094.1
  pregnancy (nephritic) (uremic) — *see* Eclampsia, pregnancy

Convulsions — *continued*
  psychomotor (*see also* Epilepsy) 345.4 ☑
  puerperal, postpartum — *see* Eclampsia,
    pregnancy
  recurrent 780.39
    epileptic — *see* Epilepsy
  reflex 781.0
  repetitive 780.39
    epileptic — *see* Epilepsy
  salaam (*see also* Epilepsy) 345.6 ☑
  scarlatinal 034.1
  spasmodic 780.39
  tetanus, tetanic (*see also* Tetanus) 037
  thymic 254.8
  uncinate 780.39
  uremic 586
Convulsive — *see also* Convulsions
  disorder or state 780.39
    epileptic — *see* Epilepsy
  equivalent, abdominal (*see also* Epilepsy)
    345.5 ☑
Cooke-Apert-Gallais syndrome (adrenogenital)
  255.2
Cooley's anemia (erythroblastic) 282.49
Coolie itch 126.9
Cooper's
  disease 610.1
  hernia — *see* Hernia, Cooper's
Coordination disturbance 781.3
Copper wire arteries, retina 362.13
Copra itch 133.8
Coprolith 560.39
Coprophilia 302.89
Coproporphyria, hereditary 277.1
Coprostasis 560.39
  with hernia — *see also* Hernia, by site, with
    obstruction
    gangrenous — *see* Hernia, by site, with
      gangrene
Cor
  biloculare 745.7
  bovinum — *see* Hypertrophy, cardiac
  bovis — *see also* Hypertrophy, cardiac
  pulmonale (chronic) 416.9
    acute 415.0
  triatriatum, triatrium 746.82
  triloculare 745.8
    biatriatum 745.3
    biventriculare 745.69
Corbus' disease 607.1
Cord — *see also* condition
  around neck (tightly) (with compression)
    affecting fetus or newborn 762.5
    complicating delivery 663.1 ☑
      without compression 663.3 ☑
        affecting fetus or newborn 762.6
  bladder NEC 344.61
    tabetic 094.0
  prolapse
    affecting fetus or newborn 762.4
    complicating delivery 663.0 ☑
Cord's angiopathy (*see also* Tuberculosis)
  017.3 ☑ *[362.18]*
Cordis ectopia 746.87
Corditis (spermatic) 608.4
Corectopia 743.46
Cori type glycogen storage disease — *see*
  Disease, glycogen storage
Cork-handlers' disease or lung 495.3
Corkscrew esophagus 530.5
Corlett's pyosis (impetigo) 684
Corn (infected) 700
Cornea — *see also* condition
  donor V59.5
  guttata (dystrophy) 371.57
  plana 743.41
Cornelia de Lange's syndrome (Amsterdam
  dwarf, mental retardation, and
  brachycephaly) 759.89
Cornual gestation or pregnancy — *see*
  Pregnancy, cornual

Cornu cutaneum 702.8
Coronary (artery) — *see also* condition
  arising from aorta or pulmonary trunk 746.85
Corpora — *see also* condition
  amylacea (prostate) 602.8
  cavernosa — *see* condition
Corpulence (*see also* Obesity) 278.0 ☑
Corpus — *see* condition
Corrigan's disease — *see* Insufficiency, aortic
Corrosive burn — *see* Burn, by site
Corsican fever (*see also* Malaria) 084.6
Cortical — *see also* condition
  blindness 377.75
  necrosis, kidney (bilateral) 583.6
Corticoadrenal — *see* condition
Corticosexual syndrome 255.2
Coryza (acute) 460
  with grippe or influenza 487.1
  syphilitic 095.8
    congenital (chronic) 090.0
Costen's syndrome or complex 524.60
Costiveness (*see also* Constipation) 564.00
Costochondritis 733.6
Cotard's syndrome (paranoia) 297.1
Cot death 798.0
Cotungo's disease 724.3
Cough 786.2
  with hemorrhage (*see also* Hemoptysis) 786.3
  affected 786.2
  bronchial 786.2
    with grippe or influenza 487.1
  chronic 786.2
  epidemic 786.2
  functional 306.1
  hemorrhagic 786.3
  hysterical 300.11
  laryngeal, spasmodic 786.2
  nervous 786.2
  psychogenic 306.1
  smokers' 491.0
  tea tasters' 112.89
Counseling NEC V65.40
  without complaint or sickness V65.49
  abuse victim NEC V62.89
    child V61.21
    partner V61.11
    spouse V61.11
  child abuse, maltreatment, or neglect V61.21
  contraceptive NEC V25.09
    device (intrauterine) V25.02
    maintenance V25.40
      intrauterine contraceptive device V25.42
      oral contraceptive (pill) V25.41
      specified type NEC V25.49
      subdermal implantable V25.43
    management NEC V25.9
    oral contraceptive (pill) V25.01
      emergency V25.03
      postcoital V25.03
    prescription NEC V25.02
      oral contraceptive (pill) V25.01
        emergency V25.03
        postcoital V25.03
        repeat prescription V25.41
      repeat prescription V25.40
    subdermal implantable V25.43
    surveillance NEC V25.40
  dietary V65.3
  excercise V65.41
  expectant mother, pediatric pre-birth visit
    V65.11
  explanation of
    investigation finding NEC V65.49
    medication NEC V65.49
  family planning V25.09
  for nonattending third party V65.19
  genetic V26.3
  gonorrhea V65.45
  health (advice) (education) (instruction) NEC
    V65.49
  HIV V65.44
  human immunodeficiency virus V65.44
  injury prevention V65.43

Counseling — *continued*
  insulin pump training V65.46
  marital V61.10
  medical (for) V65.9
    boarding school resident V60.6
    condition not demonstrated V65.5
    feared complaint and no disease found
      V65.5
    institutional resident V60.6
    on behalf of another V65.19
    person living alone V60.3
  parent-child conflict V61.20
    specified problem NEC V61.29
  partner abuse
    perpetrator V61.12
    victim V61.11
  pediatric pre-birth visit for expectant
    mother V65.11
  perpetrator of
    child abuse V62.83
      parental V61.22
    partner abuse V61.12
    spouse abuse V61.12
  procreative V65.49
  sex NEC V65.49
    transmitted disease NEC V65.45
      HIV V65.44
  specified reason NEC V65.49
  spousal abuse
    perpetrator V61.12
    victim V61.11
  substance use and abuse V65.42
  syphilis V65.45
  victim (of)
    abuse NEC V62.89
    child abuse V61.21
    partner abuse V61.11
    spousal abuse V61.11
Coupled rhythm 427.89
Couvelaire uterus (complicating delivery) — *see*
  Placenta, separation
Cowper's gland — *see* condition
Cowperitis (*see also* Urethritis) 597.89
  gonorrheal (acute) 098.0
    chronic or duration of 2 months or over
      098.2
Cowpox (abortive) 051.0
  due to vaccination 999.0
  eyelid 051.0 *[373.5]*
    postvaccination 999.0 *[373.5]*
Coxa
  plana 732.1
  valga (acquired) 736.31
    congenital 755.61
    late effect of rickets 268.1
  vara (acquired) 736.32
    congenital 755.62
    late effect of rickets 268.1
Coxae malum senilis 715.25
Coxalgia (nontuberculous) 719.45
  tuberculous (*see also* Tuberculosis) 015.1 ☑
    [730.85]
Coxalgic pelvis 736.30
Coxitis 716.65
Coxsackie (infection) (virus) 079.2
  central nervous system NEC 048
  endocarditis 074.22
  enteritis 008.67
  meningitis (aseptic) 047.0
  myocarditis 074.23
  pericarditis 074.21
  pharyngitis 074.0
  pleurodynia 074.1
  specific disease NEC 074.8
Crabs, meaning pubic lice 132.2
Crack baby 760.75
Cracked nipple 611.2
  puerperal, postpartum 676.1 ☑
Cradle cap 690.11
Craft neurosis 300.89
Craigiasis 007.8
Cramp(s) 729.82
  abdominal 789.0 ☑

Cramp(s) — *continued*
- bathing 994.1
- colic 789.0 ☑
  - psychogenic 306.4
- due to immersion 994.1
- extremity (lower) (upper) NEC 729.82
- fireman 992.2
- heat 992.2
- hysterical 300.11
- immersion 994.1
- intestinal 789.0 ☑
  - psychogenic 306.4
- linotypist's 300.89
  - organic 333.84
- muscle (extremity) (general) 729.82
  - due to immersion 994.1
  - hysterical 300.11
- occupational (hand) 300.89
  - organic 333.84
- psychogenic 307.89
- salt depletion 276.1
- stoker 992.2
- stomach 789.0 ☑
- telegraphers' 300.89
  - organic 333.84
- typists' 300.89
  - organic 333.84
- uterus 625.8
  - menstrual 625.3
- writers' 333.84
  - organic 333.84
  - psychogenic 300.89

Cranial — *see* condition

Cranioclasis, fetal 763.89

Craniocleidodysostosis 755.59

Craniofenestria (skull) 756.0

Craniolacunia (skull) 756.0

Craniopagus 759.4

Craniopathy, metabolic 733.3

Craniopharyngeal — *see* condition

Craniopharyngioma (M9350/1) 237.0

Craniorachischisis (totalis) 740.1

Cranioschisis 756.0

Craniostenosis 756.0

Craniosynostosis 756.0

Craniotabes (cause unknown) 733.3
- rachitic 268.1
- syphilitic 090.5

Craniotomy, fetal 763.89

Cranium — *see* condition

Craw-craw 125.3

Creaking joint 719.60
- ankle 719.67
- elbow 719.62
- foot 719.67
- hand 719.64
- hip 719.65
- knee 719.66
- multiple sites 719.69
- pelvic region 719.65
- shoulder (region) 719.61
- specified site NEC 719.68
- wrist 719.63

Creeping
- eruption 126.9
- palsy 335.21
- paralysis 335.21

Crenated tongue 529.8

Creotoxism 005.9

Crepitus
- caput 756.0
- joint 719.60
  - ankle 719.67
  - elbow 719.62
  - foot 719.67
  - hand 719.64
  - hip 719.65
  - knee 719.66
  - multiple sites 719.69
  - pelvic region 719.65
  - shoulder (region) 719.61
  - specified site NEC 719.68
  - wrist 719.63

Crescent or conus choroid, congenital 743.57

Cretin, cretinism (athyrotic) (congenital) (endemic) (metabolic) (nongoitrous) (sporadic) 243
- goitrous (sporadic) 246.1
- pelvis (dwarf type) (male type) 243
  - with disproportion (fetopelvic) 653.1 ☑
    - affecting fetus or newborn 763.1
    - causing obstructed labor 660.1 ☑
      - affecting fetus or newborn 763.1
- pituitary 253.3

Cretinoid degeneration 243

Creutzfeldt-Jakob disease (syndrome) 046.1
- with dementia
  - with behavioral disturbance 046.1 *[294.11]*
  - without behavioral disturbance 046.1 *[294.10]*

Crib death 798.0

Cribriform hymen 752.49

Cri-du-chat syndrome 758.31   ▲

Crigler-Najjar disease or syndrome (congenital hyperbilirubinemia) 277.4

Crimean hemorrhagic fever 065.0

Criminalism 301.7

Crisis
- abdomen 789.0 ☑
- addisonian (acute adrenocortical insufficiency) 255.4
- adrenal (cortical) 255.4
- asthmatic — *see* Asthma
- brain, cerebral (*see also* Disease, cerebrovascular, acute) 436
- celiac 579.0
- Dietl's 593.4
- emotional NEC 309.29
  - acute reaction to stress 308.0
  - adjustment reaction 309.9
  - specific to childhood ►or◄ adolescence 313.9
- gastric (tabetic) 094.0
- glaucomatocyclitic 364.22
- heart (*see also* Failure, heart) 428.9
- hypertensive — *see* Hypertension
- nitritoid
  - correct substance properly administered 458.29
  - overdose or wrong substance given or taken 961.1
- oculogyric 378.87
  - psychogenic 306.7
- Pel's 094.0
- psychosexual identity 302.6
- rectum 094.0
- renal 593.81
- sickle cell 282.62
- stomach (tabetic) 094.0
- tabetic 094.0
- thyroid (*see also* Thyrotoxicosis) 242.9 ☑
- thyrotoxic (*see also* Thyrotoxicosis) 242.9 ☑
- vascular — *see* Disease, cerebrovascular, acute

Crocq's disease (acrocyanosis) 443.89

Crohn's disease (*see also* Enteritis, regional) 555.9

Cronkhite-Canada syndrome 211.3

Crooked septum, nasal 470

Cross
- birth (of fetus) complicating delivery 652.3 ☑
  - with successful version 652.1 ☑
  - causing obstructed labor 660.0 ☑
- bite, anterior or posterior 524.20   ▲
- eye (*see also* Esotropia) 378.00

Crossed ectopia of kidney 753.3

Crossfoot 754.50

Croup, croupous (acute) (angina) (catarrhal) (infective) (inflammatory) (laryngeal) (membranous) (nondiphtheritic) (pseudomembranous) 464.4
- asthmatic (*see also* Asthma) 493.9 ☑
- bronchial 466.0
- diphtheritic (membranous) 032.3
- false 478.75
- spasmodic 478.75
  - diphtheritic 032.3

Croup, croupous — *continued*
- stridulous 478.75
  - diphtheritic 032.3

Crouzon's disease (craniofacial dysostosis) 756.0

Crowding, teeth 524.31   ▲

CRST syndrome (cutaneous systemic sclerosis) 710.1

Cruchet's disease (encephalitis lethargica) 049.8

Cruelty in children (*see also* Disturbance, conduct) 312.9

Crural ulcer (*see also* Ulcer, lower extremity) 707.10

Crush, crushed, crushing (injury) 929.9
- with
  - fracture — *see* Fracture, by site
- abdomen 926.19
  - internal — *see* Injury, internal, abdomen
- ankle 928.21
  - with other parts of foot 928.20
- arm 927.9
  - lower (and elbow) 927.10
  - upper 927.03
    - with shoulder or axillary region 927.09
- axilla 927.02
  - with shoulder or upper arm 927.09
- back 926.11
- breast 926.19
- buttock 926.12
- cheek 925.1
- chest — *see* Injury, internal, chest
- ear 925.1
- elbow 927.11
  - with forearm 927.10
- face 925.1
- finger(s) 927.3
  - with hand(s) 927.20
    - and wrist(s) 927.21
- flank 926.19
- foot, excluding toe(s) alone (with ankle) 928.20
- forearm (and elbow) 927.10
- genitalia, external (female) (male) 926.0
  - internal — *see* Injury, internal, genital organ NEC
- hand, except finger(s) alone (and wrist) 927.20
- head — *see* Fracture, skull, by site
- heel 928.20
- hip 928.01
  - with thigh 928.00
- internal organ (abdomen, chest, or pelvis) — *see* Injury, internal, by site
- knee 928.11
  - with leg, lower 928.10
- labium (majus) (minus) 926.0
- larynx 925.2
- late effect — *see* Late, effects (of), crushing
- leg 928.9
  - lower 928.10
    - and knee 928.11
  - upper 928.00
- limb
  - lower 928.9
    - multiple sites 928.8
  - upper 927.9
    - multiple sites 927.8
- multiple sites NEC 929.0
- neck 925.2
- nerve — *see* Injury, nerve, by site
- nose 802.0
  - open 802.1
- penis 926.0
- pharynx 925.2
- scalp 925.1
- scapular region 927.01
  - with shoulder or upper arm 927.09
- scrotum 926.0
- shoulder 927.00
  - with upper arm or axillary region 927.09
- skull or cranium — *see* Fracture, skull, by site
- spinal cord — *see* Injury, spinal, by site
- syndrome (complication of trauma) 958.5
- testis 926.0
- thigh (with hip) 928.00
- throat 925.2
- thumb(s) (and fingers) 927.3

Side tab: Cramp(s) — Crush, crushed, crushing

Crush, crushed, crushing — *continued*
  toe(s) 928.3
    with foot 928.20
      and ankle 928.21
  tonsil 925.2
  trunk 926.9
    chest — *see* Injury, internal, intrathoracic organs NEC
    internal organ — *see* Injury, internal, by site
    multiple sites 926.8
    specified site NEC 926.19
  vulva 926.0
  wrist 927.21
    with hand(s), except fingers alone 927.20
Crusta lactea 690.11
Crusts 782.8
Crutch paralysis 953.4
Cruveilhier's disease 335.21
Cruveilhier-Baumgarten cirrhosis, disease, or syndrome 571.5
Cruz-Chagas disease (*see also* Trypanosomiasis) 086.2
Cryoglobulinemia (mixed) 273.2
Crypt (anal) (rectal) 569.49
Cryptitis (anal) (rectal) 569.49
Cryptococcosis (European) (pulmonary) (systemic) 117.5
Cryptococcus 117.5
  epidermicus 117.5
  neoformans, infection by 117.5
Cryptopapillitis (anus) 569.49
Cryptophthalmos (eyelid) 743.06
Cryptorchid, cryptorchism, cryptorchidism 752.51
Cryptosporidiosis 007.4
Cryptotia 744.29
Crystallopathy
  calcium pyrophosphate (*see also* Arthritis) 275.49 [712.2] ☑
  dicalcium phosphate (*see also* Arthritis) 275.49 [712.1] ☑
  gouty 274.0
  pyrophosphate NEC (*see also* Arthritis) 275.49 [712.2] ☑
  uric acid 274.0
Crystalluria 791.9
Csillag's disease (lichen sclerosus or atrophicus) 701.0
Cuban itch 050.1
Cubitus
  valgus (acquired) 736.01
    congenital 755.59
    late effect of rickets 268.1
  varus (acquired) 736.02
    congenital 755.59
    late effect of rickets 268.1
Cultural deprivation V62.4
Cupping of optic disc 377.14
Curling's ulcer — *see* Ulcer, duodenum
Curling esophagus 530.5
Curschmann (-Batten) (-Steinert) disease or syndrome 359.2
Curvature
  organ or site, congenital NEC — *see* Distortion
  penis (lateral) 752.69
  Pott's (spinal) (*see also* Tuberculosis) 015.0 ☑ [737.43]
  radius, idiopathic, progressive (congenital) 755.54
  spine (acquired) (angular) (idiopathic) (incorrect) (postural) 737.9
    congenital 754.2
    due to or associated with
      Charcôt-Marie-Tooth disease 356.1 [737.40]
      mucopolysaccharidosis 277.5 [737.40]
      neurofibromatosis 237.71 [737.40]
      osteitis
        deformans 731.0 [737.40]
        fibrosa cystica 252.01 [737.40] ▲
      osteoporosis (*see also* Osteoporosis) 733.00 [737.40]

Curvature — *continued*
  spine — *continued*
    due to or associated with — *continued*
      poliomyelitis (*see also* Poliomyelitis) 138 [737.40]
      tuberculosis (Pott's curvature) (*see also* Tuberculosis) 015.0 ☑ [737.43]
    kyphoscoliotic (*see also* Kyphoscoliosis) 737.30
    kyphotic (*see also* Kyphosis) 737.10
    late effect of rickets 268.1 [737.40]
    Pott's 015.0 ☑ [737.40]
    scoliotic (*see also* Scoliosis) 737.30
    specified NEC 737.8
    tuberculous 015.0 ☑ [737.40]
Cushing's
  basophilism, disease, or syndrome (iatrogenic) (idiopathic) (pituitary basophilism) (pituitary dependent) 255.0
  ulcer — *see* Ulcer, peptic
Cushingoid due to steroid therapy
  correct substance properly administered 255.0
  overdose or wrong substance given or taken 962.0
Cut (external) — *see* Wound, open, by site
Cutaneous — *see also* condition
  hemorrhage 782.7
  horn (cheek) (eyelid) (mouth) 702.8
  larva migrans 126.9
Cutis — *see also* condition
  hyperelastic 756.83
    acquired 701.8
  laxa 756.83
    senilis 701.8
  marmorata 782.61
  osteosis 709.3
  pendula 756.83
    acquired 701.8
  rhomboidalis nuchae 701.8
  verticis gyrata 757.39
    acquired 701.8
Cyanopathy, newborn 770.83
Cyanosis 782.5
  autotoxic 289.7
  common atrioventricular canal 745.69
  congenital 770.83
  conjunctiva 372.71
  due to
    endocardial cushion defect 745.60
    nonclosure, foramen botalli 745.5
    patent foramen botalli 745.5
    persistent foramen ovale 745.5
  enterogenous 289.7
  fetus or newborn 770.83
  ostium primum defect 745.61
  paroxysmal digital 443.0
  retina, retinal 362.10
Cycle
  anovulatory 628.0
  menstrual, irregular 626.4
Cyclencephaly 759.89
Cyclical vomiting 536.2
  psychogenic 306.4
Cyclitic membrane 364.74
Cyclitis (*see also* Iridocyclitis) 364.3
  acute 364.00
    primary 364.01
    recurrent 364.02
  chronic 364.10
    in
      sarcoidosis 135 [364.11]
      tuberculosis (*see also* Tuberculosis) 017.3 ☑ [364.11]
  Fuchs' heterochromic 364.21
  granulomatous 364.10
  lens induced 364.23
  nongranulomatous 364.00
  posterior 363.21
  primary 364.01
  recurrent 364.02
  secondary (noninfectious) 364.04
    infectious 364.03
  subacute 364.00
    primary 364.01

Cyclitis (*see also* Iridocyclitis) — *continued*
  subacute — *continued*
    recurrent 364.02
Cyclokeratitis — *see* Keratitis
Cyclophoria 378.44
Cyclopia, cyclops 759.89
Cycloplegia 367.51
Cyclospasm 367.53
Cyclosporiasis 007.5
Cyclothymia 301.13
Cyclothymic personality 301.13
Cyclotropia 378.33
Cyesis — *see* Pregnancy
Cylindroma (M8200/3) — *see also* Neoplasm, by site, malignant
  eccrine dermal (M8200/0) — *see* Neoplasm, skin, benign
  skin (M8200/0) — *see* Neoplasm, skin, benign
Cylindruria 791.7
Cyllosoma 759.89
Cynanche
  diphtheritic 032.3
  tonsillaris 475
Cynorexia 783.6
Cyphosis — *see* Kyphosis
Cyprus fever (*see also* Brucellosis) 023.9
Cyriax's syndrome (slipping rib) 733.99
Cyst (mucus) (retention) (serous) (simple)

> *Note* — In general, cysts are not neoplastic and are classified to the approriate category for disease of the specified anatomical site. This generalization does not apply to certain types of cysts which are neoplastic in nature, for example, dermoid, nor does it apply to cysts of certain structures, for example, branchial cleft, which are classified as developmental anomalies.
>
> The following listing includes some of the most frequently reported sites of cysts as well as qualifiers which indicate the type of cyst. The latter qualifiers usually are not repeated under the anatomical sites. Since the code assignment for a given site may vary depending upon the type of cyst, the coder should refer to the listings under the specified type of cyst before consideration is given to the site.

  accessory, fallopian tube 752.11
  adenoid (infected) 474.8
  adrenal gland 255.8
    congenital 759.1
  air, lung 518.89
  allantoic 753.7
  alveolar process (jaw bone) 526.2
  amnion, amniotic 658.8 ☑
  anterior chamber (eye) 364.60
    exudative 364.62
    implantation (surgical) (traumatic) 364.61
    parasitic 360.13
  anterior nasopalatine 526.1
  antrum 478.1
  anus 569.49
  apical (periodontal) (tooth) 522.8
  appendix 543.9
  arachnoid, brain 348.0
  arytenoid 478.79
  auricle 706.2
  Baker's (knee) 727.51
    tuberculous (*see also* Tuberculosis) 015.2 ☑
  Bartholin's gland or duct 616.2
  bile duct (*see also* Disease, biliary) 576.8
  bladder (multiple) (trigone) 596.8
  Blessig's 362.62
  blood, endocardial (*see also* Endocarditis) 424.90
  blue dome 610.0
  bone (local) 733.20
    aneurysmal 733.22
    jaw 526.2
      developmental (odontogenic) 526.0
      fissural 526.1
      latent 526.89

Cyst — *continued*
  bone — *continued*
    solitary 733.21
    unicameral 733.21
  brain 348.0
    congenital 742.4
    hydatid (*see also* Echinococcus) 122.9
    third ventricle (colloid) 742.4
  branchial (cleft) 744.42
  branchiogenic 744.42
  breast (benign) (blue dome) (pedunculated)
      (solitary) (traumatic) 610.0
    involution 610.4
    sebaceous 610.8
  broad ligament (benign) 620.8
    embryonic 752.11
  bronchogenic (mediastinal) (sequestration)
      518.89
    congenital 748.4
  buccal 528.4
  bulbourethral gland (Cowper's) 599.89
  bursa, bursal 727.49
    pharyngeal 478.26
  calcifying odontogenic (M9301/0) 213.1
    upper jaw (bone) 213.0
  canal of Nuck (acquired) (serous) 629.1
    congenital 752.41
  canthus 372.75
  carcinomatous (M8010/3) — *see* Neoplasm, by
      site, malignant
  cartilage (joint) — *see* Derangement, joint
  cauda equina 336.8
  cavum septi pellucidi NEC 348.0
  celomic (pericardium) 746.89
  cerebellopontine (angle) — *see* Cyst, brain
  cerebellum — *see* Cyst, brain
  cerebral — *see* Cyst, brain
  cervical lateral 744.42
  cervix 622.8
    embryonal 752.41
    nabothian (gland) 616.0
  chamber, anterior (eye) 364.60
    exudative 364.62
    implantation (surgical) (traumatic) 364.61
    parasitic 360.13
  chiasmal, optic NEC (*see also* Lesion, chiasmal)
      377.54
  chocolate (ovary) 617.1
  choledochal (congenital) 751.69
    acquired 576.8
  choledochus 751.69
  chorion 658.8 ☑
  choroid plexus 348.0
  chyle, mesentery 457.8
  ciliary body 364.60
    exudative 364.64
    implantation 364.61
    primary 364.63
  clitoris 624.8
  coccyx (*see also* Cyst, bone) 733.20
  colloid
    third ventricle (brain) 742.4
    thyroid gland — *see* Goiter
  colon 569.89
  common (bile) duct (*see also* Disease, biliary)
      576.8
  congenital NEC 759.89
    adrenal glands 759.1
    epiglottis 748.3
    esophagus 750.4
    fallopian tube 752.11
    kidney 753.10
      multiple 753.19
      single 753.11
    larynx 748.3
    liver 751.62
    lung 748.4
    mediastinum 748.8
    ovary 752.0
    oviduct 752.11
    pancreas 751.7
    periurethral (tissue) 753.8
    prepuce NEC 752.69
      penis 752.69
    sublingual 750.26
    submaxillary gland 750.26
    thymus (gland) 759.2

Cyst — *continued*
  congenital NEC — *continued*
    tongue 750.19
    ureterovesical orifice 753.4
    vulva 752.41
  conjunctiva 372.75
  cornea 371.23
  corpora quadrigemina 348.0
  corpus
    albicans (ovary) 620.2
    luteum (ruptured) 620.1
  Cowper's gland (benign) (infected) 599.89
  cranial meninges 348.0
  craniobuccal pouch 253.8
  craniopharyngeal pouch 253.8
  cystic duct (*see also* Disease, gallbladder) 575.8
  Cysticercus (any site) 123.1
  Dandy-Walker 742.3
    with spina bifida (*see also* Spina bifida)
      741.0 ☑
  dental 522.8
    developmental 526.0
    eruption 526.0
    lateral periodontal 526.0
    primordial (keratocyst) 526.0
    root 522.8
  dentigerous 526.0
    mandible 526.0
    maxilla 526.0
  dermoid (M9084/0) — *see also* Neoplasm, by
      site, benign
    with malignant transformation (M9084/3)
      183.0
    implantation
      external area or site (skin) NEC 709.8
      iris 364.61
      skin 709.8
      vagina 623.8
      vulva 624.8
    mouth 528.4
    oral soft tissue 528.4
    sacrococcygeal 685.1
      with abscess 685.0
  developmental of ovary, ovarian 752.0
  dura (cerebral) 348.0
    spinal 349.2
  ear (external) 706.2
  echinococcal (*see also* Echinococcus) 122.9
  embryonal
    cervix uteri 752.41
    genitalia, female external 752.41
    uterus 752.3
    vagina 752.41
  endometrial 621.8
    ectopic 617.9
  endometrium (uterus) 621.8
    ectopic — *see* Endometriosis
  enteric 751.5
  enterogenous 751.5
  epidermal (inclusion) (*see also* Cyst, skin)
      706.2
  epidermoid (inclusion) (*see also* Cyst, skin)
      706.2
    mouth 528.4
    not of skin — *see* Cyst, by site
    oral soft tissue 528.4
  epididymis 608.89
  epiglottis 478.79
  epiphysis cerebri 259.8
  epithelial (inclusion) (*see also* Cyst, skin) 706.2
  epoophoron 752.11
  eruption 526.0
  esophagus 530.89
  ethmoid sinus 478.1
  eye (retention) 379.8
    congenital 743.03
    posterior segment, congenital 743.54
  eyebrow 706.2
  eyelid (sebaceous) 374.84
    infected 373.13
    sweat glands or ducts 374.84
  falciform ligament (inflammatory) 573.8
  fallopian tube 620.8
  female genital organs NEC 629.8
  fimbrial (congenital) 752.11
  fissural (oral region) 526.1

Cyst — *continued*
  follicle (atretic) (graafian) (ovarian) 620.0
    nabothian (gland) 616.0
  follicular (atretic) (ovarian) 620.0
    dentigerous 526.0
  frontal sinus 478.1
  gallbladder or duct 575.8
  ganglion 727.43
  Gartner's duct 752.11
  gas, of mesentery 568.89
  gingiva 523.8
  gland of moll 374.84
  globulomaxillary 526.1
  graafian follicle 620.0
  granulosal lutein 620.2
  hemangiomatous (M9121/0) (*see also*
      Hemangioma) 228.00
  hydatid (*see also* Echinococcus) 122.9
    fallopian tube (Morgagni) 752.11
    liver NEC 122.8
    lung NEC 122.9
    Morgagni 752.89
      fallopian tube 752.11
    specified site NEC 122.9
  hymen 623.8
    embryonal 752.41
  hypopharynx 478.26
  hypophysis, hypophyseal (duct) (recurrent)
      253.8
    cerebri 253.8
  implantation (dermoid)
    anterior chamber (eye) 364.61
    external area or site (skin) NEC 709.8
    iris 364.61
    vagina 623.8
    vulva 624.8
  incisor, incisive canal 526.1
  inclusion (epidermal) (epithelial) (epidermoid)
      (mucous) (squamous) (*see also* Cyst, skin)
      706.2
    not of skin — *see* Neoplasm, by site, benign
  intestine (large) (small) 569.89
  intracranial — *see* Cyst, brain
  intraligamentous 728.89
    knee 717.89
  intrasellar 253.8
  iris (idiopathic) 364.60
    exudative 364.62
    implantation (surgical) (traumatic) 364.61
    miotic pupillary 364.55
    parasitic 360.13
  Iwanoff's 362.62
  jaw (bone) (aneurysmal) (extravasation)
      (hemorrhagic) (traumatic) 526.2
    developmental (odontogenic) 526.0
    fissural 526.1
  keratin 706.2
  kidney (congenital) 753.10
    acquired 593.2
    calyceal (*see also* Hydronephrosis) 591
    multiple 753.19
    pyelogenic (*see also* Hydronephrosis) 591
    simple 593.2
    single 753.11
    solitary (not congenital) 593.2
  labium (majus) (minus) 624.8
    sebaceous 624.8
  lacrimal
    apparatus 375.43
    gland or sac 375.12
  larynx 478.79
  lens 379.39
    congenital 743.39
  lip (gland) 528.5
  liver 573.8
    congenital 751.62
    hydatid (*see also* Echinococcus) 122.8
      granulosis 122.0
      multilocularis 122.5
  lung 518.89
    congenital 748.4
    giant bullous 492.0
  lutein 620.1
  lymphangiomatous (M9173/0) 228.1
  lymphoepithelial
    mouth 528.4
    oral soft tissue 528.4

Cyst — *continued*
macula 362.54
malignant (M8000/3) — *see* Neoplasm, by site,
    malignant
mammary gland (sweat gland) (*see also* Cyst,
    breast) 610.0
mandible 526.2
    dentigerous 526.0
    radicular 522.8
maxilla 526.2
    dentigerous 526.0
    radicular 522.8
median
    anterior maxillary 526.1
    palatal 526.1
mediastinum (congenital) 748.8
meibomian (gland) (retention) 373.2
    infected 373.12
membrane, brain 348.0
meninges (cerebral) 348.0
    spinal 349.2
meniscus knee 717.5
mesentery, mesenteric (gas) 568.89
    chyle 457.8
    gas 568.89
mesonephric duct 752.89
mesothelial
    peritoneum 568.89
    pleura (peritoneal) 569.89
milk 611.5
miotic pupillary (iris) 364.55
Morgagni (hydatid) 752.89
    fallopian tube 752.11
mouth 528.4
mullerian duct 752.89
multilocular (ovary) (M8000/1) 239.5
myometrium 621.8
nabothian (follicle) (ruptured) 616.0
nasal sinus 478.1
nasoalveolar 528.4
nasolabial 528.4
nasopalatine (duct) 526.1
    anterior 526.1
nasopharynx 478.26
neoplastic (M8000/1) — *see also* Neoplasm, by
    site, unspecified nature
    benign (M8000/0) — *see* Neoplasm, by site,
        benign
    uterus 621.8
nervous system — *see* Cyst, brain
neuroenteric 742.59
neuroepithelial ventricle 348.0
nipple 610.0
nose 478.1
    skin of 706.2
odontogenic, developmental 526.0
omentum (lesser) 568.89
    congenital 751.8
oral soft tissue (dermoid) (epidermoid)
    (lymphoepithelial) 528.4
ora serrata 361.19
orbit 376.81
ovary, ovarian (twisted) 620.2
    adherent 620.2
    chocolate 617.1
    corpus
        albicans 620.2
        luteum 620.1
    dermoid (M9084/0) 220
    developmental 752.0
    due to failure of involution NEC 620.2
    endometrial 617.1
    follicular (atretic) (graafian) (hemorrhagic)
        620.0
    hemorrhagic 620.2
    in pregnancy or childbirth 654.4 ☑
        affecting fetus or newborn 763.89
        causing obstructed labor 660.2 ☑
            affecting fetus or newborn 763.1
    multilocular (M8000/1) 239.5
    pseudomucinous (M8470/0) 220
    retention 620.2
    serous 620.2
    theca lutein 620.2
    tuberculous (*see also* Tuberculosis) 016.6 ☑
    unspecified 620.2
oviduct 620.8

Cyst — *continued*
palatal papilla (jaw) 526.1
palate 526.1
    fissural 526.1
    median (fissural) 526.1
palatine, of papilla 526.1
pancreas, pancreatic 577.2
    congenital 751.7
    false 577.2
    hemorrhagic 577.2
    true 577.2
paranephric 593.2
para ovarian 752.11
paraphysis, cerebri 742.4
parasitic NEC 136.9
parathyroid (gland) 252.8
paratubal (fallopian) 620.8
paraurethral duct 599.89
paroophoron 752.11
parotid gland 527.6
    mucous extravasation or retention 527.6
parovarian 752.11
pars planus 364.60
    exudative 364.64
    primary 364.63
pelvis, female
    in pregnancy or childbirth 654.4 ☑
        affecting fetus or newborn 763.89
        causing obstructed labor 660.2 ☑
            affecting fetus or newborn 763.1
penis (sebaceous) 607.89
periapical 522.8
pericardial (congenital) 746.89
    acquired (secondary) 423.8
pericoronal 526.0
perineural (Tarlov's) 355.9
periodontal 522.8
    lateral 526.0
peripancreatic 577.2
peripelvic (lymphatic) 593.2
peritoneum 568.89
    chylous 457.8
pharynx (wall) 478.26
pilonidal (infected) (rectum) 685.1
    with abscess 685.0
    malignant (M9084/3) 173.5
pituitary (duct) (gland) 253.8
placenta (amniotic) — *see* Placenta, abnormal
pleura 519.8
popliteal 727.51
porencephalic 742.4
    acquired 348.0
postanal (infected) 685.1
    with abscess 685.0
posterior segment of eye, congenital 743.54
postmastoidectomy cavity 383.31
preauricular 744.47
prepuce 607.89
    congenital 752.69
primordial (jaw) 526.0
prostate 600.3
pseudomucinous (ovary) (M8470/0) 220
pudenda (sweat glands) 624.8
pupillary, miotic 364.55
    sebaceous 624.8
radicular (residual) 522.8
radiculodental 522.8
ranular 527.6
Rathke's pouch 253.8
rectum (epithelium) (mucous) 569.49
renal — *see* Cyst, kidney
residual (radicular) 522.8
retention (ovary) 620.2
retina 361.19
    macular 362.54
    parasitic 360.13
    primary 361.13
    secondary 361.14
retroperitoneal 568.89
sacrococcygeal (dermoid) 685.1
    with abscess 685.0
salivary gland or duct 527.6
    mucous extravasation or retention 527.6
Sampson's 617.1
sclera 379.19
scrotum (sebaceous) 706.2
    sweat glands 706.2

Cyst — *continued*
sebaceous (duct) (gland) 706.2
    breast 610.8
    eyelid 374.84
    genital organ NEC
        female 629.8
        male 608.89
    scrotum 706.2
semilunar cartilage (knee) (multiple) 717.5
seminal vesicle 608.89
serous (ovary) 620.2
sinus (antral) (ethmoidal) (frontal) (maxillary)
    (nasal) (sphenoidal) 478.1
Skene's gland 599.89
skin (epidermal) (epidermoid, inclusion)
    (epithelial) (inclusion) (retention)
    (sebaceous) 706.2
    breast 610.8
    eyelid 374.84
    genital organ NEC
        female 629.8
        male 608.89
    neoplastic 216.3
    scrotum 706.2
    sweat gland or duct 705.89
solitary
    bone 733.21
    kidney 593.2
spermatic cord 608.89
sphenoid sinus 478.1
spinal meninges 349.2
spine (*see also* Cyst, bone) 733.20
spleen NEC 289.59
    congenital 759.0
    hydatid (*see also* Echinococcus) 122.9
spring water (pericardium) 746.89
subarachnoid 348.0
    intrasellar 793.0
subdural (cerebral) 348.0
    spinal cord 349.2
sublingual gland 527.6
    mucous extravasation or retention 527.6
submaxillary gland 527.6
    mucous extravasation or retention 527.6
suburethral 599.89
suprarenal gland 255.8
suprasellar — *see* Cyst, brain
sweat gland or duct 705.89
sympathetic nervous system 337.9
synovial 727.40
    popliteal space 727.51
Tarlov's 355.9
tarsal 373.2
tendon (sheath) 727.42
testis 608.89
theca-lutein (ovary) 620.2
Thornwaldt's, Tornwaldt's 478.26
thymus (gland) 254.8
thyroglossal (duct) (infected) (persistent) 759.2
thyroid (gland) 246.2
    adenomatous — *see* Goiter, nodular
    colloid (*see also* Goiter) 240.9
thyrolingual duct (infected) (persistent) 759.2
tongue (mucous) 529.8
tonsil 474.8
tooth (dental root) 522.8
tubo-ovarian 620.8
    inflammatory 614.1
tunica vaginalis 608.89
turbinate (nose) (*see also* Cyst, bone) 733.20
Tyson's gland (benign) (infected) 607.89
umbilicus 759.89
urachus 753.7
ureter 593.89
ureterovesical orifice 593.89
    congenital 753.4
urethra 599.84
urethral gland (Cowper's) 599.89
uterine
    ligament 620.8
        embryonic 752.11
    tube 620.8
uterus (body) (corpus) (recurrent) 621.8
    embryonal 752.3
utricle (ear) 386.8
    prostatic 599.89
utriculus masculinus 599.89

☑ Additional Digit Required   ▶◀ Revised Text   ● New Line   ▲ Revised Code

Cyst — Cystitis

Cystitis — *continued*
 echinococcal
  granulosus 122.3 *[595.4]*
  multilocularis 122.6 *[595.4]*
 emphysematous 595.89
 encysted 595.81
 follicular 595.3
 following
  abortion 639.8
  ectopic or molar pregnancy 639.8
 gangrenous 595.89
 glandularis 595.89
 gonococcal (acute) 098.11
  chronic or duration of 2 months or more
   098.31
 incrusted 595.89
 interstitial 595.1
 irradiation 595.82
 irritation 595.89
 malignant 595.89
 monilial 112.2
 of trigone 595.3
 panmural 595.1
 polyposa 595.89
 prostatic 601.3
 radiation 595.82
 Reiter's (abacterial) 099.3
 specified NEC 595.89
 subacute 595.2
 submucous 595.1
 syphilitic 095.8
 trichomoniasis 131.09
 tuberculous (*see also* Tuberculosis) 016.1 ☑
 ulcerative 595.1
Cystocele (-rectocele)
 female (without uterine prolapse) 618.01 ▲
  with uterine prolapse 618.4
   complete 618.3
   incomplete 618.2
  lateral 618.02   ●
  midline 618.01   ●
  paravaginal 618.02   ●
 in pregnancy or childbirth 654.4 ☑
  affecting fetus or newborn 763.89
  causing obstructed labor 660.2 ☑
   affecting fetus or newborn 763.1
 male 596.8
Cystoid
 cicatrix limbus 372.64
 degeneration macula 362.53
Cystolithiasis 594.1
Cystoma (M8440/0) — *see also* Neoplasm, by
  site, benign
 endometrial, ovary 617.1
 mucinous (M8470/0)
  specified site — *see* Neoplasm, by site,
   benign
  unspecified site 220
 serous (M8441/0)
  specified site — *see* Neoplasm, by site,
   benign
  unspecified site 220
 simple (ovary) 620.2
Cystoplegia 596.53
Cystoptosis 596.8
Cystopyelitis (*see also* Pyelitis) 590.80
Cystorrhagia 596.8
Cystosarcoma phyllodes (M9020/1) 238.3
 benign (M9020/0) 217
 malignant (M9020/3) — *see* Neoplasm, breast,
  malignant
Cystostomy status V44.50
 appendico-vesicostomy V44.52
 cutaneous-vesicostomy V44.51
 specified type NEC V44.59
 with complication 997.5
Cystourethritis (*see also* Urethritis) 597.89
Cystourethrocele (*see also* Cystocele)
 female (without uterine prolapse) 618.09 ▲
  with uterine prolapse 618.4
   complete 618.3
   incomplete 618.2
 male 596.8

Cytomegalic inclusion disease 078.5
 congenital 771.1
Cytomycosis, reticuloendothelial (*see also*
  Histoplasmosis, American) 115.00
Cytopenia 289.9   ●

☑ Additional Digit Required   ►◄ Revised Text   ● New Line   ▲ Revised Code

D

Daae (-Finsen) disease (epidemic pleurodynia) 074.1

Dabney's grip 074.1

Da Costa's syndrome (neurocirculatory asthenia) 306.2

Dacryoadenitis, dacryadenitis 375.00
  acute 375.01
  chronic 375.02

Dacryocystitis 375.30
  acute 375.32
  chronic 375.42
  neonatal 771.6
  phlegmonous 375.33
  syphilitic 095.8
    congenital 090.0
  trachomatous, active 076.1
    late effect 139.1
  tuberculous (*see also* Tuberculosis) 017.3 ☑

Dacryocystoblenorrhea 375.42

Dacryocystocele 375.43

Dacryolith, dacryolithiasis 375.57

Dacryoma 375.43

Dacryopericystitis (acute) (subacute) 375.32
  chronic 375.42

Dacryops 375.11

Dacryosialadenopathy, atrophic 710.2

Dacryostenosis 375.56
  congenital 743.65

Dactylitis 686.9
  bone (*see also* Osteomyelitis) 730.2 ☑
  sickle cell 282.61
  syphilitic 095.5
  tuberculous (*see also* Tuberculosis) 015.5 ☑

Dactylolysis opontaned 136.0

Dactylosymphysis (*see also* Syndactylism) 755.10

Damage
  arteriosclerotic — *see* Arteriosclerosis
  brain 348.9
    anoxic, hypoxic 348.1
      during or resulting from a procedure 997.01
    child NEC 343.9
    due to birth injury 767.0
    minimal (child) (*see also* Hyperkinesia) 314.9
    newborn 767.0
  cardiac — *see also* Disease, heart
  cardiorenal (vascular) (*see also* Hypertension, cardiorenal) 404.90
  central nervous system — *see* Damage, brain
  cerebral NEC — *see* Damage, brain
  coccyx, complicating delivery 665.6 ☑
  coronary (*see also* Ischemia, heart) 414.9
  eye, birth injury 767.8
  heart — *see also* Disease, heart
    valve — *see* Endocarditis
  hypothalamus NEC 348.9
  liver 571.9
    alcoholic 571.3
  myocardium (*see also* Degeneration, myocardial) 429.1
  pelvic
    joint or ligament, during delivery 665.6 ☑
    organ NEC
      with
        abortion — *see* Abortion, by type, with damage to pelvic organs
        ectopic pregnancy (*see also* categories 633.0-633.9) 639.2
        molar pregnancy (*see also* categories 630-632) 639.2
      during delivery 665.5 ☑
      following
        abortion 639.2
        ectopic or molar pregnancy 639.2
  renal (*see also* Disease, renal) 593.9
  skin, solar 692.79
    acute 692.72
    chronic 692.74
  subendocardium, subendocardial (*see also* Degeneration, myocardial) 429.1
  vascular 459.9

Dameshek's syndrome (erythroblastic anemia) 282.49

Dana-Putnam syndrome (subacute combined sclerosis with pernicious anemia) 281.0 *[336.2]*

Danbolt (-Closs) syndrome (acrodermatitis enteropathica) 686.8

Dandruff 690.18

Dandy fever 061

Dandy-Walker deformity or syndrome (atresia, foramen of Magendie) 742.3
  with spina bifida (*see also* Spina bifida) 741.0 ☑

Dangle foot 736.79

Danielssen's disease (anesthetic leprosy) 030.1

Danlos' syndrome 756.83

Darier's disease (congenital) (keratosis follicularis) 757.39
  due to vitamin A deficiency 264.8
  meaning erythema annulare centrifugum 695.0

Darier-Roussy sarcoid 135

Darling's
  disease (*see also* Histoplasmosis, American) 115.00
  histoplasmosis (*see also* Histoplasmosis, American) 115.00

Dartre 054.9

Darwin's tubercle 744.29

Davidson's anemia (refractory) 284.9

Davies' disease 425.0

Davies-Colley syndrome (slipping rib) 733.99

Dawson's encephalitis 046.2

Day blindness (*see also* Blindness, day) 368.60

Dead
  fetus
    retained (in utero) 656.4 ☑
      early pregnancy (death before 22 completed weeks gestation) 632
      late (death after 22 completed weeks gestation) 656.4 ☑
    syndrome 641.3 ☑
  labyrinth 386.50
  ovum, retained 631

Deaf and dumb NEC 389.7

Deaf mutism (acquired) (congenital) NEC 389.7
  endemic 243
  hysterical 300.11
  syphilitic, congenital 090.0

Deafness (acquired) (bilateral) (both ears) (complete) (congenital) (hereditary) (middle ear) (partial) (unilateral) 389.9
  with blue sclera and fragility of bone 756.51
  auditory fatigue 389.9
  aviation 993.0
    nerve injury 951.5
  boilermakers' 951.5
  central 389.14
    with conductive hearing loss 389.2
  conductive (air) 389.00
    with sensorineural hearing loss 389.2
    combined types 389.08
    external ear 389.01
    inner ear 389.04
    middle ear 389.03
    multiple types 389.08
    tympanic membrane 389.02
  emotional (complete) 300.11
  functional (complete) 300.11
  high frequency 389.8
  hysterical (complete) 300.11
  injury 951.5
  low frequency 389.8
  mental 784.69
  mixed conductive and sensorineural 389.2
  nerve 389.12
    with conductive hearing loss 389.2
  neural 389.12
    with conductive hearing loss 389.2
  noise-induced 388.12
    nerve injury 951.5
  nonspeaking 389.7

Deafness — *continued*
  perceptive 389.10
    with conductive hearing loss 389.2
    central 389.14
    combined types 389.18
    multiple types 389.18
    neural 389.12
    sensory 389.11
  psychogenic (complete) 306.7
  sensorineural (*see also* Deafness, perceptive) 389.10
  sensory 389.11
    with conductive hearing loss 389.2
  specified type NEC 389.8
  sudden NEC 388.2
  syphilitic 094.89
  transient ischemic 388.02
  transmission — *see* Deafness, conductive
  traumatic 951.5
  word (secondary to organic lesion) 784.69
    developmental 315.31

Death
  after delivery (cause not stated) (sudden) 674.9 ☑
  anesthetic
    due to
      correct substance properly administered 995.4
      overdose or wrong substance given 968.4
        specified anesthetic — *see* Table of Drugs and Chemicals
    during delivery 668.9 ☑
  brain 348.8
  cardiac — *see* Disease, heart
  cause unknown 798.2
  cot (infant) 798.0
  crib (infant) 798.0
  fetus, fetal (cause not stated) (intrauterine) 779.9
    early, with retention (before 22 completed weeks gestation) 632
    from asphyxia or anoxia (before labor) 768.0
      during labor 768.1
    late, affecting management of pregnancy (after 22 completed weeks gestation) 656.4 ☑
  from pregnancy NEC 646.9 ☑
  instantaneous 798.1
  intrauterine (*see also* Death, fetus) 779.9
    complicating pregnancy 656.4 ☑
  maternal, affecting fetus or newborn 761.6
  neonatal NEC 779.9
  sudden (cause unknown) 798.1
    during delivery 669.9 ☑
      under anesthesia NEC 668.9 ☑
    infant, syndrome (SIDS) 798.0
    puerperal, during puerperium 674.9 ☑
  unattended (cause unknown) 798.9
  under anesthesia NEC
    due to
      correct substance properly administered 995.4
      overdose or wrong substance given 968.4
        specified anesthetic — *see* Table of Drugs and Chemicals
    during delivery 668.9 ☑
  violent 798.1

de Beurmann-Gougerot disease (sporotrichosis) 117.1

Debility (general) (infantile) (postinfectional) 799.3
  with nutritional difficulty 269.9
  congenital or neonatal NEC 779.9
  nervous 300.5
  old age 797
  senile 797

Débove's disease (splenomegaly) 789.2

Decalcification
  bone (*see also* Osteoporosis) 733.00
  teeth 521.8

Decapitation 874.9
  fetal (to facilitate delivery) 763.89

Decapsulation, kidney 593.89

Decay
  dental 521.00
  senile 797
  tooth, teeth 521.00

☑ Additional Digit Required   ▶◀ Revised Text   ● New Line   ▲ Revised Code

Decensus, uterus — *see* Prolapse, uterus
Deciduitis (acute)
  with
    abortion — *see* Abortion, by type, with sepsis
    ectopic pregnancy (*see also* categories
      633.0-633.9) 639.0
    molar pregnancy (*see also* categories 630-
      632) 639.0
  affecting fetus or newborn 760.8
  following
    abortion 639.0
    ectopic or molar pregnancy 639.0
  in pregnancy 646.6 ☑
  puerperal, postpartum 670.0 ☑
Deciduoma malignum (M9100/3) 181
Deciduous tooth (retained) 520.6
Decline (general) (*see also* Debility) 799.3
Decompensation
  cardiac (acute) (chronic) (*see also* Disease,
    heart) 429.9
    failure — *see* Failure, heart
  cardiorenal (*see also* Hypertension, cardiorenal)
    404.90
  cardiovascular (*see also* Disease,
    cardiovascular) 429.2
  heart (*see also* Disease, heart) 429.9
    failure — *see* Failure, heart
  hepatic 572.2
  myocardial (acute) (chronic) (*see also* Disease,
    heart) 429.9
    failure — *see* Failure, heart
  respiratory 519.9
Decompression sickness 993.3
Decrease, decreased
  blood
    platelets (*see also* Thrombocytopenia) 287.5
    pressure 796.3
      due to shock following
        injury 958.4
        operation 998.0
  cardiac reserve — *see* Disease, heart
  estrogen 256.39
    postablative 256.2
  fetal movements 655.7 ☑
  fragility of erythrocytes 289.89
  function
    adrenal (cortex) 255.4
      medulla 255.5
    ovary in hypopituitarism 253.4
    parenchyma of pancreas 577.8
    pituitary (gland) (lobe) (anterior) 253.2
      posterior (lobe) 253.8
  functional activity 780.99
  glucose 790.29
  haptoglobin (serum) NEC 273.8
  libido 799.81
  platelets (*see also* Thrombocytopenia) 287.5
  pulse pressure 785.9
  respiration due to shock following injury 958.4
  sexual desire 799.81
  tear secretion NEC 375.15
  tolerance
    fat 579.8
    salt and water 276.9
  vision NEC 369.9
Decubital gangrene 707.00 *[785.4]* ▲
Decubiti (*see also* Decubitus) 707.00 ▲
Decubitus (ulcer) 707.00 ▲
  with gangrene 707.00 *[785.4]* ▲
  ankle 707.06 ●
  back ●
    lower 707.03 ●
    upper 707.02 ●
  buttock 707.05 ●
  elbow 707.01 ●
  head 707.09 ●
  heel 707.07 ●
  hip 707.04 ●
  other site 707.09 ●
  sacrum 707.03 ●
  shoulder blades 707.02 ●
Deepening acetabulum 718.85
Defect, defective 759.9
  3-beta-hydroxysteroid dehydrogenase 255.2
  11-hydroxylase 255.2

Defect, defective — *continued*
  21-hydroxylase 255.2
  abdominal wall, congenital 756.70
  aorticopulmonary septum 745.0
  aortic septal 745.0
  atrial septal (ostium secundum type) 745.5
    acquired 429.71
    ostium primum type 745.61
    sinus venosus 745.8
  atrioventricular
    canal 745.69
    septum 745.4
      acquired 429.71
  atrium secundum 745.5
    acquired 429.71
  auricular septal 745.5
    acquired 429.71
  bilirubin excretion 277.4
  biosynthesis, testicular androgen 257.2
  bulbar septum 745.0
  butanol-insoluble iodide 246.1
  chromosome — *see* Anomaly, chromosome
  circulation (acquired) 459.9
    congenital 747.9
    newborn 747.9
  clotting NEC (*see also* Defect, coagulation)
    286.9
  coagulation (factor) (*see also* Deficiency,
    coagulation factor) 286.9
    with
      abortion — *see* Abortion, by type, with
        hemorrhage
      ectopic pregnancy (*see also* categories
        634-638) 639.1
      molar pregnancy (*see also* categories
        630-632) 639.1
    acquired (any) 286.7
    antepartum or intrapartum 641.3 ☑
      affecting fetus or newborn 762.1
    causing hemorrhage of pregnancy or delivery
      641.3 ☑
    due to
      liver disease 286.7
      vitamin K deficiency 286.7
    newborn, transient 776.3
    postpartum 666.3 ☑
    specified type NEC 286.3
  conduction (heart) 426.9
    bone (*see also* Deafness, conductive) 389.00
  congenital, organ or site NEC — *see also*
    Anomaly
    circulation 747.9
    Descemet's membrane 743.9
      specified type NEC 743.49
    diaphragm 756.6
    ectodermal 757.9
    esophagus 750.9
    pulmonic cusps — *see* Anomaly, heart valve
    respiratory system 748.9
      specified type NEC 748.8
  cushion endocardial 745.60
  dentin (hereditary) 520.5
  Descemet's membrane (congenital) 743.9
    acquired 371.30
    specific type NEC 743.49
  deutan 368.52
  developmental — *see also* Anomaly, by site
    cauda equina 742.59
    left ventricle 746.9
      with atresia or hypoplasia of aortic orifice
        or valve, with hypoplasia of
        ascending aorta 746.7
      in hypoplastic left heart syndrome 746.7
    testis 752.9
    vessel 747.9
  diaphragm
    with elevation, eventration, or hernia — *see*
      Hernia, diaphragm
    congenital 756.6
      with elevation, eventration, or hernia
        756.6
      gross (with elevation, eventration, or
        hernia) 756.6
  ectodermal, congenital 757.9
  Eisenmenger's (ventricular septal defect) 745.4
  endocardial cushion 745.60
    specified type NEC 745.69

Defect, defective — *continued*
  esophagus, congenital 750.9
  extensor retinaculum 728.9
  fibrin polymerization (*see also* Defect,
    coagulation) 286.3
  filling
    biliary tract 793.3
    bladder 793.5
    gallbladder 793.3
    kidney 793.5
    stomach 793.4
    ureter 793.5
  fossa ovalis 745.5
  gene, carrier (suspected) of V83.89
  Gerbode 745.4
  glaucomatous, without elevated tension 365.89
  Hageman (factor) (*see also* Defect, coagulation)
    286.3
  hearing (*see also* Deafness) 389.9
  high grade 317
  homogentisic acid 270.2
  interatrial septal 745.5
    acquired 429.71
  interauricular septal 745.5
    acquired 429.71
  interventricular septal 745.4
    with pulmonary stenosis or atresia,
      dextraposition of aorta, and
      hypertrophy of right ventricle 745.2
    acquired 429.71
    in tetralogy of Fallot 745.2
  iodide trapping 246.1
  iodotyrosine dehalogenase 246.1
  kynureninase 270.2
  learning, specific 315.2
  mental (*see also* Retardation, mental) 319
  osteochondral NEC 738.8
  ostium
    primum 745.61
    secundum 745.5
  pericardium 746.89
  peroxidase-binding 246.1
  placental blood supply — *see* Placenta,
    insufficiency
  platelet (qualitative) 287.1
    constitutional 286.4
  postural, spine 737.9
  protan 368.51
  pulmonic cusps, congenital 746.00
  renal pelvis 753.9
    obstructive 753.29
    specified type NEC 753.3
  respiratory system, congenital 748.9
    specified type NEC 748.8
  retina, retinal 361.30
    with detachment (*see also* Detachment,
      retina, with retinal defect) 361.00
    multiple 361.33
      with detachment 361.02
    nerve fiber bundle 362.85
    single 361.30
      with detachment 361.01
  septal (closure) (heart) NEC 745.9
    acquired 429.71
    atrial 745.5
    specified type NEC 745.8
  speech NEC 784.5
    developmental 315.39
    secondary to organic lesion 784.5
  Taussig-Bing (transposition, aorta and
    overriding pulmonary artery) 745.11
  teeth, wedge 521.20 ▲
  thyroid hormone synthesis 246.1
  tritan 368.53
  ureter 753.9
    obstructive 753.29
  vascular (acquired) (local) 459.9
    congenital (peripheral) NEC 747.60
      gastrointestinal 747.61
      lower limb 747.64
      renal 747.62
      specified NEC 747.69
      spinal 747.82
      upper limb 747.63

Decensus, uterus — Defect, defective

Defect, defective — *continued*
 ventricular septal 745.4
  with pulmonary stenosis or atresia,
   dextraposition of aorta, and
   hypertrophy of right ventricle 745.2
  acquired 429.71
  atrioventricular canal type 745.69
  between infundibulum and anterior portion
   745.4
  in tetralogy of Fallot 745.2
  isolated anterior 745.4
 vision NEC 369.9
 visual field 368.40
  arcuate 368.43
  heteronymous, bilateral 368.47
  homonymous, bilateral 368.46
 visual field — *continued*
  localized NEC 368.44
  nasal step 368.44
  peripheral 368.44
  sector 368.43
 voice 784.40
 wedge, teeth (abrasion) 521.20   ▲

Defeminization syndrome 255.2
Deferentitis 608.4
 gonorrheal (acute) 098.14
  chronic or duration of 2 months or over
   098.34
Defibrination syndrome (*see also* Fibrinolysis)
 286.6
Deficiency, deficient
 3-beta-hydroxysteroid dehydrogenase 255.2
 6-phosphogluconic dehydrogenase (anemia)
  282.2
 11-beta-hydroxylase 255.2
 17-alpha-hydroxylase 255.2
 18-hydroxysteroid dehydrogenase 255.2
 20-alpha-hydroxylase 255.2
 21-hydroxylase 255.2
 AAT (alpha-1 antitrypsin) 273.4   ●
 abdominal muscle syndrome 756.79
 accelerator globulin (Ac G) (blood) (*see also*
  Defect, coagulation) 286.3
 AC globulin (congenital) (*see also* Defect,
  coagulation) 286.3
  acquired 286.7
 activating factor (blood) (*see also* Defect,
  coagulation) 286.3
 adenohypophyseal 253.2
 adenosine deaminase 277.2
 aldolase (hereditary) 271.2
 alpha-1-antitrypsin 273.4   ▲
 alpha-1-trypsin inhibitor 273.4   ▲
 alpha-fucosidase 271.8
 alpha-lipoprotein 272.5
 alpha-mannosidase 271.8
 amino acid 270.9
 anemia — *see* Anemia, deficiency
 aneurin 265.1
  with beriberi 265.0
 antibody NEC 279.00
 antidiuretic hormone 253.5
 antihemophilic
  factor (A) 286.0
   B 286.1
   C 286.2
  globulin (AHG) NEC 286.0
 antithrombin III 289.81
 antitrypsin 273.4   ▲
 argininosuccinate synthetase or lyase 270.6
 ascorbic acid (with scurvy) 267
 autoprothrombin
  I (*see also* Defect, coagulation) 286.3
  II 286.1
  C (*see also* Defect, coagulation) 286.3
 bile salt 579.8
 biotin 266.2
 biotinidase 277.6
 bradykinase-1 277.6
 brancher enzyme (amylopectinosis) 271.0
 calciferol 268.9
  with
   osteomalacia 268.2
   rickets (*see also* Rickets) 268.0
 calcium 275.40
  dietary 269.3

Deficiency, deficient — *continued*
 calorie, severe 261
 carbamyl phosphate synthetase 270.6
 cardiac (*see also* Insufficiency, myocardial)
  428.0
 carnitine 277.81
  due to
   hemodialysis 277.83
   inborn errors of metabolism 277.82
   valproic acid therapy 277.83
  iatrogenic 277.83
  palmitoyltransferase (CPT1, CPT2) 277.85 ●
  palmityl transferase ▶(CPT1, CPT2)◀   ▲
   277.85
  primary 277.81
  secondary 277.84
 carotene 264.9
 Carr factor (*see also* Defect, coagulation) 286.9
 central nervous system 349.9
 ceruloplasmin 275.1
 cevitamic acid (with scurvy) 267
 choline 266.2
 Christmas factor 286.1
 chromium 269.3
 citrin 269.1
 clotting (blood) (*see also* Defect, coagulation)
  286.9
 coagulation factor NEC 286.9
  with
   abortion — *see* Abortion, by type, with
    hemorrhage
   ectopic pregnancy (*see also* categories
    634-638) 639.1
   molar pregnancy (*see also* categories 630-
    632) 639.1
  acquired (any) 286.7
  antepartum or intrapartum 641.3 ☑
   affecting fetus or newborn 762.1
  due to
   liver disease 286.7
   vitamin K deficiency 286.7
  newborn, transient 776.3
  postpartum 666.3 ☑
  specified type NEC 286.3
 color vision (congenital) 368.59
  acquired 368.55
 combined, two or more coagulation factors (*see
  also* Defect, coagulation) 286.9
 complement factor NEC 279.8
 contact factor (*see also* Defect, coagulation)
  286.3
 copper NEC 275.1
 corticoadrenal 255.4
 craniofacial axis 756.0
 cyanocobalamin (vitamin B_{12}) 266.2
 debrancher enzyme (limit dextrinosis) 271.0
 desmolase 255.2
 diet 269.9
 dihydrofolate reductase 281.2
 dihydropteridine reductase 270.1
 disaccharidase (intestinal) 271.3
 disease NEC 269.9
 ear(s) V48.8
 edema 262
 endocrine 259.9
 enzymes, circulating NEC (*see also* Deficiency,
  by specific enzyme) 277.6
 ergosterol 268.9
  with
   osteomalacia 268.2
   rickets (*see also* Rickets) 268.0
 erythrocytic glutathione (anemia) 282.2
 eyelid(s) V48.8
 factor (*See also* Defect, coagulation) 286.9
  I (congenital) (fibrinogen) 286.3
   antepartum or intrapartum 641.3 ☑
    affecting fetus or newborn 762.1
   newborn, transient 776.3
   postpartum 666.3 ☑
  II (congenital) (prothrombin) 286.3
  V (congenital) (labile) 286.3
  VII (congenital) (stable) 286.3
  VIII (congenital) (functional) 286.0
   with
    functional defect 286.0
    vascular defect 286.4
  IX (Christmas) (congenital) (functional) 286.1

Deficiency, deficient — *continued*
 factor (*See also* Defect, coagulation) —
  continued
  X (congenital) (Stuart-Prower) 286.3
  XI (congenital) (plasma thromboplastin
   antecedent) 286.2
  XII (congenital) (Hageman) 286.3
  XIII (congenital) (fibrin stabilizing) 286.3
  Hageman 286.3
  multiple (congenital) 286.9
   acquired 286.7
 fibrinase (*see also* Defect, coagulation) 286.3
 fibrinogen (congenital) (*see also* Defect,
  coagulation) 286.3
  acquired 286.6
 fibrin-stabilizing factor (congenital) (*see also*
  Defect, coagulation) 286.3
 finger — *see* Absence, finger
 fletcher factor (*see also* Defect, coagulation)
  286.9
 fluorine 269.3
 folate, anemia 281.2
 folic acid (vitamin B_6) 266.2
  anemia 281.2
 fructokinase 271.2
 fructose-1, 6-diphosphate 271.2
 fructose-1-phosphate aldolase 271.2
 FSH (follicle-stimulating hormone) 253.4
 fucosidase 271.8
 galactokinase 271.1
 galactose-1-phosphate uridyl transferase 271.1
 gamma globulin in blood 279.00
 glass factor (*see also* Defect, coagulation) 286.3
 glucocorticoid 255.4
 glucose-6-phosphatase 271.0
 glucose-6-phosphate dehydrogenase anemia
  282.2
 glucuronyl transferase 277.4
 glutathione-reductase (anemia) 282.2
 glycogen synthetase 271.0
 growth hormone 253.3
 Hageman factor (congenital) (*see also* Defect,
  coagulation) 286.3
 head V48.0
 hemoglobin (*see also* Anemia) 285.9
 hepatophosphorylase 271.0
 hexose monophosphate (HMP) shunt 282.2
 HGH (human growth hormone) 253.3
 HG-PRT 277.2
 homogentisic acid oxidase 270.2
 hormone — *see also* Deficiency, by specific
  hormone
  anterior pituitary (isolated) (partial) NEC
   253.4
   growth (human) 253.3
  follicle-stimulating 253.4
  growth (human) (isolated) 253.3
  human growth 253.3
  interstitial cell-stimulating 253.4
  luteinizing 253.4
  melanocyte-stimulating 253.4
  testicular 257.2
 human growth hormone 253.3
 humoral 279.00
  with
   hyper-IgM 279.05
    autosomal recessive 279.05
    X-linked 279.05
   increased IgM 279.05
  congenital hypogammaglobulinemia 279.04
  non-sex-linked 279.06
  selective immunoglobulin NEC 279.03
   IgA 279.01
   IgG 279.03
   IgM 279.02
    increased 279.05
  specified NEC 279.09
 hydroxylase 255.2
 hypoxanthine-guanine
  phosphoribosyltransferase (HG-PRT) 277.2
 ICSH (interstitial cell-stimulating hormone)
  253.4
 immunity NEC 279.3
  cell-mediated 279.10
   with
    hyperimmunoglob-ulinemia 279.2
    thrombocytopenia and eczema 279.12

Defect, defective — Deficiency, deficient

Deficiency, deficient — *continued*
  immunity NEC — *continued*
    cell-mediated — *continued*
      specified NEC 279.19
    combined (severe) 279.2
      syndrome 279.2
    common variable 279.06
    humoral NEC 279.00
    IgA (secretory) 279.01
    IgG 279.03
    IgM 279.02
  immunoglobulin, selective NEC 279.03
    IgA 279.01
    IgG 279.03
    IgM 279.02
  inositol (B complex) 266.2
  interferon 279.4
  internal organ V47.0
  interstitial cell-stimulating hormone (ICSH) 253.4
  intrinsic factor (Castle's) (congenital) 281.0
  intrinsic (urethral) sphincter (ISD) 599.82
  invertase 271.3
  iodine 269.3
  iron, anemia 280.9
  labile factor (congenital) (*see also* Defect, coagulation) 286.3
    acquired 286.7
  lacrimal fluid (acquired) 375.15
    congenital 743.64
  lactase 271.3
  Laki-Lorand factor (*see also* Defect, coagulation) 286.3
  lecithin-cholesterol acyltranferase 272.5
  LH (luteinizing hormone) 253.4
  limb V49.0
    lower V49.0
      congenital (*see also* Deficiency, lower limb, congenital) 755.30
    upper V49.0
      congenital (*see also* Deficiency, upper limb, congenital) 755.20
  lipocaic 577.8
  lipoid (high-density) 272.5
  lipoprotein (familial) (high density) 272.5
  liver phosphorylase 271.0
  long chain 3-hydroxyacyl CoA dehydrogenase (LCHAD) 277.85 ●
  long chain/very long chain acyl CoA dehydrogenase (LCAD, VLCAD) 277.85 ●
  lower limb V49.0
    congenital 755.30
      with complete absence of distal elements 755.31
      longitudinal (complete) (partial) (with distal deficiencies, incomplete) 755.32
        with complete absence of distal elements 755.31
        combined femoral, tibial, fibular (incomplete) 755.33
        femoral 755.34
        fibular 755.37
        metatarsal(s) 755.38
        phalange(s) 755.39
          meaning all digits 755.31
        tarsal(s) 755.38
        tibia 755.36
        tibiofibular 755.35
      transverse 755.31
  luteinizing hormone (LH) 253.4
  lysosomal alpha-1, 4 glucosidase 271.0
  magnesium 275.2
  mannosidase 271.8
  medium chain acyl CoA dehydrogenase (MCAD) 277.85 ●
  melanocyte-stimulating hormone (MSH) 253.4
  menadione (vitamin K) 269.0
    newborn 776.0
  mental (familial) (hereditary) (*see also* Retardation, mental) 319
  mineral NEC 269.3
  molybdenum 269.3
  moral 301.7
  multiple, syndrome 260

Deficiency, deficient — *continued*
  myocardial (*see also* Insufficiency myocardial) 428.0
  myophosphorylase 271.0
  NADH (DPNH)-methemoglobin-reductase (congenital) 289.7
  NADH-diaphorase or reductase (congenital) 289.7
  neck V48.1
  niacin (amide) (-tryptophan) 265.2
  nicotinamide 265.2
  nicotinic acid (amide) 265.2
  nose V48.8
  number of teeth (*see also* Anodontia) 520.0
  nutrition, nutritional 269.9
    specified NEC 269.8
  ornithine transcarbamylase 270.6
  ovarian 256.39
  oxygen (*see also* Anoxia) 799.0
  pantothenic acid 266.2
  parathyroid (gland) 252.1
  phenylalanine hydroxylase 270.1
  phosphoenolpyruvate carboxykinase 271.8 ●
  phosphofructokinase 271.2
  phosphoglucomutase 271.0
  phosphohexosisomerase 271.0
  phosphorylase kinase, liver 271.0
  pituitary (anterior) 253.2
    posterior 253.5
  placenta — *see* Placenta, insufficiency
  plasma
    cell 279.00
      protein (paraproteinemia) (pyroglobulinemia) 273.8
        gamma globulin 279.00
    thrombosplastin
      antecedent (PTA) 286.2
      component (PTC) 286.1
  platelet NEC 287.1
    constitutional 286.4
  polyglandular 258.9
  potassium (K) 276.8
  proaccelerin (congenital) (*see also* Defect, congenital) 286.3
    acquired 286.7
  proconvertin factor (congenital) (*see also* Defect, coagulation) 286.3
    acquired 286.7
  prolactin 253.4
  protein 260
    anemia 281.4
    C 289.81
    plasma — *see* Deficiency, plasma protein
    S 289.81
  prothrombin (congenital) (*see also* Defect coagulation) 286.3
    acquired 286.7
  Prower factor (*see also* Defect, coagulation) 286.3
  PRT 277.2
  pseudocholinesterase 289.89
  psychobiological 301.6
  PTA 286.2
  PTC 286.1
  purine nucleoside phosphorylase 277.2
  pyracin (alpha) (Beta) 266.1
  pyridoxal 266.1
  pyridoxamine 266.1
  pyridoxine (derivatives) 266.1
  pyruvate carboxylase 271.8 ●
  pyruvate dehydrogenase 271.8 ●
  pyruvate kinase (PK) 282.3
  riboflavin (vitamin B₂) 266.0
  saccadic eye movements 379.57
  salivation 527.7
  salt 276.1
  secretion
    ovary 256.39
    salivary gland (any) 527.7
    urine 788.5
  selenium 269.3
  serum
    antitrypsin, familial 273.4 ▲
    protein (congenital) 273.8
  short chain acyl CoA dehydrogenase (SCAD) 277.85 ●

Deficiency, deficient — *continued*
  smooth pursuit movements (eye) 379.58
  sodium (Na) 276.1
  SPCA (*see also* Defect, coagulation) 286.3
  specified NEC 269.8
  stable factor (congenital) (*see also* Defect, coagulation) 286.3
    acquired 286.7
  Stuart (-Prower) factor (*see also* Defect, coagulation) 286.3
  sucrase 271.3
  sucrase-isomaltase 271.3
  sulfite oxidase 270.0
  syndrome, multiple 260
  thiamine, thiaminic (chloride) 265.1
  thrombokinase (*see also* Defect, coagulation) 286.3
    newborn 776.0
  thrombopoieten 287.3
  thymolymphatic 279.2
  thyroid (gland) 244.9
  tocopherol 269.1
  toe — *see* Absence, toe
  tooth bud (*see also* Anodontia) 520.0
  trunk V48.1
  UDPG-glycogen transferase 271.0
  upper limb V49.0
    congenital 755.20
      with complete absence of distal elements 755.21
      longitudinal (complete) (partial) (with distal deficiencies, incomplete) 755.22
        carpal(s) 755.28
        combined humeral, radial, ulnar (incomplete) 755.23
        humeral 755.24
        metacarpal(s) 755.28
        phalange(s) 755.29
          meaning all digits 755.21
        radial 755.26
        radioulnar 755.25
        ulnar 755.27
      transverse (complete) (partial) 755.21
  vascular 459.9
  vasopressin 253.5
  viosterol (*see also* Deficiency, calciferol) 268.9
  vitamin (multiple) NEC 269.2
    A 264.9
      with
        Bitôt's spot 264.1
          corneal 264.2
            with corneal ulceration 264.3
        keratomalacia 264.4
        keratosis, follicular 264.8
        night blindness 264.5
        scar of cornea, xerophthalmic 264.6
        specified manifestation NEC 264.8
          ocular 264.7
        xeroderma 264.8
        xerophthalmia 264.7
        xerosis
          conjunctival 264.0
            with Bitôt's spot 264.1
          corneal 264.2
            with corneal ulceraton 264.3
    B (complex) NEC 266.9
      with
        beriberi 265.0
        pellagra 265.2
      specified type NEC 266.2
    B₁ NEC 265.1
      beriberi 265.0
    B₂ 266.0
    B₆ 266.1
    B₁₂ 266.2
    B₉ (folic acid) 266.2
    C (ascorbic acid) (with scurvy) 267
    D (calciferol) (ergosterol) 268.9
      with
        osteomalacia 268.2
        rickets (*see also* Rickets) 268.0
    E 269.1
    folic acid 266.2
    G 266.0
    H 266.2

(vertical left margin:) **Deficiency, deficient**

Deficiency, deficient — *continued*
  vitamin (multiple) NEC — *continued*
    K 269.0
      of newborn 776.0
    nicotinic acid 265.2
    P 269.1
    PP 265.2
    specified NEC 269.1
  zinc 269.3

Deficient — *see also* Deficiency
  blink reflex 374.45
  craniofacial axis 756.0
  number of teeth (*see also* Anodontia) 520.0
  secretion of urine 788.5

Deficit
  neurologic NEC 781.99
    due to
      cerebrovascular lesion (*see also* Disease, cerebrovascular, acute) 436
        late effect — *see* Late effect(s) (of) cerebrovascular disease
      transient ischemic attack 435.9
  oxygen 799.0

Deflection
  radius 736.09
  septum (acquired) (nasal) (nose) 470
  spine — *see* Curvature, spine
  turbinate (nose) 470

Defluvium
  capillorum (*see also* Alopecia) 704.00
  ciliorum 374.55
  unguium 703.8

Deformity 738.9
  abdomen, congential 759.9
  abdominal wall
    acquired 738.8
    congenital 756.70
    muscle deficiency syndrome 756.79
  acquired (unspecified site) 738.9
    specified site NEC 738.8
  adrenal gland (congenital) 759.1
  alimentary tract, congenital 751.9
    lower 751.5
      specified type NEC 751.8
    upper (any part, except tongue) 750.9
      specified type NEC 750.8
      tongue 750.10
        specified type NEC 750.19
  ankle (joint) (acquired) 736.70
    abduction 718.47
    congenital 755.69
    contraction 718.47
    specified NEC 736.79
  anus (congenital) 751.5
    acquired 569.49
  aorta (congenital) 747.20
    acquired 447.8
    arch 747.21
      acquired 447.8
    coarctation 747.10
  aortic
    arch 747.21
      acquired 447.8
    cusp or valve (congenital) 746.9
      acquired (*see also* Endocarditis, aortic) 424.1
    ring 747.21
  appendix 751.5
  arm (acquired) 736.89
    congenital 755.50
  arteriovenous (congenital) (peripheral) NEC 747.60
    gastrointestinal 747.61
    lower limb 747.64
    renal 747.62
    specified NEC 747.69
    spinal 747.82
    upper limb 747.63
  artery (congenital) (peripheral) NEC (*see also* Deformity, vascular) 747.60
    acquired 447.8
    cerebral 747.81
    coronary (congenital) 746.85
      acquired (*see also* Ischemia, heart) 414.9
    retinal 743.9
    umbilical 747.5

Deformity — *continued*
  atrial septal (congenital) (heart) 745.5
  auditory canal (congenital) (external) (*see also* Deformity, ear) 744.3
    acquired 380.50
  auricle
    ear (congenital) (*see also* Deformity, ear) 744.3
      acquired 380.32
    heart (congenital) 746.9
  back (acquired) — *see* Deformity, spine
  Bartholin's duct (congenital) 750.9
  bile duct (congenital) 751.60
    acquired 576.8
      with calculus, choledocholithiasis, or stones — *see* Choledocholithiasis
  biliary duct or passage (congenital) 751.60
    acquired 576.8
      with calculus, choledocholithiasis, or stones — *see* Choledocholithiasis
  bladder (neck) (spincter) (trigone) (acquired) 596.8
    congenital 753.9
  bone (acquired) NEC 738.9
    congenital 756.9
    turbinate 738.0
  boutonniere (finger) 736.21
  brain (congenital) 742.9
    acquired 348.8
    multiple 742.4
    reduction 742.2
    vessel (congenital) 747.81
  breast (acquired) 611.8
    congenital 757.9
  bronchus (congenital) 748.3
    acquired 519.1
  bursa, congenital 756.9
  canal of Nuck 752.9
  canthus (congenital) 743.9
    acquired 374.89
  capillary (acquired) 448.9
    congenital NEC (*see also* Deformity, vascular) 747.60
  cardiac — *see* Deformity, heart
  cardiovascular system (congenital) 746.9
  caruncle, lacrimal (congenital) 743.9
    acquired 375.69
  cascade, stomach 537.6
  cecum (congenital) 751.5
    acquired 569.89
  cerebral (congenital) 742.9
    acquired 348.8
  cervix (acquired) (uterus) 622.8
    congenital 752.40
  cheek (acquired) 738.19
    congenital 744.9
  chest (wall) (acquired) 738.3
    congenital 754.89
    late effect of rickets 268.1
  chin (acquired) 738.19
    congenital 744.9
  choroid (congenital) 743.9
    acquired 363.8
    plexus (congenital) 742.9
      acquired 349.2
  cicatricial — *see* Cicatrix
  cilia (congenital) 743.9
    acquired 374.89
  circulatory system (congenital) 747.9
  clavicle (acquired) 738.8
    congenital 755.51
  clitoris (congenital) 752.40
    acquired 624.8
  clubfoot — *see* Clubfoot
  coccyx (acquired) 738.6
    congenital 756.10
  colon (congenital) 751.5
    acquired 569.89
  concha (ear) (congenital) (*see also* Deformity, ear) 744.3
    acquired 380.32
  congenital, organ or site not listed (*see also* Anomaly) 759.9
  cornea (congenital) 743.9
    acquired 371.70
  coronary artery (congenital) 746.85
    acquired (*see also* Ischemia, heart) 414.9

Deformity — *continued*
  cranium (acquired) 738.19
    congenital (*see also* Deformity, skull, congenital) 756.0
  cricoid cartilage (congenital) 748.3
    acquired 478.79
  cystic duct (congenital) 751.60
    acquired 575.8
  Dandy-Walker 742.3
    with spina bifida (*see also* Spina bifida) 741.0 ☑
  diaphragm (congenital) 756.6
    acquired 738.8
  digestive organ(s) or system (congenital) NEC 751.9
    specified type NEC 751.8
  ductus arteriosus 747.0
  duodenal bulb 537.89
  duodenum (congenital) 751.5
    acquired 537.89
  dura 742.9
    brain 742.4
      acquired 349.2
    spinal 742.59
      acquired 349.2
  ear (congenital) 744.3
    acquired 380.32
    auricle 744.3
      causing impairment of hearing 744.02
    causing impairment of hearing 744.00
    external 744.3
      causing impairment of hearing 744.02
    internal 744.05
    lobule 744.3
    middle 744.03
      ossicles 744.04
    ossicles 744.04
  ectodermal (congenital) NEC 757.9
    specified type NEC 757.8
  ejaculatory duct (congenital) 752.9
    acquired 608.89
  elbow (joint) (acquired) 736.00
    congenital 755.50
    contraction 718.42
  endocrine gland NEC 759.2
  epididymis (congenital) 752.9
    acquired 608.89
    torsion 608.2
  epiglottis (congenital) 748.3
    acquired 478.79
  esophagus (congenital) 750.9
    acquired 530.89
  Eustachian tube (congenital) NEC 744.3
    specified type NEC 744.24
  extremity (acquired) 736.9
    congenital, except reduction deformity 755.9
      lower 755.60
      upper 755.50
    reduction — *see* Deformity, reduction
  eye (congenital) 743.9
    acquired 379.8
    muscle 743.9
  eyebrow (congenital) 744.89
  eyelid (congenital) 743.9
    acquired 374.89
    specified type NEC 743.62
  face (acquired) 738.19
    congenital (any part) 744.9
      due to intrauterine malposition and pressure 754.0
  fallopian tube (congenital) 752.10
    acquired 620.8
  femur (acquired) 736.89
    congenital 755.60
  fetal
    with fetopelvic disproportion 653.7 ☑
      affecting fetus or newborn 763.1
    causing obstructed labor 660.1 ☑
      affecting fetus or newborn 763.1
    known or suspected, affecting management of pregnancy 655.9 ☑
  finger (acquired) 736.20
    boutonniere type 736.21
    congenital 755.50
    flexion contracture 718.44
    swan neck 736.22

☑ Additional Digit Required   ▶◀ Revised Text   ● New Line   ▲ Revised Code

Deformity — continued

flexion (joint) (acquired) 736.9
  congenital NEC 755.9
  hip or thigh (acquired) 736.39
    congenital (see also Subluxation, congenital, hip) 754.32
foot (acquired) 736.70
  cavovarus 736.75
    congenital 754.59
  congenital NEC 754.70
    specified type NEC 754.79
  valgus (acquired) 736.79
    congenital 754.60
      specified type NEC 754.69
  varus (acquired) 736.79
    congenital 754.50
      specified type NEC 754.59
forearm (acquired) 736.00
  congenital 755.50
forehead (acquired) 738.19
  congenital (see also Deformity, skull, congenital) 756.0
frontal bone (acquired) 738.19
  congenital (see also Deformity, skull, congenital) 756.0
gallbladder (congenital) 751.60
  acquired 575.8
gastrointestinal tract (congenital) NEC 751.9
  acquired 569.89
  specified type NEC 751.8
genitalia, genital organ(s) or system NEC
  congenital 752.9
  female (congenital) 752.9
    acquired 629.8
    external 752.40
    internal 752.9
  male (congenital) 752.9
    acquired 608.89
globe (eye) (congenital) 743.9
  acquired 360.89
gum (congenital) 750.9
  acquired 523.9
gunstock 736.02
hand (acquired) 736.00
  claw 736.06
  congenital 755.50
  minus (and plus) (intrinsic) 736.09
  pill roller (intrinsic) 736.09
  plus (and minus) (intrinsic) 736.09
  swan neck (intrinsic) 736.09
head (acquired) 738.10
  congenital (see also Deformity, skull, congenital) 756.0
  specified NEC 738.19
heart (congenital) 746.9
  auricle (congenital) 746.9
  septum 745.9
    auricular 745.5
    specified type NEC 745.8
    ventricular 745.4
  valve (congenital) NEC 746.9
    acquired — see Endocarditis
    pulmonary (congenital) 746.00
    specified type NEC 746.89
  ventricle (congenital) 746.9
heel (acquired) 736.76
  congenital 755.67
hepatic duct (congenital) 751.60
  acquired 576.8
    with calculus, choledocholithiasis, or stones — see Choledocholithiasis
hip (joint) (acquired) 736.30
  congenital NEC 755.63
  flexion 718.45
    congenital (see also Subluxation, congenital, hip) 754.32
hourglass — see Contraction, hourglass
humerus (acquired) 736.89
  congenital 755.50
hymen (congenital) 752.40
hypophyseal (congenital) 759.2
ileocecal (coil) (valve) (congenital) 751.5
  acquired 569.89
ileum (intestine) (congenital) 751.5
  acquired 569.89
ilium (acquired) 738.6
  congenital 755.60

Deformity — continued

integument (congenital) 757.9
intervertebral cartilage or disc (acquired) — see also Displacement, intervertebral disc
  congenital 756.10
intestine (large) (small) (congenital) 751.5
  acquired 569.89
iris (acquired) 364.75
  congenital 743.9
  prolapse 364.8
ischium (acquired) 738.6
  congenital 755.60
jaw (acquired) (congenital) NEC 524.9
  due to intrauterine malposition and pressure 754.0
joint (acquired) NEC 738.8
  congenital 755.9
  contraction (abduction) (adduction) (extension) (flexion) — see Contraction, joint
kidney(s) (calyx) (pelvis) (congenital) 753.9
  acquired 593.89
  vessel 747.62
    acquired 459.9
Klippel-Feil (brevicollis) 756.16
knee (acquired) NEC 736.6
  congenital 755.64
labium (majus) (minus) (congenital) 752.40
  acquired 624.8
lacrimal apparatus or duct (congenital) 743.9
  acquired 375.69
larynx (muscle) (congenital) 748.3
  acquired 478.79
  web (glottic) (subglottic) 748.2
leg (lower) (upper) (acquired) NEC 736.89
  congenital 755.60
    reduction — see Deformity, reduction, lower limb
lens (congenital) 743.9
  acquired 379.39
lid (fold) (congenital) 743.9
  acquired 374.89
ligament (acquired) 728.9
  congenital 756.9
limb (acquired) 736.9
  congenital, except reduction deformity 755.9
    lower 755.60
      reduction (see also Deformity, reduction, lower limb) 755.30
    upper 755.50
      reduction (see also Deformity, reduction, upper limb) 755.20
  specified type NEC 736.89
lip (congenital) NEC 750.9
  acquired 528.5
  specified type NEC 750.26
liver (congenital) 751.60
  acquired 573.8
  duct (congenital) 751.60
    acquired 576.8
      with calculus, choledocholithiasis, or stones — see Choledocholithiasis
lower extremity — see Deformity, leg
lumbosacral (joint) (region) (congenital) 756.10
  acquired 738.5
lung (congenital) 748.60
  acquired 518.89
  specified type NEC 748.69
lymphatic system, congenital 759.9
Madelung's (radius) 755.54
maxilla (acquired) (congenital) 524.9
meninges or membrane (congenital) 742.9
  brain 742.4
    acquired 349.2
  spinal (cord) 742.59
    acquired 349.2
mesentery (congenital) 751.9
  acquired 568.89
metacarpus (acquired) 736.00
  congenital 755.50
metatarsus (acquired) 736.70
  congenital 754.70
middle ear, except ossicles (congenital) 744.03
  ossicles 744.04

Deformity — continued

mitral (leaflets) (valve) (congenital) 746.9
  acquired — see Endocarditis, mitral
  Ebstein's 746.89
  parachute 746.5
  specified type NEC 746.89
  stenosis, congenital 746.5
mouth (acquired) 528.9
  congenital NEC 750.9
    specified type NEC 750.26
multiple, congenital NEC 759.7
  specified type NEC 759.89
muscle (acquired) 728.9
  congenital 756.9
    specified type NEC 756.89
    sternocleidomastoid (due to intrauterine malposition and pressure) 754.1
musculoskeletal system, congenital NEC 756.9
  specified type NEC 756.9
nail (acquired) 703.9
  congenital 757.9
nasal — see Deformity, nose
neck (acquired) NEC 738.2
  congenital (any part) 744.9
    sternocleidomastoid 754.1
nervous system (congenital) 742.9
nipple (congenital) 757.9
  acquired 611.8
nose, nasal (cartilage) (acquired) 738.0
  bone (turbinate) 738.0
  congenital 748.1
    bent 754.0
    squashed 754.0
  saddle 738.0
    syphilitic 090.5
  septum 470
    congenital 748.1
  sinus (wall) (congenital) 748.1
    acquired 738.0
  syphilitic (congenital) 090.5
    late 095.8
ocular muscle (congenital) 743.9
  acquired 378.60
opticociliary vessels (congenital) 743.9
orbit (congenital) (eye) 743.9
  acquired NEC 376.40
    associated with craniofacial deformities 376.44
    due to
      bone disease 376.43
      surgery 376.47
      trauma 376.47
organ of Corti (congenital) 744.05
ovary (congenital) 752.0
  acquired 620.8
oviduct (congenital) 752.10
  acquired 620.8
palate (congenital) 750.9
  acquired 526.89
  cleft (congenital) (see also Cleft, palate) 749.00
  hard, acquired 526.89
  soft, acquired 528.9
pancreas (congenital) 751.7
  acquired 577.8
parachute, mitral valve 746.5
parathyroid (gland) 759.2
parotid (gland) (congenital) 750.9
  acquired 527.8
patella (acquired) 736.6
  congenital 755.64
pelvis, pelvic (acquired) (bony) 738.6 ☑
  with disproportion (fetopelvic) 653.0 ☑
    affecting fetus or newborn 763.1
    causing obstructed labor 660.1 ☑
      affecting fetus or newborn 763.1
  congenital 755.60
  rachitic (late effect) 268.1
penis (glans) (congenital) 752.9
  acquired 607.89
pericardium (congenital) 746.9
  acquired — see Pericarditis
pharynx (congenital) 750.9
  acquired 478.29
Pierre Robin (congenital) 756.0
pinna (acquired) 380.32
  congenital 744.3

Deformity — *continued*
  pituitary (congenital) 759.2
  pleural folds (congenital) 748.8
  portal vein (congenital) 747.40
  posture *see* Curvature, spine
  prepuce (congenital) 752.9
    acquired 607.89
  prostate (congenital) 752.9
    acquired 602.8
  pulmonary valve — *see* Endocarditis,
    pulmonary
  pupil (congenital) 743.9
    acquired 364.75
  pylorus (congenital) 750.9
    acquired 537.89
  rachitic (acquired), healed or old 268.1
  radius (acquired) 736.00
    congenital 755.50
      reduction — *see* Deformity, reduction,
        upper limb
  rectovaginal septum (congenital) 752.40
    acquired 623.8
  rectum (congenital) 751.5
    acquired 569.49
  reduction (extremity) (limb) 755.4
    brain 742.2
    lower limb 755.30
      with complete absence of distal elements
        755.31
      longitudinal (complete) (partial) (with
        distal deficiencies, incomplete)
        755.32
        with complete absence of distal
          elements 755.31
        combined femoral, tibial, fibular
          (incomplete) 755.33
        femoral 755.34
        fibular 755.37
        metatarsal(s) 755.38
        phalange(s) 755.39
          meaning all digits 755.31
        tarsal(s) 755.38
        tibia 755.36
        tibiofibular 755.35
      transverse 755.31
    upper limb 755.20
      with complete absence of distal elements
        755.21
      longitudinal (complete) (partial) (with
        distal deficiencies, incomplete)
        755.22
        with complete absence of distal
          elements 755.21
        carpal(s) 755.28
        combined humeral, radial, ulnar
          (incomplete) 755.23
        humeral 755.24
        metacarpal(s) 755.28
        phalange(s) 755.29
          meaning all digits 755.21
        radial 755.26
        radioulnar 755.25
        ulnar 755.27
      transverse (complete) (partial) 755.21
  renal — *see* Deformity, kidney
  respiratory system (congenital) 748.9
    specified type NEC 748.8
  rib (acquired) 738.3
    congenital 756.3
      cervical 756.2
  rotation (joint) (acquired) 736.9
    congenital 755.9
    hip or thigh 736.39
      congenital (*see also* Subluxation,
        congenital, hip) 754.32
  sacroiliac joint (congenital) 755.69
    acquired 738.5
  sacrum (acquired) 738.5
    congenital 756.10
  saddle
    back 737.8
    nose 738.0
      syphilitic 090.5
  salivary gland or duct (congenital) 750.9
    acquired 527.8
  scapula (acquired) 736.89
    congenital 755.50

Deformity — *continued*
  scrotum (congenital) 752.9
    acquired 608.89
  sebaceous gland, acquired 706.8
  seminal tract or duct (congenital) 752.9
    acquired 608.89
  septum (nasal) (acquired) 470
    congenital 748.1
  shoulder (joint) (acquired) 736.89
    congenital 755.50
      specified type NEC 755.59
    contraction 718.41
  sigmoid (flexure) (congenital) 751.5
    acquired 569.89
  sinus of Valsalva 747.29
  skin (congenital) 757.9
    acquired NEC 709.8
  skull (acquired) 738.19
    congenital 756.0
      with
        anencephalus 740.0
        encephalocele 742.0
        hydrocephalus 742.3
          with spina bifida (*see also* Spina
            bifida) 741.0 ☑
        microcephalus 742.1
      due to intrauterine malposition and
        pressure 754.0
  soft parts, organs or tissues (of pelvis)
    in pregnancy or childbirth NEC 654.9 ☑
      affecting fetus or newborn 763.89
      causing obstructed labor 660.2 ☑
        affecting fetus or newborn 763.1
  spermatic cord (congenital) 752.9
    acquired 608.89
      torsion 608.2
  spinal
    column — *see* Deformity, spine
    cord (congenital) 742.9
      acquired 336.8
      vessel (congenital) 747.82
    nerve root (congenital) 742.9
      acquired 724.9
  spine (acquired) NEC 738.5
    congenital 756.10
      due to intrauterine malposition and
        pressure 754.2
    kyphoscoliotic (*see also* Kyphoscoliosis)
      737.30
    kyphotic (*see also* Kyphosis) 737.10
    lordotic (*see also* Lordosis) 737.20
    rachitic 268.1
    scoliotic (*see also* Scoliosis) 737.30
  spleen
    acquired 289.59
    congenital 759.0
  Sprengel's (congenital) 755.52
  sternum (acquired) 738.3
    congenital 756.3
  stomach (congenital) 750.9
    acquired 537.89
  submaxillary gland (congenital) 750.9
    acquired 527.8
  swan neck (acquired)
    finger 736.22
    hand 736.09
  talipes — *see* Talipes
  teeth, tooth NEC 520.9
  testis (congenital) 752.9
    acquired 608.89
      torsion 608.2
  thigh (acquired) 736.89
    congenital 755.60
  thorax (acquired) (wall) 738.3
    congenital 754.89
    late effect of rickets 268.1
  thumb (acquired) 736.20
    congenital 755.50
  thymus (tissue) (congenital) 759.2
  thyroid (gland) (congenital) 759.2
    cartilage 748.3
      acquired 478.79
  tibia (acquired) 736.89
    congenital 755.60
    saber 090.5

Deformity — *continued*
  toe (acquired) 735.9
    congenital 755.66
    specified NEC 735.8
  tongue (congenital) 750.10
    acquired 529.8
  tooth, teeth NEC 520.9
  trachea (rings) (congenital) 748.3
    acquired 519.1
  transverse aortic arch (congenital) 747.21
  tricuspid (leaflets) (valve) (congenital) 746.9
    acquired — *see* Endocarditis, tricuspid
    atresia or stenosis 746.1
    specified type NEC 746.89
  trunk (acquired) 738.3
    congenital 759.9
  ulna (acquired) 736.00
    congenital 755.50
  upper extremity — *see* Deformity, arm
  urachus (congenital) 753.7
  ureter (opening) (congenital) 753.9
    acquired 593.89
  urethra (valve) (congenital) 753.9
    acquired 599.84
  urinary tract or system (congenital) 753.9
    urachus 753.7
  uterus (congenital) 752.3
    acquired 621.8
  uvula (congenital) 750.9
    acquired 528.9
  vagina (congenital) 752.40
    acquired 623.8
  valve, valvular (heart) (congenital) 746.9
    acquired — *see* Endocarditis
    pulmonary 746.00
    specified type NEC 746.89
  vascular (congenital) (peripheral) NEC 747.60
    acquired 459.9
  vas deferens (congenital) 752.9
    acquired 608.89
  vein (congenital) NEC (*see also* Deformity,
    vascular) 747.60
    brain 747.81
    coronary 746.9
    great 747.40
  vena cava (inferior) (superior) (congenital)
    747.40
  vertebra — *see* Deformity, spine
  vesicourethral orifice (acquired) 596.8
    congenital NEC 753.9
      specified type NEC 753.8
  vessels of optic papilla (congenital) 743.9
  visual field (contraction) 368.45
  vitreous humor (congenital) 743.9
    acquired 379.29
  vulva (congenital) 752.40
    acquired 624.8
  wrist (joint) (acquired) 736.00
    congenital 755.50
    contraction 718.43
    valgus 736.03
      congenital 755.59
    varus 736.04
      congenital 755.59

Degeneration, degenerative
  adrenal (capsule) (gland) 255.8
    with hypofunction 255.4
    fatty 255.8
    hyaline 255.8
    infectional 255.8
    lardaceous 277.3
  amyloid (any site) (general) 277.3
  anterior cornua, spinal cord 336.8
  aorta, aortic 440.0
    fatty 447.8
    valve (heart) (*see also* Endocarditis, aortic)
      424.1
  arteriovascular — *see* Arteriosclerosis
  artery, arterial (atheromatous) (calcareous) —
    see also Arteriosclerosis
    amyloid 277.3
    lardaceous 277.3
    medial NEC (*see also* Arteriosclerosis,
      extremities) 440.20

☑ Additional Digit Required   ▶◀ Revised Text   ● New Line   ▲ Revised Code

Degeneration, degenerative — *continued*
    articular cartilage NEC (*see also* Disorder,
        cartilage, articular) 718.0 ☑
        elbow 718.02
        knee 717.5
        patella 717.7
        shoulder 718.01
        spine (*see also* Spondylosis) 721.90
    atheromatous — *see* Arteriosclerosis
    bacony (any site) 277.3
    basal nuclei or ganglia NEC 333.0
    bone 733.90
    brachial plexus 353.0
    brain (cortical) (progressive) 331.9
        arteriosclerotic 437.0
        childhood 330.9
            specified type NEC 330.8
        congenital 742.4
        cystic 348.0
            congenital 742.4
        familial NEC 331.89
        grey matter 330.8
        heredofamilial NEC 331.89
        in
            alcoholism 303.9 ☑ [331.7]
            beriberi 265.0 [331.7]
            cerebrovascular disease 437.9 [331.7]
            congenital hydrocephalus 742.3 [331.7]
                with spina bifida (*see also* Spina
                    bifida) 741.0 ☑ [331.7]
            Fabry's disease 272.7 [330.2]
            Gaucher's disease 272.7 [330.2]
            Hunter's disease or syndrome
                277.5 [330.3]
            lipidosis
                cerebral 330.1
                generalized 272.7 [330.2]
            mucopolysaccharidosis 277.5 [330.3]
            myxedema (*see also* Myxedema)
                244.9 [331.7]
            neoplastic disease NEC (M8000/1)
                239.9 [331.7]
            Niemann-Pick disease 272.7 [330.2]
            sphingolipidosis 272.7 [330.2]
            vitamin B₁₂ deficiency 266.2 [331.7]
        motor centers 331.89
        senile 331.2
        specified type NEC 331.89
    breast — *see* Disease, breast
    Bruch's membrane 363.40
    bundle of His 426.50
        left 426.3
        right 426.4
    calcareous NEC 275.49
    capillaries 448.9
        amyloid 277.3
        fatty 448.9
        lardaceous 277.3
    cardiac (brown) (calcareous) (fatty) (fibrous)
        (hyaline) (mural) (muscular) (pigmentary)
        (senile) (with arteriosclerosis) (*see also*
        Degeneration, myocardial) 429.1
        valve, valvular — *see* Endocarditis
    cardiorenal (*see also* Hypertension, cardiorenal)
        404.90
    cardiovascular (*see also* Disease,
        cardiovascular) 429.2
        renal (*see also* Hypertension, cardiorenal)
            404.90
    cartilage (joint) — *see* Derangement, joint
    cerebellar NEC 334.9
        primary (hereditary) (sporadic) 334.2
    cerebral — *see* Degeneration, brain
    cerebromacular 330.1
    cerebrovascular 437.1
        due to hypertension 437.2
        late effect — *see* Late effect(s) (of)
            cerebrovascular disease
    cervical plexus 353.2
    cervix 622.8
        due to radiation (intended effect) 622.8
            adverse effect or misadventure 622.8
    changes, spine or vertebra (*see also*
        Spondylosis) 721.90
    chitinous 277.3
    chorioretinal 363.40
        congenital 743.53

Degeneration, degenerative — *continued*
    chorioretinal — *continued*
        hereditary 363.50
    choroid (colloid) (drusen) 363.40
        hereditary 363.50
        senile 363.41
            diffuse secondary 363.42
    cochlear 386.8
    collateral ligament (knee) (medial) 717.82
        lateral 717.81
    combined (spinal cord) (subacute) 266.2 [336.2]
        with anemia (pernicious) 281.0 [336.2]
            due to dietary deficiency 281.1 [336.2]
            due to vitamin B₁₂ deficiency anemia
                (dietary) 281.1 [336.2]
    conjunctiva 372.50
        amyloid 277.3 [372.50]
    cornea 371.40
        calcerous 371.44
        familial (hereditary) (*see also* Dystrophy,
            cornea) 371.50
            macular 371.55
            reticular 371.54
        hyaline (of old scars) 371.41
        marginal (Terrien's) 371.48
        mosaic (shagreen) 371.41
        nodular 371.46
        peripheral 371.48
        senile 371.41
    cortical (cerebellar) (parenchymatous) 334.2
        alcoholic 303.9 ☑ [334.4]
        diffuse, due to arteriopathy 437.0
    corticostriatal-spinal 334.8
    cretinoid 243
    cruciate ligament (knee) (posterior) 717.84
        anterior 717.83
    cutis 709.3
        amyloid 277.3
    dental pulp 522.2
    disc disease — *see* Degeneration, intervertebral
        disc
    dorsolateral (spinal cord) — *see* Degeration,
        combined
    endocardial 424.90
    extrapyramidal NEC 333.90
    eye NEC 360.40
        macular (*see also* Degeneration, macula)
            362.50
            congenital 362.75
            hereditary 362.76
    fatty (diffuse) (general) 272.8
        liver 571.8
            alcoholic 571.0
        localized site — *see* Degeneration, by site,
            fatty
        placenta — *see* Placenta, abnormal
    globe (eye) NEC 360.40
        macular — *see* Degeneration, macula
    grey matter 330.8
    heart (brown) (calcareous) (fatty) (fibrous)
        (hyaline) (mural) (muscular) (pigmentary)
        (senile) (with arteriosclerosis) (*see also*
        Degeneration, myocardial) 429.1
        amyloid 277.3 [425.7]
        atheromatous — *see* Arteriosclerosis,
            coronary
        gouty 274.82
        hypertensive (*see also* Hypertension, heart)
            402.90
        ischemic 414.9
        valve, valvular — *see* Endocarditis
    hepatolenticular (Wilson's) 275.1
    hepatorenal 572.4
    heredofamilial
        brain NEC 331.89
        spinal cord NEC 336.8
    hyaline (diffuse) (generalized) 728.9
        localized — *see also* Degeneration, by site
            cornea 371.41
            keratitis 371.41
    hypertensive vascular — *see* Hypertension
    infrapatellar fat pad 729.31
    internal semilunar cartilage 717.3
    intervertebral disc 722.6
        with myelopathy 722.70
            cervical, cervicothoracic 722.4
                with myelopathy 722.71

Degeneration, degenerative — *continued*
    intervertebral disc — *continued*
        lumbar, lumbosacral 722.52
            with myelopathy 722.73
        thoracic, thoracolumbar 722.51
            with myelopathy 722.72
    intestine 569.89
        amyloid 277.3
        lardaceous 277.3
    iris (generalized) (*see also* Atrophy, iris) 364.59
        pigmentary 364.53
        pupillary margin 364.54
    ischemic — *see* Ischemia
    joint disease (*see also* Osteoarthrosis) 715.9 ☑
        multiple sites 715.09
        spine (*see also* Spondylosis) 721.90
    kidney (*see also* Sclerosis, renal) 587
        amyloid 277.3 [583.81]
        cyst, cystic (multiple) (solitary) 593.2
            congenital (*see also* Cystic, disease,
                kidney) 753.10
        fatty 593.89
        fibrocystic (congenital) 753.19
        lardaceous 277.3 [583.81]
        polycystic (congenital) 753.12
            adult type (APKD) 753.13
            autosomal dominant 753.13
            autosomal recessive 753.14
            childhood type (CPKD) 753.14
            infantile type 753.14
        waxy 277.3 [583.81]
    Kuhnt-Junius (retina) 362.52
    labyrinth, osseous 386.8
    lacrimal passages, cystic 375.12
    lardaceous (any site) 277.3
    lateral column (posterior), spinal cord (*see also*
        Degeneration, combined) 266.2 [336.2]
    lattice 362.63
    lens 366.9
        infantile, juvenile, or presenile 366.00
        senile 366.10
    lenticular (familial) (progressive) (Wilson's) (with
        cirrhosis of liver) 275.1
        striate artery 437.0
    lethal ball, prosthetic heart valve 996.02
    ligament
        collateral (knee) (medial) 717.82
            lateral 717.81
        cruciate (knee) (posterior) 717.84
            anterior 717.83
    liver (diffuse) 572.8
        amyloid 277.3
        congenital (cystic) 751.62
        cystic 572.8
            congenital 751.62
        fatty 571.8
            alcoholic 571.0
        hypertrophic 572.8
        lardaceous 277.3
        parenchymatous, acute or subacute (*see
            also* Necrosis, liver) 570
        pigmentary 572.8
        toxic (acute) 573.8
        waxy 277.3
    lung 518.89
    lymph gland 289.3
        hyaline 289.3
        lardaceous 277.3
    macula (acquired) (senile) 362.50
        atrophic 362.51
        Best's 362.76
        congenital 362.75
        cystic 362.54
        cystoid 362.53
        disciform 362.52
        dry 362.51
        exudative 362.52
        familial pseudoinflammatory 362.77
        hereditary 362.76
        hole 362.54
        juvenile (Stargardt's) 362.75
        nonexudative 362.51
        pseudohole 362.54
        wet 362.52
    medullary — *see* Degeneration, brain
    membranous labyrinth, congenital (causing
        impairment of hearing) 744.05

☑ Additional Digit Required   ▶◀ Revised Text   ● New Line   ▲ Revised Code

Degeneration, degenerative — *continued*
  meniscus — *see* Derangement, joint
  microcystoid 362.62
  mitral — *see* Insufficiency, mitral
  Mönckeberg's (*see also* Arteriosclerosis,
    extremities) 440.20
  moral 301.7
  motor centers, senile 331.2
  mural (*see also* Degeneration, myocardial)
    429.1
    heart, cardiac (*see also* Degeneration,
      myocardial) 429.1
    myocardium, myocardial (*see also*
      Degeneration, myocardial) 429.1
  muscle 728.9
    fatty 728.9
    fibrous 728.9
    heart (*see also* Degeneration, myocardial)
      429.1
    hyaline 728.9
  muscular progressive 728.2
  myelin, central nervous system NEC 341.9
  myocardium, myocardial (brown) (calcareous)
    (fatty) (fibrous) (hyaline) (mural)
    (muscular) (pigmentary) (senile) (with
    arteriosclerosis) 429.1
    with rheumatic fever (conditions classifiable
      to 390) 398.0
      active, acute, or subacute 391.2
        with chorea 392.0
      inactive or quiescent (with chorea) 398.0
    amyloid 277.3 *[425.7]*
    congenital 746.89
    fetus or newborn 779.89
    gouty 274.82
    hypertensive (*see also* Hypertension, heart)
      402.90
    ischemic 414.8
    rheumatic (*see also* Degeneration,
      myocardium, with rheumatic fever)
      398.0
    syphilitic 093.82
  nasal sinus (mucosa) (*see also* Sinusitis) 473.9
    frontal 473.1
    maxillary 473.0
  nerve — *see* Disorder, nerve
  nervous system 349.89
    amyloid 277.3 *[357.4]*
    autonomic (*see also* Neuropathy, peripheral,
      autonomic) 337.9
    fatty 349.89
    peripheral autonomic NEC (*see also*
      Neuropathy, peripheral, autonomic)
      337.9
  nipple 611.9
  nose 478.1
  oculoacousticocerebral, congenital (progressive)
    743.8
  olivopontocerebellar (familial) (hereditary) 333.0
  osseous labyrinth 386.8
  ovary 620.8
    cystic 620.2
    microcystic 620.2
  pallidal, pigmentary (progressive) 333.0
  pancreas 577.8
    tuberculous (*see also* Tuberculosis) 017.9 ☑
  papillary muscle 429.81
  paving stone 362.61
  penis 607.89
  peritoneum 568.89
  pigmentary (diffuse) (general)
    localized — *see* Degeneration, by site
    pallidal (progressive) 333.0
    secondary 362.65
  pineal gland 259.8
  pituitary (gland) 253.8
  placenta (fatty) (fibrinoid) (fibroid) — *see*
    Placenta, abnormal
  popliteal fat pad 729.31
  posterolateral (spinal cord) (*see also*
    Degeneration, combined) 266.2 *[336.2]*
  pulmonary valve (heart) (*see also* Endocarditis,
    pulmonary) 424.3
  pulp (tooth) 522.2
  pupillary margin 364.54
  renal (*see also* Sclerosis, renal) 587
    fibrocystic 753.19

Degeneration, degenerative — *continued*
  renal (*see also* Sclerosis, renal) — *continued*
    polycystic 753.12
      adult type (APKD) 753.13
      autosomal dominant 753.13
      autosomal recessive 753.14
      childhood type (CPKD) 753.14
      infantile type 753.14
  reticuloendothelial system 289.89
  retina (peripheral) 362.60
    with retinal defect (*see also* Detachment,
      retina, with retinal defect) 361.00
    cystic (senile) 362.50
    cystoid 362.53
    hereditary (*see also* Dystrophy, retina)
      362.70
      cerebroretinal 362.71
      congenital 362.75
      juvenile (Stargardt's) 362.75
      macula 362.76
    Kuhnt-Junius 362.52
    lattice 362.63
    macular (*see also* Degeneration, macula)
      362.50
    microcystoid 362.62
    palisade 362.63
    paving stone 362.61
    pigmentary (primary) 362.74
      secondary 362.65
    posterior pole (*see also* Degeneration,
      macula) 362.50
    secondary 362.66
    senile 362.60
      cystic 362.53
      reticular 362.64
  saccule, congenital (causing impairment of
    hearing) 744.05
  sacculocochlear 386.8
  senile 797
    brain 331.2
    cardiac, heart, or myocardium (*see also*
      Degeneration, myocardial) 429.1
    motor centers 331.2
    reticule 362.64
    retina, cystic 362.50
    vascular — *see* Arteriosclerosis
  silicone rubber poppet (prosthetic valve) 996.02
  sinus (cystic) (*see also* Sinusitis) 473.9
    polypoid 471.1
  skin 709.3
    amyloid 277.3
    colloid 709.3
  spinal (cord) 336.8
    amyloid 277.3
    column 733.90
    combined (subacute) (*see also* Degeneration,
      combined) 266.2 *[336.2]*
      with anemia (pernicious) 281.0 *[336.2]*
    dorsolateral (*see also* Degeneration,
      combined) 266.2 *[336.2]*
    familial NEC 336.8
    fatty 336.8
    funicular (*see also* Degeneration, combined)
      266.2 *[336.2]*
    heredofamilial NEC 336.8
    posterolateral (*see also* Degeneration,
      combined) 266.2 *[336.2]*
    subacute combined — *see* Degeneration,
      combined
    tuberculous (*see also* Tuberculosis) 013.8 ☑
  spine 733.90
  spleen 289.59
    amyloid 277.3
    lardaceous 277.3
  stomach 537.89
    lardaceous 277.3
  strionigral 333.0
  sudoriparous (cystic) 705.89
  suprarenal (capsule) (gland) 255.8
    with hypofunction 255.4
  sweat gland 705.89
  synovial membrane (pulpy) 727.9
  tapetoretinal 362.74
    adult or presenile form 362.50
  testis (postinfectional) 608.89
  thymus (gland) 254.8
    fatty 254.8

Degeneration, degenerative — *continued*
  thymus (gland) — *continued*
    lardaceous 277.3
  thyroid (gland) 246.8
  tricuspid (heart) (valve) *see* Endocarditis,
    tricuspid
  tuberculous NEC (*see also* Tuberculosis)
    011.9 ☑
  turbinate 733.90
  uterus 621.8
    cystic 621.8
  vascular (senile) — *see also* Arteriosclerosis
    hypertensive — *see* Hypertension
  vitreoretinal (primary) 362.73
    secondary 362.66
  vitreous humor (with infiltration) 379.21
  wallerian NEC — *see* Disorder, nerve
  waxy (any site) 277.3
  Wilson's hepatolenticular 275.1

Deglutition
  paralysis 784.9
    hysterical 300.11
  pneumonia 507.0

Degos' disease or syndrome 447.8

**Degradation disorder, branched-chain amino
  acid** 270.3

Dehiscence
  anastomosis — *see* Complications, anastomosis
  cesarean wound 674.1 ☑
  episiotomy 674.2 ☑
  operation wound 998.32
    internal 998.31
  perineal wound (postpartum) 674.2 ☑
  postoperative 998.32
    abdomen 998.32
      internal 998.31
    internal 998.31
  uterine wound 674.1 ☑

Dehydration (cachexia) 276.5
  with
    hypernatremia 276.0
    hyponatremia 276.1
  newborn 775.5

Deiters' nucleus syndrome 386.19

Déjérine's disease 356.0

Déjérine-Klumpke paralysis 767.6

Déjérine-Roussy syndrome 348.8

Déjérine-Sottas disease or neuropathy
  (hypertrophic) 356.0

Déjérine-Thomas atrophy or syndrome 333.0

de Lange's syndrome (Amsterdam dwarf, mental
  retardation, and brachycephaly) 759.89

Delay, delayed
  adaptation, cones or rods 368.63
  any plane in pelvis
    affecting fetus or newborn 763.1
    complicating delivery 660.1 ☑
  birth or delivery NEC 662.1 ☑
    affecting fetus or newborn 763.89
    second twin, triplet, or multiple mate
      662.3 ☑
  closure — *see also* Fistula
    cranial suture 756.0
    fontanel 756.0
  coagulation NEC 790.92
  conduction (cardiac) (ventricular) 426.9
  delivery NEC 662.1 ☑
    second twin, triplet, etc. 662.3 ☑
      affecting fetus or newborn 763.89
  development
    in childhood 783.40
      physiological 783.40
    intellectual NEC 315.9
    learning NEC 315.2
    reading 315.00
    sexual 259.0
    speech 315.39
      associated with hyperkinesis 314.1
    spelling 315.09
  gastric emptying 536.8
  menarche 256.39
    due to pituitary hypofunction 253.4
  menstruation (cause unknown) 626.8
  milestone in childhood 783.42

Delay, delayed — *continued*
  motility — *see* Hypomotility
  passage of meconium (newborn) 777.1
  primary respiration 768.9
  puberty 259.0
  separation of umbilical cord 779.83
  sexual maturation, female 259.0

Del Castillo's syndrome (germinal aplasia) 606.0

Déleage's disease 359.89

Deletion syndrome   ●
  5p 758.31   ●
  22q11.2 758.32   ●
  autosomal NEC 758.39   ●

Delhi (boil) (button) (sore) 085.1

Delinquency (juvenile) 312.9
  group (*see also* Disturbance, conduct) 312.2 ☑
  neurotic 312.4

Delirium, delirious 780.09
  acute (psychotic) 293.0
  alcoholic 291.0
    acute 291.0
    chronic 291.1
  alcoholicum 291.0
  chronic (*see also* Psychosis) 293.89
    due to or associated with physical condition
      — *see* Psychosis, organic
  drug-induced 292.81
  due to conditions classified elsewhere 293.0 ●
  eclamptic (*see also* Eclampsia) 780.39
  exhaustion (*see also* Reaction, stress, acute)
    308.9
  hysterical 300.11
  in
    presenile dementia 290.11
    senile dementia 290.3
  induced by drug 292.81
  manic, maniacal (acute) (*see also* Psychosis,
    affective) 296.0
    recurrent episode 296.1 ☑
    single episode 296.0 ☑
  puerperal 293.9
  senile 290.3
  subacute (psychotic) 293.1
  thyroid (*see also* Thyrotoxicosis) 242.9 ☑
  traumatic — *see also* Injury, intracranial
    with
      lesion, spinal cord — *see* Injury, spinal,
        by site
      shock, spinal — *see* Injury, spinal, by site
  tremens (impending) 291.0
  uremic — *see* Uremia
  withdrawal
    alcoholic (acute) 291.0
      chronic 291.1
    drug 292.0

Delivery

> *Note — Use the following fifth-digit*
> *subclassification with categories 640-648, 651-*
> *676:*
>
> *0   unspecified as to episode of care*
>
> *1   delivered, with or without mention of*
> *   antepartum condition*
>
> *2   delivered, with mention of postpartum*
> *   complication*
>
> *3   antepartum condition or complication*
>
> *4   postpartum condition or complication*

  breech (assisted) (spontaneous) 652.2 ☑
    affecting fetus or newborn 763.0
    extraction NEC 669.6 ☑
  cesarean (for) 669.7 ☑
    abnormal
      cervix 654.6 ☑
      pelvic organs or tissues 654.9 ☑
      pelvis (bony) (major) NEC 653.0 ☑
      presentation or position 652.9 ☑
        in multiple gestation 652.6 ☑
      size, fetus 653.5 ☑
      soft parts (of pelvis) 654.9 ☑
      uterus, congenital 654.0 ☑
      vagina 654.7 ☑
      vulva 654.8 ☑
    abruptio placentae 641.2 ☑

Delivery — *continued*
  cesarean — *continued*
    acromion presentation 652.8 ☑
    affecting fetus or newborn 763.4
    anteversion, cervix or uterus 654.4 ☑
    atony, uterus 666.1 ☑
    bicornis or bicornuate uterus 654.0 ☑
    breech presentation 652.2 ☑
    brow presentation 652.4 ☑
    cephalopelvic disproportion (normally
      formed fetus) 653.4 ☑
    chin presentation 652.4 ☑
    cicatrix of cervix 654.6 ☑
    contracted pelvis (general) 653.1 ☑
      inlet 653.2 ☑
      outlet 653.3 ☑
    cord presentation or prolapse 663.0 ☑
    cystocele 654.4 ☑
    deformity (acquired) (congenital)
      pelvic organs or tissues NEC 654.9 ☑
      pelvis (bony) NEC 653.0 ☑
    displacement, uterus NEC 654.4 ☑
    disproportion NEC 653.9 ☑
    distress
      fetal 656.8 ☑
      maternal 669.0 ☑
    eclampsia 642.6 ☑
    face presentation 652.4 ☑
    failed
      forceps 660.7 ☑
      trial of labor NEC 660.6 ☑
      vacuum extraction 660.7 ☑
      ventouse 660.7 ☑
    fetal deformity 653.7 ☑
    fetal-maternal hemorrhage 656.0 ☑
    fetus, fetal
      distress 656.8 ☑
      prematurity 656.8 ☑
    fibroid (tumor) (uterus) 654.1 ☑
    footling 652.8 ☑
      with successful version 652.1 ☑
    hemorrhage (antepartum) (intrapartum) NEC
      641.9 ☑
    hydrocephalic fetus 653.6 ☑
    incarceration of uterus 654.3 ☑
    incoordinate uterine action 661.4 ☑
    inertia, uterus 661.2 ☑
      primary 661.0 ☑
      secondary 661.1 ☑
    lateroversion, uterus or cervix 654.4 ☑
    mal lie 652.9 ☑
    malposition
      fetus 652.9 ☑
        in multiple gestation 652.6 ☑
      pelvic organs or tissues NEC 654.9 ☑
      uterus NEC or cervix 654.4 ☑
    malpresentation NEC 652.9 ☑
      in multiple gestation 652.6 ☑
    maternal
      diabetes mellitus 648.0 ☑
      heart disease NEC 648.6 ☑
    meconium in liquor 656.8 ☑
      staining only 792.3
    oblique presentation 652.3 ☑
    oversize fetus 653.5 ☑
    pelvic tumor NEC 654.9 ☑
    placental insufficiency 656.5 ☑
    placenta previa 641.0 ☑
      with hemorrhage 641.1 ☑
    poor dilation, cervix 661.0 ☑
    preeclampsia 642.4 ☑
      severe 642.5 ☑
    previous
      cesarean delivery 654.2 ☑
      surgery (to)
        cervix 654.6 ☑
        gynecological NEC 654.9 ☑
        rectum 654.8 ☑   ●
        uterus NEC 654.9 ☑
          previous cesarean delivery 654.2 ☑
        vagina 654.7 ☑
    prolapse
      arm or hand 652.7 ☑
      uterus 654.4 ☑
    prolonged labor 662.1 ☑
    rectocele 654.4 ☑
    retroversion, uterus or cervix 654.3 ☑

Delivery — *continued*
  cesarean — *continued*
    rigid
      cervix 654.6 ☑
      pelvic floor 654.4 ☑
      perineum 654.8 ☑
      vagina 654.7 ☑
      vulva 654.8 ☑
    sacculation, pregnant uterus 654.4 ☑
    scar(s)
      cervix 654.6 ☑
      cesarean delivery 654.2 ☑
      uterus NEC 654.9 ☑
        due to previous cesarean delivery
          654.2 ☑
    Shirodkar suture in situ 654.5 ☑
    shoulder presentation 652.8 ☑
    stenosis or stricture, cervix 654.6 ☑
    transverse presentation or lie 652.3 ☑
    tumor, pelvic organs or tissues NEC
      654.4 ☑
    umbilical cord presentation or prolapse
      663.0 ☑
  completely normal case — *see* category 650
  complicated (by) NEC 669.9 ☑
    abdominal tumor, fetal 653.7 ☑
      causing obstructed labor 660.1 ☑
    abnormal, abnormality of
      cervix 654.6 ☑
        causing obstructed labor 660.2 ☑
      forces of labor 661.9 ☑
      formation of uterus 654.0 ☑
      pelvic organs or tissues 654.9 ☑
        causing obstructed labor 660.2 ☑
      pelvis (bony) (major) NEC 653.0 ☑
        causing obstructed labor 660.1 ☑
      presentation or position NEC 652.9 ☑
        causing obstructed labor 660.0 ☑
      size, fetus 653.5 ☑
        causing obstructed labor 660.1 ☑
      soft parts (of pelvis) 654.9 ☑
        causing obstructed labor 660.2 ☑
      uterine contractions NEC 661.9 ☑
      uterus (formation) 654.0 ☑
        causing obstructed labor 660.2 ☑
      vagina 654.7 ☑
        causing obstructed labor 660.2 ☑
    abnormally formed uterus (any type)
      (congenital) 654.0 ☑
      causing obstructed labor 660.2 ☑
    acromion presentation 652.8 ☑
      causing obstructed labor 660.0 ☑
    adherent placenta 667.0 ☑
      with hemorrhage 666.0 ☑
    adhesions, uterus (to abdominal wall)
      654.4 ☑
    advanced maternal age NEC 659.6 ☑
      multigravida 659.6 ☑
      primigravida 659.5 ☑
    air embolism 673.0 ☑
    amnionitis 658.4 ☑
    amniotic fluid embolism 673.1 ☑
    anesthetic death 668.9 ☑
    annular detachment, cervix 665.3 ☑
    antepartum hemorrhage — *see* Delivery,
      complicated, hemorrhage
    anteversion, cervix or uterus 654.4 ☑
      causing obstructed labor 660.2 ☑
    apoplexy 674.0 ☑
      placenta 641.2 ☑
    arrested active phase 661.1 ☑
    asymmetrical pelvis bone 653.0 ☑
      causing obstructed labor 660.1 ☑
    atony, uterus (hypotonic) (inertia) 666.1 ☑
      hypertonic 661.4 ☑
    Bandl's ring 661.4 ☑
    battledore placenta — *see* Placenta,
      abnormal
    bicornis or bicornuate uterus 654.0 ☑
      causing obstructed labor 660.2 ☑
    birth injury to mother NEC 665.9 ☑
    bleeding (*see also* Delivery, complicated,
      hemorrhage) 641.9 ☑
    breech presentation (assisted) (buttocks)
      (complete) (frank) (spontaneous)
      652.2 ☑
      with successful version 652.1 ☑

Delivery — *continued*
  complicated (by) — *continued*
    brow presentation 652.4 ✓
    cephalopelvic disproportion (normally
        formed fetus) 653.4 ✓
      causing obstructed labor 660.1 ✓
    cerebral hemorrhage 674.0 ✓
    cervical dystocia 661.0 ✓
    chin presentation 652.4 ✓
      causing obstructed labor 660.0 ✓
    cicatrix
      cervix 654.6 ✓
        causing obstructed labor 660.2 ✓
      vagina 654.7 ✓
        causing obstructed labor 660.2 ✓
    colporrhexis 665.4 ✓
      with perineal laceration 664.0 ✓
    compound presentation 652.8 ✓
      causing obstructed labor 660.0 ✓
    compression of cord (umbilical) 663.2 ✓
      around neck 663.1 ✓
      cord prolapsed 663.0 ✓
    contraction, contracted pelvis 653.1 ✓
      causing obstructed labor 660.1 ✓
      general 653.1 ✓
        causing obstructed labor 660.1 ✓
      inlet 653.2 ✓
        causing obstructed labor 660.1 ✓
      midpelvic 653.8 ✓
        causing obstructed labor 660.1 ✓
      midplane 653.8 ✓
        causing obstructed labor 660.1 ✓
      outlet 653.3 ✓
        causing obstructed labor 660.1 ✓
    contraction ring 661.4 ✓
    cord (umbilical) 663.9 ✓
      around neck, tightly or with compression
        663.1 ✓
        without compression 663.3 ✓
      bruising 663.6 ✓
      complication NEC 663.9 ✓
        specified type NEC 663.8 ✓
      compression NEC 663.2 ✓
      entanglement NEC 663.3 ✓
        with compression 663.2 ✓
      forelying 663.0 ✓
      hematoma 663.6 ✓
      marginal attachment 663.8 ✓
      presentation 663.0 ✓
      prolapse (complete) (occult) (partial)
        663.0 ✓
      short 663.4 ✓
      specified complication NEC 663.8 ✓
      thrombosis (vessels) 663.6 ✓
      vascular lesion 663.6 ✓
      velamentous insertion 663.8 ✓
    Couvelaire uterus 641.2 ✓
    cretin pelvis (dwarf type) (male type)
      653.1 ✓
      causing obstructed labor 660.1 ✓
    crossbirth 652.3 ✓
      with successful version 652.1 ✓
      causing obstructed labor 660.0 ✓
    cyst (Gartner's duct) 654.7 ✓
    cystocele 654.4 ✓
      causing obstructed labor 660.2 ✓
    death of fetus (near term) 656.4 ✓
      early (before 22 completed weeks
        gestation) 632
    deformity (acquired) (congenital)
      fetus 653.7 ✓
        causing obstructed labor 660.1 ✓
      pelvic organs or tissues NEC 654.9 ✓
        causing obstructed labor 660.2 ✓
      pelvis (bony) NEC 653.0 ✓
        causing obstructed labor 660.1 ✓
    delay, delayed
      delivery in multiple pregnancy 662.3 ✓
      due to locked mates 660.5 ✓
      following rupture of membranes
        (spontaneous) 658.2 ✓
        artificial 658.3 ✓
    depressed fetal heart tones 659.7 ✓
    diastasis recti 665.8 ✓
    dilation
      bladder 654.4 ✓
        causing obstructed labor 660.2 ✓

Delivery — *continued*
  complicated (by) — *continued*
    dilation — *continued*
      cervix, incomplete, poor or slow 661.0 ✓
    diseased placenta 656.7 ✓
    displacement uterus NEC 654.4 ✓
      causing obstructed labor 660.2 ✓
    disproportion NEC 653.9 ✓
      causing obstructed labor 660.1 ✓
    disruptio uteri — *see* Delivery, complicated,
      rupture, uterus
    distress
      fetal 656.8 ✓
      maternal 669.0 ✓
    double uterus (congenital) 654.0 ✓
      causing obstructed labor 660.2 ✓
    dropsy amnion 657.0 ✓
    dysfunction, uterus 661.9 ✓
      hypertonic 661.4 ✓
      hypotonic 661.2 ✓
        primary 661.0 ✓
        secondary 661.1 ✓
      incoordinate 661.4 ✓
    dystocia
      cervical 661.0 ✓
      fetal — *see* Delivery, complicated,
        abnormal presentation
      maternal — *see* Delivery, complicated,
        prolonged labor
      pelvic — *see* Delivery, complicated,
        contraction pelvis
      positional 652.8 ✓
      shoulder girdle 660.4 ✓
    eclampsia 642.6 ✓
    ectopic kidney 654.4 ✓
      causing obstructed labor 660.2 ✓
    edema, cervix 654.6 ✓
      causing obstructed labor 660.2 ✓
    effusion, amniotic fluid 658.1 ✓
    elderly multigravida 659.6 ✓
    elderly primigravida 659.5 ✓
    embolism (pulmonary) 673.2 ✓
      air 673.0 ✓
      amniotic fluid 673.1 ✓
      blood clot 673.2 ✓
      cerebral 674.0 ✓
      fat 673.8 ✓
      pyemic 673.3 ✓
      septic 673.3 ✓
    entanglement, umbilical cord 663.3 ✓
      with compression 663.2 ✓
      around neck (with compression) 663.1 ✓
    eversion, cervix or uterus 665.2 ✓
    excessive
      fetal growth 653.5 ✓
        causing obstructed labor 660.1 ✓
      size of fetus 653.5 ✓
        causing obstructed labor 660.1 ✓
    face presentation 652.4 ✓
      causing obstructed labor 660.0 ✓
      to pubes 660.3 ✓
    failure, fetal head to enter pelvic brim
      652.5 ✓
      causing obstructed labor 660.0 ✓
    fetal
      acid-base balance 656.8 ✓
      death (near term) NEC 656.4 ✓
        early (before 22 completed weeks
          gestation) 632
      deformity 653.7 ✓
        causing obstructed labor 660.1 ✓
      distress 656.8 ✓
      heart rate or rhythm 659.7 ✓
    fetopelvic disproportion 653.4 ✓
      causing obstructed labor 660.1 ✓
    fever during labor 659.2 ✓
    fibroid (tumor) (uterus) 654.1 ✓
      causing obstructed labor 660.2 ✓
    fibromyomata 654.1 ✓
      causing obstructed labor 660.2 ✓
    forelying umbilical cord 663.0 ✓
    fracture of coccyx 665.6 ✓
    hematoma 664.5 ✓
      broad ligament 665.7 ✓
      ischial spine 665.7 ✓
      pelvic 665.7 ✓
      perineum 664.5 ✓

Delivery — *continued*
  complicated (by) — *continued*
    hematoma — *continued*
      soft tissues 665.7 ✓
      subdural 674.0 ✓
      umbilical cord 663.6 ✓
      vagina 665.7 ✓
      vulva or perineum 664.5 ✓
    hemorrhage (uterine) (antepartum)
      (intrapartum) (pregnancy) 641.9 ✓
      accidental 641.2 ✓
      associated with
        afibrinogenemia 641.3 ✓
        coagulation defect 641.3 ✓
          hyperfibrinolysis 641.3 ✓
          hypofibrinogenemia 641.3 ✓
      cerebral 674.0 ✓
      due to
        low-lying placenta 641.1 ✓
        placenta previa 641.1 ✓
        premature separation of placenta
          (normally implanted) 641.2 ✓
        retained placenta 666.0 ✓
        trauma 641.8 ✓
        uterine leiomyoma 641.8 ✓
      marginal sinus rupture 641.2 ✓
      placenta NEC 641.9 ✓
      postpartum (atonic) (immediate) (within
        24 hours) 666.1 ✓
        with retained or trapped placenta
          666.0 ✓
        delayed 666.2 ✓
        secondary 666.2 ✓
        third stage 666.0 ✓
    hourglass contraction, uterus 661.4 ✓
    hydramnios 657.0 ✓
    hydrocephalic fetus 653.6 ✓
      causing obstructed labor 660.1 ✓
    hydrops fetalis 653.7 ✓
      causing obstructed labor 660.1 ✓
    hypertension — *see* Hypertension,
      complicating pregnancy
    hypertonic uterine dysfunction 661.4 ✓
    hypotonic uterine dysfunction 661.2 ✓
    impacted shoulders 660.4 ✓
    incarceration, uterus 654.3 ✓
      causing obstructed labor 660.2 ✓
    incomplete dilation (cervix) 661.0 ✓
    incoordinate uterus 661.4 ✓
    indication NEC 659.9 ✓
      specified type NEC 659.8 ✓
    inertia, uterus 661.2 ✓
      hypertonic 661.4 ✓
      hypotonic 661.2 ✓
      primary 661.0 ✓
      secondary 661.1 ✓
    infantile
      genitalia 654.4 ✓
        causing obstructed labor 660.2 ✓
      uterus (os) 654.4 ✓
        causing obstructed labor 660.2 ✓
    injury (to mother) NEC 665.9 ✓
    intrauterine fetal death (near term) NEC
      656.4 ✓
      early (before 22 completed weeks
        gestation) 632
    inversion, uterus 665.2 ✓
    kidney, ectopic 654.4 ✓
      causing obstructed labor 660.2 ✓
    knot (true), umbilical cord 663.2 ✓
    labor, premature (before 37 completed weeks
      gestation) 644.2 ✓
    laceration 664.9 ✓
      anus (spincter) 664.2 ✓
        with mucosa 664.3 ✓
      bladder (urinary) 665.5 ✓
      bowel 665.5 ✓
      central 664.4 ✓
      cervix (uteri) 665.3 ✓
      fourchette 664.0 ✓
      hymen 664.0 ✓
      labia (majora) (minora) 664.0 ✓
      pelvic
        floor 664.1 ✓
        organ NEC 665.5 ✓

✓ Additional Digit Required   ▶◀ Revised Text   ● New Line   ▲ Revised Code

Delivery — *continued*
  complicated (by) — *continued*
    laceration — *continued*
      perineum, perineal 664.4 ☑
        first degree 664.0 ☑
        second degree 664.1 ☑
        third degree 664.2 ☑
        fourth degree 664.3 ☑
        central 664.4 ☑
        extensive NEC 664.4 ☑
        muscles 664.1 ☑
        skin 664.0 ☑
        slight 664.0 ☑
      peritoneum 665.5 ☑
      periurethral tissue 665.5 ☑
      rectovaginal (septum) (without perineal laceration) 665.4 ☑
        with perineum 664.2 ☑
          with anal rectal mucosa 664.3 ☑
      skin (perineum) 664.0 ☑
      specified site or type NEC 664.8 ☑
      sphincter ani 664.2 ☑
        with mucosa 664.3 ☑
      urethra 665.5 ☑
      uterus 665.1 ☑
        before labor 665.0 ☑
      vagina, vaginal (deep) (high) (sulcus) (wall) (without perineal laceration) 665.4 ☑
        with perineum 664.0 ☑
        muscles, with perineum 664.1 ☑
      vulva 664.0 ☑
    lateroversion, uterus or cervix 654.4 ☑
      causing obstructed labor 660.2 ☑
    locked mates 660.5 ☑
    low implantation of placenta — *see* Delivery, complicated, placenta, previa
    mal lie 652.9 ☑
    malposition
      fetus NEC 652.9 ☑
        causing obstructed labor 660.0 ☑
      pelvic organs or tissues NEC 654.9 ☑
        causing obstructed labor 660.2 ☑
      placenta 641.1 ☑
        without hemorrhage 641.0 ☑
      uterus NEC or cervix 654.4 ☑
        causing obstructed labor 660.2 ☑
    malpresentation 652.9 ☑
      causing obstructed labor 660.0 ☑
    marginal sinus (bleeding) (rupture) 641.2 ☑
    maternal hypotension syndrome 669.2 ☑
    meconium in liquor 656.8 ☑
    membranes, retained — *see* Delivery, complicated, placenta, retained
    mentum presentation 652.4 ☑
      causing obstructed labor 660.0 ☑
    metrorrhagia (myopathia) — *see* Delivery, complicated, hemorrhage
    metrorrhexis — *see* Delivery, complicated, rupture, uterus
    multiparity (grand) 659.4 ☑
    myelomeningocele, fetus 653.7 ☑
      causing obstructed labor 660.1 ☑
    Nägele's pelvis 653.0 ☑
      causing obstructed labor 660.1 ☑
    nonengagement, fetal head 652.5 ☑
      causing obstructed labor 660.0 ☑
    oblique presentation 652.3 ☑
      causing obstructed labor 660.0 ☑
    obstetric
      shock 669.1 ☑
      trauma NEC 665.9 ☑
    obstructed labor 660.9 ☑
      due to
        abnormality pelvic organs or tissues (conditions classifiable to 654.0-654.9) 660.2 ☑
        deep transverse arrest 660.3 ☑
        impacted shoulders 660.4 ☑
        locked twins 660.5 ☑
        malposition and malpresentation of fetus (conditions classifiable to 652.0-652.9) 660.0 ☑
        persistent occipitoposterior 660.3 ☑
        shoulder dystocia 660.4 ☑
    occult prolapse of umbilical cord 663.0 ☑

Delivery — *continued*
  complicated (by) — *continued*
    oversize fetus 653.5 ☑
      causing obstructed labor 660.1 ☑
    pathological retraction ring, uterus 661.4 ☑
    pelvic
      arrest (deep) (high) (of fetal head) (transverse) 660.3 ☑
      deformity (bone) — *see also* Deformity, pelvis, with disproportion
      soft tissue 654.9 ☑
        causing obstructed labor 660.2 ☑
      tumor NEC 654.9 ☑
        causing obstructed labor 660.2 ☑
    penetration, pregnant uterus by instrument 665.1 ☑
    perforation — *see* Delivery, complicated, laceration
    persistent
      hymen 654.8 ☑
        causing obstructed labor 660.2 ☑
      occipitoposterior 660.3 ☑
    placenta, placental
      ablatio 641.2 ☑
      abnormality 656.7 ☑
        with hemorrhage 641.2 ☑
      abruptio 641.2 ☑
      accreta 667.0 ☑
        with hemorrhage 666.0 ☑
      adherent (without hemorrhage) 667.0 ☑
        with hemorrhage 666.0 ☑
      apoplexy 641.2 ☑
      battledore placenta — *see* Placenta, abnormal 663.8 ☑
      detachment (premature) 641.2 ☑
      disease 656.7 ☑
      hemorrhage NEC 641.9 ☑
      increta (without hemorrhage) 667.0 ☑
        with hemorrhage 666.0 ☑
      low (implantation) 641.0 ☑
        without hemorrhage 641.0 ☑
      malformation 656.7 ☑
        with hemorrhage 641.2 ☑
      malposition 641.1 ☑
        without hemorrhage 641.0 ☑
      marginal sinus rupture 641.2 ☑
      percreta 667.0 ☑
        with hemorrhage 666.0 ☑
      premature separation 641.2 ☑
      previa (central) (lateral) (marginal) partial) 641.1 ☑
        without hemorrhage 641.0 ☑
      retained (with hemorrhage) 666.0 ☑
        without hemorrhage 667.0 ☑
      rupture of marginal sinus 641.2 ☑
      separation (premature) 641.2 ☑
      trapped 666.0 ☑
        without hemorrhage 667.0 ☑
      vicious insertion 641.1 ☑
    polyhydramnios 657.0 ☑
    polyp, cervix 654.6 ☑
      causing obstructed labor 660.2 ☑
    precipitate labor 661.3 ☑
    premature
      labor (before 37 completed weeks gestation) 644.2 ☑
      rupture, membranes 658.1 ☑
        delayed delivery following 658.2 ☑
    presenting umbilical cord 663.0 ☑
    previous
      cesarean delivery 654.2 ☑
      surgery
        cervix 654.6 ☑
          causing obstructed labor 660.2 ☑
        gynecological NEC 654.9 ☑
          causing obstructed labor 660.2 ☑
        perineum 654.8 ☑
        rectum 654.8 ☑   ●
        uterus NEC 654.9 ☑
          due to previous cesarean delivery 654.2 ☑
        vagina 654.7 ☑
          causing obstructed labor 660.2 ☑
        vulva 654.8 ☑
    primary uterine inertia 661.0 ☑
    primipara, elderly or old 659.5 ☑

Delivery — *continued*
  complicated (by) — *continued*
    prolapse
      arm or hand 652.7 ☑
        causing obstructed labor 660.0 ☑
      cord (umbilical) 663.0 ☑
      fetal extremity 652.8 ☑
      foot or leg 652.8 ☑
        causing obstructed labor 660.0 ☑
      umbilical cord (complete) (occult) (partial) 663.0 ☑
      uterus 654.4 ☑
        causing obstructed labor 660.2 ☑
    prolonged labor 662.1 ☑
      first stage 662.0 ☑
      second stage 662.2 ☑
      active phase 661.2 ☑
      due to
        cervical dystocia 661.0 ☑
        contraction ring 661.4 ☑
        tetanic uterus 661.4 ☑
        uterine inertia 661.2 ☑
          primary 661.0 ☑
          secondary 661.1 ☑
      latent phase 661.0 ☑
    pyrexia during labor 659.2 ☑
    rachitic pelvis 653.2 ☑
      causing obstructed labor 660.1 ☑
    rectocele 654.4 ☑
      causing obstructed labor 660.2 ☑
    retained membranes or portions of placenta 666.2 ☑
      without hemorrhage 667.1 ☑
    retarded (prolonged) birth 662.1 ☑
    retention secundines (with hemorrhage) 666.2 ☑
      without hemorrhage 667.1 ☑
    retroversion, uterus or cervix 654.3 ☑
      causing obstructed labor 660.2 ☑
    rigid
      cervix 654.6 ☑
        causing obstructed labor 660.2 ☑
      pelvic floor 654.4 ☑
        causing obstructed labor 660.2 ☑
      perineum or vulva 654.8 ☑
        causing obstructed labor 660.2 ☑
      vagina 654.7 ☑
        causing obstructed labor 660.2 ☑
    Robert's pelvis 653.0 ☑
      causing obstructed labor 660.1 ☑
    rupture — *see also* Delivery, complicated, laceration
      bladder (urinary) 665.5 ☑
      cervix 665.3 ☑
      marginal sinus 641.2 ☑
      membranes, premature 658.1 ☑
      pelvic organ NEC 665.5 ☑
      perineum (without mention of other laceration) — *see* Delivery, complicated, laceration, perineum
      peritoneum 665.5 ☑
      urethra 665.5 ☑
      uterus (during labor) 665.1 ☑
        before labor 665.0 ☑
    sacculation, pregnant uterus 654.4 ☑
    sacral teratomas, fetal 653.7 ☑
      causing obstructed labor 660.1 ☑
    scar(s)
      cervix 654.6 ☑
        causing obstructed labor 660.2 ☑
      cesarean delivery 654.2 ☑
        causing obstructed labor 660.2 ☑
      perineum 654.8 ☑
        causing obstructed labor 660.2 ☑
      uterus NEC 654.9 ☑
        causing obstructed labor 660.2 ☑
        due to previous cesarean delivery 654.2 ☑
      vagina 654.7 ☑
        causing obstructed labor 660.2 ☑
      vulva 654.8 ☑
        causing obstructed labor 660.2 ☑
    scoliotic pelvis 653.0 ☑
      causing obstructed labor 660.1 ☑
    secondary uterine inertia 661.1 ☑
    secundines, retained — *see* Delivery, complicated, placenta, retained

---

☑ Additional Digit Required   ▶◀ Revised Text   ● New Line   ▲ Revised Code

Delivery — *continued*
  complicated (by) — *continued*
    separation
      placenta (premature) 641.2 ☑
      pubic bone 665.6 ☑
      symphysis pubis 665.6 ☑
    septate vagina 654.7 ☑
      causing obstructed labor 660.2 ☑
    shock (birth) (obstetric) (puerperal) 669.1 ☑
    short cord syndrome 663.4 ☑
    shoulder
      girdle dystocia 660.4 ☑
      presentation 652.8 ☑
        causing obstructed labor 660.0 ☑
    Siamese twins 653.7 ☑
      causing obstructed labor 660.1 ☑
    slow slope active phase 661.2 ☑
    spasm
      cervix 661.4 ☑
      uterus 661.4 ☑
    spondylolisthesis, pelvis 653.3 ☑
      causing obstructed labor 660.1 ☑
    spondylolysis (lumbosacral) 653.3 ☑
      causing obstructed labor 660.1 ☑
    spondylosis 653.0 ☑
      causing obstructed labor 660.1 ☑
    stenosis or stricture
      cervix 654.6 ☑
        causing obstructed labor 660.2 ☑
      vagina 654.7 ☑
        causing obstructed labor 660.2 ☑
    sudden death, unknown cause 669.9 ☑
    tear (pelvic organ) (*see also* Delivery, complicated, laceration) 664.9 ☑
    teratomas, sacral, fetal 653.7 ☑
      causing obstructed labor 660.1 ☑
    tetanic uterus 661.4 ☑
    tipping pelvis 653.0 ☑
      causing obstructed labor 660.1 ☑
    transverse
      arrest (deep) 660.3 ☑
      presentation or lie 652.3 ☑
        with successful version 652.1 ☑
        causing obstructed labor 660.0 ☑
    trauma (obstetrical) NEC 665.9 ☑
    tumor
      abdominal, fetal 653.7 ☑
        causing obstructed labor 660.1 ☑
      pelvic organs or tissues NEC 654.9 ☑
        causing obstructed labor 660.2 ☑
    umbilical cord (*see also* Delivery, complicated, cord) 663.9 ☑
      around neck tightly, or with compression 663.1 ☑
      entanglement NEC 663.3 ☑
        with compression 663.2 ☑
      prolapse (complete) (occult) (partial) 663.0 ☑
    unstable lie 652.0 ☑
      causing obstructed labor 660.0 ☑
    uterine
      inertia (*see also* Delivery, complicated, inertia, uterus) 661.2 ☑
      spasm 661.4 ☑
    vasa previa 663.5 ☑
    velamentous insertion of cord 663.8 ☑
    young maternal age 659.8 ☑
  delayed NEC 662.1 ☑
    following rupture of membranes (spontaneous) 658.2 ☑
      artificial 658.3 ☑
    second twin, triplet, etc. 662.3 ☑
  difficult NEC 669.9 ☑
    previous, affecting management of pregnancy or childbirth V23.49
    specified type NEC 669.8 ☑
  early onset (spontaneous) 644.2 ☑
  footling 652.8 ☑
    with successful version 652.1 ☑
  forceps NEC 669.5 ☑
    affecting fetus or newborn 763.2
  missed (at or near term) 656.4 ☑
  multiple gestation NEC 651.9 ☑
    with fetal loss and retention of one or more fetus(es) 651.6 ☑

Delivery — *continued*
  multiple gestation NEC — *continued*
    specified type NEC 651.8 ☑
      with fetal loss and retention of one or more fetus(es) 651.6 ☑
  nonviable infant 656.4 ☑
  normal — *see* category 650
  precipitate 661.3 ☑
    affecting fetus or newborn 763.6
  premature NEC (before 37 completed weeks gestation) 644.2 ☑
    previous, affecting management of pregnancy V23.41
  quadruplet NEC 651.2 ☑
    with fetal loss and retention of one or more fetus(es) 651.5 ☑
  quintuplet NEC 651.8 ☑
    with fetal loss and retention of one or more fetus(es) 651.6 ☑
  sextuplet NEC 651.8 ☑
    with fetal loss and retention of one or more fetus(es) 651.6 ☑
  specified complication NEC 669.8 ☑
  stillbirth (near term) NEC 656.4 ☑
    early (before 22 completed weeks gestation) 632
  term pregnancy (live birth) NEC — *see* category 650
    stillbirth NEC 656.4 ☑
  threatened premature 644.2 ☑
  triplets NEC 651.1 ☑
    with fetal loss and retention of one or more fetus(es) 651.4 ☑
    delayed delivery (one or more mates) 662.3 ☑
    locked mates 660.5 ☑
  twins NEC 651.0 ☑
    with fetal loss and retention of one fetus 651.3 ☑
    delayed delivery (one or more mates) 662.3 ☑
    locked mates 660.5 ☑
  uncomplicated — *see* category 650
  vacuum extractor NEC 669.5 ☑
    affecting fetus or newborn 763.3
  ventouse NEC 669.5 ☑
    affecting fetus or newborn 763.3

Dellen, cornea 371.41

Delusions (paranoid) 297.9
  grandiose 297.1
  parasitosis 300.29
  systematized 297.1

Dementia 294.8
  ▶alcohol-induced persisting◀ (*see also* Psychosis, alcoholic) 291.2
  Alzheimer's — *see* Alzheimer's dementia
  arteriosclerotic (simple type) (uncomplicated) 290.40
    with
      acute confusional state 290.41
      delirium 290.41
      ▶delusions◀ 290.42
      ▶depressed mood◀ 290.43
    depressed type 290.43
    paranoid type 290.42
  Binswanger's 290.12
  catatonic (acute) (*see also* Schizophrenia) 295.2 ☑
  congenital (*see also* Retardation, mental) 319
  degenerative 290.9
    presenile-onset — *see* Dementia, presenile
    senile-onset — *see* Dementia, senile
  developmental (*see also* Schizophrenia) 295.9 ☑
  dialysis 294.8
    transient 293.9
  drug-induced persisting (*see also* Psychosis, drug) 292.82 ●
  due to or associated with condition(s) classified elsewhere
    Alzheimer's
      with behavioral disturbance 331.0 [294.11]
      without behavioral disturbance 331.0 [294.10]

Dementia — *continued*
  due to or associated with condition(s) classified elsewhere — *continued*
    cerebral lipidoses
      with behavioral disturbance 330.1 [294.11]
      without behavioral disturbance 330.1 [294.10]
    epilepsy
      with behavioral disturbance 345.9 ☑ [294.11]
      without behavioral disturbance 345.9 ☑ [294.10]
    hepatolenticular degeneration
      with behavioral disturbance 275.1 [294.11]
      without behavioral disturbance 275.1 [294.10]
    HIV
      with behavioral disturbance 042 [294.11]
      without behavioral disturbance 042 [294.10]
    Huntington's chorea
      with behavioral disturbance 333.4 [294.11]
      without behavioral disturbance 333.4 [294.10]
    Jakob-Creutzfeldt disease
      with behavioral disturbance 046.1 [294.11]
      without behavioral disturbance 046.1 [294.10]
    Lewy bodies
      with behavioral disturbance 331.82 [294.11]
      without behavioral disturbance 331.82 [294.10]
    multiple sclerosis
      with behavioral disturbance 340 [294.11]
      without behavioral disturbance 340 [294.10]
    neurosyphilis
      with behavioral disturbance 094.9 [294.11]
      without behavioral disturbance 094.9 [294.10]
    Parkinsonism
      with behavioral disturbance 331.82 [294.11]
      without behavioral disturbance 331.82 [294.10]
    Pelizaeus-Merzbacher disease
      with behavioral disturbance 333.0 [294.11]
      without behavioral disturbance 333.0 [294.10]
    Pick's disease
      with behavioral disturbance 331.11 [294.11]
      without behavioral disturbance 331.11 [294.10]
    polyarteritis nodosa
      with behavioral disturbance 446.0 [294.11]
      without behavioral disturbance 446.0 [294.10]
    syphilis
      with behavioral disturbance 094.1 [294.11]
      without behavioral disturbance 094.1 [294.10]
    Wilson's disease
      with behavioral disturbance 275.1 [294.11]
      without behavioral disturbance 275.1 [294.10]
  frontal 331.19
    with behavioral disturbance 331.19 [294.11]
    without behavioral disturbance 331.19 [294.10]
  frontotemporal 331.19
    with behavioral disturbance 331.19 [294.11]
    without behavioral disturbance 331.19 [294.10]
  hebephrenic (acute) 295.1 ☑

☑ Additional Digit Required   ▶◀ Revised Text   ● New Line   ▲ Revised Code

Dementia — *continued*
  Heller's (infantile psychosis) (*see also*
    Psychosis, childhood) 299.1 ☑
  idiopathic 290.9
    presenile-onset — *see* Dementia, presenile
    senile-onset — *see* Dementia, senile
  in
    arteriosclerotic brain disease 290.40
    senility 290.0
  induced by drug 292.82
  infantile, infantilia (*see also* Psychosis,
    childhood) 299.0 ☑
  Lewy body 331.82
    with behavioral disturbance
      331.82 [294.11]
    without behavioral disturbance
      331.82 [294.10]
  multi-infarct (cerebrovascular) (*see also*
    Dementia, arteriosclerotic) 290.40
  old age 290.0
  paralytica, paralytic 094.1
    juvenilis 090.40
    syphilitic 094.1
      congenital 090.40
    tabetic form 094.1
  paranoid (*see also* Schizophrenia) 295.3 ☑
  paraphrenic (*see also* Schizophrenia) 295.3 ☑
  paretic 094.1
  praecox (*see also* Schizophrenia) 295.9 ☑
  presenile 290.10
    with
      acute confusional state 290.11
      delirium 290.11
      delusional features 290.12
      depressive features 290.13
    depressed type 290.13
    paranoid type 290.12
    simple type 290.10
    uncomplicated 290.10
  primary (acute) (*see also* Schizophrenia)
    295.0 ☑
  progressive, syphilitic 094.1
  puerperal — *see* Psychosis, puerperal
  schizophrenic (*see also* Schizophrenia) 295.9 ☑
  senile 290.0
    with
      acute confusional state 290.3
      delirium 290.3
      delusional features 290.20
      depressive features 290.21
    depressed type 290.21
    exhaustion 290.0
    paranoid type 290.20
  simple type (acute) (*see also* Schizophrenia)
    295.0 ☑
  simplex (acute) (*see also* Schizophrenia)
    295.0 ☑
  syphilitic 094.1
  uremic — *see* Uremia
  vascular 290.40
    with ●
      delirium 290.41 ●
      delusions 290.42 ●
      depressed mood 290.43 ●

Demerol dependence (*see also* Dependence)
  304.0 ☑

Demineralization, ankle (*see also* Osteoporosis)
  733.00

Demodex folliculorum (infestation) 133.8

de Morgan's spots (senile angiomas) 448.1

Demyelinating
  polyneuritis, chronic inflammatory 357.81

Demyelination, demyelinization
  central nervous system 341.9
    specified NEC 341.8
  corpus callosum (central) 341.8
  global 340

Dengue (fever) 061
  sandfly 061
  vaccination, prophylactic (against) V05.1
  virus hemorrhagic fever 065.4

Dens
  evaginatus 520.2
  in dente 520.2
  invaginatus 520.2

Density
  increased, bone (disseminated) (generalized)
    (spotted) 733.99
  lung (nodular) 518.89

Dental — *see also* condition
  examination only V72.2

Dentia praecox 520.6

Denticles (in pulp) 522.2

Dentigerous cyst 526.0

Dentin
  irregular (in pulp) 522.3
  opalescent 520.5
  secondary (in pulp) 522.3
  sensitive 521.8

Dentinogenesis imperfecta 520.5

Dentinoma (M9271/0) 213.1
  upper jaw (bone) 213.0

Dentition 520.7
  abnormal 520.6
  anomaly 520.6
  delayed 520.6
  difficult 520.7
  disorder of 520.6
  precocious 520.6
  retarded 520.6

Denture sore (mouth) 528.9

Dependence

> Note — Use the following fifth-digit
> subclassification with category 304:
>
> 0   unspecified
> 1   continuous
> 2   episodic
> 3   in remission

  with
    withdrawal symptoms
      alcohol 291.81
      drug 292.0
  14-hydroxy-dihydromorphinone 304.0 ☑
  absinthe 304.6 ☑
  acemorphan 304.0 ☑
  acetanilid(e) 304.6 ☑
  acetophenetidin 304.6 ☑
  acetorphine 304.0 ☑
  acetyldihydrocodeine 304.0 ☑
  acetyldihydrocodeinone 304.0 ☑
  Adalin 304.1 ☑
  Afghanistan black 304.3 ☑
  agrypnal 304.1 ☑
  alcohol, alcoholic (ethyl) (methyl) (wood)
    303.9 ☑
    maternal, with suspected fetal damage
      affecting management of pregnancy
      655.4 ☑
  allobarbitone 304.1 ☑
  allonal 304.1 ☑
  allylisopropylacetylurea 304.1 ☑
  alphaprodine (hydrochloride) 304.0 ☑
  Alurate 304.1 ☑
  Alvodine 304.0 ☑
  amethocaine 304.6 ☑
  amidone 304.0 ☑
  amidopyrine 304.6 ☑
  aminopyrine 304.6 ☑
  amobarbital 304.1 ☑
  amphetamine(s) (type) (drugs classifiable to
    969.7) 304.4 ☑
  amylene hydrate 304.6 ☑
  amylobarbitone 304.1 ☑
  amylocaine 304.6 ☑
  Amytal (sodium) 304.1 ☑
  analgesic (drug) NEC 304.6 ☑
    synthetic with morphine-like effect 304.0 ☑
  anesthetic (agent) (drug) (gas) (general) (local)
    NEC 304.6 ☑
  Angel dust 304.6 ☑
  anileridine 304.0 ☑
  antipyrine 304.6 ☑
  anxiolytic 304.1 ☑   ●
  aprobarbital 304.1 ☑
  aprobarbitone 304.1 ☑
  atropine 304.6 ☑
  Avertin (bromide) 304.6 ☑

Dependence — *continued*
  barbenyl 304.1 ☑
  barbital(s) 304.1 ☑
  barbitone 304.1 ☑
  barbiturate(s) (compounds) (drugs classifiable
    to 967.0) 304.1 ☑
  barbituric acid (and compounds) 304.1 ☑
  benzedrine 304.4 ☑
  benzylmorphine 304.0 ☑
  Beta-chlor 304.1 ☑
  bhang 304.3 ☑
  blue velvet 304.0 ☑
  Brevital 304.1 ☑
  bromal (hydrate) 304.1 ☑
  bromide(s) NEC 304.1 ☑
  bromine compounds NEC 304.1 ☑
  bromisovalum 304.1 ☑
  bromoform 304.1 ☑
  Bromo-seltzer 304.1 ☑
  bromural 304.1 ☑
  butabarbital (sodium) 304.1 ☑
  butabarpal 304.1 ☑
  butallylonal 304.1 ☑
  butethal 304.1 ☑
  buthalitone (sodium) 304.1 ☑
  Butisol 304.1 ☑
  butobarbitone 304.1 ☑
  butyl chloral (hydrate) 304.1 ☑
  caffeine 304.4 ☑
  cannabis (indica) (sativa) (resin) (derivatives)
    (type) 304.3 ☑
  carbamazepine 304.6 ☑
  Carbrital 304.1 ☑
  carbromal 304.1 ☑
  carisoprodol 304.6 ☑
  Catha (edulis) 304.4 ☑
  chloral (betaine) (hydrate) 304.1 ☑
  chloralamide 304.1 ☑
  chloralformamide 304.1 ☑
  chloralose 304.1 ☑
  chlordiazepoxide 304.1 ☑
  Chloretone 304.1 ☑
  chlorobutanol 304.1 ☑
  chlorodyne 304.1 ☑
  chloroform 304.6 ☑
  Cliradon 304.0 ☑
  coca (leaf) and derivatives 304.2 ☑
  cocaine 304.2 ☑
    hydrochloride 304.2 ☑
    salt (any) 304.2 ☑
  codeine 304.0 ☑
  combination of drugs (excluding morphine or
    opioid type drug) NEC 304.8 ☑
    morphine or opioid type drug with any other
      drug 304.7 ☑
  croton-chloral 304.1 ☑
  cyclobarbital 304.1 ☑
  cyclobarbitone 304.1 ☑
  dagga 304.3 ☑
  Delvinal 304.1 ☑
  Demerol 304.0 ☑
  desocodeine 304.0 ☑
  desomorphine 304.0 ☑
  desoxyephedrine 304.4 ☑
  DET 304.5 ☑
  dexamphetamine 304.4 ☑
  dexedrine 304.4 ☑
  dextromethorphan 304.0 ☑
  dextromoramide 304.0 ☑
  dextronorpseudoephedrine 304.4 ☑
  dextrorphan 304.0 ☑
  diacetylmorphine 304.0 ☑
  Dial 304.1 ☑
  diallylbarbituric acid 304.1 ☑
  diamorphine 304.0 ☑
  diazepam 304.1 ☑
  dibucaine 304.6 ☑
  dichloroethane 304.6 ☑
  diethyl barbituric acid 304.1 ☑
  diethylsulfone-diethylmethane 304.1 ☑
  difencloxazine 304.0 ☑
  dihydrocodeine 304.0 ☑
  dihydrocodeinone 304.0 ☑
  dihydrohydroxycodeinone 304.0 ☑
  dihydroisocodeine 304.0 ☑
  dihydromorphine 304.0 ☑
  dihydromorphinone 304.0 ☑

☑ Additional Digit Required   ►◄ Revised Text   ● New Line   ▲ Revised Code

Dependence — *continued*
  dihydroxcodeinone 304.0 ☑
  Dilaudid 304.0 ☑
  dimenhydrinate 304.6 ☑
  dimethylmeperidine 304.0 ☑
  dimethyltriptamine 304.5 ☑
  Dionin 304.0 ☑
  diphenoxylate 304.6 ☑
  dipipanone 304.0 ☑
  d-lysergic acid diethylamide 304.5 ☑
  DMT 304.5 ☑
  Dolophine 304.0 ☑
  DOM 304.2 ☑
  Doriden 304.1 ☑
  dormiral 304.1 ☑
  Dormison 304.1 ☑
  Dromoran 304.0 ☑
  drug NEC 304.9 ☑
    analgesic NEC 304.6 ☑
    combination (excluding morphine or opioid
        type drug) NEC 304.8 ☑
      morphine or opioid type drug with any
          other drug 304.7 ☑
    complicating pregnancy, childbirth, or
        puerperium 648.3 ☑
      affecting fetus or newborn 779.5
    hallucinogenic 304.5 ☑
    hypnotic NEC 304.1 ☑
    narcotic NEC 304.9 ☑
    psychostimulant NEC 304.4 ☑
    sedative 304.1 ☑
    soporific NEC 304.1 ☑
    specified type NEC 304.6 ☑
    suspected damage to fetus affecting
        management of pregnancy 655.5 ☑
    synthetic, with morphine-like effect 304.0 ☑
    tranquilizing 304.1 ☑
  duboisine 304.6 ☑
  ectylurea 304.1 ☑
  Endocaine 304.6 ☑
  Equanil 304.1 ☑
  Eskabarb 304.1 ☑
  ethchlorvynol 304.1 ☑
  ether (ethyl) (liquid) (vapor) (vinyl) 304.6 ☑
  ethidene 304.6 ☑
  ethinamate 304.1 ☑
  ethoheptazine 304.6 ☑
  ethyl
    alcohol 303.9 ☑
    bromide 304.6 ☑
    carbamate 304.6 ☑
    chloride 304.6 ☑
    morphine 304.0 ☑
  ethylene (gas) 304.6 ☑
    dichloride 304.6 ☑
  ethylidene chloride 304.6 ☑
  etilfen 304.1 ☑
  etorphine 304.0 ☑
  etoval 304.1 ☑
  eucodal 304.0 ☑
  euneryl 304.1 ☑
  Evipal 304.1 ☑
  Evipan 304.1 ☑
  fentanyl 304.0 ☑
  ganja 304.3 ☑
  gardenal 304.1 ☑
  gardenpanyl 304.1 ☑
  gelsemine 304.6 ☑
  Gelsemium 304.6 ☑
  Gemonil 304.1 ☑
  glucochloral 304.1 ☑
  glue (airplane) (sniffing) 304.6 ☑
  glutethimide 304.1 ☑
  hallucinogenics 304.5 ☑
  hashish 304.3 ☑
  headache powder NEC 304.6 ☑
  Heavenly Blue 304.5 ☑
  hedonal 304.1 ☑
  hemp 304.3 ☑
  heptabarbital 304.1 ☑
  Heptalgin 304.0 ☑
  heptobarbitone 304.1 ☑
  heroin 304.0 ☑
    salt (any) 304.0 ☑
  hexethal (sodium) 304.1 ☑
  hexobarbital 304.1 ☑
  Hycodan 304.0 ☑

Dependence — *continued*
  hydrocodone 304.0 ☑
  hydromorphinol 304.0 ☑
  hydromorphinone 304.0 ☑
  hydromorphone 304.0 ☑
  hydroxycodeine 304.0 ☑
  hypnotic NEC 304.1 ☑
  Indian hemp 304.3 ☑
  inhalant 304.6 ☑   ●
  intranarcon 304.1 ☑
  Kemithal 304.1 ☑
  ketobemidone 304.0 ☑
  khat 304.4 ☑
  kif 304.3 ☑
  Lactuca (virosa) extract 304.1 ☑
  lactucarium 304.1 ☑
  laudanum 304.0 ☑
  Lebanese red 304.3 ☑
  Leritine 304.0 ☑
  lettuce opium 304.1 ☑
  Levanil 304.1 ☑
  Levo-Dromoran 304.0 ☑
  levo-iso-methadone 304.0 ☑
  levorphanol 304.0 ☑
  Librium 304.1 ☑
  Lomotil 304.6 ☑
  Lotusate 304.1 ☑
  LSD (-25) (and derivatives) 304.5 ☑
  Luminal 304.1 ☑
  lysergic acid 304.5 ☑
    amide 304.5 ☑
  maconha 304.3 ☑
  magic mushroom 304.5 ☑
  marihuana 304.3 ☑
  MDA (methylene dioxyamphetamine) 304.4 ☑
  Mebaral 304.1 ☑
  Medinal 304.1 ☑
  Medomin 304.1 ☑
  megahallucinogenics 304.5 ☑
  meperidine 304.0 ☑
  mephobarbital 304.1 ☑
  meprobamate 304.1 ☑
  mescaline 304.5 ☑
  methadone 304.0 ☑
  methamphetamine(s) 304.4 ☑
  methaqualone 304.1 ☑
  metharbital 304.1 ☑
  methitural 304.1 ☑
  methobarbitone 304.1 ☑
  methohexital 304.1 ☑
  methopholine 304.6 ☑
  methyl
    alcohol 303.9 ☑
    bromide 304.6 ☑
    morphine 304.0 ☑
    sulfonal 304.1 ☑
  methylated spirit 303.9 ☑
  methylbutinol 304.6 ☑
  methyldihydromorphinone 304.0 ☑
  methylene
    chloride 304.6 ☑
    dichloride 304.6 ☑
    dioxyamphetamine (MDA) 304.4 ☑
  methylaparafynol 304.1 ☑
  methylphenidate 304.4 ☑
  methyprylone 304.1 ☑
  metopon 304.0 ☑
  Miltown 304.1 ☑
  morning glory *seeds* 304.5 ☑
  morphinan(s) 304.0 ☑
  morphine (sulfate) (sulfite) (type) (drugs
      classifiable to 965.00-965.09) 304.0 ☑
  morphine or opioid type drug (drugs classifiable
      to 965.00-965.09) with any other drug
      304.7 ☑
  morphinol(s) 304.0 ☑
  morphinon 304.0 ☑
  morpholinylethylmorphine 304.0 ☑
  mylomid 304.1 ☑
  myristicin 304.5 ☑
  narcotic (drug) NEC 304.9 ☑
  nealbarbital 304.1 ☑
  nealbarbitone 304.1 ☑
  Nembutal 304.1 ☑
  Neonal 304.1 ☑
  Neraval 304.1 ☑
  Neravan 304.1 ☑

Dependence — *continued*
  neurobarb 304.1 ☑
  nicotine 305.1
  Nisentil 304.0 ☑
  nitrous oxide 304.6 ☑
  Noctec 304.1 ☑
  Noludar 304.1 ☑
  nonbarbiturate sedatives and tranquilizers with
      similar effect 304.1 ☑
  noptil 304.1 ☑
  normorphine 304.0 ☑
  noscapine 304.0 ☑
  Novocaine 304.6 ☑
  Numorphan 304.0 ☑
  nunol 304.1 ☑
  Nupercaine 304.6 ☑
  Oblivon 304.1 ☑
  on
    aspirator V46.0
    hyperbaric chamber V46.8
    iron lung V46.11   ▲
    machine (enabling) V46.9
      specified type NEC V46.8
    Possum (Patient-Operated-Selector-
        Mechanism) V46.8
    renal dialysis machine V45.1
    respirator V46.11   ▲
      encounter during power failure   ●
          V46.12   ●
    supplemental oxygen V46.2
  opiate 304.0 ☑
  opioids 304.0 ☑
  opioid type drug 304.0 ☑
    with any other drug 304.7 ☑
  opium (alkaloids) (derivatives) (tincture)
      304.0 ☑
  ortal 304.1 ☑
  Oxazepam 304.1 ☑
  oxycodone 304.0 ☑
  oxymorphone 304.0 ☑
  Palfium 304.0 ☑
  Panadol 304.6 ☑
  pantopium 304.0 ☑
  pantopon 304.0 ☑
  papaverine 304.0 ☑
  paracetamol 304.6 ☑
  paracodin 304.0 ☑
  paraldehyde 304.1 ☑
  paregoric 304.0 ☑
  Parzone 304.0 ☑
  PCP (phencyclidine) 304.6 ☑
  Pearly Gates 304.5 ☑
  pentazocine 304.0 ☑
  pentobarbital 304.1 ☑
  pentobarbitone (sodium) 304.1 ☑
  Pentothal 304.1 ☑
  Percaine 304.6 ☑
  Percodan 304.0 ☑
  Perichlor 304.1 ☑
  Pernocton 304.1 ☑
  Pernoston 304.1 ☑
  peronine 304.0 ☑
  pethidine (hydrochloride) 304.0 ☑
  petrichloral 304.1 ☑
  peyote 304.5 ☑
  Phanodron 304.1 ☑
  phenacetin 304.6 ☑
  phenadoxone 304.0 ☑
  phenaglycodol 304.1 ☑
  phenazocine 304.0 ☑
  phencyclidine 304.6 ☑
  phenmetrazine 304.4 ☑
  phenobal 304.1 ☑
  phenobarbital 304.1 ☑
  phenobarbitone 304.1 ☑
  phenomorphan 304.0 ☑
  phenonyl 304.1 ☑
  phenoperidine 304.0 ☑
  pholcodine 304.0 ☑
  piminodine 304.0 ☑
  Pipadone 304.0 ☑
  Pitkin's solution 304.6 ☑
  Placidyl 304.1 ☑
  polysubstance 304.8 ☑
  Pontocaine 304.6 ☑
  pot 304.3 ☑
  potassium bromide 304.1 ☑

☑ Additional Digit Required   ▶◀ Revised Text   ● New Line   ▲ Revised Code

Dependence — *continued*
  Preludin 304.4 ☑
  Prinadol 304.0 ☑
  probarbital 304.1 ☑
  procaine 304.6 ☑
  propanal 304.1 ☑
  propoxyphene 304.6 ☑
  psilocibin 304.5 ☑
  psilocin 304.5 ☑
  psilocybin 304.5 ☑
  psilocyline 304.5 ☑
  psilocyn 304.5 ☑
  psychedelic agents 304.5 ☑
  psychostimulant NEC 304.4 ☑
  psychotomimetic agents 304.5 ☑
  pyrahexyl 304.3 ☑
  Pyramidon 304.6 ☑
  quinalbarbitone 304.1 ☑
  racemoramide 304.0 ☑
  racemorphan 304.0 ☑
  Rela 304.6 ☑
  scopolamine 304.6 ☑
  secobarbital 304.1 ☑
  Seconal 304.1 ☑
  sedative NEC 304.1 ☑
    nonbarbiturate with barbiturate effect 304.1 ☑
  Sedormid 304.1 ☑
  sernyl 304.1 ☑
  sodium bromide 304.1 ☑
  Soma 304.6 ☑
  Somnal 304.1 ☑
  Somnos 304.1 ☑
  Soneryl 304.1 ☑
  soporific (drug) NEC 304.1 ☑
  specified drug NEC 304.6 ☑
  speed 304.4 ☑
  spinocaine 304.6 ☑
  Stovaine 304.6 ☑
  STP 304.5 ☑
  stramonium 304.6 ☑
  Sulfonal 304.1 ☑
  sulfonethylmethane 304.1 ☑
  sulfonmethane 304.1 ☑
  Surital 304.1 ☑
  synthetic drug with morphine-like effect 304.0 ☑
  talbutal 304.1 ☑
  tetracaine 304.6 ☑
  tetrahydrocannabinol 304.3 ☑
  tetronal 304.1 ☑
  THC 304.3 ☑
  thebacon 304.0 ☑
  thebaine 304.0 ☑
  thiamil 304.1 ☑
  thiamylal 304.1 ☑
  thiopental 304.1 ☑
  tobacco 305.1
  toluene, toluol 304.6 ☑
  tranquilizer NEC 304.1 ☑
    nonbarbiturate with barbiturate effect 304.1 ☑
  tribromacetaldehyde 304.6 ☑
  tribromethanol 304.6 ☑
  tribromomethane 304.6 ☑
  trichloroethanol 304.6 ☑
  trichoroethyl phosphate 304.1 ☑
  triclofos 304.1 ☑
  Trional 304.1 ☑
  Tuinal 304.1 ☑
  Turkish Green 304.3 ☑
  urethan(e) 304.6 ☑
  Valium 304.1 ☑
  Valmid 304.1 ☑
  veganin 304.0 ☑
  veramon 304.1 ☑
  Veronal 304.1 ☑
  versidyne 304.6 ☑
  vinbarbital 304.1 ☑
  vinbarbitone 304.1 ☑
  vinyl bitone 304.1 ☑
  vitamin B_6 266.1
  wine 303.9 ☑
  Zactane 304.6 ☑
Dependency
  passive 301.6
  reactions 301.6

Depersonalization (episode, in neurotic state) (neurotic) (syndrome) 300.6
Depletion
  carbohydrates 271.9
  complement factor 279.8
  extracellular fluid 276.5
  plasma 276.5
  potassium 276.8
    nephropathy 588.89   ▲
  salt or sodium 276.1
    causing heat exhaustion or prostration 992.4
    nephropathy 593.9
  volume 276.5
    extracellular fluid 276.5
    plasma 276.5
Deposit
  argentous, cornea 371.16
  bone, in Boeck's sarcoid 135
  calcareous, calcium — *see* Calcification
  cholesterol
    retina 362.82
    skin 709.3
    vitreous (humor) 379.22
  conjunctival 372.56
  cornea, corneal NEC 371.10
    argentous 371.16
    in
      cystinosis 270.0 *[371.15]*
      mucopolysaccharidosis 277.5 *[371.15]*
  crystalline, vitreous (humor) 379.22
  hemosiderin, in old scars of cornea 371.11
  metallic, in lens 366.45
  skin 709.3
  teeth, tooth (betel) (black) (green) (materia alba) (orange) (soft) (tobacco) 523.6
  urate, in kidney (*see also* Disease, renal) 593.9
Depraved appetite 307.52
Depression 311
  acute (*see also* Psychosis, affective) 296.2 ☑
    recurrent episode 296.3 ☑
    single episode 296.2 ☑
  agitated (*see also* Psychosis, affective) 296.2 ☑
    recurrent episode 296.3 ☑
    single episode 296.2 ☑
  anaclitic 309.21
  anxiety 300.4
  arches 734
    congenital 754.61
  autogenous (*see also* Psychosis, affective) 296.2 ☑
    recurrent episode 296.3 ☑
    single episode 296.2 ☑
  basal metabolic rate (BMR) 794.7
  bone marrow 289.9
  central nervous system 799.1
    newborn 779.2
  cerebral 331.9
    newborn 779.2
  cerebrovascular 437.8
    newborn 779.2
  chest wall 738.3
  endogenous (*see also* Psychosis, affective) 296.2 ☑
    recurrent episode 296.3 ☑
    single episode 296.2 ☑
  functional activity 780.99
  hysterical 300.11
  involutional, climacteric, or menopausal (*see also* Psychosis, affective) 296.2 ☑
    recurrent episode 296.3 ☑
    single episode 296.2 ☑
  manic (*see also* Psychosis, affective) 296.80
  medullary 348.8
    newborn 779.2
  mental 300.4
  metatarsal heads — *see* Depression, arches
  metatarsus — *see* Depression, arches
  monopolar (*see also* Psychosis, affective) 296.2 ☑
    recurrent episode 296.3 ☑
    single episode 296.2 ☑
  nervous 300.4
  neurotic 300.4
  nose 738.0
  postpartum 648.4 ☑

Depression — *continued*
  psychogenic 300.4
    reactive 298.0
  psychoneurotic 300.4
  psychotic (*see also* Psychosis, affective) 296.2 ☑
    reactive 298.0
    recurrent episode 296.3 ☑
    single episode 296.2 ☑
  reactive 300.4
    neurotic 300.4
    psychogenic 298.0
    psychoneurotic 300.4
    psychotic 298.0
  recurrent 296.3 ☑
  respiratory center 348.8
    newborn 770.89
  scapula 736.89
  senile 290.21
  situational (acute) (brief) 309.0
    prolonged 309.1
  skull 754.0
  sternum 738.3
  visual field 368.40
Depressive reaction — *see also* Reaction, depressive
  acute (transient) 309.0
    with anxiety 309.28
  prolonged 309.1
  situational (acute) 309.0
    prolonged 309.1
Deprivation
  cultural V62.4
  emotional V62.89
    affecting
      adult 995.82
      infant or child 995.51
  food 994.2
    specific substance NEC 269.8
  protein (familial) (kwashiorkor) 260
  sleep V69.4   ●
  social V62.4
    affecting
      adult 995.82
      infant or child 995.51
  symptoms, syndrome
    alcohol 291.81
    drug 292.0
  vitamins (*see also* Deficiency, vitamin) 269.2
  water 994.3
de Quervain's
  disease (tendon sheath) 727.04
  thyroiditis (subacute granulomatous thyroiditis) 245.1
Derangement
  ankle (internal) 718.97
    current injury (*see also* Dislocation, ankle) 837.0
    recurrent 718.37
  cartilage (articular) NEC (*see also* Disorder, cartilage, articular) 718.0 ☑
    knee 717.9
      recurrent 718.36
    recurrent 718.3 ☑
  collateral ligament (knee) (medial) (tibial) 717.82
    current injury 844.1
      lateral (fibular) 844.0
    lateral (fibular) 717.81
      current injury 844.0
  cruciate ligament (knee) (posterior) 717.84
    anterior 717.83
      current injury 844.2
    current injury 844.2
  elbow (internal) 718.92
    current injury (*see also* Dislocation, elbow) 832.00
    recurrent 718.32
  gastrointestinal 536.9
  heart — *see* Disease, heart
  hip (joint) (internal) (old) 718.95
    current injury (*see also* Dislocation, hip) 835.00
    recurrent 718.35
  intervertebral disc — *see* Displacement, intervertebral disc

---

☑ Additional Digit Required   ►◄ Revised Text   ● New Line   ▲ Revised Code

Derangement — *continued*
joint (internal) 718.90
ankle 718.97
current injury — *see also* Dislocation, by
site
knee, meniscus or cartilage (*see also*
Tear, meniscus) 836.2
elbow 718.92
foot 718.97
hand 718.94
hip 718.95
knee 717.9
multiple sites 718.99
pelvic region 718.95
recurrent 718.30
ankle 718.37
elbow 718.32
foot 718.37
hand 718.34
hip 718.35
knee 718.36
multiple sites 718.39
pelvic region 718.35
shoulder (region) 718.31
specified site NEC 718.38
temporomandibular (old) 524.69
wrist 718.33
shoulder (region) 718.91
specified site NEC 718.98
spine NEC 724.9
temporomandibular 524.69
wrist 718.93
knee (cartilage) (internal) 717.9
current injury (*see also* Tear, meniscus)
836.2
ligament 717.89
capsular 717.85
collateral — *see* Derangement, collateral
ligament
cruciate — *see* Derangement, cruciate
ligament
specified NEC 717.85
recurrent 718.36
low back NEC 724.9
meniscus NEC (knee) 717.5
current injury (*see also* Tear, meniscus)
836.2
lateral 717.40
anterior horn 717.42
posterior horn 717.43
specified NEC 717.49
medial 717.3
anterior horn 717.1
posterior horn 717.2
recurrent 718.3 ☑
site other than knee — *see* Disorder,
cartilage, articular
mental (*see also* Psychosis) 298.9
rotator cuff (recurrent) (tear) 726.10
current 840.4
sacroiliac (old) 724.6
current — *see* Dislocation, sacroiliac
semilunar cartilage (knee) 717.5
current injury 836.2
lateral 836.1
medial 836.0
recurrent 718.3 ☑
shoulder (internal) 718.91
current injury (*see also* Dislocation,
shoulder) 831.00
recurrent 718.31
spine (recurrent) NEC 724.9
current — *see* Dislocation, spine
temporomandibular (internal) (joint) (old)
524.69
current — *see* Dislocation, jaw

Dercum's disease or syndrome (adiposis
dolorosa) 272.8

Derealization (neurotic) 300.6

Dermal — *see* condition

Dermaphytid — *see* Dermatophytosis

Dermatergosis — *see* Dermatitis

Dermatitis (allergic) (contact) (occupational)
(venenata) 692.9
ab igne 692.82
acneiform 692.9

Dermatitis — *continued*
actinic (due to sun) 692.70
acute 692.72
chronic NEC 692.74
other than from sun NEC 692.82
ambustionis
due to
burn or scald — *see* Burn, by site
sunburn (*see also* Sunburn) 692.71
amebic 006.6
ammonia 691.0
anaphylactoid NEC 692.9
arsenical 692.4
artefacta 698.4
psychogenic 316 *[698.4]*
asthmatic 691.8
atopic (allergic) (intrinsic) 691.8
psychogenic 316 *[691.8]*
atrophicans 701.8
diffusa 701.8
maculosa 701.3
berlock, berloque 692.72
blastomycetic 116.0
blister beetle 692.89
Brucella NEC 023.9
bullosa 694.9
striata pratensis 692.6
bullous 694.9
mucosynechial, atrophic 694.60
with ocular involvement 694.61
seasonal 694.8
calorica
due to
burn or scald — *see* Burn, by site
cold 692.89
sunburn (*see also* Sunburn) 692.71
caterpillar 692.89
cercarial 120.3
combustionis
due to
burn or scald — *see* Burn, by site
sunburn (*see also* Sunburn) 692.71
congelationis 991.5
contusiformis 695.2
diabetic 250.8 ☑
diaper 691.0
diphtheritica 032.85
due to
acetone 692.2
acids 692.4
adhesive plaster 692.4
alcohol (skin contact) (substances
classifiable to 980.0-980.9) 692.4
taken internally 693.8
alkalis 692.4
allergy NEC 692.9
ammonia (household) (liquid) 692.4
animal ●
dander (cat) (dog) 692.84 ●
hair (cat) (dog) 692.84 ●
arnica 692.3
arsenic 692.4
taken internally 693.8
blister beetle 692.89
cantharides 692.3
carbon disulphide 692.2
caterpillar 692.89
caustics 692.4
cereal (ingested) 693.1
contact with skin 692.5
chemical(s) NEC 692.4
internal 693.8
irritant NEC 692.4
taken internally 693.8
chlorocompounds 692.2
coffee (ingested) 693.1
contact with skin 692.5
cold weather 692.89
cosmetics 692.81
cyclohexanes 692.2
dander, animal (cat) (dog) 692.84 ●
deodorant 692.81
detergents 692.0
dichromate 692.4
drugs and medicinals (correct substance
properly administered) (internal use)
693.0

Dermatitis — *continued*
due to — *continued*
drugs and medicinals — *continued*
external (in contact with skin) 692.3
wrong substance given or taken 976.9
specified substance — *see* Table of
Drugs and Chemicals
wrong substance given or taken 977.9
specified substance — *see* Table of
Drugs and Chemicals
dyes 692.89
hair 692.89
epidermophytosis — *see* Dermatophytosis
esters 692.2
external irritant NEC 692.9
specified agent NEC 692.89
eye shadow 692.81
fish (ingested) 693.1
contact with skin 692.5
flour (ingested) 693.1
contact with skin 692.5
food (ingested) 693.1
in contact with skin 692.5
fruit (ingested) 693.1
contact with skin 692.5
fungicides 692.3
furs 692.84 ▲
glycols 692.2
greases NEC 692.1
hair dyes 692.89
hair, animal (cat) (dog) 692.84 ●
hot
objects and materials — *see* Burn, by
site
weather or places 692.89
hydrocarbons 692.2
infrared rays, except from sun 692.82
solar NEC (*see also* Dermatitis, due to,
sun) 692.70
ingested substance 693.9
drugs and medicinals (*see also*
Dermatitis, due to, drugs and
medicinals) 693.0
food 693.1
specified substance NEC 693.8
ingestion or injection of chemical 693.8
drug (correct substance properly
administered) 693.0
wrong substance given or taken 977.9
specified substance — *see* Table of
Drugs and Chemicals
insecticides 692.4
internal agent 693.9
drugs and medicinals (*see also*
Dermatitis, due to, drugs and
medicinals) 693.0
food (ingested) 693.1
in contact with skin 692.5
specified agent NEC 693.8
iodine 692.3
iodoform 692.3
irradiation 692.82
jewelry 692.83
keratolytics 692.3
ketones 692.2
lacquer tree (Rhus verniciflua) 692.6
light NEC (*see also* Dermatitis, due to, sun)
692.70
other 692.82
low temperature 692.89
mascara 692.81
meat (ingested) 693.1
contact with skin 692.5
mercury, mercurials 692.3
metals 692.83
milk (ingested) 693.1
contact with skin 692.5
Neomycin 692.3
nylon 692.4
oils NEC 692.1
paint solvent 692.2
pediculocides 692.3
petroleum products (substances classifiable
to 981) 692.4
phenol 692.3

☑ Additional Digit Required ◄► Revised Text ● New Line ▲ Revised Code

Dermatitis — Dermatosis

Dermatitis — *continued*
  due to — *continued*
    photosensitiveness, photosensitivity (sun) 692.72
      other light 692.82
    plants NEC 692.6
    plasters, medicated (any) 692.3
    plastic 692.4
    poison
      ivy (Rhus toxicodendron) 692.6
      oak (Rhus diversiloba) 692.6
      plant or vine 692.6
      sumac (Rhus venenata) 692.6
      vine (Rhus radicans) 692.6
    preservatives 692.89
    primrose (primula) 692.6
    primula 692.6
    radiation 692.82
      sun NEC (*see also* Dermatitis, due to, sun) 692.70
      tanning bed 692.82
    radioactive substance 692.82
    radium 692.82
    ragweed (Senecio jacobae) 692.6
    Rhus (diversiloba) (radicans) (toxicodendron) (venenata) (verniciflua) 692.6
    rubber 692.4
    scabicides 692.3
    Senecio jacobae 692.6
    solar radiation — *see* Dermatitis, due to, sun
    solvents (any) (substances classifiable to 982.0-982.8) 692.2
      chlorocompound group 692.2
      cyclohexane group 692.2
      ester group 692.2
      glycol group 692.2
      hydrocarbon group 692.2
      ketone group 692.2
      paint 692.2
    specified agent NEC 692.89
    sun 692.70
      acute 692.72
      chronic NEC 692.74
      specified NEC 692.79
    sunburn (*see also* Sunburn) 692.71
    sunshine NEC (*see also* Dermatitis, due to, sun) 692.70
    tanning bed 692.82
    tetrachlorethylene 692.2
    toluene 692.2
    topical medications 692.3
    turpentine 692.2
    ultraviolet rays, except from sun 692.82
      sun NEC (*see also* Dermatitis, due to, sun) 692.82
    vaccine or vaccination (correct substance properly administered) 693.0
      wrong substance given or taken
        bacterial vaccine 978.8
          specified — *see* Table of Drugs and Chemicals
        other vaccines NEC 979.9
          specified — *see* Table of Drugs and Chemicals
    varicose veins (*see also* Varicose, vein, inflamed or infected) 454.1
    x-rays 692.82
  dyshydrotic 705.81
  dysmenorrheica 625.8
  eczematoid NEC 692.9
    infectious 690.8
  eczematous NEC 692.9
  epidemica 695.89
  erysipelatosa 695.81
  escharotica — *see* Burn, by site
  exfoliativa, exfoliative 695.89
    generalized 695.89
    infantum 695.81
    neonatorum 695.81
  eyelid 373.31
    allergic 373.32
    contact 373.32
    eczematous 373.31
    herpes (zoster) 053.20
      simplex 054.41

Dermatitis — *continued*
  eyelid — *continued*
    infective 373.5
      due to
        actinomycosis 039.3 *[373.5]*
        herpes
          simplex 054.41
          zoster 053.20
        impetigo 684 *[373.5]*
        leprosy (*see also* Leprosy) 030.0 *[373.4]*
        lupus vulgaris (tuberculous) (*see also* Tuberculosis) 017.0 ☑ *[373.4]*
        mycotic dermatitis (*see also* Dermatomycosis) 111.9 *[373.5]*
        vaccinia 051.0 *[373.5]*
          postvaccination 999.0 *[373.5]*
        yaws (*see also* Yaws) 102.9 *[373.4]*
  facta, factitia 698.4
    psychogenic 316 *[698.4]*
  ficta 698.4
    psychogenic 316 *[698.4]*
  flexural 691.8
  follicularis 704.8
  friction 709.8
  fungus 111.9
    specified type NEC 111.8
  gangrenosa, gangrenous (infantum) (*see also* Gangrene) 785.4
  gestationis 646.8 ☑
  gonococcal 098.89
  gouty 274.89
  harvest mite 133.8
  heat 692.89
  herpetiformis (bullous) (erythematous) (pustular) (vesicular) 694.0
    juvenile 694.2
    senile 694.5
  hiemalis 692.89
  hypostatic, hypostatica 454.1
    with ulcer 454.2
  impetiginous 684
  infantile (acute) (chronic) (intertriginous) (intrinsic) (seborrheic) 690.12
  infectiosa eczematoides 690.8
  infectious (staphylococcal) (streptococcal) 686.9
    eczematoid 690.8
  infective eczematoid 690.8
  Jacquet's (diaper dermatitis) 691.0
  leptus 133.8
  lichenified NEC 692.9
  lichenoid, chronic 701.0
  lichenoides purpurica pigmentosa 709.1
  meadow 692.6
  medicamentosa (correct substance properly administered) (internal use) (*see also* Dermatitis, due to, drugs, or medicinals) 693.0
    due to contact with skin 692.3
  mite 133.8
  multiformis 694.0
    juvenile 694.2
    senile 694.5
  napkin 691.0
  neuro 698.3
  neurotica 694.0
  nummular NEC 692.9
  osteatosis, osteatotic 706.8
  papillaris capillitii 706.1
  pellagrous 265.2
  perioral 695.3
  perstans 696.1
  photosensitivity (sun) 692.72
    other light 692.82
  pigmented purpuric lichenoid 709.1
  polymorpha dolorosa 694.0
  primary irritant 692.9
  pruriginosa 694.0
  pruritic NEC 692.9
  psoriasiform nodularis 696.2
  psychogenic 316
  purulent 686.00
  pustular contagious 051.2
  pyococcal 686.00
  pyocyaneus 686.09
  pyogenica 686.00
  radiation 692.82

Dermatitis — *continued*
  repens 696.1
  Ritter's (exfoliativa) 695.81
  Schamberg's (progressive pigmentary dermatosis) 709.09
  schistosome 120.3
  seasonal bullous 694.8
  seborrheic 690.10
    infantile 690.12
  sensitization NEC 692.9
  septic (*see also* Septicemia) 686.00
    gonococcal 098.89
  solar, solare NEC (*see also* Dermatitis, due to, sun) 692.70
  stasis 459.81
    due to
      postphlebitic syndrome 459.12
        with ulcer 459.13
      varicose veins — *see* Varicose
    ulcerated or with ulcer (varicose) 454.2
  sunburn (*see also* Sunburn) 692.71
  suppurative 686.00
  traumatic NEC 709.8
  trophoneurotica 694.0
  ultraviolet, except from sun 692.82
    due to sun NEC (*see also* Dermatitis, due to, sun) 692.70
  varicose 454.1
    with ulcer 454.2
  vegetans 686.8
  verrucosa 117.2
  xerotic 706.8

Dermatoarthritis, lipoid 272.8 *[713.0]*

Dermatochalasia, dermatochalasis 374.87

Dermatofibroma (lenticulare) (M8832/0) — *see also* Neoplasm, skin, benign
  protuberans (M8832/1) — *see* Neoplasm, skin, uncertain behavior

Dermatofibrosarcoma (protuberans) (M8832/3) — *see* Neoplasm, skin, malignant

Dermatographia 708.3

Dermatolysis (congenital) (exfoliativa) 757.39
  acquired 701.8
  eyelids 374.34
  palpebrarum 374.34
  senile 701.8

Dermatomegaly NEC 701.8

Dermatomucomyositis 710.3

Dermatomycosis 111.9
  furfuracea 111.0
  specified type NEC 111.8

Dermatomyositis (acute) (chronic) 710.3

Dermatoneuritis of children 985.0

Dermatophiliasis 134.1

Dermatophytide — *see* Dermatophytosis

Dermatophytosis (Epidermophyton) (infection) (microsporum) (tinea) (Trichophyton) 110.9
  beard 110.0
  body 110.5
  deep seated 110.6
  fingernails 110.1
  foot 110.4
  groin 110.3
  hand 110.2
  nail 110.1
  perianal (area) 110.3
  scalp 110.0
  scrotal 110.8
  specified site NEC 110.8
  toenails 110.1
  vulva 110.8

Dermatopolyneuritis 985.0

Dermatorrhexis 756.83
  acquired 701.8

Dermatosclerosis (*see also* Scleroderma) 710.1
  localized 701.0

Dermatosis 709.9
  Andrews' 686.8
  atopic 691.8
  Bowen's (M8081/2) — *see* Neoplasm, skin, in situ
  bullous 694.9
    specified type NEC 694.8

☑ Additional Digit Required   ▶◀ Revised Text   ● New Line   ▲ Revised Code

Dermatosis — *continued*
erythematosquamous 690.8
exfoliativa 695.89
factitial 698.4
gonococcal 098.89
herpetiformis 694.0
juvenile 694.2
senile 694.5
hysterical 300.11
Linear IgA 694.8
menstrual NEC 709.8
neutrophilic, acute febrile 695.89
occupational (*see also* Dermatitis) 692.9
papulosa nigra 709.8
pigmentary NEC 709.00
progressive 709.09
Schamberg's 709.09
Siemens-Bloch 757.33
progressive pigmentary 709.09
psychogenic 316
pustular subcorneal 694.1
Schamberg's (progressive pigmentary) 709.09
senile NEC 709.3
Unna's (seborrheic dermatitis) 690.10

Dermographia 708.3

Dermographism 708.3

Dermoid (cyst) (M9084/0) — *see also* Neoplasm, by site, benign
with malignant transformation (M9084/3) 183.0

Dermopathy
infiltrative, with throtoxicosis 242.0 ☑
senile NEC 709.3

Dermophytosis — *see* Dermatophytosis

Descemet's membrane — *see* condition

Descemetocele 371.72

Descending — *see* condition

Descensus uteri (complete) (incomplete) (partial) (without vaginal wall prolapse) 618.1
with mention of vaginal wall proplapse — *see* Prolapse, uterovaginal

Desensitization to allergens V07.1

Desert
rheumatism 114.0
sore (*see also* Ulcer, skin) 707.9

Desertion (child) (newborn) 995.52
adult 995.84

Desmoid (extra-abdominal) (tumor) (M8821/1) — *see also* Neoplasm, connective tissue, uncertain behavior
abdominal (M8822/1) — *see* Neoplasm, connective tissue, uncertain behavior

Despondency 300.4

Desquamative dermatitis NEC 695.89

Destruction
articular facet (*see also* Derangement, joint) 718.9 ☑
vertebra 724.9
bone 733.90
syphilitic 095.5
joint (*see also* Derangement, joint) 718.9 ☑
sacroiliac 724.6
kidney 593.89
live fetus to facilitate birth NEC 763.89
ossicles (ear) 385.24
rectal sphincter 569.49
septum (nasal) 478.1
tuberculous NEC (*see also* Tuberculosis) 011.9 ☑
tympanic membrane 384.82
tympanum 385.89
vertebral disc — *see* Degeneration, intervertebral disc

Destructiveness (*see also* Disturbance, conduct) 312.9
adjustment reaction 309.3

Detachment
cartilage — *see also* Sprain, by site
knee — *see* Tear, meniscus
cervix, annular 622.8
complicating delivery 665.3 ☑
choroid (old) (postinfectional) (simple) (spontaneous) 363.70

Detachment — *continued*
choroid — *continued*
hemorrhagic 363.72
serous 363.71
knee, medial meniscus (old) 717.3
current injury 836.0
ligament — *see* Sprain, by site
placenta (premature) — *see* Placenta, separation
retina (recent) 361.9
with retinal defect (rhegmatogenous) 361.00
giant tear 361.03
multiple 361.02
partial
with
giant tear 361.03
multiple defects 361.02
retinal dialysis (juvenile) 361.04
single defect 361.01
retinal dialysis (juvenile) 361.04
single 361.01
subtotal 361.05
total 361.05
delimited (old) (partial) 361.06
old
delimited 361.06
partial 361.06
total or subtotal 361.07
pigment epithelium (RPE) (serous) 362.42
exudative 362.42
hemorrhagic 362.43
rhegmatogenous (*see also* Detachment, retina, with retinal defect) 361.00
serous (without retinal defect) 361.2
specified type NEC 361.89
traction (with vitreoretinal organization) 361.81
vitreous humor 379.21

Detergent asthma 507.8

Deterioration
epileptic
with behavioral disturbance 345.9 ☑ *[294.11]*
without behavioral disturbance 345.9 ☑ *[294.10]*
heart, cardiac (*see also* Degeneration, myocardial) 429.1
mental (*see also* Psychosis) 298.9
myocardium, myocardial (*see also* Degeneration, myocardial) 429.1
senile (simple) 797
transplanted organ — *see* Complications, transplant, organ, by site

de Toni-Fanconi syndrome (cystinosis) 270.0

Deuteranomaly 368.52

Deuteranopia (anomalous trichromat) (complete) (incomplete) 368.52

Deutschländer's disease — *see* Fracture, foot

Development
abnormal, bone 756.9
arrested 783.40
bone 733.91
child 783.40
due to malnutrition (protein-calorie) 263.2
fetus or newborn 764.9 ☑
tracheal rings (congenital) 748.3
defective, congenital — *see also* Anomaly
cauda equina 742.59
left ventricle 746.9
with atresia or hypoplasia of aortic orifice or valve with hypoplasia of ascending aorta 746.7
in hypoplastic left heart syndrome 746.7
delayed (*see also* Delay, development) 783.40
arithmetical skills 315.1
language (skills) 315.31
expressive 315.31
mixed receptive-expressive 315.32
learning skill, specified NEC 315.2
mixed skills 315.5
motor coordination 315.4
reading 315.00
specified
learning skill NEC 315.2
type NEC, except learning 315.8

Development — *continued*
delayed — *continued*
speech 315.39
associated with hyperkinesia 314.1
phonological 315.39
spelling 315.09
imperfect, congenital — *see also* Anomaly
heart 746.9
lungs 748.60
improper (fetus or newborn) 764.9 ☑
incomplete (fetus or newborn) 764.9 ☑
affecting management of pregnancy 656.5 ☑
bronchial tree 748.3
organ or site not listed — *see* Hypoplasia
respiratory system 748.9
sexual, precocious NEC 259.1
tardy, mental (*see also* Retardation, mental) 319
written expression 315.2

Developmental — *see* condition

Devergie's disease (pityriasis rubra pilaris) 696.4

Deviation
conjugate (eye) 378.87
palsy 378.81
spasm, spastic 378.82
esophagus 530.89
eye, skew 378.87
mandible, opening and closing 524.53 ●
midline (jaw) (teeth) 524.29 ▲
specified site NEC — *see* Malposition
occlusal plant 524.76 ●
organ or site, congenital NEC — *see* Malposition, congenital
septum (acquired) (nasal) 470
congenital 754.0
sexual 302.9
bestiality 302.9
coprophilia 302.89
ego-dystonic
homosexuality 302.0
lesbianism 302.0
erotomania 302.89
Clérambault's 297.8
exhibitionism (sexual) 302.4
fetishism 302.81
transvestic 302.3
frotteurism 302.89
homosexuality, ego-dystonic 302.0
pedophilic 302.2
lesbianism, ego-dystonic 302.0
masochism 302.83
narcissism 302.89
necrophilia 302.89
nymphomania 302.89
pederosis 302.2
pedophilia 302.2
sadism 302.84
sadomasochism 302.84
satyriasis 302.89
specified type NEC 302.89
transvestic fetishism 302.3
transvestism 302.3
voyeurism 302.82
zoophilia (erotica) 302.1
teeth, midline 524.29 ▲
trachea 519.1
ureter (congenital) 753.4

Devic's disease 341.0

Device
cerebral ventricle (communicating) in situ V45.2
contraceptive — *see* Contraceptive, device
drainage, cerebrospinal fluid V45.2

Devil's
grip 074.1
pinches (purpura simplex) 287.2

Devitalized tooth 522.9

Devonshire colic 984.9
specified type of lead — *see* Table of Drugs and Chemicals

Dextraposition, aorta 747.21
with ventricular septal defect, pulmonary stenosis or atresia, and hypertrophy of right ventricle 745.2
in tetralogy of Fallot 745.2

☑ Additional Digit Required   ▶◀ Revised Text   ● New Line   ▲ Revised Code

Dextratransposition, aorta 745.11

Dextrinosis, limit (debrancher enzyme deficiency) 271.0

Dextrocardia (corrected) (false) (isolated) (secondary) (true) 746.87
   with
      complete transposition of viscera 759.3
      situs inversus 759.3

Dextroversion, kidney (left) 753.3

Dhobie itch 110.3

Diabetes, diabetic (brittle) (congenital) (familial) (mellitus) (poorly controlled) (severe) (slight) (without complication) 250.0 ☑

Note — Use the following fifth-digit subclassification with category 250:

▶0   *type II or unspecified type, not stated as uncontrolled*

   Fifth-digit 0 is for use for type II patients, even if the patient requires insulin

1   *type I [juvenile type], not stated as uncontrolled*

2   *type II or unspecified type, uncontrolled*

   Fifth-digit 2 is for use for type II patients, even if the patient requires insulin

3   *type I [juvenile type], uncontrolled*◀

---

with
   coma (with ketoacidosis) 250.3 ☑
      hyperosmolar (nonketotic) 250.2 ☑
   complication NEC 250.9 ☑
      specified NEC 250.8 ☑
   gangrene 250.7 ☑ *[785.4]*
   hyperosmolarity 250.2 ☑
   ketosis, ketoacidosis 250.1 ☑
   osteomyelitis 250.8 ☑ *[731.8]*
   specified manisfestations NEC 250.8 ☑
acetonemia 250.1 ☑
acidosis 250.1 ☑
amyotrophy 250.6 ☑ *[358.1]*
angiopathy, peripheral 250.7 ☑ *[443.81]*
asymptomatic 790.29
autonomic neuropathy (peripheral) 250.6 ☑ *[337.1]*
bone change 250.8 ☑ *[731.8]*
bronze, bronzed 275.0
cataract 250.5 ☑ *[366.41]*
chemical 790.29
   complicating pregnancy, childbirth, or puerperium 648.8 ☑
coma (with ketoacidosis) 250.3 ☑
   hyperglycemic 250.3 ☑
   hyperosmolar (nonketotic) 250.2 ☑
   hypoglycemic 250.3 ☑
   insulin 250.3 ☑
complicating pregnancy, childbirth, or puerperium (maternal) 648.0 ☑
   affecting fetus or newborn 775.0
complication NEC 250.9 ☑
   specified NEC 250.8 ☑
dorsal sclerosis 250.6 ☑ *[340]* ☑
dwarfism-obesity syndrome 258.1
gangrene 250.7 ☑ *[785.4]*
gastroparesis 250.6 ☑ *[536.3]*
gestational 648.8 ☑
   complicating pregnancy, childbirth, or puerperium 648.8 ☑
glaucoma 250.5 ☑ *[365.44]*
glomerulosclerosis (intercapillary) 250.4 ☑ *[581.81]*
glycogenosis, secondary 250.8 ☑ *[259.8]*
hemochromatosis 275.0
hyperosmolar coma 250.2 ☑
hyperosmolarity 250.2 ☑
hypertension-nephrosis syndrome 250.4 ☑ *[581.81]*
hypoglycemia 250.8 ☑
hypoglycemic shock 250.8 ☑
insipidus 253.5
   nephrogenic 588.1
   pituitary 253.5
   vasopressin-resistant 588.1

Diabetes, diabetic — *continued*
intercapillary glomerulosclerosis 250.4 ☑ *[581.81]*
iritis 250.5 ☑ *[364.42]*
ketosis, ketoacidosis 250.1 ☑
Kimmelstiel (-Wilson) disease or syndrome (intercapillary glomerulosclerosis) 250.4 ☑ *[581.81]*
Lancereaux's (diabetes mellitus with marked emaciation) 250.8 ☑ *[261]*
latent (chemical) 790.29
   complicating pregnancy, childbirth, or puerperium 648.8 ☑
lipoidosis 250.8 ☑ *[272.7]*
macular edema 250.5 ☑ *[362.01]*
maternal
   with manifest disease in the infant 775.1
   affecting fetus or newborn 775.0
microaneurysms, retinal 250.5 ☑ *[362.01]*
mononeuropathy 250.6 ☑ *[355.9]*
neonatal, transient 775.1
nephropathy 250.4 ☑ *[583.81]*
nephrosis (syndrome) 250.4 ☑ *[581.81]*
neuralgia 250.6 ☑ *[357.2]*
neuritis 250.6 ☑ *[357.2]*
neurogenic arthropathy 250.6 ☑ *[713.5]*
neuropathy 250.6 ☑ *[357.2]*
nonclinical 790.29
osteomyelitis 250.8 ☑ *[731.8]*
peripheral autonomic neuropathy 250.6 ☑ *[337.1]*
phosphate 275.3
polyneuropathy 250.6 ☑ *[357.2]*
renal (true) 271.4
retinal
   edema 250.5 ☑ *[362.01]*
   hemorrhage 250.5 ☑ *[362.01]*
   microaneurysms 250.5 ☑ *[362.01]*
retinitis 250.5 ☑ *[362.01]*
retinopathy 250.5 ☑ *[362.01]*
   background 250.5 ☑ *[362.01]*
   proliferative 250.5 ☑ *[362.02]*
steroid induced
   correct substance properly administered 251.8
   overdose or wrong substance given or taken 962.0
stress 790.29
subclinical 790.29
subliminal 790.29
sugar 250.0 ☑
ulcer (skin) 250.8 ☑ *[707.9]*
   lower extremity 250.8 ☑ *[707.10]*
      ankle 250.8 ☑ *[707.13]*
      calf 250.8 ☑ *[707.12]*
      foot 250.8 ☑ *[707.15]*
      heel 250.8 ☑ *[707.14]*
      knee 250.8 ☑ *[707.19]*
      specified site NEC 250.8 ☑ *[707.19]*
      thigh 250.8 ☑ *[707.11]*
      toes 250.8 ☑ *[707.15]*
   specified site NEC 250.8 ☑ *[707.8]*
xanthoma 250.8 ☑ *[272.2]*

Diacyclothrombopathia 287.1

Diagnosis deferred 799.9

Dialysis (intermittent) (treatment)
anterior retinal (juvenile) (with detachment) 361.04
extracorporeal V56.0
peritoneal V56.8
renal V56.0
   status only V45.1
specified type NEC V56.8

Diamond-Blackfan anemia or syndrome (congenital hypoplastic anemia) 284.0

Diamond-Gardener syndrome (autoerythrocyte sensitization) 287.2

Diaper rash 691.0

Diaphoresis (excessive) NEC ▶(*see also* Hyperhidrosis)◀ 780.8

Diaphragm — *see* condition

Diaphragmalgia 786.52

Diaphragmitis 519.4

Diaphyseal aclasis 756.4

Diaphysitis 733.99

Diarrhea, diarrheal (acute) (autumn) (bilious) (bloody) (catarrhal) (choleraic) (chronic) (gravis) (green) (infantile) (lienteric) (noninfectious) (presumed noninfectious) (putrefactive) (secondary) (sporadic) (summer) (symptomatic) (thermic) 787.91
achlorhydric 536.0
allergic 558.3
amebic (*see also* Amebiasis) 006.9
   with abscess — *see* Abscess, amebic
   acute 006.0
   chronic 006.1
   nondysenteric 006.2
bacillary — *see* Dysentery, bacillary
bacterial NEC 008.5
balantidial — 007.0
bile salt-induced 579.8
cachectic NEC 787.91
chilomastix 007.8
choleriformis 001.1
coccidial 007.2
Cochin-China 579.1
   anguilluliasis 127.2
   psilosis 579.1
Dientamoeba 007.8
dietetic 787.91
due to
   achylia gastrica 536.8
   Aerobacter aerogenes 008.2
   Bacillus coli — *see* Enteritis, E. coli
   bacteria NEC 008.5
   bile salts 579.8
   Capillaria
      hepatica 128.8
      philippinensis 127.5
   Clostridium perfringens (C) (F) 008.46
   Enterobacter aerogenes 008.2
   enterococci 008.49
   Escherichia coli — *see* Enteritis, E. coli
   Giardia lamblia 007.1
   Heterophyes heterophyes 121.6
   irritating foods 787.91
   Metagonimus yokogawai 121.5
   Necator americanus 126.1
   Paracolobactrum arizonae 008.1
   Paracolon bacillus NEC 008.47
      Arizona 008.1
   Proteus (bacillus) (mirabilis) (Morganii) 008.3
   Pseudomonas aeruginosa 008.42
   S. japonicum 120.2
   specified organism NEC 008.8
      bacterial 008.49
      viral NEC 008.69
   Staphylococcus 008.41
   Streptococcus 008.49
      anaerobic 008.46
   Strongyloides stercoralis 127.2
   Trichuris trichiuria 127.3
   virus NEC (*see also* Enteritis, viral) 008.69
dysenteric 009.2
   due to specified organism NEC 008.8
dyspeptic 787.91
endemic 009.3
   due to specified organism NEC 008.8
epidemic 009.2
   due to specified organism NEC 008.8
fermentative 787.91
flagellate 007.9
Flexner's (ulcerative) 004.1
functional 564.5
   following gastrointestinal surgery 564.4
   psychogenic 306.4
giardial 007.1
Giardia lamblia 007.1
hill 579.1
hyperperistalsis (nervous) 306.4
infectious 009.2
   due to specified organism NEC 008.8
   presumed 009.3
inflammatory 787.91
   due to specified organism NEC 008.8
malarial (*see also* Malaria) 084.6
mite 133.8
mycotic 117.9
nervous 306.4

Diarrhea, diarrheal — *continued*
  neurogenic 564.5
  parenteral NEC 009.2
  postgastrectomy 564.4
  postvagotomy 564.4
  prostaglandin induced 579.8
  protozoal NEC 007.9
  psychogenic 306.4
  septic 009.2
    due to specified organism NEC 008.8
  specified organism NEC 008.8
    bacterial 008.49
    viral NEC 008.69
  Staphylococcus 008.41
  Streptococcus 008.49
    anaerobic 008.46
  toxic 558.2
  travelers' 009.2
    due to specified organism NEC 008.8
  trichomonal 007.3
  tropical 579.1
  tuberculous 014.8 ☑
  ulcerative (chronic) (*see also* Colitis, ulcerative)
      556.9
  viral (*see also* Enteritis, viral) 008.8
  zymotic NEC 009.2
Diastasis
  cranial bones 733.99
    congenital 756.0
  joint (traumatic) — *see* Dislocation, by site
  muscle 728.84
    congenital 756.89
  recti (abdomen) 728.84
    complicating delivery 665.8 ☑
    congenital 756.79
Diastema, teeth, tooth 524.30   ▲
Diastematomyelia 742.51
Diataxia, cerebral, infantile 343.0
Diathesis
  allergic V15.09
  bleeding (familial) 287.9
  cystine (familial) 270.0
  gouty 274.9
  hemorrhagic (familial) 287.9
    newborn NEC 776.0
  oxalic 271.8
  scrofulous (*see also* Tuberculosis) 017.2 ☑
  spasmophilic (*see also* Tetany) 781.7
  ulcer 536.9
  uric acid 274.9
Diaz's disease or osteochondrosis 732.5
Dibothriocephaliasis 123.4
  larval 123.5
Dibothriocephalus (infection) (infestation) (latus)
      123.4
  larval 123.5
Dicephalus 759.4
Dichotomy, teeth 520.2
Dichromat, dichromata (congenital) 368.59
Dichromatopsia (congenital) 368.59
Dichuchwa 104.0
Dicroceliasis 121.8
Didelphys, didelphic (*see also* Double uterus)
      752.2
Didymitis (*see also* Epididymitis) 604.90
Died — *see also* Death
  without
    medical attention (cause unknown) 798.9
    sign of disease 798.2
Dientamoeba diarrhea 007.8
Dietary
  inadequacy or deficiency 269.9
  surveillance and counseling V65.3
Dietl's crisis 593.4
Dieulafoy lesion (hemorrhagic)
  of
    duodenum 537.84
    intestine 569.86
    stomach 537.84
Difficult
  birth, affecting fetus or newborn 763.9
  delivery NEC 669.9 ☑

Difficulty
  feeding 783.3
    breast 676.8 ☑
    newborn 779.3
    nonorganic (infant) NEC 307.59
  mechanical, gastroduodenal stoma 537.89
  reading 315.00
  specific, spelling 315.09
  swallowing (*see also* Dysphagia) 787.2
  walking 719.7
Diffuse — *see* condition
Diffused ganglion 727.42
DiGeorge's syndrome (thymic hypoplasia) 279.11
Digestive — *see* condition
Di Guglielmo's disease or syndrome (M9841/3)
      207.0 ☑
Diktyoma (M9051/3) — *see* Neoplasm, by site,
      malignant
Dilaceration, tooth 520.4
Dilatation
  anus 564.89
    venule — *see* Hemorrhoids
  aorta (focal) (general) (*see also* Aneurysm,
      aorta) 441.9
    congenital 747.29
    infectional 093.0
    ruptured 441.5
    syphilitic 093.0
  appendix (cystic) 543.9
  artery 447.8
  bile duct (common) (cystic) (congenital) 751.69
    acquired 576.8
  bladder (sphincter) 596.8
    congenital 753.8
    in pregnancy or childbirth 654.4 ☑
      causing obstructed labor 660.2 ☑
        affecting fetus or newborn 763.1
  blood vessel 459.89
  bronchus, bronchi 494.0
    with acute exacerbation 494.1
  calyx (due to obstruction) 593.89
  capillaries 448.9
  cardiac (acute) (chronic) (*see also* Hypertrophy,
      cardiac) 429.3
    congenital 746.89
      valve NEC 746.89
        pulmonary 746.09
    hypertensive (*see also* Hypertension, heart)
        402.90
  cavum septi pellucidi 742.4
  cecum 564.89
    psychogenic 306.4
  cervix (uteri) — *see also* Incompetency, cervix
    incomplete, poor, slow
      affecting fetus or newborn 763.7
      complicating delivery 661.0 ☑
        affecting fetus or newborn 763.7
  colon 564.7
    congenital 751.3
    due to mechanical obstruction 560.89
    psychogenic 306.4
  common bile duct (congenital) 751.69
    acquired 576.8
      with calculus, choledocholithiasis, or
          stones — *see* Choledocholithiasis
  cystic duct 751.69
    acquired (any bile duct) 575.8
  duct, mammary 610.4
  duodenum 564.89
  esophagus 530.89
    congenital 750.4
    due to
      achalasia 530.0
      cardiospasm 530.0
  Eustachian tube, congenital 744.24
  fontanel 756.0
  gallbladder 575.8
    congenital 751.69
  gastric 536.8
    acute 536.1
    psychogenic 306.4
  heart (acute) (chronic) (*see also* Hypertrophy,
      cardiac) 429.3
    congenital 746.89

Dilatation — *continued*
  heart (*see also* Hypertrophy, cardiac) —
      continued
    hypertensive (*see also* Hypertension, heart)
        402.90
    valve — *see also* Endocarditis
      congenital 746.89
  ileum 564.89
    psychogenic 306.4
  inguinal rings — *see* Hernia, inguinal
  jejunum 564.89
    psychogenic 306.4
  kidney (calyx) (collecting structures) (cystic)
      (parenchyma) (pelvis) 593.89
  lacrimal passages 375.69
  lymphatic vessel 457.1
  mammary duct 610.4
  Meckel's diverticulum (congenital) 751.0
  meningeal vessels, congenital 742.8
  myocardium (acute) (chronic) (*see also*
      Hypertrophy, cardiac) 429.3
  organ or site, congenital NEC — *see* Distortion
  pancreatic duct 577.8
  pelvis, kidney 593.89
  pericardium — *see* Pericarditis
  pharynx 478.29
  prostate 602.8
  pulmonary
    artery (idiopathic) 417.8
      congenital 747.3
    valve, congenital 746.09
  pupil 379.43
  rectum 564.89
  renal 593.89
  saccule vestibularis, congenital 744.05
  salivary gland (duct) 527.8
  sphincter ani 564.89
  stomach 536.8
    acute 536.1
    psychogenic 306.4
  submaxillary duct 527.8
  trachea, congenital 748.3
  ureter (idiopathic) 593.89
    congenital 753.20
    due to obstruction 593.5
  urethra (acquired) 599.84
  vasomotor 443.9
  vein 459.89
  ventricular, ventricle (acute) (chronic) (*see also*
      Hypertrophy, cardiac) 429.3
    cerebral, congenital 742.4
    hypertensive (*see also* Hypertension, heart)
        402.90
  venule 459.89
    anus — *see* Hemorrhoids
  vesical orifice 596.8
Dilated, dilation — *see* Dilatation
Diminished
  hearing (acuity) (*see also* Deafness) 389.9
  pulse pressure 785.9
  vision NEC 369.9
  vital capacity 794.2
Diminuta taenia 123.6
Diminution, sense or sensation (cold) (heat)
      (tactile) (vibratory) (*see also* Disturbance,
      sensation) 782.0
Dimitri-Sturge-Weber disease
      (encephalocutaneous angiomatosis) 759.6
Dimple
  parasacral 685.1
    with abscess 685.0
  pilonidal 685.1
    with abscess 685.0
  postanal 685.1
    with abscess 685.0
Dioctophyma renale (infection) (infestation) 128.8
Dipetalonemiasis 125.4
Diphallus 752.69
Diphtheria, diphtheritic (gangrenous)
      (hemorrhagic) 032.9
  carrier (suspected) of V02.4
  cutaneous 032.85
  cystitis 032.84
  faucial 032.0
  infection of wound 032.85

☑ Additional Digit Required   ▶◀ Revised Text   ● New Line   ▲ Revised Code

Diphtheria, diphtheritic — *continued*
inoculation (anti) (not sick) V03.5
laryngeal 032.3
myocarditis 032.82
nasal anterior 032.2
nasopharyngeal 032.1
neurological complication 032.89
peritonitis 032.83
specified site NEC 032.89
Diphyllobothriasis (intestine) 123.4
larval 123.5
Diplacusis 388.41
Diplegia (upper limbs) 344.2
brain or cerebral 437.8
congenital 343.0
facial 351.0
congenital 352.6
infantile or congenital (cerebral) (spastic)
(spinal) 343.0
lower limbs 344.1
syphilitic, congenital 090.49
Diplococcus, diplococcal — *see* condition
Diplomyelia 742.59
Diplopia 368.2
refractive 368.15
Dipsomania (*see also* Alcoholism) 303.9 ☑
with psychosis (*see also* Psychosis, alcoholic)
291.9
Dipylidiasis 123.8
intestine 123.8
Direction, teeth, abnormal 524.30 ▲
Dirt-eating child 307.52
Disability
heart — *see* Disease, heart
learning NEC 315.2
special spelling 315.09
Disarticulation (*see also* Derangement, joint)
718.9 ☑
meaning
amputation
status — *see* Absence, by site
traumatic — *see* Amputation, traumatic
dislocation, traumatic or congenital — *see*
Dislocation
Disaster, cerebrovascular (*see also* Disease,
cerebrovascular, acute) 436
Discharge
anal NEC 787.99
breast (female) (male) 611.79
conjunctiva 372.89
continued locomotor idiopathic (*see also*
Epilepsy) 345.5 ☑
diencephalic autonomic idiopathic (*see also*
Epilepsy) 345.5 ☑
ear 388.60
blood 388.69
cerebrospinal fluid 388.61
excessive urine 788.42
eye 379.93
nasal 478.1
nipple 611.79
patterned motor idiopathic (*see also* Epilepsy)
345.5 ☑
penile 788.7
postnasal — *see* Sinusitis
sinus, from mediastinum 510.0
umbilicus 789.9
urethral 788.7
bloody 599.84
vaginal 623.5
Discitis 722.90
cervical, cervicothoracic 722.91
lumbar, lumbosacral 722.93
thoracic, thoracolumbar 722.92
Discogenic syndrome — *see* Displacement,
intervertebral disc
Discoid
kidney 753.3
meniscus, congenital 717.5
semilunar cartilage 717.5
Discoloration
mouth 528.9
nails 703.8

Discoloration — *continued*
teeth 521.7
due to
drugs 521.7
metals (copper) (silver) 521.7
pulpal bleeding 521.7
during formation 520.8
extrinsic 523.6 ●
▶intrinsic◀ posteruptive 521.7
Discomfort
chest 786.59
visual 368.13
Discomycosis — *see* Actinomycosis
Discontinuity, ossicles, ossicular chain 385.23
Discrepancy
centric occlusion maximum intercuspation ●
524.55 ●
leg length (acquired) 736.81
congenital 755.30
uterine size-date 646.8 ☑
Discrimination
political V62.4
racial V62.4
religious V62.4
sex V62.4
Disease, diseased — *see also* Syndrome
Abrami's (acquired hemolytic jaundice) 283.9
absorbent system 459.89
accumulation — *see* Thesaurismosis
acid-peptic 536.8
Acosta's 993.2
Adams-Stokes (-Morgagni) (syncope with heart
block) 426.9
Addison's (bronze) (primary adrenal
insufficiency) 255.4
anemia (pernicious) 281.0
tuberculous (*see also* Tuberculosis) 017.6 ☑
Addison-Gull — *see* Xanthoma
adenoids (and tonsils) (chronic) 474.9
adrenal (gland) (capsule) (cortex) 255.9
hyperfunction 255.3
hypofunction 255.4
specified type NEC 255.8
ainhum (dactylolysis spontanea) 136.0
akamushi (scrub typhus) 081.2
Akureyri (epidemic neuromyasthenia) 049.8
Albarrán's (colibacilluria) 791.9
Albers-Schönberg's (marble bones) 756.52
Albert's 726.71
Albright (-Martin) (-Bantam) 275.49
Alibert's (mycosis fungoides) (M9700/3)
202.1 ☑
Alibert-Bazin (M9700/3) 202.1 ☑
alimentary canal 569.9
alligator skin (ichthyosis congenita) 757.1
acquired 701.1
Almeida's (Brazilian blastomycosis) 116.1
Alpers' 330.8
alpine 993.2
altitude 993.2
alveoli, teeth 525.9
Alzheimer's — *see* Alzheimer's
amyloid (any site) 277.3
anarthritic rheumatoid 446.5
Anders' (adiposis tuberosa simplex) 272.8
Andersen's (glycogenosis IV) 271.0
Anderson's (angiokeratoma corporis diffusum)
272.7
Andes 993.2
Andrews' (bacterid) 686.8
angiospastic, angiospasmodic 443.9
cerebral 435.9
with transient neurologic deficit 435.9
vein 459.89
anterior
chamber 364.9
horn cell 335.9
specified type NEC 335.8
antral (chronic) 473.0
acute 461.0
anus NEC 569.49
aorta (nonsyphilitic) 447.9
syphilitic NEC 093.89
aortic (heart) (valve) (*see also* Endocarditis,
aortic) 424.1
apollo 077.4

Disease, diseased — *see also* Syndrome —
continued
aponeurosis 726.90
appendix 543.9
aqueous (chamber) 364.9
arc-welders' lung 503
Armenian 277.3
Arnold-Chiari (*see also* Spina bifida) 741.0 ☑
arterial 447.9
occlusive (*see also* Occlusion, by site)
444.22
with embolus or thrombus — *see*
Occlusion, by site
due to stricture or stenosis 447.1
specified type NEC 447.8
arteriocardiorenal (*see also* Hypertension,
cardiorenal) 404.90
arteriolar (generalized) (obliterative) 447.9
specified type NEC 447.8
arteriorenal — *see* Hypertension, kidney
arteriosclerotic — *see also* Arteriosclerosis
cardiovascular 429.2
coronary — *see* Arteriosclerosis, coronary
heart — *see* Arteriosclerosis, coronary
vascular — *see* Arteriosclerosis
artery 447.9
cerebral 437.9
coronary — *see* Arteriosclerosis, coronary
specified type NEC 447.8
arthropod-borne NEC 088.9
specified type NEC 088.89
Asboe-Hansen's (incontinentia pigmenti) 757.33
atticoantral, chronic (with posterior or superior
marginal perforation of ear drum) 382.2
auditory canal, ear 380.9
Aujeszky's 078.89
auricle, ear NEC 380.30
Australian X 062.4
autoimmune NEC 279.4
hemolytic (cold type) (warm type) 283.0
parathyroid 252.1
thyroid 245.2
aviators' (*see also* Effect, adverse, high altitude)
993.2
ax(e)-grinders' 502
Ayala's 756.89
Ayerza's (pulmonary artery sclerosis with
pulmonary hypertension) 416.0
Azorean (of the nervous system) 334.8
Babington's (familial hemorrhagic
telangiectasia) 448.0
back bone NEC 733.90
bacterial NEC 040.89
zoonotic NEC 027.9
specified type NEC 027.8
Baehr-Schiffrin (thrombotic thrombocytopenic
purpura) 446.6
Baelz's (cheilitis glandularis apostematosa)
528.5
Baerensprung's (eczema marginatum) 110.3
Balfour's (chloroma) 205.3 ☑
balloon (*see also* Effect, adverse, high altitude)
993.2
Baló's 341.1
Bamberger (-Marie) (hypertrophic pulmonary
osteoarthropathy) 731.2
Bang's (Brucella abortus) 023.1
Bannister's 995.1
Banti's (with cirrhosis) (with portal
hypertension) — *see* Cirrhosis, liver
Barcoo (*see also* Ulcer, skin) 707.9
barium lung 503
Barlow (-Möller) (infantile scurvy) 267
barometer makers' 985.0
Barraquer (-Simons) (progressive lipodystrophy)
272.6
basal ganglia 333.90
degenerative NEC 333.0
specified NEC 333.89
Basedow's (exophthalmic goiter) 242.0 ☑
basement membrane NEC 583.89
with
pulmonary hemorrhage (Goodpasture's
syndrome) 446.21 [583.81]
Bateman's 078.0
purpura (senile) 287.2
Batten's 330.1 [362.71]

Diphtheria, diphtheritic — Disease, diseased

Disease, diseased

Disease, diseased — *see also* Syndrome — *continued*

Chiari's (hepatic vein thrombosis) 453.0
Chicago (North American blastomycosis) 116.0
chignon (white piedra) 111.2
chigoe, chigo (jigger) 134.1
childhood granulomatous 288.1
Chinese liver fluke 121.1
chlamydial NEC 078.88
cholecystic (*see also* Disease, gallbladder) 575.9
choroid 363.9
  degenerative (*see also* Degeneration, choroid) 363.40
  hereditary (*see also* Dystrophy, choroid) 363.50
  specified type NEC 363.8
Christian's (chronic histiocytosis X) 277.89
Christian-Weber (nodular nonsuppurative panniculitis) 729.30
Christmas 286.1
ciliary body 364.9
circulatory (system) NEC 459.9
  chronic, maternal, affecting fetus or newborn 760.3
  specified NEC 459.89
  syphilitic 093.9
    congenital 090.5
Civatte's (poikiloderma) 709.09
climacteric 627.2
  male 608.89
coagulation factor deficiency (congenital) (*see also* Defect, coagulation) 286.9
Coats' 362.12
coccidiodal pulmonary 114.5
  acute 114.0
  chronic 114.4
  primary 114.0
  residual 114.4
Cockayne's (microcephaly and dwarfism) 759.89
Cogan's 370.52
cold
  agglutinin 283.0
    or hemoglobinuria 283.0
      paroxysmal (cold) (nocturnal) 283.2
  hemagglutinin (chronic) 283.0
collagen NEC 710.9
  nonvascular 710.9
  specified NEC 710.8
  vascular (allergic) (*see also* Angiitis, hypersensitivity) 446.20
colon 569.9
  functional 564.9
    congenital 751.3
  ischemic 557.0
combined system (of spinal cord) 266.2 *[336.2]*
  with anemia (pernicious) 281.0 *[336.2]*
compressed air 993.3
Concato's (pericardial polyserositis) 423.2
  peritoneal 568.82
  pleural — *see* Pleurisy
congenital NEC 799.89
conjunctiva 372.9
  chlamydial 077.98
    specified NEC 077.8
  specified type NEC 372.89
  viral 077.99
    specified NEC 077.8
connective tissue, diffuse (*see also* Disease, collagen) 710.9
Conor and Bruch's (boutonneuse fever) 082.1
Conradi (-Hünermann) 756.59
Cooley's (erythroblastic anemia) 282.49
Cooper's 610.1
Corbus' 607.1
cork-handlers' 495.3
cornea (*see also* Keratopathy) 371.9
coronary (*see also* Ischemia, heart) 414.9
  congenital 746.85
  ostial, syphilitic 093.20
    aortic 093.22
    mitral 093.21
    pulmonary 093.24
    tricuspid 093.23
Corrigan's — *see* Insufficiency, aortic
Cotugno's 724.3
Coxsackie (virus) NEC 074.8

Disease, diseased — *see also* Syndrome — *continued*

cranial nerve NEC 352.9
Creutzfeldt-Jakob 046.1
  with dementia
    with behavioral disturbance 046.1 *[294.11]*
    without behavioral disturbance 046.1 *[294.10]*
Crigler-Najjar (congenital hyperbilirubinemia) 277.4
Crocq's (acrocyanosis) 443.89
Crohn's (intestine) (*see also* Enteritis, regional) 555.9
Crouzon's (craniofacial dysostosis) 756.0
Cruchet's (encephalitis lethargica) 049.8
Cruveilhier's 335.21
Cruz-Chagas (*see also* Trypanosomiasis, American) 086.2
crystal deposition (*see also* Arthritis, due to, crystals) 712.9 ☑
Csillag's (lichen sclerosus et atrophicus) 701.0
Curschmann's 359.2
Cushing's (pituitary basophilism) 255.0
cystic
  breast (chronic) 610.1
  kidney, congenital (*see also* Cystic, disease, kidney) 753.10
  liver, congenital 751.62
  lung 518.89
    congenital 748.4
  pancreas 577.2
    congenital 751.7
  renal, congenital (*see also* Cystic, disease, kidney) 753.10
  semilunar cartilage 717.5
cysticercus 123.1
cystine storage (with renal sclerosis) 270.0
cytomegalic inclusion (generalized) 078.5
  with
    pneumonia 078.5 *[484.1]*
  congenital 771.1
Daae (-Finsen) (epidemic pleurodynia) 074.1
dancing 297.8
Danielssen's (anesthetic leprosy) 030.1
Darier's (congenital) (keratosis follicularis) 757.39
  erythema annulare centrifugum 695.0
  vitamin A deficiency 264.8
Darling's (histoplasmosis) (*see also* Histoplasmosis, American) 115.00
Davies' 425.0
de Beurmann-Gougerot (sporotrichosis) 117.1
Débove's (splenomegaly) 789.2
deer fly (*see also* Tularemia) 021.9
deficiency 269.9
degenerative — *see also* Degeneration
  disc — *see* Degeneration, intervertebral disc
Degos' 447.8
Déjérine (-Sottas) 356.0
Déleage's 359.89
demyelinating, demyelinizating (brain stem) (central nervous system) 341.9
  multiple sclerosis 340
  specified NEC 341.8
de Quervain's (tendon sheath) 727.04
  thyroid (subacute granulomatous thyroiditis) 245.1
Dercum's (adiposis dolorosa) 272.8
Deutschländer's — *see* Fracture, foot
Devergie's (pityriasis rubra pilaris) 696.4
Devic's 341.0
diaphorase deficiency 289.7
diaphragm 519.4
diarrheal, infectious 009.2
diatomaceous earth 502
Diaz's (osteochondrosis astragalus) 732.5
digestive system 569.9
Di Guglielmo's (erythemic myelosis) (M9841/3) 207.0 ☑
Dimitri-Sturge-Weber (encephalocutaneous angiomatosis) 759.6
disc, degenerative — *see* Degeneration, intervertebral disc
discogenic (*see also* Disease, intervertebral disc) 722.90
diverticular — *see* Diverticula

Disease, diseased — *see also* Syndrome — *continued*

Down's (mongolism) 758.0
Dubini's (electric chorea) 049.8
Dubois' (thymus gland) 090.5
Duchenne's 094.0
  locomotor ataxia 094.0
  muscular dystrophy 359.1
  paralysis 335.22
  pseudohypertrophy, muscles 359.1
Duchenne-Griesinger 359.1
ductless glands 259.9
Duhring's (dermatitis herpetiformis) 694.0
Dukes (-Filatov) 057.8
duodenum NEC 537.9
  specified NEC 537.89
Duplay's 726.2
Dupré's (meningism) 781.6
Dupuytren's (muscle contracture) 728.6
Durand-Nicolas-Favre (climatic bubo) 099.1
Duroziez's (congenital mitral stenosis) 746.5
Dutton's (trypanosomiasis) 086.9
Eales' 362.18
ear (chronic) (inner) NEC 388.9
  middle 385.9
    adhesive (*see also* Adhesions, middle ear) 385.10
    specified NEC 385.89
Eberth's (typhoid fever) 002.0
Ebstein's
  heart 746.2
  meaning diabetes 250.4 ☑ *[581.81]*
Echinococcus (*see also* Echinococcus) 122.9
ECHO virus NEC 078.89
Economo's (encephalitis lethargica) 049.8
Eddowes' (brittle bones and blue sclera) 756.51
Edsall's 992.2
Eichstedt's (pityriasis versicolor) 111.0
Ellis-van Creveld (chondroectodermal dysplasia) 756.55
endocardium — *see* Endocarditis
endocrine glands or system NEC 259.9
  specified NEC 259.8
endomyocardial, idiopathic mural 425.2
Engel-von Recklinghausen (osteitis fibrosa cystica) 252.01 ▲
Engelmann's (diaphyseal sclerosis) 756.59
English (rickets) 268.0
Engman's (infectious eczematoid dermatitis) 690.8
enteroviral, enterovirus NEC 078.89
  central nervous system NEC 048
epidemic NEC 136.9
epididymis 608.9
epigastric, functional 536.9
  psychogenic 306.4
Erb (-Landouzy) 359.1
Erb-Goldflam 358.00
Erichsen's (railway spine) 300.16
esophagus 530.9
  functional 530.5
  psychogenic 306.4
Eulenburg's (congenital paramyotonia) 359.2
Eustachian tube 381.9
Evans' (thrombocytopenic purpura) 287.3
external auditory canal 380.9
extrapyramidal NEC 333.90
eye 379.90
  anterior chamber 364.9
  inflammatory NEC 364.3
  muscle 378.9
eyeball 360.9
eyelid 374.9
eyeworm of Africa 125.2
Fabry's (angiokeratoma corporis diffusum) 272.7
facial nerve (seventh) 351.9
  newborn 767.5
Fahr-Volhard (malignant nephrosclerosis) 403.00
fallopian tube, noninflammatory 620.9
  specified NEC 620.8
familial periodic 277.3
  paralysis 359.3
Fanconi's (congenital pancytopenia) 284.0
Farber's (disseminated lipogranulomatosis) 272.8

☑ Additional Digit Required   ►◄ Revised Text   ● New Line   ▲ Revised Code

Disease, diseased — *see also* Syndrome —
continued
fascia 728.9
  inflammatory 728.9
Fauchard's (periodontitis) 523.4
Favre-Durand-Nicolas (climatic bubo) 099.1
Favre-Racouchot (elastoidosis cutanea
    nodularis) 701.8
Fede's 529.0
Feer's 985.0
Felix's (juvenile osteochondrosis, hip) 732.1
Fenwick's (gastric atrophy) 537.89
Fernels' (aortic aneurysm) 441.9
fibrocaseous, of lung (*see also* Tuberculosis,
    pulmonary) 011.9 ☑
fibrocystic — *see also* Fibrocystic, disease
    newborn 277.01
Fiedler's (leptospiral jaundice) 100.0
fifth 057.0
Filatoff's (infectious mononucleosis) 075
Filatov's (infectious mononucleosis) 075
file-cutters' 984.9
  specified type of lead — *see* Table of Drugs
    and Chemicals
filterable virus NEC 078.89
fish skin 757.1
  acquired 701.1
Flajani (-Basedow) (exophthalmic goiter)
    242.0 ☑
Flatau-Schilder 341.1
flax-dressers' 504
Fleischner's 732.3
flint 502
fluke — *see* Infestation, fluke
Følling's (phenylketonuria) 270.1
foot and mouth 078.4
foot process 581.3
Forbes' (glycogenosis III) 271.0
Fordyce's (ectopic sebaceous glands) (mouth)
    750.26
Fordyce-Fox (apocrine miliaria) 705.82
Fothergill's
  meaning scarlatina anginosa 034.1
  neuralgia (*see also* Neuralgia, trigeminal)
    350.1
Fournier's 608.83
fourth 057.8
Fox (-Fordyce) (apocrine miliaria) 705.82
Francis' (*see also* Tularemia) 021.9
Franklin's (heavy chain) 273.2
Frei's (climatic bubo) 099.1
Freiberg's (flattening metarsal) 732.5
Friedländer's (endarteritis obliterans) — *see*
    Arteriosclerosis
Friedreich's
  combined systemic or ataxia 334.0
  facial hemihypertrophy 756.0
  myoclonia 333.2
Fröhlich's (adiposogenital dystrophy) 253.8
Frommel's 676.6 ☑
frontal sinus (chronic) 473.1
  acute 461.1
Fuller's earth 502
fungus, fungous NEC 117.9
Gaisböck's (polycythemia hypertonica) 289.0
gallbladder 575.9
  congenital 751.60
Gamna's (siderotic splenomegaly) 289.51
Gamstorp's (adynamia episodica hereditaria)
    359.3
Gandy-Nanta (siderotic splenomegaly) 289.51
gannister (occupational) 502
Garré's (*see also* Osteomyelitis) 730.1 ☑
gastric (*see also* Disease, stomach) 537.9
gastrointestinal (tract) 569.9
  amyloid 277.3
  functional 536.9
    psychogenic 306.4
Gaucher's (adult) (cerebroside lipidosis)
    (infantile) 272.7
Gayet's (superior hemorrhagic
    polioencephalitis) 265.1
Gee (-Herter) (-Heubner) (-Thaysen) (nontropical
    sprue) 579.0
generalized neoplastic (M8000/6) 199.0

Disease, diseased — *see also* Syndrome —
continued
genital organs NEC
  female 629.9
    specified NEC 629.8
  male 608.9
Gerhardt's (erythromelalgia) 443.89
Gerlier's (epidemic vertigo) 078.81
Gibert's (pityriasis rosea) 696.3
Gibney's (perispondylitis) 720.9
Gierke's (glycogenosis I) 271.0
Gilbert's (familial nonhemolytic jaundice) 277.4
Gilchrist's (North American blastomycosis)
    116.0
Gilford (-Hutchinson) (progeria) 259.8
Gilles de la Tourette's (motor-verbal tic) 307.23
Giovannini's 117.9
gland (lymph) 289.9
Glanzmann's (hereditary hemorrhagic
    thrombasthenia) 287.1
glassblowers' 527.1
Glénard's (enteroptosis) 569.89
Glisson's (*see also* Rickets) 268.0
glomerular
  membranous, idiopathic 581.1
  minimal change 581.3
glycogen storage (Andersen's) (Cori types 1-7)
    (Forbes') (McArdle-Schmid-Pearson)
    (Pompe's) (types I-VII) 271.0
  cardiac 271.0 *[425.7]*
  generalized 271.0
  glucose-6-phosphatase deficiency 271.0
  heart 271.0 *[425.7]*
  hepatorenal 271.0
  liver and kidneys 271.0
  myocardium 271.0 *[425.7]*
  von Gierke's (glycogenosis I) 271.0
Goldflam-Erb 358.00
Goldscheider's (epidermolysis bullosa) 757.39
Goldstein's (familial hemorrhagic telangiectasia)
    448.0
gonococcal NEC 098.0
Goodall's (epidemic vomiting) 078.82
Gordon's (exudative enteropathy) 579.8
Gougerot's (trisymptomatic) 709.1
Gougerot-Carteaud (confluent reticulate
    papillomatosis) 701.8
Gougerot-Hailey-Hailey (benign familial chronic
    pemphigus) 757.39
graft-versus-host (bone marrow) 996.85
  due to organ transplant NEC — *see*
    Complications, transplant, organ
grain-handlers' 495.8
Grancher's (splenopneumonia) — *see*
    Pneumonia
granulomatous (childhood) (chronic) 288.1
graphite lung 503
Graves' (exophthalmic goiter) 242.0 ☑
Greenfield's 330.0
green monkey 078.89
Griesinger's (*see also* Ancylostomiasis) 126.9
grinders' 502
Grisel's 723.5
Gruby's (tinea tonsurans) 110.0
Guertin's (electric chorea) 049.8
Guillain-Barré 357.0
Guinon's (motor-verbal tic) 307.23
Gull's (thyroid atrophy with myxedema) 244.8
Gull and Sutton's — *see* Hypertension, kidney
gum NEC 523.9
Günther's (congenital erythropoietic porphyria)
    277.1
gynecological 629.9
  specified NEC 629.8
H 270.0
Haas' 732.3
Habermann's (acute parapsoriasis varioliformis)
    696.2
Haff 985.1
Hageman (congenital factor XII deficiency) (*see
    also* Defect, congenital) 286.3
Haglund's (osteochondrosis os tibiale
    externum) 732.5
Hagner's (hypertrophic pulmonary
    osteoarthropathy) 731.2
Hailey-Hailey (benign familial chronic
    pemphigus) 757.39

Disease, diseased — *see also* Syndrome —
continued
hair (follicles) NEC 704.9
  specified type NEC 704.8
Hallervorden-Spatz 333.0
Hallopeau's (lichen sclerosus et atrophicus)
    701.0
Hamman's (spontaneous mediastinal
    emphysema) 518.1
hand, foot, and mouth 074.3
Hand-Schüller-Christian (chronic
    histiocytosis X) 277.89
Hanot's — *see* Cirrhosis, biliary
Hansen's (leprosy) 030.9
  benign form 030.1
  malignant form 030.0
Harada's 363.22
Harley's (intermittent hemoglobinuria) 283.2
Hart's (pellagra-cerebellar ataxia renal
    aminoaciduria) 270.0
Hartnup (pellagra-cerebellar ataxia renal
    aminoaciduria) 270.0
Hashimoto's (struma lymphomatosa) 245.2
Hb — *see* Disease, hemoglobin
heart (organic) 429.9
  with
    acute pulmonary edema (*see also* Failure,
      ventricular, left) 428.1
      hypertensive 402.91
        with renal failure 404.91
        benign 402.11
          with renal failure 404.11
        malignant 402.01
          with renal failure 404.01
    kidney disease — *see* Hypertension,
      cardiorenal
    rheumatic fever (conditions classifiable to
      390)
      active 391.9
        with chorea 392.0
      inactive or quiescent (with chorea)
        398.90
  amyloid 277.3 *[425.7]*
  aortic (valve) (*see also* Endocarditis, aortic)
    424.1
  arteriosclerotic or sclerotic (minimal) (senile)
    — *see* Arteriosclerosis, coronary
  artery, arterial — *see* Arteriosclerosis,
    coronary
  atherosclerotic — *see* Arteriosclerosis,
    coronary
  beer drinkers' 425.5
  beriberi 265.0 *[425.7]*
  black 416.0
  congenital NEC 746.9
    cyanotic 746.9
    maternal, affecting fetus or newborn
      760.3
    specified type NEC 746.89
  congestive (*see also* Failure, heart) 428.0
  coronary 414.9
  cryptogenic 429.9
  due to
    amyloidosis 277.3 *[425.7]*
    beriberi 265.0 *[425.7]*
    cardiac glycogenosis 271.0 *[425.7]*
    Friedreich's ataxia 334.0 *[425.8]*
    gout 274.82
    mucopolysaccharidosis 277.5 *[425.7]*
    myotonia atrophica 359.2 *[425.8]*
    progressive muscular dystrophy
      359.1 *[425.8]*
    sarcoidosis 135 *[425.8]*
  fetal 746.9
    inflammatory 746.89
  fibroid (*see also* Myocarditis) 429.0
  functional 427.9
    postoperative 997.1
    psychogenic 306.2
  glycogen storage 271.0 *[425.7]*
  gonococcal NEC 098.85
  gouty 274.82
  hypertensive (*see also* Hypertension, heart)
    402.90
    benign 402.10
    malignant 402.00

Disease, diseased — *see also* Syndrome — *continued*

heart — *continued*
  hyperthyroid (*see also* Hyperthyroidism) 242.9 ☑ *[425.7]*
  incompletely diagnosed — *see* Disease, heart
  ischemic (chronic) (*see also* Ischemia, heart) 414.9
    acute (*see also* Infarct, myocardium)
      without myocardial infarction 411.89
        with coronary (artery) occlusion 411.81
    asymptomatic 412
    diagnosed on ECG or other special investigation but currently presenting no symptoms 412
  kyphoscoliotic 416.1
  mitral (*see also* Endocarditis, mitral) 394.9
  muscular (*see also* Degeneration, myocardial) 429.1
  postpartum 674.8 ☑
  psychogenic (functional) 306.2
  pulmonary (chronic) 416.9
    acute 415.0
    specified NEC 416.8
  rheumatic (chronic) (inactive) (old) (quiescent) (with chorea) 398.90
    active or acute 391.9
      with chorea (active) (rheumatic) (Sydenham's) 392.0
      specified type NEC 391.8
    maternal, affecting fetus or newborn 760.3
  rheumatoid — *see* Arthritis, rheumatoid
  sclerotic — *see* Arteriosclersis, coronary
  senile (*see also* Myocarditis) 429.0
  specified type NEC 429.89
  syphilitic 093.89
    aortic 093.1
      aneurysm 093.0
    asymptomatic 093.89
    congenital 090.5
  thyroid (gland) (*see also* Hyper-thyroidism) 242.9 ☑ *[425.7]*
  thyrotoxic (*see also* Thyrotoxicosis) 242.9 ☑ *[425.7]*
  tuberculous (*see also* Tuberculosis) 017.9 ☑ *[425.8]*
  valve, valvular (obstructive) (regurgitant) — *see also* Endocarditis
    congenital NEC (*see also* Anomaly, heart, valve) 746.9
      pulmonary 746.00
      specified type NEC 746.89
  vascular — *see* Disease, cardiovascular
heavy-chain (gamma G) 273.2
Heberden's 715.04
Hebra's
  dermatitis exfoliativa 695.89
  erythema multiforme exudativum 695.1
  pityriasis
    maculata et circinata 696.3
    rubra 695.89
      pilaris 696.4
  prurigo 698.2
Heerfordt's (uveoparotitis) 135
Heidenhain's 290.10
  with dementia 290.10
Heilmeyer-Schöner (M9842/3) 207.1 ☑
Heine-Medin (*see also* Poliomyelitis) 045.9 ☑
Heller's (*see also* Psychosis, childhood) 299.1 ☑
Heller-Döhle (syphilitic aortitis) 093.1
hematopoietic organs 289.9
hemoglobin (Hb) 282.7
  with thalassemia 282.49
  abnormal (mixed) NEC 282.7
    with thalassemia 282.49
  AS genotype 282.5
  Bart's 282.7
  C (Hb-C) 282.7
    with other abnormal hemoglobin NEC 282.7
    elliptocytosis 282.7
    Hb-S (without crisis) 282.63
      with
        crisis 282.64
        vaso-occlusive pain 282.64

Disease, diseased — *see also* Syndrome — *continued*

hemoglobin — *continued*
  C — *continued*
    sickle-cell (without crisis) 282.63
      with
        crisis 282.64
        vaso-occlusive pain 282.64
    thalassemia 282.49
  constant spring 282.7
  D (Hb-D) 282.7
    with other abnormal hemoglobin NEC 282.7
    Hb-S (without crisis) 282.68
      with crisis 282.69
    sickle-cell (without crisis) 282.68
      with crisis 282.69
    thalassemia 282.49
  E (Hb-E) 282.7
    with other abnormal hemoglobin NEC 282.7
    Hb-S (without crisis) 282.68
      with crisis 282.69
    sickle-cell (without crisis) 282.68
      with crisis 282.69
    thalassemia 282.49
  elliptocytosis 282.7
  F (Hb-F) 282.7
  G (Hb-G) 282.7
  H (Hb-H) 282.49
  hereditary persistence, fetal (HPFH) ("Swiss variety") 282.7
  high fetal gene 282.7
  I thalassemia 282.49
  M 289.7
  S — *see also* Disease, sickle-cell, Hb-S
    thalassemia (without crisis) 282.41
      with
        crisis 282.42
        vaso-occlusive pain 282.42
  spherocytosis 282.7
  unstable, hemolytic 282.7
  Zurich (Hb-Zurich) 282.7
hemolytic (fetus) (newborn) 773.2
  autoimmune (cold type) (warm type) 283.0
  due to or with
    incompatibility
      ABO (blood group) 773.1
      blood (group) (Duffy) (Kell) (Kidd) (Lewis) (M) (S) NEC 773.2
      Rh (blood group) (factor) 773.0
      Rh negative mother 773.0
  unstable hemoglobin 282.7
hemorrhagic 287.9
  newborn 776.0
Henoch (-Schönlein) (purpura nervosa) 287.0
hepatic — *see* Disease, liver
hepatolenticular 275.1
heredodegenerative NEC
  brain 331.89
  spinal cord 336.8
Hers' (glycogenosis VI) 271.0
Herter (-Gee) (-Heubner) (nontropical sprue) 579.0
Herxheimer's (diffuse idiopathic cutaneous atrophy) 701.8
Heubner's 094.89
Heubner-Herter (nontropical sprue) 579.0
high fetal gene or hemoglobin thalassemia 282.49
Hildenbrand's (typhus) 081.9
hip (joint) NEC 719.95
  congenital 755.63
  suppurative 711.05
  tuberculous (*see also* Tuberculosis) 015.1 ☑ *[730.85]*
Hippel's (retinocerebral angiomatosis) 759.6
Hirschfield's (acute diabetes mellitus) (*see also* Diabetes) 250.0 ☑
Hirschsprung's (congenital megacolon) 751.3
His (-Werner) (trench fever) 083.1
HIV 042

Disease, diseased — *see also* Syndrome — *continued*

Hodgkin's (M9650/3) 201.9 ☑

Note — *Use the following fifth-digit subclassification with category 201:*

0	*unspecifed site*
1	*lymph nodes of head, face, and neck*
2	*intrathoracic lymp nodes*
3	*intra-abdominal lymph nodes*
4	*lymph nodes of axilla and upper limb*
5	*lymph nodes of inguinal region and lower limb*
6	*intrapelvic lymph nodes*
7	*spleen*
8	*lymph nodes of multiple sites*

---

  lymphocytic
    depletion (M9653/3) 201.7 ☑
      diffuse fibrosis (M9654/3) 201.7 ☑
      reticular type (M9655/3) 201.7 ☑
    predominance (M9651/3) 201.4 ☑
  lymphocytic-histiocytic predominance (M9651/3) 201.4 ☑
  mixed cellularity (M9652/3) 201.6 ☑
  nodular sclerosis (M9656/3) 201.5 ☑
    cellular phase (M9657/3) 201.5 ☑
Hodgson's 441.9
  ruptured 441.5
Hoffa (-Kastert) (liposynovitis prepatellaris) 272.8
Holla (*see also* Spherocytosis) 282.0
homozygous-Hb-S 282.61
hoof and mouth 078.4
hookworm (*see also* Ancylostomiasis) 126.9
Horton's (temporal arteritis) 446.5
host-versus-graft (immune or nonimmune cause) 996.80
  bone marrow 996.85
  heart 996.83
  intestines 996.87
  kidney 996.81
  liver 996.82
  lung 996.84
  pancreas 996.86
  specified NEC 996.89
HPFH (hereditary persistence of fetal hemoglobin) ("Swiss variety") 282.7
Huchard's (continued arterial hypertension) 401.9
Huguier's (uterine fibroma) 218.9
human immunodeficiency (virus) 042
hunger 251.1
Hunt's
  dyssynergia cerebellaris myoclonica 334.2
  herpetic geniculate ganglionitis 053.11
Huntington's 333.4
Huppert's (multiple myeloma) (M9730/3) 203.0 ☑
Hurler's (mucopolysaccharidosis I) 277.5
Hutchinson's, meaning
  angioma serpiginosum 709.1
  cheiropompholyx 705.81
  prurigo estivalis 692.72
Hutchinson-Boeck (sarcoidosis) 135
Hutchinson-Gilford (progeria) 259.8
hyaline (diffuse) (generalized) 728.9
  membrane (lung) (newborn) 769
hydatid (*see also* Echinococcus) 122.9
Hyde's (prurigo nodularis) 698.3
hyperkinetic (*see also* Hyperkinesia) 314.9
  heart 429.82
hypertensive (*see also* Hypertension) 401.9
hypophysis 253.9
  hyperfunction 253.1
  hypofunction 253.2
Iceland (epidemic neuromyasthenia) 049.8
I cell 272.7
ill-defined 799.89
immunologic NEC 279.9
immunoproliferative 203.8 ☑
inclusion 078.5
  salivary gland 078.5
infancy, early NEC 779.9
infective NEC 136.9

☑ Additional Digit Required   ▶◀ Revised Text   ● New Line   ▲ Revised Code

Disease, diseased — *see also* Syndrome —
  continued
  inguinal gland 289.9
  internal semilunar cartilage, cystic 717.5
  intervertebral disc 722.90
    with myelopathy 722.70
    cervical, cervicothoracic 722.91
      with myelopathy 722.71
    lumbar, lumbosacral 722.93
      with myelopathy 722.73
    thoracic, thoracolumbar 722.92
      with myelopathy 722.72
  intestine 569.9
    functional 564.9
      congenital 751.3
      psychogenic 306.4
    lardaceous 277.3
    organic 569.9
    protozoal NEC 007.9
  iris 364.9
  iron
    metabolism 275.0
    storage 275.0
  Isambert's (*see also* Tuberculosis, larynx)
    012.3 ☑
  Iselin's (osteochondrosis, fifth metatarsal) 732.5
  Island (scrub typhus) 081.2
  itai-itai 985.5
  Jadassohn's (maculopapular erythroderma)
    696.2
  Jadassohn-Pellizari's (anetoderma) 701.3
  Jakob-Creutzfeldt 046.1
    with dementia
      with behavioral disturbance
        046.1 [294.11]
      without behavioral disturbance
        046.1 [294.10]
  Jaksch (-Luzet) (pseudoleukemia infantum)
    285.8
  Janet's 300.89
  Jansky-Bielschowsky 330.1
  jaw NEC 526.9
    fibrocystic 526.2
  Jensen's 363.05
  Jeune's (asphyxiating thoracic dystrophy) 756.4
  jigger 134.1
  Johnson-Stevens (erythema multiforme
    exudativum) 695.1
  joint NEC 719.9 ☑
    ankle 719.97
    Charcôt 094.0 [713.5]
    degenerative (*see also* Osteoarthrosis)
      715.9 ☑
      multiple 715.09
      spine (*see also* Spondylosis) 721.90
    elbow 719.92
    foot 719.97
    hand 719.94
    hip 719.95
    hypertrophic (chronic) (degenerative) (*see
      also* Osteoarthrosis) 715.9 ☑
      spine (*see also* Spondylosis) 721.90
    knee 719.96
    Luschka 721.90
    multiple sites 719.99
    pelvic region 719.95
    sacroiliac 724.6
    shoulder (region) 719.91
    specified site NEC 719.98
    spine NEC 724.9
      pseudarthrosis following fusion 733.82
      sacroiliac 724.6
    wrist 719.93
  Jourdain's (acute gingivitis) 523.0
  Jüngling's (sarcoidosis) 135
  Kahler (-Bozzolo) (multiple myeloma) (M9730/3)
    203.0 ☑
  Kalischer's 759.6
  Kaposi's 757.33
    lichen ruber 697.8
      acuminatus 696.4
      moniliformis 697.8
    xeroderma pigmentosum 757.33
  Kaschin-Beck (endemic polyarthritis) 716.00
    ankle 716.07
    arm 716.02
      lower (and wrist) 716.03

Disease, diseased — *see also* Syndrome —
  continued
  Kaschin-Beck — *continued*
    arm — *continued*
      upper (and elbow) 716.02
    foot (and ankle) 716.07
    forearm (and wrist) 716.03
    hand 716.04
    leg 716.06
      lower 716.06
      upper 716.05
    multiple sites 716.09
    pelvic region (hip) (thigh) 716.05
    shoulder region 716.01
    specified site NEC 716.08
  Katayama 120.2
  Kawasaki 446.1
  Kedani (scrub typhus) 081.2
  kidney (functional) (pelvis) (*see also* Disease,
    renal) 593.9
    cystic (congenital) 753.10
      multiple 753.19
      single 753.11
      specified NEC 753.19
    fibrocystic (congenital) 753.19
    in gout 274.10
    polycystic (congenital) 753.12
      adult type (APKD) 753.13
      autosomal dominant 753.13
      autosomal recessive 753.14
      childhood type (CPKD) 753.14
      infantile type 753.14
  Kienböck's (carpal lunate) (wrist) 732.3
  Kimmelstiel (-Wilson) (intercapillary
    glomerulosclerosis) 250.4 ☑ [581.81]
  Kinnier Wilson's (hepatolenticular degeneration)
    275.1
  kissing 075
  Kleb's (*see also* Nephritis) 583.9
  Klinger's 446.4
  Klippel's 723.8
  Klippel-Feil (brevicollis) 756.16
  knight's 911.1
  Köbner's (epidermolysis bullosa) 757.39
  Koenig-Wichmann (pemphigus) 694.4
  Köhler's
    first (osteoarthrosis juvenilis) 732.5
    second (Freiberg's infraction, metatarsal
      head) 732.5
    patellar 732.4
    tarsal navicular (bone) (osteoarthrosis
      juvenilis) 732.5
  Köhler-Freiberg (infraction, metatarsal head)
    732.5
  Köhler-Mouchet (osteoarthrosis juvenilis) 732.5
  Köhler-Pellegrini-Stieda (calcification, knee
    joint) 726.62
  Kok 759.89   ●
  König's (osteochondritis dissecans) 732.7
  Korsakoff's (nonalcoholic) 294.0
    alcoholic 291.1
  Kostmann's (infantile genetic agranulocytosis)
    288.0
  Krabbe's 330.0
  Kraepelin-Morel (*see also* Schizophrenia)
    295.9 ☑
  Kraft-Weber-Dimitri 759.6
  Kufs' 330.1
  Kugelberg-Welander 335.11
  Kuhnt-Junius 362.52
  Kümmell's (-Verneuil) (spondylitis) 721.7
  Kundrat's (lymphosarcoma) 200.1 ☑
  kuru 046.0
  Kussmaul (-Meier) (polyarteritis nodosa) 446.0
  Kyasanur Forest 065.2
  Kyrle's (hyperkeratosis follicularis in cutem
    penetrans) 701.1
  labia
    inflammatory 616.9
      specified NEC 616.8
    noninflammatory 624.9
      specified NEC 624.8
  labyrinth, ear 386.8
  lacrimal system (apparatus) (passages) 375.9
    gland 375.00
    specified NEC 375.89
  Lafora's 333.2

Disease, diseased — *see also* Syndrome —
  continued
  Lagleyze-von Hippel (retinocerebral
    angiomatosis) 759.6
  Lancereaux-Mathieu (leptospiral jaundice)
    100.0
  Landry's 357.0
  Lane's 569.89
  lardaceous (any site) 277.3
  Larrey-Weil (leptospiral jaundice) 100.0
  Larsen (-Johansson) (juvenile osteopathia
    patellae) 732.4
  larynx 478.70
  Lasègue's (persecution mania) 297.9
  Leber's 377.16
  Lederer's (acquired infectious hemolytic
    anemia) 283.19
  Legg's (capital femoral osteochondrosis) 732.1
  Legg-Calvé-Perthes (capital femoral
    osteochondrosis) 732.1
  Legg-Calvé-Waldenström (femoral capital
    osteochondrosis) 732.1
  Legg-Perthes (femoral capital osteochrondosis)
    732.1
  Legionnaires' 482.84
  Leigh's 330.8
  Leiner's (exfoliative dermatitis) 695.89
  Leloir's (lupus erythematosus) 695.4
  Lenegre's 426.0
  lens (eye) 379.39
  Leriche's (osteoporosis, post-traumatic) 733.7
  Letterer-Siwe (acute histiocytosis X) (M9722/3)
    202.5 ☑
  Lev's (acquired complete heart block) 426.0
  Lewandowski's (*see also* Tuberculosis) 017.0 ☑
  Lewandowski-Lutz (epidermodysplasia
    verruciformis) 078.19
  Lewy body 331.82
    with dementia
      with behavioral disturbance
        331.82 [294.11]
      without behavioral disturbance
        331.82 [294.10]
  Leyden's (periodic vomiting) 536.2
  Libman-Sacks (verrucous endocarditis)
    710.0 [424.91]
  Lichtheim's (subacute combined sclerosis with
    pernicious anemia) 281.0 [336.2]
  ligament 728.9
  light chain 203.0 ☑
  Lightwood's (renal tubular acidosis) 588.89 ▲
  Lignac's (cystinosis) 270.0
  Lindau's (retinocerebral angiomatosis) 759.6
  Lindau-von Hippel (angiomatosis
    retinocerebellosa) 759.6
  lip NEC 528.5
  lipidosis 272.7
  lipoid storage NEC 272.7
  Lipschütz's 616.50
  Little's — *see* Palsy, cerebral
  liver 573.9
    alcoholic 571.3
      acute 571.1
      chronic 571.3
    chronic 571.9
      alcoholic 571.3
    cystic, congenital 751.62
    drug-induced 573.3
    due to
      chemicals 573.3
      fluorinated agents 573.3
      hypersensitivity drugs 573.3
      isoniazids 573.3
    fibrocystic (congenital) 751.62
    glycogen storage 271.0
    organic 573.9
    polycystic (congenital) 751.62
  Lobo's (keloid blastomycosis) 116.2
  Lobstein's (brittle bones and blue sclera)
    756.51
  locomotor system 334.9
  Lorain's (pituitary dwarfism) 253.3
  Lou Gehrig's 335.20
  Lucas-Championnière (fibrinous bronchitis)
    466.0
  Ludwig's (submaxillary cellulitis) 528.3

Disease, diseased

Disease, diseased — see also Syndrome —
    continued
luetic — see Syphilis
lumbosacral region 724.6
lung NEC 518.89
    black 500
    congenital 748.60
    cystic 518.89
        congenital 748.4
    fibroid (chronic) (see also Fibrosis, lung) 515
    fluke 121.2
        Oriental 121.2
    in
        amyloidosis 277.3 [517.8]
        polymyositis 710.4 [517.8]
        sarcoidosis 135 [517.8]
        Sjögren's syndrome 710.2 [517.8]
        syphilis 095.1
        systemic lupus erythematosus
            710.0 [517.8]
        systemic sclerosis 710.1 [517.2]
    interstitial (chronic) 515
        acute 136.3
    nonspecific, chronic 496
    obstructive (chronic) (COPD) 496
        with
            acute
                bronchitis 491.22   ●
                exacerbation NEC 491.21   ●
            alveolitis, allergic (see also Alveolitis,
                allergic) 495.9
            asthma (chronic) (obstructive) 493.2 ☑
            bronchiectasis 494.0
                with acute exacerbation 494.1
            bronchitis (chronic) 491.20
                with
                    acute bronchitis 491.22   ●
                    exacerbation (acute) 491.21   ●
            emphysema NEC 492.8
        diffuse (with fibrosis) 496
    polycystic 518.89
        asthma (chronic) (obstructive) 493.2 ☑
        congenital 748.4
    purulent (cavitary) 513.0
    restrictive 518.89
    rheumatoid 714.81
        diffuse interstitial 714.81
    specified NEC 518.89
Lutembacher's (atrial septal defect with mitral
    stenosis) 745.5
Lutz-Miescher (elastosis perforans serpiginosa)
    701.1
Lutz-Splendore-de Almeida (Brazilian
    blastomycosis) 116.1
Lyell's (toxic epidermal necrolysis) 695.1
    due to drug
        correct substance properly administered
            695.1
        overdose or wrong substance given or
            taken 977.9
            specific drug — see Table of Drugs
                and Chemicals
Lyme 088.81
lymphatic (gland) (system) 289.9
    channel (noninfective) 457.9
    vessel (noninfective) 457.9
        specified NEC 457.8
lymphoproliferative (chronic) (M9970/1) 238.7
Machado-Joseph 334.8
Madelung's (lipomatosis) 272.8
Madura (actinomycotic) 039.9
    mycotic 117.4
Magitot's 526.4
Majocchi's (purpura annularis telangiectodes)
    709.1
malarial (see also Malaria) 084.6
Malassez's (cystic) 608.89
Malibu 919.8
    infected 919.9
malignant (M8000/3) — see also Neoplasm, by
    site, malignant
    previous, affecting management of
        pregnancy V23.8 ☑
Manson's 120.1
maple bark 495.6
maple syrup (urine) 270.3
Marburg (virus) 078.89

Disease, diseased — see also Syndrome —
    continued
Marchiafava (-Bignami) 341.8
Marfan's 090.49
    congenital syphilis 090.49
    meaning Marfan's syndrome 759.82
Marie-Bamberger (hypertrophic pulmonary
        osteoarthropathy) (secondary) 731.2
    primary or idiopathic (acropachyderma)
        757.39
    pulmonary (hypertrophic osteoarthropathy)
        731.2
Marie-Strümpell (ankylosing spondylitis) 720.0
Marion's (bladder neck obstruction) 596.0
Marsh's (exophthalmic goiter) 242.0 ☑
Martin's 715.27
mast cell 757.33
    systemic (M9741/3) 202.6 ☑
mastoid (see also Mastoiditis) 383.9
    process 385.9
maternal, unrelated to pregnancy NEC,
    affecting fetus or newborn 760.9
Mathieu's (leptospiral jaundice) 100.0
Mauclaire's 732.3
Mauriac's (erythema nodosum syphiliticum)
    091.3
Maxcy's 081.0
McArdle (-Schmid-Pearson) (glycogenosis V)
    271.0
mediastinum NEC 519.3
Medin's (see also Poliomyelitis) 045.9 ☑
Mediterranean (with hemoglobinopathy)
    282.49
medullary center (idiopathic) (respiratory) 348.8
Meige's (chronic hereditary edema) 757.0
Meleda 757.39
Ménétrier's (hypertrophic gastritis) 535.2 ☑
Ménière's (active) 386.00
    cochlear 386.02
    cochleovestibular 386.01
    inactive 386.04
    in remission 386.04
    vestibular 386.03
meningeal — see Meningitis
mental (see also Psychosis) 298.9
Merzbacher-Pelizaeus 330.0
mesenchymal 710.9
mesenteric embolic 557.0
metabolic NEC 277.9
metal polishers' 502
metastatic — see Metastasis
Mibelli's 757.39
microdrepanocytic 282.49
microvascular 413.9
Miescher's 709.3
Mikulicz's (dryness of mouth, absent or
    decreased lacrimation) 527.1
Milkman (-Looser) (osteomalacia with
    pseudofractures) 268.2
Miller's (osteomalacia) 268.2
Mills' 335.29
Milroy's (chronic hereditary edema) 757.0
Minamata 985.0
Minor's 336.1
Minot's (hemorrhagic disease, newborn) 776.0
Minot-von Willebrand-Jürgens
    (angiohemophilia) 286.4
Mitchell's (erythromelalgia) 443.89
mitral — see Endocarditis, mitral
Mljet (mal de Meleda) 757.39
Möbius', Moebius' 346.8 ☑
Moeller's 267
Möller (-Barlow) (infantile scurvy) 267
Mönckeberg's (see also Arteriosclerosis,
    extremities) 440.20
Mondor's (thrombophlebitis of breast) 451.89
Monge's 993.2
Morel-Kraepelin (see also Schizophrenia)
    295.9 ☑
Morgagni's (syndrome) (hyperostosis frontalis
    interna) 733.3
Morgagni-Adams-Stokes (syncope with heart
    block) 426.9
Morquio (-Brailsford) (-Ullrich)
    (mucopolysaccharidosis IV) 277.5
Morton's (with metatarsalgia) 355.6
Morvan's 336.0

Disease, diseased — see also Syndrome —
    continued
motor neuron (bulbar) (mixed type) 335.20
Mouchet's (juvenile osteochondrosis, foot)
    732.5
mouth 528.9
Moyamoya 437.5
Mucha's (acute parapsoriasis varioliformis)
    696.2
mu-chain 273.2
mucolipidosis (I) (II) (III) 272.7
Münchmeyer's (exostosis luxurians) 728.11
Murri's (intermittent hemoglobinuria) 283.2
muscle 359.9
    inflammatory 728.9
    ocular 378.9
musculoskeletal system 729.9
mushroom workers' 495.5
Myà's (congenital dilation, colon) 751.3
    mycotic 117.9
myeloproliferative (chronic) (M9960/1) 238.7
myocardium, myocardial (see also
        Degeneration, myocardial) 429.1
    hypertensive (see also Hypertension, heart)
        402.90
    primary (idiopathic) 425.4
myoneural 358.9
Naegeli's 287.1
nail 703.9
    specified type NEC 703.8
Nairobi sheep 066.1
nasal 478.1
    cavity NEC 478.1
    sinus (chronic) — see Sinusitis
navel (newborn) NEC 779.89
    delayed separation of umbilical cord
        779.83
nemaline body 359.0
neoplastic, generalized (M8000/6) 199.0
nerve — see Disorder, nerve
nervous system (central) 349.9
    autonomic, peripheral (see also Neuropathy,
        peripheral, autonomic) 337.9
    congenital 742.9
    inflammatory — see Encephalitis
    parasympathetic (see also Neuropathy,
        peripheral, autonomic) 337.9
    peripheral NEC 355.9
    specified NEC 349.89
    sympathetic (see also Neuropathy,
        peripheral, autonomic) 337.9
    vegetative (see also Neuropathy, peripheral,
        autonomic) 337.9
Nettleship's (urticaria pigmentosa) 757.33
Neumann's (pemphigus vegetans) 694.4
neurologic (central) NEC (see also Disease,
        nervous system) 349.9
    peripheral NEC 355.9
neuromuscular system NEC 358.9
Newcastle 077.8
Nicolas (-Durand) — Favre (climatic bubo)
    099.1
Niemann-Pick (lipid histiocytosis) 272.7
nipple 611.9
    Paget's (M8540/3) 174.0
Nishimoto (-Takeuchi) 437.5
nonarthropod-borne NEC 078.89
    central nervous system NEC 049.9
    enterovirus NEC 078.89
non-autoimmune hemolytic NEC 283.10
Nonne-Milroy-Meige (chronic hereditary edema)
    757.0
Norrie's (congenital progressive
        oculoacousticocerebral degeneration)
    743.8
nose 478.1
nucleus pulposus — see Disease, intervertebral
    disc
nutritional 269.9
    maternal, affecting fetus or newborn 760.4
oasthouse, urine 270.2
obliterative vascular 447.1
Odelberg's (juvenile osteochondrosis) 732.1
Oguchi's (retina) 368.61
Ohara's (see also Tularemia) 021.9
Ollier's (chondrodysplasia) 756.4
Opitz's (congestive splenomegaly) 289.51

☑ Additional Digit Required   ▶◀ Revised Text   ● New Line   ▲ Revised Code

Disease, diseased — *see also* Syndrome —
continued
Oppenheim's 358.8
Oppenheim-Urbach (necrobiosis lipoidica
diabeticorum) 250.8 ☑ *[709.3]*
optic nerve NEC 377.49
orbit 376.9
specified NEC 376.89
Oriental liver fluke 121.1
Oriental lung fluke 121.2
Ormond's 593.4
Osgood's tibia (tubercle) 732.4
Osgood-Schlatter 732.4
Osler (-Vaquez) (polycythemia vera) (M9950/1)
238.4
Osler-Rendu (familial hemorrhagic
telangiectasia) 448.0
osteofibrocystic 252.01   ▲
Otto's 715.35
outer ear 380.9
ovary (noninflammatory) NEC 620.9
cystic 620.2
polycystic 256.4
specified NEC 620.8
Owren's (congenital) (*see also* Defect,
coagulation) 286.3
Paas' 756.59
Paget's (osteitis deformans) 731.0
with infiltrating duct carcinoma of the
breast (M8541/3) — *see* Neoplasm,
breast, malignant
bone 731.0
osteosarcoma in (M9184/3) — *see*
Neoplasm, bone, malignant
breast (M8540/3) 174.0
extramammary (M8542/3) — *see also*
Neoplasm, skin, malignant
anus 154.3
skin 173.5
malignant (M8540/3)
breast 174.0
specified site NEC (M8542/3) — *see*
Neoplasm, skin, malignant
unspecified site 174.0
mammary (M8540/3) 174.0
nipple (M8540/3) 174.0
palate (soft) 528.9
Paltauf-Sternberg 201.9 ☑
pancreas 577.9
cystic 577.2
congenital 751.7
fibrocystic 277.00
Panner's 732.3
capitellum humeri 732.3
head of humerus 732.3
tarsal navicular (bone) (osteochondrosis)
732.5
panvalvular — *see* Endocarditis, mitral
parametrium 629.9
parasitic NEC 136.9
cerebral NEC 123.9
intestinal NEC 129
mouth 112.0
skin NEC 134.9
specified type — *see* Infestation
tongue 112.0
parathyroid (gland) 252.9
specified NEC 252.8
Parkinson's 332.0
parodontal 523.9
Parrot's (syphilitic osteochondritis) 090.0
Parry's (exophthalmic goiter) 242.0 ☑
Parson's (exophthalmic goiter) 242.0 ☑
Pavy's 593.6
Paxton's (white piedra) 111.2
Payr's (splenic flexure syndrome) 569.89
pearl-workers' (chronic osteomyelitis) (*see also*
Osteomyelitis) 730.1 ☑
Pel-Ebstein — *see* Disease, Hodgkin's
Pelizaeus-Merzbacher 330.0
with dementia
with behavioral disturbance
330.0 *[294.11]*
without behavioral disturbance
330.0 *[294.10]*
Pellegrini-Stieda (calcification, knee joint)
726.62

Disease, diseased — *see also* Syndrome —
continued
pelvis, pelvic
female NEC 629.9
specified NEC 629.8
gonococcal (acute) 098.19
chronic or duration of 2 months or over
098.39
infection (*see also* Disease, pelvis,
inflammatory) 614.9
inflammatory (female) (PID) 614.9
with
abortion — *see* Abortion, by type, with
sepsis
ectopic pregnancy (*see also* categories
(633.0-633.9) 639.0
molar pregnancy (*see also* categories
630-632) 639.0
acute 614.3
chronic 614.4
complicating pregnancy 646.6 ☑
affecting fetus or newborn 760.8
following
abortion 639.0
ectopic or molar pregnancy 639.0
peritonitis (acute) 614.5
chronic NEC 614.7
puerperal, postpartum, childbirth
670.0 ☑
specified NEC 614.8
organ, female NEC 629.9
specified NEC 629.8
peritoneum, female NEC 629.9
specified NEC 629.8
penis 607.9
inflammatory 607.2
peptic NEC 536.9
acid 536.8
periapical tissues NEC 522.9
pericardium 423.9
specified type NEC 423.8
perineum
female
inflammatory 616.9
specified NEC 616.8
noninflammatory 624.9
specified NEC 624.8
male (inflammatory) 682.2
periodic (familial) (Reimann's) NEC 277.3
paralysis 359.3
periodontal NEC 523.9
specified NEC 523.8
periosteum 733.90
peripheral
arterial 443.9
autonomic nervous system (*see also*
Neuropathy, autonomic) 337.9
nerve NEC (*see also* Neuropathy) 356.9
multiple — *see* Polyneuropathy
vascular 443.9
specified type NEC 443.89
peritoneum 568.9
pelvic, female 629.9
specified NEC 629.8
Perrin-Ferraton (snapping hip) 719.65
persistent mucosal (middle ear) (with posterior
or superior marginal perforation of ear
drum) 382.2
Perthes' (capital femoral osteochondrosis) 732.1
Petit's (*see also* Hernia, lumbar) 553.8
Peutz-Jeghers 759.6
Peyronie's 607.85
Pfeiffer's (infectious mononucleosis) 075
pharynx 478.20
Phocas' 610.1
photochromogenic (acid-fast bacilli)
(pulmonary) 031.0
nonpulmonary 031.9
Pick's
brain 331.11
with dementia
with behavioral disturbance
331.11 *[294.11]*
without behavioral disturbance
331.11 *[294.10]*

Disease, diseased — *see also* Syndrome —
continued
Pick's — *continued*
cerebral atrophy 331.11
with dementia
with behavioral disturbance
331.11 *[294.11]*
without behavioral disturbance
331.11 *[294.10]*
lipid histiocytosis 272.7
liver (pericardial pseudocirrhosis of liver)
423.2
pericardium (pericardial pseudocirrhosis of
liver) 423.2
polyserositis (pericardial pseudocirrhosis of
liver) 423.2
Pierson's (osteochondrosis) 732.1
pigeon fanciers' or breeders' 495.2
pineal gland 259.8
pink 985.0
Pinkus' (lichen nitidus) 697.1
pinworm 127.4
pituitary (gland) 253.9
hyperfunction 253.1
hypofunction 253.2
pituitary snuff-takers' 495.8
placenta
affecting fetus or newborn 762.2
complicating pregnancy or childbirth
656.7 ☑
pleura (cavity) (*see also* Pleurisy) 511.0
Plummer's (toxic nodular goiter) 242.3 ☑
pneumatic
drill 994.9
hammer 994.9
policeman's 729.2
Pollitzer's (hidradenitis suppurativa) 705.83
polycystic (congenital) 759.89
kidney or renal 753.12
adult type (APKD) 753.13
autosomal dominant 753.13
autosomal recessive 753.14
childhood type (CPKD) 753.14
infantile type 753.14
liver or hepatic 751.62
lung or pulmonary 518.89
congenital 748.4
ovary, ovaries 256.4
spleen 759.0
Pompe's (glycogenosis II) 271.0
Poncet's (tuberculous rheumatism) (*see also*
Tuberculosis) 015.9 ☑
Posada-Wernicke 114.9
Potain's (pulmonary edema) 514
Pott's (*see also* Tuberculosis) 015.0 ☑ *[730.88]*
osteomyelitis 015.0 ☑ *[730.88]*
paraplegia 015.0 ☑ *[730.88]*
spinal curvature 015.0 ☑ *[737.43]*
spondylitis 015.0 ☑ *[720.81]*
Potter's 753.0
Poulet's 714.2
pregnancy NEC (*see also* Pregnancy) 646.9 ☑
Preiser's (osteoporosis) 733.09
Pringle's (tuberous sclerosis) 759.5
Profichet's 729.9
prostate 602.9
specified type NEC 602.8
protozoal NEC 136.8
intestine, intestinal NEC 007.9
pseudo-Hurler's (mucolipidosis III) 272.7
psychiatric (*see also* Psychosis) 298.9
psychotic (*see also* Psychosis) 298.9
Puente's (simple glandular cheilitis) 528.5
puerperal NEC (*see also* Puerperal) 674.9 ☑
pulmonary — *see also* Disease, lung
amyloid 277.3 *[517.8]*
artery 417.9
circulation, circulatory 417.9
specified NEC 417.8
diffuse obstructive (chronic) 496
with
acute bronchitis 491.22   ●
asthma (chronic) (obstructive) 493.2 ☑
exacerbation NEC (acute) 491.21
heart (chronic) 416.9
specified NEC 416.8

Disease, diseased — *see also* Syndrome — *continued*
pulmonary — *see also* Disease, lung — *continued*
　hypertensive (vascular) 416.0
　　cardiovascular 416.0
　obstructive diffuse (chronic) 496
　　with
　　　acute bronchitis 491.22　　　●
　　　asthma (chronic) (obstructive) 493.2 ☑
　　　bronchitis (chronic) 491.20
　　　　with
　　　　　exacerbation (acute) 491.21　●
　　　　acute 491.22　　　　　　　　●
　　　　exacerbation NEC (acute) 491.21●
　valve (*see also* Endocarditis, pulmonary) 424.3
pulp (dental) NEC 522.9
pulseless 446.7
Putnam's (subacute combined sclerosis with pernicious anemia) 281.0 *[336.2]*
Pyle (-Cohn) (craniometaphyseal dysplasia) 756.89
pyramidal tract 333.90
Quervain's
　tendon sheath 727.04
　thyroid (subacute granulomatous thyroiditis) 245.1
Quincke's — *see* Edema, angioneurotic
Quinquaud (acne decalvans) 704.09
rag sorters' 022.1
Raynaud's (paroxysmal digital cyanosis) 443.0
reactive airway — *see* Asthma
Recklinghausen's (M9540/1) 237.71
　bone (osteitis fibrosa cystica) 252.01　▲
Recklinghausen-Applebaum (hemochromatosis) 275.0
Reclus' (cystic) 610.1
rectum NEC 569.49
Refsum's (heredopathia atactica polyneuritiformis) 356.3
Reichmann's (gastrosuccorrhea) 536.8
Reimann's (periodic) 277.3
Reiter's 099.3
renal (functional) (pelvis) 593.9
　with
　　edema (*see also* Nephrosis) 581.9
　　exudative nephritis 583.89
　　lesion of interstitial nephritis 583.89
　　stated generalized cause — *see* Nephritis
　acute — *see* Nephritis, acute
　basement membrane NEC 583.89
　　with
　　　pulmonary hemorrhage (Goodpasture's syndrome) 446.21 *[583.81]*
　chronic 593.9
　complicating pregnancy or puerperium NEC 646.2 ☑
　　with hypertension — *see* Toxemia, of pregnancy
　affecting fetus or newborn 760.1
　cystic, congenital (*see also* Cystic, disease, kidney) 753.10
　diabetic 250.4 ☑ *[583.81]*
　due to
　　amyloidosis 277.3 *[583.81]*
　　diabetes mellitus 250.4 ☑ *[583.81]*
　　systemic lupus erythematosis 710.0 *[583.81]*
　end-stage 585
　exudative 583.89
　fibrocystic (congenital) 753.19
　gonococcal 098.19 *[583.81]*
　gouty 274.10
　hypertensive (*see also* Hypertension, kidney) 403.90
　immune complex NEC 583.89
　interstitial (diffuse) (focal) 583.89
　lupus 710.0 *[583.81]*
　maternal, affecting fetus or newborn 760.1
　　hypertensive 760.0
　phosphate-losing (tubular) 588.0
　polycystic (congenital) 753.12
　　adult type (APKD) 753.13
　　autosomal dominant 753.13
　　autosomal recessive 753.14
　　childhood type (CPKD) 753.14

Disease, diseased — *see also* Syndrome — *continued*
renal — *continued*
　polycystic (congenital) — *continued*
　　infantile type 753.14
　specified lesion or cause NEC (*see also* Glomerulonephritis) 583.89
　subacute 581.9
　syphilitic 095.4
　tuberculous (*see also* Tuberculosis) 016.0 ☑ *[583.81]*
　tubular (*see also* Nephrosis, tubular) 584.5
Rendu-Osler-Weber (familial hemorrhagic telangiectasia) 448.0
renovascular (arteriosclerotic) (*see also* Hypertension, kidney) 403.90
respiratory (tract) 519.9
　acute or subacute (upper) NEC 465.9
　　due to fumes or vapors 506.3
　　multiple sites NEC 465.8
　　noninfectious 478.9
　　streptococcal 034.0
　chronic 519.9
　　arising in the perinatal period 770.7
　　due to fumes or vapors 506.4
　due to
　　aspiration of liquids or solids 508.9
　　external agents NEC 508.9
　　　specified NEC 508.8
　　fumes or vapors 506.9
　　　acute or subacute NEC 506.3
　　　chronic 506.4
　fetus or newborn NEC 770.9
　obstructive 496
　specified type NEC 519.8
　upper (acute) (infectious) NEC 465.9
　　multiple sites NEC 465.8
　　noninfectious NEC 478.9
　　streptococcal 034.0
retina, retinal NEC 362.9
　Batten's or Batten-Mayou 330.1 *[362.71]*
　degeneration 362.89
　vascular lesion 362.17
rheumatic (*see also* Arthritis) 716.8 ☑
　heart — *see* Disease, heart, rheumatic
rheumatoid (heart) — *see* Arthritis, rheumatoid
rickettsial NEC 083.9
　specified type NEC 083.8
Riedel's (ligneous thyroiditis) 245.3
Riga (-Fede) (cachectic aphthae) 529.0
Riggs' (compound periodontitis) 523.4
Ritter's 695.81
Rivalta's (cervicofacial actinomycosis) 039.3
Robles' (onchocerciasis) 125.3 *[360.13]*
Roger's (congenital interventricular septal defect) 745.4
Rokitansky's (*see also* Necrosis, liver) 570
Romberg's 349.89
Rosenthal's (factor XI deficiency) 286.2
Rossbach's (hyperchlorhydria) 536.8
　psychogenic 306.4
Roth (-Bernhardt) 355.1
Runeberg's (progressive pernicious anemia) 281.0
Rust's (tuberculous spondylitis) (*see also* Tuberculosis) 015.0 ☑ *[720.81]*
Rustitskii's (multiple myeloma) (M9730/3) 203.0 ☑
Ruysch's (Hirschsprung's disease) 751.3
Sachs (-Tay) 330.1
sacroiliac NEC 724.6
salivary gland or duct NEC 527.9
　inclusion 078.5
　　streptococcal 034.0
　virus 078.5
Sander's (paranoia) 297.1
Sandhoff's 330.1
sandworm 126.9
Savill's (epidemic exfoliative dermatitis) 695.89
Schamberg's (progressive pigmentary dermatosis) 709.09
Schaumann's (sarcoidosis) 135
Schenck's (sporotrichosis) 117.1
Scheuermann's (osteochondrosis) 732.0
Schilder (-Flatau) 341.1
Schimmelbusch's 610.1
Schlatter's tibia (tubercle) 732.4

Disease, diseased — *see also* Syndrome — *continued*
Schlatter-Osgood 732.4
Schmorl's 722.30
　cervical 722.39
　lumbar, lumbosacral 722.32
　specified region NEC 722.39
　thoracic, thoracolumbar 722.31
Scholz's 330.0
Schönlein (-Henoch) (purpura rheumatica) 287.0
Schottmüller's (*see also* Fever, paratyphoid) 002.9
Schüller-Christian (chronic histiocytosis X) 277.89
Schultz's (agranulocytosis) 288.0
Schwalbe-Ziehen-Oppenheimer 333.6
Schweninger-Buzzi (macular atrophy) 701.3
sclera 379.19
scrofulous (*see also* Tuberculosis) 017.2 ☑
scrotum 608.9
sebaceous glands NEC 706.9
Secretan's (posttraumatic edema) 782.3
semilunar cartilage, cystic 717.5
seminal vesicle 608.9
Senear-Usher (pemphigus erythematosus) 694.4
serum NEC 999.5
Sever's (osteochondrosis calcaneum) 732.5
Sézary's (reticulosis) (M9701/3) 202.2 ☑
Shaver's (bauxite pneumoconiosis) 503
Sheehan's (postpartum pituitary necrosis) 253.2
shimamushi (scrub typus) 081.2
shipyard 077.1
sickle cell 282.60
　with
　　crisis 282.62
　　Hb-S disease 282.61
　　other abnormal hemoglobin (Hb-D) (Hb-E) (Hb-G) (Hb-J) (Hb-K) (Hb-O) (Hb-P) (high fetal gene) (without crisis) 282.68
　　　with crisis 282.69
　elliptocytosis 282.60
　Hb-C (without crisis) 282.63
　　with
　　　crisis 282.64
　　　vaso-occlusive pain 282.64
　Hb-S 282.61
　　with
　　　crisis 282.62
　　　Hb-C (without crisis) 282.63
　　　　with
　　　　　crisis 282.64
　　　　　vaso-occlusive pain 282.64
　　　other abnormal hemoglobin (Hb-D) (Hb-E) (Hb-G) (Hb-J) (Hb-K) (Hb-O) (Hb-P) (high fetal gene) (without crisis) 282.68
　　　　with crisis 282.69
　spherocytosis 282.60
　thalassemia (without crisis) 282.41
　　with
　　　crisis 282.42
　　　vaso-occlusive pain 282.42
Siegal-Cattan-Mamou (periodic) 277.3
silo fillers' 506.9
Simian B 054.3
Simmonds' (pituitary cachexia) 253.2
Simons' (progressive lipodystrophy) 272.6
Sinding-Larsen (juvenile osteopathia patellae) 732.4
sinus — *see also* Sinusitis
　brain 437.9
　specified NEC 478.1
Sirkari's 085.0
sixth 057.8
Sjögren (-Gougerot) 710.2
　with lung involvement 710.2 *[517.8]*
Skevas-Zerfus 989.5
skin NEC 709.9
　due to metabolic disorder 277.9
　specified type NEC 709.8
sleeping ►(*see also* Narcolepsy)◄ 347.00　▲
　meaning sleeping sickness (*see also* Trypanosomiasis) 086.5

Disease, diseased — *see also* Syndrome —
continued
small vessel 443.9
Smith-Strang (oasthouse urine) 270.2
Sneddon-Wilkinson (subcorneal pustular
    dermatosis) 694.1
South African creeping 133.8
Spencer's (epidemic vomiting) 078.82
Spielmeyer-Stock 330.1
Spielmeyer-Vogt 330.1
spine, spinal 733.90
    combined system (*see also* Degeneration,
      combined) 266.2 *[336.2]*
      with pernicious anemia 281.0 *[336.2]*
    cord NEC 336.9
      congenital 742.9
    demyelinating NEC 341.8
    joint (*see also* Disease, joint, spine) 724.9
    tuberculous 015.0 ☑ *[730.8]* ☑
spinocerebellar 334.9
    specified NEC 334.8
spleen (organic) (postinfectional) 289.50
    amyloid 277.3
    lardaceous 277.3
    polycystic 759.0
    specified NEC 289.59
sponge divers' 989.5
Stanton's (melioidosis) 025
Stargardt's 362.75
Startle 759.89   ●
Steinert's 359.2
Sternberg's — *see* Disease, Hodgkin's
Stevens-Johnson (erythema multiforme
    exudativum) 695.1
Sticker's (erythema infectiosum) 057.0
Stieda's (calcification, knee joint) 726.62
Still's (juvenile rheumatoid arthritis) 714.30
Stiller's (asthenia) 780.79
Stokes' (exophthalmic goiter) 242.0 ☑
Stokes-Adams (syncope with heart block) 426.9
Stokvis (-Talma) (enterogenous cyanosis) 289.7
stomach NEC (organic) 537.9
    functional 536.9
      psychogenic 306.4
    lardaceous 277.3
stonemasons' 502
storage
    glycogen (*see also* Disease, glycogen storage)
      271.0
    lipid 272.7
    mucopolysaccharide 277.5
striatopallidal system 333.90
    specified NEC 333.89
Strümpell-Marie (ankylosing spondylitis) 720.0
Stuart's (congenital factor X deficiency) (*see*
    also Defect, coagulation) 286.3
Stuart-Prower (congenital factor X deficiency)
    (*see also* Defect, coagulation) 286.3
Sturge (-Weber) (-Dimitri) (encephalocutaneous
    angiomatosis) 759.6
Stuttgart 100.89
Sudeck's 733.7
supporting structures of teeth NEC 525.9
suprarenal (gland) (capsule) 255.9
    hyperfunction 255.3
    hypofunction 255.4
Sutton's 709.09
Sutton and Gull's — *see* Hypertension, kidney
sweat glands NEC 705.9
    specified type NEC 705.89
sweating 078.2
Sweeley-Klionsky 272.4
Swift (-Feer) 985.0
swimming pool (bacillus) 031.1
swineherd's 100.89
Sylvest's (epidemic pleurodynia) 074.1
Symmers (follicular lymphoma) (M9690/3)
    202.0 ☑
sympathetic nervous system (*see also*
    Neuropathy, peripheral, autonomic) 337.9
synovium 727.9
syphilitic — *see* Syphilis
systemic tissue mast cell (M9741/3) 202.6 ☑
Taenzer's 757.4
Takayasu's (pulseless) 446.7
Talma's 728.85

Disease, diseased — *see also* Syndrome —
continued
Tangier (familial high-density lipoprotein
    deficiency) 272.5
Tarral-Besnier (pityriasis rubra pilaris) 696.4
Tay-Sachs 330.1
Taylor's 701.8
tear duct 375.69
teeth, tooth 525.9
    hard tissues NEC 521.9
    pulp NEC 522.9
tendon 727.9
    inflammatory NEC 727.9
terminal vessel 443.9
testis 608.9
Thaysen-Gee (nontropical sprue) 579.0
Thomsen's 359.2
Thomson's (congenital poikiloderma) 757.33
Thornwaldt's, Tornwaldt's (pharyngeal bursitis)
    478.29
throat 478.20
    septic 034.0
thromboembolic (*see also* Embolism) 444.9
thymus (gland) 254.9
    specified NEC 254.8
thyroid (gland) NEC 246.9
    heart (*see also* Hyperthyroidism)
      242.9 ☑ *[425.7]*
    lardaceous 277.3
    specified NEC 246.8
Tietze's 733.6
Tommaselli's
    correct substance properly administered
      599.7
    overdose or wrong substance given or taken
      961.4
tongue 529.9
tonsils, tonsillar (and adenoids) (chronic) 474.9
    specified NEC 474.8
tooth, teeth 525.9
    hard tissues NEC 521.9
    pulp NEC 522.9
Tornwaldt's (pharyngeal bursitis) 478.29
Tourette's 307.23
trachea 519.1
tricuspid — *see* Endocarditis, tricuspid
triglyceride-storage, type I, II, III 272.7
triple vessel (coronary arteries) — *see*
    Arteriosclerosis, coronary
trisymptomatic, Gougerot's 709.1
trophoblastic (*see also* Hydatidiform mole) 630
    previous, affecting management of
      pregnancy V23.1
tsutsugamushi (scrub typhus) 081.2
tube (fallopian), noninflammatory 620.9
    specified NEC 620.8
tuberculous NEC (*see also* Tuberculosis)
    011.9 ☑
tubo-ovarian
    inflammatory (*see also* Salpingo-oophoritis)
      614.2
    noninflammatory 620.9
      specified NEC 620.8
tubotympanic, chronic (with anterior
    perforation of ear drum) 382.1
tympanum 385.9
Uhl's 746.84
umbilicus (newborn) NEC 779.89
    delayed separation 779.83
Underwood's (sclerema neonatorum) 778.1
undiagnosed 799.9
Unna's (seborrheic dermatitis) 690.18
unstable hemoglobin hemolytic 282.7
Unverricht (-Lundborg) 333.2
Urbach-Oppenheim (necrobiosis lipoidica
    diabeticorum) 250.8 ☑ *[709.3]*
Urbach-Wiethe (lipoid proteinosis) 272.8
ureter 593.9
urethra 599.9
    specified type NEC 599.84
urinary (tract) 599.9
    bladder 596.9
      specified NEC 596.8
    maternal, affecting fetus or newborn 760.1
Usher-Senear (pemphigus erythematosus)
    694.4

Disease, diseased — *see also* Syndrome —
continued
uterus (organic) 621.9
    infective (*see also* Endometritis) 615.9
    inflammatory (*see also* Endometritis) 615.9
    noninflammatory 621.9
      specified type NEC 621.8
uveal tract
    anterior 364.9
    posterior 363.9
vagabonds' 132.1
vagina, vaginal
    inflammatory 616.9
      specified NEC 616.8
    noninflammatory 623.9
      specified NEC 623.8
Valsuani's (progressive pernicious anemia,
    puerperal) 648.2 ☑
    complicating pregnancy or puerperium
      648.2 ☑
valve, valvular — *see* Endocarditis
van Bogaert-Nijssen (-Peiffer) 330.0
van Creveld-von Gierke (glycogenosis I) 271.0
van den Bergh's (enterogenous cyanosis) 289.7
van Neck's (juvenile osteochondrosis) 732.1
Vaquez (-Osler) (polycythemia vera) (M9950/1)
    238.4
vascular 459.9
    arteriosclerotic — *see* Arteriosclerosis
    hypertensive — *see* Hypertension
    obliterative 447.1
      peripheral 443.9
    occlusive 459.9
    peripheral (occlusive) 443.9
      in diabetes mellitus 250.7 ☑ *[443.81]*
      specified type NEC 443.89
vas deferens 608.9
vasomotor 443.9
vasopastic 443.9
vein 459.9
venereal 099.9
    chlamydial NEC 099.50
      anus 099.52
      bladder 099.53
      cervix 099.53
      epididymis 099.54
      genitourinary NEC 099.55
        lower 099.53
        specified NEC 099.54
      pelvic inflammatory disease 099.54
      perihepatic 099.56
      peritoneum 099.56
      pharynx 099.51
      rectum 099.52
      specified site NEC 099.54
      testis 099.54
      vagina 099.53
      vulva 099.53
    fifth 099.1
    sixth 099.1
    complicating pregnancy, childbirth, or
      puerperium 647.2 ☑
    specified nature or type NEC 099.8
      chlamydial — *see* Disease, venereal,
        chlamydial
Verneuil's (syphilitic bursitis) 095.7
Verse's (calcinosis intervertebralis)
    275.49 *[722.90]*
vertebra, vertebral NEC 733.90
    disc — *see* Disease, Intervertebral disc
vibration NEC 994.9
Vidal's (lichen simplex chronicus) 698.3
Vincent's (trench mouth) 101
Virchow's 733.99
virus (filterable) NEC 078.89
    arbovirus NEC 066.9
    arthropod-borne NEC 066.9
    central nervous system NEC 049.9
      specified type NEC 049.8
    complicating pregnancy, childbirth, or
      puerperium 647.6 ☑
    contact (with) V01.79   ▲
      varicella V01.71   ●
    exposure to V01.79   ▲
      varicella V01.71   ●
    Marburg 078.89

☑ Additional Digit Required   ►◄ Revised Text   ● New Line   ▲ Revised Code

(left margin, rotated) Disease, diseased — Dislocation

Disease, diseased — *see also* Syndrome — *continued*
  virus NEC — *continued*
    maternal
      with fetal damage affecting management of pregnancy 655.3 ☑
    nonarthropod-borne NEC 078.89
      central nervous sytem NEC 049.9
        specified NEC 049.8
    vaccination, prophylactic (against) V04.89
  vitreous 379.29
  vocal cords NEC 478.5
  Vogt's (Cecile) 333.7
  Vogt-Spielmeyer 330.1
  Volhard-Fahr (malignant nephrosclerosis) 403.00
  Volkmann's
    acquired 958.6
  von Bechterew's (ankylosing spondylitis) 720.0
  von Economo's (encephalitis lethargica) 049.8
  von Eulenburg's (congenital paramyotonia) 359.2
  von Gierke's (glycogenosis I) 271.0
  von Graefe's 378.72
  von Hippel's (retinocerebral angiomatosis) 759.6
  von Hippel-Lindau (angiomatosis retinocerebellosa) 759.6
  von Jaksch's (pseudoleukemia infantum) 285.8
  von Recklinghausen's (M9540/1) 237.71
    bone (osteitis fibrosa cystica) 252.01   ▲
  von Recklinghausen-Applebaum (hemochromatosis) 275.0
  von Willebrand (-Jürgens) (angiohemophilia) 286.4
  von Zambusch's (lichen sclerosus et atrophicus) 701.0
  Voorhoeve's (dyschondroplasia) 756.4
  Vrolik's (osteogenesis imperfecta) 756.51
  vulva
    noninflammatory 624.9
      specified NEC 624.8
  Wagner's (colloid milium) 709.3
  Waldenström's (osteochondrosis capital femoral) 732.1
  Wallgren's (obstruction of splenic vein with collateral circulation) 459.89
  Wardrop's (with lymphangitis) 681.9
    finger 681.02
    toe 681.11
  Wassilieff's (leptospiral jaundice) 100.0
  wasting NEC 799.4
    due to malnutrition 261
    paralysis 335.21
  Waterhouse-Friderichsen 036.3
  waxy (any site) 277.3
  Weber-Christian (nodular nonsuppurative panniculitis) 729.30
  Wegner's (syphilitic osteochondritis) 090.0
  Weil's (leptospral jaundice) 100.0
    of lung 100.0
  Weir Mitchell's (erythromelalgia) 443.89
  Werdnig-Hoffmann 335.0
  Werlhof's (*see also* Purpura, thrombocytopenic) 287.3
  Wermer's 258.0
  Werner's (progeria adultorum) 259.8
  Werner-His (trench fever) 083.1
  Werner-Schultz (agranulocytosis) 288.0
  Wernicke's (superior hemorrhagic polioencephalitis) 265.1
  Wernicke-Posadas 114.9
  Whipple's (intestinal lipodystrophy) 040.2
  whipworm 127.3
  white
    blood cell 288.9
      specified NEC 288.8
    spot 701.0
  White's (congenital) (keratosis follicularis) 757.39
  Whitmore's (melioidosis) 025
  Widal-Abrami (acquired hemolytic jaundice) 283.9
  Wilkie's 557.1
  Wilkinson-Sneddon (subcorneal pustular dermatosis) 694.1

Disease, diseased — *see also* Syndrome — *continued*
  Willis' (diabetes mellitus) (*see also* Diabetes) 250.0 ☑
  Wilson's (hepatolenticular degeneration) 275.1
  Wilson-Brocq (dermatitis exfoliativa) 695.89
  winter vomiting 078.82
  Wise's 696.2
  Wohlfart-Kugelberg-Welander 335.11
  Woillez's (acute idiopathic pulmonary congestion) 518.5
  Wolman's (primary familial xanthomatosis) 272.7
  wool-sorters' 022.1
  Zagari's (xerostomia) 527.7
  Zahorsky's (exanthem subitum) 057.8
  Ziehen-Oppenheim 333.6
  zoonotic, bacterial NEC 027.9
    specified type NEC 027.8

Disfigurement (due to scar) 709.2
  head V48.6
  limb V49.4
  neck V48.7
  trunk V48.7

Disgerminoma — *see* Dysgerminoma

Disinsertion, retina 361.04

Disintegration, complete, of the body 799.89
  traumatic 869.1

Disk kidney 753.3

Dislocatable hip, congenital (*see also* Dislocation, hip, congenital) 754.30

Dislocation (articulation) (closed) (displacement) (simple) (subluxation) 839.8

> *Note — "Closed" includes simple, complete, partial, uncomplicated, and unspecified dislocation.*
>
> *"Open" includes dislocation specified as infected or compound and dislocation with foreign body.*
>
> *"Chronic," "habitual," "old," or "recurrent" dislocations should be coded as indicated under the entry "Dislocation, recurrent," and "pathological" as indicated under the entry "Dislocation, pathological."*
>
> *For late effect of dislocation see Late, effect, dislocation.*

  with fracture — *see* Fracture, by site
  acromioclavicular (joint) (closed) 831.04
    open 831.14
  anatomical site (closed)
    specified NEC 839.69
      open 839.79
    unspecified or ill-defined 839.8
      open 839.9
  ankle (scaphoid bone) (closed) 837.0
    open 837.1
  arm (closed) 839.8
    open 839.9
  astragalus (closed) 837.0
    open 837.1
  atlanto-axial (closed) 839.01
    open 839.11
  atlas (closed) 839.01
    open 839.11
  axis (closed) 839.02
    open 839.12
  back (closed) 839.8
    open 839.9
  Bell-Daly 723.8
  breast bone (closed) 839.61
    open 839.71
  capsule, joint — *see* Dislocation, by site
  carpal (bone) — *see* Dislocation, wrist
  carpometacarpal (joint) (closed) 833.04
    open 833.14
  cartilage (joint) — *see also* Dislocation, by site
    knee — *see* Tear, meniscus
  cervical, cervicodorsal, or cervicothoracic (spine) (vertebra) — *see* Dislocation, vertebra, cervical
  chiropractic (*see also* Lesion, nonallopathic) 739.9
  chondrocostal — *see* Dislocation, costochondral

Dislocation — *continued*
  chronic — *see* Dislocation, recurrent
  clavicle (closed) 831.04
    open 831.14
  coccyx (closed) 839.41
    open 839.51
  collar bone (closed) 831.04
    open 831.14
  compound (open) NEC 839.9
  congenital NEC 755.8
    hip (*see also* Dislocation, hip, congenital) 754.30
    lens 743.37
    rib 756.3
    sacroiliac 755.69
    spine NEC 756.19
    vertebra 756.19
  coracoid (closed) 831.09
    open 831.19
  costal cartilage (closed) 839.69
    open 839.79
  costochondral (closed) 839.69
    open 839.79
  cricoarytenoid articulation (closed) 839.69
    open 839.79
  cricothyroid (cartilage) articulation (closed) 839.69
    open 839.79
  dorsal vertebrae (closed) 839.21
    open 839.31
  ear ossicle 385.23
  elbow (closed) 832.00
    anterior (closed) 832.01
      open 832.11
    congenital 754.89
    divergent (closed) 832.09
      open 832.19
    lateral (closed) 832.04
      open 832.14
    medial (closed) 832.03
      open 832.13
      open 832.10
    posterior (closed) 832.02
      open 832.12
    recurrent 718.32
    specified type NEC 832.09
      open 832.19
  eye 360.81
    lateral 376.36
  eyeball 360.81
    lateral 376.36
  femur
    distal end (closed) 836.50
      anterior 836.52
        open 836.62
      lateral 836.53
        open 836.63
      medial 836.54
        open 836.64
      open 836.60
      posterior 836.51
        open 836.61
    proximal end (closed) 835.00
      anterior (pubic) 835.03
        open 835.13
      obturator 835.02
        open 835.12
      open 835.10
      posterior 835.01
        open 835.11
  fibula
    distal end (closed) 837.0
      open 837.1
    proximal end (closed) 836.59
      open 836.69
  finger(s) (phalanx) (thumb) (closed) 834.00
    interphalangeal (joint) 834.02
      open 834.12
    metacarpal (bone), distal end 834.01
      open 834.11
    metacarpophalangeal (joint) 834.01
      open 834.11
    open 834.10
    recurrent 718.34
  foot (closed) 838.00
    open 838.10
    recurrent 718.37

☑ Additional Digit Required   ►◄ Revised Text   ● New Line   ▲ Revised Code

Dislocation — *continued*
  forearm (closed) 839.8
    open 839.9
  fracture — *see* Fracture, by site
  glenoid (closed) 831.09
    open 831.19
  habitual — *see* Dislocation, recurrent
  hand (closed) 839.8
    open 839.9
  hip (closed) 835.00
    anterior 835.03
      obturator 835.02
        open 835.12
      open 835.13
    congenital (unilateral) 754.30
      with subluxation of other hip 754.35
      bilateral 754.31
    developmental 718.75
    open 835.10
    posterior 835.01
      open 835.11
    recurrent 718.35
  humerus (closed) 831.00
    distal end (*see also* Dislocation, elbow) 832.00
    open 831.10
    proximal end (closed) 831.00
      anterior (subclavicular) (subcoracoid) (subglenoid) (closed) 831.01
        open 831.11
      inferior (closed) 831.03
        open 831.13
      open 831.10
      posterior (closed) 831.02
        open 831.12
  implant — *see* Complications, mechanical
  incus 385.23
  infracoracoid (closed) 831.01
    open 831.11
  innominate (pubic junction) (sacral junction) (closed) 839.69
    acetabulum (*see also* Dislocation, hip) 835.00
    open 839.79
  interphalangeal (joint)
    finger or hand (closed) 834.02
      open 834.12
    foot or toe (closed) 838.06
      open 838.16
  jaw (cartilage) (meniscus) (closed) 830.0
    open 830.1
    recurrent 524.69
  joint NEC (closed) 839.8
    developmental 718.7 ☑
    open 839.9
    pathological — *see* Dislocation, pathological
    recurrent — *see* Dislocation, recurrent
  knee (closed) 836.50
    anterior 836.51
      open 836.61
    congenital (with genu recurvatum) 754.41
    habitual 718.36
    lateral 836.54
      open 836.64
    medial 836.53
      open 836.63
    old 718.36
    open 836.60
    posterior 836.52
      open 836.62
    recurrent 718.36
    rotatory 836.59
      open 836.69
  lacrimal gland 375.16
  leg (closed) 839.8
    open 839.9
  lens (crystalline) (complete) (partial) 379.32
    anterior 379.33
    congenital 743.37
    ocular implant 996.53
    posterior 379.34
    traumatic 921.3
  ligament — *see* Dislocation, by site
  lumbar (vertebrae) (closed) 839.20
    open 839.30

Dislocation — *continued*
  lumbosacral (vertebrae) (closed) 839.20
    congenital 756.19
    open 839.30
  mandible (closed) 830.0
    open 830.1
  maxilla (inferior) (closed) 830.0
    open 830.1
  meniscus (knee) — *see also* Tear, meniscus
    other sites — *see* Dislocation, by site
  metacarpal (bone)
    distal end (closed) 834.01
      open 834.11
    proximal end (closed) 833.05
      open 833.15
  metacarpophalangeal (joint) (closed) 834.01
    open 834.11
  metatarsal (bone) (closed) 838.04
    open 838.14
  metatarsophalangeal (joint) (closed) 838.05
    open 838.15
  midcarpal (joint) (closed) 833.03
    open 833.13
  midtarsal (joint) (closed) 838.02
    open 838.12
  Monteggia's — *see* Dislocation, hip
  multiple locations (except fingers only or toes only) (closed) 839.8
    open 839.9
  navicular (bone) foot (closed) 837.0
    open 837.1
  neck (*see also* Dislocation, vertebra, cervical) 839.00
  Nélaton's — *see* Dislocation, ankle
  nontraumatic (joint) — *see* Dislocation, pathological
  nose (closed) 839.69
    open 839.79
  not recurrent, not current injury — *see* Dislocation, pathological
  occiput from atlas (closed) 839.01
    open 839.11
  old — *see* Dislocation, recurrent
  open (compound) NEC 839.9
  ossicle, ear 385.23
  paralytic (flaccid) (spastic) — *see* Dislocation, pathological
  patella (closed) 836.3
    congenital 755.64
    open 836.4
  pathological NEC 718.20
    ankle 718.27
    elbow 718.22
    foot 718.27
    hand 718.24
    hip 718.25
    knee 718.26
    lumbosacral joint 724.6
    multiple sites 718.29
    pelvic region 718.25
    sacroiliac 724.6
    shoulder (region) 718.21
    specified site NEC 718.28
    spine 724.8
      sacroiliac 724.6
    wrist 718.23
  pelvis (closed) 839.69
    acetabulum (*see also* Dislocation, hip) 835.00
    open 839.79
  phalanx
    foot or toe (closed) 838.09
      open 838.19
    hand or finger (*see also* Dislocation, finger) 834.00
  postpoliomyelitic — *see* Dislocation, pathological
  prosthesis, internal — *see* Complications, mechanical
  radiocarpal (joint) (closed) 833.02
    open 833.12
  radioulnar (joint)
    distal end (closed) 833.01
      open 833.11
    proximal end (*see also* Dislocation, elbow) 832.00

Dislocation — *continued*
  radius
    distal end (closed) 833.00
      open 833.10
    proximal end (closed) 832.01
      open 832.11
  recurrent (*see also* Derangement, joint, recurrent) 718.3 ☑
    elbow 718.32
    hip 718.35
    joint NEC 718.38
    knee 718.36
    lumbosacral (joint) 724.6
    patella 718.36
    sacroiliac 724.6
    shoulder 718.31
    temporomandibular 524.69
  rib (cartilage) (closed) 839.69
    congenital 756.3
    open 839.79
  sacrococcygeal (closed) 839.42
    open 839.52
  sacroiliac (joint) (ligament) (closed) 839.42
    congenital 755.69
    open 839.52
    recurrent 724.6
  sacrum (closed) 839.42
    open 839.52
  scaphoid (bone)
    ankle or foot (closed) 837.0
      open 837.1
    wrist (closed) (*see also* Dislocation, wrist) 833.00
      open 833.10
  scapula (closed) 831.09
    open 831.19
  semilunar cartilage, knee — *see* Tear, meniscus
  septal cartilage (nose) (closed) 839.69
    open 839.79
  septum (nasal) (old) 470
  sesamoid bone — *see* Dislocation, by site
  shoulder (blade) (ligament) (closed) 831.00
    anterior (subclavicular) (subcoracoid) (subglenoid) (closed) 831.01
      open 831.11
    chronic 718.31
    inferior 831.03
      open 831.13
    open 831.10
    posterior (closed) 831.02
      open 831.12
    recurrent 718.31
  skull — *see* Injury, intracranial
  Smith's — *see* Dislocation, foot
  spine (articular process) (*see also* Dislocation, vertebra) (closed) 839.40
    atlanto-axial (closed) 839.01
      open 839.11
      recurrent 723.8
    cervical, cervicodorsal, cervicothoracic (closed) (*see also* Dislocation, vertebrae, cervical) 839.00
      open 839.10
      recurrent 723.8
    coccyx 839.41
      open 839.51
    congenital 756.19
    due to birth trauma 767.4
    open 839.50
    recurrent 724.9
    sacroiliac 839.42
      recurrent 724.6
    sacrum (sacrococcygeal) (sacroiliac) 839.42
      open 839.52
  spontaneous — *see* Dislocation, pathological
  sternoclavicular (joint) (closed) 839.61
    open 839.71
  sternum (closed) 839.61
    open 839.71
  subastragalar — *see* Dislocation, foot
  subglenoid (closed) 831.01
    open 831.11
  symphysis
    jaw (closed) 830.0
      open 830.1
    mandibular (closed) 830.0
      open 830.1

Dislocation — Disorder

Dislocation — *continued*
  symphysis — *continued*
    pubis (closed) 839.69
      open 839.79
  tarsal (bone) (joint) 838.01
    open 838.11
  tarsometatarsal (joint) 838.03
    open 838.13
  temporomandibular (joint) (closed) 830.0
    open 830.1
    recurrent 524.69
  thigh
    distal end (*see also* Dislocation, femur, distal
      end) 836.50
    proximal end (*see also* Dislocation, hip)
      835.00
  thoracic (vertebrae) (closed) 839.21
    open 839.31
  thumb(s) (*see also* Dislocation, finger) 834.00
  thyroid cartilage (closed) 839.69
    open 839.79
  tibia
    distal end (closed) 837.0
      open 837.1
    proximal end (closed) 836.50
      anterior 836.51
        open 836.61
      lateral 836.54
        open 836.64
      medial 836.53
        open 836.63
      open 836.60
      posterior 836.52
        open 836.62
      rotatory 836.59
        open 836.69
  tibiofibular
    distal (closed) 837.0
      open 837.1
    superior (closed) 836.59
      open 836.69
  toe(s) (closed) 838.09
    open 838.19
  trachea (closed) 839.69
    open 839.79
  ulna
    distal end (closed) 833.09
      open 833.19
    proximal end — *see* Dislocation, elbow
  vertebra (articular process) (body) (closed)
    839.40
    cervical, cervicodorsal or cervicothoracic
      (closed) 839.00
      first (atlas) 839.01
        open 839.11
      second (axis) 839.02
        open 839.12
      third 839.03
        open 839.13
      fourth 839.04
        open 839.14
      fifth 839.05
        open 839.15
      sixth 839.06
        open 839.16
      seventh 839.07
        open 839.17
      congential 756.19
      multiple sites 839.08
        open 839.18
      open 839.10
    congential 756.19
    dorsal 839.21
      open 839.31
      recurrent 724.9
    lumbar, lumbosacral 839.20
      open 839.30
    open NEC 839.50
    recurrent 724.9
    specified region NEC 839.49
      open 839.59
    thoracic 839.21
      open 839.31
  wrist (carpal bone) (scaphoid) (semilunar)
    (closed) 833.00
    carpometacarpal (joint) 833.04
      open 833.14

Dislocation — *continued*
  wrist — *continued*
    metacarpal bone, proximal end 833.05
      open 833.15
    midcarpal (joint) 833.03
      open 833.13
    open 833.10
    radiocarpal (joint) 833.02
      open 833.12
    radioulnar (joint) 833.01
      open 833.11
    recurrent 718.33
    specified site NEC 833.09
      open 833.19
  xiphoid cartilage (closed) 839.61
    open 839.71

Dislodgement
  artificial skin graft 996.55
  decellularized allodermis graft 996.55

Disobedience, hostile (covert) (overt) (*see also*
  Disturbance, conduct) 312.0 ☑

Disorder — *see also* Disease
  academic underachievement, childhood and
    adolescence 313.83
  accommodation 367.51
    drug-induced 367.89
    toxic 367.89
  adjustment (*see also* Reaction, adjustment)
    309.9
    with   ●
      axiety 309.24   ●
      anxiety and depressed mood 309.28   ●
      depressed mood 309.0   ●
      disturbance of conduct 309.3   ●
      disturbance of emotions and conduct   ●
        309.4   ●
  adrenal (capsule) (cortex) (gland) 255.9
    specified type NEC 255.8
  adrenogenital 255.2
  affective (*see also* Psychosis, affective) 296.90
    atypical 296.81
  aggressive, unsocialized (*see also* Disturbance,
    conduct) 312.0 ☑
  alcohol, alcoholic (*see also* Alcohol) 291.9
  allergic — *see* Allergy
  amnestic (*see also* Amnestic syndrome)
    294.8   ▲
    alcohol-induced persisting 291.1   ●
    drug-induced persisting 292.83   ●
    in conditions classified elsewhere 294.0 ●
  amino acid (metabolic) (*see also* Disturbance,
    metabolism, amino acid) 270.9
    albinism 270.2
    alkaptonuria 270.2
    argininosuccinicaciduria 270.6
    beta-amino-isobutyricaciduria 277.2
    cystathioninuria 270.4
    cystinosis 270.0
    cystinuria 270.0
    glycinuria 270.0
    homocystinuria 270.4
    imidazole 270.5
    maple syrup (urine) disease 270.3
    neonatal, transitory 775.8
    oasthouse urine disease 270.2
    ochronosis 270.2
    phenylketonuria 270.1
    phenylpyruvic oligophrenia 270.1
    purine NEC 277.2
    pyrimidine NEC 277.2
    renal transport NEC 270.0
    specified type NEC 270.8
    transport NEC 270.0
      renal 270.0
    xanthinuria 277.2
  anaerobic glycolysis with anemia 282.3
  anxiety (*see also* Anxiety) 300.00
    due to or associated with physical condition
      293.84
  arteriole 447.9
    specified type NEC 447.8
  artery 447.9
    specified type NEC 447.8
  articulation — *see* Disorder, joint
  Asperger's 299.8 ☑

Disorder — *see also* Disease — *continued*
  attachment of infancy ►or early childhood◄
    313.89
  attention deficit 314.00
    with hyperactivity 314.01
    predominantly
      combined hyperactive/inattentive 314.01
      hyperactive/impulsive 314.01
      inattentive 314.00
    residual type 314.8
  autoimmune NEC 279.4
    hemolytic (cold type) (warm type) 283.0
    parathyroid 252.1
    thyroid 245.2
  autistic 299.0 ☑
  avoidant, childhood or adolescence 313.21
  balance
    acid-base 276.9
      mixed (with hypercapnia) 276.4
    electrolyte 276.9
    fluid 276.9
  behavior NEC (*see also* Disturbance, conduct)
    312.9
    disruptive 312.9   ●
  bilirubin excretion 277.4
  bipolar (affective) (alternating) 296.80   ▲

Note — *Use the following fifth-digit*	●
subclassification with categories 296.0-296.6:	●
0	*unspecifed*	●
1	*mild*	●
2	*moderate*	●
3	*severe, without mention of psychotic*	●
	behavior	●
4	*severe, specified as with psychotic*	●
	behavior	●
5	*in partial or unspecified remission*	●
6	*in full remission*	●

    atypical 296.7
    currently
      depressed 296.5 ☑
      hypomanic 296.4 ☑
      manic 296.4 ☑
    mixed 296.6 ☑
    specified type NEC 296.89   ●
    type I 296.7   ●
      most recent episode (or current)   ●
        depressed 296.5 ☑   ●
        hypomanic 296.4 ☑   ●
        manic 296.4 ☑   ●
        mixed 296.6 ☑   ●
        unspecified 296.7   ●
      single manic episode 296.0   ●
    type II (recurrent major depressive episodes
      with hypomania) 296.89
  bladder 596.9
    functional NEC 596.59
    specified NEC 596.8
  bone NEC 733.90
    specified NEC 733.99
  brachial plexus 353.0
  branched-chain amino-acid degradation 270.3
  breast 611.9
    puerperal, postpartum 676.3 ☑
    specified NEC 611.8
  Briquet's 300.81
  bursa 727.9
    shoulder region 726.10
  carbohydrate metabolism, congenital 271.9
  cardiac, functional 427.9
    postoperative 997.1
    psychogenic 306.2
  cardiovascular, psychogenic 306.2
  cartilage NEC 733.90
    articular 718.00
      ankle 718.07
      elbow 718.02
      foot 718.07
      hand 718.04
      hip 718.05
      knee 717.9
      multiple sites 718.09
      pelvic region 718.05
      shoulder region 718.01

☑ Additional Digit Required   ►◄ Revised Text   ● New Line   ▲ Revised Code

Disorder — see also Disease — continued
cartilage NEC — continued
  articular — continued
    specified
      site NEC 718.08
      type NEC 733.99
    wrist 718.03
catatonic — see Catatonia
cervical region NEC 723.9
cervical root (nerve) NEC 353.2
character NEC (see also Disorder, personality) 301.9
coagulation (factor) (see also Defect, coagulation) 286.9
  factor VIII (congenital) (functional) 286.0
  factor IX (congenital) (functional) 286.1
  neonatal, transitory 776.3
coccyx 724.70
  specified NEC 724.79
colon 569.9
  functional 564.9
    congenital 751.3
cognitive 294.9
communication 307.9
conduct (see also Disturbance, conduct) 312.9
  adjustment reaction 309.3
  adolescent onset type 312.82
  childhood onset type 312.81
  compulsive 312.30
    specified type NEC 312.39
  hyperkinetic 314.2
  onset unspecified 312.89
  socialized (type) 312.20
    aggressive 312.23
    unaggressive 312.21
  specified NEC 312.89
conduction, heart 426.9
  specified NEC 426.89
conflict
  sexual orientation 302.0
convulsive (secondary) (see also Convulsions) 780.39
  due to injury at birth 767.0
  idiopathic 780.39
coordination 781.3
cornea NEC 371.89
  due to contact lens 371.82
corticosteroid metabolism NEC 255.2
cranial nerve — see Disorder, nerve, cranial
cyclothymic 301.13
degradation, branched-chain amino acid 270.3
delusional 297.1
dentition 520.6
depersonalization 300.6
depressive NEC 311
  atypical 296.82
  major (see also Psychosis, affective) 296.2
    recurrent episode 296.3
    single episode 296.2
development, specific 315.9
  associated with hyperkinesia 314.1
  coordination 315.4
  language 315.31
  learning 315.2
    arithmetical 315.1
    reading 315.00
  mixed 315.5
  motor coordination 315.4
  specified type NEC 315.8
  speech 315.39
diaphragm 519.4
digestive 536.9
  fetus or newborn 777.9
    specified NEC 777.8
  psychogenic 306.4
disintegrative, childhood 299.1
dissociative 300.15
  identity 300.14
  nocturnal 307.47
drug-related 292.9
dysmorphic body 300.7
dysthymic 300.4
ear 388.9
  degenerative NEC 388.00
  external 380.9
    specified 380.89
  pinna 380.30

Disorder — see also Disease — continued
ear — continued
  specified type NEC 388.8
  vascular NEC 388.00
eating NEC 307.50
electrolyte NEC 276.9
  with
    abortion — see Abortion, by type, with metabolic disorder
    ectopic pregnancy (see also categories 633.0-633.9) 639.4
    molar pregnancy (see also categories 630-632) 639.4
  acidosis 276.2
    metabolic 276.2
    respiratory 276.2
  alkalosis 276.3
    metabolic 276.3
    respiratory 276.3
  following
    abortion 639.4
    ectopic or molar pregnancy 639.4
  neonatal, transitory NEC 775.5
emancipation as adjustment reaction 309.22
emotional (see also Disorder, mental, nonpsychotic) V40.9
endocrine 259.9
  specified type NEC 259.8
esophagus 530.9
  functional 530.5
  psychogenic 306.4
explosive
  intermittent 312.34
  isolated 312.35
expressive language 315.31
eye 379.90
  globe — see Disorder, globe
  ill-defined NEC 379.99
  limited duction NEC 378.63
  specified NEC 379.8
eyelid 374.9
  degenerative 374.50
  sensory 374.44
  specified type NEC 374.89
  vascular 374.85
factitious (with combined psychological and physical signs and symptoms) (with predominantly physical signs and symptoms) 300.19
  with predominantly psychological signs and symptoms 300.16
factor, coagulation (see also Defect, coagulation) 286.9
  VIII (congenital) (functional) 286.0
  IX (congenital) (funcitonal) 286.1
fascia 728.9
fatty acid oxidation 277.85
feeding — see Feeding
female sexual arousal 302.72
fluid NEC 276.9
gastric (functional) 536.9
  motility 536.8
  psychogenic 306.4
  secretion 536.8
gastrointestinal (functional) NEC 536.9
  newborn (neonatal) 777.9
    specified NEC 777.8
  psychogenic 306.4
gender (child) 302.6
  adult 302.85
gender identity (childhood) 302.6
  adolescents 302.85
  adults (-life) 302.85
genitourinary system, psychogenic 306.50
globe 360.9
  degenerative 360.20
    specified NEC 360.29
  specified type NEC 360.89
hearing — see also Deafness
  conductive type (air) (see also Deafness, conductive) 389.00
  mixed conductive and sensorineural 389.2
  nerve 389.12
  perceptive (see also Deafness, perceptive) 389.10
  sensorineural type NEC (see also Deafness, perceptive) 389.10

Disorder — see also Disease — continued
heart action 427.9
  postoperative 997.1
hematological, transient neonatal 776.9
  specified type NEC 776.8
hematopoietic organs 289.9
hemorrhagic NEC 287.9
  due to intrinsic circulating anticoagulants 286.5
  specified type NEC 287.8
hemostasis (see also Defect, coagulation) 286.9
homosexual conflict 302.0
hypomanic (chronic) 301.11
identity
  childhood and adolescence 313.82
    gender 302.6
  gender 302.6
immune mechanism (immunity) 279.9
  single complement (C-C) 279.8
  specified type NEC 279.8
impulse control (see also Disturbance, conduct, compulsive) 312.30
infant sialic acid storage 271.8
integument, fetus or newborn 778.9
  specified type NEC 778.8
interactional psychotic (childhood) (see also Psychosis, childhood) 299.1
intermittent explosive 312.34
intervertebral disc 722.90
  cervical, cervicothoracic 722.91
  lumbar, lumbosacral 722.93
  thoracic, thoracolumbar 722.92
intestinal 569.9
  functional NEC 564.9
    congenital 751.3
    postoperative 564.4
  psychogenic 306.4
introverted, of childhood and adolescence 313.22
iron, metabolism 275.0
isolated explosive 312.35
joint NEC 719.90
  ankle 719.97
  elbow 719.92
  foot 719.97
  hand 719.94
  hip 719.95
  knee 719.96
  multiple sites 719.99
  pelvic region 719.95
  psychogenic 306.0
  shoulder (region) 719.91
  specified site NEC 719.98
  temporomandibular 524.60
    sounds on opening or closing 524.64
    specified NEC 524.69
  wrist 719.93
kidney 593.9
  functional 588.9
    specified NEC 588.89
labyrinth, labyrinthine 386.9
  specified type NEC 386.8
lactation 676.9
language (developmental) (expressive) 315.31
  mixed receptive-expressive 315.32
learning 315.9
ligament 728.9
ligamentous attachments, peripheral — see also Enthesopathy
  spine 720.1
limb NEC 729.9
  psychogenic 306.0
lipid
  metabolism, congenital 272.9
  storage 272.7
lipoprotein deficiency (familial) 272.5
low back NEC 724.9
  psychogenic 306.0
lumbosacral
  plexus 353.1
  root (nerve) NEC 353.4
lymphoproliferative (chronic) NEC (M9970/1) 238.7
male erectile 302.72
  organic origin 607.84

Disorder — *see also* Disease — *continued*
  major depressive (*see also* Psychosis, affective) 296.2 ☑
    recurrent episode 296.3 ☑
    single episode 296.2 ☑
  manic (*see also* Psychosis, affective) 296.0 ☑
    atypical 296.81
  mathematics 315.1   ●
  meniscus NEC (*see also* Disorder, cartilage, articular) 718.0 ☑
  menopausal 627.9
    specified NEC 627.8
  menstrual 626.9
    psychogenic 306.52
    specified NEC 626.8
  mental (nonpsychotic) 300.9
    affecting management of pregnancy, childbirth, or puerperium 648.4 ☑
    drug-induced 292.9
      hallucinogen persisting perception 292.89
      specified type NEC 292.89
    due to or associated with
      alcoholism 291.9
      drug consumption NEC 292.9
        specified type NEC 292.89
      physical condition NEC 293.9
    induced by drug 292.9
      specified type NEC 292.89
    neurotic (*see also* Neurosis) 300.9
    of infancy, childhood or adolescence 313.9   ●
    persistent   ●
      other   ●
        due to conditions classified elsewhere 294.8   ●
      unspecified   ●
        due to conditions classified elsewhere 294.9   ●
    presenile 310.1
      psychotic NEC 290.10
    previous, affecting management of pregnancy V23.8 ☑
    psychoneurotic (*see also* Neurosis) 300.9
    psychotic (*see also* Psychosis) 298.9
      brief 298.8   ●
      senile 290.20
    specific, following organic brain damage 310.9
      cognitive or personality change of other type 310.1
      frontal lobe syndrome 310.0
      postconcussional syndrome 310.2
      specified type NEC 310.8
    transient   ●
      in conditions classified elsewhere 293.9   ●
  metabolism NEC 277.9
    with
      abortion — *see* Abortion, by type with metabolic disorder
      ectopic pregnancy (*see also* categories 633.0-633.9) 639.4
      molar pregnancy (*see also* categories 630-632) 639.4
    alkaptonuria 270.2
    amino acid (*see also* Disorder, amino acid) 270.9
      specified type NEC 270.8
    ammonia 270.6
    arginine 270.6
    argininosuccinic acid 270.6
    basal 794.7
    bilirubin 277.4
    calcium 275.40
    carbohydrate 271.9
      specified type NEC 271.8
    cholesterol 272.9
    citrulline 270.6
    copper 275.1
    corticosteroid 255.2
    cystine storage 270.0
    cystinuria 270.0
    fat 272.9
    fatty acid oxidation 277.85   ●
    following
      abortion 639.4
      ectopic or molar pregnancy 639.4

Disorder — *see also* Disease — *continued*
  metabolism NEC — *continued*
    fructosemia 271.2
    fructosuria 271.2
    fucosidosis 271.8
    galactose-1-phosphate uridyl transferase 271.1
    glutamine 270.7
    glycine 270.7
    glycogen storage NEC 271.0
      hepatorenal 271.0
    hemochromatosis 275.0
    in labor and delivery 669.0 ☑
    iron 275.0
    lactose 271.3
    lipid 272.9
      specified type NEC 272.8
      storage 272.7
    lipoprotein — *see also* Hyperlipemia
      deficiency (familial) 272.5
    lysine 270.7
    magnesium 275.2
    mannosidosis 271.8
    mineral 275.9
      specified type NEC 275.8
    mitochondrial 277.87   ●
    mucopolysaccharide 277.5
    nitrogen 270.9
    ornithine 270.6
    oxalosis 271.8
    pentosuria 271.8
    phenylketonuria 270.1
    phosphate 275.3
    phosphorous 275.3
    plasma protein 273.9
      specified type NEC 273.8
    porphyrin 277.1
    purine 277.2
    pyrimidine 277.2
    serine 270.7
    sodium 276.9
    specified type NEC 277.89
    steroid 255.2
    threonine 270.7
    urea cycle 270.6
    xylose 271.8
  micturition NEC 788.69
    psychogenic 306.53
  misery and unhappiness, of childhood and adolescence 313.1
  mitochondrial metabolism 277.87   ●
  mitral valve 424.0
  mood ►(*see also* Disorder, bipolar) 296.90◄   ●
    episodic 296.90   ●
      specified NEC 296.99   ●
    in conditions classified elsewhere 293.83 ●
  motor tic 307.20
    chronic 307.22
    transient ►(childhood)◄ 307.21
  movement NEC 333.90
    hysterical 300.11
    periodic limb 780.58
    sleep related 780.58   ●
    specified type NEC 333.99
    stereotypic 307.3
  mucopolysaccharide 277.5
  muscle 728.9
    psychogenic 306.0
    specified type NEC 728.3
  muscular attachments, peripheral — *see also* Enthesopathy
    spine 720.1
  musculoskeletal system NEC 729.9
    psychogenic 306.0
  myeloproliferative (chronic) NEC (M9960/1) 238.7
  myoneural 358.9
    due to lead 358.2
    specified type NEC 358.8
    toxic 358.2
  myotonic 359.2
  neck region NEC 723.9
  nerve 349.9
    abducens NEC 378.54
    accessory 352.4
    acoustic 388.5
    auditory 388.5

Disorder — *see also* Disease — *continued*
  nerve — *continued*
    auriculotemporal 350.8
    axillary 353.0
    cerebral — *see* Disorder, nerve, cranial
    cranial 352.9
      first 352.0
      second 377.49
      third
        partial 378.51
        total 378.52
      fourth 378.53
      fifth 350.9
      sixth 378.54
      seventh NEC 351.9
      eighth 388.5
      ninth 352.2
      tenth 352.3
      eleventh 352.4
      twelfth 352.5
      multiple 352.6
    entrapment — *see* Neuropathy, entrapment
    facial 351.9
      specified NEC 351.8
    femoral 355.2
    glossopharyngeal NEC 352.2
    hypoglossal 352.5
    iliohypogastric 355.79
    ilioinguinal 355.79
    intercostal 353.8
    lateral
      cutaneous of thigh 355.1
      popliteal 355.3
    lower limb NEC 355.8
    medial, popliteal 355.4
    median NEC 354.1
    obturator 355.79
    oculomotor
      partial 378.51
      total 378.52
    olfactory 352.0
    optic 377.49
      ischemic 377.41
      nutritional 377.33
      toxic 377.34
    peroneal 355.3
    phrenic 354.8
    plantar 355.6
    pneumogastric 352.3
    posterior tibial 355.5
    radial 354.3
    recurrent laryngeal 352.3
    root 353.9
      specified NEC 353.8
    saphenous 355.79
    sciatic NEC 355.0
    specified NEC 355.9
      lower limb 355.79
      upper limb 354.8
    spinal 355.9
    sympathetic NEC 337.9
    trigeminal 350.9
      specified NEC 350.8
    trochlear 378.53
    ulnar 354.2
    upper limb NEC 354.9
    vagus 352.3
  nervous system NEC 349.9
    autonomic (peripheral) (*see also* Neuropathy, peripheral, autonomic) 337.9
    cranial 352.9
    parasympathetic (*see also* Neuropathy, peripheral, autonomic) 337.9
    specified type NEC 349.89
    sympathetic (*see also* Neuropathy, peripheral, autonomic) 337.9
    vegetative (*see also* Neuropathy, peripheral, autonomic) 337.9
  neurohypophysis NEC 253.6
  neurological NEC 781.99
    peripheral NEC 355.9
  neuromuscular NEC 358.9
    hereditary NEC 359.1
    specified NEC 358.8
    toxic 358.2
  neurotic 300.9
    specified type NEC 300.89

☑ Additional Digit Required   ►◄ Revised Text   ● New Line   ▲ Revised Code

Disorder — *see also* Disease — *continued*
  neutrophil, polymorphonuclear (functional)
      288.1
  nightmare 307.47 ●
  night terror 307.46 ●
  obsessive-compulsive 300.3
  oppositional ▶defiant,◀ childhood and
      adolescence 313.81
  optic
      chiasm 377.54
        associated with
            inflammatory disorders 377.54
            neoplasm NEC 377.52
              pituitary 377.51
            pituitary disorders 377.51
            vascular disorders 377.53
      nerve 377.49
      radiations 377.63
      tracts 377.63
  orbit 376.9
      specified NEC 376.89
  orgasmic ●
      female 302.73 ●
      male 302.74 ●
  overanxious, of childhood and adolescence
      313.0
  oxidation, fatty acid 277.85 ●
  pancreas, internal secretion (other than
      diabetes mellitus) 251.9
      specified type NEC 251.8
  panic 300.01
      with agoraphobia 300.21
  papillary muscle NEC 429.81
  paranoid 297.9
      induced 297.3
      shared 297.3
  parathyroid 252.9
      specified type NEC 252.8
  paroxysmal, mixed 780.39
  pentose phosphate pathway with anemia 282.2
  periodic limb movement 780.58 ●
  peroxisomal 277.86
  personality 301.9
      affective 301.10
      aggressive 301.3
      amoral 301.7
      anancastic, anankastic 301.4
      antisocial 301.7
      asocial 301.7
      asthenic 301.6
      avoidant 301.82 ●
      boderline 301.83
      compulsive 301.4
      cyclothymic 301.13
      dependent-passive 301.6
      dyssocial 301.7
      emotional instability 301.59
      epileptoid 301.3
      explosive 301.3
      following organic brain damage 310.1
      histrionic 301.50
      hyperthymic 301.11
      hypomanic (chronic) 301.11
      hypothymic 301.12
      hysterical 301.50
      immature 301.89
      inadequate 301.6
      introverted 301.21
      labile 301.59
      moral deficiency 301.7
      narcissistic 301.81 ●
      obsessional 301.4
      ▶obsessive-compulsive◀ 301.4
      overconscientious 301.4
      paranoid 301.0
      passive (-dependent) 301.6
      passive-aggressive 301.84
      pathological NEC 301.9
      pseudosocial 301.7
      psychopathic 301.9
      schizoid 301.20
        introverted 301.21
        schizotypal 301.22
      schizotypal 301.22
      seductive 301.59
      type A 301.4
      unstable 301.59

Disorder — *see also* Disease — *continued*
  pervasive developmental 299.9 ▲
      childhood-onset 299.8 ●
      specified NEC 299.8 ●
  phonological 315.39 ●
  pigmentation, choroid (congenital) 743.53
  pinna 380.30
      specified type NEC 380.39
  pituitary, thalamic 253.9
      anterior NEC 253.4
      iatrogenic 253.7
      postablative 253.7
      specified NEC 253.8
  pityriasis-like NEC 696.8
  platelets (blood) 287.1
  polymorphonuclear neutrophils (functional)
      288.1
  porphyrin metabolism 277.1
  postmenopausal 627.9
      specified type NEC 627.8
  posttraumatic stress 309.81
      acute 309.81 ▲
      brief 309.81 ▲
      chronic 309.81
  premenstrual dysphoric (PMDD) 625.4
  psoriatic-like NEC 696.8
  psychic, with diseases classified elsewhere 316
  psychogenic NEC (*see also* condition) 300.9
      allergic NEC
        respiratory 306.1
      anxiety 300.00
        atypical 300.00
        generalized 300.02
      appetite 307.50
      articulation, joint 306.0
      asthenic 300.5
      blood 306.8
      cardiovascular (system) 306.2
      compulsive 300.3
      cutaneous 306.3
      depressive 300.4
      digestive (system) 306.4
      dysmenorrheic 306.52
      dyspneic 306.1
      eczematous 306.3
      endocrine (system) 306.6
      eye 306.7
      feeding 307.59
      functional NEC 306.9
      gastric 306.4
      gastrointestinal (system) 306.4
      genitourinary (system) 306.50
      heart (function) (rhythm) 306.2
      hemic 306.8
      hyperventilatory 306.1
      hypochondriacal 300.7
      hysterical 300.10
      intestinal 306.4
      joint 306.0
      learning 315.2
      limb 306.0
      lymphatic (system) 306.8
      menstrual 306.52
      micturition 306.53
      monoplegic NEC 306.0
      motor 307.9
      muscle 306.0
      musculoskeletal 306.0
      neurocirculatory 306.2
      obsessive 300.3
      occupational 300.89
      organ or part of body NEC 306.9
      organs of special sense 306.7
      paralytic NEC 306.0
      phobic 300.20
      physical NEC 306.9
      pruritic 306.3
      rectal 306.4
      respiratory (system) 306.1
      rheumatic 306.0
      sexual (function) 302.70
        specified type NEC 302.79
      sexual orientation conflict 302.0 ●
      skin (allergic) (eczematous) (pruritic) 306.3

Disorder — *see also* Disease — *continued*
  psychogenic NEC — *continued*
      sleep 307.40
        initiation or maintenance 307.41
            persistent 307.42
            transient 307.41
        movement 780.58 ●
        sleep terror 307.46 ●
        specified type NEC 307.49
      specified part of body NEC 306.8
      stomach 306.4
  psychomotor NEC 307.9
      hysterical 300.11
  psychoneurotic (*see also* Neurosis) 300.9
      mixed NEC 300.89
  psychophysiologic (*see also* Disorder,
      psychosomatic) 306.9
  psychosexual identity (childhood) 302.6
      adult-life 302.85
  psychosomatic NEC 306.9
      allergic NEC
        respiratory 306.1
      articulation, joint 306.0
      cardiovascular (system) 306.2
      cutaneous 306.3
      digestive (system) 306.4
      dysmenorrheic 306.52
      dyspneic 306.1
      endocrine (system) 306.6
      eye 306.7
      gastric 306.4
      gastrointestinal (system) 306.4
      genitourinary (system) 306.50
      heart (functional) (rhythm) 306.2
      hyperventilatory 306.1
      intestinal 306.4
      joint 306.0
      limb 306.0
      lymphatic (system) 306.8
      menstrual 306.52
      micturition 306.53
      monoplegic NEC 306.0
      muscle 306.0
      musculoskeletal 306.0
      neurocirculatory 306.2
      organs of special sense 306.7
      paralytic NEC 306.0
      pruritic 306.3
      rectal 306.4
      respiratory (system) 306.1
      rheumatic 306.0
      sexual (function) 302.70
      specified type NEC 302.79
      skin 306.3
      specified part of body NEC 306.8
      stomach 306.4
  psychotic ▶(*see also* Psychosis) 298.9◀ ●
      brief 298.8
  purine metabolism NEC 277.2
  pyrimidine metabolism NEC 277.2
  reactive attachment ▶of infancy or early
      childhood◀ 313.89
  reading, developmental 315.00
  reflex 796.1
  renal function, impaired 588.9
      specified type NEC 588.89 ▲
  renal transport NEC 588.89 ▲
  respiration, respiratory NEC 519.9
      due to
        aspiration of liquids or solids 508.9
        inhalation of fumes or vapors 506.9
      psychogenic 306.1
  retina 362.9
      specified type NEC 362.89
  rumination 307.53 ●
  sacroiliac joint NEC 724.6
  sacrum 724.6
  schizo-affective (*see also* Schizophrenia)
      295.7 ☑
  schizoid, childhood or adolescence 313.22
  schizophreniform 295.4 ☑
  schizotypal personality 301.22
  secretion, thyrocalcitonin 246.0
  seizure 780.39
      recurrent 780.39
        epileptic — *see* Epilepsy

☑ Additional Digit Required   ▶◀ Revised Text   ● New Line   ▲ Revised Code

Disorder — Disproportion *(side tab)*

Disorder — *see also* Disease — *continued*
  sense of smell 781.1
    psychogenic 306.7
  separation anxiety 309.21
  sexual (*see also* Deviation, sexual) 302.9
    aversion 302.79 ●
    desire, hypoactive 302.71 ●
    function, psychogenic 302.70
  shyness, of childhood and adolescence 313.21
  single complement (C-C) 279.8
  skin NEC 709.9
    fetus or newborn 778.9
      specified type 778.8
    psychogenic (allergic) (eczematous) (pruritic) 306.3
    specified type NEC 709.8
    vascular 709.1
  sleep 780.50
    with apnea — *see* Apnea, sleep
    arousal 307.46 ●
    circadian rhythm 307.45
    initiation or maintenance (*see also* Insomnia) 780.52
      nonorganic origin (transient) 307.41
        persistent 307.42
    nonorganic origin 307.40
      specified type NEC 307.49
    specified NEC 780.59
  social, of childhood and adolescence 313.22
    specified NEC 780.59
  soft tissue 729.9
  somatization 300.81
  somatoform (atypical) (undifferentiated) 300.82
    severe 300.81
    specified type NEC 300.89 ●
  speech NEC 784.5
    nonorganic origin 307.9
  spine NEC 724.9
    ligamentous or muscular attachments, peripheral 720.1
  steroid metabolism NEC 255.2
  stomach (functional) (*see also* Disorder, gastric) 536.9
    psychogenic 306.4
  storage, iron 275.0
  stress (*see also* Reaction, stress, acute) 308.3 ▲
    posttraumatic
      acute 309.81 ▲
      brief 309.81 ▲
      chronic 309.81
  substitution 300.11
  suspected — *see* Observation
  synovium 727.9
  temperature regulation, fetus or newborn 778.4
  temporomandibular joint NEC 524.60
    sounds on opening or closing 524.64 ●
    specified NEC 524.69
  tendon 727.9
    shoulder region 726.10
  thoracic root (nerve) NEC 353.3
  thyrocalcitonin secretion 246.0
  thyroid (gland) NEC 246.9
    specified type NEC 246.8
  tic 307.20
    chronic (motor or vocal) 307.22
    motor-verbal 307.23
    organic origin 333.1
    transient ▶(of childhood)◀ 307.21
  tooth NEC 525.9
    development NEC 520.9
      specified type NEC 520.8
    eruption 520.6
    specified type NEC 525.8
  Tourette's 307.23 ●
  transport, carbohydrate 271.9
    specified type NEC 271.8
  tubular, phosphate-losing 588.0
  tympanic membrane 384.9
  unaggressive, unsocialized (*see also* Disturbance, conduct) 312.1 ☑
  undersocialized, unsocialized (*see also* Disturbance, conduct)
    aggressive (type) 312.0 ☑
    unaggressive (type) 312.1 ☑
  vision, visual NEC 368.9
    binocular NEC 368.30

Disorder — *see also* Disease — *continued*
  vision, visual NEC — *continued*
    cortex 377.73
      associated with
        inflammatory disorders 377.73
        neoplasms 377.71
        vascular disorders 377.72
    pathway NEC 377.63
      associated with
        inflammatory disorders 377.63
        neoplasms 377.61
        vascular disorders 377.62
  vocal tic ●
    chronic 307.22 ●
  wakefulness (*see also* Hypersomnia) 780.54
    nonorganic origin (transient) 307.43
      persistent 307.44
  written expression 315.2 ●
Disorganized globe 360.29
Displacement, displaced

Note — For acquired displacement of bones, cartilage, joints, tendons, due to injury, see also Dislocation.

Displacements at ages under one year should be considered congenital, provided there is no indication the condition was acquired after birth.

  acquired traumatic of bone, cartilage, joint, tendon NEC (without fracture) (*see also* Dislocation) 839.8
    with fracture — *see* Fracture, by site
  adrenal gland (congenital) 759.1
  alveolus and teeth, vertical 524.75 ●
  appendix, retrocecal (congenital) 751.5
  auricle (congenital) 744.29
  bladder (acquired) 596.8
    congenital 753.8
  brachial plexus (congenital) 742.8
  brain stem, caudal 742.4
  canaliculus lacrimalis 743.65
  cardia, through esophageal hiatus 750.6
  cerebellum, caudal 742.4
  cervix (*see also* Malposition, uterus) 621.6
  colon (congenital) 751.4
  device, implant, or graft — *see* Complications, mechanical
  epithelium
    columnar of cervix 622.10 ▲
    cuboidal, beyond limits of external os (uterus) 752.49
  esophageal mucosa into cardia of stomach, congenital 750.4
  esophagus (acquired) 530.89
    congenital 750.4
  eyeball (acquired) (old) 376.36
    congenital 743.8
    current injury 871.3
    lateral 376.36
  fallopian tube (acquired) 620.4
    congenital 752.19
    opening (congenital) 752.19
  gallbladder (congenital) 751.69
  gastric mucosa 750.7
    into
      duodenum 750.7
      esophagus 750.7
      Meckel's diverticulum, congenital 750.7
  globe (acquired) (lateral) (old) 376.36
    current injury 871.3
  graft
    artificial skin graft 996.55
    decellularized allodermis graft 996.55
  heart (congenital) 746.87
    acquired 429.89
  hymen (congenital) (upward) 752.49
  internal prothesis NEC — *see* Complications, mechanical
  intervertebral disc (with neuritis, radiculitis, sciatica, or other pain) 722.2
    with myelopathy 722.70
    cervical, cervicodorsal, cervicothoracic 722.0
      with myelopathy 722.71
      due to major trauma — *see* Dislocation, vertebra, cervical
    due to major trauma — *see* Dislocation, vertebra

Displacement, displaced — *continued*
  intervertebral disc — *continued*
    lumbar, lumbosacral 722.10
      with myelopathy 722.73
      due to major trauma — *see* Dislocation, vertebra, lumbar
    thoracic, thoracolumbar 722.11
      with myelopathy 722.72
      due to major trauma — *see* Dislocation, vertebra, thoracic
  intrauterine device 996.32
  kidney (acquired) 593.0
    congenital 753.3
  lacrimal apparatus or duct (congenital) 743.65
  macula (congenital) 743.55
  Meckel's diverticulum (congenital) 751.0
  nail (congenital) 757.5
    acquired 703.8
  opening of Wharton's duct in mouth 750.26
  organ or site, congenital NEC — *see* Malposition, congenital
  ovary (acquired) 620.4
    congenital 752.0
    free in peritoneal cavity (congenital) 752.0
    into hernial sac 620.4
  oviduct (acquired) 620.4
    congenital 752.19
  parathyroid (gland) 252.8
  parotid gland (congenital) 750.26
  punctum lacrimale (congenital) 743.65
  sacroiliac (congenital) (joint) 755.69
    current injury — *see* Dislocation, sacroiliac
    old 724.6
  spine (congenital) 756.19
  spleen, congenital 759.0
  stomach (congenital) 750.7
    acquired 537.89
  subglenoid (closed) 831.01
  sublingual duct (congenital) 750.26
  teeth, tooth 524.30 ▲
    horizontal 524.33 ●
    vertical 524.34 ●
  tongue (congenital) (downward) 750.19
  trachea (congenital) 748.3
  ureter or ureteric opening or orifice (congenital) 753.4
  uterine opening of oviducts or fallopian tubes 752.19
  uterus, uterine (*see also* Malposition, uterus) 621.6
    congenital 752.3
  ventricular septum 746.89
    with rudimentary ventricle 746.89
  xyphoid bone (process) 738.3
Disproportion 653.9 ☑
  affecting fetus or newborn 763.1
  caused by
    conjoined twins 653.7 ☑
    contraction, pelvis (general) 653.1 ☑
      inlet 653.2 ☑
      midpelvic 653.8 ☑
      midplane 653.8 ☑
      outlet 653.3 ☑
    fetal
      ascites 653.7 ☑
      hydrocephalus 653.6 ☑
      hydrops 653.7 ☑
      meningomyelocele 653.7 ☑
      sacral teratoma 653.7 ☑
      tumor 653.7 ☑
    hydrocephalic fetus 653.6 ☑
    pelvis, pelvic, abnormality (bony) NEC 653.0 ☑
    unusually large fetus 653.5 ☑
  causing obstructed labor 660.1 ☑
  cephalopelvic, normally formed fetus 653.4 ☑
    causing obstructed labor 660.1 ☑
  fetal NEC 653.5 ☑
    causing obstructed labor 660.1 ☑
  fetopelvic, normally formed fetus 653.4 ☑
    causing obstructed labor 660.1 ☑
  mixed maternal and fetal origin, normally formed fetus 653.4 ☑
  pelvis, pelvic (bony) NEC 653.1 ☑
    causing obstructed labor 660.1 ☑
  specified type NEC 653.8 ☑

☑ Additional Digit Required   ▶◀ Revised Text   ● New Line   ▲ Revised Code

Disruption
cesarean wound 674.1 ☑
family V61.0
gastrointestinal anastomosis 997.4
ligament(s) — *see also* Sprain
  knee
    current injury — *see* Dislocation knee
    old 717.89
      capsular 717.85
      collateral (medial) 717.82
        lateral 717.81
      cruciate (posterior) 717.84
        anterior 717.83
      specified site NEC 717.85
marital V61.10
  involving divorce or estrangement V61.0
operation wound (external) 998.32
  internal 998.31
organ transplant, anastomosis site — *see*
    Complications, transplant, organ, by site
ossicles, ossicular chain 385.23
  traumatic — *see* Fracture, skull, base
parenchyma
  liver (hepatic) — *see* Laceration, liver, major
  spleen — *see* Laceration, spleen,
    parenchyma, massive
phase-shift, of 24-hour sleep-wake cycle
  780.55
  nonorganic origin 307.45
sleep-wake cycle (24-hour) 780.55
  circadian rhythm 307.45
  nonorganic origin 307.45
suture line (external) 998.32
  internal 998.31
wound
  cesarean operation 674.1 ☑
  episiotomy 674.2 ☑
  operation 998.32
    cesarean 674.1 ☑
    internal 998.31
  perineal (obstetric) 674.2 ☑
  uterine 674.1 ☑

Disruptio uteri — *see also* Rupture, uterus
complicating delivery — *see* Delivery,
  complicated, rupture, uterus

Dissatisfaction with
employment V62.2
school environment V62.3

Dissecting — *see* condition

Dissection
aorta 441.00
  abdominal 441.02
  thoracic 441.01
  thoracoabdominal 441.03
artery, arterial
  carotid 443.21
  coronary 414.12
  iliac 443.22
  renal 443.23
  specified NEC 443.29
  vertebral 443.24
vascular 459.9
wound — *see* Wound, open, by site

Disseminated — *see* condition

Dissociated personality NEC 300.15

Dissociation
auriculoventricular or atrioventricular (any
  degree) (AV) 426.89
  with heart block 426.0
interference 426.89
isorhythmic 426.89
rhythm
  atrioventricular (AV) 426.89
  interference 426.89

Dissociative
identity disorder 300.14
reaction NEC 300.15

Dissolution, vertebra (*see also* Osteoporosis)
733.00

Distention
abdomen (gaseous) 787.3
bladder 596.8
cecum 569.89
colon 569.89
gallbladder 575.8

Distention — *continued*
gaseous (abdomen) 787.3
intestine 569.89
kidney 593.89
liver 573.9
seminal vesicle 608.89
stomach 536.8
  acute 536.1
  psychogenic 306.4
ureter 593.5
uterus 621.8

Distichia, distichiasis (eyelid) 743.63

Distoma hepaticum infestation 121.3

Distomiasis 121.9
bile passages 121.3
  due to Clonorchis sinensis 121.1
hemic 120.9
hepatic (liver) 121.3
  due to Clonorchis sinensis (clonorchiasis)
    121.1
intestinal 121.4
liver 121.3
  due to Clonorchis sinensis 121.1
lung 121.2
pulmonary 121.2

Distomolar (fourth molar) 520.1
causing crowding 524.31   ▲

Disto-occlusion ▶(division I) (division II)◀
524.22   ▲

Distortion (congenital)
adrenal (gland) 759.1
ankle (joint) 755.69
anus 751.5
aorta 747.29
appendix 751.5
arm 755.59
artery (peripheral) NEC (*see also* Distortion,
  peripheral vascular system) 747.60
  cerebral 747.81
  coronary 746.85
  pulmonary 747.3
  retinal 743.58
  umbilical 747.5
auditory canal 744.29
  causing impairment of hearing 744.02
bile duct or passage 751.69
bladder 753.8
brain 742.4
bronchus 748.3
cecum 751.5
cervix (uteri) 752.49
chest (wall) 756.3
clavicle 755.51
clitoris 752.49
coccyx 756.19
colon 751.5
common duct 751.69
cornea 743.41
cricoid cartilage 748.3
cystic duct 751.69
duodenum 751.5
ear 744.29
  auricle 744.29
    causing impairment of hearing 744.02
  causing impairment of hearing 744.09
  external 744.29
    causing impairment of hearing 744.02
  inner 744.05
  middle, except ossicles 744.03
    ossicles 744.04
  ossicles 744.04
endocrine (gland) NEC 759.2
epiglottis 748.3
Eustachian tube 744.24
eye 743.8
  adnexa 743.69
face bone(s) 756.0
fallopian tube 752.19
femur 755.69
fibula 755.69
finger(s) 755.59
foot 755.67
gallbladder 751.69

Distortion — *continued*
genitalia, genital organ(s)
  female 752.89
    external 752.49
    internal NEC 752.89
  male 752.89
    penis 752.69
glottis 748.3
gyri 742.4
hand bone(s) 755.59
heart (auricle) (ventricle) 746.89
  valve (cusp) 746.89
hepatic duct 751.69
humerus 755.59
hymen 752.49
ileum 751.5
intestine (large) (small) 751.5
  with anomalous adhesions, fixation or
    malrotation 751.4
jaw NEC 524.89   ▲
jejunum 751.5
kidney 753.3
knee (joint) 755.64
labium (majus) (minus) 752.49
larynx 748.3
leg 755.69
lens 743.36
liver 751.69
lumbar spine 756.19
  with disproportion (fetopelvic) 653.0 ☑
    affecting fetus or newborn 763.1
    causing obstructed labor 660.1 ☑
lumbosacral (joint) (region) 756.19
lung (fissures) (lobe) 748.69
nerve 742.8
nose 748.1
organ
  of Corti 744.05
  or site not listed — *see* Anomaly, specified
    type NEC
ossicles, ear 744.04
ovary 752.0
oviduct 752.19
pancreas 751.7
parathyroid (gland) 759.2
patella 755.64
peripheral vascular system NEC 747.60
  gastrointestinal 747.61
  lower limb 747.64
  renal 747.62
  spinal 747.82
  upper limb 747.63
pituitary (gland) 759.2
radius 755.59
rectum 751.5
rib 756.3
sacroiliac joint 755.69
sacrum 756.19
scapula 755.59
shoulder girdle 755.59
site not listed — *see* Anomaly, specified type NEC
skull bone(s) 756.0
  with
    anencephalus 740.0
    encephalocele 742.0
    hydrocephalus 742.3
      with spina bifida (*see also* Spina
        bifida) 741.0 ☑
    microcephalus 742.1
spinal cord 742.59
spine 756.19
spleen 759.0
sternum 756.3
thorax (wall) 756.3
thymus (gland) 759.2
thyroid (gland) 759.2
  cartilage 748.3
tibia 755.69
toe(s) 755.66
tongue 750.19
trachea (cartilage) 748.3
ulna 755.59
ureter 753.4
  causing obstruction 753.20
urethra 753.8
  causing obstruction 753.6
uterus 752.3

☑ Additional Digit Required   ▶◀ Revised Text   ● New Line   ▲ Revised Code

Distortion — *continued*
- vagina 752.49
- vein (peripheral) NEC (*see also* Distortion, peripheral vascular system) 747.60
  - great 747.49
  - portal 747.49
  - pulmonary 747.49
- vena cava (inferior) (superior) 747.49
- vertebra 756.19
- visual NEC 368.15
  - shape or size 368.14
- vulva 752.49
- wrist (bones) (joint) 755.59

Distress
- abdomen 789.0 ☑
- colon 789.0 ☑
- emotional V40.9
- epigastric 789.0 ☑
- fetal (syndrome) 768.4
  - affecting management of pregnancy or childbirth 656.8 ☑
  - liveborn infant 768.4
    - first noted
      - before onset of labor 768.2
      - during labor or delivery 768.3
    - stillborn infant (death before onset of labor) 768.0
    - death during labor 768.1
- gastrointestinal (functional) 536.9
  - psychogenic 306.4
- intestinal (functional) NEC 564.9
  - psychogenic 306.4
- intrauterine — *see* Distress, fetal
- leg 729.5
- maternal 669.0 ☑
- mental V40.9
- respiratory 786.09
  - acute (adult) 518.82
  - adult syndrome (following shock, surgery, or trauma) 518.5
    - specified NEC 518.82
  - fetus or newborn 770.89
  - syndrome (idiopathic) (newborn) 769
- stomach 536.9
  - psychogenic 306.4

Distribution vessel, atypical NEC 747.60
- coronary artery 746.85
- spinal 747.82

Districhiasis 704.2

Disturbance — *see also* Disease
- absorption NEC 579.9
  - calcium 269.3
  - carbohydrate 579.8
  - fat 579.8
  - protein 579.8
  - specified type NEC 579.8
  - vitamin (*see also* Deficiency, vitamin) 269.2
- acid-base equilibrium 276.9
- activity and attention, simple, with hyperkinesis 314.01
- amino acid (metabolic) (*see also* Disorder, amino acid) 270.9
  - imidazole 270.5
  - maple syrup (urine) disease 270.3
  - transport 270.0
- assimilation, food 579.9
- attention, simple 314.00
  - with hyperactivity 314.01
- auditory, nerve, except deafness 388.5
- behavior (*see also* Disturbance, conduct) 312.9
- blood clotting (hypoproteinemia) (mechanism) (*see also* Defect, coagulation) 286.9
- central nervous system NEC 349.9
- cerebral nerve NEC 352.9
- circulatory 459.9
- conduct 312.9

Note — Use the following fifth-digit subclassification with categories 312.0–312.2:
- *0   unspecified*
- *1   mild*
- *2   moderate*
- *3   severe*

Disturbance — *see also* Disease — *continued*
- conduct—*continued*
  - adjustment reaction 309.3
  - adolescent onset type 312.82
  - childhood onset type 312.81
  - compulsive 312.30
    - intermittent explosive disorder 312.34
    - isolated explosive disorder 312.35
    - kleptomania 312.32
    - pathological gambling 312.31
    - pyromania 312.33
  - hyperkinetic 314.2
  - intermittent explosive 312.34
  - isolated explosive 312.35
  - mixed with emotions 312.4
  - socialized (type) 312.20
    - aggressive 312.23
    - unaggressive 312.21
  - specified type NEC 312.89
  - undersocialized, unsocialized
    - aggressive (type) 312.0 ☑
    - unaggressive (type) 312.1 ☑
- coordination 781.3
- cranial nerve NEC 352.9
- deep sensibility — *see* Disturbance, sensation
- digestive 536.9
  - psychogenic 306.4
- electrolyte — *see* Imbalance, electrolyte
- emotions specific to childhood ►or◄
  - adolescence 313.9
  - with
    - academic underachievement 313.83
    - anxiety and fearfulness 313.0
    - elective mutism 313.23
    - identity disorder 313.82
    - jealousy 313.3
    - misery and unhappiness 313.1
    - oppositional ►defiant◄ disorder 313.81
    - overanxiousness 313.0
    - sensitivity 313.21
    - shyness 313.21
    - social withdrawal 313.22
    - withdrawal reaction 313.22
  - involving relationship problems 313.3
  - mixed 313.89
  - specified type NEC 313.89
- endocrine (gland) 259.9
  - neonatal, transitory 775.9
    - specified NEC 775.8
- equilibrium 780.4
- feeding (elderly) (infant) 783.3
  - newborn 779.3
  - nonorganic origin NEC 307.59
  - psychogenic NEC 307.59
- fructose metabolism 271.2
- gait 781.2
  - hysterical 300.11
- gastric (functional) 536.9
  - motility 536.8
  - psychogenic 306.4
  - secretion 536.8
- gastrointestinal (functional) 536.9
  - psychogenic 306.4
- habit, child 307.9
- hearing, except deafness 388.40
- heart, functional (conditions classifiable to 426, 427, 428)
  - due to presence of (cardiac) prosthesis 429.4
  - postoperative (immediate) 997.1
    - long-term effect of cardiac surgery 429.4
  - psychogenic 306.2
- hormone 259.9
- innervation uterus, sympathetic, parasympathetic 621.8
- keratinization NEC
  - gingiva 523.1
  - lip 528.5
  - oral (mucosa) (soft tissue) 528.79   ▲
    - residual ridge mucosa   ●
      - excessive 528.72   ●
      - minimal 528.71   ●
  - tongue 528.79   ▲

Disturbance — *see also* Disease — *continued*
- labyrinth, labyrinthine (vestibule) 386.9
- learning, specific NEC 315.2
- memory (*see also* Amnesia) 780.93
  - mild, following organic brain damage 310.8   ▲
- mental (*see also* Disorder, mental) 300.9
  - associated with diseases classified elsewhere 316
- metabolism (acquired) (congenital) (*see also* Disorder, metabolism) 277.9
  - with
    - abortion — *see* Abortion, by type, with metabolic disorder
    - ectopic pregnancy (*see also* categories 633.0-633.9) 639.4
    - molar pregnancy (*see also* categories 630-632) 639.4
  - amino acid (*see also* Disorder, amino acid) 270.9
    - aromatic NEC 270.2
    - branched-chain 270.3
    - specified type NEC 270.8
    - straight-chain NEC 270.7
    - sulfur-bearing 270.4
    - transport 270.0
  - ammonia 270.6
  - arginine 270.6
  - argininosuccinic acid 270.6
  - carbohydrate NEC 271.9
  - cholesterol 272.9
  - citrulline 270.6
  - cystathionine 270.4
  - fat 272.9
  - following
    - abortion 639.4
    - ectopic or molar pregnancy 639.4
  - general 277.9
    - carbohydrate 271.9
    - iron 275.0
    - phosphate 275.3
    - sodium 276.9
  - glutamine 270.7
  - glycine 270.7
  - histidine 270.5
  - homocystine 270.4
  - in labor or delivery 669.0 ☑
  - iron 275.0
  - isoleucine 270.3
  - leucine 270.3
  - lipoid 272.9
    - specified type NEC 272.8
  - lysine 270.7
  - methionine 270.4
  - neonatal, transitory 775.9
    - specified type NEC 775.8
  - nitrogen 788.9
  - ornithine 270.6
  - phosphate 275.3
  - phosphatides 272.7
  - serine 270.7
  - sodium NEC 276.9
  - threonine 270.7
  - tryptophan 270.2
  - tyrosine 270.2
  - urea cycle 270.6
  - valine 270.3
- motor 796.1
- nervous functional 799.2
- neuromuscular mechanism (eye) due to syphilis 094.84
- nutritional 269.9
  - nail 703.8
- ocular motion 378.87
  - psychogenic 306.7
- oculogyric 378.87
  - psychogenic 306.7
- oculomotor NEC 378.87
  - psychogenic 306.7
- olfactory nerve 781.1
- optic nerve NEC 377.49
- oral epithelium, including tongue 528.79   ▲
  - residual ridge mucosa   ●
    - excessive 528.72   ●
    - minimal 528.71   ●

☑ Additional Digit Required   ►◄ Revised Text   ● New Line   ▲ Revised Code

Disturbance — *see also* Disease — *continued*
  personality (pattern) (trait) (*see also* Disorder,
      personality) 301.9
    following organic brain damage 310.1
  polyglandular 258.9
  psychomotor 307.9
  pupillary 379.49
  reflex 796.1
  rhythm, heart 427.9
    postoperative (immediate) 997.1
      long-term effect of cardiac surgery 429.4
    psychogenic 306.2
  salivary secretion 527.7
  sensation (cold) (heat) (localization) (tactile
      discrimination localization) (texture)
      (vibratory) NEC 782.0
    hysterical 300.11
    skin 782.0
    smell 781.1
    taste 781.1
  sensory (*see also* Disturbance, sensation) 782.0
    innervation 782.0
  situational (transient) (*see also* Reaction,
      adjustment) 309.9
    acute 308.3
  sleep 780.50
    with apnea — *see* Apnea, sleep
    initiation or maintenance (*see also*
        Insomnia) 780.52
      nonorganic origin 307.41
    nonorganic origin 307.40
      specified type NEC 307.49
    specified NEC 780.59
      nonorganic origin 307.49
    wakefulness (*see also* Hypersomnia) 780.54
      nonorganic origin 307.43
  sociopathic 301.7
  speech NEC 784.5
    developmental 315.39
      associated with hyperkinesis 314.1
    secondary to organic lesion 784.5
  stomach (functional) (*see also* Disturbance,
      gastric) 536.9
  sympathetic (nerve) (*see also* Neuropathy,
      peripheral, autonomic) 337.9
  temperature sense 782.0
    hysterical 300.11
  tooth
    eruption 520.6
    formation 520.4
    structure, hereditary NEC 520.5
  touch (*see also* Disturbance, sensation) 782.0
  vascular 459.9
    arterioslerotic — *see* Arteriosclerosis
  vasomotor 443.9
  vasospastic 443.9
  vestibular labyrinth 386.9
  vision, visual NEC 368.9
    psychophysical 368.16
    specified NEC 368.8
    subjective 368.10
  voice 784.40
  wakefulness (initiation or maintenance) (*see
      also* Hypersomnia) 780.54
    nonorganic origin 307.43
Disulfiduria, beta-mercaptolactate-cysteine
  270.0
Disuse atrophy, bone 733.7
Ditthomska syndrome 307.81
Diuresis 788.42
Divers'
  palsy or paralysis 993.3
  squeeze 993.3
Diverticula, diverticulosis, diverticulum (acute)
    (multiple) (perforated) (ruptured) 562.10
  with diverticulitis 562.11
  aorta (Kommerell's) 747.21
  appendix (noninflammatory) 543.9
  bladder (acquired) (sphincter) 596.3
    congenital 753.8
  broad ligament 620.8
  bronchus (congenital) 748.3
    acquired 494.0
      with acute exacerbation 494.1
  calyx, calyceal (kidney) 593.89
  cardia (stomach) 537.1

Diverticula, diverticulosis, diverticulum —
    continued
  cecum 562.10
    with
      diverticulitis 562.11
        with hemorrhage 562.13
      hemorrhage 562.12
    congenital 751.5
  colon (acquired) 562.10
    with
      diverticulitis 562.11
        with hemorrhage 562.13
      hemorrhage 562.12
    congenital 751.5
  duodenum 562.00
    with
      diverticulitis 562.01
        with hemorrhage 562.03
      hemorrhage 562.02
    congenital 751.5
  epiphrenic (esophagus) 530.6
  esophagus (congenital) 750.4
    acquired 530.6
    epiphrenic 530.6
    pulsion 530.6
    traction 530.6
    Zenker's 530.6
  Eustachian tube 381.89
  fallopian tube 620.8
  gallbladder (congenital) 751.69
  gastric 537.1
  heart (congenital) 746.89
  ileum 562.00
    with
      diverticulitis 562.01
        with hemorrhage 562.03
      hemorrhage 562.02
  intestine (large) 562.10
    with
      diverticulitis 562.11
        with hemorrhage 562.13
      hemorrhage 562.12
    congenital 751.5
    small 562.00
      with
        diverticulitis 562.01
          with hemorrhage 562.03
        hemorrhage 562.02
      congenital 751.5
  jejunum 562.00
    with
      diverticulitis 562.01
        with hemorrhage 562.03
      hemorrhage 562.02
  kidney (calyx) (pelvis) 593.89
    with calculus 592.0
  Kommerell's 747.21
  laryngeal ventricle (congenital) 748.3
  Meckel's (displaced) (hypertrophic) 751.0
  midthoracic 530.6
  organ or site, congenital NEC — *see* Distortion
  pericardium (congenital) (cyst) 746.89
    acquired (true) 423.8
  pharyngoesophageal (pulsion) 530.6
  pharynx (congenital) 750.27
  pulsion (esophagus) 530.6
  rectosigmoid 562.10
    with
      diverticulitis 562.11
        with hemorrhage 562.13
      hemorrhage 562.12
    congenital 751.5
  rectum 562.10
    with
      diverticulitis 562.11
        with hemorrhage 562.13
      hemorrhage 562.12
  renal (calyces) (pelvis) 593.89
    with calculus 592.0
  Rokitansky's 530.6
  seminal vesicle 608.0
  sigmoid 562.10
    with
      diverticulitis 562.11
        with hemorrhage 562.13
      hemorrhage 562.12
    congenital 751.5

Diverticula, diverticulosis, diverticulum —
    continued
  small intestine 562.00
    with
      diverticulitis 562.01
        with hemorrhage 562.03
      hemorrhage 562.02
  stomach (cardia) (juxtacardia) (juxtapyloric)
      (acquired) 537.1
    congenital 750.7
  subdiaphragmatic 530.6
  trachea (congenital) 748.3
    acquired 519.1
  traction (esophagus) 530.6
  ureter (acquired) 593.89
    congenital 753.4
  ureterovesical orifice 593.89
  urethra (acquired) 599.2
    congenital 753.8
  ventricle, left (congenital) 746.89
  vesical (urinary) 596.3
    congenital 753.8
  Zenker's (esophagus) 530.6
Diverticulitis (acute) (*see also* Diverticula) 562.11
  with hemorrhage 562.13
  bladder (urinary) 596.3
  cecum (perforated) 562.11
    with hemorrhage 562.13
  colon (perforated) 562.11
    with hemorrhage 562.13
  duodenum 562.01
    with hemorrhage 562.03
  esophagus 530.6
  ileum (perforated) 562.01
    with hemorrhage 562.03
  intestine (large) (perforated) 562.11
    with hemorrhage 562.13
    small 562.01
      with hemorrhage 562.03
  jejunum (perforated) 562.01
    with hemorrhage 562.03
  Meckel's (perforated) 751.0
  pharyngoesophageal 530.6
  rectosigmoid (perforated) 562.11
    with hemorrhage 562.13
  rectum 562.11
    with hemorrhage 562.13
  sigmoid (old) (perforated) 562.11
    with hemorrhage 562.13
  small intestine (perforated) 562.01
    with hemorrhage 562.03
  vesical (urinary) 596.3
Diverticulosis — *see* Diverticula
Division
  cervix uteri 622.8
    external os into two openings by frenum
        752.49
  external (cervical) into two openings by frenum
      752.49
  glans penis 752.69
  hymen 752.49
  labia minora (congenital) 752.49
  ligament (partial or complete) (current) — *see
      also* Sprain, by site
    with open wound — *see* Wound, open, by
        site
  muscle (partial or complete) (current) — *see
      also* Sprain, by site
    with open wound — *see* Wound, open, by
        site
  nerve — *see* Injury, nerve, by site
  penis glans 752.69
  spinal cord — *see* Injury, spinal, by site
  vein 459.9
    traumatic — *see* Injury, vascular, by site
Divorce V61.0
Dix-Hallpike neurolabyrinthitis 386.12
Dizziness 780.4
  hysterical 300.11
  psychogenic 306.9
Doan-Wiseman syndrome (primary splenic
    neutropenia) 288.0
Dog bite — *see* Wound, open, by site
Döhle-Heller aortitis 093.1
Döhle body-panmyelopathic syndrome 288.2

☑ Additional Digit Required   ▶◀ Revised Text   ● New Line   ▲ Revised Code

Dolichocephaly, dolichocephalus 754.0
Dolichocolon 751.5
Dolichostenomelia 759.82
Donohue's syndrome (leprechaunism) 259.8
Donor
blood V59.01
other blood components V59.09
stem cells V59.02
whole blood V59.01
bone V59.2
marrow V59.3
cornea V59.5
heart V59.8
kidney V59.4
liver V59.6
lung V59.8
lymphocyte V59.8
organ V59.9
specified NEC V59.8
potential, examination of V70.8
skin V59.1
specified organ or tissue NEC V59.8
sperm V59.8
stem cells V59.02
tissue V59.9
specified type NEC V59.8
Donovanosis (granuloma venereum) 099.2
DOPS (diffuse obstructive pulmonary syndrome)
496
Double
albumin 273.8
aortic arch 747.21
auditory canal 744.29
auricle (heart) 746.82
bladder 753.8
external (cervical) os 752.49
kidney with double pelvis (renal) 753.3
larynx 748.3
meatus urinarius 753.8
organ or site NEC — see Accessory
orifice
heart valve NEC 746.89
pulmonary 746.09
outlet, right ventricle 745.11
pelvis (renal) with double ureter 753.4
penis 752.69
tongue 750.13
ureter (one or both sides) 753.4
with double pelvis (renal) 753.4
urethra 753.8
urinary meatus 753.8
uterus (any degree) 752.2
with doubling of cervix and vagina 752.2
in pregnancy or childbirth 654.0 ☑
affecting fetus or newborn 763.89
vagina 752.49
with doubling of cervix and uterus 752.2
vision 368.2
vocal cords 748.3
vulva 752.49
whammy (syndrome) 360.81
Douglas' pouch, cul-de-sac — see condition
Down's disease or syndrome (mongolism) 758.0
Down-growth, epithelial (anterior chamber)
364.61
Dracontiasis 125.7
Dracunculiasis 125.7
Drancunculosis 125.7
Drainage
abscess (spontaneous) — see Abscess
anomalous pulmonary veins to hepatic veins or
right atrium 747.41
stump (amputation) (surgical) 997.62
suprapubic, bladder 596.8
Dream state, hysterical 300.13
Drepanocytic anemia (see also Disease, sickle
cell) 282.60
Dresbach's syndrome (elliptocytosis) 282.1
Dreschlera (infection) 118
hawaiiensis 117.8
Dressler's syndrome (postmyocardial infarction)
411.0
Dribbling (post-void) 788.35

Drift, ulnar 736.09
Drinking (alcohol) — see also Alcoholism
excessive, to excess NEC (see also Abuse,
drugs, nondependent) 305.0 ☑
bouts, periodic 305.0 ☑
continual 303.9 ☑
episodic 305.0 ☑
habitual 303.9 ☑
periodic 305.0 ☑
Drip, postnasal (chronic) — see Sinusitis
Drivers' license examination V70.3
Droop
Cooper's 611.8
facial 781.94
Drop
finger 736.29
foot 736.79
hematocrit (precipitous) 790.01
toe 735.8
wrist 736.05
Dropped
dead 798.1
heart beats 426.6
Dropsy, dropsical (see also Edema) 782.3
abdomen 789.5
amnion (see also Hydramnios) 657.0 ☑
brain — see Hydrocephalus
cardiac (see also Failure, heart) 428.0
cardiorenal (see also Hypertension, cardiorenal)
404.90
chest 511.9
fetus or newborn 778.0
due to isoimmunization 773.3
gangrenous (see also Gangrene) 785.4
heart (see also Failure, heart) 428.0
hepatic — see Cirrhosis, liver
infantile — see Hydrops, fetalis
kidney (see also Nephrosis) 581.9
liver — see Cirrhosis, liver
lung 514
malarial (see also Malaria) 084.9
neonatorum — see Hydrops, fetalis
nephritic 581.9
newborn — see Hydrops, fetalis
nutritional 269.9
ovary 620.8
pericardium (see also Pericarditis) 423.9
renal (see also Nephrosis) 581.9
uremic — see Uremia
Drowned, drowning 994.1
lung 518.5
Drowsiness 780.09
Drug — see also condition
addiction (see also listing under Dependence)
304.9 ☑
adverse effect NEC, correct substance properly
administered 995.2
dependence (see also listing under Dependence)
304.9 ☑
habit (see also listing under Dependence)
304.9 ☑
induced ●
mental disorder 292.9 ●
anxiety 292.89 ●
mood 292.84 ●
sexual 292.89 ●
sleep 292.89 ●
specified type 292.89 ●
persisting ●
amnestic disorder 292.83 ●
dementia 292.82 ●
psychotic disorder ●
with ●
delusions 292.11 ●
hallucinations 292.12 ●
intoxication 292.89 ●
overdose — see Table of Drugs and Chemicals
poisoning — see Table of Drugs and Chemicals
therapy (maintenance) status NEC V58.1
long-term (current) use V58.69
antibiotics V58.62
▶anticoagulants◀ V58.61
anti-inflammatories, non-steroidal
(NSAID) V58.64
▶antiplatelets◀ V58.63

Drug —see also condition— continued
therapy (maintenance) status NEC — continued
long-term (current) use — continued
▶antithrombotics◀ V58.63
aspirin V58.66 ●
insulin V58.67 ●
steroids V58.65
wrong substance given or taken in error — see
Table of Drugs and Chemicals
Drunkenness (see also Abuse, drugs,
nondependent) 305.0 ☑
acute in alcoholism (see also Alcoholism)
303.0 ☑
chronic (see also Alcoholism) 303.9 ☑
pathologic 291.4
simple (acute) 305.0 ☑
in alcoholism 303.0 ☑
sleep 307.47
Drusen
optic disc or papilla 377.21
retina (colloid) (hyaloid degeneration) 362.57
hereditary 362.77
Drusenfieber 075
Dry, dryness — see also condition
eye 375.15
syndrome 375.15
larynx 478.79
mouth 527.7
nose 478.1
skin syndrome 701.1
socket (teeth) 526.5
throat 478.29
DSAP (disseminated superficial actinic
porokeratosis) 692.75
Duane's retraction syndrome 378.71
Duane-Stilling-Türk syndrome (ocular retraction
syndrome) 378.71
Dubin-Johnson disease or syndrome 277.4
Dubini's disease (electric chorea) 049.8
Dubois' abscess or disease 090.5
Duchenne's
disease 094.0
locomotor ataxia 094.0
muscular dystrophy 359.1
pseudohypertrophy, muscles 359.1
paralysis 335.22
syndrome 335.22
Duchenne-Aran myelopathic, muscular atrophy
(nonprogressive) (progressive) 335.21
Duchenne-Griesinger disease 359.1
Ducrey's
bacillus 099.0
chancre 099.0
disease (chancroid) 099.0
Duct, ductus — see condition
Duengero 061
Duhring's disease (dermatitis herpetiformis)
694.0
Dukes (-Filatov) disease 057.8
Dullness
cardiac (decreased) (increased) 785.3
Dumb ague (see also Malaria) 084.6
Dumbness (see also Aphasia) 784.3
Dumdum fever 085.0
Dumping syndrome (postgastrectomy) 564.2
nonsurgical 536.8
Duodenitis (nonspecific) (peptic) 535.60
with hemorrhage 535.61
due to
Strongyloides stercoralis 127.2
Duodenocholangitis 575.8
Duodenum, duodenal — see condition
Duplay's disease, periarthritis, or syndrome
726.2
Duplex — see also Accessory
kidney 753.3
placenta — see Placenta, abnormal
uterus 752.2
Duplication — see also Accessory
anus 751.5
aortic arch 747.21

Dolichocephaly, dolichocephalus — Duplication

Duplication — *see also* Accessory — *continued*
appendix 751.5
biliary duct (any) 751.69
bladder 753.8
cecum 751.5
  and appendix 751.5
clitoris 752.49
cystic duct 751.69
digestive organs 751.8
duodenum 751.5
esophagus 750.4
fallopian tube 752.19
frontonasal process 756.0
gallbladder 751.69
ileum 751.5
intestine (large) (small) 751.5
jejunum 751.5
kidney 753.3
liver 751.69
nose 748.1
pancreas 751.7
penis 752.69
respiratory organs NEC 748.9
salivary duct 750.22
spinal cord (incomplete) 742.51
stomach 750.7
ureter 753.4
vagina 752.49
vas deferens 752.89
vocal cords 748.3
Dupré's disease or syndrome (meningism) 781.6
Dupuytren's
contraction 728.6
disease (muscle contracture) 728.6
fracture (closed) 824.4
  ankle (closed) 824.4
    open 824.5
  fibula (closed) 824.4
    open 824.5
  open 824.5
  radius (closed) 813.42
    open 813.52
muscle contracture 728.6
Durand-Nicolas-Favre disease (climatic bubo) 099.1
Duroziez's disease (congenital mitral stenosis) 746.5
Dust
conjunctivitis 372.05
reticulation (occupational) 504
Dutton's
disease (trypanosomiasis) 086.9
relapsing fever (West African) 087.1
Dwarf, dwarfism 259.4
with infantilism (hypophyseal) 253.3
achondroplastic 756.4
Amsterdam 759.89
bird-headed 759.89
congenital 259.4
constitutional 259.4
hypophyseal 253.3
infantile 259.4
Levi type 253.3
Lorain-Levi (pituitary) 253.3
Lorain type (pituitary) 253.3
metatropic 756.4
nephrotic-glycosuric, with hypophosphatemic rickets 270.0
nutritional 263.2
ovarian 758.6
pancreatic 577.8
pituitary 253.3
polydystrophic 277.5
primordial 253.3
psychosocial 259.4
renal 588.0
  with hypertension — *see* Hypertension, kidney
Russell's (uterine dwarfism and craniofacial dysostosis) 759.89
Dyke-Young anemia or syndrome (acquired macrocytic hemolytic anemia) (secondary) (symptomatic) 283.9
Dynia abnormality (*see also* Defect, coagulation) 286.9

Dysacousis 388.40
Dysadrenocortism 255.9
hyperfunction 255.3
hypofunction 255.4
Dysarthria 784.5
Dysautonomia (*see also* Neuropathy, peripheral, autonomic) 337.9
familial 742.8
Dysbarism 993.3
Dysbasia 719.7
angiosclerotica intermittens 443.9
  due to atherosclerosis 440.21
hysterical 300.11
lordotica (progressiva) 333.6
nonorganic origin 307.9
psychogenic 307.9
Dysbetalipoproteinemia (familial) 272.2
Dyscalculia 315.1
Dyschezia (*see also* Constipation) 564.00
Dyschondroplasia (with hemangiomata) 756.4
Voorhoeve's 756.4
Dyschondrosteosis 756.59
Dyschromia 709.00
Dyscollagenosis 710.9
Dyscoria 743.41
Dyscraniopyophalangy 759.89
Dyscrasia
blood 289.9
  with antepartum hemorrhage 641.3 ☑
  fetus or newborn NEC 776.9
  hemorrhage, subungual 287.8
  puerperal, postpartum 666.3 ☑
ovary 256.8
plasma cell 273.9
pluriglandular 258.9
polyglandular 258.9
Dysdiadochokinesia 781.3
Dysectasia, vesical neck 596.8
Dysendocrinism 259.9
Dysentery, dysenteric (bilious) (catarrhal) (diarrhea) (epidemic) (gangrenous) (hemorrhagic) (infectious) (sporadic) (tropical) (ulcerative) 009.0
abscess, liver (*see also* Abscess, amebic) 006.3
amebic (*see also* Amebiasis) 006.9
  with abscess — *see* Abscess, amebic
  acute 006.0
  carrier (suspected) of V02.2
  chronic 006.1
arthritis (*see also* Arthritis, due to, dysentery) 009.0 *[711.3]* ☑
  bacillary 004.9 *[711.3]* ☑
asylum 004.9
bacillary 004.9
  arthritis 004.9 *[711.3]* ☑
  Boyd 004.2
  Flexner 004.1
  Schmitz (-Stutzer) 004.0
  Shiga 004.0
  Shigella 004.9
    group A 004.0
    group B 004.1
    group C 004.2
    group D 004.3
    specified type NEC 004.8
  Sonne 004.3
  specified type NEC 004.8
bacterium 004.9
balantidial 007.0
Balantidium coli 007.0
Boyd's 004.2
Chilomastix 007.8
Chinese 004.9
choleriform 001.1
coccidial 007.2
Dientamoeba fragilis 007.8
due to specified organism NEC — *see* Enteritis, due to, by organism
Embadomonas 007.8
Endolimax nana — *see* Dysentery, amebic
Entamoba, entamebic — *see* Dysentery, amebic
Flexner's 004.1
Flexner-Boyd 004.2

Dysentery, dysenteric — *continued*
giardial 007.1
Giardia lamblia 007.1
Hiss-Russell 004.1
lamblia 007.1
leishmanial 085.0
malarial (*see also* Malaria) 084.6
metazoal 127.9
Monilia 112.89
protozoal NEC 007.9
Russell's 004.8
salmonella 003.0
schistosomal 120.1
Schmitz (-Stutzer) 004.0
Shiga 004.0
Shigella NEC (*see also* Dysentery, bacillary) 004.9
  boydii 004.2
  dysenteriae 004.0
    Schmitz 004.0
    Shiga 004.0
  flexneri 004.1
  Group A 004.0
  Group B 004.1
  Group C 004.2
  Group D 004.3
  Schmitz 004.0
  Shiga 004.0
  Sonnei 004.3
Sonne 004.3
strongyloidiasis 127.2
trichomonal 007.3
tuberculous (*see also* Tuberculosis) 014.8 ☑
viral (*see also* Enteritis, viral) 008.8
Dysequilibrium 780.4
Dysesthesia 782.0
hysterical 300.11
Dysfibrinogenemia (congenital) (*see also* Defect, coagulation) 286.3
Dysfunction
adrenal (cortical) 255.9
  hyperfunction 255.3
  hypofunction 255.4
associated with sleep stages or arousal from sleep 780.56
  nonorganic origin 307.47
bladder NEC 596.59
bleeding, uterus 626.8
brain, minimal (*see also* Hyperkinesia) 314.9
cerebral 348.30
colon 564.9
  psychogenic 306.4
colostomy or enterostomy 569.62
cystic duct 575.8
diastolic 429.9
  with heart failure — *see* Failure, heart
  due to
    cardiomyopathy — *see* Cardiomyopathy
    hypertension — *see* Hypertension, heart
endocrine NEC 259.9
endometrium 621.8
enteric stoma 569.62
enterostomy 569.62
esophagostomy 530.87 ●
Eustachian tube 381.81
gallbladder 575.8
gastrointestinal 536.9
gland, glandular NEC 259.9
heart 427.9
  postoperative (immediate) 997.1
    long-term effect of cardiac surgery 429.4
hemoglobin 288.8
hepatic 573.9
hepatocellular NEC 573.9
hypophysis 253.9
  hyperfunction 253.1
  hypofunction 253.2
  posterior lobe 253.6
    hypofunction 253.5
kidney (*see also* Disease, renal) 593.9
labyrinthine 386.50
  specified NEC 386.58
liver 573.9
  constitutional 277.4
minimal brain (child) (*see also* Hyperkinesia) 314.9

Dysfunction — *continued*
  ovary, ovarian 256.9
    hyperfunction 256.1
      estrogen 256.0
    hypofunction 256.39
      postablative 256.2
    postablative 256.2
    specified NEC 256.8
  papillary muscle 429.81
    with myocardial infarction 410.8 ☑
  parathyroid 252.8
    hyperfunction 252.00   ▲
    hypofunction 252.1
  pineal gland 259.8
  pituitary (gland) 253.9
    hyperfunction 253.1
    hypofunction 253.2
    posterior 253.6
      hypofunction 253.5
  placental — *see* Placenta, insufficiency
  platelets (blood) 287.1
  polyglandular 258.9
    specified NEC 258.8
  psychosexual 302.70
    with
      dyspareunia (functional) (psychogenic)
        302.76
      frigidity 302.72
      impotence 302.72
      inhibition
        orgasm
          female 302.73
          male 302.74
        sexual
          desire 302.71
          excitement 302.72
      premature ejaculation 302.75
      sexual aversion 302.79
      specified disorder NEC 302.79
      vaginismus 306.51
  pylorus 537.9
  rectum 564.9
    psychogenic 306.4
  segmental (*see also* Dysfunction, somatic)
    739.9
  senile 797
  sexual 302.70   ●
  sinoatrial node 427.81
  somatic 739.9
    abdomen 739.9
    acromioclavicular 739.7
    cervical 739.1
    cervicothoracic 739.1
    costochondral 739.8
    costovertebral 739.8
    extremities
      lower 739.6
      upper 739.7
    head 739.0
    hip 739.5
    lumbar, lumbosacral 739.3
    occipitocervical 739.0
    pelvic 739.5
    pubic 739.5
    rib cage 739.8
    sacral 739.4
    sacrococcygeal 739.4
    sacroiliac 739.4
    specified site NEC 739.9
    sternochondral 739.8
    sternoclavicular 739.7
    temporomandibular 739.0
    thoracic, thoracolumbar 739.2
  stomach 536.9
    psychogenic 306.4
  suprarenal 255.9
    hyperfunction 255.3
    hypofunction 255.4
  symbolic NEC 784.60
    specified type NEC 784.69
  temporomandibular (joint) (joint-pain-
    syndrome) NEC 524.60
    sounds on opening or closing 524.64   ●
    specified NEC 524.69
  testicular 257.9
    hyperfunction 257.0
    hypofunction 257.2

Dysfunction — *continued*
  testicular — *continued*
    specified type NEC 257.8
  thymus 254.9
  thyroid 246.9
    complicating pregnancy, childbirth or
      puerperium 648.1 ☑
    hyperfunction — *see* Hyperthyroidism
    hypofunction — *see* Hypothyroidism
  uterus, complicating delivery 661.9 ☑
    affecting fetus or newborn 763.7
    hypertonic 661.4 ☑
    hypotonic 661.2 ☑
      primary 661.0 ☑
      secondary 661.1 ☑
  velopharyngeal (acquired) 528.9
    congenital 750.29
  ventricular 429.9
    with congestive heart failure (*see also*
      Failure, heart) 428.0
    due to
      cardiomyopathy — *see* Cardiomyopathy
      hypertension — *see* Hypertension, heart
  vesicourethral NEC 596.59
  vestibular 386.50
    specified type NEC 386.58
Dysgammaglobulinemia 279.06
Dysgenesis
  gonadal (due to chromosomal anomaly) 758.6
    pure 752.7
  kidney(s) 753.0
  ovarian 758.6
  renal 753.0
  reticular 279.2
  seminiferous tubules 758.6
  tidal platelet 287.3
Dysgerminoma (M9060/3)
  specified site — *see* Neoplasm, by site,
    malignant
  unspecified site
    female 183.0
    male 186.9
Dysgeusia 781.1
Dysgraphia 781.3
Dyshidrosis 705.81
Dysidrosis 705.81
Dysinsulinism 251.8
Dyskaryotic cervical smear 795.09
Dyskeratosis (*see also* Keratosis) 701.1
  bullosa hereditaria 757.39
  cervix 622.10   ▲
  congenital 757.39
  follicularis 757.39
    vitamin A deficiency 264.8
  gingiva 523.8
  oral soft tissue NEC 528.79   ▲
  tongue 528.79   ▲
  uterus NEC 621.8
Dyskinesia 781.3
  biliary 575.8
  esophagus 530.5
  hysterical 300.11
  intestinal 564.89
  nonorganic origin 307.9
  orofacial 333.82
  psychogenic 307.9
  tardive (oral) 333.82
Dyslalia 784.5
  developmental 315.39
Dyslexia 784.61
  developmental 315.02
  secondary to organic lesion 784.61
Dyslipidemia 272.4   ●
Dysmaturity (*see also* Immaturity) 765.1 ☑
  lung 770.4
  pulmonary 770.4
Dysmenorrhea (essential) (exfoliative) (functional)
    (intrinsic) (membranous) (primary)
    (secondary) 625.3
  psychogenic 306.52
Dysmetabolic syndrome X 277.7
Dysmetria 781.3

Dysmorodystrophia mesodermalis congenita
  759.82
Dysnomia 784.3
Dysorexia 783.0
  hysterical 300.11
Dysostosis
  cleidocranial, cleidocranialis 755.59
  craniofacial 756.0
  Fairbank's (idiopathic familial generalized
    osteophytosis) 756.50
  mandibularis 756.0
  mandibulofacial, incomplete 756.0
  multiplex 277.5
  orodigitofacial 759.89
Dyspareunia (female) 625.0
  male 608.89
  psychogenic 302.76
Dyspepsia (allergic) (congenital) (fermentative)
    (flatulent) (functional) (gastric)
    (gastrointestinal) (neurogenic) (occupational)
    (reflex) 536.8
  acid 536.8
  atonic 536.3
    psychogenic 306.4
  diarrhea 787.91
    psychogenic 306.4
  intestinal 564.89
    psychogenic 306.4
  nervous 306.4
  neurotic 306.4
  psychogenic 306.4
Dysphagia 787.2
  functional 300.11
  hysterical 300.11
  nervous 300.11
  psychogenic 306.4
  sideropenic 280.8
  spastica 530.5
Dysphagocytosis, congenital 288.1
Dysphasia 784.5
Dysphonia 784.49
  clericorum 784.49
  functional 300.11
  hysterical 300.11
  psychogenic 306.1
  spastica 478.79
Dyspigmentation — *see also* Pigmentation
  eyelid (acquired) 374.52
Dyspituitarism 253.9
  hyperfunction 253.1
  hypofunction 253.2
  posterior lobe 253.6
Dysplasia — *see also* Anomaly
  artery
    fibromuscular NEC 447.8
      carotid 447.8
      renal 447.3
  bladder 596.8
  bone (fibrous) NEC 733.29
    diaphyseal, progressive 756.59
    jaw 526.89
    monostotic 733.29
    polyostotic 756.54
    solitary 733.29
  brain 742.9
  bronchopulmonary, fetus or newborn 770.7
  cervix (uteri) 622.10   ▲
    cervical intraepithelial neoplasia I [CIN I]
      622.11   ▲
    cervical intraepithelial neoplasia II [CIN II]
      622.12   ▲
    cervical intraepithelial neoplasia III [CIN III]
      233.1
    CIN I 622.11   ▲
    CIN II 622.12   ▲
    CIN III 233.1
    mild 622.11   ●
    moderate 622.12   ●
    severe 233.1   ●
  chondroectodermal 756.55
  chondromatose 756.4
  craniocarpotarsal 759.89
  craniometaphyseal 756.89
  dentinal 520.5

☑ Additional Digit Required   ►◄ Revised Text   ● New Line   ▲ Revised Code

Dysplasia — *see also* Anomaly — *continued*
　diaphyseal, progressive 756.59
　ectodermal (anhidrotic) (Bason) (Clouston's)
　　　(congenital) (Feinmesser) (hereditary)
　　　(hidrotic) (Marshall) (Robinson's) 757.31
　epiphysealis 756.9
　　multiplex 756.56
　　punctata 756.59
　epiphysis 756.9
　　multiple 756.56
　epithelial
　　epiglottis 478.79
　　uterine cervix 622.10　　　　　　　　　　　　　　▲
　erythroid NEC 289.89
　eye (*see also* Microphthalmos) 743.10
　familial metaphyseal 756.89
　fibromuscular, artery NEC 447.8
　　carotid 447.8
　　renal 447.3
　fibrous
　　bone NEC 733.29
　　diaphyseal, progressive 756.59
　　jaw 526.89
　　monostotic 733.29
　　polyostotic 756.54
　　solitary 733.29
　hip (congenital) 755.63
　　with dislocation (*see also* Dislocation, hip,
　　　congenital) 754.30
　hypohidrotic ectodermal 757.31
　joint 755.8
　kidney 753.15
　leg 755.69
　linguofacialis 759.89
　lung 748.5
　macular 743.55
　mammary (benign) (gland) 610.9
　　cystic 610.1
　　specified type NEC 610.8
　metaphyseal 756.9
　　familial 756.89
　monostotic fibrous 733.29
　muscle 756.89
　myeloid NEC 289.89
　nervous system (general) 742.9
　neuroectodermal 759.6
　oculoauriculovertebral 756.0
　oculodentodigital 759.89
　olfactogenital 253.4
　osteo-onycho-arthro (hereditary) 756.89
　periosteum 733.99
　polyostotic fibrous 756.54
　progressive diaphyseal 756.59
　prostate 602.3
　　intraepithelial neoplasia I [PIN I] 602.3
　　intraepithelial neoplasia II [PIN II] 602.3
　　intraepithelial neoplasia III [PIN III] 233.4
　renal 753.15
　renofacialis 753.0
　retinal NEC 743.56
　retrolental 362.21
　spinal cord 742.9
　thymic, with immunodeficiency 279.2
　vagina 623.0
　vocal cord 478.5
　vulva 624.8
　　intraepithelial neoplasia I [VIN I] 624.8
　　intraepithelial neoplasia II [VIN II] 624.8
　　intraepithelial neoplasia III [VIN III] 233.3
　　VIN I 624.8
　　VIN II 624.8
　　VIN III 233.3
Dyspnea (nocturnal) (paroxysmal) 786.09
　asthmatic (bronchial) (*see also* Asthma)
　　　493.9 ☑
　　with bronchitis (*see also* Asthma) 493.9 ☑
　　　chronic 493.2 ☑
　cardiac (*see also* Failure, ventricular, left)
　　　428.1
　cardiac (*see also* Failure, ventricular, left) 428.1
　functional 300.11
　hyperventilation 786.01
　hysterical 300.11
　Monday morning 504
　newborn 770.89
　psychogenic 306.1

Dyspnea — *continued*
　uremic — *see* Uremia
Dyspraxia 781.3
　syndrome 315.4
Dysproteinemia 273.8
　transient with copper deficiency 281.4
Dysprothrombinemia (constitutional) (*see also*
　　Defect, coagulation) 286.3
Dysreflexia, autonomic 337.3
Dysrhythmia
　cardiac 427.9
　　postoperative (immediate) 997.1
　　　long-term effect of cardiac surgery 429.4
　　specified type NEC 427.89
　cerebral or cortical 348.30
Dyssecretosis, mucoserous 710.2
Dyssocial reaction, without manifest
　　psychiatric disorder
　adolescent V71.02
　adult V71.01
　child V71.02
Dyssomnia NEC 780.56
　nonorganic origin 307.47
Dyssplenism 289.4
Dyssynergia
　biliary (*see also* Disease, biliary) 576.8
　cerebellaris myoclonica 334.2
　detrusor sphincter (bladder) 596.55
　ventricular 429.89
Dystasia, hereditary areflexic 334.3
Dysthymia 300.4
Dysthymic disorder 300.4
Dysthyroidism 246.9
Dystocia 660.9 ☑
　affecting fetus or newborn 763.1
　cervical 661.0 ☑
　　affecting fetus or newborn 763.7
　contraction ring 661.4 ☑
　　affecting fetus or newborn 763.7
　fetal 660.9 ☑
　　abnormal size 653.5 ☑
　　affecting fetus or newborn 763.1
　　deformity 653.7 ☑
　maternal 660.9 ☑
　　affecting fetus or newborn 763.1
　positional 660.0 ☑
　　affecting fetus or newborn 763.1
　shoulder (girdle) 660.4 ☑
　　affecting fetus or newborn 763.1
　uterine NEC 661.4 ☑
　　affecting fetus or newborn 763.7
Dystonia
　deformans progressiva 333.6
　due to drugs 333.7
　lenticularis 333.6
　musculorum deformans 333.6
　torsion (idiopathic) 333.6
　　fragments (of) 333.89
　　symptomatic 333.7
Dystonic
　movements 781.0
Dystopia kidney 753.3
Dystrophy, dystrophia 783.9
　adiposogenital 253.8
　asphyxiating thoracic 756.4
　Becker's type 359.1
　brevicollis 756.16
　Bruch's membrane 362.77
　cervical (sympathetic) NEC 337.0
　chondro-osseus with punctate epiphyseal
　　　dysplasia 756.59
　choroid (hereditary) 363.50
　　central (areolar) (partial) 363.53
　　　total (gyrate) 363.54
　　circinate 363.53
　　circumpapillary (partial) 363.51
　　　total 363.52
　　diffuse
　　　partial 363.56
　　　total 363.57
　　generalized
　　　partial 363.56
　　　total 363.57

Dystrophy, dystrophia — *continued*
　choroid (hereditary) — *continued*
　　gyrate
　　　central 363.54
　　　generalized 363.57
　　helicoid 363.52
　　peripapillary — *see* Dystrophy, choroid,
　　　circumpapillary
　　serpiginous 363.54
　cornea (hereditary) 371.50
　　anterior NEC 371.52
　　Cogan's 371.52
　　combined 371.57
　　crystalline 371.56
　　endothelial (Fuchs') 371.57
　　epithelial 371.50
　　　juvenile 371.51
　　　microscopic cystic 371.52
　　granular 371.53
　　lattice 371.54
　　macular 371.55
　　marginal (Terrien's) 371.48
　　Meesman's 371.51
　　microscopic cystic (epithelial) 371.52
　　nodular, Salzmann's 371.46
　　polymorphous 371.58
　　posterior NEC 371.58
　　ring-like 371.52
　　Salzmann's nodular 371.46
　　stromal NEC 371.56
　dermatochondrocorneal 371.50
　Duchenne's 359.1
　due to malnutrition 263.9
　Erb's 359.1
　familial
　　hyperplastic periosteal 756.59
　　osseous 277.5
　foveal 362.77
　Fuchs', cornea 371.57
　Gowers' muscular 359.1
　hair 704.2
　hereditary, progressive muscular 359.1
　hypogenital, with diabetic tendency 759.81
　Landouzy-Déjérine 359.1
　Leyden-Möbius 359.1
　mesodermalis congenita 759.82
　muscular 359.1
　　congenital (hereditary) 359.0
　　　myotonic 359.2
　　distal 359.1
　　Duchenne's 359.1
　　Erb's 359.1
　　fascioscapulohumeral 359.1
　　Gowers' 359.1
　　hereditary (progressive) 359.1
　　Landouzy-Déjérine 359.1
　　limb-girdle 359.1
　　myotonic 359.2
　　progressive (hereditary) 359.1
　　　Charcôt-Marie-Tooth 356.1
　　pseudohypertrophic (infantile) 359.1
　myocardium, myocardial (*see also*
　　　Degeneration, myocardial) 429.1
　myotonic 359.2
　myotonica 359.2
　nail 703.8
　　congenital 757.5
　neurovascular (traumatic) (*see also*
　　　Neuropathy, peripheral, autonomic) 337.9
　nutritional 263.9
　ocular 359.1
　oculocerebrorenal 270.8
　oculopharyngeal 359.1
　ovarian 620.8
　papillary (and pigmentary) 701.1
　pelvicrural atrophic 359.1
　pigmentary (*see also* Acanthosis) 701.2
　pituitary (gland) 253.8
　polyglandular 258.8
　posttraumatic sympathetic — *see* Dystrophy,
　　　sympathetic
　progressive ophthalmoplegic 359.1
　retina, retinal (hereditary) 362.70
　　albipunctate 362.74
　　Bruch's membrane 362.77
　　cone, progressive 362.75
　　hyaline 362.77

☑ Additional Digit Required　　　　　▶◀ Revised Text　　　　　● New Line　　　　　▲ Revised Code

Dystrophy, dystrophia — *continued*
 retina, retinal — *continued*
  in
   Bassen-Kornzweig syndrome
      272.5 *[362.72]*
    cerebroretinal lipidosis 330.1 *[362.71]*
    Refsum's disease 356.3 *[362.72]*
    systemic lipidosis 272.7 *[362.71]*
   juvenile (Stargardt's) 362.75
   pigmentary 362.74
   pigment epithelium 362.76
   progressive cone (-rod) 362.75
   pseudoinflammatory foveal 362.77
   rod, progressive 362.75
   sensory 362.75
   vitelliform 362.76
  Salzmann's nodular 371.46
  scapuloperoneal 359.1
  skin NEC 709.9
  sympathetic (posttraumatic) (reflex) 337.20
   lower limb 337.22
   specified NEC 337.29
   upper limb 337.21
  tapetoretinal NEC 362.74
  thoracic asphyxiating 756.4
  unguium 703.8
   congenital 757.5
  vitreoretinal (primary) 362.73
   secondary 362.66
  vulva 624.0
Dysuria 788.1
 psychogenic 306.53

E

Eagle-Barrett syndrome 756.71
Eales' disease (syndrome) 362.18
Ear — *see also* condition
 ache 388.70
  otogenic 388.71
  referred 388.72
 lop 744.29
 piercing V50.3
 swimmers' acute 380.12
 tank 380.12
 tropical 111.8 *[380.15]*
 wax 380.4
Earache 388.70
 otogenic 388.71
 referred 388.72
Early satiety 780.94
Eaton-Lambert syndrome (*see also* Neoplasm, by
   site, malignant) 199.1 *[358.1]*
Eberth's disease (typhoid fever) 002.0
Ebstein's
 anomaly or syndrome (downward displacement,
   tricuspid valve into right ventricle) 746.2
 disease (diabetes) 250.4 ☑ *[581.81]*
Eccentro-osteochondrodysplasia 277.5
Ecchondroma (M9210/0) — *see* Neoplasm, bone,
   benign
Ecchondrosis (M9210/1) 238.0
Ecchordosis physaliphora 756.0
Ecchymosis (multiple) 459.89
 conjunctiva 372.72
 eye (traumatic) 921.0
 eyelids (traumatic) 921.1
 newborn 772.6
 spontaneous 782.7
 traumatic — *see* Contusion
Echinococciasis — *see* Echinococcus
Echinococcosis — *see* Echinococcus
Echinococcus (infection) 122.9
 granulosus 122.4
  liver 122.0
  lung 122.1
  orbit 122.3 *[376.13]*
  specified site NEC 122.3
  thyroid 122.2
 liver NEC 122.8
  granulosus 122.0
  multilocularis 122.5

Echinococcus — *continued*
 lung NEC 122.9
  granulosus 122.1
  multilocularis 122.6
 multilocularis 122.7
  liver 122.5
  specified site NEC 122.6
 orbit 122.9 *[376.13]*
  granulosus 122.3 *[376.13]*
  multilocularis 122.6 *[376.13]*
 specified site NEC 122.9
  granulosus 122.3
  multilocularis 122.6 *[376.13]*
 thyroid NEC 122.9
  granulosus 122.2
  multilocularis 122.6
Echinorhynchiasis 127.7
Echinostomiasis 121.8
Echolalia 784.69
ECHO virus infection NEC 079.1
Eclampsia, eclamptic (coma) (convulsions)
   (delirium) 780.39
 female, child-bearing age NEC — *see*
    Eclampsia, pregnancy
 gravidarum — *see* Eclampsia, pregnancy
 male 780.39
 not associated with pregnancy or childbirth
    780.39
 pregnancy, childbirth, or puerperium 642.6 ☑
  with pre-existing hypertension 642.7 ☑
   affecting fetus or newborn 760.0
 uremic 586
Eclipse blindness (total) 363.31
Economic circumstance affecting care V60.9
 specified type NEC V60.8
Economo's disease (encephalitis lethargica) 049.8
Ectasia, ectasis
 aorta (*see also* Aneurysm, aorta) 441.9
  ruptured 441.5
 breast 610.4
 capillary 448.9
 cornea (marginal) (postinfectional) 371.71
 duct (mammary) 610.4
 kidney 593.89
 mammary duct (gland) 610.4
 papillary 448.9
 renal 593.89
 salivary gland (duct) 527.8
 scar, cornea 371.71
 sclera 379.11
Ecthyma 686.8
 contagiosum 051.2
 gangrenosum 686.09
 infectiosum 051.2
Ectocardia 746.87
Ectodermal dysplasia, congenital 757.31
Ectodermosis erosiva pluriorificialis 695.1
Ectopic, ectopia (congenital) 759.89
 abdominal viscera 751.8
  due to defect in anterior abdominal wall
     756.79
 ACTH syndrome 255.0
 adrenal gland 759.1
 anus 751.5
 auricular beats 427.61
 beats 427.60
 bladder 753.5
 bone and cartilage in lung 748.69
 brain 742.4
 breast tissue 757.6
 cardiac 746.87
 cerebral 742.4
 cordis 746.87
 endometrium 617.9
 gallbladder 751.69
 gastric mucosa 750.7
 gestation — *see* Pregnancy, ectopic
 heart 746.87
 hormone secretion NEC 259.3
 hyperparathyroidism 259.3
 kidney (crossed) (intrathoracic) (pelvis) 753.3
  in pregnancy or childbirth 654.4 ☑
   causing obstructed labor 660.2 ☑
 lens 743.37

Ectopic, ectopia — *continued*
 lentis 743.37
 mole — *see* Pregnancy, ectopic
 organ or site NEC — *see* Malposition,
    congenital
 ovary 752.0
 pancreas, pancreatic tissue 751.7
 pregnancy — *see* Pregnancy, ectopic
 pupil 364.75
 renal 753.3
 sebaceous glands of mouth 750.26
 secretion
  ACTH 255.0
  adrenal hormone 259.3
  adrenalin 259.3
  adrenocorticotropin 255.0
  antidiuretic hormone (ADH) 259.3
  epinephrine 259.3
  hormone NEC 259.3
  norepinephrine 259.3
  pituitary (posterior) 259.3
 spleen 759.0
 testis 752.51
 thyroid 759.2
 ureter 753.4
 ventricular beats 427.69
 vesicae 753.5
Ectrodactyly 755.4
 finger (*see also* Absence, finger, congenital)
    755.29
 toe (*see also* Absence, toe, congenital) 755.39
Ectromelia 755.4
 lower limb 755.30
 upper limb 755.20
Ectropion 374.10
 anus 569.49
 cervix 622.0
  with mention of cervicitis 616.0
 cicatricial 374.14
 congenital 743.62
 eyelid 374.10
  cicatricial 374.14
  congenital 743.62
  mechanical 374.12
  paralytic 374.12
  senile 374.11
  spastic 374.13
 iris (pigment epithelium) 364.54
 lip (congenital) 750.26
  acquired 528.5
 mechanical 374.12
 paralytic 374.12
 rectum 569.49
 senile 374.11
 spastic 374.13
 urethra 599.84
 uvea 364.54
Eczema (acute) (allergic) (chronic) (erythematous)
    (fissum) (occupational) (rubrum) (squamous)
    692.9
 asteatotic 706.8
 atopic 691.8
 contact NEC 692.9
 dermatitis NEC 692.9
 due to specified cause — *see* Dermatitis, due to
 dyshidrotic 705.81
 external ear 380.22
 flexural 691.8
 gouty 274.89
 herpeticum 054.0
 hypertrophicum 701.8
 hypostatic — *see* Varicose, vein
 impetiginous 684
 infantile (acute) (chronic) (due to any
    substance) (intertriginous) (seborrheic)
    690.12
 intertriginous NEC 692.9
  infantile 690.12
 intrinsic 691.8
 lichenified NEC 692.9
 marginatum 110.3
 nummular 692.9
 pustular 686.8
 seborrheic 690.18
  infantile 690.12
 solare 692.72

Eczema — *continued*
  stasis (lower extremity) 454.1
    ulcerated 454.2
  vaccination, vaccinatum 999.0
  varicose (lower extremity) — *see* Varicose, vein
  verrucosum callosum 698.3
Eczematoid, exudative 691.8
Eddowes' syndrome (brittle bone and blue sclera) 756.51
Edema, edematous 782.3
  with nephritis (*see also* Nephrosis) 581.9
  allergic 995.1
  angioneurotic (allergic) (any site) (with urticaria) 995.1
    hereditary 277.6
  angiospastic 443.9
  Berlin's (traumatic) 921.3
  brain 348.5
    due to birth injury 767.8
    fetus or newborn 767.8
  cardiac (*see also* Failure, heart) 428.0
  cardiovascular (*see also* Failure, heart) 428.0
  cerebral — *see* Edema, brain
  cerebrospinal vessel — *see* Edema, brain
  cervix (acute) (uteri) 622.8
    puerperal, postpartum 674.8 ☑
  chronic hereditary 757.0
  circumscribed, acute 995.1
    hereditary 277.6
  complicating pregnancy (gestational) 646.1 ☑
    with hypertension — *see* Toxemia, of pregnancy
  conjunctiva 372.73
  connective tissue 782.3
  cornea 371.20
    due to contact lenses 371.24
    idiopathic 371.21
    secondary 371.22
  due to
    lymphatic obstruction — *see* Edema, lymphatic
    salt retention 276.0
  epiglottis — *see* Edema, glottis
  essential, acute 995.1
    hereditary 277.6
  extremities, lower — *see* Edema, legs
  eyelid NEC 374.82
  familial, hereditary (legs) 757.0
  famine 262
  fetus or newborn 778.5
  genital organs
    female 629.8
    male 608.86
  gestational 646.1 ☑
    with hypertension — *see* Toxemia, of pregnancy
  glottis, glottic, glottides (obstructive) (passive) 478.6
    allergic 995.1
      hereditary 277.6
    due to external agent — *see* Condition, respiratory, acute, due to specified agent
  heart (*see also* Failure, heart) 428.0
    newborn 779.89
  heat 992.7
  hereditary (legs) 757.0
  inanition 262
  infectious 782.3
  intracranial 348.5
    due to injury at birth 767.8
  iris 364.8
  joint (*see also* Effusion, joint) 719.0 ☑
  larynx (*see also* Edema, glottis) 478.6
  legs 782.3
    due to venous obstruction 459.2
    hereditary 757.0
  localized 782.3
    due to venous obstruction 459.2
      lower extremity 459.2
  lower extremities — *see* Edema, legs
  lung 514
    acute 518.4
      with heart disease or failure (*see also* Failure, ventricular, left) 428.1
        congestive 428.0

Edema, edematous — *continued*
  lung — *continued*
    acute — *continued*
      chemical (due to fumes or vapors) 506.1
      due to
        external agent(s) NEC 508.9
          specified NEC 508.8
        fumes and vapors (chemical) (inhalation) 506.1
        radiation 508.0
    chemical (acute) 506.1
      chronic 506.4
    chronic 514
      chemical (due to fumes or vapors) 506.4
      due to
        external agent(s) NEC 508.9
          specified NEC 508.8
        fumes or vapors (chemical) (inhalation) 506.4
        radiation 508.1
    due to
      external agent 508.9
        specified NEC 508.8
      high altitude 993.2
      near drowning 994.1
    postoperative 518.4
    terminal 514
  lymphatic 457.1
    due to mastectomy operation 457.0
  macula 362.83
    cystoid 362.53
    diabetic 250.5 ☑ *[362.01]*
  malignant (*see also* Gangrene, gas) 040.0
  Milroy's 757.0
  nasopharynx 478.25
  neonatorum 778.5
  nutritional (newborn) 262
    with dyspigmentation, skin and hair 260
  optic disc or nerve — *see* Papilledema
  orbit 376.33
    circulatory 459.89
  palate (soft) (hard) 528.9
  pancrease 577.8
  penis 607.83
  periodic 995.1
    hereditary 277.6
  pharynx 478.25
  pitting 782.3
  pulmonary — *see* Edema, lung
  Quincke's 995.1
    hereditary 277.6
  renal (*see also* Nephrosis) 581.9
  retina (localized) (macular) (perepheral) 362.83
    cystoid 362.53
    diabetic 250.5 ☑ *[362.01]*
  salt 276.0
  scrotum 608.86
  seminal vesicle 608.86
  spermatic cord 608.86
  spinal cord 336.1
  starvation 262
  stasis (*see also* Hypertension, venous) 459.30
  subconjunctival 372.73
  subglottic (*see also* Edema, glottis) 478.6
  supraglottic (*see also* Edema, glottis) 478.6
  testis 608.86
  toxic NEC 782.3
  traumatic NEC 782.3
  tunica vaginalis 608.86
  vas deferens 608.86
  vocal cord — *see* Edema, glottis
  vulva (acute) 624.8
Edentia (complete) (partial) (*see also* Absence, tooth) 520.0
  acquired 525.10
    due to
      caries 525.13
      extraction 525.10
      periodontal disease 525.12
      specified NEC 525.19
      trauma 525.11
  causing malocclusion 524.30   ▲
  congenital (deficiency of tooth buds) 520.0
Edentulism 525.10
Edsall's disease 992.2
Educational handicap V62.3

Edwards' syndrome 758.2
Effect, adverse NEC
  abnormal gravitation (G) forces or states 994.9
  air pressure — *see* Effect, adverse, atmospheric pressure
  altitude (high) — *see* Effect, adverse, high altitude
  anesthetic
    in labor and delivery NEC 668.9 ☑
      affecting fetus or newborn 763.5
  antitoxin — *see* Complications, vaccination
  atmospheric pressure 993.9
    due to explosion 993.4
    high 993.3
    low — *see* Effect, adverse, high altitude
    specified effect NEC 993.8
  biological, correct substance properly administered (*see also* Effect, adverse, drug) 995.2
  blood (derivatives) (serum) (transfusion) — *see* Complications, transfusion
  chemical substance NEC 989.9
    specified — *see* Table of Drugs and Chemicals
  cobalt, radioactive (*see also* Effect, adverse, radioactive substance) 990
  cold (temperature) (weather) 991.9
    chilblains 991.5
    frostbite — *see* Frostbite
    specified effect NEC 991.8
  drugs and medicinals NEC 995.2
    correct substance properly administered 995.2
    overdose or wrong substance given or taken 977.9
      specified drug — *see* Table of Drugs and Chemicals
  electric current (shock) 994.8
    burn — *see* Burn, by site
  electricity (electrocution) (shock) 994.8
    burn — *see* Burn, by site
  exertion (excessive) 994.5
  exposure 994.9
    exhaustion 994.4
  external cause NEC 994.9
  fallout (radioactive) NEC 990
  fluoroscopy NEC 990
  foodstuffs
    allergic reaction (*see also* Allergy, food) 693.1
      anaphylactic shock due to food NEC 995.60
    noxious 988.9
      specified type NEC (*see also* Poisoning, by name of noxious foodstuff) 988.8
  gases, fumes, or vapors — *see* Table of Drugs and Chemicals
  glue (airplane) sniffing 304.6 ☑
  heat — *see* Heat
  high altitude NEC 993.2
    anoxia 993.2
    on
      ears 993.0
      sinuses 993.1
    polycythemia 289.0
  hot weather — *see* Heat
  hunger 994.2
  immersion, foot 991.4
  immunization — *see* Complications, vaccination
  immunological agents — *see* Complications, vaccination
  implantation (removable) of isotope or radium NEC 990
  infrared (radiation) (rays) NEC 990
    burn — *see* Burn, by site
    dermatitis or eczema 692.82
  infusion — *see* Complications, infusion
  ingestion or injection of isotope (therapeutic) NEC 990
  irradiation NEC (*see also* Effect, adverse, radiation) 990
  isotope (radioactive) NEC 990
  lack of care (child) (infant) (newborn) 995.52
    adult 995.84
  lightning 994.0

Effect, adverse — *continued*
  lightning — *continued*
    burn — *see* Burn, by site
  Lirugin — *see* Complications, vaccination
  medicinal substance, correct, properly
      administered (*see also* Effect, adverse,
      drugs) 995.2
  mesothorium NEC 990
  motion 994.6
  noise, inner ear 388.10
  overheated places — *see* Heat
  polonium NEC 990
  psychosocial, of work environment V62.1
  radiation (diagnostic) (fallout) (infrared) (natural
      source) (therapeutic) (tracer) (ultraviolet)
      (x-ray) NEC 990
    with pulmonary manifestations
      acute 508.0
      chronic 508.1
    dermatitis or eczema 692.82
      due to sun NEC (*see also* Dermatitis, due
        to, sun) 692.70
    fibrosis of lungs 508.1
    maternal with suspected damage to fetus
      affecting management of pregnancy
      655.6 ☑
    pneumonitis 508.0
  radioactive substance NEC 990
    dermatitis or eczema 692.82
  radioactivity NEC 990
  radiotherapy NEC 990
    dermatitis or eczema 692.82
  radium NEC 990
  reduced temperature 991.9
    frostbite — *see* Frostbite
    immersion, foot (hand) 991.4
    specified effect NEC 991.8
  roentgenography NEC 990
  roentgenoscopy NEC 990
  roentgen rays NEC 990
  serum (prophylactic) (therapeutic) NEC 999.5
  specified NEC 995.89
    external cause NEC 994.9
  strangulation 994.7
  submersion 994.1
  teletherapy NEC 990
  thirst 994.3
  transfusion — *see* Complications, transfusion
  ultraviolet (radiation) (rays) NEC 990
    burn — *see also* Burn, by site
      from sun (*see also* Sunburn) 692.71
    dermatitis or eczema 692.82
      due to sun NEC (*see also* Dermatitis, due
        to, sun) 692.70
  uranium NEC 990
  vaccine (any) — *see* Complications, vaccination
  weightlessness 994.9
  whole blood — *see also* Complications,
    transfusion
    overdose or wrong substance given (*see also*
      Table of Drugs and Chemicals) 964.7
  working environment V62.1
  x-rays NEC 990
    dermatitis or eczema 692.82
Effects, late — *see* Late, effect (of)
Effect, remote
  of cancer — *see* condition
Effluvium, telogen 704.02
Effort
  intolerance 306.2
  syndrome (aviators) (psychogenic) 306.2
Effusion
  amniotic fluid (*see also* Rupture, membranes,
    premature) 658.1 ☑
  brain (serous) 348.5
  bronchial (*see also* Bronchitis) 490
  cerebral 348.5
  cerebrospinal (*see also* Meningitis) 322.9
    vessel 348.5
  chest — *see* Effusion, pleura
  intracranial 348.5
  joint 719.00
    ankle 719.07
    elbow 719.02
    foot 719.07
    hand 719.04

Effusion — *continued*
  joint — *continued*
    hip 719.05
    knee 719.06
    multiple sites 719.09
    pelvic region 719.05
    shoulder (region) 719.01
    specified site NEC 719.08
    wrist 719.03
  meninges (*see also* Meningitis) 322.9
  pericardium, pericardial (*see also* Pericarditis)
    423.9
    acute 420.90
  peritoneal (chronic) 568.82
  pleura, pleurisy, pleuritic, pleuropericardial
    511.9
    bacterial, nontuberculous 511.1
    fetus or newborn 511.9
    malignant 197.2
    nontuberculous 511.9
      bacterial 511.1
    pneumococcal 511.1
    staphylococcal 511.1
    streptococcal 511.1
    traumatic 862.29
      with open wound 862.39
    tuberculous (*see also* Tuberculosis, pleura)
      012.0 ☑
      primary progressive 010.1 ☑
  pulmonary — *see* Effusion, pleura
  spinal (*see also* Meningitis) 322.9
  thorax, thoracic — *see* Effusion, pleura
Eggshell nails 703.8
  congenital 757.5
Ego-dystonic
  homosexuality 302.0
  lesbianism 302.0
  sexual orientation 302.0   ●
Egyptian splenomegaly 120.1
Ehlers-Danlos syndrome 756.83
Ehrlichiosis 082.40
  chaffeensis 082.41
  specified type NEC 082.49
Eichstedt's disease (pityriasis versicolor) 111.0
Eisenmenger's complex or syndrome
    (ventricular septal defect) 745.4
Ejaculation, semen
  painful 608.89
    psychogenic 306.59
  premature 302.75
  retrograde 608.87
Ekbom syndrome (restless legs) 333.99
Ekman's syndrome (brittle bones and blue sclera)
    756.51
Elastic skin 756.83
  acquired 701.8
Elastofibroma (M8820/0) — *see* Neoplasm,
    connective tissue, benign
Elastoidosis
  cutanea nodularis 701.8
  cutis cystica et comedonica 701.8
Elastoma 757.39
  juvenile 757.39
  Miescher's (elastosis perforans serpiginosa)
    701.1
Elastomyofibrosis 425.3
Elastosis 701.8
  atrophicans 701.8
  perforans serpiginosa 701.1
  reactive perforating 701.1
  senilis 701.8
  solar (actinic) 692.74
Elbow — *see* condition
Electric
  current, electricity, effects (concussion) (fatal)
    (nonfatal) (shock) 994.8
    burn — *see* Burn, by site
  feet (foot) syndrome 266.2
Electrocution 994.8
Electrolyte imbalance 276.9
  with
    abortion — *see* Abortion, by type with
      metabolic disorder

Electrolyte imbalance — *continued*
  with — *continued*
    ectopic pregnancy (*see also* categories
      633.0-633.9) 639.4
    hyperemesis gravidarum (before 22
      completed weeks gestation) 643.1 ☑
    molar pregnancy (*see also* categories 630-
      632) 639.4
  following
    abortion 639.4
    ectopic or molar pregnancy 639.4
Elephant man syndrome 237.71
Elephantiasis (nonfilarial) 457.1
  arabicum (*see also* Infestation, filarial) 125.9
  congenita hereditaria 757.0
  congenital (any site) 757.0
  due to
    Brugia (malayi) 125.1
    mastectomy operation 457.0
    Wuchereria (bancrofti) 125.0
      malayi 125.1
  eyelid 374.83
  filarial (*see also* Infestation, filarial) 125.9
  filariensis (*see also* Infestation, filarial) 125.9
  gingival 523.8
  glandular 457.1
  graecorum 030.9
  lymphangiectatic 457.1
  lymphatic vessel 457.1
    due to mastectomy operation 457.0
  neuromatosa 237.71
  postmastectomy 457.0
  scrotum 457.1
  streptococcal 457.1
  surgical 997.99
    postmastectomy 457.0
  telangiectodes 457.1
  vulva (nonfilarial) 624.8
Elevated — *see* Elevation
Elevation
  17-ketosteroids 791.9
  acid phosphatase 790.5
  alkaline phosphatase 790.5
  amylase 790.5
  antibody titers 795.79
  basal metabolic rate (BMR) 794.7
  blood pressure (*see also* Hypertension) 401.9
    reading (incidental) (isolated) (nonspecific),
      no diagnosis or hypertension 796.2
  body temperature (of unknown origin) (*see also*
    Pyrexia) 780.6
  conjugate, eye 378.81
  C-reactive protein (CRP) 790.95   ●
  CRP (C-reactive protein) 790.95   ●
  diaphragm, congenital 756.6
  glucose
    fasting 790.21
    tolerance test 790.22
  immunoglobulin level 795.79
  indolacetic acid 791.9
  lactic acid dehydrogenase (LDH) level 790.4
  lipase 790.5
  prostate specific antigen (PSA) 790.93
  renin 790.99
    in hypertension (*see also* Hypertension,
      renovascular) 405.91
  Rh titer 999.7
  scapula, congenital 755.52
  sedimentation rate 790.1
  SGOT 790.4
  SGPT 790.4
  transaminase 790.4
  vanillylmandelic acid 791.9
  venous pressure 459.89
  VMA 791.9
Elliptocytosis (congenital) (hereditary) 282.1
  Hb-C (disease) 282.7
  hemoglobin disease 282.7
  sickle-cell (disease) 282.60
    trait 282.5
Ellis-van Creveld disease or syndrome
    (chondroectodermal dysplasia) 756.55
Ellison-Zollinger syndrome (gastric
    hypersecretion with pancreatic islet cell
    tumor) 251.5

☑ Additional Digit Required   ▶◀ Revised Text   ● New Line   ▲ Revised Code

Elongation, elongated (congenital) — *see also*
     Distortion
  bone 756.9
  cervix (uteri) 752.49
     acquired 622.6
     hypertrophic 622.6
  colon 751.5
  common bile duct 751.69
  cystic duct 751.69
  frenulum, penis 752.69
  labia minora, acquired 624.8
  ligamentum patellae 756.89
  petiolus (epiglottidis) 748.3
  styloid bone (process) 733.99
  tooth, teeth 520.2
  uvula 750.26
     acquired 528.9

Elschnig bodies or pearls 366.51

El Tor cholera 001.1

Emaciation (due to malnutrition) 261

Emancipation disorder 309.22

Embadomoniasis 007.8

Embarrassment heart, cardiac — *see* Disease,
     heart

Embedded tooth, teeth 520.6
  root only 525.3

Embolic — *see* conditon

Embolism 444.9
  with
     abortion — *see* Abortion, by type, with
        embolism
     ectopic pregnancy (*see also* categories
        633.0-633.9) 639.6
     molar pregnancy (*see also* categories 630-
        632) 639.6
  air (any site) 958.0
     with
        abortion — *see* Abortion, by type, with
           embolism
        ectopic pregnancy (*see also* categories
           633.0-633.9) 639.6
        molar pregnancy (*see also* categories
           630-632) 639.6
     due to implanted device — *see*
        Complications, due to (presence of)
        any device, implant, or graft classified
        to 996.0-996.5 NEC
     following
        abortion 639.6
        ectopic or molar pregnancy 639.6
        infusion, perfusion, or transfusion 999.1
     in pregnancy, childbirth, or puerperium
        673.0 ☑
     traumatic 958.0
  amniotic fluid (pulmonary) 673.1 ☑
     with
        abortion — *see* Abortion, by type, with
           embolism
        ectopic pregnancy (*see also* categories
           633.0-633.9) 639.6
        molar pregnancy (*see also* categories 630-
           632) 639.6
     following
        abortion 639.6
        ectopic or molar pregnancy 639.6
  aorta, aortic 444.1
     abdominal 444.0
     bifurcation 444.0
     saddle 444.0
     thoracic 444.1
  artery 444.9
     auditory, internal 433.8 ☑
     basilar (*see also* Occlusion, artery, basilar)
        433.0 ☑
     bladder 444.89
     carotid (common) (internal) (*see also*
        Occlusion, artery, carotid) 433.1 ☑
     cerebellar (anterior inferior) (posterior
        inferior) (superior) 433.8 ☑
     cerebral (*see also* Embolism, brain) 434.1 ☑
     choroidal (anterior) 433.8 ☑
     communicating posterior 433.8 ☑
     coronary (*see also* Infarct, myocardium)
        410.9 ☑
        without myocardial infarction 411.81

Embolism — *continued*
  artery — *continued*
     extremity 444.22
        lower 444.22
        upper 444.21
     hypophyseal 433.8 ☑
     mesenteric (with gangrene) 557.0
     ophthalmic (*see also* Occlusion, retina)
        362.30
     peripheral 444.22
     pontine 433.8 ☑
     precerebral NEC — *see* Occlusion, artery,
        precerebral
     pulmonary — *see* Embolism, pulmonary
     renal 593.81
     retinal (*see also* Occlusion, retina) 362.30
     specified site NEC 444.89
     vertebral (*see also* Occlusion, artery,
        vertebral) 433.2 ☑
  auditory, internal 433.8 ☑
  basilar (artery) (*see also* Occlusion, artery,
     basilar) 433.0 ☑
  birth, mother — *see* Embolism, obstetrical
  blood-clot
     with
        abortion — *see* Abortion, by type, with
           embolism
        ectopic pregnancy (*see also* categories
           633.0-633.9) 639.6
        molar pregnancy (*see also* categories 630-
           632) 639.6
     following
        abortion 639.6
        ectopic or molar pregnancy 639.6
     in pregnancy, childbirth, or puerperium
        673.2 ☑
  brain 434.1 ☑
     with
        abortion — *see* Abortion, by type, with
           embolism
        ectopic pregnancy (*see also* categories
           633.0-633.9) 639.6
        molar pregnancy (*see also* categories 630-
           632) 639.6
     following
        abortion 639.6
        ectopic or molar pregnancy 639.6
     late effect — *see* Late effect(s) (of)
        cerebrovascular disease
     puerperal, postpartum, childbirth 674.0 ☑
  capillary 448.9
  cardiac (*see also* Infarct, myocardium) 410.9 ☑
  carotid (artery) (common) (internal) (*see also*
     Occlusion, artery, carotid) 433.1 ☑
  cavernous sinus (venous) — *see* Embolism,
     intracranial venous sinus
  cerebral (*see also* Embolism, brain) 434.1 ☑
  cholesterol — *see* Atheroembolism
  choroidal (anterior) (artery) 433.8 ☑
  coronary (artery or vein) (systemic) (*see also*
     Infarct, myocardium) 410.9 ☑
     without myocardial infarction 411.81
  due to (presence of) any device, implant, or
     graft classifiable to 996.0-996.5 — *see*
     Complications, due to (presence of) any
     device, implant, or graft classified to
     996.0-996.5 NEC
  encephalomalacia (*see also* Embolism, brain)
     434.1 ☑
  extremities 444.22
     lower 444.22
     upper 444.21
  eye 362.30
  fat (cerebral) (pulmonary) (systemic) 958.1
     with
        abortion — *see* Abortion, by type, with
           embolism
        ectopic pregnancy (*see also* categories
           633.0-633.9) 639.6
        molar pregnancy (*see also* categories 630-
           632) 639.6
     complicating delivery or puerperium
        673.8 ☑
     following
        abortion 639.6
        ectopic or molar pregnancy 639.6

Embolism — *continued*
  fat — *continued*
     in pregnancy, childbirth, or the puerperium
        673.8 ☑
  femoral (artery) 444.22
     vein 453.8
        deep 453.41   ●
  following
     abortion 639.6
     ectopic or molar pregnancy 639.6
     infusion, perfusion, or transfusion
        air 999.1
        thrombus 999.2
  heart (fatty) (*see also* Infarct, myocardium)
     410.9 ☑
  hepatic (vein) 453.0
  iliac (artery) 444.81
  iliofemoral 444.81
  in pregnancy, childbirth, or puerperium
     (pulmonary) — *see* Embolism, obstetrical
  intestine (artery) (vein) (with gangrene) 557.0
  intracranial (*see also* Embolism, brain)
     434.1 ☑
     venous sinus (any) 325
        late effect — *see* category 326
        nonpyogenic 437.6
           in pregnancy or puerperium 671.5 ☑
  kidney (artery) 593.81
  lateral sinus (venous) — *see* Embolism,
     intracranial venous sinus
  longitudinal sinus (venous) — *see* Embolism,
     intracranial venous sinus
  lower extremity 444.22
  lung (massive) — *see* Embolism, pulmonary
  meninges (*see also* Embolism, brain) 434.1 ☑
  mesenteric (artery) (with gangrene) 557.0
  multiple NEC 444.9
  obstetrical (pulmonary) 673.2 ☑
     air 673.0 ☑
     amniotic fluid (pulmonary) 673.1 ☑
     blood-clot 673.2 ☑
     cardiac 674.8 ☑
     fat 673.8 ☑
     heart 674.8 ☑
     pyemic 673.3 ☑
     septic 673.3 ☑
     specified NEC 674.8 ☑
  ophthalmic (*see also* Occlusion, retina) 362.30
  paradoxical NEC 444.9
  penis 607.82
  peripheral arteries NEC 444.22
     lower 444.22
     upper 444.21
  pituitary 253.8
  popliteal (artery) 444.22
  portal (vein) 452
  postoperative NEC 997.2
     cerebral 997.02
     mesenteric artery 997.71
     other vessels 997.79
     peripheral vascular 997.2
     pulmonary 415.11
     renal artery 997.72
  precerebral artery (*see also* Occlusion, artery,
     precerebral) 433.9 ☑
  puerperal — *see* Embolism, obstetrical
  pulmonary (artery) (vein) 415.1 ☑
     with
        abortion — *see* Abortion, by type, with
           embolism
        ectopic pregnancy (*see also* categories
           633.0-633.9) 639.6
        molar pregnancy (*see also* categories 630-
           632) 639.6
     following
        abortion 639.6
        ectopic or molar pregnancy 639.6
     iatrogenic 415.11
     in pregnancy, childbirth, or puerperium —
        see Embolism, obstetrical
     postoperative 415.11
  pyemic (multiple) 038.9
     with
        abortion — *see* Abortion, by type, with
           embolism
        ectopic pregnancy (*see also* categories
           633.0-633.9) 639.6

☑ Additional Digit Required   ▶◀ Revised Text   ● New Line   ▲ Revised Code

Embolism — Encephalitis

Embolism — *continued*
pyemic (multiple) — *continued*
with — *continued*
molar pregnancy (*see also* categories 630-632) 639.6
Aerobacter aerogenes 038.49
enteric gram-negative bacilli 038.40
Enterobacter aerogenes 038.49
Escherichia coli 038.42
following
abortion 639.6
ectopic or molar pregnancy 639.6
Hemophilus influenzae 038.41
pneumococcal 038.2
Proteus vulgaris 038.49
Pseudomonas (aeruginosa) 038.43
puerperal, postparztum, childbirth (any organism) 673.3 ☑
Serratia 038.44
specified organism NEC 038.8
staphylococcal 038.10
aureus 038.11
specified organism NEC 038.19
streptococcal 038.0
renal (artery) 593.81
vein 453.3
retina, retinal (*see also* Occlusion, retina) 362.30
saddle (aorta) 444.0
septicemic — *see* Embolism, pyemic
sinus — *see* Embolism, intracranial venous sinus
soap
with
abortion — *see* Abortion, by type, with embolism
ectopic pregnancy (*see also* categories 633.0-633.9) 639.6
molar pregnancy (*see also* categories 630-632) 639.6
following
abortion 639.6
ectopic or molar pregnancy 639.6
spinal cord (nonpyogenic) 336.1
in pregnancy or puerperium 671.5 ☑
pyogenic origin 324.1
late effect — *see* category 326
spleen, splenic (artery) 444.89
thrombus (thromboembolism) following infusion, perfusion, or transfusion 999.2
upper extremity 444.21
vein 453.9
with inflammation or phlebitis — *see* Thrombophlebitis
cerebral (*see also* Embolism, brain) 434.1 ☑
coronary (*see also* Infarct, myocardium) 410.9 ☑
without myocardial infarction 411.81
hepatic 453.0
lower extremity 453.8 ●
deep 453.40 ●
calf 453.42 ●
distal (lower leg) 453.42 ●
femoral 453.41 ●
iliac 453.41 ●
lower leg 453.42 ●
peroneal 453.42 ●
popliteal 453.41 ●
proximal (upper leg) 453.41 ●
thigh 453.41 ●
tibial 453.42 ●
mesenteric (with gangrene) 557.0
portal 452
pulmonary — *see* Embolism, pulmonary
renal 453.3
specified NEC 453.8
with inflammation or phlebitis — *see* Thrombophlebitis
vena cava (inferior) (superior) 453.2
vessels of brain (*see also* Embolism, brain) 434.1 ☑
Embolization — *see* Embolism
Embolus — *see* Embolism

Embryoma (M9080/1) — *see also* Neoplasm, by site, uncertain behavior
benign (M9080/0 — *see* Neoplasm, by site, benign
kidney (M8960/3) 189.0
liver (M8970/3) 155.0
malignant (M9080/3) — *see also* Neoplasm, by site, malignant
kidney (M8960/3) 189.0
liver (M8970/3) 155.0
testis (M9070/3) 186.9
undescended 186.0
testis (M9070/3) 186.9
undescended 186.0
Embryonic
circulation 747.9
heart 747.9
vas deferens 752.89
Embryopathia NEC 759.9
Embryotomy, fetal 763.89
Embryotoxon 743.43
interfering with vision 743.42
Emesis — *see also* Vomiting
gravidarum — *see* Hyperemesis, gravidarum
Emissions, nocturnal (semen) 608.89
Emotional
crisis — *see* Crisis, emotional
disorder (*see also* Disorder, mental) 300.9
instability (excessive) 301.3
overlay — *see* Reaction, adjustment
upset 300.9
Emotionality, pathological 301.3
Emotogenic disease (*see also* Disorder, psychogenic) 306.9
Emphysema (atrophic) (centriacinar) (centrilobular) (chronic) (diffuse) (essential) (hypertrophic) (interlobular) (lung) (obstructive) (panlobular) (paracicatricial) (paracinar) (postural) (pulmonary) (senile) (subpleural) (traction) (unilateral) (unilobular) (vesicular) 492.8
with bronchitis
chronic 491.20
with
acute bronchitis 491.22 ●
exacerbation (acute) 491.21 ●
bullous (giant) 492.0
cellular tissue 958.7
surgical 998.81
compensatory 518.2
congenital 770.2
conjunctiva 372.89
connective tissue 958.7
surgical 998.81
due to fumes or vapors 506.4
eye 376.89
eyelid 374.85
surgical 998.81
traumatic 958.7
fetus or newborn (interstitial) (mediastinal) (unilobular) 770.2
heart 416.9
interstitial 518.1
congenital 770.2
fetus or newborn 770.2
laminated tissue 958.7
surgical 998.81
mediastinal 518.1
fetus or newborn 770.2
newborn (interstitial) (mediastinal) (unilobular) 770.2
obstructive diffuse with fibrosis 492.8
orbit 376.89
subcutaneous 958.7
due to trauma 958.7
nontraumatic 518.1
surgical 998.81
surgical 998.81
thymus (gland) (congenital) 254.8
traumatic 958.7
tuberculous (*see also* Tuberculosis, pulmonary) 011.9 ☑
Employment examination (certification) V70.5
Empty sella (turcica) syndrome 253.8

Empyema (chest) (diaphragmatic) (double) (encapsulated) (general) (interlobar) (lung) (medial) (necessitatis) (perforating chest wall) (pleura) (pneumococcal) (residual) (sacculated) (streptococcal) (supradiaphragmatic) 510.9
with fistula 510.0
accessory sinus (chronic) (*see also* Sinusitis) 473.9
acute 510.9
with fistula 510.0
antrum (chronic) (*see also* Sinusitis, maxillary) 473.0
brain (any part) (*see also* Abcess, brain) 324.0
ethmoidal (sinus) (chronic) (*see also* Sinusitis, ethmoidal) 473.2
extradural (*see also* Abscess, extradural) 324.9
frontal (sinus) (chronic) (*see also* Sinusitis, frontal) 473.1
gallbladder (*see also* Cholecystitis, acute) 575.0
mastoid (process) (acute) (*see also* Mastoiditis, acute) 383.00
maxilla, maxillary 526.4
sinus (chronic) (*see also* Sinusitis, maxillary) 473.0
nasal sinus (chronic) (*see also* Sinusitis) 473.9
sinus (accessory) (nasal) (*see also* Sinusitis) 473.9
sphenoidal (chronic) (sinus) (*see also* Sinusitis, sphenoidal) 473.3
subarachnoid (*see also* Abscess, extradural) 324.9
subdural (*see also* Abscess, extradural) 324.9
tuberculous (*see also* Tuberculosis, pleura) 012.0 ☑
ureter (*see also* Ureteritis) 593.89
ventricular (*see also* Abscess, brain) 324.0
Enameloma 520.2
Encephalitis (bacterial) (chronic) (hemorrhagic) (idiopathic) (nonepidemic) (spurious) (subacute) 323.9
acute — *see also* Encephalitis, viral
disseminated (postinfectious) NEC 136.9 [323.6]
postimmunization or postvaccination 323.5
inclusional 049.8
inclusion body 049.8
necrotizing 049.8
arboviral, arbovirus NEC 064
arthropod-borne (*see also* Encephalitis, viral, arthropod-borne) 064
Australian X 062.4
Bwamba fever 066.3
California (virus) 062.5
Central European 063.2
Czechoslovakian 063.2
Dawson's (inclusion body) 046.2
diffuse sclerosing 046.2
due to
actinomycosis 039.8 [323.4]
cat-scratch disease 078.3 [323.0]
infectious mononucleosis 075 [323.0]
malaria (*see also* Malaria) 084.6 [323.2]
Negishi virus 064
ornithosis 073.7 [323.0]
prophylactic inoculation against smallpox 323.5
rickettsiosis (*see also* Rickettsiosis) 083.9 [323.1]
rubella 056.01
toxoplasmosis (acquired) 130.0
congenital (active) 771.2 [323.4]
typhus (fever) (*see also* Typhus) 081.9 [323.1]
vaccination (smallpox) 323.5
Eastern equine 062.2
endemic 049.8
epidemic 049.8
equine (acute) (infectious) (viral) 062.9
Eastern 062.2
Venezuelan 066.2
Western 062.1
Far Eastern 063.0
following vaccination or other immunization procedure 323.5

Encephalitis — *continued*
  herpes 054.3
  Ilheus (virus) 062.8
  inclusion body 046.2
  infectious (acute) (virus) NEC 049.8
  influenzal 487.8 *[323.4]*
    lethargic 049.8
  Japanese (B type) 062.0
  La Crosse 062.5
  Langat 063.8
  late effect — *see* Late, effect, encephalitis
  lead 984.9 *[323.7]*
  lethargic (acute) (infectious) (influenzal) 049.8
  lethargica 049.8
  louping ill 063.1
  lupus 710.0 *[323.8]*
  lymphatica 049.0
  Mengo 049.8
  meningococcal 036.1
  mumps 072.2
  Murray Valley 062.4
  myoclonic 049.8
  Negishi virus 064
  otitic NEC 382.4 *[323.4]*
  parasitic NEC 123.9 *[323.4]*
  periaxialis (concentrica) (diffusa) 341.1
  postchickenpox 052.0
  postexanthematous NEC 057.9 *[323.6]*
  postimmunization 323.5
  postinfectious NEC 136.9 *[323.6]*
  postmeasles 055.0
  posttraumatic 323.8
  postvaccinal (smallpox) 323.5
  postvaricella 052.0
  postviral NEC 079.99 *[323.6]*
    postexanthematous 057.9 *[323.6]*
      specified NEC 057.8 *[323.6]*
  Powassan 063.8
  progressive subcortical (Binswanger's) 290.12
  Rio Bravo 049.8
  rubella 056.01
  Russian
    autumnal 062.0
    spring-summer type (taiga) 063.0
  saturnine 984.9 *[323.7]*
  Semliki Forest 062.8
  serous 048
  slow-acting virus NEC 046.8
  specified cause NEC 323.8
  St. Louis type 062.3
  subacute sclerosing 046.2
  subcorticalis chronica 290.12
  summer 062.0
  suppurative 324.0
  syphilitic 094.81
    congenital 090.41
  tick-borne 063.9
  torula, torular 117.5 *[323.4]*
  toxic NEC 989.9 *[323.7]*
  toxoplasmic (acquired) 130.0
    congenital (active) 771.2 *[323.4]*
  trichinosis 124 *[323.4]*
  Trypanosomiasis (*see also* Trypanosomiasis)
    086.9 *[323.2]*
  tuberculous (*see also* Tuberculosis) 013.6 ☑
  type B (Japanese) 062.0
  type C 062.3
  van Bogaert's 046.2
  Venezuelan 066.2
  Vienna type 049.8
  viral, virus 049.9
    arthropod-borne NEC 064
      mosquito-borne 062.9
        Australian X disease 062.4
        California virus 062.5
        Eastern equine 062.2
        Ilheus virus 062.8
        Japanese (B type) 062.0
        Murray Valley 062.4
        specified type NEC 062.8
        St. Louis 062.3
        type B 062.0
        type C 062.3
        Western equine 062.1

Encephalitis — *continued*
  viral, virus — *continued*
    arthropod-borne NEC — *continued*
      tick-borne 063.9
        biundulant 063.2
        Central European 063.2
        Czechoslovakian 063.2
        diphasic meningoencephalitis 063.2
        Far Eastern 063.0
        Langat 063.8
        louping ill 063.1
        Powassan 063.8
        Russian spring-summer (taiga) 063.0
        specified type NEC 063.8
      vector unknown 064
    slow acting NEC 046.8
    specified type NEC 049.8
    vaccination, prophylactic (against) V05.0
  von Economo's 049.8
  Western equine 062.1
  West Nile type 066.41   ▲
Encephalocele 742.0
  orbit 376.81
Encephalocystocele 742.0
Encephalomalacia (brain) (cerebellar) (cerebral)
    (cerebrospinal) (*see also* Softening, brain)
    434.9 ☑
  due to
    hemorrhage (*see also* Hemorrhage, brain)
      431
    recurrent spasm of artery 435.9
  embolic (cerebral) (*see also* Embolism, brain)
    434.1 ☑
  subcorticalis chronicus arteriosclerotica 290.12
  thrombotic (*see also* thrombosis, brain)
    434.0 ☑
Encephalomeningitis — *see* Meningoencephalitis
Encephalomeningocele 742.0
Encephalomeningomyelitis — *see*
    Meningoencephalitis
Encephalomeningopathy (*see also*
    Meningoencephalitis) 349.9
Encephalomyelitis (chronic) (granulomatous)
    (hemorrhagic necrotizing, acute) (myalgic,
    benign) (*see also* Encephalitis) 323.9
  abortive disseminated 049.8
  acute disseminated (postinfectious)
    136.9 *[323.6]*
    postimmunization 323.5
  due to or resulting from vaccination (any) 323.5
  equine (acute) (infectious) 062.9
    Eastern 062.2
    Venezuelan 066.2
    Western 062.1
  funicularis infectiosa 049.8
  late effect — *see* Late, effect, encephalitis
  Munch-Peterson's 049.8
  postchickenpox 052.0
  postimmunization 323.5
  postmeasles 055.0
  postvaccinal (smallpox) 323.5
  rubella 056.01
  specified cause NEC 323.8
  syphilitic 094.81
  West Nile 066.41   ●
Encephalomyelocele 742.0
Encephalomyelomeningitis — *see*
    Meningoencephalitis
Encephalomyeloneuropathy 349.9
Encephalomyelopathy 349.9
  subacute necrotizing (infantile) 330.8
Encephalomyeloradiculitis (acute) 357.0
Encephalomyeloradiculoneuritis (acute) 357.0
Encephalomyeloradiculopathy 349.9
Encephalomyocarditis 074.23
Encephalopathia hyperbilirubinemica, newborn
    774.7
  due to isoimmunization (conditions classifiable
    to 773.0-773.2) 773.4
Encephalopathy (acute) 348.30
  alcoholic 291.2
  anoxic — *see* Damage, brain, anoxic

Encephalopathy — *continued*
  arteriosclerotic 437.0
    late effect — *see* Late effect(s) (of)
      cerebrovascular disease
  bilirubin, newborn 774.7
    due to isoimmunization 773.4
  congenital 742.9
  demyelinating (callosal) 341.8
  due to
    birth injury (intracranial) 767.8
    dialysis 294.8
      transient 293.9
    hyperinsulinism — *see* Hyperinsulinism
    influenza (virus) 487.8
    lack of vitamin (*see also* Deficiency, vitamin)
      269.2
    nicotinic acid deficiency 291.2
    serum (nontherapeutic) (therapeutic) 999.5
    syphilis 094.81
    trauma (postconcussional) 310.2
      current (*see also* Concussion, brain)
        850.9
        with skull fracture — *see* Fracture,
          skull, by site, with intracranial
          injury
    vaccination 323.5
  hepatic 572.2
  hyperbilirubinemic, newborn 774.7
    due to isoimmunization (conditions
      classifiable to 773.0-773.2) 773.4
  hypertensive 437.2
  hypoglycemic 251.2
  hypoxic — *see* Damage, brain, anoxic
  infantile cystic necrotizing (congenital) 341.8
  lead 984.9 *[323.7]*
  leukopolio 330.0
  metabolic (*see also* Delirium) 348.31
    toxic 349.82
  necrotizing, subacute 330.8
  other specified type NEC 348.39
  pellagrous 265.2
  portal-systemic 572.2
  postcontusional 310.2
  posttraumatic 310.2
  saturnine 984.9 *[323.7]*
  septic 348.31
  spongioform, subacute (viral) 046.1
  subacute
    necrotizing 330.8
    spongioform 046.1
    viral, spongioform 046.1
  subcortical progressive (Schilder) 341.1
    chronic (Binswanger's) 290.12
  toxic 349.82
    metabolic 348.31   ▲
  traumatic (postconcussional) 310.2
    current (*see also* Concussion, brain) 850.9
      with skull fracture — *see* Fracture, skull,
        by site, with intracranial injury
  vitamin B deficiency NEC 266.9
  Wernicke's (superior hemorrhagic
    polioencephalitis) 265.1
Encephalorrhagia (*see also* Hemorrhage, brain)
    432.9
  healed or old V12.59
  late effect — *see* Late effect(s) (of)
    cerebrovascular disease
Encephalosis, posttraumatic 310.2
Enchondroma (M9220/0) — *see also* Neoplasm,
    bone, benign
  multiple, congenital 756.4
Enchondromatosis (cartilaginous) (congenital)
    (multiple) 756.4
Enchondroses, multiple (cartilaginous)
    (congenital) 756.4
Encopresis (*see also* Incontinence, feces) 787.6
  nonorganic origin 307.7
Encounter for — *see also* Admission for
  administrative purpose only V68.9
    referral of patient without examination or
      treatment V68.81
    specified purpose NEC V68.89
  chemotherapy V58.1
  end-of-life care V66.7
  hospice care V66.7

☑ Additional Digit Required   ►◄ Revised Text   ● New Line   ▲ Revised Code

Encounter for — *continued*
　palliative care V66.7
　paternity testing V70.4
　radiotherapy V58.0
　respirator dependence, during power ●
　　failure V46.12 ●
　screening mammogram NEC V76.12
　　for high-risk patient V76.11
　terminal care V66.7

Encystment — *see* Cyst

End-of-life care V66.7

Endamebiasis — *see* Amebiasis

Endamoeba — *see* Amebiasis

Endarteritis (bacterial, subacute) (infective)
　　(septic) 447.6
　brain, cerebral or cerebrospinal 437.4
　　late effect — *see* Late effect(s) (of)
　　　cerebrovascular disease
　coronary (artery) — *see* Arteriosclerosis,
　　coronary
　deformans — *see* Arteriosclerosis
　embolic (*see also* Embolism) 444.9
　obliterans — *see also* Arteriosclerosis
　　pulmonary 417.8
　pulmonary 417.8
　retina 362.18
　senile — *see* Arteriosclerosis
　syphilitic 093.89
　　brain or cerebral 094.89
　　congenital 090.5
　　spinal 094.89
　tuberculous (*see also* Tuberculosis) 017.9 ☑

Endemic — *see* condition

Endocarditis (chronic) (indeterminate) (interstitial)
　　(marantis) (nonbacterial thrombotic)
　　(residual) (sclerotic) (sclerous) (senile)
　　(valvular) 424.90
　with
　　rheumatic fever (conditions classifiable to
　　　390)
　　　active — *see* Endocarditis, acute,
　　　　rheumatic
　　　inactive or quiescent (with chorea) 397.9
　acute or subacute 421.9
　　rheumatic (aortic) (mitral) (pulmonary)
　　　(tricuspid) 391.1
　　　with chorea (acute) (rheumatic)
　　　　(Sydenham's) 392.0
　aortic (heart) (nonrheumatic) (valve) 424.1
　　with
　　　mitral (valve) disease 396.9
　　　　active or acute 391.1
　　　　　with chorea (acute) (rheumatic)
　　　　　　(Sydenham's) 392.0
　　　rheumatic fever (conditions classifiable to
　　　　390)
　　　　active — *see* Endocarditis, acute,
　　　　　rheumatic
　　　　inactive or quiescent (with chorea)
　　　　　395.9
　　　　　with mitral disease 396.9
　　acute or subacute 421.9
　　arteriosclerotic 424.1
　　congenital 746.89
　　hypertensive 424.1
　　rheumatic (chronic) (inactive) 395.9
　　　with mitral (valve) disease 396.9
　　　　active or acute 391.1
　　　　　with chorea (acute) (rheumatic)
　　　　　　(Sydenham's) 392.0
　　　active or acute 391.1
　　　　with chorea (acute) (rheumatic)
　　　　　(Sydenham's) 392.0
　　specified cause, except rheumatic 424.1
　　syphilitic 093.22
　arteriosclerotic or due to arteriosclerosis
　　424.99
　atypical verrucous (Libman-Sacks)
　　710.0 *[424.91]*
　bacterial (acute) (any valve) (chronic) (subacute)
　　421.0
　blastomycotic 116.0 *[421.1]*
　candidal 112.81
　congenital 425.3
　constrictive 421.0

Endocarditis — *continued*
　Coxsackie 074.22
　due to
　　blastomycosis 116.0 *[421.1]*
　　candidiasis 112.81
　　Coxsackie (virus) 074.22
　　disseminated lupus erythematosus
　　　710.0 *[424.91]*
　　histoplasmosis (*see also* Histoplasmosis)
　　　115.94
　　hypertension (benign) 424.99
　　moniliasis 112.81
　　prosthetic cardiac valve 996.61
　　Q fever 083.0 *[421.1]*
　　serratia marcescens 421.0
　　typhoid (fever) 002.0 *[421.1]*
　fetal 425.3
　gonococcal 098.84
　hypertensive 424.99
　infectious or infective (acute) (any valve)
　　(chronic) (subacute) 421.0
　lenta (acute) (any valve) (chronic) (subacute)
　　421.0
　Libman-Sacks 710.0 *[424.91]*
　Loeffler's (parietal fibroplastic) 421.0
　malignant (acute) (any valve) (chronic)
　　(subacute) 421.0
　meningococcal 036.42
　mitral (chronic) (double) (fibroid) (heart)
　　(inactive) (valve) (with chorea) 394.9
　　with
　　　aortic (valve) disease 396.9
　　　　active or acute 391.1
　　　　　with chorea (acute) (rheumatic)
　　　　　　(Sydenham's) 392.0
　　　　rheumatic fever (conditions classifiable to
　　　　　390)
　　　　　active — *see* Endocarditis, acute,
　　　　　　rheumatic
　　　　　inactive or quiescent (with chorea)
　　　　　　394.9
　　　　　　with aortic valve disease 396.9
　　　active or acute 391.1
　　　　with chorea (acute) (rheumatic)
　　　　　(Sydenham's) 392.0
　　　bacterial 421.0
　　arteriosclerotic 424.0
　　congenital 746.89
　　hypertensive 424.0
　　nonrheumatic 424.0
　　　acute or subacute 421.9
　　syphilitic 093.21
　monilial 112.81
　mycotic (acute) (any valve) (chronic) (subacute)
　　421.0
　pneumococcic (acute) (any valve) (chronic)
　　(subacute) 421.0
　pulmonary (chronic) (heart) (valve) 424.3
　　with
　　　rheumatic fever (conditions classifiable to
　　　　390)
　　　　active — *see* Endocarditis, acute,
　　　　　rheumatic
　　　　inactive or quiescent (with chorea)
　　　　　397.1
　　acute or subacute 421.9
　　　rheumatic 391.1
　　　　with chorea (acute) (rheumatic)
　　　　　(Sydenham's) 392.0
　　arteriosclerotic or due to arteriosclerosis
　　　424.3
　　congenital 746.09
　　hypertensive or due to hypertension (benign)
　　　424.3
　　rheumatic (chronic) (inactive) (with chorea)
　　　397.1
　　　active or acute 391.1
　　　　with chorea (acute) (rheumatic)
　　　　　(Sydenham's) 392.0
　　syphilitic 093.24
　purulent (acute) (any valve) (chronic) (subacute)
　　421.0
　rheumatic (chronic) (inactive) (with chorea)
　　397.9
　　active or acute (aortic) (mitral) (pulmonary)
　　　(tricuspid) 391.1

Endocarditis — *continued*
　rheumatic — *continued*
　　active or acute — *continued*
　　　with chorea (acute) (rheumatic)
　　　　(Sydenham's) 392.0
　septic (acute) (any valve) (chronic) (subacute)
　　421.0
　specified cause, except rheumatic 424.99
　streptococcal (acute) (any valve) (chronic)
　　(subacute) 421.0
　subacute — *see* Endocarditis, acute
　suppurative (any valve) (acute) (chronic)
　　(subacute) 421.0
　syphilitic NEC 093.20
　toxic (*see also* Endocarditis, acute) 421.9
　tricuspid (chronic) (heart) (inactive) (rheumatic)
　　(valve) (with chorea) 397.0
　　with
　　　rheumatic fever (conditions classifiable to
　　　　390)
　　　　active — *see* Endocarditis, acute,
　　　　　rheumatic
　　　　inactive or quiescent (with chorea)
　　　　　397.0
　　active or acute 391.1
　　　with chorea (acute) (rheumatic)
　　　　(Sydenham's) 392.0
　　arteriosclerotic 424.2
　　congenital 746.89
　　hypertensive 424.2
　　nonrheumatic 424.2
　　　acute or subacute 421.9
　　specified cause, except rheumatic 424.2
　　syphilitic 093.23
　　tuberculous (*see also* Tuberculosis)
　　　017.9 ☑ *[424.91]*
　typhoid 002.0 *[421.1]*
　ulcerative (acute) (any valve) (chronic)
　　(subacute) 421.0
　vegetative (acute) (any valve) (chronic)
　　(subacute) 421.0
　verrucous (acute) (any valve) (chronic)
　　(subacute) NEC 710.0 *[424.91]*
　　nonbacterial 710.0 *[424.91]*
　　nonrheumatic 710.0 *[424.91]*

Endocardium, endocardial — *see also* condition
　cushion defect 745.60
　　specified type NEC 745.69

Endocervicitis (*see also* Cervicitis) 616.0
　due to
　　intrauterine (contraceptive) device 996.65
　gonorrheal (acute) 098.15
　　chronic or duration of 2 months or over
　　　098.35
　hyperplastic 616.0
　syphilitic 095.8
　trichomonal 131.09
　tuberculous (*see also* Tuberculosis) 016.7 ☑

Endocrine — *see* condition

Endocrinopathy, pluriglandular 258.9

Endodontitis 522.0

Endomastoiditis (*see also* Mastoiditis) 383.9

Endometrioma 617.9

Endometriosis 617.9
　appendix 617.5
　bladder 617.8
　bowel 617.5
　broad ligament 617.3
　cervix 617.0
　colon 617.5
　cul-de-sac (Douglas') 617.3
　exocervix 617.0
　fallopian tube 617.2
　female genital organ NEC 617.8
　gallbladder 617.8
　in scar of skin 617.6
　internal 617.0
　intestine 617.5
　lung 617.8
　myometrium 617.0
　ovary 617.1
　parametrium 617.3
　pelvic peritoneum 617.3
　peritoneal (pelvic) 617.3
　rectovaginal septum 617.4

☑ Additional Digit Required　　　　▶◀ Revised Text　　　　● New Line　　　　▲ Revised Code

Encounter for — Endometriosis

☑ Additional Digit Required   ▶◀ Revised Text   ● New Line   ▲ Revised Code

Endometriosis — Enteritis

Enteritis — *continued*
  E. coli — *continued*
    specified type NEC 008.09
  el tor 001.1
  embadomonial 007.8
  epidemic 009.0
  Eubacterium 008.46
  fermentative 558.9
  fulminant 557.0
  Fusobacterium (nucleatum) 008.46
  gangrenous (*see also* Enteritis, due to, by organism) 009.0
  giardial 007.1
  gram-negative bacteria NEC 008.47
    anaerobic NEC 008.46
  infectious NEC (*see also* Enteritis, due to, by organism) 009.0
    presumed 009.1
  influenzal 487.8
  ischemic 557.9
    acute 557.0
    chronic 557.1
    due to mesenteric artery insufficiency 557.1
  membranous 564.9
  mucous 564.9
  myxomembranous 564.9
  necrotic (*see also* Enteritis, due to, by organism) 009.0
  necroticans 005.2
  necrotizing of fetus or newborn 777.5
  neurogenic 564.9
  newborn 777.8
    necrotizing 777.5
  parasitic NEC 129
  paratyphoid (fever) (*see also* Fever, paratyphoid) 002.9
  Peptococcus 008.46
  Peptostreptococcus 008.46
  Proprionibacterium 008.46
  protozoal NEC 007.9
  radiation 558.1
  regional (of) 555.9
    intestine
      large (bowel, colon, or rectum) 555.1
        with small intestine 555.2
      small (duodenum, ileum, or jejunum) 555.0
        with large intestine 555.2
  Salmonella infection 003.0
  salmonellosis 003.0
  segmental (*see also* Enteritis, regional) 555.9
  septic (*see also* Enteritis, due to, by organism) 009.0
  Shigella 004.9
  simple 558.9
  spasmodic 564.9
  spastic 564.9
  staphylococcal 008.41
    due to food 005.0
  streptococcal 008.49
    anaerobic 008.46
  toxic 558.2
  Treponema (denticola) (macrodentium) 008.46
  trichomonal 007.3
  tuberculous (*see also* Tuberculosis) 014.8 ☑
  typhosa 002.0
  ulcerative (chronic) (*see also* Colitis, ulcerative) 556.9
  Veillonella 008.46
  viral 008.8
    adenovirus 008.62
    enterovirus 008.67
    specified virus NEC 008.69
  Yersinia enterocolitica 008.44
  zymotic 009.0
Enteroarticular syndrome 099.3
Enterobiasis 127.4
Enterobius vermicularis 127.4
Enterocele (*see also* Hernia) 553.9
  pelvis, pelvic (acquired) (congenital) 618.6
  vagina, vaginal (acquired) (congenital) 618.6
Enterocolitis — *see also* Enteritis
  fetus or newborn 777.8
    necrotizing 777.5
  fulminant 557.0
  granulomatous 555.2

Enterocolitis — *continued*
  hemorrhagic (acute) 557.0
    chronic 557.1
  necrotizing (acute) (membranous) 557.0
  primary necrotizing 777.5
  pseudomembranous 008.45
  radiation 558.1
    newborn 777.5
  ulcerative 556.0
Enterocystoma 751.5
Enterogastritis — *see* Enteritis
Enterogenous cyanosis 289.7
Enterolith, enterolithiasis (impaction) 560.39
  with hernia — *see also* Hernia, by site, with obstruction
    gangrenous — *see* Hernia, by site, with gangrene
Enteropathy 569.9
  exudative (of Gordon) 579.8
  gluten 579.0
  hemorrhagic, terminal 557.0
  protein-losing 579.8
Enteroperitonitis (*see also* Peritonitis) 567.9
Enteroptosis 569.89
Enterorrhagia 578.9
Enterospasm 564.9
  psychogenic 306.4
Enterostenosis (*see also* Obstruction, intestine) 560.9
Enterostomy status V44.4
  with complication 569.60
Enthesopathy 726.39
  ankle and tarsus 726.70
  elbow region 726.30
    specified NEC 726.39
  hip 726.5
  knee 726.60
  peripheral NEC 726.8
  shoulder region 726.10
    adhesive 726.0
  spinal 720.1
  wrist and carpus 726.4
Entrance, air into vein — *see* Embolism, air
Entrapment, nerve — *see* Neuropathy, entrapment
Entropion (eyelid) 374.00
  cicatricial 374.04
  congenital 743.62
  late effect of trachoma (healed) 139.1
  mechanical 374.02
  paralytic 374.02
  senile 374.01
  spastic 374.03
Enucleation of eye (current) (traumatic) 871.3
Enuresis 788.30
  habit disturbance 307.6
  nocturnal 788.36
    psychogenic 307.6
  nonorganic origin 307.6
  psychogenic 307.6
Enzymopathy 277.9
Eosinopenia 288.0
Eosinophilia 288.3
  allergic 288.3
  hereditary 288.3
  idiopathic 288.3
  infiltrative 518.3
  Loeffler's 518.3
  myalgia syndrome 710.5
  pulmonary (tropical) 518.3
  secondary 288.3
  tropical 518.3
Eosinophilic — *see also* condition
  fasciitis 728.89
  granuloma (bone) 277.89
  infiltration lung 518.3
Ependymitis (acute) (cerebral) (chronic) (granular) (*see also* Meningitis) 322.9
Ependymoblastoma (M9392/3)
  specified site — *see* Neoplasm, by site, malignant
  unspecified site 191.9

Ependymoma (epithelial) (malignant) (M9391/3)
  anaplastic type (M9392/3)
    specified site — *see* Neoplasm, by site, malignant
    unspecified site 191.9
  benign (M9391/0)
    specified site — *see* Neoplasm, by site, benign
    unspecified site 225.0
  myxopapillary (M9394/1) 237.5
  papillary (M9393/1) 237.5
  specified site — *see* Neoplasm, by site, malignant
  unspecified site 191.9
Ependymopathy 349.2
  spinal cord 349.2
Ephelides, ephelis 709.09
Ephemeral fever (*see also* Pyrexia) 780.6
Epiblepharon (congenital) 743.62
Epicanthus, epicanthic fold (congenital) (eyelid) 743.63
Epicondylitis (elbow) (lateral) 726.32
  medial 726.31
Epicystitis (*see also* Cystitis) 595.9
Epidemic — *see* condition
Epidermidalization, cervix — *see* condition
Epidermidization, cervix — *see* condition
Epidermis, epidermal — *see* condition
Epidermization, cervix — *see* condition
Epidermodysplasia verruciformis 078.19
Epidermoid
  cholesteatoma — *see* Cholesteatoma
  inclusion (*see also* Cyst, skin) 706.2
Epidermolysis
  acuta (combustiformis) (toxica) 695.1
  bullosa 757.39
  necroticans combustiformis 695.1
    due to drug
      correct substance properly administered 695.1
      overdose or wrong substance given or taken 977.9
      specified drug — *see* Table of Drugs and Chemicals
Epidermophytid — *see* Dermatophytosis
Epidermophytosis (infected) — *see* Dermatophytosis
Epidermosis, ear (middle) (*see also* Cholesteatoma) 385.30
Epididymis — *see* condition
Epididymitis (nonvenereal) 604.90
  with abscess 604.0
  acute 604.99
  blennorrhagic (acute) 098.0
    chronic or duration of 2 months or over 098.2
  caseous (*see also* Tuberculosis) 016.4 ☑
  chlamydial 099.54
  diphtheritic 032.89 [604.91]
  filarial 125.9 [604.91]
  gonococcal (acute) 098.0
    chronic or duration of 2 months or over 098.2
  recurrent 604.99
  residual 604.99
  syphilitic 095.8 [604.91]
  tuberculous (*see also* Tuberculosis) 016.4 ☑
Epididymo-orchitis (*see also* Epididymitis) 604.90
  with abscess 604.0
  chlamydial 099.54
  gonococcal (acute) 098.13
    chronic or duration of 2 months or over 098.33
Epidural — *see* condition
Epigastritis (*see also* Gastritis) 535.5 ☑
Epigastrium, epigastric — *see* condition
Epigastrocele (*see also* Hernia, epigastric) 553.29
Epiglottiditis (acute) 464.30
  with obstruction 464.31
  chronic 476.1
  viral 464.30
    with obstruction 464.31

Sidebar: Enteritis — Epiglottiditis

Epiglottis — *see* condition
Epiglottitis (acute) 464.30
  with obstruction 464.31
  chronic 476.1
  viral 464.30
    with obstruction 464.31
Epignathus 759.4
Epilepsia
  partialis continua (*see also* Epilepsy) 345.7 ☑
  procursiva (*see also* Epilepsy) 345.8 ☑
Epilepsy, epileptic (idiopathic) 345.9 ☑

> *Note — use the following fifth-digit subclassification with categories 345.0, 345.1, 345.4–345.9:*
>
> 0   *without mention of intractable epilepsy*
>
> 1   *with intractable epilepsy*

  abdominal 345.5 ☑
  absence (attack) 345.0 ☑
  akinetic 345.0 ☑
    psychomotor 345.4 ☑
  automatism 345.4 ☑
  autonomic diencephalic 345.5 ☑
  brain 345.9 ☑
  Bravais-Jacksonian 345.5 ☑
  cerebral 345.9 ☑
  climacteric 345.9 ☑
  clonic 345.1 ☑
  clouded state 345.9 ☑
  coma 345.3
  communicating 345.4 ☑
  congenital 345.9 ☑
  convulsions 345.9 ☑
  cortical (focal) (motor) 345.5 ☑
  cursive (running) 345.8 ☑
  cysticercosis 123.1
  deterioration
    with behavioral disturbance 345.9 ☑ *[294.11]*
    without behavioral disturbance 345.9 ☑ *[294.10]*
  due to syphilis 094.89
  equivalent 345.5 ☑
  fit 345.9 ☑
  focal (motor) 345.5 ☑
  gelastic 345.8 ☑
  generalized 345.9 ☑
    convulsive 345.1 ☑
    flexion 345.1 ☑
    nonconvulsive 345.0 ☑
  grand mal (idiopathic) 345.1 ☑
  Jacksonian (motor) (sensory) 345.5 ☑
  Kojevnikoff's, Kojevnikov's, Kojewnikoff's 345.7 ☑
  laryngeal 786.2
  limbic system 345.4 ☑
  major (motor) 345.1 ☑
  minor 345.0 ☑
  mixed (type) 345.9 ☑
  motor partial 345.5 ☑
  musicogenic 345.1 ☑
  myoclonus, myoclonic 345.1 ☑
    progressive (familial) 333.2
  nonconvulsive, generalized 345.0 ☑
  parasitic NEC 123.9
  partial (focalized) 345.5 ☑
    with
      impairment of consciousness 345.4 ☑
      memory and ideational disturbances 345.4 ☑
    abdominal type 345.5 ☑
    motor type 345.5 ☑
    psychomotor type 345.4 ☑
    psychosensory type 345.4 ☑
    secondarily generalized 345.4 ☑
    sensory type 345.5 ☑
    somatomotor type 345.5 ☑
    somatosensory type 345.5 ☑
    temporal lobe type 345.4 ☑
    visceral type 345.5 ☑
    visual type 345.5 ☑
  peripheral 345.9 ☑
  petit mal 345.0 ☑
  photokinetic 345.8 ☑

Epilepsy, epileptic — *continued*
  progresive myoclonic (familial) 333.2
  psychic equivalent 345.5 ☑
  psychomotor 345.4 ☑
  psychosensory 345.4 ☑
  reflex 345.1 ☑
  seizure 345.9 ☑
  senile 345.9 ☑
  sensory-induced 345.5 ☑
  sleep ►(*see also* Narcolepsy)◄ 347.00 ▲
  somatomotor type 345.5 ☑
  somatosensory 345.5 ☑
  specified type NEC 345.8 ☑
  status (grand mal) 345.3
    focal motor 345.7 ☑
    petit mal 345.2
    psychomotor 345.7 ☑
    temporal lobe 345.7 ☑
  symptomatic 345.9 ☑
  temporal lobe 345.4 ☑
  tonic (-clonic) 345.1 ☑
  traumatic (injury unspecified) 907.0
    injury specified — *see* Late, effect (of) specified injury
  twilight 293.0
  uncinate (gyrus) 345.4 ☑
  Unverricht (-Lundborg) (familial myoclonic) 333.2
  visceral 345.5 ☑
  visual 345.5 ☑
Epileptiform
  convulsions 780.39
  seizure 780.39
Epiloia 759.5
Epimenorrhea 626.2
Epipharyngitis (*see also* Nasopharyngitis) 460
Epiphora 375.20
  due to
    excess lacrimation 375.21
    insufficient drainage 375.22
Epiphyseal arrest 733.91
  femoral head 732.2
Epiphyseolysis, epiphysiolysis (*see also* Osteochondrosis) 732.9
Epiphysitis (*see also* Osteochondrosis) 732.9
  juvenile 732.6
  marginal (Scheuermann's) 732.0
  os calcis 732.5
  syphilitic (congenital) 090.0
  vertebral (Scheuermann's) 732.0
Epiplocele (*see also* Hernia) 553.9
Epiploitis (*see also* Peritonitis) 567.9
Epiplosarcomphalocele (*see also* Hernia, umbilicus) 553.1
Episcleritis 379.00
  gouty 274.89 *[379.09]*
  nodular 379.02
  periodica fugax 379.01
    angioneurotic — *see* Edema, angioneurotic
  specified NEC 379.09
  staphylococcal 379.00
  suppurative 379.00
  syphilitic 095.0
  tuberculous (*see also* Tuberculosis) 017.3 ☑ *[379.09]*
Episode
  brain (*see also* Disease, cerebrovascular, acute) 436
  cerebral (*see also* Disease, cerebrovascular, acute) 436
  depersonalization (in neurotic state) 300.6
  hyporesponsive 780.09
  psychotic (*see also* Psychosis) 298.9
    organic, transient 293.9
  schizophrenic (acute) NEC (*see also* Schizophrenia) 295.4 ☑
Epispadias
  female 753.8
  male 752.62
Episplenitis 289.59
Epistaxis (multiple) 784.7
  hereditary 448.0
  vicarious menstruation 625.8

Epithelioma (malignant) (M8011/3) — *see also* Neoplasm, by site, malignant
  adenoides cysticum (M8100/0) — *see* Neoplasm, skin, benign
  basal cell (M8090/3) — *see* Neoplasm, skin, malignant
  benign (M8011/0) — *see* Neoplasm, by site, benign
  Bowen's (M8081/2) — *see* Neoplasm, skin, in situ
  calcifying (benign) (Malherbe's) (M8110/0) — *see* Neoplasm, skin, benign
  external site — *see* Neoplasm, skin, malignant
  intraepidermal, Jadassohn (M8096/0) — *see* Neoplasm, skin, benign
  squamous cell (M8070/3) — *see* Neoplasm, by site, malignant
Epitheliopathy
  pigment, retina 363.15
  posterior multifocal placoid (acute) 363.15
Epithelium, epithelial — *see* condition
Epituberculosis (allergic) (with atelectasis) (*see also* Tuberculosis) 010.8 ☑
Eponychia 757.5
Epstein's
  nephrosis or syndrome (*see also* Nephrosis) 581.9
  pearl (mouth) 528.4
Epstein-Barr infection (viral) 075
  chronic 780.79 *[139.8]*
Epulis (giant cell) (gingiva) 523.8
Equinia 024
Equinovarus (congenital) 754.51
  acquired 736.71
Equivalent
  convulsive (abdominal) (*see also* Epilepsy) 345.5 ☑
  epileptic (psychic) (*see also* Epilepsy) 345.5 ☑
Erb's
  disease 359.1
  palsy, paralysis (birth) (brachial) (newborn) 767.6
    spinal (spastic) syphilitic 094.89
  pseudohypertrophic muscular dystrophy 359.1
Erb (-Duchenne) paralysis (birth injury) (newborn) 767.6
Erb-Goldflam disease or syndrome 358.00
Erdheim's syndrome (acromegalic macrospondylitis) 253.0
Erection, painful (persistent) 607.3
Ergosterol deficiency (vitamin D) 268.9
  with
    osteomalacia 268.2
    rickets (*see also* Rickets) 268.0
Ergotism (ergotized grain) 988.2
  from ergot used as drug (migraine therapy)
    correct substance properly administered 349.82
    overdose or wrong substance given or taken 975.0
Erichsen's disease (railway spine) 300.16
Erlacher-Blount syndrome (tibia vara) 732.4
Erosio interdigitalis blastomycetica 112.3
Erosion
  artery NEC 447.2
    without rupture 447.8
  arteriosclerotic plaque — *see* Arteriosclerosis, by site
  bone 733.99
  bronchus 519.1
  cartilage (joint) 733.99
  cervix (uteri) (acquired) (chronic) (congenital) 622.0
    with mention of cervicitis 616.0
  cornea (recurrent) (*see also* Keratitis) 371.42
    traumatic 918.1
  dental (idiopathic) (occupational) 521.30 ▲
    extending into ●
      dentine 521.32 ●
      pulp 521.33 ●
    generalized 521.35 ●
    limited to enamel 521.31 ●
    localized 521.34 ●

Epiglottis — Erosion

Erosion — *continued*
  duodenum, postpyloric — *see* Ulcer, duodenum
  esophagus 530.89
  gastric 535.4 ☑
  intestine 569.89
  lymphatic vessel 457.8
  pylorus, pyloric (ulcer) 535.4 ☑
  sclera 379.16
  spine, aneurysmal 094.89
  spleen 289.59
  stomach 535.4 ☑
  teeth (idiopathic) (occupational) ▶(*see also*
      Erosion, dental)◀ 521.30   ▲
    due to
      medicine 521.30   ▲
      persistent vomiting 521.30   ▲
  urethra 599.84
  uterus 621.8
  vertebra 733.99
Erotomania 302.89
  Clérambault's 297.8
Error
  in diet 269.9
  refractive 367.9
    astigmatism (*see also* Astigmatism) 367.20
    drug-induced 367.89
    hypermetropia 367.0
    hyperopia 367.0
    myopia 367.1
    presbyopia 367.4
    toxic 367.89
Eructation 787.3
  nervous 306.4
  psychogenic 306.4
Eruption
  creeping 126.9
  drug — *see* Dermatitis, due to, drug
  Hutchinson, summer 692.72
  Kaposi's varicelliform 054.0
  napkin (psoriasiform) 691.0
  polymorphous
    light (sun) 692.72
      other source 692.82
  psoriasiform, napkin 691.0
  recalcitrant pustular 694.8
  ringed 695.89
  skin (*see also* Dermatitis) 782.1
    creeping (meaning hookworm) 126.9
    due to
      chemical(s) NEC 692.4
        internal use 693.8
      drug — *see* Dermatitis, due to, drug
      prophylactic inoculation or vaccination
          against disease — *see* Dermatitis,
          due to, vaccine
      smallpox vaccination NEC — *see*
          Dermatitis, due to, vaccine
    erysipeloid 027.1
    feigned 698.4
    Hutchinson, summer 692.72
    Kaposi's, varicelliform 054.0
      vaccinia 999.0
    lichenoid, axilla 698.3
    polymorphous, due to light 692.72
    toxic NEC 695.0
    vesicular 709.8
  teeth, tooth
    accelerated 520.6
    delayed 520.6
    difficult 520.6
    disturbance of 520.6
    in abnormal sequence 520.6
    incomplete 520.6
    late 520.6
    natal 520.6
    neonatal 520.6
    obstructed 520.6
    partial 520.6
    persistent primary 520.6
    premature 520.6
  vesicular 709.8
Erysipelas (gangrenous) (infantile) (newborn)
    (phlegmonous) (suppurative) 035
  external ear 035 *[380.13]*

Erysipelas — *continued*
  puerperal, postpartum, childbirth 670.0 ☑
Erysipelatoid (Rosenbach's) 027.1
Erysipeloid (Rosenbach's) 027.1
Erythema, erythematous (generalized) 695.9
  ab igne — *see* Burn, by site, first degree
  annulare (centrifugum) (rheumaticum) 695.0
  arthriticum epidemicum 026.1
  brucellum (*see also* Brucellosis) 023.9
  bullosum 695.1
  caloricum — *see* Burn, by site, first degree
  chronicum migrans 088.81
    chronicum 088.81
  circinatum 695.1
  diaper 691.0
  due to
    chemical (contact) NEC 692.4
      internal 693.8
    drug (internal use) 693.0
      contact 692.3
  elevatum diutinum 695.89
  endemic 265.2
  epidemic, arthritic 026.1
  figuratum perstans 695.0
  gluteal 691.0
  gyratum (perstans) (repens) 695.1
  heat — *see* Burn, by site, first degree
  ichthyosiforme congenitum 757.1
  induratum (primary) (scrofulosorum) (*see also*
      Tuberculosis) 017.1 ☑
    nontuberculous 695.2
  infantum febrile 057.8
  infectional NEC 695.9
  infectiosum 057.0
  inflammation NEC 695.9
  intertrigo 695.89
  iris 695.1
  lupus (discoid) (localized) (*see also* Lupus
      erythematosus) 695.4
  marginatum 695.0
    rheumaticum — *see* Fever, rheumatic
  medicamentosum — *see* Dermatitis, due to, drug
  migrans 529.1
    chronicum 088.81
  multiforme 695.1
    bullosum 695.1
    conjunctiva 695.1
    exudativum (Hebra) 695.1
    pemphigoides 694.5
  napkin 691.0
  neonatorum 778.8
  nodosum 695.2
    tuberculous (*see also* Tuberculosis) 017.1 ☑
  nummular, nummulare 695.1
  palmar 695.0
  palmaris hereditarium 695.0
  pernio 991.5
  perstans solare 692.72
  rash, newborn 778.8
  scarlatiniform (exfoliative) (recurrent) 695.0
  simplex marginatum 057.8
  solare (*see also* Sunburn) 692.71
  streptogenes 696.5
  toxic, toxicum NEC 695.0
    newborn 778.8
  tuberculous (primary) (*see also* Tuberculosis)
      017.0 ☑
  venenatum 695.0
Erythematosus — *see* condition
Erythematous — *see* condition
Erythermalgia (primary) 443.89
Erythralgia 443.89
Erythrasma 039.0
Erythredema 985.0
  polyneuritica 985.0
  polyneuropathy 985.0
Erythremia (acute) (M9841/3) 207.0 ☑
  chronic (M9842/3) 207.1 ☑
  secondary 289.0
Erythroblastopenia (acquired) 284.8
  congenital 284.0
Erythroblastophthisis 284.0

Erythroblastosis (fetalis) (newborn) 773.2
  due to
    ABO
      antibodies 773.1
      incompatibility, maternal/fetal 773.1
      isoimmunization 773.1
    Rh
      antibodies 773.0
      incompatibility, maternal/fetal 773.0
      isoimmunization 773.0
Erythrocyanosis (crurum) 443.89
Erythrocythemia — *see* Erythremia
Erythrocytopenia 285.9
Erythrocytosis (megalosplenic)
  familial 289.6
  oval, hereditary (*see also* Elliptocytosis) 282.1
  secondary 289.0
  stress 289.0
Erythroderma (*see also* Erythema) 695.9
  desquamativa (in infants) 695.89
  exfoliative 695.89
  ichthyosiform, congenital 757.1
  infantum 695.89
  maculopapular 696.2
  neonatorum 778.8
  psoriaticum 696.1
  secondary 695.9
Erythrogenesis imperfecta 284.0
Erythroleukemia (M9840/3) 207.0 ☑
Erythromelalgia 443.89
Erythromelia 701.8
Erythropenia 285.9
Erythrophagocytosis 289.9
Erythrophobia 300.23
Erythroplakia
  oral mucosa 528.79   ▲
  tongue 528.79   ▲
Erythroplasia (Queyrat) (M8080/2)
  specified site — *see* Neoplasm, skin, in situ
  unspecified site 233.5
Erythropoiesis, idiopathic ineffective 285.0
Escaped beats, heart 427.60
  postoperative 997.1
Esoenteritis — *see* Enteritis
Esophagalgia 530.89
Esophagectasis 530.89
  due to cardiospasm 530.0
Esophagismus 530.5
Esophagitis (alkaline) (chemical) (chronic)
    (infectional) (necrotic) (peptic) (postoperative)
    (regurgitant) 530.10
  acute 530.12
  candidal 112.84
  reflux 530.11
  specified NEC 530.19
  tuberculous (*see also* Tuberculosis) 017.8 ☑
  ulcerative 530.19
Esophagocele 530.6
Esophagodynia 530.89
Esophagomalacia 530.89
Esophagoptosis 530.89
Esophagospasm 530.5
Esophagostenosis 530.3
Esophagostomiasis 127.7
Esophagostomy   ●
  complication   ●
    infection 530.86   ●
    malfunctioning 530.87   ●
    mechanical 530.87   ●
Esophagotracheal — *see* condition
Esophagus — *see* condition
Esophoria 378.41
  convergence, excess 378.84
  divergence, insufficiency 378.85
Esotropia (nonaccommodative) 378.00
  accommodative 378.35
  alternating 378.05
    with
      A pattern 378.06
      specified noncomitancy NEC 378.08
      V pattern 378.07

Esotropia — *continued*
  alternating — *continued*
    with — *continued*
      X pattern 378.08
      Y pattern 378.08
      intermittent 378.22
    intermittent 378.20
      alternating 378.22
      monocular 378.21
    monocular 378.01
      with
        A pattern 378.02
        specified noncomitancy NEC 378.04
        V pattern 378.03
        X pattern 378.04
        Y pattern 378.04
        intermittent 378.21
Espundia 085.5
Essential — *see* condition
Esterapenia 289.89
Esthesioneuroblastoma (M9522/3) 160.0
Esthesioneurocytoma (M9521/3) 160.0
Esthesioneuroepithelioma (M9523/3) 160.0
Esthiomene 099.1
Estivo-autumnal
  fever 084.0
  malaria 084.0
Estrangement V61.0
Estriasis 134.0
Ethanolaminuria 270.8
Ethanolism (*see also* Alcoholism) 303.9 ☑
Ether dependence, dependency (*see also*
  Dependence) 304.6 ☑
Etherism (*see also* Dependence) 304.6 ☑
Ethmoid, ethmoidal — *see* condition
Ethmoiditis (chronic) (nonpurulent) (purulent)
  (*see also* Sinusitis, ethmoidal) 473.2
  influenzal 487.1
  Woakes' 471.1
Ethylism (*see also* Alcoholism) 303.9 ☑
Eulenburg's disease (congenital paramyotonia)
  359.2
Eunuchism 257.2
Eunuchoidism 257.2
  hypogonadotropic 257.2
European blastomycosis 117.5
Eustachian — *see* condition
Euthyroid sick syndrome 790.94
Euthyroidism 244.9
Evaluation
  fetal lung maturity 659.8 ☑
  for suspected condition (*see also* Observation)
    V71.9
    abuse V71.81
    exposure
      anthrax V71.82
      biologic agent NEC V71.83
      SARS V71.83
    neglect V71.81
    newborn — *see* Observation, suspected,
      condition, newborn
    specified condition NEC V71.89
  mental health V70.2
    requested by authority V70.1
  nursing care V63.8
  social service V63.8
Evan's syndrome (thrombocytopenic purpura)
  287.3
Eventration
  colon into chest — *see* Hernia, diaphragm
  diaphragm (congenital) 756.6
Eversion
  bladder 596.8
  cervix (uteri) 622.0
    with mention of cervicitis 616.0
  foot NEC 736.79
    congenital 755.67
  lacrimal punctum 375.51
  punctum lacrimale (postinfectional) (senile)
    375.51
  ureter (meatus) 593.89
  urethra (meatus) 599.84

Eversion — *continued*
  uterus 618.1
    complicating delivery 665.2 ☑
      affecting fetus or newborn 763.89
    puerperal, postpartum 674.8 ☑
Evidence ●
  of malignancy ●
    cytologic ●
      without histologic confirmation ●
      795.04 ●
Evisceration
  birth injury 767.8
  bowel (congenital) — *see* Hernia, ventral
  congenital (*see also* Hernia, ventral) 553.29
  operative wound 998.32
  traumatic NEC 869.1
    eye 871.3
Evulsion — *see* Avulsion
Ewing's
  angioendothelioma (M9260/3) — *see* Neoplasm,
    bone, malignant
  sarcoma (M9260/3) — *see* Neoplasm, bone,
    malignant
  tumor (M9260/3) — *see* Neoplasm, bone,
    malignant
Exaggerated lumbosacral angle (with impinging
  spine) 756.12
Examination (general) (routine) (of) (for) V70.9
  allergy V72.7
  annual V70.0
  cardiovascular preoperative V72.81
  cervical Papanicolaou smear V76.2
    as a part of routine gynecological
      examination V72.31 ▲
    to confirm findings of recent normal ●
      smear following initial abnormal ●
      smear V72.32 ●
  child care (routine) V20.2
  clinical research investigation (normal control
    patient) (participant) V70.7
  dental V72.2
  developmental testing (child) (infant) V20.2
  donor (potential) V70.8
  ear V72.1
  eye V72.0
  following
    accident (motor vehicle) V71.4
    alleged rape or seduction (victim or culprit)
      V71.5
    inflicted injury (victim or culprit) NEC V71.6
    rape or seduction, alleged (victim or culprit)
      V71.5
    treatment (for) V67.9
      combined V67.6
      fracture V67.4
      involving high-risk medication NEC
        V67.51
      mental disorder V67.3
      specified condition NEC V67.59
  follow-up (routine) (following) V67.9
    cancer chemotherapy V67.2
    chemotherapy V67.2
    disease NEC V67.59
    high-risk medication NEC V67.51
    injury NEC V67.59
    population survey V70.6
    postpartum V24.2
    psychiatric V67.3
    psychotherapy V67.3
    radiotherapy V67.1
    specified surgery NEC V67.09
    surgery V67.00
      vaginal pap smear V67.01
  gynecological V72.31 ▲
    for contraceptive maintenance V25.40
      intrauterine device V25.42
      pill V25.41
      specified method NEC V25.49
  health (of)
    armed forces personnel V70.5
    checkup V70.0
    child, routine V20.2
    defined subpopulation NEC V70.5
    inhabitants of institutions V70.5
    occupational V70.5
    pre-employment screening V70.5

Examination — *continued*
  health (of) — *continued*
    preschool children V70.5
      for admission to school V70.3
    prisoners V70.5
      for entrance into prison V70.3
    prostitutes V70.5
    refugees V70.5
    school children V70.5
    students V70.5
  hearing V72.1
  infant V20.2
  laboratory V72.6
  lactating mother V24.1
  medical (for) (of) V70.9
    administrative purpose NEC V70.3
    admission to
      old age home V70.3
      prison V70.3
      school V70.3
    adoption V70.3
    armed forces personnel V70.5
    at health care facility V70.0
    camp V70.3
    child, routine V20.2
    clinical research investigation (control)
      (normal comparison) (participant) V70.7
    defined subpopulation NEC V70.5
    donor (potential) V70.8
    driving license V70.3
    general V70.9
      routine V70.0
      specified reason NEC V70.8
    immigration V70.3
    inhabitants of institutions V70.5
    insurance certification V70.3
    marriage V70.3
    medicolegal reasons V70.4
    naturalization V70.3
    occupational V70.5
    population survey V70.6
    pre-employment V70.5
    preschool children V70.5
      for admission to school V70.3
    prison V70.3
    prisoners V70.5
      for entrance into prison V70.3
    prostitutes V70.5
    refugees V70.5
    school children V70.5
    specified reason NEC V70.8
    sport competition V70.3
    students V70.5
  medicolegal reason V70.4
  pelvic (annual) (periodic) V72.31 ▲
  periodic (annual) (routine) V70.0
  postpartum
    immediately after delivery V24.0
    routine follow-up V24.2
  pregnancy (unconfirmed) (possible) V72.40 ▲
    negative result V72.41 ●
  prenatal V22.1
    first pregnancy V22.0
    high-risk pregnancy V23.9
      specified problem NEC V23.8 ☑
  preoperative V72.84
    cardiovascular V72.81
    respiratory V72.82
    specified NEC V72.83
  psychiatric V70.2
    follow-up not needing further care V67.3
    requested by authority V70.1
  radiological NEC V72.5
  respiratory preoperative V72.82
  screening — *see* Screening
  sensitization V72.7
  skin V72.7
    hypersensitivity V72.7
  special V72.9
  specified type or reason NEC V72.85
    preoperative V72.83
      specified NEC V72.83
  teeth V72.2
  vaginal Papanicolaou smear V76.47
    following hysterectomy for malignant
      condition V67.01

☑ Additional Digit Required   ▶◀ Revised Text   ● New Line   ▲ Revised Code

Examination — *continued*
  victim or culprit following
    alleged rape or seduction V71.5
    inflicted injury NEC V71.6
  vision V72.0
  well baby V20.2

Exanthem, exanthema (*see also* Rash) 782.1
  Boston 048
  epidemic, with meningitis 048
  lichenoid psoriasiform 696.2
  subitum 057.8
  viral, virus NEC 057.9
    specified type NEC 057.8

Excess, excessive, excessively
  alcohol level in blood 790.3
  carbohydrate tissue, localized 278.1
  carotene (dietary) 278.3
  cold 991.9
    specified effect NEC 991.8
  convergence 378.84
  crying of infant (baby) 780.92
  development, breast 611.1
  diaphoresis ▶(*see also* Hyperhidrosis)◀ 780.8
  distance, interarch 524.28 ●
  divergence 378.85
  drinking (alcohol) NEC (*see also* Abuse, drugs, nondependent) 305.0 ☑
    continual (*see also* Alcoholism) 303.9 ☑
    habitual (*see also* Alcoholism) 303.9 ☑
  eating 783.6
  eyelid fold (congenital) 743.62
  fat 278.00
    in heart (*see also* Degeneration, myocardial) 429.1
    tissue, localized 278.1
  foreskin 605
  gas 787.3
  gastrin 251.5
  glucagon 251.4
  heat (*see also* Heat) 992.9
  horizontal overlap 524.26 ●
  interarch distance 524.28 ●
  interocclusal distance of teeth 524.37 ●
  large
    colon 564.7
      congenital 751.3
    fetus or infant 766.0
      with obstructed labor 660.1 ☑
      affecting management of pregnancy 656.6 ☑
      causing disproportion 653.5 ☑
    newborn (weight of 4500 grams or more) 766.0
    organ or site, congenital NEC — *see* Anomaly, specified type NEC
  lid fold (congenital) 743.62
  long
    colon 751.5
    organ or site, congenital NEC — *see* Anomaly, specified type NEC
    umbilical cord (entangled)
      affecting fetus or newborn 762.5
      in pregnancy or childbirth 663.3 ☑
      with compression 663.2 ☑
  menstruation 626.2
  number of teeth 520.1
    causing crowding 524.31 ▲
  nutrients (dietary) NEC 783.6
  potassium (K) 276.7
  salivation (*see also* Ptyalism) 527.7
  secretion — *see also* Hypersecretion
    milk 676.6 ☑
    sputum 786.4
    sweat ▶(*see also* Hyperhidrosis)◀ 780.8
  short
    organ or site, congenital NEC — *see* Anomaly, specified type NEC
    umbilical cord
      affecting fetus or newborn 762.6
      in pregnancy or childbirth 663.4 ☑
  skin NEC 701.9
    eyelid 743.62
      acquired 374.30
  sodium (Na) 276.0
  spacing of teeth 524.32 ●
  sputum 786.4

Excess, excessive, excessively — *continued*
  sweating ▶(*see also* Hyperhidrosis)◀ 780.8
  tearing (ducts) (eye) (*see also* Epiphora) 375.20
  thirst 783.5
    due to deprivation of water 994.3
  tuberosity 524.07 ●
  vitamin
    A (dietary) 278.2
      administered as drug (chronic) (prolonged excessive intake) 278.2
      reaction to sudden overdose 963.5
    D (dietary) 278.4
      administered as drug (chronic) (prolonged excessive intake) 278.4
      reaction to sudden overdose 963.5
  weight 278.00
    gain 783.1
      of pregnancy 646.1 ☑
    loss 783.21

Excitability, abnormal, under minor stress 309.29

Excitation
  catatonic (*see also* Schizophrenia) 295.2 ☑
  psychogenic 298.1
  reactive (from emotional stress, psychological trauma) 298.1

Excitement
  manic (*see also* Psychosis, affective) 296.0 ☑
    recurrent episode 296.1 ☑
    single episode 296.0 ☑
  mental, reactive (from emotional stress, psychological trauma) 298.1
  state, reactive (from emotional stress, psychological trauma) 298.1

Excluded pupils 364.76

Excoriation (traumatic) (*see also* Injury, superficial, by site) 919.8
  neurotic 698.4

Excyclophoria 378.44

Excyclotropia 378.33

Exencephalus, exencephaly 742.0

Exercise
  breathing V57.0
  remedial NEC V57.1
  therapeutic NEC V57.1

Exfoliation, teeth due to systemic causes 525.0

Exfoliative — *see also* condition dermatitis 695.89

Exhaustion, exhaustive (physical NEC) 780.79
  battle (*see also* Reaction, stress, acute) 308.9
  cardiac (*see also* Failure, heart) 428.9
  delirium (*see also* Reaction, stress, acute) 308.9
  due to
    cold 991.8
    excessive exertion 994.5
    exposure 994.4
  fetus or newborn 779.89
  heart (*see also* Failure, heart) 428.9
  heat 992.5
    due to
      salt depletion 992.4
      water depletion 992.3
  manic (*see also* Psychosis, affective) 296.0 ☑
    recurrent episode 296.1 ☑
    single episode 296.0 ☑
  maternal, complicating delivery 669.8 ☑
    affecting fetus or newborn 763.89
  mental 300.5
  myocardium, myocardial (*see also* Failure, heart) 428.9
  nervous 300.5
  old age 797
  postinfectional NEC 780.79
  psychogenic 300.5
  psychosis (*see also* Reaction, stress, acute) 308.9
  senile 797
    dementia 290.0

Exhibitionism (sexual) 302.4

Exomphalos 756.79

Exophoria 378.42
  convergence, insufficiency 378.83
  divergence, excess 378.85

Exophthalmic
  cachexia 242.0 ☑
  goiter 242.0 ☑
  ophthalmoplegia 242.0 ☑ *[376.22]*

Exophthalmos 376.30
  congenital 743.66
  constant 376.31
  endocrine NEC 259.9 *[376.22]*
  hyperthyroidism 242.0 ☑ *[376.21]*
  intermittent NEC 376.34
  malignant 242.0 ☑ *[376.21]*
  pulsating 376.35
    endocrine NEC 259.9 *[376.22]*
  thyrotoxic 242.0 ☑ *[376.21]*

Exostosis 726.91
  cartilaginous (M9210/0) — *see* Neoplasm, bone, benign
  congenital 756.4
  ear canal, external 380.81
  gonococcal 098.89
  hip 726.5
  intracranial 733.3
  jaw (bone) 526.81
  luxurians 728.11
  multiple (cancellous) (congenital) (hereditary) 756.4
  nasal bones 726.91
  orbit, orbital 376.42
  osteocartilaginous (M9210/0) — *see* Neoplasm, bone, benign
  spine 721.8
    with spondylosis — *see* Spondylosis
  syphilitic 095.5
  wrist 726.4

Exotropia 378.10
  alternating 378.15
    with
      A pattern 378.16
      specified noncomitancy NEC 378.18
      V pattern 378.17
      X pattern 378.18
      Y pattern 378.18
      intermittent 378.24
  intermittent 378.20
    alternating 378.24
    monocular 378.23
  monocular 378.11
    with
      A pattern 378.12
      specified noncomitancy NEC 378.14
      V pattern 378.13
      X pattern 378.14
      Y pattern 378.14
      intermittent 378.23

Explanation of
  investigation finding V65.4 ☑
  medication V65.4 ☑

Exposure 994.9
  cold 991.9
    specified effect NEC 991.8
  effects of 994.9
  exhaustion due to 994.4
  to
    AIDS virus V01.79 ▲
    anthrax V01.81
    asbestos V15.84
    body fluids (hazardous) V15.85
    cholera V01.0
    communicable disease V01.9
      specified type NEC V01.89
    Escherichia coli (E. coli) V01.83 ●
    German measles V01.4
    gonorrhea V01.6
    hazardous body fluids V15.85
    HIV V01.79 ▲
    human immunodeficiency virus V01.79 ▲
    lead V15.86
    meningococcus V01.84 ●
    parasitic disease V01.89
    poliomyelitis V01.2
    potentially hazardous body fluids V15.85
    rabies V01.5
    rubella V01.4
    SARS-associated coronavirus V01.82
    smallpox V01.3
    syphilis V01.6

Examination — Exposure

Exposure — *continued*
- to — *continued*
  - tuberculosis V01.1
  - varicella V01.71   ●
  - venereal disease V01.6
  - viral disease NEC V01.79   ▲
    - varicella V01.71   ●

Exsanguination, fetal 772.0

Exstrophy
- abdominal content 751.8
- bladder (urinary) 753.5

Extensive — *see* condition

Extra — *see also* Accessory
- rib 756.3
  - cervical 756.2

Extraction
- with hook 763.89
- breech NEC 669.6 ☑
  - affecting fetus or newborn 763.0
- cataract postsurgical V45.61
- manual NEC 669.8 ☑
  - affecting fetus or newborn 763.89

Extrasystole 427.60
- atrial 427.61
- postoperative 997.1
- ventricular 427.69

Extrauterine gestation or pregnancy — *see* Pregnancy, ectopic

Extravasation
- blood 459.0
  - lower extremity 459.0
- chyle into mesentery 457.8
- pelvicalyceal 593.4
- pyelosinus 593.4
- urine 788.8
  - from ureter 788.8

Extremity — *see* condition

Extrophy — *see* Exstrophy

Extroversion
- bladder 753.5
- uterus 618.1
  - complicating delivery 665.2 ☑
    - affecting fetus or newborn 763.89
  - postpartal (old) 618.1

Extrusion
- alveolus and teeth 524.75   ●
- breast implant (prosthetic) 996.54
- device, implant, or graft — *see* Complications, mechanical
- eye implant (ball) (globe) 996.59
- intervertebral disc — *see* Displacement, intervertebral disc
- lacrimal gland 375.43
- mesh (reinforcing) 996.59
- ocular lens implant 996.53
- prosthetic device NEC — *see* Complications, mechanical
- vitreous 379.26

Exudate, pleura — *see* Effusion, pleura

Exudates, retina 362.82

Exudative — *see* condition

Eye, eyeball, eyelid — *see* condition

Eyestrain 368.13

Eyeworm disease of Africa 125.2

F

Faber's anemia or syndrome (achlorhydric anemia) 280.9

Fabry's disease (angiokeratoma corporis diffusum) 272.7

Face, facial — *see* condition

Facet of cornea 371.44

Faciocephalalgia, autonomic (*see also* Neuropathy, peripheral, autonomic) 337.9

Facioscapulohumeral myopathy 359.1

Factitious disorder, illness — *see* Illness, factitious

Factor
- deficiency — *see* Deficiency, factor
- psychic, associated with diseases classified elsewhere 316
- risk — *see* Problem

Fahr-Volhard disease (malignant nephrosclerosis) 403.00

Failure, failed
- adenohypophyseal 253.2
- attempted abortion (legal) (*see also* Abortion, failed) 638.9
- bone marrow (anemia) 284.9
  - acquired (secondary) 284.8
  - congenital 284.0
  - idiopathic 284.9
- cardiac (*see also* Failure, heart) 428.9
  - newborn 779.89
- cardiorenal (chronic) 428.9
  - hypertensive (*see also* Hypertension, cardiorenal) 404.93
- cardiorespiratory 799.1
  - specified during or due to a procedure 997.1
    - long-term effect of cardiac surgery 429.4
- cardiovascular (chronic) 428.9
- cerebrovascular 437.8
- cervical dilatation in labor 661.0 ☑
  - affecting fetus or newborn 763.7
- circulation, circulatory 799.89
  - fetus or newborn 779.89
  - peripheral 785.50
- compensation — *see* Disease, heart
- congestive (*see also* Failure, heart) 428.0
- coronary (*see also* Insufficiency, coronary) 411.89
- descent of head (at term) 652.5 ☑
  - affecting fetus or newborn 763.1
  - in labor 660.0 ☑
    - affecting fetus or newborn 763.1
- device, implant, or graft — *see* Complications, mechanical
- engagement of head NEC 652.5 ☑
  - in labor 660.0 ☑
- extrarenal 788.9
- fetal head to enter pelvic brim 652.5 ☑
  - affecting fetus or newborn 763.1
  - in labor 660.0 ☑
    - affecting fetus or newborn 763.1
- forceps NEC 660.7 ☑
  - affecting fetus or newborn 763.1
- fusion (joint) (spinal) 996.4
- growth in childhood 783.43
- heart (acute) (sudden) 428.9
  - with
    - abortion — *see* Abortion, by type, with specified complication NEC
    - acute pulmonary edema (*see also* Failure, ventricular, left) 428.1
      - with congestion (*see also* Failure, heart) 428.0
    - decompensation (*see also* Failure, heart) 428.0
    - dilation — *see* Disease, heart
    - ectopic pregnancy (*see also* categories 633.0-633.9) 639.8
    - molar pregnancy (*see also* categories 630-632) 639.8
  - arteriosclerotic 440.9
  - combined left-right sided 428.0
  - combined systolic and diastolic 428.40
    - acute 428.41
    - acute on chronic 428.43
    - chronic 428.42
  - compensated (*see also* Failure, heart) 428.0
  - complicating
    - abortion — *see* Abortion, by type, with specified complication NEC
    - delivery (cesarean) (instrumental) 669.4 ☑
    - ectopic pregnancy (*see also* categories 633.0-633.9) 639.8
    - molar pregnancy (*see also* categories 630-632) 639.8
    - obstetric anesthesia or sedation 668.1 ☑
    - surgery 997.1
  - congestive (compensated) (decompensated) (*see also* Failure, heart) 428.0
    - with rheumatic fever (conditions classifiable to 390)
      - active 391.8
      - inactive or quiescent (with chorea) 398.91

Failure, failed — *continued*
- heart — *continued*
  - congestive (*see also* Failure, heart) — *continued*
    - fetus or newborn 779.89
    - hypertensive (*see also* Hypertension, heart) 402.90
      - with renal disease (*see also* Hypertension, cardiorenal) 404.91
        - with renal failure 404.93
      - benign 402.11
      - malignant 402.01
    - rheumatic (chronic) (inactive) (with chorea) 398.91
      - active or acute 391.8
        - with chorea (Sydenham's) 392.0
  - decompensated (*see also* Failure, heart) 428.0
  - degenerative (*see also* Degeneration, myocardial) 429.1
  - diastolic 428.30
    - acute 428.31
    - acute on chronic 428.33
    - chronic 428.32
  - due to presence of (cardiac) prosthesis 429.4
  - fetus or newborn 779.89
  - following
    - abortion 639.8
    - cardiac surgery 429.4
    - ectopic or molar pregnancy 639.8
  - high output NEC 428.9
  - hypertensive (*see also* Hypertension, heart) 402.91
    - with renal disease (*see also* Hypertension, cardiorenal) 404.91
      - with renal failure 404.93
    - benign 402.11
    - malignant 402.01
  - left (ventricular) (*see also* Failure, ventricular, left) 428.1
    - with right-sided failure (see also Failure, heart) 428.0
  - low output (syndrome) NEC 428.9
  - organic — *see* Disease, heart
  - postoperative (immediate) 997.1
    - long term effect of cardiac surgery 429.4
  - rheumatic (chronic) (congestive) (inactive) 398.91
  - right (secondary to left heart failure, conditions classifiable to 428.1) (ventricular) (*see also* Failure, heart) 428.0
  - senile 797
  - specified during or due to a procedure 997.1
    - long-term effect of cardiac surgery 429.4
  - systolic 428.20
    - acute 428.21
    - acute on chronic 428.23
    - chronic 428.22
  - thyrotoxic (*see also* Thyrotoxicosis) 242.9 ☑ *[425.7]*
  - valvular — *see* Endocarditis
- hepatic 572.8
  - acute 570
  - due to a procedure 997.4
- hepatorenal 572.4
- hypertensive heart (*see also* Hypertension, heart) 402.91
  - benign 402.11
  - malignant 402.01
- induction (of labor) 659.1 ☑
  - abortion (legal) (*see also* Abortion, failed) 638.9
  - affecting fetus or newborn 763.89
  - by oxytocic drugs 659.1 ☑
  - instrumental 659.0 ☑
  - mechanical 659.0 ☑
  - medical 659.1 ☑
  - surgical 659.0 ☑
- initial alveolar expansion, newborn 770.4
- involution, thymus (gland) 254.8
- kidney — *see* Failure, renal
- lactation 676.4 ☑
- Leydig's cell, adult 257.2
- liver 572.8
  - acute 570
- medullary 799.89

Failure, failed — *continued*
mitral — *see* Endocarditis, mitral
myocardium, myocardial (*see also* Failure, heart) 428.9
  chronic (*see also* Failure, heart) 428.0
  congestive (*see also* Failure, heart) 428.0
ovarian (primary) 256.39
  iatrogenic 256.2
  postablative 256.2
  postirradiation 256.2
  postsurgical 256.2
ovulation 628.0
prerenal 788.9
renal 586
  with
    abortion — *see* Abortion, by type, with renal failure
    ectopic pregnancy (*see also* categories 633.0-633.9) 639.3
    edema (*see also* Nephrosis) 581.9
    hypertension (*see also* Hypertension, kidney) 403.91
    hypertensive heart disease (conditions classifiable to 402) 404.92
      with heart failure 404.93
      benign 404.12
        with heart failure 404.13
      malignant 404.02
        with heart failure 404.03
    molar pregnancy (*see also* categories 630-632) 639.3
    tubular necrosis (acute) 584.5
  acute 584.9
    with lesion of
      necrosis
        cortical (renal) 584.6
        medullary (renal) (papillary) 584.7
        tubular 584.5
      specified pathology NEC 584.8
  chronic 585
    hypertensive or with hypertension (*see also* Hypertension, kidney) 403.91
  due to a procedure 997.5
  following
    abortion 639.3
    crushing 958.5
    ectopic or molar pregnancy 639.3
    labor and delivery (acute) 669.3 ☑
  hypertensive (*see also* Hypertension, kidney) 403.91
  puerperal, postpartum 669.3 ☑
respiration, respiratory 518.81
  acute 518.81
  acute and chronic 518.84
  center 348.8
    newborn 770.84
  chronic 518.83
  due to trauma, surgery or shock 518.5
  newborn 770.84
rotation
  cecum 751.4
  colon 751.4
  intestine 751.4
  kidney 753.3
segmentation — *see also* Fusion
  fingers (*see also* Syndactylism, fingers) 755.11
  toes (*see also* Syndactylism, toes) 755.13
seminiferous tubule, adult 257.2
senile (general) 797
  with psychosis 290.20
testis, primary (seminal) 257.2
to progress 661.2 ☑
to thrive
  adult 783.7
  child 783.41
transplant 996.80
  bone marrow 996.85
  organ (immune or nonimmune cause) 996.80
    bone marrow 996.85
    heart 996.83
    intestines 996.87
    kidney 996.81
    liver 996.82
    lung 996.84
    pancreas 996.86
    specified NEC 996.89

Failure, failed — *continued*
transplant — *continued*
  skin 996.52
    artificial 996.55
    decellularized allodermis 996.55
    temporary allograft or pigskin graft — *omit code*
trial of labor NEC 660.6 ☑
  affecting fetus or newborn 763.1
tubal ligation 998.89 ●
urinary 586
vacuum extraction
  abortion — *see* Abortion, failed
  delivery NEC 660.7 ☑
    affecting fetus or newborn 763.1
vasectomy 998.89 ●
ventouse NEC 660.7 ☑
  affecting fetus or newborn 763.1
ventricular (*see also* Failure, heart) 428.9
  left 428.1
    with rheumatic fever (conditions classifiable to 390)
      active 391.8
        with chorea 392.0
      inactive or quiescent (with chorea) 398.91
    hypertensive (*see also* Hypertension, heart) 402.91
      benign 402.11
      malignant 402.01
    rheumatic (chronic) (inactive) (with chorea) 398.91
      active or acute 391.8
        with chorea 392.0
  right (*see also* Failure, heart) 428.0
vital centers, fetus or newborn 779.8 ☑
weight gain in childhood 783.41

Fainting (fit) (spell) 780.2
Falciform hymen 752.49
Fall, maternal, affecting fetus or newborn 760.5
Fallen arches 734
Falling, any organ or part — *see* Prolapse
Fallopian
insufflation
  fertility testing V26.21
  following sterilization reversal V26.22
tube — *see* condition
Fallot's
pentalogy 745.2
tetrad or tetralogy 745.2
triad or trilogy 746.09
Fallout, radioactive (adverse effect) NEC 990
False — *see also* condition
bundle branch block 426.50
bursa 727.89
croup 478.75
joint 733.82
labor (pains) 644.1 ☑
opening, urinary, male 752.69
passage, urethra (prostatic) 599.4
positive
  serological test for syphilis 795.6
  Wassermann reaction 795.6
pregnancy 300.11
Family, familial — *see also* condition
disruption V61.0
Li-Fraumeni (syndrome) V84.01 ●
planning advice V25.09
problem V61.9
  specified circumstance NEC V61.8
retinoblastoma (syndrome) 190.5 ●
Famine 994.2
edema 262
Fanconi's anemia (congenital pancytopenia) 284.0
Fanconi (-de Toni) (-Debré) syndrome (cystinosis) 270.0
Farber (-Uzman) syndrome or disease (disseminated lipogranulomatosis) 272.8
Farcin 024
Farcy 024

Farmers'
lung 495.0
skin 692.74
Farsightedness 367.0
Fascia — *see* condition
Fasciculation 781.0
Fasciculitis optica 377.32
Fasciitis 729.4
eosinophilic 728.89
necrotizing 728.86
nodular 728.79
perirenal 593.4
plantar 728.71
pseudosarcomatous 728.79
traumatic (old) NEC 728.79
  current — *see* Sprain, by site
Fasciola hepatica infestation 121.3
Fascioliasis 121.3
Fasciolopsiasis (small intestine) 121.4
Fasciolopsis (small intestine) 121.4
Fast pulse 785.0
Fat
embolism (cerebral) (pulmonary) (systemic) 958.1
  with
    abortion — *see* Abortion, by type, with embolism
    ectopic pregnancy (*see also* categories 633.0-633.9) 639.6
    molar pregnancy (*see also* categories 630-632) 639.6
  complicating delivery or puerperium 673.8 ☑
  following
    abortion 639.6
    ectopic or molar pregnancy 639.6
  in pregnancy, childbirth, or the puerperium 673.8 ☑
excessive 278.00
  in heart (*see also* Degeneration, myocardial) 429.1
general 278.00
hernia, herniation 729.30
  eyelid 374.34
  knee 729.31
  orbit 374.34
  retro-orbital 374.34
  retropatellar 729.31
  specified site NEC 729.39
indigestion 579.8
in stool 792.1
localized (pad) 278.1
  heart (*see also* Degeneration, myocardial) 429.1
  knee 729.31
  retropatellar 729.31
necrosis — *see also* Fatty, degeneration breast (aseptic) (segmental) 611.3
  mesentery 567.8
  omentum 567.8
pad 278.1
Fatal syncope 798.1
Fatigue 780.79
auditory deafness (*see also* Deafness) 389.9
chronic 780.7 ☑
chronic, syndrome 780.71
combat (*see also* Reaction, stress, acute) 308.9
during pregnancy 646.8 ☑
general 780.79
  psychogenic 300.5
heat (transient) 992.6
muscle 729.89
myocardium (*see also* Failure, heart) 428.9
nervous 300.5
neurosis 300.5
operational 300.89
postural 729.89
posture 729.89
psychogenic (general) 300.5
senile 797
syndrome NEC 300.5
  chronic 780.71
undue 780.79

☑ Additional Digit Required   ▶◀ Revised Text   ● New Line   ▲ Revised Code

Fatigue — *continued*
  voice 784.49
Fatness 278.00
Fatty — *see also* condition
  apron 278.1
  degeneration (diffuse) (general) NEC 272.8
    localized — *see* Degeneration, by site, fatty
    placenta — *see* Placenta, abnormal
  heart (enlarged) (*see also* Degeneration,
    myocardial) 429.1
  infiltration (diffuse) (general) (*see also*
    Degeneration, by site, fatty) 272.8
    heart (enlarged) (*see also* Degeneration,
      myocardial) 429.1
  liver 571.8
    alcoholic 571.0
  necrosis — *see* Degeneration, fatty
  phanerosis 272.8
Fauces — *see* condition
Fauchard's disease (periodontitis) 523.4
Faucitis 478.29
Faulty — *see also* condition
  position of teeth 524.30   ▲
Favism (anemia) 282.2
Favre-Racouchot disease (elastoidosis cutanea
    nodularis) 701.8
Favus 110.9
  beard 110.0
  capitis 110.0
  corporis 110.5
  eyelid 110.8
  foot 110.4
  hand 110.2
  scalp 110.0
  specified site NEC 110.8
Fear, fearfullness (complex) (reaction) 300.20
  child 313.0
  of
    animals 300.29
    closed spaces 300.29
    crowds 300.29
    eating in public 300.23
    heights 300.29
    open spaces 300.22
      with panic attacks 300.21
    public speaking 300.23
    streets 300.22
      with panic attacks 300.21
    travel 300.22
      with panic attacks 300.21
    washing in public 300.23
  transient 308.0
Feared complaint unfounded V65.5
Febricula (continued) (simple) (*see also* Pyrexia)
    780.6
Febrile (*see also* Pyrexia) 780.6
  convulsion 780.31
  seizure 780.31
Febris (*see also* Fever) 780.6
  aestiva (*see also* Fever, hay) 477.9
  flava (*see also* Fever, yellow) 060.9
  melitensis 023.0
  pestis (*see also* Plague) 020.9
  puerperalis 672.0 ☑
  recurrens (*see also* Fever, relapsing) 087.9
    pediculo vestimenti 087.0
  rubra 034.1
  typhoidea 002.0
  typhosa 002.0
Fecal — *see* condition
Fecalith (impaction) 560.39
  with hernia — *see also* Hernia, by site, with
      obstruction
    gangrenous — *see* Hernia, by site, with
        gangrene
  appendix 543.9
  congenital 777.1
Fede's disease 529.0
Feeble-minded 317
**Feeble rapid pulse due to shock following
    injury** 958.4

Feeding
  faulty (elderly) 783.3
    newborn 779.3
  formula check V20.2
  improper (elderly) (infant) 783.3
    newborn 779.3
  problem (elderly) 783.3
    infancy or early childhood 307.59   ●
    newborn 779.3
    nonorganic origin 307.59
Feer's disease 985.0
Feet — *see* condition
Feigned illness V65.2
Feil-Klippel syndrome (brevicollis) 756.16
Feinmesser's (hidrotic) **ectodermal dysplasia**
    757.31
Felix's disease (juvenile osteochondrosis, hip)
    732.1
Felon (any digit) (with lymphangitis) 681.01
  herpetic 054.6
Felty's syndrome (rheumatoid arthritis with
    splenomegaly and leukopenia) 714.1
Feminism in boys 302.6
Feminization, testicular 257.8
  with pseudohermaphroditism, male 257.8
Femoral hernia — *see* Hernia, femoral
Femora vara 736.32
Femur, femoral — *see* condition
Fenestrata placenta — *see* Placenta, abnormal
Fenestration, fenestrated — *see also* Imperfect,
    closure
  aorta-pulmonary 745.0
  aorticopulmonary 745.0
  aortopulmonary 745.0
  cusps, heart valve NEC 746.89
    pulmonary 746.09
  hymen 752.49
  pulmonic cusps 746.09
Fenwick's disease 537.89
Fermentation (gastric) (gastrointestinal)
    (stomach) 536.8
  intestine 564.89
    psychogenic 306.4
  psychogenic 306.4
Fernell's disease (aortic aneurysm) 441.9
Fertile eunuch syndrome 257.2
Fertility, meaning multiparity — *see* Multiparity
Fetal alcohol syndrome 760.71
Fetalis uterus 752.3
Fetid
  breath 784.9
  sweat 705.89
Fetishism 302.81
  transvestic 302.3
Fetomaternal hemorrhage
  affecting management of pregnancy 656.0 ☑
  fetus or newborn 772.0
Fetus, fetal — *see also* condition
  papyraceous 779.89
  type lung tissue 770.4
Fever 780.6
  with chills 780.6
    in malarial regions (*see also* Malaria) 084.6
  abortus NEC 023.9
  Aden 061
  African tick-borne 087.1
  American
    mountain tick 066.1
    spotted 082.0
  and ague (*see also* Malaria) 084.6
  aphthous 078.4
  arbovirus hemorrhagic 065.9
  Assam 085.0
  Australian A or Q 083.0
  Bangkok hemorrhagic 065.4
  biliary, Charcôt's intermittent — *see*
      Choledocholithiasis
  bilious, hemoglobinuric 084.8
  blackwater 084.8
  blister 054.9
  Bonvale Dam 780.79
  boutonneuse 082.1

Fever — *continued*
  brain 323.9
    late effect — *see* category 326
  breakbone 061
  Bullis 082.8
  Bunyamwera 066.3
  Burdwan 085.0
  Bwamba (encephalitis) 066.3
  Cameroon (*see also* Malaria) 084.6
  Canton 081.9
  catarrhal (acute) 460
    chronic 472.0
  cat-scratch 078.3
  cerebral 323.9
    late effect — *see* category 326
  cerebrospinal (meningococcal) (*see also*
      Meningitis, cerebrospinal) 036.0
  Chagres 084.0
  Chandipura 066.8
  changuinola 066.0
  Charcôt's (biliary) (hepatic) (intermittent) *see*
      Choledocholithiasis
  Chikungunya (viral) 066.3
    hemorrhagic 065.4
  childbed 670.0 ☑
  Chitral 066.0
  Colombo (*see also* Fever, paratyphoid) 002.9
  Colorado tick (virus) 066.1
  congestive
    malarial (*see also* Malaria) 084.6
    remittent (*see also* Malaria) 084.6
  Congo virus 065.0
  continued 780.6
    malarial 084.0
  Corsican (*see also* Malaria) 084.6
  Crimean hemorrhagic 065.0
  Cyprus (*see also* Brucellosis) 023.9
  dandy 061
  deer fly (*see also* Tularemia) 021.9
  dehydration, newborn 778.4
  dengue (virus) 061
    hemorrhagic 065.4
  desert 114.0
  due to heat 992.0
  Dumdum 085.0
  enteric 002.0
  ephemeral (of unknown origin) (*see also*
      Pyrexia) 780.6
  epidemic, hemorrhagic of the Far East 065.0
  erysipelatous (*see also* Erysipelas) 035
  estivo-autumnal (malarial) 084.0
  etiocholanolone 277.3
  famine — *see also* Fever, relapsing
    meaning typhus — *see* Typhus
  Far Eastern hemorrhagic 065.0
  five day 083.1
  Fort Bragg 100.89
  gastroenteric 002.0
  gastromalarial (*see also* Malaria) 084.6
  Gibraltar (*see also* Brucellosis) 023.9
  glandular 075
  Guama (viral) 066.3
  Haverhill 026.1
  hay (allergic) (with rhinitis) 477.9
    with
      asthma (bronchial) (*see also* Asthma)
        493.0 ☑
    due to
      dander, ▶animal (cat) (dog)◄ 477.2   ▲
      dust 477.8
      fowl 477.8
      hair, animal (cat) (dog) 477.2   ●
      pollen, any plant or tree 477.0
      specified allergen other than pollen 477.8
  heat (effects) 992.0
  hematuric, bilious 084.8
  hemoglobinuric (malarial) 084.8
    bilious 084.8
  hemorrhagic (arthropod-borne) NEC 065.9
    with renal syndrome 078.6
    arenaviral 078.7
    Argentine 078.7
    Bangkok 065.4
    Bolivian 078.7
    Central Asian 065.0
    chikungunya 065.4
    Crimean 065.0

Fatigue — Fever

Fever

hemorrhagic — *continued*
    dengue (virus) 065.4
    Ebola 065.8
    epidemic 078.6
        of Far East 065.0
    Far Eastern 065.0
    Junin virus 078.7
    Korean 078.6
    Kyasanur forest 065.2
    Machupo virus 078.7
    mite-borne NEC 065.8
    mosquito-borne 065.4
    Omsk 065.1
    Philippine 065.4
    Russian (Yaroslav) 078.6
    Singapore 065.4
    Southeast Asia 065.4
    Thailand 065.4
    tick-borne NEC 065.3
hepatic (*see also* Cholecystitis) 575.8
    intermittent (Charcôt's) — *see*
        Choledocholithiasis
herpetic (*see also* Herpes) 054.9
Hyalomma tick 065.0
icterohemorrhagic 100.0
inanition 780.6
    newborn 778.4
infective NEC 136.9
intermittent (bilious) (*see also* Malaria) 084.6
    hepatic (Charcôt) — *see* Choledocholithiasis
    of unknown origin (*see also* Pyrexia) 780.6
    pernicious 084.0
iodide
    correct substance properly administered
        780.6
    overdose or wrong substance given or taken
        975.5
Japanese river 081.2
jungle yellow 060.0
Junin virus, hemorrhagic 078.7
Katayama 120.2
Kedani 081.2
Kenya 082.1
Korean hemorrhagic 078.6
Lassa 078.89
Lone Star 082.8
lung — *see* Pneumonia
Machupo virus, hemorrhagic 078.7
malaria, malarial (*see also* Malaria) 084.6
Malta (*see also* Brucellosis) 023.9
Marseilles 082.1
marsh (*see also* Malaria) 084.6
Mayaro (viral) 066.3
Mediterranean (*see also* Brucellosis) 023.9
    familial 277.3
    tick 082.1
meningeal — *see* Meningitis
metal fumes NEC 985.8
Meuse 083.1
Mexican — *see* Typhus, Mexican
Mianeh 087.1
miasmatic (*see also* Malaria) 084.6
miliary 078.2
milk, female 672.0 ☑
mill 504
mite-borne hemorrhagic 065.8
Monday 504
mosquito-borne NEC 066.3
    hemorrhagic NEC 065.4
mountain 066.1
    meaning
        Rocky Mountain spotted 082.0
        undulant fever (*see also* Brucellosis)
            023.9
        tick (American) 066.1
Mucambo (viral) 066.3
mud 100.89
Neapolitan (*see also* Brucellosis) 023.9
neutropenic 288.0
nine-mile 083.0
nonexanthematous tick 066.1
North Asian tick-borne typhus 082.2
Omsk hemorrhagic 065.1
O'nyong-nyong (viral) 066.3
Oropouche (viral) 066.3
Oroya 088.0

paludal (*see also* Malaria) 084.6
Panama 084.0
pappataci 066.0
paratyphoid 002.9
    A 002.1
    B (Schottmüller's) 002.2
    C (Hirschfeld) 002.3
parrot 073.9
periodic 277.3
pernicious, acute 084.0
persistent (of unknown origin) (*see also* Pyrexia)
    780.6
petechial 036.0
pharyngoconjunctival 077.2
    adenoviral type 3 077.2
Philippine hemorrhagic 065.4
phlebotomus 066.0
Piry 066.8
Pixuna (viral) 066.3
Plasmodium ovale 084.3
pleural (*see also* Pleurisy) 511.0
pneumonic — *see* Pneumonia
polymer fume 987.8
postoperative 998.89
    due to infection 998.59
pretibial 100.89
puerperal, postpartum 672.0 ☑
putrid — *see* Septicemia
pyemic — *see* Septicemia
Q 083.0
    with pneumonia 083.0 *[484.8]*
quadrilateral 083.0
quartan (malaria) 084.2
Queensland (coastal) 083.0
    seven-day 100.89
Quintan (A) 083.1
quotidian 084.0
rabbit (*see also* Tularemia) 021.9
rat-bite 026.9
    due to
        Spirillum minor or minus 026.0
        Spirochaeta morsus muris 026.0
        Streptobacillus moniliformis 026.1
recurrent — *see* Fever, relapsing
relapsing 087.9
    Carter's (Asiatic) 087.0
    Dutton's (West African) 087.1
    Koch's 087.9
    louse-borne (epidemic) 087.0
    Novy's (American) 087.1
    Obermeyer's (European) 087.0
    spirillum NEC 087.9
    tick-borne (endemic) 087.1
remittent (bilious) (congestive) (gastric) (*see also*
    Malaria) 084.6
rheumatic (active) (acute) (chronic) (subacute)
    390
    with heart involvement 391.9
        carditis 391.9
        endocarditis (aortic) (mitral) (pulmonary)
            (tricuspid) 391.1
        multiple sites 391.8
        myocarditis 391.2
        pancarditis, acute 391.8
        pericarditis 391.0
        specified type NEC 391.8
        valvulitis 391.1
    inactive or quiescent with cardiac
        hypertrophy 398.99
        carditis 398.90
        endocarditis 397.9
            aortic (valve) 395.9
                with mitral (valve) disease 396.9
            mitral (valve) 394.9
                with aortic (valve) disease 396.9
            pulmonary (valve) 397.1
            tricuspid (valve) 397.0
        heart conditions (classifiable to 429.3,
            429.6, 429.9) 398.99
        failure (congestive) (conditions
            classifiable to 428.0, 428.9)
            398.91
        left ventricular failure (conditions
            classifiable to 428.1) 398.91
        myocardial degeneration (conditions
            classifiable to 429.1) 398.0

rheumatic — *continued*
    inactive or quiescent with cardiac —
        continued
        myocarditis (conditions classifiable to
            429.0) 398.0
        pancarditis 398.99
        pericarditis 393
Rift Valley (viral) 066.3
Rocky Mountain spotted 082.0
rose 477.0
Ross river (viral) 066.3
Russian hemorrhagic 078.6
sandfly 066.0
San Joaquin (valley) 114.0
São Paulo 082.0
scarlet 034.1
septic — *see* Septicemia
seven-day 061
    Japan 100.89
    Queensland 100.89
shin bone 083.1
Singapore hemorrhagic 065.4
solar 061
sore 054.9
South African tick-bite 087.1
Southeast Asia hemorrhagic 065.4
spinal — *see* Meningitis
spirillary 026.0
splenic (*see also* Anthrax) 022.9
spotted (Rocky Mountain) 082.0
    American 082.0
    Brazilian 082.0
    Colombian 082.0
    meaning
        cerebrospinal meningitis 036.0
        typhus 082.9
spring 309.23
steroid
    correct substance properly administered
        780.6
    overdose or wrong substance given or taken
        962.0
streptobacillary 026.1
subtertian 084.0
Sumatran mite 081.2
sun 061
swamp 100.89
sweating 078.2
swine 003.8
sylvatic yellow 060.0
Tahyna 062.5
tertian — *see* Malaria, tertian
Thailand hemorrhagic 065.4
thermic 992.0
three day 066.0
    with Coxsackie exanthem 074.8
tick
    American mountain 066.1
    Colorado 066.1
    Kemerovo 066.1
    Mediterranean 082.1
    mountain 066.1
    nonexanthematous 066.1
    Quaranfil 066.1
tick-bite NEC 066.1
tick-borne NEC 066.1
    hemorrhagic NEC 065.3
transitory of newborn 778.4
trench 083.1
tsutsugamushi 081.2
typhogastric 002.0
typhoid (abortive) (ambulant) (any site)
    (hemorrhagic) (infection) (intermittent)
    (malignant) (rheumatic) 002.0
typhomalarial (*see also* Malaria) 084.6
typhus — *see* Typhus
undulant (*see also* Brucellosis) 023.9
unknown origin (*see also* Pyrexia) 780.6
uremic — *see* Uremia
uveoparotid 135
valley (Coccidioidomycosis) 114.0
Venezuelan equine 066.2
Volhynian 083.1
Wesselsbron (viral) 066.3

☑ Additional Digit Required   ▶◀ Revised Text   ● New Line   ▲ Revised Code

Fever — *continued*
  West
    African 084.8
    Nile (viral) 066.40 ▲
      with ●
        cranial nerve disorders 066.42 ●
        encephalitis 066.41 ●
        optic neuritis 066.42 ●
        other complications 066.49 ●
        other neurologic manifestations
          066.42 ●
        polyradiculitis 066.42 ●
  Whitmore's 025
  Wolhynian 083.1
  worm 128.9
  Yaroslav hemorrhagic 078.6
  yellow 060.9
    jungle 060.0
    sylvatic 060.0
    urban 060.1
    vaccination, prophylactic (against) V04.4
  Zika (viral) 066.3
Fibrillation
  atrial (established) (paroxysmal) 427.31
  auricular (atrial) (established) 427.31
  cardiac (ventricular) 427.41
  coronary (*see also* Infarct, myocardium)
    410.9 ☑
  heart (ventricular) 427.41
  muscular 728.9
  postoperative 997.1
  ventricular 427.41
Fibrin
  ball or bodies, pleural (sac) 511.0
  chamber, anterior (eye) (gelatinous exudate)
    364.04
Fibrinogenolysis (hemorrhagic) — *see*
  Fibrinolysis
Fibrinogenopenia (congenital) (hereditary) (*see
  also* Defect, coagulation) 286.3
  acquired 286.6
Fibrinolysis (acquired) (hemorrhagic) (pathologic)
  286.6
  with
    abortion — *see* Abortion, by type, with
      hemorrhage, delayed or excessive
    ectopic pregnancy (*see also* categories
      633.0-633.9) 639.1
    molar pregnancy (*see also* categories 630-
      632) 639.1
  antepartum or intrapartum 641.3 ☑
    affecting fetus or newborn 762.1
  following
    abortion 639.1
    ectopic or molar pregnancy 639.1
  newborn, transient 776.2
  postpartum 666.3 ☑
Fibrinopenia (hereditary) (*see also* Defect,
  coagulation) 286.3
  acquired 286.6
Fibrinopurulent — *see* condition
Fibrinous — *see* condition
Fibroadenoma (M9010/0)
  cellular intracanalicular (M9020/0) 217
  giant (intracanalicular) (M9020/0) 217
  intracanalicular (M9011/0)
    cellular (M9020/0) 217
    giant (M9020/0) 217
    specified site — *see* Neoplasm, by site,
      benign
    unspecified site 217
  juvenile (M9030/0) 217
  pericanicular (M9012/0)
    specified site — *see* Neoplasm, by site,
      benign
    unspecified site 217
  phyllodes (M9020/0) 217
  prostate 600.20
    with urinary retention 600.21
  specified site — *see* Neoplasm, by site, benign
  unspecified site 217
Fibroadenosis, breast (chronic) (cystic) (diffuse)
  (periodic) (segmental) 610.2

Fibroangioma (M9160/0) — *see also* Neoplasm,
  by site, benign
  juvenile (M9160/0)
    specified site — *see* Neoplasm, by site,
      benign
    unspecified site 210.7
Fibrocellulitis progressiva ossificans 728.11
Fibrochondrosarcoma (M9220/3) — *see*
  Neoplasm, cartilage, malignant
Fibrocystic
  disease 277.00
    bone NEC 733.29
    breast 610.1
    jaw 526.2
    kidney (congenital) 753.19
    liver 751.62
    lung 518.89
      congenital 748.4
    pancreas 277.00
  kidney (congenital) 753.19
Fibrodysplasia ossificans multiplex (progressiva)
  728.11
Fibroelastosis (cordis) (endocardial)
  (endomyocardial) 425.3
Fibroid (tumor) (M8890/0) — *see also* Neoplasm,
  connective tissue, benign
  disease, lung (chronic) (*see also* Fibrosis, lung) 515
  heart (disease) (*see also* Myocarditis) 429.0
  induration, lung (chronic) (*see also* Fibrosis,
    lung) 515
  in pregnancy or childbirth 654.1 ☑
    affecting fetus or newborn 763.89
    causing obstructed labor 660.2 ☑
      affecting fetus or newborn 763.1
  liver — *see* Cirrhosis, liver
  lung (*see also* Fibrosis, lung) 515
  pneumonia (chronic) (*see also* Fibrosis, lung) 515
  uterus (M8890/0) (*see also* Leiomyoma, uterus)
    218.9
Fibrolipoma (M8851/0) (*see also* Lipoma, by site)
  214.9
Fibroliposarcoma (M8850/3) — *see* Neoplasm,
  connective tissue, malignant
Fibroma (M8810/0) — *see also* Neoplasm,
  connective tissue, benign
  ameloblastic (M9330/0) 213.1
    upper jaw (bone) 213.0
  bone (nonossifying) 733.99
    ossifying (M9262/0) — *see* Neoplasm, bone,
      benign
  cementifying (M9274/0) — *see* Neoplasm, bone,
    benign
  chondromyxoid (M9241/0) — *see* Neoplasm,
    bone, benign
  desmoplastic (M8823/1) — *see* Neoplasm,
    connective tissue, uncertain behavior
  facial (M8813/0) — *see* Neoplasm, connective
    tissue, benign
  invasive (M8821/1) — *see* Neoplasm,
    connective tissue, uncertain behavior
  molle (M8851/0) (*see also* Lipoma, by site)
    214.9
  myxoid (M8811/0) — *see* Neoplasm, connective
    tissue, benign
  nasopharynx, nasopharyngeal (juvenile)
    (M9160/0) 210.7
  nonosteogenic (nonossifying) — *see* Dysplasia,
    fibrous
  odontogenic (M9321/0) 213.1
    upper jaw (bone) 213.0
  ossifying (M9262/0) — *see* Neoplasm, bone,
    benign
  periosteal (M8812/0) — *see* Neoplasm, bone,
    benign
  prostate 600.20
    with urinary retention 600.21
  soft (M8851/0) (*see also* Lipoma, by site) 214.9
Fibromatosis
  abdominal (M8822/1) — *see* Neoplasm,
    connective tissue, uncertain behavior
  aggressive (M8821/1) — *see* Neoplasm,
    connective tissue, uncertain behavior
  Dupuytren's 728.6
  gingival 523.8
  plantar fascia 728.71

Fibromatosis — *continued*
  proliferative 728.79
  pseudosarcomatous (proliferative)
    (subcutaneous) 728.79
  subcutaneous pseudosarcomatous
    (proliferative) 728.79
Fibromyalgia 729.1
Fibromyoma (M8890/0) — *see also* Neoplasm,
  connective tissue, benign
  uterus (corpus) (*see also* Leiomyoma, uterus)
    218.9
    in pregnancy or childbirth 654.1 ☑
      affecting fetus or newborn 763.89
      causing obstructed labor 660.2 ☑
        affecting fetus or newborn 763.1
Fibromyositis (*see also* Myositis) 729.1
  scapulohumeral 726.2
Fibromyxolipoma (M8852/0) (*see also* Lipoma, by
  site) 214.9
Fibromyxoma (M8811/0) — *see* Neoplasm,
  connective tissue, benign
Fibromyxosarcoma (M8811/3) — *see* Neoplasm,
  connective tissue, malignant
Fibro-odontoma, ameloblastic (M9290/0) 213.1
  upper jaw (bone) 213.0
Fibro-osteoma (M9262/0) — *see* Neoplasm, bone,
  benign
Fibroplasia, retrolental 362.21
Fibropurulent — *see* condition
Fibrosarcoma (M8810/3) — *see also* Neoplasm,
  connective tissue, malignant
  ameloblastic (M9330/3) 170.1
    upper jaw (bone) 170.0
  congenital (M8814/3) — *see* Neoplasm,
    connective tissue, malignant
  fascial (M8813/3) — *see* Neoplasm, connective
    tissue, malignant
  infantile (M8814/3) — *see* Neoplasm,
    connective tissue, malignant
  odontogenic (M9330/3) 170.1
    upper jaw (bone) 170.0
  periosteal (M8812/3) — *see* Neoplasm, bone,
    malignant
Fibrosclerosis
  breast 610.3
  corpora cavernosa (penis) 607.89
  familial multifocal NEC 710.8
  multifocal (idiopathic) NEC 710.8
  penis (corpora cavernosa) 607.89
Fibrosis, fibrotic
  adrenal (gland) 255.8
  alveolar (diffuse) 516.3
  amnion 658.8 ☑
  anal papillae 569.49
  anus 569.49
  appendix, appendiceal, noninflammatory 543.9
  arteriocapillary — *see* Arteriosclerosis
  bauxite (of lung) 503
  biliary 576.8
    due to Clonorchis sinensis 121.1
  bladder 596.8
    interstitial 595.1
    localized submucosal 595.1
    panmural 595.1
  bone, diffuse 756.59
  breast 610.3
  capillary — *see also* Arteriosclerosis
    lung (chronic) (*see also* Fibrosis, lung) 515
  cardiac (*see also* Myocarditis) 429.0
  cervix 622.8
  chorion 658.8 ☑
  corpus cavernosum 607.89
  cystic (of pancreas) 277.00
    with
      manifestations
        gastrointestinal 277.03
        pulmonary 277.02
        specified NEC 277.09
      meconium ileus 277.01
      pulmonary exacerbation 277.02
  due to (presence of) any device, implant, or
    graft — *see* Complications, due to
    (presence of) any device, implant, or graft
    classified to 996.0-996.5 NEC

Fibrosis, fibrotic — *continued*
ejaculatory duct 608.89
endocardium (*see also* Endocarditis) 424.90
endomyocardial (African) 425.0
epididymis 608.89
eye muscle 378.62
graphite (of lung) 503
heart (*see also* Myocarditis) 429.0
hepatic — *see also* Cirrhosis, liver due to
　　Clonorchis sinensis 121.1
hepatolienal — *see* Cirrhosis, liver
hepatosplenic — *see* Cirrhosis, liver
infrapatellar fat pad 729.31
interstitial pulmonary, newborn 770.7
intrascrotal 608.89
kidney (*see also* Sclerosis, renal) 587
liver — *see* Cirrhosis, liver
lung (atrophic) (capillary) (chronic) (confluent)
　　(massive) (perialveolar) (peribronchial)
　　515
　with
　　anthracosilicosis (occupational) 500
　　anthracosis (occupational) 500
　　asbestosis (occupational) 501
　　bagassosis (occupational) 495.1
　　bauxite 503
　　berylliosis (occupational) 503
　　byssinosis (occupational) 504
　　calcicosis (occupational) 502
　　chalicosis (occupational) 502
　　dust reticulation (occupational) 504
　　farmers' lung 495.0
　　gannister disease (occupational) 502
　　graphite 503
　　pneumonoconiosis (occupational) 505
　　pneumosiderosis (occupational) 503
　　siderosis (occupational) 503
　　silicosis (occupational) 502
　　tuberculosis (*see also* Tuberculosis)
　　　011.4 ☑
　diffuse (idiopathic) (interstitial) 516.3
　due to
　　bauxite 503
　　fumes or vapors (chemical) inhalation)
　　　506.4
　　graphite 503
　following radiation 508.1
　postinflammatory 515
　silicotic (massive) (occupational) 502
　tuberculous (*see also* Tuberculosis) 011.4 ☑
lymphatic gland 289.3
median bar 600.90
　with urinary retention 600.91
mediastinum (idiopathic) 519.3
meninges 349.2
muscle NEC 728.2
　iatrogenic (from injection) 999.9
myocardium, myocardial (*see also* Myocarditis)
　　429.0
oral submucous 528.8
ovary 620.8
oviduct 620.8
pancreas 577.8
　cystic 277.00
　　with
　　　manifestations
　　　　gastrintestinal 277.03
　　　　pulmonary 277.02
　　　　specified NEC 277.09
　　　meconium ileus 277.01
　　　pulmonary exacerbation 277.02
penis 607.89
periappendiceal 543.9
periarticular (*see also* Ankylosis) 718.5 ☑
pericardium 423.1
perineum, in pregnancy or childbirth 654.8 ☑
　affecting fetus or newborn 763.89
　causing obstructed labor 660.2 ☑
　　affecting fetus or newborn 763.1
perineural NEC 355.9
　foot 355.6
periureteral 593.89
placenta — *see* Placenta, abnormal
pleura 511.0
popliteal fat pad 729.31
preretinal 362.56

Fibrosis, fibrotic — *continued*
prostate (chronic) 600.90
　with urinary retention 600.91
pulmonary (chronic) (*see also* Fibrosis, lung)
　　515
　alveolar capillary block 516.3
　interstitial
　　diffuse (idiopathic) 516.3
　　newborn 770.7
radiation — *see* Effect, adverse, radiation
rectal sphincter 569.49
retroperitoneal, idiopathic 593.4
scrotum 608.89
seminal vesicle 608.89
senile 797
skin NEC 709.2
spermatic cord 608.89
spleen 289.59
　bilharzial (*see also* Schistosomiasis) 120.9
subepidermal nodular (M8832/0) — *see*
　　Neoplasm, skin, benign
submucous NEC 709.2
　oral 528.8
　tongue 528.8
syncytium — *see* Placenta, abnormal
testis 608.89
　chronic, due to syphilis 095.8
thymus (gland) 254.8
tunica vaginalis 608.89
ureter 593.89
urethra 599.84
uterus (nonneoplastic) 621.8
　bilharzial (*see also* Schistosomiasis) 120.9
　neoplastic (*see also* Leiomyoma, uterus)
　　218.9
vagina 623.8
valve, heart (*see also* Endocarditis) 424.90
vas deferens 608.89
vein 459.89
　lower extremities 459.89
vesical 595.1
Fibrositis (periarticular) (rheumatoid) 729.0
humeroscapular region 726.2
nodular, chronic
　Jaccoud's 714.4
　rheumatoid 714.4
ossificans 728.11
scapulohumeral 726.2
Fibrothorax 511.0
Fibrotic — *see* Fibrosis
Fibrous — *see* condition
Fibroxanthoma (M8831/0) — *see also* Neoplasm,
　connective tissue, benign
atypical (M8831/1) — *see* Neoplasm,
　connective tissue, uncertain behavior
malignant (M8831/3) — *see* Neoplasm,
　connective tissue, malignant
Fibroxanthosarcoma (M8831/3) — *see* Neoplasm,
　connective tissue, malignant
Fiedler's
disease (leptospiral jaundice) 100.0
myocarditis or syndrome (acute isolated
　myocarditis) 422.91
Fiessinger-Leroy (-Reiter) syndrome 099.3
Fiessinger-Rendu syndrome (erythema
　muliforme exudativum) 695.1
Fifth disease (eruptive) 057.0
venereal 099.1
Filaria, filarial — *see* Infestation, filarial
Filariasis (*see also* Infestation, filarial) 125.9
bancroftian 125.0
Brug's 125.1
due to
　bancrofti 125.0
　Brugia (Wuchereria) (malayi) 125.1
　Loa loa 125.2
　malayi 125.1
　organism NEC 125.6
　Wuchereria (bancrofti) 125.0
　　malayi 125.1
Malayan 125.1
ozzardi 125.1
specified type NEC 125.6

Filatoff's, Filatov's, Filatow's disease (infectious
　mononucleosis) 075
File-cutters' disease 984.9
specified type of lead — *see* Table of Drugs and
　Chemicals
Filling defect
biliary tract 793.3
bladder 793.5
duodenum 793.4
gallbladder 793.3
gastrointestinal tract 793.4
intestine 793.4
kidney 793.5
stomach 793.4
ureter 793.5
Filtering bleb, eye (postglaucoma) (status) V45.69
with complication or rupture 997.99
postcataract extraction (complication) 997.99
Fimbrial cyst (congenital) 752.11
Fimbriated hymen 752.49
Financial problem affecting care V60.2
Findings, abnormal, without diagnosis
　(examination) (laboratory test) 796.4
17-ketosteroids, elevated 791.9
acetonuria 791.6
acid phosphatase 790.5
albumin-globulin ratio 790.99
albuminuria 791.0
alcohol in blood 790.3
alkaline phosphatase 790.5
amniotic fluid 792.3
amylase 790.5
anisocytosis 790.09
antenatal screening 796.5
anthrax, positive 795.31
antibody titers, elevated 795.79
anticardiolipin antibody 795.79
antigen-antibody reaction 795.79
antiphospholipid antibody 795.79
bacteriuria 791.9
ballistocardiogram 794.39
bicarbonate 276.9
bile in urine 791.4
bilirubin 277.4
bleeding time (prolonged) 790.92
blood culture, positive 790.7
blood gas level 790.91
blood sugar level 790.29
　high 790.29
　　fasting glucose 790.21
　　glucose tolerance test 790.22
　low 251.2
C-reactive protein (CRP) 790.95　　　　●
calcium 275.40
carbonate 276.9
casts, urine 791.7
catecholamines 791.9
cells, urine 791.7
cerebrospinal fluid (color) (content) (pressure)
　　792.0
cervical　　　　　　　　　　　　　　　　　●
　high risk human papillomavirus (HPV)　●
　　DNA test positive 795.05　　　　　　●
　low risk human papillomavirus (HPV)　●
　　DNA test positive 795.09　　　　　　●
chloride 276.9
cholesterol 272.9
chromosome analysis 795.2
chyluria 791.1
circulation time 794.39
cloudy dialysis effluent 792.5
cloudy urine 791.9
coagulation study 790.92
cobalt, blood 790.6
color of urine (unusual) NEC 791.9
copper, blood 790.6
crystals, urine 791.9
culture, positive NEC 795.39
　blood 790.7
　HIV V08
　human immunodeficiency virus V08
　nose 795.39
　skin lesion NEC 795.39
　spinal fluid 792.0
　sputum 795.39

Left margin (vertical): **Fibrosis, fibrotic — Findings, abnormal, without diagnosis**

Findings, abnormal, without diagnosis —
continued
  culture, positive NEC — *continued*
    stool 792.1
    throat 795.39
    urine 791.9
    viral
      human immunodeficiency V08
    wound 795.39
  echocardiogram 793.2
  echoencephalogram 794.01
  echogram NEC — *see* Findings, abnormal, structure
  electrocardiogram (ECG) (EKG) 794.31
  electroencephalogram (EEG) 794.02
  electrolyte level, urinary 791.9
  electromyogram (EMG) 794.17
    ocular 794.14
  electro-oculogram (EOG) 794.12
  electroretinogram (ERG) 794.11
  enzymes, serum NEC 790.5
  fibrinogen titer coagulation study 790.92
  filling defect — *see* Filling defect
  function study NEC 794.9
    auditory 794.15
    bladder 794.9
    brain 794.00
    cardiac 794.30
    endocrine NEC 794.6
      thyroid 794.5
    kidney 794.4
    liver 794.8
    nervous system
      central 794.00
      peripheral 794.19
    oculomotor 794.14
    pancreas 794.9
    placenta 794.9
    pulmonary 794.2
    retina 794.11
    special senses 794.19
    spleen 794.9
    vestibular 794.16
  gallbladder, nonvisualization 793.3
  glucose 790.29
    elevated
      fasting 790.21
      tolerance test 790.22
  glycosuria 791.5
  heart
    shadow 793.2
    sounds 785.3
  hematinuria 791.2
  hematocrit
    drop (precipitous) 790.01
    elevated 282.7
    low 285.9
  hematologic NEC 790.99
  hematuria 599.7
  hemoglobin
    elevated 282.7
    low 285.9
  hemoglobinuria 791.2
  histological NEC 795.4
  hormones 259.9
  immunoglobulins, elevated 795.79
  indolacetic acid, elevated 791.9
  iron 790.6
  karyotype 795.2
  ketonuria 791.6
  lactic acid dehydrogenase (LDH) 790.4
  lipase 790.5
  lipids NEC 272.9
  lithium, blood 790.6
  lung field (coin lesion) (shadow) 793.1
  magnesium, blood 790.6
  mammogram 793.80
    microcalcification 793.81
  mediastinal shift 793.2
  melanin, urine 791.9
  microbiologic NEC 795.39
  mineral, blood NEC 790.6
  myoglobinuria 791.3
  nasal swab, anthrax 795.31
  neonatal screening 796.6 ●
  nitrogen derivatives, blood 790.6
  nonvisualization of gallbladder 793.3

Findings, abnormal, without diagnosis —
continued
  nose culture, positive 795.39
  odor of urine (unusual) NEC 791.9
  oxygen saturation 790.91
  Papanicolaou (smear) 795.1
    cervix 795.00
      with ●
        ▶atypical squamous cells◄
          ▶cannot exclude high grade squamous intraepithelial lesion (ASC-H)◄ 795.02
          ▶of undetermined significance (ASC-US)◄ 795.01
        high grade squamous ●
          intraepithelial lesion ●
          (HGSIL) 795.04
        low grade squamous ●
          intraepithelial lesion ●
          (LGSIL) 795.03 ●
      dyskaryotic 795.09
      nonspecific finding NEC 795.09
    other site 795.1
  peritoneal fluid 792.9
  phonocardiogram 794.39
  phosphorus 275.3
  pleural fluid 792.9
  pneumoencephalogram 793.0
  PO₂-oxygen ratio 790.91
  poikilocytosis 790.09
  potassium
    deficiency 276.8
    excess 276.7
  PPD 795.5
  prostate specific antigen (PSA) 790.93
  protein, serum NEC 790.99
  proteinuria 791.0
  prothrombin time (partial) (prolonged) (PT) (PTT) 790.92
  pyuria 791.9
  radiologic (x-ray) 793.9
    abdomen 793.6
    biliary tract 793.3
    breast 793.89
      abnormal mammogram NOS 793.80
      mammographic microcalcification 793.81
    gastrointestinal tract 793.4
    genitourinary organs 793.5
    head 793.0
    intrathoracic organs NEC 793.2
    lung 793.1
    musculoskeletal 793.7
    placenta 793.9
    retroperitoneum 793.6
    skin 793.9
    skull 793.0
    subcutaneous tissue 793.9
  red blood cell 790.09
    count 790.09
    morphology 790.09
    sickling 790.09
    volume 790.09
  saliva 792.4
  scan NEC 794.9
    bladder 794.9
    bone 794.9
    brain 794.09
    kidney 794.4
    liver 794.8
    lung 794.2
    pancreas 794.9
    placental 794.9
    spleen 794.9
    thyroid 794.5
  sedimentation rate, elevated 790.1
  semen 792.2
  serological (for)
    human immunodeficiency virus (HIV)
      inconclusive 795.71
      positive V08
    syphilis — *see* Findings, serology for syphilis
  serology for syphilis
    false positive 795.6
    positive 097.1
      false 795.6
      follow-up of latent syphilis — *see* Syphilis, latent

Findings, abnormal, without diagnosis —
continued
  serology for syphilis**s** — *continued*
    positive — *continued*
      only finding — *see* Syphilis, latent
  serum 790.99
    blood NEC 790.99
    enzymes NEC 790.5
    proteins 790.99
  SGOT 790.4
  SGPT 790.4
  sickling of red blood cells 790.09
  skin test, positive 795.79
    tuberculin (without active tuberculosis) 795.5
  sodium 790.6
    deficiency 276.1
    excess 276.0
  spermatozoa 792.2
  spinal fluid 792.0
    culture, positive 792.0
  sputum culture, positive 795.39
    for acid-fast bacilli 795.39
  stool NEC 792.1
    bloody 578.1
      occult 792.1
    color 792.1
    culture, positive 792.1
    occult blood 792.1
  stress test 794.39
  structure, body (echogram) (thermogram) (ultrasound) (x-ray) NEC 793.9
    abdomen 793.6
    breast 793.89
      abnormal mammogram 793.80
      mammographic microcalcification 793.81
    gastrointestinal tract 793.4
    genitourinary organs 793.5
    head 793.0
      echogram (ultrasound) 794.01
    intrathoracic organs NEC 793.2
    lung 793.1
    musculoskeletal 793.7
    placenta 793.9
    retroperitoneum 793.6
    skin 793.9
    subcutaneous tissue NEC 793.9
  synovial fluid 792.9
  thermogram — *see* Finding, abnormal, structure
  throat culture, positive 795.39
  thyroid (function) 794.5
    metabolism (rate) 794.5
    scan 794.5
    uptake 794.5
  total proteins 790.99
  toxicology (drugs) (heavy metals) 796.0
  transaminase (level) 790.4
  triglycerides 272.9
  tuberculin skin test (without active tuberculosis) 795.5
  ultrasound — *see also* Finding, abnormal, structure
    cardiogram 793.2
  uric acid, blood 790.6
  urine, urinary constituents 791.9
    acetone 791.6
    albumin 791.0
    bacteria 791.9
    bile 791.4
    blood 599.7
    casts or cells 791.7
    chyle 791.1
    culture, positive 791.9
    glucose 791.5
    hemoglobin 791.2
    ketone 791.6
    protein 791.0
    pus 791.9
    sugar 791.5
  vaginal fluid 792.9
  vanillylmandelic acid, elevated 791.9
  vectorcardiogram (VCG) 794.39
  ventriculogram (cerebral) 793.0
  VMA, elevated 791.9

Findings, abnormal, without diagnosis

☑ Additional Digit Required   ▶◀ Revised Text   ● New Line   ▲ Revised Code

Findings, abnormal, without diagnosis — *continued*
  Wassermann reaction
    false positive 795.6
    positive 097.1
      follow-up of latent syphilis — *see* Syphilis, latent
      only finding — *see* Syphilis, latent
  white blood cell 288.9
    count 288.9
      elevated 288.8
      low 288.0
    differential 288.9
    morphology 288.9
  wound culture 795.39
  xerography 793.89
  zinc, blood 790.6

Finger — *see* condition

Fire, St. Anthony's (*see also* Erysipelas) 035

Fish
  hook stomach 537.89
  meal workers' lung 495.8

Fisher's syndrome 357.0

Fissure, fissured
  abdominal wall (congenital) 756.79
  anus, anal 565.0
    congenital 751.5
  buccal cavity 528.9
  clitoris (congenital) 752.49
  ear, lobule (congenital) 744.29
  epiglottis (congenital) 748.3
  larynx 478.79
    congenital 748.3
  lip 528.5
    congenital (*see also* Cleft, lip) 749.10
  nipple 611.2
    puerperal, postpartum 676.1 ☑
  palate (congenital) (*see also* Cleft, palate) 749.00
  postanal 565.0
  rectum 565.0
  skin 709.8
    streptococcal 686.9
  spine (congenital) (*see also* Spina bifida) 741.9 ☑
  sternum (congenital) 756.3
  tongue (acquired) 529.5
    congenital 750.13

Fistula (sinus) 686.9
  abdomen (wall) 569.81
    bladder 596.2
    intestine 569.81
    ureter 593.82
    uterus 619.2
  abdominorectal 569.81
  abdominosigmoidal 569.81
  abdominothoracic 510.0
  abdominouterine 619.2
    congenital 752.3
  abdominovesical 596.2
  accessory sinuses (*see also* Sinusitis) 473.9
  actinomycotic — *see* Actinomycosis
  alveolar
    antrum (*see also* Sinusitis, maxillary) 473.0
    process 522.7
  anorectal 565.1
  antrobuccal (*see also* Sinusitis, maxillary) 473.0
  antrum (*see also* Sinusitis, maxillary) 473.0
  anus, anal (infectional) (recurrent) 565.1
    congenital 751.5
    tuberculous (*see also* Tuberculosis) 014.8 ☑
  aortic sinus 747.29
  aortoduodenal 447.2
  appendix, appendicular 543.9
  arteriovenous (acquired) 447.0
    brain 437.3
      congenital 747.81
        ruptured (*see also* Hemorrhage, subarachnoid) 430
      ruptured (*see also* Hemorrhage, subarachnoid) 430
    cerebral 437.3
      congenital 747.81

Fistula — *continued*
  arteriovenous (acquired) — *continued*
    congenital (peripheral) 747.60
      brain — *see* Fistula, arteriovenous, brain, congenital
      coronary 746.85
      gastrointestinal 747.61
      lower limb 747.64
      pulmonary 747.3
      renal 747.62
      specified NEC 747.69
      upper limb 747.63
    coronary 414.19
      congenital 746.85
    heart 414.19
    pulmonary (vessels) 417.0
      congenital 747.3
    surgically created (for dialysis) V45.1
      complication NEC 996.73
        atherosclerosis — *see* Arteriosclerosis, extremities
        embolism 996.74
        infection or inflammation 996.62
        mechanical 996.1
        occlusion NEC 996.74
        thrombus 996.74
    traumatic — *see* Injury, blood vessel, by site
  artery 447.2
  aural 383.81
    congenital 744.49
  auricle 383.81
    congenital 744.49
  Bartholin's gland 619.8
  bile duct (*see also* Fistula, biliary) 576.4
  biliary (duct) (tract) 576.4
    congenital 751.69
  bladder (neck) (sphincter) 596.2
    into seminal vesicle 596.2
  bone 733.99
  brain 348.8
    arteriovenous — *see* Fistula, arteriovenous, brain
  branchial (cleft) 744.41
  branchiogenous 744.41
  breast 611.0
    puerperal, postpartum 675.1 ☑
  bronchial 510.0
  bronchocutaneous, bronchomediastinal, bronchopleural, bronchopleuromediastinal (infective) 510.0
    tuberculous (*see also* Tuberculosis) 011.3 ☑
  bronchoesophageal 530.89
    congenital 750.3
  buccal cavity (infective) 528.3
  canal, ear 380.89
  carotid-cavernous
    congenital 747.81
      with hemorrhage 430
    traumatic 900.82
      with hemorrhage (*see also* Hemorrhage, brain, traumatic) 853.0 ☑
      late effect 908.3
  cecosigmoidal 569.81
  cecum 569.81
  cerebrospinal (fluid) 349.81
  cervical, lateral (congenital) 744.41
  cervicoaural (congenital) 744.49
  cervicosigmoidal 619.1
  cervicovesical 619.0
  cervix 619.8
  chest (wall) 510.0
  cholecystocolic (*see also* Fistula, gallbladder) 575.5
  cholecystocolonic (*see also* Fistula, gallbladder) 575.5
  cholecystoduodenal (*see also* Fistula, gallbladder) 575.5
  cholecystoenteric (*see also* Fistula, gallbladder) 575.5
  cholecystogastric (*see also* Fistula, gallbladder) 575.5
  cholecystointestinal (*see also* Fistula, gallbladder) 575.5
  choledochoduodenal 576.4
  cholocolic (*see also* Fistula, gallbladder) 575.5

Fistula — *continued*
  coccyx 685.1
    with abscess 685.0
  colon 569.81
  colostomy 569.69
  colovaginal (acquired) 619.1
  common duct (bile duct) 576.4
  congenital, NEC — *see* Anomaly, specified type NEC
  cornea, causing hypotony 360.32
  coronary, arteriovenous 414.19
    congenital 746.85
  costal region 510.0
  cul-de-sac, Douglas' 619.8
  cutaneous 686.9
  cystic duct (*see also* Fistula, gallbladder) 575.5
    congenital 751.69
  dental 522.7
  diaphragm 510.0
    bronchovisceral 510.0
    pleuroperitoneal 510.0
    pulmonoperitoneal 510.0
  duodenum 537.4
  ear (canal) (external) 380.89
  enterocolic 569.81
  enterocutaneous 569.81
  enteroenteric 569.81
  entero-uterine 619.1
    congenital 752.3
  enterovaginal 619.1
    congenital 752.49
  enterovesical 596.1
  epididymis 608.89
    tuberculous (*see also* Tuberculosis) 016.4 ☑
  esophagobronchial 530.89
    congenital 750.3
  esophagocutaneous 530.89
  esophagopleurocutaneous 530.89
  esophagotracheal 530.84
    congenital 750.3
  esophagus 530.89
    congenital 750.4
  ethmoid (*see also* Sinusitis, ethmoidal) 473.2
  eyeball (cornea) (sclera) 360.32
  eyelid 373.11
  fallopian tube (external) 619.2
  fecal 569.81
    congenital 751.5
  from periapical lesion 522.7
  frontal sinus (*see also* Sinusitis, frontal) 473.1
  gallbladder 575.5
    with calculus, cholelithiasis, stones (*see also* Cholelithiasis) 574.2 ☑
    congenital 751.69
  gastric 537.4
  gastrocolic 537.4
    congenital 750.7
    tuberculous (*see also* Tuberculosis) 014.8 ☑
  gastroenterocolic 537.4
  gastroesophageal 537.4
  gastrojejunal 537.4
  gastrojejunocolic 537.4
  genital
    organs
      female 619.9
        specified site NEC 619.8
      male 608.89
    tract-skin (female) 619.2
  hepatopleural 510.0
  hepatopulmonary 510.0
  horseshoe 565.1
  ileorectal 569.81
  ileosigmoidal 569.81
  ileostomy 569.69
  ileovesical 596.1
  ileum 569.81
  in ano 565.1
    tuberculous (*see also* Tuberculosis) 014.8 ☑
  inner ear (*see also* Fistula, labyrinth) 386.40
  intestine 569.81
  intestinocolic (abdominal) 569.81
  intestinoureteral 593.82
  intestinouterine 619.1
  intestinovaginal 619.1
    congenital 752.49
  intestinovesical 596.1

☑ Additional Digit Required   ▶◀ Revised Text   ● New Line   ▲ Revised Code

Fistula — *continued*
  involving female genital tract 619.9
    digestive-genital 619.1
    genital tract-skin 619.2
    specified site NEC 619.8
    urinary-genital 619.0
  ischiorectal (fossa) 566
  jejunostomy 569.69
  jejunum 569.81
  joint 719.89
    ankle 719.87
    elbow 719.82
    foot 719.87
    hand 719.84
    hip 719.85
    knee 719.86
    multiple sites 719.89
    pelvic region 719.85
    shoulder (region) 719.81
    specified site NEC 719.88
    tuberculous — *see* Tuberculosis, joint
    wrist 719.83
  kidney 593.89
  labium (majus) (minus) 619.8
  labyrinth, labyrinthine NEC 386.40
    combined sites 386.48
    multiple sites 386.48
    oval window 386.42
    round window 386.41
    semicircular canal 386.43
  lacrimal, lachrymal (duct) (gland) (sac) 375.61
  lacrimonasal duct 375.61
  laryngotracheal 748.3
  larynx 478.79
  lip 528.5
    congenital 750.25
  lumbar, tuberculous (*see also* Tuberculosis)
    015.0 ☑ [730.8] ☑
  lung 510.0
  lymphatic (node) (vessel) 457.8
  mamillary 611.0
  mammary (gland) 611.0
    puerperal, postpartum 675.1 ☑
  mastoid (process) (region) 383.1
  maxillary (*see also* Sinusitis, maxillary) 473.0
  mediastinal 510.0
  mediastinobronchial 510.0
  mediastinocutaneous 510.0
  middle ear 385.89
  mouth 528.3
  nasal 478.1
    sinus (*see also* Sinusitis) 473.9
  nasopharynx 478.29
  nipple — *see* Fistula, breast
  nose 478.1
  oral (cutaneous) 528.3
    maxillary (*see also* Sinusitis, maxillary)
      473.0
    nasal (with cleft palate) (*see also* Cleft,
      palate) 749.00
  orbit, orbital 376.10
  oro-antral (*see also* Sinusitis, maxillary) 473.0
  oval window (internal ear) 386.42
  oviduct (external) 619.2
  palate (hard) 526.89
    soft 528.9
  pancreatic 577.8
  pancreaticoduodenal 577.8
  parotid (gland) 527.4
    region 528.3
  pelvoabdominointestinal 569.81
  penis 607.89
  perianal 565.1
  pericardium (pleura) (sac) (*see also* Pericarditis)
    423.8
  pericecal 569.81
  perineal — *see* Fistula, perineum
  perineorectal 569.81
  perineosigmoidal 569.81
  perineo-urethroscrotal 608.89
  perineum, perineal (with urethral involvement)
    NEC 599.1
    tuberculous (*see also* Tuberculosis) 017.9 ☑
    ureter 593.82
  perirectal 565.1
    tuberculous (*see also* Tuberculosis) 014.8 ☑
  peritoneum (*see also* Peritonitis) 567.2

Fistula — *continued*
  periurethral 599.1
  pharyngo-esophageal 478.29
  pharynx 478.29
    branchial cleft (congenital) 744.41
  pilonidal (infected) (rectum) 685.1
    with abscess 685.0
  pleura, pleural, pleurocutaneous,
      pleuroperitoneal 510.0
    stomach 510.0
    tuberculous (*see also* Tuberculosis) 012.0 ☑
  pleuropericardial 423.8
  postauricular 383.81
  postoperative, persistent 998.6
  preauricular (congenital) 744.46
  prostate 602.8
  pulmonary 510.0
    arteriovenous 417.0
      congenital 747.3
    tuberculous (*see also* Tuberculosis,
      pulmonary) 011.9 ☑
  pulmonoperitoneal 510.0
  rectolabial 619.1
  rectosigmoid (intercommunicating) 569.81
  rectoureteral 593.82
  rectourethral 599.1
    congenital 753.8
  rectouterine 619.1
    congenital 752.3
  rectovaginal 619.1
    congenital 752.49
    old, postpartal 619.1
    tuberculous (*see also* Tuberculosis) 014.8 ☑
  rectovesical 596.1
    congenital 753.8
  rectovesicovaginal 619.1
  rectovulvar 619.1
    congenital 752.49
  rectum (to skin) 565.1
    tuberculous (*see also* Tuberculosis) 014.8 ☑
  renal 593.89
  retroauricular 383.81
  round window (internal ear) 386.41
  salivary duct or gland 527.4
    congenital 750.24
  sclera 360.32
  scrotum (urinary) 608.89
    tuberculous (*see also* Tuberculosis) 016.5 ☑
  semicircular canals (internal ear) 386.43
  sigmoid 569.81
    vesicoabdominal 596.1
  sigmoidovaginal 619.1
    congenital 752.49
  skin 686.9
    ureter 593.82
    vagina 619.2
  sphenoidal sinus (*see also* Sinusitis,
      sphenoidal) 473.3
  splenocolic 289.59
  stercoral 569.81
  stomach 537.4
  sublingual gland 527.4
    congenital 750.24
  submaxillary
    gland 527.4
      congenital 750.24
    region 528.3
  thoracic 510.0
    duct 457.8
  thoracicoabdominal 510.0
  thoracicogastric 510.0
  thoracicointestinal 510.0
  thoracoabdominal 510.0
  thoracogastric 510.0
  thorax 510.0
  thyroglossal duct 759.2
  thyroid 246.8
  trachea (congenital) (external) (internal) 748.3
  tracheoesophageal 530.84
    congenital 750.3
    following tracheostomy 519.09
  traumatic
    arteriovenous (*see also* Injury, blood vessel,
      by site) 904.9
    brain — *see* Injury, intracranial
  tuberculous — *see* Tuberculosis, by site
  typhoid 002.0

Fistula — *continued*
  umbilical 759.89
  umbilico-urinary 753.8
  urachal, urachus 753.7
  ureter (persistent) 593.82
  ureteroabdominal 593.82
  ureterocervical 593.82
  ureterorectal 593.82
  ureterosigmoido-abdominal 593.82
  ureterovaginal 619.0
  ureterovesical 596.2
  urethra 599.1
    congenital 753.8
    tuberculous (*see also* Tuberculosis) 016.3 ☑
  urethroperineal 599.1
  urethroperineovesical 596.2
  urethrorectal 599.1
    congenital 753.8
  urethroscrotal 608.89
  urethrovaginal 619.0
  urethrovesical 596.2
  urethrovesicovaginal 619.0
  urinary (persistent) (recurrent) 599.1
  uteroabdominal (anterior wall) 619.2
    congenital 752.3
  uteroenteric 619.1
  uterofecal 619.1
  uterointestinal 619.1
    congenital 752.3
  uterorectal 619.1
    congenital 752.3
  uteroureteric 619.0
  uterovaginal 619.8
  uterovesical 619.0
    congenital 752.3
  uterus 619.8
  vagina (wall) 619.8
    postpartal, old 619.8
  vaginocutaneous (postpartal) 619.2
  vaginoileal (acquired) 619.1
  vaginoperineal 619.2
  vesical NEC 596.2
  vesicoabdominal 596.2
  vesicocervicovaginal 619.0
  vesicocolic 596.1
  vesicocutaneous 596.2
  vesicoenteric 596.1
  vesicointestinal 596.1
  vesicometrorectal 619.1
  vesicoperineal 596.2
  vesicorectal 596.1
    congenital 753.8
  vesicosigmoidal 596.1
  vesicosigmoidovaginal 619.1
  vesicoureteral 596.2
  vesicoureterovaginal 619.0
  vesicourethral 596.2
  vesicourethrorectal 596.1
  vesicouterine 619.0
    congenital 752.3
  vesicovaginal 619.0
  vulvorectal 619.1
    congenital 752.49

Fit 780.39
  apoplectic (*see also* Disease, cerebrovascular,
      acute) 436
    late effect — *see* Late effect(s) (of)
      cerebrovascular disease
  epileptic (*see also* Epilepsy) 345.9 ☑
  fainting 780.2
  hysterical 300.11
  newborn 779.0

Fitting (of)
  artificial
    arm (complete) (partial) V52.0
    breast V52.4
    eye(s) V52.2
    leg(s) (complete) (partial) V52.1
  brain neuropacemaker V53.02
  cardiac pacemaker V53.31
  carotid sinus pacemaker V53.39
  cerebral ventricle (communicating) shunt
    V53.01
  colostomy belt V53.5
  contact lenses V53.1
  cystostomy device V53.6

Fitting — *continued*
  defibrillator, automatic implantable cardiac V53.32
  dentures V52.3
  device, unspecified type V53.90
    abdominal V53.5
    cardiac
      defibrillator, automatic implantable V53.32
      pacemaker V53.31
      specified NEC V53.39
    cerebral ventricle (communicating) shunt V53.01
    insulin pump V53.91
    intrauterine contraceptive V25.1
    nervous system V53.09
    orthodontic V53.4
    orthoptic V53.1
    other device V53.99
    prosthetic V52.9
      breast V52.4
      dental V52.3
      eye V52.2
      specified type NEC V52.8
    special senses V53.09
    substitution
      auditory V53.09
      nervous system V53.09
      visual V53.09
    urinary V53.6
  diaphragm (contraceptive) V25.02
  glasses (reading) V53.1
  growth rod V54.02
  hearing aid V53.2
  ileostomy device V53.5
  intestinal appliance or device NEC V53.5
  intrauterine contraceptive device V25.1
  neuropacemaker (brain) (peripheral nerve) (spinal cord) V53.02
  orthodontic device V53.4
  orthopedic (device) V53.7
    brace V53.7
    cast V53.7
    corset V53.7
    shoes V53.7
  pacemaker (cardiac) V53.31
    brain V53.02
    carotid sinus V53.39
    peripheral nerve V53.02
    spinal cord V53.02
  prosthesis V52.9
    arm (complete) (partial) V52.0
    breast V52.4
    dental V52.3
    eye V52.2
    leg (complete) (partial) V52.1
    specified type NEC V52.8
  spectacles V53.1
  wheelchair V53.8
Fitz's syndrome (acute hemorrhagic pancreatitis) 577.0
Fitz-Hugh and Curtis syndrome 098.86
  due to
    Chlamydia trachomatis 099.56
    Neisseria gonorrhoeae (gonococcal peritonitis) 098.86
Fixation
  joint — *see* Ankylosis
  larynx 478.79
  pupil 364.76
  stapes 385.22
    deafness (*see also* Deafness, conductive) 389.04
  uterus (acquired) — *see* Malposition, uterus
  vocal cord 478.5
Flaccid — *see also* condition
  foot 736.79
  forearm 736.09
  palate, congenital 750.26
Flail
  chest 807.4
    newborn 767.3
  joint (paralytic) 718.80
    ankle 718.87
    elbow 718.82
    foot 718.87

Flail — *continued*
  joint — *continued*
    hand 718.84
    hip 718.85
    knee 718.86
    multiple sites 718.89
    pelvic region 718.85
    shoulder (region) 718.81
    specified site NEC 718.88
    wrist 718.83
Flajani (-Basedow) syndrome or disease (exophthalmic goiter) 242.0 ☑
Flap, liver 572.8
Flare, anterior chamber (aqueous) (eye) 364.04
Flashback phenomena (drug) (hallucinogenic) 292.89
Flat
  chamber (anterior) (eye) 360.34
  chest, congenital 754.89
  electroencephalogram (EEG) 348.8
  foot (acquired) (fixed type) (painful) (postural) (spastic) 734
    congenital 754.61
      rocker bottom 754.61
      vertical talus 754.61
    rachitic 268.1
    rocker bottom (congenital) 754.61
    vertical talus, congenital 754.61
  organ or site, congenital NEC — *see* Anomaly, specified type NEC
  pelvis 738.6
    with disproportion (fetopelvic) 653.2 ☑
      affecting fetus or newborn 763.1
      causing obstructed labor 660.1 ☑
        affecting fetus or newborn 763.1
    congenital 755.69
Flatau-Schilder disease 341.1
Flattening
  head, femur 736.39
  hip 736.39
  lip (congenital) 744.89
  nose (congenital) 754.0
    acquired 738.0
Flatulence 787.3
Flatus 787.3
  vaginalis 629.8
Flax dressers' disease 504
Flea bite — *see* Injury, superficial, by site
Fleischer (-Kayser) ring (corneal pigmentation) 275.1 [371.14]
Fleischner's disease 732.3
Fleshy mole 631
Flexibilitas cerea (*see also* Catalepsy) 300.11
Flexion
  cervix (*see also* Malposition, uterus) 621.6
  contracture, joint (*see also* Contraction, joint) 718.4 ☑
  deformity, joint (*see also* Contraction, joint) 718.4 ☑
    hip, congenital (*see also* Subluxation, congenital, hip) 754.32
  uterus (*see also* Malposition, uterus) 621.6
Flexner's
  bacillus 004.1
  diarrhea (ulcerative) 004.1
  dysentery 004.1
Flexner-Boyd dysentery 004.2
Flexure — *see* condition
Floater, vitreous 379.24
Floating
  cartilage (joint) (*see also* Disorder, cartilage, articular) 718.0 ☑
    knee 717.6
  gallbladder (congenital) 751.69
  kidney 593.0
    congenital 753.3
  liver (congenital) 751.69
  rib 756.3
  spleen 289.59
Flooding 626.2
Floor — *see* condition

Floppy
  infant NEC 781.99
  valve syndrome (mitral) 424.0
Flu — *see also* Influenza
  gastric NEC 008.8
Fluctuating blood pressure 796.4
Fluid
  abdomen 789.5
  chest (*see also* Pleurisy, with effusion) 511.9
  heart (*see also* Failure, heart) 428.0
  joint (*see also* Effusion, joint) 719.0 ☑
  loss (acute) 276.5
    with
      hypernatremia 276.0
      hyponatremia 276.1
  lung — *see also* Edema, lung encysted 511.8
  peritoneal cavity 789.5
  pleural cavity (*see also* Pleurisy, with effusion) 511.9
  retention 276.6
Flukes NEC (*see also* Infestation, fluke) 121.9
  blood NEC (*see also* Infestation, Schistosoma) 120.9
  liver 121.3
Fluor (albus) (vaginalis) 623.5
  trichomonal (Trichomonas vaginalis) 131.00
Fluorosis (dental) (chronic) 520.3
Flushing 782.62
  menopausal 627.2
Flush syndrome 259.2
Flutter
  atrial or auricular 427.32
  heart (ventricular) 427.42
    atrial 427.32
  impure 427.32
  postoperative 997.1
  ventricular 427.42
Flux (bloody) (serosanguineous) 009.0
Focal — *see* condition
Fochier's abscess — *see* Abscess, by site
Focus, Assmann's (*see also* Tuberculosis) 011.0 ☑
Fogo selvagem 694.4
Foix-Alajouanine syndrome 336.1
Folds, anomalous — *see also* Anomaly, specified type NEC
  Bowman's membrane 371.31
  Descemet's membrane 371.32
  epicanthic 743.63
  heart 746.89
  posterior segment of eye, congenital 743.54
Folie à deux 297.3
Follicle
  cervix (nabothian) (ruptured) 616.0
  graafian, ruptured, with hemorrhage 620.0
  nabothian 616.0
Folliclis (primary) (*see also* Tuberculosis) 017.0 ☑
Follicular — *see also* condition
  cyst (atretic) 620.0
Folliculitis 704.8
  abscedens et suffodiens 704.8
  decalvans 704.09
  gonorrheal (acute) 098.0
    chronic or duration of 2 months or more 098.2
  keloid, keloidalis 706.1
  pustular 704.8
  ulerythematosa reticulata 701.8
Folliculosis, conjunctival 372.02
Følling's disease (phenylketonuria) 270.1
Follow-up (examination) (routine) (following) V67.9
  cancer chemotherapy V67.2
  chemotherapy V67.2
  fracture V67.4
  high-risk medication V67.51
  injury NEC V67.59
  postpartum
    immediately after delivery V24.0
    routine V24.2
  psychiatric V67.3
  psychotherapy V67.3

Follow-up — *continued*
  radiotherapy V67.1
    specified condition NEC V67.59
    specified surgery NEC V67.09
  surgery V67.00
    vaginal pap smear V67.01
  treatment V67.9
    combined NEC V67.6
    fracture V67.4
    involving high-risk medication NEC V67.51
    mental disorder V67.3
    specified NEC V67.59

Fong's syndrome (hereditary
  osteoonychodysplasia) 756.89

Food
  allergy 693.1
  anaphylactic shock — *see* Anaphylactic shock,
    due to, food
  asphyxia (from aspiration or inhalation) (*see
    also* Asphyxia, food) 933.1
  choked on (*see also* Asphyxia, food) 933.1
  deprivation 994.2
    specified kind of food NEC 269.8
  intoxication (*see also* Poisoning, food) 005.9
  lack of 994.2
  poisoning (*see also* Poisoning, food) 005.9
  refusal or rejection NEC 307.59
  strangulation or suffocation (*see also* Asphyxia,
    food) 933.1
  toxemia (*see also* Poisoning, food) 005.9

Foot — *see also* condition
  and mouth disease 078.4
  process disease 581.3

Foramen ovale (nonclosure) (patent) (persistent)
  745.5

Forbes' (glycogen storage) **disease** 271.0

Forbes-Albright syndrome (nonpuerperal
  amenorrhea and lactation associated with
  pituitary tumor) 253.1

Forced birth or delivery NEC 669.8 ☑
  affecting fetus or newborn NEC 763.89

Forceps
  delivery NEC 669.5 ☑
    affecting fetus or newborn 763.2

Fordyce's disease (ectopic sebaceous glands)
  (mouth) 750.26

Fordyce-Fox disease (apocrine miliaria) 705.82

Forearm — *see* condition

Foreign body

Note — For foreign body with open wound or
other injury, see Wound, open, or the type of
injury specified.

---

  accidentally left during a procedure 998.4
  anterior chamber (eye) 871.6
    magnetic 871.5
      retained or old 360.51
    retained or old 360.61
  ciliary body (eye) 871.6
    magnetic 871.5
      retained or old 360.52
    retained or old 360.62
  entering through orifice (current) (old)
    accessory sinus 932
    air passage (upper) 933.0
      lower 934.8
    alimentary canal 938
    alveolar process 935.0
    antrum (Highmore) 932
    anus 937
    appendix 936
    asphyxia due to (*see also* Asphyxia, food)
      933.1
    auditory canal 931
    auricle 931
    bladder 939.0
    bronchioles 934.8
    bronchus (main) 934.1
    buccal cavity 935.0
    canthus (inner) 930.1
    cecum 936
    cervix (canal) uterine 939.1
    coil, ileocecal 936
    colon 936

Foreign body — *continued*
  entering through orifice — *continued*
    conjunctiva 930.1
    conjunctival sac 930.1
    cornea 930.0
    digestive organ or tract NEC 938
    duodenum 936
    ear (external) 931
    esophagus 935.1
    eye (external) 930.9
      combined sites 930.8
      intraocular — *see* Foreign body, by site
      specified site NEC 930.8
    eyeball 930.8
      intraocular — *see* Foreign body,
        intraocular
    eyelid 930.1
      retained or old 374.86
    frontal sinus 932
    gastrointestinal tract 938
    genitourinary tract 939.9
    globe 930.8
      penetrating 871.6
        magnetic 871.5
          retained or old 360.50
        retained or old 360.60
    gum 935.0
    Highmore's antrum 932
    hypopharynx 933.0
    ileocecal coil 936
    ileum 936
    inspiration (of) 933.1
    intestine (large) (small) 936
    lacrimal apparatus, duct, gland, or sac
      930.2
    larynx 933.1
    lung 934.8
    maxillary sinus 932
    mouth 935.0
    nasal sinus 932
    nasopharynx 933.0
    nose (passage) 932
    nostril 932
    oral cavity 935.0
    palate 935.0
    penis 939.3
    pharynx 933.0
    pyriform sinus 933.0
    rectosigmoid 937
      junction 937
    rectum 937
    respiratory tract 934.9
      specified part NEC 934.8
    sclera 930.1
    sinus 932
      accessory 932
      frontal 932
      maxillary 932
      nasal 932
      pyriform 933.0
    small intestine 936
    stomach (hairball) 935.2
    suffocation by (*see also* Asphyxia, food)
      933.1
    swallowed 938
      tongue 933.0
    tear ducts or glands 930.2
    throat 933.0
    tongue 935.0
      swallowed 933.0
    tonsil, tonsillar 933.0
      fossa 933.0
    trachea 934.0
    ureter 939.0
    urethra 939.0
    uterus (any part) 939.1
    vagina 939.2
    vulva 939.2
    wind pipe 934.0
  granuloma (old) 728.82
    bone 733.99
    in operative wound (inadvertently left) 998.4
      due to surgical material intentionally left
        — *see* Complications, due to
        (presence of) any device, implant, or
        graft classified to 996.0-996.5 NEC
    muscle 728.82

Foreign body — *continued*
  granuloma — *continued*
    skin 709.4
    soft tissue 709.4
    subcutaneous tissue 709.4
  in
    bone (residual) 733.99
    open wound — *see* Wound, open, by site
      complicated
    soft tissue (residual) 729.6
  inadvertently left in operation wound (causing
    adhesions, obstruction, or perforation)
    998.4
  ingestion, ingested NEC 938
  inhalation or inspiration (*see also* Asphyxia,
    food) 933.1
  internal organ, not entering through an orifice
    — *see* Injury, internal, by site, with open
    wound
  intraocular (nonmagnetic 871.6
    combined sites 871.6
      magnetic 871.5
        retained or old 360.59
      retained or old 360.69
    magnetic 871.5
      retained or old 360.50
    retained or old 360.60
    specified site NEC 871.6
      magnetic 871.5
        retained or old 360.59
      retained or old 360.69
  iris (nonmagnetic) 871.6
    magnetic 871.5
      retained or old 360.52
    retained or old 360.62
  lens (nonmagnetic) 871.6
    magnetic 871.5
      retained or old 360.53
    retained or old 360.63
  lid, eye 930.1
  ocular muscle 870.4
    retained or old 376.6
  old or residual
    bone 733.99
    eyelid 374.86
    middle ear 385.83
    muscle 729.6
      ocular 376.6
    retrobulbar 376.6
    skin 729.6
      with granuloma 709.4
    soft tissue 729.6
      with granuloma 709.4
    subcutaneous tissue 729.6
      with granuloma 709.4
  operation wound, left accidentally 998.4
  orbit 870.4
    retained or old 376.6
  posterior wall, eye 871.6
    magnetic 871.5
      retained or old 360.55
    retained or old 360.65
  respiratory tree 934.9
    specified site NEC 934.8
  retained (old) (nonmagnetic) (in)
    anterior chamber (eye) 360.61
      magnetic 360.51
    ciliary body 360.62
      magnetic 360.52
    eyelid 374.86
    globe 360.60
      magnetic 360.50
    intraocular 360.60
      magnetic 360.50
      specified site NEC 360.69
        magnetic 360.59
    iris 360.62
      magnetic 360.52
    lens 360.63
      magnetic 360.53
    muscle 729.6
    orbit 376.6
    posterior wall of globe 360.65
      magnetic 360.55
    retina 360.65
      magnetic 360.55
    retrobulbar 376.6

☑ Additional Digit Required   ▶◀ Revised Text   ● New Line   ▲ Revised Code

Foreign body — *continued*
retained — *continued*
retina — *continued*
soft tissue 729.6
vitreous 360.64
magnetic 360.54
skin 729.6
with granuloma 709.4
soft tissue 729.6
with granuloma 709.4
subcutaneous tissue 729.6
with granuloma 709.4
retina 871.6
magnetic 871.5
retained or old 360.55
retained or old 360.65
superficial, without major open wound (*see also* Injury, superficial, by site) 919.6
swallowed NEC 938
vitreous (humor) 871.6
magnetic 871.5
retained or old 360.54
retained or old 360.64
Forking, aqueduct of Sylvius 742.3
with spina bifida (*see also* Spina bifida) 741.0 ☑
Formation
bone in scar tissue (skin) 709.3
connective tissue in vitreous 379.25
Elschnig pearls (postcataract extraction) 366.51
hyaline in cornea 371.49
sequestrum in bone (due to infection) (*see also* Osteomyelitis) 730.1 ☑
valve
colon, congenital 751.5
ureter (congenital) 753.29
Formication 782.0
Fort Bragg fever 100.89
Fossa — *see also* condition
pyriform — *see* condition
Foster-Kennedy syndrome 377.04
Fothergill's
disease, meaning scarlatina anginosa 034.1
neuralgia (*see also* Neuralgia, trigeminal) 350.1
Foul breath 784.9
Found dead (cause unknown) 798.9
Foundling V20.0
Fournier's disease (idiopathic gangrene) 608.83
Fourth
cranial nerve — *see* condition
disease 057.8
molar 520.1
Foville's syndrome 344.89
Fox's
disease (apocrine miliaria) 705.82
impetigo (contagiosa) 684
Fox-Fordyce disease (apocrine miliaria) 705.82
Fracture (abduction) (adduction) (avulsion) (compression) (crush) (dislocation) (oblique) (separation) (closed) 829.0

Note — *For fracture of any of the following sites with fracture of other bones* — *see Fracture, multiple.*

"Closed" includes the following descriptions of fractures, with or without delayed healing, unless they are specified as open or compound:

comminuted	linear
depressed	simple
elevated	slipped epiphysis
fissured	spiral
greenstick	unspecified
impacted	

"Open" includes the following descriptions of fractures, with or without delayed healing:

compound	puncture
infected	with foreign body
missile	

For late effect of fracture, see Late, effect, fracture, by site.

Fracture — *continued*
with
internal injuries in same region (conditions classifiable to 860-869) — *see also* Injury, internal, by site pelvic region — *see* Fracture, pelvis
acetabulum (with visceral injury) (closed) 808.0
open 808.1
acromion (process) (closed) 811.01
open 811.11
alveolus (closed) 802.8
open 802.9
ankle (malleolus) (closed) 824.8
bimalleolar (Dupuytren's) (Pott's) 824.4
open 824.5
bone 825.21
open 825.31
lateral malleolus only (fibular) 824.2
open 824.3
medial malleolus only (tibial) 824.0
open 824.1
open 824.9
pathologic 733.16
talus 825.21
open 825.31
trimalleolar 824.6
open 824.7
antrum — *see* Fracture, skull, base
arm (closed) 818.0
and leg(s) (any bones) 828.0
open 828.1
both (any bones) (with rib(s)) (with sternum) 819.0
open 819.1
lower 813.80
open 813.90
open 818.1
upper — *see* Fracture, humerus
astragalus (closed) 825.21
open 825.31
atlas — *see* Fracture, vertebra, cervical, first
axis — *see* Fracture, vertebra, cervical, second
back — *see* Fracture, vertebra, by site
Barton's — *see* Fracture, radius, lower end
basal (skull) — *see* Fracture, skull, base
Bennett's (closed) 815.01
open 815.11
bimalleolar (closed) 824.4
open 824.5
bone (closed) NEC 829.0
birth injury NEC 767.3
open 829.1
pathologic NEC (*see also* Fracture, pathologic) 733.10
stress NEC (*see also* Fracture, stress) 733.95
boot top — *see* Fracture, fibula
boxers' — *see* Fracture, metacarpal bone(s)
breast bone — *see* Fracture, sternum
bucket handle (semilunar cartilage) — *see* Tear, meniscus
bursting — *see* Fracture, phalanx, hand, distal
calcaneus (closed) 825.0
open 825.1
capitate (bone) (closed) 814.07
open 814.17
capitellum (humerus) (closed) 812.49
open 812.59
carpal bone(s) (wrist NEC) (closed) 814.00
open 814.10
specified site NEC 814.09
open 814.19
cartilage, knee (semilunar) — *see* Tear, meniscus
cervical — *see* Fracture, vertebra, cervical
chauffeur's — *see* Fracture, ulna, lower end
chisel — *see* Fracture, radius, upper end
clavicle (interligamentous part) (closed) 810.00
acromial end 810.03
open 810.13
due to birth trauma 767.2
open 810.10
shaft (middle third) 810.02
open 810.12
sternal end 810.01
open 810.11

Fracture — *continued*
clayshovelers' — *see* Fracture, vertebra, cervical
coccyx — *see also* Fracture, vertebra, coccyx
complicating delivery 665.6 ☑
collar bone — *see* Fracture, clavicle
Colles' (reversed) (closed) 813.41
open 813.51
comminuted — *see* Fracture, by site
compression — *see also* Fracture, by site
nontraumatic — *see* Fracture, pathologic
congenital 756.9
coracoid process (closed) 811.02
open 811.12
coronoid process (ulna) (closed) 813.02
mandible (closed) 802.23
open 802.33
open 813.12
corpus cavernosum penis 959.13
costochondral junction — *see* Fracture, rib
costosternal junction — *see* Fracture, rib
cranium — *see* Fracture, skull, by site
cricoid cartilage (closed) 807.5
open 807.6
cuboid (ankle) (closed) 825.23
open 825.33
cuneiform
foot (closed) 825.24
open 825.34
wrist (closed) 814.03
open 814.13
due to
birth injury — *see* Birth injury, fracture
gunshot — *see* Fracture, by site, open
neoplasm — *see* Fracture, pathologic
osteoporosis — *see* Fracture, pathologic
Dupuytren's (ankle) (fibula) (closed) 824.4
open 824.5
radius 813.42
open 813.52
Duverney's — *see* Fracture, ilium
elbow — *see also* Fracture, humerus, lower end
olecranon (process) (closed) 813.01
open 813.11
supracondylar (closed) 812.41
open 812.51
ethmoid (bone) (sinus) — *see* Fracture, skull, base
face bone(s) (closed) NEC 802.8
with
other bone(s) — *see* Fracture, multiple, skull
skull — *see also* Fracture, skull
involving other bones — *see* Fracture, multiple, skull
open 802.9
fatigue — *see* Fracture, march
femur, femoral (closed) 821.00
cervicotrochanteric 820.03
open 820.13
condyles, epicondyles 821.21
open 821.31
distal end — *see* Fracture, femur, lower end
epiphysis (separation)
capital 820.01
open 820.11
head 820.01
open 820.11
lower 821.22
open 821.32
trochanteric 820.01
open 820.11
upper 820.01
open 820.11
head 820.09
open 820.19
lower end or extremity (distal end) (closed) 821.20
condyles, epicondyles 821.21
open 821.31
epiphysis (separation) 821.22
open 821.32
multiple sites 821.29
open 821.39
open 821.30
specified site NEC 821.29
open 821.39

Fracture

Fracture

Fracture — *continued*
  leg — *continued*
    open 827.1
    upper — *see* Fracture, femur
  limb
    lower (multiple) (closed) NEC 827.0
      open 827.1
    upper (multiple) (closed) NEC 818.0
      open 818.1
  long bones, due to birth trauma — *see* Birth
      injury, fracture
  lumbar — *see* Fracture, vertebra, lumbar
  lunate bone (closed) 814.02
    open 814.12
  malar bone (closed) 802.4
    open 802.5
  Malgaigne's (closed) 808.43
    open 808.53
  malleolus (closed) 824.8
    bimalleolar 824.4
      open 824.5
    lateral 824.2
      and medial — *see also* Fracture,
          malleolus, bimalleolar
        with lip of tibia — *see* Fracture,
            malleolus, trimalleolar
      open 824.3
    medial (closed) 824.0
      and lateral — *see also* Fracture,
          malleolus, bimalleolar
        with lip of tibia — *see* Fracture,
            malleolus, trimalleolar
      open 824.1
    open 824.9
    trimalleolar (closed) 824.6
      open 824.7
  malleus — *see* Fracture, skull, base
  malunion 733.81
  mandible (closed) 802.20
    angle 802.25
      open 802.35
    body 802.28
      alveolar border 802.27
        open 802.37
      open 802.38
      symphysis 802.26
        open 802.36
    condylar process 802.21
      open 802.31
    coronoid process 802.23
      open 802.33
    multiple sites 802.29
      open 802.39
    open 802.30
    ramus NEC 802.24
      open 802.34
    subcondylar 802.22
      open 802.32
  manubrium — *see* Fracture, sternum
  march 733.95
    fibula 733.93
    metatarsals 733.94
    tibia 733.93
  maxilla, maxillary (superior) (upper jaw)
      (closed) 802.4
    inferior — *see* Fracture, mandible
    open 802.5
  meniscus, knee — *see* Tear, meniscus
  metacarpus, metacarpal (bone(s)), of one hand
      (closed) 815.00
    with phalanx, phalanges, hand (finger(s))
        (thumb) of same hand 817.0
      open 817.1
    base 815.02
      first metacarpal 815.01
        open 815.11
      open 815.12
      thumb 815.01
        open 815.11
    multiple sites 815.09
      open 815.19
    neck 815.04
      open 815.14
    open 815.10
    shaft 815.03
      open 815.13

Fracture — *continued*
  metatarsus, metatarsal (bone(s)), of one foot
      (closed) 825.25
    with tarsal bone(s) 825.29
      open 825.39
    open 825.35
  Monteggia's (closed) 813.03
    open 813.13
  Moore's — *see* Fracture, radius, lower end
    multangular bone (closed)
      larger 814.05
        open 814.15
      smaller 814.06
        open 814.16
  multiple (closed) 829.0

> Note — *Multiple fractures of sites classifiable to
> the same three- or four-digit category are coded
> to that category, except for sites classifiable to
> 810-818 or 820-827 in different limbs.*
>
> *Multiple fractures of sites classifiable to different
> fourth-digit subdivisions within the same three-
> digit category should be dealt with according to
> coding rules.*
>
> *Multiple fractures of sites classifiable to different
> three-digit categories (identifiable from the
> listing under "Fracture"), and of sites
> classifiable to 810-818 or 820-827 in different
> limbs should be coded according to the following
> list, which should be referred to in the following
> priority order: skull or face bones, pelvis or
> vertebral column, legs, arms.*

    arm (multiple bones in same arm except in
        hand alone) (sites classifiable to 810-
        817 with sites classifiable to a
        different three-digit category in 810-
        817 in same arm) (closed) 818.0
      open 818.1
    arms, both or arm(s) with rib(s) or sternum
        (sites classifiable to 810-818 with sites
        classifiable to same range of categories
        in other limb or to 807) (closed) 819.0
      open 819.1
    bones of trunk NEC (closed) 809.0
      open 809.1
    hand, metacarpal bone(s) with phalanx or
        phalanges of same hand (sites
        classifiable to 815 with sites
        classifiable to 816 in same hand)
        (closed) 817.0
      open 817.1
    leg (multiple bones in same leg) (sites
        classifiable to 820-826 with sites
        classifiable to a different three-digit
        category in that range in same leg)
        (closed) 827.0
      open 827.1
    legs, both or leg(s) with arm(s), rib(s), or
        sternum (sites classifiable to 820-827
        with sites classifiable to same range of
        categories in other leg or to 807 or
        810-819) (closed) 828.0
      open 828.1
    open 829.1
    pelvis with other bones except skull or face
        bones (sites classifiable to 808 with
        sites classifiable to 805-807 or 810-
        829) (closed) 809.0
      open 809.1
    skull, specified or unspecified bones, or face
        bone(s) with any other bone(s) (sites
        classifiable to 800-803 with sites
        classifiable to 805-829) (closed)
        804.0 ☑

Fracture — *continued*
  multiple — *continued*
    skull, specified or unspecified bones, or face
        bone(s) with any other bone(s) —
        continued

> Note — *Use the following fifth-digit
> subclassification with categories 800, 801, 803,
> and 804:*
>
> 0   *unspecified state of consciousness*
> 1   *with no loss of consciousness*
> 2   *with brief [less than one hour] loss of
>   consciousness*
> 3   *with moderate [1-24 hours] loss of
>   consciousness*
> 4   *with prolonged [more than 24 hours]
>   loss of consciousness and return to pre-
>   existing conscious level*
> 5   *with prolonged [more than 24 hours]
>   loss of consciousness, without return to
>   pre-existing conscious level*
> *Use fifth-digit 5 to designate when a patient
> is unconscious and dies before
> regaining consciousness, regardless of
> the duration of the loss of
> consciousness*
> 6   *with loss of consciousness of
>   unspecified duration*
> 9   *with concussion, unspecified*

    with
      contusion, cerebral 804.1 ☑
      epidural hemorrhage 804.2 ☑
      extradural hemorrhage 804.2 ☑
      hemorrhage (intracranial) NEC 804.3 ☑
      intracranial injury NEC 804.4 ☑
      laceration, cerebral 804.1 ☑
      subarachnoid hemorrhage 804.2 ☑
      subdural hemorrhage 804.2 ☑
    open 804.5 ☑
      with
        contusion, cerebral 804.6 ☑
        epidural hemorrhage 804.7 ☑
        extradural hemorrhage 804.7 ☑
        hemorrhage (intracranial) NEC
            804.8 ☑
        intracranial injury NEC 804.9 ☑
        laceration, cerebral 804.6 ☑
        subarachnoid hemorrhage 804.7 ☑
        subdural hemorrhage 804.7 ☑
    vertebral column with other bones, except
        skull or face bones (sites classifiable to
        805 or 806 with sites classifiable to
        807-808 or 810-829) (closed) 809.0
      open 809.1
  nasal (bone(s)) (closed) 802.0
    open 802.1
    sinus — *see* Fracture, skull, base
  navicular
    carpal (wrist) (closed) 814.01
      open 814.11
    tarsal (ankle) (closed) 825.22
      open 825.32
  neck — *see* Fracture, vertebra, cervical
  neural arch — *see* Fracture, vertebra, by site
  nonunion 733.82
  nose, nasal, (bone) (septum) (closed) 802.0
    open 802.1
  occiput — *see* Fracture, skull, base
  odontoid process — *see* Fracture, vertebra,
      cervical
  olecranon (process) (ulna) (closed) 813.01
    open 813.11
  open 829.1
  orbit, orbital (bone) (region) (closed) 802.8
    floor (blow-out) 802.6
      open 802.7
    open 802.9
    roof — *see* Fracture, skull, base
    specified part NEC 802.8
      open 802.9
  os
    calcis (closed) 825.0
      open 825.1
    magnum (closed) 814.07
      open 814.17

Fracture — *continued*
  os — *continued*
    pubis (with visceral injury) (closed) 808.2
      open 808.3
    triquetrum (closed) 814.03
      open 814.13
  osseous
    auditory meatus — *see* Fracture, skull, base
    labyrinth — *see* Fracture, skull, base
      ossicles, auditory (incus) (malleus)
        (stapes) — *see* Fracture, skull, base
  osteoporotic — *see* Fracture, pathologic
  palate (closed) 802.8
    open 802.9
  paratrooper — *see* Fracture, tibia, lower end
  parietal bone — *see* Fracture, skull, vault
  parry — *see* Fracture, Monteggia's
  patella (closed) 822.0
    open 822.1
  pathologic (cause unknown) 733.10
    ankle 733.16
    femur (neck) 733.14
      specified NEC 733.15
    fibula 733.16
    hip 733.14
    humerus 733.11
    radius 733.12
    specified site NEC 733.19
    tibia 733.16
    ulna 733.12
    vertebrae (collapse) 733.13
    wrist 733.12
  pedicle (of vertebral arch) — *see* Fracture, vertebra, by site
  pelvis, pelvic (bone(s)) (with visceral injury) (closed) 808.8
    multiple (with disruption of pelvic circle) 808.43
      open 808.53
    open 808.9
    rim (closed) 808.49
      open 808.59
  peritrochanteric (closed) 820.20
    open 820.30
  phalanx, phalanges, of one
    foot (closed) 826.0
      with bone(s) of same lower limb 827.0
        open 827.1
      open 826.1
    hand (closed) 816.00
      with metacarpal bone(s) of same hand 817.0
        open 817.1
      distal 816.02
        open 816.12
      middle 816.01
        open 816.11
      multiple sites NEC 816.03
        open 816.13
      open 816.10
      proximal 816.01
        open 816.11
  pisiform (closed) 814.04
    open 814.14
  pond — *see* Fracture, skull, vault
  Pott's (closed) 824.4
    open 824.5
  prosthetic device, internal — *see* Complications, mechanical
  pubis (with visceral injury) (closed) 808.2
    open 808.3
  Quervain's (closed) 814.01
    open 814.11
  radius (alone) (closed) 813.81
    with ulna NEC 813.83
      open 813.93
    distal end — *see* Fracture, radius, lower end
    epiphysis
      lower — *see* Fracture, radius, lower end
      upper — *see* Fracture, radius, upper end
    head — *see* Fracture, radius, upper end
    lower end or extremity (distal end) (lower epiphysis) 813.42
      with ulna (lower end) 813.44
        open 813.54
      torus 813.45
      open 813.52

Fracture — *continued*
  radius — *continued*
    neck — *see* Fracture, radius, upper end
    open NEC 813.91
    pathologic 733.12
    proximal end — *see* Fracture, radius, upper end
    shaft (closed) 813.21
      with ulna (shaft) 813.23
        open 813.33
      open 813.31
    upper end 813.07
      with ulna (upper end) 813.08
        open 813.18
      epiphysis 813.05
        open 813.15
      head 813.05
        open 813.15
      multiple sites 813.07
        open 813.17
      neck 813.06
        open 813.16
      open 813.17
      specified site NEC 813.07
        open 813.17
  ramus
    inferior or superior (with visceral injury) (closed) 808.2
      open 808.3
    ischium — *see* Fracture, ischium
    mandible 802.24
      open 802.34
  rib(s) (closed) 807.0 ☑

Note — Use the following fifth-digit subclassification with categories 807.0-807.1:

  0   *rib(s), unspecified*
  1   *one rib*
  2   *two ribs*
  3   *three ribs*
  4   *four ribs*
  5   *five ribs*
  6   *six ribs*
  7   *seven ribs*
  8   *eight or more ribs*
  9   *multiple ribs, unspecified*

---

    with flail chest (open) 807.4
    open 807.1 ☑
  root, tooth 873.63
    complicated 873.73
  sacrum — *see* Fracture, vertebra, sacrum
  scaphoid
    ankle (closed) 825.22
      open 825.32
    wrist (closed) 814.01
      open 814.11
  scapula (closed) 811.00
    acromial, acromion (process) 811.01
      open 811.11
    body 811.09
      open 811.19
    coracoid process 811.02
      open 811.12
    glenoid (cavity) (fossa) 811.03
      open 811.13
    neck 811.03
      open 811.13
      open 811.10
  semilunar
    bone, wrist (closed) 814.02
      open 814.12
    cartilage (interior) (knee) — *see* Tear, meniscus
  sesamoid bone — *see* Fracture, by site
  Shepherd's (closed) 825.21
    open 825.31
  shoulder — *see also* Fracture, humerus, upper end
    blade — *see* Fracture, scapula
  silverfork — *see* Fracture, radius, lower end
  sinus (ethmoid) (frontal) (maxillary) (nasal) (sphenoidal) — *see* Fracture, skull, base
  Skillern's — *see* Fracture, radius, shaft

Fracture — *continued*
  skull (multiple NEC) (with face bones) (closed) 803.0 ☑

Note — Use the following fifth digit subclassification with categories 800, 801, 803, and 804:

  0   *unspecified state of consciousness*
  1   *with no loss of consciousness*
  2   *with brief [less than one hour] loss of consciousness*
  3   *with moderate [1-24 hours] loss of consciousness*
  4   *with prolonged [more than 24 hours] loss of consciousness and return to pre-existing conscious level*
  5   *with prolonged [more than 24 hours] loss of consciousness, without return to pre-existing conscious level*

    Use fifth-digit 5 to designate when a patient is unconscious and dies before regaining consciousness, regardles of the duration of loss of consciousness

  6   *with loss of consciousness of unspecified duration*
  9   *with concussion, unspecified*

---

    with
      contusion, cerebral 803.1 ☑
      epidural hemorrhage 803.2 ☑
      extradural hemorrhage 803.2 ☑
      hemorrhage (intracranial) NEC 803.3 ☑
      intracranial injury NEC 803.4 ☑
      laceration, cerebral 803.1 ☑
      other bones — *see* Fracture, multiple, skull
      subarachnoid hemorrhage 803.2 ☑
      subdural hemorrhage 803.2 ☑
    base (antrum) (ethmoid bone) (fossa) (internal ear) (nasal sinus) (occiput) (sphenoid) (temporal bone) (closed) 801.0 ☑
      with
        contusion, cerebral 801.1 ☑
        epidural hemorrhage 801.2 ☑
        extradural hemorrhage 801.2 ☑
        hemorrhage (intracranial) NEC 801.3 ☑
        intracranial injury NEC 801.4 ☑
        laceration, cerebral 801.1 ☑
        subarachnoid hemorrhage 801.2 ☑
        subdural hemorrhage 801.2 ☑
      open 801.5 ☑
        with
          contusion, cerebral 801.6 ☑
          epidural hemorrhage 801.7 ☑
          extradural hemorrhage 801.7 ☑
          hemorrhage (intracranial) NEC 801.8 ☑
          intracranial injury NEC 801.9 ☑
          laceration, cerebral 801.6 ☑
          subarachnoid hemorrhage 801.7 ☑
          subdural hemorrhage 801.7 ☑
    birth injury 767.3
    face bones — *see* Fracture, face bones
    open 803.5 ☑
      with
        contusion, cerebral 803.6 ☑
        epidural hemorrhage 803.7 ☑
        extradural hemorrhage 803.7 ☑
        hemorrhage (intracranial) NEC 803.8 ☑
        intracranial injury NEC 803.9 ☑
        laceration, cerebral 803.6 ☑
        subarachnoid hemorrhage 803.7 ☑
        subdural hemorrhage 803.7 ☑
    vault (frontal bone) (parietal bone) (vertex) (closed) 800.0 ☑
      with
        contusion, cerebral 800.1 ☑
        epidural hemorrhage 800.2 ☑
        extradural hemorrhage 800.2 ☑
        hemorrhage (intracranial) NEC 800.3 ☑
        intracranial injury NEC 800.4 ☑
        laceration, cerebral 800.1 ☑

Fracture

Fracture — *continued*
  skull — *continued*
    vault — *continued*
      with — *continued*
        subarachnoid hemorrhage 800.2 ☑
        subdural hemorrhage 800.2 ☑
        open 800.5 ☑
          with
            contusion, cerebral 800.6 ☑
            epidural hemorrhage 800.7 ☑
            extradural hemorrhage 800.7 ☑
            hemorrhage (intracranial) NEC 800.8 ☑
            intracranial injury NEC 800.9 ☑
            laceration, cerebral 800.6 ☑
            subarachnoid hemorrhage 800.7 ☑
            subdural hemorrhage 800.7 ☑
  Smith's 813.41
    open 813.51
  sphenoid (bone) (sinus) — *see* Fracture, skull, base
  spine — *see also* Fracture, vertebra, by site due to birth trauma 767.4
  spinous process — *see* Fracture, vertebra, by site
  spontaneous — *see* Fracture, pathologic
  sprinters' — *see* Fracture, ilium
  stapes — *see* Fracture, skull, base
  stave — *see also* Fracture, metacarpus, metacarpal bone(s)
    spine — *see* Fracture, tibia, upper end
  sternum (closed) 807.2
    with flail chest (open) 807.4
    open 807.3
  Stieda's — *see* Fracture, femur, lower end
  stress 733.95
    fibula 733.93
    metatarsals 733.94
    specified site NEC 733.95
    tibia 733.93
  styloid process
    metacarpal (closed) 815.02
      open 815.12
    radius — *see* Fracture, radius, lower end
    temporal bone — *see* Fracture, skull, base
    ulna — *see* Fracture, ulna, lower end
  supracondylar, elbow 812.41
    open 812.51
  symphysis pubis (with visceral injury) (closed) 808.2
    open 808.3
  talus (ankle bone) (closed) 825.21
    open 825.31
  tarsus, tarsal bone(s) (with metatarsus) of one foot (closed) NEC 825.29
    open 825.39
  temporal bone (styloid) — *see* Fracture, skull, base
  tendon — *see* Sprain, by site
  thigh — *see* Fracture, femur, shaft
  thumb (and finger(s)) of one hand (closed) (*see also* Fracture, phalanx, hand) 816.00
    with metacarpal bone(s) of same hand 817.0
      open 817.1
    metacarpal(s) — *see* Fracture, metacarpus
    open 816.10
  thyroid cartilage (closed) 807.5
    open 807.6
  tibia (closed) 823.80
    with fibula 823.82
      open 823.92
    condyles — *see* Fracture, tibia, upper end
    distal end 824.8
      open 824.9
    epiphysis
      lower 824.8
        open 824.9
      upper — *see* Fracture, tibia, upper end
    head (involving knee joint) — *see* Fracture, tibia, upper end
    intercondyloid eminence — *see* Fracture, tibia, upper end
    involving ankle 824.0
      open 824.9
    malleolus (internal) (medial) 824.0
      open 824.1
    open NEC 823.90

Fracture — *continued*
  tibia — *continued*
    pathologic 733.16
    proximal end — *see* Fracture, tibia, upper end
    shaft 823.20
      with fibula 823.22
        open 823.32
      open 823.30
    spine — *see* Fracture, tibia, upper end
    stress 733.93
    torus 823.40
      with fibula 823.42
    tuberosity — *see* Fracture, tibia, upper end
    upper end or extremity (condyle) (epiphysis) (head) (spine) (proximal end) (tuberosity) 823.00
      with fibula 823.02
        open 823.12
      open 823.10
  toe(s), of one foot (closed) 826.0
    with bone(s) of same lower limb 827.0
      open 827.1
    open 826.1
  tooth (root) 873.63
    complicated 873.73
  torus
    fibula 823.41
      with tibia 823.42
    radius 813.45
    tibia 823.40
      with fibula 823.42
  trachea (closed) 807.5
    open 807.6
  transverse process — *see* Fracture, vertebra, by site
  trapezium (closed) 814.05
    open 814.15
  trapezoid bone (closed) 814.06
    open 814.16
  trimalleolar (closed) 824.6
    open 824.7
  triquetral (bone) (closed) 814.03
    open 814.13
  trochanter (greater) (lesser) (closed) (*see also* Fracture, femur, neck, by site) 820.20
    open 820.30
  trunk (bones) (closed) 809.0
    open 809.1
  tuberosity (external) — *see* Fracture, by site
  ulna (alone) (closed) 813.82
    with radius NEC 813.83
      open 813.93
    coronoid process (closed) 813.02
      open 813.12
    distal end — *see* Fracture, ulna, lower end
    epiphysis
      lower — *see* Fracture, ulna, lower end
      upper — *see* Fracture, ulna, upper end
    head — *see* Fracture, ulna, lower end
    lower end (distal end) (head) (lower epiphysis) (styloid process) 813.43
      with radius (lower end) 813.44
        open 813.54
      open 813.53
    olecranon process (closed) 813.01
      open 813.11
    open NEC 813.92
    pathologic 733.12
    proximal end — *see* Fracture, ulna, upper end
    shaft 813.22
      with radius (shaft) 813.23
        open 813.33
      open 813.32
    styloid process — *see* Fracture, ulna, lower end
    transverse — *see* Fracture, ulna, by site
    upper end (epiphysis) 813.04
      with radius (upper end) 813.08
        open 813.18
      multiple sites 813.04
        open 813.14
      open 813.14
      specified site NEC 813.04
        open 813.14

Fracture — *continued*
  unciform (closed) 814.08
    open 814.18
  vertebra, vertebral (back) (body) (column) (neural arch) (pedicle) (spine) (spinous process) (transverse process) (closed) 805.8
    with
      hematomyelia — *see* Fracture, vertebra, by site, with spinal cord injury
      injury to
        cauda equina — *see* Fracture, vertebra, sacrum, with spinal cord injury
        nerve — *see* Fracture, vertebra, by site, with spinal cord injury
      paralysis — *see* Fracture, vertebra, by site, with spinal cord injury
      paraplegia — *see* Fracture, vertebra, by site, with spinal cord injury
      quadriplegia — *see* Fracture, vertebra, by site, with spinal cord injury
      spinal concussion — *see* Fracture, vertebra, by site, with spinal cord injury
      spinal cord injury (closed) NEC 806.8

> **Note** — *Use the following fifth-digit subclassification with categories 806.0-806.3:*
> C_1-C_4 *or unspecified level and* D_1-D_6 (T_1-T_6) *or unspecified level with:*
>   0 *unspecified spinal cord injury*
>   1 *complete lesion of cord*
>   2 *anterior cord syndrome*
>   3 *central cord syndrome*
>   4 *specified injury NEC*
> C_5-C_7 *level and* D_7-D_{12} *level with:*
>   5 *unspecified spinal cord injury*
>   6 *complete lesion of cord*
>   7 *anterior cord syndrome*
>   8 *central cord syndrome*
>   9 *specified injury NEC*

        cervical 806.0 ☑
          open 806.1 ☑
        dorsal, dorsolumbar 806.2 ☑
          open 806.3 ☑
          open 806.9
        thoracic, thoracolumbar 806.2 ☑
          open 806.3 ☑
    atlanto-axial — *see* Fracture, vertebra, cervical
    cervical (hangman) (teardrop) (closed) 805.00
      with spinal cord injury — *see* Fracture, vertebra, with spinal cord injury, cervical
      first (atlas) 805.01
        open 805.11
      second (axis) 805.02
        open 805.12
      third 805.03
        open 805.13
      fourth 805.04
        open 805.14
      fifth 805.05
        open 805.15
      sixth 805.06
        open 805.16
      seventh 805.07
        open 805.17
      multiple sites 805.08
        open 805.18
      open 805.10
    coccyx (closed) 805.6
      with spinal cord injury (closed) 806.60
        cauda equina injury 806.62
          complete lesion 806.61
            open 806.71
          open 806.72
        open 806.70
        specified type NEC 806.69
          open 806.79
      open 805.7
    collapsed 733.13
    compression, not due to trauma 733.13

☑ Additional Digit Required   ▶◀ Revised Text   ● New Line   ▲ Revised Code

Fracture — *continued*
  vertebra, vertebral — *continued*
    dorsal (closed) 805.2
      with spinal cord injury — *see* Fracture,
        vertebra, with spinal cord injury,
        dorsal
      open 805.3
    dorsolumbar (closed) 805.2
      with spinal cord injury — *see* Fracture,
        vertebra, with spinal cord injury,
        dorsal
      open 805.3
    due to osteoporosis 733.13
    fetus or newborn 767.4
    lumbar (closed) 805.4
      with spinal cord injury (closed) 806.4
        open 806.5
      open 805.5
    nontraumatic 733.13
    open NEC 805.9
    pathologic (any site) 733.13
    sacrum (closed) 805.6
      with spinal cord injury 806.60
        cauda equina injury 806.62
          complete lesion 806.61
            open 806.71
          open 806.72
        open 806.70
        specified type NEC 806.69
          open 806.79
      open 805.7
    site unspecified (closed) 805.8
      with spinal cord injury (closed) 806.8
        open 806.9
      open 805.9
    stress (any site) 733.95
    thoracic (closed) 805.2
      with spinal cord injury — *see* Fracture,
        vertebra, with spinal cord injury,
        thoracic
      open 805.3
  vertex — *see* Fracture, skull, vault
  vomer (bone) 802.0
    open 802.1
  Wagstaffe's — *see* Fracture, ankle
  wrist (closed) 814.00
    open 814.10
    pathologic 733.12
  xiphoid (process) — *see* Fracture, sternum
  zygoma (zygomatic arch) (closed) 802.4
    open 802.5
Fragile X syndrome 759.83
Fragilitas
  crinium 704.2
  hair 704.2
  ossium 756.51
    with blue sclera 756.51
  unguium 703.8
    congenital 757.5
Fragility
  bone 756.51
    with deafness and blue sclera 756.51
  capillary (hereditary) 287.8
  hair 704.2
  nails 703.8
Fragmentation — *see* Fracture, by site
Frambesia, frambesial (tropica) (*see also* Yaws)
  102.9
  initial lesion or ulcer 102.0
  primary 102.0
Frambeside
  gummatous 102.4
  of early yaws 102.2
Frambesioma 102.1
Franceschetti's syndrome (mandibulofacial
  dysostosis) 756.0
Francis' disease (*see also* Tularemia) 021.9
Frank's essential thrombocytopenia (*see also*
  Purpura, thrombocytopenic) 287.3
Franklin's disease (heavy chain) 273.2
Fraser's syndrome 759.89
Freckle 709.09
  malignant melanoma in (M8742/3) — *see*
    Melanoma

Freckle — *continued*
  melanotic (of Hutchinson) (M8742/2) — *see*
    Neoplasm, skin, in situ
Freeman-Sheldon syndrome 759.89
Freezing 991.9
  specified effect NEC 991.8
Frei's disease (climatic bubo) 099.1
Freiberg's
  disease (osteochondrosis, second metatarsal)
    732.5
  infraction of metatarsal head 732.5
  osteochondrosis 732.5
Fremitus, friction, cardiac 785.3
Frenulum linguae 750.0
Frenum
  external os 752.49
  tongue 750.0
Frequency (urinary) NEC 788.41
  micturition 788.41
  nocturnal 788.43
  psychogenic 306.53
Frey's syndrome (auriculotemporal syndrome)
  705.22   ▲
Friction
  burn (*see also* Injury, superficial, by site) 919.0
  fremitus, cardiac 785.3
  precordial 785.3
  sounds, chest 786.7
Friderichsen-Waterhouse syndrome or disease
  036.3
Friedländer's
  B (bacillus) NEC (*see also* condition) 041.3
    sepsis or septicemia 038.49
  disease (endarteritis obliterans) — *see*
    Arteriosclerosis
Friedreich's
  ataxia 334.0
  combined systemic disease 334.0
  disease 333.2
    combined systemic 334.0
  myoclonia 333.2
  sclerosis (spinal cord) 334.0
Friedrich-Erb-Arnold syndrome
  (acropachyderma) 757.39
Frigidity 302.72
  psychic or psychogenic 302.72
Fröhlich's disease or syndrome (adiposogenital
  dystrophy) 253.8
Froin's syndrome 336.8
Frommel's disease 676.6 ☑
Frommel-Chiari syndrome 676.6 ☑
Frontal — *see also* condition
  lobe syndrome 310.0
Frostbite 991.3
  face 991.0
  foot 991.2
  hand 991.1
  specified site NEC 991.3
Frotteurism 302.89
Frozen 991.9
  pelvis 620.8
  shoulder 726.0
Fructosemia 271.2
Fructosuria (benign) (essential) 271.2
Fuchs'
  black spot (myopic) 360.21
  corneal dystrophy (endothelial) 371.57
  heterochromic cyclitis 364.21
Fucosidosis 271.8
Fugue 780.99
  dissociative 300.13   ●
  hysterical (dissociative) 300.13
  reaction to exceptional stress (transient) 308.1
Fukuhara syndrome 277.87   ●
Fuller Albright's syndrome (osteitis fibrosa
  disseminata) 756.59
Fuller's earth disease 502
Fulminant, fulminating — *see* condition
Functional — see condition

Fundus — *see also* condition
  flavimaculatus 362.76
Fungemia 117.9
Fungus, fungous
  cerebral 348.8
  disease NEC 117.9
  infection — *see* Infection, fungus
  testis (*see also* Tuberculosis) 016.5 ☑ *[608.81]*
Funiculitis (acute) 608.4
  chronic 608.4
  endemic 608.4
  gonococcal (acute) 098.14
    chronic or duration of 2 months or over
      098.34
  tuberculous (*see also* Tuberculosis) 016.5 ☑
Funnel
  breast (acquired) 738.3
    congenital 754.81
    late effect of rickets 268.1
  chest (acquired) 738.3
    congenital 754.81
    late effect of rickets 268.1
  pelvis (acquired) 738.6
    with disproportion (fetopelvic) 653.3 ☑
      affecting fetus or newborn 763.1
      causing obstructed labor 660.1 ☑
        affecting fetus or newborn 763.1
    congenital 755.69
    tuberculous (*see also* Tuberculosis) 016.9 ☑
F.U.O. (*see also* Pyrexia) 780.6
Furfur 690.18
  microsporon 111.0
Furor, paroxysmal (idiopathic) (*see also* Epilepsy)
  345.8 ☑
Furriers' lung 495.8
Furrowed tongue 529.5
  congenital 750.13
Furrowing nail(s) (transverse) 703.8
  congenital 757.5
Furuncle 680.9
  abdominal wall 680.2
  ankle 680.6
  anus 680.5
  arm (any part, above wrist) 680.3
  auditory canal, external 680.0
  axilla 680.3
  back (any part) 680.2
  breast 680.2
  buttock 680.5
  chest wall 680.2
  corpus cavernosum 607.2
  ear (any part) 680.0
  eyelid 373.13
  face (any part, except eye) 680.0
  finger (any) 680.4
  flank 680.2
  foot (any part) 680.7
  forearm 680.3
  gluteal (region) 680.5
  groin 680.2
  hand (any part) 680.4
  head (any part, except face) 680.8
  heel 680.7
  hip 680.6
  kidney (*see also* Abscess, kidney) 590.2
  knee 680.6
  labium (majus) (minus) 616.4
  lacrimal
    gland (*see also* Dacryoadenitis) 375.00
    passages (duct) (sac) (*see also*
      Dacryocystitis) 375.30
  leg, any part except foot 680.6
  malignant 022.0
  multiple sites 680.9
  neck 680.1
  nose (external) (septum) 680.0
  orbit 376.01
  partes posteriores 680.5
  pectoral region 680.2
  penis 607.2
  perineum 680.2
  pinna 680.0
  scalp (any part) 680.8
  scrotum 608.4

☑ Additional Digit Required   ▶◀ Revised Text   ● New Line   ▲ Revised Code

Furuncle — *continued*
  seminal vesicle 608.0
  shoulder 680.3
  skin NEC 680.9
  specified site NEC 680.8
  spermatic cord 608.4
  temple (region) 680.0
  testis 604.90
  thigh 680.6
  thumb 680.4
  toe (any) 680.7
  trunk 680.2
  tunica vaginalis 608.4
  umbilicus 680.2
  upper arm 680.3
  vas deferens 608.4
  vulva 616.4
  wrist 680.4

Furunculosis (*see also* Furuncle) 680.9
  external auditory meatus 680.0 *[380.13]*

Fusarium (infection) 118

Fusion, fused (congenital)
  anal (with urogenital canal) 751.5
  aorta and pulmonary artery 745.0
  astragaloscaphoid 755.67
  atria 745.5
  atrium and ventricle 745.69
  auditory canal 744.02
  auricles, heart 745.5
  binocular, with defective stereopsis 368.33
  bone 756.9
  cervical spine — *see* Fusion, spine
  choanal 748.0
  commissure, mitral valve 746.5
  cranial sutures, premature 756.0
  cusps, heart valve NEC 746.89
    mitral 746.5
    tricuspid 746.89
  ear ossicles 744.04
  fingers (*see also* Syndactylism, fingers) 755.11
  hymen 752.42
  hymeno-urethral 599.89
    causing obstructed labor 660.1 ☑
      affecting fetus or newborn 763.1
  joint (acquired) — *see also* Ankylosis
    congenital 755.8
  kidneys (incomplete) 753.3
  labium (majus) (minus) 752.49
  larynx and trachea 748.3
  limb 755.8
    lower 755.69
    upper 755.59
  lobe, lung 748.5
  lumbosacral (acquired) 724.6
    congenital 756.15
    surgical V45.4
  nares (anterior) (posterior) 748.0
  nose, nasal 748.0
  nostril(s) 748.0
  organ or site NEC — *see* Anomaly, specified
    type NEC
  ossicles 756.9
    auditory 744.04
  pulmonary valve segment 746.02
  pulmonic cusps 746.02
  ribs 756.3
  sacroiliac (acquired) (joint) 724.6
    congenital 755.69
    surgical V45.4
  skull, imperfect 756.0
  spine (acquired) 724.9
    arthrodesis status V45.4
    congenital (vertebra) 756.15
    postoperative status V45.4
  sublingual duct with submaxillary duct at
    opening in mouth 750.26
  talonavicular (bar) 755.67
  teeth, tooth 520.2
  testes 752.89
  toes (*see also* Syndactylism, toes) 755.13
  trachea and esophagus 750.3
  twins 759.4
  urethral-hymenal 599.89
  vagina 752.49
  valve cusps — *see* Fusion, cusps, heart valve
  ventricles, heart 745.4

Fusion, fused — *continued*
  vertebra (arch) — *see* Fusion, spine
  vulva 752.49
Fusospirillosis (mouth) (tongue) (tonsil) 101
Fussy infant (baby) 780.91

☑ Additional Digit Required   ▶◀ Revised Text   ● New Line   ▲ Revised Code

G

Gafsa boil 085.1

Gain, weight (abnormal) (excessive) (*see also* Weight, gain) 783.1

Gaisböck's disease or syndrome (polycythemia hypertonica) 289.0

Gait
abnormality 781.2
  hysterical 300.11
ataxic 781.2
  hysterical 300.11
disturbance 781.2
  hysterical 300.11
paralytic 781.2
scissor 781.2
spastic 781.2
staggering 781.2
  hysterical 300.11

Galactocele (breast) (infected) 611.5
puerperal, postpartum 676.8 ☑

Galactophoritis 611.0
puerperal, postpartum 675.2 ☑

Galactorrhea 676.6 ☑
not associated with childbirth 611.6

Galactosemia (classic) (congenital) 271.1

Galactosuria 271.1

Galacturia 791.1
bilharziasis 120.0

Galen's vein — *see* condition

Gallbladder — *see also* condition
acute (*see also* Disease, gallbladder) 575.0

Gall duct — *see* condition

Gallop rhythm 427.89

Gallstone (cholemic) (colic) (impacted) — *see also* Cholelithiasis
causing intestinal obstruction 560.31

Gambling, pathological 312.31

Gammaloidosis 277.3

Gammopathy 273.9
macroglobulinemia 273.3
monoclonal (benign) (essential) (idiopathic) (with lymphoplasmacytic dyscrasia) 273.1

Gamna's disease (siderotic splenomegaly) 289.51

Gampsodactylia (congenital) 754.71

Gamstorp's disease (adynamia episodica hereditaria) 359.3

Gandy-Nanta disease (siderotic splenomegaly) 289.51

Gang activity, without manifest psychiatric disorder V71.09
adolescent V71.02
adult V71.01
child V71.02

Gangliocytoma (M9490/0) — *see* Neoplasm, connective tissue, benign

Ganglioglioma (M9505/1) — *see* Neoplasm, by site, uncertain behavior

Ganglion 727.43
joint 727.41
of yaws (early) (late) 102.6
periosteal (*see also* Periostitis) 730.3 ☑
tendon sheath (compound) (diffuse) 727.42
tuberculous (*see also* Tuberculosis) 015.9 ☑

Ganglioneuroblastoma (M9490/3) — *see* Neoplasm, connective tissue, malignant

Ganglioneuroma (M9490/0) — *see also* Neoplasm, connective tissue, benign
malignant (M9490/3) — *see* Neoplasm, connective tissue, malignant

Ganglioneuromatosis (M9491/0) — *see* Neoplasm, connective tissue, benign

Ganglionitis
fifth nerve (*see also* Neuralgia, trigeminal) 350.1
gasserian 350.1
geniculate 351.1
  herpetic 053.11
  newborn 767.5
herpes zoster 053.11
herpetic geniculate (Hunt's syndrome) 053.11

Gangliosidosis 330.1

Gangosa 102.5

Gangrene, gangrenous (anemia) (artery) (cellulitis) (dermatitis) (dry) (infective) (moist) (pemphigus) (septic) (skin) (stasis) (ulcer) 785.4
with
  arteriosclerosis (native artery) 440.24
    bypass graft 440.30
      autologous vein 440.31
      nonautologous biological 440.32
  diabetes (mellitus) 250.7 ☑ *[785.4]*
abdomen (wall) 785.4
adenitis 683
alveolar 526.5
angina 462
  diphtheritic 032.0
anus 569.49
appendices epiploicae — *see* Gangrene, mesentery
appendix — *see* Appendicitis, acute
arteriosclerotic — *see* Arteriosclerosis, with, gangrene
auricle 785.4
Bacillus welchii (*see also* Gangrene, gas) 040.0
bile duct (*see also* Cholangitis) 576.8
bladder 595.89
bowel — *see* Gangrene, intestine
cecum — *see* Gangrene, intestine
Clostridium perfringens or welchii (*see also* Gangrene, gas) 040.0
colon — *see* Gangrene, intestine
connective tissue 785.4
cornea 371.40
corpora cavernosa (infective) 607.2
  noninfective 607.89
cutaneous, spreading 785.4
decubital (*see also* Decubitus) 707.00 *[785.4]* ▲
diabetic (any site) 250.7 ☑ *[785.4]*
dropsical 785.4
emphysematous (*see also* Gangrene, gas) 040.0
epidemic (ergotized grain) 988.2
epididymis (infectional) (*see also* Epididymitis) 604.99
erysipelas (*see also* Erysipelas) 035
extremity (lower) (upper) 785.4
gallbladder or duct (*see also* Cholecystitis, acute) 575.0
gas (bacillus) 040.0
  with
    abortion — *see* Abortion, by type, with sepsis
    ectopic pregnancy (*see also* categories 633.0-633.9) 639.0
    molar pregnancy (*see also* categories 630-632) 639.0
  following
    abortion 639.0
    ectopic or molar pregnancy 639.0
  puerperal, postpartum, childbirth 670.0 ☑
glossitis 529.0
gum 523.8
hernia — *see* Hernia, by site, with gangrene
hospital noma 528.1
intestine, intestinal (acute) (hemorrhagic) (massive) 557.0
  with
    hernia — *see* Hernia, by site, with gangrene
    mesenteric embolism or infarction 557.0
    obstruction (*see also* Obstruction, intestine) 560.9
laryngitis 464.00
  with obstruction 464.01
liver 573.8
lung 513.0
  spirochetal 104.8
lymphangitis 457.2
Meleney's (cutaneous) 686.09
mesentery 557.0
  with
    embolism or infarction 557.0
    intestinal obstruction (*see also* Obstruction, intestine) 560.9
mouth 528.1
noma 528.1

Gangrene, gangrenous — *continued*
orchitis 604.90
ovary (*see also* Salpingo-oophoritis) 614.2
pancreas 577.0
penis (infectional) 607.2
  noninfective 607.89
perineum 785.4
pharynx 462
septic 034.0
pneumonia 513.0
Pott's 440.24
presenile 443.1
pulmonary 513.0
pulp, tooth 522.1
quinsy 475
Raynaud's (symmetric gangrene) 443.0 *[785.4]*
rectum 569.49
retropharyngeal 478.24
rupture — *see* Hernia, by site, with gangrene
scrotum 608.4
  noninfective 608.83
senile 440.24
sore throat 462
spermatic cord 608.4
  noninfective 608.89
spine 785.4
spirochetal NEC 104.8
spreading cutaneous 785.4
stomach 537.89
stomatitis 528.1
symmetrical 443.0 *[785.4]*
testis (infectional) (*see also* Orchitis) 604.99
  noninfective 608.89
throat 462
  diphtheritic 032.0
thyroid (gland) 246.8
tonsillitis (acute) 463
tooth (pulp) 522.1
tuberculous NEC (*see also* Tuberculosis) 011.9 ☑
tunica vaginalis 608.4
  noninfective 608.89
umbilicus 785.4
uterus (*see also* Endometritis) 615.9
uvulitis 528.3
vas deferens 608.4
  noninfective 608.89
vulva (*see also* Vulvitis) 616.10

Gannister disease (occupational) 502
with tuberculosis — *see* Tuberculosis, pulmonary

Ganser's syndrome, hysterical 300.16

Gardner-Diamond syndrome (autoerythrocyte sensitization) 287.2

Gargoylism 277.5

Garré's
disease (*see also* Osteomyelitis) 730.1 ☑
osteitis (sclerosing) (*see also* Osteomyelitis) 730.1 ☑
osteomyelitis (*see also* Osteomyelitis) 730.1 ☑

Garrod's pads, knuckle 728.79

Gartner's duct
cyst 752.11
persistent 752.11

Gas
asphyxia, asphyxiation, inhalation, poisoning, suffocation NEC 987.9
  specified gas — *see* Table of Drugs and Chemicals
bacillus gangrene or infection — *see* Gas, gangrene
cyst, mesentery 568.89
excessive 787.3
gangrene 040.0
  with
    abortion — *see* Abortion, by type, with sepsis
    ectopic pregnancy (*see also* categories 633.0-633.9) 639.0
    molar pregnancy (*see also* categories 630-632) 639.0
  following
    abortion 639.0
    ectopic or molar pregnancy 639.0
  puerperal, postpartum, childbirth 670.0 ☑

Gas — *continued*
on stomach 787.3
pains 787.3
Gastradenitis 535.0 ☑
Gastralgia 536.8
psychogenic 307.89
Gastrectasis, gastrectasia 536.1
psychogenic 306.4
Gastric — *see* condition
Gastrinoma (M8153/1)
malignant (M8153/3)
pancreas 157.4
specified site NEC — *see* Neoplasm, by site, malignant
unspecified site 157.4
specified site — *see* Neoplasm, by site, uncertain behavior
unspecified site 235.5
Gastritis 535.5 ☑

Note — Use the following fifth-digit subclassification for category 535:

0   *without mention of hemorrhage*
1   *with hemorrhage*

acute 535.0 ☑
alcoholic 535.3 ☑
allergic 535.4 ☑
antral 535.4 ☑
atrophic 535.1 ☑
atrophic-hyperplastic 535.1 ☑
bile-induced 535.4 ☑
catarrhal 535.0 ☑
chronic (atrophic) 535.1 ☑
cirrhotic 535.4 ☑
corrosive (acute) 535.4 ☑
dietetic 535.4 ☑
due to diet deficiency 269.9 [535.4] ☑
eosinophilic 535.4 ☑
erosive 535.4 ☑
follicular 535.4 ☑
chronic 535.1 ☑
giant hypertrophic 535.2 ☑
glandular 535.4 ☑
chronic 535.1 ☑
hypertrophic (mucosa) 535.2 ☑
chronic giant 211.1
irritant 535.4 ☑
nervous 306.4
phlegmonous 535.0 ☑
psychogenic 306.4
sclerotic 535.4 ☑
spastic 536.8
subacute 535.0 ☑
superficial 535.4 ☑
suppurative 535.0 ☑
toxic 535.4 ☑
tuberculous (*see also* Tuberculosis) 017.9 ☑
Gastrocarcinoma (M8010/3) 151.9
Gastrocolic — *see* condition
Gastrocolitis — *see* Enteritis
Gastrodisciasis 121.8
Gastroduodenitis (*see also* Gastritis) 535.5 ☑
catarrhal 535.0 ☑
infectional 535.0 ☑
virus, viral 008.8
specified type NEC 008.69
Gastrodynia 536.8
Gastroenteritis (acute) (catarrhal) (congestive) (hemorrhagic) (noninfectious) (*see also* Enteritis) 558.9
aertrycke infection 003.0
allergic 558.3
chronic 558.9
ulcerative (*see also* Colitis, ulcerative) 556.9
dietetic 558.9
due to
food poisoning (*see also* Poisoning, food) 005.9
radiation 558.1
epidemic 009.0
functional 558.9

Gastroenteritis (*see also* Enteritis) — *continued*
infectious (*see also* Enteritis, due to, by organism) 009.0
presumed 009.1
salmonella 003.0
septic (*see also* Enteritis, due to, by organism) 009.0
toxic 558.2
tuberculous (*see also* Tuberculosis) 014.8 ☑
ulcerative (*see also* Colitis, ulcerative) 556.9
viral NEC 008.8
specified type NEC 008.69
zymotic 009.0
Gastroenterocolitis — *see* Enteritis
Gastroenteropathy, protein-losing 579.8
Gastroenteroptosis 569.89
Gastroesophageal laceration-hemorrhage syndrome 530.7
Gastroesophagitis 530.19
Gastrohepatitis (*see also* Gastritis) 535.5 ☑
Gastrointestinal — *see* condition
Gastrojejunal — *see* condition
Gastrojejunitis (*see also* Gastritis) 535.5 ☑
Gastrojejunocolic — *see* condition
Gastroliths 537.89
Gastromalacia 537.89
Gastroparalysis 536.3 ▲
diabetic 250.6 ☑ [536.3]
Gastroparesis 536.3
diabetic 250.6 ☑ [536.3]
Gastropathy, exudative 579.8
Gastroptosis 537.5
Gastrorrhagia 578.0
Gastorrhea 536.8
psychogenic 306.4
Gastroschisis (congenital) 756.79
acquired 569.89
Gastrospasm (neurogenic) (reflex) 536.8
neurotic 306.4
psychogenic 306.4
Gastrostaxis 578.0
Gastrostenosis 537.89
Gastrostomy
attention to V55.1
complication 536.40
specified type 536.49
infection 536.41
malfunctioning 536.42
status V44.1
Gastrosuccorrhea (continous) (intermittent) 536.8
neurotic 306.4
psychogenic 306.4
Gaucher's
disease (adult) (cerebroside lipidosis) (infantile) 272.7
hepatomegaly 272.7
splenomegaly (cerebroside lipidosis) 272.7
Gayet's disease (superior hemorrhagic polioencephalitis) 265.1
Gayet-Wernicke's syndrome (superior hemorrhagic polioencephalitis) 265.1
Gee (-Herter) (-Heubner) (-Thaysen) disease or syndrome (nontropical sprue) 579.0
Gélineau's syndrome ▶(*see also* Narcolepsy)◀ 347.00 ▲
Gemination, teeth 520.2
Gemistocytoma (M9411/3)
specified site — *see* Neoplasm, by site, malignant
unspecified site 191.9
General, generalized — *see* condtion
Genetic
susceptibility to ●
neoplasm ●
malignant, of ●
breast V84.01 ●
endometrium V84.04 ●
other V84.09 ●
ovary V84.02 ●
prostate V84.03 ●
other disease V84.8 ●

Genital — *see* condition
Genito-anorectal syndrome 099.1
Genitourinary system — *see* condition
Genu
congenital 755.64
extrorsum (acquired) 736.42
congenital 755.64
late effects of rickets 268.1
introrsum (acquired) 736.41
congenital 755.64
late effects of rickets 268.1
rachitic (old) 268.1
recurvatum (acquired) 736.5
congenital 754.40
with dislocation of knee 754.41
late effects or rickets 268.1
valgum (acquired) (knock-knee) 736.41
congenital 755.64
late effects of rickets 268.1
varum (acquired) (bowleg) 736.42
congenital 755.64
late effect of rickets 268.1
Geographic tongue 529.1
Geophagia 307.52
Geotrichosis 117.9
intestine 117.9
lung 117.9
mouth 117.9
Gephyrophobia 300.29
Gerbode defect 745.4
Gerhardt's
disease (erythromelalgia) 443.89
syndrome (vocal cord paralysis) 478.30
Gerlier's disease (epidemic vertigo) 078.81
German measles 056.9
exposure to V01.4
Germinoblastoma (diffuse) (M9614/3) 202.8 ☑
follicular (M9692/3) 202.0 ☑
Germinoma (M9064/3) — *see* Neoplasm, by site, malignant
Gerontoxon 371.41
Gerstmann's syndrome (finger agnosia) 784.69
Gestation (period) — *see also* Pregnancy
ectopic NEC (*see also* Pregnancy, ectopic) 633.90
with intrauterine pregnancy 633.91
Gestational proteinuria 646.2 ☑
with hypertension — *see* Toxemia, of pregnancy
Ghon tubercle primary infection (*see also* Tuberculosis) 010.0 ☑
Ghost
teeth 520.4
vessels, cornea 370.64
Ghoul hand 102.3
Giant
cell
epulis 523.8
peripheral (gingiva) 523.8
tumor, tendon sheath 727.02
colon (congenital) 751.3
esophagus (congenital) 750.4
kidney 753.3
urticaria 995.1
hereditary 277.6
Giardia lamblia infestation 007.1
Giardiasis 007.1
Gibert's disease (pityriasis rosea) 696.3
Gibraltar fever — *see* Brucellosis
Giddiness 780.4
hysterical 300.11
psychogenic 306.9
Gierke's disease (glycogenosis I) 271.0
Gigantism (cerebral) (hypophyseal) (pituitary) 253.0
Gilbert's disease or cholemia (familial nonhemolytic jaundice) 277.4
Gilchrist's disease (North American blastomycosis) 116.0
Gilford (-Hutchinson) disease or syndrome (progeria) 259.8

Gilles de la Tourette's disease (motor-verbal tic) 307.23
Gillespie's syndrome (dysplasia oculodentodigitalis) 759.89
Gingivitis 523.1
  acute 523.0
    necrotizing 101
  catarrhal 523.0
  chronic 523.1
  desquamative 523.1
  expulsiva 523.4
  hyperplastic 523.1
  marginal, simple 523.1
  necrotizing, acute 101
  pellagrous 265.2
  ulcerative 523.1
    acute necrotizing 101
  Vincent's 101
Gingivoglossitis 529.0
Gingivopericementitis 523.4
Gingivosis 523.1
Gingivostomatitis 523.1
  herpetic 054.2
Giovannini's disease 117.9
GISA (glycopeptide intermediate staphylococcus aureus) V09.8
Gland, glandular — *see* condition
Glanders 024
Glanzmann (-Naegeli) disease or thrombasthenia 287.1
Glassblowers' disease 527.1
Glaucoma (capsular) (inflammatory) (noninflammatory) (primary) 365.9
  with increased episcleral venous pressure 365.82
  absolute 360.42
  acute 365.22
    narrow angle 365.22
    secondary 365.60
  angle closure 365.20
    acute 365.22
    chronic 365.23
    intermittent 365.21
    interval 365.21
    residual stage 365.24
    subacute 365.21
  borderline 365.00
  chronic 365.11
    noncongestive 365.11
    open angle 365.11
    simple 365.11
  closed angle — *see* Glaucoma, angle closure
  congenital 743.20
    associated with other eye anomalies 743.22
    simple 743.21
  congestive — *see* Glaucoma, narrow angle
  corticosteroid-induced (glaucomatous stage) 365.31
    residual stage 365.32
  hemorrhagic 365.60
  hypersecretion 365.81
  in or with
    aniridia 743.45 *[365.42]*
    Axenfeld's anomaly 743.44 *[365.41]*
    concussion of globe 921.3 *[365.65]*
    congenital syndromes NEC 759.89 *[365.44]*
    dislocation of lens
      anterior 379.33 *[365.59]*
      posterior 379.34 *[365.59]*
    disorder of lens NEC 365.59
    epithelial down-growth 364.61 *[365.64]*
    glaucomatocyclitic crisis 364.22 *[365.62]*
    hypermature cataract 366.18 *[365.51]*
    hyphema 364.41 *[365.63]*
    inflammation, ocular 365.62
    iridocyclitis 364.3 *[365.62]*
    iris
      anomalies NEC 743.46 *[365.42]*
      atrophy, essential 364.51 *[365.42]*
      bombé 364.74 *[365.61]*
      rubeosis 364.42 *[365.63]*
    microcornea 743.41 *[365.43]*
    neurofibromatosis 237.71 *[365.44]*

Glaucoma — *continued*
  in or with — *continued*
    ocular
      cysts NEC 365.64
      disorders NEC 365.60
      trauma 365.65
      tumors NEC 365.64
    postdislocation of lens
      anterior 379.33 *[365.59]*
      posterior 379.34 *[365.59]*
    pseudoexfoliation of capsule 366.11 *[365.52]*
    pupillary block or seclusion 364.74 *[365.61]*
    recession of chamber angle 364.77 *[365.65]*
    retinal vein occlusion 362.35 *[365.63]*
    Rieger's anomaly or syndrome 743.44 *[365.41]*
    rubeosis of iris 364.42 *[365.63]*
    seclusion of pupil 364.74 *[365.61]*
    spherophakia 743.36 *[365.59]*
    Sturge-Weber (-Dimitri) syndrome 759.6 *[365.44]*
    systemic syndrome NEC 365.44
    tumor of globe 365.64
    vascular disorders NEC 365.63
  infantile 365.14
    congenital 743.20
      associated with other eye anomalies 743.22
      simple 743.21
  juvenile 365.14
  low tension 365.12
  malignant 365.83
  narrow angle (primary) 365.20
    acute 365.22
    chronic 365.23
    intermittent 365.21
    interval 365.21
    residual stage 365.24
    subacute 365.21
  newborn 743.20
    associated with other eye anomalies 743.22
    simple 743.21
  noncongestive (chronic) 365.11
  nonobstructive (chronic) 365.11
  obstructive 365.60
    due to lens changes 365.59
  open angle 365.10
    with
      borderline intraocular pressure 365.01
      cupping of optic discs 365.01
    primary 365.11
    residual stage 365.15
  phacolytic 365.51
    with hypermature cataract 366.18 *[365.51]*
  pigmentary 365.13
  postinfectious 365.60
  pseudoexfoliation 365.52
    with pseudoexfoliation of capsule 366.11 *[365.52]*
  secondary NEC 365.60
  simple (chronic) 365.11
  simplex 365.11
  steroid responders 365.03
  suspect 365.00
  syphiltic 095.8
  traumatic NEC 365.65
    newborn 767.8
  tuberculous (*see also* Tuberculosis) 017.3 ☑ *[365.62]*
  wide angle (*see also* Glaucoma, open angle) 365.10
Glaucomatous flecks (subcapsular) 366.31
Glazed tongue 529.4
Gleet 098.2
Glénard's disease or syndrome (enteroptosis) 569.89
Glinski-Simmonds syndrome (pituitary cachexia) 253.2
Glioblastoma (multiforme) (M9440/3)
  with sarcomatous component (M9442/3)
    specified site — *see* Neoplasm, by site, malignant
    unspecified site 191.9
  giant cell (M9441/3)
    specified site — *see* Neoplasm, by site, malignant

Glioblastoma — *continued*
  giant cell — *continued*
    unspecified site 191.9
  specified site — *see* Neoplasm, by site, malignant
  unspecified site 191.9
Glioma (malignant) (M9380/3)
  astrocytic (M9400/3)
    specified site — *see* Neoplasm, by site, malignant
    unspecified site 191.9
  mixed (M9382/3)
    specified site — *see* Neoplasm, by site, malignant
    unspecified site 191.9
  nose 748.1
  specified site NEC — *see* Neoplasm, by site, malignant
  subependymal (M9383/1) 237.5
  unspecified site 191.9
Gliomatosis cerebri (M9381/3) 191.0
Glioneuroma (M9505/1) — *see* Neoplasm, by site, uncertain behavior
Gliosarcoma (M9380/3)
  specified site — *see* Neoplasm, by site, malignant
  unspecified site 191.9
Gliosis (cerebral) 349.89
  spinal 336.0
Glisson's
  cirrhosis — *see* Cirrhosis, portal
  disease (*see also* Rickets) 268.0
Glissonitis 573.3
Globinuria 791.2
Globus 306.4
  hystericus 300.11
Glomangioma (M8712/0) (*see also* Hemangioma) 228.00
Glomangiosarcoma (M8710/3) — *see* Neoplasm, connective tissue, malignant
Glomerular nephritis (*see also* Nephritis) 583.9
Glomerulitis (*see also* Nephritis) 583.9
Glomerulonephritis (*see also* Nephritis) 583.9
  with
    edema (*see also* Nephrosis) 581.9
    lesion of
      exudative nephritis 583.89
      interstitial nephritis (diffuse) (focal) 583.89
      necrotizing glomerulitis 583.4
        acute 580.4
        chronic 582.4
      renal necrosis 583.9
        cortical 583.6
        medullary 583.7
      specified pathology NEC 583.89
        acute 580.89
        chronic 582.89
    necrosis, renal 583.9
      cortical 583.6
      medullary (papillary) 583.7
    specified pathology or lesion NEC 583.89
  acute 580.9
    with
      exudative nephritis 580.89
      interstitial nephritis (diffuse) (focal) 580.89
      necrotizing glomerulitis 580.4
    extracapillary with epithelial crescents 580.4
    poststreptococcal 580.0
    proliferative (diffuse) 580.0
    rapidly progressive 580.4
    specified pathology NEC 580.89
  arteriolar (*see also* Hypertension, kidney) 403.90
  arteriosclerotic (*see also* Hypertension, kidney) 403.90
  ascending (*see also* Pyelitis) 590.80
  basement membrane NEC 583.89
    with
      pulmonary hemorrhage (Goodpasture's syndrome) 446.21 *[583.81]*
  chronic 582.9

Glomerulonephritis (*see also* Nephritis) — *continued*
  chronic — *continued*
    with
      exudative nephritis 582.89
      interstitial nephritis (diffuse) (focal) 582.89
      necrotizing glomerulitis 582.4
      specified pathology or lesion NEC 582.89
    endothelial 582.2
    extracapillary with epithelial crescents 582.4
    hypocomplementemic persistent 582.2
    lobular 582.2
    membranoproliferative 582.2
    membranous 582.1
      and proliferative (mixed) 582.2
      sclerosing 582.1
    mesangiocapillary 582.2
    mixed membranous and proliferative 582.2
    proliferative (diffuse) 582.0
    rapidly progressive 582.4
    sclerosing 582.1
  cirrhotic — *see* Sclerosis, renal
  desquamative — *see* Nephrosis
  due to or associated with
    amyloidosis 277.3 [583.81]
      with nephrotic syndrome 277.3 [581.81]
      chronic 277.3 [582.81]
    diabetes mellitus 250.4 ☑ [583.81]
      with nephrotic syndrome 250.4 ☑ [581.81]
    diphtheria 032.89 [580.81]
    gonococcal infection (acute) 098.19 [583.81]
      chronic or duration of 2 months or over 098.39 [583.81]
    infectious hepatitis 070.9 [580.81]
    malaria (with nephrotic syndrome) 084.9 [581.81]
    mumps 072.79 [580.81]
    polyarteritis (nodosa) (with nephrotic syndrome) 446.0 [581.81]
    specified pathology NEC 583.89
      acute 580.89
      chronic 582.89
    streptotrichosis 039.8 [583.81]
    subacute bacterial endocarditis 421.0 [580.81]
    syphilis (late) 095.4
      congenital 090.5 [583.81]
      early 091.69 [583.81]
    systemic lupus erythematosus 710.0 [583.81]
      with nephrotic syndrome 710.0 [581.81]
      chronic 710.0 [582.81]
    tuberculosis (*see also* Tuberculosis) 016.0 ☑ [583.81]
    typhoid fever 002.0 [580.81]
  extracapillary with epithelial crescents 583.4
    acute 580.4
    chronic 582.4
  exudative 583.89
    acute 580.89
    chronic 582.89
  focal (*see also* Nephritis) 583.9
    embolic 580.4
  granular 582.89
  granulomatous 582.89
  hydremic (*see also* Nephrosis) 581.9
  hypocomplementemic persistent 583.2
    with nephrotic syndrome 581.2
    chronic 582.2
  immune complex NEC 583.89
  infective (*see also* Pyelitis) 590.80
  interstitial (diffuse) (focal) 583.89
    with nephrotic syndrome 581.89
    acute 580.89
    chronic 582.89
  latent or quiescent 582.9
  lobular 583.2
    with nephrotic syndrome 581.2
    chronic 582.2
  membranoproliferative 583.2
    with nephrotic syndrome 581.2
    chronic 582.2
  membranous 583.1
    with nephrotic syndrome 581.1

Glomerulonephritis (*see also* Nephritis) — *continued*
  membranous — *continued*
    and proliferative (mixed) 583.2
      with nephrotic syndrome 581.2
      chronic 582.2
    chronic 582.1
    sclerosing 582.1
      with nephrotic syndrome 581.1
  mesangiocapillary 583.2
    with nephrotic syndrome 581.2
    chronic 582.2
  minimal change 581.3
  mixed membranous and proliferative 583.2
    with nephrotic syndrome 581.2
    chronic 582.2
  necrotizing 583.4
    acute 580.4
    chronic 582.4
  nephrotic (*see also* Nephrosis) 581.9
  old — *see* Glomerulonephritis, chronic
  parenchymatous 581.89
  poststreptococcal 580.0
  proliferative (diffuse) 583.0
    with nephrotic syndrome 581.0
    acute 580.0
    chronic 582.0
  purulent (*see also* Pyelitis) 590.80
  quiescent — *see* Nephritis, chronic
  rapidly progressive 583.4
    acute 580.4
    chronic 582.4
  sclerosing membranous (chronic) 582.1
    with nephrotic syndrome 581.1
  septic (*see also* Pyelitis) 590.80
  specified pathology or lesion NEC 583.89
    with nephrotic syndrome 581.89
    acute 580.89
    chronic 582.89
  suppurative (acute) (disseminated) (*see also* Pyelitis) 590.80
  toxic — *see* Nephritis, acute
  tubal, tubular — *see* Nephrosis, tubular
  type II (Ellis) — *see* Nephrosis
  vascular — *see* Hypertension, kidney
Glomerulosclerosis (*see also* Sclerosis, renal) 587
  focal 582.1
    with nephrotic syndrome 581.1
  intercapillary (nodular) (with diabetes) 250.4 ☑ [581.81]
Glossagra 529.6
Glossalgia 529.6
Glossitis 529.0
  areata exfoliativa 529.1
  atrophic 529.4
  benign migratory 529.1
  gangrenous 529.0
  Hunter's 529.4
  median rhomboid 529.2
  Moeller's 529.4
  pellagrous 265.2
Glossocele 529.8
Glossodynia 529.6
  exfoliativa 529.4
Glossoncus 529.8
Glossophytia 529.3
Glossoplegia 529.8
Glossoptosis 529.8
Glossopyrosis 529.6
Glossotrichia 529.3
Glossy skin 710.9
Glottis — *see* condition
Glottitis — *see* Glossitis
Glucagonoma (M8152/0)
  malignant (M8152/3)
    pancreas 157.4
    specified site NEC — *see* Neoplasm, by site, malignant
    unspecified site 157.4
  pancreas 211.7
  specified site NEC — *see* Neoplasm, by site, benign
  unspecified site 211.7
Glucoglycinuria 270.7

Glue ear syndrome 381.20
Glue sniffing (airplane glue) (*see also* Dependence) 304.6 ☑
Glycinemia (with methylmalonic acidemia) 270.7
Glycinuria (renal) (with ketosis) 270.0
Glycogen
  infiltration (*see also* Disease, glycogen storage) 271.0
  storage disease (*see also* Disease, glycogen storage) 271.0
Glycogenosis (*see also* Disease, glycogen storage) 271.0
  cardiac 271.0 [425.7]
  Cori, types I-VII 271.0
  diabetic, secondary 250.8 ☑ [259.8]
  diffuse (with hepatic cirrhosis) 271.0
  generalized 271.0
  glucose-6-phosphatase deficiency 271.0
  hepatophosphorylase deficiency 271.0
  hepatorenal 271.0
  myophosphorylase deficiency 271.0
Glycopenia 251.2
Glycopeptide ●
  intermediate staphylococcus aureus (GISA) V09.8 ●
  resistant ●
    enterococcus V09.8 ●
    staphylococcus aureus (GRSA) V09.8 ●
Glycoprolinuria 270.8
Glycosuria 791.5
  renal 271.4
Gnathostoma (spinigerum) (infection) (infestation) 128.1
  wandering swellings from 128.1
Gnathostomiasis 128.1
Goiter (adolescent) (colloid) (diffuse) (dipping) (due to iodine deficiency) (endemic) (euthyroid) (heart) (hyperplastic) (internal) (intrathoracic) (juvenile) (mixed type) (nonendemic) (parenchymatous) (plunging) (sporadic) (subclavicular) (substernal) 240.9
  with
    hyperthyroidism (recurrent) (*see also* Goiter, toxic) 242.0 ☑
    thyrotoxicosis (*see also* Goiter, toxic) 242.0 ☑
  adenomatous (*see also* Goiter, nodular) 241.9
  cancerous (M8000/3) 193
  complicating pregnancy, childbirth, or puerperium 648.1 ☑
  congenital 246.1
  cystic (*see also* Goiter, nodular) 241.9
  due to enzyme defect in synthesis of thyroid hormone (butane-insoluble iodine) (coupling) (deiodinase) (iodide trapping or organificaiton) (iodotyrosine dehalogenase) (peroxidase) 246.1
  dyshormonogenic 246.1
  exophthalmic (*see also* Goiter, toxic) 242.0 ☑
  familial (with deaf-mutism) 243
  fibrous 245.3
  lingual 759.2
  lymphadenoid 245.2
  malignant (M8000/3) 193
  multinodular (nontoxic) 241.1
    toxic or with hyperthyroidism (*see also* Goiter, toxic) 242.2 ☑
  nodular (nontoxic) 241.9
    with
      hyperthyroidism (*see also* Goiter, toxic) 242.3 ☑
      thyrotoxicosis (*see also* Goiter, toxic) 242.3 ☑
    endemic 241.9
    exophthalmic (diffuse) (*see also* Goiter, toxic) 242.0 ☑
    multinodular (nontoxic) 241.1
    sporadic 241.9
    toxic (*see also* Goiter, toxic) 242.3 ☑
    uninodular (nontoxic) 241.0
  nontoxic (nodular) 241.9
    multinodular 241.1
    uninodular 241.0
  pulsating (*see also* Goiter, toxic) 242.0 ☑

Goiter — *continued*
  simple 240.0
  toxic 242.0 ☑

> *Note — Use the following fifth-digit subclassification with category 242:*
>
> 0   *without mention of thyrotoxic crisis or storm*
> 1   *with mention of thyrotoxic crisis or storm*

    adenomatous 242.3 ☑
      multinodular 242.2 ☑
      uninodular 242.1 ☑
    multinodular 242.2 ☑
    nodular 242.3 ☑
      multinodular 242.2 ☑
      uninodular 242.1 ☑
    uninodular 242.1 ☑
    uninodular (nontoxic) 241.0
    toxic or with hyperthyroidism (*see also*
      Goiter, toxic) 242.1 ☑
Goldberg (-Maxwell) (-Morris) syndrome
  (testicular feminization) 257.8
Goldblatt's
  hypertension 440.1
  kidney 440.1
Goldenhar's syndrome (oculoauriculovertebral
  dysplasia) 756.0
Goldflam-Erb disease or syndrome 358.00
Goldscheider's disease (epidermolysis bullosa)
  757.39
Goldstein's disease (familial hemorrhagic
  telangiectasia) 448.0
Golfer's elbow 726.32
Goltz-Gorlin syndrome (dermal hypoplasia)
  757.39
Gonadoblastoma (M9073/1)
  specified site — *see* Neoplasm, by site,
    uncertain behavior
  unspecified site
    female 236.2
    male 236.4
Gonecystitis (*see also* Vesiculitis) 608.0
Gongylonemiasis 125.6
  mouth 125.6
Goniosynechiae 364.73
Gonococcemia 098.89
Gonococcus, gonococcal (disease) (infection) (*see
  also* condition) 098.0
  anus 098.7
  bursa 098.52
  chronic NEC 098.2
  complicating pregnancy, childbirth, or
    puerperium 647.1 ☑
    affecting fetus or newborn 760.2
  conjunctiva, conjunctivitis (neonatorum)
    098.40
  dermatosis 098.89
  endocardium 098.84
  epididymo-orchitis 098.13
    chronic or duration of 2 months or over
      098.33
  eye (newborn) 098.40
  fallopian tube (chronic) 098.37
    acute 098.17
  genitourinary (acute) (organ) (system) (tract)
    (*see also* Gonnorrhea) 098.0
    lower 098.0
      chronic 098.2
    upper 098.10
      chronic 098.30
  heart NEC 098.85
  joint 098.50
  keratoderma 098.81
  keratosis (blennorrhagica) 098.81
  lymphatic (gland) (node) 098.89
  meninges 098.82
  orchitis (acute) 098.13
    chronic or duration of 2 months or over
      098.33
  pelvis (acute) 098.19
    chronic or duration of 2 months or over
      098.39

Gonococcus, gonococcal (*see also* condition) —
  continued
  pericarditis 098.83
  peritonitis 098.86
  pharyngitis 098.6
  pharynx 098.6
  proctitis 098.7
  pyosalpinx (chronic) 098.37
    acute 098.17
  rectum 098.7
  septicemia 098.89
  skin 098.89
  specified site NEC 098.89
  synovitis 098.51
  tendon sheath 098.51
  throat 098.6
  urethra (acute) 098.0
    chronic or duration of 2 months or over
      098.2
  vulva (acute) 098.0
    chronic or duration of 2 months or over
      098.2
Gonocytoma (M9073/1)
  specified site — *see* Neoplasm, by site,
    uncertain behavior
  unspecified site
    female 236.2
    male 236.4
Gonorrhea 098.0
  acute 098.0
  Bartholin's gland (acute) 098.0
    chronic or duration of 2 months or over
      098.2
  bladder (acute) 098.11
    chronic or duration of 2 months or over
      098.31
  carrier (suspected of) V02.7
  cervix (acute) 098.15
    chronic or duration of 2 months or over
      098.35
  chronic 098.2
  complicating pregnancy, childbirth, or
    puerperium 647.1 ☑
    affecting fetus or newborn 760.2
  conjunctiva, conjunctivitis (neonatorum)
    098.40
  contact V01.6
  Cowper's gland (acute) 098.0
    chronic or duration of 2 months or over
      098.2
  duration of two months or over 098.2
  exposure to V01.6
  fallopian tube (chronic) 098.37
    acute 098.17
  genitourinary (acute) (organ) (system) (tract)
    098.0
    chronic 098.2
    duration of two months or over 098.2
  kidney (acute) 098.19
    chronic or duration of 2 months or over
      098.39
  ovary (acute) 098.19
    chronic or duration of 2 months or over
      098.39
  pelvis (acute) 098.19
    chronic or duration of 2 months or over
      098.39
  penis (acute) 098.0
    chronic or duration of 2 months or over
      098.2
  prostate (acute) 098.12
    chronic or duration of 2 months or over
      098.32
  seminal vesicle (acute) 098.14
    chronic or duration of 2 months or over
      098.34
  specified site NEC — *see* Gonococcus
  spermatic cord (acute) 098.14
    chronic or duration of 2 months or over
      098.34
  urethra (acute) 098.0
    chronic or duration of 2 months or over
      098.2
  vagina (acute) 098.0
    chronic or duration of 2 months or over
      098.2

Gonorrhea — *continued*
  vas deferens (acute) 098.14
    chronic or duration of 2 months or over
      098.34
  vulva (acute) 098.0
    chronic or duration of 2 months or over
      098.2
Goodpasture's syndrome (pneumorenal) 446.21
Good's syndrome 279.06   ●
Gopalan's syndrome (burning feet) 266.2
Gordon's disease (exudative enteropathy) 579.8
Gorlin-Chaudhry-Moss syndrome 759.89
Gougerot's syndrome (trisymptomatic) 709.1
Gougerot-Blum syndrome (pigmented purpuric
  lichenoid dermatitis) 709.1
Gougerot-Carteaud disease or syndrome
  (confluent reticulate papillomatosis) 701.8
Gougerot-Hailey-Hailey disease (benign familial
  chronic pemphigus) 757.39
Gougerot (-Houwer) - Sjögren syndrome
  (keratoconjunctivitis sicca) 710.2
Gouley's syndrome (constrictive pericarditis)
  423.2
Goundou 102.6
Gout, gouty 274.9
  with specified manifestations NEC 274.89
  arthritis (acute) 274.0
  arthropathy 274.0
  degeneration, heart 274.82
  diathesis 274.9
  eczema 274.89
  episcleritis 274.89 [379.09]
  external ear (tophus) 274.81
  glomerulonephritis 274.10
  iritis 274.89 [364.11]
  joint 274.0
  kidney 274.10
  lead 984.9
    specified type of lead — *see* Table of Drugs
      and Chemicals
  nephritis 274.10
  neuritis 274.89 [357.4]
  phlebitis 274.89 [451.9]
  rheumatic 714.0
  saturnine 984.9
    specified type of lead — *see* Table of Drugs
      and Chemicals
  spondylitis 274.0
  synovitis 274.0
  syphilitic 095.8
  tophi 274.0
    ear 274.81
    heart 274.82
    specified site NEC 274.82
Gowers'
  muscular dystrophy 359.1
  syndrome (vasovagal attack) 780.2
Gowers-Paton-Kennedy syndrome 377.04
Gradenigo's syndrome 383.02
Graft-versus-host disease (bone marrow) 996.85
  due to organ transplant NEC — *see*
    Complications, transplant, organ
Graham Steell's murmur (pulmonic
  regurgitation) (*see also* Endocarditis,
  pulmonary) 424.3
Grain-handlers' disease or lung 495.8
Grain mite (itch) 133.8
Grand
  mal (idiopathic) (*see also* Epilepsy) 345.1 ☑
    hysteria of Charcôt 300.11
    nonrecurrent or isolated 780.39
  multipara
    affecting management of labor and delivery
      659.4 ☑
    status only (not pregnant) V61.5
Granite workers' lung 502
Granular — *see also* condition
  inflammation, pharynx 472.1
  kidney (contracting) (*see also* Sclerosis, renal)
    587
  liver ➡ *see* Cirrhosis, liver
  nephritis — *see* Nephritis

☑ Additional Digit Required   ◄► Revised Text   ● New Line   ▲ Revised Code

Granulation tissue, abnormal — see also
  Granuloma
  abnormal or excessive 701.5
  postmastoidectomy cavity 383.33
  postoperative 701.5
  skin 701.5
Granulocytopenia, granulocytopenic (primary)
    288.0
  malignant 288.0
Granuloma NEC 686.1
  abdomen (wall) 568.89
    skin (pyogenicum) 686.1
      from residual foreign body 709.4
  annulare 695.89
  anus 569.49
  apical 522.6
  appendix 543.9
  aural 380.23
  beryllium (skin) 709.4
    lung 503
  bone (see also Osteomyelitis) 730.1 ☑
    eosinophilic 277.89
    from residual foreign body 733.99
  canaliculus lacrimalis 375.81
  cerebral 348.8
  cholesterin, middle ear 385.82
  coccidioidal (progressive) 114.3
    lung 114.4
    meninges 114.2
    primary (lung) 114.0
  colon 569.89
  conjunctiva 372.61
  dental 522.6
  ear, middle (cholesterin) 385.82
    with otitis media — see Otitis media
  eosinophilic 277.89
    bone 277.89
    lung 277.89
    oral mucosa 528.9
  exuberant 701.5
  eyelid 374.89
  facial
    lethal midline 446.3
    malignant 446.3
  faciale 701.8
  fissuratum (gum) 523.8
  foot NEC 686.1
  foreign body (in soft tissue) NEC 728.82
    bone 733.99
    in operative wound 998.4
    muscle 728.82
    skin 709.4
    subcutaneous tissue 709.4
  fungoides 202.1 ☑
  gangraenescens 446.3
  giant cell (central) (jaw) (reparative) 526.3
    gingiva 523.8
    peripheral (gingiva) 523.8
  gland (lymph) 289.3
  Hodgkin's (M9661/3) 201.1 ☑
  ileum 569.89
  infectious NEC 136.9
  inguinale (Donovan) 099.2
    venereal 099.2
  intestine 569.89
  iridocyclitis 364.10
  jaw (bone) 526.3
    reparative giant cell 526.3
  kidney (see also Infection, kidney) 590.9
  lacrimal sac 375.81
  larynx 478.79
  lethal midline 446.3
  lipid 277.89
  lipoid 277.89
  liver 572.8
  lung (infectious) (see also Fibrosis, lung) 515
    coccidioidal 114.4
    eosinophilic 277.89
  lymph gland 289.3
  Majocchi's 110.6
  malignant, face 446.3
  mandible 526.3
  mediastinum 519.3
  midline 446.3
  monilial 112.3
  muscle 728.82
    from residual foreign body 728.82

Granuloma — continued
  nasal sinus (see also Sinusitis) 473.9
  operation wound 998.59
    foreign body 998.4
    stitch (external) 998.89
      internal organ 996.7 ☑
      internal wound 998.89
    talc 998.7
  oral mucosa, eosinophilic or pyogenic 528.9
  orbit, orbital 376.11
  paracoccidiodal 116.1
  penis, venereal 099.2
  periapical 522.6
  peritoneum 568.89
      due to ova of helminths NEC (see also
          Helminthiasis) 128.9
  postmastoidectomy cavity 383.33
  postoperative — see Granuloma, operation
      wound
  prostate 601.8
  pudendi (ulcerating) 099.2
  pudendorum (ulcerative) 099.2
  pulp, internal (tooth) 521.49   ▲
  pyogenic, pyogenicum (skin) 686.1
    maxillary alveolar ridge 522.6
    oral mucosa 528.9
  rectum 569.49
  reticulohistiocytic 277.89
  rubrum nasi 705.89
  sarcoid 135
  Schistosoma 120.9
  septic (skin) 686.1
  silica (skin) 709.4
  sinus (accessory) (infectional) (nasal) (see also
      Sinusitis) 473.9
  skin (pyogenicum) 686.1
    from foreign body or material 709.4
  sperm 608.89
  spine
    syphilitic (epidural) 094.89
    tuberculous (see also Tuberculosis)
        015.0 ☑ [730.88]
  stitch (postoperative) 998.89
    internal wound 998.89
  suppurative (skin) 686.1
  suture (postoperative) 998.89
    internal wound 998.89
  swimming pool 031.1
  talc 728.82
    in operation wound 998.7
  telangiectaticum (skin) 686.1
  trichophyticum 110.6
  tropicum 102.4
  umbilicus 686.1
    newborn 771.4
  urethra 599.84
  uveitis 364.10
  vagina 099.2
  venereum 099.2
  vocal cords 478.5
  Wegener's (necrotizing respiratory
      granulomatosis) 446.4
Granulomatosis NEC 686.1
  disciformis chronica et progressiva 709.3
  infantiseptica 771.2
  lipoid 277.89
  lipohagic, intestinal 040.2
  miliary 027.0
  necrotizing, respiratory 446.4
  progressive, septic 288.1
  Wegener's (necrotizing respiratory) 446.4
Granulomatous tissue — see Granuloma
Granulosis rubra nasi 705.89
Graphite fibrosis (of lung) 503
Graphospasm 300.89
  organic 333.84
Grating scapula 733.99
Gravel (urinary) (see also Calculus) 592.9
Graves' disease (exophthalmic goiter) (see also
    Goiter, toxic) 242.0 ☑
Gravis — see condition
Grawitz's tumor (hypernephroma) (M8312/3)
    189.0
Grayness, hair (premature) 704.3
  congenital 757.4

Gray or grey syndrome (chloramphenicol)
    (newborn) 779.4
Greenfield's disease 330.0
Green sickness 280.9
Greenstick fracture — see Fracture, by site
Greig's syndrome (hypertelorism) 756.0
Griesinger's disease (see also Ancylostomiasis)
    126.9
Grinders'
  asthma 502
  lung 502
  phthisis (see also Tuberculosis) 011.4 ☑
Grinding, teeth 306.8
Grip
  Dabney's 074.1
  devil's 074.1
Grippe, grippal — see also Influenza
  Balkan 083.0
  intestinal 487.8
  summer 074.8
Grippy cold 487.1
Grisel's disease 723.5
Groin — see condition
Grooved
  nails (transverse) 703.8
  tongue 529.5
    congenital 750.13
Ground itch 126.9
Growing pains, children 781.99
Growth (fungoid) (neoplastic) (new) (M8000/1) —
    see also Neoplasm, by site, unspecified
    nature
  adenoid (vegetative) 474.12
  benign (M8000/0) — see Neoplasm, by site,
    benign
  fetal, poor 764.9 ☑
    affecting management of pregnancy 656.5 ☑
  malignant (M8000/3) — see Neoplasm, by site,
    malignant
  rapid, childhood V21.0
  secondary (M8000/6) — see Neoplasm, by site,
    malignant, secondary
GRSA (glycopeptide resistant staphylococcus   ●
    aureus) V09.8   ●
Gruber's hernia — see Hernia, Gruber's
Gruby's disease (tinea tonsurans) 110.0
G-trisomy 758.0
Guama fever 066.3
Gubler (-Millard) paralysis or syndrome 344.89
Guérin-Stern syndrome (arthorgryposis multiplex
    congenita) 754.89
Guertin's disease (electric chorea) 049.8
Guillain-Barré disease or syndrome 357.0
Guinea worms (infection) (infestation) 125.7
Guinon's disease (motor-verbal tic) 307.23
Gull's disease (thyroid atrophy with myxedema)
    244.8
Gull and Sutton's disease — see Hypertension,
    kidney
Gum — see condition
Gumboil 522.7
Gumma (syphilitic) 095.9
  artery 093.89
    cerebral or spinal 094.89
  bone 095.5
    of yaws (late) 102.6
  brain 094.89
  cauda equina 094.89
  central nervous system NEC 094.9
  ciliary body 095.8 [364.11]
  congenital 090.5
    testis 090.5
  eyelid 095.8 [373.5]
  heart 093.89
  intracranial 094.89
  iris 095.8 [364.11]
  kidney 095.4
  larynx 095.8
  leptomeninges 094.2
  liver 095.3
  meninges 094.2

Gumma — *continued*
  myocardium 093.82
  nasopharynx 095.8
  neurosyphilitic 094.9
  nose 095.8
  orbit 095.8
  palate (soft) 095.8
  penis 095.8
  pericardium 093.81
  pharynx 095.8
  pituitary 095.8
  scrofulous (*see also* Tuberculosis) 017.0 ☑
  skin 095.8
  specified site NEC 095.8
  spinal cord 094.89
  tongue 095.8
  tonsil 095.8
  trachea 095.8
  tuberculous (*see also* Tuberculosis) 017.0 ☑
  ulcerative due to yaws 102.4
  ureter 095.8
  yaws 102.4
    bone 102.6
Gunn's syndrome (jaw-winking syndrome) 742.8
Gunshot wound — *see also* Wound, open, by site
  fracture — *see* Fracture, by site, open
  internal organs (abdomen, chest, or pelvis) —
    see Injury, internal, by site, with open
    wound
  intracranial — *see* Laceration, brain, with open
    intracranial wound
Günther's disease or syndrome (congenital
  erythropoietic porphyria) 277.1
Gustatory hallucination 780.1
Gynandrism 752.7
Gynanadroblastoma (M8632/1)
  specified site — *see* Neoplasm, by site,
    uncertain behavior
  unspecified site
    female 236.2
    male 236.4
Gynandromorphism 752.7
Gynatresia (congenital) 752.49
Gynecoid pelvis, male 738.6
Gynecological examination V72.31 ▲
  for contraceptive maintenance V25.40
Gynecomastia 611.1
Gynephobia 300.29
Gyrate scalp 757.39

H

Haas' disease (osteochondrosis head of humerus)
  732.3
Habermann's disease (acute parapsoriasis
  varioliformis) 696.2
Habit, habituation
  chorea 307.22
  disturbance, child 307.9
  drug (*see also* Dependence) 304.9 ☑
  laxative (*see also* Abuse, drugs, nondependent)
    305.9 ☑
  spasm 307.20
    chronic 307.22
    transient ▶(of childhood)◀ 307.21
  tic 307.20
    chronic 307.22
    transient ▶(of childhood)◀ 307.21
  use of
    nonprescribed drugs (*see also* Abuse, drugs,
      nondependent) 305.9 ☑
    patent medicines (*see also* Abuse, drugs,
      nondependent) 305.9 ☑
  vomiting 536.2
Hadfield-Clarke syndrome (pancreatic
  infantilism) 577.8
Haff disease 985.1
Hageman factor defect, deficiency, or disease
  (*see also* Defect, coagulation) 286.3
Haglund's disease (osteochondrosis os tibiale
  externum) 732.5
Haglund-Läwen-Fründ syndrome 717.89

Hagner's disease (hypertrophic pulmonary
  osteoarthropathy) 731.2
Hag teeth, tooth 524.39 ▲
Hailey-Hailey disease (benign familial chronic
  pemphigus) 757.39
Hair — *see also* condition
  plucking 307.9
Hairball in stomach 935.2
Hairy black tongue 529.3
Half vertebra 756.14
Halitosis 784.9
Hallermann-Streiff syndrome 756.0
Hallervorden-Spatz disease or syndrome 333.0
Hallopeau's
  acrodermatitis (continua) 696.1
  disease (lichen sclerosis et atrophicus) 701.0
Hallucination (auditory) (gustatory) (olfactory)
  (tactile) 780.1
  ▶alcohol-induced◀ 291.3
  drug-induced 292.12
  visual 368.16
Hallucinosis 298.9
  ▶alcohol-induced◀ (acute) 291.3
  drug-induced 292.12
Hallus — *see* Hallux
Hallux 735.9
  malleus (acquired) 735.3
  rigidus (acquired) 735.2
    congenital 755.66
    late effects of rickets 268.1
  valgus (acquired) 735.0
    congenital 755.66
  varus (acquired) 735.1
    congenital 755.66
Halo, visual 368.15
Hamartoblastoma 759.6
Hamartoma 759.6
  epithelial (gingival), odontogenic, central, or
    peripheral (M9321/0) 213.1
    upper jaw (bone) 213.0
  vascular 757.32
Hamartosis, hamartoses NEC 759.6
Hamman's disease or syndrome (spontaneous
  mediastinal emphysema) 518.1
Hamman-Rich syndrome (diffuse interstitial
  pulmonary fibrosis) 516.3
Hammer toe (acquired) 735.4
  congenital 755.66
  late effects of rickets 268.1
Hand — *see* condition
Hand-Schüller-Christian disease or syndrome
  (chronic histiocytosis x) 277.89
Hand-foot syndrome 282.61
Hanging (asphyxia) (strangulation) (suffocation)
  994.7
Hangnail (finger) (with lymphangitis) 681.02
Hangover (alcohol) (*see also* Abuse, drugs,
  nondependent) 305.0 ☑
Hanot's cirrhosis or disease — *see* Cirrhosis,
  biliary
Hanot-Chauffard (-Troisier) syndrome (bronze
  diabetes) 275.0
Hansen's disease (leprosy) 030.9
  benign form 030.1
  malignant form 030.0
Harada's disease or syndrome 363.22
Hard chancre 091.0
Hard firm prostate 600.10
  with urinary retention 600.11
Hardening
  artery — *see* Arteriosclerosis
  brain 348.8
  liver 571.8
Hare's syndrome (M8010/3) (carcinoma,
  pulmonary apex) 162.3
Harelip (*see also* Cleft, lip) 749.10
Harlequin (fetus) 757.1
  color change syndrome 779.89

Harley's disease (intermittent hemoglobinuria)
  283.2
Harris'
  lines 733.91
  syndrome (organic hyperinsulinism) 251.1
Hart's disease or syndrome (pellagra-cerebellar
  ataxia-renal aminoaciduria) 270.0
Hartmann's pouch (abnormal sacculation of
  gallbladder neck) 575.8
  of intestine V44.3
    attention to V55.3
Hartnup disease (pellagra-cerebellar ataxia-renal
  aminoaciduria) 270.0
Harvester lung 495.0
Hashimoto's disease or struma (struma
  lymphomatosa) 245.2
Hassell-Henle bodies (corneal warts) 371.41
Haut mal (*see also* Epilepsy) 345.1 ☑
Haverhill fever 026.1
Hawaiian wood rose dependence 304.5 ☑
Hawkins' keloid 701.4
Hay
  asthma (*see also* Asthma) 493.0 ☑
  fever (allergic) (with rhinitis) 477.9
    with asthma (bronchial) (*see also* Asthma)
      493.0 ☑
    allergic, due to grass, pollen, ragweed, or
      tree 477.0
    conjunctivitis 372.05
    due to
      dander, ▶animal (cat) (dog)◀ 477.2 ▲
      dust 477.8
      fowl 477.8
      hair, animal (cat) (dog) 477.2 ●
      pollen 477.0
      specified allergen other than pollen 477.8
Hayem-Faber syndrome (achlorhydric anemia)
  280.9
Hayem-Widal syndrome (acquired hemolytic
  jaundice) 283.9
Haygarth's nodosities 715.04
Hazard-Crile tumor (M8350/3) 193
Hb (abnormal)
  disease — *see* Disease, hemoglobin
  trait — *see* Trait
H disease 270.0
Head — *see also* condition
  banging 307.3
Headache 784.0
  allergic 346.2 ☑
  cluster 346.2 ☑
  due to
    loss, spinal fluid 349.0
    lumbar puncture 349.0
    saddle block 349.0
  emotional 307.81
  histamine 346.2 ☑
  lumbar puncture 349.0
  menopausal 627.2
  migraine 346.9 ☑
  nonorganic origin 307.81
  postspinal 349.0
  psychogenic 307.81
  psychophysiologic 307.81
  sick 346.1 ☑
  spinal 349.0
    complicating labor and delivery 668.8 ☑
    postpartum 668.8 ☑
  spinal fluid loss 349.0
  tension 307.81
  vascular 784.0
    migraine type 346.9 ☑
  vasomotor 346.9 ☑
Health
  advice V65.4 ☑
  audit V70.0
  checkup V70.0
  education V65.4 ☑
  hazard (*see also* History of) V15.9
    specified cause NEC V15.89
  instruction V65.4 ☑
  services provided because (of)
    boarding school residence V60.60

☑ Additional Digit Required ▶◀ Revised Text ● New Line ▲ Revised Code

Health — *continued*
  services provided because (of) — *continued*
    holiday relief for person providing home care V60.5
    inadequate
      housing V60.1
      resources V60.2
    lack of housing V60.0
    no care available in home V60.4
    person living alone V60.3
    poverty V60.3
    residence in institution V60.6
    specified cause NEC V60.8
    vacation relief for person providing home care V60.5

Healthy
  donor (*see also* Donor) V59.9
  infant or child
    accompanying sick mother V65.0
    receiving care V20.1
  person
    accompanying sick relative V65.0
    admitted for sterilization V25.2
    receiving prophylactic inoculation or vaccination (*see also* Vaccination, prophylactic) V05.9

Hearing examination V72.1

Heart — *see* condition

Heartburn 787.1
  psychogenic 306.4

Heat (effects) 992.9
  apoplexy 992.0
  burn — *see also* Burn, by site
    from sun (*see also* Sunburn) 692.71
  collapse 992.1
  cramps 992.2
  dermatitis or eczema 692.89
  edema 992.7
  erythema — *see* Burn, by site
  excessive 992.9
    specified effect NEC 992.8
  exhaustion 992.5
    anhydrotic 992.3
    due to
      salt (and water) depletion 992.4
      water depletion 992.3
  fatigue (transient) 992.6
  fever 992.0
  hyperpyrexia 992.0
  prickly 705.1
  prostration — *see* Heat, exhaustion
  pyrexia 992.0
  rash 705.1
  specified effect NEC 992.8
  stroke 992.0
  sunburn (*see also* Sunburn) 692.71
  syncope 992.1

Heavy-chain disease 273.2

Heavy-for-dates (fetus or infant) 766.1
  4500 grams or more 766.0
  exceptionally 766.0

Hebephrenia, hebephrenic (acute) (*see also* Schizophrenia) 295.1 ☑
  dementia (praecox) (*see also* Schizophrenia) 295.1 ☑
  schizophrenia (*see also* Schizophrenia) 295.1 ☑

Heberden's
  disease or nodes 715.04
  syndrome (angina pectoris) 413.9

Hebra's disease
  dermatitis exfoliativa 695.89
  erythema multiforme exudativum 695.1
  pityriasis 695.89
    maculata et circinata 696.3
    rubra 695.89
      pilaris 696.4
  prurigo 698.2

Hebra, nose 040.1

Hedinger's syndrome (malignant carcinoid) 259.2

Heel — *see* condition

Heerfordt's disease or syndrome (uveoparotitis) 135

Hegglin's anomaly or syndrome 288.2

Heidenhain's disease 290.10
  with dementia 290.10

Heilmeyer-Schöner disease (M9842/3) 207.1 ☑

Heine-Medin disease (*see also* Poliomyelitis) 045.9 ☑

Heinz-body anemia, congenital 282.7

Heller's disease or syndrome (infantile psychosis) (*see also* Psychosis, childhood) 299.1 ☑

H.E.L.L.P 642.5 ☑

Helminthiasis (*see also* Infestation, by specific parasite) 128.9
  Ancylostoma (*see also* Ancylostoma) 126.9
  intestinal 127.9
    mixed types (types classifiable to more than one of the titles 120.0-127.7) 127.8
    specified type 127.7
  mixed types (intestinal) (types classifiable to more than one of the titles 120.0-127.7) 127.8
  Necator americanus 126.1
  specified type NEC 128.8
  Trichinella 124

Heloma 700

Hemangioblastoma (M9161/1) — *see also* Neoplasm, connective tissue, uncertain behavior
  malignant (M9161/3) — *see* Neoplasm, connective tissue, malignant

Hemangioblastomatosis, cerebelloretinal 759.6

Hemangioendothelioma (M9130/1) — *see also* Neoplasm, by site, uncertain behavior
  benign (M9130/0) 228.00
  bone (diffuse) (M9130/3) — *see* Neoplasm, bone, malignant
  malignant (M9130/3) — *see* Neoplasm, connective tissue, malignant
  nervous system (M9130/0) 228.09

Hemangioendotheliosarcoma (M9130/3) — *see* Neoplasm, connective tissue, malignant

Hemangiofibroma (M9160/0) — *see* Neoplasm, by site, benign

Hemangiolipoma (M8861/0) — *see* Lipoma

Hemangioma (M9120/0) 228.00
  arteriovenous (M9123/0) — *see* Hemangioma, by site
  brain 228.02
  capillary (M9131/0) — *see* Hemangioma, by site
  cavernous (M9121/0) — *see* Hemangioma, by site
  central nervous system NEC 228.09
  choroid 228.09
  heart 228.09
  infantile (M9131/0) — *see* Hemangioma, by site
  intra-abdominal structures 228.04
  intracranial structures 228.02
  intramuscular (M9132/0) — *see* Hemangioma, by site
  iris 228.09
  juvenile (M9131/0) — *see* Hemangioma, by site
  malignant (M9120/3) — *see* Neoplasm, connective tissue, malignant
  meninges 228.09
    brain 228.02
    spinal cord 228.09
  peritoneum 228.04
  placenta — *see* Placenta, abnormal
  plexiform (M9131/0) — *see* Hemangioma, by site
  racemose (M9123/0) — *see* Hemangioma, by site
  retina 228.03
  retroperitoneal tissue 228.04
  sclerosing (M8832/0) — *see* Neoplasm, skin, benign
  simplex (M9131/0) — *see* Hemangioma, by site
  skin and subcutaneous tissue 228.01
  specified site NEC 228.09
  spinal cord 228.09
  venous (M9122/0) — *see* Hemangioma, by site
  verrucous keratotic (M9142/0) — *see* Hemangioma, by site

Hemangiomatosis (systemic) 757.32
  involving single site — *see* Hemangioma

Hemangiopericytoma (M9150/1) — *see also* Neoplasm, connective tissue, uncertain behavior
  benign (M9150/0) — *see* Neoplasm, connective tissue, benign
  malignant (M9150/3) — *see* Neoplasm, connective tissue, malignant

Hemangiosarcoma (M9120/3) — *see* Neoplasm, connective tissue, malignant

Hemarthrosis (nontraumatic) 719.10
  ankle 719.17
  elbow 719.12
  foot 719.17
  hand 719.14
  hip 719.15
  knee 719.16
  multiple sites 719.19
  pelvic region 719.15
  shoulder (region) 719.11
  specified site NEC 719.18
  traumatic — *see* Sprain, by site
  wrist 719.13

Hematemesis 578.0
  with ulcer — *see* Ulcer, by site, with hemorrhage
  due to S. japonicum 120.2
  Goldstein's (familial hemorrhagic telangiectasia) 448.0
  newborn 772.4
    due to swallowed maternal blood 777.3

Hematidrosis 705.89

Hematinuria (*see also* Hemoglobinuria) 791.2
  malarial 084.8
  paroxysmal 283.2

Hematite miners' lung 503

Hematobilia 576.8

Hematocele (congenital) (diffuse) (idiopathic) 608.83
  broad ligament 620.7
  canal of Nuck 629.0
  cord male 608.83
  fallopian tube 620.8
  female NEC 629.0
  ischiorectal 569.89
  male NEC 608.83
  ovary 629.0
  pelvis, pelvic
    female 629.0
      with ectopic pregnancy (*see also* Pregnancy, ectopic) 633.90
        with intrauterine pregnancy 633.91
    male 608.83
  periuterine 629.0
  retrouterine 629.0
  scrotum 608.83
  spermatic cord (diffuse) 608.83
  testis 608.84
  traumatic — *see* Injury, internal, pelvis
  tunica vaginalis 608.83
  uterine ligament 629.0
  uterus 621.4
  vagina 623.6
  vulva 624.5

Hematocephalus 742.4

Hematochezia (*see also* Melena) 578.1

Hematochyluria (*see also* Infestation, filarial) 125.9

Hematocolpos 626.8

Hematocornea 371.12

Hematogenous — *see* condition

☑ Additional Digit Required   ▶◀ Revised Text   ● New Line   ▲ Revised Code

Hematoma (skin surface intact) (traumatic) — *see also* Contusion

> *Note* — *Hematomas are coded according to origin and the nature and site of the hematoma or the accompanying injury. Hematomas of unspecified origin are coded as injuries of the sites involved, except:*
>
> (a) *hematomas of genital organs which are coded as diseases of the organ involved unless they complicate pregnancy or delivery*
>
> (b) *hematomas of the eye which are coded as diseases of the eye.*
>
> *For late effect of hematoma classifiable to 920-924 see Late, effect, contusion*

with
  crush injury — *see* Crush
  fracture — *see* Fracture, by site
  injury of internal organs — *see also* Injury, internal, by site
    kidney — *see* Hematoma, kidney traumatic
    liver — *see* Hematoma, liver, traumatic
    spleen — *see* Hematoma, spleen
  nerve injury — *see* Injury, nerve
  open wound — *see* Wound, open, by site
  skin surface intact — *see* Contusion
abdomen (wall) — *see* Contusion, abdomen
amnion 658.8 ✓
aorta, dissecting 441.00
  abdominal 441.02
  thoracic 441.01
  thoracoabdominal 441.03
arterial (complicating trauma) 904.9
  specified site — *see* Injury, blood vessel, by site
auricle (ear) 380.31
birth injury 767.8
  skull 767.19
brain (traumatic) 853.0 ✓

> *Note* — *Use the following fifth-digit subclassification with categories 851-854:*
>
> 0   *unspecified state of consciousness*
> 1   *with no loss of consciousness*
> 2   *with brief [less than one hour] loss of consciousness*
> 3   *with moderate [1-24 hours] loss of consciousness*
> 4   *with prolonged [more than 24 hours] loss of consciousness and return to pre-existing conscious level*
> 5   *with prolonged [more than 24 hours] loss of consciousness, without return to pre-existing conscious level*
>   *Use fifth-digit 5 to designate when a patient is unconscious and dies before regaining consciousness, regardless of the duration of the loss of consciousness*
> 6   *with loss of consciousness of unspecified duration*
> 9   *with concussion, unspecified*

with
  cerebral
    contusion — *see* Contusion, brain
    laceration — *see* Laceration, brain
  open intracranial wound 853.1 ✓
  skull fracture — *see* Fracture, skull, by site
extradural or epidural 852.4 ✓
  with open intracranial wound 852.5 ✓
  fetus or newborn 767.0
  nontraumatic 432.0
fetus or newborn NEC 767.0
nontraumatic (*see also* Hemorrhage, brain) 431
  epidural or extradural 432.0
  newborn NEC 772.8

Hematoma — *see also* Contusion — *continued*
brain — *continued*
  nontraumatic — *continued*
    subarachnoid, arachnoid, or meningeal (*see also* Hemorrhage, subarachnoid) 430
    subdural (*see also* Hemorrhage, subdural) 432.1
  subarachnoid, arachnoid, or meningeal 852.0 ✓
    with open intracranial wound 852.1 ✓
    fetus or newborn 772.2
    nontraumatic (*see also* Hemorrhage, subarachnoid) 430
  subdural 852.2 ✓
    with open intracranial wound 852.3 ✓
    fetus or newborn (localized) 767.0
    nontraumatic (*see also* Hemorrhage, subdural) 432.1
breast (nontraumatic) 611.8
broad ligament (nontraumatic) 620.7
  complicating delivery 665.7 ✓
  traumatic — *see* Injury, internal, broad ligament
calcified NEC 959.9
capitis 920
  due to birth injury 767.19
  newborn 767.19
cerebral — *see* Hematoma, brain
cesarean section wound 674.3 ✓
chorion — *see* Placenta, abnormal
complicating delivery (perineum) (vulva) 664.5 ✓
  pelvic 665.7 ✓
  vagina 665.7 ✓
corpus
  cavernosum (nontraumatic) 607.82
  luteum (nontraumatic) (ruptured) 620.1
dura (mater) — *see* Hematoma, brain, subdural
epididymis (nontraumatic) 608.83
epidural (traumatic) — *see also* Hematoma, brain, extradural
  spinal — *see* Injury, spinal, by site
episiotomy 674.3 ✓
external ear 380.31
extradural — *see also* Hematoma, brain, extradural
  fetus or newborn 767.0
  nontraumatic 432.0
    fetus or newborn 767.0
fallopian tube 620.8
genital organ (nontraumatic)
  female NEC 629.8
  male NEC 608.83
  traumatic (external site) 922.4
    internal — *see* Injury, internal, genital organ
graafian follicle (ruptured) 620.0
internal organs (abdomen, chest, or pelvis) — *see also* Injury, internal, by site
  kidney — *see* Hematoma, kidney, traumatic
  liver — *see* Hematoma, liver, traumatic
  spleen — *see* Hematoma, brain
intracrainal — *see* Hematoma, brain
kidney, cystic 593.81
  traumatic 866.01
    with open wound into cavity 866.11
labia (nontraumatic) 624.5
lingual (and other parts of neck, scalp, or face, except eye) 920
liver (subcapsular) 573.8
  birth injury 767.8
  fetus or newborn 767.8
  traumatic NEC 864.01
    with
      laceration — *see* Laceration, liver
      open wound into cavity 864.11
mediastinum — *see* Injury, internal, mediastinum
meninges, meningeal (brain) — *see also* Hematoma, brain, subarachnoid
  spinal — *see* Injury, spinal, by site
mesosalpinx (nontraumatic) 620.8
  traumatic — *see* Injury, internal, pelvis
muscle (traumatic) — *see* Contusion, by site
nasal (septum) (and other part(s) of neck, scalp, or face, except eye) 920

Hematoma — *see also* Contusion — *continued*
obstetrical surgical wound 674.3 ✓
orbit, orbital (nontraumatic) 376.32
  traumatic 921.2
ovary (corpus luteum) (nontraumatic) 620.1
  traumatic — *see* Injury, internal, ovary
pelvis (female) (nontraumatic) 629.8
  complicating delivery 665.7 ✓
  male 608.83
  traumatic — *see also* Injury, internal, pelvis
    specified organ NEC (*see also* Injury, internal, pelvis) 867.6
penis (nontraumatic) 607.82
pericranial (and neck, or face any part, except eye) 920
  due to injury at birth 767.19
perineal wound (obstetrical) 674.3 ✓
  complicating delivery 664.5 ✓
perirenal, cystic 593.81
pinna 380.31
placenta — *see* Placenta, abnormal
postoperative 998.12
retroperitoneal (nontraumatic) 568.81
  traumatic — *see* Injury, internal, retroperitoneum
retropubic, male 568.81
scalp (and neck, or face any part, except eye) 920
  fetus or newborn 767.19
scrotum (nontraumatic) 608.83
  traumatic 922.4
seminal vesicle (nontraumatic) 608.83
  traumatic — *see* Injury, internal, seminal, vesicle
spermatic cord — *see also* Injury, internal, spermatic cord
  nontraumatic 608.83
spinal (cord) (meninges) — *see also* Injury, spinal, by site
  fetus or newborn 767.4
  nontraumatic 336.1
spleen 865.01
  with
    laceration — *see* Laceration, spleen
    open wound into cavity 865.11
sternocleidomastoid, birth injury 767.8
sternomastoid, birth injury 767.8
subarachnoid — *see also* Hematoma, brain, subarachnoid
  fetus or newborn 772.2
  nontraumatic (*see also* Hemorrhage, subarachnoid) 430
    newborn 772.2
subdural — *see also* Hematoma, brain, subdural
  fetus or newborn (localized) 767.0
  nontraumatic (*see also* Hemorrhage, subdural) 432.1
subperiosteal (syndrome) 267
  traumatic — *see* Hematoma, by site
superficial, fetus or newborn 772.6
syncytium — *see* Placenta, abnormal
testis (nontraumatic) 608.83
  birth injury 767.8
  traumatic 922.4
tunica vaginalis (nontraumatic) 608.83
umbilical cord 663.6 ✓
  affecting fetus or newborn 762.6
uterine ligament (nontraumatic) 620.7
  traumatic — *see* Injury, internal, pelvis
uterus 621.4
  traumatic — *see* Injury, internal, pelvis
vagina (nontraumatic) (ruptured) 623.6
  complicating delivery 665.7 ✓
  traumatic 922.4
vas deferens (nontraumatic) 608.83
  traumatic — *see* Injury, internal, vas deferens
vitreous 379.23
vocal cord 920
vulva (nontraumatic) 624.5
  complicating delivery 664.5 ✓
  fetus or newborn 767.8
  traumatic 922.4
Hematometra 621.4

Hematomyelia 336.1
  with fracture of vertebra (*see also* Fracture,
      vertebra, by site, with spinal cord injury)
      806.8
  fetus or newborn 767.4
Hematomyelitis 323.9
  late effect — *see* category 326
Hematoperitoneum (*see also* Hemoperitoneum)
      568.81
Hematopneumothorax (*see also* Hemothorax)
      511.8
Hematoporphyria (acquired) (congenital) 277.1
Hematoporphyrinuria (acquired) (congenital)
      277.1
Hematorachis, hematorrhachis 336.1
  fetus or newborn 767.4
Hematosalpinx 620.8
  with
      ectopic pregnancy (*see also* categories
          633.0-633.9) 639.2
      molar pregnancy (*see also* categories 630-
          632) 639.2
      infectional (*see also* Salpingo-oophoritis)
          614.2
Hematospermia 608.82
Hematothorax (*see also* Hemothorax) 511.8
Hematotympanum 381.03
Hematuria (benign) (essential) (idiopathic) 599.7
  due to S. hematobium 120.0
  endemic 120.0
  intermittent 599.7
  malarial 084.8
  paroxysmal 599.7
  sulfonamide
      correct substance properly administered
          599.7
      overdose or wrong substance given or taken
          961.0
  tropical (bilharziasis) 120.0
  tuberculous (*see also* Tuberculosis) 016.9 ☑
Hematuric bilious fever 084.8
Hemeralopia 368.10
Hemiabiotrophy 799.89
Hemi-akinesia 781.8
Hemianalgesia (*see also* Disturbance, sensation)
      782.0
Hemianencephaly 740.0
Hemianesthesia (*see also* Disturbance, sensation)
      782.0
Hemianopia, hemianopsia (altitudinal)
      (homonymous) 368.46
  binasal 368.47
  bitemporal 368.47
  heteronymous 368.47
  syphilitic 095.8
Hemiasomatognosia 307.9
Hemiathetosis 781.0
Hemiatrophy 799.89
  cerebellar 334.8
  face 349.89
      progressive 349.89
  fascia 728.9
  leg 728.2
  tongue 529.8
Hemiballism(us) 333.5
Hemiblock (cardiac) (heart) (left) 426.2
Hemicardia 746.89
Hemicephalus, hemicephaly 740.0
Hemichorea 333.5
Hemicrania 346.9 ☑
  congenital malformation 740.0
Hemidystrophy — *see* Hemiatrophy
Hemiectromelia 755.4
Hemihypalgesia (*see also* Disturbance, sensation)
      782.0
Hemihypertrophy (congenital) 759.89
  cranial 756.0
Hemihypesthesia (*see also* Disturbance,
      sensation) 782.0
Hemi-inattention 781.8

Hemimelia 755.4
  lower limb 755.30
      paraxial (complete) (incomplete) (intercalary)
          (terminal) 755.32
          fibula 755.37
          tibia 755.36
      transverse (complete) (partial) 755.31
  upper limb 755.20
      paraxial (complete) (incomplete) (intercalary)
          (terminal) 755.22
          radial 755.26
          ulnar 755.27
      transverse (complete) (partial) 755.21
Hemiparalysis (*see also* Hemiplegia) 342.9 ☑
Hemiparesis (*see also* Hemiplegia) 342.9 ☑
Hemiparesthesia (*see also* Disturbance,
      sensation) 782.0
Hemiplegia 342.9 ☑
  acute (*see also* Disease, cerebrovascular, acute)
      436
  alternans facialis 344.89
  apoplectic (*see also* Disease, cerebrovascular,
      acute) 436
      late effect or residual
          affecting
              dominant side 438.21
              nondominant side 438.22
              unspecified side 438.20
  arteriosclerotic 437.0
      late effect or residual
          affecting
              dominant side 438.21
              nondominant side 438.22
              unspecified side 438.20
  ascending (spinal) NEC 344.89
  attack (*see also* Disease, cerebrovascular,
      acute) 436
  brain, cerebral (current episode) 437.8
      congenital 343.1
  cerebral — *see* Hemiplegia, brain
  congenital (cerebral) (spastic) (spinal) 343.1
  conversion neurosis (hysterical) 300.11
  cortical — *see* Hemiplegia, brain
  due to
      arteriosclerosis 437.0
          late effect or residual
              affecting
                  dominant side 438.21
                  nondominant side 438.22
                  unspecified side 438.20
      cerebrovascular lesion (*see also* Disease,
          cerebrovascular, acute) 436
          late effect
              affecting
                  dominant side 438.21
                  nondominant side 438.22
                  unspecified side 438.20
  embolic (current) (*see also* Embolism, brain)
      434.1 ☑
      late effect
          affecting
              dominant side 438.21
              nondominant side 438.22
              unspecified side 438.20
  flaccid 342.0 ☑
  hypertensive (current episode) 437.8
  infantile (postnatal) 343.4
  late effect
      birth injury, intracranial or spinal 343.4
      cerebrovascular lesion — *see* Late effect(s)
          (of) cerebrovascular disease
      viral encephalitis 139.0
  middle alternating NEC 344.89
  newborn NEC 767.0
  seizure (current episode) (*see also* Disease,
      cerebrovascular, acute) 436
  spastic 342.1 ☑
      congenital or infantile 343.1
  specified NEC 342.8 ☑
  thrombotic (current) (*see also* Thrombosis,
      brain) 434.0 ☑
      late effect — *see* Late effect(s) (of)
          cerebrovascular disease
Hemisection, spinal cord — *see* Fracture,
      vertebra, by site, with spinal cord injury

Hemispasm 781.0
  facial 781.0
Hemispatial neglect 781.8
Hemisporosis 117.9
Hemitremor 781.0
Hemivertebra 756.14
Hemobilia 576.8
Hemocholecyst 575.8
Hemochromatosis (acquired) (diabetic)
      (hereditary) (liver) (myocardium) (primary
      idiopathic) (secondary) 275.0
  with refractory anemia 285.0
Hemodialysis V56.0
Hemoglobin — *see also* condition
  abnormal (disease) — *see* Disease, hemoglobin
  AS genotype 282.5
  fetal, hereditary persistence 282.7
  high-oxygen-affinity 289.0
  low NEC 285.9
  S (Hb-S), heterozygous 282.5
Hemoglobinemia 283.2
  due to blood transfusion NEC 999.8
      bone marrow 996.85
  paroxysmal 283.2
Hemoglobinopathy (mixed) (*see also* Disease,
      hemoblobin) 282.7
  with thalassemia 282.49
  sickle-cell 282.60
      with thalassemia (without crisis) 282.41
          with
              crisis 282.42
              vaso-occlusive pain 282.42
Hemoglobinuria, hemoglobinuric 791.2
  with anemia, hemolytic, acquired (chronic)
      NEC 283.2
  cold (agglutinin) (paroxysmal) (with Raynaud's
      syndrome) 283.2
  due to
      exertion 283.2
      hemolysis (from external causes) NEC 283.2
  exercise 283.2
  fever (malaria) 084.8
  infantile 791.2
  intermittent 283.2
  malarial 084.8
  march 283.2
  nocturnal (paroxysmal) 283.2
  paroxysmal (cold) (nocturnal) 283.2
Hemolymphangioma (M9175/0) 228.1
Hemolysis
  fetal — *see* Jaundice, fetus or newborn
  intravascular (disseminated) NEC 286.6
      with
          abortion — *see* Abortion, by type, with
              hemorrhage, delayed or excessive
          ectopic pregnancy (*see also* categories
              633.0-633.9) 639.1
          hemorrhage of pregnancy 641.3 ☑
              affecting fetus or newborn 762.1
          molar pregnancy (*see also* categories 630-
              632) 639.1
      acute 283.2
      following
          abortion 639.1
          ectopic or molar pregnancy 639.1
      neonatal — *see* Jaundice, fetus or newborn
      transfusion NEC 999.8
          bone marrow 996.85
Hemolytic — *see also* condition
  anemia — *see* Anemia, hemolytic
  uremic syndrome 283.11
Hemometra 621.4
Hemopericardium (with effusion) 423.0
  newborn 772.8
  traumatic (*see also* Hemothorax, traumatic)
      860.2
      with open wound into thorax 860.3
Hemoperitoneum 568.81
  infectional (*see also* Peritonitis) 567.2
  traumatic — *see* Injury, internal, peritoneum

Hemophilia (familial) (hereditary) 286.0
  A 286.0
    carrier (asymptomatic) V83.01
      symptomatic V83.02
  acquired 286.5
  B (Leyden) 286.1
  C 286.2
  calcipriva (*see also* Fibrinolysis) 286.7
  classical 286.0
  nonfamilial 286.7
  secondary 286.5   ●
  vascular 286.4
Hemophilus influenzae NEC 041.5
  arachnoiditis (basic) (brain) (spinal) 320.0
    late effect — *see* category 326
  bronchopneumonia 482.2
  cerebral ventriculitis 320.0
    late effect — *see* category 326
  cerebrospinal inflammation 320.0
    late effect — *see* category 326
  infection NEC 041.5
  leptomeningitis 320.0
    late effect — *see* category 326
  meningitis (cerebral) (cerebrospinal) (spinal)
    320.0
    late effect — *see* category 326
  meningomyelitis 320.0
    late effect — *see* category 326
  pachymeningitis (adhesive) (fibrous)
    (hemorrhagic) (hypertrophic) (spinal)
    320.0
    late effect — *see* category 326
  pneumonia (broncho-) 482.2
Hemophthalmos 360.43
Hemopneumothorax (*see also* Hemothorax) 511.8
  traumatic 860.4
    with open wound into thorax 860.5
Hemoptysis 786.3
  due to Paragonimus (westermani) 121.2
  newborn 770.3
  tuberculous (*see also* Tuberculosis, pulmonary)
    011.9 ☑
Hemorrhage, hemorrhagic (nontraumatic) 459.0
  abdomen 459.0
  accidental (antepartum) 641.2 ☑
    affecting fetus or newborn 762.1
  adenoid 474.8
  adrenal (capsule) (gland) (medulla) 255.4
    newborn 772.5
  after labor — *see* Hemorrhage, postpartum
  alveolar
    lung, newborn 770.3
    process 525.8
  alveolus 525.8
  amputation stump (surgical) 998.11
    secondary, delayed 997.69
  anemia (chronic) 280.0
    acute 285.1
  antepartum — *see* Hemorrhage, pregnancy
  anus (sphincter) 569.3
  apoplexy (stroke) 432.9
  arachnoid — *see* Hemorrhage, subarachnoid
  artery NEC 459.0
    brain (*see also* Hemorrhage, brain) 431
    middle meningeal — *see* Hemorrhage,
      subarachnoid
  basilar (ganglion) (*see also* Hemorrhage, brain)
    431
  bladder 596.8
  blood dyscrasia 289.9
  bowel 578.9
    newborn 772.4
  brain (miliary) (nontraumatic) 431
    with
      birth injury 767.0
      arachnoid — *see* Hemorrhage, subarachnoid
      due to
        birth injury 767.0
        rupture of aneurysm (congenital) (*see*
          also Hemorrhage, subarachnoid)
          430
          mycotic 431
          syphilis 094.89
      epidural or extradural — *see* Hemorrhage,
        extradural

Hemorrhage, hemorrhagic — *continued*
  brain — *continued*
    fetus or newborn (anoxic) (hypoxic) (due to
      birth trauma) (nontraumatic) 767.0
      intraventricular 772.10
        grade I 772.11
        grade II 772.12
        grade III 772.13
        grade IV 772.14
    iatrogenic 997.02
    postoperative 997.02
    puerperal, postpartum, childbirth 674.0 ☑
    stem 431
    subarachnoid, arachnoid, or meningeal —
      see Hemorrhage, subarachnoid
    subdural — *see* Hemorrhage, subdural
    traumatic NEC 853.0 ☑

> *Note* — *Use the following fifth-digit
> subclassification with categories 851-854:*
>
> 0   *unspecified state of consciousness*
> 1   *with no loss of consciousness*
> 2   *with brief [less than one hour] loss of
>   consciousness*
> 3   *with moderate [1-24 hours] loss of
>   consciousness*
> 4   *with prolonged [more than 24 hours]
>   loss of consciousness and return to pre-
>   existing conscious level*
> 5   *with prolonged [more than 24 hours]
>   loss of consciousness, without return to
>   pre-existing conscious level*
> *Use fifth-digit 5 to designate when a patient
> is unconscious and dies before
> regaining consciousness, regardless of
> the duration of the loss of
> consciousness*
> 6   *with loss of consciousness of
>   unspecified duration*
> 9   *with concussion, unspecified*

    with
      cerebral
        contusion — *see* Contusion, brain
        laceration — *see* Laceration, brain
      open intracranial wound 853.1 ☑
      skull fracture — *see* Fracture, skull,
        by site
    extradural or epidural 852.4 ☑
      with open intracranial wound 852.5 ☑
    subarachnoid 852.0 ☑
      with open intracranial wound 852.1 ☑
    subdural 852.2 ☑
      with open intracranial wound 852.3 ☑
  breast 611.79
  bronchial tube — *see* Hemorrhage, lung
  bronchopulmonary — *see* Hemorrhage, lung
  bronchus (cause unknown) (*see also*
    Hemorrhage, lung) 786.3
  bulbar (*see also* Hemorrhage, brain) 431
  bursa 727.89
  capillary 448.9
    primary 287.8
  capsular — *see* Hemorrhage, brain
  cardiovascular 429.89
  cecum 578.9
  cephalic (*see also* Hemorrhage, brain) 431
  cerebellar (*see also* Hemorrhage, brain) 431
  cerebellum (*see also* Hemorrhage, brain) 431
  cerebral (*see also* Hemorrhage, brain) 431
    fetus or newborn (anoxic) (traumatic) 767.0
  cerebromeningeal (*see also* Hemorrhage, brain)
    431
  cerebrospinal (*see also* Hemorrhage, brain) 431
  cerebrum (*see also* Hemorrhage, brain) 431
  cervix (stump) (uteri) 622.8
  cesarean section wound 674.3 ☑
  chamber, anterior (eye) 364.41
  childbirth — *see* Hemorrhage, complicating,
    delivery
  choroid 363.61
    expulsive 363.62
  ciliary body 364.41
  cochlea 386.8

Hemorrhage, hemorrhagic — *continued*
  colon — *see* Hemorrhage, intestine
  complicating
    delivery 641.9 ☑
      affecting fetus or newborn 762.1
      associated with
        afibrinogenemia 641.3 ☑
          affecting fetus or newborn 763.89
        coagulation defect 641.3 ☑
          affecting fetus or newborn 763.89
        hyperfibrinolysis 641.3 ☑
          affecting fetus or newborn 763.89
        hypofibrinogenemia 641.3 ☑
          affecting fetus or newborn 763.89
      due to
        low-lying placenta 641.1 ☑
          affecting fetus or newborn 762.0
        placenta previa 641.1 ☑
          affecting fetus or newborn 762.0
        premature separation of placenta
          641.2 ☑
          affecting fetus or newborn 762.1
        retained
          placenta 666.0 ☑
          secundines 666.2 ☑
        trauma 641.8 ☑
          affecting fetus or newborn 763.89
        uterine leiomyoma 641.8 ☑
          affecting fetus or newborn 763.89
    surgical procedure 998.11
  concealed NEC 459.0
  congenital 772.9
  conjunctiva 372.72
    newborn 772.8
  cord, newborn 772.0
    slipped ligature 772.3
    stump 772.3
  corpus luteum (ruptured) 620.1
  cortical (*see also* Hemorrhage, brain) 431
  cranial 432.9
  cutaneous 782.7
    newborn 772.6
  cyst, pancreas 577.2
  cystitis — *see* Cystitis
  delayed
    with
      abortion — *see* Abortion, by type, with
        hemorrhage, delayed or excessive
      ectopic pregnancy (*see also* categories
        633.0-633.9) 639.1
      molar pregnancy (*see also* categories 630-
        632) 639.1
    following
      abortion 639.1
      ectopic or molar pregnancy 639.1
    postpartum 666.2 ☑
  diathesis (familial) 287.9
    newborn 776.0
  disease 287.9
    newborn 776.0
    specified type NEC 287.8
  disorder 287.9
    due to ►intrinsic◄ circulating
      anticoagulants 286.5
    specified type NEC 287.8
  due to
    any device, implant or graft (presence of)
      classifiable to 996.0-996.5 — *see*
      Complications, due to (presence of)
      any device, implant, or graft classified
      to 996.0-996.5 NEC
    ►intrinsic◄ circulating anticoagulant 286.5
  duodenum, duodenal 537.89
    ulcer — *see* Ulcer, duodenum, with
      hemorrhage
  dura mater — *see* Hemorrhage, subdural
  endotracheal — *see* Hemorrhage, lung
  epicranial subaponeurotic (massive) 767.11
  epidural — *see* Hemorrhage, extradural
  episiotomy 674.3 ☑
  esophagus 530.82
    varix (*see also* Varix, esophagus, bleeding)
      456.0

Hemorrhage, hemorrhagic — *continued*
excessive
with
abortion — *see* Abortion, by type, with hemorrhage, delayed or excessive
ectopic pregnancy (*see also* categories 633.0-633.9) 639.1
molar pregnancy (*see also* categories 630-632) 639.1
following
abortion 639.1
ectopic or molar pregnancy 639.1
external 459.0
extradural (traumatic) — *see also* Hemorrhage, brain, traumatic, extradural
birth injury 767.0
fetus or newborn (anoxic) (traumatic) 767.0
nontraumatic 432.0
eye 360.43
chamber (anterior) (aqueous) 364.41
fundus 362.81
eyelid 374.81
fallopian tube 620.8
fetomaternal 772.0
affecting management of pregnancy or puerperium 656.0 ☑
fetus, fetal 772.0
from
cut end of co-twin's cord 772.0
placenta 772.0
ruptured cord 772.0
vasa previa 772.0
into
co-twin 772.0
mother's circulation 772.0
affecting management of pregnancy or puerperium 656.0 ☑
fever (*see also* Fever, hemorrhagic) 065.9
with renal syndrome 078.6
arthropod-borne NEC 065.9
Bangkok 065.4
Crimean 065.0
dengue virus 065.4
epidemic 078.6
Junin virus 078.7
Korean 078.6
Machupo virus 078.7
mite-borne 065.8
mosquito-borne 065.4
Philippine 065.4
Russian (Yaroslav) 078.6
Singapore 065.4
southeast Asia 065.4
Thailand 065.4
tick-borne NEC 065.3
fibrinogenolysis (*see also* Fibrinolysis) 286.6
fibrinolytic (acquired) (*see also* Fibrinolysis) 286.6
fontanel 767.19
from tracheostomy stoma 519.09
fundus, eye 362.81
funis
affecting fetus or newborn 772.0
complicating delivery 663.8 ☑
gastric (*see also* Hemorrhage, stomach) 578.9
gastroenteric 578.9
newborn 772.4
gastrointestinal (tract) 578.9
newborn 772.4
genitourinary (tract) NEC 599.89
gingiva 523.8
globe 360.43
gravidarum — *see* Hemorrhage, pregnancy
gum 523.8
heart 429.89
hypopharyngeal (throat) 784.8
intermenstrual 626.6
irregular 626.6
regular 626.5
internal (organs) 459.0
capsule (*see also* Hemorrhage, brain) 431
ear 386.8
newborn 772.8
intestine 578.9
congenital 772.4
newborn 772.4

Hemorrhage, hemorrhagic — *continued*
into
bladder wall 596.7
bursa 727.89
corpus luysii (*see also* Hemorrhage, brain) 431
intra-abdominal 459.0
during or following surgery 998.11
intra-alveolar, newborn (lung) 770.3
intracerebral (*see also* Hemorrhage, brain) 431
intracranial NEC 432.9
puerperal, postpartum, childbirth 674.0 ☑
traumatic — *see* Hemorrhage, brain, traumatic
intramedullary NEC 336.1
intraocular 360.43
intraoperative 998.11
intrapartum — *see* Hemorrhage, complicating, delivery
intrapelvic
female 629.8
male 459.0
intraperitoneal 459.0
intrapontine (*see also* Hemorrhage, brain) 431
intrauterine 621.4
complicating delivery — *see* Hemorrhage, complicating, delivery
in pregnancy or childbirth — *see* Hemorrhage, pregnancy
postpartum (*see also* Hemorrhage, postpartum) 666.1 ☑
intraventricular (*see also* Hemorrhage, brain) 431
fetus or newborn (anoxic) (traumatic) 772.10
grade I 772.11
grade II 772.12
grade III 772.13
grade IV 772.14
intravesical 596.7
iris (postinfectional) (postinflammatory) (toxic) 364.41
joint (nontraumatic) 719.10
ankle 719.17
elbow 719.12
foot 719.17
forearm 719.13
hand 719.14
hip 719.15
knee 719.16
lower leg 719.16
multiple sites 719.19
pelvic region 719.15
shoulder (region) 719.11
specified site NEC 719.18
thigh 719.15
upper arm 719.12
wrist 719.13
kidney 593.81
knee (joint) 719.16
labyrinth 386.8
leg NEC 459.0
lenticular striate artery (*see also* Hemorrhage, brain) 431
ligature, vessel 998.11
liver 573.8
lower extremity NEC 459.0
lung 786.3
newborn 770.3
tuberculous (*see also* Tuberculosis, pulmonary) 011.9 ☑
malaria 084.8
marginal sinus 641.2 ☑
massive subaponeurotic, birth injury 767.11
maternal, affecting fetus or newborn 762.1
mediastinum 786.3
medulla (*see also* Hemorrhage, brain) 431
membrane (brain) (*see also* Hemorrhage, subarachnoid) 430
spinal cord — *see* Hemorrhage, spinal cord
meninges, meningeal (brain) (middle) (*see also* Hemorrhage, subarachnoid) 430
spinal cord — *see* Hemorrhage, spinal cord
mesentery 568.81
metritis 626.8
midbrain (*see also* Hemorrhage, brain) 431
mole 631

Hemorrhage, hemorrhagic — *continued*
mouth 528.9
mucous membrane NEC 459.0
newborn 728.8 ☑
muscle 728.89
nail (subungual) 703.8
nasal turbinate 784.7
newborn 772.8
nasopharynx 478.29
navel, newborn 772.3
newborn 772.9
adrenal 772.5
alveolar (lung) 770.3
brain (anoxic) (hypoxic) (due to birth trauma) 767.0
cerebral (anoxic) (hypoxic) (due to birth trauma) 767.0
conjunctiva 772.8
cutaneous 772.6
diathesis 776.0
due to vitamin K deficiency 776.0
epicranial subaponeurotic (massive) 767.11
gastrointestinal 772.4
internal (organs) 772.8
intestines 772.4
intra-alveolar (lung) 770.3
intracranial (from any perinatal cause) 767.0
intraventricular (from any perinatal cause) 772.10
grade I 772.11
grade II 772.12
grade III 772.13
grade IV 772.14
lung 770.3
pulmonary (massive) 770.3
spinal cord, traumatic 767.4
stomach 772.4
subaponeurotic (massive) 767.11
subarachnoid (from any perinatal cause) 772.2
subconjunctival 772.8
subgaleal 767.11
umbilicus 772.0
slipped ligature 772.3
vasa previa 772.0
nipple 611.79
nose 784.7
newborn 772.8
obstetrical surgical wound 674.3 ☑
omentum 568.89
newborn 772.4
optic nerve (sheath) 377.42
orbit 376.32
ovary 620.1
oviduct 620.8
pancreas 577.8
parathyroid (gland) (spontaneous) 252.8
parturition — *see* Hemorrhage, complicating, delivery
penis 607.82
pericardium, paricarditis 423.0
perineal wound (obstetrical) 674.3 ☑
peritoneum, peritoneal 459.0
peritonsillar tissue 474.8
after operation on tonsils 998.11
due to infection 475
petechial 782.7
pituitary (gland) 253.8
placenta NEC 641.9 ☑
affecting fetus or newborn 762.1
from surgical or instrumental damage 641.8 ☑
affecting fetus or newborn 762.1
previa 641.8 ☑
affecting fetus or newborn 762.0
pleura — *see* Hemorrhage, lung
polioencephalitis, superior 265.1
polymyositis — *see* Polymyositis
pons (*see also* Hemorrhage, brain) 431
pontine (*see also* Hemorrhage, brain) 431
popliteal 459.0
postcoital 626.7
postextraction (dental) 998.11
postmenopausal 627.1
postnasal 784.7
postoperative 998.11

☑ Additional Digit Required   ▶◀ Revised Text   ● New Line   ▲ Revised Code

Hemorrhage, hemorrhagic — *continued*
　postpartum (atonic) (following delivery of
　　placenta) 666.1 ☑
　　delayed or secondary (after 24 hours)
　　　666.2 ☑
　　retained placenta 666.0 ☑
　　third stage 666.0 ☑
　pregnancy (concealed) 641.9 ☑
　　accidental 641.2 ☑
　　　affecting fetus or newborn 762.1
　　affecting fetus or newborn 762.1
　　before 22 completed weeks gestation
　　　640.9 ☑
　　　affecting fetus or newborn 762.1
　　due to
　　　abruptio placenta 641.2 ☑
　　　　affecting fetus or newborn 762.1
　　　afibrinogenemia or other coagulation
　　　　defect (conditions classifiable to
　　　　286.0-286.9) 641.3 ☑
　　　　affecting fetus or newborn 762.1
　　　coagulation defect 641.3 ☑
　　　　affecting fetus or newborn 762.1
　　　hyperfibrinolysis 641.3 ☑
　　　　affecting fetus or newborn 762.1
　　　hypofibrinogenemia 641.3 ☑
　　　　affecting fetus or newborn 762.1
　　　leiomyoma, uterus 641.8 ☑
　　　　affecting fetus or newborn 762.1
　　　low-lying placenta 641.1 ☑
　　　　affecting fetus or newborn 762.1
　　　marginal sinus (rupture) 641.2 ☑
　　　　affecting fetus or newborn 762.1
　　　placenta previa 641.1 ☑
　　　　affecting fetus or newborn 762.0
　　　premature separation of placenta
　　　　(normally implanted) 641.2 ☑
　　　　affecting fetus or newborn 762.1
　　　threatend abortion 640.0 ☑
　　　　affecting fetus or newborn 762.1
　　　trauma 641.8 ☑
　　　　affecting fetus or newborn 762.1
　　early (before 22 completed weeks gestation)
　　　640.9 ☑
　　　affecting fetus or newborn 762.1
　　previous, affecting management of
　　　pregnancy or childbirth V23.49
　　unavoidable — *see* Hemorrhage, pregnancy,
　　　due to placenta previa
　prepartum (mother) — *see* Hemorrhage,
　　pregnancy
　preretinal, cause unspecified 362.81
　prostate 602.1
　puerperal (*see also* Hemorrhage, postpartum)
　　666.1 ☑
　pulmonary — *see also* Hemorrhage, lung
　　newborn (massive) 770.3
　　renal syndrome 446.21
　purpura (primary) (*see also* Purpura,
　　thrombocytopenic) 287.3
　rectum (sphincter) 569.3
　recurring, following initial hemorrhage at time
　　of injury 958.2
　renal 593.81
　　pulmonary syndrome 446.21
　respiratory tract (*see also* Hemorrhage, lung)
　　786.3
　retina, retinal (deep) (superficial) (vessels)
　　362.81
　　diabetic 250.5 ☑ *[362.01]*
　　due to birth injury 772.8
　retrobulbar 376.89
　retroperitoneal 459.0
　retroplacental (*see also* Placenta, separation)
　　641.2 ☑
　scalp 459.0
　　due to injury at birth 767.19
　scrotum 608.83
　secondary (nontraumatic) 459.0
　　following initial hemorrhage at time of injury
　　　958.2
　seminal vesicle 608.83
　skin 782.7
　　newborn 772.6
　spermatic cord 608.83

Hemorrhage, hemorrhagic — *continued*
　spinal (cord) 336.1
　　aneurysm (ruptured) 336.1
　　　syphilitic 094.89
　　due to birth injury 767.4
　　fetus or newborn 767.4
　spleen 289.59
　spontaneous NEC 459.0
　　petechial 782.7
　stomach 578.9
　　newborn 772.4
　　ulcer — *see* Ulcer, stomach, with
　　　hemorrhage
　subaponeurotic, newborn 767.11
　　massive (birth injury) 767.11
　subarachnoid (nontraumatic) 430
　　fetus or newborn (anoxic) (traumatic) 772.2
　　puerperal, postpartum, childbirth 674.0 ☑
　　traumatic — *see* Hemorrhage, brain,
　　　traumatic, subarachnoid
　subconjunctival 372.72
　　due to birth injury 772.8
　　newborn 772.8
　subcortical (*see also* Hemorrhage, brain) 431
　subcutaneous 782.7
　subdiaphragmatic 459.0
　subdural (nontraumatic) 432.1
　　due to birth injury 767.0
　　fetus or newborn (anoxic) (hypoxic) (due to
　　　birth trauma) 767.0
　　puerperal, postpartum, childbirth 674.0 ☑
　　spinal 336.1
　　traumatic — *see* Hemorrhage, brain,
　　　traumatic, subdural
　subgaleal 767.11
　subhyaloid 362.81
　subperiosteal 733.99
　subretinal 362.81
　subtentorial (*see also* Hemorrhage, subdural)
　　432.1
　subungual 703.8
　　due to blood dyscrasia 287.8
　suprarenal (capsule) (gland) 255.4
　　fetus or newborn 772.5
　tentorium (traumatic) — *see also* Hemorrhage,
　　brain, traumatic
　　fetus or newborn 767.0
　　nontraumatic — *see* Hemorrhage, subdural
　testis 608.83
　thigh 459.0
　third stage 666.0 ☑
　thorax — *see* Hemorrhage, lung
　throat 784.8
　thrombocythemia 238.7
　thymus (gland) 254.8
　thyroid (gland) 246.3
　　cyst 246.3
　tongue 529.8
　tonsil 474.8
　　postoperative 998.11
　tooth socket (postextraction) 998.11
　trachea — *see* Hemorrhage, lung
　traumatic — *see also* nature of injury
　　brain — *see* Hemorrhage, brain, traumatic
　　recurring or secondary (following initial
　　　hemorrhage at time of injury) 958.2
　tuberculous NEC (*see also* Tuberculosis,
　　pulmonary) 011.9 ☑
　tunica vaginalis 608.83
　ulcer — *see* Ulcer, by site, with hemorrhage
　umbilicus, umbilical cord 772.0
　　after birth, newborn 772.3
　　complicating delivery 663.8 ☑
　　　affecting fetus or newborn 772.0
　　slipped ligature 772.3
　　stump 772.3
　unavoidable (due to placenta previa) 641.1 ☑
　　affecting fetus or newborn 762.0
　upper extremity 459.0
　urethra (idiopathic) 599.84
　uterus, uterine (abnormal) 626.9
　　climacteric 627.0
　　complicating delivery — *see* Hemorrhage,
　　　complicating delivery
　　due to
　　　intrauterine contraceptive device 996.76
　　　　perforating uterus 996.32

Hemorrhage, hemorrhagic — *continued*
　uterus, uterine — *continued*
　　functional or dysfunctional 626.8
　　in pregnancy — *see* Hemorrhage, pregnancy
　　intermenstrual 626.6
　　　irregular 626.6
　　　regular 626.5
　　postmenopausal 627.1
　　postpartum (*see also* Hemorrhage,
　　　postpartum) 666.1 ☑
　　prepubertal 626.8
　　pubertal 626.3
　　puerperal (immediate) 666.1 ☑
　vagina 623.8
　vasa previa 663.5 ☑
　　affecting fetus or newborn 772.0
　vas deferens 608.83
　ventricular (*see also* Hemorrhage, brain) 431
　vesical 596.8
　viscera 459.0
　　newborn 772.8
　vitreous (humor) (intraocular) 379.23
　vocal cord 478.5
　vulva 624.8

Hemorrhoids (anus) (rectum) (without
　complication) 455.6
　bleeding, prolapsed, strangulated, or ulcerated
　　NEC 455.8
　　external 455.5
　　internal 455.2
　complicated NEC 455.8
　complicating pregnancy and puerperium
　　671.8 ☑
　external 455.3
　　with complication NEC 455.5
　　　bleeding, prolapsed, strangulated, or
　　　　ulcerated 455.5
　　thrombosed 455.4
　internal 455.0
　　with complication NEC 455.2
　　　bleeding, prolapsed, strangulated, or
　　　　ulcerated 455.2
　　thrombosed 455.1
　residual skin tag 455.9
　sentinel pile 455.9
　thrombosed NEC 455.7
　　external 455.4
　　internal 455.1

Hemosalpinx 620.8

Hemosiderosis 275.0
　dietary 275.0
　pulmonary (idiopathic) 275.0 *[516.1]*
　transfusion NEC 999.8
　　bone marrow 996.85

Hemospermia 608.82

Hemothorax 511.8
　bacterial, nontuberculous 511.1
　newborn 772.8
　nontuberculous 511.8
　　bacterial 511.1
　pneumococcal 511.1
　postoperative 998.11
　staphylococcal 511.1
　streptococcal 511.1
　traumatic 860.2
　　with
　　　open wound into thorax 860.3
　　　pneumothorax 860.4
　　　　with open wound into thorax 860.5
　tuberculous (*see also* Tuberculosis, pleura)
　　012.0 ☑

Hemotympanum 385.89

Hench-Rosenberg syndrome (palindromic
　arthritis) (*see also* Rheumatism,
　palindromic) 719.3 ☑

Henle's warts 371.41

Henoch (-Schönlein)
　disease or syndrome (allergic purpura) 287.0
　purpura (allergic) 287.0

Henpue, henpuye 102.6

Heparitinuria 277.5

Hepar lobatum 095.3

Hepatalgia 573.8

Hepatic — *see also* conditon
　flexure syndrome 569.89

☑ Additional Digit Required　　　　　▶◀ Revised Text　　　　　● New Line　　　　　▲ Revised Code

Hepatitis 573.3
  acute (*see also* Necrosis, liver) 570
    alcoholic 571.1
    infective 070.1
      with hepatic coma 070.0
  alcoholic 571.1
  amebic — *see* Abscess, liver, amebic
  anicteric (acute) — *see* Hepatitis, viral
  antigen-associated (HAA) — *see* Hepatitis, viral,
      type B
  Australian antigen (positive) — *see* Hepatitis,
      viral, type B
  catarrhal (acute) 070.1
    with hepatic coma 070.0
    chronic 571.40
    newborn 070.1
      with hepatic coma 070.0
  chemical 573.3
  cholangiolitic 573.8
  cholestatic 573.8
  chronic 571.40
    active 571.49
      viral — *see* Hepatitis, viral
    aggressive 571.49
    persistent 571.41
    viral — *see* Hepatitis, viral
  cytomegalic inclusion virus 078.5 [573.1]
  diffuse 573.3
  "dirty needle" — *see* Hepatitis, viral
    with hepatic coma 070.2 ☑
  drug-induced 573.3
  due to
    Coxsackie 074.8 [573.1]
    cytomegalic inclusion virus 078.5 [573.1]
    infectious mononucleosis 075 [573.1]
    malaria 084.9 [573.2]
    mumps 072.71
    secondary syphilis 091.62
    toxoplasmosis (acquired) 130.5
      congenital (active) 771.2
  epidemic — *see* Hepatitis, viral, type A
  fetus or newborn 774.4
  fibrous (chronic) 571.49
    acute 570
  from injection, inoculation, or transfusion
      (blood) (other substance) (plasma) serum)
      (onset within 8 months after
      administration) — *see* Hepatitis, viral
  fulminant (viral) (*see also* Hepatitis, viral) 070.9
    with hepatic coma 070.6
    type A 070.1
      with hepatic coma 070.0
    type B — *see* Hepatitis, viral, type B
  giant cell (neonatal) 774.4
  hemorrhagic 573.8
  homologous serum — *see* Hepatitis, viral
  hypertrophic (chronic) 571.49
    acute 570
  infectious, infective (acute) (chronic) (subacute)
      070.1
    with hepatic coma 070.0
  inoculation — *see* Hepatitis, viral
  interstitial (chronic) 571.49
    acute 570
  lupoid 571.49
  malarial 084.9 [573.2]
  malignant (*see also* Necrosis, liver) 570
  neonatal (toxic) 774.4
  newborn 774.4
  parenchymatous (acute) (*see also* Necrosis,
      liver) 570
  peliosis 573.3
  persistent, chronic 571.41
  plasma cell 571.49
  postimmunization — *see* Hepatitis, viral
  postnecrotic 571.49
  posttransfusion — *see* Hepatitis, viral
  recurrent 571.49
  septic 573.3
  serum — *see* Hepatitis, viral
    carrier (suspected of) V02.61
  subacute (*see also* Necrosis, liver) 570
  suppurative (diffuse) 572.0
  syphilitic (late) 095.3
    congenital (early) 090.0 [573.2]
      late 090.5 [573.2]
    secondary 091.62

Hepatitis — *continued*
  toxic (noninfectious) 573.3
    fetus or newborn 774.4
  tuberculous (*see also* Tuberculosis) 017.9 ☑
  viral (acute) (anicteric) (cholangiolitic)
      (cholestatic) (chronic) (subacute) 070.9
    with hepatic coma 070.6
    AU-SH type virus — *see* Hepatitis, viral,
        type B
    Australian antigen — *see* Hepatitis, viral,
        type B
    B-antigen — *see* Hepatitis, viral, type B
    Coxsackie 074.8 [573.1]
    cytomegalic inclusion 078.5 [573.1]
    IH (virus) — *see* Hepatitis, viral, type A
    infectious hepatitis, viral, type A
    serum hepatitis virus — *see* Hepatitis, viral,
        type B
    SH — *see* Hepatitis, viral, type B
    specified type NEC 070.59
      with hepatic coma 070.49
    type A 070.1
      with hepatic coma 070.0
    type B (acute) 070.30
      with
        hepatic coma 070.20
          with hepatitis delta 070.21
        hepatitis delta 070.31
          with hepatic coma 070.21
      carrier status V02.61
      chronic 070.32
        with
          hepatic coma 070.22
            with hepatitis delta 070.23
          hepatitis delta 070.33
            with hepatic coma 070.23
    type C
      acute 070.51   ●
        ▶with hepatic coma 070.41◀
      carrier status V02.62
      chronic 070.54
        with hepatic coma 070.44
      unspecified 070.70   ●
        with hepatic coma 070.71   ●
    type delta (with hepatitis B carrier state)
        070.52
      with
        active hepatitis B disease — *see*
            Hepatitis, viral, type B
        hepatic coma 070.42
    type E 070.53
      with hepatic coma 070.43
    vaccination and inoculation (prophylactic)
        V05.3
  Waldenstrom's (lupoid hepatitis) 571.49
Hepatization, lung (acute) — *see also*
      Pneumonia, lobar
  chronic (*see also* Fibrosis, lung) 515
Hepatoblastoma (M8970/3) 155.0
Hepatocarcinoma (M8170/3) 155.0
Hepatocholangiocarcinoma (M8180/3) 155.0
Hepatocholangioma, benign (M8180/0) 211.5
Hepatocholangitis 573.8
Hepatocystitis (*see also* Cholecystitis) 575.10
Hepatodystrophy 570
Hepatolenticular degeneration 275.1
Hepatolithiasis — *see* Choledocholithiasis
Hepatoma (malignant) (M8170/3) 155.0
  benign (M8170/0) 211.5
  congenital (M8970/3) 155.0
  embryonal (M8970/3) 155.0
Hepatomegalia glycogenica diffusa 271.0
Hepatomegaly (*see also* Hypertrophy, liver) 789.1
  congenital 751.69
    syphilitic 090.0
  due to Clonorchis sinensis 121.1
  Gaucher's 272.7
  syphilitic (congenital) 090.0
Hepatoptosis 573.8
Hepatorrhexis 573.8
Hepatosis, toxic 573.8
Hepatosplenomegaly 571.8
  due to S. japonicum 120.2
  hyperlipemic (Burger-Grutz type) 272.3

Herald patch 696.3
Hereditary — *see* condition
Heredodegeneration 330.9
  macular 362.70
Heredopathia atactica polyneuritiformis 356.3
Heredosyphilis (*see also* Syphilis, congenital)
    090.9
Hermaphroditism (true) 752.7
  with specified chromosomal anomaly — *see*
      Anomaly, chromosomes, sex
Hernia, hernial (acquired) (recurrent) 553.9
  with
    gangrene (obstructed) NEC 551.9
    obstruction NEC 552.9
      and gangrene 551.9
  abdomen (wall) — *see* Hernia, ventral
  abdominal, specified site NEC 553.8
    with
      gangrene (obstructed) 551.8
      obstruction 552.8
        and gangrene 551.8
  appendix 553.8
    with
      gangrene (obstructed) 551.8
      obstruction 552.8
        and gangrene 551.8
  bilateral (inguinal) — *see* Hernia, inguinal
  bladder (sphincter)
    congenital (female) (male) 756.71
    female ▶(*see also* Cystocele, female)◀
        618.01   ▲
    male 596.8
  brain 348.4
    congenital 742.0
  broad ligament 553.8
  cartilage, vertebral — *see* Displacement,
      intervertebral disc
  cerebral 348.4
    congenital 742.0
    endaural 742.0
  ciliary body 364.8
    traumatic 871.1
  colic 553.9
    with
      gangrene (obstructed) 551.9
      obstruction 552.9
        and gangrene 551.9
  colon 553.9
    with
      gangrene (obstructed) 551.9
      obstruction 552.9
        and gangrene 551.9
  colostomy (stoma) 569.69
  Cooper's (retroperitoneal) 553.8
    with
      gangrene (obstructed) 551.8
      obstruction 552.8
        and gangrene 551.8
  crural — *see* Hernia, femoral
  diaphragm, diaphragmatic 553.3
    with
      gangrene (obstructed) 551.3
      obstruction 552.3
        and gangrene 551.3
    congenital 756.6
    due to gross defect of diaphragm 756.6
    traumatic 862.0
      with open wound into cavity 862.1
  direct (inguinal) — *see* Hernia, inguinal
  disc, intervetebral — *see* Displacement,
      intervertebral disc
  diverticulum, intestine 553.9
    with
      gangrene (obstructed) 551.9
      obstruction 552.9
        and gangrene 551.9
  double (inguinal) — *see* Hernia, inguinal
  duodenojejunal 553.8
    with
      gangrene (obstructed) 551.8
      obstruction 552.8
        and gangrene 551.8
  en glissade — *see* Hernia, inguinal
  enterostomy (stoma) 569.69

Hepatitis — Hernia, hernial

Hernia, hernial — *continued*
  epigastric 553.29
    with
      gangrene (obstruction) 551.29
      obstruction 552.29
        and gangrene 551.29
    recurrent 553.21
      with
        gangrene (obstructed) 551.21
        obstruction 552.21
          and gangrene 551.21
  esophageal hiatus (sliding) 553.3
    with
      gangrene (obstructed) 551.3
      obstruction 552.3
        and gangrene 551.3
    congenital 750.6
  external (inguinal) — *see* Hernia, inguinal
  fallopian tube 620.4
  fascia 728.89
  fat 729.30
    eyelid 374.34
    orbital 374.34
    pad 729.30
      eye, eyelid 374.34
      knee 729.31
      orbit 374.34
      popliteal (space) 729.31
      specified site NEC 729.39
  femoral (unilateral) 553.00
    with
      gangrene (obstructed) 551.00
      obstruction 552.00
        with gangrene 551.0 ☑
    bilateral 553.02
      gangrenous (obstructed) 551.02
      obstructed 552.02
        with gangrene 551.02
      recurrent 553.03
        gangrenous (obstructed) 551.03
        obstructed 552.03
          with gangrene 551.03
    recurrent (unilateral) 553.01
      bilateral 553.03
        gangrenous (obstructed) 551.03
        obstructed 552.03
          with gangrene 551.03
      gangrenous (obstructed) 551.01
      obstructed 552.01
        with gangrene
  foramen
    Bochdalek 553.3
      with
        gangrene (obstructed) 551.3
        obstruction 552.3
          and gangrene 551.3
      congenital 756.6
    magnum 348.4
    Morgagni, Morgagnian 553.3
      with
        gangrene 551.3
        obstruction 552.3
          and gangrene 551.3
      congenital 756.6
  funicular (umbilical) 553.1
    with
      gangrene (obstructed) 551.1
      obstruction 552.1
        and gangrene 551.1
    spermatic cord — *see* Hernia, inguinal
  gangrenous — *see* Hernia, by site, with
      gangrene
  gastrointestinal tract 553.9
    with
      gangrene (obstructed) 551.9
      obstruction 552.9
        and gangrene 551.9
  gluteal — *see* Hernia, femoral
  Gruber's (internal mesogastric) 553.8
    with
      gangrene (obstructed) 551.8
      obstruction 552.8
        and gangrene 551.8
  Hesselbach's 553.8
    with
      gangrene (obstructed) 551.8

Hernia, hernial — *continued*
  Hesselbach's — *continued*
    with — *continued*
      obstruction 552.8
        and gangrene 551.8
  hiatal (esophageal) (sliding) 553.3
    with
      gangrene (obstructed) 551.3
      obstruction 552.3
        and gangrene 551.3
    congenital 750.6
  incarcerated (*see also* Hernia, by site, with
      obstruction) 552.9
    gangrenous (*see also* Hernia, by site, with
      gangrene) 551.9
  incisional 553.21
    with
      gangrene (obstructed) 551.21
      obstruction 552.21
        and gangrene 551.21
    lumbar — *see* Hernia, lumbar
    recurrent 553.21
      with
        gangrene (obstructed) 551.21
        obstruction 552.21
          and gangrene 551.21
  indirect (inguinal) — *see* Hernia, inguinal
  infantile — *see* Hernia, inguinal
  infrapatellar fat pad 729.31
  inguinal (direct) (double) (encysted) (external)
      (funicular) (indirect) (infantile) (internal)
      (interstitial) (oblique) (scrotal) (sliding)
      550.9 ☑

  ┌──┐
  │ *Note — Use the following fifth-digit*   │
  │ *subclassification with category 550:*   │
  │   │
  │ *0   unilateral or unspecified (not specified*│
  │   *as recurrent)*   │
  │ *1   unilateral or unspecified, recurrent*   │
  │ *2   bilateral (not specified as recurrent)* │
  │ *3   bilateral, recurrent*   │
  └──┘

    with
      gangrene (obstructed) 550.0 ☑
      obstruction 550.1 ☑
        and gangrene 550.0 ☑
  internal 553.8
    with
      gangrene (obstructed) 551.8
      obstruction 552.8
        and gangrene 551.8
    inguinal — *see* Hernia, inguinal
  interstitial 553.9
    with
      gangrene (obstructed) 551.9
      obstruction 552.9
        and gangrene 551.9
    inguinal — *see* Hernia, inguinal
  intervertebral cartilage or disc — *see*
      Displacement, intervertebral disc
  intestine, intestinal 553.9
    with
      gangrene (obstructed) 551.9
      obstruction 552.9
        and gangrene 551.9
  intra-abdominal 553.9
    with
      gangrene (obstructed) 551.9
      obstruction 552.9
        and gangrene 551.9
  intraparietal 553.9
    with
      gangrene (obstructed) 551.9
      obstruction 552.9
        and gangrene 551.9
  iris 364.8
    traumatic 871.1
  irreducible (*see also* Hernia, by site, with
      obstruction) 552.9
    gangrenous (with obstruction) (*see also*
      Hernia, by site, with gangrene) 551.9
  ischiatic 553.8
    with
      gangrene (obstructed) 551.8
      obstruction 552.8
        and gangrene 551.8

Hernia, hernial — *continued*
  ischiorectal 553.8
    with
      gangrene (obstructed) 551.8
      obstruction 552.8
        and gangrene 551.8
  lens 379.32
    traumatic 871.1
  linea
    alba — *see* Hernia, epigastric
    semilunaris — *see* Hernia, spigelian
  Littre's (diverticular) 553.9
    with
      gangrene (obstructed) 551.9
      obstruction 552.9
        and gangrene 551.9
  lumbar 553.8
    with
      gangrene (obstructed) 551.8
      obstruction 552.8
        and gangrene 551.8
    intervertebral disc 722.10
  lung (subcutaneous) 518.89
    congenital 748.69
  mediastinum 519.3
  mesenteric (internal) 553.8
    with
      gangrene (obstructed) 551.8
      obstruction 552.8
        and gangrene 551.8
  mesocolon 553.8
    with
      gangrene (obstructed) 551.8
      obstruction 552.8
        and gangrene 551.8
  muscle (sheath) 728.89
  nucleus pulposus — *see* Displacement,
      intervertebral disc
  oblique (inguinal) — *see* Hernia, inguinal
  obstructive (*see also* Hernia, by site, with
      obstruction) 552.9
    gangrenous (with obstruction) (*see also*
      Hernia, by site, with gangrene) 551.9
  obturator 553.8
    with
      gangrene (obstructed) 551.8
      obstruction 552.8
        and gangrene 551.8
  omental 553.8
    with
      gangrene (obstructed) 551.8
      obstruction 552.8
        and gangrene 551.8
  orbital fat (pad) 374.34
  ovary 620.4
  oviduct 620.4
  paracolostomy (stoma) 569.69
  paraduodenal 553.8
    with
      gangrene (obstructed) 551.8
      obstruction 552.8
        and gangrene 551.8
  paraesophageal 553.3
    with
      gangrene (obstructed) 551.3
      obstruction 552.3
        and gangrene 551.3
    congenital 750.6
  parahiatal 553.3
    with
      gangrene (obstructed) 551.3
      obstruction 552.3
        and gangrene 551.3
  paraumbilical 553.1
    with
      gangrene (obstructed) 551.1
      obstruction 552.1
        and gangrene 551.1
  parietal 553.9
    with
      gangrene (obstructed) 551.9
      obstruction 552.9
        and gangrene 551.9
  perineal 553.8
    with
      gangrene (obstructed) 551.8

☑ Additional Digit Required   ►◄ Revised Text   ● New Line   ▲ Revised Code

Hernia, hernial — *continued*
  perineal — *continued*
    with — *continued*
      obstruction 552.8
        and gangrene 551.8
  peritoneal sac, lesser 553.8
    with
      gangrene (obstructed) 551.8
      obstruction 552.8
        and gangrene 551.8
  popliteal fat pad 729.31
  postoperative 553.21
    with
      gangrene (obstructed) 551.21
      obstruction 552.21
        and gangrene 551.21
  pregnant uterus 654.4 ☑
  prevesical 596.8
  properitoneal 553.8
    with
      gangrene (obstructed) 551.8
      obstruction 552.8
        and gangrene 551.8
  pudendal 553.8
    with
      gangrene (obstructed) 551.8
      obstruction 552.8
        and gangrene 551.8
  rectovaginal 618.6
  retroperitoneal 553.8
    with
      gangrene (obstructed) 551.8
      obstruction 552.8
        and gangrene 551.8
  Richter's (parietal) 553.9
    with
      gangrene (obstructed) 551.9
      obstruction 552.9
        and gangrene 551.9
  Rieux's, Riex's (retrocecal) 553.8
    with
      gangrene (obstructed) 551.8
      obstruction 552.8
        and gangrene 551.8
  sciatic 553.8
    with
      gangrene (obstructed) 551.8
      obstruction 552.8
        and gangrene 551.8
  scrotum, scrotal — *see* Hernia, inguinal
  sliding (inguinal) — *see also* Hernia, inguinal
    hiatus — *see* Hernia, hiatal
  spigelian 553.29
    with
      gangrene (obstructed) 551.29
      obstruction 552.29
        and gangrene 551.29
  spinal (*see also* Spina bifida) 741.9 ☑
    with hydrocephalus 741.0 ☑
  strangulated (*see also* Hernia, by site, with
      obstruction) 552.9
    gangrenous (with obstruction) (*see also*
      Hernia, by site, with gangrene) 551.9
  supraumbilicus (linea alba) — *see* Hernia,
      epigastric
  tendon 727.9
  testis (nontraumatic) 550.9 ☑
    meaning
      scrotal hernia 550.9 ☑
      symptomatic late syphilis 095.8
  Treitz's (fossa) 553.8
    with
      gangrene (obstructed) 551.8
      obstruction 552.8
        and gangrene 551.8
  tunica
    albuginea 608.89
    vaginalis 752.89
  umbilicus, umbilical 553.1
    with
      gangrene (obstructed) 551.1
      obstruction 552.1
        and gangrene 551.1
  ureter 593.89
    with obstruction 593.4

Hernia, hernial — *continued*
  uterus 621.8
    pregnant 654.4 ☑
  vaginal (posterior) 618.6
  Velpeau's (femoral) (*see also* Hernia, femoral)
      553.00
  ventral 553.20
    with
      gangrene (obstructed) 551.20
      obstruction 552.20
        and gangrene 551.20
    recurrent 553.21
      with
        gangrene (obstructed) 551.21
        obstruction 552.21
          and gangrene 551.21
  vesical
    congenital (female) (male) 756.71
    female ▶(*see also* Cystocele, female)◀
        618.01   ▲
    male 596.8
  vitreous (into anterior chamber) 379.21
    traumatic 871.1

Herniation — *see also* Hernia
  brain (stem) 348.4
  cerebral 348.4
  gastric mucosa (into duodenal bulb) 537.89
  mediastinum 519.3
  nucleus pulposus — *see* Displacement,
      intervertebral disc

Herpangina 074.0

Herpes, herpetic 054.9
  auricularis (zoster) 053.71
    simplex 054.73
  blepharitis (zoster) 053.20
    simplex 054.41
  circinate 110.5
  circinatus 110.5
    bullous 694.5
  conjunctiva (simplex) 054.43
    zoster 053.21
  cornea (simplex) 054.43
    disciform (simplex) 054.43
    zoster 053.21
  encephalitis 054.3
  eye (zoster) 053.29
    simplex 054.40
  eyelid (zoster) 053.20
    simplex 054.41
  febrilis 054.9
  fever 054.9
  geniculate ganglionitis 053.11
  genital, genitalis 054.10
    specified site NEC 054.19
  gestationis 646.8 ☑
  gingivostomatitis 054.2
  iridocyclitis (simplex) 054.44
    zoster 053.22
  iris (any site) 695.1
  iritis (simplex) 054.44
  keratitis (simplex) 054.43
    dendritic 054.42
    disciform 054.43
    interstitial 054.43
      zoster 053.21
  keratoconjunctivitis (simplex) 054.43
    zoster 053.21
  labialis 054.9
    meningococcal 036.89
  lip 054.9
  meningitis (simplex) 054.72
    zoster 053.0
  ophthalmicus (zoster) 053.20
    simplex 054.40
  otitis externa (zoster) 053.71
    simplex 054.73
  penis 054.13
  perianal 054.10
  pharyngitis 054.79
  progenitalis 054.10
  scrotum 054.19
  septicemia 054.4 ☑
  simplex 054.9
    complicated 054.8
      ophthalmic 054.40
        specified NEC 054.49

Herpes, herpetic — *continued*
  simplex — *continued*
    complicated — *continued*
      specified NEC 054.79
    congenital 771.2
    external ear 054.73
    keratitis 054.43
      dendritic 054.42
    meningitis 054.72
    neuritis 054.79
    specified complication NEC 054.79
      ophthalmic 054.49
    visceral 054.71
  stomatitis 054.2
  tonsurans 110.0
    maculosus (of Hebra) 696.3
  visceral 054.71
  vulva 054.12
  vulvovaginitis 054.11
  whitlow 054.6
  zoster 053.9
    auricularis 053.71
    complicated 053.8
      specified NEC 053.79
    conjunctiva 053.21
    cornea 053.21
    ear 053.71
    eye 053.29
    geniculate 053.11
    keratitis 053.21
      interstitial 053.21
    neuritis 053.10
    ophthalmicus(a) 053.20
    oticus 053.71
    otitis externa 053.71
    specified complication NEC 053.79
    specified site NEC 053.9
  zosteriform, intermediate type 053.9

Herrick's
  anemia (hemoglobin S disease) 282.61
  syndrome (hemoglobin S disease) 282.61

Hers' disease (glycogenosis VI) 271.0

Herter's infantilism (nontropical sprue) 579.0

Herter (-Gee) disease or syndrome (nontropical
    sprue) 579.0

Herxheimer's disease (diffuse idiopathic
    cutaneous atrophy) 701.8

Herxheimer's reaction 995.0

Hesselbach's hernia — *see* Hernia, Hesselbach's

Heterochromia (congenital) 743.46
  acquired 364.53
  cataract 366.33
  cyclitis 364.21
  hair 704.3
  iritis 364.21
  retained metallic foreign body 360.62
    magnetic 360.52
  uveitis 364.21

Heterophoria 378.40
  alternating 378.45
  vertical 378.43

Heterophyes, small intestine 121.6

Heterophyiasis 121.6

Heteropsia 368.8

Heterotopia, heterotopic — *see also* Malposition,
    congenital
  cerebralis 742.4
  pancreas, pancreatic 751.7
  spinalis 742.59

Heterotropia 378.30
  intermittent 378.20
    vertical 378.31
  vertical (constant) (intermittent) 378.31

Heubner's disease 094.89

Heubner-Herter disease or syndrome
    (nontropical sprue) 579.0

Hexadactylism 755.0 ☑

Heyd's syndrome (hepatorenal) 572.4

HGSIL (high grade squamous intraepithelial
    ▶lesion◀) 795.04   ▲

Hibernoma (M8880/0) — *see* Lipoma

Hernia, hernial — Hibernoma

Hiccough 786.8
  epidemic 078.89
  psychogenic 306.1
Hiccup (see also Hiccough) 786.8
Hicks (-Braxton) contractures 644.1 ☑
Hidden penis 752.65
Hidradenitis (axillaris) (suppurative) 705.83
Hidradenoma (nodular) (M8400/0) — see also
  Neoplasm, skin, benign
  clear cell (M8402/0) — see Neoplasm, skin,
    benign
  papillary (M8405/0) — see Neoplasm, skin,
    benign
Hidrocystoma (M8404/0) — see Neoplasm, skin,
  benign
High
  A$_2$ anemia 282.49
  altitude effects 993.2
    anoxia 993.2
    on
      ears 993.0
      sinuses 993.1
    polycythemia 289.0
  arch
    foot 755.67
    palate 750.26
  artery (arterial) tension (see also Hypertension)
    401.9
    without diagnosis of hypertension 796.2
  basal metabolic rate (BMR) 794.7
  blood pressure (see also Hypertension) 401.9
    incidental reading (isolated) (nonspecific), no
      diagnosis of hypertension 796.2
  compliance bladder 596.4
  diaphragm (congenital) 756.6
  frequency deafness (congenital) (regional) 389.8
  head at term 652.5 ☑
    affecting fetus or newborn 763.1
  output failure (cardiac) (see also Failure, heart)
    428.9
  oxygen-affinity hemoglobin 289.0
  palate 750.26
  risk
    behavior — see Problem
    cervical, human papillomavirus (HPV) ●
      DNA test positive 795.05 ●
    family situation V61.9
      specified circumstance NEC V61.8
    individual NEC V62.89
    infant NEC V20.1
    patient taking drugs (prescribed) V67.51
      nonprescribed (see also Abuse, drugs,
        nondependent) 305.9 ☑
    pregnancy V23.9
      inadequate prenatal care V23.7
      specified problem NEC V23.8 ☑
  temperature (of unknown origin) (see also
    Pyrexia) 780.6
  thoracic rib 756.3
Hildenbrand's disease (typhus) 081.9
Hilger's syndrome 337.0
Hill diarrhea 579.1
Hilliard's lupus (see also Tuberculosis) 017.0 ☑
Hilum — see condition
Hip — see condition
Hippel's disease (retinocerebral angiomatosis)
  759.6
Hippus 379.49
Hirschfeld's disease (acute diabetes mellitus) (see
  also Diabetes) 250.0 ☑
Hirschsprung's disease or megacolon
  (congenital) 751.3
Hirsuties (see also Hypertrichosis) 704.1
Hirsutism (see also Hypertrichosis) 704.1
Hirudiniasis (external) (internal) 134.2
His-Werner disease (trench fever) 083.1
Hiss-Russell dysentery 004.1
Histamine cephalgia 346.2 ☑
Histidinemia 270.5
Histidinuria 270.5

Histiocytoma (M8832/0) — see also Neoplasm,
  skin, benign
  fibrous (M8830/0) — see also Neoplasm, skin,
    benign
    atypical (M8830/1) — see Neoplasm,
      connective tissue, uncertain behavior
    malignant (M8830/3) — see Neoplasm,
      connective tissue, malignant
Histiocytosis (acute) (chronic) (subacute) 277.89
  acute differentiated progressive (M9722/3)
    202.5 ☑
  cholesterol 277.89
  essential 277.89
  lipid, lipoid (essential) 272.7
  lipochrome (familial) 288.1
  malignant (M9720/3) 202.3 ☑
  X (chronic) 277.89
    acute (progressive) (M9722/3) 202.5 ☑
Histoplasmosis 115.90
  with
    endocarditis 115.94
    meningitis 115.91
    pericarditis 115.93
    pneumonia 115.95
    retinitis 115.92
    specified manifestation NEC 115.99
  African (due to Histoplasma duboisii) 115.10
    with
      endocarditis 115.14
      meningitis 115.11
      pericarditis 115.13
      pneumonia 115.15
      retinitis 115.12
      specified manifestation NEC 115.19
  American (due to Histoplasma capsulatum)
    115.00
    with
      endocarditis 115.04
      meningitis 115.01
      pericarditis 115.03
      pneumonia 115.05
      retinitis 115.02
      specified manifestation NEC 115.09
  Darling's — see Histoplasmosis, American
  large form (see also Histoplasmosis, African)
    115.10
  lung 115.05
  small form (see also Histoplasmosis, American)
    115.00
History (personal) **of**
  abuse
    emotional V15.42
    neglect V15.42
    physical V15.41
    sexual V15.41
  affective psychosis V11.1
  alcoholism V11.3
    specified as drinking problem (see also
      Abuse, drugs, nondependent) 305.0 ☑
  allergy to
    analgesic agent NEC V14.6
    anesthetic NEC V14.4
    antibiotic agent NEC V14.1
      penicillin V14.0
    anti-infective agent NEC V14.3
    diathesis V15.09
    drug V14.9
      specified type NEC V14.8
    eggs V15.03
    food additives V15.05
    insect bite V15.06
    latex V15.07
    medicinal agents V14.9
      specified type NEC V14.8
    milk products V15.02
    narcotic agent NEC V14.5
    nuts V15.05
      peanuts V15.01
    penicillin V14.0
    radiographic dye V15.08
    seafood V15.04
    serum V14.7
    specified food NEC V15.05
    specified nonmedicinal agents NEC V15.09
    spider bite V15.06
    sulfa V14.2

History (personal) **of** — continued
  allergy to — continued
    sulfonamides V14.2
    therapeutic agent NEC V15.09
    vaccine V14.7
  anemia V12.3
  arthritis V13.4
  benign neoplasm of brain V12.41
  blood disease V12.3
  calculi, urinary V13.01
  cardiovascular disease V12.50
    myocardial infarction 412
  child abuse V15.41
  cigarette smoking V15.82
  circulatory system disease V12.50
    myocardial infarction 412
  congenital malformation V13.69
  contraception V15.7
  diathesis, allergic V15.09
  digestive system disease V12.70
    peptic ulcer V12.71
    polyps, colonic V12.72
    specified NEC V12.79
  disease (of) V13.9
    blood V12.3
    blood-forming organs V12.3
    cardiovascular system V12.50
    circulatory system V12.50
    digestive system V12.70
      peptic ulcer V12.71
      polyps, colonic V12.72
      specified NEC V12.79
    infectious V12.00
      malaria V12.03
      poliomyelitis V12.02
      specified NEC V12.09
      tuberculosis V12.01
    parasitic V12.00
      specified NEC V12.09
    respiratory system V12.6
    skin V13.3
    specified site NEC V13.8
    subcutaneous tissue V13.3
    trophoblastic V13.1
      affecting management of pregnant V23.1
  disorder (of) V13.9
    endocrine V12.2
    genital system V13.29
    hematological V12.3
    immunity V12.2
    mental V11.9
      affective type V11.1
      manic-depressive V11.1
      neurosis V11.2
      schizophrenia V11.0
      specified type NEC V11.8
    metabolic V12.2
    musculoskeletal NEC V13.5
    nervous system V12.40
      specified type NEC V12.49
    obstetric V13.29
      affecting management of current
        pregnancy V23.49
        pre-term labor V23.41
      pre-term labor V13.21
    sense organs V12.40
      specified type NEC V12.49
    specified site NEC V13.8
    urinary system V13.00
      calculi V13.01
      specified NEC V13.09
  drug use
    nonprescribed (see also Abuse, drugs,
      nondependent) 305.9 ☑
    patent (see also Abuse, drugs,
      nondependent) 305.9 ☑
  effect NEC of external cause V15.89
  embolism (pulmonary) V12.51
  emotional abuse V15.42
  endocrine disorder V12.2
  extracorporeal membrane oxygenation (ECMO)
    V15.87
  family
    allergy V19.6
    anemia V18.2
    arteriosclerosis V17.4
    arthritis V17.7

☑ Additional Digit Required   ►◄ Revised Text   ● New Line   ▲ Revised Code

History (personal) **of** — *continued*
  family — *continued*
    asthma V17.5
    blindness V19.0
    blood disorder NEC V18.3
    cardiovascular disease V17.4
    cerebrovascular disease V17.1
    chronic respiratory condition NEC V17.6
    congenital anomalies V19.5
    consanguinity V19.7
    coronary artery disease V17.3
    cystic fibrosis V18.1
    deafness V19.2
    diabetes mellitus V18.0
    digestive disorders V18.5
    disease or disorder (of)
      allergic V19.6
      blood NEC V18.3
      cardiovascular NEC V17.4
      cerebrovascular V17.1
      coronary artery V17.3
      digestive V18.5
      ear NEC V19.3
      endocrine V18.1
      eye NEC V19.1
      genitourinary NEC V18.7
      hypertensive V17.4
      infectious V18.8
      ischemic heart V17.3
      kidney V18.69
        polycystic V18.61
      mental V17.0
      metabolic V18.1
      musculoskeletal NEC V17.8
      neurological NEC V17.2
      parasitic V18.8
      psychiatric condition V17.0
      skin condition V19.4
    ear disorder NEC V19.3
    endocrine disease V18.1
    epilepsy V17.2
    eye disorder NEC V19.1
    genitourinary disease NEC V18.7
    glomerulonephritis V18.69
    gout V18.1
    hay fever V17.6
    hearing loss V19.2
    hematopoietic neoplasia V16.7
    Hodgkin's disease V16.7
    Huntington's chorea V17.2
    hydrocephalus V19.5
    hypertension V17.4
    hypospadias V13.61
    infectious disease V18.8
    ischemia heart disease V17.3
    kidney disease V18.69
      polycystic V18.61
    leukemia V16.6
    lymphatic malignant neoplasia NEC V16.7
    malignant neoplasm (of) NEC V16.9
      anorectal V16.0
      anus V16.0
      appendix V16.0
      bladder V16.59
      bone V16.8
      brain V16.8
      breast V16.3
        male V16.8
      bronchus V16.1
      cecum V16.0
      cervix V16.49
      colon V16.0
      duodenum V16.0
      esophagus V16.0
      eye V16.8
      gallbladder V16.0
      gastrointestinal tract V16.0
      genital organs V16.40
      hemopoietic NEC V16.7
      ileum V16.0
      ilium V16.8
      intestine V16.0
      intrathoracic organs NEC V16.2
      kidney V16.51
      larynx V16.2
      liver V16.0
      lung V16.1

History (personal) **of** — *continued*
  family — *continued*
    malignant neoplasm (of) — *continued*
      lymphatic NEC V16.7
      ovary V16.41
      oviduct V16.41
      pancreas V16.0
      penis V16.49
      prostate V16.42
      rectum V16.0
      respiratory organs NEC V16.2
      skin V16.8
      specified site NEC V16.8
      stomach V16.0
      testis V16.43
      trachea V16.1
      ureter V16.59
      urethra V16.59
      urinary organs V16.59
      uterus V16.49
      vagina V16.49
      vulva V16.49
    mental retardation V18.4
    metabolic disease NEC V18.1
    mongolism V19.5
    multiple myeloma V16.7
    musculoskeletal disease NEC V17.8
    nephritis V18.69
    nephrosis V18.69
    parasitic disease V18.8
    polycystic kidney disease V18.61
    psychiatric disorder V17.0
    psychosis V17.0
    retardation, mental V18.4
    retinitis pigmentosa V19.1
    schizophrenia V17.0
    skin conditions V19.4
    specified condition NEC V19.8
    stroke (cerebrovascular) V17.1
    visual loss V19.0
  genital system disorder V13.29
    pre-term labor V13.21
  health hazard V15.9
    specified cause NEC V15.89
  Hodgkin's disease V10.72
  immunity disorder V12.2
  infectious disease V12.00
    malaria V12.03
    poliomyelitis V12.02
    specified NEC V12.09
    tuberculosis V12.01
  injury NEC V15.5
  insufficient prenatal care V23.7
  irradiation V15.3
  leukemia V10.60
    lymphoid V10.61
    monocytic V10.63
    myeloid V10.62
    specified type NEC V10.69
  little or no prenatal care V23.7
  low birth weight (*see also* Status, low birth
    weight) V21.30
  lymphosarcoma V10.71
  malaria V12.03
  malignant neoplasm (of) V10.9
    accessory sinus V10.22
    adrenal V10.88
    anus V10.06
    bile duct V10.09
    bladder V10.51
    bone V10.81
    brain V10.85
    breast V10.3
    bronchus V10.11
    cervix uteri V10.41
    colon V10.05
    connective tissue NEC V10.89
    corpus uteri V10.42
    digestive system V10.00
      specified part NEC V10.09
    duodenum V10.09
    endocrine gland NEC V10.88
    epididymis V10.48
    esophagus V10.03
    eye V10.84
    fallopian tube V10.44

History (personal) **of** — *continued*
  malignant neoplasm (of) — *continued*
    female genital organ V10.40
      specified site NEC V10.44
    gallbladder V10.09
    gastrointestinal tract V10.00
    gum V10.02
    hematopoietic NEC V10.79
    hypopharynx V10.02
    ileum V10.09
    intrathoracic organs NEC V10.20
    jejunum V10.09
    kidney V10.52
    large intestine V10.05
    larynx V10.21
    lip V10.02
    liver V10.07
    lung V10.11
    lymphatic NEC V10.79
    lymph glands or nodes NEC V10.79
    male genital organ V10.45
      specified site NEC V10.49
    mediastinum V10.29
    melanoma (of skin) V10.82
    middle ear V10.22
    mouth V10.02
      specified part NEC V10.02
    nasal cavities V10.22
    nasopharynx V10.02
    nervous system NEC V10.86
    nose V10.22
    oropharynx V10.02
    ovary V10.43
    pancreas V10.09
    parathyroid V10.88
    penis V10.49
    pharynx V10.02
    pineal V10.88
    pituitary V10.88
    placenta V10.44
    pleura V10.29
    prostate V10.46
    rectosigmoid junction V10.06
    rectum V10.06
    renal pelvis V10.53
    respiratory organs NEC V10.20
    salivary gland V10.02
    skin V10.83
      melanoma V10.82
    small intestine NEC V10.09
    soft tissue NEC V10.89
    specified site NEC V10.89
    stomach V10.04
    testis V10.47
    thymus V10.29
    thyroid V10.87
    tongue V10.01
    trachea V10.12
    ureter V10.59
    urethra V10.59
    urinary organ V10.50
    uterine adnexa V10.44
    uterus V10.42
    vagina V10.44
    vulva V10.44
  manic-depressive psychosis V11.1
  mental disorder V11.9
    affective type V11.1
    manic-depressive V11.1
    neurosis V11.2
    schizophrenia V11.0
    specified type NEC V11.8
  metabolic disorder V12.2
  musculoskeletal disorder NEC V13.5
  myocardial infarction 412
  neglect (emotional) V15.42
  nervous system disorder V12.40
    specified type NEC V12.49
  neurosis V11.2
  noncompliance with medical treatment V15.81
  nutritional deficiency V12.1
  obstetric disorder V13.29
    affecting management of current pregnancy
      V23.49
      pre-term labor V13.41
    pre-term labor V13.21

☑ Additional Digit Required   ▶◀ Revised Text   ● New Line   ▲ Revised Code

History (personal) **of** — *continued*
  parasitic disease V12.00
    specified NEC V12.09
  perinatal problems V13.7
    low birth weight (*see also* Status, low birth
      weight) V21.30
  physical abuse V15.41
  poisoning V15.6
  poliomyelitis V12.02
  polyps, colonic V12.72
  poor obstetric V13.29
    affecting management of current pregnancy
      V23.49
      pre-term labor V23.41
    pre-term labor V13.21
  psychiatric disorder V11.9
    affective type V11.1
    manic-depressive V11.1
    neurosis V11.2
    schizophrenia V11.0
    specified type NEC V11.8
  psychological trauma V15.49
    emotional abuse V15.42
    neglect V15.42
    physical abuse V15.41
    rape V15.41
  psychoneurosis V11.2
  radiation therapy V15.3
  rape V15.41
  respiratory system disease V12.6
  reticulosarcoma V10.71
  schizophrenia V11.0
  skin disease V13.3
  smoking (tobacco) V15.82
  subcutaneous tissue disease V13.3
  surgery (major) to
    great vessels V15.1
    heart V15.1
    major organs NEC V15.2
  thrombophlebitis V12.52
  thrombosis V12.51
  tobacco use V15.82
  trophoblastic disease V13.1
    affecting management of pregnancy V23.1
  tuberculosis V12.01
  ulcer, peptic V12.71
  urinary system disorder V13.00
    calculi V13.01
    specified NEC V13.09
HIV infection (disease) (illness) — *see* Human
    immunodeficiency virus (disease) (illness)
    (infection)
Hives (bold) (*see also* Urticaria) 708.9
Hoarseness 784.49
Hobnail liver — *see* Cirrhosis, portal
Hobo, hoboism V60.0
Hodgkins
  disease (M9650/3) 201.9 ☑
    lymphocytic
      depletion (M9653/3) 201.7 ☑
        diffuse fibrosis (M9654/3) 201.7 ☑
        reticular type (M9655/3) 201.7 ☑
      predominance (M9651/3) 201.4 ☑
    lymphocytic-histiocytic predominance
      (M9651/3) 201.4 ☑
    mixed cellularity (M9652/3) 201.6 ☑
    nodular sclerosis (M9656/3) 201.5 ☑
      cellular phase (M9657/3) 201.5 ☑
  granuloma (M9661/3) 201.1 ☑
  lymphogranulomatosis (M9650/3) 201.9 ☑
  lymphoma (M9650/3) 201.9 ☑
  lymphosarcoma (M9650/3) 201.9 ☑
  paragranuloma (M9660/3) 201.0 ☑
  sarcoma (M9662/3) 201.2 ☑
Hodgson's disease (aneurysmal dilatation of
    aorta) 441.9
  ruptured 441.5
Hodi-potsy 111.0
Hoffa (-Kastert) disease or syndrome
    (liposynovitis prepatellaris) 272.8
Hoffman's syndrome 244.9 *[359.5]*
Hoffmann-Bouveret syndrome (paroxysmal
    tachycardia) 427.2
Hole
  macula 362.54

Hole — *continued*
  optic disc, crater-like 377.22
  retina (macula) 362.54
    round 361.31
      with detachment 361.01
Holla disease (*see also* Spherocytosis) 282.0
Holländer-Simons syndrome (progressive
    lipodystrophy) 272.6
Hollow foot (congenital) 754.71
  acquired 736.73
Holmes' syndrome (visual disorientation) 368.16
Holoprosencephaly 742.2
  due to
    trisomy 13 758.1
    trisomy 18 758.2
Holthouse's hernia — *see* Hernia, inguinal
Homesickness 309.89
Homocystinemia 270.4
Homocystinuria 270.4
Homologous serum jaundice (prophylactic)
    (therapeutic) — *see* Hepatitis, viral
Homosexuality — *omit code*
  ego-dystonic 302.0
  pedophilic 302.2
  problems with 302.0
Homozygous Hb-S disease 282.61
Honeycomb lung 518.89
  congenital 748.4
Hong Kong ear 117.3
HOOD (hereditary osteo-onychodyplasia) 756.89
Hooded
  clitoris 752.49
  penis 752.69
Hookworm (anemia) (disease) (infestation) — *see*
    Ancylostomiasis
Hoppe-Goldflam syndrome 358.00
Hordeolum (external) (eyelid) 373.11
  internal 373.12
Horn
  cutaneous 702.8
    cheek 702.8
    eyelid 702.8
    penis 702.8
  iliac 756.89
  nail 703.8
    congenital 757.5
  papillary 700
Horner's
  syndrome (*see also* Neuropathy, peripheral,
    autonomic) 337.9
    traumatic 954.0
  teeth 520.4
Horseshoe kidney (congenital) 753.3
Horton's
  disease (temporal arteritis) 446.5
  headache or neuralgia 346.2 ☑
Hospice care V66.7
Hospitalism (in children) NEC 309.83
Hourglass contraction, contracture
  bladder 596.8
  gallbladder 575.2
    congenital 751.69
  stomach 536.8
    congenital 750.7
    psychogenic 306.4
  uterus 661.4 ☑
    affecting fetus or newborn 763.7
Household circumstance affecting care V60.9
  specified type NEC V60.8
Housemaid's knee 727.2
Housing circumstance affecting care V60.9
  specified type NEC V60.8
Huchard's disease (continued arterial
    hypertension) 401.9
Hudson-Stähli lines 371.11
Huguier's disease (uterine fibroma) 218.9
Hum, venous — *omit code*
Human bite (open wound) — *see also* Wound,
    open, by site
  intact skin surface — *see* Contusion

Human immunodeficiency virus (disease)
    (illness) 042
  infection V08
    with symptoms, symptomatic 042
Human immunodeficiency virus-2 infection
    079.53
Human immunovirus (disease) (illness) (infection)
    — *see* Human immunodeficiency virus
    (disease) (illness) (infection)
Human papillomavirus 079.4 ●
  cervical
    high risk, DNA test positive 795.05 ●
    low risk, DNA test positive 795.09 ●
Human T-cell lymphotrophic virus-I infection
    079.51
Human T-cell lymphotrophic virus-II infection
    079.52
Human T-cell lymphotrophic virus-III (disease)
    (illness) (infection) — *see* Human
    immunodeficiency virus (disease) (illness)
    (infection)
HTLV-I infection 079.51
HTLV-II infection 079.52
HTLV-III (disease) (illness) (infection) — *see*
    Human immunodeficiency virus (disease)
    (illness) (infection)
HTLV-III/LAV (disease) (illness) (infection) — *see*
    Human immunodeficiency virus (disease)
    (illness) (infection)
Humpback (acquired) 737.9
  congenital 756.19
Hunchback (acquired) 737.9
  congenital 756.19
Hunger 994.2
  air, psychogenic 306.1
  disease 251.1
Hunner's ulcer (*see also* Cystitis) 595.1
Hunt's
  neuralgia 053.11
  syndrome (herpetic geniculate ganglionitis)
    053.11
    dyssynergia cerebellaris myoclonica 334.2
Hunter's glossitis 529.4
Hunter (-Hurler) syndrome
    (mucopolysaccharidosis II) 277.5
Hunterian chancre 091.0
Huntington's
  chorea 333.4
  disease 333.4
Huppert's disease (multiple myeloma) (M9730/3)
    203.0 ☑
Hurier (-Hunter) disease or syndrome
    (mucopolysaccharidosis II) 277.5
Hürthle cell
  adenocarcinoma (M8290/3) 193
  adenoma (M8290/0) 226
  carcinoma (M8290/3) 193
  tumor (M8290/0) 226
Hutchinson's
  disease meaning
    angioma serpiginosum 709.1
    cheiropompholyx 705.81
    prurigo estivalis 692.72
    summer eruption, or summer prurigo
      692.72
  incisors 090.5
  melanotic freckle (M8742/2) — *see also*
    Neoplasm, skin, in situ
    malignant melanoma in (M8742/3) — *see*
      Melanoma
  teeth or incisors (congenital syphilis) 090.5
Hutchinson-Boeck disease or syndrome
    (sarcoidosis) 135
Hutchinson-Gilford disease or syndrome
    (progeria) 259.8
Hyaline
  degeneration (diffuse) (generalized) 728.9
    localized — *see* Degeneration, by site
  membrane (disease) (lung) (newborn) 769
Hyalinosis cutis et mucosae 272.8
Hyalin plaque, sclera, senile 379.16

☑ Additional Digit Required   ▶◀ Revised Text   ● New Line   ▲ Revised Code

Sidebar: Hyalitis — Hyperaffectivity

Hyalitis (asteroid) 379.22
  syphilitic 095.8
Hydatid
  cyst or tumor — *see also* Echinococcus
    fallopian tube 752.11
  mole — *see* Hydatidiform mole
  Morgagni (congenital) 752.89
    fallopian tube 752.11
Hydatidiform mole (benign) (complicating
  pregnancy) (delivered) (undelivered) 630
  invasive (M9100/1) 236.1
  malignant (M9100/1) 236.1
  previous, affecting management of pregnancy
    V23.1
Hydatidosis — *see* Echinococcus
Hyde's disease (prurigo nodularis) 698.3
Hydradenitis 705.83
Hydradenoma (M8400/0) — *see* Hidradenoma
Hydralazine lupus or syndrome
  correct substance properly administered 695.4
  overdose or wrong substance given or taken
    972.6
Hydramnios 657.0 ☑
  affecting fetus or newborn 761.3
Hydrancephaly 742.3
  with spina bifida (*see also* Spina bifida)
    741.0 ☑
Hydranencephaly 742.3
  with spina bifida (*see also* Spina bifida)
    741.0 ☑
Hydrargyrism NEC 985.0
Hydrarthrosis (*see also* Effusion, joint) 719.0 ☑
  gonococcal 098.50
  intermittent (*see also* Rheumatism,
    palindromic) 719.3 ☑
  of yaws (early) (late) 102.6
  syphilitic 095.8
    congenital 090.5
Hydremia 285.9
Hydrencephalocele (congenital) 742.0
Hydrencephalomeningocele (congenital) 742.0
Hydroa 694.0
  aestivale 692.72
  gestationis 646.8 ☑
  herpetiformis 694.0
  pruriginosa 694.0
  vacciniforme 692.72
Hydroadenitis 705.83
Hydrocalycosis (*see also* Hydronephrosis) 591
  congenital 753.29
Hydrocalyx (*see also* Hydronephrosis) 591
Hydrocele (calcified) (chylous) (idiopathic)
  (infantile) (inguinal canal) (recurrent) (senile)
  (spermatic cord) (testis) (tunica vaginalis)
  603.9
  canal of Nuck (female) 629.1
    male 603.9
  congenital 778.6
  encysted 603.0
    congenital 778.6
  female NEC 629.8
  infected 603.1
  round ligament 629.8
  specified type NEC 603.8
    congenital 778.6
  spinalis (*see also* Spina bifida) 741.9 ☑
  vulva 624.8
Hydrocephalic fetus
  affecting management or pregnancy 655.0 ☑
  causing disproportion 653.6 ☑
    with obstructed labor 660.1 ☑
      affecting fetus or newborn 763.1
Hydrocephalus (acquired) (external) (internal)
  (malignant) (noncommunicating)
  (obstructive) (recurrent) 331.4
  aqueduct of Sylvius structure 742.3
    with spina bifida (*see also* Spina bifida)
      741.0 ☑
  chronic 742.3
    with spina bifida (*see also* Spina bifida)
      741.0 ☑
  communicating 331.3

Hydrocephalus — *continued*
  congenital (external) (internal) 742.3
    with spina bifida (*see also* Spina bifida)
      741.0 ☑
  due to
    structure of aqueduct of Sylvius 742.3
      with spina bifida (*see also* Spina bifida)
        741.0 ☑
    toxoplasmosis (congenital) 771.2
  fetal affecting management of pregnancy
    655.0 ☑
  foramen Magendie block (acquired) 331.3
    congenital 742.3
      with spina bifida (*see also* Spina bifida)
        741.0 ☑
  newborn 742.3
    with spina bifida (*see also* Spina bifida)
      741.0 ☑
  otitic 331.4
  syphilitic, congenital 090.49
  tuberculous (*see also* Tuberculosis) 013.8 ☑
Hydrocolpos (congenital) 623.8
Hydrocystoma (M8404/0) — *see* Neoplasm, skin,
  benign
Hydroencephalocele (congenital) 742.0
Hydroencephalomeningocele (congenital) 742.0
Hydrohematopneumothorax (*see also*
  Hemothorax) 511.8
Hydromeningitis — *see* Meningitis
Hydromeningocele (spinal) (*see also* Spina bifida)
  741.9 ☑
  cranial 742.0
Hydrometra 621.8
Hydrometrocolpos 623.8
Hydromicrocephaly 742.1
Hydromphalus (congenital) (since birth) 757.39
Hydromyelia 742.53
Hydromyelocele (*see also* Spina bifida) 741.9 ☑
Hydronephrosis 591
  atrophic 591
  congenital 753.29
  due to S. hematobium 120.0
  early 591
  functionless (infected) 591
  infected 591
  intermittent 591
  primary 591
  secondary 591
  tuberculous (*see also* Tuberculosis) 016.0 ☑
Hydropericarditis (*see also* Pericarditis) 423.9
Hydropericardium (*see also* Pericarditis) 423.9
Hydroperitoneum 789.5
Hydrophobia 071
Hydrophthalmos (*see also* Buphthalmia) 743.20
Hydropneumohemothorax (*see also* Hemothorax)
  511.8
Hydropneumopericarditis (*see also* Pericarditis)
  423.9
Hydropneumopericardium (*see also* Pericarditis)
  423.9
Hydropneumothorax 511.8
  nontuberculous 511.8
    bacterial 511.1
    pneumococcal 511.1
    staphylococcal 511.1
    streptococcal 511.1
  traumatic 860.0
    with open wound into thorax 860.1
  tuberculous (*see also* Tuberculosis, pleura)
    012.0 ☑
Hydrops 782.3
  abdominis 789.5
  amnii (complicating pregnancy) (*see also*
    Hydramnios) 657.0 ☑
  articulorum intermittens (*see also*
    Rheumatism, palindromic) 719.3 ☑
  cardiac (*see also* Failure, heart) 428.0
  congenital — *see* Hydrops, fetalis
  endolymphatic (*see also* Disease, Ménière's)
    386.00
  fetal(is) or newborn 778.0
    due to isoimmunization 773.3
    not due to isoimmunization 778.0

Hydrops — *continued*
  gallbladder 575.3
  idiopathic (fetus or newborn) 778.0
  joint (see also Effusion, joint) 719.0 ☑
  labyrinth (*see also* Disease, Ménière's) 386.00
  meningeal NEC 331.4
  nutritional 262
  pericardium — *see* Pericarditis
  pleura (*see also* Hydrothorax) 511.8
  renal (*see also* Nephrosis) 581.9
  spermatic cord (*see also* Hydrocele) 603.9
Hydropyonephrosis (*see also* Pyelitis) 590.80
  chronic 590.00
Hydrorachis 742.53
Hydrorrhea (nasal) 478.1
  gravidarum 658.1 ☑
  pregnancy 658.1 ☑
Hydrosadenitis 705.83
Hydrosalpinx (fallopian tube) (follicularis) 614.1
Hydrothorax (double) (pleural) 511.8
  chylous (nonfilarial) 457.8
    filaria (*see also* Infestation, filarial) 125.9
  nontuberculous 511.8
    bacterial 511.1
    pneumococcal 511.1
    staphylococcal 511.1
    streptococcal 511.1
  traumatic 862.29
    with open wound into thorax 862.39
  tuberculous (*see also* Tuberculosis, pleura)
    012.0 ☑
Hydroureter 593.5
  congenital 753.22
Hydroureteronephrosis (*see also* Hydronephrosis)
  591
Hydrourethra 599.84
Hydroxykynureninuria 270.2
Hydroxyprolinemia 270.8
Hydroxyprolinuria 270.8
Hygroma (congenital) (cystic) (M9173/0) 228.1
  prepatellar 727.3
  subdural — *see* Hematoma, subdural
Hymen — *see* condition
Hymenolepiasis (diminuta) (infection) (infestation)
  (nana) 123.6
Hymenolepis (diminuta) (infection) (infestation)
  (nana) 123.6
Hypalgesia (*see also* Disturbance, sensation)
  782.0
Hyperabduction syndrome 447.8
Hyperacidity, gastric 536.8
  psychogenic 306.4
Hyperactive, hyperactivity
  basal cell, uterine cervix 622.10   ▲
  bladder 596.51
  bowel (syndrome) 564.9
    sounds 787.5
  cervix epithelial (basal) 622.10   ▲
  child 314.01
  colon 564.9
  gastrointestinal 536.8
    psychogenic 306.4
  intestine 564.9
  labyrinth (unilateral) 386.51
    with loss of labyrinthine reactivity 386.58
    bilateral 386.52
  nasal mucous membrane 478.1
  stomach 536.8
  thyroid (gland) (*see also* Thyrotoxicosis)
    242.9 ☑
Hyperacusis 388.42
Hyperadrenalism (cortical) 255.3
  medullary 255.6
Hyperadrenocorticism 255.3
  congenital 255.2
  iatrogenic
    correct substance properly administered
      255.3
    overdose or wrong substance given or taken
      962.0
Hyperaffectivity 301.11

Hyperaldosteronism (atypical) (hyperplastic)
(normoaldosteronal) (normotensive)
(primary) 255.10
  secondary 255.14
Hyperalgesia (*see also* Disturbance, sensation)
782.0
Hyperalimentation 783.6
  carotene 278.3
  specified NEC 278.8
  vitamin A 278.2
  vitamin D 278.4
Hyperaminoaciduria 270.9
  arginine 270.6
  citrulline 270.6
  cystine 270.0
  glycine 270.0
  lysine 270.7
  ornithine 270.6
  renal (types I, II, III) 270.0
Hyperammonemia (congenital) 270.6
Hyperamnesia 780.99
Hyperamylasemia 790.5
Hyperaphia 782.0
Hyperazotemia 791.9
Hyperbetalipoproteinemia (acquired) (essential)
(familial) (hereditary) (primary) (secondary)
272.0
  with prebetalipoproteinemia 272.2
Hyperbilirubinemia 782.4
  congenital 277.4
  constitutional 277.4
  neonatal (transient) (*see also* Jaundice, fetus or
newborn) 774.6
  of prematurity 774.2
Hyperbilirubinemica encephalopathia, newborn
774.7
  due to isoimmunization 773.4
Hypercalcemia, hypercalcemic (idiopathic)
275.42
  nephropathy 588.89 ▲
Hypercalcinuria 275.40
Hypercapnia 786.09
  with mixed acid-base disorder 276.4
  fetal, affecting newborn 770.89
Hypercarotinemia 278.3
Hypercementosis 521.5
Hyperchloremia 276.9
Hyperchlorhydria 536.8
  neurotic 306.4
  psychogenic 306.4
Hypercholesterinemia — *see*
Hypercholesterolemia
Hypercholesterolemia 272.0
  with hyperglyceridemia, endogenous 272.2
  essential 272.0
  familial 272.0
  hereditary 272.0
  primary 272.0
  pure 272.0
Hypercholesterolosis 272.0
Hyperchylia gastrica 536.8
  psychogenic 306.4
Hyperchylomicronemia (familial) (with
hyperbetalipoproteinemia) 272.3
Hypercoagulation syndrome (primary) 289.81
  secondary 289.82
Hypercorticosteronism
  correct substance properly administered 255.3
  overdose or wrong substance given or taken
962.0
Hypercortisonism
  correct substance properly administered 255.3
  overdose or wrong substance given or taken
962.0
**Hyperdynamic beta-adrenergic state or
syndrome** (circulatory) 429.82
Hyperekplexia 759.89 ●
Hyperelectrolytemia 276.9
Hyperemesis 536.2
  arising during pregnancy — *see* Hyperemesis,
gravidarum

Hyperemesis — *continued*
  gravidarum (mild) (before 22 completed weeks
gestation) 643.0 ☑
    with
      carbohydrate depletion 643.1 ☑
      dehydration 643.1 ☑
      electrolyte imbalance 643.1 ☑
      metabolic disturbance 643.1 ☑
    affecting fetus or newborn 761.8
    severe (with metabolic disturbance) 643.1 ☑
  psychogenic 306.4
Hyperemia (acute) 780.99
  anal mucosa 569.49
  bladder 596.7
  cerebral 437.8
  conjunctiva 372.71
  ear, internal, acute 386.30
  enteric 564.89
  eye 372.71
  eyelid (active) (passive) 374.82
  intestine 564.89
  iris 364.41
  kidney 593.81
  labyrinth 386.30
  liver (active) (passive) 573.8
  lung 514
  ovary 620.8
  passive 780.99
  pulmonary 514
  renal 593.81
  retina 362.89
  spleen 289.59
  stomach 537.89
Hyperesthesia (body surface) (*see also*
Disturbance, sensation) 782.0
  larynx (reflex) 478.79
    hysterical 300.11
  pharynx (reflex) 478.29
Hyperestrinism 256.0
Hyperestrogenism 256.0
Hyperestrogenosis 256.0
Hyperexplexia 759.89 ●
Hyperextension, joint 718.80
  ankle 718.87
  elbow 718.82
  foot 718.87
  hand 718.84
  hip 718.85
  knee 718.86
  multiple sites 718.89
  pelvic region 718.85
  shoulder (region) 718.81
  specified site NEC 718.88
  wrist 718.83
Hyperfibrinolysis — *see* Fibrinolysis
Hyperfolliculinism 256.0
Hyperfructosemia 271.2
Hyperfunction
  adrenal (cortex) 255.3
    androgenic, acquired benign 255.3
    medulla 255.6
    virilism 255.2
  corticoadrenal NEC 255.3
  labyrinth — *see* Hyperactive, labyrinth
  medulloadrenal 255.6
  ovary 256.1
    estrogen 256.0
  pancreas 577.8
  parathyroid (gland) 252.00 ▲
  pituitary (anterior) (gland) (lobe) 253.1
  testicular 257.0
Hypergammaglobulinemia 289.89
  monoclonal, benign (BMH) 273.1
  polyclonal 273.0
  Waldenström's 273.0
Hyperglobulinemia 273.8
Hyperglycemia 790.6
  maternal
    affecting fetus or newborn 775.0
      manifest diabetes in infant 775.1
  postpancreatectomy (complete) (partial) 251.3
Hyperglyceridemia 272.1
  endogenous 272.1
  essential 272.1

Hyperglyceridemia — *continued*
  familial 272.1
  hereditary 272.1
  mixed 272.3
  pure 272.1
Hyperglycinemia 270.7
Hypergonadism
  ovarian 256.1
  testicular (infantile) (primary) 257.0
Hyperheparinemia (*see also* Circulating
anticoagulants) 286.5
Hyperhidrosis, hyperidrosis 705.21 ▲ ●
  axilla 705.21 ●
  face 705.21 ●
  focal (localized) 705.21 ●
    primary 705.21 ●
      axilla 705.21 ●
      face 705.21 ●
      palms 705.21 ●
      soles 705.21 ●
    secondary 705.22 ●
      axilla 705.22 ●
      face 705.22 ●
      palms 705.22 ●
      soles 705.22 ●
  generalized 780.8 ●
  palms 705.21 ●
  psychogenic 306.3
  secondary 780.8 ●
  soles 705.21 ●
Hyperhistidinemia 270.5
Hyperinsulinism (ectopic) (functional) (organic)
NEC 251.1
  iatrogenic 251.0
  reactive 251.2
  spontaneous 251.2
  therapeutic misadventure (from administration
of insulin) 962.3
Hyperiodemia 276.9
Hyperirritability (cerebral), in newborn 779.1
Hyperkalemia 276.7
Hyperkeratosis (*see also* Keratosis) 701.1
  cervix 622.10 ▲
  congenital 757.39
  cornea 371.89
  due to yaws (early) (late) (palmar or plantar)
102.3
  eccentrica 757.39
  figurata centrifuga atrophica 757.39
  follicularis 757.39
    in cutem penetrans 701.1
  limbic (comea) 371.89
  palmoplantaris climacterica 701.1
  pinta (carate) 103.1
  senile (with pruritus) 702.0
  tongue 528.79 ▲
  universalis congenita 757.1
  vagina 623.1
  vocal cord 478.5
  vulva 624.0
Hyperkinesia, hyperkinetic (disease) (reaction)
(syndrome) 314.9
  with
    attention deficit — *see* Disorder, attention
deficit
    conduct disorder 314.2
    developmental delay 314.1
    simple disturbance of activity and attention
314.01
    specified manifestation NEC 314.8
  heart (disease) 429.82
  of childhood or adolescence NEC 314.9
Hyperlacrimation (*see also* Epiphora) 375.20
Hyperlipemia (*see also* Hyperlipidemia) 272.4
Hyperlipidemia 272.4
  carbohydrate-induced 272.1
  combined 272.4
  endogenous 272.1
  exogenous 272.3
  fat-induced 272.3
  group
    A 272.0
    B 272.1
    C 272.2

Hyperaldosteronism — Hyperlipidemia

Hyperlipidemia — *continued*
  group — *continued*
    D 272.3
    mixed 272.2
    specified type NEC 272.4
Hyperlipidosis 272.7
  hereditary 272.7
Hyperlipoproteinemia (acquired) (essential)
    (familial) (hereditary) (primary) (secondary)
    272.4
  Fredrickson type
    I 272.3
    IIa 272.0
    IIb 272.2
    III 272.2
    IV 272.1
    V 272.3
  low-density-lipoid-type (LDL) 272.0
  very-low-density-lipoid-type (VLDL) 272.1
Hyperlucent lung, unilateral 492.8
Hyperluteinization 256.1
Hyperlysinemia 270.7
Hypermagnesemia 275.2
  neonatal 775.5
Hypermaturity (fetus or newborn)
  post-term infant 766.21
  prolonged gestation infant 766.22
Hypermenorrhea 626.2
Hypermetabolism 794.7
Hypermethioninemia 270.4
Hypermetropia (congenital) 367.0
Hypermobility
  cecum 564.9
  coccyx 724.71
  colon 564.9
    psychogenic 306.4
  ileum 564.89
  joint (acquired) 718.80
    ankle 718.87
    elbow 718.82
    foot 718.87
    hand 718.84
    hip 718.85
    knee 718.86
    multiple sites 718.89
    pelvic region 718.85
    shoulder (region) 718.81
    specified site NEC 718.88
    wrist 718.83
  kidney, congenital 753.3
  meniscus (knee) 717.5
  scapula 718.81
  stomach 536.8
    psychogenic 306.4
  syndrome 728.5
  testis, congenital 752.52
  urethral 599.81
Hypermotility
  gastrointestinal 536.8
  intestine 564.9
    psychogenic 306.4
  stomach 536.8
Hypernasality 784.49
Hypernatremia 276.0
  with water depletion 276.0
Hypernephroma (M8312/3) 189.0
Hyperopia 367.0
Hyperorexia 783.6
Hyperornithinemia 270.6
Hyperosmia (*see also* Disturbance, sensation)
    781.1
Hyperosmolality 276.0
Hyperosteogenesis 733.99
Hyperostosis 733.99
  calvarial 733.3
  cortical 733.3
    infantile 756.59
  frontal, internal of skull 733.3
  interna frontalis 733.3
  monomelic 733.99
  skull 733.3
    congenital 756.0

Hyperostosis — *continued*
  vertebral 721.8
    with spondylosis — *see* Spondylosis
    ankylosing 721.6
Hyperovarianism 256.1
Hyperovarism, hyperovaria 256.1
Hyperoxaluria (primary) 271.8
Hyperoxia 987.8
Hyperparathyroidism 252.00 ▲
  ectopic 259.3
  other 252.08 ●
  primary 252.01 ●
  secondary ▶(of renal origin)◀ 588.81 ▲
    non-renal 252.02 ●
  tertiary 252.08 ●
Hyperpathia (*see also* Disturbance, sensation)
    782.0
  psychogenic 307.80
Hyperperistalsis 787.4
  psychogenic 306.4
Hyperpermeability, capillary 448.9
Hyperphagia 783.6
Hyperphenylalaninemia 270.1
Hyperphoria 378.40
  alternating 378.45
Hyperphosphatemia 275.3
Hyperpiesia (*see also* Hypertension) 401.9
Hyperpiesis (*see also* Hypertension) 401.9
Hyperpigmentation — *see* Pigmentation
Hyperpinealism 259.8
Hyperpipecolatemia 270.7
Hyperpituitarism 253.1
Hyperplasia, hyperplastic
  adenoids (lymphoid tissue) 474.12
    and tonsils 474.10
  adrenal (capsule) (cortex) (gland) 255.8
    with
      sexual precocity (male) 255.2
      virilism, adrenal 255.2
      virilization (female) 255.2
    congenital 255.2
    due to excess ACTH (ectopic) (pituitary)
        255.0
    medulla 255.8
  alpha cells (pancreatic)
    with
      gastrin excess 251.5
      glucagon excess 251.4
  appendix (lymphoid) 543.0
  artery, fibromuscular NEC 447.8
    carotid 447.8
    renal 447.3
  bone 733.99
    marrow 289.9
  breast (*see also* Hypertrophy, breast) 611.1
  carotid artery 447.8
  cementation, cementum (teeth) (tooth) 521.5
  cervical gland 785.6
  cervix (uteri) 622.10 ▲
    basal cell 622.10 ▲
    congenital 752.49
    endometrium 622.10 ▲
    polypoid 622.10 ▲
  chin 524.05
  clitoris, congenital 752.49
  dentin 521.5
  endocervicitis 616.0
  endometrium, endometrial (adenomatous)
      (atypical) (cystic) (glandular) (polypoid)
      (uterus) 621.30 ▲
    with atypia 621.33 ●
    without atypia ●
      complex 621.32 ●
      simple 621.31 ●
  cervix 622.10 ▲
  epithelial 709.8
    focal, oral, including tongue 528.79 ▲
    mouth (focal) 528.79 ▲
    nipple 611.8
    skin 709.8
    tongue (focal) 528.79 ▲
    vaginal wall 623.0
  erythroid 289.9

Hyperplasia, hyperplastic — *continued*
  fascialis ossificans (progressiva) 728.11
  fibromuscular, artery NEC 447.8
    carotid 447.8
    renal 447.3
  genital
    female 629.8
    male 608.89
  gingiva 523.8
  glandularis
    cystica uteri 621.30 ▲
    endometrium (uterus) 621.30 ▲
    interstitialis uteri 621.30 ▲
  granulocytic 288.8
  gum 523.8
  hymen, congenital 752.49
  islands of Langerhans 251.1
  islet cell (pancreatic) 251.9
    alpha cells
      with excess
        gastrin 251.5
        glucagon 251.4
    beta cells 251.1
  juxtaglomerular (complex) (kidney) 593.89
  kidney (congenital) 753.3
  liver (congenital) 751.69
  lymph node (gland) 785.6
  lymphoid (diffuse) (nodular) 785.6
    appendix 543.0
    intestine 569.89
  mandibular 524.02
    alveolar 524.72
    unilateral condylar 526.89
  Marchand multiple nodular (liver) — *see*
      Cirrhosis, postnecrotic
  maxillary 524.01
    alveolar 524.71
  medulla, adrenal 255.8
  myometrium, myometrial 621.2
  nose (lymphoid) (polypoid) 478.1
  oral soft tissue (inflammatory) (irritative)
      (mucosa) NEC 528.9
    gingiva 523.8
    tongue 529.8
  organ or site, congenital NEC — *see* Anomaly,
      specified type NEC
  ovary 620.8
  palate, papillary 528.9
  pancreatic islet cells 251.9
    alpha
      with excess
        gastrin 251.5
        glucagon 251.4
    beta 251.1
  parathyroid (gland) 252.01 ▲
  persistent, vitreous (primary) 743.51
  pharynx (lymphoid) 478.29
  prostate 600.90
    with urinary retention 600.91
    adenofibromatous 600.20
      with urinary retention 600.21
    nodular 600.10
      with urinary retention 600.11
  renal artery (fibromuscular) 447.3
  reticuloendothelial (cell) 289.9
  salivary gland (any) 527.1
  Schimmelbusch's 610.1
  suprarenal (capsule) (gland) 255.8
  thymus (gland) (persistent) 254.0
  thyroid (*see also* Goiter) 240.9
    primary 242.0 ☑
    secondary 242.2 ☑
  tonsil (lymphoid tissue) 474.11
    and adenoids 474.10
  urethrovaginal 599.89
  uterus, uterine (myometrium) 621.2
    endometrium ▶(*see also* Hyperplasia,
        endometrium)◀ 621.30 ▲
  vitreous (humor), primary persistent 743.51
  vulva 624.3
  zygoma 738.11
Hyperpnea (*see also* Hyperventilation) 786.01
Hyperpotassemia 276.7
Hyperprebetalipoproteinemia 272.1
  with chylomicronemia 272.3
  familial 272.1

Hyperprolactinemia 253.1
Hyperprolinemia 270.8
Hyperproteinemia 273.8
Hyperprothrombinemia 289.89
Hyperpselaphesia 782.0
Hyperpyrexia 780.6
   heat (effects of) 992.0
   malarial (*see also* Malaria) 084.6
   malignant, due to anesthetic 995.86
   rheumatic — *see* Fever, rheumatic
   unknown origin (*see also* Pyrexia) 780.6
Hyperreactor, vascular 780.2
Hyperreflexia 796.1
   bladder, autonomic 596.54
      with cauda equina 344.61
   detrusor 344.61
Hypersalivation (*see also* Ptyalism) 527.7
Hypersarcosinemia 270.8
Hypersecretion
   ACTH 255.3
   androgens (ovarian) 256.1
   calcitonin 246.0
   corticoadrenal 255.3
   cortisol 255.0
   estrogen 256.0
   gastric 536.8
      psychogenic 306.4
   gastrin 251.5
   glucagon 251.4
   hormone
      ACTH 255.3
      anterior pituitary 253.1
      growth NEC 253.0
      ovarian androgen 256.1
      testicular 257.0
      thyroid stimulating 242.8 ☑
   insulin — *see* Hyperinsulinism
   lacrimal glands (*see also* Epiphora) 375.20
   medulloadrenal 255.6
   milk 676.6 ☑
   ovarian androgens 256.1
   pituitary (anterior) 253.1
   salivary gland (any) 527.7
   testicular hormones 257.0
   thyrocalcitonin 246.0
   upper respiratory 478.9
Hypersegmentation, hereditary 288.2
   eosinophils 288.2
   neutrophil nuclei 288.2
Hypersensitive, hypersensitiveness,
   hypersensitivity — *see also* Allergy
   angiitis 446.20
      specified NEC 446.29
   carotid sinus 337.0
   colon 564.9
      psychogenic 306.4
   DNA (deoxyribonucleic acid) NEC 287.2
   drug (*see also* Allergy, drug) 995.2
   esophagus 530.89
   insect bites — *see* Injury, superficial, by site
   labyrinth 386.58
   pain (*see also* Disturbance, sensation) 782.0
   pneumonitis NEC 495.9
   reaction (*see also* Allergy) 995.3
      upper respiratory tract NEC 478.8
   stomach (allergic) (nonallergic) 536.8
      psychogenic 306.4
Hypersomatotropism (classic) 253.0
Hypersomnia 780.54
   with sleep apnea 780.53
   nonorganic origin 307.43
      persistent (primary) 307.44
      transient 307.43
Hypersplenia 289.4
Hypersplenism 289.4
Hypersteatosis 706.3
Hyperstimulation, ovarian 256.1
Hypersuprarenalism 255.3
Hypersusceptibility — *see* Allergy
Hyper-TBG-nemia 246.8
Hypertelorism 756.0
   orbit, orbital 376.41

	Malignant	Benign	Unspecified
Hypertension, hypertensive (arterial) (arteriolar) (crisis) (degeneration) (disease) (essential) (fluctuating) (idiopathic) (intermittent) (labile) (low renin) (orthostatic) (paroxysmal) (primary) (systemic) (uncontrolled) (vascular)	401.0	401.1	401.9
with			
heart involvement ►(conditions classifiable to 429.0-429.3, 429.8, 429.9 due to hypertension)◄ (*see also* Hypertension, heart)	402.00	402.10	402.90
with kidney involvement — *see* Hypertension, cardiorenal			
renal involvement (only conditions classifiable to 585, 586, 587) (excludes conditions classifiable to 584) (*see also* Hypertension, kidney)	403.00	403.10	403.90
renal sclerosis or failure	403.00	403.10	403.90
with heart involvement — *see* Hypertension, cardiorenal			
failure (and sclerosis) (*see also* Hypertension, kidney)	403.01	403.11	403.91
sclerosis without failure (*see also* Hypertension, kidney)	403.00	403.10	403.90
accelerated — (*see also* Hypertension, by type, malignant)	401.0	—	—
antepartum — *see* Hypertension, complicating pregnancy, childbirth, or the puerperium			
cardiorenal (disease)	404.00	404.10	404.90
with			
heart failure	404.01	404.11	404.91
and renal failure	404.03	404.13	404.93
renal failure	404.02	404.12	404.92
and heart failure	404.03	404.13	404.93
cardiovascular disease (arteriosclerotic) (sclerotic)	402.00	402.10	402.90
with			
heart failure	402.01	402.11	402.91
renal involvement (conditions classifiable to 403) (*see also* Hypertension, cardiorenal)	404.00	404.10	404.90
cardiovascular renal (disease) (sclerosis) (*see also* Hypertension, cardiorenal)	404.00	404.10	404.90
cerebrovascular disease NEC	437.2	437.2	437.2
complicating pregnancy, childbirth, or the puerperium	642.2 ☑	642.0 ☑	642.9 ☑
with			
albuminuria (and edema) (mild)	—	—	642.4 ☑
severe	—	—	642.5 ☑
edema (mild)	—	—	642.4 ☑
severe	—	—	642.5 ☑
heart disease	642.2 ☑	642.2 ☑	642.2 ☑
and renal disease	642.2 ☑	642.2 ☑	642.2 ☑
renal disease	642.2 ☑	642.2 ☑	642.2 ☑
and heart disease	642.2 ☑	642.2 ☑	642.2 ☑
chronic	642.2 ☑	642.0 ☑	642.0 ☑
with pre-eclampsia or eclampsia	642.7 ☑	642.7 ☑	642.7 ☑
fetus or newborn	760.0	760.0	760.0
essential	—	642.0 ☑	642.0 ☑
with pre-eclampsia or eclampsia	—	642.7 ☑	642.7 ☑
fetus or newborn	760.0	760.0	760.0
fetus or newborn	760.0	760.0	760.0
gestational	—	—	642.3 ☑
pre-existing	642.2 ☑	642.0 ☑	642.0 ☑
with pre-eclampsia or eclampsia	642.7 ☑	642.7 ☑	642.7 ☑
fetus or newborn	760.0	760.0	760.0
secondary to renal disease	642.1 ☑	642.1 ☑	642.1 ☑
with pre-eclampsia or eclampsia	642.7 ☑	642.7 ☑	642.7 ☑
fetus or newborn	760.0	760.0	760.0
transient	—	—	642.3 ☑
due to			
aldosteronism, primary	405.09	405.19	405.99
brain tumor	405.09	405.19	405.99
bulbar poliomyelitis	405.09	405.19	405.99
calculus			
kidney	405.09	405.19	405.99
ureter	405.09	405.19	405.99
coarctation, aorta	405.09	405.19	405.99
Cushing's disease	405.09	405.19	405.99
glomerulosclerosis (*see also* Hypertension, kidney)	403.00	403.10	403.90
periarteritis nodosa	405.09	405.19	405.99
pheochromocytoma	405.09	405.19	405.99
polycystic kidney(s)	405.09	405.19	405.99
polycythemia	405.09	405.19	405.99
porphyria	405.09	405.19	405.99
pyelonephritis	405.09	405.19	405.99
renal (artery)			
aneurysm	405.01	405.11	405.91
anomaly	405.01	405.11	405.91
embolism	405.01	405.11	405.91
fibromuscular hyperplasia	405.01	405.11	405.91
occlusion	405.01	405.11	405.91
stenosis	405.01	405.11	405.91
thrombosis	405.01	405.11	405.91

☑ Additional Digit Required   ►◄ Revised Text   ● New Line   ▲ Revised Code

Hypertension, hypertensive — continued	Malignant	Benign	Unspecified
encephalopathy	437.2	437.2	437.2
gestational (transient) NEC	—	—	642.3 ☑
Goldblatt's	440.1	440.1	440.1
heart (disease) ▶(conditions classifiable to 429.0-429.3, 429.9 due to hypertension)◀	402.00	402.10	402.90
with heart failure	402.01	402.11	402.91
hypertensive kidney disease (conditions classifiable to 403) (see also Hypertension, cardiorenal)	404.00	404.10	404.90
renal sclerosis (see also Hypertension, cardiorenal)	404.00	404.10	404.90
intracranial, benign	—	348.2	—
intraocular	—	—	365.04
kidney	403.00	403.10	403.90
with			
heart involvement ▶(conditions classifiable to 429.0-429.3, 429.8, 429.9 due to hypertension)◀ (see also Hypertension, cardiorenal)	404.00	404.10	404.90
hypertensive heart (disease) (conditions classifiable to 402) (see also Hypertension, cardiorenal)	404.00	404.10	404.90
lesser circulation	—	—	416.0
necrotizing	401.0	—	—
ocular	—	—	365.04
portal (due to chronic liver disease)	—	—	572.3
postoperative	—	—	997.91
psychogenic	—	—	306.2
puerperal, postpartum — see Hypertension, complicating pregnancy, childbirth, or the puerperium			
pulmonary (artery)	—	—	416.8
with cor pulmonale (chronic)	—	—	416.8
acute	—	—	415.0
idiopathic	—	—	416.0
primary	—	—	416.0
of newborn	—	—	747.83
secondary	—	—	416.8
renal (disease) (see also Hypertension, kidney)	403.00	403.10	403.90
renovascular NEC	405.01	405.11	405.91
secondary NEC	405.09	405.19	405.99
due to			
aldosteronism, primary	405.09	405.19	405.99
brain tumor	405.09	405.19	405.99
bulbar poliomyelitis	405.09	405.19	405.99
calculus			
kidney	405.09	405.19	405.99
ureter	405.09	405.19	405.99
coarctation, aorta	405.09	405.19	405.99
Cushing's disease	405.09	405.19	405.99
glomerulosclerosis (see also Hypertension, kidney)	403.00	403.10	403.90
periarteritis nodosa	405.09	405.19	405.99
pheochromocytoma	405.09	405.19	405.99
polycystic kidney(s)	405.09	405.19	405.99
polycythemia	405.09	405.19	405.99
porphyria	405.09	405.19	405.99
pyelonephritis	405.09	405.19	405.99
renal (artery)			
aneurysm	405.01	405.11	405.91
anomaly	405.01	405.11	405.91
embolism	405.01	405.11	405.91
fibromuscular hyperplasia	405.01	405.11	405.91
occlusion	405.01	405.11	405.91
stenosis	405.01	405.11	405.91
thrombosis	405.01	405.11	405.91
transient	—	—	796.2
of pregnancy	—	—	642.3 ☑
venous, chronic (asymptomatic) (idiopathic)	—	—	459.30
due to			
deep vein thrombosis (see also Syndrome, postphlebetic)	—	—	459.10
with			
complication, NEC	—	—	459.39
inflammation	—	—	459.32
with ulcer	—	—	459.33
ulcer	—	—	459.31
with inflammation	—	—	459.33

Hyperthecosis, ovary 256.8

Hyperthermia (of unknown origin) (see also Pyrexia) 780.6
  malignant (due to anesthesia) 995.86
  newborn 778.4

Hyperthymergasia (see also Psychosis, affective) 296.0 ☑
  reactive (from emotional stress, psychological trauma) 298.1
  recurrent episode 296.1 ☑
  single episode 296.0 ☑

Hyperthymism 254.8

Hyperthyroid (recurrent) — see Hyperthyroidism

Hyperthyroidism (latent) (preadult) (recurrent) (without goiter) 242.9 ☑

> Note — Use the following fifth-digit subclassification with category 242:
>
> 0   without mention of thyrotoxic crisis or storm
>
> 1   with mention of thyrotoxic crisis or storm

  with
    goiter (diffuse) 242.0 ☑
      adenomatous 242.3 ☑
        multinodular 242.2 ☑
        uninodular 242.1 ☑
      nodular 242.3 ☑
        multinodular 242.2 ☑
        uninodular 242.1 ☑
    thyroid nodule 242.1 ☑
  complicating pregnancy, childbirth, or puerperium 648.1 ☑
  neonatal (transient) 775.3

Hypertonia — see Hypertonicity

Hypertonicity
  bladder 596.51
  fetus or newborn 779.89
  gastrointestinal (tract) 536.8
  infancy 779.89
    due to electrolyte imbalance 779.89
  muscle 728.85
  stomach 536.8
    psychogenic 306.4
  uterus, uterine (contractions) 661.4 ☑
    affecting fetus or newborn 763.7

Hypertony — see Hypertonicity

Hypertransaminemia 790.4

Hypertrichosis 704.1
  congenital 757.4
  eyelid 374.54
  lanuginosa 757.4
    acquired 704.1

Hypertriglyceridemia, essential 272.1

Hypertrophy, hypertrophic
  adenoids (infectional) 474.12
    and tonsils (faucial) (infective) (lingual) (lymphoid) 474.10
  adrenal 255.8
  alveolar process or ridge 525.8
  anal papillae 569.49
  apocrine gland 705.82
  artery NEC 447.8
    carotid 447.8
    congenital (peripheral) NEC 747.60
      gastrointestinal 747.61
      lower limb 747.64
      renal 747.62
      specified NEC 747.69
      spinal 747.82
      upper limb 747.63
  arthritis (chronic) (see also Osteoarthrosis) 715.9 ☑
    spine (see also Spondylosis) 721.90
  arytenoid 478.79
  asymmetrical (heart) 429.9
  auricular — see Hypertrophy, cardiac
  Bartholin's gland 624.8
  bile duct 576.8
  bladder (sphincter) (trigone) 596.8
  blind spot, visual field 368.42
  bone 733.99
  brain 348.8

Hypertrophy, hypertrophic — *continued*
  breast 611.1
    cystic 610.1
    fetus or newborn 778.7
    fibrocystic 610.1
    massive pubertal 611.1
    puerperal, postpartum 676.3 ☑
    senile (parenchymatous) 611.1
  cardiac (chronic) (idiopathic) 429.3
    with
      rheumatic fever (conditions classifiable to 390)
        active 391.8
          with chorea 392.0
        inactive or quiescent (with chorea) 398.99
    congenital NEC 746.89
    fatty (*see also* Degeneration, myocardial) 429.1
    hypertensive (*see also* Hypertension, heart) 402.90
    rheumatic (with chorea) 398.99
      active or acute 391.8
        with chorea 392.0
    valve (*see also* Endocarditis) 424.90
      congenital NEC 746.89
  cartilage 733.99
  cecum 569.89
  cervix (uteri) 622.6
    congenital 752.49
    elongation 622.6
  clitoris (cirrhotic) 624.2
    congenital 752.49
  colon 569.89
    congenital 751.3
  conjunctiva, lymphoid 372.73
  cornea 371.89
  corpora cavernosa 607.89
  duodenum 537.89
  endometrium (uterus) ▶(*see also* Hyperplasia, endometrium)◀ 621.30   ▲
    cervix 622.6
  epididymis 608.89
  esophageal hiatus (congenital) 756.6
    with hernia — *see* Hernia, diaphragm
  eyelid 374.30
  falx, skull 733.99
  fat pad 729.30
    infrapatellar 729.31
    knee 729.31
    orbital 374.34
    popliteal 729.31
    prepatellar 729.31
    retropatellar 729.31
    specified site NEC 729.39
  foot (congenital) 755.67
  frenum, frenulum (tongue) 529.8
    linguae 529.8
    lip 528.5
  gallbladder or cystic duct 575.8
  gastric mucosa 535.2 ☑
  gingiva 523.8
  gland, glandular (general) NEC 785.6
  gum (mucous membrane) 523.8
  heart (idiopathic) — *see also* Hypertrophy, cardiac
    valve — *see also* Endocarditis
      congenital NEC 746.89
  hemifacial 754.0
  hepatic — *see* Hypertrophy, liver
  hiatus (esophageal) 756.6
  hilus gland 785.6
  hymen, congenital 752.49
  ileum 569.89
  infrapatellar fat pad 729.31
  intestine 569.89
  jejunum 569.89
  kidney (compensatory) 593.1
    congenital 753.3
  labial frenulum 528.5
  labium (majus) (minus) 624.3
  lacrimal gland, chronic 375.03
  ligament 728.9
    spinal 724.8
  linguae frenulum 529.8
  lingual tonsil (infectional) 474.11
  lip (frenum) 528.5

Hypertrophy, hypertrophic — *continued*
  lip — *continued*
    congenital 744.81
  liver 789.1
    acute 573.8
    cirrhotic — *see* Cirrhosis, liver
    congenital 751.69
    fatty — *see* Fatty, liver
  lymph gland 785.6
    tuberculous — *see* Tuberculosis, lymph gland
  mammary gland — *see* Hypertrophy, breast
  maxillary frenuium 528.5
  Meckel's diverticulum (congenital) 751.0
  medial meniscus, acquired 717.3
  median bar 600.90
    with urinary retention 600.91
  mediastinum 519.3
  meibomian gland 373.2
  meniscus, knee, congenital 755.64
  metatarsal head 733.99
  metatarsus 733.99
  mouth 528.9
  mucous membrane
    alveolar process 523.8
    nose 478.1
    turbinate (nasal) 478.0
  muscle 728.9
  muscular coat, artery NEC 447.8
    carotid 447.8
    renal 447.3
  myocardium (*see also* Hypertrophy, cardiac) 429.3
    idiopathic 425.4
  myometrium 621.2
  nail 703.8
    congenital 757.5
  nasal 478.1
    alae 478.1
    bone 738.0
    cartilage 478.1
    mucous membrane (septum) 478.1
    sinus (*see also* Sinusitis) 473.9
    turbinate 478.0
  nasopharynx, lymphoid (infectional) (tissue) (wall) 478.29
  neck, uterus 622.6
  nipple 611.1
  normal aperture diaphragm (congenital) 756.6
  nose (*see also* Hypertrophy, nasal) 478.1
  orbit 376.46
  organ or site, congenital NEC — *see* Anomaly, specified type NEC
  osteoarthropathy (pulmonary) 731.2
  ovary 620.8
  palate (hard) 526.89
    soft 528.9
  pancreas (congenital) 751.7
  papillae
    anal 569.49
    tongue 529.3
  parathyroid (gland) 252.01   ▲
  parotid gland 527.1
  penis 607.89
  phallus 607.89
    female (clitoris) 624.2
  pharyngeal tonsil 474.12
  pharyngitis 472.1
  pharynx 478.29
    lymphoid (infectional) (tissue) (wall) 478.29
  pituitary (fossa) (gland) 253.8
  popliteal fat pad 729.31
  preauricular (lymph) gland (Hampstead) 785.6
  prepuce (congenital) 605
    female 624.2
  prostate (asymptomatic) (early) (recurrent) 600.90
    with urinary retention 600.91
    adenofibromatous 600.20
      with urinary retention 600.21
    benign 600.00
      with urinary retention 600.01
    congenital 752.89
  pseudoedematous hypodermal 757.0
  pseudomuscular 359.1
  pylorus (muscle) (sphincter) 537.0
    congenital 750.5

Hypertrophy, hypertrophic — *continued*
  pylorus — *continued*
    infantile 750.5
  rectal sphincter 569.49
  rectum 569.49
  renal 593.1
  rhinitis (turbinate) 472.0
  salivary duct or gland 527.1
    congenital 750.26
  scaphoid (tarsal) 733.99
  scar 701.4
  scrotum 608.89
  sella turcica 253.8
  seminal vesicle 608.89
  sigmoid 569.89
  skin condition NEC 701.9
  spermatic cord 608.89
  spinal ligament 724.8
  spleen — *see* Splenomegaly
  spondylitis (spine) (*see also* Spondylosis) 721.90
  stomach 537.89
  subaortic stenosis (idiopathic) 425.1
  sublingual gland 527.1
    congenital 750.26
  submaxillary gland 527.1
  suprarenal (gland) 255.8
  tendon 727.9
  testis 608.89
    congenital 752.89
  thymic, thymus (congenital) (gland) 254.0
  thyroid (gland) (*see also* Goiter) 240.9
    primary 242.0 ☑
    secondary 242.2 ☑
  toe (congenital) 755.65
    acquired 735.8
  tongue 529.8
    congenital 750.15
    frenum 529.8
    papillae (foliate) 529.3
  tonsil (faucial) (infective) (lingual) (lymphoid) 474.11
    with
      adenoiditis 474.01
      tonsillitis 474.00
        and adenoiditis 474.02
      and adenoids 474.10
  tunica vaginalis 608.89
  turbinate (mucous membrane) 478.0
  ureter 593.89
  urethra 599.84
  uterus 621.2
    puerperal, postpartum 674.8 ☑
  uvula 528.9
  vagina 623.8
  vas deferens 608.89
  vein 459.89
  ventricle, ventricular (heart) (left) (right) — *see also* Hypertrophy, cardiac
    congenital 746.89
    due to hypertension (left) (right) (*see also* Hypertension, heart) 402.90
      benign 402.10
      malignant 402.00
    right with ventricular septal defect, pulmonary stenosis or atresia, and dextraposition of aorta 745.2
  verumontanum 599.89
  vesical 596.8
  vocal cord 478.5
  vulva 624.3
    stasis (nonfilarial) 624.3

Hypertropia (intermittent) (periodic) 378.31
Hypertyrosinemia 270.2
Hyperuricemia 790.6
Hypervalinemia 270.3
Hyperventilation (tetany) 786.01
  hysterical 300.11
  psychogenic 306.1
  syndrome 306.1
Hyperviscidosis 277.00
Hyperviscosity (of serum) (syndrome) NEC 273.3
  polycythemic 289.0
  sclerocythemic 282.8

☑ Additional Digit Required   ▶◀ Revised Text   ● New Line   ▲ Revised Code

Hypervitaminosis (dietary) NEC 278.8
  A (dietary) 278.2
  D (dietary) 278.4
  from excessive administration or use of vitamin
    preparations (chronic) 278.8
    reaction to sudden overdose 963.5
    vitamin A 278.2
      reaction to sudden overdose 963.5
    vitamin D 278.4
      reaction to sudden overdose 963.5
    vitamin K
      correct substance properly administered
        278.8
      overdose or wrong substance given or
        taken 964.3
Hypervolemia 276.6
Hypesthesia (see also Disturbance, sensation) 782.0
  cornea 371.81
Hyphema (anterior chamber) (ciliary body) (iris) 364.41
  traumatic 921.3
Hyphemia — see Hyphema
Hypoacidity, gastric 536.8
  psychogenic 306.4
Hypoactive labyrinth (function) — see Hypofunction, labyrinth
Hypoadrenalism 255.4
  tuberculous (see also Tuberculosis) 017.6 ☑
Hypoadrenocorticism 255.4
  pituitary 253.4
Hypoalbuminemia 273.8
Hypoalphalipoproteinemia 272.5
Hypobarism 993.2
Hypobaropathy 993.2
Hypobetalipoproteinemia (familial) 272.5
Hypocalcemia 275.41
  cow's milk 775.4
  dietary 269.3
  neonatal 775.4
  phosphate-loading 775.4
Hypocalcification, teeth 520.4
Hypochloremia 276.9
Hypochlorhydria 536.8
  neurotic 306.4
  psychogenic 306.4
Hypocholesteremia 272.5
Hypochondria (reaction) 300.7
Hypochondriac 300.7
Hyponchondriasis 300.7
Hypochromasia blood cells 280.9
Hypochromic anemia 280.9
  due to blood loss (chronic) 280.0
    acute 285.1
  microcytic 280.9
Hypocoagulability (see also Defect, coagulation) 286.9
Hypocomplementemia 279.8
Hypocythemia (progressive) 284.9
Hypodontia (see also Anodontia) 520.0
Hypoeosinophilia 288.8
Hypoesthesia (see also Disturbance, sensation) 782.0
  cornea 371.81
  tactile 782.0
Hypoestrinism 256.39
Hypoestrogenism 256.39
Hypoferremia 280.9
  due to blood loss (chronic) 280.0
Hypofertility
  female 628.9
  male 606.1
Hypofibrinogenemia 286.3
  acquired 286.6
  congenital 286.3
Hypofunction
  adrenal (gland) 255.4
    cortex 255.4
    medulla 255.5
    specified NEC 255.5

Hypofunction — continued
  cerebral 331.9
  corticoadrenal NEC 255.4
  intestinal 564.89
  labyrinth (unilateral) 386.53
    with loss of labyrinthine reactivity 386.55
    bilateral 386.54
      with loss of labyrinthine reactivity 386.56
  Leydig cell 257.2
  ovary 256.39
    postablative 256.2
  pituitary (anterior) (gland) (lobe) 253.2
    posterior 253.5
  testicular 257.2
    iatrogenic 257.1
    postablative 257.1
    postirradiation 257.1
    postsurgical 257.1
Hypogammaglobulinemia 279.00
  acquired primary 279.06
  non-sex-linked, congenital 279.06
  sporadic 279.06
  transient of infancy 279.09
Hypogenitalism (congenital) (female) (male) 752.89
  penis 752.69
Hypoglycemia (spontaneous) 251.2
  coma 251.0
    diabetic 250.3 ☑
  diabetic 250.8 ☑
  due to insulin 251.0
    therapeutic misadventure 962.3
  familial (idiopathic) 251.2
  following gastrointestinal surgery 579.3
  infantile (idiopathic) 251.2
  in infant of diabetic mother 775.0
  leucine-induced 270.3
  neonatal 775.6
  reactive 251.2
  specified NEC 251.1
Hypoglycemic shock 251.0
  diabetic 250.8 ☑
  due to insulin 251.0
  functional (syndrome) 251.1
Hypogonadism
  female 256.39
  gonadotrophic (isolated) 253.4
  hypogonadotropic (isolated) (with anosmia) 253.4
  isolated 253.4
  male 257.2
  ovarian (primary) 256.39
  pituitary (secondary) 253.4
  testicular (primary) (secondary) 257.2
Hypohidrosis 705.0
Hypohidrotic ectodermal dysplasia 757.31
Hypoidrosis 705.0
Hypoinsulinemia, postsurgical 251.3
  postpancreatectomy (complete) (partial) 251.3
Hypokalemia 276.8
Hypokinesia 780.99
Hypoleukia splenica 289.4
Hypoleukocytosis 288.8
Hypolipidemia 272.5
Hypolipoproteinemia 272.5
Hypomagnesemia 275.2
  neonatal 775.4
Hypomania, hypomanic reaction (see also Psychosis, affective) 296.0 ☑
  recurrent episode 296.1 ☑
  single episode 296.0 ☑
Hypomastia (congenital) 757.6
Hypomenorrhea 626.1
Hypometabolism 783.9
Hypomotility
  gastrointestinal tract 536.8
    psychogenic 306.4
  intestine 564.89
    psychogenic 306.4
  stomach 536.8
    psychogenic 306.4
Hyponasality 784.49

Hyponatremia 276.1
Hypo-ovarianism 256.39
Hypo-ovarism 256.39
Hypoparathyroidism (idiopathic) (surgically induced) 252.1
  neonatal 775.4
Hypopharyngitis 462
Hypophoria 378.40
Hypophosphatasia 275.3
Hypophosphatemia (acquired) (congenital) (familial) 275.3
  renal 275.3
Hypophyseal, hypophysis — see also condition
  dwarfism 253.3
  gigantism 253.0
  syndrome 253.8
Hypophyseothalamic syndrome 253.8
Hypopiesis — see Hypotension
Hypopigmentation 709.00
  eyelid 374.53
Hypopinealism 259.8
Hypopituitarism (juvenile) (syndrome) 253.2
  due to
    hormone therapy 253.7
    hypophysectomy 253.7
    radiotherapy 253.7
  postablative 253.7
  postpartum hemorrhage 253.2
Hypoplasia, hypoplasis 759.89
  adrenal (gland) 759.1
  alimentary tract 751.8
    lower 751.2
    upper 750.8
  anus, anal (canal) 751.2
  aorta 747.22
  aortic
    arch (tubular) 747.10
    orifice or valve with hypoplasia of ascending aorta and defective development of left ventricle (with mitral valve atresia) 746.7
  appendix 751.2
  areola 757.6
  arm (see also Absence, arm, congenital) 755.20
  artery (congenital) (peripheral) NEC 747.60
    brain 747.81
    cerebral 747.81
    coronary 746.85
    gastrointestinal 747.61
    lower limb 747.64
    pulmonary 747.3
    renal 747.62
    retinal 743.58
    specified NEC 747.69
    spinal 747.82
    umbilical 747.5
    upper limb 747.63
  auditory canal 744.29
    causing impairment of hearing 744.02
  biliary duct (common) or passage 751.61
  bladder 753.8
  bone NEC 756.9
    face 756.0
    malar 756.0
    mandible 524.04
      alveolar 524.74
    marrow 284.9
      acquired (secondary) 284.8
      congenital 284.0
      idiopathic 284.9
    maxilla 524.03
      alveolar 524.73
    skull (see also Hypoplasia, skull) 756.0
  brain 742.1
    gyri 742.2
    specified part 742.2
  breast (areola) 757.6
  bronchus (tree) 748.3
  cardiac 746.89
    valve — see Hypoplasia, heart, valve
    vein 746.89
  carpus (see also Absence, carpal, congenital) 755.28
  cartilaginous 756.9
  cecum 751.2

(side tab: Hypervitaminosis — Hypoplasia, hypoplasis)

Hypoplasia, hypoplasis — *continued*
 cementum 520.4
  hereditary 520.5
 cephalic 742.1
 cerebellum 742.2
 cervix (uteri) 752.49
 chin 524.06
 clavicle 755.51
 coccyx 756.19
 colon 751.2
 corpus callosum 742.2
 cricoid cartilage 748.3
 dermal, focal (Goltz) 757.39
 digestive organ(s) or tract NEC 751.8
  lower 751.2
  upper 750.8
 ear 744.29
  auricle 744.23
  lobe 744.29
  middle, except ossicles 744.03
   ossicles 744.04
  ossicles 744.04
 enamel of teeth (neonatal) (postnatal) (prenatal)
   520.4
  hereditary 520.5
 endocrine (gland) NEC 759.2
 endometrium 621.8
 epididymis 752.89
 epiglottis 748.3
 erythroid, congenital 284.0
 erythropoietic, chronic acquired 284.8
 esophagus 750.3
 Eustachian tube 744.24
 eye (*see also* Microphthalmos) 743.10
  lid 743.62
 face 744.89
  bone(s) 756.0
 fallopian tube 752.19
 femur (*see also* Absence, femur, congenital)
   755.34
 fibula (*see also* Absence, fibula, congenital)
   755.37
 finger (*see also* Absence, finger, congenital)
   755.29
 focal dermal 757.39
 foot 755.31
 gallbladder 751.69
 genitalia, genital organ(s)
  female 752.89
   external 752.49
   internal NEC 752.89
  in adiposogenital dystrophy 253.8
  male 752.89
   penis 752.69
 glottis 748.3
 hair 757.4
 hand 755.21
 heart 746.89
  left (complex) (syndrome) 746.7
  valve NEC 746.89
   pulmonary 746.01
 humerus (*see also* Absence, humerus,
   congenital) 755.24
 hymen 752.49
 intestine (small) 751.1
  large 751.2
 iris 743.46
 jaw 524.09
 kidney(s) 753.0
 labium (majus) (minus) 752.49
 labyrinth, membranous 744.05
 lacrimal duct (apparatus) 743.65
 larynx 748.3
 leg (*see also* Absence, limb, congenital, lower)
   755.30
 limb 755.4
  lower (*see also* Absence, limb, congenital,
    lower) 755.30
  upper (*see also* Absence, limb, congenital,
    upper) 755.20
 liver 751.69
 lung (lobe) 748.5
 mammary (areolar) 757.6
 mandibular 524.04
  alveolar 524.74
  unilateral condylar 526.89

Hypoplasia, hypoplasis — *continued*
 maxillary 524.03
  alveolar 524.73
 medullary 284.9
 megakaryocytic 287.3
 metacarpus (*see also* Absence, metacarpal,
   congenital) 755.28
 metatarsus (*see also* Absence, metatarsal,
   congenital) 755.38
 muscle 756.89
  eye 743.69
 myocardium (congenital) (Uhl's anomaly)
   746.84
 nail(s) 757.5
 nasolacrimal duct 743.65
 nervous system NEC 742.8
 neural 742.8
 nose, nasal 748.1
 ophthalmic (*see also* Microphthalmos) 743.10
 organ
  of Corti 744.05
  or site NEC — *see* Anomaly, by site
 osseous meatus (ear) 744.03
 ovary 752.0
 oviduct 752.19
 pancreas 751.7
 parathyroid (gland) 759.2
 parotid gland 750.26
 patella 755.64
 pelvis, pelvic girdle 755.69
 penis 752.69
 peripheral vascular system (congenital)
    NEC 747.60
  gastrointestinal 747.61
  lower limb 747.64
  renal 747.62
  specified NEC 747.69
  spinal 747.82
  upper limb 747.63
 pituitary (gland) 759.2
 pulmonary 748.5
  arteriovenous 747.3
  artery 747.3
  valve 746.01
 punctum lacrimale 743.65
 radioulnar (*see also* Absence, radius,
   congenital, with ulna) 755.25
 radius (*see also* Absence, radius, congenital)
   755.26
 rectum 751.2
 respiratory system NEC 748.9
 rib 756.3
 sacrum 756.19
 scapula 755.59
 shoulder girdle 755.59
 skin 757.39
 skull (bone) 756.0
  with
   anencephalus 740.0
   encephalocele 742.0
   hydrocephalus 742.3
    with spina bifida (*see also* Spina
      bifida) 741.0 ☑
   microcephalus 742.1
 spinal (cord) (ventral horn cell) 742.59
  vessel 747.82
 spine 756.19
 spleen 759.0
 sternum 756.3
 tarsus (*see also* Absence, tarsal, congenital)
   755.38
 testis, testicle 752.89
 thymus (gland) 279.11
 thyroid (gland) 243
  cartilage 748.3
 tibiofibular (*see also* Absence, tibia, congenital,
   with fibula) 755.35
 toe (*see also* Absence, toe, congenital) 755.39
 tongue 750.16
 trachea (cartilage) (rings) 748.3
 Turner's (tooth) 520.4
 ulna (*see also* Absence, ulna, congenital)
   755.27
 umbilical artery 747.5
 ureter 753.29
 uterus 752.3
 vagina 752.49

Hypoplasia, hypoplasis — *continued*
 vascular (peripheral) NEC (*see also* Hypoplasia,
   peripheral vascular system) 747.60
  brain 747.81
 vein(s) (peripheral) NEC (*see also* Hypoplasia,
   peripheral vascular system) 747.60
  brain 747.81
  cardiac 746.89
  great 747.49
  portal 747.49
  pulmonary 747.49
 vena cava (inferior) (superior) 747.49
 vertebra 756.19
 vulva 752.49
 zonule (ciliary) 743.39
 zygoma 738.12
Hypopotassemia 276.8
Hypoproaccelerinemia (*see also* Defect,
  coagulation) 286.3
Hypoproconvertinemia (congenital) (*see also*
  Defect, coagulation) 286.3
Hypoproteinemia (essential) (hypermetabolic)
  (idiopathic) 273.8
Hypoproteinosis 260
Hypoprothrombinemia (congenital) (hereditary)
  (idiopathic) (*see also* Defect, coagulation)
  286.3
 acquired 286.7
 newborn 776.3
Hypopselaphesia 782.0
Hypopyon (anterior chamber) (eye) 364.05
 iritis 364.05
 ulcer (cornea) 370.04
Hypopyrexia 780.99
Hyporeflex 796.1
Hyporeninemia, extreme 790.99
 in primary aldosteronism 255.10
Hyporesponsive episode 780.09
Hyposecretion
 ACTH 253.4
 ovary 256.39
  postblative 256.2
 salivary gland (any) 527.7
Hyposegmentation of neutrophils, hereditary
  288.2
Hyposiderinemia 280.9
Hyposmolality 276.1
 syndrome 276.1
Hyposomatotropism 253.3
Hyposomnia (*see also* Insomnia) 780.52
Hypospadias (male) 752.61
 female 753.8
Hypospermatogenesis 606.1
Hyposphagma 372.72
Hyposplenism 289.59
Hypostasis, pulmonary 514
Hypostatic — *see* condition
Hyposthenuria 593.89
Hyposuprarenalism 255.4
Hypo-TBG-nemia 246.8
Hypotension (arterial) (constitutional) 458.9
 chronic 458.1
 iatrogenic 458.29
 maternal, syndrome (following labor and
   delivery) 669.2 ☑
 of hemodialysis 458.21
 orthostatic (chronic) 458.0
  dysautonomic-dyskinetic syndrome 333.0
 permanent idiopathic 458.1
 postoperative 458.29
 postural 458.0
 specified type NEC 458.8
 transient 796.3
Hypothermia (accidental) 991.6
 anesthetic 995.89
 newborn NEC 778.3
 not associated with low environmental
   temperature 780.99
Hypothymergasia (*see also* Psychosis, affective)
  296.2 ☑
 recurrent episode 296.3 ☑
 single episode 296.2 ☑

☑ Additional Digit Required   ▶◀ Revised Text   ● New Line   ▲ Revised Code

Hypothyroidism (acquired) 244.9
  complicating pregnancy, childbirth, or
      puerperium 648.1 ☑
  congenital 243
  due to
    ablation 244.1
      radioactive iodine 244.1
      surgical 244.0
    iodine (administration) (ingestion) 244.2
      radioactive 244.1
    irradiation therapy 244.1
    p-aminosalicylic acid (PAS) 244.3
    phenylbutazone 244.3
    resorcinol 244.3
    specified cause NEC 244.8
    surgery 244.0
  goitrous (sporadic) 246.1
  iatrogenic NEC 244.3
  iodine 244.2
  pituitary 244.8
  postablative NEC 244.1
  postsurgical 244.0
  primary 244.9
  secondary NEC 244.8
  specified cause NEC 244.8
  sporadic goitrous 246.1
Hypotonia, hypotonicity, hypotony 781.3
  benign congenital 358.8
  bladder 596.4
  congenital 779.89
    benign 358.8
  eye 360.30
    due to
      fistula 360.32
      ocular disorder NEC 360.33
    following loss of aqueous or vitreous 360.33
    primary 360.31
  infantile muscular (benign) 359.0
  muscle 728.9
  uterus, uterine (contractions) — see Inertia,
      uterus
Hypotrichosis 704.09
  congenital 757.4
  lid (congenital) 757.4
    acquired 374.55
  postinfectional NEC 704.09
Hypotropia 378.32
Hypoventilation 786.09
Hypovitaminosis (see also Deficiency, vitamin)
  269.2
Hypovolemia 276.5
  surgical shock 998.0
  traumatic (shock) 958.4
Hypoxemia (see also Anoxia) 799.0
Hypoxia (see also Anoxia) 799.0
  cerebral 348.1
    during or resulting from a procedure 997.01
    newborn 768.9
      mild or moderate 768.6
      severe 768.5
  fetal, affecting newborn 768.9
  intrauterine — see Distress, fetal
  myocardial (see also Insufficiency, coronary)
      411.89
    arteriosclerotic — see Arteriosclerosis,
        coronary
  newborn 768.9
Hypsarrhythmia (see also Epilepsy) 345.6 ☑
Hysteralgia, pregnant uterus 646.8 ☑
Hysteria, hysterical 300.10
  anxiety 300.20
  Charcôt's gland 300.11
  conversion (any manifestation) 300.11
  dissociative type NEC 300.15
  psychosis, acute 298.1
Hysteroepilepsy 300.11
Hysterotomy, affecting fetus or newborn 763.89

I

Iatrogenic syndrome of excess cortisol 255.0
Iceland disease (epidemic neuromyasthenia) 049.8

Ichthyosis (congenital) 757.1
  acquired 701.1
  fetalis gravior 757.1
  follicularis 757.1
  hystrix 757.39
  lamellar 757.1
  lingual 528.6
  palmaris and plantaris 757.39
  simplex 757.1
  vera 757.1
  vulgaris 757.1
Ichthyotoxism 988.0
  bacterial (see also Poisoning, food) 005.9
Icteroanemia, hemolytic (acquired) 283.9
  congenital (see also Spherocytosis) 282.0
Icterus (see also Jaundice) 782.4
  catarrhal — see Icterus, infectious
  conjunctiva 782.4
    newborn 774.6
  epidemic — see Icterus, infectious
  febrilis — see Icterus, infectious
  fetus or newborn — see Jaundice, fetus or
      newborn
  gravis (see also Necrosis, liver) 570
    complicating pregnancy 646.7 ☑
      affecting fetus or newborn 760.8
    fetus or newborn NEC 773.0
    obstetrical 646.7 ☑
      affecting fetus or newborn 760.8
  hematogenous (acquired) 283.9
  hemolytic (acquired) 283.9
    congenital (see also Spherocytosis) 282.0
  hemorrhagic (acute) 100.0
    leptospiral 100.0
    newborn 776.0
    spirochetal 100.0
  infectious 070.1
    with hepatic coma 070.0
    leptospiral 100.0
    spirochetal 100.0
  intermittens juvenilis 277.4
  malignant (see also Necrosis, liver) 570
  neonatorum (see also Jaundice, fetus or
      newborn) 774.6
  pernicious (see also Necrosis, liver) 570
  spirochetal 100.0
Ictus solaris, solis 992.0
Identity disorder 313.82
  dissociative 300.14
  gender role (child) 302.6
    adult 302.85
  psychosexual (child) 302.6
    adult 302.85
Idioglossia 307.9
Idiopathic — see condition
Idiosyncrasy (see also Allergy) 995.3
  drug, medicinal substance, and biological —
      see Allergy, drug
Idiot, idiocy (congenital) 318.2
  amaurotic (Bielschowsky) (-Jansky) (family)
      (infantile (late)) (juvenile (late)) (Vogt-
      Spielmeyer) 330.1
  microcephalic 742.1
  Mongolian 758.0
  oxycephalic 756.0
Id reaction (due to bacteria) 692.89
IgE asthma 493.0 ☑
Ileitis (chronic) (see also Enteritis) 558.9
  infectious 009.0
  noninfectious 558.9
  regional (ulcerative) 555.0
    with large intestine 555.2
  segmental 555.0
    with large intestine 555.2
  terminal (ulcerative) 555.0
    with large intestine 555.2
Ileocolitis (see also Enteritis) 558.9
  infectious 009.0
  regional 555.2
  ulcerative 556.1
Ileostomy status V44.2
  with complication 569.60
Ileotyphus 002.0
Ileum — see condition

Ileus (adynamic) (bowel) (colon) (inhibitory)
    (intestine) (neurogenic) (paralytic) 560.1
  arteriomesenteric duodenal 537.2
  due to gallstone (in intestine) 560.31
  duodenal, chronic 537.2
  following gastrointestinal surgery 997.4
  gallstone 560.31
  mechanical (see also Obstruction, intestine)
      560.9
  meconium 777.1
    due to cystic fibrosis 277.01
  myxedema 564.89
  postoperative 997.4
  transitory, newborn 777.4
Iliac — see condition
Iliotibial band friction syndrome 728.89
Ill, louping 063.1
Illegitimacy V61.6
Illness — see also Disease
  factitious 300.19
    with
      combined ▶psychological and physical
          signs and◀ symptoms 300.19
      predominantly   •
          ▶physical signs and symptoms◀
              300.19
          ▶psychological symptoms◀ 300.16
  chronic (with physical symptoms) 301.51
  heart — see Disease, heart
  manic-depressive (see also Psychosis, affective)
      296.80
  mental (see also Disorder, mental) 300.9
Imbalance 781.2
  autonomic (see also Neuropathy, peripheral,
      autonomic) 337.9
  electrolyte 276.9
    with
      abortion — see Abortion, by type, with
          metabolic disorder
      ectopic pregnancy (see also categories
          633.0-633.9) 639.4
      hyperemesis gravidarum (before 22
          completed weeks gestation) 643.1 ☑
      molar pregnancy (see also categories 630-
          632) 639.4
    following
      abortion 639.4
      ectopic or molar pregnancy 639.4
    neonatal, transitory NEC 775.5
  endocrine 259.9
  eye muscle NEC 378.9
    heterophoria — see Heterophoria
  glomerulotubular NEC 593.89
  hormone 259.9
  hysterical (see also Hysteria) 300.10
  labyrinth NEC 386.50
  posture 729.9
  sympathetic (see also Neuropathy, peripheral,
      autonomic) 337.9
Imbecile, imbecility 318.0
  moral 301.7
  old age 290.9
  senile 290.9
  specified IQ — see IQ
  unspecified IQ 318.0
Imbedding, intrauterine device 996.32
Imbibition, cholesterol (gallbladder) 575.6
Imerslund (-Gräsbeck) syndrome (anemia due to
    familial selective vitamin B_{12} malabsorption)
    281.1
Iminoacidopathy 270.8
Iminoglycinuria, familial 270.8
Immature — see also Immaturity
  personality 301.89
Immaturity 765.1 ☑
  extreme 765.0 ☑
  fetus or infant light-for-dates — see Light-for-
      dates
  lung, fetus or newborn 770.4
  organ or site NEC — see Hypoplasia
  pulmonary, fetus or newborn 770.4
  reaction 301.89
  sexual (female) (male) 259.0
Immersion 994.1
  foot 991.4
  hand 991.4

Hypothyroidism — Immersion

Immobile, immobility
  intestine 564.89
  joint — see Ankylosis
  syndrome (paraplegic) 728.3

Immunization
  ABO
    affecting management of pregnancy 656.2 ☑
      fetus or newborn 773.1
  complication — see Complications, vaccination
  Rh factor
    affecting management of pregnancy 656.1 ☑
      fetus or newborn 773.0
    from transfusion 999.7

Immunodeficiency 279.3
  with
    adenosine-deaminase deficiency 279.2
    defect, predominant
      B-cell 279.00
      T-cell 279.10
    hyperimmunoglobulinemia 279.2
    lymphopenia, hereditary 279.2
    thrombocytopenia and eczema 279.12
    thymic
      aplasia 279.2
      dysplasia 279.2
  autosomal recessive, Swiss-type 279.2
  common variable 279.06
  severe combined (SCID) 279.2
  to Rh factor
    affecting management of pregnancy 656.1 ☑
      fetus or newborn 773.0
  X-linked, with increased IgM 279.05

Immunotherapy, prophylactic V07.2

Impaction, impacted
  bowel, colon, rectum 560.30
    with hernia — see also Hernia, by site, with obstruction
      gangrenous — see Hernia, by site, with gangrene
    by
      calculus 560.39
      gallstone 560.31
    fecal 560.39
    specified type NEC 560.39
  calculus — see Calculus
  cerumen (ear) (external) 380.4
  cuspid 520.6
  dental 520.6
  fecal, feces 560.39
    with hernia — see also Hernia, by site, with obstruction
      gangrenous — see Hernia, by site, with gangrene
  fracture — see Fracture, by site
  gallbladder — see Cholelithiasis
  gallstone(s) — see Cholelithiasis
    in intestine (any part) 560.31
  intestine(s) 560.30
    with hernia — see also Hernia, by site, with obstruction
      grangrenous — see Hernia, by site, with gangrene
    by
      calculus 560.39
      gallstone 560.31
    fecal 560.39
    specified type NEC 560.39
  intrauterine device (IUD) 996.32
  molar 520.6
  shoulder 660.4 ☑
    affecting fetus or newborn 763.1
  tooth, teeth 520.6
  turbinate 733.99

Impaired, impairment (function)
  arm V49.1
    movement, involving
      musculoskeletal system V49.1
      nervous system V49.2
  auditory discrimination 388.43
  back V48.3
  body (entire) V49.89
  glucose
    fasting 790.21
    tolerance test (oral) 790.22
  hearing (see also Deafness) 389.9
  heart — see Disease, heart

Impaired, impairment — continued
  kidney (see also Disease, renal) 593.9
    disorder resulting from 588.9
      specified NEC 588.89 ▲
  leg V49.1
    movement, involving
      musculoskeletal system V49.1
      nervous system V49.2
  limb V49.1
    movement, involving
      musculoskeletal system V49.1
      nervous system V49.2
  liver 573.8
  mastication 524.9
  mobility
    ear ossicles NEC 385.22
    incostapedial joint 385.22
    malleus 385.21
  myocardium, myocardial (see also Insufficiency, myocardial) 428.0
  neuromusculoskeletal NEC V49.89
    back V48.3
    head V48.2
    limb V49.2
    neck V48.3
    spine V48.3
    trunk V48.3
  rectal sphincter 787.99
  renal (see also Disease, renal) 593.9
    disorder resulting from 588.9
      specified NEC 588.89 ▲
  spine V48.3
  vision NEC 369.9
    both eyes NEC 369.3
      moderate 369.74
        both eyes 369.25
          with impairment of lesser eye (specified as)
            blind, not further specified 369.15
            low vision, not further specified 369.23
            near-total 369.17
            profound 369.18
            severe 369.24
            total 369.16
        one eye 369.74
          with vision of other eye (specified as)
            near-normal 369.75
            normal 369.76
      near-total 369.64
        both eyes 369.04
          with impairment of lesser eye (specified as)
            blind, not further specified 369.02
            total 369.03
        one eye 369.64
          with vision of other eye (specified as)
            near normal 369.65
            normal 369.66
      one eye 369.60
        with low vision of other eye 369.10
      profound 369.67
        both eyes 369.08
          with impairment of lesser eye (specified as)
            blind, not further specified 369.05
            near-total 369.07
            total 369.06
        one eye 369.67
          with vision of other eye (specified as)
            near-normal 369.68
            normal 369.69
      severe 369.71
        both eyes 369.22
          with impairment of lesser eye (specified as)
            blind, not further specified 369.11
            low vision, not further specified 369.21
            near-total 369.13
            profound 369.14
            total 369.12
        one eye 369.71
          with vision of other eye (specified as)
            near-normal 369.72
            normal 369.73
    total
      both eyes 369.01

Impaired, impairment — continued
  vision — continued
    total — continued
      one eye 369.61
        with vision of other eye (specified as)
          near-normal 369.62
          normal 369.63

Impaludism — see Malaria

Impediment, speech NEC 784.5
  psychogenic 307.9
  secondary to organic lesion 784.5

Impending
  cerebrovascular accident or attack 435.9
  coronary syndrome 411.1
  delirium tremens 291.0
  myocardial infarction 411.1

Imperception, auditory (acquired) (congenital) 389.9

Imperfect
  aeration, lung (newborn) 770.5
  closure (congenital)
    alimentary tract NEC 751.8
      lower 751.5
      upper 750.8
    atrioventricular ostium 745.69
    atrium (secundum) 745.5
      primum 745.61
    branchial cleft or sinus 744.41
    choroid 743.59
    cricoid cartilage 748.3
    cusps, heart valve NEC 746.89
      pulmonary 746.09
    ductus
      arteriosus 747.0
      Botalli 747.0
    ear drum 744.29
      causing impairment of hearing 744.03
    endocardial cushion 745.60
    epiglottis 748.3
    esophagus with communication to bronchus or trachea 750.3
    Eustachian valve 746.89
    eyelid 743.62
    face, facial (see also Cleft, lip) 749.10
    foramen
      Botalli 745.5
      ovale 745.5
    genitalia, genital organ(s) or system
      female 752.89
        external 752.49
        internal NEC 752.89
        uterus 752.3
      male 752.89
        penis 752.69
    glottis 748.3
    heart valve (cusps) NEC 746.89
    interatrial ostium or septum 745.5
    interauricular ostium or septum 745.5
    interventricular ostium or septum 745.4
    iris 743.46
    kidney 753.3
    larynx 748.3
    lens 743.36
    lip (see also Cleft, lip) 749.10
    nasal septum or sinus 748.1
    nose 748.1
    omphalomesenteric duct 751.0
    optic nerve entry 743.57
    organ or site NEC — see Anomaly, specified type, by site
    ostium
      interatrial 745.5
      interauricular 745.5
      interventricular 745.4
    palate (see also Cleft, palate) 749.00
    preauricular sinus 744.46
    retina 743.56
    roof of orbit 742.0
    sclera 743.47
    septum
      aortic 745.0
      aorticopulmonary 745.0
      atrial (secundum) 745.5
        primum 745.61
      between aorta and pulmonary artery 745.0
    heart 745.9

Imperfect — *continued*
  closure — *continued*
    septum — *continued*
      interatrial (secundum) 745.5
        primum 745.61
      interauricular (secundum) 745.5
        primum 745.61
      interventricular 745.4
        with pulmonary stenosis or atresia, dextraposition of aorta, and hypertrophy of right ventricle 745.2
        in tetralogy of Fallot 745.2
      nasal 748.1
      ventricular 745.4
        with pulmonary stenosis or atresia, dextraposition of aorta, and hypertrophy of right ventricle 745.2
        in tetralogy of Fallot 745.2
    skull 756.0
      with
        anencephalus 740.0
        encephalocele 742.0
        hydrocephalus 742.3
          with spina bifida (*see also* Spina bifida) 741.0 ☑
        microcephalus 742.1
    spine (with meningocele) (*see also* Spina bifida) 741.90
    thyroid cartilage 748.3
    trachea 748.3
    tympanic membrane 744.29
      causing impairment of hearing 744.03
    uterus (with communication to bladder, intestine, or rectum) 752.3
    uvula 749.02
      with cleft lip (*see also* Cleft, palate, with cleft lip) 749.20
    vitelline duct 751.0
  development — *see* Anomaly, by site
  erection 607.84
  fusion — *see* Imperfect, closure
  inflation lung (newborn) 770.5
  intestinal canal 751.5
  poise 729.9
  rotation — *see* Malrotation
  septum, ventricular 745.4
Imperfectly descended testis 752.51
Imperforate (congenital) — *see also* Atresia
  anus 751.2
  bile duct 751.61
  cervix (uteri) 752.49
  esophagus 750.3
  hymen 752.42
  intestine (small) 751.1
    large 751.2
  jejunum 751.1
  pharynx 750.29
  rectum 751.2
  salivary duct 750.23
  urethra 753.6
  urinary meatus 753.6
  vagina 752.49
Impervious (congenital) — *see also* Atresia
  anus 751.2
  bile duct 751.61
  esophagus 750.3
  intestine (small) 751.1
    large 751.5
  rectum 751.2
  urethra 753.6
Impetiginization of other dermatoses 684
Impetigo (any organism) (any site) (bullous) (circinate) (contagiosa) (neonatorum) (simplex) 684
  Bockhart's (superficial folliculitis) 704.8
  external ear 684 [380.13]
  eyelid 684 [373.5]
  Fox's (contagiosa) 684
  furfuracea 696.5
  herpetiformis 694.3
    nonobstetrical 694.3
  staphylococcal infection 684
  ulcerative 686.8
  vulgaris 684

Impingement, soft tissue between teeth
  524.89 ▲
  anterior 524.81 ●
  posterior 524.82 ●
Implant, endometrial 617.9
Implantation
  anomalous — *see also* Anomaly, specified type, by site
    ureter 753.4
  cyst
    external area or site (skin) NEC 709.8
    iris 364.61
    vagina 623.8
    vulva 624.8
  dermoid (cyst)
    external area or site (skin) NEC 709.8
    iris 364.61
    vagina 623.8
    vulva 624.8
  placenta, low or marginal — *see* Placenta previa
Impotence (sexual) (psychogenic) 302.72
  organic origin NEC 607.84
Impoverished blood 285.9
Impression, basilar 756.0
Imprisonment V62.5
Improper
  development, infant 764.9 ☑
Improperly tied umbilical cord (causing hemorrhage) 772.3
Impulses, obsessional 300.3
Impulsive neurosis 300.3
Inaction, kidney (*see also* Disease, renal) 593.9
Inactive — *see* condition
Inadequate, inadequacy
  biologic 301.6
  cardiac and renal — *see* Hypertension, cardiorenal
  constitutional 301.6
  development
    child 783.40
    fetus 764.9 ☑
      affecting management of pregnancy 656.5 ☑
    genitalia
      after puberty NEC 259.0
      congenital — *see* Hypoplasia, genitalia
    lungs 748.5
    organ or site NEC — *see* Hypoplasia, by site
  dietary 269.9
  distance, interarch 524.28 ●
  education V62.3
  environment
    economic problem V60.2
    household condition NEC V60.1
    poverty V60.2
    unemployment V62.0
  functional 301.6
  household care, due to
    family member
      handicapped or ill V60.4
      temporarily away from home V60.4
        on vacation V60.5
    technical defects in home V60.1
    temporary absence from home of person rendering care V60.4
  housing (heating) (space) V60.1
  interarch distance 524.28 ●
  material resources V60.2
  mental (*see also* Retardation, mental) 319
  nervous system 799.2
  personality 301.6
  prenatal care in current pregnancy V23.7
  pulmonary
    function 786.09
      newborn 770.89
    ventilation, newborn 770.89
  respiration 786.09
    newborn 770.89
  sample, Papanicolaou smear 795.08 ●
  social 301.6
Inanition 263.9
  with edema 262
  due to
    deprivation of food 994.2
    malnutrition 263.9

Inanition — *continued*
  fever 780.6
Inappropriate secretion
  ACTH 255.0
  antidiuretic hormone (ADH) (excessive) 253.6
    deficiency 253.5
  ectopic hormone NEC 259.3
  pituitary (posterior) 253.6
Inattention after or at birth 995.52
Inborn errors of metabolism — *see* Disorder, metabolism
Incarceration, incarcerated
  bubonocele — *see also* Hernia, inguinal, with obstruction
    gangrenous — *see* Hernia, inguinal, with gangrene
  colon (by hernia) — *see also* Hernia, by site with obstruction
    gangrenous — *see* Hernia, by site, with gangrene
  enterocele 552.9
    gangrenous 551.9
  epigastrocele 552.29
    gangrenous 551.29
  epiplocele 552.9
    gangrenous 551.9
  exomphalos 552.1
    gangrenous 551.1
  fallopian tube 620.8
  hernia — *see also* Hernia, by site, with obstruction
    gangrenous — *see* Hernia, by site, with gangrene
  iris, in wound 871.1
  lens, in wound 871.1
  merocele (*see also* Hernia, femoral, with obstruction) 552.00
  omentum (by hernia) — *see also* Hernia, by site, with obstruction
    gangrenous — *see* Hernia, by site, with gangrene
  omphalocele 756.79
  rupture (meaning hernia) (*see also* Hernia, by site, with obstruction) 552.9
    gangrenous (*see also* Hernia, by site, with gangrene) 551.9
  sarcoepiplocele 552.9
    gangrenous 551.9
  sarcoepiplomphalocele 552.1
    with gangrene 551.1
  uterus 621.8
    gravid 654.3 ☑
      causing obstructed labor 660.2 ☑
        affecting fetus or newborn 763.1
Incident, cerebrovascular (*see also* Disease, cerebrovascular, acute) 436
Incineration (entire body) (from fire, conflagration, electricity, or lightning) — *see* Burn, multiple, specified sites
Incised wound
  external — *see* Wound, open, by site
  internal organs (abdomen, chest, or pelvis) — *see* Injury, internal, by site, with open wound
Incision, incisional
  hernia — *see* Hernia, incisional
  surgical, complication — *see* Complications, surgical procedures
  traumatic
    external — *see* Wound, open, by site
    internal organs (abdomen, chest, or pelvis) — *see* Injury, internal, by site, with open wound
Inclusion
  azurophilic leukocytic 288.2
  blennorrhea (neonatal) (newborn) 771.6
  cyst — *see* Cyst, skin
  gallbladder in liver (congenital) 751.69
Incompatibility
  ABO
    affecting management of pregnancy 656.2 ☑
    fetus or newborn 773.1
    infusion or transfusion reaction 999.6
  blood (group) (Duffy) (E) (K(ell)) (Kidd) (Lewis) (M) (N) (P) (S) NEC
    affecting management of pregnancy 656.2 ☑

☑ Additional Digit Required   ▶◀ Revised Text   ● New Line   ▲ Revised Code

Incompatibility — *continued*
　blood NEC — *continued*
　　fetus or newborn 773.2
　　infusion or transfusion reaction 999.6
　marital V61.10
　　involving divorce or estrangement V61.0
　Rh (blood group) (factor)
　　affecting management of pregnancy 656.1 ☑
　　fetus or newborn 773.0
　　infusion or transfusion reaction 999.7
　Rhesus — *see* Incompatibility, Rh
Incompetency, incompetence, incompetent
　annular
　　aortic (valve) (*see also* Insufficiency, aortic)
　　　424.1
　　mitral (valve) — (*see also* Insufficiency,
　　　mitral) 424.0
　　pulmonary valve (heart) (*see also*
　　　Endocarditis, pulmonary) 424.3
　aortic (valve) (*see also* Insufficiency, aortic)
　　424.1
　　syphilitic 093.22
　cardiac (orifice) 530.0
　　valve — *see* Endocarditis
　cervix, cervical (os) 622.5
　　in pregnancy 654.5 ☑
　　　affecting fetus or newborn 761.0
　esophagogastric (junction) (sphincter) 530.0
　heart valve, congenital 746.89
　mitral (valve) — *see* Insufficiency, mitral
　papillary muscle (heart) 429.81
　pelvic fundus
　　pubocervical tissue 618.81　　　　　　　　●
　　rectovaginal tissue 618.82　　　　　　　　●
　pulmonary valve (heart) (*see also* Endocarditis,
　　pulmonary) 424.3
　　congenital 746.09
　tricuspid (annular) (rheumatic) (valve) (*see also*
　　Endocarditis, tricuspid) 397.0
　valvular — *see* Endocarditis
　vein, venous (saphenous) (varicose) (*see also*
　　Varicose, vein) 454.9
　velopharyngeal (closure)
　　acquired 528.9
　　congenital 750.29
Incomplete — *see also* condition
　bladder emptying 788.21
　expansion lungs (newborn) 770.5
　gestation (liveborn) — *see* Immaturity
　rotation — *see* Malrotation
Incontinence 788.30
　without sensory awareness 788.34
　anal sphincter 787.6
　continuous leakage 788.37
　feces 787.6
　　due to hysteria 300.11
　　nonorganic origin 307.7
　hysterical 300.11
　mixed (male) (female) (urge and stress) 788.33
　overflow 788.38　　　　　　　　　　　　　▲
　paradoxical 788.39
　rectal 787.6
　specified NEC 788.39
　stress (female) 625.6
　　male NEC 788.32
　urethral sphincter 599.84
　urge 788.31
　　and stress (male) (female) 788.33
　urine 788.30
　　active 788.30
　　male 788.30
　　　stress 788.32
　　　　and urge 788.33
　　neurogenic 788.39
　　nonorganic origin 307.6
　　stress (female) 625.6
　　　male NEC 788.32
　　urge 788.31
　　　and stress 788.33
Incontinentia pigmenti 757.33
Incoordinate
　uterus (action) (contractions) 661.4 ☑
　　affecting fetus or newborn 763.7
Incoordination
　esophageal-pharyngeal (newborn) 787.2
　muscular 781.3
　papillary muscle 429.81

Increase, increased
　abnormal, in development 783.9
　androgens (ovarian) 256.1
　anticoagulants (antithrombin) (anti-VIIIa) (anti-
　　IXa) (anti-Xa) (anti-XIa) 286.5
　　postpartum 666.3 ☑
　cold sense (*see also* Disturbance, sensation)
　　782.0
　estrogen 256.0
　function
　　adrenal (cortex) 255.3
　　　medulla 255.6
　　pituitary (anterior) (gland) (lobe) 253.1
　　　posterior 253.6
　heat sense (*see also* Disturbance, sensation)
　　782.0
　intracranial pressure 781.99
　　injury at birth 767.8
　light reflex of retina 362.13
　permeability, capillary 448.9
　pressure
　　intracranial 781.99
　　　injury at birth 767.8
　　intraocular 365.00
　pulsations 785.9
　pulse pressure 785.9
　sphericity, lens 743.36
　splenic activity 289.4
　venous pressure 459.89
　　portal 572.3
Incrustation, cornea, lead or zinc 930.0
Incyclophoria 378.44
Incyclotropia 378.33
Indeterminate sex 752.7
India rubber skin 756.83
Indicanuria 270.2
Indigestion (bilious) (functional) 536.8
　acid 536.8
　catarrhal 536.8
　due to decomposed food NEC 005.9
　fat 579.8
　nervous 306.4
　psychogenic 306.4
Indirect — *see* condition
Indolent bubo NEC 099.8
Induced
　abortion — *see* Abortion, induced
　birth, affecting fetus or newborn 763.89
　delivery — *see* Delivery
　labor — *see* Delivery
Induration, indurated
　brain 348.8
　breast (fibrous) 611.79
　　puerperal, postpartum 676.3 ☑
　broad ligament 620.8
　chancre 091.0
　　anus 091.1
　　congenital 090.0
　　extragenital NEC 091.2
　corpora cavernosa (penis) (plastic) 607.89
　liver (chronic) 573.8
　　acute 573.8
　lung (black) (brown) (chronic) (fibroid) (*see also*
　　Fibrosis, lung) 515
　　essential brown 275.0 [516.1]
　penile 607.89
　phlebitic — *see* Phlebitis
　skin 782.8
　stomach 537.89
Induratio penis plastica 607.89
Industrial — *see* condition
Inebriety (*see also* Abuse, drugs, nondependent)
　305.0 ☑
Inefficiency
　kidney (*see also* Disease, renal) 593.9
　thyroid (acquired) (gland) 244.9
Inelasticity, skin 782.8
Inequality, leg (acquired) (length) 736.81
　congenital 755.30
Inertia
　bladder 596.4
　　neurogenic 596.54
　　　with cauda equina syndrome 344.61
　stomach 536.8
　　psychogenic 306.4

Inertia — *continued*
　uterus, uterine 661.2 ☑
　　affecting fetus or newborn 763.7
　　primary 661.0 ☑
　　secondary 661.1 ☑
　vesical 596.4
　　neurogenic 596.54
　　　with cauda equina 344.61
Infant — *see also* condition
　excessive crying of 780.92
　fussy (baby) 780.91
　held for adoption V68.89
　newborn — *see* Newborn
　post-term (gestation period over 40 completed
　　weeks to 42 completed weeks) 766.21
　prolonged gestation of (period over 42
　　completed weeks) 766.22
　syndrome of diabetic mother 775.0
"Infant Hercules" syndrome 255.2
Infantile — *see also* condition
　genitalia, genitals 259.0
　　in pregnancy or childbirth NEC 654.4 ☑
　　　affecting fetus or newborn 763.89
　　　causing obstructed labor 660.2 ☑
　　　　affecting fetus or newborn 763.1
　heart 746.9
　kidney 753.3
　lack of care 995.52
　macula degeneration 362.75
　melanodontia 521.05
　os, uterus (*see also* Infantile, genitalia) 259.0
　pelvis 738.6
　　with disproportion (fetopelvic) 653.1 ☑
　　　affecting fetus or newborn 763.1
　　　causing obstructed labor 660.1 ☑
　　　　affecting fetus or newborn 763.1
　penis 259.0
　testis 257.2
　uterus (*see also* Infantile, genitalia) 259.0
　vulva 752.49
Infantilism 259.9
　with dwarfism (hypophyseal) 253.3
　Brissaud's (infantile myxedema) 244.9
　celiac 579.0
　Herter's (nontropical sprue) 579.0
　hypophyseal 253.3
　hypothalamic (with obesity) 253.8
　idiopathic 259.9
　intestinal 579.0
　pancreatic 577.8
　pituitary 253.3
　renal 588.0
　sexual (with obesity) 259.0
Infants, healthy liveborn — *see* Newborn
Infarct, infarction
　adrenal (capsule) (gland) 255.4
　amnion 658.8 ☑
　anterior (with contiguous portion of
　　intraventricular septum) NEC (*see also*
　　Infarct, myocardium) 410.1 ☑
　appendices epiploicae 557.0
　bowel 557.0
　brain (stem) 434.91
　　embolic (*see also* Embolism, brain) 434.11
　　healed or old without residuals V12.59
　　iatrogenic 997.02
　　postoperative 997.02
　　puerperal, postpartum, childbirth 674.0 ☑
　　thrombotic (*see also* Thrombosis, brain)
　　　434.01
　breast 611.8
　Brewer's (kidney) 593.81
　cardiac (*see also* Infarct, myocardium) 410.9 ☑
　cerebellar (*see also* Infarct, brain) 434.91
　　embolic (*see also* Embolism, brain) 434.11
　cerebral (*see also* Infarct, brain) 434.91
　　embolic (*see also* Embolism, brain) 434.11
　　thrombotic (*see also* Infarct, brain)　　　●
　　　434.01　　　　　　　　　　　　　　　　　●
　chorion 658.8 ☑
　colon (acute) (agnogenic) (embolic)
　　(hemorrhagic) (nonocclusive)
　　(nonthrombotic) (occlusive) (segmental)
　　(thrombotic) (with gangrene) 557.0
　coronary artery (*see also* Infarct, myocardium)
　　410.9 ☑

☑ Additional Digit Required　　　　▶◀ Revised Text　　　　● New Line　　　　▲ Revised Code

Infarct, infarction — *continued*
  cortical 434.91 ●
  embolic (*see also* Embolism) 444.9
  fallopian tube 620.8
  gallbladder 575.8
  heart (*see also* Infarct, myocardium) 410.9 ☑
  hepatic 573.4
  hypophysis (anterior lobe) 253.8
  impending (myocardium) 411.1
  intestine (acute) (agnogenic) (embolic)
      (hemorrhagic) (nonocclusive)
      (nonthrombotic) (occlusive) (thrombotic)
      (with gangrene) 557.0
  kidney 593.81
  liver 573.4
  lung (embolic) (thrombotic) 415.1 ☑
    with
        abortion — *see* Abortion, by type, with
            embolism
        ectopic pregnancy (*see also* categories
            633.0-633.9) 639.6
        molar pregnancy (*see also* categories 630-
            632) 639.6
    following
        abortion 639.6
        ectopic or molar pregnancy 639.6
    iatrogenic 415.11
    in pregnancy, childbirth, or puerperium —
        see Embolism, obstetrical
    postoperative 415.11
  lymph node or vessel 457.8
  medullary (brain) — *see* Infarct, brain
  meibomian gland (eyelid) 374.85
  mesentery, mesenteric (embolic) (thrombotic)
      (with gangrene) 557.0
  midbrain — *see* Infarct, brain
  myocardium, myocardial (acute or with a
      stated duration of 8 weeks or less) (with
      hypertension) 410.9 ☑

---

*Note — Use the following fifth-digit
subclassification with category 410:*

  0   *episode unspecified*
  1   *initial episode*
  2   *subsequent episode without recurrence*

---

    with symptoms after 8 weeks from date of
        infarction 414.8
    anterior (wall) (with contiguous portion of
        intraventricular septum) NEC 410.1 ☑
    anteroapical (with contiguous portion of
        intraventricular septum) 410.1 ☑
    anterolateral (wall) 410.0 ☑
    anteroseptal (with contiguous portion of
        intraventricular septum) 410.1 ☑
    apical-lateral 410.5 ☑
    atrial 410.8 ☑
    basal-lateral 410.5 ☑
    chronic (with symptoms after 8 weeks from
        date of infarction) 414.8
    diagnosed on ECG, but presenting no
        symptoms 412
    diaphragmatic wall (with contiguous portion
        of intraventricular septum) 410.4 ☑
    healed or old, currently presenting no
        symptoms 412
    high lateral 410.5 ☑
    impending 411.1
    inferior (wall) (with contiguous portion of
        intraventricular septum) 410.4 ☑
    inferolateral (wall) 410.2 ☑
    inferoposterior wall 410.3 ☑
    lateral wall 410.5 ☑
    nontransmural 410.7 ☑
    papillary muscle 410.8 ☑
    past (diagnosed on ECG or other special
        investigation, but currently presenting
        no symptoms) 412
      with symptoms NEC 414.8
    posterior (strictly) (true) (wall) 410.6 ☑
    posterobasal 410.6 ☑
    posteroinferior 410.3 ☑
    posterolateral 410.5 ☑
    previous, currently presenting no symptoms
        412
    septal 410.8 ☑

Infarct, infarction — *continued*
  myocardium, myocardial — *continued*
    specified site NEC 410.8 ☑
      subendocardial 410.7 ☑
      syphilitic 093.82
    nontransmural 410.7 ☑
  omentum 557.0
  ovary 620.8
  pancreas 577.8
  papillary muscle (*see also* Infarct, myocardium)
      410.8 ☑
  parathyroid gland 252.8
  pituitary (gland) 253.8
  placenta (complicating pregnancy) 656.7 ☑
    affecting fetus or newborn 762.2
  pontine — *see* Infarct, brain
  posterior NEC (*see also* Infarct, myocardium)
      410.6 ☑
  prostate 602.8
  pulmonary (artery) (hemorrhagic) (vein)
      415.1 ☑
    with
        abortion — *see* Abortion, by type, with
            embolism
        ectopic pregnancy (*see also* categories
            633.0-633.9) 639.6
        molar pregnancy (*see also* categories 630-
            632) 639.6
    following
        abortion 639.6
        ectopic or molar pregnancy 639.6
    iatrogenic 415.11
    in pregnancy, childbirth, or puerperium —
        see Embolism, obstetrical
    postoperative 415.11
  renal 593.81
    embolic or thrombotic 593.81
  retina, retinal 362.84
    with occlusion — *see* Occlusion, retina
  spinal (acute) (cord) (embolic) (nonembolic)
      336.1
  spleen 289.59
    embolic or thrombotic 444.89
  subchorionic — *see* Infarct, placenta
  subendocardial (*see also* Infarct, myocardium)
      410.7 ☑
  suprarenal (capsule) (gland) 255.4
  syncytium — *see* Infarct, placenta
  testis 608.83
  thrombotic (*see also* Thrombosis) 453.9
    artery, arterial — *see* Embolism
  thyroid (gland) 246.3
  ventricle (heart) (*see also* Infarct, myocardium)
      410.9 ☑

Infecting — *see* condition

Infection, infected, infective (opportunistic)
      136.9
  with lymphangitis — *see* Lymphangitis
  abortion — *see* Abortion, by type, with sepsis
  abscess (skin) — *see* Abscess, by site
  Absidia 117.7
  Acanthocheilonema (perstans) 125.4
    streptocerca 125.6
  accessory sinus (chronic) (*see also* Sinusitis)
      473.9
  Achorion — *see* Dermatophytosis
  Acremonium falciforme 117.4
  acromioclavicular (joint) 711.91
  actinobacillus
    lignieresii 027.8
    mallei 024
    muris 026.1
  actinomadura — *see* Actinomycosis
  Actinomyces (israelii) — *see also* Actinomycosis
    muris-ratti 026.1
  Actinomycetales (actinomadura) (Actinomyces)
      (Nocardia) (Streptomyces) — *see*
      Actinomycosis
  actinomycotic NEC (*see also* Actinomycosis)
      039.9
  adenoid (chronic) 474.01
    acute 463
    and tonsil (chronic) 474.02
      acute or subacute 463
  adenovirus NEC 079.0
    in diseases classified elsewhere — *see*
        category 079 ☑

Infection, infected, infective — *continued*
  adenovirus NEC — *continued*
    unspecified nature or site 079.0
  Aerobacter aerogenes NEC 041.85
    enteritis 008.2
  aerogenes capsulatus (*see also* Gangrene, gas)
      040.0
  aertrycke (*see also* Infection, Salmonella) 003.9
  ajellomyces dermatitidis 116.0
  alimentary canal NEC (*see also* Enteritis, due
      to, by organism) 009.0
  Allescheria boydii 117.6
  Alternaria 118
  alveolus, alveolar (process) (pulpal origin) 522.4
  ameba, amebic (histolytica) (*see also* Amebiasis)
      006.9
    acute 006.0
    chronic 006.1
    free-living 136.2
    hartmanni 007.8
    specified
      site NEC 006.8
      type NEC 007.8
  amniotic fluid or cavity 658.4 ☑
    affecting fetus or newborn 762.7
  anaerobes (cocci) (gram-negative) (gram-
      positive) (mixed) NEC 041.84
  anal canal 569.49
  Ancylostoma braziliense 126.2
  Angiostrongylus cantonensis 128.8
  anisakiasis 127.1
  Anisakis larva 127.1
  anthrax (*see also* Anthrax) 022.9
  antrum (chronic) (*see also* Sinusitis, maxillary)
      473.0
  anus (papillae) (sphincter) 569.49
  arbor virus NEC 066.9
  arbovirus NEC 066.9
  argentophil-rod 027.0
  Ascaris lumbricoides 127.0
  ascomycetes 117.4
  Aspergillus (flavus) (fumigatus) (terreus) 117.3
  atypical
    acid-fast (bacilli) (*see also* Mycobacterium,
        atypical) 031.9
    mycobacteria (*see also* Mycobacterium,
        atypical) 031.9
  auditory meatus (circumscribed) (diffuse)
      (external) (*see also* Otitis, externa) 380.10
  auricle (ear) (*see also* Otitis, externa) 380.10
  axillary gland 683
  Babesiasis 088.82
  Babesiosis 088.82
  Bacillus NEC 041.89
    abortus 023.1
    anthracis (*see also* Anthrax) 022.9
    cereus (food poisoning) 005.89
    coli — *see* Infection, Escherichia coli
    coliform NEC 041.85
    Ducrey's (any location) 099.0
    Flexner's 004.1
    Friedländer's NEC 041.3
    fusiformis 101
    gas (gangrene) (*see also* Gangrene, gas)
        040.0
    mallei 024
    melitensis 023.0
    paratyphoid, paratyphosus 002.9
      A 002.1
      B 002.2
      C 002.3
    Schmorl's 040.3
    Shiga 004.0
    suipestifer (*see also* Infection, Salmonella)
        003.9
    swimming pool 031.1
    typhosa 002.0
    welchii (*see also* Gangrene, gas) 040.0
    Whitmore's 025
  bacterial NEC 041.9
    specified NEC 041.89
      anaerobic NEC 041.84
      gram-negative NEC 041.85
        anaerobic NEC 041.84
  Bacterium
    paratyphosum 002.9
      A 002.1

☑ Additional Digit Required   ►◄ Revised Text   ● New Line   ▲ Revised Code

Infection, infected, infective — *continued*
  Bacterium — *continued*
    paratyphosum — *continued*
      B 002.2
      C 002.3
    typhosum 002.0
  Bacteroides (fragilis) (melaninogenicus) (oralis)
      NEC 041.82 ▲
  balantidium coli 007.0
  Bartholin's gland 616.8
  Basidiobolus 117.7
  Bedsonia 079.98
    specified NEC 079.88
  bile duct 576.1
  bladder (*see also* Cystitis) 595.9
  Blastomyces, blastomycotic 116.0
    brasiliensis 116.1
    dermatitidis 116.0
    European 117.5
    Loboi 116.2
    North American 116.0
    South American 116.1
  blood stream — *see* Septicemia
  bone 730.9 ☑
    specified — *see* Osteomyelitis
  Bordetella 033.9
    bronchiseptica 033.8
    parapertussis 033.1
    pertussis 033.0
  Borrelia
    bergdorfi 088.81
    vincentii (mouth) (pharynx) (tonsil) 101
  brain (*see also* Encephalitis) 323.9
    late effect — *see* category 326
    membranes — (*see also* Meningitis) 322.9
    septic 324.0
      late effect — *see* category 326
      meninges (*see also* Meningitis) 320.9
  branchial cyst 744.42
  breast 611.0
    puerperal, postpartum 675.2 ☑
      with nipple 675.9 ☑
        specified type NEC 675.8 ☑
      nonpurulent 675.2 ☑
      purulent 675.1 ☑
  bronchus (*see also* Bronchitis) 490
    fungus NEC 117.9
  Brucella 023.9
    abortus 023.1
    canis 023.3
    melitensis 023.0
    mixed 023.8
    suis 023.2
  Brugia (Wuchereria) malayi 125.1
  bursa — *see* Bursitis
  buttocks (skin) 686.9
  Candida (albicans) (tropicalis) (*see also*
      Candidiasis) 112.9
    congenital 771.7
  Candiru 136.8
  Capillaria
    hepatica 128.8
    philippinensis 127.5
  cartilage 733.99
  cat liver fluke 121.0
  cellulitis — *see* Cellulitis, by site
  Cephalosporum falciforme 117.4
  Cercomonas hominis (intestinal) 007.3
  cerebrospinal (*see also* Meningitis) 322.9
    late effect — *see* category 326
  cervical gland 683
  cervix (*see also* Cervicitis) 616.0
  cesarean section wound 674.3 ☑
  Chilomastix (intestinal) 007.8
  Chlamydia 079.98
    specified NEC 079.88
  cholera (*see also* Cholera) 001.9
  chorionic plate 658.8 ☑
  Cladosporium
    bantianum 117.8
    carrionii 117.2
    mansoni 111.1
    trichoides 117.8
    wernecki 111.1
  Clonorchis (sinensis) (liver) 121.1
  Clostridium (haemolyticum) (novyi) NEC 041.84
    botulinum 005.1

Infection, infected, infective — *continued*
  Clostridium NEC — *continued*
    histolyticum (*see also* Gangrene, gas) 040.0
    oedematiens (*see also* Gangrene, gas) 040.0
    perfringens 041.83
      due to food 005.2
    septicum (*see also* Gangrene, gas) 040.0
    sordellii (*see also* Gangrene, gas) 040.0
    welchii (*see also* Gangrene, gas) 040.0
      due to food 005.2
  Coccidioides (immitis) (*see also*
      Coccidioidomycosis) 114.9
  coccus NEC 041.89
  colon (*see also* Enteritis, due to, by organism)
      009.0
    bacillus — *see* Infection, Escherichia coli
  colostomy or enterostomy 569.61
  common duct 576.1
  complicating pregnancy, childbirth, or
      puerperium NEC 647.9 ☑
    affecting fetus or newborn 760.2
  Condiobolus 117.7
  congenital NEC 771.89
    Candida albicans 771.7
    chronic 771.2
    cytomegalovirus 771.1
    hepatitis, viral 771.2
    herpes simplex 771.2
    listeriosis 771.2
    malaria 771.2
    poliomyelitis 771.2
    rubella 771.0
    toxoplasmosis 771.2
    tuberculosis 771.2
    urinary (tract) 771.82
    vaccinia 771.2
  coronavirus 079.89
    SARS-associated 079.82
  corpus luteum (*see also* Salpingo-oophoritis)
      614.2
  Corynebacterium diphtheriae — *see* Diphtheria
  Coxsackie (*see also* Coxsackie) 079.2
    endocardium 074.22
    heart NEC 074.20
    in diseases classified elsewhere — *see*
        category 079 ☑
    meninges 047.0
    myocardium 074.23
    pericardium 074.21
    pharynx 074.0
    specified disease NEC 074.8
    unspecified nature or site 079.2
  Cryptococcus neoformans 117.5
  Cryptosporidia 007.4
  Cunninghamella 117.7
  cyst — *see* Cyst
  Cysticercus cellulosae 123.1
  cytomegalovirus 078.5
    congenital 771.1
  dental (pulpal origin) 522.4
  deuteromycetes 117.4
  Dicrocoelium dendriticum 121.8
  Dipetalonema (perstans) 125.4
    streptocerca 125.6
  diphtherial — *see* Diphtheria
  Diphyllobothrium (adult) (latum) (pacificum)
      123.4
    larval 123.5
  Diplogonoporus (grandis) 123.8
  Dipylidium (caninum) 123.8
  Dirofilaria 125.6
  dog tapeworm 123.8
  Dracunculus medinensis 125.7
  Dreschlera 118
    hawaiiensis 117.8
  Ducrey's bacillus (any site) 099.0
  due to or resulting from
    device, implant, or graft (any) (presence of)
        — *see* Complications, infection and
        inflammation, due to (presence of) any
        device, implant, or graft classified to
        996.0-996.5 NEC
    injection, inoculation, infusion, transfusion,
        or vaccination (prophylactic)
        (therapeutic) 999.3
    injury NEC — *see* Wound, open, by site,
        complicated
    surgery 998.59

Infection, infected, infective — *continued*
  duodenum 535.6 ☑
  ear — *see also* Otitis
    external (*see also* Otitis, externa) 380.10
    inner (*see also* Labyrinthitis) 386.30
    middle — *see* Otitis, media
  Eaton's agent NEC 041.81
  Eberthella typhosa 002.0
  Ebola 065.8
  echinococcosis 122.9
  Echinococcus (*see also* Echinococcus) 122.9
  Echinostoma 121.8
  ECHO virus 079.1
    in diseases classified elsewhere — *see*
        category 079 ☑
    unspecified nature or site 079.1
  Ehrlichiosis 082.40
    chaffeensis 082.41
    specified type NEC 082.49
  Endamoeba — *see* Infection, ameba
  endocardium (*see also* Endocarditis) 421.0
  endocervix (*see also* Cervicitis) 616.0
  Entamoeba — *see* Infection, ameba
  enteric (*see also* Enteritis, due to, by organism)
      009.0
  Enterobacter aerogenes NEC 041.85
  Enterobius vermicularis 127.4
  enterococcus NEC 041.04
  enterovirus NEC 079.89
    central nervous system NEC 048
    enteritis 008.67
    meningitis 047.9
  Entomophthora 117.7
  Epidermophyton — *see* Dermatophytosis
  epidermophytosis — *see* Dermatophytosis
  episiotomy 674.3 ☑
  Epstein-Barr virus 075
    chronic 780.79 [139.8]
  erysipeloid 027.1
  Erysipelothrix (insidiosa) (rhusiopathiae) 027.1
  erythema infectiosum 057.0
  Escherichia coli NEC 041.4
    enteritis — *see* Enteritis, E. coli
    generalized 038.42
    intestinal — *see* Enteritis, E. coli
  esophagostomy 530.86 ●
  ethmoidal (chronic) (sinus) (*see also* Sinusitis,
      ethmoidal) 473.2
  Eubacterium 041.84
  Eustachian tube (ear) 381.50
    acute 381.51
    chronic 381.52
  exanthema subitum 057.8
  external auditory canal (meatus) (*see also*
      Otitis, externa) 380.10
  eye NEC 360.00
  eyelid 373.9
    specified NEC 373.8
  fallopian tube (*see also* Salpingo-oophoritis)
      614.2
  fascia 728.89
  Fasciola
    gigantica 121.3
    hepatica 121.3
  Fasciolopsis (buski) 121.4
  fetus (intra-amniotic) — *see* Infection,
      congenital
  filarial — *see* Infestation, filarial
  finger (skin) 686.9
    abscess (with lymphangitis) 681.00
      pulp 681.01
    cellulitis (with lymphangitis) 681.00
    distal closed space (with lymphangitis)
        681.00
    nail 681.02
      fungus 110.1
  fish tapeworm 123.4
    larval 123.5
  flagellate, intestinal 007.9
  fluke — *see* Infestation, fluke
  focal
    teeth (pulpal origin) 522.4
    tonsils 474.00
      and adenoids 474.02
  Fonsecaea
    compactum 117.2
    pedrosoi 117.2

☑ Additional Digit Required   ►◄ Revised Text   ● New Line   ▲ Revised Code

Infection, infected, infective — *continued*
- food (*see also* Poisoning, food) 005.9
- foot (skin) 686.9
  - fungus 110.4
- Francisella tularensis (*see also* Tularemia) 021.9
- frontal sinus (chronic) (*see also* Sinusitis, frontal) 473.1
- fungus NEC 117.9
  - beard 110.0
  - body 110.5
  - dermatiacious NEC 117.8
  - foot 110.4
  - groin 110.3
  - hand 110.2
  - nail 110.1
  - pathogenic to compromised host only 118
  - perianal (area) 110.3
  - scalp 110.0
  - scrotum 110.8
  - skin 111.9
    - foot 110.4
    - hand 110.2
  - toenails 110.1
  - trachea 117.9
- Fusarium 118
- Fusobacterium 041.84
- gallbladder (*see also* Cholecystitis, acute) 575.0
- Gardnerella vaginalis 041.89
- gas bacillus (*see also* Gas, gangrene) 040.0
- gastric (*see also* Gastritis) 535.5 ☑
- Gastrodiscoides hominis 121.8
- gastroenteric (*see also* Enteritis, due to, by organism) 009.0
- gastrointestinal (*see also* Enteritis, due to, by organism) 009.0
- gastrostomy 536.41
- generalized NEC (*see also* Septicemia) 038.9
- genital organ or tract NEC
  - female 614.9
    - with
      - abortion — *see* Abortion, by type, with sepsis
      - ectopic pregnancy (*see also* categories 633.0-633.9) 639.0
      - molar pregnancy (*see also* categories 630-632) 639.0
    - complicating pregnancy 646.6 ☑
      - affecting fetus or newborn 760.8
    - following
      - abortion 639.0
      - ectopic or molar pregnancy 639.0
    - puerperal, postpartum, childbirth 670.0 ☑
      - minor or localized 646.6 ☑
        - affecting fetus or newborn 760.8
  - male 608.4
- genitourinary tract NEC 599.0
- Ghon tubercle, primary (*see also* Tuberculosis) 010.0 ☑
- Giardia lamblia 007.1
- gingival (chronic) 523.1
  - acute 523.0
  - Vincent's 101
- glanders 024
- Glenosporopsis amazonica 116.2
- Gnathostoma spinigerum 128.1
- Gongylonema 125.6
- gonococcal NEC (*see also* Gonococcus) 098.0
- gram-negative bacilli NEC 041.85
  - anaerobic 041.84
- guinea worm 125.7
- gum (*see also* Infection, gingival) 523.1
- Hantavirus 079.81
- heart 429.89
- Helicobacter pylori (H. pylori) 041.86
- helminths NEC 128.9
  - intestinal 127.9
    - mixed (types classifiable to more than one category in 120.0-127.7) 127.8
    - specified type NEC 127.7
  - specified type NEC 128.8
- Hemophilus influenzae NEC 041.5
  - generalized 038.41
- herpes (simplex) (*see also* Herpes, simplex) 054.9
  - congenital 771.2

Infection, infected, infective — *continued*
- herpes (*see also* Herpes, simplex) — *continued*
  - zoster (*see also* Herpes, zoster) 053.9
    - eye NEC 053.29
- Heterophyes heterophyes 121.6
- Histoplasma (*see also* Histoplasmosis) 115.90
  - capsulatum (*see also* Histoplasmosis, American) 115.00
  - duboisii (*see also* Histoplasmosis, African) 115.10
- HIV V08
  - with symptoms, symptomatic 042
- hookworm (*see also* Ancylostomiasis) 126.9
- human immunodeficiency virus V08
  - with symptoms, symptomatic 042
- human papillomavirus 079.4
- hydrocele 603.1
- hydronephrosis 591
- Hymenolepis 123.6
- hypopharynx 478.29
- inguinal glands 683
  - due to soft chancre 099.0
- intestine, intestinal (*see also* Enteritis, due to, by organism) 009.0
- intrauterine (*see also* Endometritis) 615.9
  - complicating delivery 646.6 ☑
- isospora belli or hominis 007.2
- Japanese B encephalitis 062.0
- jaw (bone) (acute) (chronic) (lower) (subacute) (upper) 526.4
- joint — *see* Arthritis, infectious or infective
- kidney (cortex) (hematogenous) 590.9
  - with
    - abortion — *see* Abortion, by type, with urinary tract infection
    - calculus 592.0
    - ectopic pregnancy (*see also* categories 633.0-633.9) 639.8
    - molar pregnancy (*see also* categories 630-632) 639.8
    - complicating pregnancy or puerperium 646.6 ☑
      - affecting fetus or newborn 760.1
    - following
      - abortion 639.8
      - ectopic or molar pregnancy 639.8
    - pelvis and ureter 590.3
- Klebsiella pneumoniae NEC 041.3
- knee (skin) NEC 686.9
  - joint — *see* Arthritis, infectious
- Koch's (*see also* Tuberculosis, pulmonary) 011.9 ☑
- labia (majora) (minora) (*see also* Vulvitis) 616.10
- lacrimal
  - gland (*see also* Dacryoadenitis) 375.00
  - passages (duct) (sac) (*see also* Dacryocystitis) 375.30
- larynx NEC 478.79
- leg (skin) NEC 686.9
- Leishmania (*see also* Leishmaniasis) 085.9
  - braziliensis 085.5
  - donovani 085.0
  - Ethiopica 085.3
  - furunculosa 085.1
  - infantum 085.0
  - mexicana 085.4
  - tropica (minor) 085.1
    - major 085.2
- Leptosphaeria senegalensis 117.4
- leptospira (*see also* Leptospirosis) 100.9
  - Australis 100.89
  - Bataviae 100.89
  - pyrogenes 100.89
  - specified type NEC 100.89
- leptospirochetal NEC (*see also* Leptospirosis) 100.9
- Leptothrix — *see* Actinomycosis
- Listeria monocytogenes (listeriosis) 027.0
  - congenital 771.2
- liver fluke — *see* Infestation, fluke, liver
- Loa loa 125.2
  - eyelid 125.2 [373.6]
- Loboa loboi 116.2
- local, skin (staphylococcal) (streptococcal) NEC 686.9

Infection, infected, infective — *continued*
- local, skin NEC — *continued*
  - abscess — *see* Abscess, by site
  - cellulitis — *see* Cellulitis, by site
  - ulcer (*see also* Ulcer, skin) 707.9
- Loefflerella
  - mallei 024
  - whitmori 025
- lung 518.89
  - atypical Mycobacterium 031.0
    - tuberculous (*see also* Tuberculosis, pulmonary) 011.9 ☑
  - basilar 518.89
  - chronic 518.89
  - fungus NEC 117.9
  - spirochetal 104.8
  - virus — *see* Pneumonia, virus
- lymph gland (axillary) (cervical) (inguinal) 683
  - mesenteric 289.2
- lymphoid tissue, base of tongue or posterior pharynx, NEC 474.00
- madurella
  - grisea 117.4
  - mycetomii 117.4
- major
  - with
    - abortion — *see* Abortion, by type, with sepsis
    - ectopic pregnancy (*see also* categories 633.0-633.9) 639.0
    - molar pregnancy (*see also* categories 630-632) 639.0
  - following
    - abortion 639.0
    - ectopic or molar pregnancy 639.0
  - puerperal, postpartum, childbirth 670.0 ☑
- Malassezia furfur 111.0
- Malleomyces
  - mallei 024
  - pseudomallei 025
- mammary gland 611.0
  - puerperal, postpartum 675.2 ☑
- Mansonella (ozzardi) 125.5
- mastoid (suppurative) — *see* Mastoiditis
- maxilla, maxillary 526.4
  - sinus (chronic) (*see also* Sinusitis, maxillary) 473.0
- mediastinum 519.2
- medina 125.7
- meibomian
  - cyst 373.12
  - gland 373.12
- melioidosis 025
- meninges (*see also* Meningitis) 320.9
- meningococcal (*see also* condition) 036.9
  - brain 036.1
  - cerebrospinal 036.0
  - endocardium 036.42
  - generalized 036.2
  - meninges 036.0
  - meningococcemia 036.2
  - specified site NEC 036.89
- mesenteric lymph nodes or glands NEC 289.2
- Metagonimus 121.5
- metatarsophalangeal 711.97
- microorganism resistant to drugs — *see* Resistance (to), drugs by microorganisms
- Microsporidia 136.8
- microsporum, microsporic — *see* Dermatophytosis
- Mima polymorpha NEC 041.85
- mixed flora NEC 041.89
- Monilia (*see also* Candidiasis) 112.9
  - neonatal 771.7
- monkeypox 057.8
- Monosporium apiospermum 117.6
- mouth (focus) NEC 528.9
  - parasitic 112.0
- Mucor 117.7
- muscle NEC 728.89
- mycelium NEC 117.9
- mycetoma
  - actinomycotic NEC (*see also* Actinomycosis) 039.9
  - mycotic NEC 117.4
- Mycobacterium, mycobacterial (*see also* Mycobacterium) 031.9

☑ Additional Digit Required   ▶◀ Revised Text   ● New Line   ▲ Revised Code

Infection, infected, infective — *continued*
 mycoplasma NEC 041.81
 mycotic NEC 117.9
  pathogenic to compromised host only 118
  skin NEC 111.9
  systemic 117.9
 myocardium NEC 422.90
 nail (chronic) (with lymphangitis) 681.9
  finger 681.02
   fungus 110.1
  ingrowing 703.0
  toe 681.11
   fungus 110.1
 nasal sinus (chronic) (*see also* Sinusitis) 473.9
 nasopharynx (chronic) 478.29
  acute 460
 navel 686.9
  newborn 771.4
 Neisserian — *see* Gonococcus
 Neotestudina rosatii 117.4
 newborn, generalized 771.89
 nipple 611.0
  puerperal, postpartum 675.0 ☑
   with breast 675.9 ☑
    specified type NEC 675.8 ☑
 Nocardia — *see* Actinomycosis
 nose 478.1
 nostril 478.1
 obstetrical surgical wound 674.3 ☑
 Oesophagostomum (apiostomum) 127.7
 Oestrus ovis 134.0
 Oidium albicans (*see also* Candidiasis) 112.9
 Onchocerca (volvulus) 125.3
  eye 125.3 [360.13]
  eyelid 125.3 [373.6]
 operation wound 998.59
 Opisthorchis (felineus) (tenuicollis) (viverrini) 121.0
 orbit 376.00
  chronic 376.10
 ovary (*see also* Salpingo-oophoritis) 614.2
 Oxyuris vermicularis 127.4
 pancreas 577.0
 Paracoccidioides brasiliensis 116.1
 Paragonimus (westermani) 121.2
 parainfluenza virus 079.89
 parameningococcus NEC 036.9
  with meningitis 036.0
 parasitic NEC 136.9
 paratyphoid 002.9
  Type A 002.1
  Type B 002.2
  Type C 002.3
 paraurethral ducts 597.89
 parotid gland 527.2
 Pasteurella NEC 027.2
  multocida (cat-bite) (dog-bite) 027.2
  pestis (*see also* Plague) 020.9
  pseudotuberculosis 027.2
  septica (cat-bite) (dog-bite) 027.2
  tularensis (*see also* Tularemia) 021.9
 pelvic, female (*see also* Disease, pelvis, inflammatory) 614.9
 penis (glans) (retention) NEC 607.2
  herpetic 054.13
 Peptococcus 041.84
 Peptostreptococcus 041.84
 periapical (pulpal origin) 522.4
 peridental 523.3
 perineal wound (obstetrical) 674.3 ☑
 periodontal 523.3
 periorbital 376.00
  chronic 376.10
 perirectal 569.49
 perirenal (*see also* Infection, kidney) 590.9
 peritoneal (*see also* Peritonitis) 567.9
 periureteral 593.89
 periurethral 597.89
 Petriellidium boydii 117.6
 pharynx 478.29
  Coxsackievirus 074.0
  phlegmonous 462
  posterior, lymphoid 474.00
 Phialophora
  gougerotii 117.8
  jeanselmei 117.8
  verrucosa 117.2

Infection, infected, infective — *continued*
 Piedraia hortai 111.3
 pinna, acute 380.11
 pinta 103.9
  intermediate 103.1
  late 103.2
  mixed 103.3
  primary 103.0
 pinworm 127.4
 pityrosporum furfur 111.0
 pleuropneumonia-like organisms NEC (PPLO) 041.81
 pneumococcal NEC 041.2
  generalized (purulent) 038.2
 Pneumococcus NEC 041.2
 postoperative wound 998.59
 posttraumatic NEC 958.3
 postvaccinal 999.3
 prepuce NEC 607.1
 Proprionibacterium 041.84
 prostate (capsule) (*see also* Prostatitis) 601.9
 Proteus (mirabilis) (morganii) (vulgaris) NEC 041.6
  enteritis 008.3
 protozoal NEC 136.8
  intestinal NEC 007.9
 Pseudomonas NEC 041.7
  mallei 024
  pneumonia 482.1
  pseudomallei 025
 psittacosis 073.9
 puerperal, postpartum (major) 670.0 ☑
  minor 646.6 ☑
 pulmonary — *see* Infection, lung
 purulent — *see* Abscess
 putrid, generalized — *see* Septicemia
 pyemic — *see* Septicemia
 Pyrenochaeta romeroi 117.4
 Q fever 083.0
 rabies 071
 rectum (sphincter) 569.49
 renal (*see also* Infection, kidney) 590.9
  pelvis and ureter 590.3
 resistant to drugs — *see* Resistance (to), drugs by microorganisms
 respiratory 519.8
  chronic 519.8
  influenzal (acute) (upper) 487.1
  lung 518.89
  rhinovirus 460
  syncytial virus 079.6
  upper (acute) (infectious) NEC 465.9
   with flu, grippe, or influenza 487.1
   influenzal 487.1
   multiple sites NEC 465.8
   streptococcal 034.0
   viral NEC 465.9
 respiratory syncytial virus (RSV) 079.6
 resulting from presence of shunt or other internal prosthetic device — *see* Complications, infection and inflammation, due to (presence of) any device, implant, or graft classified to 996.0-996.5 NEC
 retrovirus 079.50
  human immunodeficiency virus type 2 [HIV 2] 079.53
  human T-cell lymphotrophic virus type I [HTLV-I] 079.51
  human T-cell lymphotrophic virus type II [HTLV-II] 079.52
  specified NEC 079.59
 Rhinocladium 117.1
 Rhinosporidium (*seeberi*) 117.0
 rhinovirus
  in diseases classified elsewhere — *see* category 079 ☑
  unspecified nature or site 079.3
 Rhizopus 117.7
 rickettsial 083.9
 rickettsialpox 083.2
 rubella (*see also* Rubella) 056.9
  congenital 771.0
 Saccharomyces (*see also* Candidiasis) 112.9
 Saksenaea 117.7
 salivary duct or gland (any) 527.2

Infection, infected, infective — *continued*
 Salmonella (aertrycke) (callinarum) (choleraesuis) (enteritidis) (suipestifer) (typhimurium) 003.9
  with
   arthritis 003.23
   gastroenteritis 003.0
   localized infection 003.20
    specified type NEC 003.29
   meningitis 003.21
   osteomyelitis 003.24
   pneumonia 003.22
   septicemia 003.1
   specified manifestation NEC 003.8
  due to food (poisoning) (any serotype) (*see also* Poisoning, food, due to, Salmonella)
  hirschfeldii 002.3
  localized 003.20
   specified type NEC 003.29
  paratyphi 002.9
   A 002.1
   B 002.2
   C 002.3
  schottmuelleri 002.2
  specified type NEC 003.8
  typhi 002.0
  typhosa 002.0
 saprophytic 136.8
 Sarcocystis, lindemanni 136.5
 SARS-associated coronavirus 079.82
 scabies 133.0
 Schistosoma — *see* Infestation, Schistosoma
 Schmorl's bacillus 040.3
 scratch or other superficial injury — *see* Injury, superficial, by site
 scrotum (acute) NEC 608.4
 secondary, burn or open wound (dislocation) (fracture) 958.3
 seminal vesicle (*see also* Vesiculitis) 608.0
 septic
  generalized — *see* Septicemia
  localized, skin (*see also* Abscess) 682.9
 septicemic — *see* Septicemia
 seroma 998.51
 Serratia (marcescens) 041.85
  generalized 038.44
 sheep liver fluke 121.3
 Shigella 004.9
  boydii 004.2
  dysenteriae 004.0
  flexneri 004.1
  group
   A 004.0
   B 004.1
   C 004.2
   D 004.3
  Schmitz (-Stutzer) 004.0
  schmitzii 004.0
  shiga 004.0
  sonnei 004.3
  specified type NEC 004.8
 Sin Nombre virus 079.81
 sinus (*see also* Sinusitis) 473.9
  pilonidal 685.1
   with abscess 685.0
  skin NEC 686.9
 Skene's duct or gland (*see also* Urethritis) 597.89
 skin (local) (staphylococcal) (streptococcal) NEC 686.9
  abscess — *see* Abscess, by site
  cellulitis — *see* Cellulitis, by site
  due to fungus 111.9
   specified type NEC 111.8
  mycotic 111.9
   specified type NEC 111.8
  ulcer (*see also* Ulcer, skin) 707.9
 slow virus 046.9
  specified condition NEC 046.8
 Sparganum (mansoni) (proliferum) 123.5
 spermatic cord NEC 608.4
 sphenoidal (chronic) (sinus) (*see also* Sinusitis, sphenoidal 473.3)
 Spherophorus necrophorus 040.3

Infection, infected, infective

Infection, infected, infective — *continued*
  spinal cord NEC (*see also* Encephalitis) 323.9
    abscess 324.1
      late effect — *see* category 326
    late effect — *see* category 326
    meninges — *see* Meningitis
    streptococcal 320.2
  Spirillum
    minus or minor 026.0
    morsus muris 026.0
    obermeieri 087.0
  spirochetal NEC 104.9
    lung 104.8
    specified nature or site NEC 104.8
  spleen 289.59
  Sporothrix schenckii 117.1
  Sporotrichum (schenckii) 117.1
  Sporozoa 136.8
  staphylococcal NEC 041.10
    aureus 041.11
    food poisoning 005.0
    generalized (purulent) 038.10
      aureus 038.11
      specified organism NEC 038.19
    pneumonia 482.40
      aureus 482.41
      specified type NEC 482.49
    septicemia 038.10
      aureus 038.11
      specified organism NEC 038.19
    specified NEC 041.19
  steatoma 706.2
  Stellantchasmus falcatus 121.6
  Streptobacillus moniliformis 026.1
  streptococcal NEC 041.00
    generalized (purulent) 038.0
    Group
      A 041.01
      B 041.02
      C 041.03
      D [enterococcus] 041.04
      G 041.05
    pneumonia — *see* Pneumonia, streptococcal
      482.3 ☑
    septicemia 038.0
    sore throat 034.0
    specified NEC 041.09
  Streptomyces — *see* Actinomycosis
  streptotrichosis — *see* Actinomycosis
  Strongyloides (stercoralis) 127.2
  stump (amputation) (posttraumatic) (surgical)
      997.62
    traumatic — *see* Amputation, traumatic, by
        site, complicated
  subcutaneous tissue, local NEC 686.9
  submaxillary region 528.9
  suipestifer (*see also* Infection, Salmonella)
      003.9
  swimming pool bacillus 031.1
  syphilitic — *see* Syphilis
  systemic — *see* Septicemia
  Taenia — *see* Infestation, Taenia
  Taeniarhynchus saginatus 123.2
  tapeworm — *see* Infestation, tapeworm
  tendon (sheath) 727.89
  Ternidens diminutus 127.7
  testis (*see also* Orchitis) 604.90
  thigh (skin) 686.9
  threadworm 127.4
  throat 478.29
    pneumococcal 462
    staphylococcal 462
    streptococcal 034.0
    viral NEC (*see also* Pharyngitis) 462
  thumb (skin) 686.9
    abscess (with lymphangitis) 681.00
      pulp 681.01
    cellulitis (with lymphangitis) 681.00
    nail 681.02
  thyroglossal duct 529.8
  toe (skin) 686.9
    abscess (with lymphangitis) 681.10
    cellulitis (with lymphangitis) 681.10
    nail 681.11
      fungus 110.1
  tongue NEC 529.0
    parasitic 112.0

Infection, infected, infective — *continued*
  tonsil (faucial) (lingual) (pharyngeal) 474.00
    acute or subacute 463
    and adenoid 474.02
    tag 474.00
  tooth, teeth 522.4
    periapical (pulpal origin) 522.4
    peridental 523.3
    periodontal 523.3
    pulp 522.0
    socket 526.5
  Torula histolytica 117.5
  Toxocara (cani) (cati) (felis) 128.0
  Toxoplasma gondii (*see also* Toxoplasmosis)
      130.9
  trachea, chronic 491.8
    fungus 117.9
  traumatic NEC 958.3
  trematode NEC 121.9
  trench fever 083.1
  Treponema
    denticola 041.84
    macrodenticum 041.84
    pallidum (*see also* Syphillis) 097.9
  Trichinella (spiralis) 124
  Trichomonas 131.9
    bladder 131.09
    cervix 131.09
    hominis 007.3
    intestine 007.3
    prostate 131.03
    specified site NEC 131.8
    urethra 131.02
    urogenitalis 131.00
    vagina 131.01
    vulva 131.01
  Trichophyton, trichophytid — *see*
      Dermatophytosis
  Trichosporon (beigelii) cutaneum 111.2
  Trichostrongylus 127.6
  Trichuris (trichiuria) 127.3
  Trombicula (irritans) 133.8
  Trypanosoma (*see also* Trypanosomiasis) 086.9
    cruzi 086.2
  tubal (*see also* Salpingo-oophoritis) 614.2
  tuberculous NEC (*see also* Tuberculosis)
      011.9 ☑
  tubo-ovarian (*see also* Salpingo-oophoritis)
      614.2
  tunica vaginalis 608.4
  tympanic membrane — *see* Myringitis
  typhoid (abortive) (ambulant) (bacillus) 002.0
  typhus 081.9
    flea-borne (endemic) 081.0
    louse-borne (epidemic) 080
    mite-borne 081.2
    recrudescent 081.1
    tick-borne 082.9
      African 082.1
      North Asian 082.2
  umbilicus (septic) 686.9
    newborn NEC 771.4
  ureter 593.89
  urethra (*see also* Urethritis) 597.80
  urinary (tract) NEC 599.0
    with
      abortion — *see* Abortion, by type, with
          urinary tract infection
      ectopic pregnancy (*see also* categories
          633.0-633.9) 639.8
      molar pregnancy (*see also* categories 630-
          632) 639.8
    candidal 112.2
    complicating pregnancy, childbirth, or
        puerperium 646.6 ☑
      affecting fetus or newborn 760.1
      asymptomatic 646.5 ☑
        affecting fetus or newborn 760.1
    diplococcal (acute) 098.0
      chronic 098.2
    due to Trichomonas (vaginalis) 131.00
    following
      abortion 639.8
      ectopic or molar pregnancy 639.8
    gonococcal (acute) 098.0
      chronic or duration of 2 months or
          over 098.2

Infection, infected, infective — *continued*
  urinary — *continued*
    newborn 771.82
    trichomonal 131.00
    tuberculous (*see also* Tuberculosis) 016.3 ☑
    uterus, uterine (*see also* Endometritis) 615.9
    utriculus masculinus NEC 597.89
    vaccination 999.3
    vagina (granulation tissue) (wall) (*see also*
        Vaginitis) 616.10
    varicella 052.9
    varicose veins — *see* Varicose, veins
    variola 050.9
      major 050.0
      minor 050.1
    vas deferens NEC 608.4
    Veillonella 041.84
    verumontanum 597.89
    vesical (*see also* Cystitis) 595.9
    Vibrio
      cholerae 001.0
        El Tor 001.1
      parahaemolyticus (food poisoning) 005.4
      vulnificus 041.85
    Vincent's (gums) (mouth) (tonsil) 101
  virus, viral 079.99
    adenovirus
      in diseases classified elsewhere — *see*
          category 079 ☑
      unspecified nature or site 079.0
    central nervous system NEC 049.9
      enterovirus 048
        meningitis 047.9
          specified type NEC 047.8
        slow virus 046.9
          specified condition NEC 046.8
    chest 519.8
    conjunctivitis 077.99
      specified type NEC 077.8
    coronavirus 079.89
      SARS-associated 079.82
    Coxsackie (*see also* Infection, Coxsackie)
        079.2
    Ebola 065.8
    ECHO
      in diseases classified elsewhere — *see*
          category 079 ☑
      unspecified nature or site 079.1
    encephalitis 049.9
      arthropod-borne NEC 064
      tick-borne 063.9
        specified type NEC 063.8
    enteritis NEC (*see also* Enteritis, viral) 008.8
    exanthem NEC 057.9
    Hantavirus 079.81
    human papilloma 079.4
    in diseases classified elsewhere — *see*
        category 079 ☑
    intestine (*see also* Enteritis, viral) 008.8
    lung — *see* Pneumonia, viral
    respiratory syncytial (RSV) 079.6
    retrovirus 079.50
    rhinovirus
      in diseases classified elsewhere — *see*
          category 079 ☑
      unspecified nature or site 079.3
    salivary gland disease 078.5
    slow 046.9
      specified condition NEC 046.8
    specified type NEC 079.89
      in diseases classified elsewhere — *see*
          category 079 ☑
    unspecified nature or site 079.99
    warts NEC 078.10
  vulva (*see also* Vulvitis) 616.10
  whipworm 127.3
  Whitmore's bacillus 025
  wound (local) (posttraumatic) NEC 958.3
    with
      dislocation — *see* Dislocation, by site,
          open
      fracture — *see* Fracture, by site, open
      open wound — *see* Wound, open, by site,
          complicated
    postoperative 998.59
    surgical 998.59

☑ Additional Digit Required   ▶◀ Revised Text   ● New Line   ▲ Revised Code

Infection, infected, infective — *continued*
  Wuchereria 125.0
    bancrofti 125.0
    malayi 125.1
  yaws — *see* Yaws
  yeast (*see also* Candidiasis) 112.9
  yellow fever (*see also* Fever, yellow) 060.9
  Yersinia pestis (*see also* Plague) 020.9
  Zeis' gland 373.12
  zoonotic bacterial NEC 027.9
  Zopfia senegalensis 117.4
Infective, infectious — *see* condition
Inferiority complex 301.9
  constitutional psychopathic 301.9
Infertility
  female 628.9
    associated with
      adhesions, peritubal 614.6 *[628.2]*
      anomaly
        cervical mucus 628.4
        congenital
          cervix 628.4
          fallopian tube 628.2
          uterus 628.3
          vagina 628.4
      anovulation 628.0
      dysmucorrhea 628.4
      endometritis, tuberculous (*see also*
        Tuberculosis) 016.7 ☑ *[628.3]*
      Stein-Leventhal syndrome 256.4 *[628.0]*
    due to
      adiposogenital dystrophy 253.8 *[628.1]*
      anterior pituitary disorder NEC
        253.4 *[628.1]*
        hyperfunction 253.1 *[628.1]*
      cervical anomaly 628.4
      fallopian tube anomaly 628.2
      ovarian failure 256.39 *[628.0]*
      Stein-Leventhal syndrome 256.4 *[628.0]*
      uterine anomaly 628.3
      vaginal anomaly 628.4
    nonimplantation 628.3
    origin
      cervical 628.4
      pituitary-hypothalamus NEC
        253.8 *[628.1]*
        anterior pituitary NEC 253.4 *[628.1]*
          hyperfunction NEC 253.1 *[628.1]*
        dwarfism 253.3 *[628.1]*
        panhypopituitarism 253.2 *[628.1]*
      specified NEC 628.8
    tubal (block) (occlusion) (stenosis) 628.2
      adhesions 614.6 *[628.2]*
    uterine 628.3
    vaginal 628.4
    previous, requiring supervision of pregnancy
      V23.0
  male 606.9
    absolute 606.0
    due to
      azoospermia 606.0
      drug therapy 606.8
      extratesticular cause NEC 606.8
      germinal cell
        aplasia 606.0
        desquamation 606.1
      hypospermatogenesis 606.1
      infection 606.8
      obstruction, afferent ducts 606.8
      oligospermia 606.1
      radiation 606.8
      spermatogenic arrest (complete) 606.0
        incomplete 606.1
      systemic disease 606.8
Infestation 134.9
  Acanthocheilonema (perstans) 125.4
    streptocerca 125.6
  Acariasis 133.9
    demodex folliculorum 133.8
    Sarcoptes scabiei 133.0
    trombiculae 133.8
  Agamofilaria streptocerca 125.6
  Ancylostoma, Ankylostoma 126.9
    americanum 126.1
    braziliense 126.2
    canium 126.8

Infestation — *continued*
  Ancylostoma, Ankylostoma — *continued*
    ceylanicum 126.3
    duodenale 126.0
    new world 126.1
    old world 126.0
  Angiostrongylus cantonensis 128.8
  anisakiasis 127.1
  Anisakis larva 127.1
  arthropod NEC 134.1
  Ascaris lumbricoides 127.0
  Bacillus fusiformis 101
  Balantidium coli 007.0
  beef tapeworm 123.2
  Bothriocephalus (latus) 123.4
    larval 123.5
  broad tapeworm 123.4
    larval 123.5
  Brugia malayi 125.1
  Candiru 136.8
  Capillaria
    hepatica 128.8
    philippinensis 127.5
  cat liver fluke 121.0
  Cercomonas hominis (intestinal) 007.3
  cestodes 123.9
    specified type NEC 123.8
  chigger 133.8
  chigoe 134.1
  Chilomastix 007.8
  Clonorchis (sinensis) (liver) 121.1
  coccidia 007.2
  complicating pregnancy, childbirth, or
    puerperium 647.9 ☑
    affecting fetus or newborn 760.8
  Cysticercus cellulosae 123.1
  Demodex folliculorum 133.8
  Dermatobia (hominis) 134.0
  Dibothriocephalus (latus) 123.4
    larval 123.5
  Dicrocoelium dendriticum 121.8
  Diphyllobothrium (adult) (intestinal) (latum)
    (pacificum) 123.4
    larval 123.5
  Diplogonoporus (grandis) 123.8
  Dipylidium (caninum) 123.8
  Distoma hepaticum 121.3
  dog tapeworm 123.8
  Dracunculus medinensis 125.7
  dragon worm 125.7
  dwarf tapeworm 123.6
  Echinococcus (*see also* Echinococcus) 122.9
  Echinostoma ilocanum 121.8
  Embadomonas 007.8
  Endamoeba (histolytica) — *see* Infection,
    ameba
  Entamoeba (histolytica) — *see* Infection, ameba
  Enterobius vermicularis 127.4
  Epidermophyton — *see* Dermatophytosis
  eyeworm 125.2
  Fasciola
    gigantica 121.3
    hepatica 121.3
  Fasciolopsis (buski) (small intestine) 121.4
    filarial 125.9
      due to
        Acanthocheilonema (perstans) 125.4
          streptocerca 125.6
        Brugia (Wuchereria) malayi 125.1
        Dracunculus medinensis 125.7
        guinea worms 125.7
        Mansonella (ozzardi) 125.5
        Onchocerca volvulus 125.3
          eye 125.3 *[360.13]*
          eyelid 125.3 *[373.6]*
        Wuchereria (bancrofti) 125.0
          malayi 125.1
      specified type NEC 125.6
    fish tapeworm 123.4
      larval 123.5
    fluke 121.9
    blood NEC (*see also* Schistosomiasis) 120.9
    cat liver 121.0
    intestinal (giant) 121.4
    liver (sheep) 121.3
      cat 121.0
      Chinese 121.1

Infestation — *continued*
  Fasciolopsis — *continued*
    liver — *continued*
      clonorchiasis 121.1
      fascioliasis 121.3
      Oriental 121.1
    lung (oriental) 121.2
    sheep liver 121.3
  fly larva 134.0
  Gasterophilus (intestinalis) 134.0
  Gastrodiscoides hominis 121.8
  Giardia lamblia 007.1
  Gnathostoma (spinigerum) 128.1
  Gongylonema 125.6
  guinea worm 125.7
  helminth NEC 128.9
    intestinal 127.9
      mixed (types classifiable to more than one
        category in 120.0-127.7) 127.8
      specified type NEC 127.7
    specified type NEC 128.8
  Heterophyes heterophyes (small intestine)
    121.6
  hookworm (*see also* Infestation, ancylostoma)
    126.9
  Hymenolepis (diminuta) (nana) 123.6
  intestinal NEC 129
  leeches (aquatic) (land) 134.2
  Leishmania — *see* Leishmaniasis
  lice (*see also* Infestation, pediculus) 132.9
  Linguatulidae, linguatula (pentastoma) (serrata)
    134.1
  Loa loa 125.2
    eyelid 125.2 *[373.6]*
  louse (*see also* Infestation, pediculus) 132.9
    body 132.1
    head 132.0
    pubic 132.2
  maggots 134.0
  Mansonella (ozzardi) 125.5
  medina 125.7
  Metagonimus yokogawai (small intestine) 121.5
  Microfilaria streptocerca 125.3
    eye 125.3 *[360.13]*
    eyelid 125.3 *[373.6]*
  Microsporon furfur 111.0
  microsporum — *see* Dermatophytosis
  mites 133.9
    scabic 133.0
    specified type NEC 133.8
  Monilia (albicans) (*see also* Candidiasis) 112.9
    vagina 112.1
    vulva 112.1
  mouth 112.0
  Necator americanus 126.1
  nematode (intestinal) 127.9
    Ancylostoma (*see also* Ancylostoma) 126.9
    Ascaris lumbricoides 127.0
    conjunctiva NEC 128.9
    Dioctophyma 128.8
    Enterobius vermicularis 127.4
    Gnathostoma spinigerum 128.1
    Oesophagostomum (apiostomum) 127.7
    Physaloptera 127.4
    specified type NEC 127.7
    Strongyloides stercoralis 127.2
    Ternidens diminutus 127.7
    Trichinella spiralis 124
    Trichostrongylus 127.6
    Trichuris (trichiuria) 127.3
  Oesophagostomum (apiostomum) 127.7
  Oestrus ovis 134.0
  Onchocerca (volvulus) 125.3
    eye 125.3 *[360.13]*
    eyelid 125.3 *[373.6]*
  Opisthorchis (felineus) (tenuicollis) (viverrini)
    121.0
  Oxyuris vermicularis 127.4
  Paragonimus (westermani) 121.2
  parasite, parasitic NEC 136.9
    eyelid 134.9 *[373.6]*
    intestinal 129
    mouth 112.0
    orbit 376.13
    skin 134.9
    tongue 112.0

☑ Additional Digit Required   ▶◀ Revised Text   ● New Line   ▲ Revised Code

Infestation — *continued*
- pediculus 132.9
  - capitis (humanus) (any site) 132.0
  - corporis (humanus) (any site) 132.1
  - eyelid 132.0 *[373.6]*
  - mixed (classifiable to more than one category in 132.0-132.2) 132.3
  - pubis (any site) 132.2
- phthirus (pubis) (any site) 132.2
  - with any infestation classifiable to 132.0, 132.1 and 132.3
- pinworm 127.4
- pork tapeworm (adult) 123.0
- protozoal NEC 136.8
- pubic louse 132.2
- rat tapeworm 123.6
- red bug 133.8
- roundworm (large) NEC 127.0
- sand flea 134.1
- saprophytic NEC 136.8
- Sarcoptes scabiei 133.0
- scabies 133.0
- Schistosoma 120.9
  - bovis 120.8
  - cercariae 120.3
  - hematobium 120.0
  - intercalatum 120.8
  - japonicum 120.2
  - mansoni 120.1
  - mattheii 120.8
  - specified
    - site — *see* Schistosomiasis
    - type NEC 120.8
  - spindale 120.8
- screw worms 134.0
- skin NEC 134.9
- Sparganum (mansoni) (proliferum) 123.5
  - larval 123.5
- specified type NEC 134.8
- Spirometra larvae 123.5
- Sporozoa NEC 136.8
- Stellantchasmus falcatus 121.6
- Strongyloides 127.2
- Strongylus (gibsoni) 127.7
- Taenia 123.3
  - diminuta 123.6
  - Echinococcus (*see also* Echinococcus) 122.9
  - mediocanellata 123.2
  - nana 123.6
  - saginata (mediocanellata) 123.2
  - solium (intestinal form) 123.0
    - larval form 123.1
- Taeniarhynchus saginatus 123.2
- tapeworm 123.9
  - beef 123.2
  - broad 123.4
    - larval 123.5
  - dog 123.8
  - dwarf 123.6
  - fish 123.4
    - larval 123.5
  - pork 123.0
  - rat 123.6
- Ternidens diminutus 127.7
- Tetranychus molestissimus 133.8
- threadworm 127.4
- tongue 112.0
- Toxocara (cani) (cati) (felis) 128.0
- trematode(s) NEC 121.9
- Trichina spiralis 124
- Trichinella spiralis 124
- Trichocephalus 127.3
- Trichomonas 131.9
  - bladder 131.09
  - cervix 131.09
  - intestine 007.3
  - prostate 131.03
  - specified site NEC 131.8
  - urethra (female) (male) 131.02
  - urogenital 131.00
  - vagina 131.01
  - vulva 131.01
- Trichophyton — *see* Dermatophytosis
- Trichostrongylus instabilis 127.6
- Trichuris (trichiuria) 127.3
- Trombicula (irritans) 133.8

Infestation — *continued*
- Trypanosoma — *see* Trypanosomiasis
- Tunga penetrans 134.1
- Uncinaria americana 126.1
- whipworm 127.3
- worms NEC 128.9
  - intestinal 127.9
- Wuchereria 125.0
  - bancrofti 125.0
  - malayi 125.1

Infiltrate, infiltration
- with an iron compound 275.0
- amyloid (any site) (generalized) 277.3
- calcareous (muscle) NEC 275.49
  - localized — *see* Degeneration, by site
- calcium salt (muscle) 275.49
- corneal (*see also* Edema, cornea) 371.20
- eyelid 373.9
- fatty (diffuse) (generalized) 272.8
  - localized — *see* Degeneration, by site, fatty
- glycogen, glycogenic (*see also* Disease, glycogen storage) 271.0
- heart, cardiac
  - fatty (*see also* Degeneration, myocardial) 429.1
  - glycogenic 271.0 *[425.7]*
- inflammatory in vitreous 379.29
- kidney (*see also* Disease, renal) 593.9
- leukemic (M9800/3) — *see* Leukemia
- liver 573.8
  - fatty — *see* Fatty, liver
  - glycogen (*see also* Disease, glycogen storage) 271.0
- lung (*see also* Infiltrate, pulmonary) 518.3
  - eosinophilic 518.3
  - x-ray finding only 793.1
- lymphatic (*see also* Leukemia, lymphatic) 204.9 ☑
  - gland, pigmentary 289.3
- muscle, fatty 728.9
- myelogenous (*see also* Leukemia, myeloid) 205.9 ☑
- myocardium, myocardial
  - fatty (*see also* Degeneration, myocardial) 429.1
  - glycogenic 271.0 *[425.7]*
- pulmonary 518.3
  - with
    - eosinophilia 518.3
    - pneumonia — *see* Pneumonia, by type
  - x-ray finding only 793.1
- Ranke's primary (*see also* Tuberculosis) 010.0 ☑
- skin, lymphocytic (benign) 709.8
- thymus (gland) (fatty) 254.8
- urine 788.8
- vitreous humor 379.29

Infirmity 799.89
- senile 797

Inflammation, inflamed, inflammatory (with exudation)
- abducens (nerve) 378.54
- accessory sinus (chronic) (*see also* Sinusitis) 473.9
- adrenal (gland) 255.8
- alimentary canal — *see* Enteritis
- alveoli (teeth) 526.5
  - scorbutic 267
- amnion — *see* Amnionitis
- anal canal 569.49
- antrum (chronic) (*see also* Sinusitis, maxillary) 473.0
- anus 569.49
- appendix (*see also* Appendicitis) 541
- arachnoid — *see* Meningitis
- areola 611.0
  - puerperal, postpartum 675.0 ☑
- areolar tissue NEC 686.9
- artery — *see* Arteritis
- auditory meatus (external) (*see also* Otitis, externa) 380.10
- Bartholin's gland 616.8
- bile duct or passage 576.1
- bladder (*see also* Cystitis) 595.9
- bone — *see* Osteomyelitis
- bowel (*see also* Enteritis) 558.9

Inflammation, inflamed, inflammatory — *continued*
- brain (*see also* Encephalitis) 323.9
  - late effect — *see* category 326
  - membrane — *see* Meningitis
- breast 611.0
  - puerperal, postpartum 675.2 ☑
- broad ligament (*see also* Disease, pelvis, inflammatory) 614.4
  - acute 614.3
- bronchus — *see* Bronchitis
- bursa — *see* Bursitis
- capsule
  - liver 573.3
  - spleen 289.59
- catarrhal (*see also* Catarrh) 460
  - vagina 616.10
- cecum (*see also* Appendicitis) 541
- cerebral (*see also* Encephalitis) 323.9
  - late effect — *see* category 326
  - membrane — *see* Meningitis
- cerebrospinal (*see also* Meningitis) 322.9
  - late effect — *see* category 326
  - meningococcal 036.0
  - tuberculous (*see also* Tuberculosis) 013.6 ☑
- cervix (uteri) (*see also* Cervicitis) 616.0
- chest 519.9
- choroid NEC (*see also* Choroiditis) 363.20
- cicatrix (tissue) — *see* Cicatrix
- colon (*see also* Enteritis) 558.9
  - granulomatous 555.1
  - newborn 558.9
- connective tissue (diffuse) NEC 728.9
- cornea (*see also* Keratitis) 370.9
  - with ulcer (*see also* Ulcer, cornea) 370.00
- corpora cavernosa (penis) 607.2
- cranial nerve — *see* Disorder, nerve, cranial
- diarrhea — *see* Diarrhea
- disc (intervertebral) (space) 722.90
  - cervical, cervicothoracic 722.91
  - lumbar, lumbosacral 722.93
  - thoracic, thoracolumbar 722.92
- Douglas' cul-de-sac or pouch (chronic) (*see also* Disease, pelvis, inflammatory) 614.4
  - acute 614.3
- due to (presence of) any device, implant, or graft classifiable to 996.0-996.5 — *see* Complications, infection and inflammation, due to (presence of) any device, implant, or graft classified to 996.0-996.5 NEC
- duodenum 535.6 ☑
- dura mater — *see* Meningitis
- ear — *see also* Otitis
  - external (*see also* Otitis, externa) 380.10
  - inner (*see also* Labyrinthitis) 386.30
  - middle — *see* Otitis media
- esophagus 530.10
- ethmoidal (chronic) (sinus) (*see also* Sinusitis, ethmoidal) 473.2
- Eustachian tube (catarrhal) 381.50
  - acute 381.51
  - chronic 381.52
- extrarectal 569.49
- eye 379.99
- eyelid 373.9
  - specified NEC 373.8
- fallopian tube (*see also* Salpingo-oophoritis) 614.2
- fascia 728.9
- fetal membranes (acute) 658.4 ☑
  - affecting fetus or newborn 762.7
- follicular, pharynx 472.1
- frontal (chronic) (sinus) (*see also* Sinusitis, frontal) 473.1
- gallbladder (*see also* Cholecystitis, acute) 575.0
- gall duct (*see also* Cholecystitis) 575.10
- gastrointestinal (*see also* Enteritis) 558.9
- genital organ (diffuse) (internal)
  - female 614.9
    - with
      - abortion — *see* Abortion, by type, with sepsis
      - ectopic pregnancy (*see also* categories 633.0-633.9) 639.0
      - molar pregnancy (*see also* categories 630-632) 639.0

Inflammation, inflamed, inflammatory —
continued
  genital organ — *continued*
    female — *continued*
      complicating pregnancy, childbirth, or
          puerperium 646.6 ☑
        affecting fetus or newborn 760.8
      following
        abortion 639.0
        ectopic or molar pregnancy 639.0
    male 608.4
  gland (lymph) (*see also* Lymphadenitis) 289.3
  glottis (*see also* Laryngitis) 464.00
    with obstruction 464.01
  granular, pharynx 472.1
  gum 523.1
  heart (*see also* Carditis) 429.89
  hepatic duct 576.8
  hernial sac — *see* Hernia, by site
  ileum (*see also* Enteritis) 558.9
    terminal or regional 555.0
      with large intestine 555.2
  intervertebral disc 722.90
    cervical, cervicothoracic 722.91
    lumbar, lumbosacral 722.93
    thoracic, thoracolumbar 722.92
  intestine (*see also* Enteritis) 558.9
  jaw (acute) (bone) (chronic) (lower) (suppurative)
    (upper) 526.4
  jejunum — *see* Enteritis
  joint NEC (*see also* Arthritis) 716.9 ☑
    sacroiliac 720.2
  kidney (*see also* Nephritis) 583.9
  knee (joint) 716.66
    tuberculous (active) (*see also* Tuberculosis)
      015.2 ☑
  labium (majus) (minus) (*see also* Vulvitis)
    616.10
  lacrimal
    gland (*see also* Dacryoadenitis) 375.00
    passages (duct) (sac) (*see also*
      Dacryocystitis) 375.30
  larynx (*see also* Laryngitis) 464.00
    with obstruction 464.01
    diphtheritic 032.3
  leg NEC 686.9
  lip 528.5
  liver (capsule) (*see also* Hepatitis) 573.3
    acute 570
    chronic 571.40
    suppurative 572.0
  lung (acute) (*see also* Pneumonia) 486
    chronic (interstitial) 518.89
  lymphatic vessel (*see also* Lymphangitis) 457.2
  lymph node or gland (*see also* Lymphadenitis)
    289.3
  mammary gland 611.0
    puerperal, postpartum 675.2 ☑
  maxilla, maxillary 526.4
    sinus (chronic) (*see also* Sinusitis, maxillary)
      473.0
  membranes of brain or spinal cord — *see*
    Meningitis
  meninges — *see* Meningitis
  mouth 528.0
  muscle 728.9
  myocardium (*see also* Myocarditis) 429.0
  nasal sinus (chronic) (*see also* Sinusitis) 473.9
  nasopharynx — *see* Nasopharyngitis
  navel 686.9
    newborn NEC 771.4
  nerve NEC 729.2
  nipple 611.0
    puerperal, postpartum 675.0 ☑
  nose 478.1
    suppurative 472.0
  oculomotor nerve 378.51
  optic nerve 377.30
  orbit (chronic) 376.10
    acute 376.00
    chronic 376.10
  ovary (*see also* Salpingo-oophoritis) 614.2
  oviduct (*see also* Salpingo-oophoritis) 614.2
  pancreas — *see* Pancreatitis
  parametrium (chronic) (*see also* Disease, pelvis,
    inflammatory) 614.4
    acute 614.3

Inflammation, inflamed, inflammatory —
continued
  parotid region 686.9
    gland 527.2
  pelvis, female (*see also* Disease, pelvis,
    inflammatory) 614.9
  penis (corpora cavernosa) 607.2
  perianal 569.49
  pericardium (*see also* Pericarditis) 423.9
  perineum (female) (male) 686.9
  perirectal 569.49
  peritoneum (*see also* Peritonitis) 567.9
  periuterine (*see also* Disease, pelvis,
    inflammatory) 614.9
  perivesical (*see also* Cystitis) 595.9
  petrous bone (*see also* Petrositis) 383.20
  pharynx (*see also* Pharyngitis) 462
    follicular 472.1
    granular 472.1
  pia mater — *see* Meningitis
  pleura — *see* Pleurisy
  postmastoidectomy cavity 383.30
    chronic 383.33
  prostate (*see also* Prostatitis) 601.9
  rectosigmoid — *see* Rectosigmoiditis
  rectum (*see also* Proctitis) 569.49
  respiratory, upper (*see also* Infection,
    respiratory, upper) 465.9
    chronic, due to external agent — *see*
      Condition, respiratory, chronic, due to,
      external agent
    due to
      fumes or vapors (chemical) (inhalation)
        506.2
      radiation 508.1
  retina (*see also* Retinitis) 363.20
  retrocecal (*see also* Appendicitis) 541
  retroperitoneal (*see also* Peritonitis) 567.9
  salivary duct or gland (any) (suppurative) 527.2
  scorbutic, alveoli, teeth 267
  scrotum 608.4
  sigmoid — *see* Enteritis
  sinus (*see also* Sinusitis) 473.9
  Skene's duct or gland (*see also* Urethritis)
    597.89
  skin 686.9
  spermatic cord 608.4
  sphenoidal (sinus) (*see also* Sinusitis,
    sphenoidal) 473.3
  spinal
    cord (*see also* Encephalitis) 323.9
      late effect — *see* category 326
    membrane — *see* Meningitis
    nerve — *see* Disorder, nerve
  spine (*see also* Spondylitis) 720.9
  spleen (capsule) 289.59
  stomach — *see* Gastritis
  stricture, rectum 569.49
  subcutaneous tissue NEC 686.9
  suprarenal (gland) 255.8
  synovial (fringe) (membrane) — *see* Bursitis
  tendon (sheath) NEC 726.90
  testis (*see also* Orchitis) 604.90
  thigh 686.9
  throat (*see also* Sore throat) 462
  thymus (gland) 254.8
  thyroid (gland) (*see also* Thyroiditis) 245.9
  tongue 529.0
  tonsil — *see* Tonsillitis
  trachea — *see* Tracheitis
  trochlear nerve 378.53
  tubal (*see also* Salpingo-oophoritis) 614.2
  tuberculous NEC (*see also* Tuberculosis)
    011.9 ☑
  tubo-ovarian (*see also* Salpingo-oophoritis)
    614.2
  tunica vaginalis 608.4
  tympanic membrane — *see* Myringitis
  umbilicus, umbilical 686.9
    newborn NEC 771.4
  uterine ligament (*see also* Disease, pelvis,
    inflammatory) 614.4
    acute 614.3
  uterus (catarrhal) (*see also* Endometritis) 615.9
  uveal tract (anterior) (*see also* Iridocyclitis)
    364.3
    posterior — *see* Chorioretinitis

Inflammation, inflamed, inflammatory —
continued
  uveal tract (*see also* Iridocyclitis) — *continued*
    sympathetic 360.11
  vagina (*see also* Vaginitis) 616.10
  vas deferens 608.4
  vein (*see also* Phlebitis) 451.9
    thrombotic 451.9
      cerebral (*see also* Thrombosis, brain)
        434.0 ☑
      leg 451.2
        deep (vessels) NEC 451.19
        superficial (vessels) 451.0
      lower extremity 451.2
        deep (vessels) NEC 451.19
        superficial (vessels) 451.0
  vocal cord 478.5
  vulva (*see also* Vulvitis) 616.10
Inflation, lung imperfect (newborn) 770.5
Influenza, influenzal 487.1
  with
    bronchitis 487.1
    bronchopneumonia 487.0
    cold (any type) 487.1
    digestive manifestations 487.8
    hemoptysis 487.1
    involvement of
      gastrointestinal tract 487.8
      nervous system 487.8
    laryngitis 487.1
    manifestations NEC 487.8
      respiratory 487.1
        pneumonia 487.0
    pharyngitis 487.1
    pneumonia (any form classifiable to 480-
      483, 485-486) 487.0
    respiratory manifestations NEC 487.1
    sinusitis 487.1
    sore throat 487.1
    tonsillitis 487.1
    tracheitis 487.1
    upper respiratory infection (acute) 487.1
  abdominal 487.8
  Asian 487.1
  bronchial 487.1
  bronchopneumonia 487.0
  catarrhal 487.1
  epidemic 487.1
  gastric 487.8
  intestinal 487.8
  laryngitis 487.1
  maternal affecting fetus or newborn 760.2
    manifest influenza in infant 771.2
  pharyngitis 487.1
  pneumonia (any form) 487.0
  respiratory (upper) 487.1
  stomach 487.8
  vaccination, prophylactic (against) V04.81
Influenza-like disease 487.1
Infraction, Freiberg's (metatarsal head) 732.5
Infraeruption, teeth 524.34   ●
Infusion complication, misadventure, or
    reaction — *see* Complication, infusion
Ingestion
  chemical — *see* Table of Drugs and Chemicals
  drug or medicinal substance
    overdose or wrong substance given or taken
      977.9
      specified drug — *see* Table of Drugs and
        Chemicals
  foreign body NEC (*see also* Foreign body) 938
Ingrowing
  hair 704.8
  nail (finger) (toe) (infected) 703.0
Inguinal — *see also* condition
  testis 752.51
Inhalation
  carbon monoxide 986
  flame
    mouth 947.0
    lung 947.1
  food or foreign body (*see also* Asphyxia, food or
    foreign body) 933.1
  gas, fumes, or vapor (noxious) 987.9
    specified agent — *see* Table of Drugs and
      Chemicals

☑ Additional Digit Required   ▶◀ Revised Text   ● New Line   ▲ Revised Code

Inhalation — *continued*
liquid or vomitus (*see also* Asphyxia, food or foreign body) 933.1
lower respiratory tract NEC 934.9
meconium (fetus or newborn) 770.1
mucus (*see also* Asphyxia, mucus) 933.1
oil (causing suffocation) (*see also* Asphyxia, food or foreign body) 933.1
pneumonia — *see* Pneumonia, aspiration
smoke 987.9
steam 987.9
stomach contents or secretions (*see also* Asphyxia, food or foreign body) 933.1
in labor and delivery 668.0 ☑

Inhibition, inhibited
academic as adjustment reaction 309.23
orgasm
female 302.73
male 302.74
sexual
desire 302.71
excitement 302.72
work as adjustment reaction 309.23

Inhibitor, systemic lupus erythematosus
(presence of) 286.5

Iniencephalus, iniencephaly 740.2

Injected eye 372.74

Injury 959.9

Note — For abrasion, insect bite (nonvenomous), blister, or scratch, see Injury, superficial.

For laceration, traumatic rupture, tear, or penetrating wound of internal organs, such as heart, lung, liver, kidney, pelvic organs, whether or not accompanied by open wound in the same region, see Injury, internal.

For nerve injury, see Injury, nerve.

For late effect of injuries classifiable to 850-854, 860-869, 900-919, 950-959, see Late, effect, injury, by type.

abdomen, abdominal (viscera) — *see also* Injury, internal, abdomen
muscle or wall 959.12
acoustic, resulting in deafness 951.5
adenoid 959.09
adrenal (gland) — *see* Injury, internal, adrenal
alveolar (process) 959.09
ankle (and foot) (and knee) (and leg, except thigh) 959.7
anterior chamber, eye 921.3
anus 959.19
aorta (thoracic) 901.0
abdominal 902.0
appendix — *see* Injury, internal, appendix
arm, upper (and shoulder) 959.2
artery (complicating trauma) (*see also* Injury, blood vessel, by site) 904.9
cerebral or meningeal (*see also* Hemorrhage, brain, traumatic, subarachnoid) 852.0 ☑
auditory canal (external) (meatus) 959.09
auricle, auris, ear 959.09
axilla 959.2
back 959.19
bile duct — *see* Injury, internal, bile duct
birth — *see also* Birth, injury
canal NEC, complicating delivery 665.9 ☑
bladder (sphincter) — *see* Injury, internal, bladder
blast (air) (hydraulic) (immersion) (underwater) NEC 869.0
with open wound into cavity NEC 869.1
abdomen or thorax — *see* Injury, internal, by site
brain — *see* Concussion, brain
ear (acoustic nerve trauma) 951.5
with perforation of tympanic membrane — *see* Wound, open, ear, drum
blood vessel NEC 904.9
abdomen 902.9
multiple 902.87
specified NEC 902.89
aorta (thoracic) 901.0
abdominal 902.0

Injury — *continued*
blood vessel NEC — *continued*
arm NEC 903.9
axillary 903.00
artery 903.01
vein 903.02
azygos vein 901.89
basilic vein 903.1
brachial (artery) (vein) 903.1
bronchial 901.89
carotid artery 900.00
common 900.01
external 900.02
internal 900.03
celiac artery 902.20
specified branch NEC 902.24
cephalic vein (arm) 903.1
colica dextra 902.26
cystic
artery 902.24
vein 902.39
deep plantar 904.6
digital (artery) (vein) 903.5
due to accidental puncture or laceration during procedure 998.2
extremity
lower 904.8
multiple 904.7
specified NEC 904.7
upper 903.9
multiple 903.8
specified NEC 903.8
femoral
artery (superficial) 904.1
above profunda origin 904.0
common 904.0
vein 904.2
gastric
artery 902.21
vein 902.39
head 900.9
intracranial — *see* Injury, intracranial
multiple 900.82
specified NEC 900.89
hemiazygos vein 901.89
hepatic
artery 902.22
vein 902.11
hypogastric 902.59
artery 902.51
vein 902.52
ileocolic
artery 902.26
vein 902.31
iliac 902.50
artery 902.53
specified branch NEC 902.59
vein 902.54
innominate
artery 901.1
vein 901.3
intercostal (artery) (vein) 901.81
jugular vein (external) 900.81
internal 900.1
leg NEC 904.8
mammary (artery) (vein) 901.82
mesenteric
artery 902.20
inferior 902.27
specified branch NEC 902.29
superior (trunk) 902.25
branches, primary 902.26
vein 902.39
inferior 902.32
superior (and primary subdivisions) 902.31
neck 900.9
multiple 900.82
specified NEC 900.89
ovarian 902.89
artery 902.81
vein 902.82
palmar artery 903.4
pelvis 902.9
multiple 902.87
specified NEC 902.89
plantar (deep) (artery) (vein) 904.6

Injury — *continued*
blood vessel NEC — *continued*
popliteal 904.40
artery 904.41
vein 904.42
portal 902.33
pulmonary 901.40
artery 901.41
vein 901.42
radial (artery) (vein) 903.2
renal 902.40
artery 902.41
specified NEC 902.49
vein 902.42
saphenous
artery 904.7
vein (greater) (lesser) 904.3
splenic
artery 902.23
vein 902.34
subclavian
artery 901.1
vein 901.3
suprarenal 902.49
thoracic 901.9
multiple 901.83
specified NEC 901.89
tibial 904.50
artery 904.50
anterior 904.51
posterior 904.53
vein 904.50
anterior 904.52
posterior 904.54
ulnar (artery) (vein) 903.3
uterine 902.59
artery 902.55
vein 902.56
vena cava
inferior 902.10
specified branches NEC 902.19
superior 901.2
brachial plexus 953.4
newborn 767.6
brain NEC (*see also* Injury, intracranial) 854.0 ☑
breast 959.19
broad ligament — *see* Injury, internal, broad ligament
bronchus, bronchi — *see* Injury, internal, bronchus
brow 959.09
buttock 959.19
canthus, eye 921.1
cathode ray 990
cauda equina 952.4
with fracture, vertebra — *see* Fracture, vertebra, sacrum
cavernous sinus (*see also* Injury, intracranial) 854.0 ☑
cecum — *see* Injury, internal, cecum
celiac ganglion or plexus 954.1
cerebellum (*see also* Injury, intracranial) 854.0 ☑
cervix (uteri) — *see* Injury, internal, cervix
cheek 959.09
chest — *see also* Injury, internal, chest wall 959.11
childbirth — *see also* Birth, injury
maternal NEC 665.9 ☑
chin 959.09
choroid (eye) 921.3
clitoris 959.14
coccyx 959.19
complicating delivery 665.6 ☑
colon — *see* Injury, internal, colon
common duct — *see* Injury, internal, common duct
conjunctiva 921.1
superficial 918.2
cord
spermatic — *see* Injury, internal, spermatic cord
spinal — *see* Injury, spinal, by site
cornea 921.3
abrasion 918.1
due to contact lens 371.82

Injury — *continued*
  cornea — *continued*
    penetrating — *see* Injury, eyeball,
      penetrating
    superficial 918.1
      due to contact lens 371.82
  cortex (cerebral) (*see also* Injury, intracranial)
    854.0 ☑
    visual 950.3
  costal region 959.11
  costochondral 959.11
  cranial
    bones — *see* Fracture, skull, by site
    cavity (*see also* Injury, intracranial) 854.0 ☑
    nerve — *see* Injury, nerve, cranial
  crushing — *see* Crush
  cutaneous sensory nerve
    lower limb 956.4
    upper limb 955.5
  delivery — *see also* Birth, injury
    maternal NEC 665.9 ☑
  Descemet's membrane — *see* Injury, eyeball,
    penetrating
  diaphragm — *see* Injury, internal, diaphragm
  duodenum — *see* Injury, internal, duodenum
  ear (auricle) (canal) (drum) (external) 959.09
  elbow (and forearm) (and wrist) 959.3
  epididymis 959.14
  epigastric region 959.12
  epiglottis 959.09
  epiphyseal, current — *see* Fracture, by site
  esophagus — *see* Injury, internal, esophagus
  Eustachian tube 959.09
  extremity (lower) (upper) NEC 959.8
  eye 921.9
    penetrating eyeball — *see* Injury, eyeball,
      penetrating
    superficial 918.9
  eyeball 921.3
    penetrating 871.7
      with
        partial loss (of intraocular tissue)
          871.2
        prolapse or exposure (of intraocular
          tissue) 871.1
        without prolapse 871.0
      foreign body (nonmagnetic) 871.6
        magnetic 871.5
    superficial 918.9
  eyebrow 959.09
  eyelid(s) 921.1
    laceration — *see* Laceration, eyelid
    superficial 918.0
  face (and neck) 959.09
  fallopian tube — *see* Injury, internal, fallopian
    tube
  finger(s) (nail) 959.5
  flank 959.19
  foot (and ankle) (and knee) (and leg except
    thigh) 959.7
  forceps NEC 767.9
    scalp 767.19
  forearm (and elbow) (and wrist) 959.3
  forehead 959.09
  gallbladder — *see* Injury, internal, gallbladder
  gasserian ganglion 951.2
  gastrointestinal tract — *see* Injury, internal,
    gastrointestinal tract
  genital organ(s)
    with
      abortion — *see* Abortion, by type, with,
        damage to pelvic organs
      ectopic pregnancy (*see also* categories
        633.0-633.9) 639.2
      molar pregnancy (*see also* categories 630-
        632) 639.2
    external 959.14
      fracture of corpus cavernosum penis
        959.13
    following
      abortion 639.2
      ectopic or molar pregnancy 639.2
    internal — *see* Injury, internal, genital
      organs
    obstetrical trauma NEC 665.9 ☑
      affecting fetus or newborn 763.89

Injury — *continued*
  gland
    lacrimal 921.1
      laceration 870.8
    parathyroid 959.09
    salivary 959.09
    thyroid 959.09
  globe (eye) (*see also* Injury, eyeball) 921.3
  grease gun — *see* Wound, open, by site,
    complicated
  groin 959.19
  gum 959.09
  hand(s) (except fingers) 959.4
  head NEC 959.01
    with
      loss of consciousness 850.5
      skull fracture — *see* Fracture, skull, by
        site
  heart — *see* Injury, internal, heart
  heel 959.7
  hip (and thigh) 959.6
  hymen 959.14
  hyperextension (cervical) (vertebra) 847.0
  ileum — *see* Injury, internal, ileum
  iliac region 959.19
  infrared rays NEC 990
  instrumental (during surgery) 998.2
    birth injury — *see* Birth, injury
    nonsurgical (*see also* Injury, by site) 959.9
    obstetrical 665.9 ☑
      affecting fetus or newborn 763.89
      bladder 665.5 ☑
      cervix 665.3 ☑
      high vaginal 665.4 ☑
      perineal NEC 664.9 ☑
      urethra 665.5 ☑
      uterus 665.5 ☑
  internal 869.0

> *Note* — For injury of internal organ(s) by foreign
> body entering through a natural orifice (e.g.,
> inhaled, ingested, or swallowed) — see Foreign
> body, entering through orifice.
>
> For internal injury of any of the following sites
> with internal injury of any other of the sites —
> see Injury, internal, multiple.

    with
      fracture
        open wound into cavity 869.1
        pelvis — *see* Fracture, pelvis
        specified site, except pelvis — *see*
          Injury, internal, by site
  abdomen, abdominal (viscera) NEC 868.00
    with
      fracture, pelvis — *see* Fracture, pelvis
      open wound into cavity 868.10
      specified site NEC 868.09
        with open wound into cavity 868.19
  adrenal (gland) 868.01
    with open wound into cavity 868.11
  aorta (thoracic) 901.0
    abdominal 902.0
  appendix 863.85
    with open wound into cavity 863.95
  bile duct 868.02
    with open wound into cavity 868.12
  bladder (sphincter) 867.0
    with
      abortion — *see* Abortion, by type, with
        damage to pelvic organs
      ectopic pregnancy (*see also* categories
        633.0-633.9) 639.2
      molar pregnancy (*see also* categories
        630-632) 639.2
      open wound into cavity 867.1
    following
      abortion 639.2
      ectopic or molar pregnancy 639.2
    obstetrical trauma 665.5 ☑
      affecting fetus or newborn 763.89
  blood vessel — *see* Injury, blood vessel, by
    site
  broad ligament 867.6
    with open wound into cavity 867.7
  bronchus, bronchi 862.21
    with open wound into cavity 862.31

Injury — *continued*
  internal — *continued*
    cecum 863.89
      with open wound into cavity 863.99
    cervix (uteri) 867.4
      with
        abortion — *see* Abortion, by type, with
          damage to pelvic organs
        ectopic pregnancy (*see also* categories
          633.0-633.9) 639.2
        molar pregnancy (*see also* categories
          630-632) 639.2
        open wound into cavity 867.5
      following
        abortion 639.2
        ectopic or molar pregnancy 639.2
      obstetrical trauma 665.3 ☑
        affecting fetus or newborn 763.89
    chest (*see also* Injury, internal, intrathoracic
      organs) 862.8
      with open wound into cavity 862.9
    colon 863.40
      with
        open wound into cavity 863.50
        rectum 863.46
          with open wound into cavity 863.56
      ascending (right) 863.41
        with open wound into cavity 863.51
      descending (left) 863.43
        with open wound into cavity 863.53
      multiple sites 863.46
        with open wound into cavity 863.56
      sigmoid 863.44
        with open wound into cavity 863.54
      specified site NEC 863.49
        with open wound into cavity 863.59
      transverse 863.42
        with open wound into cavity 863.52
    common duct 868.02
      with open wound into cavity 868.12
    complicating delivery 665.9 ☑
      affecting fetus or newborn 763.89
    diaphragm 862.0
      with open wound into cavity 862.1
    duodenum 863.21
      with open wound into cavity 863.31
    esophagus (intrathoracic) 862.22
      with open wound into cavity 862.32
      cervical region 874.4
        complicated 874.5
    fallopian tube 867.6
      with open wound into cavity 867.7
    gallbladder 868.02
      with open wound into cavity 868.12
    gastrointestinal tract NEC 863.80
      with open wound into cavity 863.90
    genital organ NEC 867.6
      with open wound into cavity 867.7
    heart 861.00
      with open wound into thorax 861.10
    ileum 863.29
      with open wound into cavity 863.39
    intestine NEC 863.89
      with open wound into cavity 863.99
      large NEC 863.40
        with open wound into cavity 863.50
      small NEC 863.20
        with open wound into cavity 863.30
    intra-abdominal (organ) 868.00
      with open wound into cavity 868.10
      multiple sites 868.09
        with open wound into cavity 868.19
      specified site NEC 868.09
        with open wound into cavity 868.19
    intrathoracic organs (multiple) 862.8
      with open wound into cavity 862.9
      diaphragm (only) — *see* Injury, internal,
        diaphragm
      heart (only) — *see* Injury, internal, heart
      lung (only) — *see* Injury, internal, lung
      specified site NEC 862.29
        with open wound into cavity 862.39
    intrauterine (*see also* Injury, internal,
      uterus) 867.4
      with open wound into cavity 867.5
    jejunum 863.29
      with open wound into cavity 863.39

☑ Additional Digit Required   ▶◀ Revised Text   ● New Line   ▲ Revised Code

Injury — *continued*
  internal — *continued*
    kidney (subcapsular) 866.00
      with
        disruption of parenchyma (complete) 866.03
          with open wound into cavity 866.13
        hematoma (without rupture of capsule) 866.01
          with open wound into cavity 866.11
        laceration 866.02
          with open wound into cavity 866.12
        open wound into cavity 866.10
    liver 864.00
      with
        contusion 864.01
          with open wound into cavity 864.11
        hematoma 864.01
          with open wound into cavity 864.11
        laceration 864.05
          with open wound into cavity 864.15
          major (disruption of hepatic parenchyma) 864.04
            with open wound into cavity 864.14
          minor (capsule only) 864.02
            with open wound into cavity 864.12
          moderate (involving parenchyma) 864.03
            with open wound into cavity 864.13
          multiple 864.04
          stellate 864.04
            with open wound into cavity 864.14
        open wound into cavity 864.10
    lung 861.20
      with open wound into thorax 861.30
      hemopneumothorax — *see* Hemopneumothorax, traumatic
      hemothorax — *see* Hemothorax, traumatic
      pneumohemothorax — *see* Pneumohemothorax, traumatic
      pneumothorax — *see* Pneumothorax, traumatic
    mediastinum 862.29
      with open wound into cavity 862.39
    mesentery 863.89
      with open wound into cavity 863.99
    mesosalpinx 867.6
      with open wound into cavity 867.7
    multiple 869.0

> *Note* — *Multiple internal injuries of sites classifiable to the same three- or four-digit category should be classified to that category.*
>
> *Multiple injuries classifiable to different fourth-digit subdivisions of 861 (heart and lung injuries) should be dealt with according to coding rules.*

    internal
      with open wound into cavity 869.1
      intra-abdominal organ (sites classifiable to 863-868)
        with
          intrathoracic organ(s) (sites classifiable to 861-862) 869.0
            with open wound into cavity 869.1
          other intra-abdominal organ(s) (sites classifiable to 863-868, except where classifiable to the same three-digit category) 868.09
            with open wound into cavity 868.19
      intrathoracic organ (sites classifiable to 861-862)
        with
          intra-abdominal organ(s) (sites classifiable to 863-868) 869.0
            with open wound into cavity 869.1

Injury — *continued*
  internal — *continued*
    multiple — *continued*
      intrathoracic organ — *continued*
        with — *continued*
          other intrathoracic organ(s) (sites classifiable to 861-862, except where classifiable to the same three-digit category) 862.8
            with open wound into cavity 862.9
      myocardium — *see* Injury, internal, heart
      ovary 867.6
        with open wound into cavity 867.7
      pancreas (multiple sites) 863.84
        with open wound into cavity 863.94
        body 863.82
          with open wound into cavity 863.92
        head 863.81
          with open wound into cavity 863.91
        tail 863.83
          with open wound into cavity 863.93
      pelvis, pelvic (organs) (viscera) 867.8
        with
          fracture, pelvis — *see* Fracture, pelvis
          open wound into cavity 867.9
        specified site NEC 867.6
          with open wound into cavity 867.7
      peritoneum 868.03
        with open wound into cavity 868.13
      pleura 862.29
        with open wound into cavity 862.39
      prostate 867.6
        with open wound into cavity 867.7
      rectum 863.45
        with
          colon 863.46
            with open wound into cavity 863.56
          open wound into cavity 863.55
      retroperitoneum 868.04
        with open wound into cavity 868.14
      round ligament 867.6
        with open wound into cavity 867.7
      seminal vesicle 867.6
        with open wound into cavity 867.7
      spermatic cord 867.6
        with open wound into cavity 867.7
        scrotal — *see* Wound, open, spermatic cord
      spleen 865.00
        with
          disruption of parenchyma (massive) 865.04
            with open wound into cavity 865.14
          hematoma (without rupture of capsule) 865.01
            with open wound into cavity 865.11
          open wound into cavity 865.10
          tear, capsular 865.02
            with open wound into cavity 865.12
            extending into parenchyma 865.03
              with open wound into cavity 865.13
      stomach 863.0
        with open wound into cavity 863.1
      suprarenal gland (multiple) 868.01
        with open wound into cavity 868.11
      thorax, thoracic (cavity) (organs) (multiple) (*see also* Injury, internal, intrathoracic organs) 862.8
        with open wound into cavity 862.9
      thymus (gland) 862.29
        with open wound into cavity 862.39
      trachea (intrathoracic) 862.29
        with open wound into cavity 862.39
        cervical region (*see also* Wound, open, trachea) 874.02
      ureter 867.2
        with open wound into cavity 867.3
      urethra (sphincter) 867.0
        with
          abortion — *see* Abortion, by type, with damage to pelvic organs
          ectopic pregnancy (*see also* categories 633.0-633.9) 639.2
          molar pregnancy (*see also* categories 630-632) 639.2
          open wound into cavity 867.1

Injury — *continued*
  internal — *continued*
    urethra — *continued*
      following
        abortion 639.2
        ectopic or molar pregnancy 639.2
        obstetrical trauma 665.5 ☑
          affecting fetus or newborn 763.89
    uterus 867.4
      with
        abortion — *see* Abortion, by type, with damage to pelvic organs
        ectopic pregnancy (*see also* categories 633.0-633.9) 639.2
        molar pregnancy (*see also* categories 630-632) 639.2
        open wound into cavity 867.5
      following
        abortion 639.2
        ectopic or molar pregnancy 639.2
        obstetrical trauma NEC 665.5 ☑
          affecting fetus or newborn 763.89
    vas deferens 867.6
      with open wound into cavity 867.7
    vesical (sphincter) 867.0
      with open wound into cavity 867.1
    viscera (abdominal) (*see also* Injury, internal, multiple) 868.00
      with
        fracture, pelvis — *see* Fracture, pelvis
        open wound into cavity 868.10
      thoracic NEC (*see also* Injury, internal, intrathoracic organs) 862.8
        with open wound into cavity 862.9
  interscapular region 959.19
  intervertebral disc 959.19
  intestine — *see* Injury, internal, intestine
  intra-abdominal (organs) NEC — *see* Injury, internal, intra-abdominal
  intracranial 854.0 ☑

> *Note* — *Use the following fifth-digit subclassification with categories 851-854:*
>
>   *0   unspecified state of consciousness*
>   *1   with no loss of consciousness*
>   *2   with brief [less than one hour] loss of consciousness*
>   *3   with moderate [1-24 hours] loss of consciousness*
>   *4   with prolonged [more than 24 hours] loss of consciousness and return to pre-existing conscious level*
>   *5   with prolonged [more than 24 hours] loss of consciousness, without return to pre-existing conscious level*
>   *Use fifth-digit 5 to designate when a patient is unconscious and dies before regaining consciousness, regardless of the duration of the loss of consciousness*
>   *6   with loss of consciousness of unspecified duration*
>   *9   with concussion, unspecified*

    with
      open intracranial wound 854.1 ☑
      skull fracture — *see* Fracture, skull, by site
    contusion 851.8 ☑
      with open intracranial wound 851.9 ☑
      brain stem 851.4 ☑
        with open intracranial wound 851.5 ☑
      cerebellum 851.4 ☑
        with open intracranial wound 851.5 ☑
      cortex (cerebral) 851.0 ☑
        with open intracranial wound 851.2 ☑
    hematoma — *see* Injury, intracranial, hemorrhage
    hemorrhage 853.0 ☑
      with
        laceration — *see* Injury, intracranial, laceration
        open intracranial wound 853.1 ☑
      extradural 852.4 ☑
        with open intracranial wound 852.5 ☑

Injury — *continued*
  intracranial — *continued*
    hemorrhage — *continued*
      subarachnoid 852.0 ☑
        with open intracranial wound 852.1 ☑
      subdural 852.2 ☑
        with open intracranial wound 852.3 ☑
    laceration 851.8 ☑
      with open intracranial wound 851.9 ☑
      brain stem 851.6 ☑
        with open intracranial wound 851.7 ☑
      cerebellum 851.6 ☑
        with open intracranial wound 851.7 ☑
      cortex (cerebral) 851.2 ☑
        with open intracranial wound 851.3 ☑
  intraocular — *see* Injury, eyeball, penetrating
  intrathoracic organs (multiple) — *see* Injury, internal, intrathoracic organs
  intrauterine — *see* Injury, internal, intrauterine
  iris 921.3
    penetrating — *see* Injury, eyeball, penetrating
  jaw 959.09
  jejunum — *see* Injury, internal, jejunum
  joint NEC 959.9
    old or residual 718.80
      ankle 718.87
      elbow 718.82
      foot 718.87
      hand 718.84
      hip 718.85
      knee 718.86
      multiple sites 718.89
      pelvic region 718.85
      shoulder (region) 718.81
      specified site NEC 718.88
      wrist 718.83
  kidney — *see* Injury, internal, kidney
  knee (and ankle) (and foot) (and leg, except thigh) 959.7
  labium (majus) (minus) 959.14
  labyrinth, ear 959.09
  lacrimal apparatus, gland, or sac 921.1
    laceration 870.8
  larynx 959.09
  late effect — *see* Late, effects (of), injury
  leg except thigh (and ankle) (and foot) (and knee) 959.7
    upper or thigh 959.6
  lens, eye 921.3
    penetrating — *see* Injury, eyeball, penetrating
  lid, eye — *see* Injury, eyelid
  lip 959.09
  liver — *see* Injury, internal, liver
  lobe, parietal — *see* Injury, intracranial
  lumbar (region) 959.19
    plexus 953.5
  lumbosacral (region) 959.19
    plexus 953.5
  lung — *see* Injury, internal, lung
  malar region 959.09
  mastoid region 959.09
  maternal, during pregnancy, affecting fetus or newborn 760.5
  maxilla 959.09
  mediastinum — *see* Injury, internal, mediastinum
  membrane
    brain (*see also* Injury, intracranial) 854.0 ☑
    tympanic 959.09
  meningeal artery — *see* Hemorrhage, brain, traumatic, subarachnoid
  meninges (cerebral) — *see* Injury, intracranial
  mesenteric
    artery — *see* Injury, blood vessel, mesenteric, artery
    plexus, inferior 954.1
    vein — *see* Injury, blood vessel, mesenteric, vein
  mesentery — *see* Injury, internal, mesentery
  mesosalpinx — *see* Injury, internal, mesosalpinx
  middle ear 959.09
  midthoracic region 959.11
  mouth 959.09

Injury — *continued*
  multiple (sites not classifiable to the same four-digit category in 959.0-959.7) 959.8
    internal 869.0
      with open wound into cavity 869.1
  musculocutaneous nerve 955.4
  nail
    finger 959.5
    toe 959.7
  nasal (septum) (sinus) 959.09
  nasopharynx 959.09
  neck (and face) 959.09
  nerve 957.9
    abducens 951.3
    abducent 951.3
    accessory 951.6
    acoustic 951.5
    ankle and foot 956.9
    anterior crural, femoral 956.1
    arm (*see also* Injury, nerve, upper limb) 955.9
    auditory 951.5
    axillary 955.0
    brachial plexus 953.4
    cervical sympathetic 954.0
    cranial 951.9
      first or olfactory 951.8
      second or optic 950.0
      third or oculomotor 951.0
      fourth or trochlear 951.1
      fifth or trigeminal 951.2
      sixth or abducens 951.3
      seventh or facial 951.4
      eighth, acoustic, or auditory 951.5
      ninth or glossopharyngeal 951.8
      tenth, pneumogastric, or vagus 951.8
      eleventh or accessory 951.6
      twelfth or hypoglossal 951.7
      newborn 767.7
    cutaneous sensory
      lower limb 956.4
      upper limb 955.5
    digital (finger) 955.6
      toe 956.5
    facial 951.4
      newborn 767.5
    femoral 956.1
    finger 955.9
    foot and ankle 956.9
    forearm 955.9
    glossopharyngeal 951.8
    hand and wrist 955.9
    head and neck, superficial 957.0
    hypoglossal 951.7
    involving several parts of body 957.8
    leg (*see also* Injury, nerve, lower limb) 956.9
    lower limb 956.9
      multiple 956.8
      specified site NEC 956.5
    lumbar plexus 953.5
    lumbosacral plexus 953.5
    median 955.1
      forearm 955.1
      wrist and hand 955.1
    multiple (in several parts of body) (sites not classifiable to the same three-digit category) 957.8
    musculocutaneous 955.4
    musculospiral 955.3
      upper arm 955.3
    oculomotor 951.0
    olfactory 951.8
    optic 950.0
    pelvic girdle 956.9
      multiple sites 956.8
      specified site NEC 956.5
    peripheral 957.9
      multiple (in several regions) (sites not classifiable to the same three-digit category) 957.8
      specified site NEC 957.1
    peroneal 956.3
      ankle and foot 956.3
      lower leg 956.3
    plantar 956.5
    plexus 957.9
      celiac 954.1

Injury — *continued*
  nerve — *continued*
    plexus — *continued*
      mesenteric, inferior 954.1
      spinal 953.9
        brachial 953.4
        lumbosacral 953.5
        multiple sites 953.8
      sympathetic NEC 954.1
    pneumogastric 951.8
    radial 955.3
      wrist and hand 955.3
    sacral plexus 953.5
    sciatic 956.0
      thigh 956.0
    shoulder girdle 955.9
      multiple 955.8
      specified site NEC 955.7
    specified site NEC 957.1
    spinal 953.9
      plexus — *see* Injury, nerve, plexus, spinal
      root 953.9
        cervical 953.0
        dorsal 953.1
        lumbar 953.2
        multiple sites 953.8
        sacral 953.3
    splanchnic 954.1
    sympathetic NEC 954.1
      cervical 954.0
    thigh 956.9
    tibial 956.5
      ankle and foot 956.2
      lower leg 956.5
      posterior 956.2
    toe 956.9
    trigeminal 951.2
    trochlear 951.1
    trunk, excluding shoulder and pelvic girdles 954.9
      specified site NEC 954.8
      sympathetic NEC 954.1
    ulnar 955.2
      forearm 955.2
      wrist (and hand) 955.2
    upper limb 955.9
      multiple 955.8
      specified site NEC 955.7
    vagus 951.8
    wrist and hand 955.9
  nervous system, diffuse 957.8
  nose (septum) 959.09
  obstetrical NEC 665.9 ☑
    affecting fetus or newborn 763.89
  occipital (region) (scalp) 959.09
    lobe (*see also* Injury, intracranial) 854.0 ☑
  optic 950.9
    chiasm 950.1
    cortex 950.3
    nerve 950.0
    pathways 950.2
  orbit, orbital (region) 921.2
    penetrating 870.3
      with foreign body 870.4
  ovary — *see* Injury, internal, ovary
  paint-gun — *see* Wound, open, by site, complicated
  palate (soft) 959.09
  pancreas — *see* Injury, internal, pancreas
  parathyroid (gland) 959.09
  parietal (region) (scalp) 959.09
    lobe — *see* Injury, intracranial
  pelvic
    floor 959.19
      complicating delivery 664.1 ☑
        affecting fetus or newborn 763.89
    joint or ligament, complicating delivery 665.6 ☑
      affecting fetus or newborn 763.89
    organs — *see also* Injury, internal, pelvis
      with
        abortion — *see* Abortion, by type, with damage to pelvic organs
        ectopic pregnancy (*see also* categories 633.0-633.9) 639.2
        molar pregnancy (*see also* categories 633.0-633.9) 639.2

☑ Additional Digit Required   ▶◀ Revised Text   ● New Line   ▲ Revised Code

Injury — *continued*
pelvic — *continued*
organs — *see also* Injury, internal, pelvis — *continued*
following
abortion 639.2
ectopic or molar pregnancy 639.2
obstetrical trauma 665.5 ☑
affecting fetus or newborn 763.89
pelvis 959.19
penis 959.14
fracture of corpus cavernosum 959.13
perineum 959.14
peritoneum — *see* Injury, internal, peritoneum
periurethral tissue
with
abortion — *see* Abortion, by type, with damage to pelvic organs
ectopic pregnancy (*see also* categories 633.0-633.9) 639.2
molar pregnancy (*see also* categories 630-632) 639.2
complicating delivery 665.5 ☑
affecting fetus or newborn 763.89
following
abortion 639.2
ectopic or molar pregnancy 639.2
phalanges
foot 959.7
hand 959.5
pharynx 959.09
pleura — *see* Injury, internal, pleura
popliteal space 959.7
prepuce 959.14
prostate — *see* Injury, internal, prostate
pubic region 959.19
pudenda 959.14
radiation NEC 990
radioactive substance or radium NEC 990
rectovaginal septum 959.14
rectum — *see* Injury, internal, rectum
retina 921.3
penetrating — *see* Injury, eyeball, penetrating
retroperitoneal — *see* Injury, internal, retroperitoneum
roentgen rays NEC 990
round ligament — *see* Injury, internal, round ligament
sacral (region) 959.19
plexus 953.5
sacroiliac ligament NEC 959.19
sacrum 959.19
salivary ducts or glands 959.09
scalp 959.09
due to birth trauma 767.19
fetus or newborn 767.19
scapular region 959.2
sclera 921.3
penetrating — *see* Injury, eyeball, penetrating
superficial 918.2
scrotum 959.14
seminal vesicle — *see* Injury, internal, seminal vesicle
shoulder (and upper arm) 959.2
sinus
cavernous (*see also* Injury, intracranial) 854.0 ☑
nasal 959.09
skeleton NEC, birth injury 767.3
skin NEC 959.9
skull — *see* Fracture, skull, by site
soft tissue (of external sites) (severe) — *see* Wound, open, by site
specified site NEC 959.8
spermatic cord — *see* Injury, internal, spermatic cord
spinal (cord) 952.9
with fracture, vertebra — *see* Fracture, vertebra, by site, with spinal cord injury
cervical (C₁-C₄) 952.00
with
anterior cord syndrome 952.02
central cord syndrome 952.03
complete lesion of cord 952.01
incomplete lesion NEC 952.04

Injury — *continued*
spinal — *continued*
cervical — *continued*
with — *continued*
posterior cord syndrome 952.04
C₅-C₇ level 952.05
with
anterior cord syndrome 952.07
central cord syndrome 952.08
complete lesion of cord 952.06
incomplete lesion NEC 952.09
posterior cord syndrome 952.09
specified type NEC 952.09
specified type NEC 952.04
dorsal (D₁-D₆) (T₁-T₆) (thoracic) 952.10
with
anterior cord syndrome 952.12
central cord syndrome 952.13
complete lesion of cord 952.11
incomplete lesion NEC 952.14
posterior cord syndrome 952.14
D₇-D₁₂ level (T₇-T₁₂) 952.15
with
anterior cord syndrome 952.17
central cord syndrome 952.18
complete lesion of cord 952.16
incomplete lesion NEC 952.19
posterior cord syndrome 952.19
specified type NEC 952.19
specified type NEC 952.14
lumbar 952.2
multiple sites 952.8
nerve (root) NEC — *see* Injury, nerve, spinal, root
plexus 953.9
brachial 953.4
lumbosacral 953.5
multiple sites 953.8
sacral 952.3
thoracic (*see also* Injury, spinal, dorsal) 952.10
spleen — *see* Injury, internal, spleen
stellate ganglion 954.1
sternal region 959.11
stomach — *see* Injury, internal, stomach
subconjunctival 921.1
subcutaneous 959.9
subdural — *see* Injury, intracranial
submaxillary region 959.09
submental region 959.09
subungual
fingers 959.5
toes 959.7
superficial 919 ☑

Note — Use the following fourth-digit subdivisions with categories 910-919:

0   *Abrasion or friction burn without mention of infection*

1   *Abrasion or friction burn, infected*

2   *Blister without mention of infection*

3   *Blister, infected*

4   *Insect bite, nonvenomous, without mention of infection*

5   *Insect bite, nonvenomous, infected*

6   *Superficial foreign body (splinter) without major open wound and without mention of infection*

7   *Superficial foreign body (splinter) without major open wound, infected*

8   *Other and unspecified superficial injury without mention of infection*

9   *Other and unspecified superficial injury, infected*

For late effects of superficial injury, see category 906.2.

---

abdomen, abdominal (muscle) (wall) (and other part(s) of trunk) 911 ☑
ankle (and hip, knee, leg, or thigh) 916 ☑
anus (and other part(s) of trunk) 911 ☑
arm 913 ☑
upper (and shoulder) 912 ☑
auditory canal (external) (meatus) (and other part(s) of face, neck, or scalp, except eye) 910 ☑

Injury — *continued*
superficial — *continued*
axilla (and upper arm) 912 ☑
back (and other part(s) of trunk) 911 ☑
breast (and other part(s) of trunk) 911 ☑
brow (and other part(s) of face, neck, or scalp) 910 ☑
buttock (and other part(s) of trunk) 911 ☑
canthus, eye 918.0
cheek(s) (and other part(s) of face, neck, or scalp, except eye) 910 ☑
chest wall (and other part(s) of trunk) 911 ☑
chin (and other part(s) of face, neck, or scalp, except eye) 910 ☑
clitoris (and other part(s) of trunk) 911 ☑
conjunctiva 918.2
cornea 918.1
due to contact lens 371.82
costal region (and other part(s) of trunk) 911 ☑
ear(s) (auricle) (canal) (drum) (external) (and other part(s) of face, neck, or scalp, except eye) 910 ☑
elbow (and forearm) (and wrist) 913 ☑
epididymis (and other part(s) of trunk) 911 ☑
epigastric region (and other part(s) of trunk) 911 ☑
epiglottis (and other part(s) of face, neck, or scalp, except eye) 910 ☑
eye(s) (and adnexa) NEC 918.9
eyelid(s) (and periocular area) 918.0
face (any part(s), except eye) (and neck or scalp) 910 ☑
finger(s) (nail) (any) 915 ☑
flank (and other part(s) of trunk) 911 ☑
foot (phalanges) (and toe(s)) 917 ☑
forearm (and elbow) (and wrist) 913 ☑
forehead (and other part(s) of face, neck, or scalp, except eye) 910 ☑
globe (eye) 918.9
groin (and other part(s) of trunk) 911 ☑
gum(s) (and other part(s) of face, neck, or scalp, except eye) 910 ☑
hand(s) (except fingers alone) 914 ☑
head (and other part(s) of face, neck, or scalp, except eye) 910 ☑
heel (and foot or toe) 917 ☑
hip (and ankle, knee, leg, or thigh) 916 ☑
iliac region (and other part(s) of trunk) 911 ☑
interscapular region (and other part(s) of trunk) 911 ☑
iris 918.9
knee (and ankle, hip, leg, or thigh) 916 ☑
labium (majus) (minus) (and other part(s) of trunk) 911 ☑
lacrimal (apparatus) (gland) (sac) 918.0
leg (lower) (upper) (and ankle, hip, knee, or thigh) 916 ☑
lip(s) (and other part(s) of face, neck, or scalp, except eye) 910 ☑
lower extremity (except foot) 916 ☑
lumbar region (and other part(s) of trunk) 911 ☑
malar region (and other part(s) of face, neck, or scalp, except eye) 910 ☑
mastoid region (and other part(s) of face, neck, or scalp, except eye) 910 ☑
midthoracic region (and other part(s) of trunk) 911 ☑
mouth (and other part(s) of face, neck, or scalp, except eye) 910 ☑
multiple sites (not classifiable to the same three-digit category) 919 ☑
nasal (septum) (and other part(s) of face, neck, or scalp, except eye) 910 ☑
neck (and face or scalp, any part(s), except eye) 910 ☑
nose (septum) (and other part(s) of face, neck, or scalp, except eye) 910 ☑
occipital region (and other part(s) of face, neck, or scalp, except eye) 910 ☑
orbital region 918.0
palate (soft) (and other part(s) of face, neck, or scalp, except eye) 910 ☑

☑ Additional Digit Required   ▶◀ Revised Text   ● New Line   ▲ Revised Code

Injury — *continued*
　superficial — *continued*
　　parietal region (and other part(s) of face, neck, or scalp, except eye) 910 ☑
　　penis (and other part(s) of trunk) 911 ☑
　　perineum (and other part(s) of trunk) 911 ☑
　　periocular area 918.0
　　pharynx (and other part(s) of face, neck, or scalp, except eye) 910 ☑
　　popliteal space (and ankle, hip, leg, or thigh) 916 ☑
　　prepuce (and other part(s) of trunk) 911 ☑
　　pubic region (and other part(s) of trunk) 911 ☑
　　pudenda (and other part(s) of trunk) 911 ☑
　　sacral region (and other part(s) of trunk) 911 ☑
　　salivary (ducts) (glands) (and other part(s) of face, neck, or scalp, except eye) 910 ☑
　　scalp (and other part(s) of face or neck, except eye) 910 ☑
　　scapular region (and upper arm) 912 ☑
　　sclera 918.2
　　scrotum (and other part(s) of trunk) 911 ☑
　　shoulder (and upper arm) 912 ☑
　　skin NEC 919 ☑
　　specified site(s) NEC 919 ☑
　　sternal region (and other part(s) of trunk) 911 ☑
　　subconjunctival 918.2
　　subcutaneous NEC 919 ☑
　　submaxillary region (and other part(s) of face, neck, or scalp, except eye) 910 ☑
　　submental region (and other part(s) of face, neck, or scalp, except eye) 910 ☑
　　supraclavicular fossa (and other part(s) of face, neck or scalp, except eye) 910 ☑
　　supraorbital 918.0
　　temple (and other part(s) of face, neck, or scalp, except eye) 910 ☑
　　temporal region (and other part(s) of face, neck, or scalp, except eye) 910 ☑
　　testis (and other part(s) of trunk) 911 ☑
　　thigh (and ankle, hip, knee, or leg) 916 ☑
　　thorax, thoracic (external) (and other part(s) of trunk) 911 ☑
　　throat (and other part(s) of face, neck, or scalp, except eye) 910 ☑
　　thumb(s) (nail) 915 ☑
　　toe(s) (nail) (subungual) (and foot) 917 ☑
　　tongue (and other part(s) of face, neck, or scalp, except eye) 910 ☑
　　tooth, teeth ▶(*see also* Abrasion, dental)◀ 521.20 ▲
　　trunk (any part(s)) 911 ☑
　　tunica vaginalis 959.14 ▲
　　tympanum, tympanic membrane (and other part(s) of face, neck, or scalp, except eye) 910 ☑
　　upper extremity NEC 913 ☑
　　uvula (and other part(s) of face, neck, or scalp, except eye) 910 ☑
　　vagina (and other part(s) of trunk) 911 ☑
　　vulva (and other part(s) of trunk) 911 ☑
　　wrist (and elbow) (and forearm) 913 ☑
　supraclavicular fossa 959.19
　supraorbital 959.09
　surgical complication (external or internal site) 998.2
　symphysis pubis 959.19
　　complicating delivery 665.6 ☑
　　　affecting fetus or newborn 763.89
　temple 959.09
　temporal region 959.09
　testis 959.14
　thigh (and hip) 959.6
　thorax, thoracic (external) 959.11
　　cavity — *see* Injury, internal, thorax
　　internal — *see* Injury, internal, intrathoracic organs
　throat 959.09
　thumb(s) (nail) 959.5
　thymus — *see* Injury, internal, thymus
　thyroid (gland) 959.09
　toe (nail) (any) 959.7
　tongue 959.09
　tonsil 959.09

Injury — *continued*
　tooth NEC 873.63
　　complicated 873.73
　trachea — *see* Injury, internal, trachea
　trunk 959.19
　tunica vaginalis 959.19
　tympanum, tympanic membrane 959.09
　ultraviolet rays NEC 990
　ureter — *see* Injury, internal, ureter
　urethra (sphincter) — *see* Injury, internal, urethra
　uterus — *see* Injury, internal, uterus
　uvula 959.09
　vagina 959.14
　vascular — *see* Injury, blood vessel
　vas deferens — *see* Injury, internal, vas deferens
　vein (*see also* Injury, blood vessel, by site) 904.9
　vena cava
　　inferior 902.10
　　superior 901.2
　vesical (sphincter) — *see* Injury, internal, vesical
　viscera (abdominal) — *see also* Injury, internal, viscera
　　with fracture, pelvis — *see* Fracture, pelvis
　visual 950.9
　　cortex 950.3
　vitreous (humor) 871.2
　vulva 959.14
　whiplash (cervical spine) 847.0
　wringer — *see* Crush, by site
　wrist (and elbow) (and forearm) 959.3
　x-ray NEC 990
Inoculation — *see also* Vaccination
　complication or reaction — *see* Complication, vaccination
Insanity, insane (*see also* Psychosis) 298.9
　adolescent (*see also* Schizophrenia) 295.9 ☑
　alternating (*see also* Psychosis, affective, circular) 296.7
　confusional 298.9
　　acute 293.0
　　subacute 293.1
　delusional 298.9
　paralysis, general 094.1
　　progressive 094.1
　paresis, general 094.1
　senile 290.20
Insect
　bite — *see* Injury, superficial, by site
　venomous, poisoning by 989.5
Insemination, artificial V26.1
Insertion
　cord (umbilical) lateral or velamentous 663.8 ☑
　　affecting fetus or newborn 762.6
　intrauterine contraceptive device V25.1
　placenta, vicious — *see* Placenta, previa
　subdermal implantable contraceptive V25.5
　velamentous, umbilical cord 663.8 ☑
　　affecting fetus or newborn 762.6
Insolation 992.0
　meaning sunstroke 992.0
Insomnia 780.52
　with sleep apnea 780.51
　nonorganic origin 307.41
　　persistent (primary) 307.42
　　transient 307.41
　subjective complaint 307.49
Inspiration
　food or foreign body (*see also* Asphyxia, food or foreign body) 933.1
　mucus (*see also* Asphyxia, mucus) 933.1
Inspissated bile syndrome, newborn 774.4
Instability
　detrusor 596.59
　emotional (excessive) 301.3
　joint (posttraumatic) 718.80
　　ankle 718.87
　　elbow 718.82
　　foot 718.87
　　hand 718.84
　　hip 718.85
　　knee 718.86

Instability — *continued*
　joint — *continued*
　　lumbosacral 724.6
　　multiple sites 718.89
　　pelvic region 718.85
　　sacroiliac 724.6
　　shoulder (region) 718.81
　　specified site NEC 718.88
　　wrist 718.83
　lumbosacral 724.6
　nervous 301.89
　personality (emotional) 301.59
　thyroid, paroxysmal 242.9 ☑
　urethral 599.83
　vasomotor 780.2
Insufficiency, insufficient
　accommodation 367.4
　adrenal (gland) (acute) (chronic) 255.4
　　medulla 255.5
　　primary 255.4
　　specified NEC 255.5
　adrenocortical 255.4
　anterior guidance 524.54　　　　●
　anus 569.49
　aortic (valve) 424.1
　　with
　　　mitral (valve) disease 396.1
　　　　insufficiency, incompetence, or regurgitation 396.3
　　　　stenosis or obstruction 396.1
　　　stenosis or obstruction 424.1
　　　　with mitral (valve) disease 396.8
　　congenital 746.4
　　rheumatic 395.1
　　　with
　　　　mitral (valve) disease 396.1
　　　　　insufficiency, incompetence, or regurgitation 396.3
　　　　　stenosis or obstruction 396.1
　　　　stenosis or obstruction 395.2
　　　　　with mitral (valve) disease 396.8
　　specified cause NEC 424.1
　　syphilitic 093.22
　arterial 447.1
　　basilar artery 435.0
　　carotid artery 435.8
　　cerebral 437.1
　　coronary (acute or subacute) 411.89
　　mesenteric 557.1
　　peripheral 443.9
　　precerebral 435.9
　　vertebral artery 435.1
　　vertebrobasilar 435.3
　arteriovenous 459.9
　basilar artery 435.0
　biliary 575.8
　cardiac (*see also* Insufficiency, myocardial) 428.0
　　complicating surgery 997.1
　　due to presence of (cardiac) prosthesis 429.4
　　postoperative 997.1
　　　long-term effect of cardiac surgery 429.4
　　specified during or due to a procedure 997.1
　　　long-term effect of cardiac surgery 429.4
　cardiorenal (*see also* Hypertension, cardiorenal) 404.90
　　nervous 301.89
　cardiovascular (*see also* Disease, cardiovascular) 429.2
　　renal (*see also* Hypertension, cardiorenal) 404.90
　carotid artery 435.8
　cerebral (vascular) 437.9
　cerebrovascular 437.9
　　with transient focal neurological signs and symptoms 435.9
　　acute 437.1
　　　with transient focal neurological signs and symptoms 435.9
　circulatory NEC 459.9
　　fetus or newborn 779.89
　convergence 378.83
　coronary (acute or subacute) 411.89
　　chronic or with a stated duration of over 8 weeks 414.8
　corticoadrenal 255.4
　dietary 269.9
　divergence 378.85

Insufficiency, insufficient — *continued*
  food 994.2
  gastroesophageal 530.89
  gonadal
    ovary 256.39
    testis 257.2
  gonadotropic hormone secretion 253.4
  heart — *see also* Insufficiency, myocardial
    fetus or newborn 779.89
    valve (*see also* Endocarditis) 424.90
      congenital NEC 746.89
  hepatic 573.8
  idiopathic autonomic 333.0
  interocclusal distance of teeth (ridge)
    524.36 ●
  kidney (acute) (chronic) 593.9
  labyrinth, labyrinthine (function) 386.53
    bilateral 386.54
    unilateral 386.53
  lacrimal 375.15
  liver 573.8
  lung (acute) (*see also* Insufficiency, pulmonary)
    518.82
    following trauma, surgery, or shock 518.5
    newborn 770.89
  mental (congenital) (*see also* Retardation,
    mental) 319
  mesenteric 557.1
  mitral (valve) 424.0
    with
      aortic (valve) disease 396.3
        insufficiency, incompetence, or
          regurgitation 396.3
        stenosis or obstruction 396.2
      obstruction or stenosis 394.2
        with aortic valve disease 396.8
    congenital 746.6
    rheumatic 394.1
      with
        aortic (valve) disease 396.3
          insufficiency, incompetence, or
            regurgitation 396.3
          stenosis or obstruction 396.2
        obstruction or stenosis 394.2
          with aortic valve disease 396.8
        active or acute 391.1
          with chorea, rheumatic (Sydenham's)
            392.0
    specified cause, except rheumatic 424.0
  muscle
    heart — *see* Insufficiency, myocardial
    ocular (*see also* Strabismus) 378.9
  myocardial, myocardium (with arteriosclerosis)
    428.0
    with rheumatic fever (conditions classifiable
      to 390)
      active, acute, or subacute 391.2
        with chorea 392.0
      inactive or quiescent (with chorea) 398.0
    congenital 746.89
    due to presence of (cardiac) prosthesis 429.4
    fetus or newborn 779.89
    following cardiac surgery 429.4
    hypertensive (*see also* Hypertension, heart)
      402.91
      benign 402.11
      malignant 402.01
    postoperative 997.1
      long-term effect of cardiac surgery 429.4
    rheumatic 398.0
      active, acute, or subacute 391.2
        with chorea (Sydenham's) 392.0
    syphilitic 093.82
  nourishment 994.2
  organic 799.89
  ovary 256.39
    postablative 256.2
  pancreatic 577.8
  parathyroid (gland) 252.1
  peripheral vascular (arterial) 443.9
  pituitary (anterior) 253.2
    posterior 253.5
  placental — *see* Placenta, insufficiency
  platelets 287.5
  prenatal care in current pregnancy V23.7
  progressive pluriglandular 258.9
  pseudocholinesterase 289.89

Insufficiency, insufficient — *continued*
  pulmonary (acute) 518.82
    following
      shock 518.5
      surgery 518.5
      trauma 518.5
    newborn 770.89
    valve (*see also* Endocarditis, pulmonary)
      424.3
      congenital 746.09
  pyloric 537.0
  renal (acute) (chronic) 593.9
    due to a procedure 997.5
  respiratory 786.09
    acute 518.82
      following shock, surgery, or trauma 518.5
    newborn 770.89
  rotation — *see* Malrotation
  suprarenal 255.4
    medulla 255.5
  tarso-orbital fascia, congenital 743.66
  tear film 375.15
  testis 257.2
  thyroid (gland) (acquired) — *see also*
    Hypothyroidism
    congenital 243
  tricuspid (*see also* Endocarditis, tricuspid)
    397.0
    congenital 746.89
    syphilitic 093.23
  urethral sphincter 599.84
  valve, valvular (heart) (*see also* Endocarditis)
    424.90
  vascular 459.9
    intestine NEC 557.9
    mesenteric 557.1
    peripheral 443.9
    renal (*see also* Hypertension, kidney) 403.90
  velopharyngeal
    acquired 528.9
    congenital 750.29
  venous (peripheral) 459.81
  ventricular — *see* Insufficiency, myocardial
  vertebral artery 435.1
  vertebrobasilar artery 435.3
  weight gain during pregnancy 646.8 ☑
  zinc 269.3
Insufflation
  fallopian
    fertility testing V26.21
    following sterilization reversal V26.22
  meconium 770.1
Insular — *see* condition
Insulinoma (M8151/0)
  malignant (M8151/3)
    pancreas 157.4
    specified site — *see* Neoplasm, by site,
      malignant
    unspecified site 157.4
  pancreas 211.7
  specified site — *see* Neoplasm, by site, benign
  unspecified site 211.7
Insuloma — *see* Insulinoma
Insult
  brain 437.9
    acute 436
  cerebral 437.9
    acute 436
  cerebrovascular 437.9
    acute 436
  vascular NEC 437.9
    acute 436
Insurance examination (certification) V70.3
Intemperance (*see also* Alcoholism) 303.9 ☑
Interception of pregnancy (menstrual extraction)
  V25.3
Intermenstrual
  bleeding 626.6
    irregular 626.6
    regular 626.5
  hemorrhage 626.6
    irregular 626.6
    regular 626.5
  pain(s) 625.2
Intermittent — *see* condition
Internal — *see* condition

Interproximal wear 521.10 ▲
Interruption
  aortic arch 747.11
  bundle of His 426.50
  fallopian tube (for sterilization) V25.2
  phase-shift, sleep cycle 307.45
  repeated REM-sleep 307.48
  sleep
    due to perceived environmental disturbances
      307.48
    phase-shift, of 24-hour sleep-wake cycle
      307.45
    repeated REM-sleep type 307.48
  vas deferens (for sterilization) V25.2
Intersexuality 752.7
Interstitial — *see* condition
Intertrigo 695.89
  labialis 528.5
Intervertebral disc — *see* condition
Intestine, intestinal — *see also* condition
  flu 487.8
Intolerance
  carbohydrate NEC 579.8
  cardiovascular exercise, with pain (at rest)
    (with less than ordinary activity) (with
    ordinary activity) V47.2
  cold 780.99
  dissacharide (hereditary) 271.3
  drug
    correct substance properly administered
      995.2
    wrong substance given or taken in error
      977.9
    specified drug — *see* Table of Drugs and
      Chemicals
  effort 306.2
  fat NEC 579.8
  foods NEC 579.8
  fructose (hereditary) 271.2
  glucose (-galactose) (congenital) 271.3
  gluten 579.0
  lactose (hereditary) (infantile) 271.3
  lysine (congenital) 270.7
  milk NEC 579.8
  protein (familial) 270.7
  starch NEC 579.8
  sucrose (-isomaltose) (congenital) 271.3
Intoxicated NEC (*see also* Alcoholism) 305.0 ☑
Intoxication
  acid 276.2
  acute
    alcoholic 305.0 ☑
      with alcoholism 303.0 ☑
      hangover effects 305.0 ☑
    caffeine 305.9 ☑
    hallucinogenic (*see also* Abuse, drugs,
      nondependent) 305.3 ☑
  alcohol (acute) 305.0 ☑
    with alcoholism 303.0 ☑
    hangover effects 305.0 ☑
    idiosyncratic 291.4
    pathological 291.4
  alimentary canal 558.2
  ammonia (hepatic) 572.2
  caffeine 305.9 ☑ ●
  chemical — *see also* Table of Drugs and
    Chemicals
    via placenta or breast milk 760.70
      alcohol 760.71
      anti-infective agents 760.74
      cocaine 760.75
      "crack" 760.75
      hallucinogenic agents NEC 760.73
      medicinal agents NEC 760.79
      narcotics 760.72
      obstetric anesthetic or analgesic drug
        763.5
      specified agent NEC 760.79
      suspected, affecting management of
        pregnancy 655.5 ☑
  cocaine, through placenta or breast milk
    760.75
  delirium
    alcohol 291.0
    drug 292.81

☑ Additional Digit Required   ◄► Revised Text   ● New Line   ▲ Revised Code

Intoxication — *continued*
drug 292.9 ▲
  with delirium 292.81
  correct substance properly administered (*see also* Allergy, drug) 995.2
  newborn 779.4
  obstetric anesthetic or sedation 668.9 ☑
    affecting fetus or newborn 763.5
  overdose or wrong substance given or taken — *see* Table of Drugs and Chemicals
  pathologic 292.2
  specific to newborn 779.4
  via placenta or breast milk 760.70
    alcohol 760.71
    anti-infective agents 760.74
    cocaine 760.75
    "crack" 760.75
    hallucinogenic agents 760.73
    medicinal agents NEC 760.79
    narcotics 760.72
    obstetric anesthetic or analgesic drug 763.5
    specified agent NEC 760.79
    suspected, affecting management of pregnancy 655.5 ☑
enteric — *see* Intoxication, intestinal
fetus or newborn, via placenta or breast milk 760.70
  alcohol 760.71
  anti-infective agents 760.74
  cocaine 760.75
  "crack" 760.75
  hallucinogenic agents 760.73
  medicinal agents NEC 760.79
  narcotics 760.72
  obstetric anesthetic or analgesic drug 763.5
  specified agent NEC 760.79
  suspected, affecting management of pregnancy 655.5 ☑
food — *see* Poisoning, food
gastrointestinal 558.2
hallucinogenic (acute) 305.3 ☑
hepatocerebral 572.2
idiosyncratic alcohol 291.4
intestinal 569.89
  due to putrefaction of food 005.9
methyl alcohol (*see also* Alcoholism) 305.0 ☑
  with alcoholism 303.0 ☑
pathologic 291.4
  drug 292.2
potassium (K) 276.7
septic
  with
    abortion — *see* Abortion, by type, with sepsis
    ectopic pregnancy (*see also* categories 633.0-633.9) 639.0
    molar pregnancy (*see also* categories 630-632) 639.0
  during labor 659.3 ☑
  following
    abortion 639.0
    ectopic or molar pregnancy 639.0
  generalized — *see* Septicemia
  puerperal, postpartum, childbirth 670.0 ☑
serum (prophylactic) (therapeutic) 999.5
uremic — *see* Uremia
water 276.6
Intracranial — *see* condition
Intrahepatic gallbladder 751.69
Intraligamentous — *see also* condition
  pregnancy — *see* Pregnancy, cornual
Intraocular — *see also* condition
  sepsis 360.00
Intrathoracic — *see also* condition
  kidney 753.3
  stomach — *see* Hernia, diaphragm
Intrauterine contraceptive device
  checking V25.42
  insertion V25.1
  in situ V45.51
  management V25.42
  prescription V25.02
    repeat V25.42
  reinsertion V25.42
  removal V25.42

Intraventricular — *see* condition
Intrinsic deformity — *see* Deformity
Intrusion, repetitive, of sleep (due to environmental disturbances) (with atypical polysomnographic features) 307.48
Intumescent, lens (eye) NEC 366.9
  senile 366.12
Intussusception (colon) (enteric) (intestine) (rectum) 560.0
  appendix 543.9
  congenital 751.5
  fallopian tube 620.8
  ileocecal 560.0
  ileocolic 560.0
  ureter (with obstruction) 593.4
Invagination
  basilar 756.0
  colon or intestine 560.0
Invalid (since birth) 799.89
Invalidism (chronic) 799.89
Inversion
  albumin-globulin (A-G) ratio 273.8
  bladder 596.8
  cecum (*see also* Intussusception) 560.0
  cervix 622.8
  nipple 611.79
    congenital 757.6
    puerperal, postpartum 676.3 ☑
  optic papilla 743.57
  organ or site, congenital NEC — *see* Anomaly, specified type NEC
  sleep rhythm 780.55
    nonorganic origin 307.45
  testis (congenital) 752.51
  uterus (postinfectional) (postpartal, old) 621.7
    chronic 621.7
    complicating delivery 665.2 ☑
      affecting fetus or newborn 763.89
  vagina — *see* Prolapse, vagina
Investigation
  allergens V72.7
  clinical research (control) (normal comparison) (participant) V70.7
Inviability — *see* Immaturity
Involuntary movement, abnormal 781.0
Involution, involutional — *see also* condition
  breast, cystic or fibrocystic 610.1
  depression (*see also* Psychosis, affective) 296.2 ☑
    recurrent episode 296.3 ☑
    single episode 296.2 ☑
  melancholia (*see also* Psychosis, affective) 296.2 ☑
    recurrent episode 296.3 ☑
    single episode 296.2 ☑
  ovary, senile 620.3
  paranoid state (reaction) 297.2
  paraphrenia (climacteric) (menopause) 297.2
  psychosis 298.8
  thymus failure 254.8
IQ
  under 20 318.2
  20-34 318.1
  35-49 318.0
  50-70 317
IRDS 769
Irideremia 743.45
Iridis rubeosis 364.42
  diabetic 250.5 ☑ *[364.42]*
Iridochoroiditis (panuveitis) 360.12
Iridocyclitis NEC 364.3
  acute 364.00
    primary 364.01
    recurrent 364.02
  chronic 364.10
    in
      lepromatous leprosy 030.0 *[364.11]*
      sarcoidosis 135 *[364.11]*
      tuberculosis (*see also* Tuberculosis) 017.3 ☑ *[364.11]*
  due to allergy 364.04
  endogenous 364.01
  gonococcal 098.41
  granulomatous 364.10

Iridocyclitis NEC — *continued*
  herpetic (simplex) 054.44
    zoster 053.22
  hypopyon 364.05
  lens induced 364.23
  nongranulomatous 364.00
  primary 364.01
  recurrent 364.02
  rheumatic 364.10
  secondary 364.04
    infectious 364.03
    noninfectious 364.04
  subacute 364.00
    primary 364.01
    recurrent 364.02
  sympathetic 360.11
  syphilitic (secondary) 091.52
  tuberculous (chronic) (*see also* Tuberculosis) 017.3 ☑ *[364.11]*
Iridocyclochoroiditis (panuveitis) 360.12
Iridodialysis 364.76
Iridodonesis 364.8
Iridoplegia (complete) (partial) (reflex) 379.49
Iridoschisis 364.52
Iris — *see* condition
Iritis 364.3
  acute 364.00
    primary 364.01
    recurrent 364.02
  chronic 364.10
    in
      sarcoidosis 135 *[364.11]*
      tuberculosis (*see also* Tuberculosis) 017.3 ☑ *[364.11]*
  diabetic 250.5 ☑ *[364.42]*
  due to
    allergy 364.04
    herpes simplex 054.44
    leprosy 030.0 *[364.11]*
  endogenous 364.01
  gonococcal 098.41
  gouty 274.89 *[364.11]*
  granulomatous 364.10
  hypopyon 364.05
  lens induced 364.23
  nongranulomatous 364.00
  papulosa 095.8 *[364.11]*
  primary 364.01
  recurrent 364.02
  rheumatic 364.10
  secondary 364.04
    infectious 364.03
    noninfectious 364.04
  subacute 364.00
    primary 364.01
    recurrent 364.02
  sympathetic 360.11
  syphilitic (secondary) 091.52
    congenital 090.0 *[364.11]*
    late 095.8 *[364.11]*
  tuberculous (*see also* Tuberculosis) 017.3 ☑ *[364.11]*
  uratic 274.89 *[364.11]*
Iron
  deficiency anemia 280.9
  metabolism disease 275.0
  storage disease 275.0
Iron-miners' lung 503
Irradiated enamel (tooth, teeth) 521.8
Irradiation
  burn — *see* Burn, by site
  effects, adverse 990
Irreducible, irreducibility — *see* condition
Irregular, irregularity
  action, heart 427.9
  alveolar process 525.8
  bleeding NEC 626.4
  breathing 786.09
  colon 569.89
  contour of cornea 743.41
    acquired 371.70
  dentin in pulp 522.3
  eye movements NEC 379.59
  menstruation (cause unknown) 626.4

Intoxication — Irregular, irregularity

Irregular, irregularity — *continued*
  periods 626.4
  prostate 602.9
  pupil 364.75
  respiratory 786.09
  septum (nasal) 470
  shape, organ or site, congenital NEC — *see* Distortion
  sleep-wake rhythm (non-24-hour) 780.55
    nonorganic origin 307.45
  vertebra 733.99
Irritability (nervous) 799.2
  bladder 596.8
    neurogenic 596.54
      with cauda equina syndrome 344.61
  bowel (syndrome) 564.1
  bronchial (*see also* Bronchitis) 490
  cerebral, newborn 779.1
  colon 564.1
    psychogenic 306.4
  duodenum 564.89
  heart (psychogenic) 306.2
  ileum 564.89
  jejunum 564.89
  myocardium 306.2
  rectum 564.89
  stomach 536.9
    psychogenic 306.4
  sympathetic (nervous system) (*see also* Neuropathy, peripheral, autonomic) 337.9
  urethra 599.84
  ventricular (heart) (psychogenic) 306.2
Irritable — *see* Irritability
Irritation
  anus 569.49
  axillary nerve 353.0
  bladder 596.8
  brachial plexus 353.0
  brain (traumatic) (*see also* Injury, intracranial) 854.0 ☑
    nontraumatic — *see* Encephalitis
  bronchial (*see also* Bronchitis) 490
  cerebral (traumatic) (*see also* Injury, intracranial) 854.0 ☑
    nontraumatic — *see* Encephalitis
  cervical plexus 353.2
  cervix (*see also* Cervicitis) 616.0
  choroid, sympathetic 360.11
  cranial nerve — *see* Disorder, nerve, cranial
  digestive tract 536.9
    psychogenic 306.4
  gastric 536.9
    psychogenic 306.4
  gastrointestinal (tract) 536.9
    functional 536.9
    psychogenic 306.4
  globe, sympathetic 360.11
  intestinal (bowel) 564.9
  labyrinth 386.50
  lumbosacral plexus 353.1
  meninges (traumatic) (*see also* Injury, intracranial) 854.0 ☑
    nontraumatic — *see* Meningitis
  myocardium 306.2
  nerve — *see* Disorder, nerve
  nervous 799.2
  nose 478.1
  penis 607.89
  perineum 709.9
  peripheral
    autonomic nervous system (*see also* Neuropathy, peripheral, autonomic) 337.9
    nerve — *see* Disorder, nerve
  peritoneum (*see also* Peritonitis) 567.9
  pharynx 478.29
  plantar nerve 355.6
  spinal (cord) (traumatic) — *see also* Injury, spinal, by site
    nerve — *see also* Disorder, nerve
      root NEC 724.9
      traumatic — *see* Injury, nerve, spinal
    nontraumatic — *see* Myelitis
  stomach 536.9
    psychogenic 306.4

Irritation — *continued*
  sympathetic nerve NEC (*see also* Neuropathy, peripheral, autonomic) 337.9
  ulnar nerve 354.2
  vagina 623.9
Isambert's disease 012.3 ☑
Ischemia, ischemic 459.9
  basilar artery (with transient neurologic deficit) 435.0
  bone NEC 733.40
  bowel (transient) 557.9
    acute 557.0
    chronic 557.1
    due to mesenteric artery insufficiency 557.1
  brain — *see also* Ischemia, cerebral
    recurrent focal 435.9
  cardiac (*see also* Ischemia, heart) 414.9
  cardiomyopathy 414.8
  carotid artery (with transient neurologic deficit) 435.8
  cerebral (chronic) (generalized) 437.1
    arteriosclerotic 437.0
    intermittent (with transient neurologic deficit) 435.9
    puerperal, postpartum, childbirth 674.0 ☑
    recurrent focal (with transient neurologic deficit) 435.9
    transient (with transient neurologic deficit) 435.9
  colon 557.9
    acute 557.0
    chronic 557.1
    due to mesenteric artery insufficiency 557.1
  coronary (chronic) (*see also* Ischemia, heart) 414.9
  heart (chronic or with a stated duration of over 8 weeks) 414.9
    acute or with a stated duration of 8 weeks or less (*see also* Infarct, myocardium) 410.9 ☑
      without myocardial infarction 411.89
        with coronary (artery) occlusion 411.81
    subacute 411.89
  intestine (transient) 557.9
    acute 557.0
    chronic 557.1
    due to mesenteric artery insufficiency 557.1
  kidney 593.81
  labyrinth 386.50
  muscles, leg 728.89
  myocardium, myocardial (chronic or with a stated duration of over 8 weeks) 414.8
    acute (*see also* Infarct, myocardium) 410.9 ☑
      without myocardial infarction 411.89
        with coronary (artery) occlusion 411.81
  renal 593.81
  retina, retinal 362.84
  small bowel 557.9
    acute 557.0
    chronic 557.1
    due to mesenteric artery insufficiency 557.1
  spinal cord 336.1
  subendocardial (*see also* Insufficiency, coronary) 411.89
  vertebral artery (with transient neurologic deficit) 435.1
Ischialgia (*see also* Sciatica) 724.3
Ischiopagus 759.4
Ischium, ischial — *see* condition
Ischomenia 626.8
Ischuria 788.5
Iselin's disease or osteochondrosis 732.5
Islands of
  parotid tissue in
    lymph nodes 750.26
    neck structures 750.26
  submaxillary glands in
    fascia 750.26
    lymph nodes 750.26
    neck muscles 750.26
Islet cell tumor, pancreas (M8150/0) 211.7

Isoimmunization NEC (*see also* Incompatibility) 656.2 ☑
  fetus or newborn 773.2
    ABO blood groups 773.1
    Rhesus (Rh) factor 773.0
Isolation V07.0
  social V62.4
Isosporosis 007.2
Issue
  medical certificate NEC V68.0
    cause of death V68.0
    fitness V68.0
    incapacity V68.0
  repeat prescription NEC V68.1
    appliance V68.1
    contraceptive V25.40
      device NEC V25.49
        intrauterine V25.42
        specified type NEC V25.49
      pill V25.41
    glasses V68.1
    medicinal substance V68.1
Itch (*see also* Pruritus) 698.9
  bakers' 692.89
  barbers' 110.0
  bricklayers' 692.89
  cheese 133.8
  clam diggers' 120.3
  coolie 126.9
  copra 133.8
  Cuban 050.1
  dew 126.9
  dhobie 110.3
  eye 379.99
  filarial (*see also* Infestation, filarial) 125.9
  grain 133.8
  grocers' 133.8
  ground 126.9
  harvest 133.8
  jock 110.3
  Malabar 110.9
    beard 110.0
    foot 110.4
    scalp 110.0
  meaning scabies 133.0
  Norwegian 133.0
  perianal 698.0
  poultrymen's 133.8
  sarcoptic 133.0
  scrub 134.1
  seven year V61.10
    meaning scabies 133.0
  straw 133.8
  swimmers' 120.3
  washerwoman's 692.4
  water 120.3
  winter 698.8
Itsenko-Cushing syndrome (pituitary basophilism) 255.0
Ivemark's syndrome (asplenia with congenital heart disease) 759.0
Ivory bones 756.52
Ixodes 134.8
Ixodiasis 134.8

J

Jaccoud's nodular fibrositis, chronic (Jaccoud's syndrome) 714.4

Jackson's
membrane 751.4
paralysis or syndrome 344.89
veil 751.4

Jacksonian
epilepsy (see also Epilepsy) 345.5 ☑
seizures (focal) (see also Epilepsy) 345.5 ☑

Jacob's ulcer (M8090/3) — see Neoplasm, skin, malignant, by site

Jacquet's dermatitis (diaper dermatitis) 691.0

Jadassohn's
blue nevus (M8780/0) — see Neoplasm, skin, benign
disease (maculopapular erythroderma) 696.2
intraepidermal epithelioma (M8096/0) — see Neoplasm, skin, benign

Jadassohn-Lewandowski syndrome (pachyonychia congenita) 757.5

Jadassohn-Pellizari's disease (anetoderma) 701.3

Jadassohn-Tièche nevus (M8780/0) — see Neoplasm, skin, benign

Jaffe-Lichtenstein (-Uehlinger) syndrome 252.01 ▲

Jahnke's syndrome (encephalocutaneous angiomatosis) 759.6

Jakob-Creutzfeldt disease or syndrome 046.1
with dementia
with behavioral disturbance 046.1 [294.11]
without behavioral disturbance 046.1 [294.10]

Jaksch (-Luzet) disease or syndrome (pseudoleukemia infantum) 285.8

Jamaican
neuropathy 349.82
paraplegic tropical ataxic-spastic syndrome 349.82

Janet's disease (psychasthenia) 300.89

Janiceps 759.4

Jansky-Bielschowsky amaurotic familial idiocy 330.1

Japanese
B type encephalitis 062.0
river fever 081.2
seven-day fever 100.89

Jaundice (yellow) 782.4
acholuric (familial) (splenomegalic) (see also Spherocytosis) 282.0
acquired 283.9
breast milk 774.39
catarrhal (acute) 070.1
with hepatic coma 070.0
chronic 571.9
epidemic — see Jaundice, epidemic
cholestatic (benign) 782.4
chronic idiopathic 277.4
epidemic (catarrhal) 070.1
with hepatic coma 070.0
leptospiral 100.0
spirochetal 100.0
febrile (acute) 070.1
with hepatic coma 070.0
leptospiral 100.0
spirochetal 100.0
fetus or newborn 774.6
due to or associated with
ABO
antibodies 773.1
incompatibility, maternal/fetal 773.1
isoimmunization 773.1
absence or deficiency of enzyme system for bilirubin conjugation (congenital) 774.39
blood group incompatibility NEC 773.2
breast milk inhibitors to conjugation 774.39
associated with preterm delivery 774.2
bruising 774.1
Crigler-Najjar syndrome 277.4 [774.31]
delayed conjugation 774.30
associated with preterm delivery 774.2

Jaundice — continued
fetus or newborn — continued
due to or associated with — continued
delayed conjugation — continued
development 774.39
drugs or toxins transmitted from mother 774.1
G-6-PD deficiency 282.2 [774.0]
galactosemia 271.1 [774.5]
Gilbert's syndrome 277.4 [774.31]
hepatocellular damage 774.4
hereditary hemolytic anemia (see also Anemia, hemolytic) 282.9 [774.0]
hypothyroidism, congenital 243 [774.31]
incompatibility, maternal/fetal NEC 773.2
infection 774.1
inspissated bile syndrome 774.4
isoimmunization NEC 773.2
mucoviscidosis 277.01 [774.5]
obliteration of bile duct, congenital 751.61 [774.5]
polycythemia 774.1
preterm delivery 774.2
red cell defect 282.9 [774.0]
Rh
antibodies 773.0
incompatibility, maternal/fetal 773.0
isoimmunization 773.0
spherocytosis (congenital) 282.0 [774.0]
swallowed maternal blood 774.1
physiological NEC 774.6
from injection, inoculation, infusion, or transfusion (blood) (plasma) (serum) (other substance) (onset within 8 months after administration) — see Hepatitis, viral
Gilbert's (familial nonhemolytic) 277.4
hematogenous 283.9
hemolytic (acquired) 283.9
congenital (see also Spherocytosis) 282.0
hemorrhagic (acute) 100.0
leptospiral 100.0
newborn 776.0
hemorrhagic
spirochetal 100.0
hepatocellular 573.8
homologous (serum) — see Hepatitis, viral
idiopathic, chronic 277.4
infectious (acute) (subacute) 070.1
with hepatic coma 070.0
leptospiral 100.0
spirochetal 100.0
leptospiral 100.0
malignant (see also Necrosis, liver) 570
newborn (physiological) (see also Jaundice, fetus or newborn) 774.6
nonhemolytic, congenital familial (Gilbert's) 277.4
nuclear, newborn (see also Kernicterus of newborn) 774.7
obstructive NEC (see also Obstruction, biliary) 576.8
postimmunization — see Hepatitis, viral
posttransfusion — see Hepatitis, viral
regurgitation (see also Obstruction, biliary) 576.8
serum (homologous) (prophylactic) (therapeutic) — see Hepatitis, viral
spirochetal (hemorrhagic) 100.0
symptomatic 782.4
newborn 774.6

Jaw — see condition

Jaw-blinking 374.43
congenital 742.8

Jaw-winking phenomenon or syndrome 742.8

Jealousy
alcoholic 291.5
childhood 313.3
sibling 313.3

Jejunitis (see also Enteritis) 558.9

Jejunostomy status V44.4

Jejunum, jejunal — see condition

Jensen's disease 363.05

Jericho boil 085.1

Jerks, myoclonic 333.2

Jeune's disease or syndrome (asphyxiating thoracic dystrophy) 756.4

Jigger disease 134.1

Job's syndrome (chronic granulomatous disease) 288.1

Jod-Basedow phenomenon 242.8 ☑

Johnson-Stevens disease (erythema multiforme exudativum) 695.1

Joint — see also condition
Charcôt's 094.0 [713.5]
false 733.82
flail — see Flail, joint
mice — see Loose, body, joint, by site
sinus to bone 730.9 ☑
von Gies' 095.8

Jordan's anomaly or syndrome 288.2

Josephs-Diamond-Blackfan anemia (congenital hypoplastic) 284.0

Joubert syndrome 759.89

Jumpers' knee 727.2

Jungle yellow fever 060.0

Jüngling's disease (sarcoidosis) 135

Junin virus hemorrhagic fever 078.7

Juvenile — see also condition
delinquent 312.9
group (see also Disturbance, conduct) 312.2 ☑
neurotic 312.4

K

Kabuki syndrome 759.89 ●

Kahler (-Bozzolo) disease (multiple myeloma) (M9730/3) 203.0 ☑

Kakergasia 300.9

Kakke 265.0

Kala-azar (Indian) (infantile) (Mediterranean) (Sudanese) 085.0

Kalischer's syndrome (encephalocutaneous angiomatosis) 759.6

Kallmann's syndrome (hypogonadotropic hypogonadism with anosmia) 253.4

Kanner's syndrome (autism) (see also Psychosis, childhood) 299.0 ☑

Kaolinosis 502

Kaposi's
disease 757.33
lichen ruber 696.4
acuminatus 696.4
moniliformis 697.8
xeroderma pigmentosum 757.33
sarcoma (M9140/3) 176.9
adipose tissue 176.1
aponeurosis 176.1
artery 176.1
blood vessel 176.1
bursa 176.1
connective tissue 176.1
external genitalia 176.8
fascia 176.1
fatty tissue 176.1
fibrous tissue 176.1
gastrointestinal tract NEC 176.3
ligament 176.1
lung 176.4
lymph
gland(s) 176.5
node(s) 176.5
lymphatic(s) NEC 176.1
muscle (skeletal) 176.1
oral cavity NEC 176.8
palate 176.2
scrotum 176.8
skin 176.0
soft tissue 176.1
specified site NEC 176.8
subcutaneous tissue 176.1
synovia 176.1
tendon (sheath) 176.1
vein 176.1
vessel 176.1

☑ Additional Digit Required   ▶◀ Revised Text   ● New Line   ▲ Revised Code

Kaposi's — *continued*
  sarcoma — *continued*
    viscera NEC 176.9
    vulva 176.8
  varicelliform eruption 054.0
  vaccinia 999.0

Kartagener's syndrome or triad (sinusitis, bronchiectasis, situs inversus) 759.3

Kasabach-Merritt syndrome (capillary hemangioma associated with thrombocytopenic purpura) 287.3

Kaschin-Beck disease (endemic polyarthritis) — *see* Disease, Kaschin-Beck

Kast's syndrome (dyschondroplasia with hemangiomas) 756.4

Katatonia (*see also* Schizophrenia) 295.2 ☑

Katayama disease or fever 120.2

Kathisophobia 781.0

Kawasaki disease 446.1

Kayser-Fleischer ring (cornea) (pseudosclerosis) 275.1 *[371.14]*

Kaznelson's syndrome (congenital hypoplastic anemia) 284.0

Kearns-Sayre syndrome 277.87   ●

Kedani fever 081.2

Kelis 701.4

Kelly (-Patterson) syndrome (sideropenic dysphagia) 280.8

Keloid, cheloid 701.4
  Addison's (morphea) 701.0
  cornea 371.00
  Hawkins' 701.4
  scar 701.4

Keloma 701.4

Kenya fever 082.1

Keratectasia 371.71
  congenital 743.41

Keratitis (nodular) (nonulcerative) (simple) (zonular) NEC 370.9
  with ulceration (*see also* Ulcer, cornea) 370.00
  actinic 370.24
  arborescens 054.42
  areolar 370.22
  bullosa 370.8
  deep — *see* Keratitis, interstitial
  dendritic(a) 054.42
  desiccation 370.34
  diffuse interstitial 370.52
  disciform(is) 054.43
    varicella 052.7 *[370.44]*
  epithelialis vernalis 372.13 *[370.32]*
  exposure 370.34
  filamentary 370.23
  gonococcal (congenital) (prenatal) 098.43
  herpes, herpetic (simplex) NEC 054.43
    zoster 053.21
  hypopyon 370.04
  in
    chickenpox 052.7 *[370.44]*
    exanthema (*see also* Exanthem) 057.9 *[370.44]*
    paravaccinia (*see also* Paravaccinia) 051.9 *[370.44]*
    smallpox (*see also* Smallpox) 050.9 *[370.44]*
    vernal conjunctivitis 372.13 *[370.32]*
  interstitial (nonsyphilitic) 370.50
    with ulcer (*see also* Ulcer, cornea) 370.00
    diffuse 370.52
    herpes, herpetic (simplex) 054.43
      zoster 053.21
    syphilitic (congenital) (hereditary) 090.3
    tuberculous (*see also* Tuberculosis) 017.3 ☑ *[370.59]*
  lagophthalmic 370.34
  macular 370.22
  neuroparalytic 370.35
  neurotrophic 370.35
  nummular 370.22
  oyster-shuckers' 370.8
  parenchymatous — *see* Keratitis, interstitial
  petrificans 370.8
  phlyctenular 370.31
  postmeasles 055.71

Keratitis NEC — *continued*
  punctata, punctate 370.21
    leprosa 030.0 *[370.21]*
    profunda 090.3
    superficial (Thygeson's) 370.21
  purulent 370.8
  pustuliformis profunda 090.3
  rosacea 695.3 *[370.49]*
  sclerosing 370.54
  specified type NEC 370.8
  stellate 370.22
  striate 370.22
  superficial 370.20
    with conjunctivitis (*see also* Keratoconjunctivitis) 370.40
    punctate (Thygeson's) 370.21
  suppurative 370.8
  syphilitic (congenital) (prenatal) 090.3
  trachomatous 076.1
    late effect 139.1
  tuberculous (phlyctenular) (*see also* Tuberculosis) 017.3 ☑ *[370.31]*
  ulcerated (*see also* Ulcer, cornea) 370.00
  vesicular 370.8
  welders' 370.24
  xerotic (*see also* Keratomalacia) 371.45
    vitamin A deficiency 264.4

Keratoacanthoma 238.2

Keratocele 371.72

Keratoconjunctivitis (*see also* Keratitis) 370.40
  adenovirus type 8 077.1
  epidemic 077.1
  exposure 370.34
  gonococcal 098.43
  herpetic (simplex) 054.43
    zoster 053.21
  in
    chickenpox 052.7 *[370.44]*
    exanthema (*see also* Exanthem) 057.9 *[370.44]*
    paravaccinia (*see also* Paravaccinia) 051.9 *[370.44]*
    smallpox (*see also* Smallpox) 050.9 *[370.44]*
  infectious 077.1
  neurotrophic 370.35
  phlyctenular 370.31
  postmeasles 055.71
  shipyard 077.1
  sicca (Sjögren's syndrome) 710.2
    not in Sjögren's syndrome 370.33
  specified type NEC 370.49
  tuberculous (phlyctenular) (*see also* Tuberculosis) 017.3 ☑ *[370.31]*

Keratoconus 371.60
  acute hydrops 371.62
  congenital 743.41
  stable 371.61

Keratocyst (dental) 526.0

Keratoderma, keratodermia (congenital) (palmaris et plantaris) (symmetrical) 757.39
  acquired 701.1
  blennorrhagica 701.1
    gonococcal 098.81
  climacterium 701.1
  eccentrica 757.39
  gonorrheal 098.81
  punctata 701.1
  tylodes, progressive 701.1

Keratodermatocele 371.72

Keratoglobus 371.70
  congenital 743.41
    associated with buphthalmos 743.22

Keratohemia 371.12

Keratoiritis (*see also* Iridocyclitis) 364.3
  syphilitic 090.3
  tuberculous (*see also* Tuberculosis) 017.3 ☑ *[364.11]*

Keratolysis exfoliativa (congenital) 757.39
  acquired 695.89
  neonatorum 757.39

Keratoma 701.1
  congenital 757.39
  malignum congenitale 757.1
  palmaris et plantaris hereditarium 757.39
  senile 702.0

Keratomalacia 371.45
  vitamin A deficiency 264.4

Keratomegaly 743.41

Keratomycosis 111.1
  nigricans (palmaris) 111.1

Keratopathy 371.40
  band (*see also* Keratitis) 371.43
  bullous (*see also* Keratitis) 371.23
  degenerative (*see also* Degeneration, cornea) 371.40
    hereditary (*see also* Dystrophy, cornea) 371.50
  discrete colliquative 371.49

Keratoscleritis, tuberculous (*see also* Tuberculosis) 017.3 ☑ *[370.31]*

Keratosis 701.1
  actinic 702.0
  arsenical 692.4
  blennorrhagica 701.1
    gonococcal 098.81
  congenital (any type) 757.39
  ear (middle) (*see also* Cholesteatoma) 385.30
  female genital (external) 629.8
  follicular, vitamin A deficiency 264.8
  follicularis 757.39
    acquired 701.1
    congenital (acneiformis) (Siemens') 757.39
    spinulosa (decalvans) 757.39
    vitamin A deficiency 264.8
  gonococcal 098.81
  larynx, laryngeal 478.79
  male genital (external) 608.89
  middle ear (*see also* Cholesteatoma) 385.30
  nigricans 701.2
    congenital 757.39
  obturans 380.21
  oral epithelium   ●
    residual ridge mucosa   ●
      excessive 528.72   ●
      minimal 528.71   ●
  palmaris et plantaris (symmetrical) 757.39
  penile 607.89
  pharyngeus 478.29
  pilaris 757.39
    acquired 701.1
  punctata (palmaris et plantaris) 701.1
  scrotal 608.89
  seborrheic 702.19
    inflamed 702.11
  senilis 702.0
  solar 702.0
  suprafollicularis 757.39
  tonsillaris 478.29
  vagina 623.1
  vegetans 757.39
  vitamin A deficiency 264.8

Kerato-uveitis (*see also* Iridocyclitis) 364.3

Keraunoparalysis 994.0

Kerion (celsi) 110.0

Kernicterus of newborn (not due to isoimmunization) 774.7
  due to isoimmunization (conditions classifiable to 773.0-773.2) 773.4

Ketoacidosis 276.2
  diabetic 250.1 ☑

Ketonuria 791.6
  branched-chain, intermittent 270.3

Ketosis 276.2
  diabetic 250.1 ☑

Kidney — *see* condition

Kienböck's
  disease 732.3
    adult 732.8
  osteochondrosis 732.3

Kimmelstiel (-Wilson) disease or syndrome (intercapillary glomerulosclerosis) 250.4 ☑ *[581.81]*

Kink, kinking
  appendix 543.9
  artery 447.1
  cystic duct, congenital 751.61
  hair (acquired) 704.2
  ileum or intestine (*see also* Obstruction, intestine) 560.9

☑ Additional Digit Required   ▶◀ Revised Text   ● New Line   ▲ Revised Code

Kink, kinking — *continued*
  Lane's (*see also* Obstruction, intestine) 560.9
  organ or site, congenital NEC — *see* Anomaly,
    specified type NEC, by site
  ureter (pelvic junction) 593.3
    congenital 753.20
  vein(s) 459.2
    caval 459.2
    peripheral 459.2
Kinnier Wilson's disease (hepatolenticular
  degeneration) 275.1
Kissing
  osteophytes 721.5
  spine 721.5
  vertebra 721.5
Klauder's syndrome (erythema multiforme,
  exudativum) 695.1
Klebs' disease (*see also* Nephritis) 583.9
Klein-Waardenburg syndrome (ptosisepicanthus)
  270.2
Kleine-Levin syndrome 349.89
Kleptomania 312.32
Klinefelter's syndrome 758.7
Klinger's disease 446.4
Klippel's disease 723.8
Klippel-Feil disease or syndrome (brevicollis)
  756.16
Klippel-Trenaunay syndrome 759.89
Klumpke (-Déjérine) palsy, paralysis (birth)
  (newborn) 767.6
Klüver-Bucy (-Terzian) syndrome 310.0
Knee — *see* condition
Knifegrinders' rot (*see also* Tuberculosis)
  011.4 ☑
Knock-knee (acquired) 736.41
  congenital 755.64
Knot
  intestinal, syndrome (volvulus) 560.2
  umbilical cord (true) 663.2 ☑
    affecting fetus or newborn 762.5
Knots, surfer 919.8
  infected 919.9
Knotting (of)
  hair 704.2
  intestine 560.2
Knuckle pads (Garrod's) 728.79
Köbner's disease (epidermolysis bullosa) 757.39
Koch's
  infection (*see also* Tuberculosis, pulmonary)
    011.9 ☑
  relapsing fever 087.9
Koch-Weeks conjunctivitis 372.03
Koenig-Wichman disease (pemphigus) 694.4
Köhler's disease (osteochondrosis) 732.5
  first (osteochondrosis juvenilis) 732.5
  second (Freiburg's infarction, metatarsal head)
    732.5
  patellar 732.4
  tarsal navicular (bone) (osteoarthrosis juvenilis)
    732.5
Köhler-Mouchet disease (osteoarthrosis juvenilis)
  732.5
Köhler-Pellegrini-Stieda disease or syndrome
  (calcification, knee joint) 726.62
Koilonychia 703.8
  congenital 757.5
Kojevnikov's, Kojewnikoff's epilepsy (*see also*
  Epilepsy) 345.7 ☑
König's
  disease (osteochondritis dissecans) 732.7
  syndrome 564.89
Koniophthisis (*see also* Tuberculosis) 011.4 ☑
Koplik's spots 055.9
Kopp's asthma 254.8
Korean hemorrhagic fever 078.6
Korsakoff (-Wernicke) disease, psychosis, or
  syndrome (nonalcoholic) 294.0
  alcoholic 291.1
Korsakov's disease — *see* Korsakoff's disease
Korsakow's disease — *see* Korsakoff's disease

Kostmann's disease or syndrome (infantile
  genetic agranulocytosis) 288.0
Krabbe's
  disease (leukodystrophy) 330.0
  syndrome
    congenital muscle hypoplasia 756.89
    cutaneocerebral angioma 759.6
Kraepelin-Morel disease (*see also* Schizophrenia)
  295.9 ☑
Kraft-Weber-Dimitri disease 759.6
Kraurosis
  ani 569.49
  penis 607.0
  vagina 623.8
  vulva 624.0
Kreotoxism 005.9
Krukenberg's
  spindle 371.13
  tumor (M8490/6) 198.6
Kufs' disease 330.1
Kugelberg-Welander disease 335.11
Kuhnt-Junius degeneration or disease 362.52
Kulchitsky's cell carcinoma (carcinoid tumor of
  intestine) 259.2
Kümmell's disease or spondylitis 721.7
Kundrat's disease (lymphosarcoma) 200.1 ☑
Kunekune — *see* Dermatophytosis
Kunkel syndrome (lupoid hepatitis) 571.49
Kupffer cell sarcoma (M9124/3) 155.0
Kuru 046.0
Kussmaul's
  coma (diabetic) 250.3 ☑
  disease (polyarteritis nodosa) 446.0
  respiration (air hunger) 786.09
Kwashiorkor (marasmus type) 260
Kyasanur Forest disease 065.2
Kyphoscoliosis, kyphoscoliotic (acquired) (*see*
  also Scoliosis) 737.30
  congenital 756.19
  due to radiation 737.33
  heart (disease) 416.1
  idiopathic 737.30
    infantile
      progressive 737.32
      resolving 737.31
  late effect of rickets 268.1 *[737.43]*
  specified NEC 737.39
  thoracogenic 737.34
  tuberculous (*see also* Tuberculosis)
    015.0 ☑ *[737.43]*
Kyphosis, kyphotic (acquired) (postural) 737.10
  adolescent postural 737.0
  congenital 756.19
  dorsalis juvenilis 732.0
  due to or associated with
    Charcôt-Marie-Tooth disease 356.1 *[737.41]*
    mucopolysaccharidosis 277.5 *[737.41]*
    neurofibromatosis 237.71 *[737.41]*
    osteitis
      deformans 731.0 *[737.41]*
      fibrosa cystica 252.01 *[737.41]*   ▲
    osteoporosis (*see also* Osteoporosis)
      733.0 ☑ *[737.41]*
    poliomyelitis (*see also* Poliomyelitis)
      138 *[737.41]*
    radiation 737.11
    tuberculosis (*see also* Tuberculosis)
      015.0 ☑ *[737.41]*
  Kümmell's 721.7
  late effect of rickets 268.1 *[737.41]*
  Morquio-Brailsford type (spinal) 277.5 *[737.41]*
  pelvis 738.6
  postlaminectomy 737.12
  specified cause NEC 737.19
  syphilitic, congenital 090.5 *[737.41]*
  tuberculous (*see also* Tuberculosis)
    015.0 ☑ *[737.41]*
Kyrle's disease (hyperkeratosis follicularis in
  cutem penetrans) 701.1

L

Labia, labium — *see* condition
Labiated hymen 752.49
Labile
  blood pressure 796.2
  emotions, emotionality 301.3
  vasomotor system 443.9
Labioglossal paralysis 335.22
Labium leporinum (*see also* Cleft, lip) 749.10
Labor (*see also* Delivery)
  with complications — *see* Delivery, complicated
  abnormal NEC 661.9 ☑
    affecting fetus or newborn 763.7
  arrested active phase 661.1 ☑
    affecting fetus or newborn 763.7
  desultory 661.2 ☑
    affecting fetus or newborn 763.7
  dyscoordinate 661.4 ☑
    affecting fetus or newborn 763.7
  early onset (22-36 weeks gestation) 644.2 ☑
  failed
    induction 659.1 ☑
      mechanical 659.0 ☑
      medical 659.1 ☑
      surgical 659.0 ☑
    trial (vaginal delivery) 660.6 ☑
  false 644.1 ☑
  forced or induced, affecting fetus or newborn
    763.89
  hypertonic 661.4 ☑
    affecting fetus or newborn 763.7
  hypotonic 661.2 ☑
    affecting fetus or newborn 763.7
    primary 661.0 ☑
      affecting fetus or newborn 763.7
    secondary 661.1 ☑
      affecting fetus or newborn 763.7
  incoordinate 661.4 ☑
    affecting fetus or newborn 763.7
  irregular 661.2 ☑
    affecting fetus or newborn 763.7
  long — *see* Labor, prolonged
  missed (at or near term) 656.4 ☑
  obstructed NEC 660.9 ☑
    affecting fetus or newborn 763.1
    specified cause NEC 660.8 ☑
      affecting fetus or newborn 763.1
  pains, spurious 644.1 ☑
  precipitate 661.3 ☑
    affecting fetus or newborn 763.6
  premature 644.2 ☑
    threatened 644.0 ☑
  prolonged or protracted 662.1 ☑
    affecting fetus or newborn 763.89
    first stage 662.0 ☑
      affecting fetus or newborn 763.89
    second stage 662.2 ☑
      affecting fetus or newborn 763.89
  threatened NEC 644.1 ☑
  undelivered 644.1 ☑
Labored breathing (*see also* Hyperventilation)
  786.09
Labyrinthitis (inner ear) (destructive) (latent)
  386.30
  circumscribed 386.32
  diffuse 386.31
  focal 386.32
  purulent 386.33
  serous 386.31
  suppurative 386.33
  syphilitic 095.8
  toxic 386.34
  viral 386.35
Laceration — *see also* Wound, open, by site
  accidental, complicating surgery 998.2
  Achilles tendon 845.09
    with open wound 892.2
  anus (sphincter) 879.6
    with
      abortion — *see* Abortion, by type, with
        damage to pelvic organs
      ectopic pregnancy (*see also* categories
        633.0-633.9) 639.2

☑ Additional Digit Required   ▶◀ Revised Text   ● New Line   ▲ Revised Code

Laceration — *see also* Wound, open, by site — *continued*
  anus — *continued*
    with — *continued*
      molar pregnancy (*see also* categories 630-632) 639.2
    complicated 879.7
    complicating delivery 664.2 ☑
      with laceration of anal or rectal mucosa 664.3 ☑
    following
      abortion 639.2
      ectopic or molar pregnancy 639.2
    nontraumatic, nonpuerperal 565.0
  bladder (urinary)
    with
      abortion — *see* Abortion, by type, with damage to pelvic organs
      ectopic pregacy (*see also* categories 633.0-633.9) 639.2
      molar pregnancy (*see also* categories 630-632) 639.2
    following
      abortion 639.2
      ectopic or molar pregnancy 639.2
    obstetrical trauma 665.5 ☑
  blood vessel — *see* Injury, blood vessel, by site
  bowel
    with
      abortion — *see* Abortion, by type, with damage to pelvic organs
      ectopic pregnancy (*see also* categories 633.0-633.9) 639.2
      molar pregnancy (*see also* categories 630-632) 639.2
    following
      abortion 639.2
      ectopic or molar pregnancy 639.2
    obstetrical trauma 665.5 ☑
  brain (with hemorrhage) (cerebral) (membrane) 851.8 ☑
  brain (cerebral) (membrane) 851.8 ☑

> *Note — Use the following fifth-digit subclassification with categories 851–854:*
>
> 0 *unspecified state of consciousness*
> 1 *with no loss of consciousness*
> 2 *with brief [less than one hour] loss of consciousness*
> 3 *with moderate [1-24 hours] loss of consciousness*
> 4 *with prolonged [more than 24 hours] loss of consciousness and return to pre-existing conscious level*
> 5 *with prolonged [more than 24 hours] loss of consciousness, without return to pre-existing conscious level*
>   *Use fifth-digit 5 to designate when a patient is unconscious and dies before regaining consciousness, regardless of the duration of the loss of consciousness*
> 6 *with loss of consciousness of unspecified duration*
> 9 *with concussion, unspecified*

    with
      open intracranial wound 851.9 ☑
      skull fracture — *see* Fracture, skull, by site
    cerebellum 851.6 ☑
      with open intracranial wound 851.7 ☑
    cortex 851.2 ☑
      with open intracranial wound 851.3 ☑
    during birth 767.0
    stem 851.6 ☑
      with open intracranial wound 851.7 ☑
  broad ligament
    with
      abortion — *see* Abortion, by type, with damage to pelvic organs
      ectopic pregnancy (*see also* categories 633.0-633.9) 639.2
      molar pregnancy (*see also* categories 630-632) 639.2

Laceration — *see also* Wound, open, by site — *continued*
  broad ligament — *continued*
    following
      abortion 639.2
      ectopic or molar pregnancy 639.2
    nontraumatic 620.6
    obstetrical trauma 665.6 ☑
    syndrome (nontraumatic) 620.6
  capsule, joint — *see* Sprain, by site
  cardiac — *see* Laceration, heart
  causing eversion of cervix uteri (old) 622.0
  central, complicating delivery 664.4 ☑
  cerebellum — *see* Laceration, brain, cerebellum
  cerebral — *see also* Laceration, brain during birth 767.0
  cervix (uteri)
    with
      abortion — *see* Abortion, by type, with damage to pelvic organs
      ectopic pregnancy (*see also* categories 633.0-633.9) 639.2
      molar pregnancy (*see also* categories 630-632) 639.2
    following
      abortion 639.2
      ectopic or molar pregnancy 639.2
    nonpuerperal, nontraumatic 622.3
    obstetrical trauma (current) 665.3 ☑
    old (postpartal) 622.3
    traumatic — *see* Injury, internal, cervix
  chordae heart 429.5
  complicated 879.9
  cornea — *see* Laceration, eyeball
    superficial 918.1
  cortex (cerebral) — *see* Laceration, brain, cortex
  esophagus 530.89
  eye(s) — *see* Laceration, ocular
  eyeball NEC 871.4
    with prolapse or exposure of intraocular tissue 871.1
    penetrating — *see* Penetrating wound, eyeball
    specified as without prolapse of intraocular tissue 871.0
  eyelid NEC 870.8
    full thickness 870.1
      involving lacrimal passages 870.2
    skin (and periocular area) 870.0
      penetrating — *see* Penetrating wound, orbit
  fourchette
    with
      abortion — *see* Abortion, by type, with damage to pelvic organs
      ectopic pregnancy (*see also* categories 633.0-633.9) 639.2
      molar pregnancy (*see also* categories 630-632) 639.2
    complicating delivery 664.0 ☑
    following
      abortion 639.2
      ectopic or molar pregnancy 639.2
  heart (without penetration of heart chambers) 861.02
    with
      open wound into thorax 861.12
      penetration of heart chambers 861.03
        with open wound into thorax 861.13
  hernial sac — *see* Hernia, by site
  internal organ (abdomen) (chest) (pelvis) NEC — *see* Injury, internal, by site
  kidney (parenchyma) 866.02
    with
      complete disruption of parenchyma (rupture) 866.03
        with open wound into cavity 866.13
      open wound into cavity 866.12
  labia
    complicating delivery 664.0 ☑
  ligament — *see also* Sprain, by site
    with open wound — *see* Wound, open, by site

Laceration — *see also* Wound, open, by site — *continued*
  liver 864.05
    with open wound into cavity 864.15
    major (disruption of hepatic parenchyma) 864.04
      with open wound into cavity 864.14
    minor (capsule only) 864.02
      with open wound into cavity 864.12
    moderate (involving parenchyma without major disruption) 864.03
      with open wound into cavity 864.13
    multiple 864.04
      with open wound into cavity 864.14
    stellate 864.04
      with open wound into cavity 864.14
  lung 861.22
    with open wound into thorax 861.32
  meninges — *see* Laceration, brain
  meniscus (knee) (*see also* Tear, meniscus) 836.2
    old 717.5
    site other than knee — *see also* Sprain, by site
      old NEC (*see also* Disorder, cartilage, articular) 718.0 ☑
  muscle — *see also* Sprain, by site
    with open wound — *see* Wound, open, by site
  myocardium — *see* Laceration, heart
  nerve — *see* Injury, nerve, by site
  ocular NEC (*see also* Laceration, eyeball) 871.4
    adnexa NEC 870.8
      penetrating 870.3
        with foreign body 870.4
  orbit (eye) 870.8
    penetrating 870.3
      with foreign body 870.4
  pelvic
    floor (muscles)
      with
        abortion — *see* Abortion, by type, with damage to pelvic organs
        ectopic pregnancy (*see also* categories 633.0-633.9) 639.2
        molar pregnancy (*see also* categories 630-632) 639.2
      complicating delivery 664.1 ☑
      following
        abortion 639.2
        ectopic or molar pregnancy 639.2
      nonpuerperal 618.7
      old (postpartal) 618.7
    organ NEC
      with
        abortion — *see* Abortion, by type, with damage to pelvic organs
        ectopic pregnancy (*see also* categories 633.0-633.9) 639.2
        molar pregnancy (*see also* categories 630-632) 639.2
      complicating delivery 665.5 ☑
        affecting fetus or newborn 763.89
      following
        abortion 639.2
        ectopic or molar pregnancy 639.2
      obstetrical trauma 665.5 ☑
  perineum, perineal (old) (postpartal) 618.7
    with
      abortion — *see* Abortion, by type, with damage to pelvic floor
      ectopic pregnancy (*see also* categories 633.0-633.9) 639.2
      molar pregnancy (*see also* categories 630-632) 639.2
    complicating delivery 664.4 ☑
      first degree 664.0 ☑
      second degree 664.1 ☑
      third degree 664.2 ☑
      fourth degree 664.3 ☑
      central 664.4 ☑
      involving
        anal sphincter 664.2 ☑
        fourchette 664.0 ☑
        hymen 664.0 ☑
        labia 664.0 ☑
        pelvic floor 664.1 ☑
        perineal muscles 664.1 ☑

☑ Additional Digit Required   ►◄ Revised Text   ● New Line   ▲ Revised Code

Laceration — *see also* Wound, open, by site — *continued*
  perineum, perineal — *continued*
    complicating delivery — *continued*
      involving — *continued*
        rectovaginal septum 664.2 ☑
          with anal mucosa 664.3 ☑
        skin 664.0 ☑
        sphincter (anal) 664.2 ☑
          with anal mucosa 664.3 ☑
        vagina 664.0 ☑
        vaginal muscles 664.1 ☑
        vulva 664.0 ☑
      secondary 674.2 ☑
    following
      abortion 639.2
      ectopic or molar pregnancy 639.2
    male 879.6
      complicated 879.7
    muscles, complicating delivery 664.1 ☑
    nonpuerperal, current injury 879.6
      complicated 879.7
    secondary (postpartal) 674.2 ☑
  peritoneum
    with
      abortion — *see* Abortion, by type, with damage to pelvic organs
      ectopic pregnancy (*see also* categories 633.0-633.9) 639.2
      molar pregnancy (*see also* categories 630-632) 639.2
    following
      abortion 639.2
      ectopic or molar pregnancy 639.2
    obstetrical trauma 665.5 ☑
  periurethral tissue
    with
      abortion — *see* Abortion, by type, with damage to pelvic organs
      ectopic pregnancy (*see also* categories 633.0-633.9) 639.2
      molar pregnancy (*see also* categories 630-632) 639.2
    following
      abortion 639.2
      ectopic or molar pregnancy 639.2
    obstetrical trauma 665.5 ☑
  rectovaginal (septum)
    with
      abortion — *see* Abortion, by type, with damage to pelvic organs
      ectopic pregnancy (*see also* categories 633.0-633.9) 639.2
      molar pregnancy (*see also* categories 630-632) 639.2
    complicating delivery 665.4 ☑
      with perineum 664.2 ☑
        involving anal or rectal mucosa 664.3 ☑
    following
      abortion 639.2
      ectopic or molar pregnancy 639.2
    nonpuerperal 623.4
    old (postpartal) 623.4
  spinal cord (meninges) — *see also* Injury, spinal, by site
    due to injury at birth 767.4
    fetus or newborn 767.4
  spleen 865.09
    with
      disruption of parenchyma (massive) 865.04
        with open wound into cavity 865.14
      open wound into cavity 865.19
    capsule (without disruption of parenchyma) 865.02
      with open wound into cavity 865.12
    parenchyma 865.03
      with open wound into cavity 865.13
      massive disruption (rupture) 865.04
        with open wound into cavity 865.14
  tendon 848.9
    with open wound — *see* Wound, open, by site
    Achilles 845.09
      with open wound 892.2

Laceration — *see also* Wound, open, by site — *continued*
  tendon — *continued*
    lower limb NEC 844.9
      with open wound NEC 894.2
    upper limb NEC 840.9
      with open wound NEC 884.2
  tentorium cerebelli — *see* Laceration, brain, cerebellum
  tongue 873.64
    complicated 873.74
  urethra
    with
      abortion — *see* Abortion, by type, with damage to pelvic organs
      ectopic pregnancy (*see also* categories 633.0-633.9) 639.2
      molar pregnancy (*see also* categories 630-632) 639.2
    following
      abortion 639.2
      ectopic or molar pregnancy 639.2
    nonpuerperal, nontraumatic 599.84
    obstetrical trauma 665.5 ☑
  uterus
    with
      abortion — *see* Abortion, by type, with damage to pelvic organs
      ectopic pregnancy (*see also* categories 633.0-633.9) 639.2
      molar pregnancy (*see also* categories 630-632) 639.2
    following
      abortion 639.2
      ectopic or molar pregnancy 639.2
    nonpuerperal, nontraumatic 621.8
    obstetrical trauma NEC 665.5 ☑
    old (postpartal) 621.8
  vagina
    with
      abortion — *see* Abortion, by type, with damage to pelvic organs
      ectopic pregnancy (*see also* categories 633.0-633.9) 639.2
      molar pregnancy (*see also* categories 630-632) 639.2
      perineal involvement, complicating delivery 664.0 ☑
    complicating delivery 665.4 ☑
      first degree 664.0 ☑
      second degree 664.1 ☑
      third degree 664.2 ☑
      fourth degree 664.3 ☑
      high 665.4 ☑
      muscles 664.1 ☑
      sulcus 665.4 ☑
      wall 665.4 ☑
    following
      abortion 639.2
      ectopic or molar pregnancy 639.2
    nonpuerperal, nontraumatic 623.4
    old (postpartal) 623.4
  valve, heart — *see* Endocarditis
  vulva
    with
      abortion — *see* Abortion, by type, with damage to pelvic organs,
      ectopic pregnancy (*see also* categories 633.0-633.9) 639.2
      molar pregnancy (*see also* categories 630-632) 639.2
    complicating delivery 664.0 ☑
    following
      abortion 639.2
      ectopic or molar pregnancy 639.2
    nonpuerperal, nontraumatic 624.4
    old (postpartal) 624.4

Lachrymal — *see* condition
Lachrymonasal duct — *see* condition
Lack of
  appetite (*see also* Anorexia) 783.0
  care
    in home V60.4
    of adut 995.84
    of infant (at or after birth) 995.52
  coordination 781.3

Lack of — *continued*
  development — *see also* Hypoplasia
    physiological in childhood 783.40
  education V62.3
  energy 780.79
  financial resources V60.2
  food 994.2
    in environment V60.8
  growth in childhood 783.43
  heating V60.1
  housing (permanent) (temporary) V60.0
    adequate V60.1
  material resources V60.2
  medical attention 799.89
  memory (*see also* Amnesia) 780.93
    mild, following organic brain damage 310.1
  ovulation 628.0
  person able to render necessary care V60.4
  physical exercise V69.0
  physiologic development in childhood 783.40
  posterior occlusal support 524.57 ●
  prenatal care in current pregnancy V23.7
  shelter V60.0
  sleep V69.4 ●
  water 994.3

Lacrimal — *see* condition
Lacrimation, abnormal (*see also* Epiphora) 375.20
Lacrimonasal duct — *see* condition
Lactation, lactating (breast) (puerperal) (postpartum)
  defective 676.4 ☑
  disorder 676.9 ☑
    specified type NEC 676.8 ☑
  excessive 676.6 ☑
  failed 676.4 ☑
  mastitis NEC 675.2 ☑
  mother (care and/or examination) V24.1
  nonpuerperal 611.6
  suppressed 676.5 ☑
Lacticemia 271.3
  excessive 276.2
Lactosuria 271.3
Lacunar skull 756.0
Laennec's cirrhosis (alcoholic) 571.2
  nonalcoholic 571.5
Lafora's disease 333.2
Lag, lid (nervous) 374.41
Lagleyze-von Hippel disease (retinocerebral angiomatosis) 759.6
Lagophthalmos (eyelid) (nervous) 374.20
  cicatricial 374.23
  keratitis (*see also* Keratitis) 370.34
  mechanical 374.22
  paralytic 374.21
La grippe — *see* Influenza
Lahore sore 085.1
Lakes, venous (cerebral) 437.8
Laki-Lorand factor deficiency (*see also* Defect, coagulation) 286.3
Lalling 307.9
Lambliasis 007.1
Lame back 724.5
Lancereaux's diabetes (diabetes mellitus with marked emaciation) 250.8 ☑ *[261]*
Landouzy-Déjérine dystrophy (fascioscapulohumeral atrophy) 359.1
Landry's disease or paralysis 357.0
Landry-Guillain-Barré syndrome 357.0
Lane's
  band 751.4
  disease 569.89
  kink (*see also* Obstruction, intestine) 560.9
Langdon Down's syndrome (mongolism) 758.0
Language abolition 784.69
Lanugo (persistent) 757.4
Laparoscopic surgical procedure converted to open procedure V64.41
Lardaceous
  degeneration (any site) 277.3
  disease 277.3

☑ Additional Digit Required   ▶◀ Revised Text   ● New Line   ▲ Revised Code

Lardaceous — *continued*
kidney 277.3 [583.81]
liver 277.3

Large
baby (regardless of gestational age) 766.1
exceptionally (weight of 4500 grams or more) 766.0
of diabetic mother 775.0
ear 744.22
fetus — *see also* Oversize, fetus
causing disproportion 653.5 ☑
with obstructed labor 660.1 ☑
for dates
fetus or newborn (regardless of gestational age) 766.1
affecting management of pregnancy656.6 ☑
exceptionally (weight of 4500 grams or more) 766.0
physiological cup 743.57
stature 783.9 ●
waxy liver 277.3
white kidney — *see* Nephrosis

Larsen's syndrome (flattened facies and multiple congenital dislocations) 755.8

Larsen-Johansson disease (juvenile osteopathia patellae) 732.4

Larva migrans
cutaneous NEC 126.9
ancylostoma 126.9
of Diptera in vitreous 128.0
visceral NEC 128.0

Laryngeal — *see also* condition syncope 786.2

Laryngismus (acute) (infectious) (stridulous) 478.75
congenital 748.3
diphtheritic 032.3

Laryngitis (acute) (edematous) (fibrinous) (gangrenous) (infective) (infiltrative) (malignant) (membranous) (phlegmonous) (pneumococcal) (pseudomembranous) (septic) (subglottic) (suppurative) (ulcerative) (viral) 464.00
with
influenza, flu, or grippe 487.1
obstruction 464.01
tracheitis (*see also* Laryngotracheitis) 464.20
with obstruction 464.21
acute 464.20
with obstruction 464.21
chronic 476.1
atrophic 476.0
Borrelia vincentii 101
catarrhal 476.0
chronic 476.0
with tracheitis (chronic) 476.1
due to external agent — *see* Condition, respiratory, chronic, due to
diphtheritic (membranous) 032.3
due to external agent — *see* Inflammation, respiratory, upper, due to
H. influenzae 464.00
with obstruction 464.01
Hemophilus influenzae 464.00
wtih obstruction 464.01
hypertrophic 476.0
influenzal 487.1
pachydermic 478.79
sicca 476.0
spasmodic 478.75
acute 464.00
with obstruction 464.01
streptococcal 034.0
stridulous 478.75
syphilitic 095.8
congenital 090.5
tuberculous (*see also* Tuberculosis, larynx) 012.3 ☑
Vincent's 101

Laryngocele (congenital) (ventricular) 748.3

Laryngofissure 478.79
congenital 748.3

Laryngomalacia (congenital) 748.3

Laryngopharyngitis (acute) 465.0
chronic 478.9
due to external agent — *see* Condition, respiratory, chronic, due to
due to external agent — *see* Inflammation, respiratory, upper, due to
septic 034.0

Laryngoplegia (*see also* Paralysis, vocal cord) 478.30

Laryngoptosis 478.79

Laryngospasm 478.75
due to external agent — *see* Condition, respiratory, acute, due to

Laryngostenosis 478.74
congenital 748.3

Laryngotracheitis (acute) (infectional) (viral) (*see also* Laryngitis) 464.20
with obstruction 464.21
atrophic 476.1
Borrelia vincenti 101
catarrhal 476.1
chronic 476.1
due to external agent — *see* Condition, respiratory, chronic, due to
diphtheritic (membranous) 032.3
due to external agent — *see* Inflammation, respiratory, upper, due to
H. influenzae 464.20
with obstruction 464.21
hypertrophic 476.1
influenzal 487.1
pachydermic 478.75
sicca 476.1
spasmodic 478.75
acute 464.20
with obstruction 464.21
streptococcal 034.0
stridulous 478.75
syphilitic 095.8
congenital 090.5
tuberculous (*see also* Tuberculosis, larynx) 012.3 ☑
Vincent's 101

Laryngotracheobronchitis (*see also* Bronchitis) 490
acute 466.0
chronic 491.8
viral 466.0

Laryngotracheobronchopneumonitis — *see* Pneumonia, broncho-

Larynx, laryngeal — *see* condition

Lasègue's disease (persecution mania) 297.9

Lassa fever 078.89

Lassitude (*see also* Weakness) 780.79

Late — *see also* condition
effect(s) (of) — *see also* condition
abscess
intracranial or intraspinal (conditions classifiable to 324) — *see* category 326
adverse effect of drug, medicinal or biological substance 909.5
amputation
postoperative (late) 997.60
traumatic (injury classifiable to 885-887 and 895-897) 905.9
burn (injury classifiable to 948-949) 906.9
extremities NEC (injury classifiable to 943 or 945) 906.7

hand or wrist (injury classifiable to 944) 906.6
eye (injury classifiable to 940) 906.5
face, head, and neck (injury classifiable to 941) 906.5
specified site NEC (injury classifiable to 942 and 946-947) 906.8
cerebrovascular disease (conditions classifiable to 430-437) 438.9
with
alterations of sensations 438.6
aphasia 438.11
apraxia 438.81
ataxia 438.84

Late — *see also* condition — *continued*
effect(s) (of) — *see also* condition — *continued*
cerebrovascular disease — *continued*
with — *continued*
cognitive deficits 438.0
disturbances of vision 438.7
dysphagia 438.82
dysphasia 438.12
facial droop 438.83
facial weakness 438.83
hemiplegia/hemiparesis
affecting
dominant side 438.21
nondominant side 438.22
unspecified side 438.20
monoplegia of lower limb
affecting
dominant side 438.41
nondominant side 438.42
unspecified side 438.40
monoplegia of upper limb
affecting
dominant side 438.31
nondominant side 438.32
unspecified side 438.30
paralytic syndrome NEC
affecting
bilateral 438.53
dominant side 438.51
nondominant side 438.52
unspecified side 438.50
speech and language deficit 438.10
vertigo 438.85
specified type NEC 438.89
childbirth complication(s) 677
complication(s) of
childbirth 677
delivery 677
pregnancy 677
puerperium 677
surgical and medical care (conditions classifiable to 996-999) 909.3
trauma (conditions classifiable to 958) 908.6
contusion (injury classifiable to 920-924) 906.3
crushing (injury classifiable to 925-929) 906.4
delivery complication(s) 677
dislocation (injury classifiable to 830-839) 905.6
encephalitis or encephalomyelitis (conditions classifiable to 323) — *see* category 326
in infectious diseases 139.8
viral (conditions classifiable to 049.8, 049.9, 062-064) 139.0
external cause NEC (conditions classifiable to 995) 909.9
certain conditions classifiable to categories 991-994 909.4
foreign body in orifice (injury classifiable to 930-939) 908.5
fracture (multiple) (injury classifiable to 828-829) 905.5
extremity
lower (injury classifiable to 821-827) 905.4
neck of femur (injury classifiable to 820) 905.3
upper (injury classifiable to 810-819) 905.2
face and skull (injury classifiable to 800-804) 905.0
skull and face (injury classifiable to 800-804) 905.0
spine and trunk (injury classifiable to 805 and 807-809) 905.1
with spinal cord lesion (injury classifiable to 806) 907.2
infection
pyogenic, intracranial — *see* category 326
infectious diseases (conditions classifiable to 001-136) NEC 139.8
injury (injury classifiable to 959) 908.9
blood vessel 908.3

☑ Additional Digit Required ▶◀ Revised Text ● New Line ▲ Revised Code

Late — *see also* condition — *continued*
 effect(s) (of) — *see also* condition — *continued*
  injury — *continued*
   blood vessel — *continued*
    abdomen and pelvis (injury classifiable to 902) 908.4
    extremity (injury classifiable to 903-904) 908.3
    head and neck (injury classifiable to 900) 908.3
     intracranial (injury classifiable to 850-854) 907.0
      with skull fracture 905.0
    thorax (injury classifiable to 901) 908.4
   internal organ NEC (injury classifiable to 867 and 869) 908.2
    abdomen (injury classifiable to 863-866 and 868) 908.1
    thorax (injury classifiable to 860-862) 908.0
   intracranial (injury classifiable to 850-854) 907.0
    with skull fracture (injury classifiable to 800-801 and 803-804) 905.0
   nerve NEC (injury classifiable to 957) 907.9
    cranial (injury classifiable to 950-951) 907.1
    peripheral NEC (injury classifiable to 957) 907.9
     lower limb and pelvic girdle (injury classifiable to 956) 907.5
     upper limb and shoulder girdle (injury classifiable to 955) 907.4
    roots and plexus(es), spinal (injury classifiable to 953) 907.3
    trunk (injury classifiable to 954) 907.3
   spinal
    cord (injury classifiable to 806 and 952) 907.2
    nerve root(s) and plexus(es) (injury classifiable to 953) 907.3
   superficial (injury classifiable to 910-919) 906.2
   tendon (tendon injury classifiable to 840-848, 880-884 with .2, and 890-894 with .2) 905.8
  meningitis
   bacterial (conditions classifiable to 320) — *see* category 326
   unspecified cause (conditions classifiable to 322) — *see* category 326
  myelitis (*see also* Late, effect(s) (of), encephalitis) — *see* category 326
  parasitic diseases (conditions classifiable to 001-136 NEC) 139.8
  phlebitis or thrombophlebitis of intracranial venous sinuses (conditions classifiable to 325) — *see* category 326
  poisoning due to drug, medicinal or biological substance (conditions classifiable to 960-979) 909.0
  poliomyelitis, acute (conditions classifiable to 045) 138
  pregnancy complication(s) 677
  puerperal complication(s) 677
  radiation (conditions classifiable to 990) 909.2
  rickets 268.1
  sprain and strain without mention of tendon injury (injury classifiable to 840-848, except tendon injury) 905.7
   tendon involvement 905.8
  toxic effect of
   drug, medicinal or biological substance (conditions classifiable to 960-979) 909.0
   nonmedical substance (conditions classifiable to 980-989) 909.1
  trachoma (conditions classifiable to 076) 139.1
  tuberculosis 137.0
   bones and joints (conditions classifiable to 015) 137.3

Late — *see also* condition — *continued*
 effect(s) (of) — *see also* condition — *continued*
  tuberculosis — *continued*
   central nervous system (conditions classifiable to 013) 137.1
   genitourinary (conditions classifiable to 016) 137.2
   pulmonary (conditions classifiable to 010-012) 137.0
   specified organs NEC (conditions classifiable to 014, 017-018) 137.4
   viral encephalitis (conditions classifiable to 049.8, 049.9, 062-064) 139.0
  wound, open
   extremity (injury classifiable to 880-884 and 890-894, except .2) 906.1
    tendon (injury classifiable to 880-884 with .2 and 890-894 with.2) 905.8
   head, neck, and trunk (injury classifiable to 870-879) 906.0
 infant
  post-term (gestation period over 40 completed weeks to 42 completed weeks) 766.21
  prolonged gestation (period over 42 completed weeks) 766.22
Latent — *see* condition
Lateral — *see* condition
Laterocession — *see* Lateroversion
Lateroflexion — *see* Lateroversion
Lateroversion
 cervix — *see* Lateroversion, uterus
 uterus, uterine (cervix) (postinfectional) (postpartal, old) 621.6
  congenital 752.3
  in pregnancy or childbirth 654.4 ☑
   affecting fetus or newborn 763.89
Lathyrism 988.2
Launois' syndrome (pituitary gigantism) 253.0
Launois-Bensaude's lipomatosis 272.8
Launois-Cléret syndrome (adiposogenital dystrophy) 253.8
Laurence-Moon-Biedl syndrome (obesity, polydactyly, and mental retardation) 759.89
LAV (disease) (illness) (infection) — *see* Human immunodeficiency virus (disease) (illness) (infection)
LAV/HTLV-III (disease) (illness) (infection) — *see* Human immunodeficiency virus (disease) (illness) (infection)
Lawford's syndrome (encephalocutaneous angiomatosis) 759.6
Lax, laxity — *see also* Relaxation
 ligament 728.4
 skin (acquired) 701.8
  congenital 756.83
Laxative habit (*see also* Abuse, drugs, nondependent) 305.9 ☑
Lazy leukocyte syndrome 288.0
LCAD (long chain/very long chain acyl CoA dehydrogenase deficiency, VLCAD) 277.85 ●
LCHAD (long chain 3-hydroxyacyl CoA dehydrogenase deficiency) 277.85 ●
Lead — *see also* condition
 exposure to V15.86
 incrustation of cornea 371.15
 poisoning 984.9
  specified type of lead — *see* Table of Drugs and Chemicals
Lead miners' lung 503
Leakage
 amniotic fluid 658.1 ☑
  with delayed delivery 658.2 ☑
  affecting fetus or newborn 761.1
 bile from drainage tube (T tube) 997.4
 blood (microscopic), fetal, into maternal circulation 656.0 ☑
  affecting management of pregnancy or puerperium 656.0 ☑
 device, implant, or graft — *see* Complications, mechanical
 spinal fluid at lumbar puncture site 997.09
 urine, continuous 788.37

Leaky heart — *see* Endocarditis
Learning defect, specific NEC (strephosymbolia) 315.2
Leather bottle stomach (M8142/3) 151.9
Leber's
 congenital amaurosis 362.76
 optic atrophy (hereditary) 377.16
Lederer's anemia or disease (acquired infectious hemolytic anemia) 283.19
Lederer-Brill syndrome (acquired infectious hemolytic anemia) 283.19
Leeches (aquatic) (land) 134.2
Left-sided neglect 781.8
Leg — *see* condition
Legal investigation V62.5
Legg (-Calvé) -Perthes disease or syndrome (osteochondrosis, femoral capital) 732.1
Legionnaires' disease 482.84
Leigh's disease 330.8
Leiner's disease (exfoliative dermatitis) 695.89
Leiofibromyoma (M8890/0) — *see also* Leiomyoma
 uterus (cervix) (corpus) (*see also* Leiomyoma, uterus) 218.9
Leiomyoblastoma (M8891/1) — *see* Neoplasm, connective tissue, uncertain behavior
Leiomyofibroma (M8890/0) — *see also* Neoplasm, connective tissue, benign
 uterus (cervix) (corpus) (*see also* Leiomyoma, uterus) 218.9
Leiomyoma (M8890/0) — *see also* Neoplasm, connective tissue, benign
 bizarre (M8893/0) — *see* Neoplasm, connective tissue, benign
 cellular (M8892/1) — *see* Neoplasm, connective tissue, uncertain behavior
 epithelioid (M8891/1) — *see* Neoplasm, connective tissue, uncertain behavior
 prostate (polypoid) 600.20
  with urinary retention 600.21
 uterus (cervix) (corpus) 218.9
  interstitial 218.1
  intramural 218.1
  submucous 218.0
  subperitoneal 218.2
  subserous 218.2
 vascular (M8894/0) — *see* Neoplasm, connective tissue, benign
Leiomyomatosis (intravascular) (M8890/1) — *see* Neoplasm, connective tissue, uncertain behavior
Leiomyosarcoma (M8890/3) — *see also* Neoplasm, connective tissue, malignant
 epithelioid (M8891/3) — *see* Neoplasm, connective tissue, malignant
Leishmaniasis 085.9
 American 085.5
  cutaneous 085.4
  mucocutaneous 085.5
 Asian desert 085.2
 Brazilian 085.5
 cutaneous 085.9
  acute necrotizing 085.2
  American 085.4
  Asian desert 085.2
  diffuse 085.3
  dry form 085.1
  Ethiopian 085.3
  eyelid 085.5 *[373.6]*
  late 085.1
  lepromatous 085.3
  recurrent 085.1
  rural 085.2
  ulcerating 085.1
  urban 085.1
  wet form 085.2
  zoonotic form 085.2
 dermal — *see also* Leishmaniasis, cutaneous
  post kala-azar 085.0
 eyelid 085.5 *[373.6]*
 infantile 085.0
 Mediterranean 085.0
 mucocutaneous (American) 085.5

☑ Additional Digit Required ▶◀ Revised Text ● New Line ▲ Revised Code

2005 ICD•9•CM

October 2004 • Volume 2 — 209

Leishmaniasis — Lesion

Leishmaniasis — *continued*
  naso-oral 085.5
  nasopharyngeal 085.5
  Old World 085.1
  tegumentaria diffusa 085.4
  vaccination, prophylactic (against) V05.2
  visceral (Indian) 085.0
Leishmanoid, dermal — *see also* Leishmaniasis,
      cutaneous
  post kala-azar 085.0
Leloir's disease 695.4
Lemiere syndrome 451.89 ●
Lenegre's disease 426.0
Lengthening, leg 736.81
Lennox-Gastaut syndrome 345.0 ☑ ●
  with tonic seizures 345.1 ☑ ●
Lennox's syndrome (*see also* Epilepsy) 345.0 ☑
Lens — *see* condition
Lenticonus (anterior) (posterior) (congenital)
      743.36
Lenticular degeneration, progressive 275.1
Lentiglobus (posterior) (congenital) 743.36
Lentigo (congenital) 709.09
  juvenile 709.09
  Maligna (M8742/2) — *see also* Neoplasm, skin,
      in situ
    melanoma (M8742/3) — *see* Melanoma
  senile 709.09
Leonine leprosy 030.0
Leontiasis
  ossium 733.3
  syphilitic 095.8
    congenital 090.5
Léopold-Lévi's syndrome (paroxysmal thyroid
      instability) 242.9 ☑
Lepore hemoglobin syndrome 282.49
Lepothrix 039.0
Lepra 030.9
  Willan's 696.1
Leprechaunism 259.8
Lepromatous leprosy 030.0
Leprosy 030.9
  anesthetic 030.1
  beriberi 030.1
  borderline (group B) (infiltrated) (neuritic) 030.3
  cornea (*see also* Leprosy, by type)
      030.9 [371.89]
  dimorphous (group B) (infiltrated) (lepromatous)
      (neuritic) (tuberculoid) 030.3
  eyelid 030.0 [373.4]
  indeterminate (group I) (macular) (neuritic)
      (uncharacteristic) 030.2
  leonine 030.0
  lepromatous (diffuse) (infiltrated) (macular)
      (neuritic) (nodular) (type L) 030.0
  macular (early) (neuritic) (simple) 030.2
  maculoanesthetic 030.1
  mixed 030.0
  neuro 030.1
  nodular 030.0
  primary neuritic 030.3
  specified type or group NEC 030.8
  tubercular 030.1
  tuberculoid (macular) (maculoanesthetic)
      (major) (minor) (neuritic) (type T) 030.1
Leptocytosis, hereditary 282.49
Leptomeningitis (chronic) (circumscribed)
      (hemorrhagic) (nonsuppurative) (*see also*
      Meningitis) 322.9
  aseptic 047.9
    adenovirus 049.1
    Coxsackie virus 047.0
    ECHO virus 047.1
    enterovirus 047.9
    lymphocytic choriomeningitis 049.0
  epidemic 036.0
  late effect — *see* category 326
  meningococcal 036.0
  pneumococcal 320.1
  syphilitic 094.2
  tuberculous (*see also* Tuberculosis, meninges)
      013.0 ☑

Leptomeningopathy (*see also* Meningitis) 322.9
Leptospiral — *see* condition
Leptospirochetal — *see* condition
Leptospirosis 100.9
  autumnalis 100.89
  canicula 100.89
  grippotyphosa 100.89
  hebdomidis 100.89
  icterohemorrhagica 100.0
  nanukayami 100.89
  pomona 100.89
  Weil's disease 100.0
Leptothricosis — *see* Actinomycosis
Leptothrix infestation — *see* Actinomycosis
Leptotricosis — *see* Actinomycosis
Leptus dermatitis 133.8
Léris pleonosteosis 756.89
Léri-Weill syndrome 756.59
Leriche's syndrome (aortic bifurcation occlusion)
      444.0
Lermoyez's syndrome (*see also* Disease,
      Ménière's) 386.00
Lesbianism — *omit code*
  ego-dystonic 302.0
  problems with 302.0
Lesch-Nyhan syndrome (hypoxanthineguanine-
      phosphoribosyltransferase deficiency) 277.2
Lesion
  abducens nerve 378.54
  alveolar process 525.8
  anorectal 569.49
  aortic (valve) — *see* Endocarditis, aortic
  auditory nerve 388.5
  basal ganglion 333.90
  bile duct (*see also* Disease, biliary) 576.8
  bladder 596.9
  bone 733.90
  brachial plexus 353.0
  brain 348.8
    congenital 742.9
    vascular (*see also* Lesion, cerebrovascular)
        437.9
      degenerative 437.1
      healed or old without residuals V12.59
      hypertensive 437.2
      late effect — *see* Late effect(s) (of)
          cerebrovascular disease
  buccal 528.9
  calcified — *see* Calcification
  canthus 373.9
  carate — *see* Pinta, lesions
  cardia 537.89
  cardiac — *see also* Disease, heart
    congenital 746.9
    valvular — *see* Endocarditis
  cauda equina 344.60
    with neurogenic bladder 344.61
  cecum 569.89
  cerebral — *see* Lesion, brain
  cerebrovascular (*see also* Disease,
      cerebrovascular NEC) 437.9
    degenerative 437.1
      healed or old without residuals V12.59
    hypertensive 437.2
    specified type NEC 437.8
  cervical root (nerve) NEC 353.2
  chiasmal 377.54
    associated with
      inflammatory disorders 377.54
      neoplasm NEC 377.52
        pituitary 377.51
      pituitary disorders 377.51
      vascular disorders 377.53
  chorda tympani 351.8
  coin, lung 793.1
  colon 569.89
  congenital — *see* Anomaly
  conjunctiva 372.9
  coronary artery (*see also* Ischemia, heart) 414.9
  cranial nerve 352.9
    first 352.0
    second 377.49
    third
      partial 378.51
      total 378.52

Lesion — *continued*
  cranial nerve — *continued*
    fourth 378.53
    fifth 350.9
    sixth 378.54
    seventh 351.9
    eighth 388.5
    ninth 352.2
    tenth 352.3
    eleventh 352.4
    twelfth 352.5
  cystic — *see* Cyst
  degenerative — *see* Degeneration
  dermal (skin) 709.9
  Dieulafoy (hemorrhagic)
    of
      duodenum 537.84
      intestine 569.86
      stomach 537.84
  duodenum 537.89
    with obstruction 537.3
  eyelid 373.9
  gasserian ganglion 350.8
  gastric 537.89
  gastroduodenal 537.89
  gastrointestinal 569.89
  glossopharyngeal nerve 352.2
  heart (organic) — *see also* Disease, heart
    vascular — *see* Disease, cardiovascular
  helix (ear) 709.9
  hyperchromic, due to pinta (carate) 103.1
  hyperkeratotic (*see also* Hyperkeratosis) 701.1
  hypoglossal nerve 352.5
  hypopharynx 478.29
  hypothalamic 253.9
  ileocecal coil 569.89
  ileum 569.89
  iliohypogastric nerve 355.79
  ilioinguinal nerve 355.79
  in continuity — *see* Injury, nerve, by site
  inflammatory — *see* Inflammation
  intestine 569.89
  intracerebral — *see* Lesion, brain
  intrachiasmal (optic) (*see also* Lesion, chiasmal)
      377.54
  intracranial, space-occupying NEC 784.2
  joint 719.90
    ankle 719.97
    elbow 719.92
    foot 719.97
    hand 719.94
    hip 719.95
    knee 719.96
    multiple sites 719.99
    pelvic region 719.95
    sacroiliac (old) 724.6
    shoulder (region) 719.91
    specified site NEC 719.98
    wrist 719.93
  keratotic (*see also* Keratosis) 701.1
  kidney (*see also* Disease, renal) 593.9
  laryngeal nerve (recurrent) 352.3
  leonine 030.0
  lip 528.5
  liver 573.8
  lumbosacral
    plexus 353.1
    root (nerve) NEC 353.4
  lung 518.89
    coin 793.1
  maxillary sinus 473.0
  mitral — *see* Endocarditis, mitral
  motor cortex 348.8
  nerve (*see also* Disorder, nerve) 355.9
  nervous system 349.9
    congenital 742.9
  nonallopathic NEC 739.9
    in region (of)
      abdomen 739.9
      acromioclavicular 739.7
      cervical, cervicothoracic 739.1
      costochondral 739.8
      costovertebral 739.8
      extremity
        lower 739.6
        upper 739.7
      head 739.0

Lesion — *continued*
　nonallopathic — *continued*
　　in region (of) — *continued*
　　　hip 739.5
　　　lower extremity 739.6
　　　lumbar, lumbosacral 739.3
　　　occipitocervical 739.0
　　　pelvic 739.5
　　　pubic 739.5
　　　rib cage 739.8
　　　sacral, sacrococcygeal, sacroiliac 739.4
　　　sternochondral 739.8
　　　sternoclavicular 739.7
　　　thoracic, thoracolumbar 739.2
　　　upper extremity 739.7
　nose (internal) 478.1
　obstructive — *see* Obstruction
　obturator nerve 355.79
　occlusive
　　artery — *see* Embolism, artery
　organ or site NEC — *see* Disease, by site
　osteolytic 733.90
　paramacular, of retina 363.32
　peptic 537.89
　periodontal, due to traumatic occlusion 523.8
　perirectal 569.49
　peritoneum (granulomatous) 568.89
　pigmented (skin) 709.00
　pinta — *see* Pinta, lesions
　polypoid — *see* Polyp
　prechiasmal (optic) (*see also* Lesion, chiasmal) 377.54
　primary — *see also* Syphilis, primary
　　carate 103.0
　　pinta 103.0
　　yaws 102.0
　pulmonary 518.89
　　valve (*see also* Endocarditis, pulmonary) 424.3
　pylorus 537.89
　radiation NEC 990
　radium NEC 990
　rectosigmoid 569.89
　retina, retinal — *see also* Retinopathy
　　vascular 362.17
　retroperitoneal 568.89
　romanus 720.1
　sacroiliac (joint) 724.6
　salivary gland 527.8
　　benign lymphoepithelial 527.8
　saphenous nerve 355.79
　secondary — *see* Syphilis, secondary
　sigmoid 569.89
　sinus (accessory) (nasal) (*see also* Sinusitis) 473.9
　skin 709.9
　　suppurative 686.00
　SLAP (superior glenoid labrum) 840.7
　space-occupying, intracranial NEC 784.2
　spinal cord 336.9
　　congenital 742.9
　　traumatic (complete) (incomplete) (transverse) — *see also* Injury, spinal, by site
　　　with
　　　　broken
　　　　　back — *see* Fracture, vertebra, by site, with spinal cord injury
　　　　　neck — *see* Fracture, vertebra, cervical, with spinal cord injury
　　　　fracture, vertebra — *see* Fracture, vertebra, by site, with spinal cord injury
　spleen 289.50
　stomach 537.89
　superior glenoid labrum (SLAP) 840.7
　syphilitic — *see* Syphilis
　tertiary — *see* Syphilis, tertiary
　thoracic root (nerve) 353.3
　tonsillar fossa 474.9
　tooth, teeth 525.8
　　white spot 521.01
　traumatic NEC (*see also* nature and site of injury) 959.9
　tricuspid (valve) — *see* Endocarditis, tricuspid
　trigeminal nerve 350.9
　ulcerated or ulcerative — *see* Ulcer

Lesion — *continued*
　uterus NEC 621.9
　vagina 623.8
　vagus nerve 352.3
　valvular — *see* Endocarditis
　vascular 459.9
　　affecting central nervous system (*see also* Lesion, cerebrovascular) 437.9
　　following trauma (*see also* Injury, blood vessel, by site) 904.9
　　retina 362.17
　　traumatic — *see* Injury, blood vessel, by site
　　umbilical cord 663.6 ☑
　　　affecting fetus or newborn 762.6
　visual
　　cortex NEC (*see also* Disorder, visual, cortex) 377.73
　　pathway NEC (*see also* Disorder, visual, pathway) 377.63
　warty — *see* Verruca
　white spot, on teeth 521.01
　x-ray NEC 990
Lethargic — *see* condition
Lethargy 780.79
Letterer-Siwe disease (acute histiocytosis X) (M9722/3) 202.5 ☑
Leucinosis 270.3
Leucocoria 360.44
Leucosarcoma (M9850/3) 207.8 ☑
Leukasmus 270.2
Leukemia, leukemic (congenital) (M9800/3) 208.9 ☑

> Note — Use the following fifth-digit subclassification for categories 203–208:
>
> 　0　without mention of remission
>
> 　1　with remission

　acute NEC (M9801/3) 208.0 ☑
　aleukemic NEC (M9804/3) 208.8 ☑
　　granulocytic (M9864/3) 205.8 ☑
　basophilic (M9870/3) 205.1 ☑
　blast (cell) (M9801/3) 208.0 ☑
　blastic (M9801/3) 208.0 ☑
　　granulocytic (M9861/3) 205.0 ☑
　chronic NEC (M9803/3) 208.1 ☑
　compound (M9810/3) 207.8 ☑
　eosinophilic (M9880/3) 205.1 ☑
　giant cell (M9910/3) 207.2 ☑
　granulocytic (M9860/3) 205.9 ☑
　　acute (M9861/3) 205.0 ☑
　　aleukemic (M9864/3) 205.8 ☑
　　blastic (M9861/3) 205.0 ☑
　　chronic (M9863/3) 205.1 ☑
　　subacute (M9862/3) 205.2 ☑
　　subleukemic (M9864/3) 205.8 ☑
　hairy cell (M9940/3) 202.4 ☑
　hemoblastic (M9801/3) 208.0 ☑
　histiocytic (M9890/3) 206.9 ☑
　lymphatic (M9820/3) 204.9 ☑
　　acute (M9821/3) 204.0 ☑
　　aleukemic (M9824/3) 204.8 ☑
　　chronic (M9823/3) 204.1 ☑
　　subacute (M9822/3) 204.2 ☑
　　subleukemic (M9824/3) 204.8 ☑
　lymphoblastic (M9821/3) 204.0 ☑
　lymphocytic (M9820/3) 204.9 ☑
　　acute (M9821/3) 204.0 ☑
　　aleukemic (M9824/3) 204.8 ☑
　　chronic (M9823/3) 204.1 ☑
　　subacute (M9822/3) 204.2 ☑
　　subleukemic (M9824/3) 204.8 ☑
　lymphogenous (M9820/3) — *see* Leukemia, lymphoid
　lymphoid (M9820/3) 204.9 ☑
　　acute (M9821/3) 204.0 ☑
　　aleukemic (M9824/3) 204.8 ☑
　　blastic (M9821/3) 204.0 ☑
　　chronic (M9823/3) 204.1 ☑
　　subacute (M9822/3) 204.2 ☑
　　subleukemic (M9824/3) 204.8 ☑
　lymphosarcoma cell (M9850/3) 207.8 ☑
　mast cell (M9900/3) 207.8 ☑
　megakaryocytic (M9910/3) 207.2 ☑
　megakaryocytoid (M9910/3) 207.2 ☑
　mixed (cell) (M9810/3) 207.8 ☑

Leukemia, leukemic — *continued*
　monoblastic (M9891/3) 206.0 ☑
　monocytic (Schilling-type) (M9890/3) 206.9 ☑
　　acute (M9891/3) 206.0 ☑
　　aleukemic (M9894/3) 206.8 ☑
　　chronic (M9893/3) 206.1 ☑
　　Naegeli-type (M9863/3) 205.1 ☑
　　subacute (M9892/3) 206.2 ☑
　　subleukemic (M9894/3) 206.8 ☑
　monocytoid (M9890/3) 206.9 ☑
　　acute (M9891/3) 206.0 ☑
　　aleukemic (M9894/3) 206.8 ☑
　　chronic (M9893/3) 206.1 ☑
　　myelogenous (M9863/3) 205.1 ☑
　　subacute (M9892/3) 206.2 ☑
　　subleukemic (M9894/3) 206.8 ☑
　monomyelocytic (M9860/3) — *see* Leukemia, myelomonocytic
　myeloblastic (M9861/3) 205.0 ☑
　myelocytic (M9863/3) 205.1 ☑
　　acute (M9861/3) 205.0 ☑
　myelogenous (M9860/3) 205.9 ☑
　　acute (M9861/3) 205.0 ☑
　　aleukemic (M9864/3) 205.8 ☑
　　chronic (M9863/3) 205.1 ☑
　　monocytoid (M9863/3) 205.1 ☑
　　subacute (M9862/3) 205.2 ☑
　　subleukemic (M9864) 205.8 ☑
　myeloid (M9860/3) 205.9 ☑
　　acute (M9861/3) 205.0 ☑
　　aleukemic (M9864/3) 205.8 ☑
　　chronic (M9863/3) 205.1 ☑
　　subacute (M9862/3) 205.2 ☑
　　subleukemic (M9864/3) 205.8 ☑
　myelomonocytic (M9860/3) 205.9 ☑
　　acute (M9861/3) 205.0 ☑
　　chronic (M9863/3) 205.1 ☑
　Naegeli-type monocytic (M9863/3) 205.1 ☑
　neutrophilic (M9865/3) 205.1 ☑
　plasma cell (M9830/3) 203.1 ☑
　plasmacytic (M9830/3) 203.1 ☑
　prolymphocytic (M9825/3) — *see* Leukemia, lymphoid
　promyelocytic, acute (M9866/3) 205.0 ☑
　Schilling-type monocytic (M9890/3) — *see* Leukemia, monocytic
　stem cell (M9801/3) 208.0 ☑
　subacute NEC (M9802/3) 208.2 ☑
　subleukemic NEC (M9804/3) 208.8 ☑
　thrombocytic (M9910/3) 207.2 ☑
　undifferentiated (M9801/3) 208.0 ☑
Leukemoid reaction (lymphocytic) (monocytic) (myelocytic) 288.8
Leukoclastic vasculitis 446.29
Leukocoria 360.44
Leukocythemia — *see* Leukemia
Leukocytosis 288.8
　basophilic 288.8
　eosinophilic 288.3
　lymphocytic 288.8
　monocytic 288.8
　neutrophilic 288.8
Leukoderma 709.09
　syphilitic 091.3
　　late 095.8
Leukodermia (*see also* Leukoderma) 709.09
Leukodystrophy (cerebral) (globoid cell) (metachromatic) (progressive) (sudanophilic) 330.0
Leukoedema, mouth or tongue 528.79 　▲
Leukoencephalitis
　acute hemorrhagic (postinfectious) NEC 136.9 *[323.6]*
　　postimmunization or postvaccinal 323.5
　subacute sclerosing 046.2
　　van Bogaert's 046.2
　van Bogaert's (sclerosing) 046.2
Leukoencephalopathy (*see also* Encephalitis) 323.9
　acute necrotizing hemorrhagic (postinfectious) 136.9 *[323.6]*
　　postimmunization or postvaccinal 323.5
　metachromatic 330.0
　multifocal (progressive) 046.3
　progressive multifocal 046.3

☑ Additional Digit Required　　　　▶◀ Revised Text　　　　● New Line　　　　▲ Revised Code

Leukoerythroblastosis — Lipogranulomatosis

Leukoerythroblastosis 289.0
Leukoerythrosis 289.0
Leukokeratosis (see also Leukoplakia) 702.8
　mouth 528.6
　nicotina palati 528.79 ▲
　tongue 528.6
Leukokoria 360.44
Leukokraurosis vulva, vulvae 624.0
Leukolymphosarcoma (M9850/3) 207.8 ☑
Leukoma (cornea) (interfering with central vision) 371.03
　adherent 371.04
Leukomalacia, periventricular 779.7
Leukomelanopathy, hereditary 288.2
Leukonychia (punctata) (striata) 703.8
　congenital 757.5
Leukopathia
　unguium 703.8
　　congenital 757.5
Leukopenia 288.0
　cyclic 288.0
　familial 288.0
　malignant 288.0
　periodic 288.0
　transitory neonatal 776.7
Leukopenic — see condition
Leukoplakia 702.8
　anus 569.49
　bladder (postinfectional) 596.8
　buccal 528.6
　cervix (uteri) 622.2
　esophagus 530.83
　gingiva 528.6
　kidney (pelvis) 593.89
　larynx 478.79
　lip 528.6
　mouth 528.6
　oral soft tissue (including tongue) (mucosa) 528.6
　palate 528.6
　pelvis (kidney) 593.89
　penis (infectional) 607.0
　rectum 569.49
　syphilitic 095.8
　tongue 528.6
　tonsil 478.29
　ureter (postinfectional) 593.89
　urethra (postinfectional) 599.84
　uterus 621.8
　vagina 623.1
　vesical 596.8
　vocal cords 478.5
　vulva 624.0
Leukopolioencephalopathy 330.0
Leukorrhea (vagina) 623.5
　due to trichomonas (vaginalis) 131.00
　trichomonal (Trichomonas vaginalis) 131.00
Leukosarcoma (M9850/3) 207.8 ☑
Leukosis (M9800/3) — see Leukemia
Lev's disease or syndrome (acquired complete heart block) 426.0
Levi's syndrome (pituitary dwarfism) 253.3
Levocardia (isolated) 746.87
　with situs inversus 759.3
Levulosuria 271.2
Lewandowski's disease (primary) (see also Tuberculosis) 017.0 ☑
Lewandowski-Lutz disease (epidermodysplasia verruciformis) 078.19
Lewy body dementia 331.82
Lewy body disease 331.82
Leyden's disease (periodic vomiting) 536.2
Leyden-Möbius dystrophy 359.1
Leydig cell
　carcinoma (M8650/3)
　　specified site — see Neoplasm, by site, malignant
　　unspecified site
　　　female 183.0
　　　male 186.9

Leydig cell — continued
　tumor (M8650/1)
　　benign (M8650/0)
　　　specified site — see Neoplasm, by site, benign
　　　unspecified site
　　　　female 220
　　　　male 222.0
　　malignant (M8650/3)
　　　specified site — see Neoplasm, by site, malignant
　　　unspecified site
　　　　female 183.0
　　　　male 186.9
　　specified site — see Neoplasm, by site, uncertain behavior
　　unspecified site
　　　female 236.2
　　　male 236.4
Leydig-Sertoli cell tumor (M8631/0)
　specified site — see Neoplasm, by site, benign
　unspecified site
　　female 220
　　male 222.0
LGSIL (low grade squamous intraepithelial ▶lesion◀) 795.03 ▲
Liar, pathologic 301.7
Libman-Sacks disease or syndrome 710.0 [424.91]
Lice (infestation) 132.9
　body (pediculus corporis) 132.1
　crab 132.2
　head (pediculus capitis) 132.0
　mixed (classifiable to more than one of the categories 132.0-132.2) 132.3
　pubic (pediculus pubis) 132.2
Lichen 697.9
　albus 701.0
　annularis 695.89
　atrophicus 701.0
　corneus obtusus 698.3
　myxedematous 701.8
　nitidus 697.1
　pilaris 757.39
　　acquired 701.1
　planopilaris 697.0
　planus (acute) (chronicus) (hypertrophic) (verrucous) 697.0
　　morphoeicus 701.0
　　sclerosus (et atrophicus) 701.0
　ruber 696.4
　　acuminatus 696.4
　　moniliformis 697.8
　　obtusus corneus 698.3
　　of Wilson 697.0
　　planus 697.0
　sclerosus (et atrophicus) 701.0
　scrofulosus (primary) (see also Tuberculosis) 017.0 ☑
　simplex (Vidal's) 698.3
　　chronicus 698.3
　　circumscriptus 698.3
　spinulosus 757.39
　　mycotic 117.9
　striata 697.8
　urticatus 698.2
Lichenification 698.3
　nodular 698.3
Lichenoides tuberculosis (primary) (see also Tuberculosis) 017.0 ☑
Lichtheim's disease or syndrome (subacute combined sclerosis with pernicious anemia) 281.0 [336.2]
Lien migrans 289.59
Lientery (see also Diarrhea) 787.91
　infectious 009.2
Life circumstance problem NEC V62.89
Li-Fraumeni cancer syndrome V84.01 ▲
Ligament — see condition
Light-for-dates (infant) 764.0 ☑
　with signs of fetal malnutrition 764.1 ☑
　affecting management of pregnancy 656.5 ☑
Light-headedness 780.4

Lightning (effects) (shock) (stroke) (struck by) 994.0
　burn — see Burn, by site
　foot 266.2
Lightwood's disease or syndrome (renal tubular acidosis) 588.89 ▲
Lignac's disease (cystinosis) 270.0
Lignac (-de Toni) (-Fanconi) (-Debré) syndrome (cystinosis) 270.0
Lignac (-Fanconi) syndrome (cystinosis) 270.0
Ligneous thyroiditis 245.3
Likoff's syndrome (angina in menopausal women) 413.9
Limb — see condition
Limitation of joint motion (see also Stiffness, joint) 719.5 ☑
　sacroiliac 724.6
Limit dextrinosis 271.0
Limited
　cardiac reserve — see Disease, heart
　duction, eye NEC 378.63
　mandibular range of motion 524.52 ●
Lindau's disease (retinocerebral angiomatosis) 759.6
Lindau (-von Hippel) disease (angiomatosis retinocerebellosa) 759.6
Linea corneae senilis 371.41
Lines
　Beau's (transverse furrows on fingernails) 703.8
　Harris' 733.91
　Hudson-Stähli 371.11
　Stähli's 371.11
Lingua
　geographical 529.1
　nigra (villosa) 529.3
　plicata 529.5
　　congenital 750.13
　tylosis 528.6
Lingual (tongue) — see also condition
　thyroid 759.2
Linitis (gastric) 535.4 ☑
　plastica (M8142/3) 151.9
Lioderma essentialis (cum melanosis et telangiectasia) 757.33
Lip — see also condition
　biting 528.9
Lipalgia 272.8
Lipedema — see Edema
Lipemia (see also Hyperlipidemia) 272.4
　retina, retinalis 272.3
Lipidosis 272.7
　cephalin 272.7
　cerebral (infantile) (juvenile) (late) 330.1
　cerebroretinal 330.1 [362.71]
　cerebroside 272.7
　cerebrospinal 272.7
　chemically-induced 272.7
　cholesterol 272.7
　diabetic 250.8 ☑ [272.7]
　dystopic (hereditary) 272.7
　glycolipid 272.7
　hepatosplenomegalic 272.3
　hereditary, dystopic 272.7
　sulfatide 330.0
Lipoadenoma (M8324/0) — see Neoplasm, by site, benign
Lipoblastoma (M8881/0) — see Lipoma, by site
Lipoblastomatosis (M8881/0) — see Lipoma, by site
Lipochondrodystrophy 277.5
Lipochrome histiocytosis (familial) 288.1
Lipodystrophia progressiva 272.6
Lipodystrophy (progressive) 272.6
　insulin 272.6
　intestinal 040.2
Lipofibroma (M8851/0) — see Lipoma, by site
Lipoglycoproteinosis 272.8
Lipogranuloma, sclerosing 709.8
Lipogranulomatosis (disseminated) 272.8
　kidney 272.8

Lipoid — *see also* condition
  histiocytosis 272.7
    essential 272.7
  nephrosis (*see also* Nephrosis) 581.3
  proteinosis of Urbach 272.8
Lipoidemia (*see also* Hyperlipidemia) 272.4
Lipoidosis (*see also* Lipidosis) 272.7
Lipoma (M8850/0) 214.9
  breast (skin) 214.1
  face 214.0
  fetal (M8881/0) — *see also* Lipoma, by site
    fat cell (M8880/0) — *see* Lipoma, by site
  infiltrating (M8856/0) — *see* Lipoma, by site
  intra-abdominal 214.3
  intramuscular (M8856/0) — *see* Lipoma, by
    site
  intrathoracic 214.2
  kidney 214.3
  mediastinum 214.2
  muscle 214.8
  peritoneum 214.3
  retroperitoneum 214.3
  skin 214.1
    face 214.0
  spermatic cord 214.4
  spindle cell (M8857/0) — *see* Lipoma, by site
  stomach 214.3
  subcutaneous tissue 214.1
    face 214.0
  thymus 214.2
  thyroid gland 214.2
Lipomatosis (dolorosa) 272.8
  epidural 214.8
  fetal (M8881/0) — *see* Lipoma, by site
  Launois-Bensaude's 272.8
Lipomyohemangioma (M8860/0)
  specified site — *see* Neoplasm, connective
    tissue, benign
  unspecified site 223.0
Lipomyoma (M8860/0)
  specified site — *see* Neoplasm, connective
    tissue, benign
  unspecified site 223.0
Lipomyxoma (M8852/0) — *see* Lipoma, by site
Lipomyxosarcoma (M8852/3) — *see* Neoplasm,
    connective tissue, malignant
Lipophagocytosis 289.89
Lipoproteinemia (alpha) 272.4
  broad-beta 272.2
  floating-beta 272.2
  hyper-pre-beta 272.1
Lipoproteinosis (Rössle-Urbach-Wiethe) 272.8
Liposarcoma (M8850/3) — *see also* Neoplasm,
    connective tissue, malignant
  differentiated type (M8851/3) — *see* Neoplasm,
    connective tissue, malignant
  embryonal (M8852/3) — *see* Neoplasm,
    connective tissue, malignant
  mixed type (M8855/3) — *see* Neoplasm,
    connective tissue, malignant
  myxoid (M8852/3) — *see* Neoplasm, connective
    tissue, malignant
  pleomorphic (M8854/3) — *see* Neoplasm,
    connective tissue, malignant
  round cell (M8853/3) — *see* Neoplasm,
    connective tissue, malignant
  well differentiated type (M8851/3) — *see*
    Neoplasm, connective tissue, malignant
Lipsynovitis prepatellaris 272.8
Lipping
  cervix 622.0
  spine (*see also* Spondylosis) 721.90
  vertebra (*see also* Spondylosis) 721.90
Lip pits (mucus), congenital 750.25
Lipschütz disease or ulcer 616.50
Lipuria 791.1
  bilharziasis 120.0
Liquefaction, vitreous humor 379.21
Lisping 307.9
Lissauer's paralysis 094.1
Lissencephalia, lissencephaly 742.2
Listerellose 027.0

Listeriose 027.0
Listeriosis 027.0
  congenital 771.2
  fetal 771.2
  suspected fetal damage affecting management
    of pregnancy 655.4 ☑
Listlessness 780.79
Lithemia 790.6
Lithiasis — *see also* Calculus
  hepatic (duct) — *see* Choledocholithiasis
  urinary 592.9
Lithopedion 779.9
  affecting management of pregnancy 656.8 ☑
Lithosis (occupational) 502
  with tuberculosis — *see* Tuberculosis,
    pulmonary
Lithuria 791.9
Litigation V62.5
Little
  league elbow 718.82
  stroke syndrome 435.9
Little's disease — *see* Palsy, cerebral
Littre's
  gland — *see* condition
  hernia — *see* Hernia, Littre's
Littritis (*see also* Urethritis) 597.89
Livedo 782.61
  annularis 782.61
  racemose 782.61
  reticularis 782.61
Live flesh 781.0
Liver — *see also* condition
  donor V59.6
Livida, asphyxia
  newborn 768.6
Living
  alone V60.3
    with handicapped person V60.4
Lloyd's syndrome 258.1
Loa loa 125.2
Loasis 125.2
Lobe, lobar — *see* condition
Lobo's disease or blastomycosis 116.2
Lobomycosis 116.2
Lobotomy syndrome 310.0
Lobstein's disease (brittle bones and blue sclera)
    756.51
Lobster-claw hand 755.58
Lobulation (congenital) — *see also* Anomaly,
    specified type NEC, by site
  kidney, fetal 753.3
  liver, abnormal 751.69
  spleen 759.0
Lobule, lobular — *see* condition
Local, localized — *see* condition
Locked bowel or intestine (*see also* Obstruction,
    intestine) 560.9
Locked-in state 344.81
Locked twins 660.5 ☑
  affecting fetus or newborn 763.1
Locking
  joint (*see also* Derangement, joint) 718.90
    knee 717.9
Lockjaw (*see also* Tetanus) 037
Locomotor ataxia (progressive) 094.0
Löffler's
  endocarditis 421.0
  eosinophilia or syndrome 518.3
  pneumonia 518.3
  syndrome (eosinophilic pneumonitis) 518.3
Löfgren's syndrome (sarcoidosis) 135
Loiasis 125.2
  eyelid 125.2 *[373.6]*
Loneliness V62.89
Lone star fever 082.8
Long labor 662.1 ☑
  affecting fetus or newborn 763.89
  first stage 662.0 ☑
  second stage 662.2 ☑

Longitudinal stripes or grooves, nails 703.8
  congenital 757.5
Long-term (current) **drug use** V58.69
  antibiotics V58.62
  anticoagulants V58.61
  anti-inflammatories, non-steroidal (NSAID)
    V58.64
  antiplatelets/antithrombotics V58.63
  aspirin V58.66   ▲
  insulin V58.67   ●
  steroids V58.65
Loop
  intestine (*see also* Volvulus) 560.2
  intrascleral nerve 379.29
  vascular on papilla (optic) 743.57
Loose — *see also* condition
  body
    in tendon sheath 727.82
    joint 718.10
      ankle 718.17
      elbow 718.12
      foot 718.17
      hand 718.14
      hip 718.15
      knee 717.6
      multiple sites 718.19
      pelvic region 718.15
      prosthetic implant — *see* Complications,
        mechanical
      shoulder (region) 718.11
      specified site NEC 718.18
      wrist 718.13
  cartilage (joint) (*see also* Loose, body, joint)
    718.1 ☑
    knee 717.6
  facet (vertebral) 724.9
  prosthetic implant — *see* Complications,
    mechanical
  sesamoid, joint (*see also* Loose, body, joint)
    718.1 ☑
  tooth, teeth 525.8
Loosening epiphysis 732.9
Looser (-Debray) -Milkman syndrome
    (osteomalacia with pseudofractures) 268.2
Lop ear (deformity) 744.29
Lorain's disease or syndrome (pituitary
    dwarfism) 253.3
Lorain-Levi syndrome (pituitary dwarfism) 253.3
Lordosis (acquired) (postural) 737.20
  congenital 754.2
  due to or associated with
    Charcôt-Marie-Tooth disease 356.1 *[737.42]*
    mucopolysaccharidosis 277.5 *[737.42]*
    neurofibromatosis 237.71 *[737.42]*
    osteitis
      deformans 731.0 *[737.42]*
      fibrosa cystica 252.01 *[737.42]*   ▲
    osteoporosis (*see also* Osteoporosis)
      733.00 *[737.42]*
    poliomyelitis (*see also* Poliomyelitis)
      138 *[737.42]*
    tuberculosis (*see also* Tuberculosis)
      015.0 ☑ *[737.42]*
  late effect of rickets 268.1 *[737.42]*
  postlaminectomy 737.21
  postsurgical NEC 737.22
  rachitic 268.1 *[737.42]*
  specified NEC 737.29
  tuberculous (*see also* Tuberculosis)
    015.0 ☑ *[737.42]*
Loss
  appetite 783.0
    hysterical 300.11
    nonorganic origin 307.59
    psychogenic 307.59
  blood — *see* Hemorrhage
  central vision 368.41
  consciousness 780.09
    transient 780.2
  control, sphincter, rectum 787.6
    nonorganic origin 307.7
  ear ossicle, partial 385.24
  elasticity, skin 782.8
  extremity or member, traumatic, current — *see*
    Amputation, traumatic

☑ Additional Digit Required   ▶◀ Revised Text   ● New Line   ▲ Revised Code

Loss — Lymph

Lymphadenitis 289.3
  with
    abortion — see Abortion, by type, with sepsis
    ectopic pregnancy (see also categories
      633.0-633.9) 639.0
    molar pregnancy (see also categories 630-
      632) 639.0
  acute 683
    mesenteric 289.2
  any site, except mesenteric 289.3
    acute 683
    chronic 289.1
    mesenteric (acute) (chronic) (nonspecific)
      (subacute) 289.2
    subacute 289.1
      mesenteric 289.2
  breast, puerperal, postpartum 675.2 ☑
  chancroidal (congenital) 099.0
  chronic 289.1
    mesenteric 289.2
  dermatopathic 695.89
  due to
    anthracosis (occupational) 500
    Brugia (Wuchereria) malayi 125.1
    diphtheria (toxin) 032.89
    lymphogranuloma venereum 099.1
    Wuchereria bancrofti 125.0
  following
    abortion 639.0
    ectopic or molar pregnancy 639.0
  generalized 289.3
  gonorrheal 098.89
  granulomatous 289.1
  infectional 683
  mesenteric (acute) (chronic) (nonspecific)
    (subacute) 289.2
    due to Bacillus typhi 002.0
    tuberculous (see also Tuberculosis) 014.8 ☑
  mycobacterial 031.8
  purulent 683
  pyogenic 683
  regional 078.3
  septic 683
  streptococcal 683
  subacute, unspecified site 289.1
  suppurative 683
  syphilitic (early) (secondary) 091.4
    late 095.8
  tuberculous — see Tuberculosis, lymph gland
  venereal 099.1
Lymphadenoid goiter 245.2
Lymphadenopathy (general) 785.6
  due to toxoplasmosis (acquired) 130.7
    congenital (active) 771.2
Lymphadenopathy-associated virus (disease)
  (illness) (infection) — see Human
  immunodeficiency virus (disease) (iliness)
  (infection)
Lymphadenosis 785.6
  acute 075
Lymphangiectasis 457.1
  conjunctiva 372.89
  postinfectional 457.1
  scrotum 457.1
Lymphangiectatic elephantiasis, nonfilarial
  457.1
Lymphangioendothelioma (M9170/0) 228.1
  malignant (M9170/3) — see Neoplasm,
    connective tissue, malignant
Lymphangioma (M9170/0) 228.1
  capillary (M9171/0) 228.1
  cavernous (M9172/0) 228.1
  cystic (M9173/0) 228.1
  malignant (M9170/3) — see Neoplasm,
    connective tissue, malignant
Lymphangiomyoma (M9174/0) 228.1
Lymphangiomyomatosis (M9174/1) — see
  Neoplasm, connective tissue, uncertain
  behavior
Lymphangiosarcoma (M9170/3) — see
  Neoplasm, connective tissue, malignant
Lymphangitis 457.2
  with
    abortion — see Abortion, by type, with sepsis

Lymphangitis — continued
  with — continued
    abscess — see Abscess, by site
    cellulitis — see Abscess, by site
    ectopic pregnancy (see also categories
      633.0-633.9) 639.0
    molar pregnancy (see also categories 630-
      632) 639.0
  acute (with abscess or cellulitis) 682.9
    specified site — see Abscess, by site
  breast, puerperal, postpartum 675.2 ☑
  chancroidal 099.0
  chronic (any site) 457.2
  due to
    Brugia (Wuchereria) malayi 125.1
    Wuchereria bancrofti 125.0
  following
    abortion 639.0
    ectopic or molar pregnancy 639.0
  gangrenous 457.2
  penis
    acute 607.2
    gonococcal (acute) 098.0
      chronic or duration of 2 months or more
      098.2
  puerperal, postpartum, childbirth 670.0 ☑
  strumous, tuberculous (see also Tuberculosis)
    017.2 ☑
  subacute (any site) 457.2
  tuberculous — see Tuberculosis, lymph gland
Lymphatic (vessel) — see condition
Lymphatism 254.8
  scrofulous (see also Tuberculosis) 017.2 ☑
Lymphectasia 457.1
Lymphedema (see also Elephantiasis) 457.1
  acquired (chronic) 457.1
  chronic hereditary 757.0
  congenital 757.0
  idiopathic hereditary 757.0
  praecox 457.1
  secondary 457.1
  surgical NEC 997.99
    postmastectomy (syndrome) 457.0
Lymph-hemangioma (M9120/0) — see
  Hemangioma, by site
Lymphoblastic — see condition
Lymphoblastoma (diffuse) (M9630/3) 200.1 ☑
  giant follicular (M9690/3) 202.0 ☑
  macrofollicular (M9690/3) 202.0 ☑
Lymphoblastosis, acute benign 075
Lymphocele 457.8
Lymphocythemia 288.8
Lymphocytic — see also condition
  chorioencephalitis (acute) (serous) 049.0
  choriomeningitis (acute) (serous) 049.0
Lymphocytoma (diffuse) (malignant) (M9620/3)
  200.1 ☑
Lymphocytomatosis (M9620/3) 200.1 ☑
Lymphocytopenia 288.8
Lymphocytosis (symptomatic) 288.8
  infectious (acute) 078.89
Lymphoepithelioma (M8082/3) — see Neoplasm,
  by site, malignant
Lymphogranuloma (malignant) (M9650/3)
  201.9 ☑
  inguinale 099.1
  venereal (any site) 099.1
    with stricture of rectum 099.1
  venereum 099.1
Lymphogranulomatosis (malignant) (M9650/3)
  201.9 ☑
  benign (Boeck's sarcoid) (Schaumann's) 135
  Hodgkin's (M9650/3) 201.9 ☑
Lymphoid — see condition
Lympholeukoblastoma (M9850/3) 207.8 ☑
Lympholeukosarcoma (M9850/3) 207.8 ☑

Lymphoma (malignant) (M9590/3) 202.8 ☑

> Note — Use the following fifth-digit
> subclassification with categories 200–202:
>
> 0   unspecified site
> 1   lymph nodes of head, face, and
>   neck
> 2   intrathoracic lymph nodes
> 3   intra-abdominal lymph nodes
> 4   lymph nodes of axilla and upper
>   limb
> 5   lymph nodes of inguinal region and
>   lower limb
> 6   intrapelvic lymph nodes
> 7   spleen
> 8   lymph nodes of multiple sites

  benign (M9590/0) — see Neoplasm, by site,
    benign
  Burkitt's type (lymphoblastic) (undifferentiated)
    (M9750/3) 200.2 ☑
  Castleman's (mediastinal lymph node
    hyperplasia) 785.6
  centroblastic-centrocytic
    diffuse (M9614/3) 202.8 ☑
    follicular (M9692/3) 202.0 ☑
  centroblastic type (diffuse) (M9632/3) 202.8 ☑
    follicular (M9697/3) 202.0 ☑
  centrocytic (M9622/3) 202.8 ☑
  compound (M9613/3) 200.8 ☑
  convoluted cell type (lymphoblastic) (M9602/3)
    202.8 ☑
  diffuse NEC (M9590/3) 202.8 ☑
  follicular (giant) (M9690/3) 202.0 ☑
    center cell (diffuse) (M9615/3) 202.8 ☑
      cleaved (diffuse) (M9623/3) 202.8 ☑
        follicular (M9695/3) 202.0 ☑
      non-cleaved (diffuse) (M9633/3) 202.8 ☑
        follicular (M9698/3) 202.0 ☑
    centroblastic-centrocytic (M9692/3) 202.0 ☑
    centroblastic type (M9697/3) 202.0 ☑
    lymphocytic
      intermediate differentiation (M9694/3)
        202.0 ☑
      poorly differentiated (M9696/3) 202.0 ☑
    mixed (cell type) (lymphocytic-histiocytic)
      (small cell and large cell) (M9691/3)
      202.0 ☑
  germinocytic (M9622/3) 202.8 ☑
  giant, follicular or follicle (M9690/3) 202.0 ☑
  histiocytic (diffuse) (M9640/3) 200.0 ☑
    nodular (M9642/3) 200.0 ☑
    pleomorphic cell type (M9641/3) 200.0 ☑
  Hodgkin's (M9650/3) (see also Disease,
    Hodgkin's) 201.9 ☑
  immunoblastic (type) (M9612/3) 200.8 ☑
  large cell (M9640/3) 200.0 ☑
    nodular (M9642/3) 200.0 ☑
    pleomorphic cell type (M9641/3) 200.0 ☑
  lymphoblastic (diffuse) (M9630/3) 200.1 ☑
    Burkitt's type (M9750/3) 200.2 ☑
    convoluted cell type (M9602/3) 202.8 ☑
  lymphocytic (cell type) (diffuse) (M9620/3)
    200.1 ☑
    with plasmacytoid differentiation, diffuse
      (M9611/3) 200.8 ☑
    intermediate differentiation (diffuse)
      (M9621/3) 200.1 ☑
      follicular (M9694/3) 202.0 ☑
      nodular (M9694/3) 202.0 ☑
    nodular (M9690/3) 202.0 ☑
    poorly differentiated (diffuse) (M9630/3)
      200.1 ☑
      follicular (M9696/3) 202.0 ☑
      nodular (M9696/3) 202.0 ☑
    well differentiated (diffuse) (M9620/3)
      200.1 ☑
      follicular (M9693/3) 202.0 ☑
      nodular (M9693/3) 202.0 ☑

☑ Additional Digit Required   ▶◀ Revised Text   ● New Line   ▲ Revised Code

Lymphoma — Malaria, malarial *(left margin vertical text)*

Lymphoma — *continued*
  lymphocytic-histiocytic, mixed (diffuse)
    (M9613/3) 200.8 ☑
    follicular (M9691/3) 202.0 ☑
    nodular (M9691/3) 202.0 ☑
  lymphoplasmacytoid type (M9611/3) 200.8 ☑
  lymphosarcoma type (M9610/3) 200.1 ☑
  macrofollicular (M9690/3) 202.0 ☑
  mixed cell type (diffuse) (M9613/3) 200.8 ☑
    follicular (M9691/3) 202.0 ☑
    nodular (M9691/3) 202.0 ☑
  nodular (M9690/3) 202.0 ☑
    histiocytic (M9642/3) 200.0 ☑
    lymphocytic (M9690/3) 202.0 ☑
      intermediate differentiation (M9694/3)
        202.0 ☑
      poorly differentiated (M9696/3) 202.0 ☑
    mixed (cell type) (lymphocytic-histiocytic)
      (small cell and large cell) (M9691/3)
      202.0 ☑
  non-Hodgkin's type NEC (M9591/3) 202.8 ☑
  reticulum cell (type) (M9640/3) 200.0 ☑
  small cell and large cell, mixed (diffuse)
    (M9613/3) 200.8 ☑
    follicular (M9691/3) 202.0 ☑
    nodular (9691/3) 202.0 ☑
  stem cell (type) (M9601/3) 202.8 ☑
  T-cell 202.1 ☑
  undifferentiated (cell type) (non-Burkitt's)
    (M9600/3) 202.8 ☑
    Burkitt's type (M9750/3) 200.2 ☑
Lymphomatosis (M9590/3) — *see also*
  Lymphoma
  granulomatous 099.1
Lymphopathia
  venereum 099.1
  veneris 099.1
Lymphopenia 288.8
  familial 279.2
Lymphoreticulosis, benign (of inoculation) 078.3
Lymphorrhea 457.8
Lymphosarcoma (M9610/3) 200.1 ☑
  diffuse (M9610/3) 200.1 ☑
    with plasmacytoid differentiation (M9611/3)
      200.8 ☑
    lymphoplasmacytic (M9611/3) 200.8 ☑
  follicular (giant) (M9690/3) 202.0 ☑
    lymphoblastic (M9696/3) 202.0 ☑
    lymphocytic, intermediate differentiation
      (M9694/3) 202.0 ☑
    mixed cell type (M9691/3) 202.0 ☑
  giant follicular (M9690/3) 202.0 ☑
  Hodgkin's (M9650/3) 201.9 ☑
  immunoblastic (M9612/3) 200.8 ☑
  lymphoblastic (diffuse) (M9630/3) 200.1 ☑
    follicular (M9696/3) 202.0 ☑
    nodular (M9696/3) 202.0 ☑
  lymphocytic (diffuse) (M9620/3) 200.1 ☑
    intermediate differentiation (diffuse)
      (M9621/3) 200.1 ☑
      follicular (M9694/3) 202.0 ☑
      nodular (M9694/3) 202.0 ☑
  mixed cell type (diffuse) (M9613/3) 200.8 ☑
    follicular (M9691/3) 202.0 ☑
    nodular (M9691/3) 202.0 ☑
  nodular (M9690/3) 202.0 ☑
    lymphoblastic (M9696/3) 202.0 ☑
    lymphocytic, intermediate differentiation
      (M9694/3) 202.0 ☑
    mixed cell type (M9691/3) 202.0 ☑
  prolymphocytic (M9631/3) 200.1 ☑
  reticulum cell (M9640/3) 200.0 ☑
Lymphostasis 457.8
Lypemania (*see also* Melancholia) 296.2 ☑
Lyssa 071

M

Macacus ear 744.29
Maceration
  fetus (cause not stated) 779.9
  wet feet, tropical (syndrome) 991.4
Machado-Joseph disease 334.8

Machupo virus hemorrhagic fever 078.7
Macleod's syndrome (abnormal transradiancy,
  one lung) 492.8
Macrocephalia, macrocephaly 756.0
Macrocheilia (congenital) 744.81
Macrochilia (congenital) 744.81
Macrocolon (congenital) 751.3
Macrocornea 743.41
  associated with buphthalmos 743.22
Macrocytic — *see* condition
Macrocytosis 289.89
Macrodactylia, macrodactylism (fingers)
  (thumbs) 755.57
  toes 755.65
Macrodontia 520.2
Macroencephaly 742.4
Macrogenia 524.05
Macrogenitosomia (female) (male) (praecox) 255.2
Macrogingivae 523.8
Macroglobulinemia (essential) (idiopathic)
  (monoclonal) (primary) (syndrome)
  (Waldenström's) 273.3
Macroglossia (congenital) 750.15
  acquired 529.8
Macrognathia, macrognathism (congenital)
  524.00
  mandibular 524.02
    alveolar 524.72
  maxillary 524.01
    alveolar 524.71
Macrogyria (congenital) 742.4
Macrohydrocephalus (*see also* Hydrocephalus)
  331.4
Macromastia (*see also* Hypertrophy, breast) 611.1
Macropsia 368.14
Macrosigmoid 564.7
  congenital 751.3
Macrospondylitis, acromegalic 253.0
Macrostomia (congenital) 744.83
Macrotia (external ear) (congenital) 744.22
Macula
  cornea, corneal
    congenital 743.43
      interfering with vision 743.42
    interfering with central vision 371.03
    not interfering with central vision 371.02
  degeneration (*see also* Degeneration, macula)
    362.50
    hereditary (*see also* Dystrophy, retina) 362.70
  edema, cystoid 362.53
Maculae ceruleae 132.1
Macules and papules 709.8
Maculopathy, toxic 362.55
Madarosis 374.55
Madelung's
  deformity (radius) 755.54
  disease (lipomatosis) 272.8
  lipomatosis 272.8
Madness (*see also* Psychosis) 298.9
  myxedema (acute) 293.0
    subacute 293.1
Madura
  disease (actinomycotic) 039.9
    mycotic 117.4
  foot (actinomycotic) 039.4
    mycotic 117.4
Maduromycosis (actinomycotic) 039.9
  mycotic 117.4
Maffucci's syndrome (dyschondroplasia with
  hemangiomas) 756.4
Magenblase syndrome 306.4
Main en griffe (acquired) 736.06
  congenital 755.59
Maintenance
  chemotherapy regimen or treatment V58.1
  dialysis regimen or treatment
    extracorporeal (renal) V56.0
    peritoneal V56.8
    renal V56.0
  drug therapy or regimen V58.1

Maintenance — *continued*
  external fixation NEC V54.89
  radiotherapy V58.0
  traction NEC V54.89
Majocchi's
  disease (purpura annularis telangiectodes)
    709.1
  granuloma 110.6
Major — *see* condition
Mal
  cerebral (idiopathic) (*see also* Epilepsy) 345.9 ☑
  comital (*see also* Epilepsy) 345.9 ☑
  de los pintos (*see also* Pinta) 103.9
  de Meleda 757.39
  de mer 994.6
  lie — *see* Presentation, fetal
  perforant (*see also* Ulcer, lower extremity)
    707.15
Malabar itch 110.9
  beard 110.0
  foot 110.4
  scalp 110.0
Malabsorption 579.9
  calcium 579.8
  carbohydrate 579.8
  disaccharide 271.3
  drug-induced 579.8
  due to bacterial overgrowth 579.8
  fat 579.8
  folate, congenital 281.2
  galactose 271.1
  glucose-galactose (congenital) 271.3
  intestinal 579.9
  isomaltose 271.3
  lactose (hereditary) 271.3
  methionine 270.4
  monosaccharide 271.8
  postgastrectomy 579.3
  postsurgical 579.3
  protein 579.8
  sucrose (-isomaltose) (congenital) 271.3
  syndrome 579.9
    postgastrectomy 579.3
    postsurgical 579.3
Malacia, bone 268.2
  juvenile (*see also* Rickets) 268.0
  Kienböck's (juvenile) (lunate) (wrist) 732.3
    adult 732.8
Malacoplakia
  bladder 596.8
  colon 569.89
  pelvis (kidney) 593.89
  ureter 593.89
  urethra 599.84
Malacosteon 268.2
  juvenile (*see also* Rickets) 268.0
Maladaptation — *see* Maladjustment
Maladie de Roger 745.4
Maladjustment
  conjugal V61.10
    involving divorce or estrangement V61.0
  educational V62.3
  family V61.9
    specified circumstance NEC V61.8
  marital V61.10
    involving divorce or estrangement V61.0
  occupational V62.2
  simple, adult (*see also* Reaction, adjustment)
    309.9
  situational acute (*see also* Reaction,
    adjustment) 309.9
  social V62.4
Malaise 780.79
Malakoplakia — *see* Malacoplakia
Malaria, malarial (fever) 084.6
  algid 084.9
  any type, with
    algid malaria 084.9
    blackwater fever 084.8
    fever
      blackwater 084.8
      hemoglobinuric (bilious) 084.8
    hemoglobinuria, malarial 084.8

☑ Additional Digit Required   ►◄ Revised Text   ● New Line   ▲ Revised Code

Malaria, malarial — *continued*
  any type, with — *continued*
    hepatitis 084.9 *[573.2]*
    nephrosis 084.9 *[581.81]*
    pernicious complication NEC 084.9
      cardiac 084.9
      cerebral 084.9
  cardiac 084.9
  carrier (suspected) of V02.9
  cerebral 084.9
  complicating pregnancy, childbirth, or
      puerperium 647.4 ☑
  congenital 771.2
  congestion, congestive 084.6
    brain 084.9
  continued 084.0
  estivo-autumnal 084.0
  falciparum (malignant tertian) 084.0
  hematinuria 084.8
  hematuria 084.8
  hemoglobinuria 084.8
  hemorrhagic 084.6
  induced (therapeutically) 084.7
    accidental — *see* Malaria, by type
  liver 084.9 *[573.2]*
  malariae (quartan) 084.2
  malignant (tertian) 084.0
  mixed infections 084.5
  monkey 084.4
  ovale 084.3
  pernicious, acute 084.0
  Plasmodium, P.
    falciparum 084.0
    malariae 084.2
    ovale 084.3
    vivax 084.1
  quartan 084.2
  quotidian 084.0
  recurrent 084.6
    induced (therapeutically) 084.7
      accidental — *see* Malaria, by type
  remittent 084.6
  specified types NEC 084.4
  spleen 084.6
  subtertian 084.0
  tertian (benign) 084.1
    malignant 084.0
  tropical 084.0
  typhoid 084.6
  vivax (benign tertian) 084.1
Malassez's disease (testicular cyst) 608.89
Malassimilation 579.9
Maldescent, testis 752.51
Maldevelopment — *see also* Anomaly, by site
  brain 742.9
  colon 751.5
  hip (joint) 755.63
    congenital dislocation (*see also* Dislocation,
      hip, congenital) 754.30
  mastoid process 756.0
  middle ear, except ossicles 744.03
    ossicles 744.04
  newborn (not malformation) 764.9 ☑
  ossicles, ear 744.04
  spine 756.10
  toe 755.66
Male type pelvis 755.69
  with disproportion (fetopelvic) 653.2 ☑
    affecting fetus or newborn 763.1
    causing obstructed labor 660.1 ☑
      affecting fetus or newborn 763.1
Malformation (congenital) — *see also* Anomaly
  bone 756.9
  bursa 756.9
  circulatory system NEC 747.9
    specified type NEC 747.89
  Chiari
    type I 348.4
    type II (*see also* Spina bifida) 741.0 ☑
    type III 742.0
    type IV 742.2
  cochlea 744.05
  digestive system NEC 751.9
    lower 751.5
    specified type NEC 751.8
    upper 750.9

Malformation — *see also* Anomaly — *continued*
  eye 743.9
  gum 750.9
  heart NEC 746.9
    specified type NEC 746.89
    valve 746.9
  internal ear 744.05
  joint NEC 755.9
    specified type NEC 755.8
  Mondini's (congenital) (malformation, cochlea)
      744.05
  muscle 756.9
  nervous system (central) 742.9
  pelvic organs or tissues
    in pregnancy or childbirth 654.9 ☑
      affecting fetus or newborn 763.89
      causing obstructed labor 660.2 ☑
        affecting fetus or newborn 763.1
  placenta (*see also* Placenta, abnormal) 656.7 ☑
  respiratory organs 748.9
    specified type NEC 748.8
  Rieger's 743.44
  sense organs NEC 742.9
    specified type NEC 742.8
  skin 757.9
    specified type NEC 757.8
  spinal cord 742.9
  teeth, tooth NEC 520.9
  tendon 756.9
  throat 750.9
  umbilical cord (complicating delivery) 663.9 ☑
    affecting fetus or newborn 762.6
  umbilicus 759.9
  urinary system NEC 753.9
    specified type NEC 753.8
Malfunction — *see also* Dysfunction
  arterial graft 996.1
  cardiac pacemaker 996.01
  catheter device — *see* Complications,
      mechanical, catheter
  colostomy 569.62
  cystostomy 997.5
  device, implant, or graft NEC — *see*
      Complications, mechanical
  enteric stoma 569.62
  enterostomy 569.62
  esophagostomy 530.87   ●
  gastroenteric 536.8
  gastrostomy 536.42
  nephrostomy 997.5
  pacemaker — *see* Complications, mechanical,
      pacemaker
  prosthetic device, internal — *see*
      Complications, mechanical
  tracheostomy 519.02
  vascular graft or shunt 996.1
Malgaigne's fracture (closed) 808.43
  open 808.53
Malherbe's
  calcifying epithelioma (M8110/0) — *see*
      Neoplasm, skin, benign
  tumor (M8110/0) — *see* Neoplasm, skin,
      benign
Malibu disease 919.8
  infected 919.9
Malignancy (M8000/3) — *see* Neoplasm, by site,
      malignant
Malignant — *see* condition
Malingerer, malingering V65.2
Mallet, finger (acquired) 736.1
  congenital 755.59
  late effect of rickets 268.1
Malleus 024
Mallory's bodies 034.1
Mallory-Weiss syndrome 530.7
Malnutrition (calorie) 263.9
  complicating pregnancy 648.9 ☑
  degree
    first 263.1
    second 263.0
    third 262
    mild 263.1
    moderate 263.0
    severe 261
      protein-calorie 262

Malnutrition — *continued*
  fetus 764.2 ☑
    "light-for-dates" 764.1 ☑
  following gastrointestinal surgery 579.3
  intrauterine or fetal 764.2 ☑
    fetus or infant "light-for-dates" 764.1 ☑
  lack of care, or neglect (child) (infant) 995.52
    adult 995.84
  malignant 260
  mild 263.1
  moderate 263.0
  protein 260
  protein-calorie 263.9
    severe 262
    specified type NEC 263.8
  severe 261
    protein-calorie NEC 262
Malocclusion (teeth) 524.4
  due to
    abnormal swallowing 524.59   ▲
    accessory teeth (causing crowding)
      524.31   ▲
    dentofacial abnormality NEC 524.89   ▲
    impacted teeth (causing crowding) 520.6 ▲
    missing teeth 524.30   ▲
    mouth breathing 524.59   ▲
    sleep postures 524.59   ●
    supernumerary teeth (causing crowding)
      524.31   ▲
    thumb sucking 524.59   ▲
    tongue, lip, or finger habits 524.59   ▲
  temporomandibular (joint) 524.69
Malposition
  cardiac apex (congenital) 746.87
  cervix — *see* Malposition, uterus
  congenital
    adrenal (gland) 759.1
    alimentary tract 751.8
      lower 751.5
      upper 750.8
    aorta 747.21
    appendix 751.5
    arterial trunk 747.29
    artery (peripheral) NEC (*see also*
        Malposition, congenital, peripheral
        vascular system) 747.60
      coronary 746.85
      pulmonary 747.3
    auditory canal 744.29
      causing impairment of hearing 744.02
    auricle (ear) 744.29
      causing impairment of hearing 744.02
      cervical 744.43
    biliary duct or passage 751.69
    bladder (mucosa) 753.8
      exteriorized or extroverted 753.5
    brachial plexus 742.8
    brain tissue 742.4
    breast 757.6
    bronchus 748.3
    cardiac apex 746.87
    cecum 751.5
    clavicle 755.51
    colon 751.5
    digestive organ or tract NEC 751.8
      lower 751.5
      upper 750.8
    ear (auricle) (external) 744.29
      ossicles 744.04
    endocrine (gland) NEC 759.2
    epiglottis 748.3
    Eustachian tube 744.24
    eye 743.8
    facial features 744.89
    fallopian tube 752.19
    finger(s) 755.59
      supernumerary 755.01
    foot 755.67
    gallbladder 751.69
    gastrointestinal tract 751.8
    genitalia, genital organ(s) or tract
      female 752.89
        external 752.49
        internal NEC 752.89
      male 752.89
        penis 752.69
        scrotal transposition 752.81

Malposition — *continued*
congenital — *continued*
  glottis 748.3
  hand 755.59
  heart 746.87
    dextrocardia 746.87
      with complete transposition of viscera 759.3
  hepatic duct 751.69
  hip (joint) (*see also* Dislocation, hip, congenital) 754.30
  intestine (large) (small) 751.5
    with anomalous adhesions, fixation, or malrotation 751.4
  joint NEC 755.8
  kidney 753.3
  larynx 748.3
  limb 755.8
    lower 755.69
    upper 755.59
  liver 751.69
  lung (lobe) 748.69
  nail(s) 757.5
  nerve 742.8
  nervous system NEC 742.8
  nose, nasal (septum) 748.1
  organ or site NEC — *see* Anomaly, specified type NEC, by site
  ovary 752.0
  pancreas 751.7
  parathyroid (gland) 759.2
  patella 755.64
  peripheral vascular system 747.60
    gastrointestinal 747.61
    lower limb 747.64
    renal 747.62
    specified NEC 747.69
    spinal 747.82
    upper limb 747.63
  pituitary (gland) 759.2
  respiratory organ or system NEC 748.9
  rib (cage) 756.3
    supernumerary in cervical region 756.2
  scapula 755.59
  shoulder 755.59
  spinal cord 742.59
  spine 756.19
  spleen 759.0
  sternum 756.3
  stomach 750.7
  symphysis pubis 755.69
  testis (undescended) 752.51
  thymus (gland) 759.2
  thyroid (gland) (tissue) 759.2
    cartilage 748.3
  toe(s) 755.66
    supernumerary 755.02
  tongue 750.19
  trachea 748.3
  uterus 752.3
  vein(s) (peripheral) NEC (*see also* Malposition, congenital, peripheral vascular system) 747.60
    great 747.49
    portal 747.49
    pulmonary 747.49
  vena cava (inferior) (superior) 747.49
device, implant, or graft — *see* Complications, mechanical
fetus NEC — (*see also* Presentation, fetal) 652.9 ☑
  with successful version 652.1 ☑
  affecting fetus or newborn 763.1
  before labor, affecting fetus or newborn 761.7
  causing obstructed labor 660.0 ☑
  in multiple gestation (one fetus or more) 652.6 ☑
    with locking 660.5 ☑
    causing obstructed labor 660.0 ☑
gallbladder — (*see also* Disease, gallbladder) 575.8
gastrointestinal tract 569.89
  congenital 751.8
heart (*see also* Malposition, congenital, heart) 746.87

Malposition — *continued*
intestine 569.89
  congenital 751.5
pelvic organs or tissues
  in pregnancy or childbirth 654.4 ☑
    affecting fetus or newborn 763.89
    causing obstructed labor 660.2 ☑
      affecting fetus or newborn 763.1
placenta — *see* Placenta, previa
stomach 537.89
  congenital 750.7
tooth, teeth 524.30   ▲
  with impaction 520.6   ●
uterus or cervix (acquired) (acute) (adherent) (any degree) (asymptomatic) (postinfectional) (postpartal, old) 621.6
  anteflexion or anteversion (*see also* Anteversion, uterus) 621.6
  congenital 752.3
  flexion 621.6
    lateral (*see also* Lateroversion, uterus) 621.6
  in pregnancy or childbirth 654.4 ☑
    affecting fetus or newborn 763.89
    causing obstructed labor 660.2 ☑
      affecting fetus or newborn 763.1
  inversion 621.6
  lateral (flexion) (version) (*see also* Lateroversion, uterus) 621.6
  lateroflexion (*see also* Lateroversion, uterus) 621.6
  lateroversion (*see also* Lateroversion, uterus) 621.6
  retroflexion or retroversion (*see also* Retroversion, uterus) 621.6

Malposture 729.9

Malpresentation, fetus — (*see also* Presentation, fetal) 652.9 ☑

Malrotation
  cecum 751.4
  colon 751.4
  intestine 751.4
  kidney 753.3

Malta fever (*see also* Brucellosis) 023.9

Maltosuria 271.3

Maltreatment (of)
  adult 995.80
    emotional 995.82
    multiple forms 995.85
    neglect (nutritional) 995.84
    physical 995.81
    psychological 995.82
    sexual 995.83
  child 995.50
    emotional 995.51
    multiple forms 995.59
    neglect (nutritional) 995.52
    physical 995.54
      shaken infant syndrome 995.55
    psychological 995.51
    sexual 995.53
  spouse 995.80 — (*see also* Maltreatment, adult)

Malt workers' lung 495.4

Malum coxae senilis 715.25

Malunion, fracture 733.81

Mammillitis (*see also* Mastitis) 611.0
  puerperal, postpartum 675.2 ☑

Mammitis (*see also* Mastitis) 611.0
  puerperal, postpartum 675.2 ☑

Mammographic microcalcification 793.81

Mammoplasia 611.1

Management
  contraceptive V25.9
    specified type NEC V25.8
  procreative V26.9
    specified type NEC V26.8

Mangled NEC (*see also* nature and site of injury) 959.9

Mania (monopolar) — (*see also* Psychosis, affective) 296.0 ☑
  alcoholic (acute) (chronic) 291.9
  Bell's — *see* Mania, chronic

Mania — (*see also* Psychosis, affective) — *continued*
  chronic 296.0 ☑
    recurrent episode 296.1 ☑
    single episode 296.0 ☑
  compulsive 300.3
  delirious (acute) 296.0 ☑
    recurrent episode 296.1 ☑
    single episode 296.0 ☑
  epileptic (*see also* Epilepsy) 345.4 ☑
  hysterical 300.10
  inhibited 296.89
  puerperal (after delivery) 296.0 ☑
    recurrent episode 296.1 ☑
    single episode 296.0 ☑
  recurrent episode 296.1 ☑
  senile 290.8
  single episode 296.0 ☑
  stupor 296.89
  stuporous 296.89
  unproductive 296.89

Manic-depressive insanity, psychosis, reaction, or syndrome (*see also* Psychosis, affective) 296.80
  circular (alternating) 296.7
    currently
      depressed 296.5 ☑
      episode unspecified 296.7
      hypomanic, previously depressed 296.4 ☑
      manic 296.4 ☑
      mixed 296.6 ☑
  depressed (type), depressive 296.2 ☑
    atypical 296.82
    recurrent episode 296.3 ☑
    single episode 296.2 ☑
  hypomanic 296.0 ☑
    recurrent episode 296.1 ☑
    single episode 296.0 ☑
  manic 296.0 ☑
    atypical 296.81
    recurrent episode 296.1 ☑
    single episode 296.0 ☑
  mixed NEC 296.89
  perplexed 296.89
  stuporous 296.89

Manifestations, rheumatoid
  lungs 714.81
  pannus — *see* Arthritis, rheumatoid
  subcutaneous nodules — *see* Arthritis, rheumatoid

Mankowsky's syndrome (familial dysplastic osteopathy) 731.2

Mannoheptulosuria 271.8

Mannosidosis 271.8

Manson's
  disease (schistosomiasis) 120.1
  pyosis (pemphigus contagiosus) 684
  schistosomiasis 120.1

Mansonellosis 125.5

Manual — *see* condition

Maple bark disease 495.6

Maple bark-strippers' lung 495.6

Maple syrup (urine) disease or syndrome 270.3

Marable's syndrome (celiac artery compression) 447.4

Marasmus 261
  brain 331.9
  due to malnutrition 261
  intestinal 569.89
  nutritional 261
  senile 797
  tuberculous NEC (*see also* Tuberculosis) 011.9 ☑

Marble
  bones 756.52
  skin 782.61

Marburg disease (virus) 078.89

March
  foot 733.94
  hemoglobinuria 283.2

Marchand multiple nodular hyperplasia (liver) 571.5

☑ Additional Digit Required   ►◄ Revised Text   ● New Line   ▲ Revised Code

Marchesani (-Weill) syndrome (brachymorphism and ectopia lentis) 759.89

Marchiafava (-Bignami) disease or syndrome 341.8

Marchiafava-Micheli syndrome (paroxysmal nocturnal hemoglobinuria) 283.2

Marcus Gunn's syndrome (jaw-winking syndrome) 742.8

Marfan's
congenital syphilis 090.49
disease 090.49
syndrome (arachnodactyly) 759.82
meaning congenital syphilis 090.49
with luxation of lens 090.49 *[379.32]*

Marginal
implantation, placenta — *see* Placenta, previa
placenta — *see* Placenta, previa
sinus (hemorrhage) (rupture) 641.2 ☑
affecting fetus or newborn 762.1

Marie's
cerebellar ataxia 334.2
syndrome (acromegaly) 253.0

Marie-Bamberger disease or syndrome (hypertrophic) (pulmonary) (secondary) 731.2
idiopathic (acropachyderma) 757.39
primary (acropachyderma) 757.39

Marie-Charcôt-Tooth neuropathic atrophy, muscle 356.1

Marie-Strümpell arthritis or disease (ankylosing spondylitis) 720.0

Marihuana, marijuana
abuse (*see also* Abuse, drugs, nondependent) 305.2 ☑
dependence (*see also* Dependence) 304.3 ☑

Marion's disease (bladder neck obstruction) 596.0

Marital conflict V61.10

Mark
port wine 757.32
raspberry 757.32
strawberry 757.32
stretch 701.3
tattoo 709.09

Maroteaux-Lamy syndrome (mucopolysaccharidosis VI) 277.5

Marriage license examination V70.3

Marrow (bone)
arrest 284.9
megakaryocytic 287.3
poor function 289.9

Marseilles fever 082.1

Marsh's disease (exophthalmic goiter) 242.0 ☑

Marshall's (hidrotic) **ectodermal dysplasia** 757.31

Marsh fever (*see also* Malaria) 084.6

Martin's disease 715.27

Martin-Albright syndrome (pseudohypoparathyroidism) 275.49

Martorell-Fabre syndrome (pulseless disease) 446.7

Masculinization, female, with adrenal hyperplasia 255.2

Masculinovoblastoma (M8670/0) 220

Masochism 302.83

Masons' lung 502

Mass
abdominal 789.3 ☑
anus 787.99
bone 733.90
breast 611.72
cheek 784.2
chest 786.6
cystic — *see* Cyst
ear 388.8
epigastric 789.3 ☑
eye 379.92
female genital organ 625.8
gum 784.2
head 784.2
intracranial 784.2

Mass — *continued*
joint 719.60
ankle 719.67
elbow 719.62
foot 719.67
hand 719.64
hip 719.65
knee 719.66
multiple sites 719.69
pelvic region 719.65
shoulder (region) 719.61
specified site NEC 719.68
wrist 719.63
kidney (*see also* Disease, kidney) 593.9
lung 786.6
lymph node 785.6
malignant (M8000/3) — *see* Neoplasm, by site, malignant
mediastinal 786.6
mouth 784.2
muscle (limb) 729.89
neck 784.2
nose or sinus 784.2
palate 784.2
pelvis, pelvic 789.3 ☑
penis 607.89
perineum 625.8
rectum 787.99
scrotum 608.89
skin 782.2
specified organ NEC — *see* Disease of specified organ or site
splenic 789.2
substernal 786.6
thyroid (*see also* Goiter) 240.9
superficial (localized) 782.2
testes 608.89
throat 784.2
tongue 784.2
umbilicus 789.3 ☑
uterus 625.8
vagina 625.8
vulva 625.8

Massive — *see* condition

Mastalgia 611.71
psychogenic 307.89

Mast cell
disease 757.33
systemic (M9741/3) 202.6 ☑
leukemia (M9900/3) 207.8 ☑
sarcoma (M9742/3) 202.6 ☑
tumor (M9740/1) 238.5
malignant (M9740/3) 202.6 ☑

Masters-Allen syndrome 620.6

Mastitis (acute) (adolescent) (diffuse) (interstitial) (lobular) (nonpuerperal) (nonsuppurative) (parenchymatous) (phlegmonous) (simple) (subacute) (suppurative) 611.0
chronic (cystic) (fibrocystic) 610.1
cystic 610.1
Schimmelbusch's type 610.1
fibrocystic 610.1
infective 611.0
lactational 675.2 ☑
lymphangitis 611.0
neonatal (noninfective) 778.7
infective 771.5
periductal 610.4
plasma cell 610.4
puerperal, postpartum, (interstitial) (nonpurulent) (parenchymatous) 675.2 ☑
purulent 675.1 ☑
stagnation 676.2 ☑
puerperalis 675.2 ☑
retromammary 611.0
puerperal, postpartum 675.1 ☑
submammary 611.0
puerperal, postpartum 675.1 ☑

Mastocytoma (M9740/1) 238.5
malignant (M9740/3) 202.6 ☑

Mastocytosis 757.33
malignant (M9741/3) 202.6 ☑
systemic (M9741/3) 202.6 ☑

Mastodynia 611.71
psychogenic 307.89

Mastoid — *see* condition

Mastoidalgia (*see also* Otalgia) 388.70

Mastoiditis (coalescent) (hemorrhagic) (pneumococcal) (streptococcal) (suppurative) 383.9
acute or subacute 383.00
with
Gradenigo's syndrome 383.02
petrositis 383.02
specified complication NEC 383.02
subperiosteal abscess 383.01
chronic (necrotic) (recurrent) 383.1
tuberculous (*see also* Tuberculosis) 015.6 ☑

Mastopathy, mastopathia 611.9
chronica cystica 610.1
diffuse cystic 610.1
estrogenic 611.8
ovarian origin 611.8

Mastoplasia 611.1

Masturbation 307.9

Maternal condition, affecting fetus or newborn
acute yellow atrophy of liver 760.8
albuminuria 760.1
anesthesia or analgesia 763.5
blood loss 762.1
chorioamnionitis 762.7
circulatory disease, chronic (conditions classifiable to 390-459, 745-747) 760.3
congenital heart disease (conditions classifiable to 745-746) 760.3
cortical necrosis of kidney 760.1
death 761.6
diabetes mellitus 775.0
manifest diabetes in the infant 775.1
disease NEC 760.9
circulatory system, chronic (conditions classifiable to 390-459, 745-747) 760.3
genitourinary system (conditions classifiable to 580-599) 760.1
respiratory (conditions classifiable to 490-519, 748) 760.3
eclampsia 760.0
hemorrhage NEC 762.1
hepatitis acute, malignant, or subacu   760.8
hyperemesis (gravidarum) 761.8
hypertension (arising during pregnancy) (conditions classifiable to 642) 760.0
infection
disease classifiable to 001-136 760.2
genital tract NEC 760.8
urinary tract 760.1
influenza 760.2
manifest influenza in the infant 771.2
injury (conditions classifiable to 800-996) 760.5
malaria 760.2
manifest malaria in infant or fetus 771.2
malnutrition 760.4
necrosis of liver 760.8
nephritis (conditions classifiable to 580-583) 760.1
nephrosis (conditions classifiable to 581) 760.1
noxious substance transmitted via breast milk or placenta 760.70
alcohol 760.71
anti-infective agents 760.74
cocaine 760.75
"crack" 760.75
diethylstilbestrol [DES] 760.76
hallucinogenic agents 760.73
medicinal agents NEC 760.79
narcotics 760.72
obstetric anesthetic or analgesic drug 760.72
specified agent NEC 760.79
nutritional disorder (conditions classifiable to 260-269) 760.4
operation unrelated to current delivery 760.6
preeclampsia 760.0
pyelitis or pyelonephritis, arising during pregnancy (conditions classifiable to 590) 760.1
renal disease or failure 760.1
respiratory disease, chronic (conditions classifiable to 490-519, 748) 760.3

☑ Additional Digit Required   ▶◀ Revised Text   ● New Line   ▲ Revised Code

Maternal condition, affecting fetus or newborn
— *continued*
rheumatic heart disease (chronic) (conditions
classifiable to 393-398) 760.3
rubella (conditions classifiable to 056) 760.2
manifest rubella in the infant or fetus 771.0
surgery unrelated to current delivery 760.6
to uterus or pelvic organs 763.89
syphilis (conditions classifiable to 090-097)
760.2
manifest syphilis in the infant or fetus 090.0
thrombophlebitis 760.3
toxemia (of pregnancy) 760.0
preeclamptic 760.0
toxoplasmosis (conditions classifiable to 130)
760.2
manifest toxoplasmosis in the infant or fetus
771.2
transmission of chemical substance through
the placenta 760.70
alcohol 760.71
anti-infective 760.74
cocaine 760.75
"crack" 760.75
diethylstilbestrol [DES] 760.76
hallucinogenic agents 760.73
narcotics 760.72
specified substance NEC 760.79
uremia 760.1
urinary tract conditions (conditions classifiable
to 580-599) 760.1
vomiting (pernicious) (persistent) (vicious)
761.8
Maternity — *see* Delivery
Matheiu's disease (leptospiral jaundice) 100.0
Mauclaire's disease or osteochondrosis 732.3
Maxcy's disease 081.0
Maxilla, maxillary — *see* condition
May (-Hegglin) anomaly or syndrome 288.2
Mayaro fever 066.3
Mazoplasia 610.8
MBD (minimal brain dysfunction), child (*see also*
Hyperkinesia) 314.9
MCAD (medium chain acyl CoA
dehydrogenase deficiency) 277.85
McArdle (-Schmid-Pearson) disease or
syndrome (glycogenosis V) 271.0
McCune-Albright syndrome (osteitis fibrosa
disseminata) 756.59
MCLS (mucocutaneous lymph node syndrome)
446.1
McQuarrie's syndrome (idiopathic familial
hypoglycemia) 251.2
Measles (black) (hemorrhagic) (suppressed) 055.9
with
encephalitis 055.0
keratitis 055.71
keratoconjunctivitis 055.71
otitis media 055.2
pneumonia 055.1
complication 055.8
specified type NEC 055.79
encephalitis 055.0
French 056.9
German 056.9
keratitis 055.71
keratoconjunctivitis 055.71
liberty 056.9
otitis media 055.2
pneumonia 055.1
specified complications NEC 055.79
vaccination, prophylactic (against) V04.2
Meatitis, urethral (*see also* Urethritis) 597.89
Meat poisoning — *see* Poisoning, food
Meatus, meatal — *see* condition
Meat-wrappers' asthma 506.9
Meckel's
diverticulitis 751.0
diverticulum (displaced) (hypertrophic) 751.0
Meconium
aspiration 770.1
delayed passage in newborn 777.1

Meconium — *continued*
ileus 777.1
due to cystic fibrosis 277.01
in liquor 792.3
noted during delivery 656.8 ☑
insufflation 770.1
obstruction
fetus or newborn 777.1
in mucoviscidosis 277.01
passage of 792.3
noted during delivery — *omit code*
peritonitis 777.6
plug syndrome (newborn) NEC 777.1
Median — *see also* condition
arcuate ligament syndrome 447.4
bar (prostate) 600.90
with urinary retention 600.91
rhomboid glossitis 529.2
vesical orifice 600.90
with urinary retention 600.91
Mediastinal shift 793.2
Mediastinitis (acute) (chronic) 519.2
actinomycotic 039.8
syphilitic 095.8
tuberculous (*see also* Tuberculosis) 012.8 ☑
Mediastinopericarditis (*see also* Pericarditis)
423.9
acute 420.90
chronic 423.8
rheumatic 393
rheumatic, chronic 393
Mediastinum, mediastinal — *see* condition
Medical services provided for — *see* Health,
services provided because (of)
Medicine poisoning (by overdose) (wrong
substance given or taken in error) 977.9
specified drug or substance — *see* Table of
Drugs and Chemicals
Medin's disease (poliomyelitis) 045.9 ☑
Mediterranean
anemia (with other hemoglobinopathy) 282.49
disease or syndrome (hemipathic) 282.49
fever (*see also* Brucellosis) 023.9
familial 277.3
kala-azar 085.0
leishmaniasis 085.0
tick fever 082.1
Medulla — *see* condition
Medullary
cystic kidney 753.16
sponge kidney 753.17
Medullated fibers
optic (nerve) 743.57
retina 362.85
Medulloblastoma (M9470/3)
desmoplastic (M9471/3) 191.6
specified site — *see* Neoplasm, by site,
malignant
unspecified site 191.6
Medulloepithelioma (M9501/3) — *see also*
Neoplasm, by site, malignant
teratoid (M9502/3) — *see* Neoplasm, by site,
malignant
Medullomyoblastoma (M9472/3)
specified site — *see* Neoplasm, by site,
malignant
unspecified site 191.6
Meekeren-Ehlers-Danlos syndrome 756.83
Megacaryocytic — *see* condition
Megacolon (acquired) (functional) (not
Hirschsprung's disease) 564.7
aganglionic 751.3
congenital, congenitum 751.3
Hirschsprung's (disease) 751.3
psychogenic 306.4
toxic (*see also* Colitis, ulcerative) 556.9
Megaduodenum 537.3
Megaesophagus (functional) 530.0
congenital 750.4
Megakaryocytic — *see* condition
Megalencephaly 742.4

Megalerythema (epidermicum) (infectiosum)
057.0
Megalia, cutis et ossium 757.39
Megaloappendix 751.5
Megalocephalus, megalocephaly NEC 756.0
Megalocornea 743.41
associated with buphthalmos 743.22
Megalocytic anemia 281.9
Megalodactylia (fingers) (thumbs) 755.57
toes 755.65
Megaloduodenum 751.5
Megaloesophagus (functional) 530.0
congenital 750.4
Megalogastria (congenital) 750.7
Megalomania 307.9
Megalophthalmos 743.8
Megalopsia 368.14
Megalosplenia (*see also* Splenomegaly) 789.2
Megaloureter 593.89
congenital 753.22
Megarectum 569.49
Megasigmoid 564.7
congenital 751.3
Megaureter 593.89
congenital 753.22
Megrim 346.9 ☑
Meibomian
cyst 373.2
infected 373.12
gland — *see* condition
infarct (eyelid) 374.85
stye 373.11
Meibomitis 373.12
Meige
-Milroy disease (chronic hereditary edema)
757.0
syndrome (blepharospasm-oromandibular
dystonia) 333.82
Melalgia, nutritional 266.2
Melancholia (*see also* Psychosis, affective) 296.90
climacteric 296.2 ☑
recurrent episode 296.3 ☑
single episode 296.2 ☑
hypochondriac 300.7
intermittent 296.2 ☑
recurrent episode 296.3 ☑
single episode 296.2 ☑
involutional 296.2 ☑
recurrent episode 296.3 ☑
single episode 296.2 ☑
menopausal 296.2 ☑
recurrent episode 296.3 ☑
single episode 296.2 ☑
puerperal 296.2 ☑
reactive (from emotional stress, psychological
trauma) 298.0
recurrent 296.3 ☑
senile 290.21
stuporous 296.2 ☑
recurrent episode 296.3 ☑
single episode 296.2 ☑
Melanemia 275.0
Melanoameloblastoma (M9363/0) — *see*
Neoplasm, bone, benign
Melanoblastoma (M8720/3) — *see* Melanoma
Melanoblastosis
Block-Sulzberger 757.33
cutis linearis sive systematisata 757.33
Melanocarcinoma (M8720/3) — *see* Melanoma
Melanocytoma, eyeball (M8726/0) 224.0
Melanoderma, melanodermia 709.09
Addison's (primary adrenal insufficiency) 255.4
Melanodontia, infantile 521.05
Melanodontoclasia 521.05
Melanoepithelioma (M8720/3) — *see* Melanoma

Melanoma (malignant) (M8720/3) 172.9

> *Note — Except where otherwise indicated,*
> *the morphological varieties of melanoma in*
> *the list below should be coded by site as for*
> *"Melanoma (malignant)". Internal sites*
> *should be coded to malignant neoplasm of*
> *those sites.*

abdominal wall 172.5
ala nasi 172.3
amelanotic (M8730/3) — *see* Melanoma, by site
ankle 172.7
anus, anal 154.3
   canal 154.2
arm 172.6
auditory canal (external) 172.2
auricle (ear) 172.2
auricular canal (external) 172.2
axilla 172.5
axillary fold 172.5
back 172.5
balloon cell (M8722/3) — *see* Melanoma, by
   site
benign (M8720/0) — *see* Neoplasm, skin,
   benign
breast (female) (male) 172.5
brow 172.3
buttock 172.5
canthus (eye) 172.1
cheek (external) 172.3
chest wall 172.5
chin 172.3
choroid 190.6
conjunctiva 190.3
ear (external) 172.2
epithelioid cell (M8771/3) — *see also*
   Melanoma, by site
   and spindle cell, mixed (M8775/3) — *see*
      Melanoma, by site
external meatus (ear) 172.2
eye 190.9
eyebrow 172.3
eyelid (lower) (upper) 172.1
face NEC 172.3
female genital organ (external) NEC 184.4
finger 172.6
flank 172.5
foot 172.7
forearm 172.6
forehead 172.3
foreskin 187.1
gluteal region 172.5
groin 172.5
hand 172.6
heel 172.7
helix 172.2
hip 172.7
in
   giant pigmented nevus (M8761/3) — *see*
      Melanoma, by site
   Hutchinson's melanotic freckle (M8742/3) —
      see Melanoma, by site
   junctional nevus (M8740/3) — *see*
      Melanoma, by site
   precancerous melanosis (M8741/3) — *see*
      Melanoma, by site
interscapular region 172.5
iris 190.0
jaw 172.3
juvenile (M8770/0) — *see* Neoplasm, skin,
   benign
knee 172.7
labium
   majus 184.1
   minus 184.2
lacrimal gland 190.2
leg 172.7
lip (lower) (upper) 172.0
liver 197.7
lower limb NEC 172.7
male genital organ (external) NEC 187.9
meatus, acoustic (external) 172.2
meibomian gland 172.1
metastatic
   of or from specified site — *see* Melanoma, by
      site

Melanoma (M8720/3) — *continued*
metastatic — *continued*
   site not of skin — *see* Neoplasm, by site,
      malignant, secondary
   to specified site — *see* Neoplasm, by site,
      malignant, secondary
   unspecified site 172.9
nail 172.9
   finger 172.6
   toe 172.7
neck 172.4
nodular (M8721/3) — *see* Melanoma, by site
nose, external 172.3
orbit 190.1
penis 187.4
perianal skin 172.5
perineum 172.5
pinna 172.2
popliteal (fossa) (space) 172.7
prepuce 187.1
pubes 172.5
pudendum 184.4
retina 190.5
scalp 172.4
scrotum 187.7
septum nasal (skin) 172.3
shoulder 172.6
skin NEC 172.8
spindle cell (M8772/3) — *see also* Melanoma,
   by site
   type A (M8773/3) 190.0
   type B (M8774/3) 190.0
submammary fold 172.5
superficial spreading (M8743/3) — *see*
   Melanoma, by site
temple 172.3
thigh 172.7
toe 172.7
trunk NEC 172.5
umbilicus 172.5
upper limb NEC 172.6
vagina vault 184.0
vulva 184.4

Melanoplakia 528.9

Melanosarcoma (M8720/3) — *see also* Melanoma
epithelioid cell (M8771/3) — *see* Melanoma

Melanosis 709.09
addisonian (primary adrenal insufficiency)
   255.4
   tuberculous (*see also* Tuberculosis) 017.6 ☑
adrenal 255.4
colon 569.89
conjunctiva 372.55
   congenital 743.49
corii degenerativa 757.33
cornea (presenile) (senile) 371.12
   congenital 743.43
      interfering with vision 743.42
   prenatal 743.43
      interfering with vision 743.42
eye 372.55
   congenital 743.49
jute spinners' 709.09
lenticularis progressiva 757.33
liver 573.8
precancerous (M8741/2) — *see also* Neoplasm,
   skin, in situ
   malignant melanoma in (M8741/3) — *see*
      Melanoma
Riehl's 709.09
sclera 379.19
   congenital 743.47
suprarenal 255.4
tar 709.09
toxic 709.09

Melanuria 791.9

MELAS ▶syndrome (mitrochondrial
   encephalopathy, lactic acidosis and stroke-
   like episodes)◄ 277.87   ▲

Melasma 709.09
adrenal (gland) 255.4
suprarenal (gland) 255.4

Melena 578.1
due to
   swallowed maternal blood 777.3

Melena — *continued*
due to — *continued*
   ulcer — *see* Ulcer, by site, with hemorrhage
newborn 772.4
   due to swallowed maternal blood 777.3

Meleney's
gangrene (cutaneous) 686.09
ulcer (chronic undermining) 686.09

Melioidosis 025

Melitensis, febris 023.0

Melitococcosis 023.0

Melkersson (-Rosenthal) syndrome 351.8

Mellitus, diabetes — *see* Diabetes

Melorheostosis (bone) (leri) 733.99

Meloschisis 744.83

Melotia 744.29

Membrana
capsularis lentis posterior 743.39
epipapillaris 743.57

Membranacea placenta — *see* Placenta,
   abnormal

Membranaceous uterus 621.8

Membrane, membranous — *see also* condition
folds, congenital — *see* Web
Jackson's 751.4
over face (causing asphyxia), fetus or newborn
   768.9
premature rupture — *see* Rupture,
   membranes, premature
pupillary 364.74
   persistent 743.46
retained (complicating delivery) (with
   hemorrhage) 666.2 ☑
   without hemorrhage 667.1 ☑
secondary (eye) 366.50
unruptured (causing asphyxia) 768.9
vitreous humor 379.25

Membranitis, fetal 658.4 ☑
affecting fetus or newborn 762.7

Memory disturbance, loss or lack (*see also*
   Amnesia) 780.93
mild, following organic brain damage 310.1

Menadione (vitamin K) **deficiency** 269.0

Menarche, precocious 259.1

Mendacity, pathologic 301.7

Mende's syndrome (ptosis-epicanthus) 270.2

Mendelson's syndrome (resulting from a
   procedure) 997.3
obstetric 668.0 ☑

Ménétrier's disease or syndrome
   (hypertrophic gastritis) 535.2 ☑

Ménière's disease, syndrome, or vertigo 386.00
cochlear 386.02
cochleovestibular 386.01
inactive 386.04
in remission 386.04
vestibular 386.03

Meninges, meningeal — *see* condition

Meningioma (M9530/0) — *see also* Neoplasm,
   meninges, benign
angioblastic (M9535/0) — *see* Neoplasm,
   meninges, benign
angiomatous (M9534/0) — *see* Neoplasm,
   meninges, benign
endotheliomatous (M9531/0) — *see* Neoplasm,
   meninges, benign
fibroblastic (M9532/0) — *see* Neoplasm,
   meninges, benign
fibrous (M9532/0) — *see* Neoplasm, meninges,
   benign
hemangioblastic (M9535/0) — *see* Neoplasm,
   meninges, benign
hemangiopericytic (M9536/0) — *see* Neoplasm,
   meninges, benign
malignant (M9530/3) — *see* Neoplasm,
   meninges, malignant
meningiothelial (M9531/0) — *see* Neoplasm,
   meninges, benign
meningotheliomatous (M9531/0) — *see*
   Neoplasm, meninges, benign
mixed (M9537/0) — *see* Neoplasm, meninges,
   benign

☑ Additional Digit Required   ▶◀ Revised Text   ● New Line   ▲ Revised Code

Meningioma (M9530/0) — *see also* Neoplasm, meninges, benign — *continued*
multiple (M9530/1) 237.6
papillary (M9538/1) 237.6
psammomatous (M9533/0) — *see* Neoplasm, meninges, benign
syncytial (M9531/0) — *see* Neoplasm, meninges, benign
transitional (M9537/0) — *see* Neoplasm, meninges, benign
Meningiomatosis (diffuse) (M9530/1) 237.6
Meningism (*see also* Meningismus) 781.6
Meningismus (infectional) (pneumococcal) 781.6
due to serum or vaccine 997.09 *[321.8]*
influenzal NEC 487.8
Meningitis (basal) (basic) (basilar) (brain) (cerebral) (cervical) (congestive) (diffuse) (hemorrhagic) (infantile) (membranous) (metastatic) (nonspecific) (pontine) (progressive) (simple) (spinal) (subacute) (sympathetica) (toxic) 322.9
abacterial NEC (*see also* Meningitis, aseptic) 047.9
actinomycotic 039.8 *[320.7]*
adenoviral 049.1
Aerobacter aerogenes 320.82
anaerobes (cocci) (gram-negative) (gram-positive) (mixed) (NEC) 320.81
arbovirus NEC 066.9 *[321.2]*
specified type NEC 066.8 *[321.2]*
aseptic (acute) NEC 047.9
adenovirus 049.1
Coxsackievirus 047.0
due to
adenovirus 049.1
Coxsackievirus 047.0
ECHO virus 047.1
enterovirus 047.9
mumps 072.1
poliovirus (*see also* Poliomyelitis) 045.2 ☑ *[321.2]*
ECHO virus 047.1
herpes (simplex) virus 054.72
zoster 053.0
leptospiral 100.81
lymphocytic choriomeningitis 049.0
noninfective 322.0
Bacillus pyocyaneus 320.89
bacterial NEC 320.9
anaerobic 320.81
gram-negative 320.82
anaerobic 320.81
Bacteroides (fragilis) (oralis) (melaninogenicus) 320.81
cancerous (M8000/6) 198.4
candidal 112.83
carcinomatous (M8010/6) 198.4
caseous (*see also* Tuberculosis, meninges) 013.0 ☑
cerebrospinal (acute) (chronic) (diplococcal) (endemic) (epidemic) (fulminant) (infectious) (malignant) (meningococcal) (sporadic) 036.0
carrier (suspected) of V02.59
chronic NEC 322.2
clear cerebrospinal fluid NEC 322.0
Clostridium (haemolyticum) (novyi) NEC 320.81
coccidioidomycosis 114.2
Coxsackievirus 047.0
cryptococcal 117.5 *[321.0]*
diplococcal 036.0
gram-negative 036.0
gram-positive 320.1
Diplococcus pneumoniae 320.1
due to
actinomycosis 039.8 *[320.7]*
adenovirus 049.1
coccidiomycosis 114.2
enterovirus 047.9
specified NEC 047.8
histoplasmosis (*see also* Histoplasmosis) 115.91
Listerosis 027.0 *[320.7]*
Lyme disease 088.81 *[320.7]*
moniliasis 112.83
mumps 072.1

Meningitis — *continued*
due to — *continued*
neurosyphilis 094.2
nonbacterial organisms NEC 321.8
oidiomycosis 112.83
poliovirus (*see also* Poliomyelitis) 045.2 ☑ *[321.2]*
preventive immunization, inoculation, or vaccination 997.09 *[321.8]*
sarcoidosis 135 *[321.4]*
sporotrichosis 117.1 *[321.1]*
syphilis 094.2
acute 091.81
congenital 090.42
secondary 091.81
trypanosomiasis (*see also* Trypanosomiasis) 086.9 *[321.3]*
whooping cough 033.9 *[320.7]*
E. coli 320.82
ECHO virus 047.1
endothelial-leukocytic, benign, recurrent 047.9
Enterobacter aerogenes 320.82
enteroviral 047.9
specified type NEC 047.8
enterovirus 047.9
specified NEC 047.8
eosinophilic 322.1
epidemic NEC 036.0
Escherichia coli (E. coli) 320.82
Eubacterium 320.81
fibrinopurulent NEC 320.9
specified type NEC 320.89
Friedländer (bacillus) 320.82
fungal NEC 117.9 *[321.1]*
Fusobacterium 320.81
gonococcal 098.82
gram-negative bacteria NEC 320.82
anaerobic 320.81
cocci 036.0
specified NEC 320.82
gram-negative cocci NEC 036.0
specified NEC 320.82
gram-positive cocci NEC 320.9
H. influenzae 320.0
herpes (simplex) virus 054.72
zoster 053.0
infectious NEC 320.9
influenzal 320.0
Klebsiella pneumoniae 320.82
late effect — *see* Late, effect, meningitis
leptospiral (aseptic) 100.81
Listerella (monocytogenes) 027.0 *[320.7]*
Listeria monocytogenes 027.0 *[320.7]*
lymphocytic (acute) (benign) (serous) 049.0
choriomeningitis virus 049.0
meningococcal (chronic) 036.0
Mima polymorpha 320.82
Mollaret's 047.9
monilial 112.83
mumps (virus) 072.1
mycotic NEC 117.9 *[321.1]*
Neisseria 036.0
neurosyphilis 094.2
nonbacterial NEC (*see also* Meningitis, aseptic) 047.9
nonpyogenic NEC 322.0
oidiomycosis 112.83
ossificans 349.2
Peptococcus 320.81
Peptostreptococcus 320.81
pneumococcal 320.1
poliovirus (*see also* Poliomyelitis) 045.2 ☑ *[321.2]*
Proprionibacterium 320.81
Proteus morganii 320.82
Pseudomonas (aeruginosa) (pyocyaneus) 320.82
purulent NEC 320.9
specified organism NEC 320.89
pyogenic NEC 320.9
specified organism NEC 320.89
Salmonella 003.21
septic NEC 320.9
specified organism NEC 320.89
serosa circumscripta NEC 322.0
serous NEC (*see also* Meningitis, aseptic) 047.9
lymphocytic 049.0
syndrome 348.2

Meningitis — *continued*
Serratia (marcescens) 320.82
specified organism NEC 320.89
sporadic cerebrospinal 036.0
sporotrichosis 117.1 *[321.1]*
staphylococcal 320.3
sterile 997.09
streptococcal (acute) 320.2
suppurative 320.9
specified organism NEC 320.89
syphilitic 094.2
acute 091.81
congenital 090.42
secondary 091.81
torula 117.5 *[321.0]*
traumatic (complication of injury) 958.8
Treponema (denticola) (Macrodenticum) 320.81
trypanosomiasis 086.1 *[321.3]*
tuberculous (*see also* Tuberculosis, meninges) 013.0 ☑
typhoid 002.0 *[320.7]*
Veillonella 320.81
Vibrio vulnificus 320.82
viral, virus NEC (*see also* Meningitis, aseptic) 047.9
Wallgren's (*see also* Meningitis, aseptic) 047.9
Meningocele (congenital) (spinal) (*see also* Spina bifida) 741.9 ☑
acquired (traumatic) 349.2
cerebral 742.0
cranial 742.0
Meningocerebritis — *see* Meningoencephalitis
Meningococcemia (acute) (chronic) 036.2
Meningococcus, meningococcal (*see also* condition) 036.9
adrenalitis, hemorrhagic 036.3
carditis 036.40
carrier (suspected) of V02.59
cerebrospinal fever 036.0
encephalitis 036.1
endocarditis 036.42
exposure to V01.84 •
infection NEC 036.9
meningitis (cerebrospinal) 036.0
myocarditis 036.43
optic neuritis 036.81
pericarditis 036.41
septicemia (chronic) 036.2
Meningoencephalitis (*see also* Encephalitis) 323.9
acute NEC 048
bacterial, purulent, pyogenic, or septic — *see* Meningitis
chronic NEC 094.1
diffuse NEC 094.1
diphasic 063.2
due to
actinomycosis 039.8 *[320.7]*
blastomycosis NEC (*see also* Blastomycosis) 116.0 *[323.4]*
free-living amebae 136.2
Listeria monocytogenes 027.0 *[320.7]*
Lyme disease 088.81 *[320.7]*
mumps 072.2
Naegleria (amebae) (gruberi) (organisms) 136.2
rubella 056.01
sporotrichosis 117.1 *[321.1]*
toxoplasmosis (acquired) 130.0
congenital (active) 771.2 *[323.4]*
Trypanosoma 086.1 *[323.2]*
epidemic 036.0
herpes 054.3
herpetic 054.3
H. influenzae 320.0
infectious (acute) 048
influenzal 320.0
late effect — *see* category 326
Listeria monocytogenes 027.0 *[320.7]*
lymphocytic (serous) 049.0
mumps 072.2
parasitic NEC 123.9 *[323.4]*
pneumococcal 320.1
primary amebic 136.2
rubella 056.01

Meningioma — Meningoencephalitis

☑ Additional Digit Required ▶◀ Revised Text ● New Line ▲ Revised Code

Meningoencephalitis (see also Encephalitis) —
  continued
  serous 048
    lymphocytic 049.0
  specific 094.2
  staphylococcal 320.3
  streptococcal 320.2
  syphilitic 094.2
  toxic NEC 989.9 [323.7]
    due to
      carbon tetrachloride 987.8 [323.7]
      hydroxyquinoline derivatives poisoning
        961.3 [323.7]
      lead 984.9 [323.7]
      mercury 985.0 [323.7]
      thallium 985.8 [323.7]
  toxoplasmosis (acquired) 130.0
  trypanosomic 086.1 [323.2]
  tuberculous (see also Tuberculosis, meninges)
    013.0 ☑
  virus NEC 048
Meningoencephalocele 742.0
  syphilitic 094.89
    congenital 090.49
Meningoencephalomyelitis (see also
  Meningoencephalitis) 323.9
  acute NEC 048
    disseminated (postinfectious) 136.9 [323.6]
      postimmunization or postvaccination
        323.5
  due to
    actinomycosis 039.8 [320.7]
    torula 117.5 [323.4]
    toxoplasma or toxoplasmosis (acquired)
      130.0
      congenital (active) 771.2 [323.4]
  late effect — see category 326
Meningoencephalomyelopathy (see also
  Meningoencephalomyelitis) 349.9
Meningoencephalopathy (see also
  Meningoencephalitis) 348.39
Meningoencephalopoliomyelitis (see also
  Poliomyelitis, bulbar) 045.0 ☑
  late effect 138
Meningomyelitis (see also Meningoencephalitis)
  323.9
  blastomycotic NEC (see also Blastomycosis)
    116.0 [323.4]
  due to
    actinomycosis 039.8 [320.7]
    blastomycosis (see also Blastomycosis)
      116.0 [323.4]
    Meningococcus 036.0
    sporotrichosis 117.1 [323.4]
    torula 117.5 [323.4]
  late effect — see category 326
  lethargic 049.8
  meningococcal 036.0
  syphilitic 094.2
  tuberculous (see also Tuberculosis, meninges)
    013.0 ☑
Meningomyelocele (see also Spina bifida)
  741.9 ☑
  syphilitic 094.89
Meningomyeloneuritis — see
  Meningoencephalitis
Meningoradiculitis — see Meningitis
Meningovascular — see condition
Meniscocytosis 282.60
Menkes' syndrome — see Syndrome, Menkes'
Menolipsis 626.0
Menometrorrhagia 626.2
Menopause, menopausal (symptoms) (syndrome)
  627.2
  arthritis (any site) NEC 716.3 ☑
  artificial 627.4
  bleeding 627.0
  crisis 627.2
  depression (see also Psychosis, affective)
    296.2 ☑
    agitated 296.2 ☑
      recurrent episode 296.3 ☑
      single episode 296.2 ☑
    psychotic 296.2 ☑
      recurrent episode 296.3 ☑

Menopause, menopausal — continued
  depression (see also Psychosis, affective) —
    continued
    psychotic — continued
      single episode 296.2 ☑
      recurrent episode 296.3 ☑
      single episode 296.2 ☑
    melancholia (see also Psychosis, affective)
      296.2 ☑
      recurrent episode 296.3 ☑
      single episode 296.2 ☑
  paranoid state 297.2
  paraphrenia 297.2
  postsurgical 627.4
  premature 256.31
    postirradiation 256.2
    postsurgical 256.2
  psychoneurosis 627.2
  psychosis NEC 298.8
  surgical 627.4
  toxic polyarthritis NEC 716.39
Menorrhagia (primary) 626.2
  climacteric 627.0
  menopausal 627.0
  postclimacteric 627.1
  postmenopausal 627.1
  preclimacteric 627.0
  premenopausal 627.0
  puberty (menses retained) 626.3
Menorrhalgia 625.3
Menoschesis 626.8
Menostaxis 626.2
Menses, retention 626.8
Menstrual — see also Menstruation
  cycle, irregular 626.4
  disorders NEC 626.9
  extraction V25.3
  fluid, retained 626.8
  molimen 625.4
  period, normal V65.5
  regulation V25.3
Menstruation
  absent 626.0
  anovulatory 628.0
  delayed 626.8
  difficult 625.3
  disorder 626.9
    psychogenic 306.52
    specified NEC 626.8
  during pregnancy 640.8 ☑
  excessive 626.2
  frequent 626.2
  infrequent 626.1
  irregular 626.4
  latent 626.8
  membranous 626.8
  painful (primary) (secondary) 625.3
    psychogenic 306.52
  passage of clots 626.2
  precocious 626.8
  protracted 626.8
  retained 626.8
  retrograde 626.8
  scanty 626.1
  suppression 626.8
  vicarious (nasal) 625.8
Mentagra (see also Sycosis) 704.8
Mental — see also condition
  deficiency (see also Retardation, mental) 319
  deterioration (see also Psychosis) 298.9
  disorder (see also Disorder, mental) 300.9
  exhaustion 300.5
  insufficiency (congenital) (see also Retardation,
    mental) 319
  observation without need for further medical
    care NEC V71.09
  retardation (see also Retardation, mental) 319
  subnormality (see also Retardation, mental)
    319
    mild 317
    moderate 318.0
    profound 318.2
    severe 318.1
  upset (see also Disorder, mental) 300.9
Meralgia paresthetica 355.1

Mercurial — see condition
Mercurialism NEC 985.0
Merergasia 300.9
Merkel cell tumor — see Neoplasm, by site,
  malignant
Merocele (see also Hernia, femoral) 553.00
Meromelia 755.4
  lower limb 755.30
    intercalary 755.32
      femur 755.34
        tibiofibular (complete) (incomplete)
          755.33
      fibula 755.37
      metatarsal(s) 755.38
      tarsal(s) 755.38
      tibia 755.36
      tibiofibular 755.35
    terminal (complete) (partial) (transverse)
      755.31
      longitudinal 755.32
        metatarsal(s) 755.38
        phalange(s) 755.39
        tarsal(s) 755.38
      transverse 755.31
  upper limb 755.20
    intercalary 755.22
      carpal(s) 755.28
      humeral 755.24
        radioulnar (complete) (incomplete)
          755.23
      metacarpal(s) 755.28
      phalange(s) 755.29
      radial 755.26
      radioulnar 755.25
      ulnar 755.27
    terminal (complete) (partial) (transverse)
      755.21
      longitudinal 755.22
        carpal(s) 755.28
        metacarpal(s) 755.28
        phalange(s) 755.29
    transverse 755.21
Merosmia 781.1
MERRF syndrome (myoclonus with epilepsy ●
  and with ragged red fibers) 277.87 ●
Merycism — see also Vomiting
  psychogenic 307.53
Merzbacher-Pelizaeus disease 330.0
Mesaortitis — see Aortitis
Mesarteritis — see Arteritis
Mesencephalitis (see also Encephalitis) 323.9
  late effect — see category 326
Mesenchymoma (M8990/1) — see also Neoplasm,
  connective tissue, uncertain behavior
  benign (M8990/0) — see Neoplasm, connective
    tissue, benign
  malignant (M8990/3) — see Neoplasm,
    connective tissue, malignant
Mesentery, mesenteric — see condition
Mesiodens, mesiodentes 520.1
  causing crowding 524.31 ▲
Mesio-occlusion 524.23 ▲
Mesocardia (with asplenia) 746.87
Mesocolon — see condition
Mesonephroma (malignant) (M9110/3) — see also
  Neoplasm, by site, malignant
  benign (M9110/0) — see Neoplasm, by site,
    benign
Mesophlebitis — see Phlebitis
Mesostromal dysgenesis 743.51
Mesothelioma (malignant) (M9050/3) — see also
  Neoplasm, by site, malignant
  benign (M9050/0) — see Neoplasm, by site,
    benign
  biphasic type (M9053/3) — see also Neoplasm,
    by site, malignant
    benign (M9053/0) — see Neoplasm, by site,
      benign
  epithelioid (M9052/3) — see also Neoplasm, by
    site, malignant
    benign (M9052/0) — see Neoplasm, by site,
      benign

☑ Additional Digit Required   ▶◀ Revised Text   ● New Line   ▲ Revised Code

Mesothelioma (M9050/3) — *see also* Neoplasm, by site, malignant — *continued*
  fibrous (M9051/3) — *see also* Neoplasm, by site, malignant
    benign (M9051/0) — *see* Neoplasm, by site, benign
Metabolic syndrome 277.7   ●
Metabolism disorder 277.9
  specified type NEC 277.89
Metagonimiasis 121.5
Metagonimus infestation (small intestine) 121.5
Metal
  pigmentation (skin) 709.00
  polishers' disease 502
Metalliferous miners' lung 503
Metamorphopsia 368.14
Metaplasia
  bone, in skin 709.3
  breast 611.8
  cervix — *omit code*
  endometrium (squamous) 621.8
  esophagus 530.85
  intestinal, of gastric mucosa 537.89
  kidney (pelvis) (squamous) (*see also* Disease, renal) 593.89
  myelogenous 289.89
  myeloid (agnogenic) (megakaryocytic) 289.89
  spleen 289.59
  squamous cell
    amnion 658.8 ☑
    bladder 596.8
    cervix — *see* condition
    trachea 519.1
    tracheobronchial tree 519.1
    uterus 621.8
      cervix — *see* condition
Metastasis, metastatic
  abscess — *see* Abscess
  calcification 275.40
  cancer, neoplasm, or disease
    from specified site (M8000/3) — *see* Neoplasm, by site, malignant
    to specified site (M8000/6) — *see* Neoplasm, by site, secondary
  deposits (in) (M8000/6) — *see* Neoplasm, by site, secondary
  pneumonia 038.8 *[484.8]*
  spread (to) (M8000/6) — *see* Neoplasm, by site, secondary
Metatarsalgia 726.70
  anterior 355.6
  due to Freiberg's disease 732.5
  Morton's 355.6
Metatarsus, metatarsal — *see also* condition
  abductus valgus (congenital) 754.60
  adductus varus (congenital) 754.53
    primus varus 754.52
  valgus (adductus) (congenital) 754.60
  varus (abductus) (congenital) 754.53
    primus 754.52
Methemoglobinemia 289.7
  acquired (with sulfhemoglobinemia) 289.7
  congenital 289.7
  enzymatic 289.7
  Hb-M disease 289.7
  hereditary 289.7
  toxic 289.7
Methemoglobinuria (*see also* Hemoglobinuria) 791.2
Methicillin-resistant staphylococcus   ●
  aureus (MRSA) V09.0   ●
Methioninemia 270.4
Metritis (catarrhal) (septic) (suppurative) (*see also* Endometritis) 615.9
  blennorrhagic 098.16
    chronic or duration of 2 months or over 098.36
  cervical (*see also* Cervicitis) 616.0
  gonococcal 098.16
    chronic or duration of 2 months or over 098.36
  hemorrhagic 626.8
  puerperal, postpartum, childbirth 670.0 ☑
  tuberculous (*see also* Tuberculosis) 016.7 ☑

Metropathia hemorrhagica 626.8
Metroperitonitis (*see also* Peritonitis, pelvic, female) 614.5
Metrorrhagia 626.6
  arising during pregnancy — *see* Hemorrhage, pregnancy
  postpartum NEC 666.2 ☑
  primary 626.6
  psychogenic 306.59
  puerperal 666.2 ☑
Metrorrhexis — *see* Rupture, uterus
Metrosalpingitis (*see also* Salpingo-oophoritis) 614.2
Metrostaxis 626.6
Metrovaginitis (*see also* Endometritis) 615.9
  gonococcal (acute) 098.16
    chronic or duration of 2 months or over 098.36
Mexican fever — *see* Typhus, Mexican
Meyenburg-Altherr-Uehlinger syndrome 733.99
Meyer-Schwickerath and Weyers syndrome (dysplasia oculodentodigitalis) 759.89
Meynert's amentia (nonalcoholic) 294.0
  alcoholic 291.1
Mibelli's disease 757.39
Mice, joint (*see also* Loose, body, joint) 718.1 ☑
  knee 717.6
Micheli-Rietti syndrome (thalassemia minor) 282.49
Michotte's syndrome 721.5
Micrencephalon, micrencephaly 742.1
Microaneurysm, retina 362.14
  diabetic 250.5 ☑ *[362.01]*
Microangiopathy 443.9
  diabetic (peripheral) 250.7 ☑ *[443.81]*
    retinal 250.5 ☑ *[362.01]*
  peripheral 443.9
    diabetic 250.7 ☑ *[443.81]*
  retinal 362.18
    diabetic 250.5 ☑ *[362.01]*
  thrombotic 446.6
    Moschcowitz's (thrombotic thrombocytopenic purpura) 446.6
Microcalcification, mammographic 793.81
Microcephalus, microcephalic, microcephaly 742.1
  due to toxoplasmosis (congenital) 771.2
Microcheilia 744.82
Microcolon (congenital) 751.5
Microcornea (congenital) 743.41
Microcytic — *see* condition
Microdeletions NEC 758.33   ●
Microdontia 520.2
Microdrepanocytosis (thalassemia-Hb-S disease) 282.49
Microembolism
  atherothrombotic — *see* Atheroembolism
  retina 362.33
Microencephalon 742.1
Microfilaria streptocerca infestation 125.3
Microgastria (congenital) 750.7
Microgenia 524.0 ☑
Microgenitalia (congenital) 752.89
  penis 752.64
Microglioma (M9710/3)
  specified site — *see* Neoplasm, by site, malignant
  unspecified site 191.9
Microglossia (congenital) 750.16
Micrognathia, micrognathism (congenital) 524.00
  mandibular 524.04
    alveolar 524.74
  maxillary 524.03
    alveolar 524.73
Microgyria (congenital) 742.2
Microinfarct, heart (*see also* Insufficiency, coronary) 411.89
Microlithiasis, alveolar, pulmonary 516.2
Micromyelia (congenital) 742.59

Micropenis 752.64
Microphakia (congenital) 743.36
Microphthalmia (congenital) (*see also* Microphthalmos) 743.10
Microphthalmos (congenital) 743.10
  associated with eye and adnexal anomalies NEC 743.12
  due to toxoplasmosis (congenital) 771.2
  isolated 743.11
  simple 743.11
  syndrome 759.89
Micropsia 368.14
Microsporidiosis 136.8
Microsporon furfur infestation 111.0
Microsporosis (*see also* Dermatophytosis) 110.9
  nigra 111.1
Microstomia (congenital) 744.84
Microthelia 757.6
Microthromboembolism — *see* Embolism
Microtia (congenital) (external ear) 744.23
Microtropia 378.34
Micturition
  disorder NEC 788.69
    psychogenic 306.53
  frequency 788.41
    psychogenic 306.53
  nocturnal 788.43
  painful 788.1
    psychogenic 306.53
Middle
  ear — *see* condition
  lobe (right) syndrome 518.0
Midplane — *see* condition
Miescher's disease 709.3
  cheilitis 351.8
  granulomatosis disciformis 709.3
Miescher-Leder syndrome or granulomatosis 709.3
Mieten's syndrome 759.89
Migraine (idiopathic) 346.9 ☑
  with aura 346.0 ☑
  abdominal (syndrome) 346.2 ☑
  allergic (histamine) 346.2 ☑
  atypical 346.1 ☑
  basilar 346.2 ☑
  classical 346.0 ☑
  common 346.1 ☑
  hemiplegic 346.8 ☑
  lower-half 346.2 ☑
  menstrual 625.4
  ophthalmic 346.8 ☑
  ophthalmoplegic 346.8 ☑
  retinal 346.2 ☑
  variant 346.2 ☑
Migrant, social V60.0
Migratory, migrating — *see also* condition
  person V60.0
  testis, congenital 752.52
Mikulicz's disease or syndrome (dryness of mouth, absent or decreased lacrimation) 527.1
Milian atrophia blanche 701.3
Miliaria (crystallina) (rubra) (tropicalis) 705.1
  apocrine 705.82
Miliary — *see* condition
Milium (*see also* Cyst, sebaceous) 706.2
  colloid 709.3
  eyelid 374.84
Milk
  crust 690.11
  excess secretion 676.6 ☑
  fever, female 672.0 ☑
  poisoning 988.8
  retention 676.2 ☑
  sickness 988.8
  spots 423.1
Milkers' nodes 051.1
Milk-leg (deep vessels) 671.4 ☑
  complicating pregnancy 671.3 ☑
  nonpuerperal 451.19
  puerperal, postpartum, childbirth 671.4 ☑

Milkman (-Looser) disease or syndrome (osteomalacia with pseudofractures) 268.2
Milky urine (*see also* Chyluria) 791.1
Millar's asthma (laryngismus stridulus) 478.75
Millard-Gubler paralysis or syndrome 344.89
Millard-Gubler-Foville paralysis 344.89
Miller's disease (osteomalacia) 268.2
Miller-Dieker syndrome 758.33   ●
Miller Fisher's syndrome 357.0
Milles' syndrome (encephalocutaneous angiomatosis) 759.6
Mills' disease 335.29
Millstone makers' asthma or lung 502
Milroy's disease (chronic hereditary edema) 757.0
Miners' — *see also* condition
   asthma 500
   elbow 727.2
   knee 727.2
   lung 500
   nystagmus 300.89
   phthisis (*see also* Tuberculosis) 011.4 ☑
   tuberculosis (see also Tuberculosis) 011.4 ☑
Minkowski-Chauffard syndrome (*see also* Spherocytosis) 282.0
Minor — *see* condition
Minor's disease 336.1
Minot's disease (hemorrhagic disease, newborn) 776.0
Minot-von Willebrand (-Jürgens) disease or syndrome (angiohemophilia) 286.4
Minus (and plus) hand (intrinsic) 736.09
Miosis (persistent) (pupil) 379.42
Mirizzi's syndrome (hepatic duct stenosis) (*see also* Obstruction, biliary) 576.2
   with calculus, cholelithiasis, or stones — *see* Choledocholithiasis
Mirror writing 315.09
   secondary to organic lesion 784.69
Misadventure (prophylactic) (therapeutic) (*see also* Complications) 999.9
   administration of insulin 962.3
   infusion — *see* Complications, infusion
   local applications (of fomentations, plasters, etc.) 999.9
      burn or scald — *see* Burn, by site
   medical care (early) (late) NEC 999.9
      adverse effect of drugs or chemicals — *see* Table of Drugs and Chemicals
      burn or scald — *see* Burn, by site
   radiation NEC 990
   radiotherapy NEC 990
   surgical procedure (early) (late) — *see* Complications, surgical procedure
   transfusion — *see* Complications, transfusion
   vaccination or other immunological procedure — *see* Complications, vaccination
Misanthropy 301.7
Miscarriage — *see* Abortion, spontaneous
Mischief, malicious, child (*see also* Disturbance, conduct) 312.0 ☑
Misdirection
   aqueous 365.83
Mismanagement, feeding 783.3
Misplaced, misplacement
   kidney (*see also* Disease, renal) 593.0
      congenital 753.3
   organ or site, congenital NEC — *see* Malposition, congenital
Missed
   abortion 632
   delivery (at or near term) 656.4 ☑
   labor (at or near term) 656.4 ☑
Missing — *see also* Absence
   teeth (acquired) 525.10
      congenital (see also Anodontia) 520.0
      due to
         caries 525.13
         extraction 525.10
         periodontal disease 525.12
         specified NEC 525.19
         trauma 525.11
   vertebrae (congenital) 756.13

Misuse of drugs NEC (*see also* Abuse, drug, nondependent) 305.9 ☑
Mitchell's disease (erythromelalgia) 443.89
Mite(s)
   diarrhea 133.8
   grain (itch) 133.8
   hair follicle (itch) 133.8
   in sputum 133.8
Mitochondrial encephalopathy, lactic acidosis and stroke-like episodes (MELAS syndrome) 277.87   ●●●
Mitochondrial neurogastrointestinal encephalopathy syndrome (MNGIE) 277.87   ●●●
Mitral — *see* condition
Mittelschmerz 625.2
Mixed — *see* condition
Mljet disease (mal de Meleda) 757.39
Mobile, mobility
   cecum 751.4
   coccyx 733.99
   excessive — *see* Hypermobility
   gallbladder 751.69
   kidney 593.0
      congenital 753.3
   organ or site, congenital NEC — *see* Malposition, congenital
   spleen 289.59
Mobitz heart block (atrioventricular) 426.10
   type I (Wenckebach's) 426.13
   type II 426.12
Möbius'
   disease 346.8 ☑
   syndrome
      congenital oculofacial paralysis 352.6
      ophthalmoplegic migraine 346.8 ☑
Moeller (-Barlow) disease (infantile scurvy) 267
   glossitis 529.4
Mohr's syndrome (types I and II) 759.89
Mola destruens (M9100/1) 236.1
Molarization, premolars 520.2
Molar pregnancy 631
   hydatidiform (delivered) (undelivered) 630
Mold(s)
   in vitreous 117.9
Molding, head (during birth) — *omit code*
Mole (pigmented) (M8720/0) — *see also* Neoplasm, skin, benign
   blood 631
   Breus' 631
   cancerous (M8720/3) — *see* Melanoma
   carneous 631
   destructive (M9100/1) 236.1
   ectopic — *see* Pregnancy, ectopic
   fleshy 631
   hemorrhagic 631
   hydatid, hydatidiform (benign) (complicating pregnancy) (delivered) (undelivered) (*see also* Hydatidiform mole) 630
      invasive (M9100/1) 236.1
      malignant (M9100/1) 236.1
      previous, affecting management of pregnancy V23.1
   invasive (hydatidiform) (M9100/1) 236.1
   malignant
      meaning
         malignant hydatidiform mole (9100/1) 236.1
         melanoma (M8720/3) — *see* Melanoma
   nonpigmented (M8730/0) — *see* Neoplasm, skin, benign
   pregnancy NEC 631
   skin (M8720/0) — *see* Neoplasm, skin, benign
   tubal — *see* Pregnancy, tubal
   vesicular (*see also* Hydatidiform mole) 630
Molimen, molimina (menstrual) 625.4
Mollaret's meningitis 047.9
Mollities (cerebellar) (cerebral) 437.8
   ossium 268.2
Molluscum
   contagiosum 078.0
   epitheliale 078.0

Molluscum — *continued*
   fibrosum (M8851/0) — *see* Lipoma, by site
   pendulum (M8851/0) — *see* Lipoma, by site
Mönckeberg's arteriosclerosis, degeneration, disease, or sclerosis (*see also* Arteriosclerosis, extremities) 440.20
Monday fever 504
Monday morning dyspnea or asthma 504
Mondini's malformation (cochlea) 744.05
Mondor's disease (thrombophlebitis of breast) 451.89
Mongolian, mongolianism, mongolism, mongoloid 758.0
   spot 757.33
Monilethrix (congenital) 757.4
Monilia infestation — *see* Candidiasis
Moniliasis — *see also* Candidiasis
   neonatal 771.7
   vulvovaginitis 112.1
Monkeypox 057.8
Monoarthritis 716.60
   ankle 716.67
   arm 716.62
      lower (and wrist) 716.63
      upper (and elbow) 716.62
   foot (and ankle) 716.67
   forearm (and wrist) 716.63
   hand 716.64
   leg 716.66
      lower 716.66
      upper 716.65
   pelvic region (hip) (thigh) 716.65
   shoulder (region) 716.61
   specified site NEC 716.68
Monoblastic — *see* condition
Monochromatism (cone) (rod) 368.54
Monocytic — *see* condition
Monocytosis (symptomatic) 288.8
Monofixation syndrome 378.34
Monomania (*see also* Psychosis) 298.9
Mononeuritis 355.9
   cranial nerve — *see* Disorder, nerve, cranial
   femoral nerve 355.2
   lateral
      cutaneous nerve of thigh 355.1
      popliteal nerve 355.3
   lower limb 355.8
      specified nerve NEC 355.79
   medial popliteal nerve 355.4
   median nerve 354.1
   multiplex 354.5
   plantar nerve 355.6
   posterior tibial nerve 355.5
   radial nerve 354.3
   sciatic nerve 355.0
   ulnar nerve 354.2
   upper limb 354.9
      specified nerve NEC 354.8
   vestibular 388.5
Mononeuropathy (*see also* Mononeuritis) 355.9
   diabetic NEC 250.6 ☑ *[355.9]*
      lower limb 250.6 ☑ *[355.8]*
      upper limb 250.6 ☑ *[354.9]*
   iliohypogastric 355.79
   ilioinguinal 355.79
   obturator 355.79
   saphenous 355.79
Mononucleosis, infectious 075
   with hepatitis 075 *[573.1]*
Monoplegia 344.5
   brain (current episode) (*see also* Paralysis, brain) 437.8
      fetus or newborn 767.8
   cerebral (current episode) (*see also* Paralysis, brain) 437.8
   congenital or infantile (cerebral) (spastic) (spinal) 343.3
   embolic (current) (*see also* Embolism, brain) 434.1 ☑
      late effect — *see* Late effect(s) (of) cerebrovascular disease
   infantile (cerebral) (spastic) (spinal) 343.3

Monoplegia — *continued*
  lower limb 344.30
    affecting
      dominant side 344.31
      nondominant side 344.32
    due to late effect of cerebrovascular accident
        — *see* Late effect(s) (of)
        cerebrovascular accident
  newborn 767.8
  psychogenic 306.0
    specified as conversion reaction 300.11
  thrombotic (current) (*see also* Thrombosis,
      brain) 434.0 ☑
    late effect — *see* Late effect(s) (of)
      cerebrovascular disease
  transient 781.4
  upper limb 344.40
    affecting
      dominant side 344.41
      nondominant side 344.42
    due to late effect of cerebrovascular accident
        — *see* Late effect(s) (of)
        cerebrovascular accident
Monorchism, monorchidism 752.89
Monteggia's fracture (closed) 813.03
  open 813.13
Mood swings
  brief compensatory 296.99
  rebound 296.99
Moore's syndrome (*see also* Epilepsy) 345.5 ☑
Mooren's ulcer (cornea) 370.07
Mooser-Neill reaction 081.0
Mooser bodies 081.0
Moral
  deficiency 301.7
  imbecility 301.7
Morax-Axenfeld conjunctivitis 372.03
Morbilli (*see also* Measles) 055.9
Morbus
  anglicus, anglorum 268.0
  Beigel 111.2
  caducus (*see also* Epilepsy) 345.9 ☑
  caeruleus 746.89
  celiacus 579.0
  comitialis (see also Epilepsy) 345.9 ☑
  cordis — *see also* Disease, heart
    valvulorum — *see* Endocarditis
  coxae 719.95
    tuberculous (*see also* Tuberculosis) 015.1 ☑
  hemorrhagicus neonatorum 776.0
  maculosus neonatorum 772.6
  renum 593.0
  senilis (*see also* Osteoarthrosis) 715.9 ☑
Morel-Kraepelin disease (*see also* Schizophrenia)
  295.9 ☑
Morel-Moore syndrome (hyperostosis frontalis
  interna) 733.3
Morel-Morgagni syndrome (hyperostosis frontalis
  interna) 733.3
Morgagni
  cyst, organ, hydatid, or appendage 752.89
    fallopian tube 752.11
  disease or syndrome (hyperostosis frontalis
    interna) 733.3
Morgagni-Adams-Stokes syndrome (syncope with
  heart block) 426.9
Morgagni-Stewart-Morel syndrome (hyperostosis
  frontalis interna) 733.3
Moria (*see also* Psychosis) 298.9
Morning sickness 643.0 ☑
Moron 317
Morphea (guttate) (linear) 701.0
Morphine dependence (*see also* Dependence)
  304.0 ☑
Morphinism (*see also* Dependence) 304.0 ☑
Morphinomania (*see also* Dependence) 304.0 ☑
Morphoea 701.0
Morquio (-Brailsford) (-Ullrich) disease or
  syndrome (mucopolysaccharidosis IV) 277.5
  kyphosis 277.5
Morris syndrome (testicular feminization) 257.8

Morsus humanus (open wound) — *see also*
    Wound, open, by site
  skin surface intact — *see* Contusion
Mortification (dry) (moist) (*see also* Gangrene)
    785.4
Morton's
  disease 355.6
  foot 355.6
  metatarsalgia (syndrome) 355.6
  neuralgia 355.6
  neuroma 355.6
  syndrome (metatarsalgia) (neuralgia) 355.6
  toe 355.6
Morvan's disease 336.0
Mosaicism, mosaic (chromosomal) 758.9
  autosomal 758.5
  sex 758.81
Moschcowitz's syndrome (thrombotic
    thrombocytopenic purpura) 446.6
Mother yaw 102.0
Motion sickness (from travel, any vehicle) (from
    roundabouts or swings) 994.6
Mottled teeth (enamel) (endemic) (nonendemic)
    520.3
Mottling enamel (endemic) (nonendemic) (teeth)
    520.3
Mouchet's disease 732.5
Mould(s) (in vitreous) 117.9
Moulders'
  bronchitis 502
  tuberculosis (*see also* Tuberculosis) 011.4 ☑
Mounier-Kuhn syndrome 494.0
  with acute exacerbation 494.1
Mountain
  fever — *see* Fever, mountain
  sickness 993.2
    with polycythemia, acquired 289.0
    acute 289.0
  tick fever 066.1
Mouse, joint (*see also* Loose, body, joint) 718.1 ☑
  knee 717.6
Mouth — *see* condition
Movable
  coccyx 724.71
  kidney (*see also* Disease, renal) 593.0
    congenital 753.3
  organ or site, congenital NEC — *see*
    Malposition, congenital
  spleen 289.59
Movement
  abnormal (dystonic) (involuntary) 781.0
  decreased fetal 655.7 ☑
  paradoxical facial 374.43
Moya Moya disease 437.5
Mozart's ear 744.29
MRSA (methicillin-resistant staphylococcus ●
    aureus) V09.0   ●
Mucha's disease (acute parapsoriasis
    varioliformis) 696.2
Mucha-Haberman syndrome (acute parapsoriasis
    varioliformis) 696.2
Mu-chain disease 273.2
Mucinosis (cutaneous) (papular) 701.8
Mucocele
  appendix 543.9
  buccal cavity 528.9
  gallbladder (*see also* Disease, gallbladder)
    575.3
  lacrimal sac 375.43
  orbit (eye) 376.81
  salivary gland (any) 527.6
  sinus (accessory) (nasal) 478.1
  turbinate (bone) (middle) (nasal) 478.1
  uterus 621.8
Mucocutaneous lymph node syndrome (acute)
    (febrile) (infantile) 446.1
Mucoenteritis 564.9
Mucolipidosis I, II, III 272.7
Mucopolysaccharidosis (types 1-6) 277.5
  cardiopathy 277.5 [425.7]
Mucormycosis (lung) 117.7

Mucositis — *see also* Inflammation by site
  necroticans agranulocytica 288.0
Mucous — *see also* condition
  patches (syphilitic) 091.3
    congenital 090.0
Mucoviscidosis 277.00
  with meconium obstruction 277.01
Mucus
  asphyxia or suffocation (*see also* Asphyxia,
    mucus) 933.1
    newborn 770.1
  in stool 792.1
  plug (*see also* Asphyxia, mucus) 933.1
    aspiration, of newborn 770.1
    tracheobronchial 519.1
      newborn 770.1
Muguet 112.0
Mulberry molars 090.5
Mullerian mixed tumor (M8950/3) — *see*
  Neoplasm, by site, malignant
Multicystic kidney 753.19
Multilobed placenta — *see* Placenta, abnormal
Multinodular prostate 600.10
  with urinary retention 600.11
Multiparity V61.5
  affecting
    fetus or newborn 763.89
    management of
      labor and delivery 659.4 ☑
      pregnancy V23.3
  requiring contraceptive management (*see also*
    Contraception) V25.9
Multipartita placenta — *see* Placenta, abnormal
Multiple, multiplex — *see also* condition
  birth
    affecting fetus or newborn 761.5
    healthy liveborn — *see* Newborn, multiple
  digits (congenital) 755.00
    fingers 755.01
    toes 755.02
  organ or site NEC — *see* Accessory
  personality 300.14
  renal arteries 747.62
Mumps 072.9
  with complication 072.8
    specified type NEC 072.79
  encephalitis 072.2
  hepatitis 072.71
  meningitis (aseptic) 072.1
  meningoencephalitis 072.2
  oophoritis 072.79
  orchitis 072.0
  pancreatitis 072.3
  polyneuropathy 072.72
  vaccination, prophylactic (against) V04.6
Mumu (*see also* Infestation, filarial) 125.9
Münchausen syndrome 301.51
Münchmeyer's disease or syndrome (exostosis
  luxurians) 728.11
Mural — *see* condition
Murmur (cardiac) (heart) (nonorganic) (organic)
    785.2
  abdominal 787.5
  aortic (valve) (*see also* Endocarditis, aortic)
    424.1
  benign — *omit code*
  cardiorespiratory 785.2
  diastolic — *see* condition
  Flint (*see also* Endocarditis, aortic) 424.1
  functional — *omit code*
  Graham Steell (pulmonic regurgitation) (*see
    also* Endocarditis, pulmonary) 424.3
  innocent — *omit code*
  insignificant — *omit code*
  midsystolic 785.2
  mitral (valve) — *see* Stenosis, mitral
  physiologic — *see* condition
  presystolic, mitral — *see* Insufficiency, mitral
  pulmonic (valve) (*see also* Endocarditis,
    pulmonary) 424.3
  Still's (vibratory) — *omit code*
  systolic (valvular) — *see* condition
  tricuspid (valve) — *see* Endocarditis, tricuspid

☑ Additional Digit Required   ►◄ Revised Text   ● New Line   ▲ Revised Code

Murmur — *continued*
  undiagnosed 785.2
  valvular — *see* condition
  vibratory — *omit code*
Murri's disease (intermittent hemoglobinuria)
  283.2
Muscae volitantes 379.24
Muscle, muscular — *see* condition
Musculoneuralgia 729.1
Mushrooming hip 718.95
Mushroom workers' (pickers') lung 495.5
Mutation
  factor V leiden 289.81
  prothrombin gene 289.81
Mutism (*see also* Aphasia) 784.3
  akinetic 784.3
  deaf (acquired) (congenital) 389.7
  hysterical 300.11
  ▶selective (elective)◀ 313.23
    adjustment reaction 309.83
Myà's disease (congenital dilation, colon) 751.3
Myalgia (intercostal) 729.1
  eosinophilia syndrome 710.5
  epidemic 074.1
    cervical 078.89
  psychogenic 307.89
  traumatic NEC 959.9
Myasthenia 358.00
  cordis — *see* Failure, heart
  gravis 358.00
    with exacerbation (acute) 358.01
    in crisis 358.01
    neonatal 775.2
    pseudoparalytica 358.00
  stomach 536.8
    psychogenic 306.4
  syndrome
    in
      botulism 005.1 *[358.1]*
      diabetes mellitus 250.6 ☑ *[358.1]*
      hypothyroidism (*see also* Hypothyroidism)
        244.9 *[358.1]*
      malignant neoplasm NEC 199.1 *[358.1]*
      pernicious anemia 281.0 *[358.1]*
      thyrotoxicosis (*see also* Thyrotoxicosis)
        242.9 ☑ *[358.1]*
Myasthenic 728.87   ●
Mycelium infection NEC 117.9
Mycetismus 988.1
Mycetoma (actinomycotic) 039.9
  bone 039.8
    mycotic 117.4
  foot 039.4
    mycotic 117.4
  madurae 039.9
    mycotic 117.4
  maduromycotic 039.9
    mycotic 117.4
  mycotic 117.4
  nocardial 039.9
Mycobacteriosis — *see* Mycobacterium
Mycobacterium, mycobacterial (infection) 031.9
  acid-fast (bacilli) 031.9
  anonymous (*see also* Mycobacterium, atypical)
    031.9
  atypical (acid-fast bacilli) 031.9
    cutaneous 031.1
    pulmonary 031.0
      tuberculous (*see also* Tuberculosis,
        pulmonary) 011.9 ☑
    specified site NEC 031.8
  avium 031.0
    intracellulare complex bacteremia (MAC)
      031.2
  balnei 031.1
  Battey 031.0
  cutaneous 031.1
  disseminated 031.2
    avium-intracellulare complex (DMAC) 031.2
  fortuitum 031.0
  intracellulare (battey bacillus) 031.0
  kakerifu 031.8
  kansasii 031.0
  kasongo 031.8

Mycobacterium, mycobacterial — *continued*
  leprae — *see* Leprosy
  luciflavum 031.0
  marinum 031.1
  pulmonary 031.0
    tuberculous (*see also* Tuberculosis,
      pulmonary) 011.9 ☑
  scrofulaceum 031.1
  tuberculosis (human, bovine) — *see also*
    Tuberculosis
    avian type 031.0
  ulcerans 031.1
  xenopi 031.0
Mycosis, mycotic 117.9
  cutaneous NEC 111.9
  ear 111.8 *[380.15]*
  fungoides (M9700/3) 202.1 ☑
  mouth 112.0
  pharynx 117.9
  skin NEC 111.9
  stomatitis 112.0
  systemic NEC 117.9
  tonsil 117.9
  vagina, vaginitis 112.1
Mydriasis (persistent) (pupil) 379.43
Myelatelia 742.59
Myelinoclasis, perivascular, acute
  (postinfectious) NEC 136.9 *[323.6]*
  postimmunization or postvaccinal 323.5
Myelinosis, central pontine 341.8
Myelitis (acute) (ascending) (cerebellar)
  (childhood) (chronic) (descending) (diffuse)
  (disseminated) (pressure) (progressive)
  (spinal cord) (subacute) (transverse) (*see also*
  Encephalitis) 323.9
  late effect — *see* category 326
  optic neuritis in 341.0
  postchickenpox 052.7
  postvaccinal 323.5
  syphilitic (transverse) 094.89
  tuberculous (*see also* Tuberculosis) 013.6 ☑
  virus 049.9
Myeloblastic — *see* condition
Myelocele (*see also* Spina bifida) 741.9 ☑
  with hydrocephalus 741.0 ☑
Myelocystocele (*see also* Spina bifida) 741.9 ☑
Myelocytic — *see* condition
Myelocytoma 205.1 ☑
Myelodysplasia (spinal cord) 742.59
  meaning myelodysplastic syndrome — *see*
    Syndrome, myelodysplastic
Myeloencephalitis — *see* Encephalitis
Myelofibrosis (osteosclerosis) 289.89
Myelogenous — *see* condition
Myeloid — *see* condition
Myelokathexis 288.0
Myeloleukodystrophy 330.0
Myelolipoma (M8870/0) — *see* Neoplasm, by site,
  benign
Myeloma (multiple) (plasma cell) (plasmacytic)
  (M9730/3) 203.0 ☑
  monostotic (M9731/1) 238.6
  solitary (M9731/1) 238.6
Myelomalacia 336.8
Myelomata, multiple (M9730/3) 203.0 ☑
Myelomatosis (M9730/3) 203.0 ☑
Myelomeningitis — *see* Meningoencephalitis
Myelomeningocele (spinal cord) (*see also* Spina
  bifida) 741.9 ☑
  fetal, causing fetopelvic disproportion 653.7 ☑
Myelo-osteo-musculodysplasia hereditaria
  756.89
Myelopathic — *see* condition
Myelopathy (spinal cord) 336.9
  cervical 721.1
  diabetic 250.6 ☑ *[336.3]*
  drug-induced 336.8
  due to or with
    carbon tetrachloride 987.8 *[323.7]*
    degeneration or displacement, intervertebral
      disc 722.70
      cervical, cervicothoracic 722.71

Myelopathy — *continued*
  due to or with — *continued*
    degeneration or displacement, intervertebral
      disc — *continued*
      lumbar, lumbosacral 722.73
      thoracic, thoracolumbar 722.72
    hydroxyquinoline derivatives 961.3 *[323.7]*
    infection — *see* Encephalitis
    intervertebral disc disorder 722.70
      cervical, cervicothoracic 722.71
      lumbar, lumbosacral 722.73
      thoracic, thoracolumbar 722.72
    lead 984.9 *[323.7]*
    mercury 985.0 *[323.7]*
    neoplastic disease (*see also* Neoplasm, by
      site) 239.9 *[336.3]*
    pernicious anemia 281.0 *[336.3]*
    spondylosis 721.91
      cervical 721.1
      lumbar, lumbosacral 721.42
      thoracic 721.41
    thallium 985.8 *[323.7]*
  lumbar, lumbosacral 721.42
  necrotic (subacute) 336.1
  radiation-induced 336.8
  spondylogenic NEC 721.91
    cervical 721.1
    lumbar, lumbosacral 721.42
    thoracic 721.41
  thoracic 721.41
  toxic NEC 989.9 *[323.7]*
  transverse (*see also* Encephalitis) 323.9
  vascular 336.1
Myeloproliferative disease (M9960/1) 238.7
Myeloradiculitis (*see also* Polyneuropathy) 357.0
Myeloradiculodysplasia (spinal) 742.59
Myelosarcoma (M9930/3) 205.3 ☑
Myelosclerosis 289.89
  with myeloid metaplasia (M9961/1) 238.7
  disseminated, of nervous system 340
  megakaryocytic (M9961/1) 238.7
Myelosis (M9860/3) (*see also* Leukemia, myeloid)
  205.9 ☑
  acute (M9861/3) 205.0 ☑
  aleukemic (M9864/3) 205.8 ☑
  chronic (M9863/3) 205.1 ☑
  erythremic (M9840/3) 207.0 ☑
    acute (M9841/3) 207.0 ☑
  megakaryocytic (M9920/3) 207.2 ☑
  nonleukemic (chronic) 288.8
  subacute (M9862/3) 205.2 ☑
Myesthenia — *see* Myasthenia
Myiasis (cavernous) 134.0
  orbit 134.0 *[376.13]*
Myoadenoma, prostate 600.20
  with urinary retention 600.21
Myoblastoma
  granular cell (M9580/0) — *see also* Neoplasm,
    connective tissue, benign
    malignant (M9580/3) — *see* Neoplasm,
      connective tissue, malignant
  tongue (M9580/0) 210.1
Myocardial — *see* condition
Myocardiopathy (congestive) (constrictive)
  (familial) (hypertrophic nonobstructive)
  (idiopathic) (infiltrative) (obstructive)
  (primary) (restrictive) (sporadic) 425.4
  alcoholic 425.5
  amyloid 277.3 *[425.7]*
  beriberi 265.0 *[425.7]*
  cobalt-beer 425.5
  due to
    amyloidosis 277.3 *[425.7]*
    beriberi 265.0 *[425.7]*
    cardiac glycogenosis 271.0 *[425.7]*
    Chagas' disease 086.0
    Friedreich's ataxia 334.0 *[425.8]*
    influenza 487.8 *[425.8]*
    mucopolysaccharidosis 277.5 *[425.7]*
    myotonia atrophica 359.2 *[425.8]*
    progressive muscular dystrophy 359.1
      [425.8]
    sarcoidosis 135 *[425.8]*
  glycogen storage 271.0 *[425.7]*

☑ Additional Digit Required   ▶◀ Revised Text   ● New Line   ▲ Revised Code

Myocardiopathy — *continued*
  hypertrophic obstructive 425.1
  metabolic NEC 277.9 *[425.7]*
  nutritional 269.9 *[425.7]*
  obscure (African) 425.2
  peripartum 674.5 ☑
  postpartum 674.5 ☑
  secondary 425.9
  thyrotoxic (*see also* Thyrotoxicosis)
    242.9 ☑ *[425.7]*
  toxic NEC 425.9

Myocarditis (fibroid) (interstitial) (old)
  (progressive) (senile) (with arteriosclerosis)
  429.0
  with
    rheumatic fever (conditions classifiable to
      390) 398.0
      active (*see also* Myocarditis, acute,
        rheumatic) 391.2
      inactive or quiescent (with chorea) 398.0
  active (nonrheumatic) 422.90
    rheumatic 391.2
      with chorea (acute) (rheumatic)
        (Sydenham's) 392.0
  acute or subacute (interstitial) 422.90
    due to Streptococcus (beta-hemolytic) 391.2
    idiopathic 422.91
    rheumatic 391.2
      with chorea (acute) (rheumatic)
        (Sydenham's) 392.0
    specified type NEC 422.99
  aseptic of newborn 074.23
  bacterial (acute) 422.92
  chagasic 086.0
  chronic (interstitial) 429.0
  congenital 746.89
  constrictive 425.4
  Coxsackie (virus) 074.23
  diphtheritic 032.82
  due to or in
    Coxsackie (virus) 074.23
    diphtheria 032.82
    epidemic louse-borne typhus 080 *[422.0]*
    influenza 487.8 *[422.0]*
    Lyme disease 088.81 *[422.0]*
    scarlet fever 034.1 *[422.0]*
    toxoplasmosis (acquired) 130.3
    tuberculosis (*see also* Tuberculosis)
      017.9 ☑ *[422.0]*
    typhoid 002.0 *[422.0]*
    typhus NEC 081.9 *[422.0]*
  eosinophilic 422.91
  epidemic of newborn 074.23
  Fiedler's (acute) (isolated) (subacute) 422.91
  giant cell (acute) (subacute) 422.91
  gonococcal 098.85
  granulomatous (idiopathic) (isolated)
    (nonspecific) 422.91
  hypertensive (*see also* Hypertension, heart)
    402.90
  idiopathic 422.91
    granulomatous 422.91
  infective 422.92
  influenzal 487.8 *[422.0]*
  isolated (diffuse) (granulomatous) 422.91
  malignant 422.99
  meningococcal 036.43
  nonrheumatic, active 422.90
  parenchymatous 422.90
  pneumococcal (acute) (subacute) 422.92
  rheumatic (chronic) (inactive) (with chorea)
    398.0
    active or acute 391.2
      with chorea (acute) (rheumatic)
        (Sydenham's) 392.0
  septic 422.92
  specific (giant cell) (productive) 422.91
  staphylococcal (acute) (subacute) 422.92
  suppurative 422.92
  syphilitic (chronic) 093.82
  toxic 422.93
    rheumatic (*see also* Myocarditis, acute,
      rheumatic) 391.2
  tuberculous (*see also* Tuberculosis)
    017.9 ☑ *[422.0]*
  typhoid 002.0 *[422.0]*

Myocarditis — *continued*
  valvular — *see* Endocarditis
  viral, except Coxsackie 422.91
    Coxsackie 074.23
    of newborn (Coxsackie) 074.23

Myocardium, myocardial — *see* condition

Myocardosis (*see also* Cardiomyopathy) 425.4

Myoclonia (essential) 333.2
  epileptica 333.2
  Friedrich's 333.2
  massive 333.2

Myoclonic
  epilepsy, familial (progressive) 333.2
  jerks 333.2

Myoclonus (familial essential) (multifocal)
  (simplex) 333.2
  with epilepsy and with ragged red fibers   ●
    (MERRF syndrome) 277.87   ●
  facial 351.8
  massive (infantile) 333.2
  pharyngeal 478.29

Myodiastasis 728.84

Myoendocarditis — *see also* Endocarditis
  acute or subacute 421.9

Myoepithelioma (M8982/0) — *see* Neoplasm, by
  site, benign

Myofascitis (acute) 729.1
  low back 724.2

Myofibroma (M8890/0) — *see also* Neoplasm,
  connective tissue, benign
  uterus (cervix) (corpus) (*see also* Leiomyoma)
    218.9

Myofibrosis 728.2
  heart (*see also* Myocarditis) 429.0
  humeroscapular region 726.2
  scapulohumeral 726.2

Myofibrositis (*see also* Myositis) 729.1
  scapulohumeral 726.2

Myogelosis (occupational) 728.89

Myoglobinuria 791.3

Myoglobulinuria, primary 791.3

Myokymia — *see also* Myoclonus
  facial 351.8

Myolipoma (M8860/0)
  specified site — *see* Neoplasm, connective
    tissue, benign
  unspecified site 223.0

Myoma (M8895/0) — *see also* Neoplasm,
  connective tissue, benign
  cervix (stump) (uterus) (*see also* Leiomyoma)
    218.9
  malignant (M8895/3) — *see* Neoplasm,
    connective tissue, malignant
  prostate 600.20
    with urinary retention 600.21
  uterus (cervix) (corpus) (*see also* Leiomyoma)
    218.9
    in pregnancy or childbirth 654.1 ☑
      affecting fetus or newborn 763.89
      causing obstructed labor 660.2 ☑
        affecting fetus or newborn 763.1

Myomalacia 728.9
  cordis, heart (*see also* Degeneration,
    myocardial) 429.1

Myometritis (*see also* Endometritis) 615.9

Myometrium — *see* condition

Myonecrosis, clostridial 040.0

Myopathy 359.9
  alcoholic 359.4
  amyloid 277.3 *[359.6]*
  benign congenital 359.0
  central core 359.0
  centronuclear 359.0
  congenital (benign) 359.0
  critical illness 359.81
  distal 359.1
  due to drugs 359.4
  endocrine 259.9 *[359.5]*
    specified type NEC 259.8 *[359.5]*
  extraocular muscles 376.82
  facioscapulohumeral 359.1

Myopathy — *continued*
  in
    Addison's disease 255.4 *[359.5]*
    amyloidosis 277.3 *[359.6]*
    cretinism 243 *[359.5]*
    Cushing's syndrome 255.0 *[359.5]*
    disseminated lupus erythematosus 710.0
      [359.6]
    giant cell arteritis 446.5 *[359.6]*
    hyperadrenocorticism NEC 255.3 *[359.5]*
    hyperparathyroidism 252.01 *[359.5]*   ▲
    hypopituitarism 253.2 *[359.5]*
    hypothyroidism (*see also* Hypothyroidism)
      244.9 *[359.5]*
    malignant neoplasm NEC (M8000/3) 199.1
      [359.6]
    myxedema (*see also* Myxedema) 244.9
      [359.5]
    polyarteritis nodosa 446.0 *[359.6]*
    rheumatoid arthritis 714.0 *[359.6]*
    sarcoidosis 135 *[359.6]*
    scleroderma 710.1 *[359.6]*
    Sjögren's disease 710.2 *[359.6]*
    thyrotoxicosis (*see also* Thyrotoxicosis)
      242.9 ☑ *[359.5]*
  inflammatory 359.89
  intensive care (ICU) 359.81
  limb-girdle 359.1
  myotubular 359.0
  necrotizing, acute 359.81
  nemaline 359.0
  ocular 359.1
  oculopharyngeal 359.1
  of critical illness 359.81
  primary 359.89
  progressive NEC 359.89
  quadriplegic, acute 359.81
  rod body 359.0
  scapulohumeral 359.1
  specified type NEC 359.89
  toxic 359.4

Myopericarditis (*see also* Pericarditis) 423.9

Myopia (axial) (congenital) (increased curvature or
  refraction, nucleus of lens) 367.1
  degenerative, malignant 360.21
  malignant 360.21
  progressive high (degenerative) 360.21

Myosarcoma (M8895/3) — *see* Neoplasm,
  connective tissue, malignant

Myosis (persistent) 379.42
  stromal (endolymphatic) (M8931/1) 236.0

Myositis 729.1
  clostridial 040.0
  due to posture 729.1
  epidemic 074.1
  fibrosa or fibrous (chronic) 728.2
    Volkmann's (complicating trauma) 958.6
  infective 728.0
  interstitial 728.81
  multiple — *see* Polymyositis
  occupational 729.1
  orbital, chronic 376.12
  ossificans 728.12
    circumscribed 728.12
    progressive 728.11
    traumatic 728.12
  progressive fibrosing 728.11
  purulent 728.0
  rheumatic 729.1
  rheumatoid 729.1
  suppurative 728.0
  syphilitic 095.6
  traumatic (old) 729.1

Myospasia impulsiva 307.23

Myotonia (acquisita) (intermittens) 728.85
  atrophica 359.2
  congenita 359.2
  dystrophica 359.2

Myotonic pupil 379.46

Myriapodiasis 134.1

Myringitis
  with otitis media — *see* Otitis media
  acute 384.00
    specified type NEC 384.09
  bullosa hemorrhagica 384.01

Myringitis — *continued*
  bullous 384.01
  chronic 384.1
Mysophobia 300.29
Mytilotoxism 988.0
Myxadenitis labialis 528.5
Myxedema (adult) (idiocy) (infantile) (juvenile)
    (thyroid gland) (*see also* Hypothyroidism)
    244.9
  circumscribed 242.9 ☑
  congenital 243
  cutis 701.8
  localized (pretibial) 242.9 ☑
  madness (acute) 293.0
    subacute 293.1
  papular 701.8
  pituitary 244.8
  postpartum 674.8 ☑
  pretibial 242.9 ☑
  primary 244.9
Myxochondrosarcoma (M9220/3) — *see*
    Neoplasm, cartilage, malignant
Myxofibroma (M8811/0) — *see also* Neoplasm,
    connective tissue, benign
  odontogenic (M9320/0) 213.1
    upper jaw (bone) 213.0
Myxofibrosarcoma (M8811/3) — *see* Neoplasm,
    connective tissue, malignant
Myxolipoma (M8852/0) (*see also* Lipoma, by site)
    214.9
Myxoliposarcoma (M8852/3) — *see* Neoplasm,
    connective tissue, malignant
Myxoma (M8840/0) — *see also* Neoplasm,
    connective tissue, benign
  odontogenic (M9320/0) 213.1
    upper jaw (bone) 213.0
Myxosarcoma (M8840/3) — *see* Neoplasm,
    connective tissue, malignant

N

Naegeli's
  disease (hereditary hemorrhagic
      thrombasthenia) 287.1
  leukemia, monocytic (M9863/3) 205.1 ☑
  syndrome (incontinentia pigmenti) 757.33
Naffziger's syndrome 353.0
Naga sore (*see also* Ulcer, skin) 707.9
Nägele's pelvis 738.6
  with disproportion (fetopelvic) 653.0 ☑
    affecting fetus or newborn 763.1
    causing obstructed labor 660.1 ☑
      affecting fetus or newborn 763.1
Nager-de Reynier syndrome (dysostosis
    mandibularis) 756.0
Nail — *see also* condition
  biting 307.9
  patella syndrome (hereditary
      osteoonychodysplasia) 756.89
Nanism, nonosomia (*see also* Dwarfism) 259.4
  hypophyseal 253.3
  pituitary 253.3
  renis, renalis 588.0
Nanukayami 100.89
Napkin rash 691.0
Narcissism 301.81
Narcolepsy 347.00   ▲
  with cataplexy 347.01   ●
  in conditions classified elsewhere 347.10   ●
    with cataplexy 347.11   ●
Narcosis
  carbon dioxide (respiratory) 786.09
  due to drug
    correct substance properly administered
        780.09
    overdose or wrong substance given or taken
        977.9
      specified drug — *see* Table of Drugs and
          Chemicals

Narcotism (chronic) (*see also* listing under
    Dependence) 304.9 ☑
  acute
    correct substance properly administered
        349.82
    overdose or wrong substance given or taken
        967.8
      specified drug — *see* Table of Drugs and
          Chemicals
NARP syndrome (neuropathy, ataxia and   ●
    retinitis pigmentosa) 277.87   ●
Narrow
  anterior chamber angle 365.02
  pelvis (inlet) (outlet) — *see* Contraction, pelvis
Narrowing
  artery NEC 447.1
    auditory, internal 433.8 ☑
      basilar 433.0 ☑
        with other precerebral artery 433.3 ☑
          bilateral 433.3 ☑
      carotid 433.1 ☑
        with other precerebral artery 433.3 ☑
          bilateral 433.3 ☑
      cerebellar 433.8 ☑
      choroidal 433.8 ☑
      communicating posterior 433.8 ☑
      coronary — *see also* Arteriosclerosis,
          coronary
        congenital 746.85
          due to syphilis 090.5
      hypophyseal 433.8 ☑
      pontine 433.8 ☑
      precerebral NEC 433.9 ☑
        multiple or bilateral 433.3 ☑
        specified NEC 433.8 ☑
      vertebral 433.2 ☑
        with other precerebral artery 433.3 ☑
          bilateral 433.3 ☑
    auditory canal (external) (*see also* Stricture, ear
        canal, acquired) 380.50
    cerebral arteries 437.0
    cicatricial — *see* Cicatrix
    congenital — *see* Anomaly, congenital
    coronary artery — *see* Narrowing, artery,
        coronary
    ear, middle 385.22
    Eustachian tube (*see also* Obstruction,
        Eustachian tube) 381.60
    eyelid 374.46
      congenital 743.62
    intervertebral disc or space NEC — *see*
        Degeneration, intervertebral disc
    joint space, hip 719.85
    larynx 478.74
    lids 374.46
      congenital 743.62
    mesenteric artery (with gangrene) 557.0
    palate 524.89   ▲
    palpebral fissure 374.46
    retinal artery 362.13
    ureter 593.3
    urethra (*see also* Stricture, urethra) 598.9
Narrowness, abnormal, eyelid 743.62
Nasal — *see* condition
Nasolacrimal — *see* condition
Nasopharyngeal — *see also* condition
  bursa 478.29
  pituitary gland 759.2
  torticollis 723.5
Nasopharyngitis (acute) (infective) (subacute) 460
  chronic 472.2
    due to external agent — *see* Condition,
        respiratory, chronic, due to
  due to external agent — *see* Condition,
      respiratory, due to
  septic 034.0
  streptococcal 034.0
  suppurative (chronic) 472.2
  ulcerative (chronic) 472.2
Nasopharynx, nasopharyngeal — *see* condition
Natal tooth, teeth 520.6
Nausea (*see also* Vomiting) 787.02
  with vomiting 787.01
  epidemic 078.82

Nausea (*see also* Vomiting) — *continued*
  gravidarum — *see* Hyperemesis, gravidarum
  marina 994.6
Navel — *see* condition
Neapolitan fever (*see also* Brucellosis) 023.9
Nearsightedness 367.1
Near-syncope 780.2
Nebécourt's syndrome 253.3
Nebula, cornea (eye) 371.01
  congenital 743.43
    interfering with vision 743.42
Necator americanus infestation 126.1
Necatoriasis 126.1
Neck — *see* condition
Necrencephalus (*see also* Softening, brain) 437.8
Necrobacillosis 040.3
Necrobiosis 799.89
  brain or cerebral (*see also* Softening, brain)
      437.8
  lipoidica 709.3
    diabeticorum 250.8 ☑ [709.3]
Necrodermolysis 695.1
Necrolysis, toxic epidermal 695.1
  due to drug
    correct substance properly administered
        695.1
    overdose or wrong substance given or taken
        977.9
      specified drug — *see* Table of Drugs and
          Chemicals
Necrophilia 302.89
Necrosis, necrotic
  adrenal (capsule) (gland) 255.8
  antrum, nasal sinus 478.1
  aorta (hyaline) (*see also* Aneurysm, aorta)
      441.9
    cystic medial 441.00
      abdominal 441.02
      thoracic 441.01
      thoracoabdominal 441.03
    ruptured 441.5
  arteritis 446.0
  artery 447.5
  aseptic, bone 733.40
    femur (head) (neck) 733.42
      medial condyle 733.43
    humoral head 733.41
    medial femoral condyle 733.43
    specific site NEC 733.49
    talus 733.44
  avascular, bone NEC (*see also* Necrosis,
      aseptic, bone) 733.40
  bladder (aseptic) (sphincter) 596.8
  bone (*see also* Osteomyelitis) 730.1 ☑
    acute 730.0 ☑
    aseptic or avascular 733.40
      femur (head) (neck) 733.42
        medial condyle 733.43
      humoral head 733.41
      medial femoral condyle 733.43
      specified site NEC 733.49
      talus 733.44
    ethmoid 478.1
    ischemic 733.40
    jaw 526.4
    marrow 289.89
    Paget's (osteitis deformans) 731.0
    tuberculous — *see* Tuberculosis, bone
  brain (softening) (*see also* Softening, brain)
      437.8
  breast (aseptic) (fat) (segmental) 611.3
  bronchus, bronchi 519.1
  central nervous system NEC (*see also*
      Softening, brain) 437.8
  cerebellar (*see also* Softening, brain) 437.8
  cerebral (softening) (*see also* Softening, brain)
      437.8
  cerebrospinal (softening) (*see also* Softening,
      brain) 437.8
  cornea (*see also* Keratitis) 371.40
  cortical, kidney 583.6
  cystic medial (aorta) 441.00
    abdominal 441.02
    thoracic 441.01

☑ Additional Digit Required   ►◄ Revised Text   ● New Line   ▲ Revised Code

Necrosis, necrotic — *continued*
cystic medial — *continued*
thoracoabdominal 441.03
dental 521.09
pulp 522.1
due to swallowing corrosive substance — *see*
Burn, by site
ear (ossicle) 385.24
esophagus 530.89
ethmoid (bone) 478.1
eyelid 374.50
fat, fatty (generalized) (*see also* Degeneration,
fatty) 272.8
abdominal wall 567.8 ●
breast (aseptic) (segmental) 611.3
intestine 569.89
localized — *see* Degeneration, by site, fatty
mesentery 567.8
omentum 567.8
pancreas 577.8
peritoneum 567.8
skin (subcutaneous) 709.3
newborn 778.1
femur (aseptic) (avascular) 733.42
head 733.42
medial condyle 733.43
neck 733.42
gallbladder (*see also* Cholecystitis, acute) 575.0
gangrenous 785.4
gastric 537.89
glottis 478.79
heart (myocardium) — *see* Infarct, myocardium
hepatic (*see also* Necrosis, liver) 570
hip (aseptic) (avascular) 733.42
intestine (acute) (hemorrhagic) (massive) 557.0
ischemic 785.4
jaw 526.4
kidney (bilateral) 583.9
acute 584.9
cortical 583.6
acute 584.6
with
abortion — *see* Abortion, by type,
with renal failure
ectopic pregnancy (*see also*
categories 633.0-633.9) 639.3
molar pregnancy (*see also*
categories 630-632) 639.3
complicating pregnancy 646.2 ☑
affecting fetus or newborn 760.1
following labor and delivery 669.3 ☑
medullary (papillary) (*see also* Pyelitis)
590.80
in
acute renal failure 584.7
nephritis, nephropathy 583.7
papillary (*see also* Pyelitis) 590.80
in
acute renal failure 584.7
nephritis, nephropathy 583.7
tubular 584.5
with
abortion — *see* Abortion, by type, with
renal failure
ectopic pregnancy (*see also* categories
633.0-633.9) 639.3
molar pregnancy (*see also* categories
630-632) 639.3
complicating
abortion 639.3
ectopic or molar pregnancy 639.3
pregnancy 646.2 ☑
affecting fetus or newborn 760.1
following labor and delivery 669.3 ☑
traumatic 958.5
larynx 478.79
liver (acute) (congenital) (diffuse) (massive)
(subacute) 570
with
abortion — *see* Abortion, by type, with
specified complication NEC
ectopic pregnancy (*see also* categories
633.0-633.9) 639.8
molar pregnancy (*see also* categories 630-
632) 639.8
complicating pregnancy 646.7 ☑
affecting fetus or newborn 760.8

Necrosis, necrotic — *continued*
liver — *continued*
following
abortion 639.8
ectopic or molar pregnancy 639.8
obstetrical 646.7 ☑
postabortal 639.8
puerperal, postpartum 674.8 ☑
toxic 573.3
lung 513.0
lymphatic gland 683
mammary gland 611.3
mastoid (chronic) 383.1
mesentery 557.0
fat 567.8
mitral valve — *see* Insufficiency, mitral
myocardium, myocardial — *see* Infarct,
myocardium
nose (septum) 478.1
omentum 557.0
with mesenteric infarction 557.0
fat 567.8
orbit, orbital 376.10
ossicles, ear (aseptic) 385.24
ovary (*see also* Salpingo-oophoritis) 614.2
pancreas (aseptic) (duct) (fat) 577.8
acute 577.0
infective 577.0
papillary, kidney (*see also* Pyelitis) 590.80
peritoneum 557.0
with mesenteric infarction 557.0
fat 567.8
pharynx 462
in granulocytopenia 288.0
phosphorus 983.9
pituitary (gland) (postpartum) (Sheehan) 253.2
placenta (*see also* Placenta, abnormal) 656.7 ☑
pneumonia 513.0
pulmonary 513.0
pulp (dental) 522.1
pylorus 537.89
radiation — *see* Necrosis, by site
radium — *see* Necrosis, by site
renal — *see* Necrosis, kidney
sclera 379.19
scrotum 608.89
skin or subcutaneous tissue 709.8
due to burn — *see* Burn, by site
gangrenous 785.4
spine, spinal (column) 730.18
acute 730.18
cord 336.1
spleen 289.59
stomach 537.89
stomatitis 528.1
subcutaneous fat 709.3
fetus or newborn 778.1
subendocardial — *see* Infarct, myocardium
suprarenal (capsule) (gland) 255.8
teeth, tooth 521.09
testis 608.89
thymus (gland) 254.8
tonsil 474.8
trachea 519.1
tuberculous NEC — *see* Tuberculosis
tubular (acute) (anoxic) (toxic) 584.5
due to a procedure 997.5
umbilical cord, affecting fetus or newborn
762.6
vagina 623.8
vertebra (lumbar) 730.18
acute 730.18
tuberculous (*see also* Tuberculosis)
015.0 ☑ *[730.8]* ☑
vesical (aseptic) (bladder) 596.8
x-ray — *see* Necrosis, by site
Necrospermia 606.0
Necrotizing angiitis 446.0
Negativism 301.7
Neglect (child) (newborn) NEC 995.52
adult 995.84
after or at birth 995.52
hemispatial 781.8
left-sided 781.8
sensory 781.8
visuospatial 781.8

Negri bodies 071
Neill-Dingwall syndrome (microcephaly and
dwarfism) 759.89
Neisserian infection NEC — *see* Gonococcus
Nematodiasis NEC (*see also* Infestation,
Nematode) 127.9
ancylostoma (*see also* Ancylostomiasis) 126.9
Neoformans cryptococcus infection 117.5
Neonatal — *see also* condition
adrenoleukodystrophy 277.86 ●
teeth, tooth 520.6
Neonatorum — *see* condition

	Malignant					
	Primary	Secondary	Ca in situ	Benign	Uncertain Behavior	Unspecified
Neoplasm, neoplastic	199.1	199.1	234.9	229.9	238.9	239.9

Notes — 1. The list below gives the code numbers for neoplasms by anatomical site. For each site there are six possible code numbers according to whether the neoplasm in question is malignant, benign, in situ, of uncertain behavior, or of unspecified nature. The description of the neoplasm will often indicate which of the six columns is appropriate; e.g., malignant melanoma of skin, benign fibroadenoma of breast, carcinoma in situ of cervix uteri.

Where such descriptors are not present, the remainder of the Index should be consulted where guidance is given to the appropriate column for each morphological (histological) variety listed; e.g., Mesonephroma — see Neoplasm, malignant; Embryoma — see also Neoplasm, uncertain behavior; Disease, Bowen's — see Neoplasm, skin, in situ. However, the guidance in the Index can be overridden if one of the descriptors mentioned above is present; e.g., malignant adenoma of colon is coded to 153.9 and not to 211.3 as the adjective "malignant" overrides the Index entry "Adenoma — see also Neoplasm, benign."

2. Sites marked with the sign * (e.g., face NEC*) should be classified to malignant neoplasm of skin of these sites if the variety of neoplasm is a squamous cell carcinoma or an epidermoid carcinoma, and to benign neoplasm of skin of these sites if the variety of neoplasm is a papilloma (any type).

	Primary	Secondary	Ca in situ	Benign	Uncertain Behavior	Unspecified
abdomen, abdominal	195.2	198.89	234.8	229.8	238.8	239.8
cavity	195.2	198.89	234.8	229.8	238.8	239.8
organ	195.2	198.89	234.8	229.8	238.8	239.8
viscera	195.2	198.89	234.8	229.8	238.8	239.8
wall	173.5	198.2	232.5	216.5	238.2	239.2
connective tissue	171.5	198.89	—	215.5	238.1	239.2
abdominopelvic	195.8	198.89	234.8	229.8	238.8	239.8
accessory sinus — see Neoplasm, sinus						
acoustic nerve	192.0	198.4	—	225.1	237.9	239.7
acromion (process)	170.4	198.5	—	213.4	238.0	239.2
adenoid (pharynx) (tissue)	147.1	198.89	230.0	210.7	235.1	239.0
adipose tissue (see also Neoplasm, connective tissue)	171.9	198.89	—	215.9	238.1	239.2
adnexa (uterine)	183.9	198.82	233.3	221.8	236.3	239.5
adrenal (cortex) (gland) (medulla)	194.0	198.7	234.8	227.0	237.2	239.7
ala nasi (external)	173.3	198.2	232.3	216.3	238.2	239.2
alimentary canal or tract NEC	159.9	197.8	230.9	211.9	235.5	239.0
alveolar	143.9	198.89	230.0	210.4	235.1	239.0
mucosa	143.9	198.89	230.0	210.4	235.1	239.0
lower	143.1	198.89	230.0	210.4	235.1	239.0
upper	143.0	198.89	230.0	210.4	235.1	239.0
ridge or process	170.1	198.5	—	213.1	238.0	239.2
carcinoma	143.9	—	—	—	—	—
lower	143.1	—	—	—	—	—
upper	143.0	—	—	—	—	—
lower	170.1	198.5	—	213.1	238.0	239.2
mucosa	143.9	198.89	230.0	210.4	235.1	239.0
lower	143.1	198.89	230.0	210.4	235.1	239.0
upper	143.0	198.89	230.0	210.4	235.1	239.0
upper	170.0	198.5	—	213.0	238.0	239.2
sulcus	145.1	198.89	230.0	210.4	235.1	239.0
alveolus	143.9	198.89	230.0	210.4	235.1	239.0
lower	143.1	198.89	230.0	210.4	235.1	239.0
upper	143.0	198.89	230.0	210.4	235.1	239.0
ampulla of Vater	156.2	197.8	230.8	211.5	235.3	239.0
ankle NEC*	195.5	198.89	232.7	229.8	238.8	239.8
anorectum, anorectal (junction)	154.8	197.5	230.7	211.4	235.2	239.0
antecubital fossa or space*	195.4	198.89	232.6	229.8	238.8	239.8
antrum (Highmore) (maxillary)	160.2	197.3	231.8	212.0	235.9	239.1
pyloric	151.2	197.8	230.2	211.1	235.2	239.0
tympanicum	160.1	197.3	231.8	212.0	235.9	239.1
anus, anal	154.3	197.5	230.6	211.4	235.5	239.0
canal	154.2	197.5	230.5	211.4	235.5	239.0
contiguous sites with rectosigmoid junction or rectum	154.8	—	—	—	—	—
margin	173.5	198.2	232.5	216.5	238.2	239.2
skin	173.5	198.2	232.5	216.5	238.2	239.2
sphincter	154.2	197.5	230.5	211.4	235.5	239.0
aorta (thoracic)	171.4	198.89	—	215.4	238.1	239.2
abdominal	171.5	198.89	—	215.5	238.1	239.2

	Malignant					
Neoplasm, neoplastic — continued	Primary	Secondary	Ca in situ	Benign	Uncertain Behavior	Unspecified
aortic body	194.6	198.89	—	227.6	237.3	239.7
aponeurosis	171.9	198.89	—	215.9	238.1	239.2
palmar	171.2	198.89	—	215.2	238.1	239.2
plantar	171.3	198.89	—	215.3	238.1	239.2
appendix	153.5	197.5	230.3	211.3	235.2	239.0
arachnoid (cerebral)	192.1	198.4	—	225.2	237.6	239.7
spinal	192.3	198.4	—	225.4	237.6	239.7
areola (female)	174.0	198.81	233.0	217	238.3	239.3
male	175.0	198.81	233.0	217	238.3	239.3
arm NEC*	195.4	198.89	232.6	229.8	238.8	239.8
artery — see Neoplasm, connective tissue						
aryepiglottic fold	148.2	198.89	230.0	210.8	235.1	239.0
hypopharyngeal aspect	148.2	198.89	230.0	210.8	235.1	239.0
laryngeal aspect	161.1	197.3	231.0	212.1	235.6	239.1
marginal zone	148.2	198.89	230.0	210.8	235.1	239.0
arytenoid (cartilage)	161.3	197.3	231.0	212.1	235.6	239.1
fold — see Neoplasm, aryepiglottic						
atlas	170.2	198.5	—	213.2	238.0	239.2
atrium, cardiac	164.1	198.89	—	212.7	238.8	239.8
auditory						
canal (external) (skin)	173.2	198.2	232.2	216.2	238.2	239.2
internal	160.1	197.3	231.8	212.0	235.9	239.1
nerve	192.0	198.4	—	225.1	237.9	239.7
tube	160.1	197.3	231.8	212.0	235.9	239.1
opening	147.2	198.89	230.0	210.7	235.1	239.0
auricle, ear	173.2	198.2	232.2	216.2	238.2	239.2
cartilage	171.0	198.89	—	215.0	238.1	239.2
auricular canal (external)	173.2	198.2	232.2	216.2	238.2	239.2
internal	160.1	197.3	231.8	212.0	235.9	239.1
autonomic nerve or nervous system NEC	171.9	198.89	—	215.9	238.1	239.2
axilla, axillary	195.1	198.89	234.8	229.8	238.8	239.8
fold	173.5	198.2	232.5	216.5	238.2	239.2
back NEC*	195.8	198.89	232.5	229.8	238.8	239.8
Bartholin's gland	184.1	198.82	233.3	221.2	236.3	239.5
basal ganglia	191.0	198.3	—	225.0	237.5	239.6
basis pedunculi	191.7	198.3	—	225.0	237.5	239.6
bile or biliary (tract)	156.9	197.8	230.8	211.5	235.3	239.0
canaliculi (biliferi) (intrahepatic)	155.1	197.8	230.8	211.5	235.3	239.0
canals, interlobular	155.1	197.8	230.8	211.5	235.3	239.0
contiguous sites	156.8	—	—	—	—	—
duct or passage (common) (cystic) (extrahepatic)	156.1	197.8	230.8	211.5	235.3	239.0
contiguous sites with gallbladder	156.8	—	—	—	—	—
interlobular	155.1	197.8	230.8	211.5	235.3	239.0
intrahepatic	155.1	197.8	230.8	211.5	235.3	239.0
and extrahepatic	156.9	197.8	230.8	211.5	235.3	239.0
bladder (urinary)	188.9	198.1	233.7	223.3	236.7	239.4
contiguous sites	188.8	—	—	—	—	—
dome	188.1	198.1	233.7	223.3	236.7	239.4
neck	188.5	198.1	233.7	223.3	236.7	239.4
orifice	188.9	198.1	233.7	223.3	236.7	239.4
ureteric	188.6	198.1	233.7	223.3	236.7	239.4
urethral	188.5	198.1	233.7	223.3	236.7	239.4
sphincter	188.8	198.1	233.7	223.3	236.7	239.4
trigone	188.0	198.1	233.7	223.3	236.7	239.4
urachus	188.7	—	233.7	223.3	236.7	239.4
wall	188.9	198.1	233.7	223.3	236.7	239.4
anterior	188.3	198.1	233.7	223.3	236.7	239.4
lateral	188.2	198.1	233.7	223.3	236.7	239.4
posterior	188.4	198.1	233.7	223.3	236.7	239.4
blood vessel — see Neoplasm, connective tissue						
bone (periosteum)	170.9	198.5	—	213.9	238.0	239.2

Note — Carcinomas and adenocarcinomas, of any type other than intraosseous or odontogenic, of the sites listed under "Neoplasm, bone" should be considered as constituting metastatic spread from an unspecified primary site and coded to 198.5 for morbidity coding and to 199.1 for underlying cause of death coding.

	Primary	Secondary	Ca in situ	Benign	Uncertain Behavior	Unspecified
acetabulum	170.6	198.5	—	213.6	238.0	239.2
acromion (process)	170.4	198.5	—	213.4	238.0	239.2
ankle	170.8	198.5	—	213.8	238.0	239.2
arm NEC	170.4	198.5	—	213.4	238.0	239.2
astragalus	170.8	198.5	—	213.8	238.0	239.2

Neoplasm, abdomen, abdominal — Neoplasm, bone

Neoplasm, neoplastic — continued	Malignant Primary	Malignant Secondary	Ca in situ	Benign	Uncertain Behavior	Unspecified
bone — continued						
atlas	170.2	198.5	—	213.2	238.0	239.2
axis	170.2	198.5	—	213.2	238.0	239.2
back NEC	170.2	198.5	—	213.2	238.0	239.2
calcaneus	170.8	198.5	—	213.8	238.0	239.2
calvarium	170.0	198.5	—	213.0	238.0	239.2
carpus (any)	170.5	198.5	—	213.5	238.0	239.2
cartilage NEC	170.9	198.5	—	213.9	238.0	239.2
clavicle	170.3	198.5	—	213.3	238.0	239.2
clivus	170.0	198.5	—	213.0	238.0	239.2
coccygeal vertebra	170.6	198.5	—	213.6	238.0	239.2
coccyx	170.6	198.5	—	213.6	238.0	239.2
costal cartilage	170.3	198.5	—	213.3	238.0	239.2
costovertebral joint	170.3	198.5	—	213.3	238.0	239.2
cranial	170.0	198.5	—	213.0	238.0	239.2
cuboid	170.8	198.5	—	213.8	238.0	239.2
cuneiform	170.9	198.5	—	213.9	238.0	239.2
ankle	170.8	198.5	—	213.8	238.0	239.2
wrist	170.5	198.5	—	213.5	238.0	239.2
digital	170.9	198.5	—	213.9	238.0	239.2
finger	170.5	198.5	—	213.5	238.0	239.2
toe	170.8	198.5	—	213.8	238.0	239.2
elbow	170.4	198.5	—	213.4	238.0	239.2
ethmoid (labyrinth)	170.0	198.5	—	213.0	238.0	239.2
face	170.0	198.5	—	213.0	238.0	239.2
lower jaw	170.1	198.5	—	213.1	238.0	239.2
femur (any part)	170.7	198.5	—	213.7	238.0	239.2
fibula (any part)	170.7	198.5	—	213.7	238.0	239.2
finger (any)	170.5	198.5	—	213.5	238.0	239.2
foot	170.8	198.5	—	213.8	238.0	239.2
forearm	170.4	198.5	—	213.4	238.0	239.2
frontal	170.0	198.5	—	213.0	238.0	239.2
hand	170.5	198.5	—	213.5	238.0	239.2
heel	170.8	198.5	—	213.8	238.0	239.2
hip	170.6	198.5	—	213.6	238.0	239.2
humerus (any part)	170.4	198.5	—	213.4	238.0	239.2
hyoid	170.0	198.5	—	213.0	238.0	239.2
ilium	170.6	198.5	—	213.6	238.0	239.2
innominate	170.6	198.5	—	213.6	238.0	239.2
intervertebral cartilage or disc	170.2	198.5	—	213.2	238.0	239.2
ischium	170.6	198.5	—	213.6	238.0	239.2
jaw (lower)	170.1	198.5	—	213.1	238.0	239.2
upper	170.0	198.5	—	213.0	238.0	239.2
knee	170.7	198.5	—	213.7	238.0	239.2
leg NEC	170.7	198.5	—	213.7	238.0	239.2
limb NEC	170.9	198.5	—	213.9	238.0	239.2
lower (long bones)	170.7	198.5	—	213.7	238.0	239.2
short bones	170.8	198.5	—	213.8	238.0	239.2
upper (long bones)	170.4	198.5	—	213.4	238.0	239.2
short bones	170.5	198.5	—	213.5	238.0	239.2
long	170.9	198.5	—	213.9	238.0	239.2
lower limbs NEC	170.7	198.5	—	213.7	238.0	239.2
upper limbs NEC	170.4	198.5	—	213.4	238.0	239.2
malar	170.0	198.5	—	213.0	238.0	239.2
mandible	170.1	198.5	—	213.1	238.0	239.2
marrow NEC	202.9 ☑	198.5	—	—	—	238.7
mastoid	170.0	198.5	—	213.0	238.0	239.2
maxilla, maxillary (superior)	170.0	198.5	—	213.0	238.0	239.2
inferior	170.1	198.5	—	213.1	238.0	239.2
metacarpus (any)	170.5	198.5	—	213.5	238.0	239.2
metatarsus (any)	170.8	198.5	—	213.8	238.0	239.2
navicular (ankle)	170.8	198.5	—	213.8	238.0	239.2
hand	170.5	198.5	—	213.5	238.0	239.2
nose, nasal	170.0	198.5	—	213.0	238.0	239.2
occipital	170.0	198.5	—	213.0	238.0	239.2
orbit	170.0	198.5	—	213.0	238.0	239.2
parietal	170.0	198.5	—	213.0	238.0	239.2
patella	170.8	198.5	—	213.8	238.0	239.2
pelvic	170.6	198.5	—	213.6	238.0	239.2
phalanges	170.9	198.5	—	213.9	238.0	239.2
foot	170.8	198.5	—	213.8	238.0	239.2
hand	170.5	198.5	—	213.5	238.0	239.2
pubic	170.6	198.5	—	213.6	238.0	239.2
radius (any part)	170.4	198.5	—	213.4	238.0	239.2
rib	170.3	198.5	—	213.3	238.0	239.2
sacral vertebra	170.6	198.5	—	213.6	238.0	239.2
sacrum	170.6	198.5	—	213.6	238.0	239.2
scaphoid (of hand)	170.5	198.5	—	213.5	238.0	239.2
of ankle	170.8	198.5	—	213.8	238.0	239.2
scapula (any part)	170.4	198.5	—	213.4	238.0	239.2
sella turcica	170.0	198.5	—	213.0	238.0	239.2
short	170.9	198.5	—	213.9	238.0	239.2
lower limb	170.8	198.5	—	213.8	238.0	239.2
upper limb	170.5	198.5	—	213.5	238.0	239.2
shoulder	170.4	198.5	—	213.4	238.0	239.2
skeleton, skeletal NEC	170.9	198.5	—	213.9	238.0	239.2
skull	170.0	198.5	—	213.0	238.0	239.2
sphenoid	170.0	198.5	—	213.0	238.0	239.2
spine, spinal (column)	170.2	198.5	—	213.2	238.0	239.2
coccyx	170.6	198.5	—	213.6	238.0	239.2
sacrum	170.6	198.5	—	213.6	238.0	239.2
sternum	170.3	198.5	—	213.3	238.0	239.2
tarsus (any)	170.8	198.5	—	213.8	238.0	239.2
temporal	170.0	198.5	—	213.0	238.0	239.2
thumb	170.5	198.5	—	213.5	238.0	239.2
tibia (any part)	170.7	198.5	—	213.7	238.0	239.2
toe (any)	170.8	198.5	—	213.8	238.0	239.2
trapezium	170.5	198.5	—	213.5	238.0	239.2
trapezoid	170.5	198.5	—	213.5	238.0	239.2
turbinate	170.0	198.5	—	213.0	238.0	239.2
ulna (any part)	170.4	198.5	—	213.4	238.0	239.2
unciform	170.5	198.5	—	213.5	238.0	239.2
vertebra (column)	170.2	198.5	—	213.2	238.0	239.2
coccyx	170.6	198.5	—	213.6	238.0	239.2
sacrum	170.6	198.5	—	213.6	238.0	239.2
vomer	170.0	198.5	—	213.0	238.0	239.2
wrist	170.5	198.5	—	213.5	238.0	239.2
xiphoid process	170.3	198.5	—	213.3	238.0	239.2
zygomatic	170.0	198.5	—	213.0	238.0	239.2
book-leaf (mouth)	145.8	198.89	230.0	210.4	235.1	239.0
bowel — see Neoplasm, intestine						
brachial plexus	171.2	198.89	—	215.2	238.1	239.2
brain NEC	191.9	198.3	—	225.0	237.5	239.6
basal ganglia	191.0	198.3	—	225.0	237.5	239.6
cerebellopontine angle	191.6	198.3	—	225.0	237.5	239.6
cerebellum NOS	191.6	198.3	—	225.0	237.5	239.6
cerebrum	191.0	198.3	—	225.0	237.5	239.6
choroid plexus	191.5	198.3	—	225.0	237.5	239.6
contiguous sites	191.8	—	—	—	—	—
corpus callosum	191.8	198.3	—	225.0	237.5	239.6
corpus striatum	191.0	198.3	—	225.0	237.5	239.6
cortex (cerebral)	191.0	198.3	—	225.0	237.5	239.6
frontal lobe	191.1	198.3	—	225.0	237.5	239.6
globus pallidus	191.0	198.3	—	225.0	237.5	239.6
hippocampus	191.2	198.3	—	225.0	237.5	239.6
hypothalamus	191.0	198.3	—	225.0	237.5	239.6
internal capsule	191.0	198.3	—	225.0	237.5	239.6
medulla oblongata	191.7	198.3	—	225.0	237.5	239.6
meninges	192.1	198.4	—	225.2	237.6	239.7
midbrain	191.7	198.3	—	225.0	237.5	239.6
occipital lobe	191.4	198.3	—	225.0	237.5	239.6
parietal lobe	191.3	198.3	—	225.0	237.5	239.6
peduncle	191.7	198.3	—	225.0	237.5	239.6
pons	191.7	198.3	—	225.0	237.5	239.6
stem	191.7	198.3	—	225.0	237.5	239.6
tapetum	191.8	198.3	—	225.0	237.5	239.6
temporal lobe	191.2	198.3	—	225.0	237.5	239.6
thalamus	191.0	198.3	—	225.0	237.5	239.6
uncus	191.2	198.3	—	225.0	237.5	239.6
ventricle (floor)	191.5	198.3	—	225.0	237.5	239.6
branchial (cleft) (vestiges)	146.8	198.89	230.0	210.6	235.1	239.0
breast (connective tissue) (female) (glandular tissue) (soft parts)	174.9	198.81	233.0	217	238.3	239.3
areola	174.0	198.81	233.0	217	238.3	239.3
male	175.0	198.81	233.0	217	238.3	239.3
axillary tail	174.6	198.81	233.0	217	238.3	239.3
central portion	174.1	198.81	233.0	217	238.3	239.3
contiguous sites	174.8	—	—	—	—	—
ectopic sites	174.8	198.81	233.0	217	238.3	239.3
inner	174.8	198.81	233.0	217	238.3	239.3
lower	174.8	198.81	233.0	217	238.3	239.3

☑ Additional Digit Required   ►◄ Revised Text   ● New Line   ▲ Revised Code

Neoplasm, neoplastic — continued	Malignant Primary	Malignant Secondary	Malignant Ca in situ	Benign	Uncertain Behavior	Unspecified
breast — continued						
lower-inner quadrant	174.3	198.81	233.0	217	238.3	239.3
lower-outer quadrant	174.5	198.81	233.0	217	238.3	239.3
male	175.9	198.81	233.0	217	238.3	239.3
areola	175.0	198.81	233.0	217	238.3	239.3
ectopic tissue	175.9	198.81	233.0	217	238.3	239.3
nipple	175.0	198.81	233.0	217	238.3	239.3
mastectomy site (skin)	173.5	198.2	—	—	—	—
specified as breast tissue	174.8	198.81	—	—	—	—
midline	174.8	198.81	233.0	217	238.3	239.3
nipple	174.0	198.81	233.0	217	238.3	239.3
male	175.0	198.81	233.0	217	238.3	239.3
outer	174.8	198.81	233.0	217	238.3	239.3
skin	173.5	198.2	232.5	216.5	238.2	239.2
tail (axillary)	174.6	198.81	233.0	217	238.3	239.3
upper	174.8	198.81	233.0	217	238.3	239.3
upper-inner quadrant	174.2	198.81	233.0	217	238.3	239.3
upper-outer quadrant	174.4	198.81	233.0	217	238.3	239.3
broad ligament	183.3	198.82	233.3	221.0	236.3	239.5
bronchiogenic, bronchogenic (lung)	162.9	197.0	231.2	212.3	235.7	239.1
bronchiole	162.9	197.0	231.2	212.3	235.7	239.1
bronchus	162.9	197.0	231.2	212.3	235.7	239.1
carina	162.2	197.0	231.2	212.3	235.7	239.1
contiguous sites with lung or trachea	162.8	—	—	—	—	—
lower lobe of lung	162.5	197.0	231.2	212.3	235.7	239.1
main	162.2	197.0	231.2	212.3	235.7	239.1
middle lobe of lung	162.4	197.0	231.2	212.3	235.7	239.1
upper lobe of lung	162.3	197.0	231.2	212.3	235.7	239.1
brow	173.3	198.2	232.3	216.3	238.2	239.2
buccal (cavity)	145.9	198.89	230.0	210.4	235.1	239.0
commissure	145.0	198.89	230.0	210.4	235.1	239.0
groove (lower) (upper)	145.1	198.89	230.0	210.4	235.1	239.0
mucosa	145.0	198.89	230.0	210.4	235.1	239.0
sulcus (lower) (upper)	145.1	198.89	230.0	210.4	235.1	239.0
bulbourethral gland	189.3	198.1	233.9	223.81	236.99	239.5
bursa — see Neoplasm, connective tissue						
buttock NEC*	195.3	198.89	232.5	229.8	238.8	239.8
calf*	195.5	198.89	232.7	229.8	238.8	239.8
calvarium	170.0	198.5	—	213.0	238.0	239.2
calyx, renal	189.1	198.0	233.9	223.1	236.91	239.5
canal						
anal	154.2	197.5	230.5	211.4	235.5	239.0
auditory (external)	173.2	198.2	232.2	216.2	238.2	239.2
auricular (external)	173.2	198.2	232.2	216.2	238.2	239.2
canaliculi, biliary (biliferi) (intrahepatic)	155.1	197.8	230.8	211.5	235.3	239.0
canthus (eye) (inner) (outer)	173.1	198.2	232.1	216.1	238.2	239.2
capillary — see Neoplasm, connective tissue						
caput coli	153.4	197.5	230.3	211.3	235.2	239.0
cardia (gastric)	151.0	197.8	230.2	211.1	235.2	239.0
cardiac orifice (stomach)	151.0	197.8	230.2	211.1	235.2	239.0
cardio-esophageal junction	151.0	197.8	230.2	211.1	235.2	239.0
cardio-esophagus	151.0	197.8	230.2	211.1	235.2	239.0
carina (trachea) (bronchus)	162.2	197.0	231.2	212.3	235.7	239.1
carotid (artery)	171.0	198.89	—	215.0	238.1	239.2
body	194.5	198.89	—	227.5	237.3	239.7
carpus (any bone)	170.5	198.5	—	213.5	238.0	239.2
cartilage (articular) (joint) NEC — see also Neoplasm, bone	170.9	198.5	—	213.9	238.0	239.2
arytenoid	161.3	197.3	231.0	212.1	235.6	239.1
auricular	171.0	198.89	—	215.0	238.1	239.2
bronchi	162.2	197.3	—	212.3	235.7	239.1
connective tissue — see Neoplasm, connective tissue						
costal	170.3	198.5	—	213.3	238.0	239.2
cricoid	161.3	197.3	231.0	212.1	235.6	239.1
cuneiform	161.3	197.3	231.0	212.1	235.6	239.1
ear (external)	171.0	198.89	—	215.0	238.1	239.2
ensiform	170.3	198.5	—	213.3	238.0	239.2
epiglottis	161.1	197.3	231.0	212.1	235.6	239.1
anterior surface	146.4	198.89	230.0	210.6	235.1	239.0
eyelid	171.0	198.89	—	215.0	238.1	239.2
intervertebral	170.2	198.5	—	213.2	238.0	239.2
larynx, laryngeal	161.3	197.3	231.0	212.1	235.6	239.1
nose, nasal	160.0	197.3	231.8	212.0	235.9	239.1
pinna	171.0	198.89	—	215.0	238.1	239.2
cartilage NEC — see also Neoplasm, bone — continued						
rib	170.3	198.5	—	213.3	238.0	239.2
semilunar (knee)	170.7	198.5	—	213.7	238.0	239.2
thyroid	161.3	197.3	231.0	212.1	235.6	239.1
trachea	162.0	197.3	231.1	212.2	235.7	239.1
cauda equina	192.2	198.3	—	225.3	237.5	239.7
cavity						
buccal	145.9	198.89	230.0	210.4	235.1	239.0
nasal	160.0	197.3	231.8	212.0	235.9	239.1
oral	145.9	198.89	230.0	210.4	235.1	239.0
peritoneal	158.9	197.6	—	211.8	235.4	239.0
tympanic	160.1	197.3	231.8	212.0	235.9	239.1
cecum	153.4	197.5	230.3	211.3	235.2	239.0
central						
nervous system — see Neoplasm, nervous system						
white matter	191.0	198.3	—	225.0	237.5	239.6
cerebellopontine (angle)	191.6	198.3	—	225.0	237.5	239.6
cerebellum, cerebellar	191.6	198.3	—	225.0	237.5	239.6
cerebrum, cerebral (cortex) (hemisphere) (white matter)	191.0	198.3	—	225.0	237.5	239.6
meninges	192.1	198.4	—	225.2	237.6	239.7
peduncle	191.7	198.3	—	225.0	237.5	239.6
ventricle (any)	191.5	198.3	—	225.0	237.5	239.6
cervical region	195.0	198.89	234.8	229.8	238.8	239.8
cervix (cervical) (uteri) (uterus)	180.9	198.82	233.1	219.0	236.0	239.5
canal	180.0	198.82	233.1	219.0	236.0	239.5
contiguous sites	180.8	—	—	—	—	—
endocervix (canal) (gland)	180.0	198.82	233.1	219.0	236.0	239.5
exocervix	180.1	198.82	233.1	219.0	236.0	239.5
external os	180.1	198.82	233.1	219.0	236.0	239.5
internal os	180.0	198.82	233.1	219.0	236.0	239.5
nabothian gland	180.0	198.82	233.1	219.0	236.0	239.5
squamocolumnar junction	180.8	198.82	233.1	219.0	236.0	239.5
stump	180.8	198.82	233.1	219.0	236.0	239.5
cheek	195.0	198.89	234.8	229.8	238.8	239.8
external	173.3	198.2	232.3	216.3	238.2	239.2
inner aspect	145.0	198.89	230.0	210.4	235.1	239.0
internal	145.0	198.89	230.0	210.4	235.1	239.0
mucosa	145.0	198.89	230.0	210.4	235.1	239.0
chest (wall) NEC	195.1	198.89	234.8	229.8	238.8	239.8
chiasma opticum	192.0	198.4	—	225.1	237.9	239.7
chin	173.3	198.2	232.3	216.3	238.2	239.2
choana	147.3	198.89	230.0	210.7	235.1	239.0
cholangiole	155.1	197.8	230.8	211.5	235.3	239.0
choledochal duct	156.1	197.8	230.8	211.5	235.3	239.0
choroid	190.6	198.4	234.0	224.6	238.8	239.8
plexus	191.5	198.3	—	225.0	237.5	239.6
ciliary body	190.0	198.4	234.0	224.0	238.8	239.8
clavicle	170.3	198.5	—	213.3	238.0	239.2
clitoris	184.3	198.82	233.3	221.2	236.3	239.5
clivus	170.0	198.5	—	213.0	238.0	239.2
cloacogenic zone	154.8	197.5	230.7	211.4	235.5	239.0
coccygeal						
body or glomus	194.6	198.89	—	227.6	237.3	239.7
vertebra	170.6	198.5	—	213.6	238.0	239.2
coccyx	170.6	198.5	—	213.6	238.0	239.2
colon — see also Neoplasm, intestine, large						
and rectum	154.0	197.5	230.4	211.4	235.2	239.0
column, spinal — see Neoplasm, spine						
columnella	173.3	198.2	232.3	216.3	238.2	239.2
commissure						
labial, lip	140.6	198.89	230.0	210.4	235.1	239.0
laryngeal	161.0	197.3	231.0	212.1	235.6	239.1
common (bile) duct	156.1	197.8	230.8	211.5	235.3	239.0
concha	173.2	198.2	232.2	216.2	238.2	239.2
nose	160.0	197.3	231.8	212.0	235.9	239.1
conjunctiva	190.3	198.4	234.0	224.3	238.8	239.8

☑ Additional Digit Required ▶◀ Revised Text ● New Line ▲ Revised Code

Neoplasm, neoplastic — continued	Malignant			Benign	Uncertain Behavior	Unspecified
	Primary	Secondary	Ca in situ			
connective tissue NEC	171.9	198.89	—	215.9	238.1	239.2

Note — For neoplasms of connective tissue (blood vessel, bursa, fascia, ligament, muscle, peripheral nerves, sympathetic and parasympathetic nerves and ganglia, synovia, tendon, etc.) or of morphological types that indicate connective tissue, code according to the list under "Neoplasm, connective tissue"; for sites that do not appear in this list, code to neoplasm of that site; e.g.,

> liposarcoma, shoulder 171.2
> leiomyosarcoma, stomach 151.9
> neurofibroma, chest wall 215.4

Morphological types that indicate connective tissue appear in the proper place in the alphabetic index with the instruction "see Neoplasm, connective tissue..."

Neoplasm, neoplastic — continued	Malignant			Benign	Uncertain Behavior	Unspecified
	Primary	Secondary	Ca in situ			
abdomen	171.5	198.89	—	215.5	238.1	239.2
abdominal wall	171.5	198.89	—	215.5	238.1	239.2
ankle	171.3	198.89	—	215.3	238.1	239.2
antecubital fossa or space	171.2	198.89	—	215.2	238.1	239.2
arm	171.2	198.89	—	215.2	238.1	239.2
auricle (ear)	171.0	198.89	—	215.0	238.1	239.2
axilla	171.4	198.89	—	215.4	238.1	239.2
back	171.7	198.89	—	215.7	238.1	239.2
breast (female) (*see also* Neoplasm, breast)	174.9	198.81	233.0	217	238.3	239.3
male	175.9	198.81	233.0	217	238.3	239.3
buttock	171.6	198.89	—	215.6	238.1	239.2
calf	171.3	198.89	—	215.3	238.1	239.2
cervical region	171.0	198.89	—	215.0	238.1	239.2
cheek	171.0	198.89	—	215.0	238.1	239.2
chest (wall)	171.4	198.89	—	215.4	238.1	239.2
chin	171.0	198.89	—	215.0	238.1	239.2
contiguous sites	171.8	—	—	—	—	—
diaphragm	171.4	198.89	—	215.4	238.1	239.2
ear (external)	171.0	198.89	—	215.0	238.1	239.2
elbow	171.2	198.89	—	215.2	238.1	239.2
extrarectal	171.6	198.89	—	215.6	238.1	239.2
extremity	171.8	198.89	—	215.8	238.1	239.2
lower	171.3	198.89	—	215.3	238.1	239.2
upper	171.2	198.89	—	215.2	238.1	239.2
eyelid	171.0	198.89	—	215.0	238.1	239.2
face	171.0	198.89	—	215.0	238.1	239.2
finger	171.2	198.89	—	215.2	238.1	239.2
flank	171.7	198.89	—	215.7	238.1	239.2
foot	171.3	198.89	—	215.3	238.1	239.2
forearm	171.2	198.89	—	215.2	238.1	239.2
forehead	171.0	198.89	—	215.0	238.1	239.2
gastric ●	171.5	198.89	—	215.5	238.1	—
gastrointestinal ●	171.5	198.89	—	215.5	238.1	—
gluteal region	171.6	198.89	—	215.6	238.1	239.2
great vessels NEC	171.4	198.89	—	215.4	238.1	239.2
groin	171.6	198.89	—	215.6	238.1	239.2
hand	171.2	198.89	—	215.2	238.1	239.2
head	171.0	198.89	—	215.0	238.1	239.2
heel	171.3	198.89	—	215.3	238.1	239.2
hip	171.3	198.89	—	215.3	238.1	239.2
hypochondrium	171.5	198.89	—	215.5	238.1	239.2
iliopsoas muscle	171.6	198.89	—	215.6	238.1	239.2
infraclavicular region	171.4	198.89	—	215.4	238.1	239.2
inguinal (canal) (region)	171.6	198.89	—	215.6	238.1	239.2
intrathoracic	171.4	198.89	—	215.4	238.1	239.2
intestine ●	171.5	198.89	—	215.5	238.1	—
ischorectal fossa	171.6	198.89	—	215.6	238.1	239.2
jaw	143.9	198.89	230.0	210.4	235.1	239.0
knee	171.3	198.89	—	215.3	238.1	239.2
leg	171.3	198.89	—	215.3	238.1	239.2
limb NEC	171.9	198.89	—	215.8	238.1	239.2
lower	171.3	198.89	—	215.3	238.1	239.2
upper	171.2	198.89	—	215.2	238.1	239.2
nates	171.6	198.89	—	215.6	238.1	239.2
neck	171.0	198.89	—	215.0	238.1	239.2
orbit	190.1	198.4	234.0	224.1	238.8	239.8
pararectal	171.6	198.89	—	215.6	238.1	239.2
para-urethral	171.6	198.89	—	215.6	238.1	239.2
paravaginal	171.6	198.89	—	215.6	238.1	239.2
connective tissue NEC — continued						
pelvis (floor)	171.6	198.89	—	215.6	238.1	239.2
pelvo-abdominal	171.8	198.89	—	215.8	238.1	239.2
perineum	171.6	198.89	—	215.6	238.1	239.2
perirectal (tissue)	171.6	198.89	—	215.6	238.1	239.2
periurethral (tissue)	171.6	198.89	—	215.6	238.1	239.2
popliteal fossa or space	171.3	198.89	—	215.3	238.1	239.2
presacral	171.6	198.89	—	215.6	238.1	239.2
psoas muscle	171.5	198.89	—	215.5	238.1	239.2
pterygoid fossa	171.0	198.89	—	215.0	238.1	239.2
rectovaginal septum or wall	171.6	198.89	—	215.6	238.1	239.2
rectovesical	171.6	198.89	—	215.6	238.1	239.2
retroperitoneum	158.0	197.6	—	211.8	235.4	239.0
sacrococcygeal region	171.6	198.89	—	215.6	238.1	239.2
scalp	171.0	198.89	—	215.0	238.1	239.2
scapular region	171.4	198.89	—	215.4	238.1	239.2
shoulder	171.2	198.89	—	215.2	238.1	239.2
skin (dermis) NEC	173.9	198.2	232.9	216.9	238.2	239.2
stomach ●	171.5	198.89	—	215.5	238.1	—
submental	171.0	198.89	—	215.0	238.1	239.2
supraclavicular region	171.0	198.89	—	215.0	238.1	239.2
temple	171.0	198.89	—	215.0	238.1	239.2
temporal region	171.0	198.89	—	215.0	238.1	239.2
thigh	171.3	198.89	—	215.3	238.1	239.2
thoracic (duct) (wall)	171.4	198.89	—	215.4	238.1	239.2
thorax	171.4	198.89	—	215.4	238.1	239.2
thumb	171.2	198.89	—	215.2	238.1	239.2
toe	171.3	198.89	—	215.3	238.1	239.2
trunk	171.7	198.89	—	215.7	238.1	239.2
umbilicus	171.5	198.89	—	215.5	238.1	239.2
vesicorectal	171.6	198.89	—	215.6	238.1	239.2
wrist	171.2	198.89	—	215.2	238.1	239.2
conus medullaris	192.2	198.3	—	225.3	237.5	239.7
cord (true) (vocal)	161.0	197.3	231.0	212.1	235.6	239.1
false	161.1	197.3	231.0	212.1	235.6	239.1
spermatic	187.6	198.82	233.6	222.8	236.6	239.5
spinal (cervical) (lumbar) (thoracic)	192.2	198.3	—	225.3	237.5	239.7
cornea (limbus)	190.4	198.4	234.0	224.4	238.8	239.8
corpus						
albicans	183.0	198.6	233.3	220	236.2	239.5
callosum, brain	191.8	198.3	—	225.0	237.5	239.6
cavernosum	187.3	198.82	233.5	222.1	236.6	239.5
gastric	151.4	197.8	230.2	211.1	235.2	239.0
penis	187.3	198.82	233.5	222.1	236.6	239.5
striatum, cerebrum	191.0	198.3	—	225.0	237.5	239.6
uteri	182.0	198.82	233.2	219.1	236.0	239.5
isthmus	182.1	198.82	233.2	219.1	236.0	239.5
cortex						
adrenal	194.0	198.7	234.8	227.0	237.2	239.7
cerebral	191.0	198.3	—	225.0	237.5	239.6
costal cartilage	170.3	198.5	—	213.3	238.0	239.2
costovertebral joint	170.3	198.5	—	213.3	238.0	239.2
Cowper's gland	189.3	198.1	233.9	223.81	236.99	239.5
cranial (fossa, any)	191.9	198.3	—	225.0	237.5	239.6
meninges	192.1	198.4	—	225.2	237.6	239.7
nerve (any)	192.0	198.4	—	225.1	237.9	239.7
craniobuccal pouch	194.3	198.89	234.8	227.3	237.0	239.7
craniopharyngeal (duct) (pouch)	194.3	198.89	234.8	227.3	237.0	239.7
cricoid	148.0	198.89	230.0	210.8	235.1	239.0
cartilage	161.3	197.3	231.0	212.1	235.6	239.1
cricopharynx	148.0	198.89	230.0	210.8	235.1	239.0
crypt of Morgagni	154.8	197.5	230.7	211.4	235.2	239.0
crystalline lens	190.0	198.4	234.0	224.0	238.8	239.8
cul-de-sac (Douglas')	158.8	197.6	—	211.8	235.4	239.0
cuneiform cartilage	161.3	197.3	231.0	212.1	235.6	239.1
cutaneous — *see* Neoplasm, skin						
cutis — *see* Neoplasm, skin						
cystic (bile) duct (common)	156.1	197.8	230.8	211.5	235.3	239.0
dermis — *see* Neoplasm, skin						
diaphragm	171.4	198.89	—	215.4	238.1	239.2
digestive organs, system, tube, or tract NEC	159.9	197.8	230.9	211.9	235.5	239.0
contiguous sites with peritoneum	159.8	—	—	—	—	—
disc, intervertebral	170.2	198.5	—	213.2	238.0	239.2
disease, generalized	199.0	199.0	234.9	229.9	238.9	199.0
disseminated	199.0	199.0	234.9	229.9	238.9	199.0

☑ Additional Digit Required   ▶◀ Revised Text   ● New Line   ▲ Revised Code

Neoplasm, neoplastic — continued	Malignant Primary	Malignant Secondary	Malignant Ca in situ	Benign	Uncertain Behavior	Unspecified
Douglas' cul-de-sac or pouch	158.8	197.6	—	211.8	235.4	239.0
duodenojejunal junction	152.8	197.4	230.7	211.2	235.2	239.0
duodenum	152.0	197.4	230.7	211.2	235.2	239.0
dura (cranial) (mater)	192.1	198.4	—	225.2	237.6	239.7
cerebral	192.1	198.4	—	225.2	237.6	239.7
spinal	192.3	198.4	—	225.4	237.6	239.7
ear (external)	173.2	198.2	232.2	216.2	238.2	239.2
auricle or auris	173.2	198.2	232.2	216.2	238.2	239.2
canal, external	173.2	198.2	232.2	216.2	238.2	239.2
cartilage	171.0	198.89	—	215.0	238.1	239.2
external meatus	173.2	198.2	232.2	216.2	238.2	239.2
inner	160.1	197.3	231.8	212.0	235.9	239.8
lobule	173.2	198.2	232.2	216.2	238.2	239.2
middle	160.1	197.3	231.8	212.0	235.9	239.8
contiguous sites with accessory sinuses or nasal cavities	160.8	—	—	—	—	—
skin	173.2	198.2	232.2	216.2	238.2	239.2
earlobe	173.2	198.2	232.2	216.2	238.2	239.2
ejaculatory duct	187.8	198.82	233.6	222.8	236.6	239.5
elbow NEC*	195.4	198.89	232.6	229.8	238.8	239.8
endocardium	164.1	198.89	—	212.7	238.8	239.8
endocervix (canal) (gland)	180.0	198.82	233.1	219.0	236.0	239.5
endocrine gland NEC	194.9	198.89	—	227.9	237.4	239.7
pluriglandular NEC	194.8	198.89	234.8	227.8	237.4	239.7
endometrium (gland) (stroma)	182.0	198.82	233.2	219.1	236.0	239.5
ensiform cartilage	170.3	198.5	—	213.3	238.0	239.2
enteric — see Neoplasm, intestine						
ependyma (brain)	191.5	198.3	—	225.0	237.5	239.6
epicardium	164.1	198.89	—	212.7	238.8	239.8
epididymis	187.5	198.82	233.6	222.3	236.6	239.5
epidural	192.9	198.4	—	225.9	237.9	239.7
epiglottis	161.1	197.3	231.0	212.1	235.6	239.1
anterior aspect or surface	146.4	198.89	230.0	210.6	235.1	239.0
cartilage	161.3	197.3	231.0	212.1	235.6	239.1
free border (margin)	146.4	198.89	230.0	210.6	235.1	239.0
junctional region	146.5	198.89	230.0	210.6	235.1	239.0
posterior (laryngeal) surface	161.1	197.3	231.0	212.1	235.6	239.1
suprahyoid portion	161.1	197.3	231.0	212.1	235.6	239.1
esophagogastric junction	151.0	197.8	230.2	211.1	235.2	239.0
esophagus	150.9	197.8	230.1	211.0	235.5	239.0
abdominal	150.2	197.8	230.1	211.0	235.5	239.0
cervical	150.0	197.8	230.1	211.0	235.5	239.0
contiguous sites	150.8	—	—	—	—	—
distal (third)	150.5	197.8	230.1	211.0	235.5	239.0
lower (third)	150.5	197.8	230.1	211.0	235.5	239.0
middle (third)	150.4	197.8	230.1	211.0	235.5	239.0
proximal (third)	150.3	197.8	230.1	211.0	235.5	239.0
specified part NEC	150.8	197.8	230.1	211.0	235.5	239.0
thoracic	150.1	197.8	230.1	211.0	235.5	239.0
upper (third)	150.3	197.8	230.1	211.0	235.5	239.0
ethmoid (sinus)	160.3	197.3	231.8	212.0	235.9	239.1
bone or labyrinth	170.0	198.5	—	213.0	238.0	239.2
Eustachian tube	160.1	197.3	231.8	212.0	235.9	239.1
exocervix	180.1	198.82	233.1	219.0	236.0	239.5
external						
meatus (ear)	173.2	198.2	232.2	216.2	238.2	239.2
os, cervix uteri	180.1	198.82	233.1	219.0	236.0	239.5
extradural	192.9	198.4	—	225.9	237.9	239.7
extrahepatic (bile) duct	156.1	197.8	230.8	211.5	235.3	239.0
contiguous sites with gallbladder	156.8	—	—	—	—	—
extraocular muscle	190.1	198.4	234.0	224.1	238.8	239.8
extrarectal	195.3	198.89	234.8	229.8	238.8	239.8
extremity*	195.8	198.89	232.8	229.8	238.8	239.8
lower*	195.5	198.89	232.7	229.8	238.8	239.8
upper*	195.4	198.89	232.6	229.8	238.8	239.8
eye NEC	190.9	198.4	234.0	224.9	238.8	239.8
contiguous sites	190.8	—	—	—	—	—
specified sites NEC	190.8	198.4	234.0	224.8	238.8	239.8
eyeball	190.0	198.4	234.0	224.0	238.8	239.8
eyebrow	173.3	198.2	232.3	216.3	238.2	239.2
eyelid (lower) (skin) (upper)	173.1	198.2	232.1	216.1	238.2	239.2
cartilage	171.0	198.89	—	215.0	238.1	239.2
face NEC*	195.0	198.89	232.3	229.8	238.8	239.8
fallopian tube (accessory)	183.2	198.82	233.3	221.0	236.3	239.5
falx (cerebelli) (cerebri)	192.1	198.4	—	225.2	237.6	239.7

Neoplasm, neoplastic — continued	Malignant Primary	Malignant Secondary	Malignant Ca in situ	Benign	Uncertain Behavior	Unspecified
fascia — see also Neoplasm, connective tissue						
palmar	171.2	198.89	—	215.2	238.1	239.2
plantar	171.3	198.89	—	215.3	238.1	239.2
fatty tissue — see Neoplasm, connective tissue						
fauces, faucial NEC	146.9	198.89	230.0	210.6	235.1	239.0
pillars	146.2	198.89	230.0	210.6	235.1	239.0
tonsil	146.0	198.89	230.0	210.5	235.1	239.0
femur (any part)	170.7	198.5	—	213.7	238.0	239.2
fetal membrane	181	198.82	233.2	219.8	236.1	239.5
fibrous tissue — see Neoplasm, connective tissue						
fibula (any part)	170.7	198.5	—	213.7	238.0	239.2
filum terminale	192.2	198.3	—	225.3	237.5	239.7
finger NEC*	195.4	198.89	232.6	229.8	238.8	239.8
flank NEC*	195.8	198.89	232.5	229.8	238.8	239.8
follicle, nabothian	180.0	198.82	233.1	219.0	236.0	239.5
foot NEC*	195.5	198.89	232.7	229.8	238.8	239.8
forearm NEC*	195.4	198.89	232.6	229.8	238.8	239.8
forehead (skin)	173.3	198.2	232.3	216.3	238.2	239.2
foreskin	187.1	198.82	233.5	222.1	236.6	239.5
fornix						
pharyngeal	147.3	198.89	230.0	210.7	235.1	239.0
vagina	184.0	198.82	233.3	221.1	236.3	239.5
fossa (of)						
anterior (cranial)	191.9	198.3	—	225.0	237.5	239.6
cranial	191.9	198.3	—	225.0	237.5	239.6
ischiorectal	195.3	198.89	234.8	229.8	238.8	239.8
middle (cranial)	191.9	198.3	—	225.0	237.5	239.6
pituitary	194.3	198.89	234.8	227.3	237.0	239.7
posterior (cranial)	191.9	198.3	—	225.0	237.5	239.6
pterygoid	171.0	198.89	—	215.0	238.1	239.2
pyriform	148.1	198.89	230.0	210.8	235.1	239.0
Rosenmüller	147.2	198.89	230.0	210.7	235.1	239.0
tonsillar	146.1	198.89	230.0	210.6	235.1	239.0
fourchette	184.4	198.82	233.3	221.2	236.3	239.5
frenulum						
labii — see Neoplasm, lip, internal						
linguae	141.3	198.89	230.0	210.1	235.1	239.0
frontal						
bone	170.0	198.5	—	213.0	238.0	239.2
lobe, brain	191.1	198.3	—	225.0	237.5	239.6
meninges	192.1	198.4	—	225.2	237.6	239.7
pole	191.1	198.3	—	225.0	237.5	239.6
sinus	160.4	197.3	231.8	212.0	235.9	239.1
fundus						
stomach	151.3	197.8	230.2	211.1	235.2	239.0
uterus	182.0	198.82	233.2	219.1	236.0	239.5
gall duct (extrahepatic)	156.1	197.8	230.8	211.5	235.3	239.0
intrahepatic	155.1	197.8	230.8	211.5	235.3	239.0
gallbladder	156.0	197.8	230.8	211.5	235.3	239.0
contiguous sites with extrahepatic bile ducts	156.8	—	—	—	—	—
ganglia (see also Neoplasm, connective tissue)	171.9	198.89	—	215.9	238.1	239.2
basal	191.0	198.3	—	225.0	237.5	239.6
ganglion (see also Neoplasm, connective tissue)	171.9	198.89	—	215.9	238.1	239.2
cranial nerve	192.0	198.4	—	225.1	237.9	239.7
Gartner's duct	184.0	198.82	233.3	221.1	236.3	239.5
gastric — see Neoplasm, stomach						
gastrocolic	159.8	197.8	230.9	211.9	235.5	239.0
gastroesophageal junction	151.0	197.8	230.2	211.1	235.2	239.0
gastrointestinal (tract) NEC	159.9	197.8	230.9	211.9	235.5	239.0
generalized	199.0	199.0	234.9	229.9	238.9	199.0
genital organ or tract						
female NEC	184.9	198.82	233.3	221.9	236.3	239.5
contiguous sites	184.8	—	—	—	—	—
specified site NEC	184.8	198.82	233.3	221.8	236.3	239.5
male NEC	187.9	198.82	233.6	222.9	236.6	239.5
contiguous sites	187.8	—	—	—	—	—
specified site NEC	187.8	198.82	233.6	222.8	236.6	239.5
genitourinary tract						
female	184.9	198.82	233.3	221.9	236.3	239.5
male	187.9	198.82	233.6	222.9	236.6	239.5

Neoplasm, Douglas' cul-de-sac or pouch — Neoplasm, genitourinary tract

Neoplasm, gingiva — Neoplasm, kidney

Neoplasm, neoplastic — continued	Malignant Primary	Secondary	Ca in situ	Benign	Uncertain Behavior	Unspecified
gingiva (alveolar) (marginal)	143.9	198.89	230.0	210.4	235.1	239.0
lower	143.1	198.89	230.0	210.4	235.1	239.0
mandibular	143.1	198.89	230.0	210.4	235.1	239.0
maxillary	143.0	198.89	230.0	210.4	235.1	239.0
upper	143.0	198.89	230.0	210.4	235.1	239.0
gland, glandular (lymphatic) (system) — see also Neoplasm, lymph gland						
endocrine NEC	194.9	198.89	—	227.9	237.4	239.7
salivary — see Neoplasm, salivary, gland						
glans penis	187.2	198.82	233.5	222.1	236.6	239.5
globus pallidus	191.0	198.3	—	225.0	237.5	239.6
glomus						
coccygeal	194.6	198.89	—	227.6	237.3	239.7
jugularis	194.6	198.89	—	227.6	237.3	239.7
glosso-epiglottic fold(s)	146.4	198.89	230.0	210.6	235.1	239.0
glossopalatine fold	146.2	198.89	230.0	210.6	235.1	239.0
glossopharyngeal sulcus	146.1	198.89	230.0	210.6	235.1	239.0
glottis	161.0	197.3	231.0	212.1	235.6	239.1
gluteal region*	195.3	198.89	232.5	229.8	238.8	239.8
great vessels NEC	171.4	198.89	—	215.4	238.1	239.2
groin NEC*	195.3	198.89	232.5	229.8	238.8	239.8
gum	143.9	198.89	230.0	210.4	235.1	239.0
contiguous sites	143.8	—	—	—	—	—
lower	143.1	198.89	230.0	210.4	235.1	239.0
upper	143.0	198.89	230.0	210.4	235.1	239.0
hand NEC*	195.4	198.89	232.6	229.8	238.8	239.8
head NEC*	195.0	198.89	232.4	229.8	238.8	239.8
heart	164.1	198.89	—	212.7	238.8	239.8
contiguous sites with mediastinum or thymus	164.8	—	—	—	—	—
heel NEC*	195.5	198.89	232.7	229.8	238.8	239.8
helix	173.2	198.2	232.2	216.2	238.2	239.2
hematopoietic, hemopoietic tissue NEC	202.8 ☑	198.89	—	—	—	238.7
hemisphere, cerebral	191.0	198.3	—	225.0	237.5	239.6
hemorrhoidal zone	154.2	197.5	230.5	211.4	235.5	239.0
hepatic	155.2	197.7	230.8	211.5	235.3	239.0
duct (bile)	156.1	197.8	230.8	211.5	235.3	239.0
flexure (colon)	153.0	197.5	230.3	211.3	235.2	239.0
primary	155.0	—	—	—	—	—
hilus of lung	162.2	197.0	231.2	212.3	235.7	239.1
hip NEC*	195.5	198.89	232.7	229.8	238.8	239.8
hippocampus, brain	191.2	198.3	—	225.0	237.5	239.6
humerus (any part)	170.4	198.5	—	213.4	238.0	239.2
hymen	184.0	198.82	233.3	221.1	236.3	239.5
hypopharynx, hypopharyngeal NEC	148.9	198.89	230.0	210.8	235.1	239.0
contiguous sites	148.8	—	—	—	—	—
postcricoid region	148.0	198.89	230.0	210.8	235.1	239.0
posterior wall	148.3	198.89	230.0	210.8	235.1	239.0
pyriform fossa (sinus)	148.1	198.89	230.0	210.8	235.1	239.0
specified site NEC	148.8	198.89	230.0	210.8	235.1	239.0
wall	148.9	198.89	230.0	210.8	235.1	239.0
posterior	148.3	198.89	230.0	210.8	235.1	239.0
hypophysis	194.3	198.89	234.8	227.3	237.0	239.7
hypothalamus	191.0	198.3	—	225.0	237.5	239.6
ileocecum, ileocecal (coil) (junction) (valve)	153.4	197.5	230.3	211.3	235.2	239.0
ileum	152.2	197.4	230.7	211.2	235.2	239.0
ilium	170.6	198.5	—	213.6	238.0	239.2
immunoproliferative NEC	203.8 ☑	—	—	—	—	—
infraclavicular (region)*	195.1	198.89	232.5	229.8	238.8	239.8
inguinal (region)*	195.3	198.89	232.5	229.8	238.8	239.8
insula	191.0	198.3	—	225.0	237.5	239.6
insular tissue (pancreas)	157.4	197.8	230.9	211.7	235.5	239.0
brain	191.0	198.3	—	225.0	237.5	239.6
interarytenoid fold	148.2	198.89	230.0	210.8	235.1	239.0
hypopharyngeal aspect	148.2	198.89	230.0	210.8	235.1	239.0
laryngeal aspect	161.1	197.3	231.0	212.1	235.6	239.1
marginal zone	148.2	198.89	230.0	210.8	235.1	239.0
interdental papillae	143.9	198.89	230.0	210.4	235.1	239.0
lower	143.1	198.89	230.0	210.4	235.1	239.0
upper	143.0	198.89	230.0	210.4	235.1	239.0
internal						
capsule	191.0	198.3	—	225.0	237.5	239.6
os (cervix)	180.0	198.82	233.1	219.0	236.0	239.5
intervertebral cartilage or disc	170.2	198.5	—	213.2	238.0	239.2

Neoplasm, neoplastic — continued	Malignant Primary	Secondary	Ca in situ	Benign	Uncertain Behavior	Unspecified
intestine, intestinal	159.0	197.8	230.7	211.9	235.2	239.0
large	153.9	197.5	230.3	211.3	235.2	239.0
appendix	153.5	197.5	230.3	211.3	235.2	239.0
caput coli	153.4	197.5	230.3	211.3	235.2	239.0
cecum	153.4	197.5	230.3	211.3	235.2	239.0
colon	153.9	197.5	230.3	211.3	235.2	239.0
and rectum	154.0	197.5	230.4	211.4	235.2	239.0
ascending	153.6	197.5	230.3	211.3	235.2	239.0
caput	153.4	197.5	230.3	211.3	235.2	239.0
contiguous sites	153.8	—	—	—	—	—
descending	153.2	197.5	230.3	211.3	235.2	239.0
distal	153.2	197.5	230.3	211.3	235.2	239.0
left	153.2	197.5	230.3	211.3	235.2	239.0
pelvic	153.3	197.5	230.3	211.3	235.2	239.0
right	153.6	197.5	230.3	211.3	235.2	239.0
sigmoid (flexure)	153.3	197.5	230.3	211.3	235.2	239.0
transverse	153.1	197.5	230.3	211.3	235.2	239.0
contiguous sites	153.8	—	—	—	—	—
hepatic flexure	153.0	197.5	230.3	211.3	235.2	239.0
ileocecum, ileocecal (coil) (valve)	153.4	197.5	230.3	211.3	235.2	239.0
sigmoid flexure (lower) (upper)	153.3	197.5	230.3	211.3	235.2	239.0
splenic flexure	153.7	197.5	230.3	211.3	235.2	239.0
small	152.9	197.4	230.7	211.2	235.2	239.0
contiguous sites	152.8	—	—	—	—	—
duodenum	152.0	197.4	230.7	211.2	235.2	239.0
ileum	152.2	197.4	230.7	211.2	235.2	239.0
jejunum	152.1	197.4	230.7	211.2	235.2	239.0
tract NEC	159.0	197.8	230.7	211.9	235.2	239.0
intra-abdominal	195.2	198.89	234.8	229.8	238.8	239.8
intracranial NEC	191.9	198.3	—	225.0	237.5	239.6
intrahepatic (bile) duct	155.1	197.8	230.8	211.5	235.3	239.0
intraocular	190.0	198.4	234.0	224.0	238.8	239.8
intraorbital	190.1	198.4	234.0	224.1	238.8	239.8
intrasellar	194.3	198.89	234.8	227.3	237.0	239.7
intrathoracic (cavity) (organs NEC)	195.1	198.89	234.8	229.8	238.8	239.8
contiguous sites with respiratory organs	165.8	—	—	—	—	—
iris	190.0	198.4	234.0	224.0	238.8	239.8
ischiorectal (fossa)	195.3	198.89	234.8	229.8	238.8	239.8
ischium	170.6	198.5	—	213.6	238.0	239.2
island of Reil	191.0	198.3	—	225.0	237.5	239.6
islands or islets of Langerhans	157.4	197.8	230.9	211.7	235.5	239.0
isthmus uteri	182.1	198.82	233.2	219.1	236.0	239.5
jaw	195.0	198.89	234.8	229.8	238.8	239.8
bone	170.1	198.5	—	213.1	238.0	239.2
carcinoma	143.9	—	—	—	—	—
lower	143.1	—	—	—	—	—
upper	143.0	—	—	—	—	—
lower	170.1	198.5	—	213.1	238.0	239.2
upper	170.0	198.5	—	213.0	238.0	239.2
carcinoma (any type) (lower) (upper)	195.0	—	—	—	—	—
skin	173.3	198.2	232.3	216.3	238.2	239.2
soft tissues	143.9	198.89	230.0	210.4	235.1	239.0
lower	143.1	198.89	230.0	210.4	235.1	239.0
upper	143.0	198.89	230.0	210.4	235.1	239.0
jejunum	152.1	197.4	230.7	211.2	235.2	239.0
joint NEC (see also Neoplasm, bone)	170.9	198.5	—	213.9	238.0	239.2
acromioclavicular	170.4	198.5	—	213.4	238.0	239.2
bursa or synovial membrane — see Neoplasm, connective tissue						
costovertebral	170.3	198.5	—	213.3	238.0	239.2
sternocostal	170.3	198.5	—	213.3	238.0	239.2
temporomandibular	170.1	198.5	—	213.1	238.0	239.2
junction						
anorectal	154.8	197.5	230.7	211.4	235.5	239.0
cardioesophageal	151.0	197.8	230.2	211.1	235.2	239.0
esophagogastric	151.0	197.8	230.2	211.1	235.2	239.0
gastroesophageal	151.0	197.8	230.2	211.1	235.2	239.0
hard and soft palate	145.5	198.89	230.0	210.4	235.1	239.0
ileocecal	153.4	197.5	230.3	211.3	235.2	239.0
pelvirectal	154.0	197.5	230.4	211.4	235.2	239.0
pelviureteric	189.1	198.0	233.9	223.1	236.91	239.5
rectosigmoid	154.0	197.5	230.4	211.4	235.2	239.0
squamocolumnar, of cervix	180.8	198.82	233.1	219.0	236.0	239.5
kidney (parenchyma)	189.0	198.0	233.9	223.0	236.91	239.5
calyx	189.1	198.0	233.9	223.1	236.91	239.5

☑ Additional Digit Required   ◄ Revised Text   ● New Line   ▲ Revised Code

Neoplasm, neoplastic — continued	Malignant Primary	Malignant Secondary	Malignant Ca in situ	Benign	Uncertain Behavior	Unspecified
kidney — continued						
hilus	189.1	198.0	233.9	223.1	236.91	239.5
pelvis	189.1	198.0	233.9	223.1	236.91	239.5
knee NEC*	195.5	198.89	232.7	229.8	238.8	239.8
labia (skin)	184.4	198.82	233.3	221.2	236.3	239.5
majora	184.1	198.82	233.3	221.2	236.3	239.5
minora	184.2	198.82	233.3	221.2	236.3	239.5
labial — see also Neoplasm, lip						
sulcus (lower) (upper)	145.1	198.89	230.0	210.4	235.1	239.0
labium (skin)	184.4	198.82	233.3	221.2	236.3	239.5
majus	184.1	198.82	233.3	221.2	236.3	239.5
minus	184.2	198.82	233.3	221.2	236.3	239.5
lacrimal						
canaliculi	190.7	198.4	234.0	224.7	238.8	239.8
duct (nasal)	190.7	198.4	234.0	224.7	238.8	239.8
gland	190.2	198.4	234.0	224.2	238.8	239.8
punctum	190.7	198.4	234.0	224.7	238.8	239.8
sac	190.7	198.4	234.0	224.7	238.8	239.8
Langerhans, islands or islets	157.4	197.8	230.9	211.7	235.5	239.0
laryngopharynx	148.9	198.89	230.0	210.8	235.1	239.0
larynx, laryngeal NEC	161.9	197.3	231.0	212.1	235.6	239.1
aryepiglottic fold	161.1	197.3	231.0	212.1	235.6	239.1
cartilage (arytenoid) (cricoid) (cuneiform) (thyroid)	161.3	197.3	231.0	212.1	235.6	239.1
commissure (anterior) (posterior)	161.0	197.3	231.0	212.1	235.6	239.1
contiguous sites	161.8	—	—	—	—	—
extrinsic NEC	161.1	197.3	231.0	212.1	235.6	239.1
meaning hypopharynx	148.9	198.89	230.0	210.8	235.1	239.0
interarytenoid fold	161.1	197.3	231.0	212.1	235.6	239.1
intrinsic	161.0	197.3	231.0	212.1	235.6	239.1
ventricular band	161.1	197.3	231.0	212.1	235.6	239.1
leg NEC*	195.5	198.89	232.7	229.8	238.8	239.8
lens, crystalline	190.0	198.4	234.0	224.0	238.8	239.8
lid (lower) (upper)	173.1	198.2	232.1	216.1	238.2	239.2
ligament — see also Neoplasm, connective tissue						
broad	183.3	198.82	233.3	221.0	236.3	239.5
Mackenrodt's	183.8	198.82	233.3	221.8	236.3	239.5
non-uterine — see Neoplasm, connective tissue						
round	183.5	198.82	—	221.0	236.3	239.5
sacro-uterine	183.4	198.82	—	221.0	236.3	239.5
uterine	183.4	198.82	—	221.0	236.3	239.5
utero-ovarian	183.8	198.82	233.3	221.8	236.3	239.5
uterosacral	183.4	198.82	—	221.0	236.3	239.5
limb*	195.8	198.89	232.8	229.8	238.8	239.8
lower*	195.5	198.89	232.7	229.8	238.8	239.8
upper*	195.4	198.89	232.6	229.8	238.8	239.8
limbus of cornea	190.4	198.4	234.0	224.4	238.8	239.8
lingual NEC (see also Neoplasm, tongue)	141.9	198.89	230.0	210.1	235.1	239.0
lingula, lung	162.3	197.0	231.2	212.3	235.7	239.1
lip (external) (lipstick area) (vermillion border)	140.9	198.89	230.0	210.0	235.1	239.0
buccal aspect — see Neoplasm, lip, internal						
commissure	140.6	198.89	230.0	210.4	235.1	239.0
contiguous sites	140.8	—	—	—	—	—
with oral cavity or pharynx	149.8	—	—	—	—	—
frenulum — see Neoplasm, lip, internal						
inner aspect — see Neoplasm, lip, internal						
internal (buccal) (frenulum) (mucosa) (oral)	140.5	198.89	230.0	210.0	235.1	239.0
lower	140.4	198.89	230.0	210.0	235.1	239.0
upper	140.3	198.89	230.0	210.0	235.1	239.0
lower	140.1	198.89	230.0	210.0	235.1	239.0
internal (buccal) (frenulum) (mucosa) (oral)	140.4	198.89	230.0	210.0	235.1	239.0
mucosa — see Neoplasm, lip, internal						
oral aspect — see Neoplasm, lip, internal						
skin (commissure) (lower) (upper)	173.0	198.2	232.0	216.0	238.2	239.2
upper	140.0	198.89	230.0	210.0	235.1	239.0
internal (buccal) (frenulum) (mucosa) (oral)	140.3	198.89	230.0	210.0	235.1	239.0

Neoplasm, neoplastic — continued	Malignant Primary	Malignant Secondary	Malignant Ca in situ	Benign	Uncertain Behavior	Unspecified
liver	155.2	197.7	230.8	211.5	235.3	239.0
primary	155.0	—	—	—	—	—
lobe						
azygos	162.3	197.0	231.2	212.3	235.7	239.1
frontal	191.1	198.3	—	225.0	237.5	239.6
lower	162.5	197.0	231.2	212.3	235.7	239.1
middle	162.4	197.0	231.2	212.3	235.7	239.1
occipital	191.4	198.3	—	225.0	237.5	239.6
parietal	191.3	198.3	—	225.0	237.5	239.6
temporal	191.2	198.3	—	225.0	237.5	239.6
upper	162.3	197.0	231.2	212.3	235.7	239.1
lumbosacral plexus	171.6	198.4	—	215.6	238.1	239.2
lung	162.9	197.0	231.2	212.3	235.7	239.1
azgos lobe	162.3	197.0	231.2	212.3	235.7	239.1
carina	162.2	197.0	231.2	212.3	235.7	239.1
contiguous sites with bronchus or trachea	162.8	—	—	—	—	—
hilus	162.2	197.0	231.2	212.3	235.7	239.1
lingula	162.3	197.0	231.2	212.3	235.7	239.1
lobe NEC	162.9	197.0	231.2	212.3	235.7	239.1
lower lobe	162.5	197.0	231.2	212.3	235.7	239.1
main bronchus	162.2	197.0	231.2	212.3	235.7	239.1
middle lobe	162.4	197.0	231.2	212.3	235.7	239.1
upper lobe	162.3	197.0	231.2	212.3	235.7	239.1
lymph, lymphatic						
channel NEC (see also Neoplasm, connective tissue)	171.9	198.89	—	215.9	238.1	239.2
gland (secondary)	—	196.9	—	229.0	238.8	239.8
abdominal	—	196.2	—	229.0	238.8	239.8
aortic	—	196.2	—	229.0	238.8	239.8
arm	—	196.3	—	229.0	238.8	239.8
auricular (anterior) (posterior)	—	196.0	—	229.0	238.8	239.8
axilla, axillary	—	196.3	—	229.0	238.8	239.8
brachial	—	196.3	—	229.0	238.8	239.8
bronchial	—	196.1	—	229.0	238.8	239.8
bronchopulmonary	—	196.1	—	229.0	238.8	239.8
celiac	—	196.2	—	229.0	238.8	239.8
cervical	—	196.0	—	229.0	238.8	239.8
cervicofacial	—	196.0	—	229.0	238.8	239.8
Cloquet	—	196.5	—	229.0	238.8	239.8
colic	—	196.2	—	229.0	238.8	239.8
common duct	—	196.2	—	229.0	238.8	239.8
cubital	—	196.3	—	229.0	238.8	239.8
diaphragmatic	—	196.1	—	229.0	238.8	239.8
epigastric, inferior	—	196.6	—	229.0	238.8	239.8
epitrochlear	—	196.3	—	229.0	238.8	239.8
esophageal	—	196.1	—	229.0	238.8	239.8
face	—	196.0	—	229.0	238.8	239.8
femoral	—	196.5	—	229.0	238.8	239.8
gastric	—	196.2	—	229.0	238.8	239.8
groin	—	196.5	—	229.0	238.8	239.8
head	—	196.0	—	229.0	238.8	239.8
hepatic	—	196.2	—	229.0	238.8	239.8
hilar (pulmonary)	—	196.1	—	229.0	238.8	239.8
splenic	—	196.2	—	229.0	238.8	239.8
hypogastric	—	196.6	—	229.0	238.8	239.8
ileocolic	—	196.2	—	229.0	238.8	239.8
iliac	—	196.6	—	229.0	238.8	239.8
infraclavicular	—	196.3	—	229.0	238.8	239.8
inguina, inguinal	—	196.5	—	229.0	238.8	239.8
innominate	—	196.1	—	229.0	238.8	239.8
intercostal	—	196.1	—	229.0	238.8	239.8
intestinal	—	196.2	—	229.0	238.8	239.8
intra-abdominal	—	196.2	—	229.0	238.8	239.8
intrapelvic	—	196.6	—	229.0	238.8	239.8
intrathoracic	—	196.1	—	229.0	238.8	239.9
jugular	—	196.0	—	229.0	238.8	239.8
leg	—	196.5	—	229.0	238.8	239.8
limb						
lower	—	196.5	—	229.0	238.8	239.8
upper	—	196.3	—	229.0	238.8	239.8
lower limb	—	196.5	—	229.0	238.8	239.9
lumbar	—	196.2	—	229.0	238.8	239.8
mandibular	—	196.0	—	229.0	238.8	239.8
mediastinal	—	196.1	—	229.0	238.8	239.8
mesenteric (inferior) (superior)	—	196.2	—	229.0	238.8	239.8

☑ Additional Digit Required   ▶◀ Revised Text   ● New Line   ▲ Revised Code

Neoplasm, kidney — Neoplasm, lymph, lymphatic

Neoplasm, lymph, lymphatic — Neoplasm, nasolacrimal duct

Neoplasm, neoplastic — continued	Malignant Primary	Malignant Secondary	Malignant Ca in situ	Benign	Uncertain Behavior	Unspecified
lymph, lymphatic — continued						
gland — continued						
midcolic	—	196.2	—	229.0	238.8	239.8
multiple sites in categories 196.0-196.6	—	196.8	—	229.0	238.8	239.8
neck	—	196.0	—	229.0	238.8	239.8
obturator	—	196.6	—	229.0	238.8	239.8
occipital	—	196.0	—	229.0	238.8	239.8
pancreatic	—	196.2	—	229.0	238.8	239.8
para-aortic	—	196.2	—	229.0	238.8	239.8
paracervical	—	196.6	—	229.0	238.8	239.8
parametrial	—	196.6	—	229.0	238.8	239.8
parasternal	—	196.1	—	229.0	238.8	239.8
parotid	—	196.0	—	229.0	238.8	239.8
pectoral	—	196.3	—	229.0	238.8	239.8
pelvic	—	196.6	—	229.0	238.8	239.8
peri-aortic	—	196.2	—	229.0	238.8	239.8
peripancreatic	—	196.2	—	229.0	238.8	239.8
popliteal	—	196.5	—	229.0	238.8	239.8
porta hepatis	—	196.2	—	229.0	238.8	239.8
portal	—	196.2	—	229.0	238.8	239.8
preauricular	—	196.0	—	229.0	238.8	239.8
prelaryngeal	—	196.0	—	229.0	238.8	239.8
presymphysial	—	196.6	—	229.0	238.8	239.8
pretracheal	—	196.0	—	229.0	238.8	239.8
primary (any site) NEC	202.9 ☑	—	—	—	—	—
pulmonary (hiler)	—	196.1	—	229.0	238.8	239.8
pyloric	—	196.2	—	229.0	238.8	239.8
retroperitoneal	—	196.2	—	229.0	238.8	239.8
retropharyngeal	—	196.0	—	229.0	238.8	239.8
Rosenmüller's	—	196.5	—	229.0	238.8	239.8
sacral	—	196.6	—	229.0	238.8	239.8
scalene	—	196.0	—	229.0	238.8	239.8
site NEC	—	196.9	—	229.0	238.8	239.8
splenic (hilar)	—	196.2	—	229.0	238.8	239.8
subclavicular	—	196.3	—	229.0	238.8	239.8
subinguinal	—	196.5	—	229.0	238.8	239.8
sublingual	—	196.0	—	229.0	238.8	239.8
submandibular	—	196.0	—	229.0	238.8	239.8
submaxillary	—	196.0	—	229.0	238.8	239.8
submental	—	196.0	—	229.0	238.8	239.8
subscapular	—	196.3	—	229.0	238.8	239.8
supraclavicular	—	196.0	—	229.0	238.8	239.8
thoracic	—	196.1	—	229.0	238.8	239.8
tibial	—	196.5	—	229.0	238.8	239.8
tracheal	—	196.1	—	229.0	238.8	239.8
tracheobronchial	—	196.1	—	229.0	238.8	239.8
upper limb	—	196.3	—	229.0	238.8	239.8
Virchow's	—	196.0	—	229.0	238.8	239.8
node — see also Neoplasm, lymph gland						
primary NEC	202.9 ☑	—	—	—	—	—
vessel (see also Neoplasm, connective tissue)	171.9	198.89	—	215.9	238.1	239.2
Nackenrodt's ligament	183.8	198.82	233.3	221.8	236.3	239.5
malar	170.0	198.5	—	213.0	238.0	239.2
region — see Neoplasm, cheek						
mammary gland — see Neoplasm, breast						
mandible	170.1	198.5	—	213.1	238.0	239.2
alveolar						
mucose	143.1	198.89	230.0	210.4	235.1	239.0
ridge or process	170.1	198.5	—	213.1	238.0	239.2
carcinoma	143.1	—	—	—	—	—
carcinoma	143.1	—	—	—	—	—
marrow (bone) NEC	202.9 ☑	198.5	—	—	—	238.7
mastectomy site (skin)	173.5	198.2	—	—	—	—
specified as breast tissue	174.8	198.81	—	—	—	—
mastoid (air cells) (antrum) (cavity)	160.1	197.3	231.8	212.0	235.9	239.1
bone or process	170.0	198.5	—	213.0	238.0	239.2
maxilla, maxillary (superior)	170.0	198.5	—	213.0	238.0	239.2
alveolar						
mucosa	143.0	198.89	230.0	210.4	235.1	239.0
ridge or process	170.0	198.5	—	213.0	238.0	239.2
carcinoma	143.0	—	—	—	—	—
antrum	160.2	197.3	231.8	212.0	235.9	239.1
carcinoma	143.0	—	—	—	—	—

Neoplasm, neoplastic — continued	Malignant Primary	Malignant Secondary	Malignant Ca in situ	Benign	Uncertain Behavior	Unspecified
maxilla, maxillary — continued						
inferior — see Neoplasm, mandible						
sinus	160.2	197.3	231.8	212.0	235.9	239.1
meatus						
external (ear)	173.2	198.2	232.2	216.2	238.2	239.2
Meckel's diverticulum	152.3	197.4	230.7	211.2	235.2	239.0
mediastinum, mediastinal	164.9	197.1	—	212.5	235.8	239.8
anterior	164.2	197.1	—	212.5	235.8	239.8
contiguous sites with heart and thymus	164.8	—	—	—	—	—
posterior	164.3	197.1	—	212.5	235.8	239.8
medulla						
adrenal	194.0	198.7	234.8	227.0	237.2	239.7
oblongata	191.7	198.3	—	225.0	237.5	239.6
meibomian gland	173.1	198.2	232.1	216.1	238.2	239.2
melanoma — see Melanoma						
meninges (brain) (cerebral) (cranial) (intracranial)	192.1	198.4	—	225.2	237.6	239.7
spinal (cord)	192.3	198.4	—	225.4	237.6	239.7
meniscus, knee joint (lateral) (medial)	170.7	198.5	—	213.7	238.0	239.2
mesentery, mesenteric	158.8	197.6	—	211.8	235.4	239.0
mesoappendix	158.8	197.6	—	211.8	235.4	239.0
mesocolon	158.8	197.6	—	211.8	235.4	239.0
mesopharynx — see Neoplasm, oropharynx						
mesosalpinx	183.3	198.82	233.3	221.0	236.3	239.5
mesovarium	183.3	198.82	233.3	221.0	236.3	239.5
metacarpus (any bone)	170.5	198.5	—	213.5	238.0	239.2
metastatic NEC — see also Neoplasm, by site, secondary	—	199.1	—	—	—	—
metatarsus (any bone)	170.8	198.5	—	213.8	238.0	239.2
midbrain	191.7	198.3	—	225.0	237.5	239.6
milk duct — see Neoplasm, breast						
mons						
pubis	184.4	198.82	233.3	221.2	236.3	239.5
veneris	184.4	198.82	233.3	221.2	236.3	239.5
motor tract	192.9	198.4	—	225.9	237.9	239.7
brain	191.9	198.3	—	225.0	237.5	239.6
spinal	192.3	198.3	—	225.3	237.5	239.7
mouth	145.9	198.89	230.0	210.4	235.1	239.0
contiguous sites	145.8	—	—	—	—	—
floor	144.9	198.89	230.0	210.3	235.1	239.0
anterior portion	144.0	198.89	230.0	210.3	235.1	239.0
contiguous sites	144.8	—	—	—	—	—
lateral portion	144.1	198.89	230.0	210.3	235.1	239.0
roof	145.5	198.89	230.0	210.4	235.1	239.0
specified part NEC	145.8	198.89	230.0	210.4	235.1	239.0
vestibule	145.1	198.89	230.0	210.4	235.1	239.0
mucosa						
alveolar (ridge or process)	143.9	198.89	230.0	210.4	235.1	239.0
lower	143.1	198.89	230.0	210.4	235.1	239.0
upper	143.0	198.89	230.0	210.4	235.1	239.0
buccal	145.0	198.89	230.0	210.4	235.1	239.0
cheek	145.0	198.89	230.0	210.4	235.1	239.0
lip — see Neoplasm, lip, internal						
nasal	160.0	197.3	231.8	212.0	235.9	239.1
oral	145.0	198.89	230.0	210.4	235.1	239.0
Müllerian duct						
female	184.8	198.82	233.3	221.8	236.3	239.5
male	187.8	198.82	233.6	222.8	236.6	239.5
multiple sites NEC	199.0	199.0	234.9	229.9	238.9	199.0
muscle — see also Neoplasm, connective tissue						
extraocular	190.1	198.4	234.0	224.1	238.8	239.8
myocardium	164.1	198.89	—	212.7	238.8	239.8
myometrium	182.0	198.82	233.2	219.1	236.0	239.5
myopericardium	164.1	198.89	—	212.7	238.8	239.8
nabothian gland (follicle)	180.0	198.82	233.1	219.0	236.0	239.5
nail	173.9	198.2	232.9	216.9	238.2	239.2
finger	173.6	198.2	232.6	216.6	238.2	239.2
toe	173.7	198.2	232.7	216.7	238.2	239.2
nares, naris (anterior) (posterior)	160.0	197.3	231.8	212.0	235.9	239.1
nasal — see Neoplasm, nose						
nasolabial groove	173.3	198.2	232.3	216.3	238.2	239.2
nasolacrimal duct	190.7	198.4	234.0	224.7	238.8	239.8

Neoplasm, neoplastic — continued	Malignant Primary	Malignant Secondary	Malignant Ca in situ	Benign	Uncertain Behavior	Unspecified
nasopharynx, nasopharyngeal	147.9	198.89	230.0	210.7	235.1	239.0
contiguous sites	147.8	—	—	—	—	—
floor	147.3	198.89	230.0	210.7	235.1	239.0
roof	147.0	198.89	230.0	210.7	235.1	239.0
specified site NEC	147.8	198.89	230.0	210.7	235.1	239.0
wall	147.9	198.89	230.0	210.7	235.1	239.0
anterior	147.3	198.89	230.0	210.7	235.1	239.0
lateral	147.2	198.89	230.0	210.7	235.1	239.0
posterior	147.1	198.89	230.0	210.7	235.1	239.0
superior	147.0	198.89	230.0	210.7	235.1	239.0
nates	173.5	198.2	232.5	216.5	238.2	239.2
neck NEC*	195.0	198.89	234.8	229.8	238.8	239.8
nerve (autonomic) (ganglion) (parasympathetic) (peripheral) (sympathetic) — see also Neoplasm, connective tissue						
abducens	192.0	198.4	—	225.1	237.9	239.7
accessory (spinal)	192.0	198.4	—	225.1	237.9	239.7
acoustic	192.0	198.4	—	225.1	237.9	239.7
auditory	192.0	198.4	—	225.1	237.9	239.7
brachial	171.2	198.89	—	215.2	238.1	239.2
cranial (any)	192.0	198.4	—	225.1	237.9	239.7
facial	192.0	198.4	—	225.1	237.9	239.7
femoral	171.3	198.89	—	215.3	238.1	239.2
glossopharyngeal	192.0	198.4	—	225.1	237.9	239.7
hypoglossal	192.0	198.4	—	225.1	237.9	239.7
intercostal	171.4	198.89	—	215.4	238.1	239.2
lumbar	171.7	198.89	—	215.7	238.1	239.2
median	171.2	198.89	—	215.2	238.1	239.2
obturator	171.3	198.89	—	215.3	238.1	239.2
oculomotor	192.0	198.4	—	225.1	237.9	239.7
olfactory	192.0	198.4	—	225.1	237.9	239.7
optic	192.0	198.4	—	225.1	237.9	239.7
peripheral NEC	171.9	198.89	—	215.9	238.1	239.2
radial	171.2	198.89	—	215.2	238.1	239.2
sacral	171.6	198.89	—	215.6	238.1	239.2
sciatic	171.3	198.89	—	215.3	238.1	239.2
spinal NEC	171.9	198.89	—	215.9	238.1	239.2
trigeminal	192.0	198.4	—	225.1	237.9	239.7
trochlear	192.0	198.4	—	225.1	237.9	239.7
ulnar	171.2	198.89	—	215.2	238.1	239.2
vagus	192.0	198.4	—	225.1	237.9	239.7
nervous system (central) NEC	192.9	198.4	—	225.9	237.9	239.7
autonomic NEC	171.9	198.89	—	215.9	238.1	239.2
brain — see also Neoplasm, brain						
membrane or meninges	192.1	198.4	—	225.2	237.6	239.7
contiguous sites	192.8	—	—	—	—	—
parasympathetic NEC	171.9	198.89	—	215.9	238.1	239.2
sympathetic NEC	171.9	198.89	—	215.9	238.1	239.2
nipple (female)	174.0	198.81	233.0	217	238.3	239.3
male	175.0	198.81	233.0	217	238.3	239.3
nose, nasal	195.0	198.89	234.8	229.8	238.8	239.8
ala (external)	173.3	198.2	232.3	216.3	238.2	239.2
bone	170.0	198.5	—	213.0	238.0	239.2
cartilage	160.0	197.3	231.8	212.0	235.9	239.1
cavity	160.0	197.3	231.8	212.0	235.9	239.1
contiguous sites with accessory sinuses or middle ear	160.8	—	—	—	—	—
choana	147.3	198.89	230.0	210.7	235.1	239.0
external (skin)	173.3	198.2	232.3	216.3	238.2	239.2
fossa	160.0	197.3	231.8	212.0	235.9	239.1
internal	160.0	197.3	231.8	212.0	235.9	239.1
mucosa	160.0	197.3	231.8	212.0	235.9	239.1
septum	160.0	197.3	231.8	212.0	235.9	239.1
posterior margin	147.3	198.89	230.0	210.7	235.1	239.0
sinus — see Neoplasm, sinus						
skin	173.3	198.2	232.3	216.3	238.2	239.2
turbinate (mucosa)	160.0	197.3	231.8	212.0	235.9	239.1
bone	170.0	198.5	—	213.0	238.0	239.2
vestibule	160.0	197.3	231.8	212.0	235.9	239.1
nostril	160.0	197.3	231.8	212.0	235.9	239.1
nucleus pulposus	170.2	198.5	—	213.2	238.0	239.2
occipital						
bone	170.0	198.5	—	213.0	238.0	239.2
lobe or pole, brain	191.4	198.3	—	225.0	237.5	239.6
odontogenic — see Neoplasm, jaw bone						
oesophagus — see Neoplasm, esophagus						
olfactory nerve or bulb	192.0	198.4	—	225.1	237.9	239.7
olive (brain)	191.7	198.3	—	225.0	237.5	239.6
omentum	158.8	197.6	—	211.8	235.4	239.0
operculum (brain)	191.0	198.3	—	225.0	237.5	239.6
optic nerve, chiasm, or tract	192.0	198.4	—	225.1	237.9	239.7
oral (cavity)	145.9	198.89	230.0	210.4	235.1	239.0
contiguous sites with lip or pharynx	149.8	—	—	—	—	—
ill-defined	149.9	198.89	230.0	210.4	235.1	239.0
mucosa	145.9	198.89	230.0	210.4	235.1	239.0
orbit	190.1	198.4	234.0	224.1	238.8	239.8
bone	170.0	198.5	—	213.0	238.0	239.2
eye	190.1	198.4	234.0	224.1	238.8	239.8
soft parts	190.1	198.4	234.0	224.1	238.8	239.8
organ of Zuckerkandl	194.6	198.89	—	227.6	237.3	239.7
oropharynx	146.9	198.89	230.0	210.6	235.1	239.0
branchial cleft (vestige)	146.8	198.89	230.0	210.6	235.1	239.0
contiguous sites	146.8	—	—	—	—	—
junctional region	146.5	198.89	230.0	210.6	235.1	239.0
lateral wall	146.6	198.89	230.0	210.6	235.1	239.0
pillars of fauces	146.2	198.89	230.0	210.6	235.1	239.0
posterior wall	146.7	198.89	230.0	210.6	235.1	239.0
specified part NEC	146.8	198.89	230.0	210.6	235.1	239.0
vallecula	146.3	198.89	230.0	210.6	235.1	239.0
os						
external	180.1	198.82	233.1	219.0	236.0	239.5
internal	180.0	198.82	233.1	219.0	236.0	239.5
ovary	183.0	198.6	233.3	220	236.2	239.5
oviduct	183.2	198.82	233.3	221.0	236.3	239.5
palate	145.5	198.89	230.0	210.4	235.1	239.0
hard	145.2	198.89	230.0	210.4	235.1	239.0
junction of hard and soft palate	145.5	198.89	230.0	210.4	235.1	239.0
soft	145.3	198.89	230.0	210.4	235.1	239.0
nasopharyngeal surface	147.3	198.89	230.0	210.7	235.1	239.0
posterior surface	147.3	198.89	230.0	210.7	235.1	239.0
superior surface	147.3	198.89	230.0	210.7	235.1	239.0
palatoglossal arch	146.2	198.89	230.0	210.6	235.1	239.0
palatopharyngeal arch	146.2	198.89	230.0	210.6	235.1	239.0
pallium	191.0	198.3	—	225.0	237.5	239.6
palpebra	173.1	198.2	232.1	216.1	238.2	239.2
pancreas	157.9	197.8	230.9	211.6	235.5	239.0
body	157.1	197.8	230.9	211.6	235.5	239.0
contiguous sites	157.8	—	—	—	—	—
duct (of Santorini) (of Wirsung)	157.3	197.8	230.9	211.6	235.5	239.0
ectopic tissue	157.8	197.8	230.9	211.6	235.5	239.0
head	157.0	197.8	230.9	211.6	235.5	239.0
islet cells	157.4	197.8	230.9	211.7	235.5	239.0
neck	157.8	197.8	230.9	211.6	235.5	239.0
tail	157.2	197.8	230.9	211.6	235.5	239.0
para-aortic body	194.6	198.89	—	227.6	237.3	239.7
paraganglion NEC	194.6	198.89	—	227.6	237.3	239.7
parametrium	183.4	198.82	—	221.0	236.3	239.5
paranephric	158.0	197.6	—	211.8	235.4	239.0
pararectal	195.3	198.89	—	229.8	238.8	239.8
parasagittal (region)	195.0	198.89	234.8	229.8	238.8	239.8
parasellar	192.9	198.4	—	225.9	237.9	239.7
parathyroid (gland)	194.1	198.89	234.8	227.1	237.4	239.7
paraurethral	195.3	198.89	—	229.8	238.8	239.8
gland	189.4	198.1	233.9	223.89	236.99	239.5
paravaginal	195.3	198.89	—	229.8	238.8	239.8
parenchyma, kidney	189.0	198.0	233.9	223.0	236.91	239.5
parietal						
bone	170.0	198.5	—	213.0	238.0	239.2
lobe, brain	191.3	198.3	—	225.0	237.5	239.6
paroophoron	183.3	198.82	233.3	221.0	236.3	239.5
parotid (duct) (gland)	142.0	198.89	230.0	210.2	235.0	239.0
parovarium	183.3	198.82	233.3	221.0	236.3	239.5
patella	170.8	198.5	—	213.8	238.0	239.2
peduncle, cerebral	191.7	198.3	—	225.0	237.5	239.6
pelvirectal junction	154.0	197.5	230.4	211.4	235.2	239.0
pelvis, pelvic	195.3	198.89	234.8	229.8	238.8	239.8
bone	170.6	198.5	—	213.6	238.0	239.2
floor	195.3	198.89	234.8	229.8	238.8	239.8
renal	189.1	198.0	233.9	223.1	236.91	239.5
viscera	195.3	198.89	234.8	229.8	238.8	239.8
wall	195.3	198.89	234.8	229.8	238.8	239.8

☑ Additional Digit Required　　▶◀ Revised Text　　● New Line　　▲ Revised Code

Neoplasm, neoplastic — continued	Malignant Primary	Malignant Secondary	Malignant Ca in situ	Benign	Uncertain Behavior	Unspecified
pelvo-abdominal	195.8	198.89	234.8	229.8	238.8	239.8
penis	187.4	198.82	233.5	222.1	236.6	239.5
body	187.3	198.82	233.5	222.1	236.6	239.5
corpus (cavernosum)	187.3	198.82	233.5	222.1	236.6	239.5
glans	187.2	198.82	233.5	222.1	236.6	239.5
skin NEC	187.4	198.82	233.5	222.1	236.6	239.5
periadrenal (tissue)	158.0	197.6	—	211.8	235.4	239.0
perianal (skin)	173.5	198.2	232.5	216.5	238.2	239.2
pericardium	164.1	198.89	—	212.7	238.8	239.8
perinephric	158.0	197.6	—	211.8	235.4	239.0
perineum	195.3	198.89	234.8	229.8	238.8	239.8
periodontal tissue NEC	143.9	198.89	230.0	210.4	235.1	239.0
periosteum — see Neoplasm, bone						
peripancreatic	158.0	197.6	—	211.8	235.4	239.0
peripheral nerve NEC	171.9	198.89	—	215.9	238.1	239.2
perirectal (tissue)	195.3	198.89	—	229.8	238.8	239.8
perirenal (tissue)	158.0	197.6	—	211.8	235.4	239.0
peritoneum, peritoneal (cavity)	158.9	197.6	—	211.8	235.4	239.0
contiguous sites	158.8	—	—	—	—	—
with digestive organs	159.8	—	—	—	—	—
parietal	158.8	197.6	—	211.8	235.4	239.0
pelvic	158.8	197.6	—	211.8	235.4	239.0
specified part NEC	158.8	197.6	—	211.8	235.4	239.0
peritonsillar (tissue)	195.0	198.89	234.8	229.8	238.8	239.8
periurethral tissue	195.3	198.89	—	229.8	238.8	239.8
phalanges	170.9	198.5	—	213.9	238.0	239.2
foot	170.8	198.5	—	213.8	238.0	239.2
hand	170.5	198.5	—	213.5	238.0	239.2
pharynx, pharyngeal	149.0	198.89	230.0	210.9	235.1	239.0
bursa	147.1	198.89	230.0	210.7	235.1	239.0
fornix	147.3	198.89	230.0	210.7	235.1	239.0
recess	147.2	198.89	230.0	210.7	235.1	239.0
region	149.0	198.89	230.0	210.9	235.1	239.0
tonsil	147.1	198.89	230.0	210.7	235.1	239.0
wall (lateral) (posterior)	149.0	198.89	230.0	210.9	235.1	239.0
pia mater (cerebral) (cranial)	192.1	198.4	—	225.2	237.6	239.7
spinal	192.3	198.4	—	225.4	237.6	239.7
pillars of fauces	146.2	198.89	230.0	210.6	235.1	239.0
pineal (body) (gland)	194.4	198.89	234.8	227.4	237.1	239.7
pinna (ear) NEC	173.2	198.2	232.2	216.2	238.2	239.2
cartilage	171.0	198.89	—	215.0	238.1	239.2
piriform fossa or sinus	148.1	198.89	230.0	210.8	235.1	239.0
pituitary (body) (fossa) (gland) (lobe)	194.3	198.89	234.8	227.3	237.0	239.7
placenta	181	198.82	233.2	219.8	236.1	239.5
pleura, pleural (cavity)	163.9	197.2	—	212.4	235.8	239.1
contiguous sites	163.8	—	—	—	—	—
parietal	163.0	197.2	—	212.4	235.8	239.1
visceral	163.1	197.2	—	212.4	235.8	239.1
plexus						
brachial	171.2	198.89	—	215.2	238.1	239.2
cervical	171.0	198.89	—	215.0	238.1	239.2
choroid	191.5	198.3	—	225.0	237.5	239.6
lumbosacral	171.6	198.89	—	215.6	238.1	239.2
sacral	171.6	198.89	—	215.6	238.1	239.2
pluri-endocrine	194.8	198.89	234.8	227.8	237.4	239.7
pole						
frontal	191.1	198.3	—	225.0	237.5	239.6
occipital	191.4	198.3	—	225.0	237.5	239.6
pons (varolii)	191.7	198.3	—	225.0	237.5	239.6
popliteal fossa or space*	195.5	198.89	234.8	229.8	238.8	239.8
postcricoid (region)	148.0	198.89	230.0	210.8	235.1	239.0
posterior fossa (cranial)	191.6	198.3	—	225.0	237.5	239.6
postnasal space	147.9	198.89	230.0	210.7	235.1	239.0
prepuce	187.1	198.82	233.5	222.1	236.6	239.5
prepylorus	151.1	197.8	230.2	211.1	235.2	239.0
presacral (region)	195.3	198.89	—	229.8	238.8	239.8
prostate (gland)	185	198.82	233.4	222.2	236.5	239.5
utricle	189.3	198.1	233.9	223.81	236.99▲	239.5
pterygoid fossa	171.0	198.89	—	215.0	238.1	239.2
pubic bone	170.6	198.5	—	213.6	238.0	239.2
pudenda, pudendum (female)	184.4	198.82	233.3	221.2	236.3	239.5
pulmonary	162.9	197.0	231.2	212.3	235.7	239.1
putamen	191.0	198.3	—	225.0	237.5	239.6
pyloric						
antrum	151.2	197.8	230.2	211.1	235.2	239.0
canal	151.1	197.8	230.2	211.1	235.2	239.0

Neoplasm, neoplastic — continued	Malignant Primary	Malignant Secondary	Malignant Ca in situ	Benign	Uncertain Behavior	Unspecified
pylorus	151.1	197.8	230.2	211.1	235.2	239.0
pyramid (brain)	191.7	198.3	—	225.0	237.5	239.6
pyriform fossa or sinus	148.1	198.89	230.0	210.8	235.1	239.0
radius (any part)	170.4	198.5	—	213.4	238.0	239.2
Rathke's pouch	194.3	198.89	234.8	227.3	237.0	239.7
rectosigmoid (colon) (junction)	154.0	197.5	230.4	211.4	235.2	239.0
contiguous sites with anus or rectum	154.8	—	—	—	—	—
rectouterine pouch	158.8	197.6	—	211.8	235.4	239.0
rectovaginal septum or wall	195.3	198.89	234.8	229.8	238.8	239.8
rectovesical septum	195.3	198.89	234.8	229.8	238.8	239.8
rectum (ampulla)	154.1	197.5	230.4	211.4	235.2	239.0
and colon	154.0	197.5	230.4	211.4	235.2	239.0
contiguous sites with anus or rectosigmoid junction	154.8	—	—	—	—	—
renal	189.0	198.0	233.9	223.0	236.91	239.5
calyx	189.1	198.0	233.9	223.1	236.91	239.5
hilus	189.1	198.0	233.9	223.1	236.91	239.5
parenchyma	189.0	198.0	233.9	223.0	236.91	239.5
pelvis	189.1	198.0	233.9	223.1	236.91	239.5
respiratory						
organs or system NEC	165.9	197.3	231.9	212.9	235.9	239.1
contiguous sites with intrathoracic organs	165.8	—	—	—	—	—
specified sites NEC	165.8	197.3	231.8	212.8	235.9	239.1
tract NEC	165.9	197.3	231.9	212.9	235.9	239.1
upper	165.0	197.3	231.9	212.9	235.9	239.1
retina	190.5	198.4	234.0	224.5	238.8	239.8
retrobulbar	190.1	198.4	—	224.1	238.8	239.8
retrocecal	158.0	197.6	—	211.8	235.4	239.0
retromolar (area) (triangle) (trigone)	145.6	198.89	230.0	210.4	235.1	239.0
retro-orbital	195.0	198.89	234.8	229.8	238.8	239.8
retroperitoneal (space) (tissue)	158.0	197.6	—	211.8	235.4	239.0
contiguous sites	158.8	—	—	—	—	—
retroperitoneum	158.0	197.6	—	211.8	235.4	239.0
contiguous sites	158.8	—	—	—	—	—
retropharyngeal	149.0	198.89	230.0	210.9	235.1	239.0
retrovesical (septum)	195.3	198.89	234.8	229.8	238.8	239.8
rhinencephalon	191.0	198.3	—	225.0	237.5	239.6
rib	170.3	198.5	—	213.3	238.0	239.2
Rosenmüller's fossa	147.2	198.89	230.0	210.7	235.1	239.0
round ligament	183.5	198.82	—	221.0	236.3	239.5
sacrococcyx, sacrococcygeal	170.6	198.5	—	213.6	238.0	239.2
region	195.3	198.89	234.8	229.8	238.8	239.8
sacrouterine ligament	183.4	198.82	—	221.0	236.3	239.5
sacrum, sacral (vertebra)	170.6	198.5	—	213.6	238.0	239.2
salivary gland or duct (major)	142.9	198.89	230.0	210.2	235.0	239.0
contiguous sites	142.8	—	—	—	—	—
minor NEC	145.9	198.89	230.0	210.4	235.1	239.0
parotid	142.0	198.89	230.0	210.2	235.0	239.0
pluriglandular	142.8	198.89	230.0	210.2	235.0	239.0
sublingual	142.2	198.89	230.0	210.2	235.0	239.0
submandibular	142.1	198.89	230.0	210.2	235.0	239.0
submaxillary	142.1	198.89	230.0	210.2	235.0	239.0
salpinx (uterine)	183.2	198.82	233.3	221.0	236.3	239.5
Santorini's duct	157.3	197.8	230.9	211.6	235.5	239.0
scalp	173.4	198.2	232.4	216.4	238.2	239.2
scapula (any part)	170.4	198.5	—	213.4	238.0	239.2
scapular region	195.1	198.89	234.8	229.8	238.8	239.8
scar NEC (see also Neoplasm, skin)	173.9	198.2	232.9	216.9	238.2	239.2
sciatic nerve	171.3	198.89	—	215.3	238.1	239.2
sclera	190.0	198.4	234.0	224.0	238.8	239.8
scrotum (skin)	187.7	198.82	233.6	222.4	236.6	239.5
sebaceous gland — see Neoplasm, skin						
sella turcica	194.3	198.89	234.8	227.3	237.0	239.7
bone	170.0	198.5	—	213.0	238.0	239.2
semilunar cartilage (knee)	170.7	198.5	—	213.7	238.0	239.2
seminal vesicle	187.8	198.82	233.6	222.8	236.6	239.5
septum						
nasal	160.0	197.3	231.8	212.0	235.9	239.1
posterior margin	147.3	198.89	230.0	210.7	235.1	239.0
rectovaginal	195.3	198.89	234.8	229.8	238.8	239.8
rectovesical	195.3	198.89	234.8	229.8	238.8	239.8
urethrovaginal	184.9	198.82	233.3	221.9	236.3	239.5
vesicovaginal	184.9	198.82	233.3	221.9	236.3	239.5
shoulder NEC*	195.4	198.89	232.6	229.8	238.8	239.8
sigmoid flexure (lower) (upper)	153.3	197.5	230.3	211.3	235.2	239.0

Neoplasm, neoplastic — continued	Malignant Primary	Malignant Secondary	Malignant Ca in situ	Benign	Uncertain Behavior	Unspecified
sinus (accessory)	160.9	197.3	231.8	212.0	235.9	239.1
bone (any)	170.0	198.5	—	213.0	238.0	239.2
contiguous sites with middle ear or nasal cavities	160.8	—	—	—	—	—
ethmoidal	160.3	197.3	231.8	212.0	235.9	239.1
frontal	160.4	197.3	231.8	212.0	235.9	239.1
maxillary	160.2	197.3	231.8	212.0	235.9	239.1
nasal, paranasal NEC	160.9	197.3	231.8	212.0	235.9	239.1
pyriform	148.1	198.89	230.0	210.8	235.1	239.0
sphenoidal	160.5	197.3	231.8	212.0	235.9	239.1
skeleton, skeletal NEC	170.9	198.5	—	213.9	238.0	239.2
Skene's gland	189.4	198.1	233.9	223.89	236.99	239.5
skin NEC	173.9	198.2	232.9	216.9	238.2	239.2
abdominal wall	173.5	198.2	232.5	216.5	238.2	239.2
ala nasi	173.3	198.2	232.3	216.3	238.2	239.2
ankle	173.7	198.2	232.7	216.7	238.2	239.2
antecubital space	173.6	198.2	232.6	216.6	238.2	239.2
anus	173.5	198.2	232.5	216.5	238.2	239.2
arm	173.6	198.2	232.6	216.6	238.2	239.2
auditory canal (external)	173.2	198.2	232.2	216.2	238.2	239.2
auricle (ear)	173.2	198.2	232.2	216.2	238.2	239.2
auricular canal (external)	173.2	198.2	232.2	216.2	238.2	239.2
axilla, axillary fold	173.5	198.2	232.5	216.5	238.2	239.2
back	173.5	198.2	232.5	216.5	238.2	239.2
breast	173.5	198.2	232.5	216.5	238.2	239.2
brow	173.3	198.2	232.3	216.3	238.2	239.2
buttock	173.5	198.2	232.5	216.5	238.2	239.2
calf	173.7	198.2	232.7	216.7	238.2	239.2
canthus (eye) (inner) (outer)	173.1	198.2	232.1	216.1	238.2	239.2
cervical region	173.4	198.2	232.4	216.4	238.2	239.2
cheek (external)	173.3	198.2	232.3	216.3	238.2	239.2
chest (wall)	173.5	198.2	232.5	216.5	238.2	239.2
chin	173.3	198.2	232.3	216.3	238.2	239.2
clavicular area	173.5	198.2	232.5	216.5	238.2	239.2
clitoris	184.3	198.82	233.3	221.2	236.3	239.5
columnella	173.3	198.2	232.3	216.3	238.2	239.2
concha	173.2	198.2	232.2	216.2	238.2	239.2
contiguous sites	173.8	—	—	—	—	—
ear (external)	173.2	198.2	232.2	216.2	238.2	239.2
elbow	173.6	198.2	232.6	216.6	238.2	239.2
eyebrow	173.3	198.2	232.3	216.3	238.2	239.2
eyelid	173.1	198.2	232.1	216.1	238.2	239.2
face NEC	173.3	198.2	232.3	216.3	238.2	239.2
female genital organs (external)	184.4	198.82	233.3	221.2	236.3	239.5
clitoris	184.3	198.82	233.3	221.2	236.3	239.5
labium NEC	184.4	198.82	233.3	221.2	236.3	239.5
majus	184.1	198.82	233.3	221.2	236.3	239.5
minus	184.2	198.82	233.3	221.2	236.3	239.5
pudendum	184.4	198.82	233.3	221.2	236.3	239.5
vulva	184.4	198.82	233.3	221.2	236.3	239.5
finger	173.6	198.2	232.6	216.6	238.2	239.2
flank	173.5	198.2	232.5	216.5	238.2	239.2
foot	173.7	198.2	232.7	216.7	238.2	239.2
forearm	173.6	198.2	232.6	216.6	238.2	239.2
forehead	173.3	198.2	232.3	216.3	238.2	239.2
glabella	173.3	198.2	232.3	216.3	238.2	239.2
gluteal region	173.5	198.2	232.5	216.5	238.2	239.2
groin	173.5	198.2	232.5	216.5	238.2	239.2
hand	173.6	198.2	232.6	216.6	238.2	239.2
head NEC	173.4	198.2	232.4	216.4	238.2	239.2
heel	173.7	198.2	232.7	216.7	238.2	239.2
helix	173.2	198.2	232.2	216.2	238.2	239.2
hip	173.7	198.2	232.7	216.7	238.2	239.2
infraclavicular region	173.5	198.2	232.5	216.5	238.2	239.2
inguinal region	173.5	198.2	232.5	216.5	238.2	239.2
jaw	173.3	198.2	232.3	216.3	238.2	239.2
knee	173.7	198.2	232.7	216.7	238.2	239.2
labia						
majora	184.1	198.82	233.3	221.2	236.3	239.5
minora	184.2	198.82	233.3	221.2	236.3	239.5
leg	173.7	198.2	232.7	216.7	238.2	239.2
lid (lower) (upper)	173.1	198.2	232.1	216.1	238.2	239.2
limb NEC	173.9	198.2	232.9	216.9	238.2	239.5
lower	173.7	198.2	232.7	216.7	238.2	239.2
upper	173.6	198.2	232.6	216.6	238.2	239.2
lip (lower) (upper)	173.0	198.2	232.0	216.0	238.2	239.2

Neoplasm, neoplastic — continued	Malignant Primary	Malignant Secondary	Malignant Ca in situ	Benign	Uncertain Behavior	Unspecified
skin NEC — continued						
male genital organs	187.9	198.82	233.6	222.9	236.6	239.5
penis	187.4	198.82	233.5	222.1	236.6	239.5
prepuce	187.1	198.82	233.5	222.1	236.6	239.5
scrotum	187.7	198.82	233.6	222.4	236.6	239.5
mastectomy site	173.5	198.2	—	—	—	—
specified as breast tissue	174.8	198.81	—	—	—	—
meatus, acoustic (external)	173.2	198.2	232.2	216.2	238.2	239.2
melanoma — see Melanoma						
nates	173.5	198.2	232.5	216.5	238.2	239.0
neck	173.4	198.2	232.4	216.4	238.2	239.2
nose (external)	173.3	198.2	232.3	216.3	238.2	239.2
palm	173.6	198.2	232.6	216.6	238.2	239.2
palpebra	173.1	198.2	232.1	216.1	238.2	239.2
penis NEC	187.4	198.82	233.5	222.1	236.6	239.5
perianal	173.5	198.2	232.5	216.5	238.2	239.2
perineum	173.5	198.2	232.5	216.5	238.2	239.2
pinna	173.2	198.2	232.2	216.2	238.2	239.2
plantar	173.7	198.2	232.7	216.7	238.2	239.2
popliteal fossa or space	173.7	198.2	232.7	216.7	238.2	239.2
prepuce	187.1	198.82	233.5	222.1	236.6	239.5
pubes	173.5	198.2	232.5	216.5	238.2	239.2
sacrococcygeal region	173.5	198.2	232.5	216.5	238.2	239.2
scalp	173.4	198.2	232.4	216.4	238.2	239.2
scapular region	173.5	198.2	232.5	216.5	238.2	239.2
scrotum	187.7	198.82	233.6	222.4	236.6	239.5
shoulder	173.6	198.2	232.6	216.6	238.2	239.2
sole (foot)	173.7	198.2	232.7	216.7	238.2	239.2
specified sites NEC	173.8	198.2	232.8	216.8	232.8	239.2
submammary fold	173.5	198.2	232.5	216.5	238.2	239.2
supraclavicular region	173.4	198.2	232.4	216.4	238.2	239.2
temple	173.3	198.2	232.3	216.3	238.2	239.2
thigh	173.7	198.2	232.7	216.7	238.2	239.2
thoracic wall	173.5	198.2	232.5	216.5	238.2	239.2
thumb	173.6	198.2	232.6	216.6	238.2	239.2
toe	173.7	198.2	232.7	216.7	238.2	239.2
tragus	173.2	198.2	232.2	216.2	238.2	239.2
trunk	173.5	198.2	232.5	216.5	238.2	239.2
umbilicus	173.5	198.2	232.5	216.5	238.2	239.2
vulva	184.4	198.82	233.3	221.2	236.3	239.5
wrist	173.6	198.2	232.6	216.6	238.2	239.2
skull	170.0	198.5	—	213.0	238.0	239.2
soft parts or tissues — see Neoplasm, connective tissue						
specified site NEC	195.8	198.89	234.8	229.8	238.8	239.8
spermatic cord	187.6	198.82	233.6	222.8	236.6	239.5
sphenoid	160.5	197.3	231.8	212.0	235.9	239.1
bone	170.0	198.5	—	213.0	238.0	239.2
sinus	160.5	197.3	231.8	212.0	235.9	239.1
sphincter						
anal	154.2	197.5	230.5	211.4	235.5	239.0
of Oddi	156.1	197.8	230.8	211.5	235.3	239.0
spine, spinal (column)	170.2	198.5	—	213.2	238.0	239.2
bulb	191.7	198.3	—	225.0	237.5	239.6
coccyx	170.6	198.5	—	213.6	238.0	239.2
cord (cervical) (lumbar) (sacral) (thoracic)	192.2	198.3	—	225.3	237.5	239.7
dura mater	192.3	198.4	—	225.4	237.6	239.7
lumbosacral	170.2	198.5	—	213.2	238.0	239.2
membrane	192.3	198.4	—	225.4	237.6	239.7
meninges	192.3	198.4	—	225.4	237.6	239.7
nerve (root)	171.9	198.89	—	215.9	238.1	239.2
pia mater	192.3	198.4	—	225.4	237.6	239.7
root	171.9	198.89	—	215.9	238.1	239.2
sacrum	170.6	198.5	—	213.6	238.0	239.2
spleen, splenic NEC	159.1	197.8	230.9	211.9	235.5	239.0
flexure (colon)	153.7	197.5	230.3	211.3	235.2	239.0
stem, brain	191.7	198.3	—	225.0	237.5	239.6
Stensen's duct	142.0	198.89	230.0	210.2	235.0	239.0
sternum	170.3	198.5	—	213.3	238.0	239.2
stomach	151.9	197.8	230.2	211.1	235.2	239.0
antrum (pyloric)	151.2	197.8	230.2	211.1	235.2	239.0
body	151.4	197.8	230.2	211.1	235.2	239.0
cardia	151.0	197.8	230.2	211.1	235.2	239.0
cardiac orifice	151.0	197.8	230.2	211.1	235.2	239.0
contiguous sites	151.8	—	—	—	—	—

☑ Additional Digit Required   ▶◀ Revised Text   ● New Line   ▲ Revised Code

Neoplasm, neoplastic — continued	Malignant			Benign	Uncertain Behavior	Unspecified
	Primary	Secondary	Ca in situ			
stomach — continued						
corpus	151.4	197.8	230.2	211.1	235.2	239.0
fundus	151.3	197.8	230.2	211.1	235.2	239.0
greater curvature NEC	151.6	197.8	230.2	211.1	235.2	239.0
lesser curvature NEC	151.5	197.8	230.2	211.1	235.2	239.0
prepylorus	151.1	197.8	230.2	211.1	235.2	239.0
pylorus	151.1	197.8	230.2	211.1	235.2	239.0
wall NEC	151.9	197.8	230.2	211.1	235.2	239.0
anterior NEC	151.8	197.8	230.2	211.1	235.2	239.0
posterior NEC	151.8	197.8	230.2	211.1	235.2	239.0
stroma, endometrial	182.0	198.82	233.2	219.1	236.0	239.5
stump, cervical	180.8	198.82	233.1	219.0	236.0	239.5
subcutaneous (nodule) (tissue) NEC — see Neoplasm, connective tissue						
subdural	192.1	198.4	—	225.2	237.6	239.7
subglottis, subglottic	161.2	197.3	231.0	212.1	235.6	239.1
sublingual	144.9	198.89	230.0	210.3	235.1	239.0
gland or duct	142.2	198.89	230.0	210.2	235.0	239.0
submandibular gland	142.1	198.89	230.0	210.2	235.0	239.0
submaxillary gland or duct	142.1	198.89	230.0	210.2	235.0	239.0
submental	195.0	198.89	234.8	229.8	238.8	239.8
subpleural	162.9	197.0	—	212.3	235.7	239.1
substernal	164.2	197.1	—	212.5	235.8	239.8
sudoriferous, sudoriparous gland, site unspecified	173.9	198.2	232.9	216.9	238.2	239.2
specified site — see Neoplasm, skin						
supraclavicular region	195.0	198.89	234.8	229.8	238.8	239.8
supraglottis	161.1	197.3	231.0	212.1	235.6	239.1
suprarenal (capsule) (cortex) (gland) (medulla)	194.0	198.7	234.8	227.0	237.2	239.7
suprasellar (region)	191.9	198.3	—	225.0	237.5	239.6
sweat gland (apocrine) (eccrine), site unspecified	173.9	198.2	232.9	216.9	238.2	239.2
specified site — see Neoplasm, skin						
sympathetic nerve or nervous system NEC	171.9	198.89	—	215.9	238.1	239.2
symphysis pubis	170.6	198.5	—	213.6	238.0	239.2
synovial membrane — see Neoplasm, connective tissue						
tapetum, brain	191.8	198.3	—	225.0	237.5	239.6
tarsus (any bone)	170.8	198.5	—	213.8	238.0	239.2
temple (skin)	173.3	198.2	232.3	216.3	238.2	239.2
temporal						
bone	170.0	198.5	—	213.0	238.0	239.2
lobe or pole	191.2	198.3	—	225.0	237.5	239.6
region	195.0	198.89	234.8	229.8	238.8	239.8
skin	173.3	198.2	232.3	216.3	238.2	239.2
tendon (sheath) — see Neoplasm, connective tissue						
tentorium (cerebelli)	192.1	198.4	—	225.2	237.6	239.7
testis, testes (descended) (scrotal)	186.9	198.82	233.6	222.0	236.4	239.5
ectopic	186.0	198.82	233.6	222.0	236.4	239.5
retained	186.0	198.82	233.6	222.0	236.4	239.5
undescended	186.0	198.82	233.6	222.0	236.4	239.5
thalamus	191.0	198.3	—	225.0	237.5	239.6
thigh NEC*	195.5	198.89	234.8	229.8	238.8	239.8
thorax, thoracic (cavity) (organs NEC)	195.1	198.89	234.8	229.8	238.8	239.8
duct	171.4	198.89	—	215.4	238.1	239.2
wall NEC	195.1	198.89	234.8	229.8	238.8	239.8
throat	149.0	198.89	230.0	210.9	235.1	239.0
thumb NEC*	195.4	198.89	232.6	229.8	238.8	239.8
thymus (gland)	164.0	198.89	—	212.6	235.8	239.8
contiguous sites with heart and mediastinum	164.8	—	—	—	—	—
thyroglossal duct	193	198.89	234.8	226	237.4	239.7
thyroid (gland)	193	198.89	234.8	226	237.4	239.7
cartilage	161.3	197.3	231.0	212.1	235.6	239.1
tibia (any part)	170.7	198.5	—	213.7	238.0	239.2
toe NEC*	195.5	198.89	232.7	229.8	238.8	239.8
tongue	141.9	198.89	230.0	210.1	235.1	239.0
anterior (two-thirds) NEC	141.4	198.89	230.0	210.1	235.1	239.0
dorsal surface	141.1	198.89	230.0	210.1	235.1	239.0
ventral surface	141.3	198.89	230.0	210.1	235.1	239.0
base (dorsal surface)	141.0	198.89	230.0	210.1	235.1	239.0
border (lateral)	141.2	198.89	230.0	210.1	235.1	239.0
contiguous sites	141.8	—	—	—	—	—

Neoplasm, neoplastic — continued	Malignant			Benign	Uncertain Behavior	Unspecified
	Primary	Secondary	Ca in situ			
tongue — continued						
dorsal surface NEC	141.1	198.89	230.0	210.1	235.1	239.0
fixed part NEC	141.0	198.89	230.0	210.1	235.1	239.0
foreamen cecum	141.1	198.89	230.0	210.1	235.1	239.0
frenulum linguae	141.3	198.89	230.0	210.1	235.1	239.0
junctional zone	141.5	198.89	230.0	210.1	235.1	239.0
margin (lateral)	141.2	198.89	230.0	210.1	235.1	239.0
midline NEC	141.1	198.89	230.0	210.1	235.1	239.0
mobile part NEC	141.4	198.89	230.0	210.1	235.1	239.0
posterior (third)	141.0	198.89	230.0	210.1	235.1	239.0
root	141.0	198.89	230.0	210.1	235.1	239.0
surface (dorsal)	141.1	198.89	230.0	210.1	235.1	239.0
base	141.0	198.89	230.0	210.1	235.1	239.0
ventral	141.3	198.89	230.0	210.1	235.1	239.0
tip	141.2	198.89	230.0	210.1	235.1	239.0
tonsil	141.6	198.89	230.0	210.1	235.1	239.0
tonsil	146.0	198.89	230.0	210.5	235.1	239.0
fauces, faucial	146.0	198.89	230.0	210.5	235.1	239.0
lingual	141.6	198.89	230.0	210.1	235.1	239.0
palatine	146.0	198.89	230.0	210.5	235.1	239.0
pharyngeal	147.1	198.89	230.0	210.7	235.1	239.0
pillar (anterior) (posterior)	146.2	198.89	230.0	210.6	235.1	239.0
tonsillar fossa	146.1	198.89	230.0	210.6	235.1	239.0
tooth socket NEC	143.9	198.89	230.0	210.4	235.1	239.0
trachea (cartilage) (mucosa)	162.0	197.3	231.1	212.2	235.7	239.1
contiguous sites with bronchus or lung	162.8	—	—	—	—	—
tracheobronchial	162.8	197.3	231.1	212.2	235.7	239.1
contiguous sites with lung	162.8	—	—	—	—	—
tragus	173.2	198.2	232.2	216.2	238.2	239.2
trunk NEC*	195.8	198.89	232.5	229.8	238.8	239.8
tubo-ovarian	183.8	198.82	233.3	221.8	236.3	239.5
tunica vaginalis	187.8	198.82	233.6	222.8	236.6	239.5
turbinate (bone)	170.0	198.5	—	213.0	238.0	239.2
nasal	160.0	197.3	231.8	212.0	235.9	239.1
tympanic cavity	160.1	197.3	231.8	212.0	235.9	239.1
ulna (any part)	170.4	198.5	—	213.4	238.0	239.2
umbilicus, umbilical	173.5	198.2	232.5	216.5	238.2	239.2
uncus, brain	191.2	198.3	—	225.0	237.5	239.6
unknown site or unspecified	199.1	199.1	234.9	229.9	238.9	239.9
urachus	188.7	198.1	233.7	223.3	236.7	239.4
ureter, ureteral	189.2	198.1	233.9	223.2	236.91	239.5
orifice (bladder)	188.6	198.1	233.7	223.3	236.7	239.4
ureter-bladder junction	188.6	198.1	233.7	223.3	236.7	239.4
urethra, urethral (gland)	189.3	198.1	233.9	223.81	236.99	239.5
orifice, internal	188.5	198.1	233.7	223.3	236.7	239.4
urethrovaginal (septum)	184.9	198.82	233.3	221.9	236.3	239.5
urinary organ or system NEC	189.9	198.1	233.9	223.9	236.99	239.5
bladder — see Neoplasm, bladder						
contiguous sites	189.8	—	—	—	—	—
specified sites NEC	189.8	198.1	233.9	223.89	236.99	239.5
utero-ovarian	183.8	198.82	233.3	221.8	236.3	239.5
ligament	183.3	198.82	—	221.0	236.3	239.5
uterosacral ligament	183.4	198.82	—	221.0	236.3	239.5
uterus, uteri, uterine	179	198.82	233.2	219.9	236.0	239.5
adnexa NEC	183.9	198.82	233.3	221.8	236.3	239.5
contiguous sites	183.8	—	—	—	—	—
body	182.0	198.82	233.2	219.1	236.0	239.5
contiguous sites	182.8	—	—	—	—	—
cervix	180.9	198.82	233.1	219.0	236.0	239.5
tornu	182.0	198.82	233.2	219.1	236.0	239.5
corpus	182.0	198.82	233.2	219.1	236.0	239.5
endocervix (canal) (gland)	180.0	198.82	233.1	219.0	236.0	239.5
endometrium	182.0	198.82	233.2	219.1	236.0	239.5
exocervix	180.1	198.82	233.1	219.0	236.0	239.5
external os	180.1	198.82	233.1	219.0	236.0	239.5
fundus	182.0	198.82	233.2	219.1	236.0	239.5
internal os	180.0	198.82	233.1	219.0	236.0	239.5
isthmus	182.1	198.82	233.2	219.1	236.0	239.5
ligament	183.4	198.82	—	221.0	236.3	239.5
broad	183.3	198.82	233.3	221.0	236.3	239.5
round	183.5	198.82	—	221.0	236.3	239.5
lower segment	182.1	198.82	233.2	219.1	236.0	239.5
myometrium	182.0	198.82	233.2	219.1	236.0	239.5
squamocolumnar junction	180.8	198.82	233.1	219.0	236.0	239.5
tube	183.2	198.82	233.3	221.0	236.3	239.5

☑ Additional Digit Required ◄► Revised Text ● New Line ▲ Revised Code

Neoplasm, neoplastic — *continued*	Malignant			Benign	Uncertain Behavior	Unspecified
	Primary	Secondary	Ca in situ			
utricle, prostatic	189.3	198.1	233.9	223.81	236.99	239.5
uveal tract	190.0	198.4	234.0	224.0	238.8	239.8
uvula	145.4	198.89	230.0	210.4	235.1	239.0
vagina, vaginal (fornix) (vault) (wall)	184.0	198.82	233.3	221.1	236.3	239.5
vaginovesical	184.9	198.82	233.3	221.9	236.3	239.5
septum	194.9	198.82	233.3	221.9	236.3	239.5
vallecula (epiglottis)	146.3	198.89	230.0	210.6	235.1	239.0
vascular — *see* Neoplasm, connective tissue						
vas deferens	187.6	198.82	233.6	222.8	236.6	239.5
Vater's ampulla	156.2	197.8	230.8	211.5	235.3	239.0
vein, venous — *see* Neoplasm, connective tissue						
vena cava (abdominal) (inferior)	171.5	198.89	—	215.5	238.1	239.2
superior	171.4	198.89	—	215.4	238.1	239.2
ventricle (cerebral) (floor) (fourth) (lateral) (third)	191.5	198.3	—	225.0	237.5	239.6
cardiac (left) (right)	164.1	198.89	—	212.7	238.8	239.8
ventricular band of larynx	161.1	197.3	231.0	212.1	235.6	239.1
ventriculus — see Neoplasm, stomach						
vermillion border — *see* Neoplasm, lip						
vermis, cerebellum	191.6	198.3	—	225.0	237.5	239.6
vertebra (column)	170.2	198.5	—	213.2	238.0	239.2
coccyx	170.6	198.5	—	213.6	238.0	239.2
sacrum	170.6	198.5	—	213.6	238.0	239.2
vesical — *see* Neoplasm, bladder						
vesicle, seminal	187.8	198.82	233.6	222.8	236.6	239.5
vesicocervical tissue	184.9	198.82	233.3	221.9	236.3	239.5
vesicorectal	195.3	198.89	234.8	229.8	238.8	239.8
vesicovaginal	184.9	198.82	233.3	221.9	236.3	239.5
septum	184.9	198.82	233.3	221.9	236.3	239.5

Neoplasm, neoplastic — *continued*	Malignant			Benign	Uncertain Behavior	Unspecified
	Primary	Secondary	Ca in situ			
vessel (blood) — *see* Neoplasm, connective tissue						
vestibular gland, greater	184.1	198.82	233.3	221.2	236.3	239.5
vestibule						
mouth	145.1	198.89	230.0	210.4	235.1	239.0
nose	160.0	197.3	231.8	212.0	235.9	239.1
Virchow's gland	—	196.0	—	229.0	238.8	239.8
viscera NEC	195.8	198.89	234.8	229.8	238.8	239.8
vocal cords (true)	161.0	197.3	231.0	212.1	235.6	239.1
false	161.1	197.3	231.0	212.1	235.6	239.1
vomer	170.0	198.5	—	213.0	238.0	239.2
vulva	184.4	198.82	233.3	221.2	236.3	239.5
vulvovaginal gland	184.4	198.82	233.3	221.2	236.3	239.5
Waldeyer's ring	149.1	198.89	230.0	210.9	235.1	239.0
Wharton's duct	142.1	198.89	230.0	210.2	235.0	239.0
white matter (central) (cerebral)	191.0	198.3	—	225.0	237.5	239.6
windpipe	162.0	197.3	231.1	212.2	235.7	239.1
Wirsung's duct	157.3	197.8	230.9	211.6	235.5	239.0
wolffian (body) (duct)						
female	184.8	198.82	233.3	221.8	236.3	239.5
male	187.8	198.82	233.6	222.8	236.6	239.5
womb — *see* Neoplasm, uterus						
wrist NEC*	195.4	198.89	232.6	229.8	238.8	239.8
xiphoid process	170.3	198.5	—	213.3	238.0	239.2
Zuckerkandl's organ	194.6	198.89	—	227.6	237.3	239.7

Neovascularization
  choroid 362.16
  ciliary body 364.42
  cornea 370.60
    deep 370.63
    localized 370.61
  iris 364.42
  retina 362.16
  subretinal 362.16
Nephralgia 788.0
Nephritis, nephritic (albuminuric) (azotemic) (congenital) (degenerative) (diffuse) (disseminated) (epithelial) (familial) (focal) (granulomatous) (hemorrhagic) (infantile) (nonsuppurative, excretory) (uremic) 583.9
  with
    edema — *see* Nephrosis
    lesion of
      glomerulonephritis
        hypocomplementemic persistent 583.2
          with nephrotic syndrome 581.2
          chronic 582.2
        lobular 583.2
          with nephrotic syndrome 581.2
          chronic 582.2
        membranoproliferative 583.2
          with nephrotic syndrome 581.2
          chronic 582.2
        membranous 583.1
          with nephrotic syndrome 581.1
          chronic 582.1
        mesangiocapillary 583.2
          with nephrotic syndrome 581.2
          chronic 582.2
        mixed membranous and proliferative 583.2
          with nephrotic syndrome 581.2
          chronic 582.2
        proliferative (diffuse) 583.0
          with nephrotic syndrome 581.0
          acute 580.0
          chronic 582.0

Nephritis, nephritic — *continued*
  with — *continued*
    lesion of — *continued*
      glomerulonephritis — *continued*
        rapidly progressive 583.4
          acute 580.4
          chronic 582.4
      interstitial nephritis (diffuse) (focal) 583.89
        with nephrotic syndrome 581.89
        acute 580.89
        chronic 582.89
      necrotizing glomerulitis 583.4
        acute 580.4
        chronic 582.4
      renal necrosis 583.9
        cortical 583.6
        medullary 583.7
      specified pathology NEC 583.89
        with nephrotic syndrome 581.89
        acute 580.89
        chronic 582.89
    necrosis, renal 583.9
      cortical 583.6
      medullary (papillary) 583.7
    nephrotic syndrome (*see also* Nephrosis) 581.9
    papillary necrosis 583.7
    specified pathology NEC 583.89
  acute 580.9
    extracapillary with epithelial crescents 580.4
    hypertensive (*see also* Hypertension, kidney) 403.90
    necrotizing 580.4
    poststreptococcal 580.0
    proliferative (diffuse) 580.0
    rapidly progressive 580.4
    specified pathology NEC 580.89
  amyloid 277.3 [583.81]
    chronic 277.3 [582.81]
  arteriolar (*see also* Hypertension, kidney) 403.90
  arteriosclerotic (*see also* Hypertension, kidney) 403.90

Nephritis, nephritic — *continued*
  ascending (*see also* Pyelitis) 590.80
  atrophic 582.9
  basement membrane NEC 583.89
    with
      pulmonary hemorrhage (Goodpasture's syndrome) 446.21 [583.81]
  calculous, calculus 592.0
  cardiac (*see also* Hypertension, kidney) 403.90
  cardiovascular (*see also* Hypertension, kidney) 403.90
  chronic 582.9
    arteriosclerotic (*see also* Hypertension, kidney) 403.90
    hypertensive (*see also* Hypertension, kidney) 403.90
  cirrhotic (*see also* Sclerosis, renal) 587
  complicating pregnancy, childbirth, or puerperium 646.2 ☑
    with hypertension 642.1 ☑
      affecting fetus or newborn 760.0
    affecting fetus or newborn 760.1
  croupous 580.9
  desquamative — *see* Nephrosis
  due to
    amyloidosis 277.3 [583.81]
      chronic 277.3 [582.81]
    arteriosclerosis (*see also* Hypertension, kidney) 403.90
    diabetes mellitus 250.4 ☑ [583.81]
      with nephrotic syndrome 250.4 ☑ [581.81]
    diphtheria 032.89 [580.81]
    gonococcal infection (acute) 098.19 [583.81]
      chronic or duration of 2 months or over 098.39 [583.81]
    gout 274.10
    infectious hepatitis 070.9 [580.81]
    mumps 072.79 [580.81]
    specified kidney pathology NEC 583.89
      acute 580.89
      chronic 582.89
    streptotrichosis 039.8 [583.81]
    subacute bacterial endocarditis 421.0

Nephritis, nephritic — continued

- due to — *continued*
  - systemic lupus erythematosus 710.0 *[583.81]*
    - chronic 710.0 *[582.81]*
  - typhoid fever 002.0 *[580.81]*
- endothelial 582.2
- end stage (chronic) (terminal) NEC 585
- epimembranous 581.1
- exudative 583.89
  - with nephrotic syndrome 581.89
  - acute 580.89
  - chronic 582.89
- gonococcal (acute) 098.19 *[583.81]*
  - chronic or duration of 2 months or over 098.39 *[583.81]*
- gouty 274.10
- hereditary (Alport's syndrome) 759.89
- hydremic — *see* Nephrosis
- hypertensive (*see also* Hypertension, kidney) 403.90
- hypocomplementemic persistent 583.2
  - with nephrotic syndrome 581.2
  - chronic 582.2
- immune complex NEC 583.89
- infective (*see also* Pyelitis) 590.80
- interstitial (diffuse) (focal) 583.89
  - with nephrotic syndrome 581.89
  - acute 580.89
  - chronic 582.89
- latent or quiescent — *see* Nephritis, chronic
- lead 984.9
  - specified type of lead — *see* Table of Drugs and Chemicals
- lobular 583.2
  - with nephrotic syndrome 581.2
  - chronic 582.2
- lupus 710.0 *[583.81]*
  - acute 710.0 *[580.81]*
  - chronic 710.0 *[582.81]*
- membranoproliferative 583.2
  - with nephrotic syndrome 581.2
  - chronic 582.2
- membranous 583.1
  - with nephrotic syndrome 581.1
  - chronic 582.1
- mesangiocapillary 583.2
  - with nephrotic syndrome 581.2
  - chronic 582.2
- minimal change 581.3
- mixed membranous and proliferative 583.2
  - with nephrotic syndrome 581.2
  - chronic 582.2
- necrotic, necrotizing 583.4
  - acute 580.4
  - chronic 582.4
- nephrotic — *see* Nephrosis
- old — *see* Nephritis, chronic
- parenchymatous 581.89
- polycystic 753.12
  - adult type (APKD) 753.13
  - autosomal dominant 753.13
  - autosomal recessive 753.14
  - childhood type (CPKD) 753.14
  - infantile type 753.14
- poststreptococcal 580.0
- pregnancy — *see* Nephritis, complicating pregnancy
- proliferative 583.0
  - with nephrotic syndrome 581.0
  - acute 580.0
  - chronic 582.0
- purulent (*see also* Pyelitis) 590.80
- rapidly progressive 583.4
  - acute 580.4
  - chronic 582.4
- salt-losing or salt-wasting (*see also* Disease, renal) 593.9
- saturnine 984.9
  - specified type of lead — *see* Table of Drugs and Chemicals
- septic (*see also* Pyelitis) 590.80
- specified pathology NEC 583.89
  - acute 580.89
  - chronic 582.89
- staphylococcal (*see also* Pyelitis) 590.80
- streptotrichosis 039.8 *[583.81]*

Nephritis, nephritic — *continued*

- subacute (*see also* Nephrosis) 581.9
- suppurative (*see also* Pyelitis) 590.80
- syphilitic (late) 095.4
  - congenital 090.5 *[583.81]*
  - early 091.69 *[583.81]*
- terminal (chronic) (end-stage) NEC 585
- toxic — *see* Nephritis, acute
- tubal, tubular — *see* Nephrosis, tubular
- tuberculous (*see also* Tuberculosis) 016.0 ☑ *[583.81]*
- type II (Ellis) — *see* Nephrosis
- vascular — *see* Hypertension, kidney
- war 580.9

Nephroblastoma (M8960/3) 189.0
- epithelial (M8961/3) 189.0
- mesenchymal (M8962/3) 189.0

Nephrocalcinosis 275.49

Nephrocystitis, pustular (*see also* Pyelitis) 590.80

Nephrolithiasis (congenital) (pelvis) (recurrent) 592.0
- uric acid 274.11

Nephroma (M8960/3) 189.0
- mesoblastic (M8960/1) 236.9 ☑

Nephronephritis (*see also* Nephrosis) 581.9

Nephronophthisis 753.16

Nephropathy (*see also* Nephritis) 583.9
- with
  - exudative nephritis 583.89
  - interstitial nephritis (diffuse) (focal) 583.89
  - medullary necrosis 583.7
  - necrosis 583.9
    - cortical 583.6
    - medullary or papillary 583.7
  - papillary necrosis 583.7
  - specified lesion or cause NEC 583.89
- analgesic 583.89
  - with medullary necrosis, acute 584.7
- arteriolar (*see also* Hypertension, kidney) 403.90
- arteriosclerotic (*see also* Hypertension, kidney) 403.90
- complicating pregnancy 646.2 ☑
- diabetic 250.4 ☑ *[583.81]*
- gouty 274.10
  - specified type NEC 274.19
- hypercalcemic 588.89 ▲
- hypertensive (*see also* Hypertension, kidney) 403.90
- hypokalemic (vacuolar) 588.89 ▲
- IgA 583.9 ●
- obstructive 593.89
  - congenital 753.20
- phenacetin 584.7
- phosphate-losing 588.0
- potassium depletion 588.89 ▲
- proliferative (*see also* Nephritis, proliferative) 583.0
- protein-losing 588.89 ▲
- salt-losing or salt-wasting (*see also* Disease, renal) 593.9
- sickle-cell (*see also* Disease, sickle-cell) 282.60 *[583.81]*
- toxic 584.5
- vasomotor 584.5
- water-losing 588.89 ▲

Nephroptosis (*see also* Disease, renal) 593.0
- congenital (displaced) 753.3

Nephropyosis (*see also* Abscess, kidney) 590.2

Nephrorrhagia 593.81

Nephrosclerosis (arteriolar) (arteriosclerotic) (chronic) (hyaline) (*see also* Hypertension, kidney) 403.90
- gouty 274.10
- hyperplastic (arteriolar) (*see also* Hypertension, kidney) 403.90
- senile (*see also* Sclerosis, renal) 587

Nephrosis, nephrotic (Epstein's) (syndrome) 581.9
- with
  - lesion of
    - focal glomerulosclerosis 581.1
    - glomerulonephritis
      - endothelial 581.2

Nephrosis, nephrotic — *continued*

- with — *continued*
  - lesion of — *continued*
    - glomerulonephritis — *continued*
      - hypocomplementemic persistent 581.2
      - lobular 581.2
      - membranoproliferative 581.2
      - membranous 581.1
      - mesangiocapillary 581.2
      - minimal change 581.3
      - mixed membranous and proliferative 581.2
      - proliferative 581.0
    - segmental hyalinosis 581.1
    - specified pathology NEC 581.89
- acute — *see* Nephrosis, tubular
- anoxic — *see* Nephrosis, tubular
- arteriosclerotic (*see also* Hypertension, kidney) 403.90
- chemical — *see* Nephrosis, tubular
- cholemic 572.4
- complicating pregnancy, childbirth, or puerperium — *see* Nephritis, complicating pregnancy
- diabetic 250.4 ☑ *[581.81]*
- hemoglobinuric — *see* Nephrosis, tubular
- in
  - amyloidosis 277.3 *[581.81]*
  - diabetes mellitus 250.4 ☑ *[581.81]*
  - epidemic hemorrhagic fever 078.6
  - malaria 084.9 *[581.81]*
  - polyarteritis 446.0 *[581.81]*
  - systemic lupus erythematosus 710.0 *[581.81]*
- ischemic — *see* Nephrosis, tubular
- lipoid 581.3
- lower nephron — *see* Nephrosis, tubular
- lupoid 710.0 *[581.81]*
- lupus 710.0 *[581.81]*
- malarial 084.9 *[581.81]*
- minimal change 581.3
- necrotizing — *see* Nephrosis, tubular
- osmotic (sucrose) 588.89 ▲
- polyarteritic 446.0 *[581.81]*
- radiation 581.9
- specified lesion or cause NEC 581.89
- syphilitic 095.4
- toxic — *see* Nephrosis, tubular
- tubular (acute) 584.5
  - due to a procedure 997.5
  - radiation 581.9

Nephrosonephritis hemorrhagic (endemic) 078.6

Nephrostomy status V44.6
- with complication 997.5

Nerve — *see* condition

Nerves 799.2

Nervous (*see also* condition) 799.2
- breakdown 300.9
- heart 306.2
- stomach 306.4
- tension 799.2

Nervousness 799.2

Nesidioblastoma (M8150/0)
- pancreas 211.7
- specified site NEC — *see* Neoplasm, by site, benign
- unspecified site 211.7

Netherton's syndrome (ichthyosiform erythroderma) 757.1

Nettle rash 708.8

Nettleship's disease (urticaria pigmentosa) 757.33

Neumann's disease (pemphigus vegetans) 694.4

Neuralgia, neuralgic (acute) (*see also* Neuritis) 729.2
- accessory (nerve) 352.4
- acoustic (nerve) 388.5
- ankle 355.8
- anterior crural 355.8
- anus 787.99
- arm 723.4
- auditory (nerve) 388.5
- axilla 353.0
- bladder 788.1

Nephritis, nephritic — Neuralgia, neuralgic

☑ Additional Digit Required   ►◄ Revised Text   ● New Line   ▲ Revised Code

244 — Volume 2 • October 2004

2005 ICD•9•CM

Neuralgia, neuralgic (*see also* Neuritis) — *continued*
brachial 723.4
brain — *see* Disorder, nerve, cranial
broad ligament 625.9
cerebral — *see* Disorder, nerve, cranial
ciliary 346.2 ☑
cranial nerve — *see* also Disorder, nerve, cranial
  fifth or trigeminal (*see also* Neuralgia, trigeminal) 350.1
ear 388.71
  middle 352.1
facial 351.8
finger 354.9
flank 355.8
foot 355.8
forearm 354.9
Fothergill's (*see also* Neuralgia, trigeminal) 350.1
  postherpetic 053.12
glossopharyngeal (nerve) 352.1
groin 355.8
hand 354.9
heel 355.8
Horton's 346.2 ☑
Hunt's 053.11
hypoglossal (nerve) 352.5
iliac region 355.8
infraorbital (*see also* Neuralgia, trigeminal) 350.1
inguinal 355.8
intercostal (nerve) 353.8
  postherpetic 053.19
jaw 352.1
kidney 788.0
knee 355.8
loin 355.8
malarial (*see also* Malaria) 084.6
mastoid 385.89
maxilla 352.1
median thenar 354.1
metatarsal 355.6
middle ear 352.1
migrainous 346.2 ☑
Morton's 355.6
nerve, cranial — *see* Disorder, nerve, cranial
nose 352.0
occipital 723.8
ophthalmic 377.30
  postherpetic 053.19
optic (nerve) 377.30
penis 607.9
perineum 355.8
pleura 511.0
postherpetic NEC 053.19
  geniculate ganglion 053.11
  ophthalmic 053.19
  trifacial 053.12
  trigeminal 053.12
pubic region 355.8
radial (nerve) 723.4
rectum 787.99
sacroiliac joint 724.3
sciatic (nerve) 724.3
scrotum 608.9
seminal vesicle 608.9
shoulder 354.9
Sluder's 337.0
specified nerve NEC — *see* Disorder, nerve
spermatic cord 608.9
sphenopalatine (ganglion) 337.0
subscapular (nerve) 723.4
suprascapular (nerve) 723.4
testis 608.89
thenar (median) 354.1
thigh 355.8
tongue 352.5
trifacial (nerve) (*see also* Neuralgia, trigeminal) 350.1
trigeminal (nerve) 350.1
  postherpetic 053.12
tympanic plexus 388.71
ulnar (nerve) 723.4
vagus (nerve) 352.3
wrist 354.9

Neuralgia, neuralgic (*see also* Neuritis) — *continued*
writers' 300.89
  organic 333.84
Neurapraxia — *see* Injury, nerve, by site
Neurasthenia 300.5
cardiac 306.2
gastric 306.4
heart 306.2
postfebrile 780.79
postviral 780.79
Neurilemmoma (M9560/0) — *see also* Neoplasm, connective tissue, benign
acoustic (nerve) 225.1
malignant (M9560/3) — *see also* Neoplasm, connective tissue, malignant
  acoustic (nerve) 192.0
Neurilemmosarcoma (M9560/3) — *see* Neoplasm, connective tissue, malignant
Neurilemoma — *see* Neurilemmoma
Neurinoma (M9560/0) — *see* Neurilemmoma
Neurinomatosis (M9560/1) — *see also* Neoplasm, connective tissue, uncertain behavior
centralis 759.5
Neuritis (*see also* Neuralgia) 729.2
abducens (nerve) 378.54
accessory (nerve) 352.4
acoustic (nerve) 388.5
  syphilitic 094.86
alcoholic 357.5
  with psychosis 291.1
amyloid, any site 277.3 [357.4]
anterior crural 355.8
arising during pregnancy 646.4 ☑
arm 723.4
ascending 355.2
auditory (nerve) 388.5
brachial (nerve) NEC 723.4
  due to displacement, intervertebral disc 722.0
cervical 723.4
chest (wall) 353.8
costal region 353.8
cranial nerve — *see also* Disorder, nerve, cranial
  first or olfactory 352.0
  second or optic 377.30
  third or oculomotor 378.52
  fourth or trochlear 378.53
  fifth or trigeminal (*see also* Neuralgia, trigeminal) 350.1
  sixth or abducens 378.54
  seventh or facial 351.8
    newborn 767.5
  eighth or acoustic 388.5
  ninth or glossopharyngeal 352.1
  tenth or vagus 352.3
  eleventh or accessory 352.4
  twelfth or hypoglossal 352.5
Déjérine-Sottas 356.0
diabetic 250.6 ☑ [357.2]
diphtheritic 032.89 [357.4]
due to
  beriberi 265.0 [357.4]
  displacement, prolapse, protrusion, or rupture of intervertebral disc 722.2
    cervical 722.0
    lumbar, lumbosacral 722.10
    thoracic, thoracolumbar 722.11
  herniation, nucleus pulposus 722.2
    cervical 722.0
    lumbar, lumbosacral 722.10
    thoracic, thoracolumbar 722.11
endemic 265.0 [357.4]
facial (nerve) 351.8
  newborn 767.5
general — *see* Polyneuropathy
geniculate ganglion 351.1
  due to herpes 053.11
glossopharyngeal (nerve) 352.1
gouty 274.89 [357.4]
hypoglossal (nerve) 352.5
ilioinguinal (nerve) 355.8
in diseases classified elsewhere — *see* Polyneuropathy, in
infectious (multiple) 357.0

Neuritis (*see also* Neuralgia) — *continued*
intercostal (nerve) 353.8
interstitial hypertrophic progressive NEC 356.9
leg 355.8
lumbosacral NEC 724.4
median (nerve) 354.1
  thenar 354.1
multiple (acute) (infective) 356.9
  endemic 265.0 [357.4]
multiplex endemica 265.0 [357.4]
nerve root (*see also* Radiculitis) 729.2
oculomotor (nerve) 378.52
olfactory (nerve) 352.0
optic (nerve) 377.30
  in myelitis 341.0
  meningococcal 036.81
pelvic 355.8
peripheral (nerve) — *see also* Neuropathy, peripheral
  complicating pregnancy or puerperium 646.4 ☑
  specified nerve NEC — *see* Mononeuritis
pneumogastric (nerve) 352.3
postchickenpox 052.7
postherpetic 053.19
progressive hypertrophic interstitial NEC 356.9
puerperal, postpartum 646.4 ☑
radial (nerve) 723.4
retrobulbar 377.32
  syphilitic 094.85
rheumatic (chronic) 729.2
sacral region 355.8
sciatic (nerve) 724.3
  due to displacement of intervertebral disc 722.10
serum 999.5
specified nerve NEC — *see* Disorder, nerve
spinal (nerve) 355.9
  root (*see also* Radiculitis) 729.2
subscapular (nerve) 723.4
suprascapular (nerve) 723.4
syphilitic 095.8
thenar (median) 354.1
thoracic NEC 724.4
toxic NEC 357.7
trochlear (nerve) 378.53
ulnar (nerve) 723.4
vagus (nerve) 352.3
Neuroangiomatosis, encephalofacial 759.6
Neuroastrocytoma (M9505/1) — *see* Neoplasm, by site, uncertain behavior
Neuro-avitaminosis 269.2
Neuroblastoma (M9500/3)
olfactory (M9522/3) 160.0
specified site — *see* Neoplasm, by site, malignant
unspecified site 194.0
Neurochorioretinitis (*see also* Chorioretinitis) 363.20
Neurocirculatory asthenia 306.2
Neurocytoma (M9506/0) — *see* Neoplasm, by site, benign
Neurodermatitis (circumscribed) (circumscripta) (local) 698.3
atopic 691.8
diffuse (Brocq) 691.8
disseminated 691.8
nodulosa 698.3
Neuroencephalomyelopathy, optic 341.0
Neuroepithelioma (M9503/3) — *see also* Neoplasm, by site, malignant
olfactory (M9521/3) 160.0
Neurofibroma (M9540/0) — *see also* Neoplasm, connective tissue, benign
melanotic (M9541/0) — *see* Neoplasm, connective tissue, benign
multiple (M9540/1) 237.70
  type 1 237.71
  type 2 237.72
plexiform (M9550/0) — *see* Neoplasm, connective tissue, benign
Neurofibromatosis (multiple) (M9540/1) 237.70
acoustic 237.72
malignant (M9540/3) — *see* Neoplasm, connective tissue, malignant

Neurofibromatosis (M9540/1) — *continued*
  type 1 237.71
  type 2 237.72
  von Recklinghausen's 237.71
Neurofibrosarcoma (M9540/3) — *see* Neoplasm, connective tissue, malignant
Neurogenic — *see also* condition
  bladder (atonic) (automatic) (autonomic) (flaccid) (hypertonic) (hypotonic) (inertia) (infranuclear) (irritable) (motor) (nonreflex) (nuclear) (paralysis) (reflex) (sensory) (spastic) (supranuclear) (uninhibited) 596.54
    with cauda equina syndrome 344.61
  bowel 564.81
  heart 306.2
Neuroglioma (M9505/1) — *see* Neoplasm, by site, uncertain behavior
Neurolabyrinthitis (of Dix and Hallpike) 386.12
Neurolathyrism 988.2
Neuroleprosy 030.1
Neuroleptic malignant syndrome 333.92
Neurolipomatosis 272.8
Neuroma (M9570/0) — *see also* Neoplasm, connective tissue, benign
  acoustic (nerve) (M9560/0) 225.1
  amputation (traumatic) — *see also* Injury, nerve, by site
    surgical complication (late) 997.61
  appendix 211.3
  auditory nerve 225.1
  digital 355.6
    toe 355.6
  interdigital (toe) 355.6
  intermetatarsal 355.6
  Morton's 355.6
  multiple 237.70
    type 1 237.71
    type 2 237.72
  nonneoplastic 355.9
    arm NEC 354.9
    leg NEC 355.8
    lower extremity NEC 355.8
    specified site NEC — *see* Mononeuritis, by site
    upper extremity NEC 354.9
  optic (nerve) 225.1
  plantar 355.6
  plexiform (M9550/0) — *see* Neoplasm, connective tissue, benign
  surgical (nonneoplastic) 355.9
    arm NEC 354.9
    leg NEC 355.8
    lower extremity NEC 355.8
    upper extremity NEC 354.9
  traumatic — *see also* Injury, nerve, by site
    old — *see* Neuroma, nonneoplastic
Neuromyalgia 729.1
Neuromyasthenia (epidemic) 049.8
Neuromyelitis 341.8
  ascending 357.0
  optica 341.0
Neuromyopathy NEC 358.9
Neuromyositis 729.1
Neuronevus (M8725/0) — *see* Neoplasm, skin, benign
Neuronitis 357.0
  ascending (acute) 355.2
  vestibular 386.12
Neuroparalytic — *see* condition
Neuropathy, neuropathic (*see also* Disorder, nerve) 355.9
  acute motor 357.82
  alcoholic 357.5
    with psychosis 291.1
  arm NEC 354.9
  ataxia and retinitis pigmentosa (NARP syndrome) 277.87
  autonomic (peripheral) — *see* Neuropathy, peripheral, autonomic
  axillary nerve 353.0
  brachial plexus 353.0
  cervical plexus 353.2

Neuropathy, neuropathic (*see also* Disorder, nerve) — *continued*
  chronic
    progressive segmentally demyelinating 357.89
    relapsing demyelinating 357.89
  congenital sensory 356.2
  Déjérine-Sottas 356.0
  diabetic 250.6 ☑ *[357.2]*
  entrapment 355.9
    iliohypogastric nerve 355.79
    ilioinguinal nerve 355.79
    lateral cutaneous nerve of thigh 355.1
    median nerve 354.0
    obturator nerve 355.79
    peroneal nerve 355.3
    posterior tibial nerve 355.5
    saphenous nerve 355.79
    ulnar nerve 354.2
  facial nerve 351.9
  hereditary 356.9
    peripheral 356.0
    sensory (radicular) 356.2
  hypertrophic
    Charcôt-Marie-Tooth 356.1
    Déjérine-Sottas 356.0
    interstitial 356.9
    Refsum 356.3
  intercostal nerve 354.8
  ischemic — *see* Disorder, nerve
  Jamaican (ginger) 357.7
  leg NEC 355.8
  lower extremity NEC 355.8
  lumbar plexus 353.1
  median nerve 354.1
  motor
    acute 357.82
  multiple (acute) (chronic) (*see also* Polyneuropathy) 356.9
  optic 377.39
    ischemic 377.41
    nutritional 377.33
    toxic 377.34
  peripheral (nerve) (*see also* Polyneuropathy) 356.9
    arm NEC 354.9
    autonomic 337.9
      amyloid 277.3 *[337.1]*
      idiopathic 337.0
      in
        amyloidosis 277.3 *[337.1]*
        diabetes (mellitus) 250.6 ☑ *[337.1]*
        diseases classified elsewhere 337.1
        gout 274.89 *[337.1]*
        hyperthyroidism 242.9 ☑ *[337.1]*
    due to
      antitetanus serum 357.6
      arsenic 357.7
      drugs 357.6
      lead 357.7
      organophosphate compounds 357.7
      toxic agent NEC 357.7
    hereditary 356.0
    idiopathic 356.9
      progresive 356.4
      specified type NEC 356.8
    in diseases classified elsewhere — *see* Polyneuropathy, in
    leg NEC 355.8
    lower extremity NEC 355.8
    upper extremity NEC 354.9
  plantar nerves 355.6
  progressive hypertrophic interstitial 356.9
  radicular NEC 729.2
    brachial 723.4
    cervical NEC 723.4
    hereditary sensory 356.2
    lumbar 724.4
    lumbosacral 724.4
    thoracic NEC 724.4
  sacral plexus 353.1
  sciatic 355.0
  spinal nerve NEC 355.9
    root (*see also* Radiculitis) 729.2
  toxic 357.7
  trigeminal sensory 350.8
  ulnar nerve 354.2
  upper extremity NEC 354.9

Neuropathy, neuropathic (*see also* Disorder, nerve) — *continued*
  uremic 585 *[357.4]*
  vitamin B₁₂ 266.2 *[357.4]*
    with anemia (pernicious) 281.0 *[357.4]*
      due to dietary deficiency 281.1 *[357.4]*
Neurophthisis — (*see also* Disorder, nerve peripheral) 356.9
  diabetic 250.6 ☑ *[357.2]*
Neuropraxia — *see* Injury, nerve
Neuroretinitis 363.05
  syphilitic 094.85
Neurosarcoma (M9540/3) — *see* Neoplasm, connective tissue, malignant
Neurosclerosis — *see* Disorder, nerve
Neurosis, neurotic 300.9
  accident 300.16
  anancastic, anankastic 300.3
  anxiety (state) 300.00
    generalized 300.02
    panic type 300.01
  asthenic 300.5
  bladder 306.53
  cardiac (reflex) 306.2
  cardiovascular 306.2
  climacteric, unspecified type 627.2
  colon 306.4
  compensation 300.16
  compulsive, compulsion 300.3
  conversion 300.11
  craft 300.89
  cutaneous 306.3
  depersonalization 300.6
  depressive (reaction) (type) 300.4
  endocrine 306.6
  environmental 300.89
  fatigue 300.5
  functional (*see also* Disorder, psychosomatic) 306.9
  gastric 306.4
  gastrointestinal 306.4
  genitourinary 306.50
  heart 306.2
  hypochondriacal 300.7
  hysterical 300.10
    conversion type 300.11
    dissociative type 300.15
  impulsive 300.3
  incoordination 306.0
    larynx 306.1
    vocal cord 306.1
  intestine 306.4
  larynx 306.1
    hysterical 300.11
    sensory 306.1
  menopause, unspecified type 627.2
  mixed NEC 300.89
  musculoskeletal 306.0
  obsessional 300.3
    phobia 300.3
  obsessive-compulsive 300.3
  occupational 300.89
  ocular 306.7
  oral 307.0
  organ (*see also* Disorder, psychosomatic) 306.9
  pharynx 306.1
  phobic 300.20
  posttraumatic (acute) (situational) 309.81 ▲
    chronic 309.81
  psychasthenic (type) 300.89
  railroad 300.16
  rectum 306.4
  respiratory 306.1
  rumination 306.4
  senile 300.89
  sexual 302.70
  situational 300.89
  specified type NEC 300.89
  state 300.9
    with depersonalization episode 300.6
  stomach 306.4
  vasomotor 306.2
  visceral 306.4
  war 300.16
Neurospongioblastosis diffusa 759.5

Neurosyphilis (arrested) (early) (inactive) (late) (latent) (recurrent) 094.9
  with ataxia (cerebellar) (locomotor) (spastic) (spinal) 094.0
  acute meningitis 094.2
  aneurysm 094.89
  arachnoid (adhesive) 094.2
  arteritis (any artery) 094.89
  asymptomatic 094.3
  congenital 090.40
  dura (mater) 094.89
  general paresis 094.1
  gumma 094.9
  hemorrhagic 094.9
  juvenile (asymptomatic) (meningeal) 090.40
  leptomeninges (aseptic) 094.2
  meningeal 094.2
  meninges (adhesive) 094.2
  meningovascular (diffuse) 094.2
  optic atrophy 094.84
  parenchymatous (degenerative) 094.1
  paresis (see also Paresis, general) 094.1
  paretic (see also Paresis, general) 094.1
  relapse 094.9
  remission in (sustained) 094.9
  serological 094.3
  specified nature or site NEC 094.89
  tabes (dorsalis) 094.0
    juvenile 090.40
  tabetic 094.0
    juvenile 090.40
  taboparesis 094.1
    juvenile 090.40
  thrombosis 094.89
  vascular 094.89
Neurotic (see also Neurosis) 300.9
  excoriation 698.4
    psychogenic 306.3
Neurotmesis — see Injury, nerve, by site
Neurotoxemia — see Toxemia
▶**Neutro-occlusion**◀ 524.21 ▲
Neutropenia, neutropenic (chronic) (cyclic) (drug-induced) (genetic) (idiopathic) (immune) (infantile) (malignant) (periodic) (pernicious) (primary) (splenic) (splenomegaly) (toxic) 288.0
  chronic hypoplastic 288.0
  congenital (nontransient) 288.0
  fever 288.0
  neonatal, transitory (isoimmune) (maternal transfer) 776.7
Neutrophilia, hereditary giant 288.2
Nevocarcinoma (M8720/3) — see Melanoma
Nevus (M8720/0) — see also Neoplasm, skin, benign

Note — Except where otherwise indicated, varieties of nevus in the list below that are followed by a morphology code number (M----/0) should be coded by site as for "Neoplasm, skin, benign."

  acanthotic 702.8
  achromic (M8730/0)
  amelanotic (M8730/0)
  anemic, anemicus 709.09
  angiomatous (M9120/0) (see also Hemangioma) 228.00
  araneus 448.1
  avasculosus 709.09
  balloon cell (M8722/0)
  bathing trunk (M8761/1) 238.2
  blue (M8780/0)
    cellular (M8790/0)
    giant (M8790/0)
    Jadassohn's (M8780/0)
    malignant (M8780/3) — see Melanoma
  capillary (M9131/0) (see also Hemangioma) 228.00
  cavernous (M9121/0) (see also Hemangioma) 228.00
  cellular (M8720/0)
    blue (M8790/0)
  comedonicus 757.33
  compound (M8760/0)
  conjunctiva (M8720/0) 224.3

Nevus (M8720/0) — see also Neoplasm, skin, benign — continued
  dermal (M8750/0)
    and epidermal (M8760/0)
  epithelioid cell (and spindle cell) (M8770/0)
  flammeus 757.32
    osteohypertrophic 759.89
  hairy (M8720/0)
  halo (M8723/0)
  hemangiomatous (M9120/0) (see also Hemangioma) 228.00
  intradermal (M8750/0)
  intraepidermal (M8740/0)
  involuting (M8724/0)
  Jadassohn's (blue) (M8780/0)
  junction, junctional (M8740/0)
    malignant melanoma in (M8740/3) — see Melanoma
  juvenile (M8770/0)
  lymphatic (M9170/0) 228.1
  magnocellular (M8726/0)
    specified site — see Neoplasm, by site, benign
    unspecified site 224.0
  malignant (M8720/3) — see Melanoma
  meaning hemangioma (M9120/0) (see also Hemangioma) 228.00
  melanotic (pigmented) (M8720/0)
  multiplex 759.5
  nonneoplastic 448.1
  nonpigmented (M8730/0)
  nonvascular (M8720/0)
  oral mucosa, white sponge 750.26
  osteohypertrophic, flammeus 759.89
  papillaris (M8720/0)
  papillomatosus (M8720/0)
  pigmented (M8720/0)
    giant (M8761/1) — see also Neoplasm, skin, uncertain behavior
      malignant melanoma in (M8761/3) — see Melanoma
    systematicus 757.33
  pilosus (M8720/0)
  port wine 757.32
  sanguineous 757.32
  sebaceous (senile) 702.8
  senile 448.1
  spider 448.1
  spindle cell (and epithelioid cell) (M8770/0)
  stellar 448.1
  strawberry 757.32
  syringocystadenomatous papilliferous (M8406/0)
  unius lateris 757.33
  Unna's 757.32
  vascular 757.32
  verrucous 757.33
  white sponge (oral mucosa) 750.26
Newborn (infant) (liveborn)
  affected by maternal abuse of drugs (gestational) (via placenta) (via breast milk) 760.70
  gestation
    24 completed weeks 765.22
    25-26 completed weeks 765.23
    27-28 completed weeks 765.24
    29-30 completed weeks 765.25
    31-32 completed weeks 765.26
    33-34 completed weeks 765.27
    35-36 completed weeks 765.28
    37 or more completed weeks 765.29
    less than 24 completed weeks 765.21
    unspecified completed weeks 765.20
  multiple NEC
    born in hospital (without mention of cesarean delivery or section) V37.00
      with cesarean delivery or section V37.01
    born outside hospital
      hospitalized V37.1
      not hospitalized V37.2
    mates all liveborn
      born in hospital (without mention of cesarean delivery or section) V34.00
        with cesarean delivery or section V34.01

Newborn — continued
  multiple NEC — continued
    mates all liveborn — continued
      born outside hospital
        hospitalized V34.1
        not hospitalized V34.2
    mates all stillborn
      born in hospital (without mention of cesarean delivery or section) V35.00
        with cesarean delivery or section V35.01
      born outside hospital
        hospitalized V35.1
        not hospitalized V35.2
    mates liveborn and stillborn
      born in hospital (without mention of cesarean delivery or section) V36.00
        with cesarean delivery or section V36.01
      born outside hospital
        hospitalized V36.1
        not hospitalized V36.2
  single
    born in hospital (without mention of cesarean delivery or section) V30.00
      with cesarean delivery or section V30.01
    born outside hospital
      hospitalized V30.1
      not hospitalized V30.2
  twin NEC
    born in hospital (without mention of cesarean delivery or section) V33.00
      with cesarean delivery or section V33.01
    born outside hospital
      hospitalized V33.1
      not hospitalized V33.2
    mate liveborn
      born in hospital V31.0 ☑
      born outside hospital
        hospitalized V31.1
        not hospitalized V31.2
    mate stillborn
      born in hospital V32.0 ☑
      born outside hospital
        hospitalized V32.1
        not hospitalized V32.2
  unspecified as to single or multiple birth
    born in hospital (without mention of cesarean delivery or section) V39.00
      with cesarean delivery or section V39.01
    born outside hospital
      hospitalized V39.1
      not hospitalized V39.2
Newcastle's conjunctivitis or disease 077.8
Nezelof's syndrome (pure alymphocytosis) 279.13
Niacin (amide) **deficiency** 265.2
Nicolas-Durand-Favre disease (climatic bubo) 099.1
Nicolas-Favre disease (climatic bubo) 099.1
Nicotinic acid (amide) **deficiency** 265.2
Niemann-Pick disease (lipid histiocytosis) (splenomegaly) 272.7
Night
  blindness (see also Blindness, night) 368.60
    congenital 368.61
    vitamin A deficiency 264.5
  cramps 729.82
  sweats 780.8
  terrors, child 307.46
Nightmare 307.47
  REM-sleep type 307.47
Nipple — see condition
Nisbet's chancre 099.0
Nishimoto (-Takeuchi) disease 437.5
Nitritoid crisis or reaction — see Crisis, nitritoid
Nitrogen retention, extrarenal 788.9
Nitrosohemoglobinemia 289.89
Njovera 104.0
No
  diagnosis 799.9
  disease (found) V71.9
  room at the inn V65.0
Nocardiasis — see Nocardiosis

Nocardiosis 039.9
  with pneumonia 039.1
  lung 039.1
  specified type NEC 039.8
Nocturia 788.43
  psychogenic 306.53
Nocturnal — *see also* condition
  dyspnea (paroxysmal) 786.09
  emissions 608.89
  enuresis 788.36
    psychogenic 307.6
  frequency (micturition) 788.43
    psychogenic 306.53
Nodal rhythm disorder 427.89
Nodding of head 781.0
Node(s) — *see also* Nodule
  Heberden's 715.04
  larynx 478.79
  lymph — *see* condition
  milkers' 051.1
  Osler's 421.0
  rheumatic 729.89
  Schmorl's 722.30
    lumbar, lumbosacral 722.32
    specified region NEC 722.39
    thoracic, thoracolumbar 722.31
  singers' 478.5
  skin NEC 782.2
  tuberculous — *see* Tuberculosis, lymph gland
  vocal cords 478.5
Nodosities, Haygarth's 715.04
Nodule(s), nodular
  actinomycotic (*see also* Actinomycosis) 039.9
  arthritic — *see* Arthritis, nodosa
  cutaneous 782.2
  Haygarth's 715.04
  inflammatory — *see* Inflammation
  juxta-articular 102.7
    syphilitic 095.7
    yaws 102.7
  larynx 478.79
  lung, solitary 518.89
    emphysematous 492.8
  milkers' 051.1
  prostate 600.10
    with urinary retention 600.11
  rheumatic 729.89
  rheumatoid — *see* Arthritis, rheumatoid
  scrotum (inflammatory) 608.4
  singers' 478.5
  skin NEC 782.2
  solitary, lung 518.89
    emphysematous 492.8
  subcutaneous 782.2
  thyroid (gland) (nontoxic) (uninodular) 241.0
    with
      hyperthyroidism 242.1 ☑
      thyrotoxicosis 242.1 ☑
    toxic or with hyperthyroidism 242.1 ☑
  vocal cords 478.5
Noma (gangrenous) (hospital) (infective) 528.1
  auricle (*see also* Gangrene) 785.4
  mouth 528.1
  pudendi (*see also* Vulvitis) 616.10
  vulvae (*see also* Vulvitis) 616.10
Nomadism V60.0
Non-adherence
  artificial skin graft 996.55
  decellularized allodermis graft 996.55
Non-autoimmune hemolytic anemia NEC
  283.10
Nonclosure — *see also* Imperfect, closure
  ductus
    arteriosus 747.0
    Botalli 747.0
  Eustachian valve 746.89
  foramen
    Botalli 745.5
    ovale 745.5
Noncompliance with medical treatment V15.81
Nondescent (congenital) — *see also* Malposition,
    congenital
  cecum 751.4
  colon 751.4
  testis 752.51

Nondevelopment
  brain 742.1
    specified part 742.2
  heart 746.89
  organ or site, congenital NEC — *see* Hypoplasia
Nonengagement
  head NEC 652.5 ☑
    in labor 660.1 ☑
      affecting fetus or newborn 763.1
Nonexanthematous tick fever 066.1
Nonexpansion, lung (newborn) NEC 770.4
Nonfunctioning
  cystic duct (*see also* Disease, gallbladder) 575.8
  gallbladder (*see also* Disease, gallbladder)
    575.8
  kidney (*see also* Disease, renal) 593.9
  labyrinth 386.58
Nonhealing
  stump (surgical) 997.69
  wound, surgical 998.83
Nonimplantation of ovum, causing infertility
  628.3
Noninsufflation, fallopian tube 628.2
Nonne-Milroy-Meige syndrome (chronic
    hereditary edema) 757.0
Nonovulation 628.0
Nonpatent fallopian tube 628.2
Nonpneumatization, lung NEC 770.4
Nonreflex bladder 596.54
  with cauda equina 344.61
Nonretention of food — *see* Vomiting
Nonrotation — *see* Malrotation
Nonsecretion, urine (*see also* Anuria) 788.5
  newborn 753.3
Nonunion
  fracture 733.82
  organ or site, congenital NEC — *see* Imperfect,
    closure
  symphysis pubis, congenital 755.69
  top sacrum, congenital 756.19
Nonviability 765.0 ☑
Nonvisualization, gallbladder 793.3
Nonvitalized tooth 522.9
Non-working side interference 524.56   ●
Normal
  delivery — *see* category 650
  menses V65.5
  state (feared complaint unfounded) V65.5
Normoblastosis 289.89
Normocytic anemia (infectional) 285.9
  due to blood loss (chronic) 280.0
    acute 285.1
Norrie's disease (congenital) (progressive
    oculoacousticocerebral degeneration) 743.8
North American blastomycosis 116.0
Norwegian itch 133.0
Nose, nasal — *see* condition
Nosebleed 784.7
Nosomania 298.9
Nosophobia 300.29
Nostalgia 309.89
Notch of iris 743.46
Notched lip, congenital (*see also* Cleft, lip)
  749.10
Notching nose, congenital (tip) 748.1
Nothnagel's
  syndrome 378.52
  vasomotor acroparesthesia 443.89
Novy's relapsing fever (American) 087.1
Noxious
  foodstuffs, poisoning by
    fish 988.0
    fungi 988.1
    mushrooms 988.1
    plants (food) 988.2
    shellfish 988.0
    specified type NEC 988.8
    toadstool 988.1

Noxious — *continued*
  substances transmitted through placenta or
      breast milk ▶(affecting fetus or
      newborn)◀ 760.70
    alcohol 760.71
    anti-infective agents 760.74
    cocaine 760.75
    "crack" 760.75
    diethylstilbestrol (DES) 760.76
    hallucinogenic agents NEC 760.73
    medicinal agents NEC 760.79
    narcotics 760.72
    obstetric anesthetic or analgesic 763.5
    specified agent NEC 760.79
    suspected, affecting management of
        pregnancy 655.5 ☑
Nuchal hitch (arm) 652.8 ☑
Nucleus pulposus — *see* condition
Numbness 782.0
Nuns' knee 727.2
Nursemaid's
  elbow 832.0 ☑
  shoulder 831.0 ☑
Nutmeg liver 573.8
Nutrition, deficient or insufficient (particular
    kind of food) 269.9
  due to
    insufficient food 994.2
    lack of
      care (child) (infant) 995.52
        adult 995.84
      food 994.2
Nyctalopia (*see also* Blindness, night) 368.60
  vitamin A deficiency 264.5
Nycturia 788.43
  psychogenic 306.53
Nymphomania 302.89
Nystagmus 379.50
  associated with vestibular system disorders
      379.54
  benign paroxysmal positional 386.11
  central positional 386.2
  congenital 379.51
  deprivation 379.53
  dissociated 379.55
  latent 379.52
  miners' 300.89
  positional
    benign paroxysmal 386.11
    central 386.2
  specified NEC 379.56
  vestibular 379.54
  visual deprivation 379.53

O

Oasthouse urine disease 270.2
Obermeyer's relapsing fever (European) 087.0
Obesity (constitutional) (exogenous) (familial) (nutritional) (simple) 278.00
  adrenal 255.8
  due to hyperalimentation 278.00
  endocrine NEC 259.9
  endogenous 259.9
  Fröhlich's (adiposogenital dystrophy) 253.8
  glandular NEC 259.9
  hypothyroid (see also Hypothyroidism) 244.9
  morbid 278.01
  of pregnancy 646.1 ☑
  pituitary 253.8
  severe 278.01
  thyroid (see also Hypothyroidism) 244.9
Oblique — see also condition
  lie before labor, affecting fetus or newborn 761.7
Obliquity, pelvis 738.6
Obliteration
  abdominal aorta 446.7
  appendix (lumen) 543.9
  artery 447.1
  ascending aorta 446.7
  bile ducts 576.8
    with calculus, choledocholithiasis, or stones — see Choledocholithiasis
    congenital 751.61
      jaundice from 751.61 [774.5]
  common duct 576.8
    with calculus, choledocholithiasis, or stones — see Choledocholithiasis
    congenital 751.61
  cystic duct 575.8
    with calculus, choledocholithiasis, or stones — see Choledocholithiasis
  disease, arteriolar 447.1
  endometrium 621.8
  eye, anterior chamber 360.34
  fallopian tube 628.2
  lymphatic vessel 457.1
    postmastectomy 457.0
  organ or site, congenital NEC — see Atresia
  placental blood vessels — see Placenta, abnormal
  supra-aortic branches 446.7
  ureter 593.89
  urethra 599.84
  vein 459.9
  vestibule (oral) 525.8
Observation (for) V71.9
  without need for further medical care V71.9
  accident NEC V71.4
    at work V71.3
  criminal V71.6
  deleterious agent ingestion V71.89
  disease V71.9
    cardiovascular V71.7
      heart V71.7
    mental V71.09
    specified condition NEC V71.89
  foreign body ingestion V71.89
  growth and development variations V21.8
  injuries (accidental) V71.4
    inflicted NEC V71.6
      during alleged rape or seduction V71.5
  malignant neoplasm, suspected V71.1
  postpartum
    immediately after delivery V24.0
    routine follow-up V24.2
  pregnancy
    high-risk V23.9
      specified problem NEC V23.8 ☑
    normal (without complication) V22.1
      with nonobstetric complication V22.2
      first V22.0
  rape or seduction, alleged V71.5
    injury during V71.5
  suicide attempt, alleged V71.89
  suspected (undiagnosed) (unproven)
    abuse V71.81
    cardiovascular disease V71.7
    child or wife battering victim V71.6
    concussion (cerebral) V71.6

Observation — continued
  suspected — continued
    condition NEC V71.89
      infant — see Observation, suspected, condition, newborn
      newborn V29.9
        cardiovascular disease V29.8
        congenital anomaly V29.8
        genetic V29.3
        infectious V29.0
        ingestion foreign object V29.8
        injury V29.8
        metabolic V29.3
        neoplasm V29.8
        neurological V29.1
        poison, poisoning V29.8
        respiratory V29.2
        specified NEC V29.8
    exposure
      anthrax V71.82
      biologic agent NEC V71.83
      SARS V71.83
    infectious disease not requiring isolation V71.89
    malignant neoplasm V71.1 ☑
    mental disorder V71.09
    neglect V71.81
    neoplasm
      benign V71.89
      malignant V71.1
    specified condition NEC V71.89
    tuberculosis V71.2
  tuberculosis, suspected V71.2
Obsession, obsessional 300.3
  ideas and mental images 300.3
  impulses 300.3
  neurosis 300.3
  phobia 300.3
  psychasthenia 300.3
  ruminations 300.3
  state 300.3
  syndrome 300.3
Obsessive-compulsive 300.3
  neurosis 300.3
  personality 301.4   ●
  reaction 300.3
Obstetrical trauma NEC (complicating delivery) 665.9 ☑
  with
    abortion — see Abortion, by type, with damage to pelvic organs
    ectopic pregnancy (see also categories 633.0-633.9) 639.2
    molar pregnancy (see also categories 630-632) 639.2
  affecting fetus or newborn 763.89
  following
    abortion 639.2
    ectopic or molar pregnancy 639.2
Obstipation (see also Constipation) 564.00
  psychogenic 306.4
Obstruction, obstructed, obstructive
  airway NEC 519.8
    with
      allergic alveolitis NEC 495.9
      asthma NEC (see also Asthma) 493.9 ☑
      bronchiectasis 494.0
        with acute exacerbation 494.1
      bronchitis (chronic) (see also Bronchitis, with, obstruction) 491.20
      emphysema NEC 492.8
    chronic 496
      with
        allergic alveolitis NEC 495.5
        asthma NEC (see also Asthma) 493.2 ☑
        bronchiectasis 494.0
          with acute exacerbation 494.1
        bronchitis (chronic) (see also Bronchitis, with, obstruction) 491.20
        emphysema NEC 492.8
    due to
      bronchospasm 519.1
      foreign body 934.9
      inhalation of fumes or vapors 506.9

Obstruction, obstructed, obstructive — continued
  airway NEC — continued
    due to — continued
      laryngospasm 478.75
  alimentary canal (see also Obstruction, intestine) 560.9
  ampulla of Vater 576.2
    with calculus, cholelithiasis, or stones — see Choledocholithiasis
  aortic (heart) (valve) (see also Stenosis, aortic) 424.1
    rheumatic (see also Stenosis, aortic, rheumatic) 395.0
  aortoiliac 444.0
  aqueduct of Sylvius 331.4
    congenital 742.3
      with spina bifida (see also Spina bifida) 741.0 ☑
  Arnold-Chiari (see also Spina bifida) 741.0 ☑
  artery (see also Embolism, artery) 444.9
    basilar (complete) (partial) (see also Occlusion, artery, basilar) 433.0 ☑
    carotid (complete) (partial) (see also Occlusion, artery, carotid) 433.1 ☑
    precerebral — see Occlusion, artery, precerebral NEC
    retinal (central) (see also Occlusion, retina) 362.30
    vertebral (complete) (partial) (see also Occlusion, artery, vertebral) 433.2 ☑
  asthma (chronic) (with obstructive pulmonary disease) 493.2 ☑
  band (intestinal) 560.81
  bile duct or passage (see also Obstruction, biliary) 576.2
    congenital 751.61
      jaundice from 751.61 [774.5]
  biliary (duct) (tract) 576.2
    with calculus 574.51
      with cholecystitis (chronic) 574.41
        acute 574.31
    congenital 751.61
      jaundice from 751.61 [774.5]
    gallbladder 575.2
      with calculus 574.21
        with cholecystitis (chronic) 574.11
          acute 574.01
  bladder neck (acquired) 596.0
    congenital 753.6
  bowel (see also Obstruction, intestine) 560.9
  bronchus 519.1
  canal, ear (see also Stricture, ear canal, acquired) 380.50
  cardia 537.89
  caval veins (inferior) (superior) 459.2
  cecum (see also Obstruction, intestine) 560.9
  circulatory 459.9
  colon (see also Obstruction, intestine) 560.9
    sympathicotonic 560.89
  common duct (see also Obstruction, biliary) 576.2
    congenital 751.61
  coronary (artery) (heart) — see also Arteriosclerosis, coronary
    acute (see also Infarct, myocardium) 410.9 ☑
      without myocardial infarction 411.81
  cystic duct (see also Obstruction, gallbladder) 575.2
    congenital 751.61
  device, implant, or graft — see Complications, due to (presence of) any device, implant, or graft classified to 996.0-996.5 NEC
  due to foreign body accidentally left in operation wound 998.4
  duodenum 537.3
    congenital 751.1
    due to
      compression NEC 537.3
      cyst 537.3
      intrinsic lesion or disease NEC 537.3
      scarring 537.3
      torsion 537.3
      ulcer 532.91
      volvulus 537.3
  ejaculatory duct 608.89

Oasthouse urine disease — Obstruction, obstructed, obstructive

Obstruction, obstructed, obstructive — Occlusion (vertical side text)

Obstruction, obstructed, obstructive —
continued
  endocardium 424.90
    arteriosclerotic 424.99
    specified cause, except rheumatic 424.99
  esophagus 530.3
  eustachian tube (complete) (partial) 381.60
    cartilaginous
      extrinsic 381.63
      intrinsic 381.62
    due to
      cholesteatoma 381.61
      osseous lesion NEC 381.61
      polyp 381.61
    osseous 381.61
  fallopian tube (bilateral) 628.2
  fecal 560.39
    with hernia — *see also* Hernia, by site, with
      obstruction
      gangrenous — *see* Hernia, by site, with
        gangrene
  foramen of Monro (congenital) 742.3
    with spina bifida (*see also* Spina bifida)
      741.0 ☑
  foreign body — *see* Foreign body
  gallbladder 575.2
    with calculus, cholelithiasis, or stones
      574.21
      with cholecystitis (chronic) 574.11
        acute 574.01
    congenital 751.69
      jaundice from 751.69 *[774.5]*
  gastric outlet 537.0
  gastrointestinal (*see also* Obstruction,
    intestine) 560.9
  glottis 478.79
  hepatic 573.8
    duct (*see also* Obstruction, biliary) 576.2
      congenital 751.61
  icterus (*see also* Obstruction, biliary) 576.8
    congenital 751.61
  ileocecal coil (*see also* Obstruction, intestine)
    560.9
  ileum (*see also* Obstruction, intestine) 560.9
  iliofemoral (artery) 444.81
  internal anastomosis — *see* Complications,
    mechanical, graft
  intestine (mechanical) (neurogenic)
    (paroxysmal) (postinfectional) (reflex)
    560.9
    with
      adhesions (intestinal) (peritoneal) 560.81
      hernia — *see also* Hernia, by site, with
        obstruction
        gangrenous — *see* Hernia, by site,
          with gangrene
    adynamic (*see also* Ileus) 560.1
    by gallstone 560.31
    congenital or infantile (small) 751.1
      large 751.2
    due to
      Ascaris lumbricoides 127.0
      mural thickening 560.89
      procedure 997.4
        involving urinary tract 997.5
    impaction 560.39
    infantile — *see* Obstruction, intestine,
      congenital
    newborn
      due to
        fecaliths 777.1
        inspissated milk 777.2
        meconium (plug) 777.1
          in mucoviscidosis 277.01
        transitory 777.4
    specified cause NEC 560.89
    transitory, newborn 777.4
    volvulus 560.2
  intracardiac ball valve prosthesis 996.02
  jaundice (*see also* Obstruction, biliary) 576.8
    congenital 751.61
  jejunum (*see also* Obstruction, intestine) 560.9
  kidney 593.89
  labor 660.9 ☑
    affecting fetus or newborn 763.1

Obstruction, obstructed, obstructive —
continued
  labor — *continued*
    by
      bony pelvis (conditions classifiable to
        653.0-653.9) 660.1 ☑
      deep transverse arrest 660.3 ☑
      impacted shoulder 660.4 ☑
      locked twins 660.5 ☑
      malposition (fetus) (conditions classifiable
        to 652.0-652.9) 660.0 ☑
        head during labor 660.3 ☑
      persistent occipitoposterior position
        660.3 ☑
      soft tissue, pelvic (conditions classifiable
        to 654.0-654.9) 660.2 ☑
  lacrimal
    canaliculi 375.53
    congenital 743.65
    punctum 375.52
    sac 375.54
  lacrimonasal duct 375.56
    congenital 743.65
    neonatal 375.55
  lacteal, with steatorrhea 579.2
  laryngitis (*see also* Laryngitis) 464.01
  larynx 478.79
    congenital 748.3
  liver 573.8
    cirrhotic (*see also* Cirrhosis, liver) 571.5
  lung 518.89
    with
      asthma — *see* Asthma
      bronchitis (chronic) 491.20
      emphysema NEC 492.8
    airway, chronic 496
    chronic NEC 496
      with
        asthma (chronic) (obstructive) 493.2 ☑
    disease, chronic 496
      with
        asthma (chronic) (obstructive) 493.2 ☑
    emphysematous 492.8
  lymphatic 457.1
  meconium
    fetus or newborn 777.1
      in mucoviscidosis 277.01
    newborn due to fecaliths 777.1
  mediastinum 519.3
  mitral (rheumatic) — *see* Stenosis, mitral
  nasal 478.1
    duct 375.56
      neonatal 375.55
    sinus — *see* Sinusitis
  nasolacrimal duct 375.56
    congenital 743.65
    neonatal 375.55
  nasopharynx 478.29
  nose 478.1
  organ or site, congenital NEC — *see* Atresia
  pancreatic duct 577.8
  parotid gland 527.8
  pelviureteral junction (*see also* Obstruction,
    ureter) 593.4
  pharynx 478.29
  portal (circulation) (vein) 452
  prostate 600.90
    with urinary retention 600.91
    valve (urinary) 596.0
  pulmonary
    valve (heart) (*see also* Endocarditis,
      pulmonary) 424.3
    vein, isolated 747.49
  pyemic — *see* Septicemia
  pylorus (acquired) 537.0
    congenital 750.5
    infantile 750.5
  rectosigmoid (*see also* Obstruction, intestine)
    560.9
  rectum 569.49
  renal 593.89
  respiratory 519.8
    chronic 496
  retinal (artery) (vein) (central) (*see also*
    Occlusion, retina) 362.30
  salivary duct (any) 527.8
    with calculus 527.5

Obstruction, obstructed, obstructive —
continued
  sigmoid (*see also* Obstruction, intestine) 560.9
  sinus (accessory) (nasal) (*see also* Sinusitis)
    473.9
  Stensen's duct 527.8
  stomach 537.89
    acute 536.1
    congenital 750.7
  submaxillary gland 527.8
    with calculus 527.5
  thoracic duct 457.1
  thrombotic — *see* Thrombosis
  tooth eruption 520.6
  trachea 519.1
  tracheostomy airway 519.09
  tricuspid — *see* Endocarditis, tricuspid
  upper respiratory, congenital 748.8
  ureter (functional) 593.4
    congenital 753.20
    due to calculus 592.1
  ureteropelvic junction, congenital 753.21
  ureterovesical junction, congenital 753.22
  urethra 599.6
    congenital 753.6
  urinary (moderate) 599.6
    organ or tract (lower) 599.6
    prostatic valve 596.0
  uropathy 599.6
  uterus 621.8
  vagina 623.2
  valvular — *see* Endocarditis
  vascular graft or shunt 996.1
    atherosclerosis — *see* Arteriosclerosis,
      coronary
    embolism 996.74
    occlusion NEC 996.74
    thrombus 996.74
  vein, venous 459.2
    caval (inferior) (superior) 459.2
    thrombotic — *see* Thrombosis
  vena cava (inferior) (superior) 459.2
  ventricular shunt 996.2
  vesical 596.0
  vesicourethral orifice 596.0
  vessel NEC 459.9

Obturator — *see* condition

Occlusal
  plane deviation 524.76 ●
  wear, teeth 521.10 ●

Occlusion
  anus 569.49
    congenital 751.2
    infantile 751.2
  aortoiliac (chronic) 444.0
  aqueduct of Sylvius 331.4
    congenital 742.3
      with spina bifida (*see also* Spina bifida)
        741.0 ☑
  arteries of extremities, lower 444.22
    without thrombus or embolus (*see also*
      Arteriosclerosis, extremities) 440.20
    due to stricture or stenosis 447.1
    upper 444.21
      without thrombus or embolus (*see also*
        Arteriosclerosis, extremities) 440.20
      due to stricture or stenosis 447.1
  artery NEC (*see also* Embolism, artery) 444.9
    auditory, internal 433.8 ☑
    basilar 433.0 ☑
      with other precerebral artery 433.3 ☑
      bilateral 433.3 ☑
    brain or cerebral (*see also* Infarct, brain)
      434.9 ☑
    carotid 433.1 ☑
      with other precerebral artery 433.3 ☑
      bilateral 433.3 ☑
    cerebellar (anterior inferior) (posterior
      inferior) (superior) 433.8 ☑
    cerebral (*see also* Infarct, brain) 434.9 ☑
    choroidal (anterior) 433.8 ☑
    communicating posterior 433.8 ☑
    coronary (thrombotic) (*see also* Infarct,
      myocardium) 410.9 ☑
      acute 410.9 ☑
        without myocardial infarction 411.81

Occlusion — *continued*
  artery (*see also* Embolism, artery) — *continued*
    coronary — *continued*
      healed or old 412
    hypophyseal 433.8 ☑
    iliac 444.81
    mesenteric (embolic) (thrombotic) (with
        gangrene) 557.0
    pontine 433.8 ☑
    precerebral NEC 433.9 ☑
      late effect — *see* Late effect(s) (of)
          cerebrovascular disease
      multiple or bilateral 433.3 ☑
      puerperal, postpartum, childbirth
          674.0 ☑
      specified NEC 433.8 ☑
    renal 593.81
    retinal — *see* Occlusion, retina, artery
    spinal 433.8 ☑
    vertebral 433.2 ☑
      with other precerebral artery 433.3 ☑
      bilateral 433.3 ☑
  basilar (artery) — *see* Occlusion, artery, basilar
  bile duct (any) (*see also* Obstruction, biliary)
      576.2
  bowel (*see also* Obstruction, intestine) 560.9
  brain (artery) (vascular) (*see also* Infarct, brain)
      434.9 ☑
  breast (duct) 611.8
  carotid (artery) (common) (internal) — *see*
      Occlusion, artery, carotid
  cerebellar (anterior inferior) (artery) (posterior
      inferior) (superior) 433.8 ☑
  cerebral (artery) (*see also* Infarct, brain)
      434.9 ☑
  cerebrovascular (*see also* Infarct, brain)
      434.9 ☑
    diffuse 437.0
  cervical canal (*see also* Stricture, cervix) 622.4
    by falciparum malaria 084.0
  cervix (uteri) (*see also* Stricture, cervix) 622.4
  choanal 748.0
  choroidal (artery) 433.8 ☑
  colon (*see also* Obstruction, intestine) 560.9
  communicating posterior artery 433.8 ☑
  coronary (artery) (thrombotic) (*see also* Infarct,
      myocardium) 410.9 ☑
    acute 410.9 ☑
      without myocardial infarction 411.81
    healed or old 412
      without myocardial infarction 411.81
  cystic duct (*see also* Obstruction, gallbladder)
      575.2
    congenital 751.69
  disto
    division I 524.22   ●
    division II 524.22   ●
  embolic — *see* Embolism
  fallopian tube 628.2
    congenital 752.19
  gallbladder (*see also* Obstruction, gallbladder)
      575.2
    congenital 751.69
      jaundice from 751.69 [774.5]
  gingiva, traumatic 523.8
  hymen 623.3
    congenital 752.42
  hypophyseal (artery) 433.8 ☑
  iliac artery 444.81
  intestine (*see also* Obstruction, intestine) 560.9
  kidney 593.89
  lacrimal apparatus — *see* Stenosis, lacrimal
  lung 518.89
  lymph or lymphatic channel 457.1
  mammary duct 611.8
  mesenteric artery (embolic) (thrombotic) (with
      gangrene) 557.0
  nose 478.1
    congenital 748.0
  organ or site, congenital NEC — *see* Atresia
  oviduct 628.2
    congenital 752.19
  periodontal, traumatic 523.8
  peripheral arteries (lower extremity) 444.22
    without thrombus or embolus (*see also*
        Arteriosclerosis, extremities) 440.20
    due to stricture or stenosis 447.1

Occlusion — *continued*
  peripheral arteries — *continued*
    upper extremity 444.21
      without thrombus or embolus (*see also*
          Arteriosclerosis, extremities 440.20
      due to stricture or stenosis 447.1
  pontine (artery) 433.8 ☑
  posterior lingual, of mandibular teeth
      524.29   ▲
  precerebral artery — *see* Occlusion, artery,
      precerebral
  puncta lacrimalia 375.52
  pupil 364.74
  pylorus (*see also* Stricture, pylorus) 537.0
  renal artery 593.81
  retina, retinal (vascular) 362.30
    artery, arterial 362.30
      branch 362.32
      central (total) 362.31
      partial 362.33
      transient 362.34
      tributary 362.32
    vein 362.30
      branch 362.36
      central (total) 362.35
      incipient 362.37
      partial 362.37
      tributary 362.36
  spinal artery 433.8 ☑
  stent
    coronary 996.72
  teeth (mandibular) (posterior lingual)
      524.29   ▲
  thoracic duct 457.1
  tubal 628.2
  ureter (complete) (partial) 593.4
    congenital 753.29
  urethra (*see also* Stricture, urethra) 598.9
    congenital 753.6
  uterus 621.8
  vagina 623.2
  vascular NEC 459.9
  vein — *see* Thrombosis
  vena cava (inferior) (superior) 453.2
  ventricle (brain) NEC 331.4
  vertebral (artery) — *see* Occlusion, artery,
      vertebral
  vessel (blood) NEC 459.9
  vulva 624.8
Occlusio pupillae 364.74
Occupational
  problems NEC V62.2
  therapy V57.21
Ochlophobia 300.29
Ochronosis (alkaptonuric) (congenital)
    (endogenous) 270.2
  with chloasma of eyelid 270.2
Ocular muscle — *see also* condition
  myopathy 359.1
  torticollis 781.93
Oculoauriculovertebral dysplasia 756.0
Oculogyric
  crisis or disturbance 378.87
    psychogenic 306.7
Oculomotor syndrome 378.81
Oddi's sphincter spasm 576.5
Odelberg's disease (juvenile osteochondrosis)
    732.1
Odontalgia 525.9
Odontoameloblastoma (M9311/0) 213.1
  upper jaw (bone) 213.0
Odontoclasia 521.05
Odontoclasis 873.63
  complicated 873.73
Odontodysplasia, regional 520.4
Odontogenesis imperfecta 520.5
Odontoma (M9280/0) 213.1
  ameloblastic (M9311/0) 213.1
    upper jaw (bone) 213.0
  calcified (M9280/0) 213.1
    upper jaw (bone) 213.0
  complex (M9282/0) 213.1
    upper jaw (bone) 213.0

Odontoma — *continued*
  compound (M9281/0) 213.1
    upper jaw (bone) 213.0
  fibroameloblastic (M9290/0) 213.1
    upper jaw (bone) 213.0
  follicular 526.0
    upper jaw (bone) 213.0
Odontomyelitis (closed) (open) 522.0
Odontonecrosis 521.09
Odontorrhagia 525.8
Odontosarcoma, ameloblastic (M9290/3) 170.1
    upper jaw (bone) 170.0
Odynophagia 787.2
Oesophagostomiasis 127.7
Oesophagostomum infestation 127.7
Oestriasis 134.0
Ogilvie's syndrome (sympathicotonic colon
    obstruction) 560.89
Oguchi's disease (retina) 368.61
Ohara's disease (*see also* Tularemia) 021.9
Oidiomycosis (*see also* Candidiasis) 112.9
Oidiomycotic meningitis 112.83
Oidium albicans infection (*see also* Candidiasis)
    112.9
Old age 797
  dementia (of) 290.0
Olfactory — *see* condition
Oligemia 285.9
Oligergasia (*see also* Retardation, mental) 319
Oligoamnios 658.0 ☑
  affecting fetus or newborn 761.2
Oligoastrocytoma, mixed (M9382/3)
  specified site — *see* Neoplasm, by site,
      malignant
  unspecified site 191.9
Oligocythemia 285.9
Oligodendroblastoma (M9460/3)
  specified site — *see* Neoplasm, by site,
      malignant
  unspecified site 191.9
Oligodendroglioma (M9450/3)
  anaplastic type (M9451/3)
    specified site — *see* Neoplasm, by site,
        malignant
    unspecified site 191.9
  specified site — *see* Neoplasm, by site,
      malignant
  unspecified site 191.9
Oligodendroma — *see* Oligodendroglioma
Oligodontia (*see also* Anodontia) 520.0
Oligoencephalon 742.1
Oligohydramnios 658.0 ☑
  affecting fetus or newborn 761.2
  due to premature rupture of membranes
      658.1 ☑
    affecting fetus or newborn 761.2
Oligohydrosis 705.0
Oligomenorrhea 626.1
Oligophrenia (*see also* Retardation, mental) 319
  phenylpyruvic 270.1
Oligospermia 606.1
Oligotrichia 704.09
  congenita 757.4
Oliguria 788.5
  with
    abortion — *see* Abortion, by type, with renal
        failure
    ectopic pregnancy (*see also* categories
        633.0-633.9) 639.3
    molar pregnancy (*see also* categories 630-
        632) 639.3
  complicating
    abortion 639.3
    ectopic or molar pregnancy 639.3
    pregnancy 646.2 ☑
      with hypertension — *see* Toxemia, of
          pregnancy
  due to a procedure 997.5
  following labor and delivery 669.3 ☑
  heart or cardiac — *see* Failure, heart
  puerperal, postpartum 669.3 ☑

Occlusion — Oliguria

Oliguria — *continued*
  specified due to a procedure 997.5
Ollier's disease (chondrodysplasia) 756.4
Omentitis (*see also* Peritonitis) 567.9
Omentocele (*see also* Hernia, omental) 553.8
Omentum, omental — *see* condition
Omphalitis (congenital) (newborn) 771.4
  not of newborn 686.9
  tetanus 771.3
Omphalocele 756.79
Omphalomesenteric duct, persistent 751.0
Omphalorrhagia, newborn 772.3
Omsk hemorrhagic fever 065.1
Onanism 307.9
Onchocerciasis 125.3
  eye 125.3 *[360.13]*
Onchocercosis 125.3
Oncocytoma (M8290/0) — *see* Neoplasm, by site,
  benign
Ondine's curse 348.8
Oneirophrenia (*see also* Schizophrenia) 295.4 ☑
Onychauxis 703.8
  congenital 757.5
Onychia (with lymphangitis) 681.9
  dermatophytic 110.1
  finger 681.02
  toe 681.11
Onychitis (with lymphangitis) 681.9
  finger 681.02
  toe 681.11
Onychocryptosis 703.0
Onychodystrophy 703.8
  congenital 757.5
Onychogryphosis 703.8
Onychogryposis 703.8
Onycholysis 703.8
Onychomadesis 703.8
Onychomalacia 703.8
Onychomycosis 110.1
  finger 110.1
  toe 110.1
Onycho-osteodysplasia 756.89
Onychophagy 307.9
Onychoptosis 703.8
Onychorrhexis 703.8
  congenital 757.5
Onychoschizia 703.8
Onychotrophia (*see also* Atrophy, nail) 703.8
O'nyong-nyong fever 066.3
Onyxis (finger) (toe) 703.0
Onyxitis (with lymphangitis) 681.9
  finger 681.02
  toe 681.11
Oophoritis (cystic) (infectional) (interstitial) (*see
  also* Salpingo-oophoritis) 614.2
  complicating pregnancy 646.6 ☑
  fetal (acute) 752.0
  gonococcal (acute) 098.19
    chronic or duration of 2 months or over
    098.39
  tuberculous (*see also* Tuberculosis) 016.6 ☑
Opacity, opacities
  cornea 371.00
    central 371.03
    congenital 743.43
      interfering with vision 743.42
    degenerative (*see also* Degeneration, cornea)
      371.40
    hereditary (*see also* Dystrophy, cornea)
      371.50
    inflammatory (*see also* Keratitis) 370.9
    late effect of trachoma (healed) 139.1
    minor 371.01
    peripheral 371.02
  enamel (fluoride) (nonfluoride) (teeth) 520.3
  lens (*see also* Cataract) 366.9
  snowball 379.22
  vitreous (humor) 379.24
    congenital 743.51
Opalescent dentin (hereditary) 520.5

Open, opening
  abnormal, organ or site, congenital — *see*
    Imperfect, closure
  angle with
    borderline intraocular pressure 365.01
    cupping of discs 365.01
  bite (anterior) (posterior) 524.29   ▲
  false — *see* Imperfect, closure
  wound — *see* Wound, open, by site
Operation
  causing mutilation of fetus 763.89
  destructive, on live fetus, to facilitate birth
    763.89
  for delivery, fetus or newborn 763.89
  maternal, unrelated to current delivery,
    affecting fetus or newborn 760.6
Operational fatigue 300.89
Operative — *see* condition
Operculitis (chronic) 523.4
  acute 523.3
Operculum, retina 361.32
  with detachment 361.01
Ophiasis 704.01
Ophthalmia (*see also* Conjunctivitis) 372.30
  actinic rays 370.24
  allergic (acute) 372.05
    chronic 372.14
  blennorrhagic (neonatorum) 098.40
  catarrhal 372.03
  diphtheritic 032.81
  Egyptian 076.1
  electric, electrica 370.24
  gonococcal (neonatorum) 098.40
  metastatic 360.11
  migraine 346.8 ☑
  neonatorum, newborn 771.6
    gonococcal 098.40
  nodosa 360.14
  phlyctenular 370.31
    with ulcer (*see also* Ulcer, cornea) 370.00
  sympathetic 360.11
Ophthalmitis — *see* Ophthalmia
Ophthalmocele (congenital) 743.66
Ophthalmoneuromyelitis 341.0
**Ophthalmopathy, infiltrative with
  thyrotoxicosis** 242.0 ☑
Ophthalmoplegia (*see also* Strabismus) 378.9
  anterior internuclear 378.86
  ataxia-areflexia syndrome 357.0
  bilateral 378.9
  diabetic 250.5 ☑ *[378.86]*
  exophthalmic 242.0 ☑ *[376.22]*
  external 378.55
    progressive 378.72
    total 378.56
  interna(l) (complete) (total) 367.52
  internuclear 378.86
  migraine 346.8 ☑
  painful 378.55
  Parinaud's 378.81
  progressive external 378.72
  supranuclear, progressive 333.0
  total (external) 378.56
    internal 367.52
  unilateral 378.9
Opisthognathism 524.00
Opisthorchiasis (felineus) (tenuicollis) (viverrini)
  121.0
Opisthotonos, opisthotonus 781.0
Opitz's disease (congestive splenomegaly) 289.51
Opiumism (*see also* Dependence) 304.0 ☑
Oppenheim's disease 358.8
Oppenheim-Urbach disease or syndrome
  (necrobiosis lipoidica diabeticorum)
  250.8 ☑ *[709.3]*
Opsoclonia 379.59
Optic nerve — *see* condition
Orbit — *see* condition
Orchioblastoma (M9071/3) 186.9
Orchitis (nonspecific) (septic) 604.90
  with abscess 604.0

Orchitis — *continued*
  blennorrhagic (acute) 098.13
    chronic or duration of 2 months or over
    098.33
  diphtheritic 032.89 *[604.91]*
  filarial 125.9 *[604.91]*
  gangrenous 604.99
  gonococcal (acute) 098.13
    chronic or duration of 2 months or over
    098.33
  mumps 072.0
  parotidea 072.0
  suppurative 604.99
  syphilitic 095.8 *[604.91]*
  tuberculous (*see also* Tuberculosis)
    016.5 ☑ *[608.81]*
Orf 051.2
Organic — *see also* condition
  heart — *see* Disease, heart
  insufficiency 799.89
Oriental
  bilharziasis 120.2
  schistosomiasis 120.2
  sore 085.1
Orientation   ●
  ego-dystonic sexual 302.0   ●
Orifice — *see* condition
Origin, both great vessels from right ventricle
  745.11
Ormond's disease or syndrome 593.4
Ornithosis 073.9
  with
    complication 073.8
      specified NEC 073.7
    pneumonia 073.0
    pneumonitis (lobular) 073.0
Orodigitofacial dysostosis 759.89
Oropouche fever 066.3
Orotaciduria, oroticaciduria (congenital)
  (hereditary) (pyrimidine deficiency) 281.4
Oroya fever 088.0
Orthodontics V58.5
  adjustment V53.4
  aftercare V58.5
  fitting V53.4
Orthopnea 786.02
Orthoptic training V57.4
Os, uterus — *see* condition
Osgood-Schlatter
  disease 732.4
  osteochondrosis 732.4
Osler's
  disease (M9950/1) (polycythemia vera) 238.4
  nodes 421.0
Osler-Rendu disease (familial hemorrhagic
  telangiectasia) 448.0
Osler-Vaquez disease (M9950/1) (polycythemia
  vera) 238.4
Osler-Weber-Rendu syndrome (familial
  hemorrhagic telangiectasia) 448.0
Osmidrosis 705.89
Osseous — *see* condition
Ossification
  artery — *see* Arteriosclerosis
  auricle (ear) 380.39
  bronchus 519.1
  cardiac (*see also* Degeneration, myocardial)
    429.1
  cartilage (senile) 733.99
  coronary (artery) — *see* Arteriosclerosis,
    coronary
  diaphragm 728.10
  ear 380.39
    middle (*see also* Otosclerosis) 387.9
  falx cerebri 349.2
  fascia 728.10
  fontanel
    defective or delayed 756.0
    premature 756.0
  heart (*see also* Degeneration, myocardial) 429.1
    valve — *see* Endocarditis
  larynx 478.79

☑ Additional Digit Required   ▶◀ Revised Text   ● New Line   ▲ Revised Code

Ossification — *continued*
  ligament
    posterior longitudinal 724.8
      cervical 723.7
  meninges (cerebral) 349.2
    spinal 336.8
  multiple, eccentric centers 733.99
  muscle 728.10
    heterotopic, postoperative 728.13
  myocardium, myocardial (*see also*
    Degeneration, myocardial) 429.1
  penis 607.81
  periarticular 728.89
  sclera 379.16
  tendon 727.82
  trachea 519.1
  tympanic membrane (*see also*
    Tympanosclerosis) 385.00
  vitreous (humor) 360.44
Osteitis (*see also* Osteomyelitis) 730.2 ✓
  acute 730.0 ✓
  alveolar 526.5
  chronic 730.1 ✓
  condensans (ilii) 733.5
  deformans (Paget's) 731.0
    due to or associated with malignant
      neoplasm (*see also* Neoplasm, bone,
      malignant) 170.9 *[731.1]*
  due to yaws 102.6
  fibrosa NEC 733.29
    cystica (generalisata) 252.01   ▲
    disseminata 756.59
    osteoplastica 252.01   ▲
  fragilitans 756.51
  Garré's (sclerosing) 730.1 ✓
  infectious (acute) (subacute) 730.0 ✓
    chronic or old 730.1 ✓
  jaw (acute) (chronic) (lower) (neonatal)
    (suppurative) (upper) 526.4
  parathyroid 252.01   ▲
  petrous bone (*see also* Petrositis) 383.20
  pubis 733.5
  sclerotic, nonsuppurative 730.1 ✓
  syphilitic 095.5
  tuberculosa
    cystica (of Jüngling) 135
    multiplex cystoides 135
Osteoarthritica spondylitis (spine) (*see also*
  Spondylosis) 721.90
Osteoarthritis (*see also* Osteoarthrosis) 715.9 ✓
  distal interphalangeal 715.9 ✓
  hyperplastic 731.2
  interspinalis (*see also* Spondylosis) 721.90
  spine, spinal NEC (*see also* Spondylosis)
    721.90
Osteoarthropathy (*see also* Osteoarthrosis)
  715.9 ✓
  chronic idiopathic hypertrophic 757.39
  familial idiopathic 757.39
  hypertrophic pulmonary 731.2
    secondary 731.2
  idiopathic hypertrophic 757.39
  primary hypertrophic 731.2
  pulmonary hypertrophic 731.2
  secondary hypertrophic 731.2
Osteoarthrosis (degenerative) (hypertrophic)
  (rheumatoid) 715.9 ✓

*Note — Use the following fifth-digit
subclassification with category 715:*

  0   site unspecified
  1   shoulder region
  2   upper arm
  3   forearm
  4   hand
  5   pelvic region and thigh
  6   lower leg
  7   ankle and foot
  8   other specified sites except spine
  9   multiple sites

  Deformans alkaptonurica 270.2
  generalized 715.09
  juvenilis (Köhler's) 732.5

Osteoarthrosis — *continued*
  localized 715.3 ✓
    idiopathic 715.1 ✓
    primary 715.1 ✓
    secondary 715.2 ✓
  multiple sites, not specified as generalized
    715.89
  polyarticular 715.09
  spine (*see also* Spondylosis) 721.90
  temporomandibular joint 524.69
Osteoblastoma (M9200/0) — *see* Neoplasm,
  bone, benign
Osteochondritis (*see also* Osteochondrosis) 732.9
  dissecans 732.7
    hip 732.7
  ischiopubica 732.1
  multiple 756.59
  syphilitic (congenital) 090.0
Osteochondrodermodysplasia 756.59
Osteochondrodystrophy 277.5
  deformans 277.5
  familial 277.5
  fetalis 756.4
Osteochondrolysis 732.7
Osteochondroma (M9210/0) — *see also*
  Neoplasm, bone, benign
  multiple, congenital 756.4
Osteochondromatosis (M9210/1) 238.0
  synovial 727.82
Osteochondromyxosarcoma (M9180/3) — *see*
  Neoplasm, bone, malignant
Osteochondropathy NEC 732.9
Osteochondrosarcoma (M9180/3) — *see*
  Neoplasm, bone, malignant
Osteochondrosis 732.9
  acetabulum 732.1
  adult spine 732.8
  astragalus 732.5
  Blount's 732.4
  Buchanan's (juvenile osteochondrosis of iliac
    crest) 732.1
  Buchman's (juvenile osteochondrosis) 732.1
  Burns' 732.3
  calcaneus 732.5
  capitular epiphysis (femur) 732.1
  carpal
    lunate (wrist) 732.3
    scaphoid 732.3
  coxae juvenilis 732.1
  deformans juvenilis (coxae) (hip) 732.1
    Scheuermann's 732.0
    spine 732.0
    tibia 732.4
    vertebra 732.0
  Diaz's (astragalus) 732.5
  dissecans (knee) (shoulder) 732.7
  femoral capital epiphysis 732.1
  femur (head) (juvenile) 732.1
  foot (juvenile) 732.5
  Freiberg's (disease) (second metatarsal) 732.5
  Haas' 732.3
  Haglund's (os tibiale externum) 732.5
  hand (juvenile) 732.3
  head of
    femur 732.1
    humerus (juvenile) 732.3
  hip (juvenile) 732.1
  humerus (juvenile) 732.3
  iliac crest (juvenile) 732.1
  ilium (juvenile) 732.1
  ischiopubic synchondrosis 732.1
  Iselin's (osteochondrosis fifth metatarsal) 732.5
  juvenile, juvenilis 732.6
    arm 732.3
    capital femoral epiphysis 732.1
    capitellum humeri 732.3
    capitular epiphysis 732.1
    carpal scaphoid 732.3
    clavicle, sternal epiphysis 732.6
    coxae 732.1
    deformans 732.1
    foot 732.5
    hand 732.3
    hip and pelvis 732.1
    lower extremity, except foot 732.4

Osteochondrosis — *continued*
  juvenile, juvenilis — *continued*
    lunate, wrist 732.3
    medial cuneiform bone 732.5
    metatarsal (head) 732.5
    metatarsophalangeal 732.5
    navicular, ankle 732.5
    patella 732.4
    primary patellar center (of Köhler) 732.4
    specified site NEC 732.6
    spine 732.0
    tarsal scaphoid 732.5
    tibia (epiphysis) (tuberosity) 732.4
    upper extremity 732.3
    vertebra (body) (Calvé) 732.0
      epiphyseal plates (of Scheuermann) 732.0
  Kienböck's (disease) 732.3
  Köhler's (disease) (navicular, ankle) 732.5
    patellar 732.4
    tarsal navicular 732.5
  Legg-Calvé-Perthes (disease) 732.1
  lower extremity (juvenile) 732.4
  lunate bone 732.3
  Mauclaire's 732.3
  metacarpal heads (of Mauclaire) 732.3
  metatarsal (fifth) (head) (second) 732.5
  navicular, ankle 732.5
  os calcis 732.5
  Osgood-Schlatter 732.4
  os tibiale externum 732.5
  Panner's 732.3
  patella (juvenile) 732.4
  patellar center
    primary (of Köhler) 732.4
    secondary (of Sinding-Larsen) 732.4
  pelvis (juvenile) 732.1
  Pierson's 732.1
  radial head (juvenile) 732.3
  Scheuermann's 732.0
  Sever's (calcaneum) 732.5
  Sinding-Larsen (secondary patellar center)
    732.4
  spine (juvenile) 732.0
    adult 732.8
  symphysis pubis (of Pierson) (juvenile) 732.1
  syphilitic (congenital) 090.0
  tarsal (navicular) (scaphoid) 732.5
  tibia (proximal) (tubercle) 732.4
  tuberculous — *see* Tuberculosis, bone
  ulna 732.3
  upper extremity (juvenile) 732.3
  van Neck's (juvenile osteochondrosis) 732.1
  vertebral (juvenile) 732.0
    adult 732.8
Osteoclastoma (M9250/1) 238.0
  malignant (M9250/3) — *see* Neoplasm, bone,
    malignant
Osteocopic pain 733.90
Osteodynia 733.90
Osteodystrophy
  azotemic 588.0
  chronica deformans hypertrophica 731.0
  congenital 756.50
    specified type NEC 756.59
  deformans 731.0
  fibrosa localisata 731.0
  parathyroid 252.01   ▲
  renal 588.0
Osteofibroma (M9262/0) — *see* Neoplasm, bone,
  benign
Osteofibrosarcoma (M9182/3) — *see* Neoplasm,
  bone, malignant
Osteogenesis imperfecta 756.51
Osteogenic — *see* condition
Osteoma (M9180/0) — *see also* Neoplasm, bone,
  benign
  osteoid (M9191/0) — *see also* Neoplasm, bone,
    benign
    giant (M9200/0) — *see* Neoplasm, bone,
      benign
Osteomalacia 268.2
  chronica deformans hypertrophica 731.0
  due to vitamin D deficiency 268.2
  infantile (*see also* Rickets) 268.0
  juvenile (*see also* Rickets) 268.0

✓ Additional Digit Required   ►◄ Revised Text   ● New Line   ▲ Revised Code

Osteomalacia — *continued*
　pelvis 268.2
　vitamin D-resistant 275.3
Osteomalacic bone 268.2
Osteomalacosis 268.2
Osteomyelitis (general) (infective) (localized)
　　(neonatal) (purulent) (pyogenic) (septic)
　　(staphylococcal) (streptococcal) (suppurative)
　　(with periostitis) 730.2 ☑

> *Note* — *Use the following fifth-digit*
> *subclassification with category 730:*
>
> 　0　　*site unspecified*
> 　1　　*shoulder region*
> 　2　　*upper arm*
> 　3　　*forearm*
> 　4　　*hand*
> 　5　　*pelvic region and thigh*
> 　6　　*lower leg*
> 　7　　*ankle and foot*
> 　8　　*other specified sites*
> 　9　　*multiple sites*

　acute or subacute 730.0 ☑
　chronic or old 730.1 ☑
　due to or associated with
　　diabetes mellitus 250.8 ☑ *[731.8]*
　　tuberculosis (*see also* Tuberculosis, bone)
　　　015.9 ☑ *[730.8]* ☑
　　　limb bones 015.5 ☑ *[730.8]* ☑
　　　specified bones NEC 015.7 ☑ *[730.8]* ☑
　　　spine 015.0 ☑ *[730.8]* ☑
　　typhoid 002.0 *[730.8]* ☑
　Garré's 730.1 ☑
　jaw (acute) (chronic) (lower) (neonatal)
　　(suppurative) (upper) 526.4
　nonsuppurating 730.1 ☑
　orbital 376.03
　petrous bone (*see also* Petrositis) 383.20
　Salmonella 003.24
　sclerosing, nonsuppurative 730.1 ☑
　sicca 730.1 ☑
　syphilitic 095.5
　　congenital 090.0 *[730.8]* ☑
　tuberculous — *see* Tuberculosis, bone
　typhoid 002.0 *[730.8]* ☑
Osteomyelofibrosis 289.89
Osteomyelosclerosis 289.89
Osteonecrosis 733.40
　meaning osteomyelitis 730.1 ☑
Osteo-onycho-arthro dysplasia 756.89
Osteo-onychodysplasia, hereditary 756.89
Osteopathia
　condensans disseminata 756.53
　hyperostotica multiplex infantilis 756.59
　hypertrophica toxica 731.2
　striata 756.4
Osteopathy resulting from poliomyelitis (*see*
　　also Poliomyelitis) 045.9 ☑ *[730.7]*
　familial dysplastic 731.2
Osteopecilia 756.53
Osteopenia 733.90
Osteoperiostitis (*see also* Osteomyelitis) 730.2 ☑
　ossificans toxica 731.2
　toxica ossificans 731.2
Osteopetrosis (familial) 756.52
Osteophyte — *see* Exostosis
Osteophytosis — *see* Exostosis
Osteopoikilosis 756.53
Osteoporosis (generalized) 733.00
　circumscripta 731.0
　disuse 733.03
　drug-induced 733.09
　idiopathic 733.02
　postmenopausal 733.01
　posttraumatic 733.7
　screening V82.81
　senile 733.01
　specified type NEC 733.09
Osteoporosis-osteomalacia syndrome 268.2
Osteopsathyrosis 756.51
Osteoradionecrosis, jaw 526.89

Osteosarcoma (M9180/3) — *see also* Neoplasm,
　　bone, malignant
　chondroblastic (M9181/3) — *see* Neoplasm,
　　bone, malignant
　fibroblastic (M9182/3) — *see* Neoplasm, bone,
　　malignant
　in Paget's disease of bone (M9184/3) — *see*
　　Neoplasm, bone, malignant
　juxtacortical (M9190/3) — *see* Neoplasm, bone,
　　malignant
　parosteal (M9190/3) — *see* Neoplasm, bone,
　　malignant
　telangiectatic (M9183/3) — *see* Neoplasm,
　　bone, malignant
Osteosclerosis 756.52
　fragilis (generalisata) 756.52
　myelofibrosis 289.89
Osteosclerotic anemia 289.89
Osteosis
　acromegaloid 757.39
　cutis 709.3
　parathyroid 252.01　　　　　　　　　　▲
　renal fibrocystic 588.0
Österreicher-Turner syndrome 756.89
Ostium
　atrioventriculare commune 745.69
　primum (arteriosum) (defect) (persistent)
　　745.61
　secundum (arteriosum) (defect) (patent)
　　(persistent) 745.5
Ostrum-Furst syndrome 756.59
Otalgia 388.70
　otogenic 388.71
　referred 388.72
Othematoma 380.31
Otitic hydrocephalus 348.2
Otitis 382.9
　with effusion 381.4
　　purulent 382.4
　　secretory 381.4
　　serous 381.4
　　suppurative 382.4
　acute 382.9
　adhesive (*see also* Adhesions, middle ear)
　　385.10
　chronic 382.9
　　with effusion 381.3
　　mucoid, mucous (simple) 381.20
　　purulent 382.3
　　secretory 381.3
　　serous 381.10
　　suppurative 382.3
　diffuse parasitic 136.8
　externa (acute) (diffuse) (hemorrhagica) 380.10
　　actinic 380.22
　　candidal 112.82
　　chemical 380.22
　　chronic 380.23
　　　mycotic — *see* Otitis, externa, mycotic
　　　specified type NEC 380.23
　　circumscribed 380.10
　　contact 380.22
　　due to
　　　erysipelas 035 *[380.13]*
　　　impetigo 684 *[380.13]*
　　　seborrheic dermatitis 690.10 *[380.13]*
　　eczematoid 380.22
　　furuncular 680.0 *[380.13]*
　　infective 380.10
　　　chronic 380.16
　　malignant 380.14
　　mycotic (chronic) 380.15
　　　due to
　　　　aspergillosis 117.3 *[380.15]*
　　　　moniliasis 112.82
　　　　otomycosis 111.8 *[380.15]*
　　reactive 380.22
　　specified type NEC 380.22
　　tropical 111.8 *[380.15]*
　insidiosa (*see also* Otosclerosis) 387.9
　interna (*see also* Labyrinthitis) 386.30
　media (hemorrhagic) (staphylococcal)
　　(streptococcal) 382.9
　　acute 382.9
　　　with effusion 381.00

Otitis — *continued*
　media — *continued*
　　acute — *continued*
　　　allergic 381.04
　　　　mucoid 381.05
　　　　sanguineous 381.06
　　　　serous 381.04
　　　catarrhal 381.00
　　　exudative 381.00
　　　mucoid 381.02
　　　　allergic 381.05
　　　necrotizing 382.00
　　　　with spontaneous rupture of ear drum
　　　　　382.01
　　　　in
　　　　　influenza 487.8 *[382.02]*
　　　　　measles 055.2
　　　　　scarlet fever 034.1 *[382.02]*
　　　nonsuppurative 381.00
　　　purulent 382.00
　　　　with spontaneous rupture of ear drum
　　　　　382.01
　　　sanguineous 381.03
　　　　allergic 381.06
　　　secretory 381.01
　　　seromucinous 381.02
　　　serous 381.01
　　　　allergic 381.04
　　　suppurative 382.00
　　　　with spontaneous rupture of ear drum
　　　　　382.01
　　　　due to
　　　　　influenza 487.8 *[382.02]*
　　　　　scarlet fever 034.1 *[382.02]*
　　　transudative 381.00
　　adhesive (*see also* Adhesions, middle ear)
　　　385.10
　　allergic 381.4
　　　acute 381.04
　　　　mucoid 381.05
　　　　sanguineous 381.06
　　　　serous 381.04
　　　chronic 381.3
　　catarrhal 381.4
　　　acute 381.00
　　　chronic (simple) 381.10
　　chronic 382.9
　　　with effusion 381.3
　　　adhesive (*see also* Adhesions, middle ear)
　　　　385.10
　　　allergic 381.3
　　　atticoantral, suppurative (with posterior
　　　　or superior marginal perforation of
　　　　ear drum) 382.2
　　　benign suppurative (with anterior
　　　　perforation of ear drum) 382.1
　　　catarrhal 381.10
　　　exudative 381.3
　　　mucinous 381.20
　　　mucoid, mucous (simple) 381.20
　　　mucosanguineous 381.29
　　　nonsuppurative 381.3
　　　purulent 382.3
　　　secretory 381.3
　　　seromucinous 381.3
　　　serosanguineous 381.19
　　　serous (simple) 381.10
　　　suppurative 382.3
　　　　atticoantral (with posterior or superior
　　　　　marginal perforation of ear
　　　　　drum) 382.2
　　　　benign (with anterior perforation of ear
　　　　　drum) 382.1
　　　　tuberculous (*see also* Tuberculosis)
　　　　　017.4 ☑
　　　　tubotympanic 382.1
　　　transudative 381.3
　　exudative 381.4
　　　acute 381.00
　　　chronic 381.3
　　fibrotic (*see also* Adhesions, middle ear)
　　　385.10
　　mucoid, mucous 381.4
　　　acute 381.02
　　　chronic (simple) 381.20
　　mucosanguineous, chronic 381.29

Otitis — *continued*
  media — *continued*
    nonsuppurative 381.4
      acute 381.00
      chronic 381.3
    postmeasles 055.2
    purulent 382.4
      acute 382.00
        with spontaneous rupture of ear drum
          382.01
      chronic 382.3
    sanguineous, acute 381.03
      allergic 381.06
    secretory 381.4
      acute or subacute 381.01
      chronic 381.3
    seromucinous 381.4
      acute or subacute 381.02
      chronic 381.3
    serosanguineous, chronic 381.19
    serous 381.4
      acute or subacute 381.01
      chronic (simple) 381.10
    subacute — *see* Otitis, media, acute
    suppurative 382.4
      acute 382.00
        with spontaneous rupture of ear drum
          382.01
      chronic 382.3
        atticoantral 382.2
        benign 382.1
        tuberculous (*see also* Tuberculosis)
          017.4 ☑
        tubotympanic 382.1
    transudative 381.4
      acute 381.00
      chronic 381.3
    tuberculous (*see also* Tuberculosis) 017.4 ☑
  postmeasles 055.2
Otoconia 386.8
Otolith syndrome 386.19
Otomycosis 111.8 *[380.15]*
  in
    aspergillosis 117.3 *[380.15]*
    moniliasis 112.82
Otopathy 388.9
Otoporosis (*see also* Otosclerosis) 387.9
Otorrhagia 388.69
  traumatic — *see* nature of injury
Otorrhea 388.60
  blood 388.69
  cerebrospinal (fluid) 388.61
Otosclerosis (general) 387.9
  cochlear (endosteal) 387.2
  involving
    otic capsule 387.2
    oval window
      nonobliterative 387.0
      obliterative 387.1
    round window 387.2
  nonobliterative 387.0
  obliterative 387.1
  specified type NEC 387.8
Otospongiosis (*see also* Otosclerosis) 387.9
Otto's disease or pelvis 715.35
Outburst, aggressive (*see also* Disturbance,
    conduct) 312.0 ☑
  in children ►or◄ adolescents 313.9
Outcome of delivery
  multiple birth NEC V27.9
    all liveborn V27.5
    all stillborn V27.7
    some liveborn V27.6
    unspecified V27.9
  single V27.9
    liveborn V27.0
    stillborn V27.1
  twins V27.9
    both liveborn V27.2
    both stillborn V27.4
    one liveborn, one stillborn V27.3
Outlet — *see also* condition
  syndrome (thoracic) 353.0
Outstanding ears (bilateral) 744.29

Ovalocytosis (congenital) (hereditary) (*see also*
    Elliptocytosis) 282.1
Ovarian — *see also* condition
  pregnancy — *see* Pregnancy, ovarian
  remnant syndrome 620.8
  vein syndrome 593.4
Ovaritis (cystic) (*see also* Salpingo-oophoritis)
    614.2
Ovary, ovarian — *see* condition
Overactive — *see also* Hyperfunction
  bladder 596.51
  eye muscle (*see also* Strabismus) 378.9
  hypothalamus 253.8
  thyroid (*see also* Thyrotoxicosis) 242.9 ☑
Overactivity, child 314.01
Overbite (deep) (excessive) (horizontal) (vertical)
    524.29   ▲
Overbreathing (*see also* Hyperventilation) 786.01
Overconscientious personality 301.4
Overdevelopment — *see also* Hypertrophy
  breast (female) (male) 611.1
  nasal bones 738.0
  prostate, congenital 752.89
Overdistention — *see* Distention
Overdose, overdosage (drug) 977.9
  specified drug or substance — *see* Table of
    Drugs and Chemicals
Overeating 783.6
  with obesity 278.0 ☑
  nonorganic origin 307.51
Overexertion (effects) (exhaustion) 994.5
Overexposure (effects) 994.9
  exhaustion 994.4
Overfeeding (*see also* Overeating) 783.6
Overgrowth, bone NEC 733.99
Overheated (effects) (places) — *see* Heat
Overinhibited child 313.0
Overjet 524.29   ▲
Overlaid, overlying (suffocation) 994.7
Overlap   ●
  excessive horizontal 524.26   ●
Overlapping toe (acquired) 735.8
  congenital (fifth toe) 755.66
Overload
  fluid 276.6
  potassium (K) 276.7
  sodium (Na) 276.0
Overnutrition (*see also* Hyperalimentation) 783.6
Overproduction — *see also* Hypersecretion
  ACTH 255.3
  cortisol 255.0
  growth hormone 253.0
  thyroid-stimulating hormone (TSH) 242.8 ☑
Overriding
  aorta 747.21
  finger (acquired) 736.29
    congenital 755.59
  toe (acquired) 735.8
    congenital 755.66
Oversize
  fetus (weight of 4500 grams or more) 766.0
    affecting management of pregnancy 656.6 ☑
    causing disproportion 653.5 ☑
      with obstructed labor 660.1 ☑
    affecting fetus or newborn 763.1
Overstimulation, ovarian 256.1
Overstrained 780.79
  heart — *see* Hypertrophy, cardiac
Overweight (*see also* Obesity) 278.00
Overwork 780.79
Oviduct — *see* condition
Ovotestis 752.7
Ovulation (cycle)
  failure or lack of 628.0
  pain 625.2
Ovum
  blighted 631
  dropsical 631
  pathologic 631

Owren's disease or syndrome (parahemophilia)
    (*see also* Defect, coagulation) 286.3
Oxalosis 271.8
Oxaluria 271.8
Ox heart — *see* Hypertrophy, cardiac
OX syndrome 758.6
Oxycephaly, oxycephalic 756.0
  syphilitic, congenital 090.0
Oxyuriasis 127.4
Oxyuris vermicularis (infestation) 127.4
Ozena 472.0

P

Pacemaker syndrome 429.4
Pachyderma, pachydermia 701.8
  laryngis 478.5
  laryngitis 478.79
  larynx (verrucosa) 478.79
Pachydermatitis 701.8
Pachydermatocele (congenital) 757.39
  acquired 701.8
Pachydermatosis 701.8
Pachydermoperiostitis
  secondary 731.2
Pachydermoperiostosis
  primary idiopathic 757.39
  secondary 731.2
Pachymeningitis (adhesive) (basal) (brain)
    (cerebral) (cervical) (chronic) (circumscribed)
    (external) (fibrous) (hemorrhagic)
    (hypertrophic) (internal) (purulent) (spinal)
    (suppurative) (*see also* Meningitis) 322.9
  gonococcal 098.82
Pachyonychia (congenital) 757.5
  acquired 703.8
Pachyperiosteodermia
  primary or idiopathic 757.39
  secondary 731.2
Pachyperiostosis
  primary or idiopathic 757.39
  secondary 731.2
Pacinian tumor (M9507/0) — *see* Neoplasm,
  skin, benign
Pads, knuckle or Garrod's 728.79
Paget's disease (osteitis deformans) 731.0
  with infiltrating duct carcinoma of the breast
    (M8541/3) — *see* Neoplasm, breast,
    malignant
  bone 731.0
    osteosarcoma in (M9184/3) — *see*
      Neoplasm, bone, malignant
  breast (M8540/3) 174.0
  extramammary (M8542/3) — *see also*
    Neoplasm, skin, malignant
    anus 154.3
    skin 173.5
  malignant (M8540/3)
    breast 174.0
    specified site NEC (M8542/3) — *see*
      Neoplasm, skin, malignant
    unspecified site 174.0
  mammary (M8540/3) 174.0
  necrosis of bone 731.0
  nipple (M8540/3) 174.0
  osteitis deformans 731.0
Paget-Schroetter syndrome (intermittent venous
    claudication) 453.8
Pain(s)
  abdominal 789.0 ☑
  adnexa (uteri) 625.9
  alimentary, due to vascular insufficiency 557.9
  anginoid (*see also* Pain, precordial) 786.51
  anus 569.42
  arch 729.5
  arm 729.5
  back (postural) 724.5
    low 724.2
    psychogenic 307.89
  bile duct 576.9
  bladder 788.9
  bone 733.90

Pain(s) — Palsy

Pain(s) — continued
- breast 611.71
  - psychogenic 307.89
- broad ligament 625.9
- cartilage NEC 733.90
- cecum 789.0 ☑
- cervicobrachial 723.3
- chest (central) 786.50
  - atypical 786.59
  - midsternal 786.51
  - musculoskeletal 786.59
  - noncardiac 786.59
  - substernal 786.51
  - wall (anterior) 786.52
- coccyx 724.79
- colon 789.0 ☑
- common duct 576.9
- coronary — see Angina
- costochondral 786.52
- diaphragm 786.52
- due to (presence of) any device, implant, or graft classifiable to 996.0-996.5 — see Complications, due to (presence of) any device, implant, or graft classified to 996.0-996.5 NEC
- ear (see also Otalgia) 388.70
- epigastric, epigastrium 789.0 ☑
- extremity (lower) (upper) 729.5
- eye 379.91
- face, facial 784.0
  - atypical 350.2
  - nerve 351.8
- false (labor) 644.1 ☑
- female genital organ NEC 625.9
  - psychogenic 307.89
- finger 729.5
- flank 789.0 ☑
- foot 729.5
- gallbladder 575.9
- gas (intestinal) 787.3
- gastric 536.8
- generalized 780.99
- genital organ
  - female 625.9
  - male 608.9
  - psychogenic 307.89
- groin 789.0 ☑
- growing 781.99
- hand 729.5
- head (see also Headache) 784.0
- heart (see also Pain, precordial) 786.51
- infraorbital (see also Neuralgia, trigeminal) 350.1
- intermenstrual 625.2
- jaw 526.9
- joint 719.40
  - ankle 719.47
  - elbow 719.42
  - foot 719.47
  - hand 719.44
  - hip 719.45
  - knee 719.46
  - multiple sites 719.49
  - pelvic region 719.45
  - psychogenic 307.89
  - shoulder (region) 719.41
  - specified site NEC 719.48
  - wrist 719.43
- kidney 788.0
- labor, false or spurious 644.1 ☑
- laryngeal 784.1
- leg 729.5
- limb 729.5
- low back 724.2
- lumbar region 724.2
- mastoid (see also Otalgia) 388.70
- maxilla 526.9
- metacarpophalangeal (joint) 719.44
- metatarsophalangeal (joint) 719.47
- mouth 528.9
- muscle 729.1
  - intercostal 786.59
- nasal 478.1
- nasopharynx 478.29
- neck NEC 723.1
  - psychogenic 307.89
- nerve NEC 729.2

Pain(s) — continued
- neuromuscular 729.1
- nose 478.1
- ocular 379.91
- ophthalmic 379.91
- orbital region 379.91
- osteocopic 733.90
- ovary 625.9
  - psychogenic 307.89
- over heart (see also Pain, precordial) 786.51
- ovulation 625.2
- pelvic (female) 625.9
  - male NEC 789.0 ☑
    - psychogenic 307.89
  - psychogenic 307.89
- penis 607.9
  - psychogenic 307.89
- pericardial (see also Pain, precordial) 786.51
- perineum
  - female 625.9
  - male 608.9
- pharynx 478.29
- pleura, pleural, pleuritic 786.52
- post-operative — see Pain, by site
- preauricular 388.70
- precordial (region) 786.51
  - psychogenic 307.89
- psychogenic 307.80
  - cardiovascular system 307.89
  - gastrointestinal system 307.89
  - genitourinary system 307.89
  - heart 307.89
  - musculoskeletal system 307.89
  - respiratory system 307.89
  - skin 306.3
- radicular (spinal) (see also Radiculitis) 729.2
- rectum 569.42
- respiration 786.52
- retrosternal 786.51
- rheumatic NEC 729.0
  - muscular 729.1
- rib 786.50
- root (spinal) (see also Radiculitis) 729.2
- round ligament (stretch) 625.9
- sacroiliac 724.6
- sciatic 724.3
- scrotum 608.9
  - psychogenic 307.89
- seminal vesicle 608.9
- sinus 478.1
- skin 782.0
- spermatic cord 608.9
- spinal root (see also Radiculitis) 729.2
- stomach 536.8
  - psychogenic 307.89
- substernal 786.51
- temporomandibular (joint) 524.62
- temporomaxillary joint 524.62
- testis 608.9
  - psychogenic 307.89
- thoracic spine 724.1
  - with radicular and visceral pain 724.4
- throat 784.1
- tibia 733.90
- toe 729.5
- tongue 529.6
- tooth 525.9
- trigeminal (see also Neuralgia, trigeminal) 350.1
- umbilicus 789.0 ☑
- ureter 788.0
- urinary (organ) (system) 788.0
- uterus 625.9
  - psychogenic 307.89
- vagina 625.9
- vertebrogenic (syndrome) 724.5
- vesical 788.9
- vulva 625.9
- xiphoid 733.90

Painful — see also Pain
- arc syndrome 726.19
- coitus
  - female 625.0
  - male 608.89
  - psychogenic 302.76

Painful — see also Pain — continued
- ejaculation (semen) 608.89
  - psychogenic 302.79
- erection 607.3
- feet syndrome 266.2
- menstruation 625.3
  - psychogenic 306.52
- micturition 788.1
- ophthalmoplegia 378.55
- respiration 786.52
- scar NEC 709.2
- urination 788.1
- wire sutures 998.89

Painters' colic 984.9
- specified type of lead — see Table of Drugs and Chemicals

Palate — see condition

Palatoplegia 528.9

Palatoschisis (see also Cleft, palate) 749.00

Palilalia 784.69

Palindromic arthritis (see also Rheumatism, palindromic) 719.3 ☑

Palliative care V66.7

Pallor 782.61
- temporal, optic disc 377.15

Palmar — see also condition
- fascia — see condition

Palpable
- cecum 569.89
- kidney 593.89
- liver 573.9
- lymph nodes 785.6
- ovary 620.8
- prostate 602.9
- spleen (see also Splenomegaly) 789.2
- uterus 625.8

Palpitation (heart) 785.1
- psychogenic 306.2

Palsy (see also Paralysis) 344.9
- atrophic diffuse 335.20
- Bell's 351.0
  - newborn 767.5
- birth 767.7
- brachial plexus 353.0
  - fetus or newborn 767.6
- brain — see also Palsy, cerebral
  - noncongenital or noninfantile 344.89
    - due to vascular lesion — see category 438 ☑
    - late effect — see Late effect(s) (of) cerebrovascular disease
  - syphilitic 094.89
    - congenital 090.49
- bulbar (chronic) (progressive) 335.22
  - pseudo NEC 335.23
  - supranuclear NEC 344.8 ☑
- cerebral (congenital) (infantile) (spastic) 343.9
  - athetoid 333.7
  - diplegic 343.0
    - due to previous vascular lesion — see category 438 ☑
    - late effect — see Late effect(s) (of) cerebrovascular disease
  - hemiplegic 343.1
  - monoplegic 343.3
  - noncongenital or noninfantile 437.8
    - due to previous vascular lesion — see category 438 ☑
    - late effect — see Late effect(s) (of) cerebrovascular disease
  - paraplegic 343.0
  - quadriplegic 343.2
  - spastic, not congenital or infantile 344.8 ☑
  - syphilitic 094.89
    - congenital 090.49
  - tetraplegic 343.2
- cranial nerve — see also Disorder, nerve, cranial
  - multiple 352.6
- creeping 335.21
- divers' 993.3
- Erb's (birth injury) 767.6
- facial 351.0
  - newborn 767.5

Palsy (*see also* Paralysis) — *continued*
  glossopharyngeal 352.2
  Klumpke (-Déjérine) 767.6
  lead 984.9
    specified type of lead — *see* Table of Drugs
      and Chemicals
  median nerve (tardy) 354.0
  peroneal nerve (acute) (tardy) 355.3
  progressive supranuclear 333.0
  pseudobulbar NEC 335.23
  radial nerve (acute) 354.3
  seventh nerve 351.0
    newborn 767.5
  shaking (*see also* Parkinsonism) 332.0
  spastic (cerebral) (spinal) 343.9
    hemiplegic 343.1
  specified nerve NEC — *see* Disorder, nerve
  supranuclear NEC 356.8
    progressive 333.0
  ulnar nerve (tardy) 354.2
  wasting 335.21
Paltauf-Sternberg disease 201.9 ☑
Paludism — *see* Malaria
Panama fever 084.0
Panaris (with lymphangitis) 681.9
  finger 681.02
  toe 681.11
Panaritium (with lymphangitis) 681.9
  finger 681.02
  toe 681.11
Panarteritis (nodosa) 446.0
  brain or cerebral 437.4
Pancake heart 793.2
  with cor pulmonale (chronic) 416.9
Pancarditis (acute) (chronic) 429.89
  with
    rheumatic
      fever (active) (acute) (chronic) (subacute)
        391.8
        inactive or quiescent 398.99
  rheumatic, acute 391.8
    chronic or inactive 398.99
Pancoast's syndrome or tumor (carcinoma,
  pulmonary apex) (M8010/3) 162.3
Pancoast-Tobias syndrome (M8010/3)
  (carcinoma, pulmonary apex) 162.3
Pancolitis 556.6
Pancreas, pancreatic — *see* condition
Pancreatitis 577.0
  acute (edematous) (hemorrhagic) (recurrent)
    577.0
  annular 577.0
  apoplectic 577.0
  calcercous 577.0
  chronic (infectious) 577.1
    recurrent 577.1
  cystic 577.2
  fibrous 577.8
  gangrenous 577.0
  hemorrhagic (acute) 577.0
  interstitial (chronic) 577.1
    acute 577.0
  malignant 577.0
  mumps 072.3
  painless 577.1
  recurrent 577.1
  relapsing 577.1
  subacute 577.0
  suppurative 577.0
  syphilitic 095.8
Pancreatolithiasis 577.8
Pancytolysis 289.9
Pancytopenia (acquired) 284.8
  with malformations 284.0
  congenital 284.0
Panencephalitis — *see also* Encephalitis
  subacute, sclerosing 046.2
Panhematopenia 284.8
  congenital 284.0
  constitutional 284.0
  splenic, primary 289.4
Panhemocytopenia 284.8
  congenital 284.0

Panhemocytopenia — *continued*
  constitutional 284.0
Panhypogonadism 257.2
Panhypopituitarism 253.2
  prepubertal 253.3
Panic (attack) (state) 300.01
  reaction to exceptional stress (transient) 308.0
Panmyelopathy, familial constitutional 284.0
Panmyelophthisis 284.9
  acquired (secondary) 284.8
  congenital 284.0
  idiopathic 284.9
Panmyelosis (acute) (M9951/1) 238.7
Panner's disease 732.3
  capitellum humeri 732.3
  head of humerus 732.3
  tarsal navicular (bone) (osteochondrosis) 732.5
Panneuritis endemica 265.0 [357.4]
Panniculitis 729.30
  back 724.8
  knee 729.31
  neck 723.6
  nodular, nonsuppurative 729.30
  sacral 724.8
  specified site NEC 729.39
Panniculus adiposus (abdominal) 278.1
Pannus 370.62
  allergic eczematous 370.62
  degenerativus 370.62
  keratic 370.62
  rheumatoid — *see* Arthritis, rheumatoid
  trachomatosus, trachomatous (active) 076.1
    [370.62]
    late effect 139.1
Panophthalmitis 360.02
Panotitis — *see* Otitis media
Pansinusitis (chronic) (hyperplastic) (nonpurulent)
  (purulent) 473.8
  acute 461.8
  due to fungus NEC 117.9
  tuberculous (*see also* Tuberculosis) 012.8 ☑
Panuveitis 360.12
  sympathetic 360.11
Panvalvular disease — *see* Endocarditis, mitral
Papageienkrankheit 073.9
Papanicolaou smear
  cervix (screening test) V76.2
    as part of gynecological examination
      V72.31   ▲
    for suspected malignant neoplasm V76.2
      no disease found V71.1
    inadequate sample 795.08   ●
    nonspecific abnormal finding 795.00   ●
      with   ●
        ►atypical squamous cells◄ changes of
          undetermined significance
        ►cannot exclude high grade
          squamous intraepithelial
          lesion (ASC-H)◄ 795.02
        ►of undetermined significance (ASC-
          US)◄ 795.01
      high grade squamous   ●
        intraepithelial lesion   ●
        (HGSIL) 795.04   ●
      low grade squamous   ●
        intraepithelial lesion   ●
        (LGSIL) 795.03   ●
      nonspecific finding NEC 795.09
      to confirm findings of recent normal   ●
        smear following initial   ●
        abnormal smear V72.32   ●
    ►unsatisfactory◄ 795.08   ▲
    other specified site — *see also* Screening,
      malignant neoplasm
      for suspected malignant neoplasm — *see*
        also Screening, malignant neoplasm
      no disease found V71.1
      nonspecific abnormal finding 795.1
    vagina V76.47
      following hysterectomy for malignant
        condition V67.01

Papilledema 377.00
  associated with
    decreased ocular pressure 377.02
    increased intracranial pressure 377.01
    retinal disorder 377.03
  choked disc 377.00
  infectional 377.00
Papillitis 377.31
  anus 569.49
  chronic lingual 529.4
  necrotizing, kidney 584.7
  optic 377.31
  rectum 569.49
  renal, necrotizing 584.7
  tongue 529.0
Papilloma (M8050/0) — *see also* Neoplasm, by
  site, benign

> *Note — Except where otherwise indicated, the*
> *morphological varieties of papilloma in the list*
> *below should be coded by site as for "Neoplasm,*
> *benign."*

  acuminatum (female) (male) 078.1 ☑
  bladder (urinary) (transitional cell) (M8120/1)
    236.7
    benign (M8120/0) 223.3
  choroid plexus (M9390/0) 225.0
    anaplastic type (M9390/3) 191.5
    malignant (M9390/3) 191.5
  ductal (M8503/0)
  dyskeratotic (M8052/0)
  epidermoid (M8052/0)
  hyperkeratotic (M8052/0)
  intracystic (M8504/0)
  intraductal (M8503/0)
  inverted (M8053/0)
  keratotic (M8052/0)
  parakeratotic (M8052/0)
  pinta (primary) 103.0
  renal pelvis (transitional cell) (M8120/1) 236.99
    benign (M8120/0) 223.1
  Schneiderian (M8121/0)
    specified site — *see* Neoplasm, by site,
      benign
    unspecified site 212.0
  serous surface (M8461/0)
    borderline malignancy (M8461/1)
      specified site — *see* Neoplasm, by site,
        uncertain behavior
      unspecified site 236.2
    specified site — *see* Neoplasm, by site,
      benign
    unspecified site 220
  squamous (cell) (M8052/0)
  transitional (cell) (M8120/0)
    bladder (urinary) (M8120/1) 236.7
    inverted type (M8121/1) — *see* Neoplasm,
      by site, uncertain behavior
    renal pelvis (M8120/1) 236.91
    ureter (M8120/1) 236.91
  ureter (transitional cell) (M8120/1) 236.91
    benign (M8120/0) 223.2
  urothelial (M8120/1) — *see* Neoplasm, by site,
    uncertain behavior
  verrucous (M8051/0)
  villous (M8261/1) — *see* Neoplasm, by site,
    uncertain behavior
  yaws, plantar or palmar 102.1
Papillomata, multiple, of yaws 102.1
Papillomatosis (M8060/0) — *see also* Neoplasm,
  by site, benign
  confluent and reticulate 701.8
  cutaneous 701.8
  ductal, breast 610.1
  Gougerot-Carteaud (confluent reticulate) 701.8
  intraductal (diffuse) (M8505/0) — *see*
    Neoplasm, by site, benign
  subareolar duct (M8506/0) 217
Papillon-Léage and Psaume syndrome
  (orodigitofacial dysostosis) 759.89
Papule 709.8
  carate (primary) 103.0
  fibrous, of nose (M8724/0) 216.3
  pinta (primary) 103.0

☑ Additional Digit Required   ►◄ Revised Text   ● New Line   ▲ Revised Code

Papulosis, malignant 447.8
Papyraceous fetus 779.89
  complicating pregnancy 646.0 ☑
Paracephalus 759.7
Parachute mitral valve 746.5
Paracoccidioidomycosis 116.1
  mucocutaneous-lymphangitic 116.1
  pulmonary 116.1
  visceral 116.1
Paracoccidiomycosis — *see*
  Paracoccidioidomycosis
Paracusis 388.40
Paradentosis 523.5
Paradoxical facial movements 374.43
Paraffinoma 999.9
Paraganglioma (M8680/1)
  adrenal (M8700/0) 227.0
    malignant (M8700/3) 194.0
  aortic body (M8691/1) 237.3
    malignant (M8691/3) 194.6
  carotid body (M8692/1) 237.3
    malignant (M8692/3) 194.5
  chromaffin (M8700/0) — *see also* Neoplasm, by
    site, benign
    malignant (M8700/3) — *see* Neoplasm, by
      site, malignant
  extra-adrenal (M8693/1)
    malignant (M8693/3)
      specified site — *see* Neoplasm, by site,
        malignant
      unspecified site 194.6
    specified site — *see* Neoplasm, by site,
      uncertain behavior
    unspecified site 237.3
  glomus jugulare (M8690/1) 237.3
    malignant (M8690/3) 194.6
  jugular (M8690/1) 237.3
    malignant (M8680/3)
      specified site — *see* Neoplasm, by site,
        malignant
      unspecified site 194.6
  nonchromaffin (M8693/1)
    malignant (M8693/3)
      specified site — *see* Neoplasm, by site,
        malignant
      unspecified site 194.6
    specified site — *see* Neoplasm, by site,
      uncertain behavior
    unspecified site 237.3
  parasympathetic (M8682/1)
    specified site — *see* Neoplasm, by site,
      uncertain behavior
    unspecified site 237.3
  specified site — *see* Neoplasm, by site,
    uncertain behavior
  sympathetic (M8681/1)
    specified site — *see* Neoplasm, by site,
      uncertain behavior
    unspecified site 237.3
  unspecified site 237.3
Parageusia 781.1
  psychogenic 306.7
Paragonimiasis 121.2
Paragranuloma, Hodgkin's (M9660/3) 201.0 ☑
Parahemophilia (*see also* Defect, coagulation)
  286.3
Parakeratosis 690.8
  psoriasiformis 696.2
  variegata 696.2
Paralysis, paralytic (complete) (incomplete) 344.9
  with
    broken
      back — *see* Fracture, vertebra, by site,
        with spinal cord injury
      neck — *see* Fracture, vertebra, cervical,
        with spinal cord injury
    fracture, vertebra — *see* Fracture, vertebra,
      by site, with spinal cord injury
    syphilis 094.89
  abdomen and back muscles 355.9
  abdominal muscles 355.9
  abducens (nerve) 378.54
  abductor 355.9
    lower extremity 355.8

Paralysis, paralytic — *continued*
  abductor — *continued*
    upper extremity 354.9
  accessory nerve 352.4
  accommodation 367.51
    hysterical 300.11
  acoustic nerve 388.5
  agitans 332.0
    arteriosclerotic 332.0
  alternating 344.89
    oculomotor 344.89
  amyotrophic 335.20
  ankle 355.8
  anterior serratus 355.9
  anus (sphincter) 569.49
  apoplectic (current episode) (*see also* Disease,
    cerebrovascular, acute) 436
    late effect — *see* Late effect(s) (of)
      cerebrovascular disease
  arm 344.40
    affecting
      dominant side 344.41
      nondominant side 344.42
    both 344.2
    due to old CVA — *see* category 438 ☑
    hysterical 300.11
    late effect — *see* Late effect(s) (of)
      cerebrovascular disease
    psychogenic 306.0
      transient 781.4
      traumatic NEC (*see also* Injury, nerve,
        upper limb) 955.9
  arteriosclerotic (current episode) 437.0
    late effect — *see* Late effect(s) (of)
      cerebrovascular disease
  ascending (spinal), acute 357.0
  associated, nuclear 344.89
  asthenic bulbar 358.00
  ataxic NEC 334.9
    general 094.1
  athetoid 333.7
  atrophic 356.9
    infantile, acute (*see also* Poliomyelitis, with
      paralysis) 045.1 ☑
    muscle NEC 355.9
    progressive 335.21
    spinal (acute) (*see also* Poliomyelitis, with
      paralysis) 045.1 ☑
  attack (*see also* Disease, cerebrovascular,
    acute) 436
  axillary 353.0
  Babinski-Nageotte's 344.89
  Bell's 351.0
    newborn 767.5
  Benedikt's 344.89
  birth (injury) 767.7
    brain 767.0
    intracranial 767.0
    spinal cord 767.4
  bladder (sphincter) 596.53
    neurogenic 596.54
      with cauda equina syndrome 344.61
    puerperal, postpartum, childbirth 665.5 ☑
    sensory 344.61
      with cauda equina 344.61
    spastic 344.61
      with cauda equina 344.61
  bowel, colon, or intestine (*see also* Ileus) 560.1
  brachial plexus 353.0
    due to birth injury 767.6
    newborn 767.6
  brain
    congenital — *see* Palsy, cerebral
    current episode 437.8
    diplegia 344.2
    due to previous vascular lesion — *see*
      category 438 ☑
    hemiplegia 342.9 ☑
      due to previous vascular lesion — *see*
        category 438 ☑
      late effect — *see* Late effect(s) (of)
        cerebrovascular disease
    infantile — *see* Palsy, cerebral
    late effect — *see* Late effect(s) (of)
      cerebrovascular disease

Paralysis, paralytic — *continued*
  brain — *continued*
    monoplegia — *see also* Monoplegia
      due to previous vascular lesion — *see*
        category 438 ☑
      late effect — *see* Late effect(s) (of)
        cerebrovascular disease
    paraplegia 344.1
    quadriplegia — *see* Quadriplegia
    syphilitic, congenital 090.49
    triplegia 344.89
  bronchi 519.1
  Brown-Séquard's 344.89
  bulbar (chronic) (progressive) 335.22
    infantile (*see also* Poliomyelitis, bulbar)
      045.0 ☑
    poliomyelitic (*see also* Poliomyelitis, bulbar)
      045.0 ☑
    pseudo 335.23
    supranuclear 344.89
  bulbospinal 358.00
  cardiac (*see also* Failure, heart) 428.9
  cerebral
    current episode 437.8
    spastic, infantile — *see* Palsy, cerebral
  cerebrocerebellar 437.8
    diplegic infantile 343.0
  cervical
    plexus 353.2
    sympathetic NEC 337.0
  Céstan-Chenais 344.89
  Charcôt-Marie-Tooth type 356.1
  childhood — *see* Palsy, cerebral
  Clark's 343.9
  colon (*see also* Ileus) 560.1
  compressed air 993.3
  compression
    arm NEC 354.9
    cerebral — *see* Paralysis, brain
    leg NEC 355.8
    lower extremity NEC 355.8
    upper extremity NEC 354.9
  congenital (cerebral) (spastic) (spinal) — *see*
    Palsy, cerebral
  conjugate movement (of eye) 378.81
    cortical (nuclear) (supranuclear) 378.81
  convergence 378.83
  cordis (*see also* Failure, heart) 428.9
  cortical (*see also* Paralysis, brain) 437.8
  cranial or cerebral nerve (*see also* Disorder,
    nerve, cranial) 352.9
  creeping 335.21
  crossed leg 344.89
  crutch 953.4
  deglutition 784.9
    hysterical 300.11
  dementia 094.1
  descending (spinal) NEC 335.9
  diaphragm (flaccid) 519.4
    due to accidental section of phrenic nerve
      during procedure 998.2
  digestive organs NEC 564.89
  diplegic — *see* Diplegia
  divergence (nuclear) 378.85
  divers' 993.3
  Duchenne's 335.22
  due to intracranial or spinal birth injury — *see*
    Palsy, cerebral
  embolic (current episode) (*see also* Embolism,
    brain) 434.1 ☑
    late effect — *see* Late effect(s) (of)
      cerebrovascular disease
  enteric (*see also* Ileus) 560.1
    with hernia — *see* Hernia, by site, with
      obstruction
  Erb's syphilitic spastic spinal 094.89
  Erb (-Duchenne) (birth) (newborn) 767.6
  esophagus 530.8 ☑
  essential, infancy (*see also* Poliomyelitis)
    045.9 ☑
  extremity
    lower — *see* Paralysis, leg
    spastic (hereditary) 343.3
      noncongenital or noninfantile 344.1
    transient (cause unknown) 781.4
    upper — *see* Paralysis, arm

Paralysis, paralytic — *continued*
- eye muscle (extrinsic) 378.55
  - intrinsic 367.51
- facial (nerve) 351.0
  - birth injury 767.5
  - congenital 767.5
  - following operation NEC 998.2
  - newborn 767.5
- familial 359.3
  - periodic 359.3
  - spastic 334.1
- fauces 478.29
- finger NEC 354.9
- foot NEC 355.8
- gait 781.2
- gastric nerve 352.3
- gaze 378.81
- general 094.1
  - ataxic 094.1
  - insane 094.1
  - juvenile 090.40
  - progressive 094.1
  - tabetic 094.1
- glossopharyngeal (nerve) 352.2
- glottis (*see also* Paralysis, vocal cord) 478.30
- gluteal 353.4
- Gubler (-Millard) 344.89
- hand 354.9
  - hysterical 300.11
  - psychogenic 306.0
- heart (*see also* Failure, heart) 428.9
- hemifacial, progressive 349.89
- hemiplegic — *see* Hemiplegia
- hyperkalemic periodic (familial) 359.3
- hypertensive (current episode) 437.8
- hypoglossal (nerve) 352.5
- hypokalemic periodic 359.3
- Hyrtl's sphincter (rectum) 569.49
- hysterical 300.11
- ileus (*see also* Ileus) 560.1
- infantile (*see also* Poliomyelitis) 045.9 ☑
  - atrophic acute 045.1 ☑
  - bulbar 045.0 ☑
  - cerebral — *see* Palsy, cerebral
  - paralytic 045.1 ☑
  - progressive acute 045.9 ☑
  - spastic — *see* Palsy, cerebral
  - spinal 045.9 ☑
- infective (*see also* Poliomyelitis) 045.9 ☑
- inferior nuclear 344.9
- insane, general or progressive 094.1
- internuclear 378.86
- interosseous 355.9
- intestine (*see also* Ileus) 560.1
- intracranial (current episode) (*see also* Paralysis, brain) 437.8
  - due to birth injury 767.0
- iris 379.49
  - due to diphtheria (toxin) 032.81 [379.49]
- ischemic, Volkmann's (complicating trauma) 958.6
- Jackson's 344.8 ☑
- jake 357.7
- Jamaica ginger (jake) 357.7
- juvenile general 090.40
- Klumpke (-Déjérine) (birth) (newborn) 767.6
- labioglossal (laryngeal) (pharyngeal) 335.22
- Landry's 357.0
- laryngeal nerve (recurrent) (superior) (*see also* Paralysis, vocal cord) 478.30
- larynx (*see also* Paralysis, vocal cord) 478.30
  - due to diphtheria (toxin) 032.3
- late effect
  - due to
    - birth injury, brain or spinal (cord) — *see* Palsy, cerebral
    - edema, brain or cerebral — *see* Paralysis, brain
    - lesion
      - cerebrovascular — *see* category 438 ☑
      - late effect — *see* Late effect(s) (of) cerebrovascular disease
      - spinal (cord) — *see* Paralysis, spinal
- lateral 335.24
- lead 984.9
  - specified type of lead — *see* Table of Drugs and Chemicals

Paralysis, paralytic — *continued*
- left side — *see* Hemiplegia
- leg 344.30
  - affecting
    - dominant side 344.31
    - nondominant side 344.32
  - both (*see also* Paraplegia) 344.1
  - crossed 344.89
  - hysterical 300.11
  - psychogenic 306.0
  - transient or transitory 781.4
    - traumatic NEC (*see also* Injury, nerve, lower limb) 956.9
- levator palpebrae superioris 374.31
- limb NEC 344.5
  - all four — *see* Quadriplegia
  - quadriplegia — *see* Quadriplegia
- lip 528.5
- Lissauer's 094.1
- local 355.9
- lower limb — *see also* Paralysis, leg
  - both (*see also* Paraplegia) 344.1
- lung 518.89
  - newborn 770.89
- median nerve 354.1
- medullary (tegmental) 344.89
- mesencephalic NEC 344.89
  - tegmental 344.89
- middle alternating 344.89
- Millard-Gubler-Foville 344.89
- monoplegic — *see* Monoplegia
- motor NEC 344.9
  - cerebral — *see* Paralysis, brain
  - spinal — *see* Paralysis, spinal
- multiple
  - cerebral — *see* Paralysis, brain
  - spinal — *see* Paralysis, spinal
- muscle (flaccid) 359.9
  - due to nerve lesion NEC 355.9
  - eye (extrinsic) 378.55
    - intrinsic 367.51
    - oblique 378.51
  - iris sphincter 364.8
  - ischemic (complicating trauma) (Volkmann's) 958.6
  - pseudohypertrophic 359.1
- muscular (atrophic) 359.9
  - progressive 335.21
- musculocutaneous nerve 354.9
- musculospiral 354.9
- nerve — *see also* Disorder, nerve
  - third or oculomotor (partial) 378.51
    - total 378.52
  - fourth or trochlear 378.53
  - sixth or abducens 378.54
  - seventh or facial 351.0
    - birth injury 767.5
    - due to
      - injection NEC 999.9
      - operation NEC 997.09
    - newborn 767.5
  - accessory 352.4
  - auditory 388.5
  - birth injury 767.7
  - cranial or cerebral (*see also* Disorder, nerve, cranial) 352.9
  - facial 351.0
    - birth injury 767.5
    - newborn 767.5
  - laryngeal (*see also* Paralysis, vocal cord) 478.30
  - newborn 767.7
  - phrenic 354.8
    - newborn 767.7
  - radial 354.3
    - birth injury 767.6
    - newborn 767.6
  - syphilitic 094.89
  - traumatic NEC (*see also* Injury, nerve, by site) 957.9
  - trigeminal 350.9
  - ulnar 354.2
- newborn NEC 767.0
- normokalemic periodic 359.3
- obstetrical, newborn 767.7
- ocular 378.9
- oculofacial, congenital 352.6

Paralysis, paralytic — *continued*
- oculomotor (nerve) (partial) 378.51
  - alternating 344.89
  - external bilateral 378.55
  - total 378.52
- olfactory nerve 352.0
- palate 528.9
- palatopharyngolaryngeal 352.6
- paratrigeminal 350.9
- periodic (familial) (hyperkalemic) (hypokalemic) (normokalemic) (secondary) 359.3
- peripheral
  - autonomic nervous system — *see* Neuropathy, peripheral, autonomic
  - nerve NEC 355.9
- peroneal (nerve) 355.3
- pharynx 478.29
- phrenic nerve 354.8
- plantar nerves 355.6
- pneumogastric nerve 352.3
- poliomyelitis (current) (*see also* Poliomyelitis, with paralysis) 045.1 ☑
  - bulbar 045.0 ☑
- popliteal nerve 355.3
- pressure (*see also* Neuropathy, entrapment) 355.9
- progressive 335.21
  - atrophic 335.21
  - bulbar 335.22
  - general 094.1
  - hemifacial 349.89
  - infantile, acute (*see also* Poliomyelitis) 045.9 ☑
  - multiple 335.20
- pseudobulbar 335.23
- pseudohypertrophic 359.1
  - muscle 359.1
- psychogenic 306.0
- pupil, pupillary 379.49
- quadriceps 355.8
- quadriplegic (*see also* Quadriplegia) 344.0 ☑
- radial nerve 354.3
  - birth injury 767.6
- rectum (sphincter) 569.49
- rectus muscle (eye) 378.55
- recurrent laryngeal nerve (*see also* Paralysis, vocal cord) 478.30
- respiratory (muscle) (system) (tract) 786.09
  - center NEC 344.89
    - fetus or newborn 770.89
  - congenital 768.9
  - newborn 768.9
- right side — *see* Hemiplegia
- Saturday night 354.3
- saturnine 984.9
  - specified type of lead — *see* Table of Drugs and Chemicals
- sciatic nerve 355.0
- secondary — *see* Paralysis, late effect
- seizure (cerebral) (current episode) (*see also* Disease, cerebrovascular, acute) 436
  - late effect — *see* Late effect(s) (of) cerebrovascular disease
- senile NEC 344.9
- serratus magnus 355.9
- shaking (*see also* Parkinsonism) 332.0
- shock (*see also* Disease, cerebrovascular, acute) 436
  - late effect — *see* Late effect(s) (of) cerebrovascular disease
- shoulder 354.9
- soft palate 528.9
- spasmodic — *see* Paralysis, spastic
- spastic 344.9
  - cerebral infantile — *see* Palsy, cerebral
  - congenital (cerebral) — *see* Palsy, cerebral
  - familial 334.1
  - hereditary 334.1
  - infantile 343.9
  - noncongenital or noninfantile, cerebral 344.9
  - syphilitic 094.0
  - spinal 094.89
- sphincter, bladder (*see also* Paralysis, bladder) 596.53
- spinal (cord) NEC 344.1
  - accessory nerve 352.4

Paralysis, paralytic — *continued*
  spinal — *continued*
    acute (*see also* Poliomyelitis) 045.9 ☑
    ascending acute 357.0
    atrophic (acute) (*see also* Poliomyelitis, with
        paralysis) 045.1 ☑
      spastic, syphilitic 094.89
    congenital NEC 343.9
    hemiplegic — *see* Hemiplegia
    hereditary 336.8
    infantile (*see also* Poliomyelitis) 045.9 ☑
    late effect NEC 344.89
    monoplegic — *see* Monoplegia
    nerve 355.9
    progressive 335.10
    quadriplegic — *see* Quadriplegia
    spastic NEC 343.9
    traumatic — *see* Injury, spinal, by site
  sternomastoid 352.4
  stomach 536.3
    nerve 352.3
  stroke (current episode) ►— *see* Infarct, brain◄
    late effect — *see* Late effect(s) (of)
        cerebrovascular disease
  subscapularis 354.8
  superior nuclear NEC 334.9
  supranuclear 356.8
  sympathetic
    cervical NEC 337.0
    nerve NEC (*see also* Neuropathy, peripheral,
        autonomic) 337.9
    nervous system — *see* Neuropathy,
        peripheral, autonomic
  syndrome 344.9
    specified NEC 344.89
  syphilitic spastic spinal (Erb's) 094.89
  tabetic general 094.1
  thigh 355.8
  throat 478.29
    diphtheritic 032.0
    muscle 478.29
  thrombotic (current episode) (*see also*
        Thrombosis, brain) 434.0 ☑
    late effect — *see* Late effect(s) (of)
        cerebrovascular disease
    old — *see* category 438 ☑
  thumb NEC 354.9
  tick (-bite) 989.5
  Todd's (postepileptic transitory paralysis) 344.89
  toe 355.6
  tongue 529.8
  transient
    arm or leg NEC 781.4
    traumatic NEC (*see also* Injury, nerve, by
        site) 957.9
  trapezius 352.4
  traumatic, transient NEC (*see also* Injury,
        nerve, by site) 957.9
  trembling (*see also* Parkinsonism) 332.0
  triceps brachii 354.9
  trigeminal nerve 350.9
  trochlear nerve 378.53
  ulnar nerve 354.2
  upper limb — *see also* Paralysis, arm
    both (*see also* Diplegia) 344.2
  uremic — *see* Uremia
  uveoparotitic 135
  uvula 528.9
    hysterical 300.11
    postdiphtheritic 032.0
  vagus nerve 352.3
  vasomotor NEC 337.9
  velum palati 528.9
  vesical (*see also* Paralysis, bladder) 596.53
  vestibular nerve 388.5
  visual field, psychic 368.16
  vocal cord 478.30
    bilateral (partial) 478.33
      complete 478.34
    complete (bilateral) 478.34
    unilateral (partial) 478.31
      complete 478.32
  Volkmann's (complicating trauma) 958.6
  wasting 335.21
  Weber's 344.89
  wrist NEC 354.9

Paramedial orifice, urethrovesical 753.8
Paramenia 626.9
Parametritis (chronic) (*see also* Disease, pelvis,
    inflammatory) 614.4
  acute 614.3
  puerperal, postpartum, childbirth 670.0 ☑
Parametrium, parametric — *see* condition
Paramnesia (*see also* Amnesia) 780.93
Paramolar 520.1
  causing crowding 524.31   ▲
Paramyloidosis 277.3
Paramyoclonus multiplex 333.2
Paramyotonia 359.2
  congenita 359.2
Paraneoplastic syndrome — *see* condition
Parangi (*see also* Yaws) 102.9
Paranoia 297.1
  alcoholic 291.5
  querulans 297.8
  senile 290.20
Paranoid
  dementia (*see also* Schizophrenia) 295.3 ☑
    praecox (acute) 295.3 ☑
    senile 290.20
  personality 301.0
  psychosis 297.9
    alcoholic 291.5
    climacteric 297.2
    drug-induced 292.11
    involutional 297.2
    menopausal 297.2
    protracted reactive 298.4
    psychogenic 298.4
      acute 298.3
    senile 290.20
  reaction (chronic) 297.9
    acute 298.3
  schizophrenia (acute) (*see also* Schizophrenia)
        295.3 ☑
  state 297.9
    alcohol-induced 291.5
    climacteric 297.2
    drug-induced 292.11
    due to or associated with
      arteriosclerosis (cerebrovascular) 290.42
      presenile brain disease 290.12
      senile brain disease 290.20
    involutional 297.2
    menopausal 297.2
    senile 290.20
    simple 297.0
    specified type NEC 297.8
  tendencies 301.0
  traits 301.0
  trends 301.0
  type, psychopathic personality 301.0
Paraparesis (*see also* Paralysis) 344.9
Paraphasia 784.3
Paraphilia (*see also* Deviation, sexual) 302.9
Paraphimosis (congenital) 605
  chancroidal 099.0
Paraphrenia, paraphrenic (late) 297.2
  climacteric 297.2
  dementia (*see also* Schizophrenia) 295.3 ☑
  involutional 297.2
  menopausal 297.2
  schizophrenia (acute) (*see also* Schizophrenia)
        295.3 ☑
Paraplegia 344.1
  with
    broken back — *see* Fracture, vertebra, by
        site, with spinal cord injury
    fracture, vertebra — *see* Fracture, vertebra,
        by site, with spinal cord injury
  ataxic — *see* Degeneration, combined, spinal
        cord
  brain (current episode) (*see also* Paralysis,
        brain) 437.8
  cerebral (current episode) (*see also* Paralysis,
        brain) 437.8
  congenital or infantile (cerebral) (spastic)
        (spinal) 343.0
  cortical — *see* Paralysis, brain

Paraplegia — *continued*
  familial spastic 334.1
  functional (hysterical) 300.11
  hysterical 300.11
  infantile 343.0
  late effect 344.1
  Pott's (*see also* Tuberculosis) 015.0 ☑ *[730.88]*
  psychogenic 306.0
  spastic
    Erb's spinal 094.89
    hereditary 334.1
    not infantile or congenital 344.1
  spinal (cord)
    traumatic NEC — *see* Injury, spinal, by site
  syphilitic (spastic) 094.89
  traumatic NEC — *see* Injury, spinal, by site
Paraproteinemia 273.2
  benign (familial) 273.1
  monoclonal 273.1
  secondary to malignant or inflammatory
        disease 273.1
Parapsoriasis 696.2
  en plaques 696.2
  guttata 696.2
  lichenoides chronica 696.2
  retiformis 696.2
  varioliformis (acuta) 696.2
Parascarlatina 057.8
Parasitic — *see also* condition
  disease NEC (*see also* Infestation, parasitic)
        136.9
    contact V01.89
    exposure to V01.89
    intestinal NEC 129
    skin NEC 134.9
  stomatitis 112.0
  sycosis 110.0
    beard 110.0
    scalp 110.0
  twin 759.4
Parasitism NEC 136.9
  intestinal NEC 129
  skin NEC 134.9
  specified — *see* Infestation
Parasitophobia 300.29
Parasomnia 780.59
  nonorganic origin 307.47
Paraspadias 752.69
Paraspasm facialis 351.8
Parathyroid gland — *see* condition
Parathyroiditis (autoimmune) 252.1
Parathyroprival tetany 252.1
Paratrachoma 077.0
Paratyphilitis (*see also* Appendicitis) 541
Paratyphoid (fever) — *see* Fever, paratyphoid
Paratyphus — *see* Fever, paratyphoid
Paraurethral duct 753.8
Para-urethritis 597.89
  gonococcal (acute) 098.0
    chronic or duration of 2 months or over
        098.2
Paravaccinia NEC 051.9
  milkers' node 051.1
Paravaginitis (*see also* Vaginitis) 616.10
Parencephalitis (*see also* Encephalitis) 323.9
  late effect — *see* category 326
Parergasia 298.9
Paresis (*see also* Paralysis) 344.9
  accommodation 367.51
  bladder (spastic) (sphincter) (*see also* Paralysis,
        bladder) 596.53
    tabetic 094.0
  bowel, colon, or intestine (*see also* Ileus) 560.1
  brain or cerebral — *see* Paralysis, brain
  extrinsic muscle, eye 378.55
  general 094.1
    arrested 094.1
    brain 094.1
    cerebral 094.1
    insane 094.1
    juvenile 090.40
      remission 090.49

Paresis (*see also* Paralysis) — *continued*
  general — *continued*
    progressive 094.1
      remission (sustained) 094.1
      tabetic 094.1
  heart (*see also* Failure, heart) 428.9 ☑
  infantile (*see also* Poliomyelitis) 045.9 ☑
  insane 094.1
  juvenile 090.40
  late effect — *see* Paralysis, late effect
  luetic (general) 094.1
  peripheral progressive 356.9
  pseudohypertrophic 359.1
  senile NEC 344.9
  stomach 536.3
  syphilitic (general) 094.1
    congenital 090.40
  transient, limb 781.4
  vesical (sphincter) NEC 596.53
Paresthesia (*see also* Disturbance, sensation) 782.0
  Berger's (paresthesia of lower limb) 782.0
  Bernhardt 355.1
  Magnan's 782.0
Paretic — *see* condition
Parinaud's
  conjunctivitis 372.02
  oculoglandular syndrome 372.02
  ophthalmoplegia 378.81
  syndrome (paralysis of conjugate upward gaze) 378.81
Parkes Weber and Dimitri syndrome (encephalocutaneous angiomatosis) 759.6
Parkinson's disease, syndrome, or tremor — *see* Parkinsonism
Parkinsonism (arteriosclerotic) (idiopathic) (primary) 332.0
  associated with orthostatic hypotension (idiopathic) (symptomatic) 333.0
  due to drugs 332.1
  secondary 332.1
  syphilitic 094.82
Parodontitis 523.4
Parodontosis 523.5
Paronychia (with lymphangitis) 681.9
  candidal (chronic) 112.3
  chronic 681.9
    candidal 112.3
    finger 681.02
    toe 681.11
  finger 681.02
  toe 681.11
  tuberculous (primary) (*see also* Tuberculosis) 017.0 ☑
Parorexia NEC 307.52
  hysterical 300.11
Parosmia 781.1
  psychogenic 306.7
Parotid gland — *see* condition
Parotiditis (*see also* Parotitis) 527.2
  epidemic 072.9
  infectious 072.9
Parotitis 527.2
  allergic 527.2
  chronic 527.2
  epidemic (*see also* Mumps) 072.9
  infectious (*see also* Mumps) 072.9
  noninfectious 527.2
  nonspecific toxic 527.2
  not mumps 527.2
  postoperative 527.2
  purulent 527.2
  septic 527.2
  suppurative (acute) 527.2
  surgical 527.2
  toxic 527.2
Paroxysmal — *see also* condition
  dyspnea (nocturnal) 786.09
Parrot's disease (syphilitic osteochondritis) 090.0
Parrot fever 073.9
Parry's disease or syndrome (exophthalmic goiter) 242.0 ☑
Parry-Romberg syndrome 349.89

Parson's disease (exophthalmic goiter) 242.0 ☑
Parsonage-Aldren-Turner syndrome 353.5
Parsonage-Turner syndrome 353.5
Pars planitis 363.21
Particolored infant 757.39
Parturition — *see* Delivery
Passage
  false, urethra 599.4
  of sounds or bougies (*see also* Attention to artificial opening) V55.9
Passive — *see* condition
Pasteurella septica 027.2
Pasteurellosis (*see also* Infection, Pasteurella) 027.2
PAT (paroxysmal atrial tachycardia) 427.0
Patau's syndrome (trisomy D) 758.1
Patch
  herald 696.3
Patches
  mucous (syphilitic) 091.3
    congenital 090.0
  smokers' (mouth) 528.6
Patellar — *see* condition
Patellofemoral syndrome 719.46
Patent — *see also* Imperfect closure
  atrioventricular ostium 745.69
  canal of Nuck 752.41
  cervix 622.5
    complicating pregnancy 654.5 ☑
      affecting fetus or newborn 761.0
  ductus arteriosus or Botalli 747.0
  Eustachian
    tube 381.7
    valve 746.89
  foramen
    Botalli 745.5
    ovale 745.5
  interauricular septum 745.5
  interventricular septum 745.4
  omphalomesenteric duct 751.0
  os (uteri) — *see* Patent, cervix
  ostium secundum 745.5
  urachus 753.7
  vitelline duct 751.0
Paternity testing V70.4
Paterson's syndrome (sideropenic dysphagia) 280.8
Paterson (-Brown) (-Kelly) syndrome (sideropenic dysphagia) 280.8
Paterson-Kelly syndrome or web (sideropenic dysphagia) 280.8
Pathologic, pathological — *see also* condition
  asphyxia 799.0
  drunkenness 291.4
  emotionality 301.3
  liar 301.7
  personality 301.9
  resorption, tooth 521.40 ▲
    external 521.42 ●
    internal 521.41 ●
    specified NEC 521.49 ●
  sexuality (*see also* Deviation, sexual) 302.9
Pathology (of) — *see* Disease
Patterned motor discharge, idiopathic (*see also* Epilepsy) 345.5 ☑
Patulous — *see also* Patent
  anus 569.49
  Eustachian tube 381.7
Pause, sinoatrial 427.81
Pavor nocturnus 307.46
Pavy's disease 593.6
Paxton's disease (white piedra) 111.2
Payr's disease or syndrome (splenic flexure syndrome) 569.89
Pearls
  Elschnig 366.51
  enamel 520.2
Pearl-workers' disease (chronic osteomyelitis) (*see also* Osteomyelitis) 730.1 ☑
Pectenitis 569.49
Pectenosis 569.49

Pectoral — *see* condition
Pectus
  carinatum (congenital) 754.82
    acquired 738.3
    rachitic (*see also* Rickets) 268.0
  excavatum (congenital) 754.81
    acquired 738.3
    rachitic (*see also* Rickets) 268.0
  recurvatum (congenital) 754.81
    acquired 738.3
Pedatrophia 261
Pederosis 302.2
Pediculosis (infestation) 132.9
  capitis (head louse) (any site) 132.0
  corporis (body louse) (any site) 132.1
  eyelid 132.0 [373.6]
  mixed (classifiable to more than one category in 132.0-132.2) 132.3
  pubis (pubic louse) (any site) 132.2
  vestimenti 132.1
  vulvae 132.2
Pediculus (infestation) — *see* Pediculosis
Pedophilia 302.2
Peg-shaped teeth 520.2
Pel's crisis 094.0
Pel-Ebstein disease — *see* Disease, Hodgkin's
Pelade 704.01
Pelger-Huât anomaly or syndrome (hereditary hyposegmentation) 288.2
Peliosis (rheumatica) 287.0
Pelizaeus-Merzbacher
  disease 330.0
  sclerosis, diffuse cerebral 330.0
Pellagra (alcoholic or with alcoholism) 265.2
  with polyneuropathy 265.2 [357.4]
Pellagra-cerebellar-ataxia-renal aminoaciduria syndrome 270.0
Pellegrini's disease (calcification, knee joint) 726.62
Pellegrini (-Stieda) disease or syndrome (calcification, knee joint) 726.62
Pellizzi's syndrome (pineal) 259.8
Pelvic — *see also* condition
  congestion-fibrosis syndrome 625.5
  kidney 753.3
Pelvioectasis 591
Pelviolithiasis 592.0
Pelviperitonitis
  female (*see also* Peritonitis, pelvic, female) 614.5
  male (*see also* Peritonitis) 567.2
Pelvis, pelvic — *see also* condition or type
  infantile 738.6
  Nägele's 738.6
  obliquity 738.6
  Robert's 755.69
Pemphigoid 694.5
  benign, mucous membrane 694.60
    with ocular involvement 694.61
  bullous 694.5
  cicatricial 694.60
    with ocular involvement 694.61
  juvenile 694.2
Pemphigus 694.4
  benign 694.5
    chronic familial 757.39
  Brazilian 694.4
  circinatus 694.0
  congenital, traumatic 757.39
  conjunctiva 694.61
  contagiosus 684
  erythematodes 694.4
  erythematosus 694.4
  foliaceus 694.4
  frambesiodes 694.4
  gangrenous (*see also* Gangrene) 785.4
  malignant 694.4
  neonatorum, newborn 684
  ocular 694.61
  papillaris 694.4
  seborrheic 694.4
  South American 694.4

☑ Additional Digit Required   ▶◀ Revised Text   ● New Line   ▲ Revised Code

Pemphigus — *continued*
  syphilitic (congenital) 090.0
  vegetans 694.4
  vulgaris 694.4
  wildfire 694.4
Pendred's syndrome (familial goiter with deaf-mutism) 243
Pendulous
  abdomen 701.9
    in pregnancy or childbirth 654.4 ☑
      affecting fetus or newborn 763.89
  breast 611.8
Penetrating wound — *see also* Wound, open, by site
  with internal injury — *see* Injury, internal, site, with open wound
  eyeball 871.7
    with foreign body (nonmagnetic) 871.6
      magnetic 871.5
    ocular (*see also* Penetrating wound, eyeball) 871.7
      adnexa 870.3
        with foreign body 870.4
      orbit 870.3
        with foreign body 870.4
Penetration, pregnant uterus by instrument
  with
    abortion — *see* Abortion, by type, with damage to pelvic organs
    ectopic pregnancy (*see also* categories 633.0-633.9) 639.2
    molar pregnancy (*see also* categories 630-632) 639.2
  complication of delivery 665.1 ☑
    affecting fetus or newborn 763.89
  following
    abortion 639.2
    ectopic or molar pregnancy 639.2
Penfield's syndrome (*see also* Epilepsy) 345.5 ☑
Penicilliosis of lung 117.3
Penis — *see* condition
Penitis 607.2
Penta X syndrome 758.81
Pentalogy (of Fallot) 745.2
Pentosuria (benign) (essential) 271.8
Peptic acid disease 536.8
Peregrinating patient V65.2
Perforated — *see* Perforation
Perforation, perforative (nontraumatic)
  antrum (*see also* Sinusitis, maxillary) 473.0
  appendix 540.0
    with peritoneal abscess 540.1
  atrial septum, multiple 745.5
  attic, ear 384.22
    healed 384.81
  bile duct, except cystic (*see also* Disease, biliary) 576.3
    cystic 575.4
  bladder (urinary) 596.6
    with
      abortion — *see* Abortion, by type, with damage to pelvic organs
      ectopic pregnancy (*see also* categories 633.0-633.9) 639.2
      molar pregnancy (*see also* categories 630-632) 639.2
    following
      abortion 639.2
      ectopic or molar pregnancy 639.2
    obstetrical trauma 665.5 ☑
  bowel 569.83
    with
      abortion — *see* Abortion, by type, with damage to pelvic organs
      ectopic pregnancy (*see also* categories 633.0-633.9) 639.2
      molar pregnancy (*see also* categories 630-632) 639.2
    fetus or newborn 777.6
    following
      abortion 639.2
      ectopic or molar pregnancy 639.2
    obstetrical trauma 665.5 ☑

Perforation, perforative — *continued*
  broad ligament
    with
      abortion — *see* Abortion, by type, with damage to pelvic organs
      ectopic pregnancy (*see also* categories 633.0-633.9) 639.2
      molar pregnancy (*see also* categories 630-632) 639.2
    following
      abortion 639.2
      ectopic or molar pregnancy 639.2
    obstetrical trauma 665.6 ☑
  by
    device, implant, or graft — *see* Complications, mechanical
    foreign body left accidentally in operation wound 998.4
    instrument (any) during a procedure, accidental 998.2
  cecum 540.0
    with peritoneal abcess 540.1
  cervix (uteri) — *see also* Injury, internal, cervix
    with
      abortion — *see* Abortion, by type, with damage to pelvic organs
      ectopic pregnancy (*see also* categories 633.0-633.9) 639.2
      molar pregnancy (*see also* categories 630-632) 639.2
    following
      abortion 639.2
      ectopic or molar pregnancy 639.2
    obstetrical trauma 665.3 ☑
  colon 569.83
  common duct (bile) 576.3
  cornea (*see also* Ulcer, cornea) 370.00
    due to ulceration 370.06
  cystic duct 575.4
  diverticulum (*see also* Diverticula) 562.10
    small intestine 562.00
  duodenum, duodenal (ulcer) — *see* Ulcer, duodenum, with perforation
  ear drum — *see* Perforation, tympanum
  enteritis — *see* Enteritis
  esophagus 530.4
  ethmoidal sinus (*see also* Sinusitis, ethmoidal) 473.2
  foreign body (external site) — *see also* Wound, open, by site, complicated
    internal site, by ingested object — *see* Foreign body
  frontal sinus (*see also* Sinusitis, frontal) 473.1
  gallbladder or duct (*see also* Disease, gallbladder) 575.4
  gastric (ulcer) — *see* Ulcer, stomach, with perforation
  heart valve — *see* Endocarditis
  ileum (*see also* Perforation, intestine) 569.83
  instrumental
    external — *see* Wound, open, by site
    pregnant uterus, complicating delivery 665.9 ☑
    surgical (accidental) (blood vessel) (nerve) (organ) 998.2
  intestine 569.83
    with
      abortion — *see* Abortion, by type, with damage to pelvic organs
      ectopic pregnancy (*see also* categories 633.0-633.9) 639.2
      molar pregnancy (*see also* categories 630-632) 639.2
    fetus or newborn 777.6
    obstetrical trauma 665.5 ☑
    ulcerative NEC 569.83
  jejunum, jejunal 569.83
    ulcer — *see* Ulcer, gastrojejunal, with perforation
  mastoid (antrum) (cell) 383.89
  maxillary sinus (*see also* Sinusitis, maxillary) 473.0
  membrana tympani — *see* Perforation, tympanum
  nasal
    septum 478.1

Perforation, perforative — *continued*
  nasal — *continued*
    septum — *continued*
      congenital 748.1
      syphilitic 095.8
    sinus (*see also* Sinusitis) 473.9
      congenital 748.1
  palate (hard) 526.89
    soft 528.9
      syphilitic 095.8
        syphilitic 095.8
  palatine vault 526.89
    syphilitic 095.8
      congenital 090.5
  pelvic
    floor
      with
        abortion — *see* Abortion, by type, with damage to pelvic organs
        ectopic pregnancy (*see also* categories 633.0-633.9) 639.2
        molar pregnancy (*see also* categories 630-632) 639.2
      obstetrical trauma 664.1 ☑
    organ
      with
        abortion — *see* Abortion, by type, with damage to pelvic organs
        ectopic pregnancy (*see also* categories 633.0-633.9) 639.2
        molar pregnancy (*see also* categories 630-632) 639.2
      following
        abortion 639.2
        ectopic or molar pregnancy 639.2
      obstetrical trauma 665.5 ☑
  perineum — *see* Laceration, perineum
  periurethral tissue
    with
      abortion — *see* Abortion, by type, with damage to pelvic organs
      ectopic pregnancy (*see also* categories 630-632) 639.2
      molar pregnancy (*see also* categories 630-632) 639.2
  pharynx 478.29
  pylorus, pyloric (ulcer) — *see* Ulcer, stomach, with perforation
  rectum 569.49
  sigmoid 569.83
  sinus (accessory) (chronic) (nasal) (*see also* Sinusitis) 473.9
  sphenoidal sinus (*see also* Sinusitis, sphenoidal) 473.3
  stomach (due to ulcer) — *see* Ulcer, stomach, with perforation
  surgical (accidental) (by instrument) (blood vessel) (nerve) (organ) 998.2
  traumatic
    external — *see* Wound, open, by site
    eye (*see also* Penetrating wound, ocular) 871.7
    internal organ — *see* Injury, internal, by site
  tympanum (membrane) (persistent posttraumatic) (postinflammatory) 384.20
    with
      otitis media — *see* Otitis media
    attic 384.22
    central 384.21
    healed 384.81
    marginal NEC 384.23
    multiple 384.24
    pars flaccida 384.22
    total 384.25
    traumatic — *see* Wound, open, ear, drum
  typhoid, gastrointestinal 002.0
  ulcer — *see* Ulcer, by site, with perforation
  ureter 593.89
  urethra
    with
      abortion — *see* Abortion, by type, with damage to pelvic organs
      ectopic pregnancy (*see also* categories 633.0-633.9) 639.2
      molar pregnancy (*see also* categories 630-632) 639.2

☑ Additional Digit Required   ►◄ Revised Text   ● New Line   ▲ Revised Code

Perforation, perforative — *continued*
  urethra — *continued*
    following
      abortion 639.2
      ectopic or molar pregnancy 639.2
    obstetrical trauma 665.5 ☑
  uterus — *see also* Injury, internal, uterus
    with
      abortion — *see* Abortion, by type, with
        damage to pelvic organs
      ectopic pregnancy (*see also* categories
        633.0-633.9) 639.2
      molar pregnancy (*see also* categories 630-
        632) 639.2
    by intrauterine contraceptive device 996.32
    following
      abortion 639.2
      ectopic or molar pregnancy 639.2
    obstetrical trauma — *see* Injury, internal,
      uterus, obstetrical trauma
  uvula 528.9
    syphilitic 095.8
  vagina — *see* Laceration, vagina
  viscus NEC 799.89
    traumatic 868.00
      with open wound into cavity 868.10
Periadenitis mucosa necrotica recurrens 528.2
Periangiitis 446.0
Periantritis 535.4 ☑
Periappendicitis (acute) (*see also* Appendicitis)
  541
Periarteritis (disseminated) (infectious)
  (necrotizing) (nodosa) 446.0
Periarthritis (joint) 726.90
  Duplay's 726.2
  gonococcal 098.50
  humeroscapularis 726.2
  scapulohumeral 726.2
  shoulder 726.2
  wrist 726.4
Periarthrosis (angioneural) — *see* Periarthritis
Peribronchitis 491.9
  tuberculous (*see also* Tuberculosis) 011.3 ☑
Pericapsulitis, adhesive (shoulder) 726.0
Pericarditis (granular) (with decompensation)
  (with effusion) 423.9
  with
    rheumatic fever (conditions classifiable to
      390)
      active (*see also* Pericarditis, rheumatic)
        391.0
      inactive or quiescent 393
  actinomycotic 039.8 *[420.0]*
  acute (nonrheumatic) 420.90
    with chorea (acute) (rheumatic)
      (Sydenham's) 392.0
    bacterial 420.99
    benign 420.91
    hemorrhagic 420.90
    idiopathic 420.91
    infective 420.90
    nonspecific 420.91
    rheumatic 391.0
      with chorea (acute) (rheumatic)
        (Sydenham's) 392.0
    sicca 420.90
    viral 420.91
  adhesive or adherent (external) (internal) 423.1
    acute — *see* Pericarditis, acute
    rheumatic (external) (internal) 393
  amebic 006.8 *[420.0]*
  bacterial (acute) (subacute) (with serous or
    seropurulent effusion) 420.99
  calcareous 423.2
  cholesterol (chronic) 423.8
    acute 420.90
  chronic (nonrheumatic) 423.8
    rheumatic 393
  constrictive 423.2
  Coxsackie 074.21
  due to
    actinomycosis 039.8 *[420.0]*
    amebiasis 006.8 *[420.0]*
    Coxsackie (virus) 074.21

Pericarditis — *continued*
  due to — *continued*
    histoplasmosis (*see also* Histoplasmosis)
      115.93
    nocardiosis 039.8 *[420.0]*
    tuberculosis (*see also* Tuberculosis)
      017.9 ☑ *[420.0]*
  fibrinocaseous (*see also* Tuberculosis)
    017.9 ☑ *[420.0]*
  fibrinopurulent 420.99
  fibrinous — *see* Pericarditis, rheumatic
  fibropurulent 420.99
  fibrous 423.1
  gonococcal 098.83
  hemorrhagic 423.0
  idiopathic (acute) 420.91
  infective (acute) 420.90
  meningococcal 036.41
  neoplastic (chronic) 423.8
    acute 420.90
  nonspecific 420.91
  obliterans, obliterating 423.1
  plastic 423.1
  pneumococcal (acute) 420.99
  postinfarction 411.0
  purulent (acute) 420.99
  rheumatic (active) (acute) (with effusion) (with
    pneumonia) 391.0
    with chorea (acute) (rheumatic)
      (Sydenham's) 392.0
    chronic or inactive (with chorea) 393
  septic (acute) 420.99
  serofibrinous — *see* Pericarditis, rheumatic
  staphylococcal (acute) 420.99
  streptococcal (acute) 420.99
  suppurative (acute) 420.99
  syphilitic 093.81
  tuberculous (acute) (chronic) (*see also*
    Tuberculosis) 017.9 ☑ *[420.0]*
  uremic 585 *[420.0]*
  viral (acute) 420.91
Pericardium, pericardial — *see* condition
Pericellulitis (*see also* Cellulitis) 682.9
Pericementitis 523.4
  acute 523.3
  chronic (suppurative) 523.4
Pericholecystitis (*see also* Cholecystitis) 575.10
Perichondritis
  auricle 380.00
    acute 380.01
    chronic 380.02
  bronchus 491.9
  ear (external) 380.00
    acute 380.01
    chronic 380.02
  larynx 478.71
    syphilitic 095.8
    typhoid 002.0 *[478.71]*
  nose 478.1
  pinna 380.00
    acute 380.01
    chronic 380.02
  trachea 478.9
Periclasia 523.5
Pericolitis 569.89
Pericoronitis (chronic) 523.4
  acute 523.3
Pericystitis (*see also* Cystitis) 595.9
Pericytoma (M9150/1) — *see also* Neoplasm,
  connective tissue, uncertain behavior
  benign (M9150/0) — *see* Neoplasm, connective
    tissue, benign
  malignant (M9150/3) — *see* Neoplasm,
    connective tissue, malignant
Peridacryocystitis, acute 375.32
Peridiverticulitis (*see also* Diverticulitis) 562.11
Periduodenitis 535.6 ☑
Periendocarditis (*see also* Endocarditis) 424.90
  acute or subacute 421.9
Periepididymitis (*see also* Epididymitis) 604.90
Perifolliculitis (abscedens) 704.8
  capitis, abscedens et suffodiens 704.8
  dissecting, scalp 704.8
  scalp 704.8

Perifolliculitis — *continued*
  superficial pustular 704.8
Perigastritis (acute) 535.0 ☑
Perigastrojejunitis (acute) 535.0 ☑
Perihepatitis (acute) 573.3
  chlamydial 099.56
  gonococcal 098.86
Peri-ileitis (subacute) 569.89
Perilabyrinthitis (acute) — *see* Labyrinthitis
Perimeningitis — *see* Meningitis
Perimetritis (*see also* Endometritis) 615.9
Perimetrosalpingitis (*see also* Salpingo-
  oophoritis) 614.2
Perineocele 618.05   ●
Perinephric — *see* condition
Perinephritic — *see* condition
Perinephritis (*see also* Infection, kidney) 590.9
  purulent (*see also* Abscess, kidney) 590.2
Perineum, perineal — *see* condition
Perineuritis NEC 729.2
Periodic — *see also* condition
  disease (familial) 277.3
  edema 995.1
    hereditary 277.6
  fever 277.3
  limb movement disorder 780.58   ●
  paralysis (familial) 359.3
  peritonitis 277.3
  polyserositis 277.3
  somnolence ▶(*see also* Narcolepsy)◀ 347.00▲
Periodontal
  cyst 522.8
  pocket 523.8
Periodontitis (chronic) (complex) (compound)
  (local) (simplex) 523.4
  acute 523.3
  apical 522.6
    acute (pulpal origin) 522.4
Periodontoclasia 523.5
Periodontosis 523.5
Periods — *see also* Menstruation
  heavy 626.2
  irregular 626.4
Perionychia (with lymphangitis) 681.9
  finger 681.02
  toe 681.11
Perioophoritis (*see also* Salpingo-oophoritis)
  614.2
Periorchitis (*see also* Orchitis) 604.90
Periosteum, periosteal — *see* condition
Periostitis (circumscribed) (diffuse) (infective)
  730.3 ☑

> *Note — Use the following fifth-digit*
> *subclassification with category 730:*
>
> 0   *site unspecified*
> 1   *shoulder region*
> 2   *upper arm*
> 3   *forearm*
> 4   *hand*
> 5   *pelvic region and thigh*
> 6   *lower leg*
> 7   *ankle and foot*
> 8   *other specified sites*
> 9   *multiple sites*

  with osteomyelitis (*see also* Osteomyelitis)
    730.2 ☑
    acute or subacute 730.0 ☑
    chronic or old 730.1 ☑
  albuminosa, albuminosus 730.3 ☑
  alveolar 526.5
  alveolodental 526.5
  dental 526.5
  gonorrheal 098.89
  hyperplastica, generalized 731.2
  jaw (lower) (upper) 526.4
  monomelic 733.99
  orbital 376.02

Periostitis — continued
  syphilitic 095.5
    congenital 090.0 *[730.8]* ☑
    secondary 091.61
  tuberculous (see also Tuberculosis, bone)
    015.9 ☑ *[730.8]* ☑
  yaws (early) (hypertrophic) (late) 102.6
Periostosis (see also Periostitis) 730.3 ☑
  with osteomyelitis (see also Osteomyelitis)
    730.2 ☑
    acute or subacute 730.0 ☑
    chronic or old 730.1 ☑
  hyperplastic 756.59
Peripartum cardiomyopathy 674.5 ☑
Periphlebitis (see also Phlebitis) 451.9
  lower extremity 451.2
    deep (vessels) 451.19
    superficial (vessels) 451.0
  portal 572.1
  retina 362.18
  superficial (vessels) 451.0
  tuberculous (see also Tuberculosis) 017.9 ☑
    retina 017.3 ☑ *[362.18]*
Peripneumonia — see Pneumonia
Periproctitis 569.49
Periprostatitis (see also Prostatitis) 601.9
Perirectal — see condition
Perirenal — see condition
Perisalpingitis (see also Salpingo-oophoritis)
  614.2
Perisigmoiditis 569.89
Perisplenitis (infectional) 289.59
Perispondylitis — see Spondylitis
Peristalsis reversed or visible 787.4
Peritendinitis (see also Tenosynovitis) 726.90
  adhesive (shoulder) 726.0
Perithelioma (M9150/1) — see Pericytoma
Peritoneum, peritoneal — see also condition
  equilibration test V56.32
Peritonitis (acute) (adhesive) (fibrinous)
  (hemorrhagic) (idiopathic) (localized)
  (perforative) (primary) (with adhesions) (with
  effusion) 567.9
  with or following
    abortion — see Abortion, by type, with
      sepsis
    abscess 567.2
    appendicitis 540.0
      with peritoneal abcess 540.1
    ectopic pregnancy (see also categories
      633.0-633.9) 639.0
    molar pregnancy (see also categories 630-
      632) 639.0
  aseptic 998.7
  bacterial 567.2
  bile, biliary 567.8
  chemical 998.7
  chlamydial 099.56
  chronic proliferative 567.8
  congenital NEC 777.6
  diaphragmatic 567.2
  diffuse NEC 567.2
  diphtheritic 032.83
  disseminated NEC 567.2
  due to
    bile 567.8
    foreign
      body or object accidentally left during a
        procedure (instrument) (sponge)
        (swab) 998.4
      substance accidentally left during a
        procedure (chemical) (powder) (talc)
        998.7
    talc 998.7
    urine 567.8
  fibrinopurulent 567.2
  fibrinous 567.2
  fibrocaseous (see also Tuberculosis) 014.0 ☑
  fibropurulent 567.2
  general, generalized (acute) 567.2
  gonococcal 098.86
  in infective disease NEC 136.9 *[567.0]*
  meconium (newborn) 777.6
  pancreatic 577.8

Peritonitis — continued
  paroxysmal, benign 277.3
  pelvic
    female (acute) 614.5
      chronic NEC 614.7
        with adhesions 614.6
      puerperal, postpartum, childbirth
        670.0 ☑
    male (acute) 567.2
  periodic (familial) 277.3
  phlegmonous 567.2
  pneumococcal 567.1
  postabortal 639.0
  proliferative, chronic 567.8
  puerperal, postpartum, childbirth 670.0 ☑
  purulent 567.2
  septic 567.2
  staphylococcal 567.2
  streptococcal 567.2
  subdiaphragmatic 567.2
  subphrenic 567.2
  suppurative 567.2
  syphilitic 095.2
    congenital 090.0 *[567.0]*
  talc 998.7
  tuberculous (see also Tuberculosis) 014.0 ☑
  urine 567.8
Peritonsillar — see condition
Peritonsillitis 475
Perityphlitis (see also Appendicitis) 541
Periureteritis 593.89
Periurethral — see condition
Periurethritis (gangrenous) 597.89
Periuterine — see condition
Perivaginitis (see also Vaginitis) 616.10
Perivasculitis, retinal 362.18
Perivasitis (chronic) 608.4
Periventricular leukomalacia 779.7
Perivesiculitis (seminal) (see also Vesiculitis)
  608.0
Perlèche 686.8
  due to
    moniliasis 112.0
    riboflavin deficiency 266.0
Pernicious — see condition
Pernio, perniosis 991.5
Persecution
  delusion 297.9
  social V62.4
Perseveration (tonic) 784.69
Persistence, persistent (congenital) 759.89
  anal membrane 751.2
  arteria stapedia 744.04
  atrioventricular canal 745.69
  bloody ejaculate 792.2
  branchial cleft 744.41
  bulbus cordis in left ventricle 745.8
  canal of Cloquet 743.51
  capsule (opaque) 743.51
  cilioretinal artery or vein 743.51
  cloaca 751.5
  communication — see Fistula, congenital
  convolutions
    aortic arch 747.21
    fallopian tube 752.19
    oviduct 752.19
    uterine tube 752.19
  double aortic arch 747.21
  ductus
    arteriosus 747.0
    Botalli 747.0
  fetal
    circulation 747.83
    form of cervix (uteri) 752.49
    hemoglobin (hereditary) ("Swiss variety")
      282.7
    pulmonary hypertension 747.83
  foramen
    Botalli 745.5
    ovale 745.5
  Gartner's duct 752.11
  hemoglobin, fetal (hereditary) (HPFH) 282.7

Persistence, persistent — continued
  hyaloid
    artery (generally incomplete) 743.51
    system 743.51
  hymen (tag)
    in pregnancy or childbirth 654.8 ☑
      causing obstructed labor 660.2 ☑
  lanugo 757.4
  left
    posterior cardinal vein 747.49
    root with right arch of aorta 747.21
    superior vena cava 747.49
  Meckel's diverticulum 751.0
  mesonephric duct 752.89
    fallopian tube 752.11
  mucosal disease (middle ear) (with posterior or
    superior marginal perforation of ear
    drum) 382.2
  nail(s), anomalous 757.5
  occiput, anterior or posterior 660.3 ☑
    fetus or newborn 763.1
  omphalomesenteric duct 751.0
  organ or site NEC — see Anomaly, specified
    type NEC
  ostium
    atrioventriculare commune 745.69
    primum 745.61
    secundum 745.5
  ovarian rests in fallopian tube 752.19
  pancreatic tissue in intestinal tract 751.5
  primary (deciduous)
    teeth 520.6
    vitreous hyperplasia 743.51
  pulmonary hypertension 747.83
  pupillary membrane 743.46
    iris 743.46
  Rhesus (Rh) titer 999.7
  right aortic arch 747.21
  sinus
    urogenitalis 752.89
    venosus with imperfect incorporation in
      right auricle 747.49
  thymus (gland) 254.8
    hyperplasia 254.0
  thyroglossal duct 759.2
  thyrolingual duct 759.2
  truncus arteriosus or communis 745.0
  tunica vasculosa lentis 743.39
  umbilical sinus 753.7
  urachus 753.7
  vegetative state 780.03
  vitelline duct 751.0
  wolffian duct 752.89
Person (with)
  admitted for clinical research, as participant or
    control subject V70.7
  awaiting admission to adequate facility
    elsewhere V63.2
    undergoing social agency investigation V63.8
  concern (normal) about sick person in family
    V61.49
  consulting on behalf of another V65.19
    pediatric pre-birth visit for expectant
      mother V65.11
  feared
    complaint in whom no diagnosis was made
      V65.5
    condition not demonstrated V65.5
  feigning illness V65.2
  healthy, accompanying sick person V65.0
  living (in)
    alone V60.3
    boarding school V60.6
    residence remote from hospital or medical
      care facility V63.0
    residential institution V60.6
    without
      adequate
        financial resources V60.2
        housing (heating) (space) V60.1
      housing (permanent) (temporary) V60.0
      material resources V60.2
      person able to render necessary care
        V60.4
      shelter V60.0
  medical services in home not available V63.1

☑ Additional Digit Required   ►◄ Revised Text   ● New Line   ▲ Revised Code

Person — *continued*
on waiting list V63.2
undergoing social agency investigation V63.8
sick or handicapped in family V61.49
"worried well" V65.5
Personality
affective 301.10
aggressive 301.3
amoral 301.7
anancastic, anankastic 301.4
antisocial 301.7
asocial 301.7
asthenic 301.6
avoidant 301.82
borderline 301.83
change 310.1
compulsive 301.4
cycloid 301.13
cyclothymic 301.13
dependent 301.6
depressive (chronic) 301.12
disorder, disturbance NEC 301.9
with
antisocial disturbance 301.7
pattern disturbance NEC 301.9
sociopathic disturbance 301.7
trait disturbance 301.9
dual 300.14
dyssocial 301.7
eccentric 301.89
"haltlose" type 301.89
emotionally unstable 301.59
epileptoid 301.3
explosive 301.3
fanatic 301.0
histrionic 301.50
hyperthymic 301.11
hypomanic 301.11
hypothymic 301.12
hysterical 301.50
immature 301.89
inadequate 301.6
labile 301.59
masochistic 301.89
morally defective 301.7
multiple 300.14
narcissistic 301.81
obsessional 301.4
▶obsessive-compulsive◀ 301.4
overconscientious 301.4
paranoid 301.0
passive (-dependent) 301.6
passive-aggressive 301.84
pathologic NEC 301.9
pattern defect or disturbance 301.9
pseudosocial 301.7
psychoinfantile 301.59
psychoneurotic NEC 301.89
psychopathic 301.9
with
amoral trend 301.7
antisocial trend 301.7
asocial trend 301.7
pathologic sexuality (*see also* Deviation, sexual) 302.9
mixed types 301.9
schizoid 301.20
introverted 301.21
schizotypal 301.22
with sexual deviation (*see also* Deviation, sexual) 302.9
antisocial 301.7
dyssocial 301.7
type A 301.4
unstable (emotional) 301.59
Perthes' disease (capital femoral osteochondrosis) 732.1
Pertussis (*see also* Whooping cough) 033.9
vaccination, prophylactic (against) V03.6
Peruvian wart 088.0
Perversion, perverted
appetite 307.52
hysterical 300.11
function
pineal gland 259.8

Perversion, perverted — *continued*
function — *continued*
pituitary gland 253.9
anterior lobe
deficient 253.2
excessive 253.1
posterior lobe 253.6
placenta — *see* Placenta, abnormal
sense of smell or taste 781.1
psychogenic 306.7
sexual (*see also* Deviation, sexual) 302.9
Pervious, congenital — *see also* Imperfect, closure
ductus arteriosus 747.0
Pes (congenital) (*see also* Talipes) 754.70
abductus (congenital) 754.60
acquired 736.79
acquired NEC 736.79
planus 734
adductus (congenital) 754.79
acquired 736.79
cavus 754.71
acquired 736.73
planovalgus (congenital) 754.69
acquired 736.79
planus (acquired) (any degree) 734
congenital 754.61
rachitic 268.1
valgus (congenital) 754.61
acquired 736.79
varus (congenital) 754.50
acquired 736.79
Pest (*see also* Plague) 020.9
Pestis (*see also* Plague) 020.9
bubonica 020.0
fulminans 020.0
minor 020.8
pneumonica — *see* Plague, pneumonic
Petechia, petechiae 782.7
fetus or newborn 772.6
Petechial
fever 036.0
typhus 081.9
Petges-Cléjat or Petges-Clégat syndrome (poikilodermatomyositis) 710.3
Petit's
disease (*see also* Hernia, lumbar) 553.8
Petit mal (idiopathic) (*see also* Epilepsy) 345.0 ☑
status 345.2
Petrellidosis 117.6
Petrositis 383.20
acute 383.21
chronic 383.22
Peutz-Jeghers disease or syndrome 759.6
Peyronie's disease 607.85
Pfeiffer's disease 075
Phacentocele 379.32
traumatic 921.3
Phacoanaphylaxis 360.19
Phacocele (old) 379.32
traumatic 921.3
Phaehyphomycosis 117.8
Phagedena (dry) (moist) (*see also* Gangrene) 785.4
arteriosclerotic 440.2 ☑ *[785.4]*
geometric 686.09
penis 607.89
senile 440.2 ☑ *[785.4]*
sloughing 785.4
tropical (*see also* Ulcer, skin) 707.9
vulva 616.50
Phagedenic — *see also* condition
abscess — *see also* Abscess
chancroid 099.0
bubo NEC 099.8
chancre 099.0
ulcer (tropical) (*see also* Ulcer, skin) 707.9
Phagomania 307.52
Phakoma 362.89
Phantom limb (syndrome) 353.6
Pharyngeal — *see also* condition
arch remnant 744.41
pouch syndrome 279.11

Pharyngitis (acute) (catarrhal) (gangrenous) (infective) (malignant) (membranous) (phlegmonous) (pneumococcal) (pseudomembranous) (simple) (staphylococcal) (subacute) (suppurative) (ulcerative) (viral) 462
with influenza, flu, or grippe 487.1
aphthous 074.0
atrophic 472.1
chronic 472.1
chlamydial 099.51
coxsackie virus 074.0
diphtheritic (membranous) 032.0
follicular 472.1
fusospirochetal 101
gonococcal 098.6
granular (chronic) 472.1
herpetic 054.79
hypertrophic 472.1
infectional, chronic 472.1
influenzal 487.1
lymphonodular, acute 074.8
septic 034.0
streptococcal 034.0
tuberculous (*see also* Tuberculosis) 012.8 ☑
vesicular 074.0
Pharyngoconjunctival fever 077.2
Pharyngoconjunctivitis, viral 077.2
Pharyngolaryngitis (acute) 465.0
chronic 478.9
septic 034.0
Pharyngoplegia 478.29
Pharyngotonsillitis 465.8
tuberculous 012.8 ☑
Pharyngotracheitis (acute) 465.8
chronic 478.9
Pharynx, pharyngeal — *see* condition
Phase of life problem NEC V62.89
Phenomenon
Arthus' — *see* Arthus' phenomenon
flashback (drug) 292.89
jaw-winking 742.8
Jod-Basedow 242.8 ☑
L. E. cell 710.0
lupus erythematosus cell 710.0
Pelger-Huët (hereditary hyposegmentation) 288.2
Raynaud's (paroxysmal digital cyanosis) (secondary) 443.0
Reilly's (*see also* Neuropathy, peripheral, autonomic) 337.9
vasomotor 780.2
vasospastic 443.9
vasovagal 780.2
Wenckebach's, heart block (second degree) 426.13
Phenylketonuria (PKU) 270.1
Phenylpyruvicaciduria 270.1
Pheochromoblastoma (M8700/3)
specified site — *see* Neoplasm, by site, malignant
unspecified site 194.0
Pheochromocytoma (M8700/0)
malignant (M8700/3)
specified site — *see* Neoplasm, by site, malignant
unspecified site 194.0
specified site — *see* Neoplasm, by site, benign
unspecified site 227.0
Phimosis (congenital) 605
chancroidal 099.0
due to infection 605
Phlebectasia (*see also* Varicose, vein) 454.9
congenital 747.6 ☑
esophagus (*see also* Varix, esophagus) 456.1
with hemorrhage (*see also* Varix, esophagus, bleeding) 456.0
Phlebitis (infective) (pyemic) (septic) (suppurative) 451.9
antecubital vein 451.82
arm NEC 451.84
axillary vein 451.89
basilic vein 451.82
deep 451.83
superficial 451.82
basilic vein 451.82

Person — Phlebitis

☑ Additional Digit Required ▶◀ Revised Text ● New Line ▲ Revised Code

Phlebitis — *continued*
  blue 451.19
  brachial vein 451.83
  breast, superficial 451.89
  cavernous (venous) sinus — *see* Phlebitis,
      intracranial sinus
  cephalic vein 451.82
  cerebral (venous) sinus — *see* Phlebitis,
      intracranial sinus
  chest wall, superficial 451.89
  complicating pregnancy or puerperium
      671.9 ☑
      affecting fetus or newborn 760.3
  cranial (venous) sinus — *see* Phlebitis,
      intracranial sinus
  deep (vessels) 451.19
      femoral vein 451.11
      specified vessel NEC 451.19
  due to implanted device — *see* Complications,
      due to (presence of) any device, implant
      or graft classified to 996.0-996.5 NEC
  during or resulting from a procedure 997.2
  femoral vein (deep) 451.11
  femoropopliteal 451.0
  following infusion, perfusion, or transfusion
      999.2
  gouty 274.89 *[451.9]*
  hepatic veins 451.89
  iliac vein 451.81
  iliofemoral 451.11
  intracranial sinus (any) (venous) 325
      late effect — *see* category 326
      nonpyogenic 437.6
          in pregnancy or puerperium 671.5 ☑
  jugular vein 451.89
  lateral (venous) sinus — *see* Phlebitis,
      intracranial sinus
  leg 451.2
      deep (vessels) 451.19
          femoral vein 451.11
          specified vessel NEC 451.19
      superficial (vessels) 451.0
          femoral vein 451.11
  longitudinal sinus — *see* Phlebitis, intracranial
      sinus
  lower extremity 451.2
      deep (vessels) 451.19
          femoral vein 451.11
          specified vessel NEC 451.19
      superficial (vessels) 451.0
          femoral vein 451.11
  migrans, migrating (superficial) 453.1
  pelvic
      with
          abortion — *see* Abortion, by type, with
              sepsis
          ectopic pregnancy (*see also* categories
              633.0-633.9) 639.0
          molar pregnancy (*see also* categories 630-
              632) 639.0
      following
          abortion 639.0
          ectopic or molar pregnancy 639.0
      puerperal, postpartum 671.4 ☑
  popliteal vein 451.19
  portal (vein) 572.1
  postoperative 997.2
  pregnancy 671.9 ☑
      deep 671.3 ☑
      specified type NEC 671.5 ☑
      superficial 671.2 ☑
  puerperal, postpartum, childbirth 671.9 ☑
      deep 671.4 ☑
      lower extremities 671.2 ☑
      pelvis 671.4 ☑
      specified site NEC 671.5 ☑
      superficial 671.2 ☑
  radial vein 451.83
  retina 362.18
  saphenous (great) (long) 451.0
      accessory or small 451.0
  sinus (meninges) — *see* Phlebitis, intracranial
      sinus
  specified site NEC 451.89
  subclavian vein 451.89
  syphilitic 093.89

Phlebitis — *continued*
  tibial vein 451.19
  ulcer, ulcerative 451.9
      leg 451.2
          deep (vessels) 451.19
              femoral vein 451.11
              specified vessel NEC 451.19
          superficial (vessels) 451.0
              femoral vein 451.11
      lower extremity 451.2
          deep (vessels) 451.19
              femoral vein 451.11
              specified vessel NEC 451.19
          superficial (vessels) 451.0
  ulnar vein 451.83
  upper extremity — *see* Phlebitis, arm
  umbilicus 451.89
  uterus (septic) (*see also* Endometritis) 615.9
  varicose (leg) (lower extremity) (*see also*
      Varicose, vein) 454.1
Phlebofibrosis 459.89
Pleboliths 459.89
Phlebosclerosis 459.89
Phlebothrombosis — *see* Thrombosis
Phlebotomus fever 066.0
Phlegm, choked on 933.1
Phlegmasia
  alba dolens (deep vessels) 451.19
      complicating pregnancy 671.3 ☑
      nonpuerperal 451.19
      puerperal, postpartum, childbirth 671.4 ☑
  cerulea dolens 451.19
Phlegmon (*see also* Abscess) 682.9
  erysipelatous (*see also* Erysipelas) 035
  iliac 682.2
      fossa 540.1
  throat 478.29
Phlegmonous — *see* condition
Phlyctenulosis (allergic) (keratoconjuctivitis)
      (nontuberculous) 370.31
  cornea 370.31
      with ulcer (*see also* Ulcer, cornea) 370.00
  tuberculous (*see also* Tuberculosis) 017.3 ☑
      [370.31]
Phobia, phobic (reaction) 300.20
  animal 300.29
  isolated NEC 300.29
  obsessional 300.3
  simple NEC 300.29
  social 300.23
  specified NEC 300.29
  state 300.20
Phocas' disease 610.1
Phocomelia 755.4
  lower limb 755.32
      complete 755.33
      distal 755.35
      proximal 755.34
  upper limb 755.22
      complete 755.23
      distal 755.25
      proximal 755.24
Phoria (*see also* Heterophoria) 378.40
Phosphate-losing tubular disorder 588.0
Phosphatemia 275.3
Phosphaturia 275.3
Photoallergic response 692.72
Photocoproporphyria 277.1
Photodermatitis (sun) 692.72
  light other than sun 692.82
Photokeratitis 370.24
Photo-ophthalmia 370.24
Photophobia 368.13
Photopsia 368.15
Photoretinitis 363.31
Photoretinopathy 363.31
Photosensitiveness (sun) 692.72
  light other than sun 692.82
Photosensitization (sun) skin 692.72
  light other than sun 692.82
Phototoxic response 692.72
Phrenitis 323.9
Phrynoderma 264.8

Phthiriasis (pubis) (any site) 132.2
  with any infestation classifiable to 132.0, 132.1
      and 132.3
Phthirus infestation — *see* Phthiriasis
Phthisis (*see also* Tuberculosis) 011.9 ☑
  bulbi (infectional) 360.41
  colliers' 011.4 ☑
  cornea 371.05
  eyeball (due to infection) 360.41
  millstone makers' 011.4 ☑
  miners' 011.4 ☑
  potters' 011.4 ☑
  sandblasters' 011.4 ☑
  stonemasons' 011.4 ☑
Phycomycosis 117.7
Physalopteriasis 127.7
Physical therapy NEC V57.1
  breathing exercises V57.0
Physiological cup, optic papilla
  borderline, glaucoma suspect 365.00
  enlarged 377.14
  glaucomatous 377.14
Phytobezoar 938
  intestine 936
  stomach 935.2
Pian (*see also* Yaws) 102.9
Pianoma 102.1
Piarhemia, piarrhemia (*see also* Hyperlipemia)
      272.4
  bilharziasis 120.9
Pica 307.52
  hysterical 300.11
Pick's
  cerebral atrophy 331.11
      with dementia
          with behavioral disturbance
              331.11 *[294.11]*
          without behavioral disturbance
              331.11 *[294.10]*
  disease
      brain 331.11
          dementia in
              with behavioral disturbance
                  331.11 *[294.11]*
              without behavioral disturbance
                  331.11 *[294.10]*
      lipid histiocytosis 272.7
      liver (pericardial pseudocirrhosis of liver) 423.2
      pericardium (pericardial pseudocirrhosis of
          liver) 423.2
      polyserositis (pericardial pseudocirrhosis of
          liver) 423.2
      syndrome
          heart (pericardial pseudocirrhosis of liver)
              423.2
          liver (pericardial pseudocirrhosis of liver)
              423.2
      tubular adenoma (M8640/0)
          specified site — *see* Neoplasm, by site,
              benign
          unspecified site
              female 220
              male 222.0
Pick-Herxheimer syndrome (diffuse idiopathic
      cutaneous atrophy) 701.8
Pick-Niemann disease (lipid histiocytosis) 272.7
Pickwickian syndrome (cardiopulmonary obesity)
      278.8
Piebaldism, classic 709.09
Piedra 111.2
  beard 111.2
      black 111.3
      white 111.2
  black 111.3
  scalp 111.3
      black 111.3
      white 111.2
  white 111.2
Pierre Marie's syndrome (pulmonary
      hypertrophic osteoarthropathy) 731.2
Pierre Marie-Bamberger syndrome (hypertrophic
      pulmonary osteoarthropathy) 731.2

☑ Additional Digit Required   ►◄ Revised Text   ● New Line   ▲ Revised Code

Pierre Mauriac's syndrome (diabetes-dwarfism-obesity) 258.1
Pierre Robin deformity or syndrome (congenital) 756.0
Pierson's disease or osteochondrosis 732.1
Pigeon
  breast or chest (acquired) 738.3
    congenital 754.82
    rachitic (see also Rickets) 268.0
  breeders' disease or lung 495.2
  fanciers' disease or lung 495.2
  toe 735.8
Pigmentation (abnormal) 709.00
  anomaly 709.00
    congenital 757.33
    specified NEC 709.09
  conjunctiva 372.55
  cornea 371.10
    anterior 371.11
    posterior 371.13
    stromal 371.12
  lids (congenital) 757.33
    acquired 374.52
  limbus corneae 371.10
  metals 709.00
  optic papilla, congenital 743.57
  retina (congenital) (grouped) (nevoid) 743.53
    acquired 362.74
  scrotum, congenital 757.33
Piles — see Hemorrhoids
Pili
  annulati or torti (congenital) 757.4
  incarnati 704.8
Pill roller hand (intrinsic) 736.09
Pilomatrixoma (M8110/0) — see Neoplasm, skin, benign
Pilonidal — see condition
Pimple 709.8
PIN I (prostatic intraepithelial neoplasia I) 602.3
PIN II (prostatic intraepithelial neoplasia II) 602.3
PIN III (prostatic intraepithelial neoplasia III) 233.4
Pinched nerve — see Neuropathy, entrapment
Pineal body or gland — see condition
Pinealoblastoma (M9362/3) 194.4
Pinealoma (M9360/1) 237.1
  malignant (M9360/3) 194.4
Pineoblastoma (M9362/3) 194.4
Pineocytoma (M9361/1) 237.1
Pinguecula 372.51
Pinhole meatus (see also Stricture, urethra) 598.9
Pink
  disease 985.0
  eye 372.03
  puffer 492.8
Pinkus' disease (lichen nitidus) 697.1
Pinpoint
  meatus (see also Stricture, urethra) 598.9
  os uteri (see also Stricture, cervix) 622.4
Pinselhaare (congenital) 757.4
Pinta 103.9
  cardiovascular lesions 103.2
  chancre (primary) 103.0
  erythematous plaques 103.1
  hyperchromic lesions 103.1
  hyperkeratosis 103.1
  lesions 103.9
    cardiovascular 103.2
    hyperchromic 103.1
    intermediate 103.1
    late 103.2
    mixed 103.3
    primary 103.0
    skin (achromic) (cicatricial) (dyschromic) 103.2
      hyperchromic 103.1
      mixed (achromic and hyperchromic) 103.3
  papule (primary) 103.0

Pinta — continued
  skin lesions (achromic) (cicatricial) (dyschromic) 103.2
    hyperchromic 103.1
    mixed (achromic and hyperchromic) 103.3
  vitiligo 103.2
Pintid 103.0
Pinworms (disease) (infection) (infestation) 127.4
Piry fever 066.8
Pistol wound — see Gunshot wound
Pit, lip (mucus), congenital 750.25
Pitchers' elbow 718.82
Pithecoid pelvis 755.69
  with disproportion (fetopelvic) 653.2 ✓
    affecting fetus or newborn 763.1
    causing obstructed labor 660.1 ✓
Pithiatism 300.11
Pitted — see also Pitting
  teeth 520.4
Pitting (edema) (see also Edema) 782.3
  lip 782.3
  nail 703.8
    congenital 757.5
Pituitary gland — see condition
Pituitary snuff-takers' disease 495.8
Pityriasis 696.5
  alba 696.5
  capitis 690.11
  circinata (et maculata) 696.3
  Hebra's (exfoliative dermatitis) 695.89
  lichenoides et varioliformis 696.2
  maculata (et circinata) 696.3
  nigra 111.1
  pilaris 757.39
    acquired 701.1
    Hebra's 696.4
  rosea 696.3
  rotunda 696.3
  rubra (Hebra) 695.89
    pilaris 696.4
  sicca 690.18
  simplex 690.18
  specified type NEC 696.5
  streptogenes 696.5
  versicolor 111.0
    scrotal 111.0
Placenta, placental
  ablatio 641.2 ✓
    affecting fetus or newborn 762.1
  abnormal, abnormality 656.7 ✓
    with hemorrhage 641.8 ✓
      affecting fetus or newborn 762.1
    affecting fetus or newborn 762.2
  abruptio 641.2 ✓
    affecting fetus or newborn 762.1
  accessory lobe — see Placenta, abnormal
  accreta (without hemorrhage) 667.0 ✓
    with hemorrhage 666.0 ✓
  adherent (without hemorrhage) 667.0 ✓
    with hemorrhage 666.0 ✓
  apoplexy — see Placenta, separation
  battledore — see Placenta, abnormal
  bilobate — see Placenta, abnormal
  bipartita — see Placenta, abnormal
  carneous mole 631
  centralis — see Placenta, previa
  circumvallata — see Placenta, abnormal
  cyst (amniotic) — see Placenta, abnormal
  deficiency — see Placenta, insufficiency
  degeneration — see Placenta, insufficiency
  detachment (partial) (premature) (with hemorrhage) 641.2 ✓
    affecting fetus or newborn 762.1
  dimidiata — see Placenta, abnormal
  disease 656.7 ✓
    affecting fetus or newborn 762.2
  duplex — see Placenta, abnormal
  dysfunction — see Placenta, insufficiency
  fenestrata — see Placenta, abnormal
  fibrosis — see Placenta, abnormal
  fleshy mole 631
  hematoma — see Placenta, abnormal
  hemorrhage NEC — see Placenta, separation

Placenta, placental — continued
  hormone disturbance or malfunction — see Placenta, abnormal
  hyperplasia — see Placenta, abnormal
  increta (without hemorrhage) 667.0 ✓
    with hemorrhage 666.0 ✓
  infarction 656.7 ✓
    affecting fetus or newborn 762.2
  insertion, vicious — see Placenta, previa
  insufficiency
    affecting
      fetus or newborn 762.2
      management of pregnancy 656.5 ✓
  lateral — see Placenta, previa
  low implantation or insertion — see Placenta, previa
  low-lying — see Placenta, previa
  malformation — see Placenta, abnormal
  malposition — see Placenta, previa
  marginalis, marginata — see Placenta, previa
  marginal sinus (hemorrhage) (rupture) 641.2 ✓
    affecting fetus or newborn 762.1
  membranacea — see Placenta, abnormal
  multilobed — see Placenta, abnormal
  multipartita — see Placenta, abnormal
  necrosis — see Placenta, abnormal
  percreta (without hemorrhage) 667.0 ✓
    with hemorrhage 666.0 ✓
  polyp 674.4 ✓
  previa (central) (centralis) (complete) (lateral) (marginal) (marginalis) (partial) (partialis) (total) (with hemorrhage) 641.1 ✓
    affecting fetus or newborn 762.0
    noted
      before labor, without hemorrhage (with cesarean delivery) 641.0 ✓
      during pregnancy (without hemorrhage) 641.0 ✓
    without hemorrhage (before labor and delivery) (during pregnancy) 641.0 ✓
  retention (with hemorrhage) 666.0 ✓
    fragments, complicating puerperium (delayed hemorrhage) 666.2 ✓
      without hemorrhage 667.1 ✓
    postpartum, puerperal 666.2 ✓
    without hemorrhage 667.0 ✓
  separation (normally implanted) (partial) (premature) (with hemorrhage) 641.2 ✓
    affecting fetus or newborn 762.1
  septuplex — see Placenta, abnormal
  small — see Placenta, insufficiency
  softening (premature) — see Placenta, abnormal
  spuria — see Placenta, abnormal
  succenturiata — see Placenta, abnormal
  syphilitic 095.8
  transfusion syndromes 762.3
  transmission of chemical substance — see Absorption, chemical, through placenta
  trapped (with hemorrhage) 666.0 ✓
    without hemorrhage 667.0 ✓
  trilobate — see Placenta, abnormal
  tripartita — see Placenta, abnormal
  triplex — see Placenta, abnormal
  varicose vessel — see Placenta, abnormal
  vicious insertion — see Placenta, previa
Placentitis
  affecting fetus or newborn 762.7
  complicating pregnancy 658.4 ✓
Plagiocephaly (skull) 754.0
Plague 020.9
  abortive 020.8
  ambulatory 020.8
  bubonic 020.0
  cellulocutaneous 020.1
  lymphatic gland 020.0
  pneumonic 020.5
    primary 020.3
    secondary 020.4
  pulmonary — see Plague, pneumonic
  pulmonic — see Plague, pneumonic
  septicemic 020.2
  tonsillar 020.9
    septicemic 020.2
  vaccination, prophylactic (against) V03.3

Planning, family V25.09
  contraception V25.9
  procreation V26.4
Plaque
  artery, arterial — *see* Arteriosclerosis
  calcareous — *see* Calcification
  Hollenhorst's (retinal) 362.33
  tongue 528.6
Plasma cell myeloma 203.0 ☑
Plasmacytoma, plasmocytoma (solitary)
    (M9731/1) 238.6
  benign (M9731/0) — *see* Neoplasm, by site,
    benign
  malignant (M9731/3) 203.8 ☑
Plasmacytosis 288.8
Plaster ulcer (*see also* Decubitus) 707.00   ▲
Platybasia 756.0
Platyonychia (congenital) 757.5
  acquired 703.8
Platypelloid pelvis 738.6
  with disproportion (fetopelvic) 653.2 ☑
    affecting fetus or newborn 763.1
    causing obstructed labor 660.1 ☑
      affecting fetus or newborn 763.1
  congenital 755.69
Platyspondylia 756.19
Plethora 782.62
  newborn 776.4
Pleura, pleural — *see* condition
Pleuralgia 786.52
Pleurisy (acute) (adhesive) (chronic) (costal)
    (diaphragmatic) (double) (dry) (fetid)
    (fibrinous) (fibrous) (interlobar) (latent) (lung)
    (old) (plastic) (primary) (residual) (sicca)
    (sterile) (subacute) (unresolved) (with
    adherent pleura) 511.0
  with
    effusion (without mention of cause) 511.9
      bacterial, nontuberculous 511.1
      nontuberculous NEC 511.9
        bacterial 511.1
      pneumococcal 511.1
      specified type NEC 511.8
      staphylococcal 511.1
      streptococcal 511.1
      tuberculous (*see also* Tuberculosis,
        pleura) 012.0 ☑
        primary, progressive 010.1 ☑
    influenza, flu, or grippe 487.1
    tuberculosis — *see* Pleurisy, tuberculous
  encysted 511.8
  exudative (*see also* Pleurisy, with effusion)
    511.9
    bacterial, nontuberculous 511.1
  fibrinopurulent 510.9
    with fistula 510.0
  fibropurulent 510.9
    with fistula 510.0
  hemorrhagic 511.8
  influenzal 487.1
  pneumococcal 511.0
    with effusion 511.1
  purulent 510.9
    with fistula 510.0
  septic 510.9
    with fistula 510.0
  serofibrinous (*see also* Pleurisy, with effusion)
    511.9
    bacterial, nontuberculous 511.1
  seropurulent 510.9
    with fistula 510.0
  serous (*see also* Pleurisy, with effusion) 511.9
    bacterial, nontuberculous 511.1
  staphylococcal 511.0
    with effusion 511.1
  streptococcal 511.0
    with effusion 511.1
  suppurative 510.9
    with fistula 510.0
  traumatic (post) (current) 862.29
    with open wound into cavity 862.39
  tuberculous (with effusion) (*see also*
    Tuberculosis, pleura) 012.0 ☑
    primary, progressive 010.1 ☑

Pleuritis sicca — *see* Pleurisy
Pleurobronchopneumonia (*see also* Pneumonia,
  broncho-) 485
Pleurodynia 786.52
  epidemic 074.1
  viral 074.1
Pleurohepatitis 573.8
Pleuropericarditis (*see also* Pericarditis) 423.9
  acute 420.90
Pleuropneumonia (acute) (bilateral) (double)
    (septic) (*see also* Pneumonia) 486
  chronic (*see also* Fibrosis, lung) 515
Pleurorrhea (*see also* Hydrothorax) 511.8
Plexitis, brachial 353.0
Plica
  knee 727.83
  polonica 132.0
  tonsil 474.8
Plicae dysphonia ventricularis 784.49
Plicated tongue 529.5
  congenital 750.13
Plug
  bronchus NEC 519.1
  meconium (newborn) NEC 777.1
  mucus — *see* Mucus, plug
Plumbism 984.9
  specified type of lead — *see* Table of Drugs and
    Chemicals
Plummer's disease (toxic nodular goiter) 242.3 ☑
Plummer-Vinson syndrome (sideropenic
  dysphagia) 280.8
Pluricarential syndrome of infancy 260
Plurideficiency syndrome of infancy 260
Plus (and minus) hand (intrinsic) 736.09
PMDD (premenstrual dysphoric disorder)
  625.4
PMS 625.4
Pneumathemia — see Air, embolism, by type
Pneumatic drill or hammer disease 994.9
Pneumatocele (lung) 518.89
  intracranial 348.8
  tension 492.0
Pneumatosis
  cystoides intestinalis 569.89
  peritonei 568.89
  pulmonum 492.8
Pneumaturia 599.84
Pneumoblastoma (M8981/3) — *see* Neoplasm,
  lung, malignant
Pneumocephalus 348.8
Pneumococcemia 038.2
Pneumococcus, pneumococcal — *see* condition
Pneumoconiosis (due to) (inhalation of) 505
  aluminum 503
  asbestos 501
  bagasse 495.1
  bauxite 503
  beryllium 503
  carbon electrode makers' 503
  coal
    miners' (simple) 500
    workers' (simple) 500
  cotton dust 504
  diatomite fibrosis 502
  dust NEC 504
    inorganic 503
    lime 502
    marble 502
    organic NEC 504
  fumes or vapors (from silo) 506.9
  graphite 503
  hard metal 503
  mica 502
  moldy hay 495.0
  rheumatoid 714.81
  silica NEC 502
    and carbon 500
  silicate NEC 502
  talc 502
Pneumocystis carinii pneumonia 136.3

Pneumocystosis 136.3
  with pneumonia 136.3
Pneumoenteritis 025
Pneumohemopericardium (*see also* Pericarditis)
  423.9
Pneumohemothorax (*see also* Hemothorax) 511.8
  traumatic 860.4
    with open wound into thorax 860.5
Pneumohydropericardium (*see also* Pericarditis)
  423.9
Pneumohydrothorax (*see also* Hydrothorax)
  511.8
Pneumomediastinum 518.1
  congenital 770.2
  fetus or newborn 770.2
Pneumomycosis 117.9
Pneumonia (acute) (Alpenstich) (benign) (bilateral)
    (brain) (cerebral) (circumscribed) (congestive)
    (creeping) (delayed resolution) (double)
    (epidemic) (fever) (flash) (fulminant) (fungoid)
    (granulomatous) (hemorrhagic) (incipient)
    (infantile) (infectious) (infiltration) (insular)
    (intermittent) (latent) (lobe) (migratory)
    (newborn) (organized) (overwhelming)
    (primary) (progressive) (pseudolobar)
    (purulent) (resolved) (secondary) (senile)
    (septic) (suppurative) (terminal) (true)
    (unresolved) (vesicular) 486
  with influenza, flu, or grippe 487.0
  adenoviral 480.0
  adynamic 514
  alba 090.0
  allergic 518.3
  alveolar — *see* Pneumonia, lobar
  anaerobes 482.81
  anthrax 022.1 *[484.5]*
  apex, apical — *see* Pneumonia, lobar
  ascaris 127.0 *[484.8]*
  aspiration 507.0
    due to
      aspiration of microorganisms
        bacterial 482.9
          specified type NEC 482.89
        specified organism NEC 483.8
          bacterial NEC 482.89
        viral 480.9
          specified type NEC 480.8
      food (regurgitated) 507.0
      gastric secretions 507.0
      milk 507.0
      oils, essences 507.1
      solids, liquids NEC 507.8
      vomitus 507.0
    newborn 770.1
  asthenic 514
  atypical (disseminated, focal) (primary) 486
    with influenza 487.0
  bacillus 482.9
    specified type NEC 482.89
  bacterial 482.9
    specified type NEC 482.89
  Bacteroides (fragilis) (oralis) (melaninogenicus)
    482.81
  basal, basic, basilar — *see* Pneumonia, lobar
  broncho-, bronchial (confluent) (croupous)
    (diffuse) (disseminated) (hemorrhagic)
    (involving lobes) (lobar) (terminal) 485
    with influenza 487.0
    allergic 518.3
    aspiration (*see also* Pneumonia, aspiration)
      507.0
    bacterial 482.9
      specified type NEC 482.89
    capillary 466.19
      with bronchospasm or obstruction
        466.19
    chronic (*see also* Fibrosis, lung) 515
  congenital (infective) 770.0
  diplococcal 481
  Eaton's agent 483.0
  Escherichia coli (E. coli) 482.82
  Friedländer's bacillus 482.0
  Hemophilus influenzae 482.2
  hiberno-vernal 083.0 *[484.8]*
  hypostatic 514
  influenzal 487.0

☑ Additional Digit Required   ▶◀ Revised Text   ● New Line   ▲ Revised Code

Pneumonia — *continued*
 broncho-, bronchial — *continued*
  inhalation (*see also* Pneumonia, aspiration) 507.0
   due to fumes or vapors (chemical) 506.0
  Klebsiella 482.0
  lipid 507.1
   endogenous 516.8
  Mycoplasma (pneumoniae) 483.0
  ornithosis 073.0
  pleuropneumonia-like organisms (PPLO) 483.0
  pneumococcal 481
  Proteus 482.83
  pseudomonas 482.1
  specified organism NEC 483.8
   bacterial NEC 482.89
  staphylococcal 482.40
   aureus 482.41
   specified type NEC 482.49
  streptococcal — *see* Pneumonia, streptococcal
  typhoid 002.0 *[484.8]*
  viral, virus (*see also* Pneumonia, viral) 480.9
 butyrivibrio (fibriosolvens) 482.81
 Candida 112.4
 capillary 466.19
  with bronchospasm or obstruction 466.19
 caseous (*see also* Tuberculosis) 011.6 ☑
 catarrhal — *see* Pneumonia, broncho-central — *see* Pneumonia, lobar
 Chlamydia, chlamydial 483.1
  pneumoniae 483.1
  psittaci 073.0
  specified type NEC 483.1
  trachomatis 483.1
 cholesterol 516.8
 chronic (*see also* Fibrosis, lung) 515
 Clostridium (haemolyticum) (novyi) NEC 482.81
 confluent — *see* Pneumonia, broncho-
 congenital (infective) 770.0
  aspiration 770.1
 croupous — *see* Pneumonia, lobar
 cytomegalic inclusion 078.5 *[484.1]*
 deglutition (*see also* Pneumonia, aspiration) 507.0
 desquamative interstitial 516.8
 diffuse — *see* Pneumonia, broncho-
 diplococcal, diplococcus (broncho-) (lobar) 481
 disseminated (focal) — *see* Pneumonia, broncho-
 due to
  adenovirus 480.0
  Bacterium anitratum 482.83
  Chlamydia, chlamydial 483.1
   pneumoniae 483.1
   psittaci 073.0
   specified type NEC 483.1
   trachomatis 483.1
  coccidioidomycosis 114.0
  Diplococcus (pneumoniae) 481
  Eaton's agent 483.0
  Escherichia coli (E. coli) 482.82
  Friedländer's bacillus 482.0
  fumes or vapors (chemical) (inhalation) 506.0
  fungus NEC 117.9 *[484.7]*
   coccidioidomycosis 114.0
  Hemophilus influenzae (H. influenzae) 482.2
  Herellea 482.83
  influenza 487.0
  Klebsiella pneumoniae 482.0
  Mycoplasma (pneumoniae) 483.0
  parainfluenza virus 480.2
  pleuropneumonia-like organism (PPLO) 483.0
  Pneumococcus 481
  Pneumocystis carinii 136.3
  Proteus 482.83
  pseudomonas 482.1
  respiratory syncytial virus 480.1
  rickettsia 083.9 *[484.8]*
  SARS-associated coronavirus 480.3
  specified
   bacteria NEC 482.89
   organism NEC 483.8
   virus NEC 480.8

Pneumonia — *continued*
 due to — *continued*
  Staphylococcus 482.40
   aureus 482.41
   specified type NEC 482.49
  Streptococcus — *see also* Pneumonia, streptococcal
   pneumoniae 481
  virus (*see also* Pneumonia, viral) 480.9
 Eaton's agent 483.0
 embolic, embolism (*see also* Embolism, pulmonary) 415.1 ☑
 eosinophilic 518.3
 Escherichia coli (E. coli) 482.82
 Eubacterium 482.81
 fibrinous — *see* Pneumonia, lobar
 fibroid (chronic)(*see also* Fibrosis, lung) 515
 fibrous (*see also* Fibrosis, lung) 515
 Friedländer's bacillus 482.0
 Fusobacterium (nucleatum) 482.81
 gangrenous 513.0
 giant cell (*see also* Pneumonia, viral) 480.9
 gram-negative bacteria NEC 482.83
  anaerobic 482.81
 grippal 487.0
 Hemophilus influenzae (bronchial) (lobar) 482.2
 hypostatic (broncho-) (lobar) 514
 in
  actinomycosis 039.1
  anthrax 022.1 *[484.5]*
  aspergillosis 117.3 *[484.6]*
  candidiasis 112.4
  coccidioidomycosis 114.0
  cytomegalic inclusion disease 078.5 *[484.1]*
  histoplasmosis (*see also* Histoplasmosis) 115.95
  infectious disease NEC 136.9 *[484.8]*
  measles 055.1
  mycosis, systemic NEC 117.9 *[484.7]*
  nocardiasis, nocardiosis 039.1
  ornithosis 073.0
  pneumocystosis 136.3
  psittacosis 073.0
  Q fever 083.0 *[484.8]*
  salmonellosis 003.22
  toxoplasmosis 130.4
  tularemia 021.2
  typhoid (fever) 002.0 *[484.8]*
  varicella 052.1
  whooping cough (*see also* Whooping cough) 033.9 *[484.3]*
 infective, acquired prenatally 770.0
 influenzal (broncho) (lobar) (virus) 487.0
 inhalation (*see also* Pneumonia, aspiration) 507.0
  fumes or vapors (chemical) 506.0
 interstitial 516.8
  with influenzal 487.0
  acute 136.3
  chronic (*see also* Fibrosis, lung) 515
  desquamative 516.8
  hypostatic 514
  lipoid 507.1
  lymphoid 516.8
  plasma cell 136.3
  pseudomonas 482.1
 intrauterine (infective) 770.0
  aspiration 770.1
 Klebsiella pneumoniae 482.0
 Legionnaires' 482.84
 lipid, lipoid (exogenous) (interstitial) 507.1
  endogenous 516.8
 lobar (diplococcal) (disseminated) (double) (interstitial) (pneumococcal, any type) 481
  with influenza 487.0
  bacterial 482.9
   specified type NEC 482.89
  chronic (*see also* Fibrosis, lung) 515
  Escherichia coli (E. coli) 482.82
  Friedländer's bacillus 482.0
  Hemophilus influenzae (H. influenzae) 482.2
  hypostatic 514
  influenzal 487.0
  Klebsiella 482.0
  ornithosis 073.0
  Proteus 482.83
  pseudomonas 482.1

Pneumonia — *continued*
 lobar — *continued*
  psittacosis 073.0
  specified organism NEC 483.8
   bacterial NEC 482.89
  staphylococcal 482.40
   aureus 482.41
   specified type NEC 482.49
  streptococcal — *see* Pneumonia, streptococcal
  viral, virus (*see also* Pneumonia, viral) 480.9
 lobular (confluent) — *see* Pneumonia, broncho-
 Löffler's 518.3
 massive — *see* Pneumonia, lobar
 meconium 770.1
 metastatic NEC 038.8 *[484.8]*
 Mycoplasma (pneumoniae) 483.0
 necrotic 513.0
 nitrogen dioxide 506.9
 orthostatic 514
 parainfluenza virus 480.2
 parenchymatous (*see also* Fibrosis, lung) 515
 passive 514
 patchy — *see* Pneumonia, broncho-
 Peptococcus 482.81
 Peptostreptococcus 482.81
 plasma cell 136.3
 pleurolobar — *see* Pneumonia, lobar
 pleuropneumonia-like organism (PPLO) 483.0
 pneumococcal (broncho) (lobar) 481
 Pneumocystis (carinii) 136.3
 postinfectional NEC 136.9 *[484.8]*
 postmeasles 055.1
 postoperative 997.3
 primary atypical 486
 Proprionibacterium 482.81
 Proteus 482.83
 pseudomonas 482.1
 psittacosis 073.0
 radiation 508.0
 respiratory syncytial virus 480.1
 resulting from a procedure 997.3
 rheumatic 390 *[517.1]*
 Salmonella 003.22
 SARS-associated coronavirus 480.3
 segmented, segmental — *see* Pneumonia, broncho-
 Serratia (marcescens) 482.83
 specified
  bacteria NEC 482.89
  organism NEC 483.8
  virus NEC 480.8
 spirochetal 104.8 *[484.8]*
 staphylococcal (broncho) (lobar) 482.40
  aureus 482.41
  specified type NEC 482.49
 static, stasis 514
 streptococcal (broncho) (lobar) NEC 482.30
  Group
   A 482.31
   B 482.32
   specified NEC 482.39
  pneumoniae 481
  specified type NEC 482.39
 Streptococcus pneumoniae 481
 traumatic (complication) (early) (secondary) 958.8
 tuberculous (any) (*see also* Tuberculosis) 011.6 ☑
 tularemic 021.2
 TWAR agent 483.1
 varicella 052.1
 Veillonella 482.81
 viral, virus (broncho) (interstitial) (lobar) 480.9
  with influenza, flu, or grippe 487.0
  adenoviral 480.0
  parainfluenza 480.2
  respiratory syncytial 480.1
  SARS-associated coronavirus 480.3
  specified type NEC 480.8
 white (congenital) 090.0
Pneumonic — *see* condition
Pneumonitis (acute) (primary) (*see also* Pneumonia) 486
 allergic 495.9
  specified type NEC 495.8

Pneumonitis (see also Pneumonia) — continued
  aspiration 507.0
    due to fumes or gases 506.0
    newborn 770.1
    obstetric 668.0 ☑
  chemical 506.0
    due to fumes or gases 506.0
  cholesterol 516.8
  chronic (see also Fibrosis, lung) 515
  congenital rubella 771.0
  crack 506.0   ●
  due to
    crack (cocaine) 506.0   ●
    fumes or vapors 506.0
    inhalation
      food (regurgitated), milk, vomitus 507.0
      oils, essences 507.1
      saliva 507.0
      solids, liquids NEC 507.8
    toxoplasmosis (acquired) 130.4
      congenital (active) 771.2 [484.8]
  eosinophilic 518.3
  fetal aspiration 770.1
  hypersensitivity 495.9
  interstitial (chronic) (see also Fibrosis, lung) 515
    lymphoid 516.8
  lymphoid, interstitial 516.8
  meconium 770.1
  postanesthetic
    correct substance properly administered 507.0
    obstetric 668.0 ☑
    overdose or wrong substance given 968.4
      specified anesthetic — see Table of Drugs and Chemicals
  postoperative 997.3
    obstetric 668.0 ☑
  radiation 508.0
  rubella, congenital 771.0
  "ventilation" 495.7
  wood-dust 495.8

Pneumonoconiosis — see Pneumoconiosis

Pneumoparotid 527.8

Pneumopathy NEC 518.89
  alveolar 516.9
    specified NEC 516.8
  due to dust NEC 504
  parietoalveolar 516.9
    specified condition NEC 516.8

Pneumopericarditis (see also Pericarditis) 423.9
  acute 420.90

Pneumopericardium — see also Pericarditis
  congenital 770.2
  fetus or newborn 770.2
  traumatic (post) (see also Pneumothorax, traumatic) 860.0
    with open wound into thorax 860.1

Pneumoperitoneum 568.89
  fetus or newborn 770.2

Pneumophagia (psychogenic) 306.4

Pneumopleurisy, pneumopleuritis (see also Pneumonia) 486

Pneumopyopericardium 420.99

Pneumopyothorax (see also Pyopneumothorax) 510.9
  with fistula 510.0

Pneumorrhagia 786.3
  newborn 770.3
  tuberculous (see also Tuberculosis, pulmonary) 011.9 ☑

Pneumosiderosis (occupational) 503

Pneumothorax (acute) (chronic) 512.8
  congenital 770.2
  due to operative injury of chest wall or lung 512.1
    accidental puncture or laceration 512.1
  fetus or newborn 770.2
  iatrogenic 512.1
  postoperative 512.1
  spontaneous 512.8
    fetus or newborn 770.2
    tension 512.0
  sucking 512.8
    iatrogenic 512.1
    postoperative 512.1

Pneumothorax — continued
  tense valvular, infectional 512.0
  tension 512.0
    iatrogenic 512.1
    postoperative 512.1
    spontaneous 512.0
  traumatic 860.0
    with
      hemothorax 860.4
        with open wound into thorax 860.5
      open wound into thorax 860.1
    tuberculous (see also Tuberculosis) 011.7 ☑

Pocket(s)
  endocardial (see also Endocarditis) 424.90
  periodontal 523.8

Podagra 274.9

Podencephalus 759.89

Poikilocytosis 790.09

Poikiloderma 709.09
  Civatte's 709.09
  congenital 757.33
  vasculare atrophicans 696.2

Poikilodermatomyositis 710.3

Pointed ear 744.29

Poise imperfect 729.9

Poisoned — see Poisoning

Poisoning (acute) — see also Table of Drugs and Chemicals
  Bacillus, B.
    aertrycke (see also Infection, Salmonella) 003.9
    botulinus 005.1
    cholerae (suis) (see also Infection, Salmonella) 003.9
    paratyphosus (see also Infection, Salmonella) 003.9
    suipestifer (see also Infection, Salmonella) 003.9
  bacterial toxins NEC 005.9
  berries, noxious 988.2
  blood (general) — see Septicemia
  botulism 005.1
  bread, moldy, mouldy — see Poisoning, food
  damaged meat — see Poisoning, food
  death-cap (Amanita phalloides) (Amanita verna) 988.1
  decomposed food — see Poisoning, food
  diseased food — see Poisoning, food
  drug — see Table of Drugs and Chemicals
  epidemic, fish, meat, or other food — see Poisoning, food
  fava bean 282.2
  fish (bacterial) — see also Poisoning, food
    noxious 988.0
  food (acute) (bacterial) (diseased) (infected) NEC 005.9
    due to
      bacillus
        aertrycke (see also Poisoning, food, due to Salmonella) 003.9
        botulinus 005.1
        cereus 005.89
        choleraesuis (see also Poisoning, food, due to Salmonella) 003.9
        paratyphosus (see also Poisoning, food, due to Salmonella) 003.9
        suipestifer (see also Poisoning, food, due to Salmonella) 003.9
      Clostridium 005.3
        botulinum 005.1
        perfringens 005.2
        welchii 005.2
      Salmonella (aertrycke) (callinarum) (choleraesuis) (enteritidis) (paratyphi) (suipestifer) 003.9
        with
          gastroenteritis 003.0
          localized infection(s) (see also Infection, Salmonella) 003.20
          septicemia 003.1
          specified manifestation NEC 003.8
      specified bacterium NEC 005.89
      Staphylococcus 005.0
      Streptococcus 005.8 ☑
      Vibrio parahaemolyticus 005.4
      Vibrio vulnificus 005.81

Poisoning — see also Table of Drugs and Chemicals — continued
  food — continued
    noxious or naturally toxic 988.0
      berries 988.2
      fish 988.0
      mushroom 988.1
      plants NEC 988.2
  ice cream — see Poisoning, food
  ichthyotoxism (bacterial) 005.9
  kreotoxism, food 005.9
  malarial — see Malaria
  meat — see Poisoning, food
  mushroom (noxious) 988.1
  mussel — see also Poisoning, food
    noxious 988.0
  noxious foodstuffs (see also Poisoning, food, noxious) 988.9
    specified type NEC 988.8
  plants, noxious 988.2
  pork — see also Poisoning, food
    specified NEC 988.8
    Trichinosis 124
  ptomaine — see Poisoning, food
  putrefaction, food — see Poisoning, food
  radiation 508.0
  Salmonella (see also Infection, Salmonella) 003.9
  sausage — see also Poisoning, food
    Trichinosis 124
  saxitoxin 988.0
  shellfish — see also Poisoning, food
    noxious 988.0
  Staphylococcus, food 005.0
  toxic, from disease NEC 799.89
  truffles — see Poisoning, food
  uremic — see Uremia
  uric acid 274.9

Poison ivy, oak, sumac or other plant dermatitis 692.6

Poker spine 720.0

Policeman's disease 729.2

Polioencephalitis (acute) (bulbar) (see also Poliomyelitis, bulbar) 045.0 ☑
  inferior 335.22
  influenzal 487.8
  superior hemorrhagic (acute) (Wernicke's) 265.1
  Wernicke's (superior hemorrhagic) 265.1

Polioencephalomyelitis (acute) (anterior) (bulbar) (see also Polioencephalitis) 045.0 ☑

Polioencephalopathy, superior hemorrhagic 265.1
  with
    beriberi 265.0
    pellagra 265.2

Poliomeningoencephalitis — see Meningoencephalitis

Poliomyelitis (acute) (anterior) (epidemic) 045.9 ☑

Note — Use the following fifth-digit subclassification with category 045:

  0   poliovirus, unspecified type
  1   poliovirus, type I
  2   poliovirus, type II
  3   poliovirus, type III

  with
    paralysis 045.1 ☑
      bulbar 045.0 ☑
  abortive 045.2 ☑
  ascending 045.9 ☑
    progressive 045.9 ☑
  bulbar 045.0 ☑
  cerebral 045.0 ☑
  chronic 335.21
  congenital 771.2
  contact V01.2
  deformities 138
  exposure to V01.2
  late effect 138
  nonepidemic 045.9 ☑
  nonparalytic 045.2 ☑
  old with deformity 138

☑ Additional Digit Required   ►◄ Revised Text   ● New Line   ▲ Revised Code

Poliomyelitis — *continued*
  posterior, acute 053.19
  residual 138
  sequelae 138
  spinal, acute 045.9 ☑
  syphilitic (chronic) 094.89
  vaccination, prophylactic (against) V04.0
Poliosis (eyebrow) (eyelashes) 704.3
  circumscripta (congenital) 757.4
    acquired 704.3
  congenital 757.4
Pollakiuria 788.4 ☑
  psychogenic 306.53
Pollinosis 477.0
Pollitzer's disease (hidradenitis suppurativa) 705.83
Polyadenitis (*see also* Adenitis) 289.3
  malignant 020.0
Polyalgia 729.9
Polyangiitis (essential) 446.0
Polyarteritis (nodosa) (renal) 446.0
Polyarthralgia 719.49
  psychogenic 306.0
Polyarthritis, polyarthropathy NEC 716.59
  due to or associated with other specified
    conditions — *see* Arthritis, due to or
    associated with
  endemic (*see also* Disease, Kaschin-Beck) 716.0 ☑
  inflammatory 714.9
    specified type NEC 714.89
  juvenile (chronic) 714.30
    acute 714.31
  migratory — *see* Fever, rheumatic
  rheumatic 714.0
    fever (acute) — *see* Fever, rheumatic
Polycarential syndrome of infancy 260
Polychondritis (atrophic) (chronic) (relapsing) 733.99
Polycoria 743.46
Polycystic (congenital) (disease) 759.89
  degeneration, kidney — *see* Polycystic, kidney
  kidney (congenital) 753.12
    adult type (APKD) 753.13
    autosomal dominant 753.13
    autosomal recessive 753.14
    childhood type (CPKD) 753.14
    infantile type 753.14
  liver 751.62
  lung 518.89
    congenital 748.4
  ovary, ovaries 256.4
  spleen 759.0
Polycythemia (primary) (rubra) (vera) (M9950/1) 238.4
  acquired 289.0
  benign 289.0
    familial 289.6
  due to
    donor twin 776.4
    fall in plasma volume 289.0
    high altitude 289.0
    maternal-fetal transfusion 776.4
    stress 289.0
  emotional 289.0
  erythropoietin 289.0
  familial (benign) 289.6
  Gaisböck's (hypertonica) 289.0
  high altitude 289.0
  hypertonica 289.0
  hypoxemic 289.0
  neonatorum 776.4
  nephrogenous 289.0
  relative 289.0
  secondary 289.0
  spurious 289.0
  stress 289.0
Polycytosis cryptogenica 289.0
Polydactylism, polydactyly 755.00
  fingers 755.01
  toes 755.02
Polydipsia 783.5
Polydystrophic oligophrenia 277.5

Polyembryoma (M9072/3) — *see* Neoplasm, by site, malignant
Polygalactia 676.6 ☑
Polyglandular
  deficiency 258.9
  dyscrasia 258.9
  dysfunction 258.9
  syndrome 258.8
Polyhydramnios (*see also* Hydramnios) 657.0 ☑
Polymastia 757.6
Polymenorrhea 626.2
Polymicrogyria 742.2
Polymyalgia 725
  arteritica 446.5
  rheumatica 725
Polymyositis (acute) (chronic) (hemorrhagic) 710.4
  with involvement of
    lung 710.4 [517.8]
    skin 710.3
  ossificans (generalisata) (progressiva) 728.19
  Wagner's (dermatomyositis) 710.3
Polyneuritis, polyneuritic (*see also* Polyneuropathy) 356.9
  alcoholic 357.5
    with psychosis 291.1
  cranialis 352.6
  diabetic 250.6 ☑ [357.2]
  demyelinating, chronic inflammatory 357.81
  due to lack of vitamin NEC 269.2 [357.4]
  endemic 265.0 [357.4]
  erythredema 985.0
  febrile 357.0
  hereditary ataxic 356.3
  idiopathic, acute 357.0
  infective (acute) 357.0
  nutritional 269.9 [357.4]
  postinfectious 357.0
Polyneuropathy (peripheral) 356.9
  alcoholic 357.5
  amyloid 277.3 [357.4]
  arsenical 357.7
  critical illness 357.82
  diabetic 250.6 ☑ [357.2]
  due to
    antitetanus serum 357.6
    arsenic 357.7
    drug or medicinal substance 357.6
      correct substance properly administered 357.6
      overdose or wrong substance given or taken 977.9
        specified drug — *see* Table of Drugs and Chemicals
    lack of vitamin NEC 269.2 [357.4]
    lead 357.7
    organophosphate compounds 357.7
    pellagra 265.2 [357.4]
    porphyria 277.1 [357.4]
    serum 357.6
    toxic agent NEC 357.7
  hereditary 356.0
  idiopathic 356.9
    progressive 356.4
  in
    amyloidosis 277.3 [357.4]
    avitaminosis 269.2 [357.4]
      specified NEC 269.1 [357.4]
    beriberi 265.0 [357.4]
    collagen vascular disease NEC 710.9 [357.1]
    deficiency
      B-complex NEC 266.2 [357.4]
      vitamin B 266.9 [357.4]
      vitamin B 266.1 [357.4]
    diabetes 250.6 ☑ [357.2]
    diphtheria (*see also* Diphtheria) 032.89 [357.4]
    disseminated lupus erythematosus 710.0 [357.1]
    herpes zoster 053.13
    hypoglycemia 251.2 [357.4]
    malignant neoplasm (M8000/3) NEC 199.1 [357.4]
    mumps 072.72
    pellagra 265.2 [357.4]

Polyneuropathy — *continued*
  in — *continued*
    polyarteritis nodosa 446.0 [357.1]
    porphyria 277.1 [357.4]
    rheumatoid arthritis 714.0 [357.1]
    sarcoidosis 135 [357.4]
    uremia 585 [357.4]
  lead 357.7
  nutritional 269.9 [357.4]
    specified NEC 269.8 [357.4]
  postherpetic 053.13
  progressive 356.4
  sensory (hereditary) 356.2
Polyonychia 757.5
Polyopia 368.2
  refractive 368.15
Polyorchism, polyorchidism (three testes) 752.89
Polyorrhymenitis (peritoneal) (*see also* Polyserositis) 568.82
  pericardial 423.2
Polyostotic fibrous dysplasia 756.54
Polyotia 744.1
Polyp, polypus

> *Note* — Polyps of organs or sites that do not appear in the list below should be coded to the residual category for diseases of the organ or site concerned.

  accessory sinus 471.8
  adenoid tissue 471.0
  adenomatous (M8210/0) — *see also* Neoplasm, by site, benign
    adenocarcinoma in (M8210/3) — *see* Neoplasm, by site, malignant
    carcinoma in (M8210/3) — *see* Neoplasm, by site, malignant
    multiple (M8221/0) — *see* Neoplasm, by site, benign
  antrum 471.8
  anus, anal (canal) (nonadenomatous) 569.0
    adenomatous 211.4
  Bartholin's gland 624.6
  bladder (M8120/1) 236.7
  broad ligament 620.8
  cervix (uteri) 622.7
    adenomatous 219.0
    in pregnancy or childbirth 654.6 ☑
      affecting fetus or newborn 763.89
      causing obstructed labor 660.2 ☑
    mucous 622.7
    nonneoplastic 622.7
  choanal 471.0
  cholesterol 575.6
  clitoris 624.6
  colon (M8210/0) (*see also* Polyp, adenomatous) 211.3
  corpus uteri 621.0
  dental 522.0
  ear (middle) 385.30
  endometrium 621.0
  ethmoidal (sinus) 471.8
  fallopian tube 620.8
  female genital organs NEC 624.8
  frontal (sinus) 471.8
  gallbladder 575.6
  gingiva 523.8
  gum 523.8
  labia 624.6
  larynx (mucous) 478.4
  malignant (M8000/3) — *see* Neoplasm, by site, malignant
  maxillary (sinus) 471.8
  middle ear 385.30
  myometrium 621.0
  nares
    anterior 471.9
    posterior 471.0
  nasal (mucous) 471.9
    cavity 471.0
    septum 471.9
  nasopharyngeal 471.0
  neoplastic (M8210/0) — *see* Neoplasm, by site, benign
  nose (mucous) 471.9

☑ Additional Digit Required   ▶◀ Revised Text   ● New Line   ▲ Revised Code

Polyp, polypus — *continued*
  oviduct 620.8
  paratubal 620.8
  pharynx 478.29
    congenital 750.29
  placenta, placental 674.4 ☑
  prostate 600.20
    with urinary retention 600.21
  pudenda 624.6
  pulp (dental) 522.0
  rectosigmoid 211.4
  rectum (nonadenomatous) 569.0
    adenomatous 211.4
  septum (nasal) 471.9
  sinus (accessory) (ethmoidal) (frontal)
    (maxillary) (sphenoidal) 471.8
  sphenoidal (sinus) 471.8
  stomach (M8210/0) 211.1
  tube, fallopian 620.8
  turbinate, mucous membrane 471.8
  ureter 593.89
  urethra 599.3
  uterine
    ligament 620.8
    tube 620.8
  uterus (body) (corpus) (mucous) 621.0
    in pregnancy or childbirth 654.1 ☑
      affecting fetus or newborn 763.89
      causing obstructed labor 660.2 ☑
  vagina 623.7
  vocal cord (mucous) 478.4
  vulva 624.6
Polyphagia 783.6
Polypoid — *see* condition
Polyposis — *see also* Polyp
  coli (adenomatous) (M8220/0) 211.3
    adenocarcinoma in (M8220/3) 153.9
    carcinoma in (M8220/3) 153.9
  familial (M8220/0) 211.3
  intestinal (adenomatous) (M8220/0) 211.3
  multiple (M8221/0) — *see* Neoplasm, by site,
    benign
Polyradiculitis (acute) 357.0
Polyradiculoneuropathy (acute) (segmentally
  demyelinating) 357.0
Polysarcia 278.00
Polyserositis (peritoneal) 568.82
  due to pericarditis 423.2
  paroxysmal (familial) 277.3
  pericardial 423.2
  periodic 277.3
  pleural — *see* Pleurisy
  recurrent 277.3
  tuberculous (*see also* Tuberculosis,
    polyserositis) 018.9 ☑
Polysialia 527.7
Polysplenia syndrome 759.0
Polythelia 757.6
Polytrichia (*see also* Hypertrichosis) 704.1
Polyunguia (congenital) 757.5
  acquired 703.8
Polyuria 788.42
Pompe's disease (glycogenosis II) 271.0
Pompholyx 705.81
Poncet's disease (tuberculous rheumatism) (*see
  also* Tuberculosis) 015.9 ☑
Pond fracture — *see* Fracture, skull, vault
Ponos 085.0
Pons, pontine — *see* condition
Poor
  contractions, labor 661.2 ☑
    affecting fetus or newborn 763.7
  fetal growth NEC 764.9 ☑
    affecting management of pregnancy 656.5 ☑
  incorporation
    artificial skin graft 996.55
    decellularized allodermis graft 996.55
  obstetrical history V13.29
    affecting management of current pregnancy
      V23.49
        pre-term labor V23.41
        pre-term labor V13.21
  sucking reflex (newborn) 796.1

Poor — *continued*
  vision NEC 369.9
Poradenitis, nostras 099.1
Porencephaly (congenital) (developmental) (true)
  742.4
  acquired 348.0
  nondevelopmental 348.0
  traumatic (post) 310.2
Porocephaliasis 134.1
Porokeratosis 757.39
  disseminated superficial actinic (DSAP) 692.75
Poroma, eccrine (M8402/0) — *see* Neoplasm,
  skin, benign
Porphyria (acute) (congenital) (constitutional)
  (erythropoietic) (familial) (hepatica)
  (idiopathic) (idiosyncratic) (intermittent)
  (latent) (mixed hepatic) (photosensitive)
  (South African genetic) (Swedish) 277.1
  acquired 277.1
  cutaneatarda
    hereditaria 277.1
    symptomatica 277.1
  due to drugs
    correct substance properly administered
      277.1
    overdose or wrong substance given or taken
      977.9
      specified drug — *see* Table of Drugs and
        Chemicals
  secondary 277.1
  toxic NEC 277.1
  variegata 277.1
Porphyrinuria (acquired) (congenital) (secondary)
  277.1
Porphyruria (acquired) (congenital) 277.1
Portal — *see* condition
Port wine nevus or mark 757.32
Posadas-Wernicke disease 114.9
Position
  fetus, abnormal (*see also* Presentation, fetal)
    652.9 ☑
  teeth, faulty ▶(*see also* Anomaly, position
    tooth)◀ 524.30   ▲
Positive
  culture (nonspecific) 795.39
    AIDS virus V08
    blood 790.7
    HIV V08
    human immunodeficiency virus V08
    nose 795.39
    skin lesion NEC 795.39
    spinal fluid 792.0
    sputum 795.39
    stool 792.1
    throat 795.39
    urine 791.9
    wound 795.39
  findings, anthrax 795.31
  HIV V08
  human immunodeficiency virus (HIV) V08
  PPD 795.5
  serology
    AIDS virus V08
      inconclusive 795.71
    HIV V08
      inconclusive 795.71
    human immunodeficiency virus (HIV) V08
      inconclusive 795.71
    syphilis 097.1
      with signs or symptoms — *see* Syphilis,
        by site and stage
      false 795.6
  skin test 795.7 ☑
    tuberculin (without active tuberculosis)
      795.5
  VDRL 097.1
    with signs or symptoms — *see* Syphilis, by
      site and stage
    false 795.6
  Wassermann reaction 097.1
    false 795.6
Postcardiotomy syndrome 429.4
Postcaval ureter 753.4

Postcholecystectomy syndrome 576.0
Postclimacteric bleeding 627.1
Postcommissurotomy syndrome 429.4
Postconcussional syndrome 310.2
Postcontusional syndrome 310.2
Postcricoid region — *see* condition
Post-dates (pregnancy) — *see* Pregnancy
Postencephalitic — *see also* condition
  syndrome 310.8
Posterior — *see* condition
Posterolateral sclerosis (spinal cord) — *see*
  Degeneration, combined
Postexanthematous — *see* condition
Postfebrile — *see* condition
Postgastrectomy dumping syndrome 564.2
Posthemiplegic chorea 344.89
Posthemorrhagic anemia (chronic) 280.0
  acute 285.1
  newborn 776.5
Posthepatitis syndrome 780.79
Postherpetic neuralgia (intercostal) (syndrome)
  (zoster) 053.19
  geniculate ganglion 053.11
  ophthalmica 053.19
  trigeminal 053.12
Posthitis 607.1
Postimmunization complication or reaction —
  see Complications, vaccination
Postinfectious — *see* condition
Postinfluenzal syndrome 780.79
Postlaminectomy syndrome 722.80
  cervical, cervicothoracic 722.81
  kyphosis 737.12
  lumbar, lumbosacral 722.83
  thoracic, thoracolumbar 722.82
Postleukotomy syndrome 310.0
Postlobectomy syndrome 310.0
Postmastectomy lymphedema (syndrome) 457.0
Postmaturity, postmature (fetus or newborn)
  (gestation period over 42 completed weeks)
  766.22
  affecting management of pregnancy
    post-term pregnancy 645.1 ☑
    prolonged pregnancy 645.2 ☑
  syndrome 766.22
Postmeasles — *see also* condition
  complication 055.8
    specified NEC 055.79
Postmenopausal
  endometrium (atrophic) 627.8
    suppurative (see also Endometritis) 615.9
  hormone replacement V07.4
  status (age related) (natural) V49.81
Postnasal drip — *see* Sinusitis
Postnatal — *see* condition
Postoperative — *see also* condition
  confusion state 293.9
  psychosis 293.9
  status NEC (*see also* Status (post)) V45.89
Postpancreatectomy hyperglycemia 251.3
Postpartum — *see also* condition
  anemia 648.2 ☑
  cardiomyopathy 674.5 ☑
  observation
    immediately after delivery V24.0
    routine follow-up V24.2
Postperfusion syndrome NEC 999.8
  bone marrow 996.85
Postpoliomyelitic — *see* condition
Postsurgery status NEC (*see also* Status (post))
  V45.89
Post-term (pregnancy) 645.1 ☑
  infant (gestation period over 40 completed
    weeks to 42 completed weeks)
    766.21
Posttraumatic — *see* condition
Posttraumatic brain syndrome, nonpsychotic
  310.2
Post-typhoid abscess 002.0
Postures, hysterical 300.11

☑ Additional Digit Required   ▶◀ Revised Text   ● New Line   ▲ Revised Code

Postvaccinal reaction or complication — *see* Complications, vaccination
Postvagotomy syndrome 564.2
Postvalvulotomy syndrome 429.4
Postvasectomy sperm count V25.8
Potain's disease (pulmonary edema) 514
Potain's syndrome (gastrectasis with dyspepsia) 536.1
Pott's
  curvature (spinal) (*see also* Tuberculosis) 015.0 ☑ [737.43]
  disease or paraplegia (*see also* Tuberculosis) 015.0 ☑ [730.88]
  fracture (closed) 824.4
    open 824.5
  gangrene 440.24
  osteomyelitis (*see also* Tuberculosis) 015.0 ☑ [730.88]
  spinal curvature (*see also* Tuberculosis) 015.0 ☑ [737.43]
  tumor, puffy (*see also* Osteomyelitis) 730.2 ☑
Potter's
  asthma 502
  disease 753.0
  facies 754.0
  lung 502
  syndrome (with renal agenesis) 753.0
Pouch
  bronchus 748.3
  Douglas' — *see* condition
  esophagus, esophageal (congenital) 750.4
    acquired 530.6
  gastric 537.1
  Hartmann's (abnormal sacculation of gallbladder neck) 575.8
    of intestine V44.3
      attention to V55.3
  pharynx, pharyngeal (congenital) 750.27
Poulet's disease 714.2
Poultrymen's itch 133.8
Poverty V60.2
Prader-Labhart-Willi-Fanconi syndrome (hypogenital dystrophy with diabetic tendency) 759.81
Prader-Willi syndrome (hypogenital dystrophy with diabetic tendency) 759.81
Preachers' voice 784.49
Pre-AIDS — *see* Human immunodeficiency virus (disease) (illness) (infection)
Preauricular appendage 744.1
Prebetalipoproteinemia (acquired) (essential) (familial) (hereditary) (primary) (secondary) 272.1
  with chylomicronemia 272.3
Precipitate labor 661.3 ☑
  affecting fetus or newborn 763.6
Preclimacteric bleeding 627.0
  menorrhagia 627.0
Precocious
  adrenarche 259.1
  menarche 259.1
  menstruation 626.8
  pubarche 259.1
  puberty NEC 259.1
  sexual development NEC 259.1
  thelarche 259.1
Precocity, sexual (constitutional) (cryptogenic) (female) (idiopathic) (male) NEC 259.1
  with adrenal hyperplasia 255.2
Precordial pain 786.51
  psychogenic 307.89
Predeciduous teeth 520.2
Prediabetes, prediabetic 790.29
  complicating pregnancy, childbirth, or puerperium 648.8 ☑
    fetus or newborn 775.8
Predislocation status of hip, at birth (*see also* Subluxation, congenital, hip) 754.32
Preeclampsia (mild) 642.4 ☑
  with pre-existing hypertension 642.7 ☑
  affecting fetus or newborn 760.0
  severe 642.5 ☑

Preeclampsia — *continued*
  superimposed on pre-existing hypertensive disease 642.7 ☑
Preeruptive color change, teeth, tooth 520.8
Preexcitation 426.7
  atrioventricular conduction 426.7
  ventricular 426.7
Preglaucoma 365.00
Pregnancy (single) (uterine) (without sickness) V22.2

> *Note — Use the following fifth-digit subclassification with categories 640-648, 651-676:*
>
> 0   *unspecified as to episode of care*
> 1   *delivered, with or without mention of antepartum condition*
> 2   *delivered, with mention of postpartum complication*
> 3   *antepartum condition or complication*
> 4   *postpartum condition or complication*

  abdominal (ectopic) 633.00
    with intrauterine pregnancy 633.01
    affecting fetus or newborn 761.4
  abnormal NEC 646.9 ☑
  ampullar — *see* Pregnancy, tubal
  broad ligament — *see* Pregnancy, cornual
  cervical — *see* Pregnancy, cornual
  combined (extrauterine and intrauterine) — *see* Pregnancy, cornual
  complicated (by)
    abnormal, abnormality NEC 646.9 ☑
      cervix 654.6 ☑
      cord (umbilical) 663.9 ☑
      glucose tolerance (conditions classifiable to 790.21-790.29) 648.8 ☑
      injury 648.9 ☑
        obstetrical NEC 665.9 ☑
      obstetrical trauma NEC 665.9 ☑
      pelvic organs or tissues NEC 654.9 ☑
      pelvis (bony) 653.0 ☑
      perineum or vulva 654.8 ☑
      placenta, placental (vessel) 656.7 ☑
      position
        cervix 654.4 ☑
        placenta 641.1 ☑
          without hemorrhage 641.0 ☑
        uterus 654.4 ☑
      size, fetus 653.5 ☑
      uterus (congenital) 654.0 ☑
    abscess or cellulitis
      bladder 646.6 ☑
      genitourinary tract (conditions classifiable to 590, 595, 597, 599.0, 614.0-614.5, 614.7-614.9, 615) 646.6 ☑
      kidney 646.6 ☑
      urinary tract NEC 646.6 ☑
    adhesion, pelvic peritoneal 648.9 ☑
    air embolism 673.0 ☑
    albuminuria 646.2 ☑
      with hypertension — *see* Toxemia, of pregnancy
    amnionitis 658.4 ☑
    amniotic fluid embolism 673.1 ☑
    anemia (conditions classifiable to 280-285) 648.2 ☑
    atrophy, yellow (acute) (liver) (subacute) 646.7 ☑
    bacilluria, asymptomatic 646.5 ☑
    bacteriuria, asymptomatic 646.5 ☑
    bicornis or bicornuate uterus 654.0 ☑
    biliary problems 646.8 ☑ ●
    bone and joint disorders (conditions classifiable to 720-724 or conditions affecting lower limbs classifiable to 711-719, 725-738) 648.7 ☑
    breech presentation 652.2 ☑
      with successful version 652.1 ☑
    cardiovascular disease (conditions classifiable to 390-398, 410-429) 648.6 ☑
      congenital (conditions classifiable to 745-747) 648.5 ☑

Pregnancy — *continued*
  complicated (by) — *continued*
    cerebrovascular disorders (conditions classifiable to 430-434, 436-437) 674.0 ☑
    cervicitis (conditions classifiable to 616.0) 646.6 ☑
    chloasma (gravidarum) 646.8 ☑
    chorea (gravidarum) — *see* Eclampsia, pregnancy
    cholelithiasis 646.8 ☑
    contraction, pelvis (general) 653.1 ☑
      inlet 653.2 ☑
      outlet 653.3 ☑
    convulsions (eclamptic) (uremic) 642.6 ☑
      with pre-existing hypertension 642.7 ☑
    current disease or condition (nonobstetric)
      abnormal glucose tolerance 648.8 ☑
      anemia 648.2 ☑
      bone and joint (lower limb) 648.7 ☑
      cardiovascular 648.6 ☑
        congenital 648.5 ☑
      cerebrovascular 674.0 ☑
      diabetic 648.0 ☑
      drug dependence 648.3 ☑
      genital organ or tract 646.6 ☑
      gonorrheal 647.1 ☑
      hypertensive 642.2 ☑
        renal 642.1 ☑
      infectious 647.9 ☑
        specified type NEC 647.8 ☑
      liver 646.7 ☑
      malarial 647.4 ☑
      nutritional deficiency 648.9 ☑
      parasitic NEC 647.8 ☑
      periodontal disease 648.9 ☑ ●
      renal 646.2 ☑
        hypertensive 642.1 ☑
      rubella 647.5 ☑
      specified condition NEC 648.9 ☑
      syphilitic 647.0 ☑
      thyroid 648.1 ☑
      tuberculous 647.3 ☑
      urinary 646.6 ☑
      venereal 647.2 ☑
      viral NEC 647.6 ☑
    cystitis 646.6 ☑
    cystocele 654.4 ☑
    death of fetus (near term) 656.4 ☑
      early pregnancy (before 22 completed weeks gestation) 632
    deciduitis 646.6 ☑
    decreased fetal movements 655.7 ☑
    diabetes (mellitus) (conditions classifiable to 250) 648.0 ☑
    disorders of liver 646.7 ☑
    displacement, uterus NEC 654.4 ☑
    disproportion — *see* Disproportion
    double uterus 654.0 ☑
    drug dependence (conditions classifiable to 304) 648.3 ☑
    dysplasia, cervix 654.6 ☑
    early onset of delivery (spontaneous) 644.2 ☑
    eclampsia, eclamptic (coma) (convulsions) (delirium) (nephritis) (uremia) 642.6 ☑
      with pre-existing hypertension 642.7 ☑
    edema 646.1 ☑
      with hypertension — *see* Toxemia, of pregnancy
    effusion, amniotic fluid 658.1 ☑
      delayed delivery following 658.2 ☑
    embolism
      air 673.0 ☑
      amniotic fluid 673.1 ☑
      blood-clot 673.2 ☑
      cerebral 674.0 ☑
      pulmonary NEC 673.2 ☑
      pyemic 673.3 ☑
      septic 673.3 ☑
    emesis (gravidarum) — *see* Pregnancy, complicated, vomiting
    endometritis (conditions classifiable to 615.0-615.9) 646.6 ☑
      decidual 646.6 ☑
    excessive weight gain NEC 646.1 ☑
    face presentation 652.4 ☑

☑ Additional Digit Required   ▶◀ Revised Text   ● New Line   ▲ Revised Code

Pregnancy

☑ Additional Digit Required   ▶◀ Revised Text   ● New Line   ▲ Revised Code

Pregnancy — *continued*
  complicated (by) — *continued*
    viral disease NEC (conditions classifiable to
      042, 050-055, 057-079) 647.6 ☑
    vomiting (incoercible) (pernicious)
      (persistent) (uncontrollable) (vicious)
      643.9 ☑
      due to organic disease or other cause
        643.8 ☑
      early — *see* Hyperemesis, gravidarum
      late (after 22 completed weeks gestation)
        643.2 ☑
    young maternal age 659.8 ☑
  complications NEC 646.9 ☑
  cornual 633.80
    with intrauterine pregnancy 633.81
    affecting fetus or newborn 761.4
  death, maternal NEC 646.9 ☑
  delivered — *see* Delivery
  ectopic (ruptured) NEC 633.90
    with intrauterine pregnancy 633.91
    abdominal — *see* Pregnancy, abdominal
    affecting fetus or newborn 761.4
    combined (extrauterine and intrauterine) —
      see Pregnancy, cornual
    ovarian — *see* Pregnancy, ovarian
    specified type NEC 633.80
      with intrauterine pregnancy 633.81
      affecting fetus or newborn 761.4
    tubal — *see* Pregnancy, tubal
  examination, pregnancy
    negative result V72.41   ●
    not confirmed V72.40   ●
  extrauterine — *see* Pregnancy, ectopic
  fallopian — *see* Pregnancy, tubal
  false 300.11
    labor (pains) 644.1 ☑
  fatigue 646.8 ☑
  illegitimate V61.6
  incidental finding V22.2
  in double uterus 654.0 ☑
  interstitial — *see* Pregnancy, cornual
  intraligamentous — *see* Pregnancy, cornual
  intramural — *see* Pregnancy, cornual
  intraperitoneal — *see* Pregnancy, abdominal
  isthmian — *see* Pregnancy, tubal
  management affected by
    abnormal, abnormality
      fetus (suspected) 655.9 ☑
        specified NEC 655.8 ☑
      placenta 656.7 ☑
    advanced maternal age NEC 659.6 ☑
      multigravida 659.6 ☑
      primigravida 659.5 ☑
    antibodies (maternal)
      anti-c 656.1 ☑
      anti-d 656.1 ☑
      anti-e 656.1 ☑
      blood group (ABO) 656.2 ☑
        Rh(esus) 656.1 ☑
    elderly multigravida 659.6 ☑
    elderly primigravida 659.5 ☑
    fetal (suspected)
      abnormality 655.9 ☑
        acid-base balance 656.8 ☑
        heart rate or rhythm 659.7 ☑
        specified NEC 655.8 ☑
      acidemia 656.3 ☑
      anencephaly 655.0 ☑
      bradycardia 659.7 ☑
      central nervous system malformation
        655.0 ☑
      chromosomal abnormalities (conditions
        classifiable to 758.0-758.9) 655.1 ☑
      damage from
        drugs 655.5 ☑
          obstetric, anesthetic, or sedative
            655.5 ☑
        environmental toxins 655.8 ☑
        intrauterine contraceptive device
          655.8 ☑
        maternal
          alcohol addiction 655.4 ☑
          disease NEC 655.4 ☑
          drug use 655.5 ☑
          listeriosis 655.4 ☑
          rubella 655.3 ☑

Pregnancy — *continued*
  management affected by — *continued*
    fetal — *continued*
      damage from — *continued*
        maternal — *continued*
          toxoplasmosis 655.4 ☑
          viral infection 655.3 ☑
        radiation 655.6 ☑
      death (near term) 656.4 ☑
        early (before 22 completed weeks'
          gestation) 632
      distress 656.8 ☑
      excessive growth 656.6 ☑
      growth retardation 656.5 ☑
      hereditary disease 655.2 ☑
      hydrocephalus 655.0 ☑
      intrauterine death 656.4 ☑
      poor growth 656.5 ☑
      spina bifida (with myelomeningocele)
        655.0 ☑
    fetal-maternal hemorrhage 656.0 ☑
    hereditary disease in family (possibly)
      affecting fetus 655.2 ☑
    incompatibility, blood groups (ABO)
      656.2 ☑
      rh(esus) 656.1 ☑
    insufficient prenatal care V23.7
    intrauterine death 656.4 ☑
    isoimmunization (ABO) 656.2 ☑
      rh(esus) 656.1 ☑
    large-for-dates fetus 656.6 ☑
    light-for-dates fetus 656.5 ☑
    meconium in liquor 656.8 ☑
    mental disorder (conditions classifiable to
      290-303, 305-316, 317-319) 648.4 ☑
    multiparity (grand) 659.4 ☑
    poor obstetric history V23.49
      pre-term labor V23.41
    postmaturity
      post-term 645.1 ☑
      prolonged 645.2 ☑
    post-term pregnancy 645.1 ☑
    previous
      abortion V23.2
        habitual 646.3 ☑
      cesarean delivery 654.2 ☑
      difficult delivery V23.49
      forceps delivery V23.49
      habitual abortions 646.3 ☑
      hemorrhage, antepartum or postpartum
        V23.49
      hydatidiform mole V23.1
      infertility V23.0
      malignancy NEC V23.8 ☑
      nonobstetrical conditions V23.8 ☑
      premature delivery V23.41
      trophoblastic disease (conditions in 630)
        V23.1
      vesicular mole V23.1
    prolonged pregnancy 645.2 ☑
    small-for-dates fetus 656.5 ☑
    young maternal age 659.8 ☑
  maternal death NEC 646.9 ☑
  mesometric (mural) — *see* Pregnancy, cornual
  molar 631
    hydatidiform (*see also* Hydatidiform mole)
      630
      previous, affecting management of
        pregnancy V23.1
    previous, affecting management of
      pregnancy V23.49
  multiple NEC 651.9 ☑
    with fetal loss and retention of one or more
      fetus(es) 651.6 ☑
    affecting fetus or newborn 761.5
    specified type NEC 651.8 ☑
      with fetal loss and retention of one or
        more fetus(es) 651.6 ☑
  mural — *see* Pregnancy, cornual
  observation NEC V22.1
    first pregnancy V22.0
    high-risk V23.9
      specified problem NEC V23.8 ☑
  ovarian 633.20
    with intrauterine pregnancy 633.21
    affecting fetus or newborn 761.4

Pregnancy — *continued*
  possible, not (yet) confirmed V72.40   ●
  postmature
    post-term 645.1 ☑
    prolonged 645.2 ☑
  post-term 645.1 ☑
  prenatal care only V22.1
    first pregnancy V22.0
    high-risk V23.9
      specified problem NEC V23.8 ☑
  prolonged 645.2 ☑
  quadruplet NEC 651.2 ☑
    with fetal loss and retention of one or more
      fetus(es) 651.5 ☑
    affecting fetus or newborn 761.5
  quintuplet NEC 651.8 ☑
    with fetal loss and retention of one or more
      fetus(es) 651.6 ☑
    affecting fetus or newborn 761.5
  sextuplet NEC 651.8 ☑
    with fetal loss and retention of one or more
      fetus(es) 651.6 ☑
    affecting fetus or newborn 761.5
  spurious 300.11
  superfecundation NEC 651.9 ☑
    with fetal loss and retention of one or more
      fetus(es) 651.6 ☑
  superfetation NEC 651.9 ☑
    with fetal loss and retention of one or more
      fetus(es) 651.6 ☑
  supervision (of) (for) — *see also* Pregnancy,
    management affected by
    elderly
      multigravida V23.82
      primigravida V23.81
    high-risk V23.9
      insufficient prenatal care V23.7
      specified problem NEC V23.8 ☑
    multiparity V23.3
    normal NEC V22.1
      first V22.0
    poor
      obstetric history V23.49
        pre-term labor V23.41
      reproductive history V23.5
    previous
      abortion V23.2
      hydatidiform mole V23.1
      infertility V23.0
      neonatal death V23.5
      stillbirth V23.5
      trophoblastic disease V23.1
      vesicular mole V23.1
    specified problem NEC V23.8 ☑
    young
      multigravida V23.84
      primigravida V23.83
  triplet NEC 651.1 ☑
    with fetal loss and retention of one or more
      fetus(es) 651.4 ☑
    affecting fetus or newborn 761.5
  tubal (with rupture) 633.10
    with intrauterine pregnancy 633.11
    affecting fetus or newborn 761.4
  twin NEC 651.0 ☑
    with fetal loss and retention of one fetus
      651.3 ☑
    affecting fetus or newborn 761.5
  unconfirmed V72.40   ▲
  undelivered (no other diagnosis) V22.2
    with false labor 644.1 ☑
    high-risk V23.9
      specified problem NEC V23.8 ☑
  unwanted NEC V61.7

Pregnant uterus — *see* condition

Preiser's disease (osteoporosis) 733.09

Prekwashiorkor 260

Preleukemia 238.7

Preluxation of hip, congenital (*see also*
  Subluxation, congenital, hip) 754.32

Premature — *see also* condition
  beats (nodal) 427.60
    atrial 427.61
    auricular 427.61
    postoperative 997.1
    specified type NEC 427.69

☑ Additional Digit Required   ▶◀ Revised Text   ● New Line   ▲ Revised Code

Premature — *see also* condition — *continued*
  beats — *continued*
    supraventricular 427.61
    ventricular 427.69
  birth NEC 765.1 ☑
  closure
    cranial suture 756.0
    fontanel 756.0
    foramen ovale 745.8
  contractions 427.60
    atrial 427.61
    auricular 427.61
    auriculoventricular 427.61
    heart (extrasystole) 427.60
    junctional 427.60
    nodal 427.60
    postoperative 997.1
    ventricular 427.69
  ejaculation 302.75
  infant NEC 765.1 ☑
    excessive 765.0 ☑
    light-for-dates — *see* Light-for-dates
  labor 644.2 ☑
    threatened 644.0 ☑
  lungs 770.4
  menopause 256.31
  puberty 259.1
  rupture of membranes or amnion 658.1 ☑
    affecting fetus or newborn 761.1
    delayed delivery following 658.2 ☑
  senility (syndrome) 259.8
  separation, placenta (partial) — *see* Placenta, separation
  ventricular systole 427.69
Prematurity NEC 765.1 ☑
  extreme 765.0 ☑
Premenstrual syndrome 625.4
Premenstrual tension 625.4
Premolarization, cuspids 520.2
Premyeloma 273.1
Prenatal
  care, normal pregnancy V22.1
    first V22.0
  death, cause unknown — *see* Death, fetus
  screening — *see* Antenatal, screening
Prepartum — *see* condition
Preponderance, left or right ventricular 429.3
Prepuce — *see* condition
Presbycardia 797
  hypertensive (*see also* Hypertension, heart) 402.90
Presbycusis 388.01
Presbyesophagus 530.89
Presbyophrenia 310.1
Presbyopia 367.4
Prescription of contraceptives NEC V25.02
  diaphragm V25.02
  oral (pill) V25.01
    emergency V25.03
    postcoital V25.03
    repeat V25.41
  repeat V25.40
    oral (pill) V25.41
Presenile — *see also* condition
  aging 259.8
  dementia (*see also* Dementia, presenile) 290.10
Presenility 259.8
Presentation, fetal
  abnormal 652.9 ☑
    with successful version 652.1 ☑
    before labor, affecting fetus or newborn 761.7
    causing obstructed labor 660.0 ☑
      affecting fetus or newborn, any, except breech 763.1
    in multiple gestation (one or more) 652.6 ☑
    specified NEC 652.8 ☑
  arm 652.7 ☑
    causing obstructed labor 660.0 ☑
  breech (buttocks) (complete) (frank) 652.2 ☑
    with successful version 652.1 ☑
      before labor, affecting fetus or newborn 761.7

Presentation, fetal — *continued*
  breech — *continued*
    before labor, affecting fetus or newborn 761.7
  brow 652.4 ☑
    causing obstructed labor 660.0 ☑
  buttocks 652.2 ☑
  chin 652.4 ☑
  complete 652.2 ☑
  compound 652.8 ☑
  cord 663.0 ☑
  extended head 652.4 ☑
  face 652.4 ☑
    to pubes 652.8 ☑
  footling 652.8 ☑
  frank 652.2 ☑
  hand, leg, or foot NEC 652.8 ☑
  incomplete 652.8 ☑
  mentum 652.4 ☑
  multiple gestation (one fetus or more) 652.6 ☑
  oblique 652.3 ☑
    with successful version 652.1 ☑
  shoulder 652.8 ☑
    affecting fetus or newborn 763.1
  transverse 652.3 ☑
    with successful version 652.1 ☑
  umbilical cord 663.0 ☑
  unstable 652.0 ☑
Prespondylolisthesis (congenital) (lumbosacral) 756.11
Pressure
  area, skin ulcer (*see also* Decubitus) 707.00▲
  atrophy, spine 733.99
  birth, fetus or newborn NEC 767.9
  brachial plexus 353.0
  brain 348.4
    injury at birth 767.0
  cerebral — *see* Pressure, brain
  chest 786.59
  cone, tentorial 348.4
    injury at birth 767.0
  funis — *see* Compression, umbilical cord
  hyposystolic (*see also* Hypotension) 458.9
  increased
    intracranial 781.99
      due to
        benign intracranial hypertension 348.2
        hydrocephalus — *see* hydrocephalus
        injury at birth 767.8
    intraocular 365.00
  lumbosacral plexus 353.1
  mediastinum 519.3
  necrosis (chronic) (skin) (*see also* Decubitus) 707.00   ▲
  nerve — *see* Compression, nerve
  paralysis (*see also* Neuropathy, entrapment) 355.9
  sore (chronic) (*see also* Decubitus) 707.00 ▲
  spinal cord 336.9
  ulcer (chronic) (*see also* Decubitus) 707.00 ▲
  umbilical cord — *see* Compression, umbilical cord
  venous, increased 459.89
Pre-syncope 780.2
Preterm infant NEC 765.1 ☑
  extreme 765.0 ☑
Priapism (penis) 607.3
Prickling sensation (*see also* Disturbance, sensation) 782.0
Prickly heat 705.1
Primary — *see* condition
Primigravida, elderly
  affecting
    fetus or newborn 763.89
    management of pregnancy, labor, and delivery 659.5 ☑
Primipara, old
  affecting
    fetus or newborn 763.89
    management of pregnancy, labor, and delivery 659.5 ☑
Primula dermatitis 692.6
Primus varus (bilateral) (metatarsus) 754.52
P.R.I.N.D. 436

Pringle's disease (tuberous sclerosis) 759.5
Prinzmetal's angina 413.1
Prinzmetal-Massumi syndrome (anterior chest wall) 786.52
Prizefighter ear 738.7
Problem (with) V49.9
  academic V62.3
  acculturation V62.4
  adopted child V61.29
  aged
    in-law V61.3
    parent V61.3
    person NEC V61.8
  alcoholism in family V61.41
  anger reaction (*see also* Disturbance, conduct) 312.0 ☑
  behavior, child 312.9
  behavioral V40.9
    specified NEC V40.3
  betting V69.3
  cardiorespiratory NEC V47.2
  care of sick or handicapped person in family or household V61.49
  career choice V62.2
  communication V40.1
  conscience regarding medical care V62.6
  delinquency (juvenile) 312.9
  diet, inappropriate V69.1
  digestive NEC V47.3
  ear NEC V41.3
  eating habits, inappropriate V69.1
  economic V60.2
    affecting care V60.9
      specified type NEC V60.8
  educational V62.3
  enuresis, child 307.6
  exercise, lack of V69.0
  eye NEC V41.1
  family V61.9
    specified circumstance NEC V61.8
  fear reaction, child 313.0
  feeding (elderly) (infant) 783.3
    newborn 779.3
    nonorganic 307.50
  fetal, affecting management of pregnancy 656.9 ☑
    specified type NEC 656.8 ☑
  financial V60.2
  foster child V61.29
    specified NEC V41.8
  functional V41.9
    specified type NEC V41.8
  gambling V69.3
  genital NEC V47.5
  head V48.9
    deficiency V48.0
    disfigurement V48.6
    mechanical V48.2
    motor V48.2
    movement of V48.2
    sensory V48.4
    specified condition NEC V48.8
  hearing V41.2
  high-risk sexual behavior V69.2
  identity 313.82   ●
  influencing health status NEC V49.89
  internal organ NEC V47.9
    deficiency V47.0
    mechanical or motor V47.1
  interpersonal NEC V62.81
  jealousy, child 313.3
  learning V40.0
  legal V62.5
  life circumstance NEC V62.89
  lifestyle V69.9
    specified NEC V69.8
  limb V49.9
    deficiency V49.0
    disfigurement V49.4
    mechanical V49.1
    motor V49.2
    movement, involving
      musculoskeletal system V49.1
      nervous system V49.2
    sensory V49.3
    specified condition NEC V49.5

☑ Additional Digit Required   ▶◀ Revised Text   ● New Line   ▲ Revised Code

Problem (with) — *continued*
  litigation V62.5
  living alone V60.3
  loneliness NEC V62.89
  marital V61.10
    involving
      divorce V61.0
      estrangement V61.0
      psychosexual disorder 302.9
      sexual function V41.7
  mastication V41.6
  medical care, within family V61.49
  mental V40.9
    specified NEC V40.2
  mental hygiene, adult V40.9
  multiparity V61.5
  nail biting, child 307.9
  neck V48.9
    deficiency V48.1
    disfigurement V48.7
    mechanical V48.3
    motor V48.3
    movement V48.3
    sensory V48.5
    specified condition NEC V48.8
  neurological NEC 781.99
  none (feared complaint unfounded) V65.5
  occupational V62.2
  parent-child V61.20
  partner V61.10
  personal NEC V62.89
    interpersonal conflict NEC V62.81
  personality (*see also* Disorder, personality) 301.9
  phase of life V62.89
  placenta, affecting managment of pregnancy 656.9 ☑
    specified type NEC 656.8 ☑
  poverty V60.2
  presence of sick or handicapped person in family or household V61.49
  psychiatric 300.9
  psychosocial V62.9
    specified type NEC V62.89
  relational NEC V62.81
  relationship, childhood 313.3
  religious or spiritual belief
    other than medical care V62.89
    regarding medical care V62.6
  self-damaging behavior V69.8
  sexual
    behavior, high-risk V69.2
    function NEC V41.7
  sibling relational V61.8
  sight V41.0
  sleep, lack of V69.4 ●
  sleep disorder, child 307.40
  smell V41.5
  speech V40.1
  spite reaction, child (*see also* Disturbance, conduct) 312.0 ☑
  spoiled child reaction (*see also* Disturbance, conduct) 312.1 ☑
  swallowing V41.6
  tantrum, child (*see also* Disturbance, conduct) 312.1 ☑
  taste V41.5
  thumb sucking, child 307.9
  tic ►(child)◄ 307.21
  trunk V48.9
    deficiency V48.1
    disfigurement V48.7
    mechanical V48.3
    motor V48.3
    movement V48.3
    sensory V48.5
    specified condition NEC V48.8
  unemployment V62.0
  urinary NEC V47.4
  voice production V41.4
Procedure (surgical) **not done** NEC V64.3
  because of
    contraindication V64.1
    patient's decision V64.2
      for reasons of conscience or religion V62.6
    specified reason NEC V64.3

Procidentia
  anus (sphincter) 569.1
  rectum (sphincter) 569.1
  stomach 537.89
  uteri 618.1
Proctalgia 569.42
  fugax 564.6
  spasmodic 564.6
    psychogenic 307.89
Proctitis 569.49
  amebic 006.8
  chlamydial 099.52
  gonococcal 098.7
  granulomatous 555.1
  idiopathic 556.2
    with ulcerative sigmoiditis 556.3
  tuberculous (*see also* Tuberculosis) 014.8 ☑
  ulcerative (chronic) (nonspecific) 556.2
    with ulcerative sigmoiditis 556.3
Proctocele
  female (without uterine prolapse) 618.04 ▲
    with uterine prolapse 618.4
      complete 618.3
      incomplete 618.2
  male 569.49
Proctocolitis, idiopathic 556.2
  with ulcerative sigmoiditis 556.3
Proctoptosis 569.1
Proctosigmoiditis 569.89
  ulcerative (chronic) 556.3
Proctospasm 564.6
  psychogenic 306.4
Prodromal-AIDS — *see* Human immunodeficiency virus (disease) (illness) (infection)
Profichet's disease or syndrome 729.9
Progeria (adultorum) (syndrome) 259.8
Prognathism (mandibular) (maxillary) 524.00
Progonoma (melanotic) (M9363/0) — *see* Neoplasm, by site, benign
Progressive — *see* condition
Prolapse, prolapsed
  anus, anal (canal) (sphincter) 569.1
  arm or hand, complicating delivery 652.7 ☑
    causing obstructed labor 660.0 ☑
      affecting fetus or newborn 763.1
    fetus or newborn 763.1
  bladder (acquired) (mucosa) (sphincter)
    congenital (female) (male) 756.71
    female ►(*see also* Cystocele, female)◄ 618.01 ▲
    male 596.8
  breast implant (prosthetic) 996.54
  cecostomy 569.69
  cecum 569.89
  cervix, cervical (stump) (hypertrophied) 618.1
    anterior lip, obstructing labor 660.2 ☑
      affecting fetus or newborn 763.1
    congenital 752.49
    postpartal (old) 618.1
  ciliary body 871.1
  colon (pedunculated) 569.89
  colostomy 569.69
  conjunctiva 372.73
  cord — *see* Prolapse, umbilical cord
  disc (intervertebral) — *see* Displacement, intervertebral disc
  duodenum 537.89
  eye implant (orbital) 996.59
    lens (ocular) 996.53
  fallopian tube 620.4
  fetal extremity, complicating delivery 652.8 ☑
    causing obstructed labor 660.0 ☑
    fetus or newborn 763.1
  funis — *see* Prolapse, umbilical cord
  gastric (mucosa) 537.89
  genital, female 618.9
    specified NEC 618.89 ▲
  globe 360.81
  ileostomy bud 569.69
  intervertebral disc — *see* Displacement, intervertebral disc
  intestine (small) 569.89
  iris 364.8
    traumatic 871.1

Prolapse, prolapsed — *continued*
  kidney (*see also* Disease, renal) 593.0
    congenital 753.3
  laryngeal muscles or ventricle 478.79
  leg, complicating delivery 652.8 ☑
    causing obstructed labor 660.0 ☑
    fetus or newborn 763.1
  liver 573.8
  meatus urinarius 599.5
  mitral valve 424.0
  ocular lens implant 996.53
  organ or site, congenital NEC — *see* Malposition, congenital
  ovary 620.4
  pelvic (floor), female 618.89 ▲
  perineum, female 618.89 ▲
  pregnant uterus 654.4 ☑
  rectum (mucosa) (sphincter) 569.1
    due to Trichuris trichiuria 127.3
  spleen 289.59
  stomach 537.89
  umbilical cord
    affecting fetus or newborn 762.4
    complicating delivery 663.0 ☑
  ureter 593.89
    with obstruction 593.4
  ureterovesical orifice 593.89
  urethra (acquired) (infected) (mucosa) 599.5
    congenital 753.8
  uterovaginal 618.4
    complete 618.3
    incomplete 618.2
    specified NEC 618.89 ▲
  uterus (first degree) (second degree) (third degree) (complete) (without vaginal wall prolapse) 618.1
    with mention of vaginal wall prolapse — *see* Prolapse, uterovaginal
    congenital 752.3
    in pregnancy or childbirth 654.4 ☑
      affecting fetus or newborn 763.1
      causing obstructed labor 660.2 ☑
        affecting fetus or newborn 763.1
    postpartal (old) 618.1
  uveal 871.1
  vagina (anterior) (posterior) (vault) (wall) (without uterine prolapse) 618.00 ▲
    with uterine prolapse 618.4
      complete 618.3
      incomplete 618.2
    paravaginal 618.02 ●
    posthysterectomy 618.5
    specified NEC 618.09 ●
  vitreous (humor) 379.26
    traumatic 871.1
  womb — *see* Prolapse, uterus
Prolapsus, female 618.9
Proliferative — *see* condition
Prolinemia 270.8
Prolinuria 270.8
Prolonged, prolongation
  bleeding time (*see also* Defect, coagulation) 790.92
    "idiopathic" (in von Willebrand's disease) 286.4
  coagulation time (*see also* Defect, coagulation) 790.92
  gestation syndrome 766.22
  labor 662.1 ☑
    affecting fetus or newborn 763.89
    first stage 662.0 ☑
    second stage 662.2 ☑
  pregnancy 645.2 ☑
  PR interval 426.11
  prothrombin time (*see also* Defect, coagulation) 790.92
  rupture of membranes (24 hours or more prior to onset of labor) 658.2 ☑
  uterine contractions in labor 661.4 ☑
    affecting fetus or newborn 763.7
Prominauris 744.29
Prominence
  auricle (ear) (congenital) 744.29
    acquired 380.32

Prominence — *continued*
ischial spine or sacral promontory
with disproportion (fetopelvic) 653.3 ☑
affecting fetus or newborn 763.1
causing obstructed labor 660.1 ☑
affecting fetus or newborn 763.1
nose (congenital) 748.1
acquired 738.0
Pronation
ankle 736.79
foot 736.79
congenital 755.67
Prophylactic
administration of
antibiotics V07.39
antitoxin, any V07.2
antivenin V07.2
chemotherapeutic agent NEC V07.39
fluoride V07.31
diphtheria antitoxin V07.2
gamma globulin V07.2
immune sera (gamma globulin) V07.2
RhoGAM V07.2
tetanus antitoxin V07.2
chemotherapy NEC V07.39
fluoride V07.31
hormone replacement (postmenopausal)   ●
V07.4   ●
immunotherapy V07.2
measure V07.9
specified type NEC V07.8
postmenopausal hormone replacement V07.4
sterilization V25.2
Proptosis (ocular) (*see also* Exophthalmos) 376.30
thyroid 242.0 ☑
Propulsion
eyeball 360.81
Prosecution, anxiety concerning V62.5
Prostate, prostatic — *see* condition
Prostatism 600.90
with urinary retention 600.91
Prostatitis (congestive) (suppurative) 601.9
acute 601.0
cavitary 601.8
chlamydial 099.54
chronic 601.1
diverticular 601.8
due to Trichomonas (vaginalis) 131.03
fibrous 600.90
with urinary retention 600.91
gonococcal (acute) 098.12
chronic or duration of 2 months or over
098.32
granulomatous 601.8
hypertrophic 600.00
with urinary retention 600.01
specified type NEC 601.8
subacute 601.1
trichomonal 131.03
tuberculous (*see also* Tuberculosis)
016.5 ☑ [601.4]
Prostatocystitis 601.3
Prostatorrhea 602.8
Prostatoseminovesiculitis, trichomonal 131.03
Prostration 780.79
heat 992.5
anhydrotic 992.3
due to
salt (and water) depletion 992.4
water depletion 992.3
nervous 300.5
newborn 779.89
senile 797
Protanomaly 368.51
Protanopia (anomalous trichromat) (complete)
(incomplete) 368.51
Protein
deficiency 260
malnutrition 260
sickness (prophylactic) (therapeutic) 999.5
Proteinemia 790.99
Proteinosis
alveolar, lung or pulmonary 516.0
lipid 272.8

Proteinosis — *continued*
lipoid (of Urbach) 272.8
Proteinuria (*see also* Albuminuria) 791.0
Bence-Jones NEC 791.0
gestational 646.2 ☑
with hypertension — *see* Toxemia, of
pregnancy
orthostatic 593.6
postural 593.6
Proteolysis, pathologic 286.6
Protocoproporphyria 277.1
Protoporphyria (erythrohepatic) (erythropoietic)
277.1
Protrusio acetabuli 718.65
Protrusion
acetabulum (into pelvis) 718.65
device, implant, or graft — *see*
Complications, mechanical
ear, congenital 744.29
intervertebral disc — *see* Displacement,
intervertebral disc
nucleus pulposus — *see* Displacement,
intervertebral disc
Proud flesh 701.5
Prune belly (syndrome) 756.71
Prurigo (ferox) (gravis) (Hebra's) (hebrae) (mitis)
(simplex) 698.2
agria 698.3
asthma syndrome 691.8
Besnier's (atopic dermatitis) (infantile eczema)
691.8
eczematodes allergicum 691.8
estivalis (Hutchinson's) 692.72
Hutchinson's 692.72
nodularis 698.3
psychogenic 306.3
Pruritus, pruritic 698.9
ani 698.0
psychogenic 306.3
conditions NEC 698.9
psychogenic 306.3
due to Onchocerca volvulus 125.3
ear 698.9
essential 698.9
genital organ(s) 698.1
psychogenic 306.3
gravidarum 646.8 ☑
hiemalis 698.8
neurogenic (any site) 306.3
perianal 698.0
psychogenic (any site) 306.3
scrotum 698.1
psychogenic 306.3
senile, senilis 698.8
Trichomonas 131.9
vulva, vulvae 698.1
psychogenic 306.3
Psammocarcinoma (M8140/3) — *see* Neoplasm,
by site, malignant
Pseudarthrosis, pseudoarthrosis (bone) 733.82
joint following fusion V45.4
Pseudoacanthosis
nigricans 701.8
Pseudoaneurysm — *see* Aneurysm
Pseudoangina (pectoris) — *see* Angina
Pseudoangioma 452
Pseudo-Argyll-Robertson pupil 379.45
Pseudoarteriosus 747.89
Pseudoarthrosis — *see* Pseudarthrosis
Pseudoataxia 799.89
Pseudobursa 727.89
Pseudocholera 025
Pseudochromidrosis 705.89
Pseudocirrhosis, liver, pericardial 423.2
Pseudocoarctation 747.21
Pseudocowpox 051.1
Pseudocoxalgia 732.1
Pseudocroup 478.75
Pseudocyesis 300.11
Pseudocyst
lung 518.89

Pseudocyst — *continued*
pancreas 577.2
retina 361.19
Pseudodementia 300.16
Pseudoelephantiasis neuroarthritica 757.0
Pseudoemphysema 518.89
Pseudoencephalitis
superior (acute) hemorrhagic 265.1
Pseudoerosion cervix, congenital 752.49
Pseudoexfoliation, lens capsule 366.11
Pseudofracture (idiopathic) (multiple)
(spontaneous) (symmetrical) 268.2
Pseudoglanders 025
Pseudoglioma 360.44
Pseudogout — *see* Chondrocalcinosis
Pseudohallucination 780.1
Pseudohemianesthesia 782.0
Pseudohemophilia (Bernuth's) (hereditary)
(type B) 286.4
type A 287.8
vascular 287.8
Pseudohermaphroditism 752.7
with chromosomal anomaly — *see* Anomaly,
chromosomal
adrenal 255.2
female (without adrenocortical disorder) 752.7
with adrenocortical disorder 255.2
adrenal 255.2
male (without gonadal disorder) 752.7
with
adrenocortical disorder 255.2
cleft scrotum 752.7
feminizing testis 257.8
gonadal disorder 257.9
adrenal 255.2
Pseudohole, macula 362.54
Pseudo-Hurler's disease (mucolipidosis III) 272.7
Pseudohydrocephalus 348.2
Pseudohypertrophic muscular dystrophy (Erb's)
359.1
Pseudohypertrophy, muscle 359.1
Pseudohypoparathyroidism 275.49
Pseudoinfluenza 487.1
Pseudoinsomnia 307.49
Pseudoleukemia 288.8
infantile 285.8
Pseudomembranous — *see* condition
Pseudomeningocele (cerebral) (infective) (surgical)
349.2
spinal 349.2
Pseudomenstruation 626.8
Pseudomucinous
cyst (ovary) (M8470/0) 220
peritoneum 568.89
Pseudomyeloma 273.1
Pseudomyxoma peritonei (M8480/6) 197.6
Pseudoneuritis optic (nerve) 377.24
papilla 377.24
congenital 743.57
Pseudoneuroma — *see* Injury, nerve, by site
Pseudo-obstruction
intestine ▶(chronic) (idiopathic) (intermittent
secondary) (primary)◀ 564.89   ●
acute 560.89
Pseudopapilledema 377.24
Pseudoparalysis
arm or leg 781.4
atonic, congenital 358.8
Pseudopelade 704.09
Pseudophakia V43.1
Pseudopolycythemia 289.0
Pseudopolyposis, colon 556.4
Pseudoporencephaly 348.0
Pseudopseudohypoparathyroidism 275.49
Pseudopsychosis 300.16
Pseudopterygium 372.52
Pseudoptosis (eyelid) 374.34
Pseudorabies 078.89

Pseudoretinitis, pigmentosa 362.65
Pseudorickets 588.0
　senile (Pozzi's) 731.0
Pseudorubella 057.8
Pseudoscarlatina 057.8
Pseudosclerema 778.1
Pseudosclerosis (brain)
　Jakob's 046.1
　of Westphal (-Strümpell) (hepatolenticular
　　degeneration) 275.1
　spastic 046.1
　　with dementia
　　　with behavioral disturbance 046.1
　　　　[294.11]
　　　without behavioral disturbance 046.1
　　　　[294.10]
Pseudoseizure 780.39
　non-psychiatric 780.39
　psychiatric 300.11
Pseudotabes 799.89
　diabetic 250.6 ☑ [337.1]
Pseudotetanus (see also Convulsions) 780.39
Pseudotetany 781.7
　hysterical 300.11
Pseudothalassemia 285.0
Pseudotrichinosis 710.3
Pseudotruncus arteriosus 747.29
Pseudotuberculosis, pasteurella (infection) 027.2
Pseudotumor
　cerebri 348.2
　orbit (inflammatory) 376.11
Pseudo-Turner's syndrome 759.89
Pseudoxanthoma elasticum 757.39
Psilosis (sprue) (tropical) 579.1
　Monilia 112.89
　nontropical 579.0
　not sprue 704.00
Psittacosis 073.9
Psoitis 728.89
Psora NEC 696.1
Psoriasis 696.1
　any type, except arthropathic 696.1
　arthritic, arthropathic 696.0
　buccal 528.6
　flexural 696.1
　follicularis 696.1
　guttate 696.1
　inverse 696.1
　mouth 528.6
　nummularis 696.1
　psychogenic 316 [696.1]
　punctata 696.1
　pustular 696.1
　rupioides 696.1
　vulgaris 696.1
Psorospermiasis 136.4
Psorospermosis 136.4
　follicularis (vegetans) 757.39
Psychalgia 307.80
Psychasthenia 300.89
　compulsive 300.3
　mixed compulsive states 300.3
　obsession 300.3
Psychiatric disorder or problem NEC 300.9
Psychogenic — see also condition
　factors associated with physical conditions 316
Psychoneurosis, psychoneurotic (see also
　　Neurosis) 300.9
　anxiety (state) 300.00
　climacteric 627.2
　compensation 300.16
　compulsion 300.3
　conversion hysteria 300.11
　depersonalization 300.6
　depressive type 300.4
　dissociative hysteria 300.15
　hypochondriacal 300.7
　hysteria 300.10
　　conversion type 300.11
　　dissociative type 300.15
　mixed NEC 300.89
　neurasthenic 300.5

Psychoneurosis, psychoneurotic — continued
　obsessional 300.3
　obsessive-compulsive 300.3
　occupational 300.89
　personality NEC 301.89
　phobia 300.20
　senile NEC 300.89
Psychopathic — see also condition
　constitution, posttraumatic 310.2
　　with psychosis 293.9
　personality 301.9
　　amoral trends 301.7
　　antisocial trends 301.7
　　asocial trends 301.7
　　mixed types 301.7
　state 301.9
Psychopathy, sexual (see also Deviation, sexual)
　302.9
Psychophysiologic, psychophysiological
　condition — see Reaction,
　psychophysiologic
Psychose passionelle 297.8
Psychosexual identity disorder 302.6
　adult-life 302.85
　childhood 302.6
Psychosis 298.9
　acute hysterical 298.1
　affecting management of pregnancy, childbirth,
　　or puerperium 648.4 ☑
　affective ▶(see also Disorder, mood)◀ 296.90

> Note — Use the following fifth-digit
> subclassification with categories 296.0-296.6:
>
> 　0　unspecified
> 　1　mild
> 　2　moderate
> 　3　severe, without mention of psychotic
> 　　behavior
> 　4　severe, specified as with psychotic
> 　　behavior
> 　5　in partial or unspecified remission
> 　6　in full remission

　　drug-induced 292.84
　　due to or associated with physical condition
　　　293.83
　　involutional 296.2 ☑
　　　recurrent episode 296.3 ☑
　　　single episode 296.2 ☑
　　manic-depressive 296.80
　　　circular (alternating) 296.7
　　　　currently depressed 296.5 ☑
　　　　currently manic 296.4 ☑
　　　depressed type 296.2 ☑
　　　　atypical 296.82
　　　　recurrent episode 296.3 ☑
　　　　single episode 296.2 ☑
　　　manic 296.0 ☑
　　　　atypical 296.81
　　　　recurrent episode 296.1 ☑
　　　　single episode 296.0 ☑
　　　mixed type NEC 296.89
　　　specified type NEC 296.89
　　senile 290.21
　　specified type NEC 296.99
　alcoholic 291.9
　　with
　　　anxiety 291.89
　　　delirium tremens 291.0
　　　delusions 291.5
　　　dementia 291.2
　　　hallucinosis 291.3
　　　mood disturbance 291.89
　　　jealousy 291.5
　　　paranoia 291.5
　　　persisting amnesia 291.1
　　　sexual dysfunction 291.89
　　　sleep disturbance 291.89
　　amnestic confabulatory 291.1
　　delirium tremens 291.0
　　hallucinosis 291.3
　　Korsakoff's, Korsakov's, Korsakow's 291.1
　　paranoid type 291.5
　　pathological intoxication 291.4

Psychosis — continued
　alcoholic — continued
　　polyneuritic 291.1
　　specified type NEC 291.89
　alternating (see also Psychosis, manic-
　　depressive, circular) 296.7
　anergastic (see also Psychosis, organic) 294.9
　arteriosclerotic 290.40
　　with
　　　acute confusional state 290.41
　　　delirium 290.41
　　　▶delusions◀ 290.42
　　　▶depressed mood◀ 290.43
　　　depressed type 290.43
　　　paranoid type 290.42
　　　simple type 290.40
　　　uncomplicated 290.40
　atypical 298.9
　　depressive 296.82
　　manic 296.81
　borderline (schizophrenia) (see also
　　Schizophrenia) 295.5
　　of childhood (see also Psychosis, childhood)
　　　299.8 ☑
　　prepubertal 299.8 ☑
　brief reactive 298.8
　childhood, with origin specific to 299.9 ☑

> Note — Use the following fifth-digit
> subclassification with category 299:
>
> 　0　current or active state
> 　1　residual state

　　atypical 299.8 ☑
　　specified type NEC 299.8 ☑
　circular (see also Psychosis, manic-depressive,
　　circular) 296.7
　climacteric (see also Psychosis, involutional)
　　298.8
　confusional 298.9
　　acute 293.0
　　reactive 298.2
　　subacute 293.1
　depressive (see also Psychosis, affective)
　　296.2 ☑
　　atypical 296.82
　　involutional 296.2 ☑
　　　recurrent episode 296.3 ☑
　　　single episode 296.2 ☑
　　psychogenic 298.0
　　reactive (emotional stress) (psychological
　　　trauma) 298.0
　　recurrent episode 296.3 ☑
　　　with hypomania (bipolar II) 296.89
　　single episode 296.2 ☑
　disintegrative, ▶childhood◀ (see also
　　Psychosis, childhood) 299.1 ☑
　drug 292.9
　　with
　　　affective syndrome 292.84
　　　amnestic syndrome 292.83
　　　anxiety 292.89
　　　delirium 292.81
　　　　withdrawal 292.0
　　　▶delusions◀ 292.11
　　　dementia 292.82
　　　depressive state 292.84
　　　hallucinations 292.12　　　　　　　●
　　　hallucinosis 292.12
　　　mood disorder 292.84　　　　　　　●
　　　mood disturbance 292.84
　　　organic personality syndrome NEC
　　　　292.89
　　　sexual dysfunction 292.89
　　　sleep disturbance 292.89
　　　withdrawal syndrome (and delirium)
　　　　292.0
　　affective syndrome 292.84
　　▶delusions◀ 292.11
　　hallucinatory state 292.12
　　hallucinosis 292.12
　　paranoid state 292.11
　　specified type NEC 292.89
　　withdrawal syndrome (and delirium) 292.0
　due to or associated with physical condition
　　(see also Psychosis, organic) 293.9

Psychosis — *continued*
  epileptic NEC 294.8
  excitation (psychogenic) (reactive) 298.1
  exhaustive (*see also* Reaction, stress, acute)
    308.9
  hypomanic (*see also* Psychosis, affective) 296.0 ☑
    recurrent episode 296.1 ☑
    single episode 296.0 ☑
  hysterical 298.8
    acute 298.1
  incipient 298.8
    schizophrenic (*see also* Schizophrenia)
      295.5 ☑
  induced 297.3
  infantile (*see also* Psychosis, childhood)
    299.0 ☑
  infective 293.9
    acute 293.0
    subacute 293.1
  in
    conditions classified elsewhere   ●
      with   ●
        delusions 293.81   ●
        hallucinations 293.82   ●
    pregnancy, childbirth, or puerperium
      648.4 ☑   ●
  interactional (childhood) (*see also* Psychosis,
    childhood) 299.1 ☑
  involutional 298.8
    depressive (*see also* Psychosis, affective)
      296.2 ☑
      recurrent episode 296.3 ☑
      single episode 296.2 ☑
    melancholic 296.2 ☑
      recurrent episode 296.3 ☑
      single episode 296.2 ☑
    paranoid state 297.2
    paraphrenia 297.2
  Korsakoff's, Korakov's, Korsakow's
    (nonalcoholic) 294.0
    alcoholic 291.1
  mania (phase) (*see also* Psychosis, affective)
    296.0 ☑
    recurrent episode 296.1 ☑
    single episode 296.0 ☑
  manic (*see also* Psychosis, affective) 296.0 ☑
    atypical 296.81
    recurrent episode 296.1 ☑
    single episode 296.0 ☑
  manic-depressive 296.80
    circular 296.7
      currently
        depressed 296.5 ☑
        manic 296.4 ☑
      mixed 296.6 ☑
    depressive 296.2 ☑
      recurrent episode 296.3 ☑
        with hypomania (bipolar II) 296.89
      single episode 296.2 ☑
    hypomanic 296.0 ☑
      recurrent episode 296.1 ☑
      single episode 296.0 ☑
    manic 296.0 ☑
      atypical 296.81
      recurrent episode 296.1 ☑
      single episode 296.0 ☑
    mixed NEC 296.89
    perplexed 296.89
    stuporous 296.89
  menopausal (*see also* Psychosis, involutional)
    298.8
  mixed schizophrenic and affective (*see also*
    Schizophrenia) 295.7 ☑
  multi-infarct (cerebrovascular) (*see also*
    Psychosis, arteriosclerotic) 290.40
  organic NEC 294.9
    due to or associated with
      addiction
        alcohol (*see also* Psychosis, alcoholic)
          291.9
        drug (*see also* Psychosis, drug) 292.9
      alcohol intoxication, acute (*see also*
        Psychosis, alcoholic) 291.9
      alcoholism (*see also* Psychosis, alcoholic)
        291.9
      arteriosclerosis (cerebral) (*see also*
        Psychosis, arteriosclerotic) 290.40

Psychosis — *continued*
  organic NEC — *continued*
    due to or associated with — *continued*
      cerebrovascular disease
        acute (psychosis) 293.0
        arteriosclerotic (*see also* Psychosis,
          arteriosclerotic) 290.40
      childbirth — *see* Psychosis, puerperal
      dependence
        alcohol (*see also* Psychosis, alcoholic)
          291.9
        drug 292.9
      disease
        alcoholic liver (*see also* Psychosis,
          alcoholic) 291.9
        brain
          arteriosclerotic (*see also* Psychosis,
            arteriosclerotic) 290.40
        cerebrovascular
          acute (psychosis) 293.0
          arteriosclerotic (*see also* Psychosis,
            arteriosclerotic) 290.40
        endocrine or metabolic 293.9
          acute (psychosis) 293.0
          subacute (psychosis) 293.1
        Jakob-Creutzfeldt
          with behavioral disturbance 046.1
            [294.11]
          without behavioral disturbance
            046.1 *[294.10]*
        liver, alcoholic (*see also* Psychosis,
          alcoholic) 291.9
      disorder
        cerebrovascular
          acute (psychosis) 293.0
        endocrine or metabolic 293.9
          acute (psychosis) 293.0
          subacute (psychosis) 293.1
      epilepsy
        with behavioral disturbance
          345.9 ☑ *[294.11]*
        without behavioral disturbance
          345.9 ☑ *[294.10]*
        transient (acute) 293.0
      Huntington's chorea
        with behavioral disturbance
          333.4 *[294.11]*
        without behavioral disturbance
          333.4 *[294.10]*
      infection
        brain 293.9
          acute (psychosis) 293.0
          chronic 294.8
          subacute (psychosis) 293.1
        intracranial NEC 293.9
          acute (psychosis) 293.0
          chronic 294.8
          subacute (psychosis) 293.1
      intoxication
        alcoholic (acute) (*see also* Psychosis,
          alcoholic) 291.9
        pathological 291.4
        drug (*see also* Psychosis, drug) 292.2
      ischemia
        cerebrovascular (generalized) (*see also*
          Psychosis, arteriosclerotic)
          290.40
      Jakob-Creutzfeldt disease or syndrome
        with behavioral disturbance
          046.1 *[294.11]*
        without behavioral disturbance
          046.1 *[294.10]*
      multiple sclerosis
        with behavioral disturbance
          340 *[294.11]*
        without behavioral disturbance
          340 *[294.10]*
      physical condition NEC 293.9
        with
          delusions 293.81
          hallucinations 293.82
      presenility 290.10
      puerperium — *see* Psychosis, puerperal
      sclerosis, multiple
        with behavioral disturbance
          340 *[294.11]*

Psychosis — *continued*
  organic NEC — *continued*
    due to or associated with — *continued*
      sclerosis, multiple — *continued*
        without behavioral disturbance
          340 *[294.10]*
      senility 290.20
      status epilepticus
        with behavioral disturbance
          345.3 *[294.11]*
        without behavioral disturbance
          345.3 *[294.10]*
      trauma
        brain (birth) (from electrical current)
          (surgical) 293.9
          acute (psychosis) 293.0
          chronic 294.8
          subacute (psychosis) 293.1
          unspecified physical condition
            294.9
    infective 293.9
      acute (psychosis) 293.0
      subacute 293.1
    posttraumatic 293.9
      acute 293.0
      subacute 293.1
    specified type NEC 294.8
    transient 293.9
      with
        anxiety 293.84
        delusions 293.81
        depression 293.83
        hallucinations 293.82
      depressive type 293.83
      hallucinatory type 293.82
      paranoid type 293.81
      specified type NEC 293.89
  paranoic 297.1
  paranoid (chronic) 297.9
    alcoholic 291.5
    chronic 297.1
    climacteric 297.2
    involutional 297.2
    menopausal 297.2
    protracted reactive 298.4
    psychogenic 298.4
      acute 298.3
    schizophrenic (*see also* Schizophrenia)
      295.3 ☑
    senile 290.20
  paroxysmal 298.9
    senile 290.20
  polyneuritic, alcoholic 291.1
  postoperative 293.9
  postpartum — *see* Psychosis, puerperal
  prepsychotic (*see also* Schizophrenia) 295.5 ☑
  presbyophrenic (type) 290.8
  presenile (*see also* Dementia, presenile) 290.10
  prison 300.16
  psychogenic 298.8
    depressive 298.0
    paranoid 298.4
      acute 298.3
  puerperal
    specified type — *see* categories 295-298 ☑
    unspecified type 293.89
      acute 293.0
      chronic 293.89
      subacute 293.1
  reactive (emotional stress) (psychological
    trauma) 298.8
    brief 298.8
    confusion 298.2
    depressive 298.0
    excitation 298.1
  schizo-affective (depressed) (excited) (*see also*
    Schizophrenia) 295.7 ☑
  schizophrenia, schizophrenic (*see also*
    Schizophrenia) 295.9 ☑
    borderline type 295.5 ☑
      of childhood (*see also* Psychosis,
        childhood) 299.8 ☑
    catatonic (excited) (withdrawn) 295.2 ☑
    childhood type (*see also* Psychosis,
      childhood) 299.9 ☑
    hebephrenic 295.1 ☑

☑ Additional Digit Required   ▶◀ Revised Text   ● New Line   ▲ Revised Code

Psychosis — *continued*
schizophrenia, schizophrenic — *continued*
incipient 295.5 ☑
latent 295.5 ☑
paranoid 295.3 ☑
prepsychotic 295.5 ☑
prodromal 295.5 ☑
pseudoneurotic 295.5 ☑
pseudopsychopathic 295.5 ☑
schizophreniform 295.4 ☑
simple 295.0 ☑
undifferentiated type 295.9 ☑ ●
schizophreniform 295.4 ☑
senile NEC 290.20
with
delusional features 290.20
depressive features 290.21
depressed type 290.21
paranoid type 290.20
simple deterioration 290.20
specified type — *see* categories 295-298 ☑
shared 297.3
situational (reactive) 298.8
symbiotic (childhood) (*see also* Psychosis,
childhood) 299.1 ☑
toxic (acute) 293.9
Psychotic (*see also* condition) 298.9
episode 298.9
due to or associated with physical
conditions (*see also* Psychosis,
organic) 293.9
Pterygium (eye) 372.40
central 372.43
colli 744.5
double 372.44
peripheral (stationary) 372.41
progressive 372.42
recurrent 372.45
Ptilosis 374.55
Ptomaine (poisoning) (*see also* Poisoning, food)
005.9
Ptosis (adiposa) 374.30
breast 611.8
cecum 569.89
colon 569.89
congenital (eyelid) 743.61
specified site NEC — *see* Anomaly, specified
type NEC
epicanthus syndrome 270.2
eyelid 374.30
congenital 743.61
mechanical 374.33
myogenic 374.32
paralytic 374.31
gastric 537.5
intestine 569.89
kidney (*see also* Disease, renal) 593.0
congenital 753.3
liver 573.8
renal (*see also* Disease, renal) 593.0
congenital 753.3
splanchnic 569.89
spleen 289.59
stomach 537.5
viscera 569.89
Ptyalism 527.7
hysterical 300.11
periodic 527.2
pregnancy 646.8 ☑
psychogenic 306.4
Ptyalolithiasis 527.5
Pubalgia 848.8
Pubarche, precocious 259.1
Pubertas praecox 259.1
Puberty V21.1
abnormal 259.9
bleeding 626.3
delayed 259.0
precocious (constitutional) (cryptogenic)
(idiopathic) NEC 259.1
due to
adrenal
cortical hyperfunction 255.2
hyperplasia 255.2
cortical hyperfunction 255.2

Puberty — *continued*
precocious — *continued*
due to — *continued*
ovarian hyperfunction 256.1
estrogen 256.0
pineal tumor 259.8
testicular hyperfunction 257.0
premature 259.1
due to
adrenal cortical hyperfunction 255.2
pineal tumor 259.8
pituitary (anterior) hyperfunction 253.1
Puckering, macula 362.56
Pudenda, pudendum — *see* condition
Puente's disease (simple glandular cheilitis)
528.5
Puerperal
abscess
areola 675.1 ☑
Bartholin's gland 646.6 ☑
breast 675.1 ☑
cervix (uteri) 670.0 ☑
fallopian tube 670.0 ☑
genital organ 670.0 ☑
kidney 646.6 ☑
mammary 675.1 ☑
mesosalpinx 670.0 ☑
nabothian 646.6 ☑
nipple 675.0 ☑
ovary, ovarian 670.0 ☑
oviduct 670.0 ☑
parametric 670.0 ☑
para-uterine 670.0 ☑
pelvic 670.0 ☑
perimetric 670.0 ☑
periuterine 670.0 ☑
retro-uterine 670.0 ☑
subareolar 675.1 ☑
suprapelvic 670.0 ☑
tubal (ruptured) 670.0 ☑
tubo-ovarian 670.0 ☑
urinary tract NEC 646.6 ☑
uterine, uterus 670.0 ☑
vagina (wall) 646.6 ☑
vaginorectal 646.6 ☑
vulvovaginal gland 646.6 ☑
accident 674.9 ☑
adnexitis 670.0 ☑
afibrinogenemia, or other coagulation defect
666.3 ☑
albuminuria (acute) (subacute) 646.2 ☑
pre-eclamptic 642.4 ☑
anemia (conditions classifiable to 280-285)
648.2 ☑
anuria 669.3 ☑
apoplexy 674.0 ☑
asymptomatic bacteriuria 646.5 ☑
atrophy, breast 676.3 ☑
blood dyscrasia 666.3 ☑
caked breast 676.2 ☑
cardiomyopathy 674.5 ☑
cellulitis — *see* Puerperal, abscess
cerebrovascular disorder (conditions
classifiable to 430-434, 436-437) 674.0 ☑
cervicitis (conditions classifiable to 616.0)
646.6 ☑
coagulopathy (any) 666.3 ☑
complications 674.9 ☑
specified type NEC 674.8 ☑
convulsions (eclamptic) (uremic) 642.6 ☑
with pre-existing hypertension 642.7 ☑
cracked nipple 676.1 ☑
cystitis 646.6 ☑
cystopyelitis 646.6 ☑
deciduitis (acute) 670.0 ☑
delirium NEC 293.9
diabetes (mellitus) (conditions classifiable to
250) 648.0 ☑
disease 674.9 ☑
breast NEC 676.3 ☑
cerebrovascular (acute) 674.0 ☑
nonobstetric NEC (*see also* Pregnancy,
complicated, current disease or
condition) 648.9 ☑
pelvis inflammatory 670.0 ☑
renal NEC 646.2 ☑

Puerperal — *continued*
disease — *continued*
tubo-ovarian 670.0 ☑
Valsuani's (progressive pernicious anemia)
648.2 ☑
disorder
lactation 676.9 ☑
specified type NEC 676.8 ☑
nonobstetric NEC (*see also* Pregnancy,
complicated, current disease or
condition) 648.9 ☑
disruption
cesarean wound 674.1 ☑
episiotomy wound 674.2 ☑
perineal laceration wound 674.2 ☑
drug dependence (conditions classifiable to
304) 648.3 ☑
eclampsia 642.6 ☑
with pre-existing hypertension 642.7 ☑
embolism (pulmonary) 673.2 ☑
air 673.0 ☑
amniotic fluid 673.1 ☑
blood-clot 673.2 ☑
brain or cerebral 674.0 ☑
cardiac 674.8 ☑
fat 673.8 ☑
intracranial sinus (venous) 671.5 ☑
pyemic 673.3 ☑
septic 673.3 ☑
spinal cord 671.5 ☑
endometritis (conditions classifiable to 615.0-
615.9) 670.0 ☑
endophlebitis — *see* Puerperal, phlebitis
endotrachelitis 646.6 ☑
engorgement, breasts 676.2 ☑
erysipelas 670.0 ☑
failure
lactation 676.4 ☑
renal, acute 669.3 ☑
fever 670.0 ☑
meaning pyrexia (of unknown origin)
672.0 ☑
meaning sepsis 670.0 ☑
fissure, nipple 676.1 ☑
fistula
breast 675.1 ☑
mammary gland 675.1 ☑
nipple 675.0 ☑
galactophoritis 675.2 ☑
galactorrhea 676.6 ☑
gangrene
gas 670.0 ☑
uterus 670.0 ☑
gonorrhea (conditions classifiable to 098)
647.1 ☑
hematoma, subdural 674.0 ☑
hematosalpinx, infectional 670.0 ☑
hemiplegia, cerebral 674.0 ☑
hemorrhage 666.1 ☑
brain 674.0 ☑
bulbar 674.0 ☑
cerebellar 674.0 ☑
cerebral 674.0 ☑
cortical 674.0 ☑
delayed (after 24 hours) (uterine) 666.2 ☑
extradural 674.0 ☑
internal capsule 674.0 ☑
intracranial 674.0 ☑
intrapontine 674.0 ☑
meningeal 674.0 ☑
pontine 674.0 ☑
subarachnoid 674.0 ☑
subcortical 674.0 ☑
subdural 674.0 ☑
uterine, delayed 666.2 ☑
ventricular 674.0 ☑
hemorrhoids 671.8 ☑
hepatorenal syndrome 674.8 ☑
hypertrophy
breast 676.3 ☑
mammary gland 676.3 ☑
induration breast (fibrous) 676.3 ☑
infarction
lung — *see* Puerperal, embolism
pulmonary — *see* Puerperal, embolism

Psychosis — Puerperal

Puerperal — *continued*
  infection
    Bartholin's gland 646.6 ☑
    breast 675.2 ☑
      with nipple 675.9 ☑
        specified type NEC 675.8 ☑
    cervix 646.6 ☑
    endocervix 646.6 ☑
    fallopian tube 670.0 ☑
    generalized 670.0 ☑
    genital tract (major) 670.0 ☑
      minor or localized 646.6 ☑
    kidney (bacillus coli) 646.6 ☑
    mammary gland 675.2 ☑
      with nipple 675.9 ☑
        specified type NEC 675.8 ☑
    nipple 675.0 ☑
      with breast 675.9 ☑
        specified type NEC 675.8 ☑
    ovary 670.0 ☑
    pelvic 670.0 ☑
    peritoneum 670.0 ☑
    renal 646.6 ☑
    tubo-ovarian 670.0 ☑
    urinary (tract) NEC 646.6 ☑
      asymptomatic 646.5 ☑
    uterus, uterine 670.0 ☑
    vagina 646.6 ☑
  inflammation — *see also* Puerperal, infection
    areola 675.1 ☑
    Bartholin's gland 646.6 ☑
    breast 675.2 ☑
    broad ligament 670.0 ☑
    cervix (uteri) 646.6 ☑
    fallopian tube 670.0 ☑
    genital organs 670.0 ☑
      localized 646.6 ☑
    mammary gland 675.2 ☑
    nipple 675.0 ☑
    ovary 670.0 ☑
    oviduct 670.0 ☑
    pelvis 670.0 ☑
    periuterine 670.0 ☑
    tubal 670.0 ☑
    vagina 646.6 ☑
    vein — *see* Puerperal, phlebitis
  inversion, nipple 676.3 ☑
  ischemia, cerebral 674.0 ☑
  lymphangitis 670.0 ☑
    breast 675.2 ☑
  malaria (conditions classifiable to 084) 647.4 ☑
  malnutrition 648.9 ☑
  mammillitis 675.0 ☑
  mammitis 675.2 ☑
  mania 296.0 ☑
    recurrent episode 296.1 ☑
    single episode 296.0 ☑
  mastitis 675.2 ☑
    purulent 675.1 ☑
    retromammary 675.1 ☑
    submammary 675.1 ☑
  melancholia 296.2 ☑
    recurrent episode 296.3 ☑
    single episode 296.2 ☑
  mental disorder (conditions classifiable to 290-303, 305-316, 317-319) 648.4 ☑
  metritis (septic) (suppurative) 670.0 ☑
  metroperitonitis 670.0 ☑
  metrorrhagia 666.2 ☑
  metrosalpingitis 670.0 ☑
  metrovaginitis 670.0 ☑
  milk leg 671.4 ☑
  monoplegia, cerebral 674.0 ☑
  necrosis
    kidney, tubular 669.3 ☑
    liver (acute) (subacute) (conditions classifiable to 570) 674.8 ☑
    ovary 670.0 ☑
    renal cortex 669.3 ☑
  nephritis or nephrosis (conditions classifiable to 580-589) 646.2 ☑
    with hypertension 642.1 ☑
  nutritional deficiency (conditions classifiable to 260-269) 648.9 ☑
  occlusion, precerebral artery 674.0 ☑
  oliguria 669.3 ☑
  oophoritis 670.0 ☑

Puerperal — *continued*
  ovaritis 670.0 ☑
  paralysis
    bladder (sphincter) 665.5 ☑
    cerebral 674.0 ☑
  paralytic stroke 674.0 ☑
  parametritis 670.0 ☑
  paravaginitis 646.6 ☑
  pelviperitonitis 670.0 ☑
  perimetritis 670.0 ☑
  perimetrosalpingitis 670.0 ☑
  perinephritis 646.6 ☑
  perioophoritis 670.0 ☑
  periphlebitis — *see* Puerperal, phlebitis
  perisalpingitis 670.0 ☑
  peritoneal infection 670.0 ☑
  peritonitis (pelvic) 670.0 ☑
  perivaginitis 646.6 ☑
  phlebitis 671.9 ☑
    deep 671.4 ☑
    intracranial sinus (venous) 671.5 ☑
    pelvic 671.4 ☑
    specified site NEC 671.5 ☑
    superficial 671.2 ☑
  phlegmasia alba dolens 671.4 ☑
  placental polyp 674.4 ☑
  pneumonia, embolic — *see* Puerperal, embolism
  prediabetes 648.8 ☑
  pre-eclampsia (mild) 642.4 ☑
    with pre-existing hypertension 642.7 ☑
    severe 642.5 ☑
  psychosis, unspecified (*see also* Psychosis, puerperal) 293.89
  pyelitis 646.6 ☑
  pyelocystitis 646.6 ☑
  pyelohydronephrosis 646.6 ☑
  pyelonephritis 646.6 ☑
  pyelonephrosis 646.6 ☑
  pyemia 670.0 ☑
  pyocystitis 646.6 ☑
  pyohemia 670.0 ☑
  pyometra 670.0 ☑
  pyonephritis 646.6 ☑
  pyonephrosis 646.6 ☑
  pyo-oophoritis 670.0 ☑
  pyosalpingitis 670.0 ☑
  pyosalpinx 670.0 ☑
  pyrexia (of unknown origin) 672.0 ☑
  renal
    disease NEC 646.2 ☑
    failure, acute 669.3 ☑
  retention
    decidua (fragments) (with delayed hemorrhage) 666.2 ☑
      without hemorrhage 667.1 ☑
    placenta (fragments) (with delayed hemorrhage) 666.2 ☑
      without hemorrhage 667.1 ☑
    secundines (fragments) (with delayed hemorrhage) 666.2 ☑
      without hemorrhage 667.1 ☑
  retracted nipple 676.0 ☑
  rubella (conditions classifiable to 056) 647.5 ☑
  salpingitis 670.0 ☑
  salpingo-oophoritis 670.0 ☑
  salpingo-ovaritis 670.0 ☑
  salpingoperitonitis 670.0 ☑
  sapremia 670.0 ☑
  secondary perineal tear 674.2 ☑
  sepsis (pelvic) 670.0 ☑
  septicemia 670.0 ☑
  subinvolution (uterus) 674.8 ☑
  sudden death (cause unknown) 674.9 ☑
  suppuration — *see* Puerperal, abscess
  syphilis (conditions classifiable to 090-097) 647.0 ☑
  tetanus 670.0 ☑
  thelitis 675.0 ☑
  thrombocytopenia 666.3 ☑
  thrombophlebitis (superficial) 671.2 ☑
    deep 671.4 ☑
    pelvic 671.4 ☑
    specified site NEC 671.5 ☑
  thrombosis (venous) — *see* Thrombosis, puerperal

Puerperal — *continued*
  thyroid dysfunction (conditions classifiable to 240-246) 648.1 ☑
  toxemia (*see also* Toxemia, of pregnancy) 642.4 ☑
    eclamptic 642.6 ☑
      with pre-existing hypertension 642.7 ☑
    pre-eclamptic (mild) 642.4 ☑
      with
        convulsions 642.6 ☑
        pre-existing hypertension 642.7 ☑
      severe 642.5 ☑
  tuberculosis (conditions classifiable to 010-018) 647.3 ☑
  uremia 669.3 ☑
  vaginitis (conditions classifiable to 616.1) 646.6 ☑
  varicose veins (legs) 671.0 ☑
    vulva or perineum 671.1 ☑
  vulvitis (conditions classifiable to 616.1) 646.6 ☑
  vulvovaginitis (conditions classifiable to 616.1) 646.6 ☑
  white leg 671.4 ☑
Pulled muscle — *see* Sprain, by site
Pulmolithiasis 518.89
Pulmonary — *see* condition
Pulmonitis (unknown etiology) 486
Pulpitis (acute) (anachoretic) (chronic) (hyperplastic) (putrescent) (suppurative) (ulcerative) 522.0
Pulpless tooth 522.9
Pulse
  alternating 427.89
    psychogenic 306.2
  bigeminal 427.89
  fast 785.0
  feeble, rapid, due to shock following injury 958.4
  rapid 785.0
  slow 427.89
  strong 785.9
  trigeminal 427.89
  water-hammer (*see also* Insufficiency, aortic) 424.1
  weak 785.9
Pulseless disease 446.7
Pulsus
  alternans or trigeminy 427.89
    psychogenic 306.2
Punch drunk 310.2
Puncta lacrimalia occlusion 375.52
Punctiform hymen 752.49
Puncture (traumatic) — *see also* Wound, open, by site
  accidental; complicating surgery 998.2
  bladder, nontraumatic 596.6
  by
    device, implant, or graft — *see* Complications, mechanical
    foreign body
      internal organs — *see also* Injury, internal, by site
        by ingested object — *see* Foreign body
      left accidentally in operation wound 998.4
    instrument (any) during a procedure, accidental 998.2
  internal organs, abdomen, chest, or pelvis — *see* Injury, internal, by site
  kidney, nontraumatic 593.89
Pupil — *see* condition
Pupillary membrane 364.74
  persistent 743.46
Pupillotonia 379.46
  pseudotabetic 379.46
Purpura 287.2
  abdominal 287.0
  allergic 287.0
  anaphylactoid 287.0
  annularis telangiectodes 709.1
  arthritic 287.0
  autoerythrocyte sensitization 287.2
  autoimmune 287.0

☑ Additional Digit Required   ▶◀ Revised Text   ● New Line   ▲ Revised Code

Purpura — *continued*
  bacterial 287.0
  Bateman's (senile) 287.2
  capillary fragility (hereditary) (idiopathic) 287.8
  cryoglobulinemic 273.2
  devil's pinches 287.2
  fibrinolytic (*see also* Fibrinolysis) 286.6
  fulminans, fulminous 286.6
  gangrenous 287.0
  hemorrhagic (*see also* Purpura,
      thrombocytopenic) 287.3
    nodular 272.7
    nonthrombocytopenic 287.0
    thrombocytopenic 287.3
  Henoch's (purpura nervosa) 287.0
  Henoch-Schönlein (allergic) 287.0
  hypergammaglobulinemic (benign primary)
      (Waldenström's) 273.0
  idiopathic 287.3
    nonthrombocytopenic 287.0
    thrombocytopenic 287.3
  infectious 287.0
  malignant 287.0
  neonatorum 772.6
  nervosa 287.0
  newborn NEC 772.6
  nonthrombocytopenic 287.2
    hemorrhagic 287.0
    idiopathic 287.0
  nonthrombopenic 287.2
  peliosis rheumatica 287.0
  pigmentaria, progressiva 709.09
  posttransfusion 287.4
  primary 287.0
  primitive 287.0
  red cell membrane sensitivity 287.2
  rheumatica 287.0
  Schönlein (-Henoch) (allergic) 287.0
  scorbutic 267
  senile 287.2
  simplex 287.2
  symptomatica 287.0
  telangiectasia annularis 709.1
  thrombocytopenic (congenital) (essential)
        (hereditary) (idiopathic) (primary) (*see
        also* Thrombocytopenia) 287.3
    neonatal, transitory (*see also*
        Thrombocytopenia, neonatal
        transitory) 776.1
    puerperal, postpartum 666.3 ☑
    thrombotic 446.6
  thrombohemolytic (*see also* Fibrinolysis) 286.6
  thrombopenic (congenital) (essential) (*see also*
      Thrombocytopenia) 287.3
    thrombotic 446.6
      thrombocytic 446.6
      thrombocytopenic 446.6
  toxic 287.0
  variolosa 050.0
  vascular 287.0
  visceral symptoms 287.0
  Werlhof's (*see also* Purpura, thrombocytopenic)
      287.3
Purpuric spots 782.7
Purulent — *see* condition
Pus
  absorption, general — *see* Septicemia
  in
    stool 792.1
    urine 791.9
  tube (rupture) (*see also* Salpingo-oophoritis)
      614.2
Pustular rash 782.1
Pustule 686.9
  malignant 022.0
  nonmalignant 686.9
Putnam's disease (subacute combined sclerosis
    with pernicious anemia) 281.0 *[336.2]*
Putnam-Dana syndrome (subacute combined
    sclerosis with pernicious anemia) 281.0
    [336.2]
Putrefaction, intestinal 569.89
Putrescent pulp (dental) 522.1
Pyarthritis — *see* Pyarthrosis
Pyarthrosis (*see also* Arthritis, pyogenic) 711.0 ☑
  tuberculous — *see* Tuberculosis, joint

Pycnoepilepsy, pycnolepsy (idiopathic) (*see also*
    Epilepsy) 345.0 ☑
Pyelectasia 593.89
Pyelectasis 593.89
Pyelitis (congenital) (uremic) 590.80
  with
    abortion — *see* Abortion, by type, with
        specified complication NEC
    contracted kidney 590.00
    ectopic pregnancy (*see also* categories
        633.0-633.9) 639.8
    molar pregnancy (*see also* categories 630-
        632) 639.8
  acute 590.10
    with renal medullary necrosis 590.11
  chronic 590.00
    with
      renal medullary necrosis 590.01
  complicating pregnancy, childbirth, or
      puerperium 646.6 ☑
    affecting fetus or newborn 760.1
  cystica 590.3
    following
      abortion 639.8
      ectopic or molar pregnancy 639.8
  gonococcal 098.19
    chronic or duration of 2 months or over
        098.39
  tuberculous (*see also* Tuberculosis) 016.0 ☑
    [590.81]
Pyelocaliectasis 593.89
Pyelocystitis (*see also* Pyelitis) 590.80
Pyelohydronephrosis 591
Pyelonephritis (*see also* Pyelitis) 590.80
  acute 590.10
    with renal medullary necrosis 590.11
  chronic 590.00
  syphilitic (late) 095.4
  tuberculous (*see also* Tuberculosis) 016.0 ☑
    [590.81]
Pyelonephrosis (*see also* Pyelitis) 590.80
  chronic 590.00
Pyelophlebitis 451.89
Pyelo-ureteritis cystica 590.3
Pyemia, pyemic (purulent) (*see also* Septicemia)
    038.9
  abscess — *see* Abscess
  arthritis (*see also* Arthritis, pyogenic) 711.0 ☑
  Bacillus coli 038.42
  embolism — *see* Embolism, pyemic
  fever 038.9
  infection 038.9
  joint (*see also* Arthritis, pyogenic) 711.0 ☑
  liver 572.1
  meningococcal 036.2
  newborn 771.81
  phlebitis — *see* Phlebitis
  pneumococcal 038.2
  portal 572.1
  postvaccinal 999.3
  specified organism NEC 038.8
  staphylococcal 038.10
    aureus 038.11
    specified organism NEC 038.19
  streptococcal 038.0
  tuberculous — *see* Tuberculosis, miliary
Pygopagus 759.4
Pykno-epilepsy, pyknolepsy (idiopathic) (*see also*
    Epilepsy) 345.0 ☑
Pyle (-Cohn) disease (craniometaphyseal
    dysplasia) 756.89
Pylephlebitis (suppurative) 572.1
Pylethrombophlebitis 572.1
Pylethrombosis 572.1
Pyloritis (*see also* Gastritis) 535.5 ☑
Pylorospasm (reflex) 537.81
  congenital or infantile 750.5
  neurotic 306.4
  newborn 750.5
  psychogenic 306.4
Pylorus, pyloric — *see* condition
Pyoarthrosis — *see* Pyarthrosis
Pyocele
  mastoid 383.00
  sinus (accessory) (nasal) (*see also* Sinusitis) 473.9
  turbinate (bone) 473.9
  urethra (*see also* Urethritis) 597.0

Pyococcal dermatitis 686.00
Pyococcide, skin 686.00
Pyocolpos (*see also* Vaginitis) 616.10
Pyocyaneus dermatitis 686.09
Pyocystitis (*see also* Cystitis) 595.9
Pyoderma, pyodermia 686.00
  gangrenosum 686.01
  specified type NEC 686.09
  vegetans 686.8
Pyodermatitis 686.00
  vegetans 686.8
Pyogenic — *see* condition
Pyohemia — *see* Septicemia
Pyohydronephrosis (*see also* Pyelitis) 590.80
Pyometra 615.9
Pyometritis (*see also* Endometritis) 615.9
Pyometrium (*see also* Endometritis) 615.9
Pyomyositis 728.0
  ossificans 728.19
  tropical (bungpagga) 040.81
Pyonephritis (*see also* Pyelitis) 590.80
  chronic 590.00
Pyonephrosis (congenital) (*see also* Pyelitis)
    590.80
  acute 590.10
Pyo-oophoritis (*see also* Salpingo-oophoritis)
    614.2
Pyo-ovarium (*see also* Salpingo-oophoritis) 614.2
Pyopericarditis 420.99
Pyopericardium 420.99
Pyophlebitis — *see* Phlebitis
Pyopneumopericardium 420.99
Pyopneumothorax (infectional) 510.9
  with fistula 510.0
  subdiaphragmatic (*see also* Peritonitis) 567.2
  subphrenic (*see also* Peritonitis) 567.2
  tuberculous (*see also* Tuberculosis, pleura)
      012.0 ☑
Pyorrhea (alveolar) (alveolaris) 523.4
  degenerative 523.5
Pyosalpingitis (*see also* Salpingo-oophoritis)
    614.2
Pyosalpinx (*see also* Salpingo-oophoritis) 614.2
Pyosepticemia — *see* Septicemia
Pyosis
  Corlett's (impetigo) 684
  Manson's (pemphigus contagiosus) 684
Pyothorax 510.9
  with fistula 510.0
  tuberculous (*see also* Tuberculosis, pleura)
      012.0 ☑
Pyoureter 593.89
  tuberculous (*see also* Tuberculosis) 016.2 ☑
Pyramidopallidonigral syndrome 332.0
Pyrexia (of unknown origin) (P.U.O.) 780.6
  atmospheric 992.0
  during labor 659.2 ☑
  environmentally-induced newborn 778.4
  heat 992.0
  newborn, environmentally-induced 778.4
  puerperal 672.0 ☑
Pyroglobulinemia 273.8
Pyromania 312.33
Pyrosis 787.1
Pyrroloporphyria 277.1
Pyuria (bacterial) 791.9

Q

Q fever 083.0
  with pneumonia 083.0 *[484.8]*
Quadricuspid aortic valve 746.89
Quadrilateral fever 083.0
Quadriparesis — *see* Quadriplegia
Quadriplegia 344.00
  with fracture, vertebra (process) — *see*
      Fracture, vertebra, cervical, with spinal
      cord injury
  brain (current episode) 437.8

☑ Additional Digit Required   ▶◀ Revised Text   ● New Line   ▲ Revised Code

Quadriplegia — *continued*
- C1-C4
  - complete 344.01
  - incomplete 344.02
- C5-C7
  - complete 344.03
  - incomplete 344.04
- cerebral (current episode) 437.8
- congenital or infantile (cerebral) (spastic) (spinal) 343.2
- cortical 437.8
- embolic (current episode) (*see also* Embolism, brain) 434.1 ☑
- infantile (cerebral) (spastic) (spinal) 343.2
- newborn NEC 767.0
- specified NEC 344.09
- thrombotic (current episode) (*see also* Thrombosis, brain) 434.0 ☑
- traumatic — *see* Injury, spinal, cervical

Quadruplet
- affected by maternal complications of pregnancy 761.5
- healthy liveborn — *see* Newborn, multiple
- pregnancy (complicating delivery) NEC 651.8 ☑
  - with fetal loss and retention of one or more fetus(es) 651.5 ☑

Quarrelsomeness 301.3

Quartan
- fever 084.2
- malaria (fever) 084.2

Queensland fever 083.0
- coastal 083.0
- seven-day 100.89

Quervain's disease 727.04
- thyroid (subacute granulomatous thyroiditis) 245.1

Queyrat's erythroplasia (M8080/2)
- specified site — *see* Neoplasm, skin, in situ
- unspecified site 233.5

Quincke's disease or edema — *see* Edema, angioneurotic

Quinquaud's disease (acne decalvans) 704.09

Quinsy (gangrenous) 475

Quintan fever 083.1

Quintuplet
- affected by maternal complications of pregnancy 761.5
- healthy liveborn — *see* Newborn, multiple
- pregnancy (complicating delivery) NEC 651.2 ☑
  - with fetal loss and retention of one or more fetus(es) 651.6 ☑

Quotidian
- fever 084.0
- malaria (fever) 084.0

R

Rabbia 071

Rabbit fever (*see also* Tularemia) 021.9

Rabies 071
- contact V01.5
- exposure to V01.5
- inoculation V04.5
  - reaction — *see* Complications, vaccination
- vaccination, prophylactic (against) V04.5

Rachischisis (*see also* Spina bifida) 741.9 ☑

Rachitic — *see also* condition
- deformities of spine 268.1
- pelvis 268.1
  - with disproportion (fetopelvic) 653.2 ☑
    - affecting fetus or newborn 763.1
    - causing obstructed labor 660.1 ☑
      - affecting fetus or newborn 763.1

Rachitis, rachitism — *see also* Rickets
- acute 268.0
- fetalis 756.4
- renalis 588.0
- tarda 268.0

Racket nail 757.5

Radial nerve — *see* condition

Radiation effects or sickness — *see also* Effect, adverse, radiation
- cataract 366.46

Radiation effects or sickness — *see also* Effect, adverse, radiation — *continued*
- dermatitis 692.82
  - sunburn (*see also* Sunburn) 692.71

Radiculitis (pressure) (vertebrogenic) 729.2
- accessory nerve 723.4
- anterior crural 724.4
- arm 723.4
- brachial 723.4
- cervical NEC 723.4
- due to displacement of intervertebral disc — *see* Neuritis, due to, displacement intervertebral disc
- leg 724.4
- lumbar 724.4
- lumbosacral 724.4
- rheumatic 729.2
- syphilitic 094.89
- thoracic (with visceral pain) 724.4

Radiculomyelitis 357.0
- toxic, due to
  - Clostridium tetani 037
  - Corynebacterium diphtheriae 032.89

Radiculopathy (*see also* Radiculitis) 729.2

Radioactive substances, adverse effect — *see* Effect, adverse, radioactive substance

Radiodermal burns (acute) (chronic) (occupational) — *see* Burn, by site

Radiodermatitis 692.82

Radionecrosis — *see* Effect, adverse, radiation

Radiotherapy session V58.0

Radium, adverse effect — *see* Effect, adverse, radioactive substance

Raeder-Harbitz syndrome (pulseless disease) 446.7

Rage (*see also* Disturbance, conduct) 312.0 ☑
- meaning rabies 071

Rag sorters' disease 022.1

Raillietiniasis 123.8

Railroad neurosis 300.16

Railway spine 300.16

Raised — *see* Elevation

Raiva 071

Rake teeth, tooth 524.39 ▲

Rales 786.7

Ramifying renal pelvis 753.3

Ramsay Hunt syndrome (herpetic geniculate ganglionitis) 053.11
- meaning dyssynergia cerebellaris myoclonica 334.2

Ranke's primary infiltration (*see also* Tuberculosis) 010.0 ☑

Ranula 527.6
- congenital 750.26

Rape — *see* Injury, by site
- alleged, observation or examination V71.5

Rapid
- feeble pulse, due to shock, following injury 958.4
- heart (beat) 785.0
  - psychogenic 306.2
- respiration 786.06
  - psychogenic 306.1
- second stage (delivery) 661.3 ☑
  - affecting fetus or newborn 763.6
- time-zone change syndrome 307.45

Rarefaction, bone 733.99

Rash 782.1
- canker 034.1
- diaper 691.0
- drug (internal use) 693.0
  - contact 692.3
- ECHO 9 virus 078.89
- enema 692.89
- food (*see also* Allergy, food) 693.1
- heat 705.1
- napkin 691.0
- nettle 708.8
- pustular 782.1
- rose 782.1
  - epidemic 056.9
  - of infants 057.8

Rash — *continued*
- scarlet 034.1
- serum (prophylactic) (therapeutic) 999.5
- toxic 782.1
- wandering tongue 529.1

Rasmussen's aneurysm (*see also* Tuberculosis) 011.2 ☑

Rat-bite fever 026.9
- due to Streptobacillus moniliformis 026.1 ☑
- spirochetal (morsus muris) 026.0 ☑

Rathke's pouch tumor (M9350/1) 237.0

Raymond (-Céstan) syndrome 433.8 ☑

Raynaud's
- disease or syndrome (paroxysmal digital cyanosis) 443.0
- gangrene (symmetric) 443.0 [785.4]
- phenomenon (paroxysmal digital cyanosis) (secondary) 443.0

RDS 769

Reaction
- acute situational maladjustment (*see also* Reaction, adjustment) 309.9
- adaptation (*see also* Reaction, adjustment) 309.9
- adjustment 309.9
  - with
    - anxious mood 309.24
      - with depressed mood 309.28
    - conduct disturbance 309.3
      - combined with disturbance of emotions 309.4
    - depressed mood 309.0
      - brief 309.0
        - with anxious mood 309.28
      - prolonged 309.1
    - elective mutism 309.83
    - mixed emotions and conduct 309.4
    - mutism, elective 309.83
    - physical symptoms 309.82
    - predominant disturbance (of)
      - conduct 309.3
      - emotions NEC 309.29
        - mixed 309.28
      - mixed, emotions and conduct 309.4
      - specified type NEC 309.89
    - specific academic or work inhibition 309.23
    - withdrawal 309.83
  - depressive 309.0
    - with conduct disturbance 309.4
    - brief 309.0
    - prolonged 309.1
    - specified type NEC 309.89
- adverse food NEC 995.7
- affective (*see also* Psychosis, affective) 296.90
  - specified type NEC 296.99
- aggressive 301.3
  - unsocialized (*see also* Disturbance, conduct) 312.0 ☑
- allergic (*see also* Allergy) 995.3
  - drug, medicinal substance, and biological — *see* Allergy, drug
  - food — *see* Allergy, food
  - serum 999.5
- anaphylactic — *see* Shock, anaphylactic
- anesthesia — *see* Anesthesia, complication
- anger 312.0 ☑
- antisocial 301.7
- antitoxin (prophylactic) (therapeutic) — *see* Complications, vaccination
- anxiety 300.00
- asthenic 300.5
- compulsive 300.3
- conversion (anesthetic) (autonomic) (hyperkinetic) (mixed paralytic) (paresthetic) 300.11
- deoxyribonuclease (DNA) (DNase) hypersensitivity NEC 287.2
- depressive 300.4
  - acute 309.0
  - affective (*see also* Psychosis, affective) 296.2 ☑
    - recurrent episode 296.3 ☑
    - single episode 296.2 ☑
  - brief 309.0

Reaction — *continued*
  depressive — *continued*
    manic (*see also* Psychosis, affective) 296.80
    neurotic 300.4
    psychoneurotic 300.4
    psychotic 298.0
  dissociative 300.15
  drug NEC (*see also* Table of Drugs and
    Chemicals) 995.2
    allergic — *see* Allergy, drug
    correct substance properly administered
      995.2
    obstetric anesthetic or analgesic NEC
      668.9 ☑
      affecting fetus or newborn 763.5
      specified drug — *see* Table of Drugs and
        Chemicals
    overdose or poisoning 977.9
      specified drug — *see* Table of Drugs and
        Chemicals
    specific to newborn 779.4
    transmitted via placenta or breast milk —
      see Absorption, drug, through
      placenta
    withdrawal NEC 292.0
      infant of dependent mother 779.5
    wrong substance given or taken in error
      977.9
      specified drug — *see* Table of Drugs and
        Chemicals
  dyssocial 301.7
  erysipeloid 027.1
  fear 300.20
    child 313.0
  fluid loss, cerebrospinal 349.0
  food — *see also* Allergy, food
    adverse NEC 995.7
    anaphylactic shock — *see* Anaphylactic
      shock, due to, food
  foreign
    body NEC 728.82
      in operative wound (inadvertently left)
        998.4
        due to surgical material intentionally
          left — *see* Complications, due to
          (presence of) any device, implant,
          or graft classified to 996.0-996.5
          NEC
      substance accidentally left during a
        procedure (chemical) (powder) (talc)
        998.7
      body or object (instrument) (sponge)
        (swab) 998.4
  graft-versus-host (GVH) 996.85
  grief (acute) (brief) 309.0
    prolonged 309.1
  gross stress (*see also* Reaction, stress, acute)
    308.9
  group delinquent (*see also* Disturbance,
    conduct) 312.2 ☑
  Herxheimer's 995.0
  hyperkinetic (*see also* Hyperkinesia) 314.9
  hypochondriacal 300.7
  hypoglycemic, due to insulin 251.0
    therapeutic misadventure 962.3
  hypomanic (*see also* Psychosis, affective)
    296.0 ☑
    recurrent episode 296.1 ☑
    single episode 296.0 ☑
  hysterical 300.10
    conversion type 300.11
    dissociative 300.15
  id (bacterial cause) 692.89
  immaturity NEC 301.89
    aggressive 301.3
    emotional instability 301.59
  immunization — *see* Complications,
    vaccination
  incompatibility
    blood group (ABO) (infusion) (transfusion)
      999.6
    Rh (factor) (infusion) (transfusion) 999.7
  inflammatory — *see* Infection
  infusion — *see* Complications, infusion
  inoculation (immune serum) — *see*
    Complications, vaccination
  insulin 995.2

Reaction — *continued*
  involutional
    paranoid 297.2
    psychotic (*see also* Psychosis, affective,
      depressive) 296.2 ☑
  leukemoid (lymphocytic) (monocytic)
    (myelocytic) 288.8
  LSD (*see also* Abuse, drugs, nondependent)
    305.3 ☑
  lumbar puncture 349.0
  manic-depressive (*see also* Psychosis, affective)
    296.80
    depressed 296.2 ☑
      recurrent episode 296.3 ☑
      single episode 296.2 ☑
    hypomanic 296.0 ☑
  neurasthenic 300.5
  neurogenic (*see also* Neurosis) 300.9
  neurotic NEC 300.9
  neurotic-depressive 300.4
  nitritoid — *see* Crisis, nitritoid
  obsessive (-compulsive) 300.3
  organic 293.9
    acute 293.0
    subacute 293.1
  overanxious, child or adolescent 313.0
  paranoid (chronic) 297.9
    acute 298.3
    climacteric 297.2
    involutional 297.2
    menopausal 297.2
    senile 290.20
    simple 297.0
  passive
    aggressive 301.84
    dependency 301.6
  personality (*see also* Disorder, personality)
    301.9
  phobic 300.20
  postradiation — *see* Effect, adverse, radiation
  psychogenic NEC 300.9
  psychoneurotic (*see also* Neurosis) 300.9
    anxiety 300.00
    compulsive 300.3
    conversion 300.11
    depersonalization 300.6
    depressive 300.4
    dissociative 300.15
    hypochondriacal 300.7
    hysterical 300.10
      conversion type 300.11
      dissociative type 300.15
    neurasthenic 300.5
    obsessive 300.3
    obsessive-compulsive 300.3
    phobic 300.20
    tension state 300.9
  psychophysiologic NEC (*see also* Disorder,
    psychosomatic) 306.9
    cardiovascular 306.2
    digestive 306.4
    endocrine 306.6
    gastrointestinal 306.4
    genitourinary 306.50
    heart 306.2
    hemic 306.8
    intestinal (large) (small) 306.4
    laryngeal 306.1
    lymphatic 306.8
    musculoskeletal 306.0
    pharyngeal 306.1
    respiratory 306.1
    skin 306.3
    special sense organs 306.7
  psychosomatic (*see also* Disorder,
    psychosomatic) 306.9
  psychotic (*see also* Psychosis) 298.9
    depressive 298.0
    due to or associated with physical condition
      (*see also* Psychosis, organic) 293.9
    involutional (*see also* Psychosis, affective)
      296.2 ☑
      recurrent episode 296.3 ☑
      single episode 296.2 ☑
  pupillary (myotonic) (tonic) 379.46
  radiation — *see* Effect, adverse, radiation

Reaction — *continued*
  runaway — *see also* Disturbance, conduct
    socialized 312.2 ☑
    undersocialized, unsocialized 312.1 ☑
  scarlet fever toxin — *see* Complications,
    vaccination
  schizophrenic (*see also* Schizophrenia) 295.9 ☑
    latent 295.5 ☑
  serological for syphilis — *see* Serology for
    syphilis
  serum (prophylactic) (therapeutic) 999.5
    immediate 999.4
  situational (*see also* Reaction, adjustment)
    309.9
    acute, to stress 308.3
    adjustment (*see also* Reaction, adjustment)
      309.9
  somatization (*see also* Disorder, psychosomatic)
    306.9
  spinal puncture 349.0
  spite, child (*see also* Disturbance, conduct)
    312.0 ☑
  stress, acute 308.9
    with predominant disturbance (of)
      consciousness 308.1
      emotions 308.0
      mixed 308.4
      psychomotor 308.2
      specified type NEC 308.3
    bone or cartilage — *see* Fracture, stress
  surgical procedure — *see* Complications,
    surgical procedure
  tetanus antitoxin — *see* Complications,
    vaccination
  toxin-antitoxin — *see* Complications,
    vaccination
  transfusion (blood) (bone marrow)
    (lymphocytes) (allergic) — *see*
    Complications, transfusion
  tuberculin skin test, nonspecific (without active
    tuberculosis) 795.5
    positive (without active tuberculosis) 795.5
  ultraviolet — *see* Effect, adverse, ultraviolet
  undersocialized, unsocialized — *see also*
    Disturbance, conduct
    aggressive (type) 312.0 ☑
    unaggressive (type) 312.1 ☑
  vaccination (any) — *see* Complications,
    vaccination
  white graft (skin) 996.52
  withdrawing, child or adolescent 313.22
  x-ray — *see* Effect, adverse, x-rays
Reactive depression (*see also* Reaction,
  depressive) 300.4
  neurotic 300.4
  psychoneurotic 300.4
  psychotic 298.0
Rebound tenderness 789.6 ☑
Recalcitrant patient V15.81
Recanalization, thrombus — *see* Thrombosis
Recession, receding
  chamber angle (eye) 364.77
  chin 524.06
  gingival (postinfective) (postoperative)
    523.20   ▲
    generalized 523.25   ●
    localized 523.24   ●
    minimal 523.21   ●
    moderate 523.22   ●
    severe 523.23   ●
Recklinghausen's disease (M9540/1) 237.71
  bones (osteitis fibrosa cystica) 252.01   ▲
Recklinghausen-Applebaum disease
  (hemochromatosis) 275.0
Reclus' disease (cystic) 610.1
Recrudescent typhus (fever) 081.1
Recruitment, auditory 388.44
Rectalgia 569.42
Rectitis 569.49
Rectocele
  female (without uterine prolapse) 618.04   ▲
    with uterine prolapse 618.4
      complete 618.3
      incomplete 618.2

☑ Additional Digit Required   ▶◀ Revised Text   ● New Line   ▲ Revised Code

Rectocele — *continued*
  in pregnancy or childbirth 654.4 ☑
    causing obstructed labor 660.2 ☑
      affecting fetus or newborn 763.1
  male 569.49
  vagina, vaginal (outlet) 618.04   ▲
Rectosigmoiditis 569.89
  ulcerative (chronic) 556.3
Rectosigmoid junction — *see* condition
Rectourethral — *see* condition
Rectovaginal — *see* condition
Rectovesical — *see* condition
Rectum, rectal — *see* condition
Recurrent — *see* condition
Red bugs 133.8
Red cedar asthma 495.8
Redness
  conjunctiva 379.93
  eye 379.93
  nose 478.1
Reduced ventilatory or vital capacity 794.2
Reduction
  function
    kidney (*see also* Disease, renal) 593.9
    liver 573.8
  ventilatory capacity 794.2
  vital capacity 794.2
Redundant, redundancy
  abdomen 701.9
  anus 751.5
  cardia 537.89
  clitoris 624.2
  colon (congenital) 751.5
  foreskin (congenital) 605
  intestine 751.5
  labia 624.3
  organ or site, congenital NEC — *see* Accessory
  panniculus (abdominal) 278.1
  prepuce (congenital) 605
  pylorus 537.89
  rectum 751.5
  scrotum 608.89
  sigmoid 751.5
  skin (of face) 701.9
    eyelids 374.30
  stomach 537.89
  uvula 528.9
  vagina 623.8
Reduplication — *see* Duplication
Referral
  adoption (agency) V68.89
  nursing care V63.8
  patient without examination or treatment
    V68.81
  social services V63.8
Reflex — *see also* condition
  blink, deficient 374.45
  hyperactive gag 478.29
  neurogenic bladder NEC 596.54
    atonic 596.54
      with cauda equina syndrome 344.61
  vasoconstriction 443.9
  vasovagal 780.2
Reflux
  esophageal 530.81
  esophagitis 530.11
  gastroesophageal 530.81
  mitral — *see* Insufficiency, mitral
  ureteral — *see* Reflux, vesicoureteral
  vesicoureteral 593.70
    with
      reflux nephropathy 593.73
        bilateral 593.72
        unilateral 593.71
Reformed gallbladder 576.0
Reforming, artificial openings (*see also*
  Attention to, artificial, opening) V55.9
Refractive error (*see also* Error, refractive) 367.9
Refsum's disease or syndrome (heredopathia
  atactica polyneuritiformis) 356.3
Refusal of
  food 307.59
    hysterical 300.11

Refusal of — *continued*
  treatment because of, due to
    patient's decision NEC V64.2
    reason of conscience or religion V62.6
Regaud
  tumor (M8082/3) — *see* Neoplasm,
    nasopharynx, malignant
  type carcinoma (M8082/3) — *see* Neoplasm,
    nasopharynx, malignant
Regional — *see* condition
Regulation feeding (elderly) (infant) 783.3
  newborn 779.3
Regurgitated
  food, choked on 933.1
  stomach contents, choked on 933.1
Regurgitation
  aortic (valve) (*see also* Insufficiency, aortic)
    424.1
    congenital 746.4
    syphilitic 093.22
  food — *see also* Vomiting
    with reswallowing — *see* Rumination
    newborn 779.3
  gastric contents — *see* Vomiting
  heart — *see* Endocarditis
  mitral (valve) (*see also* Insufficiency, mitral)
    congenital 746.6
  myocardial — *see* Endocarditis
  pulmonary (heart) (valve) (*see also*
    Endocarditis, pulmonary) 424.3
  stomach — *see* Vomiting
  tricuspid — *see* Endocarditis, tricuspid
  valve, valvular — *see* Endocarditis
  vesicoureteral — *see* Reflux, vesicoureteral
Rehabilitation V57.9
  multiple types V57.89
  occupational V57.21
  specified type NEC V57.89
  speech V57.3
  vocational V57.22
Reichmann's disease or syndrome
  (gastrosuccorrhea) 536.8
Reifenstein's syndrome (hereditary familial
  hypogonadism, male) 257.2
Reilly's syndrome or phenomenon (*see also*
  Neuropathy, peripheral, autonomic) 337.9
Reimann's periodic disease 277.3
Reinsertion, contraceptive device V25.42
Reiter's disease, syndrome, or urethritis
  099.3 *[711.1]* ☑
Rejection
  food, hysterical 300.11
  transplant 996.80
    bone marrow 996.85
    corneal 996.51
    organ (immune or nonimmune cause)
      996.80
      bone marrow 996.85
      heart 996.83
      intestines 996.87
      kidney 996.81
      liver 996.82
      lung 996.84
      pancreas 996.86
      specified NEC 996.89
    skin 996.52
      artificial 996.55
      decellularized allodermis 996.55
Relapsing fever 087.9
  Carter's (Asiatic) 087.0
  Dutton's (West African) 087.1
  Koch's 087.9
  louse-borne (epidemic) 087.0
  Novy's (American) 087.1
  Obermeyer's (European) 087.0
  Spirillum 087.9
  tick-borne (endemic) 087.1
Relaxation
  anus (sphincter) 569.49
    due to hysteria 300.11
  arch (foot) 734
    congenital 754.61
  back ligaments 728.4
  bladder (sphincter) 596.59

Relaxation — *continued*
  cardio-esophageal 530.89
  cervix (*see also* Incompetency, cervix) 622.5
  diaphragm 519.4
  inguinal rings — *see* Hernia, inguinal
  joint (capsule) (ligament) (paralytic) (*see also*
    Derangement, joint) 718.90
    congenital 755.8
  lumbosacral joint 724.6
  pelvic floor 618.89   ▲
  pelvis 618.89   ▲
  perineum 618.89   ▲
  posture 729.9
  rectum (sphincter) 569.49
  sacroiliac (joint) 724.6
  scrotum 608.89
  urethra (sphincter) 599.84
  uterus (outlet) 618.89   ▲
  vagina (outlet) 618.89   ▲
  vesical 596.59
Remains
  canal of Cloquet 743.51
  capsule (opaque) 743.51
Remittent fever (malarial) 084.6
Remnant
  canal of Cloquet 743.51
  capsule (opaque) 743.51
  cervix, cervical stump (acquired) (postoperative)
    622.8
  cystic duct, postcholecystectomy 576.0
  fingernail 703.8
    congenital 757.5
  meniscus, knee 717.5
  thyroglossal duct 759.2
  tonsil 474.8
    infected 474.00
  urachus 753.7
Remote effect of cancer — *see* condition
Removal (of)
  catheter (urinary) (indwelling) V53.6
    from artificial opening — *see* Attention to,
      artificial, opening
    non-vascular V58.82
    vascular V58.81
  cerebral ventricle (communicating) shunt
    V53.01
  device — *see also* Fitting (of)
    contraceptive V25.42
    fixation
      external V54.89
      internal V54.01
    traction V54.89
  dressing V58.3
  ileostomy V55.2
  Kirschner wire V54.89
  nonvascular catheter V58.82
  pin V54.01
  plaster cast V54.89
  plate (fracture) V54.01
  rod V54.01
  screw V54.01
  splint, external V54.89
  subdermal implantable contraceptive V25.43
  suture V58.3
  traction device, external V54.89
  vascular catheter V58.81
Ren
  arcuatus 753.3
  mobile, mobilis (*see also* Disease, renal) 593.0
    congenital 753.3
  unguliformis 753.3
Renal — *see also* condition
  glomerulohyalinosis-diabetic syndrome
    250.4 ☑ *[581.81]*
Rendu-Osler-Weber disease or syndrome
  (familial hemorrhagic telangiectasia) 448.0
Reninoma (M8361/1) 236.91
Rénon-Delille syndrome 253.8
Repair
  pelvic floor, previous, in pregnancy or
    childbirth 654.4 ☑
    affecting fetus or newborn 763.89
  scarred tissue V51

☑ Additional Digit Required   ►◄ Revised Text   ● New Line   ▲ Revised Code

Replacement by artificial or mechanical device
or prosthesis of (see also Fitting (of))
artificial skin V43.83
bladder V43.5
blood vessel V43.4
breast V43.82
eye globe V43.0
heart
  with
    assist device V43.21
    fully implantable artificial heart V43.22
  valve V43.3
intestine V43.89
joint V43.60
  ankle V43.66
  elbow V43.62
  finger V43.69
  hip (partial) (total) V43.64
  knee V43.65
  shoulder V43.61
  specified NEC V43.69
  wrist V43.63
kidney V43.89
larynx V43.81
lens V43.1
limb(s) V43.7
liver V43.89
lung V43.89
organ NEC V43.89
pancreas V43.89
skin (artificial) V43.83
tissue NEC V43.89

Reprogramming
cardiac pacemaker V53.31

Request for expert evidence V68.2

Reserve, decreased or low
cardiac — see Disease, heart
  kidney (see also Disease, renal) 593.9

Residual — see also condition
bladder 596.8
foreign body — see Retention, foreign body
state, schizophrenic (see also Schizophrenia)
  295.6 ☑
urine 788.69

Resistance, resistant (to)
activated protein C 289.81

Note — use the following subclassification for
categories V09.5, V09.7, V09.8, V09.9:

  0   without mention of resistance to
       multiple drugs

  1   with resistance to multiple drugs
      V09.5   quinolones and
              fluoroquinolones
      V09.7   antimycobacterial agents
      V09.8   specified drugs NEC
      V09.9   unspecified drugs
---

drugs by microorganisms V09.9 ☑
Amikacin V09.4
aminoglycosides V09.4
Amodiaquine V09.5 ☑
Amoxicillin V09.0
Ampicillin V09.0
antimycobacterial agents V09.7 ☑
Azithromycin V09.2
Azlocillin V09.0
Aztreonam V09.1
B-lactam antibiotics V09.1
bacampicillin V09.0
Bacitracin V09.8 ☑
Benznidazole V09.8 ☑
Capreomycin V09.7 ☑
Carbenicillin V09.0
Cefaclor V09.1
Cefadroxil V09.1
Cefamandole V09.1
Cefatetan V09.1
Cefazolin V09.1
Cefixime V09.1
Cefonicid V09.1
Cefoperazone V09.1
Ceforanide V09.1

Resistance, resistant — continued
drugs by microorganisms — continued
Cefotaxime V09.1
Cefoxitin V09.1
Ceftazidime V09.1
Ceftizoxime V09.1
Ceftriaxone V09.1
Cefuroxime V09.1
Cephalexin V09.1
Cephaloglycin V09.1
Cephaloridine V09.1
Cephalosporins V09.1
Cephalothin V09.1
Cephapirin V09.1
Cephradine V09.1
Chloramphenicol V09.8 ☑
Chloraquine V09.5 ☑
Chlorguanide V09.8 ☑
Chlorproguanil V09.8 ☑
Chlortetracyline V09.3
Cinoxacin V09.5 ☑
Ciprofloxacin V09.5 ☑
Clarithromycin V09.2
Clindamycin V09.8 ☑
Clioquinol V09.5 ☑
Clofazimine V09.7 ☑
Cloxacillin V09.0
Cyclacillin V09.0
Cycloserine V09.7 ☑
Dapsone [DZ] V09.7 ☑
Demeclocycline V09.3
Dicloxacillin V09.0
Doxycycline V09.3
Enoxacin V09.5 ☑
Erythromycin V09.2
Ethambutol [EMB] V09.7 ☑
Ethionamide [ETA] V09.7 ☑
fluoroquinolones V09.5 ☑
Gentamicin V09.4
Halofantrine V09.8 ☑
Imipenem V09.1
Iodoquinol V09.5 ☑
Isoniazid [INH] V09.7 ☑
Kanamycin V09.4
macrolides V09.2
Mafenide V09.6
MDRO (multiple drug resistant ●
  organisms) NOS V09.91 ●
Mefloquine V09.8 ☑
Melasoprol V09.8 ☑
Methacycline V09.3
Methenamine V09.8 ☑
Methicillin V09.0
Metronidazole V09.8 ☑
Mezlocillin V09.0
Minocycline V09.3
multiple drug resistant organisms ●
  NOS V09.91 ●
Nafcillin V09.0
Nalidixic acid V09.5 ☑
Natamycin V09.2
Neomycin V09.4
Netilmicin V09.4
Nifurtimox V09.8 ☑
Nimorazole V09.8 ☑
Nitrofurantoin V09.8 ☑
Norfloxacin V09.5 ☑
Nystatin V09.2
Ofloxacin V09.5 ☑
Oleandomycin V09.2
Oxacillin V09.0
Oxytetracycline V09.3
Para-amino salicylic acid [PAS] V09.7 ☑
Paromomycin V09.4
Penicillin (G) (V) (VK) V09.0
penicillins V09.0
Pentamidine V09.8 ☑
Piperacillin V09.0
Primaquine V09.5 ☑
Proguanil V09.8 ☑
Pyrazinamide [PZA] V09.7 ☑
Pyrimethamine/sulfalene V09.8 ☑
Pyrimethamine/sulfodoxine V09.8 ☑
Quinacrine V09.5 ☑
Quinidine V09.8 ☑
Quinine V09.8 ☑
quinolones V09.5 ☑

Resistance, resistant — continued
drugs by microorganisms — continued
Rifabutin V09.7 ☑
Rifampin [RIF] V09.7 ☑
Rifamycin V09.7 ☑
Rolitetracycline V09.3
Specified drugs NEC V09.8 ☑
Spectinomycin V09.8 ☑
Spiramycin V09.2
Streptomycin [SM] V09.4
Sulfacetamide V09.6
Sulfacytine V09.6
Sulfadiazine V09.6
Sulfadoxine V09.6
Sulfamethoxazole V09.6
Sulfapyridine V09.6
Sulfasalizine V09.6
Sulfasoxazone V09.6
sulfonamides V09.6
Sulfoxone V09.7 ☑
tetracycline V09.3
tetracyclines V09.3
Thiamphenicol V09.8 ☑
Ticarcillin V09.0
Tinidazole V09.8 ☑
Tobramycin V09.4
Triamphenicol V09.8 ☑
Trimethoprim V09.8 ☑
Vancomycin V09.8 ☑
insulin 277.7 ●

Resorption
biliary 576.8
  purulent or putrid (see also Cholecystitis)
    576.8
dental (roots) 521.40 ▲
  alveoli 525.8
  pathological ●
    external 521.42 ●
    internal 521.41 ●
    specified NEC 521.49 ●
septic — see Septicemia
teeth (roots) 521.40 ▲
  pathological ●
    external 521.42 ●
    internal 521.41 ●
    specified NEC 521.49 ●

Respiration
asymmetrical 786.09
bronchial 786.09
Cheyne-Stokes (periodic respiration) 786.04
decreased, due to shock following injury 958.4
disorder of 786.00
  psychogenic 306.1
  specified NEC 786.09
failure 518.81
  acute 518.81
  acute and chronic 518.84
  chronic 518.83
  newborn 770.84
insufficiency 786.09
  acute 518.82
  newborn NEC 770.89
Kussmaul (air hunger) 786.09
painful 786.52
periodic 786.09
poor 786.09
  newborn NEC 770.89
sighing 786.7
  psychogenic 306.1
wheezing 786.07

Respiratory — see also condition
distress 786.09
  acute 518.82
  fetus or newborn NEC 770.89
  syndrome (newborn) 769
    adult (following shock, surgery, or
      trauma) 518.5
    specified NEC 518.82
failure 518.81
  acute 518.81
  acute and chronic 518.8
  chronic 518.83

Respiratory syncytial virus (RSV) 079.6
bronchiolitis 466.11
pneumonia 480.1
vaccination, prophylactic (against) V04.82

☑ Additional Digit Required   ▶◀ Revised Text   ● New Line   ▲ Revised Code

Response
  photoallergic 692.72
  phototoxic 692.72
Rest, rests
  mesonephric duct 752.89
    fallopian tube 752.11
  ovarian, in fallopian tubes 752.19
  wolffian duct 752.89
Restless leg (syndrome) 333.99
Restlessness 799.2
Restoration of organ continuity from previous sterilization (tuboplasty) (vasoplasty) V26.0
Restriction of housing space V60.1
Restzustand, schizophrenic (*see also* Schizophrenia) 295.6 ☑
Retained — *see* Retention
Retardation
  development, developmental, specific (*see also* Disorder, development, specific) 315.9
    learning, specific 315.2
      arithmetical 315.1
      language (skills) 315.31
        expressive 315.31
        mixed receptive-expressive 315.32
      mathematics 315.1
      reading 315.00
        phonological 315.39
      written expression 315.2
    motor 315.4
  endochondral bone growth 733.91
  growth (physical) in childhood 783.43
    due to malnutrition 263.2
    fetal (intrauterine) 764.9 ☑
      affecting management of pregnancy 656.5 ☑
  intrauterine growth 764.9 ☑
    affecting management of pregnancy 656.5 ☑
  mental 319
    borderline V62.89
    mild, IQ 50-70 317
    moderate, IQ 35-49 318.0
    profound, IQ under 20 318.2
    severe, IQ 20-34 318.1
  motor, specific 315.4
  physical 783.43
    child 783.43
    due to malnutrition 263.2
    fetus (intrauterine) 764.9 ☑
      affecting management of pregnancy 656.5 ☑
  psychomotor NEC 307.9
  reading 315.00
Retching — *see* Vomiting
Retention, retained
  bladder NEC (*see also* Retention, urine) 788.20
    psychogenic 306.53
  carbon dioxide 276.2
  cyst — *see* Cyst
  dead
    fetus (after 22 completed weeks gestation) 656.4 ☑
      early fetal death (before 22 completed weeks gestation) 632
    ovum 631
  decidua (following delivery) (fragments) (with hemorrhage) 666.2 ☑
    without hemorrhage 667.1 ☑
  deciduous tooth 520.6
  dental root 525.3
  fecal (*see also* Constipation) 564.00
  fluid 276.6
  foreign body — *see also* Foreign body, retained
    bone 733.99
    current trauma — *see* Foreign body, by site or type
    middle ear 385.83
    muscle 729.6
    soft tissue NEC 729.6
  gastric 536.8
  membranes (following delivery) (with hemorrhage) 666.2 ☑
    with abortion — *see* Abortion, by type
    without hemorrhage 667.1 ☑
  menses 626.8
  milk (puerperal) 676.2 ☑

Retention, retained — *continued*
  nitrogen, extrarenal 788.9
  placenta (total) (with hemorrhage) 666.0 ☑
    with abortion — *see* Abortion, by type
    portions or fragments 666.2 ☑
      without hemorrhage 667.1 ☑
    without hemorrhage 667.0 ☑
  products of conception
    early pregnancy (fetal death before 22 completed weeks gestation) 632
    following
      abortion — *see* Abortion, by type
      delivery 666.2 ☑
        with hemorrhage 666.2 ☑
        without hemorrhage 667.1 ☑
  secundines (following delivery) (with hemorrhage) 666.2 ☑
    with abortion — *see* Abortion, by type
    complicating puerperium (delayed hemorrhage) 666.2 ☑
    without hemorrhage 667.1 ☑
  smegma, clitoris 624.8
  urine NEC 788.20
    bladder, incomplete emptying 788.21
    psychogenic 306.53
    specified NEC 788.29
  water (in tissue) (*see also* Edema) 782.3
Reticulation, dust (occupational) 504
Reticulocytosis NEC 790.99
Reticuloendotheliosis
  acute infantile (M9722/3) 202.5 ☑
  leukemic (M9940/3) 202.4 ☑
  malignant (M9720/3) 202.3 ☑
  nonlipid (M9722/3) 202.5 ☑
Reticulohistiocytoma (giant cell) 277.89
Reticulohistiocytosis, multicentric 272.8
Reticulolymphosarcoma (diffuse) (M9613/3) 200.8 ☑
  follicular (M9691/3) 202.0 ☑
  nodular (M9691/3) 202.0 ☑
Reticulosarcoma (M9640/3) 200.0 ☑
  nodular (M9642/3) 200.0 ☑
  pleomorphic cell type (M9641/3) 200.0 ☑
Reticulosis (skin)
  acute of infancy (M9722/3) 202.5 ☑
  histiocytic medullary (M9721/3) 202.3 ☑
  lipomelanotic 695.89
  malignant (M9720/3) 202.3 ☑
  Sézary's (M9701/3) 202.2 ☑
Retina, retinal — *see* condition
Retinitis (*see also* Chorioretinitis) 363.20
  albuminurica 585 [363.10]
  arteriosclerotic 440.8 [362.13]
  central angiospastic 362.41
  Coat's 362.12
  diabetic 250.5 ☑ [362.01]
  disciformis 362.52
  disseminated 363.10
    metastatic 363.14
    neurosyphilitic 094.83
    pigment epitheliopathy 363.15
  exudative 362.12
  focal 363.00
    in histoplasmosis 115.92
      capsulatum 115.02
      duboisii 115.12
    juxtapapillary 363.05
    macular 363.06
    paramacular 363.06
    peripheral 363.08
    posterior pole NEC 363.07
  gravidarum 646.8 ☑
  hemorrhagica externa 362.12
  juxtapapillary (Jensen's) 363.05
  luetic — *see* Retinitis, syphilitic
  metastatic 363.14
  pigmentosa 362.74
  proliferans 362.29
  proliferating 362.29
  punctata albescens 362.76
  renal 585 [363.13]
  syphilitic (secondary) 091.51
    congenital 090.0 [363.13]
    early 091.51
    late 095.8 [363.13]

Retinitis (*see also* Chorioretinitis) — *continued*
  syphilitica, central, recurrent 095.8 [363.13]
  tuberculous (*see also* Tuberculous) 017.3 ☑ [363.13]
Retinoblastoma (M9510/3) 190.5
  differentiated type (M9511/3) 190.5
  undifferentiated type (M9512/3) 190.5
Retinochoroiditis (*see also* Chorioretinitis) 363.20
  central angiospastic 362.41
  disseminated 363.10
    metastatic 363.14
    neurosyphilitic 094.83
    pigment epitheliopathy 363.15
    syphilitic 094.83
  due to toxoplasmosis (acquired) (focal) 130.2
  focal 363.00
    in histoplasmosis 115.92
      capsulatum 115.02
      duboisii 115.12
    juxtapapillary (Jensen's) 363.05
    macular 363.06
    paramacular 363.06
    peripheral 363.08
    posterior pole NEC 363.07
  juxtapapillaris 363.05
  syphilitic (disseminated) 094.83
Retinopathy (background) 362.10
  arteriosclerotic 440.8 [362.13]
  atherosclerotic 440.8 [362.13]
  central serous 362.41
  circinate 362.10
  Coat's 362.12
  diabetic 250.5 ☑ [362.01]
    proliferative 250.5 ☑ [362.02]
  exudative 362.12
  hypertensive 362.11
  of prematurity 362.21
  pigmentary, congenital 362.74
  proliferative 362.29
    diabetic 250.5 [362.02]
    sickle-cell 282.60 [362.29]
  solar 363.31
Retinoschisis 361.10
  bullous 361.12
  congenital 743.56
  flat 361.11
  juvenile 362.73
Retractile testis 752.52
Retraction
  cervix (*see also* Retroversion, uterus) 621.6
  drum (membrane) 384.82
  eyelid 374.41
  finger 736.29
  head 781.0
  lid 374.41
  lung 518.89
  mediastinum 519.3
  nipple 611.79
    congenital 757.6
    puerperal, postpartum 676.0 ☑
  palmar fascia 728.6
  pleura (*see also* Pleurisy) 511.0
  ring, uterus (Bandl's) (pathological) 661.4 ☑
    affecting fetus or newborn 763.7
  sternum (congenital) 756.3
    acquired 738.3
    during respiration 786.9
  substernal 738.3
  supraclavicular 738.8
  syndrome (Duane's) 378.71
  uterus (*see also* Retroversion, uterus) 621.6
  valve (heart) — *see* Endocarditis
Retrobulbar — *see* condition
Retrocaval ureter 753.4
Retrocecal — *see also* condition
  appendix (congenital) 751.5
Retrocession — *see* Retroversion
Retrodisplacement — *see* Retroversion
Retroflection, retroflexion — *see* Retroversion
Retrognathia, retrognathism (mandibular) (maxillary) 524.06

☑ Additional Digit Required   ▶◀ Revised Text   ● New Line   ▲ Revised Code

Retrograde
ejaculation 608.87
menstruation 626.8

Retroiliac ureter 753.4

Retroperineal — *see* condition

Retroperitoneal — *see* condition

Retroperitonitis (*see also* Peritonitis) 567.9

Retropharyngeal — *see* condition

Retroplacental — *see* condition

Retroposition — *see* Retroversion

Retrosternal thyroid (congenital) 759.2

Retroversion, retroverted
cervix (*see also* Retroversion, uterus) 621.6
female NEC (*see also* Retroversion, uterus)
621.6
iris 364.70
testis (congenital) 752.51
uterus, uterine (acquired) (acute) (adherent)
(any degree) (asymptomatic) (cervix)
(postinfectional) (postpartal, old) 621.6
congenital 752.3
in pregnancy or childbirth 654.3 ☑
affecting fetus or newborn 763.89
causing obstructed labor 660.2 ☑
affecting fetus or newborn 763.1

Retrusion, premaxilla (developmental) 524.04

Rett's syndrome 330.8

Reverse, reversed
peristalsis 787.4

Reye's syndrome 331.81

Reye-Sheehan syndrome (postpartum pituitary
necrosis) 253.2

Rh (factor)
hemolytic disease 773.0
incompatibility, immunization, or sensitization
affecting management of pregnancy 656.1 ☑
fetus or newborn 773.0
transfusion reaction 999.7
negative mother, affecting fetus or newborn
773.0
titer elevated 999.7
transfusion reaction 999.7

Rhabdomyolysis (idiopathic) 728.88

Rhabdomyoma (M8900/0) — *see also* Neoplasm,
connective tissue, benign
adult (M8904/0) — *see* Neoplasm, connective
tissue, benign
fetal (M8903/0) — *see* Neoplasm, connective
tissue, benign
glycogenic (M8904/0) — *see* Neoplasm,
connective tissue, benign

Rhabdomyosarcoma (M8900/3) — *see also*
Neoplasm, connective tissue, malignant
alveolar (M8920/3) — *see* Neoplasm,
connective tissue, malignant
embryonal (M8910/3) — *see* Neoplasm,
connective tissue, malignant
mixed type (M8902/3) — *see* Neoplasm,
connective tissue, malignant
pleomorphic (M8901/3) — *see* Neoplasm,
connective tissue, malignant

Rhabdosarcoma (M8900/3) — *see*
Rhabdomyosarcoma

Rhesus (factor) (Rh) incompatibility — *see* Rh,
incompatibility

Rheumaticosis — *see* Rheumatism

Rheumatism, rheumatic (acute NEC) 729.0
adherent pericardium 393
arthritis
acute or subacute — *see* Fever, rheumatic
chronic 714.0
spine 720.0
articular (chronic) NEC (*see also* Arthritis)
716.9 ☑
acute or subacute — *see* Fever, rheumatic
back 724.9
blennorrhagic 098.59
carditis — *see* Disease, heart, rheumatic
cerebral — *see* Fever, rheumatic
chorea (acute) — *see* Chorea, rheumatic
chronic NEC 729.0
coronary arteritis 391.9
chronic 398.99

Rheumatism, rheumatic — *continued*
degeneration, myocardium (*see also*
Degeneration, myocardium, with
rheumatic fever) 398.0
desert 114.0
febrile — *see* Fever, rheumatic
fever — *see* Fever, rheumatic
gonococcal 098.59
gout 274.0
heart
disease (*see also* Disease, heart, rheumatic)
398.90
failure (chronic) (congestive) (inactive)
398.91
hemopericardium — *see* Rheumatic,
pericarditis
hydropericardium — *see* Rheumatic,
pericarditis
inflammatory (acute) (chronic) (subacute) — *see*
Fever, rheumatic
intercostal 729.0
meaning Tietze's disease 733.6
joint (chronic) NEC (*see also* Arthritis) 716.9 ☑
acute — *see* Fever, rheumatic
mediastinopericarditis — *see* Rheumatic,
pericarditis
muscular 729.0
myocardial degeneration (*see also*
Degeneration, myocardium, with
rheumatic fever) 398.0
myocarditis (chronic) (inactive) (with chorea)
398.0
active or acute 391.2
with chorea (acute) (rheumatic)
(Sydenham's) 392.0
myositis 729.1
neck 724.9
neuralgic 729.0
neuritis (acute) (chronic) 729.2
neuromuscular 729.0
nodose — *see* Arthritis, nodosa
nonarticular 729.0
palindromic 719.30
ankle 719.37
elbow 719.32
foot 719.37
hand 719.34
hip 719.35
knee 719.36
multiple sites 719.39
pelvic region 719.35
shoulder (region) 719.31
specified site NEC 719.38
wrist 719.33
pancarditis, acute 391.8
with chorea (acute) (rheumatic)
(Sydenham's) 392.0
chronic or inactive 398.99
pericarditis (active) (acute) (with effusion) (with
pneumonia) 391.0
with chorea (acute) (rheumatic)
(Sydenham's) 392.0
chronic or inactive 393
pericardium — *see* Rheumatic, pericarditis
pleuropericarditis — *see* Rheumatic,
pericarditis
pneumonia 390 [517.1]
pneumonitis 390 [517.1]
pneumopericarditis — *see* Rheumatic,
pericarditis
polyarthritis
acute or subacute — *see* Fever, rheumatic
chronic 714.0
polyarticular NEC (*see also* Arthritis) 716.9 ☑
psychogenic 306.0
radiculitis 729.2
sciatic 724.3
septic — *see* Fever, rheumatic
spine 724.9
subacute NEC 729.0
torticollis 723.5
tuberculous NEC (*see also* Tuberculosis)
015.9 ☑
typhoid fever 002.0

Rheumatoid — *see also* condition
lungs 714.81

Rhinitis (atrophic) (catarrhal) (chronic) (croupous)
(fibrinous) (hyperplastic) (hypertrophic)
(membranous) (purulent) (suppurative)
(ulcerative) 472.0
with
hay fever (*see also* Fever, hay) 477.9
with asthma (bronchial) 493.0 ☑
sore throat — *see* Nasopharyngitis
acute 460
allergic (nonseasonal) (seasonal) (*see also* Fever,
hay) 477.9
with asthma (*see also* Asthma) 493.0 ☑
due to food 477.1
granulomatous 472.0
infective 460
obstructive 472.0
pneumococcal 460
syphilitic 095.8
congenital 090.0
tuberculous (*see also* Tuberculosis) 012.8 ☑
vasomotor (*see also* Fever, hay) 477.9

Rhinoantritis (chronic) 473.0
acute 461.0

Rhinodacryolith 375.57

Rhinolalia (aperta) (clausa) (open) 784.49

Rhinolith 478.1
nasal sinus (*see also* Sinusitis) 473.9

Rhinomegaly 478.1

Rhinopharyngitis (acute) (subacute) (*see also*
Nasopharyngitis) 460
chronic 472.2
destructive ulcerating 102.5
mutilans 102.5

Rhinophyma 695.3

Rhinorrhea 478.1
cerebrospinal (fluid) 349.81
paroxysmal (*see also* Fever, hay) 477.9
spasmodic (*see also* Fever, hay) 477.9

Rhinosalpingitis 381.50
acute 381.51
chronic 381.52

Rhinoscleroma 040.1

Rhinosporidiosis 117.0

Rhinovirus infection 079.3

Rhizomelic chrondrodysplasia punctata ●
277.86 ●

Rhizomelique, pseudopolyarthritic 446.5

Rhoads and Bomford anemia (refractory) 284.9

Rhus
diversiloba dermatitis 692.6
radicans dermatitis 692.6
toxicodendron dermatitis 692.6
venenata dermatitis 692.6
verniciflua dermatitis 692.6

Rhythm
atrioventricular nodal 427.89
disorder 427.9
coronary sinus 427.89
ectopic 427.89
nodal 427.89
escape 427.89
heart, abnormal 427.9
fetus or newborn — *see* Abnormal, heart
rate
idioventricular 426.89
accelerated 427.89
nodal 427.89
sleep, inversion 780.55
nonorganic origin 307.45

Rhytidosis facialis 701.8

Rib — *see also* condition
cervical 756.2

Riboflavin deficiency 266.0

Rice bodies (*see also* Loose, body, joint) 718.1 ☑
knee 717.6

Richter's hernia — *see* Hernia, Richter's

Ricinism 988.2

Rickets (active) (acute) (adolescent) (adult) (chest
wall) (congenital) (current) (infantile)
(intestinal) 268.0
celiac 579.0
fetal 756.4

Retrograde — Rickets

Rickets — *continued*
  hemorrhagic 267
  hypophosphatemic with nephroticglycosuric dwarfism 270.0
  kidney 588.0
  late effect 268.1
  renal 588.0
  scurvy 267
  vitamin D-resistant 275.3
Rickettsial disease 083.9
  specified type NEC 083.8
Rickettsialpox 083.2
Rickettsiosis NEC 083.9
  specified type NEC 083.8
  tick-borne 082.9
    specified type NEC 082.8
  vesicular 083.2
Ricord's chancre 091.0
Riddoch's syndrome (visual disorientation) 368.16
Rider's
  bone 733.99
  chancre 091.0
Ridge, alveolus — *see also* condition
  edentulous ●
    atrophy 525.20 ●
      mandible 525.20 ●
        minimal 525.21 ●
        moderate 525.22 ●
        severe 525.23 ●
      maxilla 525.20 ●
        minimal 525.24 ●
        moderate 525.25 ●
        severe 525.26 ●
  flabby 525.20 ▲
Ridged ear 744.29
Riedel's
  disease (ligneous thyroiditis) 245.3
  lobe, liver 751.69
  struma (ligneous thyroiditis) 245.3
  thyroiditis (ligneous) 245.3
Rieger's anomaly or syndrome (mesodermal dysgenesis, anterior ocular segment) 743.44
Riehl's melanosis 709.09
Rietti-Greppi-Micheli anemia or syndrome 282.49
Rieux's hernia — *see* Hernia, Rieux's
Rift Valley fever 066.3
Riga's disease (cachectic aphthae) 529.0
Riga-Fede disease (cachectic aphthae) 529.0
Riggs' disease (compound periodontitis) 523.4
Right middle lobe syndrome 518.0
Rigid, rigidity — *see also* condition
  abdominal 789.4 ☑
  articular, multiple congenital 754.89
  back 724.8
  cervix uteri
    in pregnancy or childbirth 654.6 ☑
      affecting fetus or newborn 763.89
      causing obstructed labor 660.2 ☑
        affecting fetus or newborn 763.1
  hymen (acquired) (congenital) 623.3
  nuchal 781.6
  pelvic floor
    in pregnancy or childbirth 654.4 ☑
      affecting fetus or newborn 763.89
      causing obstructed labor 660.2 ☑
        affecting fetus or newborn 763.1
  perineum or vulva
    in pregnancy or childbirth 654.8 ☑
      affecting fetus or newborn 763.89
      causing obstructed labor 660.2 ☑
        affecting fetus or newborn 763.1
  spine 724.8
  vagina
    in pregnancy or childbirth 654.7 ☑
      affecting fetus or newborn 763.89
      causing obstructed labor 660.2 ☑
        affecting fetus or newborn 763.1
Rigors 780.99
Riley-Day syndrome (familial dysautonomia) 742.8

Ring(s)
  aorta 747.21
  Bandl's, complicating delivery 661.4 ☑
    affecting fetus or newborn 763.7
  contraction, complicating delivery 661.4 ☑
    affecting fetus or newborn 763.7
  esophageal (congenital) 750.3
  Fleischer (-Kayser) (cornea) 275.1 *[371.14]*
  hymenal, tight (acquired) (congenital) 623.3
  Kayser-Fleischer (cornea) 275.1 *[371.14]*
  retraction, uterus, pathological 661.4 ☑
    affecting fetus or newborn 763.7
  Schatzki's (esophagus) (congenital) (lower) 750.3
    acquired 530.3
  Soemmering's 366.51
  trachea, abnormal 748.3
  vascular (congenital) 747.21
  Vossius' 921.3
    late effect 366.21
Ringed hair (congenital) 757.4
Ringing in the ear (*see also* Tinnitus) 388.30
Ringworm 110.9
  beard 110.0
  body 110.5
  Burmese 110.9
  corporeal 110.5
  foot 110.4
  groin 110.3
  hand 110.2
  honeycomb 110.0
  nails 110.1
  perianal (area) 110.3
  scalp 110.0
  specified site NEC 110.8
  Tokelau 110.5
Rise, venous pressure 459.89
Risk
  factor — *see* Problem
  suicidal 300.9
Ritter's disease (dermatitis exfoliativa neonatorum) 695.81
Rivalry, sibling 313.3
Rivalta's disease (cervicofacial actinomycosis) 039.3
River blindness 125.3 *[360.13]*
Robert's pelvis 755.69
  with disproportion (fetopelvic) 653.0 ☑
    affecting fetus or newborn 763.1
    causing obstructed labor 660.1 ☑
      affecting fetus or newborn 763.1
Robin's syndrome 756.0
Robinson's (hidrotic) **ectodermal dysplasia** 757.31
Robles' disease (onchocerciasis) 125.3 *[360.13]*
Rochalimea — *see* Rickettsial disease
Rocky Mountain fever (spotted) 082.0
Rodent ulcer (M8090/3) — *see also* Neoplasm, skin, malignant
  cornea 370.07
Roentgen ray, adverse effect — *see* Effect, adverse, x-ray
Roetheln 056.9
Roger's disease (congenital interventricular septal defect) 745.4
Rokitansky's
  disease (*see also* Necrosis, liver) 570
  tumor 620.2
Rokitansky-Aschoff sinuses (mucosal outpouching of gallbladder) (*see also* Disease, gallbladder) 575.8
Rokitansky-Kuster-Hauser syndrome (congenital absence vagina) 752.49
Rollet's chancre (syphilitic) 091.0
Rolling of head 781.0
Romano-Ward syndrome (prolonged Q-T interval) 794.31
Romanus lesion 720.1
Romberg's disease or syndrome 349.89
Roof, mouth — *see* condition

Rosacea 695.3
  acne 695.3
  keratitis 695.3 *[370.49]*
Rosary, rachitic 268.0
Rose
  cold 477.0
  fever 477.0
  rash 782.1
    epidemic 056.9
    of infants 057.8
Rosen-Castleman-Liebow syndrome (pulmonary proteinosis) 516.0
Rosenbach's erysipelatoid or erysipeloid 027.1
Rosenthal's disease (factor XI deficiency) 286.2
Roseola 057.8
  infantum, infantilis 057.8
Rossbach's disease (hyperchlorhydria) 536.8
  psychogenic 306.4
Rössle-Urbach-Wiethe lipoproteinosis 272.8
Ross river fever 066.3
Rostan's asthma (cardiac) (*see also* Failure, ventricular, left) 428.1
Rot
  Barcoo (*see also* Ulcer, skin) 707.9
  knife-grinders' (*see also* Tuberculosis) 011.4 ☑
Rot-Bernhardt disease 355.1
Rotation
  anomalous, incomplete or insufficient — *see* Malrotation
  cecum (congenital) 751.4
  colon (congenital) 751.4
  manual, affecting fetus or newborn 763.89
  spine, incomplete or insufficient 737.8
  tooth, teeth 524.35 ▲
  vertebra, incomplete or insufficient 737.8
Röteln 056.9
Roth's disease or meralgia 355.1
Roth-Bernhardt disease or syndrome 355.1
Rothmund (-Thomson) syndrome 757.33
Rotor's disease or syndrome (idiopathic hyperbilirubinemia) 277.4
Rotundum ulcus — *see* Ulcer, stomach
Round
  back (with wedging of vertebrae) 737.10
    late effect of rickets 268.1
  hole, retina 361.31
    with detachment 361.01
  ulcer (stomach) — *see* Ulcer, stomach
  worms (infestation) (large) NEC 127.0
Roussy-Lévy syndrome 334.3
Routine postpartum follow-up V24.2
Roy (-Jutras) syndrome (acropachyderma) 757.39
Rubella (German measles) 056.9
  complicating pregnancy, childbirth, or puerperium 647.5 ☑
  complication 056.8
    neurological 056.00
      encephalomyelitis 056.01
      specified type NEC 056.09
    specified type NEC 056.79
  congenital 771.0
  contact V01.4
  exposure to V01.4
  maternal
    with suspected fetal damage affecting management of pregnancy 655.3 ☑
    affecting fetus or newborn 760.2
      manifest rubella in infant 771.0
  specified complications NEC 056.79
  vaccination, prophylactic (against) V04.3
Rubeola (measles) (*see also* Measles) 055.9
  complicated 055.8
  meaning rubella (*see also* Rubella) 056.9
  scarlatinosis 057.8
Rubeosis iridis 364.42
  diabetica 250.5 ☑ *[364.42]*
Rubinstein-Taybi's syndrome (brachydactylia, short stature, and mental retardation) 759.89
Rud's syndrome (mental deficiency, epilepsy, and infantilism) 759.89

Rickets — Rud's syndrome

Rudimentary (congenital) — *see also* Agenesis
arm 755.22
bone 756.9
cervix uteri 752.49
eye (*see also* Microphthalmos) 743.10
fallopian tube 752.19
leg 755.32
lobule of ear 744.21
patella 755.64
respiratory organs in thoracopagus 759.4
tracheal bronchus 748.3
uterine horn 752.3
uterus 752.3
in male 752.7
solid or with cavity 752.3
vagina 752.49

Ruiter-Pompen (-Wyers) syndrome
(angiokeratoma corporis diffusum) 272.7

Ruled out condition (*see also* Observation, suspected) V71.9

Rumination — *see also* Vomiting ●
disorder 307.53
neurotic 300.3
obsessional 300.3
psychogenic 307.53

Runaway reaction — *see also* Disturbance, conduct
socialized 312.2 ☑
undersocialized, unsocialized 312.1 ☑

Runeberg's disease (progressive pernicious anemia) 281.0

Runge's syndrome (postmaturity) 766.22

Rupia 091.3
congenital 090.0
tertiary 095.9

Rupture, ruptured 553.9
abdominal viscera NEC 799.89
obstetrical trauma 665.5 ☑
abscess (spontaneous) — *see* Abscess, by site
amnion — *see* Rupture, membranes
aneurysm — *see* Aneurysm
anus (sphincter) — *see* Laceration, anus
aorta, aortic 441.5
abdominal 441.3
arch 441.1
ascending 441.1
descending 441.5
abdominal 441.3
thoracic 441.1
syphilitic 093.0
thoracoabdominal 441.6
thorax, thoracic 441.1
transverse 441.1
traumatic (thoracic) 901.0
abdominal 902.0
valve or cusp (*see also* Endocarditis, aortic) 424.1
appendix (with peritonitis) 540.0
with peritoneal abscess 540.1
traumatic — *see* Injury, internal, gastrointestinal tract
arteriovenous fistula, brain (congenital) 430
artery 447.2
brain (*see also* Hemorrhage, brain) 431
coronary (*see also* Infarct, myocardium) 410.9 ☑
heart (*see also* Infarct, myocardium) 410.9 ☑
pulmonary 417.8
traumatic (complication) (*see also* Injury, blood vessel, by site) 904.9
bile duct, except cystic (*see also* Disease, biliary) 576.3
cystic 575.4
traumatic — *see* Injury, internal, intra-abdominal
bladder (sphincter) 596.6
with
abortion — *see* Abortion, by type, with damage to pelvic organs
ectopic pregnancy (*see also* categories 633.0-633.9) 639.2
molar pregnancy (*see also* categories 630-632) 639.2

Rupture, ruptured — *continued*
bladder — *continued*
following
abortion 639.2
ectopic or molar pregnancy 639.2
nontraumatic 596.6
obstetrical trauma 665.5 ☑
spontaneous 596.6
traumatic — *see* Injury, internal, bladder
blood vessel (*see also* Hemorrhage) 459.0
brain (*see also* Hemorrhage, brain) 431
heart (*see also* Infarct, myocardium) 410.9 ☑
traumatic (complication) (*see also* Injury, blood vessel, by site) 904.9
bone — *see* Fracture, by site
bowel 569.89
traumatic — *see* Injury, internal, intestine
Bowman's membrane 371.31
brain
aneurysm (congenital) (*see also* Hemorrhage, subarachnoid) 430
late effect — *see* Late effect(s) (of) cerebrovascular disease
syphilitic 094.87
hemorrhagic (*see also* Hemorrhage, brain) 431
injury at birth 767.0
syphilitic 094.89
capillaries 448.9
cardiac (*see also* Infarct, myocardium) 410.9 ☑
cartilage (articular) (current) — *see also* Sprain, by site
knee — *see* Tear, meniscus
semilunar — *see* Tear, meniscus
cecum (with peritonitis) 540.0
with peritoneal abscess 540.1
traumatic 863.89
with open wound into cavity 863.99
cerebral aneurysm (congenital) (*see also* Hemorrhage, subarachnoid) 430
late effect — *see* Late effect(s) (of) cerebrovascular disease
cervix (uteri)
with
abortion — *see* Abortion, by type, with damage to pelvic organs
ectopic pregnancy (*see also* categories 633.0-633.9) 639.2
molar pregnancy (*see also* categories 630-632) 639.2
following
abortion 639.2
ectopic or molar pregnancy 639.2
obstetrical trauma 665.3 ☑
traumatic — *see* Injury, internal, cervix
chordae tendineae 429.5
choroid (direct) (indirect) (traumatic) 363.63
circle of Willis (*see also* Hemorrhage, subarachnoid) 430
late effect — *see* Late effect(s) (of) cerebrovascular disease
colon 569.89
traumatic — *see* Injury, internal, colon
cornea (traumatic) — *see also* Rupture, eye
due to ulcer 370.00
coronary (artery) (thrombotic) (*see also* Infarct, myocardium) 410.9 ☑
corpus luteum (infected) (ovary) 620.1
cyst — *see* Cyst
cystic duct (*see also* Disease, gallbladder) 575.4
Descemet's membrane 371.33
traumatic — *see* Rupture, eye
diaphragm — *see also* Hernia, diaphragm
traumatic — *see* Injury, internal, diaphragm
diverticulum
bladder 596.3
intestine (large) (*see also* Diverticula) 562.10
small 562.00
duodenal stump 537.89
duodenum (ulcer) — *see* Ulcer, duodenum, with perforation
ear drum (*see also* Perforation, tympanum) 384.20
with otitis media — *see* Otitis media
traumatic — *see* Wound, open, ear

Rupture, ruptured — *continued*
esophagus 530.4
traumatic 862.22
with open wound into cavity 862.32
cervical region — *see* Wound, open, esophagus
eye (without prolapse of intraocular tissue) 871.0
with
exposure of intraocular tissue 871.1
partial loss of intraocular tissue 871.2
prolapse of intraocular tissue 871.1
due to burn 940.5
fallopian tube 620.8
due to pregnancy — *see* Pregnancy, tubal
traumatic — *see* Injury, internal, fallopian tube
fontanel 767.3
free wall (ventricle) (*see also* Infarct, myocardium) 410.9 ☑
gallbladder or duct (*see also* Disease, gallbladder) 575.4
traumatic — *see* Injury, internal, gallbladder
gastric (*see also* Rupture, stomach) 537.89
vessel 459.0
globe (eye) (traumatic) — *see* Rupture, eye
graafian follicle (hematoma) 620.0
heart (auricle) (ventricle) (*see also* Infarct, myocardium) 410.9 ☑
infectional 422.90
traumatic — *see* Rupture, myocardium, traumatic
hymen 623.8
internal
organ, traumatic — *see also* Injury, internal, by site
heart — *see* Rupture, myocardium, traumatic
kidney — *see* Rupture, kidney
liver — *see* Rupture, liver
spleen — *see* Rupture, spleen, traumatic
semilunar cartilage — *see* Tear, meniscus
intervertebral disc — *see* Displacement, intervertebral disc
traumatic (current) — *see* Dislocation, vertebra
intestine 569.89
traumatic — *see* Injury, internal, intestine
intracranial, birth injury 767.0
iris 364.76
traumatic — *see* Rupture, eye
joint capsule — *see* Sprain, by site
kidney (traumatic) 866.03
with open wound into cavity 866.13
due to birth injury 767.8
nontraumatic 593.89
lacrimal apparatus (traumatic) 870.2
lens (traumatic) 366.20
ligament — *see also* Sprain, by site
with open wound — *see* Wound, open, by site
old (*see also* Disorder, cartilage, articular) 718.0 ☑
liver (traumatic) 864.04
with open wound into cavity 864.14
due to birth injury 767.8
nontraumatic 573.8
lymphatic (node) (vessel) 457.8
marginal sinus (placental) (with hemorrhage) 641.2 ☑
affecting fetus or newborn 762.1
meaning hernia — *see* Hernia
membrana tympani (*see also* Perforation, tympanum) 384.20
with otitis media — *see* Otitis media
traumatic — *see* Wound, open, ear
membranes (spontaneous)
artificial
delayed delivery following 658.3 ☑
affecting fetus or newborn 761.1
fetus or newborn 761.1
delayed delivery following 658.2 ☑
affecting fetus or newborn 761.1
premature (less than 24 hours prior to onset of labor) 658.1 ☑
affecting fetus or newborn 761.1
delayed delivery following 658.2 ☑
affecting fetus or newborn 761.1

Rupture, ruptured — *continued*
- meningeal artery (*see also* Hemorrhage, subarachnoid) 430
  - late effect — *see* Late effect(s) (of) cerebrovascular diseas
- meniscus (knee) — *see also* Tear, meniscus
  - old (*see also* Derangement, meniscus) 717.5
    - site other than knee — *see* Disorder, cartilage, articular
    - site other than knee — *see* Sprain, by site
- mesentery 568.89
  - traumatic — *see* Injury, internal, mesentery
- mitral — *see* Insufficiency, mitral
- muscle (traumatic) NEC — *see also* Sprain, by site
  - with open wound — *see* Wound, open, by site
  - nontraumatic 728.83
- musculotendinous cuff (nontraumatic) (shoulder) 840.4
- mycotic aneurysm, causing cerebral hemorrhage (*see also* Hemorrhage, subarachnoid) 430
  - late effect — *see* Late effect(s) (of) cerebrovascular disease
- myocardium, myocardial (*see also* Infarct, myocardium) 410.9 ☑
  - traumatic 861.03
    - with open wound into thorax 861.13
- nontraumatic (meaning hernia) (*see also* Hernia, by site) 553.9
- obstructed (*see also* Hernia, by site, with obstruction) 552.9
  - gangrenous (*see also* Hernia, by site, with gangrene) 551.9
- operation wound 998.32
  - internal 998.31
- ovary, ovarian 620.8
  - corpus luteum 620.1
  - follicle (graafian) 620.0
- oviduct 620.8
  - due to pregnancy — *see* Pregnancy, tubal
- pancreas 577.8
  - traumatic — *see* Injury, internal, pancreas
- papillary muscle (ventricular) 429.6
- pelvic
  - floor, complicating delivery 664.1 ☑
  - organ NEC — *see* Injury, pelvic, organs
- penis (traumatic) — *see* Wound, open, penis
- perineum 624.8
  - during delivery (*see also* Laceration, perineum, complicating delivery) 664.4 ☑ ,
- pharynx (nontraumatic) (spontaneous) 478.29
- pregnant uterus (before onset of labor) 665.0 ☑
- prostate (traumatic) — *see* Injury, internal, prostate
- pulmonary
  - artery 417.8
  - valve (heart) (*see also* Endocarditis, pulmonary) 424.3
  - vein 417.8
  - vessel 417.8
- pupil, sphincter 364.75
- pus tube (*see also* Salpingo-oophoritis) 614.2
- pyosalpinx (*see also* Salpingo-oophoritis) 614.2
- rectum 569.49
  - traumatic — *see* Injury, internal, rectum
- retina, retinal (traumatic) (without detachment) 361.30
  - with detachment (*see also* Detachment, retina, with retinal defect) 361.00
- rotator cuff (capsule) (traumatic) 840.4
  - nontraumatic, complete 727.61
- sclera 871.0
- semilunar cartilage, knee (*see also* Tear, meniscus) 836.2
  - old (*see also* Derangement, meniscus) 717.5
- septum (cardiac) 410.8 ☑
- sigmoid 569.89
  - traumatic — *see* Injury, internal, colon, sigmoid
- sinus of Valsalva 747.29
- spinal cord — *see also* Injury, spinal, by site
  - due to injury at birth 767.4
  - fetus or newborn 767.4
  - syphilitic 094.89

Rupture, ruptured — *continued*
- spinal cord — *see also* Injury, spinal, by site — *continued*
  - traumatic — *see also* Injury, spinal, by site
    - with fracture — *see* Fracture, vertebra, by site, with spinal cord injury
- spleen 289.59
  - congenital 767.8
  - due to injury at birth 767.8
  - malarial 084.9
  - nontraumatic 289.59
  - spontaneous 289.59
  - traumatic 865.04
    - with open wound into cavity 865.14
- splenic vein 459.0
- stomach 537.89
  - due to injury at birth 767.8
  - traumatic — *see* Injury, internal, stomach
  - ulcer — *see* Ulcer, stomach, with perforation
- synovium 727.50
  - specified site NEC 727.59
- tendon (traumatic) — *see also* Sprain, by site
  - with open wound — *see* Wound, open, by site
  - Achilles 845.09
    - nontraumatic 727.67
  - ankle 845.09
    - nontraumatic 727.68
  - biceps (long head) 840.8
    - nontraumatic 727.62
  - foot 845.10
    - interphalangeal (joint) 845.13
    - metatarsophalangeal (joint) 845.12
    - nontraumatic 727.68
    - specified site NEC 845.19
    - tarsometatarsal (joint) 845.11
  - hand 842.10
    - carpometacarpal (joint) 842.11
    - interphalangeal (joint) 842.13
    - metacarpophalangeal (joint) 842.12
    - nontraumatic 727.63
      - extensors 727.63
      - flexors 727.64
    - specified site NEC 842.19
  - nontraumatic 727.60
    - specified site NEC 727.69
  - patellar 844.8
    - nontraumatic 727.66
  - quadriceps 844.8
    - nontraumatic 727.65
  - rotator cuff (capsule) 840.4
    - nontraumatic, complete 727.61
  - wrist 842.00
    - carpal (joint) 842.01
    - nontraumatic 727.63
      - extensors 727.63
      - flexors 727.64
    - radiocarpal (joint) (ligament) 842.02
    - radioulnar (joint), distal 842.09
    - specified site NEC 842.09
- testis (traumatic) 878.2
  - complicated 878.3
  - due to syphilis 095.8
- thoracic duct 457.8
- tonsil 474.8
- traumatic
  - with open wound — *see* Wound, open, by site
  - aorta — *see* Rupture, aorta, traumatic
  - ear drum — *see* Wound, open, ear, drum
  - external site — *see* Wound, open, by site
  - eye 871.2
  - globe (eye) — *see* Wound, open, eyeball
  - internal organ (abdomen, chest, or pelvis) — *see also* Injury, internal, by site
    - heart — *see* Rupture, myocardium, traumatic
    - kidney — *see* Rupture, kidney
    - liver — *see* Rupture, liver
    - spleen — *see* Rupture, spleen, traumatic
  - ligament, muscle, or tendon — *see also* Sprain, by site
    - with open wound — *see* Wound, open, by site
  - meaning hernia — *see* Hernia
  - tricuspid (heart) (valve) — *see* Endocarditis, tricuspid

Rupture, ruptured — *continued*
- tube, tubal 620.8
  - abscess (*see also* Salpingo-oophoritis) 614.2
  - due to pregnancy — *see* Pregnancy, tubal
- tympanum, tympanic (membrane) (*see also* Perforation, tympanum) 384.20
  - with otitis media — *see* Otitis media
  - traumatic — *see* Wound, open, ear, drum
- umbilical cord 663.8 ☑
  - fetus or newborn 772.0
- ureter (traumatic) (*see also* Injury, internal, ureter) 867.2
  - nontraumatic 593.89
- urethra 599.84
  - with
    - abortion — *see* Abortion, by type, with damage to pelvic organs
    - ectopic pregnancy (*see also* categories 633.0-633.9) 639.2
    - molar pregnancy (*see also* categories 630-632) 639.2
  - following
    - abortion 639.2
    - ectopic or molar pregnancy 639.2
  - obstetrical trauma 665.5 ☑
  - traumatic — *see* Injury, internal urethra
- uterosacral ligament 620.8
- uterus (traumatic) — *see also* Injury, internal uterus
  - affecting fetus or newborn 763.89
  - during labor 665.1 ☑
  - nonpuerperal, nontraumatic 621.8
  - nontraumatic 621.8
  - pregnant (during labor) 665.1 ☑
    - before labor 665.0 ☑
- vagina 878.6
  - complicated 878.7
  - complicating delivery — *see* Laceration, vagina, complicating delivery
- valve, valvular (heart) — *see* Endocarditis
- varicose vein — *see* Varicose, vein
- varix — *see* Varix
- vena cava 459.0
- ventricle (free wall) (left) (*see also* Infarct, myocardium) 410.9 ☑
- vesical (urinary) 596.6
  - traumatic — *see* Injury, internal, bladder
- vessel (blood) 459.0
  - pulmonary 417.8
- viscus 799.89
- vulva 878.4
  - complicated 878.5
  - complicating delivery 664.0 ☑

Russell's dwarf (uterine dwarfism and craniofacial dysostosis) 759.89

Russell's dysentery 004.8

Russell (-Silver) syndrome (congenital hemihypertrophy and short stature) 759.89

Russian spring-summer type encephalitis 063.0

Rust's disease (tuberculous spondylitis) 015.0 ☑ *[720.81]*

Rustitskii's disease (multiple myeloma) (M9730/3) 203.0 ☑

Ruysch's disease (Hirschsprung's disease) 751.3

Rytand-Lipsitch syndrome (complete atrioventricular bloc) 426.0

☑ Additional Digit Required   ►◄ Revised Text   ● New Line   ▲ Revised Code

Rupture, ruptured — Rytand-Lipsitch syndrome

S

Saber
shin 090.5
tibia 090.5

Sac, lacrimal — *see* condition

Saccharomyces infection (*see also* Candidiasis) 112.9

Saccharopinuria 270.7

Saccular — *see* condition

Sacculation
aorta (nonsyphilitic) (*see also* Aneurysm, aorta) 441.9
ruptured 441.5
syphilitic 093.0
bladder 596.3
colon 569.89
intralaryngeal (congenital) (ventricular) 748.3
larynx (congenital) (ventricular) 748.3
organ or site, congenital — *see* Distortion
pregnant uterus, complicating delivery 654.4 ☑
affecting fetus or newborn 763.1
causing obstructed labor 660.2 ☑
affecting fetus or newborn 763.1
rectosigmoid 569.89
sigmoid 569.89
ureter 593.89
urethra 599.2
vesical 596.3

Sachs (-Tay) disease (amaurotic familial idiocy) 330.1

Sacks-Libman disease 710.0 [424.91]

Sacralgia 724.6

Sacralization
fifth lumbar vertebra 756.15
incomplete (vertebra) 756.15

Sacrodynia 724.6

Sacroiliac joint — *see* condition

Sacroiliitis NEC 720.2

Sacrum — *see* condition

Saddle
back 737.8
embolus, aorta 444.0
nose 738.0
congenital 754.0
due to syphilis 090.5

Sadism (sexual) 302.84

Saemisch's ulcer 370.04

Saenger's syndrome 379.46

Sago spleen 277.3

Sailors' skin 692.74

Saint
Anthony's fire (*see also* Erysipelas) 035
Guy's dance — *see* Chorea
Louis-type encephalitis 062.3
triad (*see also* Hernia, diaphragm) 553.3
Vitus' dance — *see* Chorea

Salicylism
correct substance properly administered 535.4 ☑
overdose or wrong substance given or taken 965.1

Salivary duct or gland — *see also* condition
virus disease 078.5

Salivation (excessive) (*see also* Ptyalism) 527.7

Salmonella (aertrycke) (choleraesuis) (enteritidis) (gallinarum) (suipestifer) (typhimurium) (*see also* Infection, Salmonella) 003.9
arthritis 003.23
carrier (suspected) of V02.3
meningitis 003.21
osteomyelitis 003.24
pneumonia 003.22
septicemia 003.1
typhosa 002.0
carrier (suspected) of V02.1

Salmonellosis 003.0
with pneumonia 003.22

Salpingitis (catarrhal) (fallopian tube) (nodular) (pseudofollicular) (purulent) (septic) (*see also* Salpingo-oophoritis) 614.2

Salpingitis (*see also* Salpingo-oophoritis) — *continued*
ear 381.50
acute 381.51
chronic 381.52

Salpingitis
Eustachian (tube) 381.50
acute 381.51
chronic 381.52
follicularis 614.1
gonococcal (chronic) 098.37
acute 098.17
interstitial, chronic 614.1
isthmica nodosa 614.1
old — *see* Salpingo-oophoritis, chronic
puerperal, postpartum, childbirth 670.0 ☑
specific (chronic) 098.37
acute 098.17
tuberculous (acute) (chronic) (*see also* Tuberculosis) 016.6 ☑
venereal (chronic) 098.37
acute 098.17

Salpingocele 620.4

Salpingo-oophoritis (catarrhal) (purulent) (ruptured) (septic) (suppurative) 614.2
acute 614.0
with
abortion — *see* Abortion, by type, with sepsis
ectopic pregnancy (*see also* categories 633.0-633.9) 639.0
molar pregnancy (*see also* categories 630-632) 639.0
following
abortion 639.0
ectopic or molar pregnancy 639.0
gonococcal 098.17
puerperal, postpartum, childbirth 670.0 ☑
tuberculous (*see also* Tuberculosis) 016.6 ☑
chronic 614.1
gonococcal 098.37
tuberculous (see also Tuberculosis) 016.6 ☑
complicating pregnancy 646.6 ☑
affecting fetus or newborn 760.8
gonococcal (chronic) 098.37
acute 098.17
old — *see* Salpingo-oophoritis, chronic
puerperal 670.0 ☑
specific — *see* Salpingo-oophoritis, gonococcal
subacute (*see also* Salpingo-oophoritis, acute) 614.0
tuberculous (acute) (chronic) (*see also* Tuberculosis) 016.6 ☑
venereal — *see* Salpingo-oophoritis, gonococcal

Salpingo-ovaritis (*see also* Salpingo-oophoritis) 614.2

Salpingoperitonitis (*see also* Salpingo-oophoritis) 614.2

Salt-losing
nephritis (*see also* Disease, renal) 593.9
syndrome (*see also* Disease, renal) 593.9

Salt-rheum (*see also* Eczema) 692.9

Salzmann's nodular dystrophy 371.46

Sampson's cyst or tumor 617.1

Sandblasters'
asthma 502
lung 502

Sander's disease (paranoia) 297.1

Sandfly fever 066.0

Sandhoff's disease 330.1

Sanfilippo's syndrome (mucopolysaccharidosis III) 277.5

Sanger-Brown's ataxia 334.2

San Joaquin Valley fever 114.0

Sao Paulo fever or typhus 082.0

Saponification, mesenteric 567.8

Sapremia — *see* Septicemia

Sarcocele (benign)
syphilitic 095.8
congenital 090.5

Sarcoepiplocele (*see also* Hernia) 553.9

Sarcoepiplomphalocele (*see also* Hernia, umbilicus) 553.1

Sarcoid (any site) 135
with lung involvement 135 [517.8]
Boeck's 135
Darier-Roussy 135
Spiegler-Fendt 686.8

Sarcoidosis 135
cardiac 135 [425.8]
lung 135 [517.8]

Sarcoma (M8800/3) — *see also* Neoplasm, connective tissue, malignant
alveolar soft part (M9581/3) — *see* Neoplasm, connective tissue, malignant
ameloblastic (M9330/3) 170.1
upper jaw (bone) 170.0
botryoid (M8910/3) — *see* Neoplasm, connective tissue, malignant
botryoides (M8910/3) — *see* Neoplasm, connective tissue, malignant
cerebellar (M9480/3) 191.6
circumscribed (arachnoidal) (M9471/3) 191.6
circumscribed (arachnoidal) cerebellar (M9471/3) 191.6
clear cell, of tendons and aponeuroses (M9044/3) — *see* Neoplasm, connective tissue, malignant
embryonal (M8991/3) — *see* Neoplasm, connective tissue, malignant
endometrial (stromal) (M8930/3) 182.0
isthmus 182.1
endothelial (M9130/3) — *see also* Neoplasm, connective tissue, malignant
bone (M9260/3) — *see* Neoplasm, bone, malignant
epithelioid cell (M8804/3) — *see* Neoplasm, connective tissue, malignant
Ewing's (M9260/3) — *see* Neoplasm, bone, malignant
follicular dendritic cell 202.9 ☑
germinoblastic (diffuse) (M9632/3) 202.8 ☑
follicular (M9697/3) 202.0 ☑
giant cell (M8802/3) — *see also* Neoplasm, connective tissue, malignant
bone (M9250/3) — *see* Neoplasm, bone, malignant
glomoid (M8710/3) — *see* Neoplasm, connective tissue, malignant
granulocytic (M9930/3) 205.3 ☑
hemangioendothelial (M9130/3) — *see* Neoplasm, connective tissue, malignant
hemorrhagic, multiple (M9140/3) — *see* Kaposi's, sarcoma
Hodgkin's (M9662/3) 201.2 ☑
immunoblastic (M9612/3) 200.8 ☑
interdigitating dendritic cell 202.9 ☑
Kaposi's (M9140/3) — *see* Kaposi's, sarcoma
Kupffer cell (M9124/3) 155.0
Langerhans cell 202.9 ☑
leptomeningeal (M9530/3) — *see* Neoplasm, meninges, malignant
lymphangioendothelial (M9170/3) — *see* Neoplasm, connective tissue, malignant
lymphoblastic (M9630/3) 200.1 ☑
lymphocytic (M9620/3) 200.1 ☑
mast cell (M9740/3) 202.6 ☑
melanotic (M8720/3) — *see* Melanoma
meningeal (M9530/3) — *see* Neoplasm, meninges, malignant
meningothelial (M9530/3) — *see* Neoplasm, meninges, malignant
mesenchymal (M8800/3) — *see also* Neoplasm, connective tissue, malignant
mixed (M8990/3) — *see* Neoplasm, connective tissue, malignant
mesothelial (M9050/3) — *see* Neoplasm, by site, malignant
monstrocellular (M9481/3)
specified site — *see* Neoplasm, by site, malignant
unspecified site 191.9
myeloid (M9930/3) 205.3 ☑
neurogenic (M9540/3) — *see* Neoplasm, connective tissue, malignant

---

☑ Additional Digit Required   ►◄ Revised Text   ● New Line   ▲ Revised Code

Sarcoma (M8800/3) — *see also* Neoplasm, connective tissue, malignant — *continued*
  odontogenic (M9270/3) 170.1
    upper jaw (bone) 170.0
  osteoblastic (M9180/3) — *see* Neoplasm, bone, malignant
  osteogenic (M9180/3) — *see also* Neoplasm, bone, malignant
    juxtacortical (M9190/3) — *see* Neoplasm, bone, malignant
    periosteal (M9190/3) — *see* Neoplasm, bone, malignant
  periosteal (M8812/3) — *see also* Neoplasm, bone, malignant
  osteogenic (M9190/3) — *see* Neoplasm, bone, malignant
  plasma cell (M9731/3) 203.8 ☑
  pleomorphic cell (M8802/3) — *see* Neoplasm, connective tissue, malignant
  reticuloendothelial (M9720/3) 202.3 ☑
  reticulum cell (M9640/3) 200.0 ☑
    nodular (M9642/3) 200.0 ☑
    pleomorphic cell type (M9641/3) 200.0 ☑
  round cell (M8803/3) — *see* Neoplasm, connective tissue, malignant
  small cell (M8803/3) — *see* Neoplasm, connective tissue, malignant
  spindle cell (M8801/3) — *see* Neoplasm, connective tissue, malignant
  stromal (endometrial) (M8930/3) 182.0
    isthmus 182.1
  synovial (M9040/3) — *see also* Neoplasm, connective tissue, malignant
    biphasic type (M9043/3) — *see* Neoplasm, connective tissue, malignant
    epithelioid cell type (M9042/3) — *see* Neoplasm, connective tissue, malignant
    spindle cell type (M9041/3) — *see* Neoplasm, connective tissue, malignant

Sarcomatosis
  meningeal (M9539/3) — *see* Neoplasm, meninges, malignant
  specified site NEC (M8800/3) — *see* Neoplasm, connective tissue, malignant
  unspecified site (M8800/6) 171.9

Sarcosinemia 270.8
Sarcosporidiosis 136.5
Satiety, early 780.94
Saturnine — *see* condition
Saturnism 984.9
  specified type of lead — *see* Table of Drugs and Chemicals
Satyriasis 302.89
Sauriasis — *see* Ichthyosis
Sauriderma 757.39
Sauriosis — *see* Ichthyosis
Savill's disease (epidemic exfoliative dermatitis) 695.89
SBE (subacute bacterial endocarditis) 421.0
Scabies (any site) 133.0
Scabs 782.8
Scaglietti-Dagnini syndrome (acromegalic macrospondylitis) 253.0
Scald, scalded — *see also* Burn, by site
  skin syndrome 695.1
Scalenus anticus (anterior) syndrome 353.0
Scales 782.8
Scalp — *see* condition
Scaphocephaly 756.0
Scaphoiditis, tarsal 732.5
Scapulalgia 733.90
Scapulohumeral myopathy 359.1
Scar, scarring (*see also* Cicatrix) 709.2
  adherent 709.2
  atrophic 709.2
  cervix
    in pregnancy or childbirth 654.6 ☑
      affecting fetus or newborn 763.89
      causing obstructed labor 660.2 ☑
        affecting fetus or newborn 763.1

Scar, scarring (*see also* Cicatrix) — *continued*
  cheloid 701.4
  chorioretinal 363.30
    disseminated 363.35
    macular 363.32
    peripheral 363.34
    posterior pole NEC 363.33
  choroid (*see also* Scar, chorioretinal) 363.30
  compression, pericardial 423.9
  congenital 757.39
  conjunctiva 372.64
  cornea 371.00
    xerophthalmic 264.6
  due to previous cesarean delivery, complicating pregnancy or childbirth 654.2 ☑
    affecting fetus or newborn 763.89
  duodenal (bulb) (cap) 537.3
  hypertrophic 701.4
  keloid 701.4
  labia 624.4
  lung (base) 518.89
  macula 363.32
    disseminated 363.35
    peripheral 363.34
  muscle 728.89
  myocardium, myocardial 412
  painful 709.2
  papillary muscle 429.81
  posterior pole NEC 363.33
    macular — *see* Scar, macula
  postnecrotic (hepatic) (liver) 571.9
  psychic V15.49
  retina (*see also* Scar, chorioretinal) 363.30
  trachea 478.9
  uterus 621.8
    in pregnancy or childbirth NEC 654.9 ☑
      affecting fetus or newborn 763.89
      due to previous cesarean delivery 654.2 ☑
  vulva 624.4
Scarabiasis 134.1
Scarlatina 034.1
  anginosa 034.1
  maligna 034.1
  myocarditis, acute 034.1 [422.0]
    old (*see also* Myocarditis) 429.0
  otitis media 034.1 [382.02]
  ulcerosa 034.1
Scarlatinella 057.8
Scarlet fever (albuminuria) (angina) (convulsions) (lesions of lid) (rash) 034.1
Schamberg's disease, dermatitis, or dermatosis (progressive pigmentary dermatosis) 709.09
Schatzki's ring (esophagus) (lower) (congenital) 750.3
  acquired 530.3
Schaufenster krankheit 413.9
Schaumann's
  benign lymphogranulomatosis 135
  disease (sarcoidosis) 135
  syndrome (sarcoidosis) 135
Scheie's syndrome (mucopolysaccharidosis IS) 277.5
Schenck's disease (sporotrichosis) 117.1
Scheuermann's disease or osteochondrosis 732.0
Scheuthauer-Marie-Sainton syndrome (cleidocranialis dysostosis) 755.59
Schilder (-Flatau) disease 341.1
Schilling-type monocytic leukemia (M9890/3) 206.9 ☑
Schimmelbusch's disease, cystic mastitis, or hyperplasia 610.1
Schirmer's syndrome (encephalocutaneous angiomatosis) 759.6
Schistocelia 756.79
Schistoglossia 750.13
Schistosoma infestation — *see* Infestation, Schistosoma
Schistosomiasis 120.9
  Asiatic 120.2
  bladder 120.0
  chestermani 120.8

Schistosomiasis — *continued*
  colon 120.1
  cutaneous 120.3
  due to
    S. hematobium 120.0
    S. japonicum 120.2
    S. mansoni 120.1
    S. mattheii 120.8
  eastern 120.2
  genitourinary tract 120.0
  intestinal 120.1
  lung 120.2
  Manson's (intestinal) 120.1
  Oriental 120.2
  pulmonary 120.2
  specified type NEC 120.8
  vesical 120.0
Schizencephaly 742.4
Schizo-affective psychosis (*see also* Schizophrenia) 295.7 ☑
Schizodontia 520.2
Schizoid personality 301.20
  introverted 301.21
  schizotypal 301.22
Schizophrenia, schizophrenic (reaction) 295.9 ☑

> *Note* — Use the following fifth-digit subclassification with category 295:
>
> 0   *unspecified*
> 1   *subchronic*
> 2   *chronic*
> 3   *subchronic with acute exacerbation*
> 4   *chronic with acute exacerbation*
> 5   *in remission*

  acute (attack) NEC 295.8 ☑
    episode 295.4 ☑
  atypical form 295.8 ☑
  borderline 295.5 ☑
  catalepsy 295.2 ☑
  catatonic (type) (acute) (excited) (withdrawn) 295.2 ☑
  childhood (type) (*see also* Psychosis, childhood) 299.9 ☑
  chronic NEC 295.6 ☑
  coenesthesiopathic 295.8 ☑
  cyclic (type) 295.7 ☑
  disorganized (type) 295.1 ☑
  flexibilitas cerea 295.2 ☑
  hebephrenic (type) (acute) 295.1 ☑
  incipient 295.5 ☑
  latent 295.5 ☑
  paranoid (type) (acute) 295.3 ☑
  paraphrenic (acute) 295.3 ☑
  prepsychotic 295.5 ☑
  primary (acute) 295.0 ☑
  prodromal 295.5 ☑
  pseudoneurotic 295.5 ☑
  pseudopsychopathic 295.5 ☑
  reaction 295.9 ☑
  residual ▶type◀ (state) 295.6 ☑
  restzustand 295.6 ☑
  schizo-affective (type) (depressed) (excited) 295.7 ☑
  schizophreniform type 295.4 ☑
  simple (type) (acute) 295.0 ☑
  simplex (acute) 295.0 ☑
  specified type NEC 295.8 ☑
  syndrome of childhood NEC (*see also* Psychosis, childhood) 299.9 ☑
  undifferentiated ▶type◀ 295.9 ☑
    acute 295.8 ☑
    chronic 295.6 ☑
Schizothymia 301.20
  introverted 301.21
  schizotypal 301.22
Schlafkrankheit 086.5
Schlatter's tibia (osteochondrosis) 732.4
Schlatter-Osgood disease (osteochondrosis, tibial tubercle) 732.4
Schloffer's tumor (*see also* Peritonitis) 567.2
Schmidt's syndrome
  sphallo-pharyngo-laryngeal hemiplegia 352.6

☑ Additional Digit Required   ▶◀ Revised Text   ● New Line   ▲ Revised Code

Schmidt's syndrome — *continued*
  thyroid-adrenocortical insufficiency 258.1
  vagoaccessory 352.6
Schmincke
  carcinoma (M8082/3) — *see* Neoplasm,
    nasopharynx, malignant
  tumor (M8082/3) — *see* Neoplasm,
    nasopharynx, malignant
Schmitz (-Stutzer) dysentery 004.0
Schmorl's disease or nodes 722.30
  lumbar, lumbosacral 722.32
  specified region NEC 722.39
  thoracic, thoracolumbar 722.31
Schneider's syndrome 047.9
Schneiderian
  carcinoma (M8121/3)
    specified site — *see* Neoplasm, by site,
      malignant
    unspecified site 160.0
  papilloma (M8121/0)
    specified site — *see* Neoplasm, by site,
      benign
    unspecified site 212.0
Schnitzler syndrome 273.1 ●
Schoffer's tumor (*see also* Peritonitis) 567.2
Scholte's syndrome (malignant carcinoid) 259.2
Scholz's disease 330.0
Scholz (-Bielschowsky-Henneberg) syndrome
  330.0
Schönlein (-Henoch) disease (primary) (purpura)
  (rheumatic) 287.0
School examination V70.3
Schottmüller's disease (*see also* Fever,
  paratyphoid) 002.9
Schroeder's syndrome (endocrine-hypertensive)
  255.3
Schüller-Christian disease or syndrome (chronic
  histiocytosis X) 277.89
Schultz's disease or syndrome (agranulocytosis)
  288.0
Schultze's acroparesthesia, simple 443.89
Schwalbe-Ziehen-Oppenheimer disease 333.6
Schwannoma (M9560/0) — *see also* Neoplasm,
  connective tissue, benign
  malignant (M9560/3) — *see* Neoplasm,
    connective tissue, malignant
Schwartz (-Jampel) syndrome 756.89
Schwartz-Bartter syndrome (inappropriate
  secretion of antidiuretic hormone) 253.6
Schweninger-Buzzi disease (macular atrophy)
  701.3
Sciatic — *see* condition
Sciatica (infectional) 724.3
  due to
    displacement of intervertebral disc 722.10
    herniation, nucleus pulposus 722.10
Scimitar syndrome (anomalous venous drainage,
  right lung to inferior vena cava) 747.49
Sclera — *see* condition
Sclerectasia 379.11
Scleredema
  adultorum 710.1
  Buschke's 710.1
  newborn 778.1
Sclerema
  adiposum (newborn) 778.1
  adultorum 710.1
  edematosum (newborn) 778.1
  neonatorum 778.1
  newborn 778.1
Scleriasis — *see* Scleroderma
Scleritis 379.00
  with corneal involvement 379.05
  anterior (annular) (localized) 379.03
  brawny 379.06
  granulomatous 379.09
  posterior 379.07
  specified NEC 379.09
  suppurative 379.09
  syphilitic 095.0

Scleritis — *continued*
  tuberculous (nodular) (*see also* Tuberculosis)
    017.3 ☑ *[379.09]*
Sclerochoroiditis (*see also* Scleritis) 379.00
Scleroconjunctivitis (*see also* Scleritis) 379.00
Sclerocystic ovary (syndrome) 256.4
Sclerodactylia 701.0
Scleroderma, sclerodermia (acrosclerotic)
  (diffuse) (generalized) (progressive)
  (pulmonary) 710.1
  circumscribed 701.0
  linear 701.0
  localized (linear) 701.0
  newborn 778.1
Sclerokeratitis 379.05
  meaning sclerosing keratitis 370.54
  tuberculous (*see also* Tuberculosis)
    017.3 ☑ *[379.09]*
Scleroma, trachea 040.1
Scleromalacia
  multiple 731.0
  perforans 379.04
Scleromyxedema 701.8
Scleroperikeratitis 379.05
Sclerose en plaques 340
Sclerosis, sclerotic
  adrenal (gland) 255.8
  Alzheimer's 331.0
    with dementia — *see* Alzheimer's, dementia
  amyotrophic (lateral) 335.20
  annularis fibrosi
    aortic 424.1
    mitral 424.0
  aorta, aortic 440.0
    valve (*see also* Endocarditis, aortic) 424.1
  artery, arterial, arteriolar, arteriovascular —
    see Arteriosclerosis
  ascending multiple 340
  Baló's (concentric) 341.1
  basilar — *see* Sclerosis, brain
  bone (localized) NEC 733.99
  brain (general) (lobular) 341.9
    Alzheimer's — *see* Alzheimer's, dementia
    artery, arterial 437.0
    atrophic lobar 331.0
      with dementia
        with behavioral disturbance 331.0
          [294.11]
        without behavioral disturbance 331.0
          [294.10]
    diffuse 341.1
      familial (chronic) (infantile) 330.0
      infantile (chronic) (familial) 330.0
      Pelizaeus-Merzbacher type 330.0
    disseminated 340
    hereditary 334.2
    infantile, (degenerative) (diffuse) 330.0
    insular 340
    Krabbe's 330.0
    miliary 340
    multiple 340
    Pelizaeus-Merzbacher 330.0
    progressive familial 330.0
    senile 437.0
    tuberous 759.5
  bulbar, progressive 340
  bundle of His 426.50
    left 426.3
    right 426.4
  cardiac — *see* Arteriosclerosis, coronary
  cardiorenal (*see also* Hypertension, cardiorenal)
    404.90
  cardiovascular (*see also* Disease,
    cardiovascular) 429.2
    renal (*see also* Hypertension, cardiorenal)
      404.90
  centrolobar, familial 330.0
  cerebellar — *see* Sclerosis, brain
  cerebral — *see* Sclerosis, brain
  cerebrospinal 340
    disseminated 340
    multiple 340
  cerebrovascular 437.0

Sclerosis, sclerotic — *continued*
  choroid 363.40
    diffuse 363.56
  combined (spinal cord) — *see also*
    Degeneration, combined
    multiple 340
  concentric, Baló's 341.1
  cornea 370.54
  coronary (artery) — *see* Arteriosclerosis,
    coronary
  corpus cavernosum
    female 624.8
    male 607.89
  Dewitzky's
    aortic 424.1
    mitral 424.0
  diffuse NEC 341.1
  disease, heart — *see* Arteriosclerosis, coronary
  disseminated 340
  dorsal 340
  dorsolateral (spinal cord) — *see* Degeneration,
    combined
  endometrium 621.8
  extrapyramidal 333.90
  eye, nuclear (senile) 366.16
  Friedreich's (spinal cord) 334.0
  funicular (spermatic cord) 608.89
  gastritis 535.4 ☑
  general (vascular) — *see* Arteriosclerosis
  gland (lymphatic) 457.8
  hepatic 571.9
  hereditary
    cerebellar 334.2
    spinal 334.0
  idiopathic cortical (Garré's) (*see also*
    Osteomyelitis) 730.1 ☑
  ilium, piriform 733.5
  insular 340
    pancreas 251.8
  Islands of Langerhans 251.8
  kidney — *see* Sclerosis, renal
  larynx 478.79
  lateral 335.24
    amyotrophic 335.20
    descending 335.24
    primary 335.24
    spinal 335.24
  liver 571.9
  lobar, atrophic (of brain) 331.0
    with dementia
      with behavioral disturbance 331.0
        [294.11]
      without behavioral disturbance 331.0
        [294.10]
  lung (*see also* Fibrosis, lung) 515
  mastoid 383.1
  mitral — *see* Endocarditis, mitral
  Mönckeberg's (medial) (*see also*
    Arteriosclerosis, extremities) 440.20
  multiple (brain stem) (cerebral) (generalized)
    (spinal cord) 340
  myocardium, myocardial — *see*
    Arteriosclerosis, coronary
  nuclear (senile), eye 366.16
  ovary 620.8
  pancreas 577.8
  penis 607.89
  peripheral arteries NEC (*see also*
    Arteriosclerosis, extremities) 440.20
  plaques 340
  pluriglandular 258.8
  polyglandular 258.8
  posterior (spinal cord) (syphilitic) 094.0
  posterolateral (spinal cord) — *see* Degeneration,
    combined
  prepuce 607.89
  primary lateral 335.24
  progressive systemic 710.1
  pulmonary (*see also* Fibrosis, lung) 515
    artery 416.0
    valve (heart) (*see also* Endocarditis,
      pulmonary) 424.3
  renal 587
    with
      cystine storage disease 270.0
      hypertension (*see also* Hypertension,
        kidney) 403.90

Sclerosis, sclerotic — *continued*
  renal — *continued*
    with — *continued*
      hypertensive heart disease (conditions
        classifiable to 402) (*see also*
        Hypertension, cardiorenal) 404.90
      arteriolar (hyaline) (*see also* Hypertension,
        kidney) 403.90
      hyperplastic (*see also* Hypertension,
        kidney) 403.90
  retina (senile) (vascular) 362.17
  rheumatic
    aortic valve 395.9
    mitral valve 394.9
  Schilder's 341.1
  senile — *see* Arteriosclerosis
  spinal (cord) (general) (progressive) (transverse)
    336.8
    ascending 357.0
    combined — *see also* Degeneration,
      combined
      multiple 340
      syphilitic 094.89
    disseminated 340
    dorsolateral — *see* Degeneration, combined
    hereditary (Friedreich's) (mixed form) 334.0
    lateral (amyotrophic) 335.24
    multiple 340
    posterior (syphilitic) 094.0
  stomach 537.89
  subendocardial, congenital 425.3
  systemic (progressive) 710.1
    with lung involvement 710.1 [517.2]
  tricuspid (heart) (valve) — *see* Endocarditis,
    tricuspid
  tuberous (brain) 759.5
  tympanic membrane (*see also*
    Tympanosclerosis) 385.00
  valve, valvular (heart) — *see* Endocarditis
  vascular — *see* Arteriosclerosis
  vein 459.89

Sclerotenonitis 379.07

Sclerotitis (*see also* Scleritis) 379.00
  syphilitic 095.0
  tuberculous (*see also* Tuberculosis)
    017.3 ☑ [379.09]

Scoliosis (acquired) (postural) 737.30
  congenital 754.2
  due to or associated with
    Charcôt-Marie-Tooth disease 356.1 [737.43]
    mucopolysaccharidosis 277.5 [737.43]
    neurofibromatosis 237.71 [737.43]
    osteitis
      deformans 731.0 [737.43]
      fibrosa cystica 252.01 [737.43] ▲
    osteoporosis (*see also* Osteoporosis) 733.00
      [737.43]
    poliomyelitis 138 [737.43]
    radiation 737.33
    tuberculosis (*see also* Tuberculosis)
      015.0 ☑ [737.43]
  idiopathic 737.30
    infantile
      progressive 737.32
      resolving 737.31
  paralytic 737.39
  rachitic 268.1
  sciatic 724.3
  specified NEC 737.39
  thoracogenic 737.34
  tuberculous (*see also* Tuberculosis)
    015.0 ☑ [737.43]

Scoliotic pelvis 738.6
  with disproportion (fetopelvic) 653.0 ☑
    affecting fetus or newborn 763.1
    causing obstructed labor 660.1 ☑
      affecting fetus or newborn 763.1

Scorbutus, scorbutic 267
  anemia 281.8

Scotoma (ring) 368.44
  arcuate 368.43
  Bjerrum 368.43
  blind spot area 368.42
  central 368.41
  centrocecal 368.41
  paracecal 368.42

Scotoma — *continued*
  paracentral 368.41
  scintillating 368.12
  Seidel 368.43

Scratch — *see* Injury, superficial, by site

Screening (for) V82.9
  alcoholism V79.1
  anemia, deficiency NEC V78.1
    iron V78.0
  anomaly, congenital V82.89
  antenatal V28.9
    alphafetoprotein levels, raised V28.1
    based on amniocentesis V28.2
      chromosomal anomalies V28.0
      raised alphafetoprotein levels V28.1
    fetal growth retardation using
      ultrasonics V28.4
    isoimmunization V28.5
    malformations using ultrasonics V28.3
    raised alphafetoprotein levels V28.1
    specified condition NEC V28.8
    Streptococcus B V28.6
  arterial hypertension V81.1
  arthropod-borne viral disease NEC V73.5
  asymptomatic bacteriuria V81.5
  bacterial
    conjunctivitis V74.4
    disease V74.9
      specified condition NEC V74.8
  bacteriuria, asymptomatic V81.5
  blood disorder NEC V78.9
    specified type NEC V78.8
  bronchitis, chronic V81.3
  brucellosis V74.8
  cancer — *see* Screening, malignant neoplasm
  cardiovascular disease NEC V81.2
  cataract V80.2
  Chagas' disease V75.3
  chemical poisoning V82.5
  cholera V74.0
  cholesterol level V77.91
  chromosomal
    anomalies
      by amniocentesis, antenatal V28.0
      maternal postnatal V82.4
    athletes V70.3
  condition
    cardiovascular NEC V81.2
    eye NEC V80.2
    genitourinary NEC V81.6
    neurological V80.0
    respiratory NEC V81.4
    skin V82.0
    specified NEC V82.89
  congenital
    anomaly V82.89
      eye V80.2
    dislocation of hip V82.3
    eye condition or disease V80.2
  conjunctivitis, bacterial V74.4
  contamination NEC (*see also* Poisoning) V82.5
  coronary artery disease V81.0
  cystic fibrosis V77.6
  deficiency anemia NEC V78.1
    iron V78.0
  dengue fever V73.5
  depression V79.0
  developmental handicap V79.9
    in early childhood V79.3
    specified type NEC V79.8
  diabetes mellitus V77.1
  diphtheria V74.3
  disease or disorder V82.9
    bacterial V74.9
      specified NEC V74.8
    blood V78.9
      specified type NEC V78.8
    blood-forming organ V78.9
      specified type NEC V78.8
    cardiovascular NEC V81.2
      hypertensive V81.1
      ischemic V81.0
    Chagas' V75.3
    chlamydial V73.98
      specified NEC V73.88
    ear NEC V80.3

Screening (for) — *continued*
  disease or disorder — *continued*
    endocrine NEC V77.99
    eye NEC V80.2
    genitourinary NEC V81.6
    heart NEC V81.2
      hypertensive V81.1
      ischemic V81.0
    immunity NEC V77.99
    infectious NEC V75.9
    lipoid NEC V77.91
    mental V79.9
      specified type NEC V79.8
    metabolic NEC V77.99
      inborn NEC V77.7
    neurological V80.0
    nutritional NEC V77.99
    rheumatic NEC V82.2
    rickettsial V75.0
    sickle-cell V78.2
      trait V78.2
    specified type NEC V82.89
    thyroid V77.0
    vascular NEC V81.2
      ischemic V81.0
    venereal V74.5
    viral V73.99
      arthropod-borne NEC V73.5
      specified type NEC V73.89
  dislocation of hip, congenital V82.3
  drugs in athletes V70.3
  emphysema (chronic) V81.3
  encephalitis, viral (mosquito or tick borne)
    V73.5
  endocrine disorder NEC V77.99
  eye disorder NEC V80.2
    congenital V80.2
  fever
    dengue V73.5
    hemorrhagic V73.5
    yellow V73.4
  filariasis V75.6
  galactosemia V77.4
  genitourinary condition NEC V81.6
  glaucoma V80.1
  gonorrhea V74.5
  gout V77.5
  Hansen's disease V74.2
  heart disease NEC V81.2
    hypertensive V81.1
    ischemic V81.0
  heavy metal poisoning V82.5
  helminthiasis, intestinal V75.7
  hematopoietic malignancy V76.89
  hemoglobinopathies NEC V78.3
  hemorrhagic fever V73.5
  Hodgkin's disease V76.89
  hormones in athletes V70.3
  hypercholesterolemia V77.91
  hyperlipidemia V77.91
  hypertension V81.1
  immunity disorder NEC V77.99
  inborn errors of metabolism NEC V77.7
  infection
    bacterial V74.9
      specified type NEC V74.8
    mycotic V75.4
    parasitic NEC V75.8
  infectious disease V75.9
    specified type NEC V75.8
  ingestion of radioactive substance V82.5
  intestinal helminthiasis V75.7
  iron deficiency anemia V78.0
  ischemic heart disease V81.0
  lead poisoning V82.5
  leishmaniasis V75.2
  leprosy V74.2
  leptospirosis V74.8
  leukemia V76.89
  lipoid disorder NEC V77.91
  lymphoma V76.89
  malaria V75.1
  malignant neoplasm (of) V76.9
    bladder V76.3
    blood V76.89

☑ Additional Digit Required   ▶◀ Revised Text   ● New Line   ▲ Revised Code

Screening (for) — *continued*
  malignant neoplasm (of) — *continued*
    breast V76.10
      mammogram NEC V76.12
        for high-risk patient V76.11
      specified type NEC V76.19
    cervix V76.2
    colon V76.51
    colorectal V76.51
    hematopoietic system V76.89
    intestine V76.50
      colon V76.51
      small V76.52
    lymph (glands) V76.89
    nervous system V76.81
    oral cavity V76.42
    other specified neoplasm NEC V76.89
    ovary V76.46
    prostate V76.44
    rectum V76.41
    respiratory organs V76.0
    skin V76.43
    specified sites NEC V76.49
    testis V76.45
    vagina V76.47
      following hysterectomy for malignant
        condition V67.01
  maternal postnatal chromosomal anomalies
    V82.4
  malnutrition V77.2
  mammogram NEC V76.12
    for high-risk patient V76.11
  measles V73.2
  mental
    disorder V79.9
      specified type NEC V79.8
    retardation V79.2
  metabolic disorder NEC V77.99
  metabolic errors, inborn V77.7
  mucoviscidosis V77.6
  multiphasic V82.6
  mycosis V75.4
  mycotic infection V75.4
  nephropathy V81.5
  neurological condition V80.0
  nutritional disorder V77.99
  obesity V77.8
  osteoporosis V82.81
  parasitic infection NEC V75.8
  phenylketonuria V77.3
  plague V74.8
  poisoning
    chemical NEC V82.5
      contaminated water supply V82.5
      heavy metal V82.5
  poliomyelitis V73.0
  postnatal chromosomal anomalies, maternal
    V82.4
  prenatal — *see* Screening, antenatal
  pulmonary tuberculosis V74.1
  radiation exposure V82.5
  renal disease V81.5
  respiratory condition NEC V81.4
  rheumatic disorder NEC V82.2
  rheumatoid arthritis V82.1
  rickettsial disease V75.0
  rubella V73.3
  schistosomiasis V75.5
  senile macular lesions of eye V80.2
  sickle-cell anemia, disease, or trait V78.2
  skin condition V82.0
  sleeping sickness V75.3
  smallpox V73.1
  special V82.9
    specified condition NEC V82.89
  specified type NEC V82.89
  spirochetal disease V74.9
    specified type NEC V74.8
  stimulants in athletes V70.3
  syphilis V74.5
  tetanus V74.8
  thyroid disorder V77.0
  trachoma V73.6
  trypanosomiasis V75.3
  tuberculosis, pulmonary V74.1
  venereal disease V74.5

Screening (for) — *continued*
  viral encephalitis
    mosquito-borne V73.5
    tick-borne V73.5
  whooping cough V74.8
  worms, intestinal V75.7
  yaws V74.6
  yellow fever V73.4
Scrofula (*see also* Tuberculosis) 017.2 ☑
Scrofulide (primary) (*see also* Tuberculosis)
  017.0 ☑
Scrofuloderma, scrofulodermia (any site)
  (primary) (*see also* Tuberculosis) 017.0 ☑
Scrofulosis (universal) (*see also* Tuberculosis)
  017.2 ☑
Scrofulosis lichen (primary) (*see also*
  Tuberculosis) 017.0 ☑
Scrofulous — *see* condition
Scrotal tongue 529.5
  congenital 750.13
Scrotum — *see* condition
Scurvy (gum) (infantile) (rickets) (scorbutic) 267
Sea-blue histiocyte syndrome 272.7
Seabright-Bantam syndrome
  (pseudohypoparathyroidism) 275.49
Seasickness 994.6
Seatworm 127.4
Sebaceous
  cyst (*see also* Cyst, sebaceous) 706.2
  gland disease NEC 706.9
Sebocystomatosis 706.2
Seborrhea, seborrheic 706.3
  adiposa 706.3
  capitis 690.11
  congestiva 695.4
  corporis 706.3
  dermatitis 690.10
    infantile 690.12
  diathesis in infants 695.89
  eczema 690.18
    infantile 691.12
  keratosis 702.19
    inflamed 702.11
  nigricans 705.89
  sicca 690.18
  wart 702.19
    inflamed 702.11
Seckel's syndrome 759.89
Seclusion pupil 364.74
Seclusiveness, child 313.22
Secondary — *see also* condition
  neoplasm — *see* Neoplasm, by site, malignant,
    secondary
Secretan's disease or syndrome (posttraumatic
  edema) 782.3
Secretion
  antidiuretic hormone, inappropriate (syndrome)
    253.6
  catecholamine, by pheochromocytoma 255.6
  hormone
    antidiuretic, inappropriate (syndrome) 253.6
    by
      carcinoid tumor 259.2
      pheochromocytoma 255.6
    ectopic NEC 259.3
  urinary
    excessive 788.42
    suppression 788.5
Section
  cesarean
    affecting fetus or newborn 763.4
    post mortem, affecting fetus or newborn
      761.6
    previous, in pregnancy or childbirth
      654.2 ☑
      affecting fetus or newborn 763.89
  nerve, traumatic — *see* Injury, nerve, by site
Seeligmann's syndrome (ichthyosis congenita)
  757.1
Segmentation, incomplete (congenital) — *see*
  also Fusion
  bone NEC 756.9

Segmentation, incomplete — *see also* Fusion —
  continued
  lumbosacral (joint) 756.15
  vertebra 756.15
    lumbosacral 756.15
Seizure 780.39
  akinetic (idiopathic) (*see also* Epilepsy) 345.0 ☑
    psychomotor 345.4 ☑
  apoplexy, apoplectic (*see also* Disease,
    cerebrovascular, acute) 436
  atonic (*see also* Epilepsy) 345.0 ☑
  autonomic 300.11
  brain or cerebral (*see also* Disease,
    cerebrovascular, acute) 436
  convulsive (*see also* Convulsions) 780.39
  cortical (focal) (motor) (*see also* Epilepsy)
    345.5 ☑
  epilepsy, epileptic (cryptogenic) (*see also*
    Epilepsy) 345.9 ☑
  epileptiform, epileptoid 780.39
    focal (*see also* Epilepsy) 345.5 ☑
  febrile 780.31
  heart — *see* Disease, heart
  hysterical 300.11
  Jacksonian (focal) (*see also* Epilepsy) 345.5 ☑
    motor type 345.5 ☑
    sensory type 345.5 ☑
  newborn 779.0
  paralysis (*see also* Disease, cerebrovascular,
    acute) 436
  recurrent 780.39
    epileptic — *see* Epilepsy
  repetitive 780.39
    epileptic — *see* Epilepsy
  salaam (*see also* Epilepsy) 345.6 ☑
  uncinate (*see also* Epilepsy) 345.4 ☑
Self-mutilation 300.9
Semicoma 780.09
Semiconsciousness 780.09
Seminal
  vesicle — *see* condition
  vesiculitis (*see also* Vesiculitis) 608.0
Seminoma (M9061/3)
  anaplastic type (M9062/3)
    specified site — *see* Neoplasm, by site,
      malignant
    unspecified site 186.9
  specified site — *see* Neoplasm, by site,
    malignant
  spermatocytic (M9063/3)
    specified site — *see* Neoplasm, by site,
      malignant
    unspecified site 186.9
  unspecified site 186.9
Semliki Forest encephalitis 062.8
Senear-Usher disease or syndrome (pemphigus
  erythematosus) 694.4
Senecio jacobae dermatitis 692.6
Senectus 797
Senescence 797
Senile (*see also* condition) 797
  cervix (atrophic) 622.8
  degenerative atrophy, skin 701.3
  endometrium (atrophic) 621.8
  fallopian tube (atrophic) 620.3
  heart (failure) 797
  lung 492.8
  ovary (atrophic) 620.3
  syndrome 259.8
  vagina, vaginitis (atrophic) 627.3
  wart 702.0
Senility 797
  with
    acute confusional state 290.3
    delirium 290.3
    mental changes 290.9
    psychosis NEC (*see also* Psychosis, senile)
      290.20
  premature (syndrome) 259.8
Sensation
  burning (*see also* Disturbance, sensation)
    782.0
  tongue 529.6

☑ Additional Digit Required   ▶◀ Revised Text   ● New Line   ▲ Revised Code

Sensation — *continued*
- choking 784.9
- loss of (*see also* Disturbance, sensation) 782.0
- prickling (*see also* Disturbance, sensation) 782.0
- tingling (*see also* Disturbance, sensation) 782.0

Sense loss (touch) (*see also* Disturbance, sensation) 782.0
- smell 781.1
- taste 781.1

Sensibility disturbance NEC (cortical) (deep) (vibratory) (*see also* Disturbance, sensation) 782.0

Sensitive dentine 521.8

Sensitiver Beziehungswahn 297.8

Sensitivity, sensitization — *see also* Allergy
- autoerythrocyte 287.2
- carotid sinus 337.0
- child (excessive) 313.21
- cold, autoimmune 283.0
- methemoglobin 289.7
- suxamethonium 289.89
- tuberculin, without clinical or radiological symptoms 795.5

Sensory
- extinction 781.8
- neglect 781.8

Separation
- acromioclavicular — *see* Dislocation, acromioclavicular
- anxiety, abnormal 309.21
- apophysis, traumatic — *see* Fracture, by site
- choroid 363.70
  - hemorrhagic 363.72
  - serous 363.71
- costochondral (simple) (traumatic) — *see* Dislocation, costochondral
- delayed
  - umbilical cord 779.83
- epiphysis, epiphyseal
  - nontraumatic 732.9
    - upper femoral 732.2
  - traumatic — *see* Fracture, by site
- fracture — *see* Fracture, by site
- infundibulum cardiac from right ventricle by a partition 746.83
- joint (current) (traumatic) — *see* Dislocation, by site
- placenta (normally implanted) — *see* Placenta, separation
- pubic bone, obstetrical trauma 665.6 ☑
- retina, retinal (*see also* Detachment, retina) 361.9
  - layers 362.40
    - sensory (*see also* Retinoschisis) 361.10
  - pigment epithelium (exudative) 362.42
    - hemorrhagic 362.43
- sternoclavicular (traumatic) — *see* Dislocation, sternoclavicular
- symphysis pubis, obstetrical trauma 665.6 ☑
- tracheal ring, incomplete (congenital) 748.3

Sepsis (generalized) 995.91
- with
  - abortion — *see* Abortion, by type, with sepsis
  - ectopic pregnancy (*see also* categories 633.0-633.9) 639.0
  - molar pregnancy (*see also* categories 630-632) 639.0
- buccal 528.3
- complicating labor 659.3 ☑
- dental (pulpal origin) 522.4
- female genital organ NEC 614.9
- fetus (intrauterine) 771.81
- following
  - abortion 639.0
  - ectopic or molar pregnancy 639.0
  - infusion, perfusion, or transfusion 999.3
- Friedländer's 038.49
- intraocular 360.00
- localized
  - in operation wound 998.59
  - skin (*see also* Abscess) 682.9
- malleus 024

Sepsis (*see also* Septicemia) — *continued*
- nadir 038.9
- newborn (organism unspecified) NEC 771.81
- oral 528.3
- puerperal, postpartum, childbirth (pelvic) 670.0 ☑
- resulting from infusion, injection, transfusion, or vaccination 999.3
- severe 995.92
- skin, localized (*see also* Abscess) 682.9
- umbilical (newborn) (organism unspecified) 771.89
  - tetanus 771.3
- urinary 599.0
  - meaning sepsis 995.91
  - meaning urinary tract infection 599.0   ▲

Septate — *see also* Septum

Septic — *see also* condition
- adenoids 474.01
  - and tonsils 474.02
- arm (with lymphangitis) 682.3
- embolus — *see* Embolism
- finger (with lymphangitis) 681.00
- foot (with lymphangitis) 682.7
- gallbladder (*see also* Cholecystitis) 575.8
- hand (with lymphangitis) 682.4
- joint (*see also* Arthritis, septic) 711.0 ☑
- kidney (*see also* Infection, kidney) 590.9
- leg (with lymphangitis) 682.6
- mouth 528.3
- nail 681.9
  - finger 681.02
  - toe 681.11
- shock (endotoxic) 785.52
- sore (*see also* Abscess) 682.9
  - throat 034.0
    - milk-borne 034.0
    - streptococcal 034.0
- spleen (acute) 289.59
- teeth (pulpal origin) 522.4
- throat 034.0
- thrombus — *see* Thrombosis
- toe (with lymphangitis) 681.10
- tonsils 474.00
  - and adenoids 474.02
- umbilical cord (newborn) (organism unspecified) 771.89
- uterus (*see also* Endometritis) 615.9

Septicemia, septicemic (generalized) (suppurative) 038.9
- with
  - abortion — *see* Abortion, by type, with sepsis
  - ectopic pregnancy (*see also* categories 633.0-633.9) 639.0
  - molar pregnancy (*see also* categories 630-632) 639.0
- Aerobacter aerogenes 038.49
- anaerobic 038.3
- anthrax 022.3
- Bacillus coli 038.42
- Bacteroides 038.3
- Clostridium 038.3
- complicating labor 659.3 ☑
- cryptogenic 038.9
- enteric gram-negative bacilli 038.40
- Enterobacter aerogenes 038.49
- Erysipelothrix (insidiosa) (rhusiopathiae) 027.1
- Escherichia coli 038.42
- following
  - abortion 639.0
  - ectopic or molar pregnancy 639.0
  - infusion, injection, transfusion, or vaccination 999.3
- Friedländer's (bacillus) 038.49
- gangrenous 038.9
- gonococcal 098.89
- gram-negative (organism) 038.40
  - anaerobic 038.3
- Hemophilus influenzae 038.41
- herpes (simplex) 054.5
- herpetic 054.5
- Listeria monocytogenes 027.0
- meningeal — *see* Meningitis
- meningococcal (chronic) (fulminating) 036.2
- navel, newborn (organism unspecified) 771.89

Septicemia, septicemic — *continued*
- newborn (organism unspecified) 771.81
- plague 020.2
- pneumococcal 038.2
- postabortal 639.0
- postoperative 998.59
- Proteus vulgaris 038.49
- Pseudomonas (aeruginosa) 038.43
- puerperal, postpartum 670.0 ☑
- Salmonella (aertrycke) (callinarum) (choleraesuis) (enteritidis) (suipestifer) 003.1
- Serratia 038.44
- Shigella (*see also* Dysentery, bacillary) 004.9
- specified organism NEC 038.8
- staphylococcal 038.10
  - aureus 038.11
  - specified organism NEC 038.19
- streptococcal (anaerobic) 038.0
- suipestifer 003.1
- umbilicus, newborn (organism unspecified) 771.89
- viral 079.99
- Yersinia enterocolitica 038.49

Septum, septate (congenital) — *see also* Anomaly, specified type NEC
- anal 751.2
- aqueduct of Sylvius 742.3
  - with spina bifida (*see also* Spina bifida) 741.0 ☑
- hymen 752.49
- uterus (*see also* Double, uterus) 752.2
- vagina 752.49
  - in pregnancy or childbirth 654.7 ☑
    - affecting fetus or newborn 763.89
    - causing obstructed labor 660.2 ☑
      - affecting fetus or newborn 763.1

Sequestration
- lung (congenital) (extralobar) (intralobar) 748.5
- orbit 376.10
- pulmonary artery (congenital) 747.3
- splenic 289.52

Sequestrum
- bone (*see also* Osteomyelitis) 730.1 ☑
  - jaw 526.4
- dental 525.8
- jaw bone 526.4
- sinus (accessory) (nasal) (*see also* Sinusitis) 473.9
  - maxillary 473.0

Sequoiosis asthma 495.8

Serology for syphilis
- doubtful
  - with signs or symptoms — *see* Syphilis, by site and stage
  - follow-up of latent syphilis — *see* Syphilis, latent
- false positive 795.6
- negative, with signs or symptoms — *see* Syphilis, by site and stage
- positive 097.1
  - with signs or symptoms — *see* Syphilis, by site and stage
  - false 795.6
  - follow-up of latent syphilis — *see* Syphilis, latent
  - only finding — *see* Syphilis, latent
- reactivated 097.1

Seroma (postoperative) (non-infected) 998.13
- infected 998.51

Seropurulent — *see* condition

Serositis, multiple 569.89
- pericardial 423.2
- peritoneal 568.82
- pleural — *see* Pleurisy

Serotonin syndrome 333.99

Serous — *see* condition

Sertoli cell
- adenoma (M8640/0)
  - specified site — *see* Neoplasm, by site, benign
  - unspecified site
    - female 220
    - male 222.0

Sertoli cell — *continued*
  carcinoma (M8640/3)
    specified site — *see* Neoplasm, by site,
      malignant
    unspecified site 186.9
  syndrome (germinal aplasia) 606.0
  tumor (M8640/0)
    with lipid storage (M8641/0)
      specified site — *see* Neoplasm, by site,
        benign
      unspecified site
        female 220
        male 222.0
    specified site — *see* Neoplasm, by site,
      benign
    unspecified site
      female 220
      male 222.0
Sertoli-Leydig cell tumor (M8631/0)
  specified site — *see* Neoplasm, by site, benign
  unspecified site
    female 220
    male 222.0
Serum
  allergy, allergic reaction 999.5
    shock 999.4
  arthritis 999.5 *[713.6]*
  complication or reaction NEC 999.5
  disease NEC 999.5
  hepatitis 070.3 ☑
  intoxication 999.5
  jaundice (homologous) — *see* Hepatitis, viral
  neuritis 999.5
  poisoning NEC 999.5
  rash NEC 999.5
  reaction NEC 999.5
  sickness NEC 999.5
Sesamoiditis 733.99
Seven-day fever 061
  of
    Japan 100.89
    Queensland 100.89
Sever's disease or osteochondrosis (calcaneum)
  732.5
Sex chromosome mosaics 758.81
Sextuplet
  affected by maternal complications of
    pregnancy 761.5
  healthy liveborn — *see* Newborn, multiple
  pregnancy (complicating delivery) NEC 651.8 ☑
    with fetal loss and retention of one or more
      fetus(es) 651.6 ☑
Sexual
  anesthesia 302.72
  deviation (*see also* Deviation, sexual) 302.9
  disorder (*see also* Deviation, sexual) 302.9
  frigidity (female) 302.72
  function, disorder of (psychogenic) 302.70
    specified type NEC 302.79
  immaturity (female) (male) 259.0
  impotence (psychogenic) 302.72
    organic origin NEC 607.84
  precocity (constitutional) (cryptogenic) (female)
    (idiopathic) (male) NEC 259.1
    with adrenal hyperplasia 255.2
  sadism 302.84
Sexuality, pathological (*see also* Deviation,
  sexual) 302.9
Sézary's disease, reticulosis, or syndrome
  (M9701/3) 202.2 ☑
Shadow, lung 793.1
Shaken infant syndrome 995.55
Shaking
  head (tremor) 781.0
  palsy or paralysis (*see also* Parkinsonism)
    332.0
Shallowness, acetabulum 736.39
Shaver's disease or syndrome (bauxite
  pneumoconiosis) 503
Shearing
  artificial skin graft 996.55
  decellularized allodermis graft 996.55
Sheath (tendon) — *see* condition

Shedding
  nail 703.8
  teeth, premature, primary (deciduous) 520.6
Sheehan's disease or syndrome (postpartum
  pituitary necrosis) 253.2
Shelf, rectal 569.49
Shell
  shock (current) (*see also* Reaction, stress,
    acute) 308.9
    lasting state 300.16
  teeth 520.5
Shield kidney 753.3
Shift, mediastinal 793.2
Shifting
  pacemaker 427.89
  sleep-work schedule (affecting sleep) 307.45
Shiga's
  bacillus 004.0
  dysentery 004.0
Shigella (dysentery) (*see also* Dysentery, bacillary)
  004.9
  carrier (suspected) of V02.3
Shigellosis (*see also* Dysentery, bacillary) 004.9
Shingles (*see also* Herpes, zoster) 053.9
  eye NEC 053.29
Shin splints 844.9
Shipyard eye or disease 077.1
Shirodkar suture, in pregnancy 654.5 ☑
Shock 785.50
  with
    abortion — *see* Abortion, by type, with
      shock
    ectopic pregnancy (*see also* categories
      633.0-633.9) 639.5
    molar pregnancy (*see also* categories 630-
      632) 639.5
  allergic — *see* Shock, anaphylactic
  anaclitic 309.21
  anaphylactic 995.0
    chemical — *see* Table of Drugs and
      Chemicals
    correct medicinal substance properly
      administered 995.0
    drug or medicinal substance
      correct substance properly administered
        995.0
      overdose or wrong substance given or
        taken 977.9
        specified drug — *see* Table of Drugs
          and Chemicals
    following sting(s) 989.5
    food — *see* Anaphylactic shock, due to, food
    immunization 999.4
    serum 999.4
  anaphylactoid — *see* Shock, anaphylactic
  anesthetic
    correct substance properly administered
      995.4
    overdose or wrong substance given 968.4
      specified anesthetic — *see* Table of Drugs
        and Chemicals
  birth, fetus or newborn NEC 779.89
  cardiogenic 785.51
  chemical substance — *see* Table of Drugs and
    Chemicals
  circulatory 785.59
  complicating
    abortion — *see* Abortion, by type, with
      shock
    ectopic pregnancy (*see also* categories
      633.0-633.9) 639.5
    labor and delivery 669.1 ☑
    molar pregnancy (*see also* categories 630-
      632) 639.5
  culture 309.29
  due to
    drug 995.0
      correct substance properly administered
        995.0
      overdose or wrong substance given or
        taken 977.9
        specified drug — *see* Table of Drugs
          and Chemicals
    food — *see* Anaphylactic shock, due to, food

Shock — *continued*
  during labor and delivery 669.1 ☑
  electric 994.8
  endotoxic 785.52
    due to surgical procedure 998.0
  following
    abortion 639.5
    ectopic or molar pregnancy 639.5
    injury (immediate) (delayed) 958.4
    labor and delivery 669.1 ☑
  gram-negative 785.52
  hematogenic 785.59
  hemorrhagic
    due to
      disease 785.59
      surgery (intraoperative) (postoperative)
        998.0
      trauma 958.4
  hypovolemic NEC 785.59
    surgical 998.0
    traumatic 958.4
  insulin 251.0
    therapeutic misadventure 962.3
  kidney 584.5
    traumatic (following crushing) 958.5
  lightning 994.0
  lung 518.5
  nervous (*see also* Reaction, stress, acute) 308.9
  obstetric 669.1 ☑
    with
      abortion — *see* Abortion, by type, with
        shock
      ectopic pregnancy (*see also* categories
        633.0-633.9) 639.5
      molar pregnancy (*see also* categories 630-
        632) 639.5
    following
      abortion 639.5
      ectopic or molar pregnancy 639.5
  paralysis, paralytic (*see also* Disease,
    cerebrovascular, acute) 436
    late effect — *see* Late effect(s) (of)
      cerebrovascular disease
  pleural (surgical) 998.0
    due to trauma 958.4
  postoperative 998.0
    with
      abortion — *see* Abortion, by type, with
        shock
      ectopic pregnancy (*see also* categories
        633.0-633.9) 639.5
      molar pregnancy (*see also* categories 630-
        632) 639.5
    following
      abortion 639.5
      ectopic or molar pregnancy 639.5
  psychic (*see also* Reaction, stress, acute) 308.9
    past history (of) V15.49
  psychogenic (*see also* Reaction, stress, acute)
    308.9
  septic 785.52
    with
      abortion — *see* Abortion, by type, with
        shock
      ectopic pregnancy (categories 633.0-
        633.9) 639.5
      molar pregnancy (*see also* categories 630-
        632) 639.5
    due to
      surgical procedure 998.0
      transfusion NEC 999.8
        bone marrow 996.85
    following
      abortion 639.5
      ectopic or molar pregnancy 639.5
      surgical procedure 998.0
      transfusion NEC 999.8
        bone marrow 996.85
  spinal — *see also* Injury, spinal, by site
    with spinal bone injury — *see* Fracture,
      vertebra, by site, with spinal cord
      injury
  surgical 998.0
  therapeutic misadventure NEC (*see also*
    Complications) 998.89
  thyroxin 962.7
  toxic 040.82

Shock — *continued*
- transfusion — *see* Complications, transfusion
- traumatic (immediate) (delayed) 958.4

Shoemakers' chest 738.3
Short, shortening, shortness
- Achilles tendon (acquired) 727.81
- arm 736.89
  - congenital 755.20
- back 737.9
- bowel syndrome 579.3
- breath 786.05
- chain acyl CoA dehydrogenase deficiency ●
  - (SCAD) 277.85 ●
- common bile duct, congenital 751.69
- cord (umbilical) 663.4 ☑
  - affecting fetus or newborn 762.6
- cystic duct, congenital 751.69
- esophagus (congenital) 750.4
- femur (acquired) 736.81
  - congenital 755.34
- frenulum linguae 750.0
- frenum, lingual 750.0
- hamstrings 727.81
- hip (acquired) 736.39
  - congenital 755.63
- leg (acquired) 736.81
  - congenital 755.30
- metatarsus (congenital) 754.79
  - acquired 736.79
- organ or site, congenital NEC — *see* Distortion
- palate (congenital) 750.26
- P-R interval syndrome 426.81
- radius (acquired) 736.09
  - congenital 755.26
- round ligament 629.8
- sleeper 307.49
- stature, constitutional (hereditary) 783.43
- tendon 727.81
  - Achilles (acquired) 727.81
    - congenital 754.79
  - congenital 756.89
- thigh (acquired) 736.81
  - congenital 755.34
- tibialis anticus 727.81
- umbilical cord 663.4 ☑
  - affecting fetus or newborn 762.6
- urethra 599.84
- uvula (congenital) 750.26
- vagina 623.8

Shortsightedness 367.1
Shoshin (acute fulminating beriberi) 265.0
Shoulder — *see* condition
Shovel-shaped incisors 520.2
Shower, thromboembolic — *see* Embolism
Shunt (status)
- aortocoronary bypass V45.81
- arterial-venous (dialysis) V45.1
- arteriovenous, pulmonary (acquired) 417.0
  - congenital 747.3
  - traumatic (complication) 901.40
- cerebral ventricle (communicating) in situ V45.2
- coronary artery bypass V45.81
- surgical, prosthetic, with complications — *see* Complications, shunt
- vascular NEC V45.89

Shutdown
- renal 586
  - with
    - abortion — *see* Abortion, by type, with renal failure
    - ectopic pregnancy (*see also* categories 633.0-633.9) 639.3
    - molar pregnancy (*see also* categories 630-632) 639.3
  - complicating
    - abortion 639.3
    - ectopic or molar pregnancy 639.3
  - following labor and delivery 669.3 ☑

Shwachman's syndrome 288.0
Shy-Drager syndrome (orthostatic hypotension with multisystem degeneration) 333.0

Sialadenitis (any gland) (chronic) (suppurative) 527.2
- epidemic — *see* Mumps
Sialadenosis, periodic 527.2
Sialaporia 527.7
Sialectasia 527.8
Sialitis 527.2
Sialoadenitis (*see also* Sialadenitis) 527.2
Sioloangitis 527.2
Sialodochitis (fibrinosa) 527.2
Sialodocholithiasis 527.5
Sialolithiasis 527.5
Sialorrhea (*see also* Ptyalism) 527.7
- periodic 527.2
Sialosis 527.8
- rheumatic 710.2
Siamese twin 759.4
Sicard's syndrome 352.6
Sicca syndrome (keratoconjunctivitis) 710.2
Sick 799.9
- cilia syndrome 759.89
- or handicapped person in family V61.49
Sickle-cell
- anemia (*see also* Disease, sickle-cell) 282.60
- disease (*see also* Disease, sickle-cell) 282.60
- hemoglobin
  - C disease (without crisis) 282.63
    - with
      - crisis 282.64
        - vaso-occlusive pain 282.64
  - D disease (without crisis) 282.68
    - with crisis 282.69
  - E disease (without crisis) 282.68
    - with crisis 282.69
  - thalassemia (without crisis) 282.41
    - with
      - crisis 282.42
        - vaso-occlusive pain 282.42
  - trait 282.5
Sicklemia (*see also* Disease, sickle-cell) 282.60
- trait 282.5
Sickness
- air (travel) 994.6
- airplane 994.6
- alpine 993.2
- altitude 993.2
- Andes 993.2
- aviators' 993.2
- balloon 993.2
- car 994.6
- compressed air 993.3
- decompression 993.3
- green 280.9
- harvest 100.89
- milk 988.8
- morning 643.0 ☑
- motion 994.6
- mountain 993.2
  - acute 289.0
- protein (*see also* Complications, vaccination) 999.5
- radiation NEC 990
- roundabout (motion) 994.6
- sea 994.6
- serum NEC 999.5
- sleeping (African) 086.5
  - by Trypanosoma 086.5
    - gambiense 086.3
    - rhodesiense 086.4
  - Gambian 086.3
  - late effect 139.8
  - Rhodesian 086.4
- sweating 078.2
- swing (motion) 994.6
- train (railway) (travel) 994.6
- travel (any vehicle) 994.6
Sick sinus syndrome 427.81
Sideropenia (*see also* Anemia, iron deficiency) 280.9
Siderosis (lung) (occupational) 503
- cornea 371.15
- eye (bulbi) (vitreous) 360.23
- lens 360.23

Siegal-Cattan-Mamou disease (periodic) 277.3
Siemens' syndrome
- ectodermal dysplasia 757.31
- keratosis follicularis spinulosa (decalvans) 757.39
Sighing respiration 786.7
Sigmoid
- flexure — *see* condition
- kidney 753.3
Sigmoiditis — *see* Enteritis
Silfverskiöld's syndrome 756.5 ☑
Silicosis, silicotic (complicated) (occupational) (simple) 502
- fibrosis, lung (confluent) (massive) (occupational) 502
- non-nodular 503
- pulmonum 502
Silicotuberculosis (*see also* Tuberculosis) 011.4 ☑
Silo fillers' disease 506.9
Silver's syndrome (congenital hemihypertrophy and short stature) 759.89
Silver wire arteries, retina 362.13
Silvestroni-Bianco syndrome (thalassemia minima) 282.49
Simian crease 757.2
Simmonds' cachexia or disease (pituitary cachexia) 253.2
Simons' disease or syndrome (progressive lipodystrophy) 272.6
Simple, simplex — *see* condition
Sinding-Larsen disease (juvenile osteopathia patellae) 732.4
Singapore hemorrhagic fever 065.4
Singers' node or nodule 478.5
Single
- atrium 745.69
- coronary artery 746.85
- umbilical artery 747.5
- ventricle 745.3
Singultus 786.8
- epidemicus 078.89
Sinus — *see also* Fistula
- abdominal 569.81
- arrest 426.6
- arrhythmia 427.89
- bradycardia 427.89
  - chronic 427.81
- branchial cleft (external) (internal) 744.41
- coccygeal (infected) 685.1
  - with abscess 685.0
- dental 522.7
- dermal (congenital) 685.1
  - with abscess 685.0
- draining — *see* Fistula
- infected, skin NEC 686.9
- marginal, ruptured or bleeding 641.2 ☑
  - affecting fetus or newborn 762.1
- pause 426.6
- pericranii 742.0
- pilonidal (infected) (rectum) 685.1
  - with abscess 685.0
- preauricular 744.46
- rectovaginal 619.1
- sacrococcygeal (dermoid) (infected) 685.1
  - with abscess 685.0
- skin
  - infected NEC 686.9
  - noninfected — *see* Ulcer, skin
- tachycardia 427.89
- tarsi syndrome 726.79
- testis 608.89
- tract (postinfectional) — *see* Fistula
- urachus 753.7
Sinuses, Rokitansky-Aschoff (*see also* Disease, gallbladder) 575.8
Sinusitis (accessory) (nasal) (hyperplastic) (nonpurulent) (purulent) (chronic) 473.9
- with influenza, flu, or grippe 487.1
- acute 461.9
  - ethmoidal 461.2
  - frontal 461.1
  - maxillary 461.0
  - specified type NEC 461.8

Sinusitis — *continued*
  acute — *continued*
    sphenoidal 461.3
  allergic (*see also* Fever, hay) 477.9
  antrum — *see* Sinusitis, maxillary
  due to
    fungus, any sinus 117.9
    high altitude 993.1
  ethmoidal 473.2
    acute 461.2
  frontal 473.1
    acute 461.1
  influenzal 478.1
  maxillary 473.0
    acute 461.0
  specified site NEC 473.8
  sphenoidal 473.3
    acute 461.3
  syphilitic, any sinus 095.8
  tuberculous, any sinus (*see also* Tuberculosis) 012.8 ☑
Sinusitis-bronchiectasis-situs inversus (syndrome) (triad) 759.3
Sipple's syndrome (medullary thyroid carcinoma-pheochromocytoma) 193
Sirenomelia 759.89
Siriasis 992.0
Sirkari's disease 085.0
SIRS (systemic inflammatory response syndrome) 995.90
  due to
    infectious process 995.91
      with organ dysfunction 995.92
    non-infectious process 995.93
      with organ dysfunction 995.94
Siti 104.0
Sitophobia 300.29
Situation, psychiatric 300.9
Situational
  disturbance (transient) (*see also* Reaction, adjustment) 309.9
    acute 308.3
  maladjustment, acute (*see also* Reaction, adjustment) 309.9
  reaction (*see also* Reaction, adjustment) 309.9
    acute 308.3
Situs inversus or transversus 759.3
  abdominalis 759.3
  thoracis 759.3
Sixth disease 057.8
Sjögren (-Gougerot) syndrome or disease (keratoconjunctivitis sicca) 710.2
  with lung involvement 710.2 [517.8]
Sjögren-Larsson syndrome (ichthyosis congenita) 757.1
Skeletal — *see* condition
Skene's gland — *see* condition
Skenitis (*see also* Urethritis) 597.89
  gonorrheal (acute) 098.0
    chronic or duration of 2 months or over 098.2
Skerljevo 104.0
Skevas-Zerfus disease 989.5
Skin — *see also* condition
  donor V59.1
  hidebound 710.9
SLAP lesion (superior glenoid labrum) 840.7
Slate-dressers' lung 502
Slate-miners' lung 502
Sleep
  deprivation V69.4 ●
  disorder 780.50
    with apnea — *see* Apnea, sleep
    child 307.40
    movement 780.58 ●
    nonorganic origin 307.40
      specified type NEC 307.49
  disturbance 780.50
    with apnea — *see* Apnea, sleep
    nonorganic origin 307.40
      specified type NEC 307.49
  drunkenness 307.47
  movement disorder 780.58 ●

Sleep — *continued*
  paroxysmal ▶(*see also* Narcolepsy)◀ 347.00 ▲
  related movement disorder 780.58 ●
  rhythm inversion 780.55
    nonorganic origin 307.45
  walking 307.46
    hysterical 300.13
Sleeping sickness 086.5
  late effect 139.8
Sleeplessness (*see also* Insomnia) 780.52
  menopausal 627.2
  nonorganic origin 307.41
Slipped, slipping
  epiphysis (postinfectional) 732.9
    traumatic (old) 732.9
      current — *see* Fracture, by site
    upper femoral (nontraumatic) 732.2
  intervertebral disc — *see* Displacement, intervertebral disc
  ligature, umbilical 772.3
  patella 717.89
  rib 733.99
  sacroiliac joint 724.6
  tendon 727.9
  ulnar nerve, nontraumatic 354.2
  vertebra NEC (*see also* Spondylolisthesis) 756.12
Slocumb's syndrome 255.3
Sloughing (multiple) (skin) 686.9
  abscess — *see* Abscess, by site
  appendix 543.9
  bladder 596.8
  fascia 728.9
  graft — *see* Complications, graft
  phagedena (*see also* Gangrene) 785.4
  reattached extremity (*see also* Complications, reattached extremity) 996.90
  rectum 569.49
  scrotum 608.89
  tendon 727.9
  transplanted organ (*see also* Rejection, transplant, organ, by site) 996.80
  ulcer (*see also* Ulcer, skin) 707.9
Slow
  feeding newborn 779.3
  fetal, growth NEC 764.9 ☑
    affecting management of pregnancy 656.5 ☑
Slowing
  heart 427.89
  urinary stream 788.62
Sluder's neuralgia or syndrome 337.0
Slurred, slurring, speech 784.5
Small, smallness
  cardiac reserve — *see* Disease, heart
  for dates
    fetus or newborn 764.0 ☑
      with malnutrition 764.1 ☑
      affecting management of pregnancy 656.5 ☑
  infant, term 764.0 ☑
    with malnutrition 764.1 ☑
    affecting management of pregnancy 656.5 ☑
  introitus, vagina 623.3
  kidney, unknown cause 589.9
    bilateral 589.1
    unilateral 589.0
  ovary 620.8
  pelvis
    with disproportion (fetopelvic) 653.1 ☑
      affecting fetus or newborn 763.1
    causing obstructed labor 660.1 ☑
      affecting fetus or newborn 763.1
  placenta — *see* Placenta, insufficiency
  uterus 621.8
  white kidney 582.9
Small-for-dates (*see also* Light-for-dates) 764.0 ☑
  affecting management of pregnancy 656.5 ☑
Smallpox 050.9
  contact V01.3
  exposure to V01.3
  hemorrhagic (pustular) 050.0
  malignant 050.0
  modified 050.2

Smallpox — *continued*
  vaccination
    complications — *see* Complications, vaccination
    prophylactic (against) V04.1
Smith's fracture (separation) (closed) 813.41
  open 813.51
Smith-Lemli Opitz syndrome (cerebrohepatorenal syndrome) 759.89
Smith-Magenis syndrome 758.33 ●
Smith-Strang disease (oasthouse urine) 270.2
Smokers'
  bronchitis 491.0
  cough 491.0
  syndrome (*see also* Abuse, drugs, nondependent) 305.1
  throat 472.1
  tongue 528.6
Smothering spells 786.09
Snaggle teeth, tooth 524.39 ▲
Snapping
  finger 727.05
  hip 719.65
  jaw 524.69
    temporomandibular joint sounds on opening or closing 524.64 ●●
  knee 717.9
  thumb 727.05
Sneddon-Wilkinson disease or syndrome (subcorneal pustular dermatosis) 694.1
Sneezing 784.9
  intractable 478.1
Sniffing
  cocaine (*see also* Dependence) 304.2 ☑
  ether (*see also* Dependence) 304.6 ☑
  glue (airplane) (*see also* Dependence) 304.6 ☑
Snoring 786.09
Snow blindness 370.24
Snuffles (nonsyphilitic) 460
  syphilitic (infant) 090.0
Social migrant V60.0
Sodoku 026.0
Soemmering's ring 366.51
Soft — *see also* condition
  enlarged prostate 600.00
    with urinary retention 600.01
  nails 703.8
Softening
  bone 268.2
  brain (necrotic) (progressive) 434.9 ☑
    arteriosclerotic 437.0
    congenital 742.4
    embolic (*see also* Embolism, brain) 434.1 ☑
    hemorrhagic (*see also* Hemorrhage, brain) 431
    occlusive 434.9 ☑
    thrombotic (*see also* Thrombosis, brain) 434.0 ☑
  cartilage 733.92
  cerebellar — *see* Softening, brain
  cerebral — *see* Softening, brain
  cerebrospinal — *see* Softening, brain
  myocardial, heart (*see also* Degeneration, myocardial) 429.1
  nails 703.8
  spinal cord 336.8
  stomach 537.89
Solar fever 061
Soldier's
  heart 306.2
  patches 423.1
Solitary
  cyst
    bone 733.21
    kidney 593.2
  kidney (congenital) 753.0
  tubercle, brain (*see also* Tuberculosis, brain) 013.2 ☑
  ulcer, bladder 596.8
Somatization reaction, somatic reaction (*see also* Disorder, psychosomatic) 306.9
  disorder 300.81

☑ Additional Digit Required   ▶◀ Revised Text   ● New Line   ▲ Revised Code

Somatoform disorder 300.82
  atypical 300.82
  severe 300.81
  undifferentiated 300.82
Somnambulism 307.46
  hysterical 300.13
Somnolence 780.09
  nonorganic origin 307.43
  periodic 349.89
Sonne dysentery 004.3
Soor 112.0
Sore
  Delhi 085.1
  desert (see also Ulcer, skin) 707.9
  eye 379.99
  Lahore 085.1
  mouth 528.9
    canker 528.2
    due to dentures 528.9
  muscle 729.1
  Naga (see also Ulcer, skin) 707.9
  oriental 085.1
  pressure ▶(see also Decubitus)◀ 707.00 ▲
    with gangrene ▶(see also Decubitus)◀
      707.00 [785.4] ▲
  skin NEC 709.9
  soft 099.0
  throat 462
    with influenza, flu, or grippe 487.1
    acute 462
    chronic 472.1
    clergyman's 784.49
    coxsackie (virus) 074.0
    diphtheritic 032.0
    epidemic 034.0
    gangrenous 462
    herpetic 054.79
    influenzal 487.1
    malignant 462
    purulent 462
    putrid 462
    septic 034.0
    streptococcal (ulcerative) 034.0
    ulcerated 462
    viral NEC 462
      Coxsackie 074.0
  tropical (see also Ulcer, skin) 707.9
  veldt (see also Ulcer, skin) 707.9
Sotos' syndrome (cerebral gigantism) 253.0
Sounds
  friction, pleural 786.7
  succussion, chest 786.7
  temporomandibular joint ●
    on opening or closing 524.64 ●
South African cardiomyopathy syndrome 425.2
South American
  blastomycosis 116.1
  trypanosomiasis — see Trypanosomiasis
Southeast Asian hemorrhagic fever 065.4
Spacing, teeth, abnormal 524.30 ▲
  excessive 524.32 ●
Spade-like hand (congenital) 754.89
Spading nail 703.8
  congenital 757.5
Spanemia 285.9
Spanish collar 605
Sparganosis 123.5
Spasm, spastic, spasticity (see also condition)
    781.0
  accommodation 367.53
  ampulla of Vater (see also Disease, gallbladder)
    576.8
  anus, ani (sphincter) (reflex) 564.6
    psychogenic 306.4
  artery NEC 443.9
    basilar 435.0
    carotid 435.8
    cerebral 435.9
      specified artery NEC 435.8
    retinal (see also Occlusion, retinal, artery)
      362.30
    vertebral 435.1
    vertebrobasilar 435.3
  Bell's 351.0

Spasm, spastic, spasticity (see also condition) —
    continued
  bladder (sphincter, external or internal) 596.8
  bowel 564.9
    psychogenic 306.4
  bronchus, bronchiole 519.1
  cardia 530.0
  cardiac — see Angina
  carpopedal (see also Tetany) 781.7
  cecum 564.9
    psychogenic 306.4
  cerebral (arteries) (vascular) 435.9
    specified artery NEC 435.8
  cerebrovascular 435.9
  cervix, complicating delivery 661.4 ☑
    affecting fetus or newborn 763.7
  ciliary body (of accommodation) 367.53
  colon 564.1
    psychogenic 306.4
  common duct (see also Disease, biliary) 576.8
  compulsive 307.22
  conjugate 378.82
  convergence 378.84
  coronary (artery) — see Angina
  diaphragm (reflex) 786.8
    psychogenic 306.4
  duodenum, duodenal (bulb) 564.89
  esophagus (diffuse) 530.5
    psychogenic 306.4
  facial 351.8
  fallopian tube 620.8
  gait 781.2
  gastrointestinal (tract) 536.8
    psychogenic 306.4
  glottis 478.75
    hysterical 300.11
    psychogenic 306.1
      specified as conversion reaction 300.11
    reflex through recurrent laryngeal nerve
      478.75
  habit 307.20
    chronic 307.22
    transient ▶(of childhood)◀ 307.21
  heart — see Angina
  hourglass — see Contraction, hourglass
  hysterical 300.11
  infantile (see also Epilepsy) 345.6 ☑
  internal oblique, eye 378.51
  intestinal 564.9
    psychogenic 306.4
  larynx, laryngeal 478.75
    hysterical 300.11
    psychogenic 306.1
      specified as conversion reaction 300.11
  levator palpebrae superioris 333.81
  lightning (see also Epilepsy) 345.6 ☑
  mobile 781.0
  muscle 728.85
    back 724.8
    psychogenic 306.0
  nerve, trigeminal 350.1
  nervous 306.0
  nodding 307.3
    infantile (see also Epilepsy) 345.6 ☑
  occupational 300.89
  oculogyric 378.87
  ophthalmic artery 362.30
  orbicularis 781.0
  perineal 625.8
  peroneo-extensor (see also Flat, foot) 734
  pharynx (reflex) 478.29
    hysterical 300.11
    psychogenic 306.1
      specified as conversion reaction 300.11
  pregnant uterus, complicating delivery 661.4 ☑
  psychogenic 306.0
  pylorus 537.81
    adult hypertrophic 537.0
    congenital or infantile 750.5
    psychogenic 306.4
  rectum (sphincter) 564.6
    psychogenic 306.4
  retinal artery NEC (see also Occlusion, retina,
    artery) 362.30
  sacroiliac 724.6
  salaam (infantile) (see also Epilepsy) 345.6 ☑
  saltatory 781.0

Spasm, spastic, spasticity (see also condition) —
    continued
  sigmoid 564.9
    psychogenic 306.4
  sphincter of Oddi (see also Disease,
    gallbladder) 576.5
  stomach 536.8
    neurotic 306.4
  throat 478.29
    hysterical 300.11
    psychogenic 306.1
      specified as conversion reaction 300.11
  tic 307.20
    chronic 307.22
    transient ▶(of childhood)◀ 307.21
  tongue 529.8
  torsion 333.6
  trigeminal nerve 350.1
    postherpetic 053.12
  ureter 593.89
  urethra (sphincter) 599.84
  uterus 625.8
    complicating labor 661.4 ☑
      affecting fetus or newborn 763.7
  vagina 625.1
    psychogenic 306.51
  vascular NEC 443.9
  vasomotor NEC 443.9
  vein NEC 459.89
  vesical (sphincter, external or internal) 596.8
  viscera 789.0 ☑
Spasmodic — see condition
Spasmophilia (see also Tetany) 781.7
Spasmus nutans 307.3
Spastic — see also Spasm
  child 343.9
Spasticity — see also Spasm
  cerebral, child 343.9
Speakers' throat 784.49
Specific, specified — see condition
Speech
  defect, disorder, disturbance, impediment NEC
    784.5
    psychogenic 307.9
  therapy V57.3
Spells 780.39
  breath-holding 786.9
Spencer's disease (epidemic vomiting) 078.82
Spens' syndrome (syncope with heart block)
    426.9
Spermatic cord — see condition
Spermatocele 608.1
  congenital 752.89
Spermatocystitis 608.4
Spermatocytoma (M9063/3)
  specified site — see Neoplasm, by site,
    malignant
  unspecified site 186.9
Spermatorrhea 608.89
Sperm counts
  fertility testing V26.21
  following sterilization reversal V26.22
  postvasectomy V25.8
Sphacelus (see also Gangrene) 785.4
Sphenoidal — see condition
Sphenoiditis (chronic) (see also Sinusitis,
    sphenoidal) 473.3
Sphenopalatine ganglion neuralgia 337.0
Sphericity, increased, lens 743.36
Spherocytosis (congenital) (familial) (hereditary)
    282.0
  hemoglobin disease 282.7
  sickle-cell (disease) 282.60
Spherophakia 743.36
Sphincter — see condition
Sphincteritis, sphincter of Oddi (see also
    Cholecystitis) 576.8
Sphingolipidosis 272.7
Sphingolipodystrophy 272.7
Sphingomyelinosis 272.7
Spicule tooth 520.2

Spider
finger 755.59
nevus 448.1
vascular 448.1
Spiegler-Fendt sarcoid 686.8
Spielmeyer-Stock disease 330.1
Spielmeyer-Vogt disease 330.1
Spina bifida (aperta) 741.9 ☑

> Note — Use the following fifth-digit
> subclassification with category 741:
>
> 0   unspecified region
> 1   cervical region
> 2   dorsal [thoracic] region
> 3   lumbar region

with hydrocephalus 741.0 ☑
   fetal (suspected), affecting management of
     pregnancy 655.0 ☑
occulta 756.17
Spindle, Krukenberg's 371.13
Spine, spinal — see condition
Spiradenoma (eccrine) (M8403/0) — see
   Neoplasm, skin, benign
Spirillosis NEC (see also Fever, relapsing) 087.9
Spirillum minus 026.0
Spirillum obermeieri infection 087.0
Spirochetal — see condition
Spirochetosis 104.9
arthritic, arthritica 104.9 [711.8] ☑
bronchopulmonary 104.8
icterohemorrhagica 100.0
lung 104.8
Spitting blood (see also Hemoptysis) 786.3
Splanchnomegaly 569.89
Splanchnoptosis 569.89
Spleen, splenic — see also condition
agenesis 759.0
flexure syndrome 569.89
neutropenia syndrome 288.0
sequestration syndrome 289.52
Splenectasis (see also Splenomegaly) 789.2
Splenitis (interstitial) (malignant) (nonspecific)
   289.59
malarial (see also Malaria) 084.6
tuberculous (see also Tuberculosis) 017.7 ☑
Splenocele 289.59
Splenomegalia — see Splenomegaly
Splenomegalic — see condition
Splenomegaly 789.2
Bengal 789.2
cirrhotic 289.51
congenital 759.0
congestive, chronic 289.51
cryptogenic 789.2
Egyptian 120.1
Gaucher's (cerebroside lipidosis) 272.7
idiopathic 789.2
malarial (see also Malaria) 084.6
neutropenic 288.0
Niemann-Pick (lipid histiocytosis) 272.7
siderotic 289.51
syphilitic 095.8
   congenital 090.0
tropical (Bengal) (idiopathic) 789.2
Splenopathy 289.50
Splenopneumonia — see Pneumonia
Splenoptosis 289.59
Splinter — see Injury, superficial, by site
Split, splitting
heart sounds 427.89
lip, congenital (see also Cleft, lip) 749.10
nails 703.8
urinary stream 788.61
Spoiled child reaction (see also Disturbance,
   conduct) 312.1 ☑
Spondylarthritis (see also Spondylosis) 721.90
Spondylarthrosis (see also Spondylosis) 721.90
Spondylitis 720.9
ankylopoietica 720.0
ankylosing (chronic) 720.0
atrophic 720.9
ligamentous 720.9

Spondylitis — continued
chronic (traumatic) (see also Spondylosis)
   721.90
deformans (chronic) (see also Spondylosis)
   721.90
gonococcal 098.53
gouty 274.0
hypertrophic (see also Spondylosis) 721.90
infectious NEC 720.9
juvenile (adolescent) 720.0
Kümmell's 721.7
Marie-Strümpell (ankylosing) 720.0
muscularis 720.9
ossificans ligamentosa 721.6
osteoarthritica (see also Spondylosis) 721.90
posttraumatic 721.7
proliferative 720.0
rheumatoid 720.0
rhizomelica 720.0
sacroiliac NEC 720.2
senescent (see also Spondylosis) 721.90
senile (see also Spondylosis) 721.90
static (see also Spondylosis) 721.90
traumatic (chronic) (see also Spondylosis)
   721.90
tuberculous (see also Tuberculosis)
   015.0 ☑ [720.81]
typhosa 002.0 [720.81]
Spondyloarthrosis (see also Spondylosis) 721.90
Spondylolisthesis (congenital) (lumbosacral)
   756.12
with disproportion (fetopelvic) 653.3 ☑
   affecting fetus or newborn 763.1
   causing obstructed labor 660.1 ☑
     affecting fetus or newborn 763.1
acquired 738.4
degenerative 738.4
traumatic 738.4
   acute (lumbar) — see Fracture, vertebra,
     lumbar
   site other than lumbosacral — see
     Fracture, vertebra, by site
Spondylolysis (congenital) 756.11
acquired 738.4
cervical 756.19
lumbosacral region 756.11
   with disproportion (fetopelvic) 653.3 ☑
     affecting fetus or newborn 763.1
     causing obstructed labor 660.1 ☑
       affecting fetus or newborn 763.1
Spondylopathy
inflammatory 720.9
   specified type NEC 720.89
traumatic 721.7
Spondylose rhizomelique 720.0
Spondylosis 721.90
with
   disproportion 653.3 ☑
     affecting fetus or newborn 763.1
     causing obstructed labor 660.1 ☑
       affecting fetus or newborn 763.1
   myelopathy NEC 721.91
cervical, cervicodorsal 721.0
   with myelopathy 721.1
inflammatory 720.9
lumbar, lumbosacral 721.3
   with myelopathy 721.42
sacral 721.3
   with myelopathy 721.42
thoracic 721.2
   with myelopathy 721.41
traumatic 721.7
Sponge
divers' disease 989.5
inadvertently left in operation wound 998.4
kidney (medullary) 753.17
Spongioblastoma (M9422/3)
multiforme (M9440/3)
   specified site — see Neoplasm, by site,
     malignant
   unspecified site 191.9
polare (M9423/3)
   specified site — see Neoplasm, by site,
     malignant
   unspecified site 191.9

Spongioblastoma (M9422/3) — continued
primitive polar (M9443/3)
   specified site — see Neoplasm, by site,
     malignant
   unspecified site 191.9
specified site — see Neoplasm, by site,
   malignant
unspecified site 191.9
Spongiocytoma (M9400/3)
specified site — see Neoplasm, by site,
   malignant
unspecified site 191.9
Spongioneuroblastoma (M9504/3) — see
   Neoplasm, by site, malignant
Spontaneous — see also condition
fracture — see Fracture, pathologic
Spoon nail 703.8
congenital 757.5
Sporadic — see condition
Sporotrichosis (bones) (cutaneous) (disseminated)
   (epidermal) (lymphatic) (lymphocutaneous)
   (mucous membranes) (pulmonary) (skeletal)
   (visceral) 117.1
Sporotrichum schenckii infection 117.1
Spots, spotting
atrophic (skin) 701.3
Bitôt's (in the young child) 264.1
café au lait 709.09
cayenne pepper 448.1
cotton wool (retina) 362.83
de Morgan's (senile angiomas) 448.1
Fúchs' black (myopic) 360.21
intermenstrual
   irregular 626.6
   regular 626.5
interpalpebral 372.53
Koplik's 055.9
liver 709.09
Mongolian (pigmented) 757.33
of pregnancy 641.9 ☑
purpuric 782.7
ruby 448.1
Spotted fever — see Fever, spotted
Sprain, strain (joint) (ligament) (muscle) (tendon)
   848.9
abdominal wall (muscle) 848.8
Achilles tendon 845.09
acromioclavicular 840.0
ankle 845.00
   and foot 845.00
anterior longitudinal, cervical 847.0
arm 840.9
   upper 840.9
     and shoulder 840.9
astragalus 845.00
atlanto-axial 847.0
atlanto-occipital 847.0
atlas 847.0
axis 847.0
back (see also Sprain, spine) 847.9
breast bone 848.40
broad ligament — see Injury, internal, broad
   ligament
calcaneofibular 845.02
carpal 842.01
carpometacarpal 842.11
cartilage
   costal, without mention of injury to sternum
     848.3
     involving sternum 848.42
   ear 848.8
   knee 844.9
     with current tear (see also Tear,
       meniscus) 836.2
     semilunar (knee) 844.8
       with current tear (see also Tear,
         meniscus) 836.2
   septal, nose 848.0
   thyroid region 848.2
   xiphoid 848.49
cervical, cervicodorsal, cervicothoracic 847.0
chondrocostal, without mention of injury to
   sternum 848.3
   involving sternum 848.42
chondrosternal 848.42

Sprain, strain — Staggering gait

Sprain, strain — *continued*
chronic (joint) — *see* Derangement, joint
clavicle 840.9
coccyx 847.4
collar bone 840.9
collateral, knee (medial) (tibial) 844.1
  lateral (fibular) 844.0
  recurrent or old 717.89
    lateral 717.81
    medial 717.82
coracoacromial 840.8
coracoclavicular 840.1
coracohumeral 840.2
coracoid (process) 840.9
coronary, knee 844.8
costal cartilage, without mention of injury to
  sternum 848.3
  involving sternum 848.42
cricoarytenoid articulation 848.2
cricothyroid articulation 848.2
cruciate
  knee 844.2
  old 717.89
    anterior 717.83
    posterior 717.84
deltoid
  ankle 845.01
  shoulder 840.8
dorsal (spine) 847.1
ear cartilage 848.8
elbow 841.9
  and forearm 841.9
  specified site NEC 841.8
femur (proximal end) 843.9
  distal end 844.9
fibula (proximal end) 844.9
  distal end 845.00
fibulocalcaneal 845.02
finger(s) 842.10
foot 845.10
  and ankle 845.00
forearm 841.9
  and elbow 841.9
  specified site NEC 841.8
glenoid (shoulder) (*see also* SLAP lesion) 840.8
hand 842.10
hip 843.9
  and thigh 843.9
humerus (proximal end) 840.9
  distal end 841.9
iliofemoral 843.0
infraspinatus 840.3
innominate
  acetabulum 843.9
  pubic junction 848.5
  sacral junction 846.1
internal
  collateral, ankle 845.01
  semilunar cartilage 844.8
    with current tear (*see also* Tear,
      meniscus) 836.2
    old 717.5
interphalangeal
  finger 842.13
  toe 845.13
ischiocapsular 843.1
jaw (cartilage) (meniscus) 848.1
  old 524.69
knee 844.9
  and leg 844.9
  old 717.5
    collateral
      lateral 717.81
      medial 717.82
    cruciate
      anterior 717.83
      posterior 717.84
late effect — *see* Late, effects (of), sprain
lateral collateral, knee 844.0
  old 717.81
leg 844.9
  and knee 844.9
ligamentum teres femoris 843.8
low back 846.9
lumbar (spine) 847.2
lumbosacral 846.0
  chronic or old 724.6

Sprain, strain — *continued*
mandible 848.1
  old 524.69
maxilla 848.1
medial collateral, knee 844.1
  old 717.82
meniscus
  jaw 848.1
    old 524.69
  knee 844.8
    with current tear (*see also* Tear,
      meniscus) 836.2
    old 717.5
  mandible 848.1
    old 524.69
  specified site NEC 848.8
metacarpal 842.10
  distal 842.12
  proximal 842.11
metacarpophalangeal 842.12
metatarsal 845.10
metatarsophalangeal 845.12
midcarpal 842.19
midtarsal 845.19
multiple sites, except fingers alone or toes
  alone 848.8
neck 847.0
nose (septal cartilage) 848.0
occiput from atlas 847.0
old — *see* Derangement, joint
orbicular, hip 843.8
patella(r) 844.9
  old 717.89
pelvis 848.5
phalanx
  finger 842.10
  toe 845.10
radiocarpal 842.02
radiohumeral 841.2
radioulnar 841.9
  distal 842.09
radius, radial (proximal end) 841.9
  and ulna 841.9
    distal 842.09
  collateral 841.0
  distal end 842.00
recurrent — *see* Sprain, by site
rib (cage), without mention of injury to sternum
  848.3
  involving sternum 848.42
rotator cuff (capsule) 840.4
round ligament — *see also* Injury, internal,
  round ligament
  femur 843.8
sacral (spine) 847.3
sacrococcygeal 847.3
sacroiliac (region) 846.9
  chronic or old 724.6
  ligament 846.1
  specified site NEC 846.8
sacrospinatus 846.2
sacrospinous 846.2
sacrotuberous 846.3
scaphoid bone, ankle 845.00
scapula(r) 840.9
semilunar cartilage (knee) 844.8
  with current tear (*see also* Tear, meniscus)
    836.2
  old 717.5
septal cartilage (nose) 848.0
shoulder 840.9
  and arm, upper 840.9
  blade 840.9
specified site NEC 848.8
spine 847.9
  cervical 847.0
  coccyx 847.4
  dorsal 847.1
  lumbar 847.2
  lumbosacral 846.0
    chronic or old 724.6
  sacral 847.3
  sacroiliac (*see also* Sprain, sacroiliac) 846.9
    chronic or old 724.6
  thoracic 847.1
sternoclavicular 848.41
sternum 848.40

Sprain, strain — *continued*
subglenoid (*see also* SLAP lesion) 840.8
subscapularis 840.5
supraspinatus 840.6
symphysis
  jaw 848.1
    old 524.69
  mandibular 848.1
    old 524.69
  pubis 848.5
talofibular 845.09
tarsal 845.10
tarsometatarsal 845.11
temporomandibular 848.1
  old 524.69
teres
  ligamentum femoris 843.8
  major or minor 840.8
thigh (proximal end) 843.9
  and hip 843.9
  distal end 844.9
thoracic (spine) 847.1
thorax 848.8
thumb 842.10
thyroid cartilage or region 848.2
tibia (proximal end) 844.9
  distal end 845.00
tibiofibular
  distal 845.03
  superior 844.3
toe(s) 845.10
trachea 848.8
trapezoid 840.8
ulna, ulnar (proximal end) 841.9
  collateral 841.1
  distal end 842.00
ulnohumeral 841.3
vertebrae (*see also* Sprain, spine) 847.9
  cervical, cervicodorsal, cervicothoracic 847.0
wrist (cuneiform) (scaphoid) (semilunar) 842.00
xiphoid cartilage 848.49
Sprengel's deformity (congenital) 755.52
Spring fever 309.23
Sprue 579.1
celiac 579.0
idiopathic 579.0
meaning thrush 112.0
nontropical 579.0
tropical 579.1
Spur — *see also* Exostosis
bone 726.91
  calcaneal 726.73
calcaneal 726.73
iliac crest 726.5
nose (septum) 478.1
  bone 726.91
septal 478.1
Spuria placenta — *see* Placenta, abnormal
Spurway's syndrome (brittle bones and blue
  sclera) 756.51
Sputum, abnormal (amount) (color) (excessive)
  (odor) (purulent) 786.4
bloody 786.3
Squamous — *see also* condition
cell metaplasia
  bladder 596.8
  cervix — *see* condition
epithelium in
  cervical canal (congenital) 752.49
  uterine mucosa (congenital) 752.3
metaplasia
  bladder 596.8
  cervix — *see* condition
Squashed nose 738.0
congenital 754.0
Squeeze, divers' 993.3
Squint (*see also* Strabismus) 378.9
accommodative (*see also* Esotropia) 378.00
concomitant (*see also* Heterotropia) 378.30
Stab — *see also* Wound, open, by site
internal organs — *see* Injury, internal, by site,
  with open wound
Staggering gait 781.2
hysterical 300.11

☑ Additional Digit Required   ▶◀ Revised Text   ● New Line   ▲ Revised Code

Staghorn calculus 592.0

Stälh's
  ear 744.29
  pigment line (cornea) 371.11

Stälhi's pigment lines (cornea) 371.11

Stain
  port wine 757.32
  tooth, teeth (hard tissues) 521.7
    due to
      accretions 523.6
      deposits (betel) (black) (green) (materia
        alba) (orange) (tobacco) 523.6
      metals (copper) (silver) 521.7
      nicotine 523.6
      pulpal bleeding 521.7
      tobacco 523.6

Stammering 307.0

Standstill
  atrial 426.6
  auricular 426.6
  cardiac (see also Arrest, cardiac) 427.5
  sinoatrial 429.6
  sinus 426.6
  ventricular (see also Arrest, cardiac) 427.5

Stannosis 503

Stanton's disease (melioidosis) 025

Staphylitis (acute) (catarrhal) (chronic)
  (gangrenous) (membranous) (suppurative)
  (ulcerative) 528.3

Staphylococcemia 038.10
  aureus 038.11
  specified organism NEC 038.19

Staphylococcus, staphylococcal — see condition

Staphyloderma (skin) 686.00

Staphyloma 379.11
  anterior, localized 379.14
  ciliary 379.11
  cornea 371.73
  equatorial 379.13
  posterior 379.12
  posticum 379.12
  ring 379.15
  sclera NEC 379.11

Starch eating 307.52

Stargardt's disease 362.75

Starvation (inanition) (due to lack of food) 994.2
  edema 262
  voluntary NEC 307.1

Stasis
  bile (duct) (see also Disease, biliary) 576.8
  bronchus (see also Bronchitis) 490
  cardiac (see also Failure, heart) 428.0
  cecum 564.89
  colon 564.89
  dermatitis (see also Varix, with stasis
    dermatitis) 454.1
  duodenal 536.8
  eczema (see also Varix, with stasis dermatitis)
    454.1
  edema (see also Hypertension, venous) 459.30
  foot 991.4
  gastric 536.3
  ileocecal coil 564.89
  ileum 564.89
  intestinal 564.89
  jejunum 564.89
  kidney 586
  liver 571.9
    cirrhotic — see Cirrhosis, liver
  lymphatic 457.8
  pneumonia 514
  portal 571.9
  pulmonary 514
  rectal 564.89
  renal 586
    tubular 584.5
  stomach 536.3
  ulcer
    with varicose veins 454.0
    without varicose veins 459.81
  urine NEC (see also Retention, urine) 788.20
  venous 459.81

State
  affective and paranoid, mixed, organic
    psychotic 294.8
  agitated 307.9
    acute reaction to stress 308.2
  anxiety (neurotic) (see also Anxiety) 300.00
    specified type NEC 300.09
  apprehension (see also Anxiety) 300.00
    specified type NEC 300.09
  climacteric, female 627.2
    following induced menopause 627.4
  clouded
    epileptic (see also Epilepsy) 345.9 ☑
    paroxysmal (idiopathic) (see also Epilepsy)
      345.9 ☑
  compulsive (mixed) (with obsession) 300.3
  confusional 298.9
    acute 293.0
      with
        arteriosclerotic dementia 290.41
        presenile brain disease 290.11
        senility 290.3
      alcoholic 291.0
      drug-induced 292.81
    epileptic 293.0
    postoperative 293.9
    reactive (emotional stress) (psychological
      trauma) 298.2
    subacute 293.1
  constitutional psychopathic 301.9
  convulsive (see also Convulsions) 780.39
  depressive NEC 311
    induced by drug 292.84
    neurotic 300.4
  dissociative 300.15
  hallucinatory 780.1
    induced by drug 292.12
  hypercoagulable (primary) 289.81
    secondary 289.82
  hyperdynamic beta-adrenergic circulatory
    429.82
  locked-in 344.81
  menopausal 627.2
    artificial 627.4
    following induced menopause 627.4
  neurotic NEC 300.9
    with depersonalization episode 300.6
  obsessional 300.3
  oneiroid (see also Schizophrenia) 295.4 ☑
  panic 300.01
  paranoid 297.9
    alcohol-induced 291.5
    arteriosclerotic 290.42
    climacteric 297.2
    drug-induced 292.11
    in
      presenile brain disease 290.12
      senile brain disease 290.20
    involutional 297.2
    menopausal 297.2
    senile 290.20
    simple 297.0
  postleukotomy 310.0
  pregnant (see also Pregnancy) V22.2
  psychogenic, twilight 298.2
  psychotic, organic (see also Psychosis, organic)
    294.9
    mixed paranoid and affective 294.8
    senile or presenile NEC 290.9
    transient NEC 293.9
      with
        anxiety 293.84
        delusions 293.81
        depression 293.83
        hallucinations 293.82
  residual schizophrenic (see also Schizophrenia)
    295.6 ☑
  tension (see also Anxiety) 300.9
  transient organic psychotic 293.9
    anxiety type 293.84
    depressive type 293.83
    hallucinatory type 293.83
    paranoid type 293.81
    specified type NEC 293.89
  twilight
    epileptic 293.0
    psychogenic 298.2

State — continued
  vegetative (persistent) 780.03

Status (post)
  absence
    epileptic (see also Epilepsy) 345.2
    of organ, acquired (postsurgical) — see
      Absence, by site, acquired
  anastomosis of intestine (for bypass) V45.3
  angioplasty, percutaneous transluminal
    coronary V45.82
  anginosus 413.9
  ankle prosthesis V43.66
  aortocoronary bypass or shunt V45.81
  arthrodesis V45.4
  artificially induced condition NEC V45.89
  artificial opening (of) V44.9
    gastrointestinal tract NEC V44.4
    specified site NEC V44.8
    urinary tract NEC V44.6
    vagina V44.7
  aspirator V46.0
  awaiting organ transplant V49.83   ●
  asthmaticus (see also Asthma) 493.9 ☑
  breast implant removal V45.83
  cardiac
    device (in situ) V45.00
      carotid sinus V45.09
        fitting or adjustment V53.39
      defibrillator, automatic implantable
        V45.02
      pacemaker V45.01
        fitting or adjustmanet V53.31
  carotid sinus stimulator V45.09
  cataract extraction V45.61
  chemotherapy V66.2
    current V58.69
  circumcision, female 629.20   ●
  clitorectomy (female genital mutilation   ●
    type I) 629.21   ●
    with excision of labia minora (female   ●
      gental mutilation type II) 629.22   ●
  colostomy V44.3
  contraceptive device V45.59
    intrauterine V45.51
    subdermal V45.52
  convulsivus idiopathicus (see also Epilepsy)
    345.3
  coronary artery bypass or shunt V45.81
  cystostomy V44.50
    appendico-vesicostomy V44.52
    cutaneous-vesicostomy V44.51
    specified type NEC V44.59
  defibrillator, automatic implant-able cardiac
    V45.02
  dental crowns V45.84
  dental fillings V45.84
  dental restoration V45.84
  dental sealant V49.82
  dialysis V45.1
  donor V59.9
  drug therapy or regimen V67.59
    high-risk medication NEC V67.51
  elbow prosthesis V43.62
  enterostomy V44.4
  epileptic, epilepticus (absence) (grand mal) (see
    also Epilepsy) 345.3
    focal motor 345.7 ☑
    partial 345.7 ☑
    petit mal 345.2
    psychomotor 345.7 ☑
    temporal lobe 345.7 ☑
  eye (adnexa) surgery V45.69
  female genital mutilation 629.20   ●
    type I 629.21   ●
    type II 629.22   ●
    type III 629.23   ●
  filtering bleb (eye) (postglaucoma) V45.69
    with rupture or complication 997.99
    pastcataract extraction (complication)
      997.99
  finger joint prosthesis V43.69
  gastrostomy V44.1
  grand mal 345.3
  heart valve prosthesis V43.3
  hip prosthesis (joint) (partial) (total) V43.64
  ileostomy V44.2

☑ Additional Digit Required   ▶◀ Revised Text   ● New Line   ▲ Revised Code

Status — *continued*
- infibulation (female genital mutilation type III) 629.23 ●
- insulin pump V45.85
- intestinal bypass V45.3
- intrauterine contraceptive device V45.51
- jejunostomy V44.4
- knee joint prosthesis V43.65
- lacunaris 437.8
- lacunosis 437.8
- low birth weight V21.30
  - less than 500 grams V21.31
  - 500-999 grams V21.32
  - 1000-1499 grams V21.33
  - 1500-1999 grams V21.34
  - 2000-2500 grams V21.35
- lymphaticus 254.8
- malignant neoplasm, ablated or excised — *see* History, malignant neoplasm
- marmoratus 333.7
- mutilation, female 629.20 ●
  - type I 629.21 ●
  - type II 629.22 ●
  - type III 629.23 ●
- nephrostomy V44.6
- neuropacemaker NEC V45.89
  - brain V45.89
  - carotid sinus V45.09
  - neurologic NEC V45.89
- organ replacement
  - by artificial or mechanical device or prosthesis of
    - artery V43.4
    - artificial skin V43.83
    - bladder V43.5
    - blood vessel V43.4
    - breast V43.82
    - eye globe V43.0
    - heart
      - assist device V43.21
      - fully implantable artificial heart V43.22
      - valve V43.3
    - intestine V43.89
    - joint V43.60
      - ankle V43.66
      - elbow V43.62
      - finger V43.69
      - hip (partial) (total) V43.64
      - knee V43.65
      - shoulder V43.61
      - specified NEC V43.69
      - wrist V43.63
    - kidney V43.89
    - larynx V43.81
    - lens V43.1
    - limb(s) V43.7
    - liver V43.89
    - lung V43.89
    - organ NEC V43.89
    - pancreas V43.89
    - skin (artificial) V43.83
    - tissue NEC V43.89
    - vein V43.4
  - by organ transplant (heterologous) (homologous) — *see* Status, transplant
- pacemaker
  - brain V45.89
  - cardiac V45.01
  - carotid sinus V45.09
  - neurologic NEC V45.89
  - specified site NEC V45.89
- percutaneous transluminal coronary angioplasty V45.82
- petit mal 345.2
- postcommotio cerebri 310.2
- postmenopausal (age related) (natural) V49.81
- postoperative NEC V45.89
- postpartum NEC V24.2
  - care immediately following delivery V24.0
  - routine follow-up V24.2
- postsurgical NEC V45.89
- renal dialysis V45.1
- respirator V46.11 ▲
  - encounter during power failure V46.12 ●
- reversed jejunal transposition (for bypass) V45.3

Status — *continued*
- shoulder prosthesis V43.61
- shunt
  - aortocoronary bypass V45.81
  - arteriovenous (for dialysis) V45.1
  - cerebrospinal fluid V45.2
  - vascular NEC V45.89
    - aortocoronary (bypass) V45.81
  - ventricular (communicating) (for drainage) V45.2
- sterilization
  - tubal ligation V26.51
  - vasectomy V26.52
- subdermal contraceptive device V45.52
- thymicolymphaticus 254.8
- thymicus 254.8
- thymolymphaticus 254.8
- tooth extraction 525.10
- tracheostomy V44.0
- transplant
  - blood vessel V42.89
  - bone V42.4
    - marrow V42.81
  - cornea V42.5
  - heart V42.1
    - valve V42.2
  - intestine V42.84
  - kidney V42.0
  - liver V42.7
  - lung V42.6
  - organ V42.9
    - specified site NEC V42.89
  - pancreas V42.83
  - peripheral stem cells V42.82
  - skin V42.3
  - stem cells, peripheral V42.82
  - tissue V42.9
    - specified type NEC V42.89
  - vessel, blood V42.89
- tubal ligation V26.51
- ureterostomy V44.6
- urethrostomy V44.6
- vagina, artificial V44.7
- vascular shunt NEC V45.89
  - aortocoronary (bypass) V45.81
- vasectomy V26.52
- ventilator V46.11 ●
  - encounter during power failure V46.12 ●
- wrist prosthesis V43.63

Stave fracture — *see* Fracture, metacarpus, metacarpal bone(s)

Steal
- subclavian artery 435.2
- vertebral artery 435.1

Stealing, solitary, child problem (*see also* Disturbance, conduct) 312.1 ☑

Steam burn — *see* Burn, by site

Steatocystoma multiplex 706.2

Steatoma (infected) 706.2
- eyelid (cystic) 374.84
  - infected 373.13

Steatorrhea (chronic) 579.8
- with lacteal obstruction 579.2
- idiopathic 579.0
  - adult 579.0
  - infantile 579.0
- pancreatic 579.4
- primary 579.0
- secondary 579.8
- specified cause NEC 579.8
- tropical 579.1

Steatosis 272.8
- heart (*see also* Degeneration, myocardial) 429.1
- kidney 593.89
- liver 571.8

Steele-Richardson (-Olszewski) Syndrome 333.0

Stein's syndrome (polycystic ovary) 256.4

Stein-Leventhal syndrome (polycystic ovary) 256.4

Steinbrocker's syndrome (*see also* Neuropathy, peripheral, autonomic) 337.9

Steinert's disease 359.2

Stenocardia (*see also* Angina) 413.9

Stenocephaly 756.0

Stenosis (cicatricial) — *see also* Stricture
- ampulla of Vater 576.2
  - with calculus, cholelithiasis, or stones — *see* Choledocholithiasis
- anus, anal (canal) (sphincter) 569.2
  - congenital 751.2
- aorta (ascending) 747.22
  - arch 747.10
  - arteriosclerotic 440.0
  - calcified 440.0
- aortic (valve) 424.1
  - with
    - mitral (valve)
      - insufficiency or incompetence 396.2
      - stenosis or obstruction 396.0
  - atypical 396.0
  - congenital 746.3
  - rheumatic 395.0
    - with
      - insufficiency, incompetency or regurgitation 395.2
        - with mitral (valve) disease 396.8
      - mitral (valve)
        - disease (stenosis) 396.0
        - insufficiency or incompetence 396.2
        - stenosis or obstruction 396.0
  - specified cause, except rheumatic 424.1
  - syphilitic 093.22
- aqueduct of Sylvius (congenital) 742.3
  - with spina bifida (*see also* Spina bifida) 741.0 ☑
  - acquired 331.4
- artery NEC 447.1
  - basilar — *see* Narrowing, artery, basilar
  - carotid (common) (internal) — *see* Narrowing, artery, carotid
  - celiac 447.4
  - cerebral 437.0
    - due to
      - embolism (*see also* Embolism, brain) 434.1 ☑
      - thrombus (*see also* Thrombosis, brain) 434.0 ☑
  - precerebral — *see* Narrowing, artery, precerebral
  - pulmonary (congenital) 747.3
    - acquired 417.8
  - renal 440.1
  - vertebral — *see* Narrowing, artery, vertebral
- bile duct or biliary passage (*see also* Obstruction, biliary) 576.2
  - congenital 751.61
- bladder neck (acquired) 596.0
  - congenital 753.6
- brain 348.8
- bronchus 519.1
  - syphilitic 095.8
- cardia (stomach) 537.89
  - congenital 750.7
- cardiovascular (*see also* Disease, cardiovascular) 429.2
- carotid artery — *see* Narrowing, artery, carotid
- cervix, cervical (canal) 622.4
  - congenital 752.49
  - in pregnancy or childbirth 654.6 ☑
    - affecting fetus or newborn 763.89
    - causing obstructed labor 660.2 ☑
      - affecting fetus or newborn 763.1
- colon (*see also* Obstruction, intestine) 560.9
  - congenital 751.2
- colostomy 569.62
- common bile duct (*see also* Obstruction, biliary) 576.2
  - congenital 751.61
- coronary (artery) —*see* Arteriosclerosis, coronary
- cystic duct (*see also* Obstruction, gallbladder) 575.2
  - congenital 751.61
- due to (presence of) any device, implant, or graft classifiable to 996.0-996.5 — *see* Complications, due to (presence of) any device, implant, or graft classified to 996.0-996.5 NEC
- duodenum 537.3
  - congenital 751.1
- ejaculatory duct NEC 608.89

☑ Additional Digit Required   ►◄ Revised Text   ● New Line   ▲ Revised Code

Stenosis — *see also* Stricture — *continued*
  endocervical os — *see* Stenosis, cervix
  enterostomy 569.62
  esophagostomy 530.87 ●
  esophagus 530.3
    congenital 750.3
    syphilitic 095.8
      congenital 090.5
  external ear canal 380.50
    secondary to
      inflammation 380.53
      surgery 380.52
      trauma 380.51
  gallbladder (*see also* Obstruction, gallbladder) 575.2
  glottis 478.74
  heart valve (acquired) — *see also* Endocarditis
    congenital NEC 746.89
      aortic 746.3
      mitral 746.5
      pulmonary 746.02
      tricuspid 746.1
  hepatic duct (*see also* Obstruction, biliary) 576.2
  hymen 623.3
  hypertrophic subaortic (idiopathic) 425.1
  infundibulum cardiac 746.83
  intestine (*see also* Obstruction, intestine) 560.9
    congenital (small) 751.1
      large 751.2
  lacrimal
    canaliculi 375.53
    duct 375.56
      congenital 743.65
    punctum 375.52
      congenital 743.65
    sac 375.54
      congenital 743.65
  lacrimonasal duct 375.56
    congenital 743.65
    neonatal 375.55
  larynx 478.74
    congenital 748.3
    syphilitic 095.8
      congenital 090.5
  mitral (valve) (chronic) (inactive) 394.0
    with
      aortic (valve)
        disease (insufficiency) 396.1
        insufficiency or incompetence 396.1
        stenosis or obstruction 396.0
      incompetency, insufficiency or regurgitation 394.2
        with aortic valve disease 396.8
    active or acute 391.1
      with chorea (acute) (rheumatic) (Sydenham's) 392.0
    congenital 746.5
    specified cause, except rheumatic 424.0
    syphilitic 093.21
  myocardium, myocardial (*see also* Degeneration, myocardial) 429.1
    hypertrophic subaortic (idiopathic) 425.1
  nares (anterior) (posterior) 478.1
    congenital 748.0
  nasal duct 375.56
    congenital 743.65
  nasolacrimal duct 375.56
    congenital 743.65
    neonatal 375.55
  organ or site, congenital NEC — *see* Atresia
  papilla of Vater 576.2
    with calculus, cholelithiasis, or stones — *see* Choledocholithiasis
  pulmonary (artery) (congenital) 747.3
    with ventricular septal defect, dextraposition of aorta and hypertrophy of right ventricle 745.2
    acquired 417.8
    infundibular 746.83
    in tetralogy of Fallot 745.2
    subvalvular 746.83
    valve (*see also* Endocarditis, pulmonary) 424.3
      congenital 746.02
    vein 747.49
      acquired 417.8

Stenosis — *see also* Stricture — *continued*
  pulmonary — *continued*
    vessel NEC 417.8
  pulmonic (congenital) 746.02
    infundibular 746.83
    subvalvular 746.83
  pylorus (hypertrophic) 537.0
    adult 537.0
    congenital 750.5
    infantile 750.5
  rectum (sphincter) (*see also* Stricture, rectum) 569.2
  renal artery 440.1
  salivary duct (any) 527.8
  sphincter of Oddi (*see also* Obstruction, biliary) 576.2
  spinal 724.00
    cervical 723.0
    lumbar, lumbosacral 724.02
    nerve (root) NEC 724.9
    specified region NEC 724.09
    thoracic, thoracolumbar 724.01
  stomach, hourglass 537.6
  subaortic 746.81
    hypertrophic (idiopathic) 425.1
  supra (valvular)-aortic 747.22
  trachea 519.1
    congenital 748.3
    syphilitic 095.8
    tuberculous (*see also* Tuberculosis) 012.8 ☑
  tracheostomy 519.02
  tricuspid (valve) (*see also* Endocarditis, tricuspid) 397.0
    congenital 746.1
    nonrheumatic 424.2
  tubal 628.2
  ureter (*see also* Stricture, ureter) 593.3
    congenital 753.29
  urethra (*see also* Stricture, urethra) 598.9
  vagina 623.2
    congenital 752.49
    in pregnancy or childbirth 654.7 ☑
      affecting fetus or newborn 763.89
      causing obstructed labor 660.2 ☑
        affecting fetus or newborn 763.1
  valve (cardiac) (heart) (*see also* Endocarditis) 424.90
    congenital NEC 746.89
      aortic 746.3
      mitral 746.5
      pulmonary 746.02
      tricuspid 746.1
      urethra 753.6
  valvular (*see also* Endocarditis) 424.90
    congenital NEC 746.89
    urethra 753.6
  vascular graft or shunt 996.1
    atherosclerosis — *see* Arteriosclerosis, extremitites
    embolism 996.74
    occlusion NEC 996.74
    thrombus 996.74
  vena cava (inferior) (superior) 459.2
    congenital 747.49
  ventricular shunt 996.2
  vulva 624.8

Stercolith (*see also* Fecalith) 560.39
  appendix 543.9

Stercoraceous, stercoral ulcer 569.82
  anus or rectum 569.41

Stereopsis, defective
  with fusion 368.33
  without fusion 368.32

Stereotypes NEC 307.3

Sterility
  female — *see* Infertility, female
  male (*see also* Infertility, male) 606.9

Sterilization, admission for V25.2
  status
    tubal ligation V26.51
    vasectomy V26.52

Sternalgia (*see also* Angina) 413.9

Sternopagus 759.4

Sternum bifidum 756.3

Sternutation 784.9

Steroid
  effects (adverse) (iatrogenic)
    cushingoid
      correct substance properly administered 255.0
      overdose or wrong substance given or taken 962.0
    diabetes
      correct substance properly administered 251.8
      overdose or wrong substance given or taken 962.0
    due to
      correct substance properly administered 255.8
      overdose or wrong substance given or taken 962.0
    fever
      correct substance properly administered 780.6
      overdose or wrong substance given or taken 962.0
    withdrawal
      correct substance properly administered 255.4
      overdose or wrong substance given or taken 962.0
  responder 365.03

Stevens-Johnson disease or syndrome (erythema multiforme exudativum) 695.1

Stewart-Morel syndrome (hyperostosis frontalis interna) 733.3

Sticker's disease (erythema infectiosum) 057.0

Sticky eye 372.03

Stieda's disease (calcification, knee joint) 726.62

Stiff
  back 724.8
  neck (*see also* Torticollis) 723.5

Stiff-baby 759.89 ●

Stiff-man syndrome 333.91

Stiffness, joint NEC 719.50
  ankle 719.57
  back 724.8
  elbow 719.52
  finger 719.54
  hip 719.55
  knee 719.56
  multiple sites 719.59
  sacroiliac 724.6
  shoulder 719.51
  specified site NEC 719.58
  spine 724.9
  surgical fusion V45.4
  wrist 719.53

Stigmata, congenital syphilis 090.5

Still's disease or syndrome 714.30

Still-Felty syndrome (rheumatoid arthritis with splenomegaly and leukopenia) 714.1

Stillbirth, stillborn NEC 779.9

Stiller's disease (asthenia) 780.79

Stilling-Türk-Duane syndrome (ocular retraction syndrome) 378.71

Stimulation, ovary 256.1

Sting (animal) (bee) (fish) (insect) (jellyfish) (Portuguese man-o-war) (wasp) (venomous) 989.5
  anaphylactic shock or reaction 989.5
  plant 692.6

Stippled epiphyses 756.59

Stitch
  abscess 998.59
  burst (in external operation wound) 998.32
    internal 998.31
  in back 724.5

Stojano's (subcostal) **syndrome** 098.86

Stokes' disease (exophthalmic goiter) 242.0 ☑

Stokes-Adams syndrome (syncope with heart block) 426.9

Stokvis' (-Talma) disease (enterogenous cyanosis) 289.7

Stomach — *see* condition

☑ Additional Digit Required   ►◄ Revised Text   ● New Line   ▲ Revised Code

Stoma malfunction
  colostomy 569.62
  cystostomy 997.5
  enterostomy 569.62
  esophagostomy 530.87
  gastrostomy 536.42
  ileostomy 569.62
  nephrostomy 997.5
  tracheostomy 519.02
  ureterostomy 997.5
Stomatitis 528.0
  angular 528.5
    due to dietary or vitamin deficiency 266.0
  aphthous 528.2
  candidal 112.0
  catarrhal 528.0
  denture 528.9
  diphtheritic (membranous) 032.0
  due to
    dietary deficiency 266.0
    thrush 112.0
    vitamin deficiency 266.0
  epidemic 078.4
  epizootic 078.4
  follicular 528.0
  gangrenous 528.1
  herpetic 054.2
  herpetiformis 528.2
  malignant 528.0
  membranous acute 528.0
  monilial 112.0
  mycotic 112.0
  necrotic 528.1
    ulcerative 101
  necrotizing ulcerative 101
  parasitic 112.0
  septic 528.0
  spirochetal 101
  suppurative (acute) 528.0
  ulcerative 528.0
    necrotizing 101
  ulceromembranous 101
  vesicular 528.0
    with exanthem 074.3
  Vincent's 101
Stomatocytosis 282.8
Stomatomycosis 112.0
Stomatorrhagia 528.9
Stone(s) — see also Calculus
  bladder 594.1
    diverticulum 594.0
  cystine 270.0
  heart syndrome (see also Failure, ventricular, left) 428.1
  kidney 592.0
  prostate 602.0
  pulp (dental) 522.2
  renal 592.0
  salivary duct or gland (any) 527.5
  ureter 592.1
  urethra (impacted) 594.2
  urinary (duct) (impacted) (passage) 592.9
    bladder 594.1
      diverticulum 594.0
    lower tract NEC 594.9
    specified site 594.8
  xanthine 277.2
Stonecutters' lung 502
  tuberculous (see also Tuberculosis) 011.4 ☑
Stonemasons'
  asthma, disease, or lung 502
    tuberculous (see also Tuberculosis) 011.4 ☑
  phthisis (see also Tuberculosis) 011.4 ☑
Stoppage
  bowel (see also Obstruction, intestine) 560.9
  heart (see also Arrest, cardiac) 427.5
  intestine (see also Obstruction, intestine) 560.9
  urine NEC (see also Retention, urine) 788.20
Storm, thyroid (apathetic) (see also Thyrotoxicosis) 242.9 ☑
Strabismus (alternating) (congenital) (nonparalytic) 378.9
  concomitant (see also Heterotropia) 378.30
    convergent (see also Esotropia) 378.00
    divergent (see also Exotropia) 378.10

Strabismus — continued
  convergent (see also Esotropia) 378.00
  divergent (see also Exotropia) 378.10
  due to adhesions, scars — see Strabismus, mechanical
  in neuromuscular disorder NEC 378.73
    intermittent 378.20
      vertical 378.31
  latent 378.40
    convergent (esophoria) 378.41
    divergent (exophoria) 378.42
    vertical 378.43
  mechanical 378.60
    due to
      Brown's tendon sheath syndrome 378.61
      specified musculofascial disorder NEC 378.62
  paralytic 378.50
    third or oculomotor nerve (partial) 378.51
      total 378.52
    fourth or trochlear nerve 378.53
    sixth or abducens nerve 378.54
  specified type NEC 378.73
  vertical (hypertropia) 378.31
Strain — see also Sprain, by site
  eye NEC 368.13
  heart — see Disease, heart
  meaning gonorrhea — see Gonorrhea
  physical NEC V62.89
  postural 729.9
  psychological NEC V62.89
Strands
  conjunctiva 372.62
  vitreous humor 379.25
Strangulation, strangulated 994.7
  appendix 543.9
  asphyxiation or suffocation by 994.7
  bladder neck 596.0
  bowel — see Strangulation, intestine
  colon — see Strangulation, intestine
  cord (umbilical) — see Compression, umbilical cord
  due to birth injury 767.8
  food or foreign body (see also Asphyxia, food) 933.1
  hemorrhoids 455.8
    external 455.5
    internal 455.2
  hernia — see also Hernia, by site, with obstruction
    gangrenous — see Hernia, by site, with gangrene
  intestine (large) (small) 560.2
    with hernia — see also Hernia, by site, with obstruction
      gangrenous — see Hernia, by site, with gangrene
    congenital (small) 751.1
      large 751.2
  mesentery 560.2
  mucus (see also Asphyxia, mucus) 933.1
    newborn 770.1
  omentum 560.2
  organ or site, congenital NEC — see Atresia
  ovary 620.8
    due to hernia 620.4
  penis 607.89
    foreign body 939.3
  rupture (see also Hernia, by site, with obstruction) 552.9
    gangrenous (see also Hernia, by site, with gangrene) 551.9
  stomach, due to hernia (see also Hernia, by site, with obstruction) 552.9
    with gangrene (see also Hernia, by site, with gangrene) 551.9
  umbilical cord — see Compression, umbilical cord
  vesicourethral orifice 596.0
Strangury 788.1
Strawberry
  gallbladder (see also Disease, gallbladder) 575.6
  mark 757.32
  tongue (red) (white) 529.3
Straw itch 133.8
Streak, ovarian 752.0

Strephosymbolia 315.01
  secondary to organic lesion 784.69
Streptobacillary fever 026.1
Streptobacillus moniliformis 026.1
Streptococcemia 038.0
Streptococcicosis — see Infection, streptococcal
Streptococcus, streptococcal — see condition
Streptoderma 686.00
Streptomycosis — see Actinomycosis
Streptothricosis — see Actinomycosis
Streptothrix — see Actinomycosis
Streptotrichosis — see Actinomycosis
Stress
  fracture — see Fracture, stress
  polycythemia 289.0
  reaction (gross) (see also Reaction, stress, acute) 308.9
Stretching, nerve — see Injury, nerve, by site
Striae (albicantes) (atrophicae) (cutis distensae) (distensae) 701.3
Striations of nails 703.8
Stricture (see also Stenosis) 799.89
  ampulla of Vater 576.2
    with calculus, cholelithiasis, or stones — see Choledocholithiasis
  anus (sphincter) 569.2
    congenital 751.2
    infantile 751.2
  aorta (ascending) 747.22
    arch 747.10
    arteriosclerotic 440.0
    calcified 440.0
  aortic (valve) (see also Stenosis, aortic) 424.1
    congenital 746.3
  aqueduct of Sylvius (congenital) 742.3
    with spina bifida (see also Spina bifida) 741.0 ☑
    acquired 331.4
  artery 447.1
    basilar — see Narrowing, artery, basilar
    carotid (common) (internal) — see Narrowing, artery, carotid
    celiac 447.4
    cerebral 437.0
      congenital 747.81
      due to
        embolism (see also Embolism, brain) 434.1 ☑
        thrombus (see also Thrombosis, brain) 434.0 ☑
    congenital (peripheral) 747.60
      cerebral 747.81
      coronary 746.85
      gastrointestinal 747.61
      lower limb 747.64
      renal 747.62
      retinal 743.58
      specified NEC 747.69
      spinal 747.82
      umbilical 747.5
      upper limb 747.63
    coronary — see Arteriosclerosis, coronary
      congenital 746.85
    precerebral — see Narrowing, artery, precerebral NEC
    pulmonary (congenital) 747.3
      acquired 417.8
    renal 440.1
    vertebral — see Narrowing, artery, vertebral
  auditory canal (congenital) (external) 744.02
    acquired (see also Stricture, ear canal, acquired) 380.50
  bile duct or passage (any) (postoperative) (see also Obstruction, biliary) 576.2
    congenital 751.61
  bladder 596.8
    congenital 753.6
    neck 596.0
      congenital 753.6
  bowel (see also Obstruction, intestine) 560.9
  brain 348.8
  bronchus 519.1
    syphilitic 095.8

Stricture (*see also* Stenosis) — *continued*
  cardia (stomach) 537.89
    congenital 750.7
  cardiac — *see also* Disease, heart
    orifice (stomach) 537.89
  cardiovascular (*see also* Disease,
    cardiovascular) 429.2
  carotid artery — *see* Narrowing, artery, carotid
  cecum (*see also* Obstruction, intestine) 560.9
  cervix, cervical (canal) 622.4
    congenital 752.49
    in pregnancy or childbirth 654.6 ☑
      affecting fetus or newborn 763.89
      causing obstructed labor 660.2 ☑
        affecting fetus or newborn 763.1
  colon (*see also* Obstruction, intestine) 560.9
    congenital 751.2
  colostomy 569.62
  common bile duct (*see also* Obstruction,
    biliary) 576.2
    congenital 751.61
  coronary (artery) — *see* Arteriosclerosis,
    coronary
    congenital 746.85
  cystic duct (*see also* Obstruction, gallbladder)
    575.2
    congenital 751.61
  cystostomy 997.5
  digestive organs NEC, congenital 751.8
  duodenum 537.3
    congenital 751.1
  ear canal (external) (congenital) 744.02
    acquired 380.50
      secondary to
        inflammation 380.53
        surgery 380.52
        trauma 380.51
  ejaculatory duct 608.85
  enterostomy 569.62
  esophagostomy 530.87   ●
  esophagus (corrosive) (peptic) 530.3
    congenital 750.3
    syphilitic 095.8
      congenital 090.5
  eustachian tube (*see also* Obstruction,
    Eustachian tube) 381.60
    congenital 744.24
  fallopian tube 628.2
    gonococcal (chronic) 098.37
      acute 098.17
    tuberculous (*see also* Tuberculosis) 016.6 ☑
  gallbladder (*see also* Obstruction, gallbladder)
    575.2
    congenital 751.69
  glottis 478.74
  heart — *see also* Disease, heart
    congenital NEC 746.89
    valve — *see also* Endocarditis
      congenital NEC 746.89
        aortic 746.3
        mitral 746.5
        pulmonary 746.02
        tricuspid 746.1
  hepatic duct (*see also* Obstruction, biliary)
    576.2
  hourglass, of stomach 537.6
  hymen 623.3
  hypopharynx 478.29
  intestine (*see also* Obstruction, intestine) 560.9
    congenital (small) 751.1
      large 751.2
    ischemic 557.1
  lacrimal
    canaliculi 375.53
      congenital 743.65
    punctum 375.52
      congenital 743.65
    sac 375.54
      congenital 743.65
  lacrimonasal duct 375.56
    congenital 743.65
    neonatal 375.55
  larynx 478.79
    congenital 748.3
    syphilitic 095.8
      congenital 090.5
  lung 518.89

Stricture (*see also* Stenosis) — *continued*
  meatus
    ear (congenital) 744.02
      acquired (*see also* Stricture, ear canal,
        acquired) 380.50
      osseous (congenital) (ear) 744.03
        acquired (*see also* Stricture, ear canal,
          acquired) 380.50
    urinarius (*see also* Stricture, urethra) 598.9
      congenital 753.6
  mitral (valve) (*see also* Stenosis, mitral) 394.0
    congenital 746.5
    specified cause, except rheumatic 424.0
  myocardium, myocardial (*see also*
    Degeneration, myocardial) 429.1
    hypertrophic subaortic (idiopathic) 425.1
  nares (anterior) (posterior) 478.1
    congenital 748.0
  nasal duct 375.56
    congenital 743.65
    neonatal 375.55
  nasolacrimal duct 375.56
    congenital 743.65
    neonatal 375.55
  nasopharynx 478.29
    syphilitic 095.8
  nephrostomy 997.5
  nose 478.1
    congenital 748.0
  nostril (anterior) (posterior) 478.1
    congenital 748.0
  organ or site, congenital NEC — *see* Atresia
  osseous meatus (congenital) (ear) 744.03
    acquired (*see also* Stricture, ear canal,
      acquired) 380.50
  os uteri (*see also* Stricture, cervix) 622.4
  oviduct — *see* Stricture, fallopian tube
  pelviureteric junction 593.3
  pharynx (dilation) 478.29
  prostate 602.8
  pulmonary, pulmonic
    artery (congenital) 747.3
      acquired 417.8
      noncongenital 417.8
    infundibulum (congenital) 746.83
    valve (*see also* Endocarditis, pulmonary)
      424.3
      congenital 746.02
    vein (congenital) 747.49
      acquired 417.8
    vessel NEC 417.8
  punctum lacrimale 375.52
    congenital 743.65
  pylorus (hypertrophic) 537.0
    adult 537.0
    congenital 750.5
    infantile 750.5
  rectosigmoid 569.89
  rectum (sphincter) 569.2
    congenital 751.2
    due to
      chemical burn 947.3
      irradiation 569.2
      lymphogranuloma venereum 099.1
    gonococcal 098.7
    inflammatory 099.1
    syphilitic 095.8
    tuberculous (*see also* Tuberculosis) 014.8 ☑
  renal artery 440.1
  salivary duct or gland (any) 527.8
  sigmoid (flexure) (*see also* Obstruction,
    intestine) 560.9
  spermatic cord 608.85
  stoma (following) (of)
    colostomy 569.62
    cystostomy 997.5
    enterostomy 569.62
    esophagostomy 530.87   ●
    gastrostomy 536.42
    ileostomy 569.62
    nephrostomy 997.5
    tracheostomy 519.02
    ureterostomy 997.5
  stomach 537.89
    congenital 750.7
    hourglass 537.6

Stricture (*see also* Stenosis) — *continued*
  subaortic 746.81
    hypertrophic (acquired) (idiopathic) 425.1
  subglottic 478.74
  syphilitic NEC 095.8
  tendon (sheath) 727.81
  trachea 519.1
    congenital 748.3
    syphilitic 095.8
    tuberculous (*see also* Tuberculosis) 012.8 ☑
  tracheostomy 519.02
  tricuspid (valve) (*see also* Endocarditis,
    tricuspid) 397.0
    congenital 746.1
    nonrheumatic 424.2
  tunica vaginalis 608.85
  ureter (postoperative) 593.3
    congenital 753.29
    tuberculous (*see also* Tuberculosis) 016.2 ☑
  ureteropelvic junction 593.3
    congenital 753.21
  ureterovesical orifice 593.3
    congenital 753.22
  urethra (anterior) (meatal) (organic) (posterior)
    (spasmodic) 598.9
    associated with schistosomiasis (*see also*
      Schistosomiasis) 120.9 *[598.01]*
    congenital (valvular) 753.6
    due to
      infection 598.00
        syphilis 095.8 *[598.01]*
      trauma 598.1
    gonococcal 098.2 *[598.01]*
    gonorrheal 098.2 *[598.01]*
    infective 598.00
    late effect of injury 598.1
    postcatheterization 598.2
    postobstetric 598.1
    postoperative 598.2
    specified cause NEC 598.8
    syphilitic 095.8 *[598.01]*
    traumatic 598.1
    valvular, congenital 753.6
  urinary meatus (*see also* Stricture, urethra)
    598.9
    congenital 753.6
  uterus, uterine 621.5
    os (external) (internal) — *see* Stricture,
      cervix
  vagina (outlet) 623.2
    congenital 752.49
  valve (cardiac) (heart) (*see also* Endocarditis)
    424.90
    congenital (cardiac) (heart) NEC 746.89
      aortic 746.3
      mitral 746.5
      pulmonary 746.02
      tricuspid 746.1
      urethra 753.6
  valvular (*see also* Endocarditis) 424.90
  vascular graft or shunt 996.1
    atherosclerosis — *see* Arteriosclersis,
      extremities
    embolism 996.74
    occlusion NEC 996.74
    thrombus 996.74
  vas deferens 608.85
    congenital 752.89
  vein 459.2
  vena cava (inferior) (superior) NEC 459.2
    congenital 747.49
  ventricular shunt 996.2
  vesicourethral orifice 596.0
    congenital 753.6
  vulva (acquired) 624.8

Stridor 786.1
  congenital (larynx) 748.3

Stridulous — *see* condition

Strippling of nails 703.8

Stroke 434.91   ▲
  apoplectic (*see also* Disease, cerebrovascular,
    acute) 436
  brain ▶— *see* Infarct, brain◀
  embolic 434.11   ●
  epileptic — *see* Epilepsy
  healed or old V12.59

Stricture — Stroke

☑ Additional Digit Required   ▶◀ Revised Text   ● New Line   ▲ Revised Code

Stroke — *continued*
  heart — *see* Disease, heart
  heat 992.0
  iatrogenic 997.02
  in evolution 435.9
  ischemic 434.91   ●
  late effect — *see* Late effect(s) (of)
    cerebrovascular disease
  lightning 994.0
  paralytic ▶— *see* Infarct, brain◀
  postoperative 997.02
  progressive 435.9
  thrombotic 434.01   ●
Stromatosis, endometrial (M8931/1) 236.0
Strong pulse 785.9
Strongyloides stercoralis infestation 127.2
Strongyloidiasis 127.2
Strongyloidosis 127.2
Strongylus (gibsoni) infestation 127.7
Strophulus (newborn) 779.89
  pruriginosus 698.2
Struck by lightning 994.0
Struma (*see also* Goiter) 240.9
  fibrosa 245.3
  Hashimoto (struma lymphomatosa) 245.2
  lymphomatosa 245.2
  nodosa (simplex) 241.9
    endemic 241.9
    multinodular 241.1
    sporadic 241.9
    toxic or with hyperthyroidism 242.3 ☑
      multinodular 242.2 ☑
      uninodular 242.1 ☑
    toxicosa 242.3 ☑
      multinodular 242.2 ☑
      uninodular 242.1 ☑
    uninodular 241.0
  ovarii (M9090/0) 220
    and carcinoid (M9091/1) 236.2
    malignant (M9090/3) 183.0
  Riedel's (ligneous thyroiditis) 245.3
  scrofulous (*see also* Tuberculosis) 017.2 ☑
  tuberculous (*see also* Tuberculosis) 017.2 ☑
    abscess 017.2 ☑
    adenitis 017.2 ☑
    lymphangitis 017.2 ☑
    ulcer 017.2 ☑
Strumipriva cachexia (*see also* Hypothyroidism)
  244.9
Strümpell-Marie disease or spine (ankylosing
  spondylitis) 720.0
Strümpell-Westphal pseudosclerosis
  (hepatolenticular degeneration) 275.1
Stuart's disease (congenital factor X deficiency)
  (*see also* Defect, coagulation) 286.3
Stuart-Prower factor deficiency (congenital
  factor X deficiency) (*see also* Defect,
  coagulation) 286.3
Students' elbow 727.2
Stuffy nose 478.1
Stump — *see also* Amputation
  cervix, cervical (healed) 622.8
Stupor 780.09
  catatonic (*see also* Schizophrenia) 295.2 ☑
  circular (*see also* Psychosis, manic-depressive,
    circular) 296.7
  manic 296.89
  manic-depressive (*see also* Psychosis, affective)
    296.89
  mental (anergic) (delusional) 298.9
  psychogenic 298.8
  reaction to exceptional stress (transient) 308.2
  traumatic NEC — *see also* Injury, intracranial
    with spinal (cord)
      lesion — *see* Injury, spinal, by site
      shock — *see* Injury, spinal, by site
Sturge (-Weber) (-Dimitri) disease or syndrome
  (encephalocutan-eous angiomatosis) 759.6
Sturge-Kalischer-Weber syndrome
  (encephalocutaneous angiomatosis) 759.6
Stuttering 307.0

Sty, stye 373.11
  external 373.11
  internal 373.12
  meibomian 373.12
Subacidity, gastric 536.8
  psychogenic 306.4
Subacute — *see* condition
Subarachnoid — *see* condition
Subclavian steal syndrome 435.2
Subcortical — *see* condition
Subcostal syndrome 098.86
  nerve compression 354.8
Subcutaneous, subcuticular — *see* condition
Subdelirium 293.1
Subdural — *see* condition
Subendocardium — *see* condition
Subependymoma (M9383/1) 237.5
Suberosis 495.3
Subglossitis — *see* Glossitis
Subhemophilia 286.0
Subinvolution (uterus) 621.1
  breast (postlactational) (postpartum) 611.8
  chronic 621.1
  puerperal, postpartum 674.8 ☑
Sublingual — *see* condition
Sublinguitis 527.2
Subluxation — *see also* Dislocation, by site
  congenital NEC — *see also* Malposition,
    congenital
    hip (unilateral) 754.32
      with dislocation of other hip 754.35
      bilateral 754.33
    joint
      lower limb 755.69
      shoulder 755.59
      upper limb 755.59
    lower limb (joint) 755.69
    shoulder (joint) 755.59
    upper limb (joint) 755.59
  lens 379.32
    anterior 379.33
    posterior 379.34
  rotary, cervical region of spine — *see* Fracture,
    vertebra, cervical
Submaxillary — *see* condition
Submersion (fatal) (nonfatal) 994.1
Submissiveness (undue), in child 313.0
Submucous — *see* condition
Subnormal, subnormality
  accommodation (*see also* Disorder,
    accommodation) 367.9
  mental (*see also* Retardation, mental) 319
    mild 317
    moderate 318.0
    profound 318.2
    severe 318.1
  temperature (accidental) 991.6
    not associated with low environmental
      temperature 780.99
Subphrenic — *see* condition
Subscapular nerve — *see* condition
Subseptus uterus 752.3
Subsiding appendicitis 542
Substernal thyroid (*see also* Goiter) 240.9
  congenital 759.2
Substitution disorder 300.11
Subtentorial — *see* condition
Subtertian
  fever 084.0
  malaria (fever) 084.0
Subthyroidism (acquired) (*see also*
  Hypothyroidism) 244.9
  congenital 243
Succenturiata placenta — *see* Placenta,
  abnormal
Succussion sounds, chest 786.7
Sucking thumb, child 307.9
Sudamen 705.1
Sudamina 705.1
Sudanese kala-azar 085.0

Sudden
  death, cause unknown (less than 24 hours)
    798.1
    during childbirth 669.9 ☑
    infant 798.0
    puerperal, postpartum 674.9 ☑
  hearing loss NEC 388.2
  heart failure (*see also* Failure, heart) 428.9
  infant death syndrome 798.0
Sudeck's atrophy, disease, or syndrome 733.7
SUDS (sudden unexplained death) 798.2
Suffocation (*see also* Asphyxia) 799.0
  by
    bed clothes 994.7
    bunny bag 994.7
    cave-in 994.7
    constriction 994.7
    drowning 994.1
    inhalation
      food or foreign body (*see also* Asphyxia,
        food or foreign body) 933.1
      oil or gasoline (*see also* Asphyxia, food or
        foreign body) 933.1
    overlying 994.7
    plastic bag 994.7
    pressure 994.7
    strangulation 994.7
  during birth 768.1
  mechanical 994.7
Sugar
  blood
    high 790.29
    low 251.2
  in urine 791.5
Suicide, suicidal (attempted)
  by poisoning — *see* Table of Drugs and
    Chemicals
  risk 300.9
  tendencies 300.9
  trauma NEC (*see also* nature and site of injury)
    959.9
Suipestifer infection (*see also* Infection,
  Salmonella) 003.9
Sulfatidosis 330.0
Sulfhemoglobinemia, sulphemoglobinemia
  (acquired) (congenital) 289.7
Sumatran mite fever 081.2
Summer — *see* condition
Sunburn 692.71
  dermatitis 692.71
  due to
    other ultraviolet radiation 692.82
    tanning bed 692.82
  first degree 692.71
  second degree 692.76
  third degree 692.77
Sunken
  acetabulum 718.85
  fontanels 756.0
Sunstroke 992.0
Superfecundation 651.9 ☑
  with fetal loss and retention of one or more
    fetus(es) 651.6 ☑
Superfetation 651.9 ☑
  with fetal loss and retention of one or more
    fetus(es) 651.6 ☑
Superinvolution uterus 621.8
Supernumerary (congenital)
  aortic cusps 746.89
  auditory ossicles 744.04
  bone 756.9
  breast 757.6
  carpal bones 755.56
  cusps, heart valve NEC 746.89
    mitral 746.5
    pulmonary 746.09
  digit(s) 755.00
    finger 755.01
    toe 755.02
  ear (lobule) 744.1
  fallopian tube 752.19
  finger 755.01
  hymen 752.49
  kidney 753.3

Supernumerary — *continued*
  lacrimal glands 743.64
  lacrimonasal duct 743.65
  lobule (ear) 744.1
  mitral cusps 746.5
  muscle 756.82
  nipples 757.6
  organ or site NEC — *see* Accessory
  ossicles, auditory 744.04
  ovary 752.0
  oviduct 752.19
  pulmonic cusps 746.09
  rib 756.3
    cervical or first 756.2
      syndrome 756.2
  roots (of teeth) 520.2
  spinal vertebra 756.19
  spleen 759.0
  tarsal bones 755.67
  teeth 520.1
    causing crowding 524.31   ▲
  testis 752.89
  thumb 755.01
  toe 755.02
  uterus 752.2
  vagina 752.49
  vertebra 756.19
Supervision (of)
  contraceptive method previously prescribed
      V25.40
    intrauterine device V25.42
    oral contraceptive (pill) V25.41
    specified type NEC V25.49
    subdermal implantable contraceptive V25.43
  dietary (for) V65.3
    allergy (food) V65.3
    colitis V65.3
    diabetes mellitus V65.3
    food allergy intolerance V65.3
    gastritis V65.3
    hypercholesterolemia V65.3
    hypoglycemia V65.3
    intolerance (food) V65.3
    obesity V65.3
    specified NEC V65.3
  lactation V24.1
  pregnancy — *see* Pregnancy, supervision of
Supplemental teeth 520.1
  causing crowding 524.31   ▲
Suppression
  binocular vision 368.31
  lactation 676.5 ☑
  menstruation 626.8
  ovarian secretion 256.39
  renal 586
  urinary secretion 788.5
  urine 788.5
Suppuration, suppurative — *see also* condition
  accessory sinus (chronic) (*see also* Sinusitis)
      473.9
  adrenal gland 255.8
  antrum (chronic) (*see also* Sinusitis, maxillary)
      473.0
  bladder (*see also* Cystitis) 595.89
  bowel 569.89
  brain 324.0
    late effect 326
  breast 611.0
    puerperal, postpartum 675.1 ☑
  dental periosteum 526.5
  diffuse (skin) 686.00
  ear (middle) (*see also* Otitis media) 382.4
    external (*see also* Otitis, externa) 380.10
    internal 386.33
  ethmoidal (sinus) (chronic) (*see also* Sinusitis,
      ethmoidal) 473.2
  fallopian tube (*see also* Salpingo-oophoritis)
      614.2
  frontal (sinus) (chronic) (*see also* Sinusitis,
      frontal) 473.1
  gallbladder (*see also* Cholecystitis, acute) 575.0
  gum 523.3
  hernial sac — *see* Hernia, by site
  intestine 569.89
  joint (*see also* Arthritis, suppurative) 711.0 ☑
  labyrinthine 386.33

Suppuration, suppurative — *see also* condition
    — *continued*
  lung 513.0
  mammary gland 611.0
    puerperal, postpartum 675.1 ☑
  maxilla, maxillary 526.4
    sinus (chronic) (*see also* Sinusitis, maxillary)
      473.0
  muscle 728.0
  nasal sinus (chronic) (*see also* Sinusitis) 473.9
  pancreas 577.0
  parotid gland 527.2
  pelvis, pelvic
    female (*see also* Disease, pelvis,
      inflammatory) 614.4
      acute 614.3
    male (*see also* Peritonitis) 567.2
  pericranial (*see also* Osteomyelitis) 730.2 ☑
  salivary duct or gland (any) 527.2
  sinus (nasal) (*see also* Sinusitis) 473.9
  sphenoidal (sinus) (chronic) (*see also* Sinusitis,
      sphenoidal) 473.3
  thymus (gland) 254.1
  thyroid (gland) 245.0
  tonsil 474.8
  uterus (*see also* Endometritis) 615.9
  vagina 616.10
  wound — *see also* Wound, open, by site,
      complicated
    dislocation — *see* Dislocation, by site,
      compound
    fracture — *see* Fracture, by site, open
    scratch or other superficial injury — *see*
      Injury, superficial, by site
Supraeruption, teeth 524.34   ●
Supraglottitis 464.50
  with obstruction 464.51
Suprapubic drainage 596.8
Suprarenal (gland) — *see* condition
Suprascapular nerve — *see* condition
Suprasellar — *see* condition
Supraspinatus syndrome 726.10
Surfer knots 919.8
  infected 919.9
Surgery
  cosmetic NEC V50.1
    following healed injury or operation V51
    hair transplant V50.0
  elective V50.9
    breast augmentation or reduction V50.1
    circumcision, ritual or routine (in absence of
      medical indication) V50.2
    cosmetic NEC V50.1
    ear piercing V50.3
    face-lift V50.1
    following healed injury or operation V51
    hair transplant V50.0
  not done because of
    contraindication V64.1
    patient's decision V64.2
    specified reason NEC V64.3
  plastic
    breast augmentation or reduction V50.1
    cosmetic V50.1
    face-lift V50.1
    following healed injury or operation V51
    repair of scarred tissue (following healed
      injury or operation) V51
    specified type NEC V50.8
  previous, in pregnancy or childbirth
    cervix 654.6 ☑
      affecting fetus or newborn 763.89
      causing obstructed labor 660.2 ☑
        affecting fetus or newborn 763.1
    pelvic soft tissues NEC 654.9 ☑
      affecting fetus or newborn 763.89
      causing obstructed labor 660.2 ☑
        affecting fetus or newborn 763.1
    perineum or vulva 654.8 ☑
    uterus NEC 654.9 ☑
      affecting fetus or newborn 763.89
      causing obstructed labor 660.2 ☑
        affecting fetus or newborn 763.1
      due to previous cesarean delivery
        654.2 ☑
    vagina 654.7 ☑

Surgical
  abortion — *see* Abortion, legal
  emphysema 998.81
  kidney (*see also* Pyelitis) 590.80
  operation NEC 799.9
  procedures, complication or misadventure —
      see Complications, surgical procedure
  shock 998.0
Susceptibility   ●
  genetic   ●
    to   ●
      neoplasm   ●
        malignant, of   ●
          breast V84.01   ●
          endometrium V84.04   ●
          other V84.09   ●
          ovary V84.02   ●
          prostate V84.03   ●
      other disease V84.8   ●
Suspected condition, ruled out (*see also*
      Observation, suspected) V71.9
  specified condition NEC V71.89
Suspended uterus, in pregnancy or childbirth
      654.4 ☑
  affecting fetus or newborn 763.89
  causing obstructed labor 660.2 ☑
    affecting fetus or newborn 763.1
Sutton's disease 709.09
Sutton and Gull's disease (arteriolar
      nephrosclerosis) (*see also* Hypertension,
      kidney) 403.90
Suture
  burst (in external operation wound) 998.32
    internal 998.31
  inadvertently left in operation wound 998.4
  removal V58.3
  Shirodkar, in pregnancy (with or without
      cervical incompetence) 654.5 ☑
Swab inadvertently left in operation wound
      998.4
Swallowed, swallowing
  difficulty (*see also* Dysphagia) 787.2
  foreign body NEC (*see also* Foreign body) 938
Swamp fever 100.89
Swan neck hand (intrinsic) 736.09
Sweat(s), sweating
  disease or sickness 078.2
  excessive ▶(*see also* Hyperhidrosis)◀ 780.8
  fetid 705.89
  fever 078.2
  gland disease 705.9
    specified type NEC 705.89
  miliary 078.2
  night 780.8
Sweeley-Klionsky disease (angiokeratoma
      corporis diffusum) 272.7
Sweet's syndrome (acute febrile neutrophilic
      dermatosis) 695.89
Swelling
  abdominal (not referable to specific organ)
      789.3 ☑
  adrenal gland, cloudy 255.8
  ankle 719.07
  anus 787.99
  arm 729.81
  breast 611.72
  Calabar 125.2
  cervical gland 785.6
  cheek 784.2
  chest 786.6
  ear 388.8
  epigastric 789.3 ☑
  extremity (lower) (upper) 729.81
  eye 379.92
  female genital organ 625.8
  finger 729.81
  foot 729.81
  glands 785.6
  gum 784.2
  hand 729.81
  head 784.2
  inflammatory — *see* Inflammation
  joint (*see also* Effusion, joint) 719.0 ☑
    tuberculous — *see* Tuberculosis, joint

Swelling — *continued*
  kidney, cloudy 593.89
  leg 729.81
  limb 729.81
  liver 573.8
  lung 786.6
  lymph nodes 785.6
  mediastinal 786.6
  mouth 784.2
  muscle (limb) 729.81
  neck 784.2
  nose or sinus 784.2
  palate 784.2
  pelvis 789.3 ☑
  penis 607.83
  perineum 625.8
  rectum 787.99
  scrotum 608.86
  skin 782.2
  splenic (*see also* Splenomegaly) 789.2
  substernal 786.6
  superficial, localized (skin) 782.2
  testicle 608.86
  throat 784.2
  toe 729.81
  tongue 784.2
  tubular (*see also* Disease, renal) 593.9
  umbilicus 789.3 ☑
  uterus 625.8
  vagina 625.8
  vulva 625.8
  wandering, due to Gnathostoma (spinigerum) 128.1
  white — *see* Tuberculosis, arthritis
Swift's disease 985.0
Swimmers'
  ear (acute) 380.12
  itch 120.3
Swimming in the head 780.4
Swollen — *see also* Swelling
  glands 785.6
Swyer-James syndrome (unilateral hyperlucent lung) 492.8
Swyer's syndrome (XY pure gonadal dysgenesis) 752.7
Sycosis 704.8
  barbae (not parasitic) 704.8
  contagiosa 110.0
  lupoid 704.8
  mycotic 110.0
  parasitic 110.0
  vulgaris 704.8
Sydenham's chorea — *see* Chorea, Sydenham's
Sylvatic yellow fever 060.0
Sylvest's disease (epidemic pleurodynia) 074.1
Symblepharon 372.63
  congenital 743.62
Symonds' syndrome 348.2
Sympathetic — *see* condition
Sympatheticotonia (*see also* Neuropathy, peripheral, autonomic) 337.9
Sympathicoblastoma (M9500/3)
  specified site — *see* Neoplasm, by site, malignant
  unspecified site 194.0
Sympathicogonioma (M9500/3) — *see* Sympathicoblastoma
Sympathoblastoma (M9500/3) — *see* Sympathicoblastoma
Sympathogonioma (M9500/3) — *see* Sympathicoblastoma
Symphalangy (*see also* Syndactylism) 755.10
Symptoms, specified (general) NEC 780.99
  abdomen NEC 789.9
  bone NEC 733.90
  breast NEC 611.79
  cardiac NEC 785.9
  cardiovascular NEC 785.9
  chest NEC 786.9
  development NEC 783.9
  digestive system NEC 787.99
  eye NEC 379.99
  gastrointestinal tract NEC 787.99

Symptoms, specified NEC — *continued*
  genital organs NEC
    female 625.9
    male 608.9
  head and neck NEC 784.9
  heart NEC 785.9
  joint NEC 719.60
    ankle 719.67
    elbow 719.62
    foot 719.67
    hand 719.64
    hip 719.65
    knee 719.66
    multiple sites 719.69
    pelvic region 719.65
    shoulder (region) 719.61
    specified site NEC 719.68
    wrist 719.63
  larynx NEC 784.9
  limbs NEC 729.89
  lymphatic system NEC 785.9
  menopausal 627.2
  metabolism NEC 783.9
  mouth NEC 528.9
  muscle NEC 728.9
  musculoskeletal NEC 781.99
    limbs NEC 729.89
  nervous system NEC 781.99
  neurotic NEC 300.9
  nutrition, metabolism, and development NEC 783.9
  pelvis NEC 789.9
    female 625.9
  peritoneum NEC 789.9
  respiratory system NEC 786.9
  skin and integument NEC 782.9
  subcutaneous tissue NEC 782.9
  throat NEC 784.9
  tonsil NEC 784.9
  urinary system NEC 788.9
  vascular NEC 785.9
Sympus 759.89
Synarthrosis 719.80
  ankle 719.87
  elbow 719.82
  foot 719.87
  hand 719.84
  hip 719.85
  knee 719.86
  multiple sites 719.89
  pelvic region 719.85
  shoulder (region) 719.81
  specified site NEC 719.88
  wrist 719.83
Syncephalus 759.4
Synchondrosis 756.9
  abnormal (congenital) 756.9
  ischiopubic (van Neck's) 732.1
Synchysis (senile) (vitreous humor) 379.21
  scintillans 379.22
Syncope (near) (pre-) 780.2
  anginosa 413.9
  bradycardia 427.89
  cardiac 780.2
  carotid sinus 337.0
  complicating delivery 669.2 ☑
  due to lumbar puncture 349.0
  fatal 798.1
  heart 780.2
  heat 992.1
  laryngeal 786.2
  tussive 786.2
  vasoconstriction 780.2
  vasodepressor 780.2
  vasomotor 780.2
  vasovagal 780.2
Syncytial infarct — *see* Placenta, abnormal
Syndactylism, syndactyly (multiple sites) 755.10
  fingers (without fusion of bone) 755.11
    with fusion of bone 755.12
  toes (without fusion of bone) 755.13
    with fusion of bone 755.14
Syndrome — *see also* Disease
  abdominal
    acute 789.0 ☑

Syndrome — *see also* Disease — *continued*
  abdominal — *continued*
    migraine 346.2 ☑
    muscle deficiency 756.79
  Abercrombie's (amyloid degeneration) 277.3
  abnormal innervation 374.43
  abstinence
    alcohol 291.81
    drug 292.0
  Abt-Letterer-Siwe (acute histiocytosis X) (M9722/3) 202.5 ☑
  Achard-Thiers (adrenogenital) 255.2
  acid pulmonary aspiration 997.3
    obstetric (Mendelson's) 668.0 ☑
  acquired immune deficiency 042
  acquired immunodeficiency 042
  acrocephalosyndactylism 755.55
  acute abdominal 789.0 ☑
  acute chest 517.3
  acute coronary 411.1
  Adair-Dighton (brittle bones and blue sclera, deafness) 756.51
  Adams-Stokes (-Morgagni) (syncope with heart block) 426.9
  addisonian 255.4
  Adie (-Holmes) (pupil) 379.46
  adiposogenital 253.8
  adrenal
    hemorrhage 036.3
    meningococcic 036.3
  adrenocortical 255.3
  adrenogenital (acquired) (congenital) 255.2
    feminizing 255.2
    iatrogenic 760.79
    virilism (acquired) (congenital) 255.2
  affective organic NEC 293.89
    drug-induced 292.84
  afferent loop NEC 537.89
  African macroglobulinemia 273.3
  Ahumada-Del Castillo (nonpuerperal galactorrhea and amenorrhea) 253.1
  air blast concussion — *see* Injury, internal, by site
  Albright (-Martin) (pseudohypoparathyroidism) 275.49
  Albright-McCune-Sternberg (osteitis fibrosa disseminata) 756.59
  alcohol withdrawal 291.81
  Alder's (leukocyte granulation anomaly) 288.2
  Aldrich (-Wiskott) (eczema-thrombocytopenia) 279.12
  Alibert-Bazin (mycosis fungoides) (M9700/3) 202.1 ☑
  Alice in Wonderland 293.89
  Allen-Masters 620.6
  Alligator baby (ichthyosis congenita) 757.1
  Alport's (hereditary hematuria-nephropathy-deafness) 759.89
  Alvarez (transient cerebral ischemia) 435.9
  alveolar capillary block 516.3
  Alzheimer's 331.0
    with dementia — *see* Alzheimer's, dementia
  amnestic (confabulatory) 294.0
    ▶alcohol-induced persisting◀ 291.1
    drug-induced 292.83
    posttraumatic 294.0
  amotivational 292.89
  amyostatic 275.1
  amyotrophic lateral sclerosis 335.20
  Angelman 759.89
  angina (*see also* Angina) 413.9
  ankyloglossia superior 750.0
  anterior
    chest wall 786.52
    compartment (tibial) 958.8
    spinal artery 433.8 ☑
      compression 721.1
    tibial (compartment) 958.8
  antibody deficiency 279.00
    agammaglobulinemic 279.00
    congenital 279.04
    hypogammaglobulinemic 279.00
  anticardiolipin antibody 795.79
  antimongolism 758.39   ▲
  antiphospholipid antibody 795.79
  Anton (-Babinski) (hemiasomatognosia) 307.9

☑ Additional Digit Required   ▶◀ Revised Text   ● New Line   ▲ Revised Code

Syndrome — *see also* Disease — *continued*
  anxiety (*see also* Anxiety) 300.00
    organic 293.84
  aortic
    arch 446.7
    bifurcation (occlusion) 444.0
    ring 747.21
  Apert's (acrocephalosyndactyly) 755.55
  Apert-Gallais (adrenogenital) 255.2
  aphasia-apraxia-alexia 784.69
  "approximate answers" 300.16
  arcuate ligament (-celiac axis) 447.4
  arcus aortae 446.7
  arc-welders' 370.24
  argentaffin, argintaffinoma 259.2
  Argonz-Del Castillo (nonpuerperal galactorrhea
    and amenorrhea) 253.1
  Argyll Robertson's (syphilitic) 094.89
    nonsyphilitic 379.45
  arm-shoulder (*see also* Neuropathy, peripheral,
    autonomic) 337.9
  Arnold-Chiari (*see also* Spina bifida) 741.0 ☑
    type I 348.4
    type II 741.0 ☑
    type III 742.0
    type IV 742.2
  Arrillaga-Ayerza (pulmonary artery sclerosis
    with pulmonary hypertension) 416.0
  arteriomesenteric duodenum occlusion 537.89
  arteriovenous steal 996.73
  arteritis, young female (obliterative
    brachiocephalic) 446.7
  aseptic meningitis — *see* Meningitis, aseptic
  Asherman's 621.5
  Asperger's 299.8 ●
  asphyctic (*see also* Anxiety) 300.00
  aspiration, of newborn, massive or meconium
    770.1
  ataxia-telangiectasia 334.8
  Audry's (acropachyderma) 757.39
  auriculotemporal 350.8
  autosomal — *see also* Abnormal, autosomes
    NEC
    deletion 758.39 ▲
      5p 758.31 ●
      22q11.2 758.32 ●
  Avellis' 344.89
  Axenfeld's 743.44
  Ayerza (-Arrillaga) (pulmonary artery sclerosis
    with pulmonary hypertension) 416.0
  Baader's (erythema multiforme exudativum)
    695.1
  Baastrup's 721.5
  Babinski (-Vaquez) (cardiovascular syphilis)
    093.89
  Babinski-Fröhlich (adiposogenital dystrophy)
    253.8
  Babinski-Nageotte 344.89
  Bagratuni's (temporal arteritis) 446.5
  Bakwin-Krida (craniometaphyseal dysplasia)
    756.89
  Balint's (psychic paralysis of visual
    disorientation) 368.16
  Ballantyne (-Runge) (postmaturity) 766.22
  ballooning posterior leaflet 424.0
  Banti's — *see* Cirrhosis, liver
  Bard-Pic's (carcinoma, head of pancreas) 157.0
  Bardet-Biedl (obesity, polydactyly, and mental
    retardation) 759.89
  Barlow's (mitral valve prolapse) 424.0
  Barlow (-Möller) (infantile scurvy) 267
  Baron Munchausen's 301.51
  Barré-Guillain 357.0
  Barré-Liéou (posterior cervical sympathetic)
    723.2
  Barrett's (chronic peptic ulcer of esophagus)
    530.85
  Bársony-Polgár (corkscrew esophagus) 530.5
  Bársony-Teschendorf (corkscrew esophagus)
    530.5
  Bartter's (secondary hyperaldosteronism with
    juxtaglomerular hyperplasia) 255.13
  Basedow's (exophthalmic goiter) 242.0 ☑
  basilar artery 435.0
  basofrontal 377.04
  Bassen-Kornzweig (abetalipoproteinemia) 272.5
  Batten-Steinert 359.2

Syndrome — *see also* Disease — *continued*
  battered
    adult 995.81
    baby or child 995.54
    spouse 995.81
  Baumgarten-Cruveilhier (cirrhosis of liver)
    571.5
  Beals 759.82 ●
  Bearn-Kunkel (-Slater) (lupoid hepatitis) 571.49
  Beau's (*see also* Degeneration, myocardial)
    429.1
  Bechterew-Strümpell-Marie (ankylosing
    spondylitis) 720.0
  Beck's (anterior spinal artery occlusion)
    433.8 ☑
  Beckwith (-Wiedemann) 759.89
  Behçet's 136.1
  Bekhterev-Strümpell-Marie (ankylosing
    spondylitis) 720.0
  Benedikt's 344.89
  Béquez César (-Steinbrinck-Chédiak- Higashi)
    (congenital gigantism of peroxidase
    granules) 288.2
  Bernard-Horner (*see also* Neuropathy,
    peripheral, autonomic) 337.9
  Bernard-Sergent (acute adrenocortical
    insufficiency) 255.4
  Bernhardt-Roth 355.1
  Bernheim's (*see also* Failure, heart) 428.0
  Bertolotti's (sacralization of fifth lumbar
    vertebra) 756.15
  Besnier-Boeck-Schaumann (sarcoidosis) 135
  Bianchi's (aphasia-apraxia-alexia syndrome)
    784.69
  Biedl-Bardet (obesity, polydactyly, and mental
    retardation) 759.89
  Biemond's (obesity, polydactyly, and mental
    retardation) 759.89
  big spleen 289.4
  bilateral polycystic ovarian 256.4
  Bing-Horton's 346.2 ☑
  Biörck (-Thorson) (malignant carcinoid) 259.2
  Blackfan-Diamond (congenital hypoplastic
    anemia) 284.0
  black lung 500
  black widow spider bite 989.5
  bladder neck (*see also* Incontinence, urine)
    788.30
  blast (concussion) — *see* Blast, injury
  blind loop (postoperative) 579.2
  Bloch-Siemens (incontinentia pigmenti) 757.33
  Bloch-Sulzberger (incontinentia pigmenti)
    757.33
  Bloom (-Machacek) (-Torre) 757.39
  Blount-Barber (tibia vara) 732.4
  blue
    bloater 491.20
      with
        acute bronchitis 491.22 ●
        exacerbation (acute) 491.21 ●
    diaper 270.0
    drum 381.02
    sclera 756.51
    toe 445.02
  Boder-Sedgwick (ataxia-telangiectasia) 334.8
  Boerhaave's (spontaneous esophageal rupture)
    530.4
  Bonnevie-Ullrich 758.6
  Bonnier's 386.19
  Bouillaud's (rheumatic heart disease) 391.9
  Bourneville (-Pringle) (tuberous sclerosis) 759.5
  Bouveret (-Hoffmann) (paroxysmal tachycardia)
    427.2
  brachial plexus 353.0
  Brachman-de Lange (Amsterdam dwarf, mental
    retardation, and brachycephaly) 759.89
  bradycardia-tachycardia 427.81
  Brailsford-Morquio (dystrophy)
    (mucopolysaccharidosis IV) 277.5
  brain (acute) (chronic) (nonpsychotic) (organic)
    (with behavioral reaction) (with neurotic
    reaction) 310.9
    with
      presenile brain disease (*see also*
        Dementia, presenile) 290.10
      psychosis, psychotic reaction (*see also*
        Psychosis, organic) 294.9

Syndrome — *see also* Disease — *continued*
  brain — *continued*
    chronic alcoholic 291.2
    congenital (*see also* Retardation, mental)
      319
    postcontusional 310.2
    posttraumatic
      nonpsychotic 310.2
      psychotic 293.9
        acute 293.0
        chronic (*see also* Psychosis, organic)
          294.8
        subacute 293.1
    psycho-organic (*see also* Syndrome, psycho-
      organic) 310.9
    psychotic (*see also* Psychosis, organic) 294.9
    senile (*see also* Dementia, senile) 290.0
  branchial arch 744.41
  Brandt's (acrodermatitis enteropathica) 686.8
  Brennemann's 289.2
  Briquet's 300.81
  Brissaud-Meige (infantile myxedema) 244.9
  broad ligament laceration 620.6
  Brock's (atelectasis due to enlarged lymph
    nodes) 518.0
  Brown's tendon sheath 378.61
  Brown-Séquard 344.89
  brown spot 756.59
  Brugada 746.89
  Brugsch's (acropachyderma) 757.39
  bubbly lung 770.7
  Buchem's (hyperostosis corticalis) 733.3
  Budd-Chiari (hepatic vein thrombosis) 453.0
  Büdinger-Ludloff-Läwen 717.89
  bulbar 335.22
    lateral (*see also* Disease, cerebrovascular,
      acute) 436
  Bullis fever 082.8
  bundle of Kent (anomalous atrioventricular
    excitation) 426.7
  Bürger-Grütz (essential familial hyperlipemia)
    272.3
  Burke's (pancreatic insufficiency and chronic
    neutropenia) 577.8
  Burnett's (milk-alkali) 275.42
  Burnier's (hypophyseal dwarfism) 253.3
  burning feet 266.2
  Bywaters' 958.5
  Caffey's (infantile cortical hyperostosis) 756.59
  Calvé-Legg-Perthes (osteochondrosis, femoral
    capital) 732.1
  Caplan (-Colinet) syndrome 714.81
  capsular thrombosis (*see also* Thrombosis,
    brain) 434.0 ☑
  carcinogenic thrombophlebitis 453.1
  carcinoid 259.2
  cardiac asthma (*see also* Failure, ventricular,
    left) 428.1
  cardiacos negros 416.0
  cardiopulmonary obesity 278.8
  cardiorenal (*see also* Hypertension, cardiorenal)
    404.90
  cardiorespiratory distress (idiopathic), newborn
    769
  cardiovascular renal (*see also* Hypertension,
    cardiorenal) 404.90
  cardiovasorenal 272.7
  Carini's (ichthyosis congenita) 757.1
  carotid
    artery (internal) 435.8
    body or sinus 337.0
  carpal tunnel 354.0
  Carpenter's 759.89
  Cassidy (-Scholte) (malignant carcinoid) 259.2
  cat-cry 758.31 ▲
  cauda equina 344.60
  causalgia 355.9
    lower limb 355.71
    upper limb 354.4
  cavernous sinus 437.6
  celiac 579.0
    artery compression 447.4
    axis 447.4
  cerebellomedullary malformation (*see also*
    Spina bifida) 741.0 ☑
  cerebral gigantism 253.0
  cerebrohepatorenal 759.89

Syndrome (vertical text, right margin)

Syndrome — *see also* Disease — *continued*
  cervical (root) (spine) NEC 723.8
    disc 722.71
    posterior, sympathetic 723.2
    rib 353.0
    sympathetic paralysis 337.0
    traumatic (acute) NEC 847.0
  cervicobrachial (diffuse) 723.3
  cervicocranial 723.2
  cervicodorsal outlet 353.2
  Céstan's 344.89
  Céstan (-Raymond) 433.8 ☑
  Céstan-Chenais 344.89
  chancriform 114.1
  Charcôt's (intermittent claudication) 443.9
    angina cruris 443.9
    due to atherosclerosis 440.21
  Charcôt-Marie-Tooth 356.1
  Charcôt-Weiss-Baker 337.0
  CHARGE association 759.89   ●
  Cheadle (-Möller) (-Barlow) (infantile scurvy)
      267
  Chédiak-Higashi (-Steinbrinck) (congenital
      gigantism of peroxidase granules) 288.2
  chest wall 786.52
  Chiari's (hepatic vein thrombosis) 453.0
  Chiari-Frommel 676.6 ☑
  chiasmatic 368.41
  Chilaiditi's (subphrenic displacement, colon)
      751.4
  chondroectodermal dysplasia 756.55
  chorea-athetosis-agitans 275.1
  Christian's (chronic histiocytosis X) 277.89
  chromosome 4 short arm deletion 758.39   ▲
  Churg-Strauss 446.4
  Clarke-Hadfield (pancreatic infantilism) 577.8
  Claude's 352.6
  Claude Bernard-Horner (*see also* Neuropathy,
      peripheral, autonomic) 337.9
  Clérambault's
    automatism 348.8
    erotomania 297.8
  Clifford's (postmaturity) 766.22
  climacteric 627.2
  Clouston's (hidrotic ectodermal dysplasia)
      757.31
  clumsiness 315.4
  Cockayne's (microcephaly and dwarfism)
      759.89
  Cockayne-Weber (epidermolysis bullosa) 757.39
  Coffin-Lowry 759.89
  Cogan's (nonsyphilitic interstitial keratitis)
      370.52
  cold injury (newborn) 778.2
  Collet (-Sicard) 352.6
  combined immunity deficiency 279.2
  compartment(al) (anterior) (deep) (posterior)
      (tibial) 958.8
    nontraumatic 729.9
  compression 958.5
    cauda equina 344.60
      with neurogenic bladder 344.61
  concussion 310.2
  congenital
    affecting more than one system 759.7
      specified type NEC 759.89
    facial diplegia 352.6
    muscular hypertrophy-cerebral 759.89
  congestion-fibrosis (pelvic) 625.5
  conjunctivourethrosynovial 099.3
  Conn (-Louis) (primary aldosteronism)
      255.12
  Conradi (-Hünermann) (chondrodysplasia
      calcificans congenita) 756.59
  conus medullaris 336.8
  Cooke-Apert-Gallais (adrenogenital) 255.2
  Cornelia de Lange's (Amsterdam dwarf, mental
      retardation, and brachycephaly) 759.8 ☑
  coronary insufficiency or intermediate 411.1
  cor pulmonale 416.9
  corticosexual 255.2
  Costen's (complex) 524.60
  costochondral junction 733.6
  costoclavicular 353.0
  costovertebral 253.0
  Cotard's (paranoia) 297.1
  Cowden 759.6

Syndrome — *see also* Disease — *continued*
  craniovertebral 723.2
  Creutzfeldt-Jakob 046.1
    with dementia
      with behavioral disturbance 046.1
        [294.11]
      without behavioral disturbance 046.1
        [294.10]
  crib death 798.0
  cricopharyngeal 787.2
  cri-du-chat 758.31   ▲
  Crigler-Najjar (congenital hyperbilirubinemia)
      277.4
  crocodile tears 351.8
  Cronkhite-Canada 211.3
  croup 464.4
  CRST (cutaneous systemic sclerosis) 710.1
  crush 958.5
  crushed lung (*see also* Injury, internal, lung)
      861.20
  Cruveilhier-Baumgarten (cirrhosis of liver)
      571.5
  cubital tunnel 354.2
  Cuiffini-Pancoast (M8010/3) (carcinoma,
      pulmonary apex) 162.3
  Curschmann (-Batten) (-Steinert) 359.2
  Cushing's (iatrogenic) (idiopathic) (pituitary
      basophilism) (pituitary-dependent) 255.0
    overdose or wrong substance given or taken
      962.0
  Cyriax's (slipping rib) 733.99
  cystic duct stump 576.0
  Da Costa's (neurocirculatory asthenia) 306.2
  Dameshek's (erythroblastic anemia) 282.49
  Dana-Putnam (subacute combined sclerosis
      with pernicious anemia) 281.0 [336.2]
  Danbolt (-Closs) (acrodermatitis enteropathica)
      686.8
  Dandy-Walker (atresia, foramen of Magendie)
      742.3
    with spina bifida (*see also* Spina bifida)
      741.0 ☑
  Danlos' 756.83
  Davies-Colley (slipping rib) 733.99
  dead fetus 641.3 ☑
  defeminization 255.2
  defibrination (*see also* Fibrinolysis) 286.6
  Degos' 447.8
  Deiters' nucleus 386.19
  Déjérine-Roussy 348.8
  Déjérine-Thomas 333.0
  de Lange's (Amsterdam dwarf, mental
      retardation, and brachycephaly)
      (Cornelia) 759.89
  Del Castillo's (germinal aplasia) 606.0
  deletion chromosomes 758.39   ▲
  delusional
    induced by drug 292.11
  dementia-aphonia, of childhood (*see also*
      Psychosis, childhood) 299.1 ☑
  demyelinating NEC 341.9
  denial visual hallucination 307.9
  depersonalization 300.6
  Dercum's (adiposis dolorosa) 272.8
  de Toni-Fanconi (-Debré) (cystinosis) 270.0
  diabetes-dwarfism-obesity (juvenile) 258.1
  diabetes mellitus-hypertension-nephrosis
      250.4 ☑ [581.81]
  diabetes mellitus in newborn infant 775.1
  diabetes-nephrosis 250.4 ☑ [581.81]
  diabetic amyotrophy 250.6 ☑ [358.1]
  Diamond-Blackfan (congenital hypoplastic
      anemia) 284.0
  Diamond-Gardner (autoerythrocyte
      sensitization) 287.2
  DIC (diffuse or disseminated intravascular
      coagulopathy) (*see also* Fibrinolysis)
      286.6
  diencephalohypophyseal NEC 253.8
  diffuse cervicobrachial 723.3
  diffuse obstructive pulmonary 496
  DiGeorge's (thymic hypoplasia) 279.11
  Dighton's 756.51
  Di Guglielmo's (erythremic myelosis) (M9841/3)
      207.0 ☑
  disc — *see* Displacement, intervertebral disc

Syndrome — *see also* Disease — *continued*
  discogenic — *see* Displacement, intervertebral
      disc
  disequilibrium 276.9
  disseminated platelet thrombosis 446.6
  Ditthomska 307.81
  Doan-Wiseman (primary splenic neutropenia)
      288.0
  Döhle body-panmyelopathic 288.2
  Donohue's (leprechaunism) 259.8
  dorsolateral medullary (*see also* Disease,
      cerebrovascular, acute) 436
  double whammy 360.81
  Down's (mongolism) 758.0
  Dresbach's (elliptocytosis) 282.1
  Dressler's (postmyocardial infarction) 411.0
    hemoglobinuria 283.2
  drug withdrawal, infant, of dependent mother
      779.5
  dry skin 701.1
    eye 375.15
  DSAP (disseminated superficial actinic
      porokeratosis) 692.75
  Duane's (retraction) 378.71
  Duane-Stilling-Türk (ocular retraction
      syndrome) 378.71
  Dubin-Johnson (constitutional
      hyperbilirubinemia) 277.4
  Dubin-Sprinz (constitutional
      hyperbilirubinemia) 277.4
  Duchenne's 335.22
  due to abnormality
    autosomal NEC (*see also* Abnormal,
        autosomes NEC) 758.5
      13 758.1
      18 758.2
      21 or 22 758.0
      D 758.1
      E 758.2
      G 758.0
    chromosomal 758.89
      sex 758.81
  dumping 564.2
    nonsurgical 536.8
  Duplay's 726.2
  Dupré's (meningism) 781.6
  Dyke-Young (acquired macrocytic hemolytic
      anemia) 283.9
  dyspraxia 315.4
  dystocia, dystrophia 654.9 ☑
  Eagle-Barret 756.71
  Eales' 362.18
  Eaton-Lambert (*see also* Neoplasm, by site,
      malignant) 199.1 [358.1]
  Ebstein's (downward displacement, tricuspid
      valve into right ventricle) 746.2
  ectopic ACTH secretion 255.0
  eczema-thrombocytopenia 279.12
  Eddowes' (brittle bones and blue sclera) 756.51
  Edwards' 758.2
  efferent loop 537.89
  effort (aviators') (psychogenic) 306.2
  Ehlers-Danlos 756.83
  Eisenmenger's (ventricular septal defect) 745.4
  Ekbom's (restless legs) 333.99
  Ekman's (brittle bones and blue sclera) 756.51
  electric feet 266.2
  Elephant man 237.71
  Ellison-Zollinger (gastric hypersecretion with
      pancreatic islet cell tumor) 251.5
  Ellis-van Creveld (chondroectodermal
      dysplasia) 756.55
  embryonic fixation 270.2
  empty sella (turcica) 253.8
  endocrine-hypertensive 255.3
  Engel-von Recklinghausen (osteitis fibrosa
      cystica) 252.01   ▲
  enteroarticular 099.3
  entrapment — *see* Neuropathy, entrapment
  eosinophilia myalgia 710.5
  epidemic vomiting 078.82
  Epstein's — *see* Nephrosis
  Erb (-Oppenheim)-Goldflam 358.00
  Erdheim's (acromegalic macrospondylitis) 253.0
  Erlacher-Blount (tibia vara) 732.4
  erythrocyte fragmentation 283.19
  euthyroid sick 790.94

☑ Additional Digit Required   ▶◀ Revised Text   ● New Line   ▲ Revised Code

Syndrome — *see also* Disease — *continued*
Evans' (thrombocytopenic purpura) 287.3
excess cortisol, iatrogenic 255.0
exhaustion 300.5
extrapyramidal 333.90
eyelid-malar-mandible 756.0
eye retraction 378.71
Faber's (achlorhydric anemia) 280.9
Fabry (-Anderson) (angiokeratoma corporis
    diffusum) 272.7
facet 724.8
Fallot's 745.2
falx (*see also* Hemorrhage, brain) 431
familial eczema-thrombocytopenia 279.12
Fanconi's (anemia) (congenital pancytopenia)
    284.0
Fanconi (-de Toni) (-Debré) (cystinosis) 270.0
Farber (-Uzman) (disseminated
    lipogranulomatosis) 272.8
fatigue NEC 300.5
    chronic 780.71
faulty bowel habit (idiopathic megacolon) 564.7
FDH (focal dermal hypoplasia) 757.39
fecal reservoir 560.39
Feil-Klippel (brevicollis) 756.16
Felty's (rheumatoid arthritis with splenomegaly
    and leukopenia) 714.1
fertile eunuch 257.2
fetal alcohol 760.71
    late effect 760.71
fibrillation-flutter 427.32
fibrositis (periarticular) 729.0
Fiedler's (acute isolated myocarditis) 422.91
Fiessinger-Leroy (-Reiter) 099.3
Fiessinger-Rendu (erythema multiforme
    exudativum) 695.1
first arch 756.0
Fisher's 357.0
Fitz's (acute hemorrhagic pancreatitis) 577.0
Fitz-Hugh and Curtis 098.86
    due to
        Chlamydia trachomatis 099.56
        Neisseria gonorrhoeae (gonococcal
            peritonitis) 098.86
Flajani (-Basedow) (exophthalmic goiter)
    242.0 ☑
floppy
    infant 781.99
    valve (mitral) 424.0
flush 259.2
Foix-Alajouanine 336.1
Fong's (hereditary osteo-onychodysplasia)
    756.89
foramen magnum 348.4
Forbes-Albright (nonpuerperal amenorrhea and
    lactation associated with pituitary tumor)
    253.1
Foster-Kennedy 377.04
Foville's (peduncular) 344.89
fragile X 759.83
Franceschetti's (mandibulofacial dysostosis)
    756.0
Fraser's 759.89
Freeman-Sheldon 759.89
Frey's (auriculotemporal) 705.22   ▲
Friderichsen-Waterhouse 036.3
Friedrich-Erb-Arnold (acropachyderma) 757.39
Fröhlich's (adiposogenital dystrophy) 253.8
Froin's 336.8
Frommel-Chiari 676.6 ☑
frontal lobe 310.0
Fukuhara 277.87   ●
Fuller Albright's (osteitis fibrosa disseminata)
    756.59
functional
    bowel 564.9
    prepubertal castrate 752.89
Gaisböck's (polycythemia hypertonica) 289.0
ganglion (basal, brain) 333.90
    geniculi 351.1
Ganser's, hysterical 300.16
Gardner-Diamond (autoerythrocyte
    sensitization) 287.2
gastroesophageal junction 530.0
gastroesophageal laceration-hemorrhage 530.7
gastrojejunal loop obstruction 537.89

Syndrome — *see also* Disease — *continued*
Gayet-Wernicke's (superior hemorrhagic
    polioencephalitis) 265.1
Gee-Herter-Heubner (nontropical sprue) 579.0
Gélineau's ▶(*see also* Narcolepsy)◀ 347.00 ▲
genito-anorectal 099.1
Gerhardt's (vocal cord paralysis) 478.30
Gerstmann's (finger agnosia) 784.69
Gilbert's 277.4
Gilford (-Hutchinson) (progeria) 259.8
Gilles de la Tourette's 307.23
Gillespie's (dysplasia oculodentodigitalis)
    759.89
Glénard's (enteroptosis) 569.89
Glinski-Simmonds (pituitary cachexia) 253.2
glucuronyl transferase 277.4
glue ear 381.20
Goldberg (-Maxwell) (-Morris) (testicular
    feminization) 257.8
Goldenhar's (oculoauriculovertebral dysplasia)
    756.0
Goldflam-Erb 358.00
Goltz-Gorlin (dermal hypoplasia) 757.39
Good's 279.06   ●
Goodpasture's (pneumorenal) 446.21
Gopalan's (burning feet) 266.2
Gorlin-Chaudhry-Moss 759.89
Gougerot (-Houwer)-Sjögren
    (keratoconjunctivitis sicca) 710.2
Gougerot-Blum (pigmented purpuric lichenoid
    dermatitis) 709.1
Gougerot-Carteaud (confluent reticulate
    papillomatosis) 701.8
Gouley's (constrictive pericarditis) 423.2
Gowers' (vasovagal attack) 780.2
Gowers-Paton-Kennedy 377.04
Gradenigo's 383.02
gray or grey (chloramphenicol) (newborn) 779.4
Greig's (hypertelorism) 756.0
Gubler-Millard 344.89
Guérin-Stern (arthrogryposis multiplex
    congenita) 754.89
Guillain-Barré (-Strohl) 357.0
Gunn's (jaw-winking syndrome) 742.8
Günther's (congenital erythropoietic porphyria)
    277.1
gustatory sweating 350.8
H₃O 759.81
Hadfield-Clarke (pancreatic infantilism) 577.8
Haglund-Läwen-Fründ 717.89
hair tourniquet — *see also* Injury,
    superficial, by site
    finger 915.8
        infected 915.9
    penis 911.8
        infected 911.9
    toe 917.8
        infected 917.9
hairless women 257.8
Hallermann-Streiff 756.0
Hallervorden-Spatz 333.0
Hamman's (spontaneous mediastinal
    emphysema) 518.1
Hamman-Rich (diffuse interstitial pulmonary
    fibrosis) 516.3
Hand-Schüller-Christian (chronic histiocytosis
    X) 277.89
hand-foot 282.61
Hanot-Chauffard (-Troisier) (bronze diabetes)
    275.0
Harada's 363.22
Hare's (M8010/3) (carcinoma, pulmonary apex)
    162.3
Harkavy's 446.0
harlequin color change 779.89
Harris' (organic hyperinsulinism) 251.1
Hart's (pellagra-cerebellar ataxia-renal
    aminoaciduria) 270.0
Hayem-Faber (achlorhydric anemia) 280.9
Hayem-Widal (acquired hemolytic jaundice)
    283.9
Heberden's (angina pectoris) 413.9
Hedinger's (malignant carcinoid) 259.2
Hegglin's 288.2
Heller's (infantile psychosis) (*see also*
    Psychosis, childhood) 299.1 ☑
H.E.L.L.P 642.5 ☑

Syndrome — *see also* Disease — *continued*
hemolytic-uremic (adult) (child) 283.11
Hench-Rosenberg (palindromic arthritis) (*see
    also* Rheumatism, palindromic) 719.3 ☑
Henoch-Schönlein (allergic purpura) 287.0
hepatic flexure 569.89
hepatorenal 572.4
    due to a procedure 997.4
    following delivery 674.8 ☑
hepatourologic 572.4
Herrick's (hemoglobin S disease) 282.61
Herter (-Gee) (nontropical sprue) 579.0
Heubner-Herter (nontropical sprue) 579.0
Heyd's (hepatorenal) 572.4
HHHO 759.81
Hilger's 337.0
Hoffa (-Kastert) (liposynovitis prepatellaris)
    272.8
Hoffmann's 244.9 *[359.5]*
Hoffmann-Bouveret (paroxysmal tachycardia)
    427.2
Hoffmann-Werdnig 335.0
Holländer-Simons (progressive lipodystrophy)
    272.6
Holmes' (visual disorientation) 368.16
Holmes-Adie 379.46
Hoppe-Goldflam 358.00
Horner's (*see also* Neuropathy, peripheral,
    autonomic) 337.9
    traumatic — *see* Injury, nerve, cervical
        sympathetic
hospital addiction 301.51
Hunt's (herpetic geniculate ganglionitis) 053.11
    dyssynergia cerebellaris myoclonica 334.2
Hunter (-Hurler) (mucopolysaccharidosis II)
    277.5
hunterian glossitis 529.4
Hurler (-Hunter) (mucopolysaccharidosis II)
    277.5
Hutchinson's incisors or teeth 090.5
Hutchinson-Boeck (sarcoidosis) 135
Hutchinson-Gilford (progeria) 259.8
hydralazine
    correct substance properly administered
        695.4
    overdose or wrong substance given or taken
        972.6
hydraulic concussion (abdomen) (*see also*
    Injury, internal, abdomen) 868.00
hyperabduction 447.8
hyperactive bowel 564.9
hyperaldosteronism with hypokalemic alkalosis
    (Bartter's) 255.13
hypercalcemic 275.42
hypercoagulation NEC 289.89
hypereosinophilic (idiopathic) 288.3
hyperkalemic 276.7
hyperkinetic — *see also* Hyperkinesia
    heart 429.82
hyperlipemia-hemolytic anemia-icterus 571.1
hypermobility 728.5
hypernatremia 276.0
hyperosmolarity 276.0
hypersomnia-bulimia 349.89
hypersplenic 289.4
hypersympathetic (*see also* Neuropathy,
    peripheral, autonomic) 337.9
hypertransfusion, newborn 776.4
hyperventilation, psychogenic 306.1
hyperviscosity (of serum) NEC 273.3
    polycythemic 289.0
    sclerothymic 282.8
hypoglycemic (familial) (neonatal) 251.2
    functional 251.1
hypokalemic 276.8
hypophyseal 253.8
hypophyseothalamic 253.8
hypopituitarism 253.2
hypoplastic left heart 746.7
hypopotassemia 276.8
hyposmolality 276.1
hypotension, maternal 669.2 ☑
hypotonia-hypomentia-hypogonadism-obesity
    759.81
ICF (intravascular coagulation-fibrinolysis) (*see
    also* Fibrinolysis) 286.6

☑ Additional Digit Required   ▶◀ Revised Text   ● New Line   ▲ Revised Code

Syndrome — *see also* Disease — *continued*
  idiopathic cardiorespiratory distress, newborn
    769
  idiopathic nephrotic (infantile) 581.9
  Imerslund (-Gräsbeck) (anemia due to familial
    selective vitamin B$_{12}$ malabsorption)
    281.1
  immobility (paraplegic) 728.3
  immunity deficiency, combined 279.2
  impending coronary 411.1
  impingement
    shoulder 726.2
    vertebral bodies 724.4
  inappropriate secretion of antidiuretic hormone
    (ADH) 253.6
  incomplete
    mandibulofacial 756.0
  infant
    death, sudden (SIDS) 798.0
    Hercules 255.2
    of diabetic mother 775.0
    shaken 995.55
  infantilism 253.3
  inferior vena cava 459.2
  influenza-like 487.1
  inspissated bile, newborn 774.4
  intermediate coronary (artery) 411.1
  internal carotid artery (*see also* Occlusion,
    artery, carotid) 433.1 ☑
  interspinous ligament 724.8
  intestinal
    carcinoid 259.2
    gas 787.3
    knot 560.2
  intravascular
    coagulation-fibrinolysis (ICF) (*see also*
      Fibrinolysis) 286.6
    coagulopathy (*see also* Fibrinolysis) 286.6
  inverted Marfan's 759.89
  IRDS (idiopathic respiratory distress, newborn)
    769
  irritable
    bowel 564.1
    heart 306.2
    weakness 300.5
  ischemic bowel (transient) 557.9
    chronic 557.1
    due to mesenteric artery insufficiency 557.1
  Itsenko-Cushing (pituitary basophilism) 255.0
  IVC (intravascular coagulopathy) (*see also*
    Fibrinolysis) 286.6
  Ivemark's (asplenia with congenital heart
    disease) 759.0
  Jaccoud's 714.4
  Jackson's 344.89
  Jadassohn-Lewandowski (pachyonchia
    congenita) 757.5
  Jaffe-Lichtenstein (-Uehlinger) 252.01   ▲
  Jahnke's (encephalocutaneous angiomatosis)
    759.6
  Jakob-Creutzfeldt 046.1
    with dementia
      with behavioral disturbance 046.1
        [294.11]
      without behavioral disturbance 046.1
        [294.10]
  Jaksch's (pseudoleukemia infantum) 285.8
  Jaksch-Hayem (-Luzet) (pseudoleukemia
    infantum) 285.8
  jaw-winking 742.8
  jejunal 564.2
  jet lag 307.45
  Jeune's (asphyxiating thoracic dystrophy of
    newborn) 756.4
  Job's (chronic granulomatous disease) 288.1
  Jordan's 288.2
  Joseph-Diamond-Blackfan (congenital
    hypoplastic anemia) 284.0
  Joubert 759.89
  jugular foramen 352.6
  Kabuki 759.89   ●
  Kahler's (multiple myeloma) (M9730/3)
    203.0 ☑
  Kalischer's (encephalocutaneous angiomatosis)
    759.6
  Kallmann's (hypogonadotropic hypogonadism
    with anosmia) 253.4

  Kanner's (autism) (*see also* Psychosis,
    childhood) 299.0 ☑
  Kartagener's (sinusitis, bronchiectasis, situs
    inversus) 759.3
  Kasabach-Merritt (capillary hemangioma
    associated with thrombocytopenic
    purpura) 287.3
  Kast's (dyschondroplasia with hemangiomas)
    756.4
  Kaznelson's (congenital hypoplastic anemia)
    284.0
  Kearns-Sayer 277.87   ●
  Kelly's (sideropenic dysphagia) 280.8
  Kimmelstiel-Wilson (intercapillary
    glomerulosclerosis) 250.4 ☑ [581.81]
  Klauder's (erythema multiforme exudativum)
    695.1
  Klein-Waardenburg (ptosis-epicanthus) 270.2
  Kleine-Levin 349.89
  Klinefelter's 758.7
  Klippel-Feil (brevicollis) 756.16
  Klippel-Trenaunay 759.89
  Klumpke (-Déjérine) (injury to brachial plexus
    at birth) 767.6
  Klüver-Bucy (-Terzian) 310.0
  Köhler-Pellegrini-Stieda (calcification, knee
    joint) 726.62
  König's 564.89
  Korsakoff's (nonalcoholic) 294.0
    alcoholic 291.1
  Korsakoff (-Wernicke) (nonalcoholic) 294.0
    alcoholic 291.1
  Kostmann's (infantile genetic agranulocytosis)
    288.0
  Krabbe's
    congenital muscle hypoplasia 756.89
    cutaneocerebral angioma 759.6
  Kunkel (lupoid hepatitis) 571.49
  labyrinthine 386.50
  laceration, broad ligament 620.6
  Langdon Down (mongolism) 758.0
  Larsen's (flattened facies and multiple
    congenital dislocations) 755.8
  lateral
    cutaneous nerve of thigh 355.1
    medullary (*see also* Disease, cerebrovascular
      acute) 436
  Launois' (pituitary gigantism) 253.0
  Launois-Cléret (adiposogenital dystrophy) 253.8
  Laurence-Moon (-Bardet)-Biedl (obesity,
    polydactyly, and mental retardation)
    759.89
  Lawford's (encephalocutaneous angiomatosis)
    759.6
  lazy
    leukocyte 288.0
    posture 728.3
  Lederer-Brill (acquired infectious hemolytic
    anemia) 283.19
  Legg-Calvé-Perthes (osteochondrosis capital
    femoral) 732.1
  Lemiere 451.89   ●
  Lennox-Gastaut syndrome 345.0 ☑   ●
    with tonic seizures 345.1 ☑   ●
  Lennox's (*see also* Epilepsy) 345.0 ☑
  lenticular 275.1
  Léopold-Lévi's (paroxysmal thyroid instability)
    242.9 ☑
  Lepore hemoglobin 282.49
  Léri-Weill 756.59
  Leriche's (aortic bifurcation occlusion) 444.0
  Lermoyez's (*see also* Disease, Ménière's) 386.00
  Lesch-Nyhan (hypoxanthine-guanine-
    phosphoribosyltransferase deficiency)
    277.2
  Lev's (acquired complete heart block) 426.0
  Levi's (pituitary dwarfism) 253.3
  Lévy-Roussy 334.3
  Lichtheim's (subacute combined sclerosis with
    pernicious anemia) 281.0 [336.2]
  Li-Fraumeni V84.01   ▲
  Lightwood's (renal tubular acidosis) 588.89 ▲
  Lignac (-de Toni) (-Fanconi) (-Debré) (cystinosis)
    270.0
  Likoff's (angina in menopausal women) 413.9
  liver-kidney 572.4

  Lloyd's 258.1
  lobotomy 310.0
  Löffler's (eosinophilic pneumonitis) 518.3
  Löfgren's (sarcoidosis) 135
  long arm 18 or 21 deletion 758.39   ▲
  Looser (-Debray)-Milkman (osteomalacia with
    pseudofractures) 268.2
  Lorain-Levi (pituitary dwarfism) 253.3
  Louis-Bar (ataxia-telangiectasia) 334.8
  low
    atmospheric pressure 993.2
    back 724.2
      psychogenic 306.0
    output (cardiac) (*see also* Failure, heart)
      428.9
  Lowe's (oculocerebrorenal dystrophy) 270.8
  Lowe-Terrey-MacLachlan (oculocerebrorenal
    dystrophy) 270.8
  lower radicular, newborn 767.4
  Lown (-Ganong)-Levine (short P-R interval,
    normal QRS complex, and
    supraventricular tachycardia) 426.81
  Lucey-Driscoll (jaundice due to delayed
    conjugation) 774.30
  Luetscher's (dehydration) 276.5
  lumbar vertebral 724.4
  Lutembacher's (atrial septal defect with mitral
    stenosis) 745.5
  Lyell's (toxic epidermal necrolysis) 695.1
    due to drug
      correct substance properly administered
        695.1
      overdose or wrong substance given or
        taken 977.9
        specified drug — *see* Table of Drugs
          and Chemicals
  MacLeod's 492.8
  macrogenitosomia praecox 259.8
  macroglobulinemia 273.3
  Maffucci's (dyschondroplasia with
    hemangiomas) 756.4
  Magenblase 306.4
  magnesium-deficiency 781.7
  Mal de Debarquement 780.4
  malabsorption 579.9
    postsurgical 579.3
    spinal fluid 331.3
  malignant carcinoid 259.2
  Mallory-Weiss 530.7
  mandibulofacial dysostosis 756.0
  manic-depressive (*see also* Psychosis, affective)
    296.80
  Mankowsky's (familial dysplastic osteopathy)
    731.2
  maple syrup (urine) 270.3
  Marable's (celiac artery compression) 447.4
  Marchesani (-Weill) (brachymorphism and
    ectopia lentis) 759.89
  Marchiafava-Bignami 341.8
  Marchiafava-Micheli (paroxysmal nocturnal
    hemoglobinuria) 283.2
  Marcus Gunn (jaw-winking syndrome) 742.8
  Marfan's (arachnodactyly) 759.82
    meaning congenital syphilis 090.49
      with luxation of lens 090.49 [379.32]
  Marie's (acromegaly) 253.0
    primary or idiopathic (acropachyderma)
      757.39
    secondary (hypertrophic pulmonary
      osteoarthropathy) 731.2
  Markus-Adie 379.46
  Maroteaux-Lamy (mucopolysaccharidosis VI)
    277.5
  Martin's 715.27
  Martin-Albright (pseudohypoparathyroidism)
    275.49
  Martorell-Fabré (pulseless disease) 446.7
  massive aspiration of newborn 770.1
  Masters-Allen 620.6
  mastocytosis 757.33
  maternal hypotension 669.2 ☑
  maternal obesity 646.1 ☑
  May (-Hegglin) 288.2
  McArdle (-Schmid) (-Pearson) (glycogenosis V)
    271.0

☑ Additional Digit Required   ►◄ Revised Text   ● New Line   ▲ Revised Code

Syndrome — *see also* Disease — *continued*
McCune-Albright (osteitis fibrosa disseminata) 756.59
McQuarrie's (idiopathic familial hypoglycemia) 251.2
meconium
 aspiration 770.1
 plug (newborn) NEC 777.1
median arcuate ligament 447.4
mediastinal fibrosis 519.3
Meekeren-Ehlers-Danlos 756.83
Meige (blepharospasm-oromandibular dystonia) 333.82
 -Milroy (chronic hereditary edema) 757.0
MELAS ▶(mitochondrial encephalopathy, lactic acidosis and stroke-like episodes)◀ 277.87   ▲
Melkersson (-Rosenthal) 351.8
Mende's (ptosis-epicanthus) 270.2
Mendelson's (resulting from a procedure) 997.3
 during labor 668.0 ☑
 obstetric 668.0 ☑
Ménétrier's (hypertrophic gastritis) 535.2 ☑
Ménière's (*see also* Disease, Ménière's) 386.00
meningo-eruptive 047.1
Menkes' 759.89
 glutamic acid 759.89
 maple syrup (urine) disease 270.3
menopause 627.2
 postartificial 627.4
menstruation 625.4
MERRF (myoclonus with epilepsy and   ●
  with ragged red fibers) 277.87   ●
mesenteric
 artery, superior 557.1
 vascular insufficiency (with gangrene) 557.1
metabolic 277.7   ●
metastatic carcinoid 259.2
Meyenburg-Altherr-Uehlinger 733.99
Meyer-Schwickerath and Weyers (dysplasia oculodentodigitalis) 759.89
Micheli-Rietti (thalassemia minor) 282.49
Michotte's 721.5
micrognathia-glossoptosis 756.0
microphthalmos (congenital) 759.89
midbrain 348.8
middle
 lobe (lung) (right) 518.0
 radicular 353.0
Miescher's
 familial acanthosis nigricans 701.2
 granulomatosis disciformis 709.3
Mieten's 759.89
migraine 346.0 ☑
Mikity-Wilson (pulmonary dysmaturity) 770.7
Mikulicz's (dryness of mouth, absent or decreased lacrimation) 527.1
milk alkali (milk drinkers') 275.42
Milkman (-Looser) (osteomalacia with pseudofractures) 268.2
Millard-Gubler 344.89
Miller-Dieker 758.33   ●
Miller Fisher's 357.0
Milles' (encephalocutaneous angiomatosis) 759.6
Minkowski-Chauffard (*see also* Spherocytosis) 282.0
Mirizzi's (hepatic duct stenosis) 576.2
 with calculus, cholelithiasis, or stones — *see* Choledocholithiasis
mitochondrial neurogastrointestinal   ●
 encephalopathy (MNGIE) 277.87   ●
mitral
 click (-murmur) 785.2
 valve prolapse 424.0
MNGIE (mitochondrial   ●
 neurogastrointestinal   ●
 encephalopathy) 277.87   ●
Möbius'
 congenital oculofacial paralysis 352.6
 ophthalmoplegic migraine 346.8 ☑
Mohr's (types I and II) 759.89
monofixation 378.34
Moore's (*see also* Epilepsy) 345.5 ☑
Morel-Moore (hyperostosis frontalis interna) 733.3

Syndrome — *see also* Disease — *continued*
Morel-Morgagni (hyperostosis frontalis interna) 733.3
Morgagni (-Stewart-Morel) (hyperostosis frontalis interna) 733.3
Morgagni-Adams-Stokes (syncope with heart block) 426.9
Morquio (-Brailsford) (-Ullrich) (mucopolysaccharidosis IV) 277.5
Morris (testicular feminization) 257.8
Morton's (foot) (metatarsalgia) (metatarsal neuralgia) (neuralgia) (neuroma) (toe) 355.6
Moschcowitz (-Singer-Symmers) (thrombotic thrombocytopenic purpura) 446.6
Mounier-Kuhn 494.0
 with acute exacerbation 494.1
Mucha-Haberman (acute parapsoriasis varioliformis) 696.2
mucocutaneous lymph node (acute) (febrile) (infantile) (MCLS) 446.1
multiple
 deficiency 260
 operations 301.51
Munchausen's 301.51
Münchmeyer's (exostosis luxurians) 728.11
Murchison-Sanderson — *see* Disease, Hodgkin's
myasthenic — *see* Myasthenia, syndrome
myelodysplastic 238.7
myeloproliferative (chronic) (M9960/1) 238.7
myofascial pain NEC 729.1
Naffziger's 353.0
Nager-de Reynier (dysostosis mandibularis) 756.0
nail-patella (hereditary osteo-onychodysplasia) 756.89
NARP (neuropathy, ataxia and retinitis   ●
 pigmentosa) 277.87   ●
Nebécourt's 253.3
Neill-Dingwall (microencephaly and dwarfism) 759.89
nephrotic (*see also* Nephrosis) 581.9
 diabetic 250.4 ☑ [581.81]
Netherton's (ichthyosiform erythroderma) 757.1
neurocutaneous 759.6
neuroleptic malignant 333.92
Nezelof's (pure alymphocytosis) 279.13
Niemann-Pick (lipid histiocytosis) 272.7
Nonne-Milroy-Meige (chronic hereditary edema) 757.0
nonsense 300.16
Noonan's 759.89
Nothnagel's
 ophthalmoplegia-cerebellar ataxia 378.52
 vasomotor acroparesthesia 443.89
nucleus ambiguous-hypoglossal 352.6
OAV (oculoauriculovertebral dysplasia) 756.0
obsessional 300.3
oculocutaneous 364.24
oculomotor 378.81
oculourethroarticular 099.3
Ogilvie's (sympathicotonic colon obstruction) 560.89
ophthalmoplegia-cerebellar ataxia 378.52
Oppenheim-Urbach (necrobiosis lipoidica diabeticorum) 250.8 ☑ [709.3]
oral-facial-digital 759.89
organic
 affective NEC 293.83
  drug-induced 292.84
 anxiety 293.84
 delusional 293.81
  alcohol-induced 291.5
  drug-induced 292.11
  due to or associated with
   arteriosclerosis 290.42
    presenile brain disease 290.12
    senility 290.20
 depressive 293.83
  drug-induced 292.84
  due to or associated with
   arteriosclerosis 290.43
    presenile brain disease 290.13
    senile brain disease 290.21
 hallucinosis 293.82
  drug-induced 292.84

Syndrome — *see also* Disease — *continued*
organic affective 293.83
 induced by drug 292.84
organic personality 310.1
 induced by drug 292.89
Ormond's 593.4
orodigitofacial 759.89
orthostatic hypotensive-dysautonomic dyskinetic 333.0
Osler-Weber-Rendu (familial hemorrhagic telangiectasia) 448.0
osteodermopathic hyperostosis 757.39
osteoporosis-osteomalacia 268.2
Österreicher-Turner (hereditary osteo-onychodysplasia) 756.89
Ostrum-Furst 756.59
otolith 386.19
otopalatodigital 759.89
outlet (thoracic) 353.0
ovarian remnant 620.8
ovarian vein 593.4
Owren's (*see also* Defect, coagulation) 286.3
OX 758.6
pacemaker 429.4
Paget-Schroetter (intermittent venous claudication) 453.8
pain — *see* Pain
painful
 apicocostal vertebral (M8010/3) 162.3
 arc 726.19
 bruising 287.2
 feet 266.2
Pancoast's (carcinoma, pulmonary apex) (M8010/3) 162.3
panhypopituitary (postpartum) 253.2
papillary muscle 429.81
 with myocardial infarction 410.8 ☑
Papillon-Léage and Psaume (orodigitofacial dysostosis) 759.89
parabiotic (transfusion)
 donor (twin) 772.0
 recipient (twin) 776.4
paralysis agitans 332.0
paralytic 344.9
 specified type NEC 344.89
paraneoplastic — *see* condition
Parinaud's (paralysis of conjugate upward gaze) 378.81
 oculoglandular 372.02
Parkes Weber and Dimitri (encephalocutaneous angiomatosis) 759.6
Parkinson's (*see also* Parkinsonism) 332.0
parkinsonian (*see also* Parkinsonism) 332.0
Parry's (exophthalmic goiter) 242.0 ☑
Parry-Romberg 349.89
Parsonage-Aldren-Turner 353.5
Parsonage-Turner 353.5
Patau's (trisomy D) 758.1
patellofemoral 719.46
Paterson (-Brown) (-Kelly) (sideropenic dysphagia) 280.8
Payr's (splenic flexure syndrome) 569.89
pectoral girdle 447.8
pectoralis minor 447.8
Pelger-Huët (hereditary hyposegmentation) 288.2
pellagra-cerebellar ataxia-renal aminoaciduria 270.0
Pellegrini-Stieda 726.62
pellagroid 265.2
Pellizzi's (pineal) 259.8
pelvic congestion (-fibrosis) 625.5
Pendred's (familial goiter with deaf-mutism) 243
Penfield's (*see also* Epilepsy) 345.5 ☑
Penta X 758.81
peptic ulcer — *see* Ulcer, peptic 533.9 ☑
perabduction 447.8
periodic 277.3
periurethral fibrosis 593.4
persistent fetal circulation 747.83
Petges-Cléjat (poikilodermatomyositis) 710.3
Peutz-Jeghers 759.6
Pfeiffer (acrocephalosyndactyly) 755.55
phantom limb 353.6
pharyngeal pouch 279.11

Syndrome (right margin, vertical)

☑ Additional Digit Required   ▶◀ Revised Text   ● New Line   ▲ Revised Code

Syndrome — *see also* Disease — *continued*
  Pick's (pericardial pseudocirrhosis of liver) 423.2
    heart 423.2
    liver 423.2
  Pick-Herxheimer (diffuse idiopathic cutaneous atrophy) 701.8
  Pickwickian (cardiopulmonary obesity) 278.8
  PIE (pulmonary infiltration with eosinophilia) 518.3
  Pierre Marie-Bamberger (hypertrophic pulmonary osteoarthropathy) 731.2
  Pierre Mauriac's (diabetes-dwarfism-obesity) 258.1
  Pierre Robin 756.0
  pigment dispersion, iris 364.53
  pineal 259.8
  pink puffer 492.8
  pituitary 253.0
  placental
    dysfunction 762.2
    insufficiency 762.2
    transfusion 762.3
  plantar fascia 728.71
  plica knee 727.83
  Plummer-Vinson (sideropenic dysphagia) 280.8
  pluricarential of infancy 260
  plurideficiency of infancy 260
  pluriglandular (compensatory) 258.8
  polycarential of infancy 260
  polyglandular 258.8
  polysplenia 759.0
  pontine 433.8 ☑
  popliteal
    artery entrapment 447.8
    web 756.89
  postartificial menopause 627.4
  postcardiotomy 429.4
  postcholecystectomy 576.0
  postcommissurotomy 429.4
  postconcussional 310.2
  postcontusional 310.2
  postencephalitic 310.8
  posterior
    cervical sympathetic 723.2
    fossa compression 348.4
    inferior cerebellar artery (*see also* Disease, cerebrovascular, acute) 436
  postgastrectomy (dumping) 564.2
  post-gastric surgery 564.2
  posthepatitis 780.79
  postherpetic (neuralgia) (zoster) 053.19
    geniculate ganglion 053.11
    ophthalmica 053.19
  postimmunization — *see* Complications, vaccination
  postinfarction 411.0
  postinfluenza (asthenia) 780.79
  postirradiation 990
  postlaminectomy 722.80
    cervical, cervicothoracic 722.81
    lumbar, lumbosacral 722.83
    thoracic, thoracolumbar 722.82
  postleukotomy 310.0
  postlobotomy 310.0
  postmastectomy lymphedema 457.0
  postmature (of newborn) 766.22
  postmyocardial infarction 411.0
  postoperative NEC 998.9
    blind loop 579.2
  postpartum panhypopituitary 253.2
  postperfusion NEC 999.8
    bone marrow 996.85
  postpericardiotomy 429.4
  postphlebitic (asymptomatic) 459.10
    with
      complications NEC 459.19
      inflammation 459.12
        and ulcer 459.13
      stasis dermatitis 459.12
        with ulcer 459.13
      ulcer 459.11
        with inflammation 459.13
  postpolio (myelitis) 138
  postvagotomy 564.2
  postvalvulotomy 429.4
  postviral (asthenia) NEC 780.79

Syndrome — *see also* Disease — *continued*
  Potain's (gastrectasis with dyspepsia) 536.1
  potassium intoxication 276.7
  Potter's 753.0
  Prader (-Labhart) -Willi (-Fanconi) 759.81
  preinfarction 411.1
  preleukemic 238.7
  premature senility 259.8
  premenstrual 625.4
  premenstrual tension 625.4
  pre ulcer 536.9
  Prinzmetal-Massumi (anterior chest wall syndrome) 786.52
  Profichet's 729.9
  progeria 259.8
  progressive pallidal degeneration 333.0
  prolonged gestation 766.22
  Proteus (dermal hypoplasia) 757.39
  prune belly 756.71
  prurigo-asthma 691.8
  pseudocarpal tunnel (sublimis) 354.0
  pseudohermaphroditism-virilism-hirsutism 255.2
  pseudoparalytica 358.00
  pseudo-Turner's 759.89
  psycho-organic 293.9
    acute 293.0
    anxiety type 293.84
    depressive type 293.83
    hallucinatory type 293.82
    nonpsychotic severity 310.1
      specified focal (partial) NEC 310.8
    paranoid type 293.81
    specified type NEC 293.89
    subacute 293.1
  pterygolymphangiectasia 758.6
  ptosis-epicanthus 270.2
  pulmonary 660.1 ☑
    arteriosclerosis 416.0
    hypoperfusion (idiopathic) 769
    renal (hemorrhagic) 446.21
  pulseless 446.7
  Putnam-Dana (subacute combined sclerosis with pernicious anemia) 281.0 *[336.2]*
  pyloroduodenal 537.89
  pyramidopallidonigral 332.0
  pyriformis 355.0
  Q-T interval prolongation 794.31
  radicular NEC 729.2
    lower limbs 724.4
    upper limbs 723.4
      newborn 767.4
  Raeder-Harbitz (pulseless disease) 446.7
  Ramsay Hunt's
    dyssynergia cerebellaris myoclonica 334.2
    herpetic geniculate ganglionitis 053.11
  rapid time-zone change 307.45
  Raymond (-Céstan) 433.8 ☑
  Raynaud's (paroxysmal digital cyanosis) 443.0
  RDS (respiratory distress syndrome, newborn) 769
  Refsum's (heredopathia atactica polyneuritiformis) 356.3
  Reichmann's (gastrosuccorrhea) 536.8
  Reifenstein's (hereditary familial hypogonadism, male) 257.2
  Reilly's (*see also* Neuropathy, peripheral, autonomic) 337.9
  Reiter's 099.3
  renal glomerulohyalinosis-diabetic 250.4 ☑ *[581.81]*
  Rendu-Osler-Weber (familial hemorrhagic telangiectasia) 448.0
  renofacial (congenital biliary fibroangiomatosis) 753.0
  Rénon-Delille 253.8
  respiratory distress (idiopathic) (newborn) 769
    adult (following shock, surgery, or trauma) 518.5
    specified NEC 518.82
  restless leg 333.99
  retinoblastoma (familial) 190.5 ●
  retraction (Duane's) 378.71
  retroperitoneal fibrosis 593.4
  Rett's 330.8
  Reye's 331.81

Syndrome — *see also* Disease — *continued*
  Reye-Sheehan (postpartum pituitary necrosis) 253.2
  Riddoch's (visual disorientation) 368.16
  Ridley's (*see also* Failure, ventricular, left) 428.1
  Rieger's (mesodermal dysgenesis, anterior ocular segment) 743.44
  Rietti-Greppi-Micheli (thalassemia minor) 282.49
  right ventricular obstruction — *see* Failure, heart
  Riley-Day (familial dysautonomia) 742.8
  Robin's 756.0
  Rokitansky-Kuster-Hauser (congenital absence, vagina) 752.49
  Romano-Ward (prolonged Q-T interval) 794.31
  Romberg's 349.89
  Rosen-Castleman-Liebow (pulmonary proteinosis) 516.0
  rotator cuff, shoulder 726.10
  Roth's 355.1
  Rothmund's (congenital poikiloderma) 757.33
  Rotor's (idiopathic hyperbilirubinemia) 277.4
  Roussy-Lévy 334.3
  Roy (-Jutras) (acropachyderma) 757.39
  rubella (congenital) 771.0
  Rubinstein-Taybi's (brachydactylia, short stature, and mental retardation) 759.89
  Rud's (mental deficiency, epilepsy, and infantilism) 759.89
  Ruiter-Pompen (-Wyers) (angiokeratoma corporis diffusum) 272.7
  Runge's (postmaturity) 766.22
  Russell (-Silver) (congenital hemihypertrophy and short stature) 759.89
  Rytand-Lipsitch (complete atrioventricular block) 426.0
  sacralization-scoliosis-sciatica 756.15
  sacroiliac 724.6
  Saenger's 379.46
  salt
    depletion (*see also* Disease, renal) 593.9
      due to heat NEC 992.8
        causing heat exhaustion or prostration 992.4
    low (*see also* Disease, renal) 593.9
  salt-losing (*see also* Disease, renal) 593.9
  Sanfilippo's (mucopolysaccharidosis III) 277.5
  Scaglietti-Dagnini (acromegalic macrospondylitis) 253.0
  scalded skin 695.1
  scalenus anticus (anterior) 353.0
  scapulocostal 354.8
  scapuloperoneal 359.1
  scapulovertebral 723.4
  Schaumann's (sarcoidosis) 135
  Scheie's (mucopolysaccharidosis IS) 277.5
  Scheuthauer-Marie-Sainton (cleidocranialis dysostosis) 755.59
  Schirmer's (encephalocutaneous angiomatosis) 759.6
  schizophrenic, of childhood NEC (*see also* Psychosis, childhood) 299.9 ☑
  Schmidt's
    sphallo-pharyngo-laryngeal hemiplegia 352.6
    thyroid-adrenocortical insufficiency 258.1
    vagoaccessory 352.6
  Schneider's 047.9
  Schnitzler 273.1 ●
  Scholte's (malignant carcinoid) 259.2
  Scholz (-Bielschowsky-Henneberg) 330.0
  Schroeder's (endocrine-hypertensive) 255.3
  Schüller-Christian (chronic histiocytosis X) 277.89
  Schultz's (agranulocytosis) 288.0
  Schwartz (-Jampel) 756.89
  Schwartz-Bartter (inappropriate secretion of antidiuretic hormone) 253.6
  Scimitar (anomalous venous drainage, right lung to inferior vena cava) 747.49
  sclerocystic ovary 256.4
  sea-blue histiocyte 272.7
  Seabright-Bantam (pseudohypoparathyroidism) 275.49
  Seckel's 759.89
  Secretan's (posttraumatic edema) 782.3

☑ Additional Digit Required   ►◄ Revised Text   ● New Line   ▲ Revised Code

Syndrome — see also Disease — continued
  secretoinhibitor (keratoconjunctivitis sicca) 710.2
  Seeligmann's (ichthyosis congenita) 757.1
  Senear-Usher (pemphigus erythematosus) 694.4
  senilism 259.8
  serotonin 333.99
  serous meningitis 348.2
  Sertoli cell (germinal aplasia) 606.0
  sex chromosome mosaic 758.81
  Sézary's (reticulosis) (M9701/3) 202.2 ☑
  shaken infant 995.55
  Shaver's (bauxite pneumoconiosis) 503
  Sheehan's (postpartum pituitary necrosis) 253.2
  shock (traumatic) 958.4
    kidney 584.5
      following crush injury 958.5
    lung 518.5
    neurogenic 308.9
    psychic 308.9
  short
    bowel 579.3
    P-R interval 426.81
  shoulder-arm (see also Neuropathy, peripheral, autonomic) 337.9
  shoulder-girdle 723.4
  shoulder-hand (see also Neuropathy, peripheral, autonomic) 337.9
  Shwachman's 288.0
  Shy-Drager (orthostatic hypotension with multisystem degeneration) 333.0
  Sicard's 352.6
  sicca (keratoconjunctivitis) 710.2
  sick
    cell 276.1
    cilia 759.89
    sinus 427.81
  sideropenic 280.8
  Siemens'
    ectodermal dysplasia 757.31
    keratosis follicularis spinulosa (decalvans) 757.39
  Silfverskiöld's (osteochondrodystrophy, extremities) 756.50
  Silver's (congenital hemihypertrophy and short stature) 759.89
  Silvestroni-Bianco (thalassemia minima) 282.49
  Simons' (progressive lipodystrophy) 272.6
  sinus tarsi 726.79
  sinusitis-bronchiectasis-situs inversus 759.3
  Sipple's (medullary thyroid carcinoma-pheochromocytoma) 193
  Sjögren (-Gougerot) (keratoconjunctivitis sicca) 710.2
    with lung involvement 710.2 [517.8]
  Sjögren-Larsson (ichthyosis congenita) 757.1
  Slocumb's 255.3
  Sluder's 337.0
  Smith-Lemli-Opitz (cerebrohepatorenal syndrome) 759.89
  Smith-Magenis 758.33   ▲
  smokers' 305.1
  Sneddon-Wilkinson (subcorneal pustular dermatosis) 694.1
  Sotos' (cerebral gigantism) 253.0
  South African cardiomyopathy 425.2
  spasmodic
    upward movement, eye(s) 378.82
    winking 307.20
  Spens' (syncope with heart block) 426.9
  spherophakia-brachymorphia 759.89
  spinal cord injury — see also Injury, spinal, by site
    with fracture, vertebra — see Fracture, vertebra, by site, with spinal cord injury
    cervical — see Injury, spinal, cervical
    fluid malabsorption (acquired) 331.3
  splenic
    agenesis 759.0
    flexure 569.89
    neutropenia 288.0
    sequestration 289.52

Syndrome — see also Disease — continued
  Spurway's (brittle bones and blue sclera) 756.51
  staphylococcal scalded skin 695.1
  Stein's (polycystic ovary) 256.4
  Stein-Leventhal (polycystic ovary) 256.4
  Steinbrocker's (see also Neuropathy, peripheral, autonomic) 337.9
  Stevens-Johnson (erythema multiforme exudativum) 695.1
  Stewart-Morel (hyperostosis frontalis interna) 733.3
  stiff-baby 759.89   ●
  stiff-man 333.91
  Still's (juvenile rheumatoid arthritis) 714.30
  Still-Felty (rheumatoid arthritis with splenomegaly and leukopenia) 714.1
  Stilling-Türk-Duane (ocular retraction syndrome) 378.71
  Stojano's (subcostal) 098.86
  Stokes (-Adams) (syncope with heart block) 426.9
  Stokvis-Talma (enterogenous cyanosis) 289.7
  stone heart (see also Failure, ventricular, left) 428.1
  straight-back 756.19
  stroke (see also Disease, cerebrovascular, acute) 436
    little 435.9
  Sturge-Kalischer-Weber (encephalotrigeminal angiomatosis) 759.6
  Sturge-Weber (-Dimitri) (encephalocutaneous angiomatosis) 759.6
  subclavian-carotid obstruction (chronic) 446.7
  subclavian steal 435.2
  subcoracoid-pectoralis minor 447.8
  subcostal 098.86
    nerve compression 354.8
  subperiosteal hematoma 267
  subphrenic interposition 751.4
  sudden infant death (SIDS) 798.0
  Sudeck's 733.7
  Sudeck-Leriche 733.7
  superior
    cerebellar artery (see also Disease, cerebrovascular, acute) 436
    mesenteric artery 557.1
    pulmonary sulcus (tumor) (M8010/3) 162.3
    vena cava 459.2
  suprarenal cortical 255.3
  supraspinatus 726.10
  swallowed blood 777.3
  sweat retention 705.1
  Sweet's (acute febrile neutrophilic dermatosis) 695.89
  Swyer-James (unilateral hyperlucent lung) 492.8
  Swyer's (XY pure gonadal dysgenesis) 752.7
  Symonds' 348.2
  sympathetic
    cervical paralysis 337.0
    pelvic 625.5
  syndactylic oxycephaly 755.55
  syphilitic-cardiovascular 093.89
  systemic
    fibrosclerosing 710.8
    inflammatory response (SIRS) 995.90
      due to
        infectious process 995.91
          with organ dysfunction 995.92
        non-infectious process 995.93
          with organ dysfunction 995.94
  systolic click (-murmur) 785.2
  Tabagism 305.1
  tachycardia-bradycardia 427.81
  Takayasu (-Onishi) (pulseless disease) 446.7
  Tapia's 352.6
  tarsal tunnel 355.5
  Taussig-Bing (transposition, aorta and overriding pulmonary artery) 745.11
  Taybi's (otopalatodigital) 759.89
  Taylor's 625.5
  teething 520.7
  tegmental 344.89
  telangiectasis-pigmentation-cataract 757.33
  temporal 383.02
    lobectomy behavior 310.0

Syndrome — see also Disease — continued
  temporomandibular joint-pain-dysfunction [TMJ] NEC 524.60
    specified NEC 524.69
  Terry's 362.21
  testicular feminization 257.8
  testis, nonvirilizing 257.8
  tethered (spinal) cord 742.59
  thalamic 348.8
  Thibierge-Weissenbach (cutaneous systemic sclerosis) 710.1
  Thiele 724.6
  thoracic outlet (compression) 353.0
  thoracogenous rheumatic (hypertrophic pulmonary osteoarthropathy) 731.2
  Thorn's (see also Disease, renal) 593.9
  Thorson-Biörck (malignant carcinoid) 259.2
  thrombopenia-hemangioma 287.3
  thyroid-adrenocortical insufficiency 258.1
  Tietze's 733.6
  time-zone (rapid) 307.45
  Tobias' (carcinoma, pulmonary apex) (M8010/3) 162.3
  toilet seat 926.0
  Tolosa-Hunt 378.55
  Toni-Fanconi (cystinosis) 270.0
  Touraine's (hereditary osteo-onychodysplasia) 756.89
  Touraine-Solente-Golé (acropachyderma) 757.39
  toxic
    oil 710.5
    shock 040.82
  transfusion
    fetal-maternal 772.0
    twin
      donor (infant) 772.0
      recipient (infant) 776.4
  Treacher Collins' (incomplete mandibulofacial dysostosis) 756.0
  trigeminal plate 259.8
  triple X female 758.81
  trisomy NEC 758.5
    13 or D₁ 758.1
    16-18 or E 758.2
    18 or E₃ 758.2
    20 758.5
    21 or G (mongolism) 758.0
    22 or G (mongolism) 758.0
    G 758.0
  Troisier-Hanot-Chauffard (bronze diabetes) 275.0
  tropical wet feet 991.4
  Trousseau's (thrombophlebitis migrans visceral cancer) 453.1
  Türk's (ocular retraction syndrome) 378.71
  Turner's 758.6
  Turner-Varny 758.6
  twin-to-twin transfusion 762.3
    recipient twin 776.4
  Uehlinger's (acropachyderma) 757.39
  Ullrich (-Bonnevie) (-Turner) 758.6
  Ullrich-Feichtiger 759.89
  underwater blast injury (abdominal) (see also Injury, internal, abdomen) 868.00
  universal joint, cervix 620.6
  Unverricht (-Lundborg) 333.2
  Unverricht-Wagner (dermatomyositis) 710.3
  upward gaze 378.81
  Urbach-Oppenheim (necrobiosis lipoidica diabeticorum) 250.8 ☑ [709.3]
  Urbach-Wiethe (lipoid proteinosis) 272.8
  uremia, chronic 585
  urethral 597.81
  urethro-oculoarticular 099.3
  urethro-oculosynovial 099.3
  urohepatic 572.4
  uveocutaneous 364.24
  uveomeningeal, uveomeningitis 363.22
  vagohypoglossal 352.6
  vagovagal 780.2
  van Buchem's (hyperostosis corticalis) 733.3
  van der Hoeve's (brittle bones and blue sclera, deafness) 756.51
  van der Hoeve-Halbertsma-Waardenburg (ptosis-epicanthus) 270.2

Syndrome — *see also* Disease — *continued*
van der Hoeve-Waardenburg-Gualdi (ptosis-epicanthus) 270.2
van Neck-Odelberg (juvenile osteochondrosis) 732.1
vanishing twin 651.33
vascular splanchnic 557.0
vasomotor 443.9
vasovagal 780.2
VATER 759.89
Velo-cardio-facial 758.32 ▲
vena cava (inferior) (superior) (obstruction) 459.2
Verbiest's (claudicatio intermittens spinalis) 435.1
Vernet's 352.6
vertebral
  artery 435.1
    compression 721.1
    lumbar 724.4
    steal 435.1
vertebrogenic (pain) 724.5
vertiginous NEC 386.9
video display tube 723.8
Villaret's 352.6
Vinson-Plummer (sideropenic dysphagia) 280.8
virilizing adrenocortical hyperplasia, congenital 255.2
virus, viral 079.99
visceral larval migrans 128.0
visual disorientation 368.16
vitamin B₆ deficiency 266.1
vitreous touch 997.99
Vogt's (corpus striatum) 333.7
Vogt-Koyanagi 364.24
Volkmann's 958.6
von Bechterew-Strümpell (ankylosing spondylitis) 720.0
von Graefe's 378.72
von Hippel-Lindau (angiomatosis retinocerebellosa) 759.6
von Schroetter's (intermittent venous claudication) 453.8
von Willebrand (-Jürgens) (angiohemophilia) 286.4
Waardenburg-Klein (ptosis epicanthus) 270.2
Wagner (-Unverricht) (dermatomyositis) 710.3
Waldenström's (macroglobulinemia) 273.3
Waldenström-Kjellberg (sideropenic dysphagia) 280.8
Wallenberg's (posterior inferior cerebellar artery) (*see also* Disease, cerebrovascular, acute) 436
Waterhouse (-Friderichsen) 036.3
water retention 276.6
Weber's 344.89
Weber-Christian (nodular nonsuppurative panniculitis) 729.30
Weber-Cockayne (epidermolysis bullosa) 757.39
Weber-Dimitri (encephalocutaneous angiomatosis) 759.6
Weber-Gubler 344.89
Weber-Leyden 344.89
Weber-Osler (familial hemorrhagic telangiectasia) 448.0
Wegener's (necrotizing respiratory granulomatosis) 446.4
Weill-Marchesani (brachymorphism and ectopia lentis) 759.89
Weingarten's (tropical eosinophilia) 518.3
Weiss-Baker (carotid sinus syncope) 337.0
Weissenbach-Thibierge (cutaneous systemic sclerosis) 710.1
Werdnig-Hoffmann 335.0
Werlhof-Wichmann (*see also* Purpura, thrombocytopenic) 287.3
Wermer's (polyendocrine adenomatosis) 258.0
Werner's (progeria adultorum) 259.8
Wernicke's (nonalcoholic) (superior hemorrhagic polioencephalitis) 265.1
Wernicke-Korsakoff (nonalcoholic) 294.0
  alcoholic 291.1
Westphal-Strümpell (hepatolenticular degeneration) 275.1
wet
  brain (alcoholic) 303.9 ☑
  feet (maceration) (tropical) 991.4

Syndrome — *see also* Disease — *continued*
wet — *continued*
  lung
    adult 518.5
    newborn 770.6
whiplash 847.0
Whipple's (intestinal lipodystrophy) 040.2
"whistling face" (craniocarpotarsal dystrophy) 759.89
Widal (-Abrami) (acquired hemolytic jaundice) 283.9
Wilkie's 557.1
Wilkinson-Sneddon (subcorneal pustular dermatosis) 694.1
Willan-Plumbe (psoriasis) 696.1
Willebrand (-Jürgens) (angiohemophilia) 286.4
Willi-Prader (hypogenital dystrophy with diabetic tendency) 759.81
Wilson's (hepatolenticular degeneration) 275.1
Wilson-Mikity 770.7
Wiskott-Aldrich (eczema-thrombocytopenia) 279.12
withdrawal
  alcohol 291.81
  drug 292.0
    infant of dependent mother 779.5
Woakes' (ethmoiditis) 471.1
Wolff-Parkinson-White (anomalous atrioventricular excitation) 426.7
Wright's (hyperabduction) 447.8
X
  cardiac 413.9
  dysmetabolic 277.7
xiphoidalgia 733.99
XO 758.6
XXX 758.81
XXXXY 758.81
XXY 758.7
yellow vernix (placental dysfunction) 762.2
Zahorsky's 074.0
Zellweger 277.86 ●
Zieve's (jaundice, hyperlipemia and hemolytic anemia) 571.1
Zollinger-Ellison (gastric hypersecretion with pancreatic islet cell tumor) 251.5
Zuelzer-Ogden (nutritional megaloblastic anemia) 281.2

Synechia (iris) (pupil) 364.70
anterior 364.72
  peripheral 364.73
intrauterine (traumatic) 621.5
posterior 364.71
vulvae, congenital 752.49

Synesthesia (*see also* Disturbance, sensation) 782.0

Synodontia 520.2

Synophthalmus 759.89

Synorchidism 752.89

Synorchism 752.89

Synostosis (congenital) 756.59
astragaloscaphoid 755.67
radioulnar 755.53
talonavicular (bar) 755.67
tarsal 755.67

Synovial — *see* condition

Synovioma (M9040/3) — *see also* Neoplasm, connective tissue, malignant
benign (M9040/0) — *see* Neoplasm, connective tissue, benign

Synoviosarcoma (M9040/3) — *see* Neoplasm, connective tissue, malignant

Synovitis 727.00
chronic crepitant, wrist 727.2
due to crystals — *see* Arthritis, due to crystals
gonococcal 098.51
gouty 274.0
syphilitic 095.7
  congenital 090.0
traumatic, current — *see* Sprain, by site
tuberculous — *see* Tuberculosis, synovitis
villonodular 719.20
  ankle 719.27
  elbow 719.22
  foot 719.27
  hand 719.24

Synovitis — *continued*
villonodular — *continued*
  hip 719.25
  knee 719.26
  multiple sites 719.29
  pelvic region 719.25
  shoulder (region) 719.21
  specified site NEC 719.28
  wrist 719.23

Syphilide 091.3
congenital 090.0
newborn 090.0
tubercular 095.8
  congenital 090.0

Syphilis, syphilitic (acquired) 097.9
with lung involvement 095.1
abdomen (late) 095.2
acoustic nerve 094.86
adenopathy (secondary) 091.4
adrenal (gland) 095.8
  with cortical hypofunction 095.8
age under 2 years NEC (*see also* Syphilis, congenital) 090.9
  acquired 097.9
alopecia (secondary) 091.82
anemia 095.8
aneurysm (artery) (ruptured) 093.89
  aorta 093.0
  central nervous system 094.89
  congenital 090.5
anus 095.8
  primary 091.1
  secondary 091.3
aorta, aortic (arch) (abdominal) (insufficiency) (pulmonary) (regurgitation) (stenosis) (thoracic) 093.89
  aneurysm 093.0
arachnoid (adhesive) 094.2
artery 093.89
  cerebral 094.89
  spinal 094.89
arthropathy (neurogenic) (tabetic) 094.0 [713.5]
asymptomatic — *see* Syphilis, latent
ataxia, locomotor (progressive) 094.0
atrophoderma maculatum 091.3
auricular fibrillation 093.89
Bell's palsy 094.89
bladder 095.8
bone 095.5
  secondary 091.61
brain 094.89
breast 095.8
bronchus 095.8
bubo 091.0
bulbar palsy 094.89
bursa (late) 095.7
cardiac decompensation 093.89
cardiovascular (early) (late) (primary) (secondary) (tertiary) 093.9
  specified type and site NEC 093.89
causing death under 2 years of age (*see also* Syphilis, congenital) 090.9
  stated to be acquired NEC 097.9
central nervous system (any site) (early) (late) (latent) (primary) (recurrent) (relapse) (secondary) (tertiary) 094.9
  with
    ataxia 094.0
    paralysis, general 094.1
      juvenile 090.40
    paresis (general) 094.1
      juvenile 090.40
    tabes (dorsalis) 094.0
      juvenile 090.40
    taboparesis 094.1
      juvenile 090.40
  aneurysm (ruptured) 094.87
  congenital 090.40
  juvenile 090.40
  remission in (sustained) 094.9
  serology doubtful, negative, or positive 094.9
  specified nature or site NEC 094.89
  vascular 094.89
cerebral 094.89
  meningovascular 094.2
  nerves 094.89
  sclerosis 094.89
  thrombosis 094.89

Syndrome — Syphilis, syphilitic

Syphilis, syphilitic — *continued*
  cerebrospinal 094.89
    tabetic 094.0
  cerebrovascular 094.89
  cervix 095.8
  chancre (multiple) 091.0
    extragenital 091.2
    Rollet's 091.0
  Charcôt's joint 094.0 [713.5]
  choked disc 094.89 [377.00]
  chorioretinitis 091.51
    congenital 090.0 [363.13]
    late 094.83
  choroiditis 091.51
    congenital 090.0 [363.13]
    late 094.83
    prenatal 090.0 [363.13]
  choroidoretinitis (secondary) 091.51
    congenital 090.0 [363.13]
    late 094.83
  ciliary body (secondary) 091.52
    late 095.8 [364.11]
  colon (late) 095.8
  combined sclerosis 094.89
  complicating pregnancy, childbirth or
    puerperium 647.0 ☑
    affecting fetus or newborn 760.2
  condyloma (latum) 091.3
  congenital 090.9
    with
      encephalitis 090.41
      paresis (general) 090.40
      tabes (dorsalis) 090.40
      taboparesis 090.40
    chorioretinitis, choroiditis 090.0 [363.13]
    early or less than 2 years after birth NEC
      090.2
      with manifestations 090.0
      latent (without manifestations) 090.1
        negative spinal fluid test 090.1
        serology, positive 090.1
      symptomatic 090.0
    interstitial keratitis 090.3
    juvenile neurosyphilis 090.40
    late or 2 years or more after birth NEC
      090.7
      chorioretinitis, choroiditis 090.5 [363.13]
      interstitial keratitis 090.3
      juvenile neurosyphilis NEC 090.40
      latent (without manifestations) 090.6
        negative spinal fluid test 090.6
        serology, positive 090.6
      symptomatic or with manifestations NEC
        090.5
        interstitial keratitis 090.3
  conjugal 097.9
    tabes 094.0
  conjunctiva 095.8 [372.10]
  contact V01.6
  cord, bladder 094.0
  cornea, late 095.8 [370.59]
  coronary (artery) 093.89
    sclerosis 093.89
  coryza 095.8
    congenital 090.0
  cranial nerve 094.89
  cutaneous — *see* Syphilis, skin
  dacryocystitis 095.8
  degeneration, spinal cord 094.89
  d'emblée 095.8
  dementia 094.1
    paralytica 094.1
      juvenilis 090.40
  destruction of bone 095.5
  dilatation, aorta 093.0
  due to blood transfusion 097.9
  dura mater 094.89
  ear 095.8
    inner 095.8
      nerve (eighth) 094.86
      neurorecurrence 094.86
  early NEC 091.0
    cardiovascular 093.9
    central nervous system 094.9
      paresis 094.1
      tabes 094.0
    latent (without manifestations) (less than 2
      years after infection) 092.9

Syphilis, syphilitic — *continued*
  early NEC — *continued*
    latent — *continued*
      negative spinal fluid test 092.9
      serological relapse following treatment
        092.0
      serology positive 092.9
    paresis 094.1
    relapse (treated, untreated) 091.7
    skin 091.3
    symptomatic NEC 091.89
      extragenital chancre 091.2
      primary, except extragenital chancre
        091.0
      secondary (*see also* Syphilis, secondary)
        091.3
        relapse (treated, untreated) 091.7
    tabes 094.0
    ulcer 091.3
  eighth nerve 094.86
  endemic, nonvenereal 104.0
  endocarditis 093.20
    aortic 093.22
    mitral 093.21
    pulmonary 093.24
    tricuspid 093.23
  epididymis (late) 095.8
  epiglottis 095.8
  epiphysitis (congenital) 090.0
  esophagus 095.8
  Eustachian tube 095.8
  exposure to V01.6
  eye 095.8 [363.13]
    neuromuscular mechanism 094.85
  eyelid 095.8 [373.5]
    with gumma 095.8 [373.5]
    ptosis 094.89
  fallopian tube 095.8
  fracture 095.5
  gallbladder (late) 095.8
  gastric 095.8
    crisis 094.0
    polyposis 095.8
  general 097.9
    paralysis 094.1
      juvenile 090.40
  genital (primary) 091.0
  glaucoma 095.8
  gumma (late) NEC 095.9
    cardiovascular system 093.9
    central nervous system 094.9
    congenital 090.5
    heart or artery 093.89
  heart 093.89
    block 093.89
    decompensation 093.89
    disease 093.89
    failure 093.89
    valve (*see also* Syphilis, endocarditis) 093.20
  hemianesthesia 094.89
  hemianopsia 095.8
  hemiparesis 094.89
  hemiplegia 094.89
  hepatic artery 093.89
  hepatitis 095.3
  hepatomegaly 095.3
    congenital 090.0
  hereditaria tarda (*see also* Syphilis, congenital,
    late) 090.7
  hereditary (*see also* Syphilis, congenital) 090.9
    interstitial keratitis 090.3
  Hutchinson's teeth 090.5
  hyalitis 095.8
  inactive — *see* Syphilis, latent
  infantum NEC (*see also* Syphilis, congenital)
    090.9
  inherited — *see* Syphilis, congenital
  internal ear 095.8
  intestine (late) 095.8
  iris, iritis (secondary) 091.52
    late 095.8 [364.11]
  joint (late) 095.8
  keratitis (congenital) (early) (interstitial) (late)
    (parenchymatous) (punctata profunda)
    090.3
  kidney 095.4
  lacrimal apparatus 095.8

Syphilis, syphilitic — *continued*
  laryngeal paralysis 095.8
  larynx 095.8
  late 097.0
    cardiovascular 093.9
    central nervous system 094.9
    latent or 2 years or more after infection
      (without manifestations) 096
      negative spinal fluid test 096
      serology positive 096
    paresis 094.1
    specified site NEC 095.8
    symptomatic or with symptoms 095.9
    tabes 094.0
  latent 097.1
    central nervous system 094.9
    date of infection unspecified 097.1
    early or less than 2 years after infection
      092.9
    late or 2 years or more after infection 096
    serology
      doubtful
        follow-up of latent syphilis 097.1
          central nervous system 094
          date of infection unspecified 097.1
          early or less than 2 years after
            infection 092
          late or 2 years or more after
            infection 096
      positive, only finding 097.1
        date of infection unspecified 097.1
        early or less than 2 years after
          infection 097.1
        late or 2 years or more after infection
          097.1
  lens 095.8
  leukoderma 091.3
    late 095.8
  lienis 095.8
  lip 091.3
    chancre 091.2
    late 095.8
    primary 091.2
  Lissauer's paralysis 094.1
  liver 095.3
    secondary 091.62
  locomotor ataxia 094.0
  lung 095.1
  lymphadenitis (secondary) 091.4
  lymph gland (early) (secondary) 091.4
    late 095.8
  macular atrophy of skin 091.3
    striated 095.8
  maternal, affecting fetus or newborn 760.2
    manifest syphilis in newborn — *see* Syphilis,
      congenital
  mediastinum (late) 095.8
  meninges (adhesive) (basilar) (brain) (spinal
    cord) 094.2
  meningitis 094.2
    acute 091.81
    congenital 090.42
  meningoencephalitis 094.2
  meningovascular 094.2
    congenital 090.49
  mesarteritis 093.89
    brain 094.89
    spine 094.89
  middle ear 095.8
  mitral stenosis 093.21
  monoplegia 094.89
  mouth (secondary) 091.3
    late 095.8
  mucocutaneous 091.3
    late 095.8
  mucous
    membrane 091.3
      late 095.8
    patches 091.3
      congenital 090.0
  mulberry molars 090.5
  muscle 095.6
  myocardium 093.82
  myositis 095.6
  nasal sinus 095.8
  neonatorum NEC (*see also* Syphilis, congenital)
    090.9

Syphilis, syphilitic — continued
  nerve palsy (any cranial nerve) 094.89
  nervous system, central 094.9
  neuritis 095.8
    acoustic nerve 094.86
  neurorecidive of retina 094.83
  neuroretinitis 094.85
  newborn (see also Syphilis, congenital) 090.9
  nodular superficial 095.8
  nonvenereal, endemic 104.0
  nose 095.8
    saddle back deformity 090.5
    septum 095.8
      perforated 095.8
  occlusive arterial disease 093.89
  ophthalmic 095.8 [363.13]
  ophthalmoplegia 094.89
  optic nerve (atrophy) (neuritis) (papilla) 094.84
  orbit (late) 095.8
  orchitis 095.8
  organic 097.9
  osseous (late) 095.5
  osteochondritis (congenital) 090.0
  osteoporosis 095.5
  ovary 095.8
  oviduct 095.8
  palate 095.8
    gumma 095.8
    perforated 090.5
  pancreas (late) 095.8
  pancreatitis 095.8
  paralysis 094.89
    general 094.1
    juvenile 090.40
  paraplegia 094.89
  paresis (general) 094.1
    juvenile 090.40
  paresthesia 094.89
  Parkinson's disease or syndrome 094.82
  paroxysmal tachycardia 093.89
  pemphigus (congenital) 090.0
  penis 091.0
    chancre 091.0
    late 095.8
  pericardium 093.81
  perichondritis, larynx 095.8
  periosteum 095.5
    congenital 090.0
    early 091.61
    secondary 091.61
  peripheral nerve 095.8
  petrous bone (late) 095.5
  pharynx 095.8
    secondary 091.3
  pituitary (gland) 095.8
  placenta 095.8
  pleura (late) 095.8
  pneumonia, white 090.0
  pontine (lesion) 094.89
  portal vein 093.89
  primary NEC 091.2
    anal 091.1
    and secondary (see also Syphilis, secondary) 091.9
    cardiovascular 093.9
    central nervous system 094.9
    extragenital chancre NEC 091.2
    fingers 091.2
    genital 091.0
    lip 091.2
    specified site NEC 091.2
    tonsils 091.2
  prostate 095.8
  psychosis (intracranial gumma) 094.89
  ptosis (eyelid) 094.89
  pulmonary (late) 095.1
    artery 093.89
  pulmonum 095.1
  pyelonephritis 095.4
  recently acquired, symptomatic NEC 091.89
  rectum 095.8
  respiratory tract 095.8
  retina
    late 094.83
    neurorecidive 094.83
  retrobulbar neuritis 094.85
  salpingitis 095.8

Syphilis, syphilitic — continued
  sclera (late) 095.0
  sclerosis
    cerebral 094.89
    coronary 093.89
    multiple 094.89
    subacute 094.89
  scotoma (central) 095.8
  scrotum 095.8
  secondary (and primary) 091.9
    adenopathy 091.4
    anus 091.3
    bone 091.61
    cardiovascular 093.9
    central nervous system 094.9
    chorioretinitis, choroiditis 091.51
    hepatitis 091.62
    liver 091.62
    lymphadenitis 091.4
    meningitis, acute 091.81
    mouth 091.3
    mucous membranes 091.3
    periosteum 091.61
    periostitis 091.61
    pharynx 091.3
    relapse (treated) (untreated) 091.7
    skin 091.3
    specified form NEC 091.89
    tonsil 091.3
    ulcer 091.3
    viscera 091.69
    vulva 091.3
  seminal vesicle (late) 095.8
  seronegative
    with signs or symptoms — see Syphilis, by site and stage
  seropositive
    with signs or symptoms — see Syphilis, by site and stage
    follow-up of latent syphilis — see Syphilis, latent
    only finding — see Syphilis, latent
  seventh nerve (paralysis) 094.89
  sinus 095.8
  sinusitis 095.8
  skeletal system 095.5
  skin (early) (secondary) (with ulceration) 091.3
    late or tertiary 095.8
  small intestine 095.8
  spastic spinal paralysis 094.0
  spermatic cord (late) 095.8
  spinal (cord) 094.89
    with
      paresis 094.1
      tabes 094.0
  spleen 095.8
  splenomegaly 095.8
  spondylitis 095.5
  staphyloma 095.8
  stigmata (congenital) 090.5
  stomach 095.8
  synovium (late) 095.7
  tabes dorsalis (early) (late) 094.0
    juvenile 090.40
  tabetic type 094.0
    juvenile 090.40
  taboparesis 094.1
    juvenile 090.40
  tachycardia 093.89
  tendon (late) 095.7
  tertiary 097.0
    with symptoms 095.8
    cardiovascular 093.9
    central nervous system 094.9
    multiple NEC 095.8
    specified site NEC 095.8
  testis 095.8
  thorax 095.8
  throat 095.8
  thymus (gland) 095.8
  thyroid (late) 095.8
  tongue 095.8
  tonsil (lingual) 095.8
    primary 091.2
    secondary 091.3
  trachea 095.8
  tricuspid valve 093.23

Syphilis, syphilitic — continued
  tumor, brain 094.89
  tunica vaginalis (late) 095.8
  ulcer (any site) (early) (secondary) 091.3
    late 095.9
    perforating 095.9
      foot 094.0
  urethra (stricture) 095.8
  urogenital 095.8
  uterus 095.8
  uveal tract (secondary) 091.50
    late 095.8 [363.13]
  uveitis (secondary) 091.50
    late 095.8 [363.13]
  uvula (late) 095.8
    perforated 095.8
  vagina 091.0
    late 095.8
  valvulitis NEC 093.20
  vascular 093.89
    brain or cerebral 094.89
  vein 093.89
    cerebral 094.89
  ventriculi 095.8
  vesicae urinariae 095.8
  viscera (abdominal) 095.2
    secondary 091.69
  vitreous (hemorrhage) (opacities) 095.8
  vulva 091.0
    late 095.8
    secondary 091.3
Syphiloma 095.9
  cardiovascular system 093.9
  central nervous system 094.9
  circulatory system 093.9
  congenital 090.5
Syphilophobia 300.29
Syringadenoma (M8400/0) — see also Neoplasm, skin, benign
  papillary (M8406/0) — see Neoplasm, skin, benign
Syringobulbia 336.0
Syringocarcinoma (M8400/3) — see Neoplasm, skin, malignant
Syringocystadenoma (M8400/0) — see also Neoplasm, skin, benign
  papillary (M8406/0) — see Neoplasm, skin, benign
Syringocystoma (M8407/0) — see Neoplasm, skin, benign
Syringoma (M8407/0) — see also Neoplasm, skin, benign
  chondroid (M8940/0) — see Neoplasm, by site, benign
Syringomyelia 336.0
Syringomyelitis 323.9
  late effect — see category 326
Syringomyelocele (see also Spina bifida) 741.9 ☑
Syringopontia 336.0
  disease, combined — see Degeneration, combined
  fibrosclerosing syndrome 710.8
  inflammatory response syndrome (SIRS) 995.90
    due to
      infectious process 995.91
        with organ dsfunction 995.92
      non-infectious process 995.93
        with organ dysfunction 995.94
  lupus erythematosus 710.0
    inhibitor 286.5

T

Tab — see Tag
Tabacism 989.8 ☑
Tabacosis 989.8 ☑
Tabardillo 080
  flea-borne 081.0
  louse-borne 080
Tabes, tabetic
  with
    central nervous system syphilis 094.0
    Charcôt's joint 094.0 [713.5]
    cord bladder 094.0

Tabes, tabetic — *continued*
  with — *continued*
    crisis, viscera (any) 094.0
    paralysis, general 094.1
    paresis (general) 094.1
    perforating ulcer 094.0
  arthropathy 094.0 *[713.5]*
  bladder 094.0
  bone 094.0
  cerebrospinal 094.0
  congenital 090.40
  conjugal 094.0
  dorsalis 094.0
    neurosyphilis 094.0
  early 094.0
  juvenile 090.40
  latent 094.0
  mesenterica (*see also* Tuberculosis) 014.8 ☑
  paralysis insane, general 094.1
  peripheral (nonsyphilitic) 799.89
  spasmodic 094.0
    not dorsal or dorsalis 343.9
  syphilis (cerebrospinal) 094.0
Taboparalysis 094.1
Taboparesis (remission) 094.1
  with
    Charcôt's joint 094.1 *[713.5]*
    cord bladder 094.1
    perforating ulcer 094.1
  juvenile 090.40
Tachyalimentation 579.3
Tachyarrhythmia, tachyrhythmia — *see also*
  Tachycardia
  paroxysmal with sinus bradycardia 427.81
Tachycardia 785.0
  atrial 427.89
  auricular 427.89
  newborn 779.82
  nodal 427.89
    nonparoxysmal atrioventricular 426.89
  nonparoxysmal atrioventricular (nodal) 426.89
  paroxysmal 427.2
    with sinus bradycardia 427.81
    atrial (PAT) 427.0
      psychogenic 316 *[427.0]*
    atrioventricular (AV) 427.0
      psychogenic 316 *[427.0]*
    essential 427.2
    junctional 427.0
    nodal 427.0
    psychogenic 316 *[427.2]*
      atrial 316 *[427.0]*
      supraventricular 316 *[427.0]*
      ventricular 316 *[427.1]*
    supraventricular 427.0
      psychogenic 316 *[427.0]*
    ventricular 427.1
      psychogenic 316 *[427.1]*
  postoperative 997.1
  psychogenic 306.2
  sick sinus 427.81
  sinoauricular 427.89
  sinus 427.89
  supraventricular 427.89
  ventricular (paroxysmal) 427.1
    psychogenic 316 *[427.1]*
Tachypnea 786.06
  hysterical 300.11
  newborn (idiopathic) (transitory) 770.6
  psychogenic 306.1
  transitory, of newborn 770.6
Taenia (infection) (infestation) (*see also*
  Infestation, taenia) 123.3
  diminuta 123.6
  echinococcal infestation (*see also*
    Echinococcus) 122.9
  nana 123.6
  saginata infestation 123.2
  solium (intestinal form) 123.0
    larval form 123.1
Taeniasis (intestine) (*see also* Infestation, Taenia)
  123.3
  saginata 123.2
  solium 123.0
Taenzer's disease 757.4

Tag (hypertrophied skin) (infected) 701.9
  adenoid 474.8
  anus 455.9
  endocardial (*see also* Endocarditis) 424.90
  hemorrhoidal 455.9
  hymen 623.8
  perineal 624.8
  preauricular 744.1
  rectum 455.9
  sentinel 455.9
  skin 701.9
    accessory 757.39
    anus 455.9
    congenital 757.39
    preauricular 744.1
    rectum 455.9
  tonsil 474.8
  urethra, urethral 599.84
  vulva 624.8
Tahyna fever 062.5
Takayasu (-Onishi) disease or syndrome
  (pulseless disease) 446.7
Talc granuloma 728.82
Talcosis 502
Talipes (congenital) 754.70
  acquired NEC 736.79
    planus 734
  asymmetric 754.79
    acquired 736.79
  calcaneovalgus 754.62
    acquired 736.76
  calcaneovarus 754.59
    acquired 736.76
  calcaneus 754.79
    acquired 736.76
  cavovarus 754.59
    acquired 736.75
  cavus 754.71
    acquired 736.73
  equinovalgus 754.69
    acquired 736.72
  equinovarus 754.51
    acquired 736.71
  equinus 754.79
    acquired, NEC 736.72
  percavus 754.71
    acquired 736.73
  planovalgus 754.69
    acquired 736.79
  planus (acquired) (any degree) 734
    congenital 754.61
    due to rickets 268.1
  valgus 754.60
    acquired 736.79
  varus 754.50
    acquired 736.79
Talma's disease 728.85
Tamponade heart (Rose's) (*see also* Pericarditis)
  423.9
Tanapox 078.89
Tangier disease (familial high-density lipoprotein
  deficiency) 272.5
Tank ear 380.12
Tantrum (childhood) (*see also* Disturbance,
  conduct) 312.1 ☑
Tapeworm (infection) (infestation) (*see also*
  Infestation, tapeworm) 123.9
Tapia's syndrome 352.6
Tarantism 297.8
Target-oval cell anemia 282.49
Tarlov's cyst 355.9
Tarral-Besnier disease (pityriasis rubra pilaris)
  696.4
Tarsalgia 729.2
Tarsal tunnel syndrome 355.5
Tarsitis (eyelid) 373.00
  syphilitic 095.8 *[373.00]*
  tuberculous (*see also* Tuberculosis)
    017.0 ☑ *[373.4]*
Tartar (teeth) 523.6
Tattoo (mark) 709.09
Taurodontism 520.2

Taussig-Bing defect, heart, or syndrome
  (transposition, aorta and overriding
  pulmonary artery) 745.11
Tay's choroiditis 363.41
Tay-Sachs
  amaurotic familial idiocy 330.1
  disease 330.1
Taybi's syndrome (otopalatodigital) 759.89
Taylor's
  disease (diffuse idiopathic cutaneous atrophy)
    701.8
  syndrome 625.5
Tear, torn (traumatic) — *see also* Wound, open,
  by site
  anus, anal (sphincter) 863.89
    with open wound in cavity 863.99
    complicating delivery 664.2 ☑
      with mucosa 664.3 ☑
    nontraumatic, nonpuerperal 565.0
  articular cartilage, old (*see also* Disorder,
    cartilage, articular) 718.0 ☑
  bladder
    with
      abortion — *see* Abortion, by type, with
        damage to pelvic organs
      ectopic pregnancy (*see also* categories
        633.0-633.9) 639.2
      molar pregnancy (*see also* categories 630-
        632) 639.2
    following
      abortion 639.2
      ectopic or molar pregnancy 639.2
    obstetrical trauma 665.5 ☑
  bowel
    with
      abortion — *see* Abortion, by type, with
        damage to pelvic organs
      ectopic pregnancy (*see also* categories
        633.0-633.9) 639.2
      molar pregnancy (*see also* categories 630-
        632) 639.2
    following
      abortion 639.2
      ectopic or molar pregnancy 639.2
    obstetrical trauma 665.5 ☑
  broad ligament
    with
      abortion — *see* Abortion, by type, with
        damage to pelvic organs
      ectopic pregnancy (*see also* categories
        633.0-633.9) 639.2
      molar pregnancy (*see also* categories 630-
        632) 639.2
    following
      abortion 639.2
      ectopic or molar pregnancy 639.2
    obstetrical trauma 665.6 ☑
  bucket handle (knee) (meniscus) — *see* Tear,
    meniscus
  capsule
    joint — *see* Sprain, by site
    spleen — *see* Laceration, spleen, capsule
  cartilage — *see also* Sprain, by site
    articular, old (*see also* Disorder, cartilage,
      articular) 718.0 ☑
    knee — *see* Tear, meniscus
    semilunar (knee) (current injury) — *see*
      Tear, meniscus
  cervix
    with
      abortion — *see* Abortion, by type, with
        damage to pelvic organs
      ectopic pregnancy (*see also* categories
        633.0-633.9) 639.2
      molar pregnancy (*see also* categories 630-
        632) 639.2
    following
      abortion 639.2
      ectopic or molar pregnancy 639.2
    obstetrical trauma (current) 665.3 ☑
    old 622.3
  internal organ (abdomen, chest, or pelvis) —
    see Injury, internal, by site
  ligament — *see also* Sprain, by site
    with open wound — *see* Wound, open by
      site

☑ Additional Digit Required   ▶◀ Revised Text   ● New Line   ▲ Revised Code

Tear, torn — *see also* Wound, open, by site — *continued*
  meniscus (knee) (current injury) 836.2
    bucket handle 836.0
      old 717.0
    lateral 836.1
      anterior horn 836.1
        old 717.42
      bucket handle 836.1
        old 717.41
      old 717.40
      posterior horn 836.1
        old 717.43
      specified site NEC 836.1
        old 717.49
    medial 836.0
      anterior horn 836.0
        old 717.1
      bucket handle 836.0
        old 717.0
      old 717.3
      posterior horn 836.0
        old 717.2
    old NEC 717.5
    site other than knee — *see* Sprain, by site
  muscle — *see also* Sprain, by site
    with open wound — *see* Wound, open by site
  pelvic
    floor, complicating delivery 664.1 ☑
    organ NEC
      with
        abortion — *see* Abortion, by type, with damage to pelvic organs
        ectopic pregnancy (*see also* categories 633.0-633.9) 639.2
        molar pregnancy (*see also* categories 630-632) 639.2
      following
        abortion 639.2
        ectopic or molar pregnancy 639.2
      obstetrical trauma 665.5 ☑
  perineum — *see also* Laceration, perineum
    obstetrical trauma 665.5 ☑
  periurethral tissue
    with
      abortion — *see* Abortion, by type, with damage to pelvic organs
      ectopic pregnancy (*see also* categories 633.0-633.9) 639.2
      molar pregnancy (*see also* categories 630-632) 639.2
    following
      abortion 639.2
      ectopic or molar pregnancy 639.2
    obstetrical trauma 665.5 ☑
  rectovaginal septum — *see* Laceration, rectovaginal septum
  retina, retinal (recent) (with detachment) 361.00
    without detachment 361.30
    dialysis (juvenile) (with detachment) 361.04
    giant (with detachment) 361.03
    horseshoe (without detachment) 361.32
    multiple (with detachment) 361.02
      without detachment 361.33
    old
      delimited (partial) 361.06
      partial 361.06
      total or subtotal 361.07
    partial (without detachment)
      giant 361.03
      multiple defects 361.02
      old (delimited) 361.06
      single defect 361.01
    round hole (without detachment) 361.31
    single defect (with detachment) 361.01
    total or subtotal (recent) 361.05
      old 361.07
  rotator cuff (traumatic) 840.4
    current injury 840.4
    degenerative 726.10
    nontraumatic 727.61
  semilunar cartilage, knee (*see also* Tear, meniscus) 836.2
    old 717.5

Tear, torn — *see also* Wound, open, by site — *continued*
  tendon — *see also* Sprain, by site
    with open wound — *see* Wound, open by site
  tentorial, at birth 767.0
  umbilical cord
    affecting fetus or newborn 772.0
    complicating delivery 663.8 ☑
  urethra
    with
      abortion — *see* Abortion, by type, with damage to pelvic organs
      ectopic pregnancy (*see also* categories 633.0-633.9) 639.2
      molar pregnancy (*see also* categories 630-632) 639.2
    following
      abortion 639.2
      ectopic or molar pregnancy 639.2
    obstetrical trauma 665.5 ☑
  uterus — *see* Injury, internal, uterus
  vagina — *see* Laceration, vagina
  vessel, from catheter 998.2
  vulva, complicating delivery 664.0 ☑

Tear stone 375.57

Teeth, tooth — *see also* condition
  grinding 306.8

Teething 520.7
  syndrome 520.7

Tegmental syndrome 344.89

Telangiectasia, telangiectasis (verrucous) 448.9
  ataxic (cerebellar) 334.8
  familial 448.0
  hemorrhagic, hereditary (congenital) (senile) 448.0
  hereditary hemorrhagic 448.0
  retina 362.15
  spider 448.1

Telecanthus (congenital) 743.63

Telescoped bowel or intestine (*see also* Intussusception) 560.0

Teletherapy, adverse effect NEC 990

Telogen effluvium 704.02

Temperature
  body, high (of unknown origin) (*see also* Pyrexia) 780.6
  cold, trauma from 991.9
    newborn 778.2
    specified effect NEC 991.8
  high
    body (of unknown origin) (*see also* Pyrexia) 780.6
    trauma from — *see* Heat

Temper tantrum (childhood) (*see also* Disturbance, conduct) 312.1 ☑

Temple — *see* condition

Temporal — *see also* condition
  lobe syndrome 310.0

Temporomandibular joint-pain-dysfunction syndrome 524.60

Temporosphenoidal — *see* condition

Tendency
  bleeding (*see also* Defect, coagulation) 286.9
  homosexual, ego-dystonic 302.0
  paranoid 301.0
  suicide 300.9

Tenderness
  abdominal (generalized) (localized) 789.6 ☑
  rebound 789.6 ☑
  skin 782.0

Tendinitis, tendonitis (*see also* Tenosynovitis) 726.90
  Achilles 726.71
  adhesive 726.90
    shoulder 726.0
  calcific 727.82
    shoulder 726.11
  gluteal 726.5
  patellar 726.64
  peroneal 726.79
  pes anserinus 726.61
  psoas 726.5

Tendinitis, tendonitis (*see also* Tenosynovitis) — *continued*
  tibialis (anterior) (posterior) 726.72
  trochanteric 726.5

Tendon — *see* condition

Tendosynovitis — *see* Tenosynovitis

Tendovaginitis — *see* Tenosynovitis

Tenesmus 787.99
  rectal 787.99
  vesical 788.9

Tenia — *see* Taenia

Teniasis — *see* Taeniasis

Tennis elbow 726.32

Tenonitis — *see also* Tenosynovitis
  eye (capsule) 376.04

Tenontosynovitis — *see* Tenosynovitis

Tenontothecitis — *see* Tenosynovitis

Tenophyte 727.9

Tenosynovitis 727.00
  adhesive 726.90
    shoulder 726.0
  ankle 727.06
  bicipital (calcifying) 726.12
  buttock 727.09
  due to crystals — *see* Arthritis, due to crystals
  elbow 727.09
  finger 727.05
  foot 727.06
  gonococcal 098.51
  hand 727.05
  hip 727.09
  knee 727.09
  radial styloid 727.04
  shoulder 726.10
    adhesive 726.0
  spine 720.1
  supraspinatus 726.10
  toe 727.06
  tuberculous — *see* Tuberculosis, tenosynovitis
  wrist 727.05

Tenovaginitis — *see* Tenosynovitis

Tension
  arterial, high (*see also* Hypertension) 401.9
    without diagnosis of hypertension 796.2
  headache 307.81
  intraocular (elevated) 365.00
  nervous 799.2
  ocular (elevated) 365.00
  pneumothorax 512.0
    iatrogenic 512.1
    postoperative 512.1
    spontaneous 512.0
  premenstrual 625.4
  state 300.9

Tentorium — *see* condition

Teratencephalus 759.89

Teratism 759.7

Teratoblastoma (malignant) (M9080/3) — *see* Neoplasm, by site, malignant

Teratocarcinoma (M9081/3) — *see also* Neoplasm, by site, malignant
  liver 155.0

Teratoma (solid) (M9080/1) — *see also* Neoplasm, by site, uncertain behavior
  adult (cystic) (M9080/0) — *see* Neoplasm, by site, benign
  and embryonal carcinoma, mixed (M9081/3) — *see* Neoplasm, by site, malignant
  benign (M9080/0) — *see* Neoplasm, by site, benign
  combined with choriocarcinoma (M9101/3) — *see* Neoplasm, by site, malignant
  cystic (adult) (M9080/0) — *see* Neoplasm, by site, benign
  differentiated type (M9080/0) — *see* Neoplasm, by site, benign
  embryonal (M9080/3) — *see also* Neoplasm, by site, malignant
    liver 155.0
  fetal
    sacral, causing fetopelvic disproportion 653.7 ☑

Teratoma (M9080/1) — *see also* Neoplasm, by
    site, uncertain behavior — *continued*
  immature (M9080/3) — *see* Neoplasm, by site,
      malignant
  liver (M9080/3) 155.0
    adult, benign, cystic, differentiated type or
        mature (M9080/0) 211.5
  malignant (M9080/3) — *see also* Neoplasm, by
      site, malignant
    anaplastic type (M9082/3) — *see* Neoplasm,
        by site, malignant
    intermediate type (M9083/3) — *see*
        Neoplasm, by site, malignant
      liver (M9080/3) 155.0
    trophoblastic (M9102/3)
      specified site — *see* Neoplasm, by site,
          malignant
      unspecified site 186.9
    undifferentiated type (M9082/3) — *see*
        Neoplasm, by site, malignant
  mature (M9080/0) — *see* Neoplasm, by site,
      benign
  ovary (M9080/0) 220
    embryonal, immature, or malignant
        (M9080/3) 183.0
  suprasellar (M9080/3) — *see* Neoplasm, by
      site, malignant
  testis (M9080/3) 186.9
    adult, benign, cystic, differentiated type or
        mature (M9080/0) 222.0
    undescended 186.0
Terminal care V66.7
Termination
  anomalous — *see also* Malposition, congenital
    portal vein 747.49
    right pulmonary vein 747.42
  pregnancy (legal) (therapeutic) (*see* Abortion,
      legal) 635.9 ☑
    fetus NEC 779.6
    illegal (*see also* Abortion, illegal) 636.9 ☑
Ternidens diminutus infestation 127.7
Terrors, night (child) 307.46
Terry's syndrome 362.21
Tertiary — *see* condition
Tessellated fundus, retina (tigroid) 362.89
Test(s)
  AIDS virus V72.6
  adequacy
    hemodialysis V56.31
    peritoneal dialysis V56.32
  allergen V72.7
  bacterial disease NEC (*see also* Screening, by
      name of disease) V74.9
  basal metabolic rate V72.6
  blood-alcohol V70.4
  blood-drug V70.4
    for therapeutic drug monitoring V58.83
  developmental, infant or child V20.2
  Dick V74.8
  fertility V26.21
  genetic V26.3
  hearing V72.1
  HIV V72.6
  human immunodeficiency virus V72.6
  Kveim V82.89
  laboratory V72.6
    for medicolegal reason V70.4
  Mantoux (for tuberculosis) V74.1
  mycotic organism V75.4
  parasitic agent NEC V75.8
  paternity V70.4
  peritoneal equilibration V56.32
  pregnancy
    negative result V72.41   ●
    positive V22.1
      first pregnancy V22.0
    unconfirmed V72.40   ▲
  preoperative V72.84
    cardiovascular V72.81
    respiratory V72.82
    specified NEC V72.83
  procreative management NEC V26.29
  sarcoidosis V82.89
  Schick V74.3
  Schultz-Charlton V74.8

Test(s) — *continued*
  skin, diagnostic
    allergy V72.7
    bacterial agent NEC (*see also* Screening, by
        name of disease) V74.9
    Dick V74.8
    hypersensitivity V72.7
    Kveim V82.89
    Mantoux V74.1
    mycotic organism V75.4
    parasitic agent NEC V75.8
    sarcoidosis V82.89
    Schick V74.3
    Schultz-Charlton V74.8
    tuberculin V74.1
  specified type NEC V72.8 ☑
  tuberculin V74.1
  vision V72.0
  Wassermann
    positive (*see also* Serology for syphilis,
        positive) 097.1
    false 795.6
Testicle, testicular, testis — *see also* condition
  feminization (syndrome) 257.8
Tetanus, tetanic (cephalic) (convulsions) 037
  with
    abortion — *see* Abortion, by type, with
        sepsis
    ectopic pregnancy (*see also* categories
        633.0-633.9) 639.0
    molar pregnancy (*see* categories 630-632)
        639.0
  following
    abortion 639.0
    ectopic or molar pregnancy 639.0
  inoculation V03.7
    reaction (due to serum) — *see*
        Complications, vaccination
  neonatorum 771.3
  puerperal, postpartum, childbirth 670.0 ☑
Tetany, tetanic 781.7
  alkalosis 276.3
  associated with rickets 268.0
  convulsions 781.7
    hysterical 300.11
  functional (hysterical) 300.11
  hyperkinetic 781.7
    hysterical 300.11
  hyperpnea 786.01
    hysterical 300.11
    psychogenic 306.1
  hyperventilation 786.01
    hysterical 300.11
    psychogenic 306.1
  hypocalcemic, neonatal 775.4
  hysterical 300.11
  neonatal 775.4
  parathyroid (gland) 252.1
  parathyroprival 252.1
  postoperative 252.1
  postthyroidectomy 252.1
  pseudotetany 781.7
    hysterical 300.11
  psychogenic 306.1
    specified as conversion reaction 300.11
Tetralogy of Fallot 745.2
Tetraplegia — *see* Quadriplegia
Thailand hemorrhagic fever 065.4
Thalassanemia 282.49
Thalassemia (alpha) (beta) (disease) (Hb-C) (Hb-D)
    (Hb-E) (Hb-H) (Hb-I) (high fetal gene) (high
    fetal hemoglobin) (intermedia) (major)
    (minima) (minor) (mixed) (trait) (with other
    hemoglobinopathy) 282.49
  HB-S (without crisis) 282.41
    with
      crisis 282.42
      vaso-occlusive pain 282.42
  sickle-cell (without crisis) 282.41
    with
      crisis 282.42
      vaso-occlusive pain 282.42
Thalassemic variants 282.49
Thaysen-Gee disease (nontropical sprue) 579.0

Thecoma (M8600/0) 220
  malignant (M8600/3) 183.0
Thelarche, precocious 259.1
Thelitis 611.0
  puerperal, postpartum 675.0 ☑
Therapeutic — *see* condition
Therapy V57.9
  blood transfusion, without reported diagnosis
      V58.2
  breathing V57.0
  chemotherapy V58.1
    fluoride V07.31
    prophylactic NEC V07.39
  dialysis (intermittent) (treatment)
    extracorporeal V56.0
    peritoneal V56.8
    renal V56.0
    specified type NEC V56.8
  exercise NEC V57.1
    breathing V57.0
  extracorporeal dialysis (renal) V56.0
  fluoride prophylaxis V07.31
  hemodialysis V56.0
  hormone replacement (postmenopausal)   ●
      V07.4   ●
  long term oxygen therapy V46.2
  occupational V57.21
  orthoptic V57.4
  orthotic V57.81
  peritoneal dialysis V56.8
  physical NEC V57.1
  postmenopausal hormone replacement V07.4
  radiation V58.0
  speech V57.3
  vocational V57.22
Thermalgesia 782.0
Thermalgia 782.0
Thermanalgesia 782.0
Thermanesthesia 782.0
Thermic — *see* condition
Thermography (abnormal) 793.9
  breast 793.89
Thermoplegia 992.0
Thesaurismosis
  amyloid 277.3
  bilirubin 277.4
  calcium 275.40
  cystine 270.0
  glycogen (*see also* Disease, glycogen storage)
      271.0
  kerasin 272.7
  lipoid 272.7
  melanin 255.4
  phosphatide 272.7
  urate 274.9
Thiaminic deficiency 265.1
  with beriberi 265.0
Thibierge-Weissenbach syndrome (cutaneous
    systemic sclerosis) 710.1
Thickened endometrium 793.5
Thickening
  bone 733.99
    extremity 733.99
  breast 611.79
  hymen 623.3
  larynx 478.79
  nail 703.8
    congenital 757.5
  periosteal 733.99
  pluera (*see also* Pleurisy) 511.0
  skin 782.8
  subepiglottic 478.79
  tongue 529.8
  valve, heart — *see* Endocarditis
Thiele syndrome 724.6
Thigh — *see* condition
Thinning vertebra (*see also* Osteoporosis) 733.00
Thirst, excessive 783.5
  due to deprivation of water 994.3
Thomsen's disease 359.2
Thomson's disease (congenital poikiloderma)
    757.33

☑ Additional Digit Required   ►◄ Revised Text   ● New Line   ▲ Revised Code

Thoracic — *see also* condition
  kidney 753.3
  outlet syndrome 353.0
  stomach — *see* Hernia, diaphragm
Thoracogastroschisis (congenital) 759.89
Thoracopagus 759.4
Thoracoschisis 756.3
Thoracoscopic surgical procedure converted to open procedure V64.42
Thorax — *see* condition
Thorn's syndrome (*see also* Disease, renal) 593.9
Thornwaldt's, Tornwaldt's
  bursitis (pharyngeal) 478.29
  cyst 478.26
  disease (pharyngeal bursitis) 478.29
Thorson-Biörck syndrome (malignant carcinoid) 259.2
Threadworm (infection) (infestation) 127.4
Threatened
  abortion or miscarriage 640.0 ☑
    with subsequent abortion (*see also* Abortion, spontaneous) 634.9 ☑
    affecting fetus 762.1
  labor 644.1 ☑
    affecting fetus or newborn 761.8
    premature 644.0 ☑
  miscarriage 640.0 ☑
    affecting fetus 762.1
  premature
    delivery 644.2 ☑
      affecting fetus or newborn 761.8
    labor 644.0 ☑
      before 22 completed weeks gestation 640.0 ☑
Three-day fever 066.0
Threshers' lung 495.0
Thrix annulata (congenital) 757.4
Throat — *see* condition
Thrombasthenia (Glanzmann's) (hemorrhagic) (hereditary) 287.1
Thromboangiitis 443.1
  obliterans (general) 443.1
    cerebral 437.1
    vessels
      brain 437.1
      spinal cord 437.1
Thromboarteritis — *see* Arteritis
Thromboasthenia (Glanzmann's) (hemorrhagic) (hereditary) 287.1
Thrombocytasthenia (Glanzmann's) 287.1
Thrombocythemia (essential) (hemorrhagic) (primary) (M9962/1) 238.7
  idiopathic (M9962/1) 238.7
Thrombocytopathy (dystrophic) (granulopenic) 287.1
Thrombocytopenia, thrombocytopenic 287.5
  with giant hemangioma 287.3
  amegakaryocytic, congenital 287.3
  congenital 287.3
  cyclic 287.3
  dilutional 287.4
  due to
    drugs 287.4
    extracorporeal circulation of blood 287.4
    massive blood transfusion 287.4
    platelet alloimmunization 287.4
  essential 287.3
  hereditary 287.3
  Kasabach-Merritt 287.3
  neonatal, transitory 776.1
    due to
      exchange transfusion 776.1
      idiopathic maternal thrombocytopenia 776.1
      isoimmunization 776.1
  primary 287.3
  puerperal, postpartum 666.3 ☑
  purpura (*see also* Purpura, thrombocytopenic) 287.3
    thrombotic 446.6
  secondary 287.4
  sex-linked 287.3

Thrombocytosis, essential 289.9
Thromboembolism — *see* Embolism
Thrombopathy (Bernard-Soulier) 287.1
  constitutional 286.4
  Willebrand-Jürgens (angiohemophilia) 286.4
Thrombopenia (*see also* Thrombocytopenia) 287.5
Thrombophlebitis 451.9
  antecubital vein 451.82
  antepartum (superficial) 671.2 ☑
    affecting fetus or newborn 760.3
    deep 671.3 ☑
  arm 451.89
    deep 451.83
    superficial 451.82
  breast, superficial 451.89
  cavernous (venous) sinus — *see* Thrombophlebitis, intracranial venous sinus
  cephalic vein 451.82
  cerebral (sinus) (vein) 325
    late effect — *see* category 326
    nonpyogenic 437.6
      in pregnancy or puerperium 671.5 ☑
      late effect — *see* Late effect(s) (of) cerebrovascular disease
  due to implanted device — *see* Complications, due to (presence of) any device, implant or graft classified to 996.0-996.5 NEC
  during or resulting from a procedure NEC 997.2
  femoral 451.11
  femoropopliteal 451.19
  following infusion, perfusion, or transfusion 999.2
  hepatic (vein) 451.89
  idiopathic, recurrent 453.1
  iliac vein 451.81
  iliofemoral 451.11
  intracranial venous sinus (any) 325
    late effect — *see* category 326
    nonpyogenic 437.6
      in pregnancy or puerperium 671.5 ☑
      late effect — *see* Late effect(s) (of) cerebrovascular disease
  jugular vein 451.89
  lateral (venous) sinus — *see* Thrombophlebitis, intracranial venous sinus
  leg 451.2
    deep (vessels) 451.19
      femoral vein 451.11
      specified vessel NEC 451.19
    superficial (vessels) 451.0
      femoral vein 451.11
  longitudinal (venous) sinus — *see* Thrombophlebitis, intracranial venous sinus
  lower extremity 451.2
    deep (vessels) 451.19
      femoral vein 451.11
      specified vessel NEC 451.19
    superficial (vessels) 451.0
  migrans, migrating 453.1
  pelvic
    with
      abortion — *see* Abortion, by type, with sepsis
      ectopic pregnancy — (*see also* categories 633.0-633.9) 639.0
      molar pregnancy — (*see also* categories 630-632) 639.0
    following
      abortion 639.0
      ectopic or molar pregnancy 639.0
    puerperal 671.4 ☑
  popliteal vein 451.19
  portal (vein) 572.1
  postoperative 997.2
  pregnancy (superficial) 671.2 ☑
    affecting fetus or newborn 760.3
    deep 671.3 ☑
  puerperal, postpartum, childbirth (extremities) (superficial) 671.2 ☑
    deep 671.4 ☑
    pelvic 671.4 ☑
    specified site NEC 671.5 ☑
  radial vein 451.83

Thrombophlebitis — *continued*
  saphenous (greater) (lesser) 451.0
  sinus (intracranial) — *see* Thrombophlebitis, intracranial venous sinus
    specified site NEC 451.89
    tibial vein 451.19
Thrombosis, thrombotic (marantic) (multiple) (progressive) (septic) (vein) (vessel) 453.9
  with childbirth or during the puerperium — *see* Thrombosis, puerperal, postpartum
  antepartum — *see* Thrombosis, pregnancy
  aorta, aortic 444.1
    abdominal 444.0
    bifurcation 444.0
    saddle 444.0
    terminal 444.0
    thoracic 444.1
    valve — *see* Endocarditis, aortic
  apoplexy (*see also* Thrombosis, brain) 434.0 ☑
    late effect — *see* Late effect(s) (of) cerebrovascular disease
  appendix, septic — *see* Appendicitis, acute
  arteriolar-capillary platelet, disseminated 446.6
  artery, arteries (postinfectional) 444.9
    auditory, internal 433.8 ☑
    basilar (*see also* Occlusion, artery, basilar) 433.0 ☑
    carotid (common) (internal) (*see also* Occlusion, artery, carotid) 433.1 ☑
      with other precerebral artery 433.3 ☑
    cerebellar (anterior inferior) (posterior inferior) (superior) 433.8 ☑
    cerebral (*see also* Thrombosis, brain) 434.0 ☑
    choroidal (anterior) 433.8 ☑
    communicating posterior 433.8 ☑
    coronary (*see also* Infarct, myocardium) 410.9 ☑
      without myocardial infarction 411.81
      due to syphilis 093.89
      healed or specified as old 412
    extremities 444.22
      lower 444.22
      upper 444.21
    femoral 444.22
    hepatic 444.89
    hypophyseal 433.8 ☑
    meningeal, anterior or posterior 433.8 ☑
    mesenteric (with gangrene) 557.0
    ophthalmic (*see also* Occlusion, retina) 362.30
    pontine 433.8 ☑
    popliteal 444.22
    precerebral — *see* Occlusion, artery, precerebral NEC
    pulmonary 415.19
      iatrogenic 415.11
      postoperative 415.11
    renal 593.81
    retinal (*see also* Occlusion, retina) 362.30
    specified site NEC 444.89
    spinal, anterior or posterior 433.8 ☑
    traumatic (complication) (early) (*see also* Injury, blood vessel, by site) 904.9
    vertebral (*see also* Occlusion, artery, vertebral) 433.2 ☑
      with other precerebral artery 433.3 ☑
  atrial (endocardial) 424.90
    due to syphilis 093.89
  auricular (*see also* Infarct, myocardium) 410.9 ☑
  axillary (vein) 453.8
  basilar (artery) (*see also* Occlusion, artery, basilar) 433.0 ☑
  bland NEC 453.9
  brain (artery) (stem) 434.0 ☑
    due to syphilis 094.89
    iatrogenic 997.02
    late effect — *see* Late effect(s) (of) cerebrovascular disease
    postoperative 997.02
    puerperal, postpartum, childbirth 674.0 ☑
    sinus (*see also* Thrombosis, intracranial venous sinus) 325
  capillary 448.9
    arteriolar, generalized 446.6

☑ Additional Digit Required   ▶◀ Revised Text   ● New Line   ▲ Revised Code

Thrombosis, thrombotic — *continued*
  cardiac (*see also* Infarct, myocardium) 410.9 ☑
    due to syphilis 093.89
    healed or specified as old 412
    valve — *see* Endocarditis
  carotid (artery) (common) (internal) (*see also*
      Occlusion, artery, carotid) 433.1 ☑
    with other precerebral artery 433.3 ☑
  cavernous sinus (venous) — *see* Thrombosis,
      intracranial venous sinus
  cerebellar artery (anterior inferior) (posterior
      inferior) (superior) 433.8 ☑
    late effect — *see* Late effect(s) (of)
        cerebrovascular disease
  cerebral (arteries) (*see also* Thrombosis, brain)
      434.0 ☑
    late effect — *see* Late effect(s) (of)
        cerebrovascular disese
  coronary (artery) (*see also* Infarct, myocardium)
      410.9 ☑
    without myocardial infarction 411.81
    due to syphilis 093.89
    healed or specified as old 412
  corpus cavernosum 607.82
  cortical (*see also* Thrombosis, brain) 434.0 ☑
  due to (presence of) any device, implant, or
      graft classifiable to 996.0-996.5— *see*
      Complications, due to (presence of) any
      device, implant, or graft classified to
      996.0-996.5 NEC
  effort 453.8
  endocardial — *see* Infarct, myocardium
  eye (*see also* Occlusion, retina) 362.30
  femoral (vein) 453.8
    with inflammation or phlebitis 451.11
    artery 444.22
    deep 453.41   ●
  genital organ, male 608.83
  heart (chamber) (*see also* Infarct, myocardium)
      410.9 ☑
  hepatic (vein) 453.0
    artery 444.89
    infectional or septic 572.1
  iliac (vein) 453.8
    with inflammation or phlebitis 451.81
    artery (common) (external) (internal) 444.81
  inflammation, vein — *see* Thrombophlebitis
  internal carotid artery (*see also* Occlusion,
      artery, carotid) 433.1 ☑
    with other precerebral artery 433.3 ☑
  intestine (with gangrene) 557.0
  intracranial (*see also* Thrombosis, brain)
      434.0 ☑
    venous sinus (any) 325
      nonpyogenic origin 437.6
        in pregnancy or puerperium 671.5 ☑
  intramural (*see also* Infarct, myocardium)
      410.9 ☑
    without
      cardiac condition 429.89
      coronary artery disease 429.89
      myocardial infarction 429.89
    healed or specified as old 412
  jugular (bulb) 453.8
  kidney 593.81
    artery 593.81
  lateral sinus (venous) — *see* Thrombosis,
      intracranial venous sinus
  leg 453.8
    with inflammation or phlebitis — *see*
        Thrombophlebitis
    deep (vessels) 453.40   ▲
      lower (distal) 453.42   ●
      upper (proximal) 453.41   ●
    superficial (vessels) 453.8
  liver (venous) 453.0
    artery 444.89
    infectional or septic 572.1
    portal vein 452
  longitudinal sinus (venous) — *see* Thrombosis,
      intracranial venous sinus
  lower extremity 453.8   ▲
    deep vessels 453.40   ●
      calf 453.42   ●
      distal (lower leg) 453.42   ●
      femoral 453.41   ●
      iliac 453.41   ●

Thrombosis, thrombotic — *continued*
  lower extremity — *continued*
    deep vessels — *continued*
      lower leg 453.42   ●
      peroneal 453.42   ●
      popliteal 453.41   ●
      proximal (upper leg) 453.41   ●
      thigh 453.41   ●
      tibial 453.42   ●
  lung 415.19
    iatrogenic 415.11
    postoperative 415.11
  marantic, dural sinus 437.6
  meninges (brain) (*see also* Thrombosis, brain)
      434.0 ☑
  mesenteric (artery) (with gangrene) 557.0
    vein (inferior) (superior) 557.0
  mitral — *see* Insufficiency, mitral
  mural (heart chamber) (*see also* Infarct,
      myocardium) 410.9 ☑
    without
      cardiac condition 429.89
      coronary artery disease 429.89
      myocardial infarction 429.89
    due to syphilis 093.89
    following myocardial infarction 429.79
    healed or specified as old 412
  omentum (with gangrene) 557.0
  ophthalmic (artery) (*see also* Occlusion, retina)
      362.30
  pampiniform plexus (male) 608.83
    female 620.8
  parietal (*see also* Infarct, myocardium) 410.9 ☑
  penis, penile 607.82
  peripheral arteries 444.22
    lower 444.22
    upper 444.21
  platelet 446.6
  portal 452
    due to syphilis 093.89
    infectional or septic 572.1
  precerebral artery — *see also* Occlusion, artery,
      precerebral NEC
  pregnancy 671.9 ☑
    deep (vein) 671.3 ☑
    superficial (vein) 671.2 ☑
  puerperal, postpartum, childbirth 671.9 ☑
    brain (artery) 674.0 ☑
      venous 671.5 ☑
    cardiac 674.8 ☑
    cerebral (artery) 674.0 ☑
      venous 671.5 ☑
    deep (vein) 671.4 ☑
    intracranial sinus (nonpyogenic) (venous)
        671.5 ☑
    pelvic 671.4 ☑
    pulmonary (artery) 673.2 ☑
    specified site NEC 671.5 ☑
    superficial 671.2 ☑
  pulmonary (artery) (vein) 415.19
    iatrogenic 415.11
    postoperative 415.11
  renal (artery) 593.81
    vein 453.3
  resulting from presence of shunt or other
      internal prosthetic device — *see*
      Complications, due to (presence of) any
      device, implant, or graft classified to
      996.0-996.5 NEC
  retina, retinal (artery) 362.30
    arterial branch 362.32
    central 362.31
    partial 362.33
    vein
      central 362.35
      tributary (branch) 362.36
  scrotum 608.83
  seminal vesicle 608.83
  sigmoid (venous) sinus (*see* Thrombosis,
      intracranial venous sinus) 325
  silent NEC 453.9
  sinus, intracranial (venous) (any) (*see also*
      Thrombosis, intracranial venous sinus)
      325
  softening, brain (*see also* Thrombosis, brain)
      434.0 ☑
  specified site NEC 453.8

Thrombosis, thrombotic — *continued*
  spermatic cord 608.83
  spinal cord 336.1
    due to syphilis 094.89
    in pregnancy or puerperium 671.5 ☑
    pyogenic origin 324.1
      late effect — *see* category 326
  spleen, splenic 289.59
    artery 444.89
  testis 608.83
  traumatic (complication) (early) (*see also* Injury,
      blood vessel, by site) 904.9
  tricuspid — *see* Endocarditis, tricuspid
  tunica vaginalis 608.83
  umbilical cord (vessels) 663.6 ☑
    affecting fetus or newborn 762.6
  vas deferens 608.83
  vein
    deep 453.8   ●
    lower extremity — *see* Thrombosis,   ●
        lower extremity   ●
  vena cava (inferior) (superior) 453.2

Thrombus — *see* Thrombosis

Thrush 112.0
  newborn 771.7

Thumb — *see also* condition
  gamekeeper's 842.12
  sucking (child problem) 307.9

Thygeson's superficial punctate keratitis
    370.21

Thymergasia (*see also* Psychosis, affective)
    296.80

Thymitis 254.8

Thymoma (benign) (M8580/0) 212.6
  malignant (M8580/3) 164.0

Thymus, thymic (gland) — *see* condition

Thyrocele (*see also* Goiter) 240.9

Thyroglossal — *see also* condition
  cyst 759.2
  duct, persistent 759.2

Thyroid (body) (gland) — *see also* condition
  lingual 759.2

Thyroiditis 245.9
  acute (pyogenic) (suppurative) 245.0
    nonsuppurative 245.0
  autoimmune 245.2
  chronic (nonspecific) (sclerosing) 245.8
    fibrous 245.3
    lymphadenoid 245.2
    lymphocytic 245.2
    lymphoid 245.2
  complicating pregnancy, childbirth, or
      puerperium 648.1 ☑
  de Quervain's (subacute granulomatous) 245.1
  fibrous (chronic) 245.3
  giant (cell) (follicular) 245.1
  granulomatous (de Quervain's) (subacute)
      245.1
  Hashimoto's (struma lymphomatosa) 245.2
  iatrogenic 245.4
  invasive (fibrous) 245.3
  ligneous 245.3
  lymphocytic (chronic) 245.2
  lymphoid 245.2
  lymphomatous 245.2
  pseudotuberculous 245.1
  pyogenic 245.0
  radiation 245.4
  Riedel's (ligneous) 245.3
  subacute 245.1
  suppurative 245.0
  tuberculous (*see also* Tuberculosis) 017.5 ☑
  viral 245.1
  woody 245.3

Thyrolingual duct, persistent 759.2

Thyromegaly 240.9

Thyrotoxic
  crisis or storm (*see also* Thyrotoxicosis)
      242.9 ☑
  heart failure (*see also* Thyrotoxicosis)
      242.9 ☑ [425.7]

☑ Additional Digit Required   ►◄ Revised Text   ● New Line   ▲ Revised Code

Thyrotoxicosis 242.9 ☑

> Note — Use the following fifth-digit
> subclassification with category 242:
>
> 0   without mention of thyrotoxic crisis or
>   storm
> 1   with mention of thyrotoxic crisis or
>   storm

with
 goiter (diffuse) 242.0 ☑
  adenomatous 242.3 ☑
   multinodular 242.2 ☑
   uninodular 242.1 ☑
  nodular 242.3 ☑
   multinodular 242.2 ☑
   uninodular 242.1 ☑
 infiltrative
  dermopathy 242.0 ☑
  ophthalmopathy 242.0 ☑
 thyroid acropachy 242.0 ☑
complicating pregnancy, childbirth, or
  puerperium 648.1 ☑
due to
 ectopic thyroid nodule 242.4 ☑
 ingestion of (excessive) thyroid material
  242.8 ☑
 specified cause NEC 242.8 ☑
factitia 242.8 ☑
heart 242.9 ☑ *[425.7]*
neonatal (transient) 775.3

TIA (transient ischemic attack) 435.9
 with transient neurologic deficit 435.9
 late effect — *see* Late effect(s) (of)
  cerebrovascular disease

Tibia vara 732.4

Tic 307.20
 breathing 307.20
 child problem 307.21
 compulsive 307.22
 convulsive 307.20
 degenerative (generalized) (localized) 333.3
  facial 351.8
 douloureux (*see also* Neuralgia, trigeminal)
  350.1
  atypical 350.2
 habit 307.20
  chronic (motor or vocal) 307.22
  transient ▶(of childhood)◀ 307.21
 lid 307.20
  transient ▶(of childhood)◀ 307.21
 motor-verbal 307.23
 occupational 300.89
 orbicularis 307.20
  transient ▶(of childhood)◀ 307.21
 organic origin 333.3
 postchoreic — *see* Chorea
 psychogenic 307.20
  compulsive 307.22
 salaam 781.0
 spasm 307.20
  chronic (motor or vocal) 307.22
  transient ▶(of childhood)◀ 307.21

Tick (-borne) fever NEC 066.1
 American mountain 066.1
 Colorado 066.1
 hemorrhagic NEC 065.3
  Crimean 065.0
  Kyasanur Forest 065.2
  Omsk 065.1
 mountain 066.1
 nonexanthematous 066.1

Tick-bite fever NEC 066.1
 African 087.1
 Colorado (virus) 066.1
 Rocky Mountain 082.0

Tick paralysis 989.5

Tics and spasms, compulsive 307.22

Tietze's disease or syndrome 733.6

Tight, tightness
 anus 564.89
 chest 786.59
 fascia (lata) 728.9
 foreskin (congenital) 605
 hymen 623.3

Tight, tightness — *continued*
 introitus (acquired) (congenital) 623.3
 rectal sphincter 564.89
 tendon 727.81
  Achilles (heel) 727.81
 urethral sphincter 598.9

Tilting vertebra 737.9

Timidity, child 313.21

Tinea (intersecta) (tarsi) 110.9
 amiantacea 110.0
 asbestina 110.0
 barbae 110.0
 beard 110.0
 black dot 110.0
 blanca 111.2
 capitis 110.0
 corporis 110.5
 cruris 110.3
 decalvans 704.09
 flava 111.0
 foot 110.4
 furfuracea 111.0
 imbricata (Tokelau) 110.5
 lepothrix 039.0
 manuum 110.2
 microsporic (*see also* Dermatophytosis) 110.9
 nigra 111.1
 nodosa 111.2
 pedis 110.4
 scalp 110.0
 specified site NEC 110.8
 sycosis 110.0
 tonsurans 110.0
 trichophytic (*see also* Dermatophytosis) 110.9
 unguium 110.1
 versicolor 111.0

Tingling sensation (*see also* Disturbance,
  sensation) 782.0

Tin-miners' lung 503

Tinnitus (aurium) 388.30
 audible 388.32
 objective 388.32
 subjective 388.31

Tipping
 pelvis 738.6 ●
  ▶with disproportion (fetopelvic) 653.0 ☑◀
   ▶affecting fetus or newborn 763.1◀
   ▶causing obstructed labor 660.1 ☑◀
    ▶affecting fetus or newborn 763.1◀
 teeth 524.33 ●

Tiredness 780.79

Tissue — *see* condition

Tobacco
 abuse (affecting health) NEC (*see also* Abuse,
  drugs, nondependent) 305.1
 heart 989.8 ☑

Tobias' syndrome (carcinoma, pulmonary apex)
  (M8010/3) 162.3

Tocopherol deficiency 269.1

Todd's
 cirrhosis — *see* Cirrhosis, biliary
 paralysis (postepileptic transitory paralysis)
  344.8 ☑

Toe — *see* condition

Toilet, artificial opening (*see also* Attention to,
  artificial, opening) V55.9

Tokelau ringworm 110.5

Tollwut 071

Tolosa-Hunt syndrome 378.55

Tommaselli's disease
 correct substance properly administered 599.7
 overdose or wrong substance given or taken
  961.4

Tongue — *see also* condition
 worms 134.1

Tongue tie 750.0

Toni-Fanconi syndrome (cystinosis) 270.0

Tonic pupil 379.46

Tonsil — *see* condition

Tonsillitis (acute) (catarrhal) (croupous)
  (follicular) (gangrenous) (infective) (lacunar)
  (lingual) (malignant) (membranous)
  (phlegmonous) (pneumococcal)
  (pseudomembranous) (purulent) (septic)
  (staphylococcal) (subacute) (suppurative)
  (toxic) (ulcerative) (vesicular) (viral) 463
 with influenza, flu, or grippe 487.1
 chronic 474.00
 diphtheritic (membranous) 032.0
 hypertrophic 474.00
 influenzal 487.1
 parenchymatous 475
 streptococcal 034.0
 tuberculous (*see also* Tuberculosis) 012.8 ☑
 Vincent's 101

Tonsillopharyngitis 465.8

Tooth, teeth — *see* condition

Toothache 525.9

Topagnosis 782.0

Tophi (gouty) 274.0
 ear 274.81
 heart 274.82
 specified site NEC 274.82

Torn — *see* Tear, torn

Tornwaldt's bursitis (disease) (pharyngeal
  bursitis) 478.29
 cyst 478.26

Torpid liver 573.9

Torsion
 accessory tube 620.5
 adnexa (female) 620.5
 aorta (congenital) 747.29
  acquired 447.1
 appendix epididymis 608.2
 bile duct 576.8
  with calculus, choledocholithiasis or stones
   — *see* Choledocholithiasis
  congenital 751.69
 bowel, colon, or intestine 560.2
 cervix (*see also* Malposition, uterus) 621.6
 duodenum 537.3
 dystonia — *see* Dystonia, torsion
 epididymis 608.2
  appendix 608.2
 fallopian tube 620.5
 gallbladder (*see also* Disease, gallbladder)
  575.8
  congenital 751.69
 gastric 537.89
 hydatid of Morgagni (female) 620.5
 kidney (pedicle) 593.89
 Meckel's diverticulum (congenital) 751.0
 mesentery 560.2
 omentum 560.2
 organ or site, congenital NEC — *see* Anomaly,
  specified type NEC
 ovary (pedicle) 620.5
  congenital 752.0
 oviduct 620.5
 penis 607.89
  congenital 752.69
 renal 593.89
 spasm — *see* Dystonia, torsion
 spermatic cord 608.2
 spleen 289.59
 testicle, testis 608.2
 tibia 736.89
 umbilical cord — *see* Compression, umbilical
  cord
 uterus (*see also* Malposition, uterus) 621.6

Torticollis (intermittent) (spastic) 723.5
 congenital 754.1
  sternomastoid 754.1
 due to birth injury 767.8
 hysterical 300.11
 ocular 781.93
 psychogenic 306.0
  specified as conversion reaction 300.11
 rheumatic 723.5
 rheumatoid 714.0
 spasmodic 333.83
 traumatic, current NEC 847.0

☑ Additional Digit Required   ▶◀ Revised Text   ● New Line   ▲ Revised Code

Tortuous
　artery 447.1
　fallopian tube 752.19
　organ or site, congenital NEC — *see* Distortion
　renal vessel, congenital 747.62
　retina vessel (congenital) 743.58
　　acquired 362.17
　ureter 593.4
　urethra 599.84
　vein — *see* Varicose, vein
Torula, torular (infection) 117.5
　histolytica 117.5
　lung 117.5
Torulosis 117.5
Torus
　fracture
　　fibula 823.41
　　　with tibia 823.42
　　radius 813.45
　　tibia 823.40
　　　with fibula 823.42
　mandibularis 526.81
　palatinus 526.81
Touch, vitreous 997.99
Touraine's syndrome (hereditary osteo-onychodysplasia) 756.89
Touraine-Solente-Golé syndrome (acropachyderma) 757.39
Tourette's disease (motor-verbal tic) 307.23
Tower skull 756.0
　with exophthalmos 756.0
Toxemia 799.89
　with
　　abortion — *see* Abortion, by type, with toxemia
　bacterial — *see* Septicemia
　biliary (*see also* Disease, biliary) 576.8
　burn — *see* Burn, by site
　congenital NEC 779.89
　eclamptic 642.6 ☑
　　with pre-existing hypertension 642.7 ☑
　erysipelatous (*see also* Erysipelas) 035
　fatigue 799.89
　fetus or newborn NEC 779.89
　food (*see also* Poisoning, food) 005.9
　gastric 537.89
　gastrointestinal 558.2
　intestinal 558.2
　kidney (*see also* Disease, renal) 593.9
　lung 518.89
　malarial NEC (*see also* Malaria) 084.6
　maternal (of pregnancy), affecting fetus or newborn 760.0
　myocardial — *see* Myocarditis, toxic
　of pregnancy (mild) (pre-eclamptic) 642.4 ☑
　　with
　　　convulsions 642.6 ☑
　　　pre-existing hypertension 642.7 ☑
　　affecting fetus or newborn 760.0
　　severe 642.5 ☑
　pre-eclamptic — *see* Toxemia, of pregnancy
　puerperal, postpartum — *see* Toxemia, of pregnancy
　pulmonary 518.89
　renal (*see also* Disease, renal) 593.9
　septic (*see also* Septicemia) 038.9
　small intestine 558.2
　staphylococcal 038.10
　　aureus 038.11
　　due to food 005.0
　　specified organism NEC 038.19
　stasis 799.89
　stomach 537.89
　uremic (*see also* Uremia) 586
　urinary 586
Toxemica cerebropathia psychica (nonalcoholic) 294.0
　alcoholic 291.1
Toxic (poisoning) — *see also* condition
　from drug or poison — *see* Table of Drugs and Chemicals
　oil syndrome 710.5
　shock syndrome 040.82
　thyroid (gland) (*see also* Thyrotoxicosis) 242.9 ☑

Toxicemia — *see* Toxemia
Toxicity
　dilantin
　　asymptomatic 796.0
　　symptomatic — *see* Table of Drugs and Chemicals
　drug
　　asymptomatic 796.0
　　symptomatic — *see* Table of Drugs and Chemicals
　fava bean 282.2
　from drug or poison
　　asymptomatic 796.0
　　symptomatic — *see* Table of Drugs and Chemicals
Toxicosis (*see also* Toxemia) 799.89
　capillary, hemorrhagic 287.0
Toxinfection 799.89
　gastrointestinal 558.2
Toxocariasis 128.0
Toxoplasma infection, generalized 130.9
Toxoplasmosis (acquired) 130.9
　with pneumonia 130.4
　congenital, active 771.2
　disseminated (multisystemic) 130.8
　maternal
　　with suspected damage to fetus affecting management of pregnancy 655.4 ☑
　　affecting fetus or newborn 760.2
　　　manifest toxoplasmosis in fetus or newborn 771.2
　multiple sites 130.8
　multisystemic disseminated 130.8
　specified site NEC 130.7
Trabeculation, bladder 596.8
Trachea — *see* condition
Tracheitis (acute) (catarrhal) (infantile) (membranous) (plastic) (pneumococcal) (septic) (suppurative) (viral) 464.10
　with
　　bronchitis 490
　　　acute or subacute 466.0
　　　chronic 491.8
　　　tuberculosis — *see* Tuberculosis, pulmonary
　　laryngitis (acute) 464.20
　　　with obstruction 464.21
　　　chronic 476.1
　　　tuberculous (*see also* Tuberculosis, larynx) 012.3 ☑
　　obstruction 464.11
　chronic 491.8
　　with
　　　bronchitis (chronic) 491.8
　　　laryngitis (chronic) 476.1
　　due to external agent — *see* Condition, respiratory, chronic, due to
　diphtheritic (membranous) 032.3
　due to external agent — *see* Inflammation, respiratory, upper, due to
　edematous 464.11
　influenzal 487.1
　streptococcal 034.0
　syphilitic 095.8
　tuberculous (*see also* Tuberculosis) 012.8 ☑
Trachelitis (nonvenereal) (*see also* Cervicitis) 616.0
　trichomonal 131.09
Tracheobronchial — *see* condition
Tracheobronchitis (*see also* Bronchitis) 490
　acute or subacute 466.0
　　with bronchospasm or obstruction 466.0
　chronic 491.8
　influenzal 487.1
　senile 491.8
Tracheobronchomegaly (congenital) 748.3
Tracheobronchopneumonitis — *see* Pneumonia, broncho
Tracheocele (external) (internal) 519.1
　congenital 748.3
Tracheomalacia 519.1
　congenital 748.3

Tracheopharyngitis (acute) 465.8
　chronic 478.9
　due to external agent — *see* Condition, respiratory, chronic, due to
　due to external agent — *see* Inflammation, respiratory, upper, due to
Tracheostenosis 519.1
　congenital 748.3
Tracheostomy
　attention to V55.0
　complication 519.00
　hemorrhage 519.09
　infection 519.01
　malfunctioning 519.02
　obstruction 519.09
　sepsis 519.01
　status V44.0
　stenosis 519.02
Trachoma, trachomatous 076.9
　active (stage) 076.1
　contraction of conjunctiva 076.1
　dubium 076.0
　healed or late effect 139.1
　initial (stage) 076.0
　Türck's (chronic catarrhal laryngitis) 476.0
Trachyphonia 784.49
Training
　insulin pump V65.46
　orthoptic V57.4
　orthotic V57.81
Train sickness 994.6
Trait
　hemoglobin
　　abnormal NEC 282.7
　　　with thalassemia 282.49
　　C (*see also* Disease, hemoglobin, C) 282.7
　　　with elliptocytosis 282.7
　　S (Hb-S) 282.5
　　Lepore 282.49
　　with other abnormal hemoglobin NEC 282.49
　paranoid 301.0
　sickle-cell 282.5
　　with
　　　elliptocytosis 282.5
　　　spherocytosis 282.5
Traits, paranoid 301.0
Tramp V60.0
Trance 780.09
　hysterical 300.13
Transaminasemia 790.4
Transfusion, blood
　donor V59.01
　　stem cells V59.02
　incompatible 999.6
　reaction or complication — *see* Complications, transfusion
　syndrome
　　fetomaternal 772.0
　　twin-to-twin
　　　blood loss (donor twin) 772.0
　　　recipient twin 776.4
　without reported diagnosis V58.2
Transient — *see also* condition
　alteration of awareness 780.02
　blindness 368.12
　deafness (ischemic) 388.02
　global amnesia 437.7
　person (homeless) NEC V60.0
Transitional, lumbosacral joint of vertebra 756.19
Translocation
　autosomes NEC 758.5
　　13-15 758.1
　　16-18 758.2
　　21 or 22 758.0
　　balanced in normal individual 758.4
　　D₁ 758.1
　　E₃ 758.2
　　G 758.0
　balanced autosomal in normal individual 758.4
　chromosomes NEC 758.89
　Down's syndrome 758.0
Translucency, iris 364.53

☑ Additional Digit Required　　　　　▶◀ Revised Text　　　　　● New Line　　　　　▲ Revised Code

Transmission of chemical substances through the placenta (affecting fetus or newborn) 760.70
  alcohol 760.71
  anti-infective agents 760.74
  cocaine 760.75
  "crack" 760.75
  diethylstilbestrol [DES] 760.76
  hallucinogenic agents 760.73
  medicinal agents NEC 760.79
  narcotics 760.72
  obstetric anesthetic or analgesic drug 763.5
  specified agent NEC 760.79
  suspected, affecting management of pregnancy 655.5 ☑

Transplant(ed)
  bone V42.4
    marrow V42.81
  complication — *see also* Complications, due to (presence of) any device, implant, or graft classified to 996.0-996.5 NEC
    bone marrow 996.85
    corneal graft NEC 996.79
      infection or inflammation 996.69
      reaction 996.51
      rejection 996.51
    organ (failure) (immune or nonimmune cause) (infection) (rejection) 996.87
      bone marrow 996.85
      heart 996.83
      intestines 996.87
      kidney 996.81
      liver 996.82
      lung 996.84
      pancreas 996.86
      specified NEC 996.89
    skin NEC 996.79
      infection or inflammation 996.69
      rejection 996.52
        artificial 996.55
        decellularized allodermis 996.55
  cornea V42.5
  hair V50.0
  heart V42.1
    valve V42.2
  intestine V42.84
  kidney V42.0
  liver V42.7
  lung V42.6
  organ V42.9
    specified NEC V42.89
  pancreas V42.83
  peripheral stem cells V42.82
  skin V42.3
  stem cells, peripheral V42.82
  tissue V42.9
    specified NEC V42.89

Transplants, ovarian, endometrial 617.1

Transposed — *see* Transposition

Transposition (congenital) — *see also* Malposition, congenital
  abdominal viscera 759.3
  aorta (dextra) 745.11
  appendix 751.5
  arterial trunk 745.10
  colon 751.5
  great vessels (complete) 745.10
    both originating from right ventricle 745.11
    corrected 745.12
    double outlet right ventricle 745.11
    incomplete 745.11
    partial 745.11
    specified type NEC 745.19
  heart 746.87
    with complete transposition of viscera 759.3
  intestine (large) (small) 751.5
  pulmonary veins 747.49
  reversed jejunal (for bypass) (status) V45.3
  scrotal 752.81
  stomach 750.7
    with general transposition of viscera 759.3
  teeth, tooth 524.30 ▲
  vessels (complete) 745.10
    partial 745.11
  viscera (abdominal) (thoracic) 759.3

Trans-sexualism 302.50
  with
    asexual history 302.51
    heterosexual history 302.53
    homosexual history 302.52
Transverse — *see also* condition
  arrest (deep), in labor 660.3 ☑
    affecting fetus or newborn 763.1
  lie 652.3 ☑
    before labor, affecting fetus or newborn 761.7
    causing obstructed labor 660.0 ☑
      affecting fetus or newborn 763.1
    during labor, affecting fetus or newborn 763.1
Transvestism, transvestitism (transvestic fetishism) 302.3
Trapped placenta (with hemorrhage) 666.0 ☑
  without hemorrhage 667.0 ☑
Trauma, traumatism (*see also* Injury, by site) 959.9
  birth — *see* Birth, injury NEC
  causing hemorrhage of pregnancy or delivery 641.8 ☑
  complicating
    abortion — *see* Abortion, by type, with damage to pelvic organs
    ectopic pregnancy (*see also* categories 633.0-633.9) 639.2
    molar pregnancy (*see also* categories 630-632) 639.2
  during delivery NEC 665.9 ☑
  following
    abortion 639.2
    ectopic or molar pregnancy 639.2
  maternal, during pregnancy, affecting fetus or newborn 760.5
  neuroma — *see* Injury, nerve, by site
  previous major, affecting management of pregnancy, childbirth, or puerperium V23.8 ☑
  psychic (current) — *see also* Reaction, adjustment
    previous (history) V15.49
  psychologic, previous (affecting health) V15.49
  transient paralysis — *see* Injury, nerve, by site
Traumatic — *see* condition
Treacher Collins' syndrome (incomplete facial dysostosis) 756.0
Treitz's hernia — *see* Hernia, Treitz's
Trematode infestation NEC 121.9
Trematodiasis NEC 121.9
Trembles 988.8
Trembling paralysis (*see also* Parkinsonism) 332.0
Tremor 781.0
  essential (benign) 333.1
  familial 333.1
  flapping (liver) 572.8
  hereditary 333.1
  hysterical 300.11
  intention 333.1
  mercurial 985.0
  muscle 728.85
  Parkinson's (*see also* Parkinsonism) 332.0
  psychogenic 306.0
    specified as conversion reaction 300.11
  senilis 797
  specified type NEC 333.1
Trench
  fever 083.1
  foot 991.4
  mouth 101
  nephritis — *see* Nephritis, acute
Treponema pallidum infection (*see also* Syphilis) 097.9
Treponematosis 102.9
  due to
    T. pallidum — *see* Syphilis
    T. pertenue (yaws) (*see also* Yaws) 102.9
Triad
  Kartagener's 759.3
  Reiter's (complete) (incomplete) 099.3
  Saint's (*see also* Hernia, diaphragm) 553.3

Trichiasis 704.2
  cicatricial 704.2
  eyelid 374.05
    with entropion (*see also* Entropion) 374.00
Trichinella spiralis (infection) (infestation) 124
Trichinelliasis 124
Trichinellosis 124
Trichiniasis 124
Trichinosis 124
Trichobezoar 938
  intestine 936
  stomach 935.2
Trichocephaliasis 127.3
Trichocephalosis 127.3
Trichocephalus infestation 127.3
Trichoclasis 704.2
Trichoepithelioma (M8100/0) — *see also* Neoplasm, skin, benign
  breast 217
  genital organ NEC — *see* Neoplasm, by site, benign
  malignant (M8100/3) — *see* Neoplasm, skin, malignant
Trichofolliculoma (M8101/0) — *see* Neoplasm, skin, benign
Tricholemmoma (M8102/0) — *see* Neoplasm, skin, benign
Trichomatosis 704.2
Trichomoniasis 131.9
  bladder 131.09
  cervix 131.09
  intestinal 007.3
  prostate 131.03
  seminal vesicle 131.09
  specified site NEC 131.8
  urethra 131.02
  urogenitalis 131.00
  vagina 131.01
  vulva 131.01
  vulvovaginal 131.01
Trichomycosis 039.0
  axillaris 039.0
  nodosa 111.2
  nodularis 111.2
  rubra 039.0
Trichonocardiosis (axillaris) (palmellina) 039.0
Trichonodosis 704.2
Trichophytid, trichophyton infection (*see also* Dermatophytosis) 110.9
Trichophytide — *see* Dermatophytosis
Trichophytobezoar 938
  intestine 936
  stomach 935.2
Trichophytosis — *see* Dermatophytosis
Trichoptilosis 704.2
Trichorrhexis (nodosa) 704.2
Trichosporosis nodosa 111.2
Trichostasis spinulosa (congenital) 757.4
Trichostrongyliasis (small intestine) 127.6
Trichostrongylosis 127.6
Trichostrongylus (instabilis) infection 127.6
Trichotillomania 312.39
Trichromat, anomalous (congenital) 368.59
Trichromatopsia, anomalous (congenital) 368.59
Trichuriasis 127.3
Trichuris trichiuria (any site) (infection) (infestation) 127.3
Tricuspid (valve) — *see* condition
Trifid — *see also* Accessory
  kidney (pelvis) 753.3
  tongue 750.13
Trigeminal neuralgia (*see also* Neuralgia, trigeminal) 350.1
Trigeminoencephaloangiomatosis 759.6
Trigeminy 427.89
  postoperative 997.1
Trigger finger (acquired) 727.03
  congenital 756.89

Trigonitis (bladder) (chronic) (pseudomembranous) 595.3
  tuberculous (see also Tuberculosis) 016.1 ☑
Trigonocephaly 756.0
Trihexosidosis 272.7
Trilobate placenta — see Placenta, abnormal
Trilocular heart 745.8
Tripartita placenta — see Placenta, abnormal
Triple — see also Accessory
  kidneys 753.3
  uteri 752.2
  X female 758.81
Triplegia 344.89
  congenital or infantile 343.8
Triplet
  affected by maternal complications of pregnancy 761.5
  healthy liveborn — see Newborn, multiple
  pregnancy (complicating delivery) NEC 651.1 ☑
    with fetal loss and retention of one or more fetus(es) 651.4 ☑
Triplex placenta — see Placenta, abnormal
Triplication — see Accessory
Trismus 781.0
  neonatorum 771.3
  newborn 771.3
Trisomy (syndrome) NEC 758.5
  13 (partial) 758.1
  16-18 758.2
  18 (partial) 758.2
  21 (partial) 758.0
  22 758.0
  autosomes NEC 758.5
  D₁ 758.1
  E₃ 758.2
  G (group) 758.0
  group D₁ 758.1
  group E 758.2
  group G 758.0
Tritanomaly 368.53
Tritanopia 368.53
Troisier-Hanot-Chauffard syndrome (bronze diabetes) 275.0
Trombidiosis 133.8
Trophedema (hereditary) 757.0
  congenital 757.0
Trophoblastic disease (see also Hydatidiform mole) 630
  previous, affecting management of pregnancy V23.1
Tropholymphedema 757.0
Trophoneurosis NEC 356.9
  arm NEC 354.9
  disseminated 710.1
  facial 349.89
  leg NEC 355.8
  lower extremity NEC 355.8
  upper extremity NEC 354.9
Tropical — see also condition
  maceration feet (syndrome) 991.4
  wet foot (syndrome) 991.4
Trouble — see also Disease
  bowel 569.9
  heart — see Disease, heart
  intestine 569.9
  kidney (see also Disease, renal) 593.9
  nervous 799.2
  sinus (see also Sinusitis) 473.9
Trousseau's syndrome (thrombophlebitis migrans) 453.1
Truancy, childhood — see also Disturbance, conduct
  socialized 312.2 ☑
  undersocialized, unsocialized 312.1 ☑
Truncus
  arteriosus (persistent) 745.0
  common 745.0
  communis 745.0
Trunk — see condition
Trychophytide — see Dermatophytosis
Trypanosoma infestation — see Trypanosomiasis

Trypanosomiasis 086.9
  with meningoencephalitis 086.9 [323.2]
  African 086.5
    due to Trypanosoma 086.5
      gambiense 086.3
      rhodesiense 086.4
  American 086.2
    with
      heart involvement 086.0
      other organ involvement 086.1
    without mention of organ involvement 086.2
  Brazilian — see Trypanosomiasis, American
  Chagas' — see Trypanosomiasis, American
  due to Trypanosoma
    cruzi — see Trypanosomiasis, American
    gambiense 086.3
    rhodesiense 086.4
  gambiensis, Gambian 086.3
  North American — see Trypanosomiasis, American
  rhodesiensis, Rhodesian 086.4
  South American — see Trypanosomiasis, American
T-shaped incisors 520.2
Tsutsugamushi fever 081.2
Tube, tubal, tubular — see also condition
  ligation, admission for V25.2
Tubercle — see also Tuberculosis
  brain, solitary 013.2 ☑
  Darwin's 744.29
  epithelioid noncaseating 135
  Ghon, primary infection 010.0 ☑
Tuberculid, tuberculide (indurating) (lichenoid) (miliary) (papulonecrotic) (primary) (skin) (subcutaneous) (see also Tuberculosis) 017.0 ☑
Tuberculoma — see also Tuberculosis
  brain (any part) 013.2 ☑
  meninges (cerebral) (spinal) 013.1 ☑
  spinal cord 013.4 ☑
Tuberculosis, tubercular, tuberculous (calcification) (calcified) (caseous) (chromogenic acid-fast bacilli) (congenital) (degeneration) (disease) (fibrocaseous) (fistula) (gangrene) (interstitial) (isolated circumscribed lesions) (necrosis) (parenchymatous) (ulcerative) 011.9 ☑

> Note — Use the following fifth-digit subclassification with categories 010-018:
>
> 0   unspecified
> 1   bacteriological or histological examination not done
> 2   bacteriological or histological examination unknown (at present)
> 3   tubercle bacilli found (in sputum) by microscopy
> 4   tubercle bacilli not found (in sputum) by microscopy, but found by bacterial culture
> 5   tubercle bacilli not found by bacteriological exam-ination, but tuberculosis confirmed histologically
> 6   tubercle bacilli not found by bacteriological or histological examination, but tuberculosis confirmed by other methods [inoculation of animals]
>
> For tuberculous conditions specified as late effects or sequelae, see category 137.

  abdomen 014.8 ☑
    lymph gland 014.8 ☑
  abscess 011.9 ☑
    arm 017.9 ☑
    bone (see also Osteomyelitis, due to, tuberculosis) 015.9 ☑ [730.8]
      hip 015.1 ☑ [730.85]
      knee 015.2 ☑ [730.96]
      sacrum 015.0 ☑ [730.88]
      specified site NEC 015.7 ☑ [730.88]
      spinal 015.0 ☑ [730.88]
      vertebra 015.0 ☑ [730.88]

Tuberculosis, tubercular, tuberculous — continued
  abscess — continued
    brain 013.3 ☑
    breast 017.9 ☑
    Cowper's gland 016.5 ☑
    dura (mater) 013.8 ☑
      brain 013.3 ☑
      spinal cord 013.5 ☑
    epidural 013.8 ☑
      brain 013.3 ☑
      spinal cord 013.5 ☑
    frontal sinus — see Tuberculosis, sinus
    genital organs NEC 016.9 ☑
      female 016.7 ☑
      male 016.5 ☑
    genitourinary NEC 016.9 ☑
    gland (lymphatic) — see Tuberculosis, lymph gland
    hip 015.1 ☑
    iliopsoas 015.0 ☑ [730.88]
    intestine 014.8 ☑
    ischiorectal 014.8 ☑
    joint 015.9 ☑
      hip 015.1 ☑
      knee 015.2 ☑
      specified joint NEC 015.8 ☑
      vertebral 015.0 ☑ [730.88]
    kidney 016.0 ☑ [590.81]
    knee 015.2 ☑
    lumbar 015.0 ☑ [730.88]
    lung 011.2 ☑
      primary, progressive 010.8 ☑
    meninges (cerebral) (spinal) 013.0 ☑
    pelvic 016.9 ☑
      female 016.7 ☑
      male 016.5 ☑
    perianal 014.8 ☑
      fistula 014.8 ☑
    perinephritic 016.0 ☑ [590.81]
    perineum 017.9 ☑
    perirectal 014.8 ☑
    psoas 015.0 ☑ [730.88]
    rectum 014.8 ☑
    retropharyngeal 012.8 ☑
    sacrum 015.0 ☑ [730.88]
    scrofulous 017.2 ☑
    scrotum 016.5 ☑
    skin 017.0 ☑
      primary 017.0 ☑
    spinal cord 013.5 ☑
    spine or vertebra (column) 015.0 ☑ [730.88]
    strumous 017.2 ☑
    subdiaphragmatic 014.8 ☑
    testis 016.5 ☑
    thigh 017.9 ☑
    urinary 016.3 ☑
      kidney 016.0 ☑ [590.81]
    uterus 016.7 ☑
  accessory sinus — see Tuberculosis, sinus
  Addison's disease 017.6 ☑
  adenitis (see also Tuberculosis, lymph gland) 017.2 ☑
  adenoids 012.8 ☑
  adenopathy (see also Tuberculosis, lymph gland) 017.2 ☑
    tracheobronchial 012.1 ☑
      primary progressive 010.8 ☑
  adherent pericardium 017.9 ☑ [420.0]
  adnexa (uteri) 016.7 ☑
  adrenal (capsule) (gland) 017.6 ☑
  air passage NEC 012.8 ☑
  alimentary canal 014.8 ☑
  anemia 017.9 ☑
  ankle (joint) 015.8 ☑
    bone 015.5 ☑ [730.87]
  anus 014.8 ☑
  apex (see also Tuberculosis, pulmonary) 011.9 ☑
  apical (see also Tuberculosis, pulmonary) 011.9 ☑
  appendicitis 014.8 ☑
  appendix 014.8 ☑
  arachnoid 013.0 ☑
  artery 017.9 ☑
  arthritis (chronic) (synovial) 015.9 ☑ [711.40]
    ankle 015.8 ☑ [730.87]

Tuberculosis, tubercular, tuberculous —
  continued
  arthritis — *continued*
    hip 015.1 ☑ *[711.45]*
    knee 015.2 ☑ *[711.46]*
    specified site NEC 015.8 ☑ *[711.48]*
    spine or vertebra (column) 015.0 ☑ *[720.81]*
    wrist 015.8 ☑ *[730.83]*
  articular — *see* Tuberculosis, joint
  ascites 014.0 ☑
  asthma (*see also* Tuberculosis, pulmonary)
    011.9 ☑
  axilla, axillary 017.2 ☑
    gland 017.2 ☑
  bilateral (*see also* Tuberculosis, pulmonary)
    011.9 ☑
  bladder 016.1 ☑
  bone (*see also* Osteomyelitis, due to,
    tuberculosis) 015.9 ☑ *[730.8]* ☑
    hip 015.1 ☑ *[730.85]*
    knee 015.2 ☑ *[730.86]*
    limb NEC 015.5 ☑ *[730.88]*
    sacrum 015.0 ☑ *[730.88]*
    specified site NEC 015.7 ☑ *[730.88]*
    spinal or vertebral column 015.0 ☑ *[730.88]*
  bowel 014.8 ☑
    miliary 018.9 ☑
  brain 013.2 ☑
  breast 017.9 ☑
  broad ligament 016.7 ☑
  bronchi, bronchial, bronchus 011.3 ☑
    ectasia, ectasis 011.5 ☑
    fistula 011.3 ☑
      primary, progressive 010.8 ☑
    gland 012.1 ☑
      primary, progressive 010.8 ☑
    isolated 012.2 ☑
    lymph gland or node 012.1 ☑
      primary, progressive 010.8 ☑
  bronchiectasis 011.5 ☑
  bronchitis 011.3 ☑
  bronchopleural 012.0 ☑
  bronchopneumonia, bronchopneumonic
    011.6 ☑
  bronchorrhagia 011.3 ☑
  bronchotracheal 011.3 ☑
    isolated 012.2 ☑
  bronchus — *see* Tuberculosis, bronchi
  bronze disease (Addison's) 017.6 ☑
  buccal cavity 017.9 ☑
  bulbourethral gland 016.5 ☑
  bursa (*see also* Tuberculosis, joint) 015.9 ☑
  cachexia NEC (*see also* Tuberculosis,
    pulmonary) 011.9 ☑
  cardiomyopathy 017.9 ☑ *[425.8]*
  caries (*see also* Tuberculosis, bone)
    015.9 ☑ *[730.8]* ☑
  cartilage (*see also* Tuberculosis, bone)
    015.9 ☑ *[730.8]* ☑
    intervertebral 015.0 ☑ *[730.88]*
  catarrhal (*see also* Tuberculosis, pulmonary)
    011.9 ☑
  cecum 014.8 ☑
  cellular tissue (primary) 017.0 ☑
  cellulitis (primary) 017.0 ☑
  central nervous system 013.9 ☑
    specified site NEC 013.8 ☑
  cerebellum (current) 013.2 ☑
  cerebral (current) 013.2 ☑
    meninges 013.0 ☑
  cerebrospinal 013.6 ☑
    meninges 013.0 ☑
  cerebrum (current) 013.2 ☑
  cervical 017.2 ☑
    gland 017.2 ☑
    lymph nodes 017.2 ☑
  cervicitis (uteri) 016.7 ☑
  cervix 016.7 ☑
  chest (*see also* Tuberculosis, pulmonary)
    011.9 ☑
  childhood type or first infection 010.0 ☑
  choroid 017.3 ☑ *[363.13]*
  choroiditis 017.3 ☑ *[363.13]*
  ciliary body 017.3 ☑ *[364.11]*
  colitis 014.8 ☑
  colliers' 011.4 ☑
  colliquativa (primary) 017.0 ☑

Tuberculosis, tubercular, tuberculous —
  continued
  colon 014.8 ☑
    ulceration 014.8 ☑
  complex, primary 010.0 ☑
  complicating pregnancy, childbirth, or
    puerperium 647.3 ☑
    affecting fetus or newborn 760.2
  congenital 771.2
  conjunctiva 017.3 ☑ *[370.31]*
  connective tissue 017.9 ☑
    bone — *see* Tuberculosis, bone
  contact V01.1
  converter (tuberculin test) (without disease)
    795.5
  cornea (ulcer) 017.3 ☑ *[370.31]*
  Cowper's gland 016.5 ☑
  coxae 015.1 ☑ *[730.85]*
  coxalgia 015.1 ☑ *[730.85]*
  cul-de-sac of Douglas 014.8 ☑
  curvature, spine 015.0 ☑ *[737.40]*
  cutis (colliquativa) (primary) 017.0 ☑
  cyst, ovary 016.6 ☑
  cystitis 016.1 ☑
  dacryocystitis 017.3 ☑ *[375.32]*
  dactylitis 015.5 ☑
  diarrhea 014.8 ☑
  diffuse (*see also* Tuberculosis, miliary) 018.9 ☑
    lung — *see* Tuberculosis, pulmonary
    meninges 013.0 ☑
  digestive tract 014.8 ☑
  disseminated (*see also* Tuberculosis, miliary)
    018.9 ☑
    meninges 013.0 ☑
  duodenum 014.8 ☑
  dura (mater) 013.9 ☑
    abscess 013.8 ☑
      cerebral 013.3 ☑
      spinal 013.5 ☑
  dysentery 014.8 ☑
  ear (inner) (middle) 017.4 ☑
    bone 015.6 ☑
    external (primary) 017.0 ☑
    skin (primary) 017.0 ☑
  elbow 015.8 ☑
  emphysema — *see* Tuberculosis, pulmonary
  empyema 012.0 ☑
  encephalitis 013.6 ☑
  endarteritis 017.9 ☑
  endocarditis (any valve) 017.9 ☑ *[424.91]*
  endocardium (any valve) 017.9 ☑ *[424.91]*
  endocrine glands NEC 017.9 ☑
  endometrium 016.7 ☑
  enteric, enterica 014.8 ☑
  enteritis 014.8 ☑
  enterocolitis 014.8 ☑
  epididymis 016.4 ☑
  epididymitis 016.4 ☑
  epidural abscess 013.8 ☑
    brain 013.3 ☑
    spinal cord 013.5 ☑
  epiglottis 012.3 ☑
  episcleritis 017.3 ☑ *[379.00]*
  erythema (induratum) (nodosum) (primary)
    017.1 ☑
  esophagus 017.8 ☑
  Eustachian tube 017.4 ☑
  exposure to V01.1
  exudative 012.0 ☑
    primary, progressive 010.1 ☑
  eye 017.3 ☑
    glaucoma 017.3 ☑ *[365.62]*
  eyelid (primary) 017.0 ☑
    lupus 017.0 ☑ *[373.4]*
  fallopian tube 016.6 ☑
  fascia 017.9 ☑
  fauces 012.8 ☑
  finger 017.9 ☑
  first infection 010.0 ☑
  fistula, perirectal 014.8 ☑
  Florida 011.6 ☑
  foot 017.9 ☑
  funnel pelvis 137.3
  gallbladder 017.9 ☑
  galloping (*see also* Tuberculosis, pulmonary)
    011.9 ☑
  ganglionic 015.9 ☑

Tuberculosis, tubercular, tuberculous —
  continued
  gastritis 017.9 ☑
  gastrocolic fistula 014.8 ☑
  gastroenteritis 014.8 ☑
  gastrointestinal tract 014.8 ☑
  general, generalized 018.9 ☑
    acute 018.0 ☑
    chronic 018.8 ☑
  genital organs NEC 016.9 ☑
    female 016.7 ☑
    male 016.5 ☑
  genitourinary NEC 016.9 ☑
  genu 015.2 ☑
  glandulae suprarenalis 017.6 ☑
  glandular, general 017.2 ☑
  glottis 012.3 ☑
  grinders' 011.4 ☑
  groin 017.2 ☑
  gum 017.9 ☑
  hand 017.9 ☑
  heart 017.9 ☑ *[425.8]*
  hematogenous — *see* Tuberculosis, miliary
  hemoptysis (*see also* Tuberculosis, pulmonary)
    011.9 ☑
  hemorrhage NEC (*see also* Tuberculosis,
    pulmonary) 011.9 ☑
  hemothorax 012.0 ☑
  hepatitis 017.9 ☑
  hilar lymph nodes 012.1 ☑
    primary, progressive 010.8 ☑
  hip (disease) (joint) 015.1 ☑
    bone 015.1 ☑ *[730.85]*
  hydrocephalus 013.8 ☑
  hydropneumothorax 012.0 ☑
  hydrothorax 012.0 ☑
  hypoadrenalism 017.6 ☑
  hypopharynx 012.8 ☑
  ileocecal (hyperplastic) 014.8 ☑
  ileocolitis 014.8 ☑
  ileum 014.8 ☑
  iliac spine (superior) 015.0 ☑ *[730.88]*
  incipient NEC (*see also* Tuberculosis,
    pulmonary) 011.9 ☑
  indurativa (primary) 017.1 ☑
  infantile 010.0 ☑
  infection NEC 011.9 ☑
    without clinical manifestation 010.0 ☑
  infraclavicular gland 017.2 ☑
  inguinal gland 017.2 ☑
  inguinalis 017.2 ☑
  intestine (any part) 014.8 ☑
  iris 017.3 ☑ *[364.11]*
  iritis 017.3 ☑ *[364.11]*
  ischiorectal 014.8 ☑
  jaw 015.7 ☑ *[730.88]*
  jejunum 014.8 ☑
  joint 015.9 ☑
    hip 015.1 ☑
    knee 015.2 ☑
    specified site NEC 015.8 ☑
    vertebral 015.0 ☑ *[730.88]*
  keratitis 017.3 ☑ *[370.31]*
    interstitial 017.3 ☑ *[370.59]*
  keratoconjunctivitis 017.3 ☑ *[370.31]*
  kidney 016.0 ☑
  knee (joint) 015.2 ☑
  kyphoscoliosis 015.0 ☑ *[737.43]*
  kyphosis 015.0 ☑ *[737.41]*
  lacrimal apparatus, gland 017.3 ☑
  laryngitis 012.3 ☑
  larynx 012.3 ☑
  leptomeninges, leptomeningitis (cerebral)
    (spinal) 013.0 ☑
  lichenoides (primary) 017.0 ☑
  linguae 017.9 ☑
  lip 017.9 ☑
  liver 017.9 ☑
  lordosis 015.0 ☑ *[737.42]*
  lung — *see* Tuberculosis, pulmonary
  luposa 017.0 ☑
    eyelid 017.0 ☑ *[373.4]*
  lymphadenitis — *see* Tuberculosis, lymph
    gland
  lymphangitis — *see* Tuberculosis, lymph gland
  lymphatic (gland) (vessel) — *see* Tuberculosis,
    lymph gland

Tuberculosis, tubercular, tuberculous —
continued
  lymph gland or node (peripheral) 017.2 ☑
    abdomen 014.8 ☑
    bronchial 012.1 ☑
      primary, progressive 010.8 ☑
    cervical 017.2 ☑
    hilar 012.1 ☑
      primary, progressive 010.8 ☑
    intrathoracic 012.1 ☑
      primary, progressive 010.8 ☑
    mediastinal 012.1 ☑
      primary, progressive 010.8 ☑
    mesenteric 014.8 ☑
    peripheral 017.2 ☑
    retroperitoneal 014.8 ☑
    tracheobronchial 012.1 ☑
      primary, progressive 010.8 ☑
  malignant NEC (*see also* Tuberculosis, pulmonary) 011.9 ☑
  mammary gland 017.9 ☑
  marasmus NEC (*see also* Tuberculosis, pulmonary) 011.9 ☑
  mastoiditis 015.6 ☑
  maternal, affecting fetus or newborn 760.2
  mediastinal (lymph) gland or node 012.1 ☑
    primary, progressive 010.8 ☑
  mediastinitis 012.8 ☑
    primary, progressive 010.8 ☑
  mediastinopericarditis 017.9 ☑ *[420.0]*
  mediastinum 012.8 ☑
    primary, progressive 010.8 ☑
  medulla 013.9 ☑
    brain 013.2 ☑
    spinal cord 013.4 ☑
  melanosis, Addisonian 017.6 ☑
  membrane, brain 013.0 ☑
  meninges (cerebral) (spinal) 013.0 ☑
  meningitis (basilar) (brain) (cerebral) (cerebrospinal) (spinal) 013.0 ☑
  meningoencephalitis 013.0 ☑
  mesentery, mesenteric 014.8 ☑
    lymph gland or node 014.8 ☑
  miliary (any site) 018.9 ☑
    acute 018.0 ☑
    chronic 018.8 ☑
    specified type NEC 018.8 ☑
  millstone makers' 011.4 ☑
  miners' 011.4 ☑
  moulders' 011.4 ☑
  mouth 017.9 ☑
  multiple 018.9 ☑
    acute 018.0 ☑
    chronic 018.8 ☑
  muscle 017.9 ☑
  myelitis 013.6 ☑
  myocarditis 017.9 ☑ *[422.0]*
  myocardium 017.9 ☑ *[422.0]*
  nasal (passage) (sinus) 012.8 ☑
  nasopharynx 012.8 ☑
  neck gland 017.2 ☑
  nephritis 016.0 ☑ *[583.81]*
  nerve 017.9 ☑
  nose (septum) 012.8 ☑
  ocular 017.3 ☑
  old NEC 137.0
    without residuals V12.01
  omentum 014.8 ☑
  oophoritis (acute) (chronic) 016.6 ☑
  optic 017.3 ☑ *[377.39]*
    nerve trunk 017.3 ☑ *[377.39]*
    papilla, papillae 017.3 ☑ *[377.39]*
  orbit 017.3 ☑
  orchitis 016.5 ☑ *[608.81]*
  organ, specified NEC 017.9 ☑
  orificialis (primary) 017.0 ☑
  osseous (*see also* Tuberculosis, bone) 015.9 ☑ *[730.8]*
  osteitis (*see also* Tuberculosis, bone) 015.9 ☑ *[730.8]*
  osteomyelitis (*see also* Tuberculosis, bone) 015.9 ☑ *[730.8]*
  otitis (media) 017.4 ☑
  ovaritis (acute) (chronic) 016.6 ☑
  ovary (acute) (chronic) 016.6 ☑
  oviducts (acute) (chronic) 016.6 ☑
  pachymeningitis 013.0 ☑

Tuberculosis, tubercular, tuberculous —
continued
  palate (soft) 017.9 ☑
  pancreas 017.9 ☑
  papulonecrotic (primary) 017.0 ☑
  parathyroid glands 017.9 ☑
  paronychia (primary) 017.0 ☑
  parotid gland or region 017.9 ☑
  pelvic organ NEC 016.9 ☑
    female 016.7 ☑
    male 016.5 ☑
  pelvis (bony) 015.7 ☑ *[730.85]*
  penis 016.5 ☑
  peribronchitis 011.3 ☑
  pericarditis 017.9 ☑ *[420.0]*
  pericardium 017.9 ☑ *[420.0]*
  perichondritis, larynx 012.3 ☑
  perineum 017.9 ☑
  periostitis (*see also* Tuberculosis, bone) 015.9 ☑ *[730.8]* ☑
  periphlebitis 017.9 ☑
    eye vessel 017.3 ☑ *[362.18]*
    retina 017.3 ☑ *[362.18]*
  perirectal fistula 014.8 ☑
  peritoneal gland 014.8 ☑
  peritoneum 014.0 ☑
  peritonitis 014.0 ☑
  pernicious NEC (*see also* Tuberculosis, pulmonary) 011.9 ☑
  pharyngitis 012.8 ☑
  pharynx 012.8 ☑
  phlyctenulosis (conjunctiva) 017.3 ☑ *[370.31]*
  phthisis NEC (*see also* Tuberculosis, pulmonary) 011.9 ☑
  pituitary gland 017.9 ☑
  placenta 016.7 ☑
  pleura, pleural, pleurisy, pleuritis (fibrinous) (obliterative) (purulent) (simple plastic) (with effusion) 012.0 ☑
    primary, progressive 010.1 ☑
  pneumonia, pneumonic 011.6 ☑
  pneumothorax 011.7 ☑
  polyserositis 018.9 ☑
    acute 018.0 ☑
    chronic 018.8 ☑
  potters' 011.4 ☑
  prepuce 016.5 ☑
  primary 010.9 ☑
    complex 010.0 ☑
    complicated 010.8 ☑
      with pleurisy or effusion 010.1 ☑
    progressive 010.8 ☑
      with pleurisy or effusion 010.1 ☑
    skin 017.0 ☑
  proctitis 014.8 ☑
  prostate 016.5 ☑ *[601.4]*
  prostatitis 016.5 ☑ *[601.4]*
  pulmonaris (*see also* Tuberculosis, pulmonary) 011.9 ☑
  pulmonary (artery) (incipient) (malignant) (multiple round foci) (pernicious) (reinfection stage) 011.9 ☑
    cavitated or with cavitation 011.2 ☑
      primary, progressive 010.8 ☑
    childhood type or first infection 010.0 ☑
    chromogenic acid-fast bacilli 795.39
    fibrosis or fibrotic 011.4 ☑
    infiltrative 011.0 ☑
      primary, progressive 010.9 ☑
    nodular 011.1 ☑
    specified NEC 011.8 ☑
    sputum positive only 795.39
    status following surgical collapse of lung NEC 011.9 ☑
  pyelitis 016.0 ☑ *[590.81]*
  pyelonephritis 016.0 ☑ *[590.81]*
  pyemia — *see* Tuberculosis, miliary
  pyonephrosis 016.0 ☑
  pyopneumothorax 012.0 ☑
  pyothorax 012.0 ☑
  rectum (with abscess) 014.8 ☑
    fistula 014.8 ☑
  reinfection stage (*see also* Tuberculosis, pulmonary) 011.9 ☑
  renal 016.0 ☑
  renis 016.0 ☑
  reproductive organ 016.7 ☑

Tuberculosis, tubercular, tuberculous —
continued
  respiratory NEC (*see also* Tuberculosis, pulmonary) 011.9 ☑
    specified site NEC 012.8 ☑
  retina 017.3 ☑ *[363.13]*
  retroperitoneal (lymph gland or node) 014.8 ☑
    gland 014.8 ☑
  retropharyngeal abscess 012.8 ☑
  rheumatism 015.9 ☑
  rhinitis 012.8 ☑
  sacroiliac (joint) 015.8 ☑
  sacrum 015.0 ☑ *[730.88]*
  salivary gland 017.9 ☑
  salpingitis (acute) (chronic) 016.6 ☑
  sandblasters' 011.4 ☑
  sclera 017.3 ☑ *[379.09]*
  scoliosis 015.0 ☑ *[737.43]*
  scrofulous 017.2 ☑
  scrotum 016.5 ☑
  seminal tract or vesicle 016.5 ☑ *[608.81]*
  senile NEC (*see also* Tuberculosis, pulmonary) 011.9 ☑
  septic NEC (*see also* Tuberculosis, miliary) 018.9 ☑
  shoulder 015.8 ☑
    blade 015.7 ☑ *[730.8]*
  sigmoid 014.8 ☑
  sinus (accessory) (nasal) 012.8 ☑
    bone 015.7 ☑ *[730.88]*
    epididymis 016.4 ☑
  skeletal NEC (*see also* Osteomyelitis, due to tuberculosis) 015.9 ☑ *[730.8]* ☑
  skin (any site) (primary) 017.0 ☑
  small intestine 014.8 ☑
  soft palate 017.9 ☑
  spermatic cord 016.5 ☑
  spinal
    column 015.0 ☑ *[730.88]*
    cord 013.4 ☑
    disease 015.0 ☑ *[730.88]*
    medulla 013.4 ☑
    membrane 013.0 ☑
    meninges 013.0 ☑
  spine 015.0 ☑ *[730.88]*
  spleen 017.7 ☑
  splenitis 017.7 ☑
  spondylitis 015.0 ☑ *[720.81]*
  spontaneous pneumothorax — *see* Tuberculosis, pulmonary
  sternoclavicular joint 015.8 ☑
  stomach 017.9 ☑
  stonemasons' 011.4 ☑
  struma 017.2 ☑
  subcutaneous tissue (cellular) (primary) 017.0 ☑
  subcutis (primary) 017.0 ☑
  subdeltoid bursa 017.9 ☑
  submaxillary 017.9 ☑
    region 017.9 ☑
  supraclavicular gland 017.2 ☑
  suprarenal (capsule) (gland) 017.6 ☑
  swelling, joint (*see also* Tuberculosis, joint) 015.9 ☑
  symphysis pubis 015.7 ☑ *[730.88]*
  synovitis 015.9 ☑ *[727.01]*
    hip 015.1 ☑ *[727.01]*
    knee 015.2 ☑ *[727.01]*
    specified site NEC 015.8 ☑ *[727.01]*
    spine or vertebra 015.0 ☑ *[727.01]*
  systemic — *see* Tuberculosis, miliary
  tarsitis (eyelid) 017.0 ☑ *[373.4]*
    ankle (bone) 015.5 ☑ *[730.87]*
  tendon (sheath) — *see* Tuberculosis, tenosynovitis
  tenosynovitis 015.9 ☑ *[727.01]*
    hip 015.1 ☑ *[727.01]*
    knee 015.2 ☑ *[727.01]*
    specified site NEC 015.8 ☑ *[727.01]*
    spine or vertebra 015.0 ☑ *[727.01]*
  testis 016.5 ☑ *[608.81]*
  throat 012.8 ☑
  thymus gland 017.9 ☑
  thyroid gland 017.5 ☑
  toe 017.9 ☑
  tongue 017.9 ☑
  tonsil (lingual) 012.8 ☑

☑ Additional Digit Required   ▶◀ Revised Text   ● New Line   ▲ Revised Code

Tuberculosis, tubercular, tuberculous — *continued*

tonsillitis 012.8 ☑

trachea, tracheal 012.8 ☑
gland 012.1 ☑
primary, progressive 010.8 ☑
isolated 012.2 ☑

tracheobronchial 011.3 ☑
glandular 012.1 ☑
primary, progressive 010.8 ☑
isolated 012.2 ☑
lymph gland or node 012.1 ☑
primary, progressive 010.8 ☑

tubal 016.6 ☑

tunica vaginalis 016.5 ☑

typhlitis 014.8 ☑

ulcer (primary) (skin) 017.0 ☑
bowel or intestine 014.8 ☑
specified site NEC — *see* Tuberculosis, by site

unspecified site — *see* Tuberculosis, pulmonary

ureter 016.2 ☑

urethra, urethral 016.3 ☑

urinary organ or tract 016.3 ☑
kidney 016.0 ☑

uterus 016.7 ☑

uveal tract 017.3 ☑ *[363.13]*

uvula 017.9 ☑

vaccination, prophylactic (against) V03.2

vagina 016.7 ☑

vas deferens 016.5 ☑

vein 017.9 ☑

verruca (primary) 017.0 ☑

verrucosa (cutis) (primary) 017.0 ☑

vertebra (column) 015.0 ☑ *[730.88]*

vesiculitis 016.5 ☑ *[608.81]*

viscera NEC 014.8 ☑

vulva 016.7 ☑ *[616.51]*

wrist (joint) 015.8 ☑
bone 015.5 ☑ *[730.83]*

Tuberculum
auriculae 744.29
occlusal 520.2
paramolare 520.2

Tuberous sclerosis (brain) 759.5

Tubo-ovarian — *see* condition

Tuboplasty, after previous sterilization V26.0

Tubotympanitis 381.10

Tularemia 021.9
with
conjunctivitis 021.3
pneumonia 021.2
bronchopneumonic 021.2
conjunctivitis 021.3
cryptogenic 021.1
disseminated 021.8
enteric 021.1
generalized 021.8
glandular 021.8
intestinal 021.1
oculoglandular 021.3
ophthalmic 021.3
pneumonia 021.2
pulmonary 021.2
specified NEC 021.8
typhoidal 021.1
ulceroglandular 021.0
vaccination, prophylactic (against) V03.4

Tularensis conjunctivitis 021.3

Tumefaction — *see also* Swelling
liver (*see also* Hypertrophy, liver) 789.1

Tumor (M8000/1) — *see also* Neoplasm, by site, unspecified nature
Abrikossov's (M9580/0) — *see also* Neoplasm, connective tissue, benign
malignant (M9580/3) — *see* Neoplasm, connective tissue, malignant
acinar cell (M8550/1) — *see* Neoplasm, by site, uncertain behavior
acinic cell (M8550/1) — *see* Neoplasm, by site, uncertain behavior
adenomatoid (M9054/0) — *see also* Neoplasm, by site, benign
odontogenic (M9300/0) 213.1
upper jaw (bone) 213.0

Tumor (M8000/1) — *see also* Neoplasm, by site, unspecified nature — *continued*
adnexal (skin) (M8390/0) — *see* Neoplasm, skin, benign
adrenal
cortical (benign) (M8370/0) 227.0
malignant (M8370/3) 194.0
rest (M8671/0) — *see* Neoplasm, by site, benign
alpha cell (M8152/0)
malignant (M8152/3)
pancreas 157.4
specified site NEC — *see* Neoplasm, by site, malignant
unspecified site 157.4
pancreas 211.7
specified site NEC — *see* Neoplasm, by site, benign
unspecified site 211.7
aneurysmal (*see also* Aneurysm) 442.9
aortic body (M8691/1) 237.3
malignant (M8691/3) 194.6
argentaffin (M8241/1) — *see* Neoplasm, by site, uncertain behavior
basal cell (M8090/1) — *see also* Neoplasm, skin, uncertain behavior
benign (M8000/0) — *see* Neoplasm, by site, benign
beta cell (M8151/0)
malignant (M8151/3)
pancreas 157.4
specified site — *see* Neoplasm, by site, malignant
unspecified site 157.4
pancreas 211.7
specified site NEC — *see* Neoplasm, by site, benign
unspecified site 211.7
blood — *see* Hematoma
Brenner (M9000/0) 220
borderline malignancy (M9000/1) 236.2
malignant (M9000/3) 183.0
proliferating (M9000/1) 236.2
Brooke's (M8100/0) — *see* Neoplasm, skin, benign
brown fat (M8880/0) — *see* Lipoma, by site
Burkitt's (M9750/3) 200.2 ☑
calcifying epithelial odontogenic (M9340/0) 213.1
upper jaw (bone) 213.0
carcinoid (M8240/1) — *see* Carcinoid
carotid body (M8692/1) 237.3
malignant (M8692/3) 194.5
Castleman's (mediastinal lymph node hyperplasia) 785.6
cells (M8001/1) — *see also* Neoplasm, by site, unspecified nature
benign (M8001/0) — *see* Neoplasm, by site, benign
malignant (M8001/3) — *see* Neoplasm, by site, malignant
uncertain whether benign or malignant (M8001/1) — *see* Neoplasm, by site, uncertain nature
cervix
in pregnancy or childbirth 654.6 ☑
affecting fetus or newborn 763.89
causing obstructed labor 660.2 ☑
affecting fetus or newborn 763.1
chondromatous giant cell (M9230/0) — *see* Neoplasm, bone, benign
chromaffin (M8700/0) — *see also* Neoplasm, by site, benign
malignant (M8700/3) — *see* Neoplasm, by site, malignant
Cock's peculiar 706.2
Codman's (benign chondroblastoma) (M9230/0) — *see* Neoplasm, bone, benign
dentigerous, mixed (M9282/0) 213.1
upper jaw (bone) 213.0
dermoid (M9084/0) — *see* Neoplasm, by site, benign
with malignant transformation (M9084/3) 183.0

Tumor (M8000/1) — *see also* Neoplasm, by site, unspecified nature — *continued*
desmoid (extra-abdominal) (M8821/1) — *see also* Neoplasm, connective tissue, uncertain behavior
abdominal (M8822/1) — *see* Neoplasm, connective tissue, uncertain behavior
embryonal (mixed) (M9080/1) — *see also* Neoplasm, by site, uncertain behavior
liver (M9080/3) 155.0
endodermal sinus (M9071/3)
specified site — *see* Neoplasm, by site, malignant
unspecified site
female 183.0
male 186.9
epithelial
benign (M8010/0) — *see* Neoplasm, by site, benign
malignant (M8010/3) — *see* Neoplasm, by site, malignant
Ewing's (M9260/3) — *see* Neoplasm, bone, malignant
fatty — *see* Lipoma
fetal, causing disproportion 653.7 ☑
causing obstructed labor 660.1 ☑
fibroid (M8890/0) — *see* Leiomyoma
G cell (M8153/1)
malignant (M8153/3)
pancreas 157.4
specified site NEC — *see* Neoplasm, by site, malignant
unspecified site 157.4
specified site — *see* Neoplasm, by site, uncertain behavior
unspecified site 235.5
giant cell (type) (M8003/1) — *see also* Neoplasm, by site, unspecified nature
bone (M9250/1) 238.0
malignant (M9250/3) — *see* Neoplasm, bone, malignant
chondromatous (M9230/0) — *see* Neoplasm, bone, benign
malignant (M8003/3) — *see* Neoplasm, by site, malignant
peripheral (gingiva) 523.8
giant cell — *see also* Neoplasm, by site, unspecified nature — *continued*
soft parts (M9251/1) — *see also* Neoplasm, connective tissue, uncertain behavior
malignant (M9251/3) — *see* Neoplasm, connective tissue, malignant
tendon sheath 727.02
glomus (M8711/0) — *see also* Hemangioma, by site
jugulare (M8690/1) 237.3
malignant (M8690/3) 194.6
gonadal stromal (M8590/1) — *see* Neoplasm, by site, uncertain behavior
granular cell (M9580/0) — *see also* Neoplasm, connective tissue, benign
malignant (M9580/3) — *see* Neoplasm, connective tissue, malignant
granulosa cell (M8620/1) 236.2
malignant (M8620/3) 183.0
granulosa cell-theca cell (M8621/1) 236.2
malignant (M8621/3) 183.0
Grawitz's (hypernephroma) (M8312/3) 189.0
hazard-crile (M8350/3) 193
hemorrhoidal — *see* Hemorrhoids
hilar cell (M8660/0) 220
Hürthle cell (benign) (M8290/0) 226
malignant (M8290/3) 193
hydatid (*see also* Echinococcus) 122.9
hypernephroid (M8311/1) — *see also* Neoplasm, by site, uncertain behavior
interstitial cell (M8650/1) — *see also* Neoplasm, by site, uncertain behavior
benign (M8650/0) — *see* Neoplasm, by site, benign
malignant (M8650/3) — *see* Neoplasm, by site, malignant
islet cell (M8150/0)
malignant (M8150/3)
pancreas 157.4
specified site — *see* Neoplasm, by site, malignant

☑ Additional Digit Required   ▶◀ Revised Text   ● New Line   ▲ Revised Code

Tumor (M8000/1) — *see also* Neoplasm, by site, unspecified nature — *continued*
    islet cell (M8150/0) — *continued*
        malignant (M8150/3) — *continued*
            unspecified site 157.4
        pancreas 211.7
        specified site NEC — *see* Neoplasm, by site, benign
        unspecified site 211.7
    juxtaglomerular (M8361/1) 236.91
    Krukenberg's (M8490/6) 198.6
    Leydig cell (M8650/1)
        benign (M8650/0)
            specified site — *see* Neoplasm, by site, benign
            unspecified site
                female 220
                male 222.0
        malignant (M8650/3)
            specified site — *see* Neoplasm, by site, malignant
            unspecified site
                female 183.0
                male 186.9
        specified site — *see* Neoplasm, by site, uncertain behavior
        unspecified site
            female 236.2
            male 236.4
    lipid cell, ovary (M8670/0) 220
    lipoid cell, ovary (M8670/0) 220
    lymphomatous, benign (M9590/0) — *see also* Neoplasm, by site, benign
    Malherbe's (M8110/0) — *see* Neoplasm, skin, benign
    malignant (M8000/3) — *see also* Neoplasm, by site, malignant
        fusiform cell (type) (M8004/3) — *see* Neoplasm, by site, malignant
        giant cell (type) (M8003/3) — *see* Neoplasm, by site, malignant
        mixed NEC (M8940/3) — *see* Neoplasm, by site, malignant
        small cell (type) (M8002/3) — *see* Neoplasm, by site, malignant
        spindle cell (type) (M8004/3) — *see* Neoplasm, by site, malignant
    mast cell (M9740/1) 238.5
        malignant (M9740/3) 202.6 ☑
    melanotic, neuroectodermal (M9363/0) — *see* Neoplasm, by site, benign
    Merkel cell — *see* Neoplasm, by site, malignant
    mesenchymal
        malignant (M8800/3) — *see* Neoplasm, connective tissue, malignant
        mixed (M8990/1) — *see* Neoplasm, connective tissue, uncertain behavior
    mesodermal, mixed (M8951/3) — *see also* Neoplasm, by site, malignant
        liver 155.0
    mesonephric (M9110/1) — *see also* Neoplasm, by site, uncertain behavior
        malignant (M9110/3) — *see* Neoplasm, by site, malignant
    metastatic
        from specified site (M8000/3) — *see* Neoplasm, by site, malignant
        to specified site (M8000/6) — *see* Neoplasm, by site, malignant, secondary
    mixed NEC (M8940/0) — *see also* Neoplasm, by site, benign
        malignant (M8940/3) — *see* Neoplasm, by site, malignant
    mucocarcinoid, malignant (M8243/3) — *see* Neoplasm, by site, malignant
    mucoepidermoid (M8430/1) — *see* Neoplasm, by site, uncertain behavior
    Mullerian, mixed (M8950/3) — *see* Neoplasm, by site, malignant
    myoepithelial (M8982/0) — *see* Neoplasm, by site, benign
    neurogenic olfactory (M9520/3) 160.0
    nonencapsulated sclerosing (M8350/3) 193
    odontogenic (M9270/1) 238.0
        adenomatoid (M9300/0) 213.1
            upper jaw (bone) 213.0

Tumor (M8000/1) — *see also* Neoplasm, by site, unspecified nature — *continued*
    odontogenic (M9270/1) — *continued*
        benign (M9270/0) 213.1
            upper jaw (bone) 213.0
        calcifying epithelial (M9340/0) 213.1
            upper jaw (bone) 213.0
        malignant (M9270/3) 170.1
            upper jaw (bone) 170.0
        squamous (M9312/0) 213.1
            upper jaw (bone) 213.0
    ovarian stromal (M8590/1) 236.2
    ovary
        in pregnancy or childbirth 654.4 ☑
            affecting fetus or newborn 763.89
            causing obstructed labor 660.2 ☑
                affecting fetus or newborn 763.1
    pacinian (M9507/0) — *see* Neoplasm, skin, benign
    Pancoast's (M8010/3) 162.3
    papillary — *see* Papilloma
    pelvic, in pregnancy or childbirth 654.9 ☑
        affecting fetus or newborn 763.89
        causing obstructed labor 660.2 ☑
            affecting fetus or newborn 763.1
    phantom 300.11
    plasma cell (M9731/1) 238.6
        benign (M9731/0) — *see* Neoplasm, by site, benign
        malignant (M9731/3) 203.8 ☑
    polyvesicular vitelline (M9071/3)
        specified site — *see* Neoplasm, by site, malignant
        unspecified site
            female 183.0
            male 186.9
    Pott's puffy (*see also* Osteomyelitis) 730.2 ☑
    Rathke's pouch (M9350/1) 237.0
    regaud's (M8082/3) — *see* Neoplasm, nasopharynx, malignant
    rete cell (M8140/0) 222.0
    retinal anlage (M9363/0) — *see* Neoplasm, by site, benign
    Rokitansky's 620.2
    salivary gland type, mixed (M8940/0) — *see also* Neoplasm, by site, benign
        malignant (M8940/3) — *see* Neoplasm, by site, malignant
    Sampson's 617.1
    Schloffer's (*see also* Peritonitis) 567.2
    Schmincke (M8082/3) — *see* Neoplasm, nasopharynx, malignant
    sebaceous (*see also* Cyst, sebaceous) 706.2
    secondary (M8000/6) — *see* Neoplasm, by site, secondary
    Sertoli cell (M8640/0)
        with lipid storage (M8641/0)
            specified site — *see* Neoplasm, by site, benign
            unspecified site
                female 220
                male 222.0
        specified site — *see* Neoplasm, by site, benign
        unspecified site
            female 220
            male 222.0
    Sertoli-Leydig cell (M8631/0)
        specified site, — *see* Neoplasm, by site, benign
        unspecified site
            female 220
            male 222.0
    sex cord (-stromal) (M8590/1) — *see* Neoplasm, by site, uncertain behavior
    skin appendage (M8390/0) — *see* Neoplasm, skin, benign
    soft tissue
        benign (M8800/0) — *see* Neoplasm, connective tissue, benign
        malignant (M8800/3) — *see* Neoplasm, connective tissue, malignant
    sternomastoid 754.1
    stromal   ●
        gastric 238.1   ●
            benign 215.5   ●
            malignant 171.5   ●
            uncertain behavior 238.1   ●

Tumor (M8000/1) — *see also* Neoplasm, by site, unspecified nature — *continued*
    stromal — *continued*
        gastrointestinal 238.1   ●
            benign 215.5   ●
            malignant 171.5   ●
            uncertain behavior 238.1   ●
        intestine 238.1   ●
            benign 215.5   ●
            malignant 171.5   ●
            uncertain behavior 238.1   ●
        stomach 238.1   ●
            benign 215.5   ●
            malignant 171.5   ●
            uncertain behavior 238.1   ●
    superior sulcus (lung) (pulmonary) (syndrome) (M8010/3) 162.3
    suprasulcus (M8010/3) 162.3
    sweat gland (M8400/1) — *see also* Neoplasm, skin, uncertain behavior
        benign (M8400/0) — *see* Neoplasm, skin, benign
        malignant (M8400/3) — *see* Neoplasm, skin, malignant
    syphilitic brain 094.89
        congenital 090.49
    testicular stromal (M8590/1) 236.4
    theca cell (M8600/0) 220
    theca cell-granulosa cell (M8621/1) 236.2
    theca-lutein (M8610/0) 220
    turban (M8200/0) 216.4
    uterus
        in pregnancy or childbirth 654.1 ☑
            affecting fetus or newborn 763.89
            causing obstructed labor 660.2 ☑
                affecting fetus or newborn 763.1
    vagina
        in pregnancy or childbirth 654.7 ☑
            affecting fetus or newborn 763.89
            causing obstructed labor 660.2 ☑
                affecting fetus or newborn 763.1
    varicose (*see also* Varicose, vein) 454.9
    von Recklinghausen's (M9540/1) 237.71
    vulva
        in pregnancy or childbirth 654.8 ☑
            affecting fetus or newborn 763.89
            causing obstructed labor 660.2 ☑
                affecting fetus or newborn 763.1
    Warthin's (salivary gland) (M8561/0) 210.2
    white — *see also* Tuberculosis, arthritis
    White-Darier 757.39
    Wilms' (nephroblastoma) (M8960/3) 189.0
    yolk sac (M9071/3)
        specified site — *see* Neoplasm, by site, malignant
        unspecified site
            female 183.0
            male 186.9

Tumorlet (M8040/1) — *see* Neoplasm, by site, uncertain behavior

Tungiasis 134.1

Tunica vasculosa lentis 743.39

Tunnel vision 368.45

Turban tumor (M8200/0) 216.4

Türck's trachoma (chronic catarrhal laryngitis) 476.0

Türk's syndrome (ocular retraction syndrome) 378.71

Turner's
    hypoplasia (tooth) 520.4
    syndrome 758.6
    tooth 520.4

Turner-Kieser syndrome (hereditary osteo-onychodysplasia) 756.89

Turner-Varny syndrome 758.6

Turricephaly 756.0

Tussis convulsiva (*see also* Whooping cough) 033.9

Twin
    affected by maternal complications of pregnancy 761.5
    conjoined 759.4
    healthy liveborn — *see* Newborn, twin

☑ Additional Digit Required   ▶◀ Revised Text   ● New Line   ▲ Revised Code

Twin — *continued*
  pregnancy (complicating delivery) NEC 651.0 ☑
    with fetal loss and retention of one fetus 651.3 ☑
Twinning, teeth 520.2
Twist, twisted
  bowel, colon, or intestine 560.2
  hair (congenital) 757.4
  mesentery 560.2
  omentum 560.2
  organ or site, congenital NEC — *see* Anomaly, specified type NEC
  ovarian pedicle 620.5
    congenital 752.0
  umbilical cord — *see* Compression, umbilical cord
Twitch 781.0
Tylosis 700
  buccalis 528.6
  gingiva 523.8
  linguae 528.6
  palmaris et plantaris 757.39
Tympanism 787.3
Tympanites (abdominal) (intestine) 787.3
Tympanitis — *see* Myringitis
Tympanosclerosis 385.00
  involving
    combined sites NEC 385.09
      with tympanic membrane 385.03
    tympanic membrane 385.01
      with ossicles 385.02
        and middle ear 385.03
Tympanum — *see* condition
Tympany
  abdomen 787.3
  chest 786.7
Typhlitis (*see also* Appendicitis) 541
Typhoenteritis 002.0
Typhogastric fever 002.0
Typhoid (abortive) (ambulant) (any site) (fever) (hemorrhagic) (infection) (intermittent) (malignant) (rheumatic) 002.0
  with pneumonia 002.0 [484.8]
  abdominal 002.0
  carrier (suspected) of V02.1
  cholecystitis (current) 002.0
  clinical (Widal and blood test negative) 002.0
  endocarditis 002.0 [421.1]
  inoculation reaction — *see* Complications, vaccination
  meningitis 002.0 [320.7]
  mesenteric lymph nodes 002.0
  myocarditis 002.0 [422.0]
  osteomyelitis (*see also* Osteomyelitis, due to, typhoid) 002.0 [730.8] ☑
  perichondritis, larynx 002.0 [478.71]
  pneumonia 002.0 [484.8]
  spine 002.0 [720.81]
  ulcer (perforating) 002.0
  vaccination, prophylactic (against) V03.1
  Widal negative 002.0
Typhomalaria (fever) (*see also* Malaria) 084.6
Typhomania 002.0
Typhoperitonitis 002.0
Typhus (fever) 081.9
  abdominal, abdominalis 002.0
  African tick 082.1
  amarillic (*see also* Fever, Yellow) 060.9
  brain 081.9
  cerebral 081.9
  classical 080
  endemic (flea-borne) 081.0
  epidemic (louse-borne) 080
  exanthematic NEC 080
  exanthematicus SAI 080
    brillii SAI 081.1
    Mexicanus SAI 081.0
    pediculo vestimenti causa 080
    typhus murinus 081.0
  flea-borne 081.0
  Indian tick 082.1
  Kenya tick 082.1
  louse-borne 080

Typhus — *continued*
  Mexican 081.0
    flea-borne 081.0
    louse-borne 080
    tabardillo 080
  mite-borne 081.2
  murine 081.0
  North Asian tick-borne 082.2
  petechial 081.9
  Queensland tick 082.3
  rat 081.0
  recrudescent 081.1
  recurrent (*see also* Fever, relapsing) 087.9
  São Paulo 082.0
  scrub (China) (India) (Malaya) (New Guinea) 081.2
  shop (of Malaya) 081.0
  Siberian tick 082.2
  tick-borne NEC 082.9
  tropical 081.2
  vaccination, prophylactic (against) V05.8
Tyrosinemia 270.2
  neonatal 775.8
Tyrosinosis (Medes) (Sakai) 270.2
Tyrosinuria 270.2
Tyrosyluria 270.2

U

Uehlinger's syndrome (acropachyderma) 757.39
Uhl's anomaly or disease (hypoplasia of myocardium, right ventricle) 746.84
Ulcer, ulcerated, ulcerating, ulceration, ulcerative 707.9
  with gangrene 707.9 [785.4]
  abdomen (wall) (*see also* Ulcer, skin) 707.8
  ala, nose 478.1
  alveolar process 526.5
  amebic (intestine) 006.9
    skin 006.6
  anastomotic — *see* Ulcer, gastrojejunal
  anorectal 569.41
  antral — *see* Ulcer, stomach
  anus (sphincter) (solitary) 569.41
    varicose — *see* Varicose, ulcer, anus
  aphthous (oral) (recurrent) 528.2
    genital organ(s)
      female 616.8
      male 608.89
    mouth 528.2
  arm (*see also* Ulcer, skin) 707.8
  arteriosclerotic plaque — *see* Arteriosclerosis, by site
  artery NEC 447.2
    without rupture 447.8
  atrophic NEC — *see* Ulcer, skin
  Barrett's (chronic peptic ulcer of esophagus) 530.85
  bile duct 576.8
  bladder (solitary) (sphincter) 596.8
    bilharzial (*see also* Schistosomiasis) 120.9 [595.4]
    submucosal (*see also* Cystitis) 595.1
    tuberculous (*see also* Tuberculosis) 016.1 ☑
  bleeding NEC — *see* Ulcer, peptic, with hemorrhage
  bone 730.9 ☑
  bowel (*see also* Ulcer, intestine) 569.82
  breast 611.0
  bronchitis 491.8
  bronchus 519.1
  buccal (cavity) (traumatic) 528.9
  burn (acute) — *see* Ulcer, duodenum
  Buruli 031.1
  buttock (*see also* Ulcer, skin) 707.8
    decubitus (*see also* Ulcer, decubitus) 707.00 ▲
  cancerous (M8000/3) — *see* Neoplasm, by site, malignant
  cardia — *see* Ulcer, stomach
  cardio-esophageal (peptic) 530.20
    with bleeding 530.21
  cecum (*see also* Ulcer, intestine) 569.82
  cervix (uteri) (trophic) 622.0
    with mention of cervicitis 616.0

Ulcer, ulcerated, ulcerating, ulceration, ulcerative — *continued*
  chancroidal 099.0
  chest (wall) (*see also* Ulcer, skin) 707.8
  Chiclero 085.4
  chin (pyogenic) (*see also* Ulcer, skin) 707.8
  chronic (cause unknown) — *see also* Ulcer, skin
    penis 607.89
  Cochin-China 085.1
  colitis — *see* Colitis, ulcerative
  colon (*see also* Ulcer, intestine) 569.82
  conjunctiva (acute) (postinfectional) 372.00
  cornea (infectional) 370.00
    with perforation 370.06
    annular 370.02
    catarrhal 370.01
    central 370.03
    dendritic 054.42
    marginal 370.01
    mycotic 370.05
    phlyctenular, tuberculous (*see also* Tuberculosis) 017.3 ☑ [370.31]
    ring 370.02
    rodent 370.07
    serpent, serpiginous 370.04
    superficial marginal 370.01
    tuberculous (*see also* Tuberculosis) 017.3 ☑ [370.31]
  corpus cavernosum (chronic) 607.89
  crural — *see* Ulcer, lower extremity
  Curling's — *see* Ulcer, duodenum
  Cushing's — *see* Ulcer, peptic
  cystitis (interstitial) 595.1
  decubitus (▶unspecified◀ site) 707.00 ▲
    with gangrene 707.00 [785.4] ▲
    ankle 707.06 ●
    back ●
      lower 707.03 ●
      upper 707.02 ●
    buttock 707.05 ●
    elbow 707.01 ●
    head 707.09 ●
    heel 707.07 ●
    hip 707.04 ●
    other site 707.09 ●
    sacrum 707.03 ●
    shoulder blades 707.02 ●
  dendritic 054.42
  diabetes, diabetic (mellitus) 250.8 ☑ [707.9]
    lower limb 250.8 ☑ [707.10]
      ankle 250.8 ☑ [707.13]
      calf 250.8 ☑ [707.12]
      foot 250.8 ☑ [707.15]
      heel 250.8 ☑ [707.14]
      knee 250.8 ☑ [707.19]
      specified site NEC 250.8 ☑ [707.19]
      thigh 250.8 ☑ [707.11]
      toes 250.8 ☑ [707.15]
    specified site NEC 250.8 ☑ [707.8]
  Dieulafoy — *see* Lesion, Dieulafoy
  due to
    infection NEC — *see* Ulcer, skin
    radiation, radium — *see* Ulcer, by site
    trophic disturbance (any region) — *see* Ulcer, skin
    x-ray — *see* Ulcer, by site
  duodenum, duodenal (eroded) (peptic) 532.9 ☑

Note — *Use the following fifth-digit subclassification with categories 531-534:*

0	*without mention of obstruction*
1	*with obstruction*

  with
    hemorrhage (chronic) 532.4 ☑
      and perforation 532.6 ☑
    perforation (chronic) 532.5 ☑
      and hemorrhage 532.6 ☑
  acute 532.3 ☑
    with
      hemorrhage 532.0 ☑
        and perforation 532.2 ☑
      perforation 532.1 ☑
        and hemorrhage 532.2 ☑

Ulcer, ulcerated, ulcerating, ulceration, ulcerative — *continued*
duodenum, duodenal — *continued*
    bleeding (recurrent) — *see* Ulcer, duodenum, with hemorrhage
    chronic 532.7 ☑
      with
        hemorrhage 532.4 ☑
          and perforation 532.6 ☑
        perforation 532.5 ☑
          and hemorrhage 532.6 ☑
    penetrating — *see* Ulcer, duodenum, with perforation
    perforating — *see* Ulcer, duodenum, with perforation
  dysenteric NEC 009.0
  elusive 595.1
  endocarditis (any valve) (acute) (chronic) (subacute) 421.0
  enteritis — *see* Colitis, ulcerative
  enterocolitis 556.0
  epiglottis 478.79
  esophagus (peptic) 530.20
    with bleeding 530.21
    due to ingestion
      aspirin 530.20
      chemicals 530.20
      medicinal agents 530.20
    fungal 530.20
    infectional 530.20
    varicose (*see also* Varix, esophagus) 456.1
      bleeding (*see also* Varix, esophagus, bleeding) 456.0
  eye NEC 360.00
    dendritic 054.42
  eyelid (region) 373.01
  face (*see also* Ulcer, skin) 707.8
  fauces 478.29
  Fenwick (-Hunner) (solitary) (*see also* Cystitis) 595.1
  fistulous NEC — *see* Ulcer, skin
  foot (indolent) (*see also* Ulcer, lower extremity) 707.15
    perforating 707.15
      leprous 030.1
      syphilitic 094.0
    trophic 707.15
    varicose 454.0
      inflamed or infected 454.2
  frambesial, initial or primary 102.0
  gallbladder or duct 575.8
  gall duct 576.8
  gangrenous (*see also* Gangrene) 785.4
  gastric — *see* Ulcer, stomach
  gastrocolic — *see* Ulcer, gastrojejunal
  gastroduodenal — *see* Ulcer, peptic
  gastroesophageal — *see* Ulcer, stomach
  gastrohepatic — *see* Ulcer, stomach
  gastrointestinal — *see* Ulcer, gastrojejunal
  gastrojejunal (eroded) (peptic) 534.9 ☑

Note — *Use the following fifth-digit subclassification with categories 531-534:*	
0	*without mention of obstruction*
1	*with obstruction*

    with
      hemorrhage (chronic) 534.4 ☑
        and perforation 534.6 ☑
      perforation 534.5 ☑
        and hemorrhage 534.6 ☑
    acute 534.3 ☑
      with
        hemorrhage 534.0 ☑
          and perforation 534.2 ☑
        perforation 534.1 ☑
          and hemorrhage 534.2 ☑
    bleeding (recurrent) — *see* Ulcer, gastrojejunal, with hemorrhage
    chronic 534.7 ☑
      with
        hemorrhage 534.4 ☑
          and perforation 534.6 ☑
        perforation 534.5 ☑
          and hemorrhage 534.6 ☑

Ulcer, ulcerated, ulcerating, ulceration, ulcerative — *continued*
gastrojejunal — *continued*
    penetrating — *see* Ulcer, gastrojejunal, with perforation
    perforating — *see* Ulcer, gastrojejunal, with perforation
  gastrojejunocolic — *see* Ulcer, gastrojejunal
  genital organ
    female 629.8
    male 608.89
  gingiva 523.8
  gingivitis 523.1
  glottis 478.79
  granuloma of pudenda 099.2
  groin (*see also* Ulcer, skin) 707.8
  gum 523.8
  gumma, due to yaws 102.4
  hand (*see also* Ulcer, skin) 707.8
  hard palate 528.9
  heel (*see also* Ulcer, lower extremity) 707.14
    decubitus (*see also* Ulcer, decubitus) 707.07 ▲
  hemorrhoids 455.8
    external 455.5
    internal 455.2
  hip (*see also* Ulcer, skin) 707.8
    decubitus (*see also* Ulcer, decubitus) 707.04 ▲
  Hunner's 595.1
  hypopharynx 478.29
  hypopyon (chronic) (subacute) 370.04
  hypostaticum — *see* Ulcer, varicose
  ileocolitis 556.1
  ileum (*see also* Ulcer, intestine) 569.82
  intestine, intestinal 569.82
    with perforation 569.83
    amebic 006.9
    duodenal — *see* Ulcer, duodenum
    granulocytopenic (with hemorrhage) 288.0
    marginal 569.82
    perforating 569.83
    small, primary 569.82
    stercoraceous 569.82
    stercoral 569.82
    tuberculous (*see also* Tuberculosis) 014.8 ☑
    typhoid (fever) 002.0
    varicose 456.8
  ischemic 707.9
    lower extremity (*see also* Ulcer, lower extremity) 707.10
      ankle 707.13
      calf 707.12
      foot 707.15
      heel 707.14
      knee 707.19
      specified site NEC 707.19
      thigh 707.11
      toes 707.15
  jejunum, jejunal — *see* Ulcer, gastrojejunal
  keratitis (*see also* Ulcer, cornea) 370.00
  knee — *see* Ulcer, lower extremity
  labium (majus) (minus) 616.50
  laryngitis (*see also* Laryngitis) 464.00
    with obstruction 464.01
  larynx (aphthous) (contact) 478.79
    diphtheritic 032.3
  leg — *see* Ulcer, lower extremity
  lip 528.5
  Lipschütz's 616.50
  lower extremity (atrophic) (chronic) (neurogenic) (perforating) (pyogenic) (trophic) (tropical) 707.10
    with gangrene (*see also* Ulcer, lower extremity) 707.10 [785.4]
      arteriosclerotic 440.24
    ankle 707.13
      arteriosclerotic 440.23
        with gangrene 440.24
    calf 707.12
    decubitus 707.00 ▲
      with gangrene 707.00 [785.4] ▲
      ankle 707.06 ●
      buttock 707.05 ●
      heel 707.07 ●
      hip 707.04 ●
    foot 707.15
    heel 707.14

Ulcer, ulcerated, ulcerating, ulceration, ulcerative — *continued*
lower extremity — *continued*
    knee 707.19
    specified site NEC 707.19
    thigh 707.11
    toes 707.15
    varicose 454.0
      inflamed or infected 454.2
  luetic — *see* Ulcer, syphilitic
  lung 518.89
    tuberculous (*see also* Tuberculosis) 011.2 ☑
  malignant (M8000/3) — *see* Neoplasm, by site, malignant
  marginal NEC — *see* Ulcer, gastrojejunal
  meatus (urinarius) 597.89
  Meckel's diverticulum 751.0
  Meleney's (chronic undermining) 686.09
  Mooren's (cornea) 370.07
  mouth (traumatic) 528.9
  mycobacterial (skin) 031.1
  nasopharynx 478.29
  navel cord (newborn) 771.4
  neck (*see also* Ulcer, skin) 707.8
    uterus 622.0
  neurogenic NEC — *see* Ulcer, skin
  nose, nasal (infectional) (passage) 478.1
    septum 478.1
      varicose 456.8
    skin — *see* Ulcer, skin
    spirochetal NEC 104.8
  oral mucosa (traumatic) 528.9
  palate (soft) 528.9
  penetrating NEC — *see* Ulcer, peptic, with perforation
  penis (chronic) 607.89
  peptic (site unspecified) 533.9 ☑

Note — *Use the following fifth-digit subclassification with categories 531-534:*	
0	*without mention of obstruction*
1	*with obstruction*

    with
      hemorrhage 533.4 ☑
        and perforation 533.6 ☑
      perforation (chronic) 533.5 ☑
        and hemorrhage 533.6 ☑
    acute 533.3 ☑
      with
        hemorrhage 533.0 ☑
          and perforation 533.2 ☑
        perforation 533.1 ☑
          and hemorrhage 533.2 ☑
    bleeding (recurrent) — *see* Ulcer, peptic, with hemorrhage
    chronic 533.7 ☑
      with
        hemorrhage 533.4 ☑
          and perforation 533.6 ☑
        perforation 533.5 ☑
          and hemorrhage 533.6 ☑
    penetrating — *see* Ulcer, peptic, with perforation
    perforating NEC (*see also* Ulcer, peptic, with perforation) 533.5 ☑
    skin 707.9
  perineum (*see also* Ulcer, skin) 707.8
  peritonsillar 474.8
  phagedenic (tropical) NEC — *see* Ulcer, skin
  pharynx 478.29
  phlebitis — *see* Phlebitis
  plaster (*see also* Ulcer, decubitus) 707.00 ▲
  popliteal space — *see* Ulcer, lower extremity
  postpyloric — *see* Ulcer, duodenum
  prepuce 607.89
  prepyloric — *see* Ulcer, stomach
  pressure (*see also* Ulcer, decubitus) 707.00 ▲
  primary of intestine 569.82
    with perforation 569.83
  proctitis 556.2
    with ulcerative sigmoiditis 556.3
  prostate 601.8
  pseudopeptic — *see* Ulcer, peptic
  pyloric — *see* Ulcer, stomach
  rectosigmoid 569.82
    with perforation 569.83

☑ Additional Digit Required   ▶◀ Revised Text   ● New Line   ▲ Revised Code

Ulcer, ulcerated, ulcerating, ulceration, ulcerative — *continued*
  rectum (sphincter) (solitary) 569.41
    stercoraceous, stercoral 569.41
    varicose — *see* Varicose, ulcer, anus
  retina (*see also* Chorioretinitis) 363.20
  rodent (M8090/3) — *see also* Neoplasm, skin, malignant
    cornea 370.07
  round — *see* Ulcer, stomach
  sacrum (region) (*see also* Ulcer, skin) 707.8
  Saemisch's 370.04
  scalp (*see also* Ulcer, skin) 707.8
  sclera 379.09
  scrofulous (*see also* Tuberculosis) 017.2 ☑
  scrotum 608.89
    tuberculous (*see also* Tuberculosis) 016.5 ☑
    varicose 456.4
  seminal vesicle 608.89
  sigmoid 569.82
    with perforation 569.83
  skin (atrophic) (chronic) (neurogenic) (non-healing) (perforating) (pyogenic) (trophic) 707.9
    with gangrene 707.9 *[785.4]*
    amebic 006.6
    decubitus ►(*see also* Ulcer, decubitus)◄ 707.00 ▲
      with gangrene 707.00 *[785.4]* ▲
    in granulocytopenia 288.0
    lower extremity (*see also* Ulcer, lower extremity) 707.10
      with gangrene 707.10 *[785.4]*
        arteriosclerotic 440.24
      ankle 707.13
      arteriosclerotic 440.23
        with gangrene 440.24
      calf 707.12
      foot 707.15
      heel 707.14
      knee 707.19
      specified site NEC 707.19
      thigh 707.11
      toes 707.15
    mycobacterial 031.1
    syphilitic (early) (secondary) 091.3
    tuberculous (primary) (*see also* Tuberculosis) 017.0 ☑
    varicose — *see* Ulcer, varicose
  sloughing NEC — *see* Ulcer, skin
  soft palate 528.9
  solitary, anus or rectum (sphincter) 569.41
  sore throat 462
    streptococcal 034.0
  spermatic cord 608.89
  spine (tuberculous) 015.0 ☑ *[730.88]*
  stasis (leg) (venous) 454.0
    inflamed or infected 454.2
    without varicose veins 459.81
  stercoral, stercoraceous 569.82
    with perforation 569.83
    anus or rectum 569.41
  stoma, stomal — *see* Ulcer, gastrojejunal
  stomach (eroded) (peptic) (round) 531.9 ☑

> *Note* — Use the following fifth-digit subclassification with categories 531-534:
>
> 0   *without mention of obstruction*
> 1   *with obstruction*

    with
      hemorrhage 531.4 ☑
        and perforation 531.6 ☑
      perforation (chronic) 531.5 ☑
        and hemorrhage 531.6 ☑
      acute 531.3 ☑
        with
          hemorrhage 531.0 ☑
            and perforation 531.2 ☑
          perforation 531.1 ☑
            and hemorrhage 531.2 ☑
      bleeding (recurrent) — *see* Ulcer, stomach, with hemorrhage

Ulcer, ulcerated, ulcerating, ulceration, ulcerative — *continued*
  stomach — *continued*
    chronic 531.7 ☑
      with
        hemorrhage 531.4 ☑
          and perforation 531.6 ☑
        perforation 531.5 ☑
          and hemorrhage 531.6 ☑
    penetrating — *see* Ulcer, stomach, with perforation
    perforating — *see* Ulcer, stomach, with perforation
  stomatitis 528.0
  stress — *see* Ulcer, peptic
  strumous (tuberculous) (*see also* Tuberculosis) 017.2 ☑
  submental (*see also* Ulcer, skin) 707.8
  submucosal, bladder 595.1
  syphilitic (any site) (early) (secondary) 091.3
    late 095.9
    perforating 095.9
      foot 094.0
  testis 608.89
  thigh — *see* Ulcer, lower extremity
  throat 478.29
    diphtheritic 032.0
  toe — *see* Ulcer, lower extremity
  tongue (traumatic) 529.0
  tonsil 474.8
    diphtheritic 032.0
  trachea 519.1
  trophic — *see* Ulcer, skin
  tropical NEC (*see also* Ulcer, skin) 707.9
  tuberculous — *see* Tuberculosis, ulcer
  tunica vaginalis 608.89
  turbinate 730.9 ☑
  typhoid (fever) 002.0
    perforating 002.0
  umbilicus (newborn) 771.4
  unspecified site NEC — *see* Ulcer, skin
  urethra (meatus) (*see also* Urethritis) 597.89
  uterus 621.8
    cervix 622.0
      with mention of cervicitis 616.0
    neck 622.0
      with mention of cervicitis 616.0
  vagina 616.8
  valve, heart 421.0
  varicose (lower extremity, any part) 454.0
    anus — *see* Varicose, ulcer, anus
    broad ligament 456.5
    esophagus (*see also* Varix, esophagus) 456.1
      bleeding (*see also* Varix, esophagus, bleeding) 456.0
    inflamed or infected 454.2
    nasal septum 456.8
    perineum 456.6
    rectum — *see* Varicose, ulcer, anus
    scrotum 456.4
    specified site NEC 456.8
    sublingual 456.3
    vulva 456.6
  vas deferens 608.89
  vesical (*see also* Ulcer, bladder) 596.8
  vulva (acute) (infectional) 616.50
    Behçet's syndrome 136.1 *[616.51]*
    herpetic 054.12
    tuberculous 016.7 ☑ *[616.51]*
  vulvobuccal, recurring 616.50
  x-ray — *see* Ulcer, by site
  yaws 102.4
Ulcerosa scarlatina 034.1
Ulcus — *see also* Ulcer
  cutis tuberculosum (*see also* Tuberculosis) 017.0 ☑
  duodeni — *see* Ulcer, duodenum
  durum 091.0
    extragenital 091.2
  gastrojejunale — *see* Ulcer, gastrojejunal
  hypostaticum — *see* Ulcer, varicose
  molle (cutis) (skin) 099.0
  serpens corneae (pneumococcal) 370.04
  ventriculi — *see* Ulcer, stomach
Ulegyria 742.4

Ulerythema
  acneiforma 701.8
  centrifugum 695.4
  ophryogenes 757.4
Ullrich (-Bonnevie) (-Turner) syndrome 758.6
Ullrich-Feichtiger syndrome 759.89
Ulnar — *see* condition
Ulorrhagia 523.8
Ulorrhea 523.8
Umbilicus, umbilical — *see also* condition
  cord necrosis, affecting fetus or newborn 762.6
Unavailability of medical facilities (at) V63.9
  due to
    investigation by social service agency V63.8
    lack of services at home V63.1
    remoteness from facility V63.0
    waiting list V63.2
  home V63.1
  outpatient clinic V63.0
  specified reason NEC V63.8
Uncinaria americana infestion 126.1
Uncinariasis (*see also* Ancylostomiasis) 126.9
Unconscious, unconsciousness 780.09
Underdevelopment — *see also* Undeveloped
  sexual 259.0
Undernourishment 269.9
Undernutrition 269.9
Under observation — *see* Observation
Underweight 783.22
  for gestational age — *see* Light-for-dates
Underwood's disease (sclerema neonatorum) 778.1
Undescended — *see also* Malposition, congenital
  cecum 751.4
  colon 751.4
  testis 752.51
Undetermined diagnosis or cause 799.9
Undeveloped, undevelopment — *see also* Hypoplasia
  brain (congenital) 742.1
  cerebral (congenital) 742.1
  fetus or newborn 764.9 ☑
  heart 746.89
  lung 748.5
  testis 257.2
  uterus 259.0
Undiagnosed (disease) 799.9
Undulant fever (*see also* Brucellosis) 023.9
Unemployment, anxiety concerning V62.0
Unequal leg (acquired) (length) 736.81
  congenital 755.30
Unerupted teeth, tooth 520.6
Unextracted dental root 525.3
Unguis incarnatus 703.0
Unicornis uterus 752.3
Unicorporeus uterus 752.3
Uniformis uterus 752.3
Unilateral — *see also* condition
  development, breast 611.8
  organ or site, congenital NEC — *see* Agenesis
  vagina 752.49
Unilateralis uterus 752.3
Unilocular heart 745.8
Uninhibited bladder 596.54
  with cauda equina syndrome 344.61
  neurogenic — *see* Neurogenic, bladder 596.54
Union, abnormal — *see also* Fusion
  divided tendon 727.89
  larynx and trachea 748.3
Universal
  joint, cervix 620.6
  mesentery 751.4
Unknown
  cause of death 799.9
  diagnosis 799.9
Unna's disease (seborrheic dermatitis) 690.10
Unresponsiveness, adrenocorticotropin (ACTH) 255.4
Unsatisfactory smear 795.08   ●

☑ Additional Digit Required   ►◄ Revised Text   ● New Line   ▲ Revised Code

Unsoundness of mind (*see also* Psychosis) 298.9
Unspecified cause of death 799.9
Unstable
   back NEC 724.9
   colon 569.89
   joint — *see* Instability, joint
   lie 652.0 ☑
      affecting fetus or newborn (before labor) 761.7
      causing obstructed labor 660.0 ☑
         affecting fetus or newborn 763.1
   lumbosacral joint (congenital) 756.19
      acquired 724.6
   sacroiliac 724.6
   spine NEC 724.9
Untruthfulness, child problem (*see also* Disturbance, conduct) 312.0 ☑
Unverricht (-Lundborg) disease, syndrome, or epilepsy 333.2
Unverricht-Wagner syndrome (dermatomyositis) 710.3
Upper respiratory — *see* condition
Upset
   gastric 536.8
      psychogenic 306.4
   gastrointestinal 536.8
      psychogenic 306.4
      virus (*see also* Enteritis, viral) 008.8
   intestinal (large) (small) 564.9
      psychogenic 306.4
   menstruation 626.9
   mental 300.9
   stomach 536.8
      psychogenic 306.4
Urachus — *see also* condition
   patent 753.7
   persistent 753.7
Uratic arthritis 274.0
Urbach's lipoid proteinosis 272.8
Urbach-Oppenheim disease or syndrome (necrobiosis lipoidica diabeticorum) 250.8 ☑ [709.3]
Urbach-Wiethe disease or syndrome (lipoid proteinosis) 272.8
Urban yellow fever 060.1
Urea, blood, high — *see* Uremia
Uremia, uremic (absorption) (amaurosis) (amblyopia) (aphasia) (apoplexy) (coma) (delirium) (dementia) (dropsy) (dyspnea) (fever) (intoxication) (mania) (paralysis) (poisoning) (toxemia) (vomiting) 586
   with
      abortion — *see* Abortion, by type, with renal failure
      ectopic pregnancy (*see also* categories 633.0-633.9) 639.3
      hypertension (*see also* Hypertension, kidney) 403.91
      molar pregnancy (*see also* categories 630-632) 639.3
   chronic 585
   complicating
      abortion 639.3
      ectopic or molar pregnancy 639.3
      hypertension (*see also* Hypertension, kidney) 403.91
      labor and delivery 669.3 ☑
   congenital 779.89
   extrarenal 788.9
   hypertensive (chronic) (*see also* Hypertension, kidney) 403.91
   maternal NEC, affecting fetus or newborn 760.1
   neuropathy 585 [357.4]
   pericarditis 585 [420.0]
   prerenal 788.9
   pyelitic (*see also* Pyelitis) 590.80
Ureter, ureteral — *see* condition
Ureteralgia 788.0
Ureterectasis 593.89
Ureteritis 593.89
   cystica 590.3
   due to calculus 592.1

Ureteritis — *continued*
   gonococcal (acute) 098.19
      chronic or duration of 2 months or over 098.39
   nonspecific 593.89
Ureterocele (acquired) 593.89
   congenital 753.23
Ureterolith 592.1
Ureterolithiasis 592.1
Ureterostomy status V44.6
   with complication 997.5
Urethra, urethral — *see* condition
Urethralgia 788.9
Urethritis (abacterial) (acute) (allergic) (anterior) (chronic) (nonvenereal) (posterior) (recurrent) (simple) (subacute) (ulcerative) (undifferentiated) 597.80
   diplococcal (acute) 098.0
      chronic or duration of 2 months or over 098.2
   due to Trichomonas (vaginalis) 131.02
   gonococcal (acute) 098.0
      chronic or duration of 2 months or over 098.2
   nongonococcal (sexually transmitted) 099.40
      Chlamydia trachomatis 099.41
      Reiter's 099.3
      specified organism NEC 099.49
   nonspecific (sexually transmitted) (*see also* Urethritis, nongonococcal) 099.40
   not sexually transmitted 597.80
   Reiter's 099.3
   trichomonal or due to Trichomonas (vaginalis) 131.02
   tuberculous (*see also* Tuberculosis) 016.3 ☑
   venereal NEC (*see also* Urethritis, nongonococcal) 099.40
Urethrocele
   female 618.03 ▲
      with uterine prolapse 618.4
         complete 618.3
         incomplete 618.2
   male 599.5
Urethrolithiasis 594.2
Urethro-oculoarticular syndrome 099.3
Urethro-oculosynovial syndrome 099.3
Urethrorectal — *see* condition
Urethrorrhagia 599.84
Urethrorrhea 788.7
Urethrostomy status V44.6
   with complication 997.5
Urethrotrigonitis 595.3
Urethrovaginal — *see* condition
Urhidrosis, uridrosis 705.89
Uric acid
   diathesis 274.9
   in blood 790.6
Uricacidemia 790.6
Uricemia 790.6
Uricosuria 791.9
Urination
   frequent 788.41
   painful 788.1
   urgency 788.63
Urine, urinary — *see also* condition
   abnormality NEC 788.69
   blood in (*see also* Hematuria) 599.7
   discharge, excessive 788.42
   enuresis 788.30
      nonorganic origin 307.6
   extravasation 788.8
   frequency 788.41
   incontinence 788.30
      active 788.30
      female 788.30
         stress 625.6
            and urge 788.33
      male 788.30
         stress 788.32
            and urge 788.33
      mixed (stress and urge) 788.33
      neurogenic 788.39

Urine, urinary — *see also* condition — *continued*
   incontinence — *continued*
      nonorganic origin 307.6
      overflow 788.38 ●
      stress (female) 625.6
         male NEC 788.32
   intermittent stream 788.61
   pus in 791.9
   retention or stasis NEC 788.20
      bladder, incomplete emptying 788.21
      psychogenic 306.53
      specified NEC 788.29
   secretion
      deficient 788.5
      excessive 788.42
      frequency 788.41
   stream
      intermittent 788.61
      slowing 788.62
      splitting 788.61
      weak 788.62
   urgency 788.63
Urinemia — *see* Uremia
Urinoma NEC 599.9
   bladder 596.8
   kidney 593.89
   renal 593.89
   ureter 593.89
   urethra 599.84
Uroarthritis, infectious 099.3
Urodialysis 788.5
Urolithiasis 592.9
Uronephrosis 593.89
Uropathy 599.9
   obstructive 599.6
Urosepsis 599.0
   meaning sepsis 995.91 ▲
   meaning urinary tract infection 599.0
Urticaria 708.9
   with angioneurotic edema 995.1
      hereditary 277.6
   allergic 708.0
   cholinergic 708.5
   chronic 708.8
   cold, familial 708.2
   dermatographic 708.3
   due to
      cold or heat 708.2
      drugs 708.0
      food 708.0
      inhalants 708.0
      plants 708.8
      serum 999.5
   factitial 708.3
   giant 995.1
      hereditary 277.6
   gigantea 995.1
      hereditary 277.6
   idiopathic 708.1
   larynx 995.1
      hereditary 277.6
   neonatorum 778.8
   nonallergic 708.1
   papulosa (Hebra) 698.2
   perstans hemorrhagica 757.39
   pigmentosa 757.33
   recurrent periodic 708.8
   serum 999.5
   solare 692.72
   specified type NEC 708.8
   thermal (cold) (heat) 708.2
   vibratory 708.4
Urticarioides acarodermatitis 133.9
Use of
   nonprescribed drugs (*see also* Abuse, drugs, nondependent) 305.9 ☑
   patent medicines (*see also* Abuse, drugs, nondependent) 305.9 ☑
Usher-Senear disease (pemphigus erythematosus) 694.4
Uta 085.5
Uterine size-date discrepancy 646.8 ☑
Uteromegaly 621.2
Uterovaginal — *see* condition

☑ Additional Digit Required   ▶◀ Revised Text   ● New Line   ▲ Revised Code

Uterovesical — *see* condition

Uterus — *see* condition

Utriculitis (utriculus prostaticus) 597.89

Uveal — *see* condition

Uveitis (anterior) (*see also* Iridocyclitis) 364.3
   acute or subacute 364.00
      due to or associated with
         gonococcal infection 098.41
         herpes (simplex) 054.44
            zoster 053.22
      primary 364.01
      recurrent 364.02
      secondary (noninfectious) 364.04
         infectious 364.03
   allergic 360.11
   chronic 364.10
      due to or associated with
         sarcoidosis 135 *[364.11]*
         tuberculosis (*see also* Tuberculosis)
            017.3 ☑ *[364.11]*
   due to
      operation 360.11
      toxoplasmosis (acquired) 130.2
         congenital (active) 771.2
   granulomatous 364.10
   heterochromic 364.21
   lens-induced 364.23
   nongranulomatous 364.00
   posterior 363.20
      disseminated — *see* Chorioretinitis,
         disseminated
      focal — *see* Chorioretinitis, focal
   recurrent 364.02
   sympathetic 360.11
   syphilitic (secondary) 091.50
      congenital 090.0 *[363.13]*
      late 095.8 *[363.13]*
   tuberculous (*see also* Tuberculosis)
      017.3 ☑ *[364.11]*

Uveoencephalitis 363.22

Uveokeratitis (*see also* Iridocyclitis) 364.3

Uveoparotid fever 135

Uveoparotitis 135

Uvula — *see* condition

Uvulitis (acute) (catarrhal) (chronic) (gangrenous)
   (membranous) (suppurative) (ulcerative)
   528.3

V

Vaccination
complication or reaction — *see* Complications, vaccination
not done (contraindicated) V64.0
  because of patient's decision V64.2
prophylactic (against) V05.9
  arthropod-borne viral
    disease NEC V05.1
    encephalitis V05.0
  chickenpox V05.4
  cholera (alone) V03.0
    with typhoid-paratyphoid (cholera + TAB) V06.0
  common cold V04.7
  diphtheria (alone) V03.5
    with
      poliomyelitis (DTP+ polio) V06.3
      tetanus V06.5
        pertussis combined (DTP) (DTaP) V06.1
        typhoid-paratyphoid (DTP + TAB) V06.2
  disease (single) NEC V05.9
    bacterial NEC V03.9
      specified type NEC V03.89
    combinations NEC V06.9
      specified type NEC V06.8
    specified type NEC V05.8
  encephalitis, viral, arthropod-borne V05.0
  Hemophilus influenzae, type B [Hib] V03.81
  hepatitis, viral V05.3
  influenza V04.81
    with
      Streptococcus pneumoniae [pneumococcus] V06.6
  ▶leishmaniasis◀ V05.2
  measles (alone) V04.2
    with mumps-rubella (MMR) V06.4
  mumps (alone) V04.6
    with measles and rubella (MMR) V06.4
  pertussis alone V03.6
  plague V03.3
  poliomyelitis V04.0
    with diphtheria-tetanus-pertussis (DTP + polio) V06.3
  rabies V04.5
  respiratory syncytial virus (RSV) V04.82
  rubella (alone) V04.3
    with measles and mumps (MMR) V06.4
  smallpox V04.1
  Streptococcus pneumoniae [pneumococcus] V03.82
    with
      influenza V06.6
  tetanus toxoid (alone) V03.7
    with diphtheria [Td] [DT] V06.5
      with
        pertussis (DTP) (DTaP) V06.1
          with poliomyelitis (DTP+polio) V06.3
  tuberculosis (BCG) V03.2
  tularemia V03.4
  typhoid-paratyphoid (TAB) (alone) V03.1
    with diphtheria-tetanus-pertussis (TAB + DTP) V06.2
  varicella V05.4
  viral
    disease NEC V04.89
    encephalitis, arthropod-borne V05.0
    hepatitis V05.3
  yellow fever V04.4
Vaccinia (generalized) 999.0
congenital 771.2
conjunctiva 999.3
eyelids 999.0 *[373.5]*
localized 999.3
nose 999.3
not from vaccination 051.0
  eyelid 051.0 *[373.5]*
sine vaccinatione 051.0
without vaccination 051.0
Vacuum
extraction of fetus or newborn 763.3

Vacuum — *continued*
in sinus (accessory) (nasal) (*see also* Sinusitis) 473.9
Vagabond V60.0
Vagabondage V60.0
Vagabonds' disease 132.1
Vagina, vaginal — *see* condition
Vaginalitis (tunica) 608.4
Vaginismus (reflex) 625.1
functional 306.51
hysterical 300.11
psychogenic 306.51
Vaginitis (acute) (chronic) (circumscribed) (diffuse) (emphysematous) (Hemophilus vaginalis) (nonspecific) (nonvenereal) (ulcerative) 616.10
with
  abortion — *see* Abortion, by type, with sepsis
  ectopic pregnancy (*see also* categories 633.0-633.9) 639.0
  molar pregnancy (*see also* categories 630-632) 639.0
adhesive, congenital 752.49
atrophic, postmenopausal 627.3
bacterial 616.10
blennorrhagic (acute) 098.0
  chronic or duration of 2 months or over 098.2
candidal 112.1
chlamydial 099.53
complicating pregnancy or puerperium 646.6 ☑
  affecting fetus or newborn 760.8
congenital (adhesive) 752.49
due to
  C. albicans 112.1
  Trichomonas (vaginalis) 131.01
following
  abortion 639.0
  ectopic or molar pregnancy 639.0
gonococcal (acute) 098.0
  chronic or duration of 2 months or over 098.2
granuloma 099.2
Monilia 112.1
mycotic 112.1
pinworm 127.4 *[616.11]*
postirradiation 616.10
postmenopausal atrophic 627.3
senile (atrophic) 627.3
syphilitic (early) 091.0
  late 095.8
trichomonal 131.01
tuberculous (*see also* Tuberculosis) 016.7 ☑
venereal NEC 099.8
Vaginosis — *see* Vaginitis
Vagotonia 352.3
Vagrancy V60.0
Vallecula — *see* condition
Valley fever 114.0
Valsuani's disease (progressive pernicious anemia, puerperal) 648.2 ☑
Valve, valvular (formation) — *see also* condition
cerebral ventricle (communicating) in situ V45.2
cervix, internal os 752.49
colon 751.5
congenital NEC — *see* Atresia
formation, congenital NEC — *see* Atresia
heart defect — *see* Anomaly, heart, valve
ureter 753.29
  pelvic junction 753.21
  vesical orifice 753.22
urethra 753.6
Valvulitis (chronic) (*see also* Endocarditis) 424.90
rheumatic (chronic) (inactive) (with chorea) 397.9
  active or acute (aortic) (mitral) (pulmonary) (tricuspid) 391.1
syphilitic NEC 093.20
  aortic 093.22
  mitral 093.21
  pulmonary 093.24

Valvulitis (*see also* Endocarditis) — *continued*
syphilitic — *continued*
  tricuspid 093.23
Valvulopathy — *see* Endocarditis
van Bogaert's leukoencephalitis (sclerosing) (subacute) 046.2
van Bogaert-Nijssen (-Peiffer) disease 330.0
van Buchem's syndrome (hyperostosis corticalis) 733.3
van Creveld-von Gierke disease (glycogenosis I) 271.0
van den Bergh's disease (enterogenous cyanosis) 289.7
van der Hoeve's syndrome (brittle bones and blue sclera, deafness) 756.51
van der Hoeve-Halbertsma-Waardenburg syndrome (ptosis-epicanthus) 270.2
van der Hoeve-Waardenburg-Gualdi syndrome (ptosis epicanthus) 270.2
Vancomycin (glycopeptide) ●
intermediate staphylococcus aureus (VISA/GISA) V09.8 ●
resistant ●
  enterococcus (VRE) V09.8 ●
  staphylococcus aureus (VRSA/GRSA) V09.8 ●
Vanillism 692.89
Vanishing lung 492.0
van Neck (-Odelberg) disease or syndrome (juvenile osteochondrosis) 732.1
Vanishing twin 651.33
Vapor asphyxia or suffocation NEC 987.9
specified agent — *see* Table of Drugs and Chemicals
Vaquez's disease (M9950/1) 238.4
Vaquez-Osler disease (polycythemia vera) (M9950/1) 238.4
Variance, lethal ball, prosthetic heart valve 996.02
Variants, thalassemic 282.49
Variations in hair color 704.3
Varicella 052.9
with
  complication 052.8
    specified NEC 052.7
  pneumonia 052.1
  vaccination and inoculation (prophylactic) V05.4
exposure to V01.71 ●
Varices — *see* Varix
Varicocele (scrotum) (thrombosed) 456.4
ovary 456.5
perineum 456.6
spermatic cord (ulcerated) 456.4
Varicose
aneurysm (ruptured) (*see also* Aneurysm) 442.9
dermatitis (lower extremity) — *see* Varicose, vein, inflamed or infected
eczema — *see* Varicose, vein
phlebitis — *see* Varicose, vein, inflamed or infected
placental vessel — *see* Placenta, abnormal
tumor — *see* Varicose, vein
ulcer (lower extremity, any part) 454.0
  anus 455.8
    external 455.5
    internal 455.2
  esophagus (*see also* Varix, esophagus) 456.1
    bleeding (*see also* Varix, esophagus, bleeding) 456.0
  inflamed or infected 454.2
  nasal septum 456.8
  perineum 456.6
  rectum — *see* Varicose, ulcer, anus
  scrotum 456.4
  specified site NEC 456.8
vein (lower extremity) (ruptured) (*see also* Varix) 454.9
  with
    complications NEC 454.8
    edema 454.8

Varicose — Verruca (side tab)

Varicose — *continued*
vein (*see also* Varix) — *continued*
with — *continued*
inflammation or infection 454.1
ulcerated 454.2
pain 454.8
stasis dermatitis 454.1
with ulcer 454.2
swelling 454.8
ulcer 454.0
inflamed or infected 454.2
anus — *see* Hemorrhoids
broad ligament 456.5
congenital (peripheral) NEC 747.60
gastrointestinal 747.61
lower limb 747.64
renal 747.62
specified NEC 747.69
upper limb 747.63
esophagus (ulcerated) (*see also* Varix, esophagus) 456.1
bleeding (*see also* Varix, esophagus, bleeding) 456.0
inflamed or infected 454.1
with ulcer 454.2
in pregnancy or puerperium 671.0 ☑
vulva or perineum 671.1 ☑
nasal septum (with ulcer) 456.8
pelvis 456.5
perineum 456.6
in pregnancy, childbirth, or puerperium 671.1 ☑
rectum — *see* Hemorrhoids
scrotum (ulcerated) 456.4
specified site NEC 456.8
sublingual 456.3
ulcerated 454.0
inflamed or infected 454.2
umbilical cord, affecting fetus or newborn 762.6
urethra 456.8
vulva 456.6
in pregnancy, childbirth, or puerperium 671.1 ☑
vessel — *see also* Varix
placenta — *see* Placenta, abnormal
Varicosis, varicosities, varicosity (*see also* Varix) 454.9
Variola 050.9
hemorrhagic (pustular) 050.0
major 050.0
minor 050.1
modified 050.2
Varioloid 050.2
Variolosa, purpura 050.0
Varix (lower extremity) (ruptured) 454.9
with
complications NEC 454.8
edema 454.8
inflammation or infection 454.1
with ulcer 454.2
pain 454.8
stasis dermatitis 454.1
with ulcer 454.2
swelling 454.8
ulcer 454.0
with inflammation or infection 454.2
aneurysmal (*see also* Aneurysm) 442.9
anus — *see* Hemorrhoids
arteriovenous (congenital) (peripheral) NEC 747.60
gastrointestinal 747.61
lower limb 747.64
renal 747.62
specified NEC 747.69
spinal 747.82
upper limb 747.63
bladder 456.5
broad ligament 456.5
congenital (peripheral) NEC 747.60
esophagus (ulcerated) 456.1
bleeding 456.0
in
cirrhosis of liver 571.5 *[456.20]*
portal hypertension 572.3 *[456.20]*

Varix — *continued*
esophagus — *continued*
congenital 747.69
in
cirrhosis of liver 571.5 *[456.21]*
with bleeding 571.5 *[456.20]*
portal hypertension 572.3 *[456.21]*
with bleeding 572.3 *[456.20]*
gastric 456.8
inflamed or infected 454.1
ulcerated 454.2
in pregnancy or puerperium 671.0 ☑
perineum 671.1 ☑
vulva 671.1 ☑
labia (majora) 456.6
orbit 456.8
congenital 747.69
ovary 456.5
papillary 448.1
pelvis 456.5
perineum 456.6
in pregnancy or puerperium 671.1 ☑
pharynx 456.8
placenta — *see* Placenta, abnormal
prostate 456.8
rectum — *see* Hemorrhoids
renal papilla 456.8
retina 362.17
scrotum (ulcerated) 456.4
sigmoid colon 456.8
specified site NEC 456.8
spinal (cord) (vessels) 456.8
spleen, splenic (vein) (with phlebolith) 456.8
sublingual 456.3
ulcerated 454.0
inflamed or infected 454.2
umbilical cord, affecting fetus or newborn 762.6
uterine ligament 456.5
vocal cord 456.8
vulva 456.6
in pregnancy, childbirth, or puerperium 671.1 ☑
Vasa previa 663.5 ☑
affecting fetus or newborn 762.6
hemorrhage from, affecting fetus or newborn 772.0
Vascular — *see also* condition
loop on papilla (optic) 743.57
sheathing, retina 362.13
spasm 443.9
spider 448.1
Vascularity, pulmonary, congenital 747.3
Vascularization
choroid 362.16
cornea 370.60
deep 370.63
localized 370.61
retina 362.16
subretinal 362.16
Vasculitis 447.6
allergic 287.0
cryoglobulinemic 273.2
disseminated 447.6
kidney 447.8
leukocytoclastic 446.29
nodular 695.2
retinal 362.18
rheumatic — *see* Fever, rheumatic
Vasculopathy
cardiac allograft 996.83
Vas deferens — *see* condition
Vas deferentitis 608.4
Vasectomy, admission for V25.2
Vasitis 608.4
nodosa 608.4
scrotum 608.4
spermatic cord 608.4
testis 608.4
tuberculous (*see also* Tuberculosis) 016.5 ☑
tunica vaginalis 608.4
vas deferens 608.4
Vasodilation 443.9
Vasomotor — *see* condition

Vasoplasty, after previous sterilization V26.0
Vasoplegia, splanchnic (*see also* Neuropathy, peripheral, autonomic) 337.9
Vasospasm 443.9
cerebral (artery) 435.9
with transient neurologic deficit 435.9
nerve
arm NEC 354.9
autonomic 337.9
brachial plexus 353.0
cervical plexus 353.2
Vasospasm — *continued*
nerve — *continued*
leg NEC 355.8
lower extremity NEC 355.8
peripheral NEC 355.9
spinal NEC 355.9
sympathetic 337.9
upper extremity NEC 354.9
peripheral NEC 443.9
retina (artery) (*see also* Occlusion, retinal, artery) 362.30
Vasospastic — *see* condition
Vasovagal attack (paroxysmal) 780.2
psychogenic 306.2
Vater's ampulla — *see* condition
VATER syndrome 759.89
Vegetation, vegetative
adenoid (nasal fossa) 474.2
consciousness (persistent) 780.03
endocarditis (acute) (any valve) (chronic) (subacute) 421.0
heart (mycotic) (valve) 421.0
state (persistent) 780.03
Veil
Jackson's 751.4
over face (causing asphyxia) 768.9
Vein, venous — *see* condition
Veldt sore (*see also* Ulcer, skin) 707.9
Velo-cardio-facial syndrome 758.32 ●
Velpeau's hernia — *see* Hernia, femoral
Venereal
balanitis NEC 099.8
bubo 099.1
disease 099.9
specified nature or type NEC 099.8
granuloma inguinale 099.2
lymphogranuloma (Durand-Nicolas-Favre), any site 099.1
salpingitis 098.37
urethritis (*see also* Urethritis, nongonococcal) 099.40
vaginitis NEC 099.8
warts 078.19
Vengefulness, in child (*see also* Disturbance, conduct) 312.0 ☑
Venofibrosis 459.89
Venom, venomous
bite or sting (animal or insect) 989.5
poisoning 989.5
Venous — *see* condition
Ventouse delivery NEC 669.5 ☑
affecting fetus or newborn 763.3
Ventral — *see* condition
Ventricle, ventricular — *see also* condition
escape 427.69
standstill (*see also* Arrest, cardiac) 427.5
Ventriculitis, cerebral (*see also* Meningitis) 322.9
Ventriculostomy status V45.2
Verbiest's syndrome (claudicatio intermittens spinalis) 435.1
Vernet's syndrome 352.6
Verneuil's disease (syphilitic bursitis) 095.7
Verruca (filiformis) 078.10
acuminata (any site) 078.11
necrogenica (primary) (*see also* Tuberculosis) 017.0 ☑
plana (juvenilis) 078.19
peruana 088.0
peruviana 088.0
plantaris 078.19

☑ Additional Digit Required   ►◄ Revised Text   ● New Line   ▲ Revised Code

Verruca — *continued*
  seborrheica 702.19
    inflamed 702.11
  senilis 702.0
  tuberculosa (primary) (*see also* Tuberculosis) 017.0 ☑
  venereal 078.19
  viral NEC 078.10
Verrucosities (*see also* Verruca) 078.10
Verrucous endocarditis (acute) (any valve) (chronic) (subacute) 710.0 *[424.91]*
  nonbacterial 710.0 *[424.91]*
Verruga
  peruana 088.0
  peruviana 088.0
Verse's disease (calcinosis intervertebralis) 275.49 *[722.90]*
Version
  before labor, affecting fetus or newborn 761.7
  cephalic (correcting previous malposition) 652.1 ☑
    affecting fetus or newborn 763.1
  cervix (*see also* Malposition, uterus) 621.6
  uterus (postinfectional) (postpartal, old) (*see also* Malposition, uterus) 621.6
    forward — *see* Anteversion, uterus
    lateral — *see* Lateroversion, uterus
Vertebra, vertebral — *see* condition
Vertigo 780.4
  auditory 386.19
  aural 386.19
  benign paroxysmal positional 386.11
  central origin 386.2
  cerebral 386.2
  Dix and Hallpike (epidemic) 386.12
  endemic paralytic 078.81
  epidemic 078.81
    Dix and Hallpike 386.12
    Gerlier's 078.81
    Pedersen's 386.12
    vestibular neuronitis 386.12
  epileptic — *see* Epilepsy
  Gerlier's (epidemic) 078.81
  hysterical 300.11
  labyrinthine 386.10
  laryngeal 786.2
  malignant positional 386.2
  Ménière's (*see also* Disease, Ménière's) 386.00
  menopausal 627.2
  otogenic 386.19
  paralytic 078.81
  paroxysmal positional, benign 386.11
  Pedersen's (epidemic) 386.12
  peripheral 386.10
    specified type NEC 386.19
  positional
    benign paroxysmal 386.11
    malignant 386.2
Verumontanitis (chronic) (*see also* Urethritis) 597.89
Vesania (*see also* Psychosis) 298.9
Vesical — *see* condition
Vesicle
  cutaneous 709.8
  seminal — *see* condition
  skin 709.8
Vesicocolic — *see* condition
Vesicoperineal — *see* condition
Vesicorectal — *see* condition
Vesicourethrorectal — *see* condition
Vesicovaginal — *see* condition
Vesicular — *see* condition
Vesiculitis (seminal) 608.0
  amebic 006.8
  gonorrheal (acute) 098.14
    chronic or duration of 2 months or over 098.34
  trichomonal 131.09
  tuberculous (*see also* Tuberculosis) 016.5 ☑ *[608.81]*
Vestibulitis (ear) (*see also* Labyrinthitis) 386.30
  nose (external) 478.1
  vulvar 616.10

Vestibulopathy, acute peripheral (recurrent) 386.12
Vestige, vestigial — *see also* Persistence
  branchial 744.41
  structures in vitreous 743.51
Vibriosis NEC 027.9
Vidal's disease (lichen simplex chronicus) 698.3
Video display tube syndrome 723.8
Vienna type encephalitis 049.8
Villaret's syndrome 352.6
Villous — *see* condition
VIN I (vulvar intraepithelial neoplasia I) 624.8
VIN II (vulvar intraepithelial neoplasia II) 624.8
VIN III (vulvar intraepithelial neoplasia III) 233.3
Vincent's
  angina 101
  bronchitis 101
  disease 101
  gingivitis 101
  infection (any site) 101
  laryngitis 101
  stomatitis 101
  tonsillitis 101
Vinson-Plummer syndrome (sideropenic dysphagia) 280.8
Viosterol deficiency (*see also* Deficiency, calciferol) 268.9
Virchow's disease 733.99
Viremia 790.8
Virilism (adrenal) (female) NEC 255.2
  with
    3-beta-hydroxysteroid dehydrogenase defect 255.2
    11-hydroxylase defect 255.2
    21-hydroxylase defect 255.2
    adrenal
      hyperplasia 255.2
      insufficiency (congenital) 255.2
    cortical hyperfunction 255.2
Virilization (female) (suprarenal) (*see also* Virilism) 255.2
  isosexual 256.4
Virulent bubo 099.0
Virus, viral — *see also* condition
  infection NEC (*see also* Infection, viral) 079.99
  septicemia 079.99
VISA (vancomycin intermediate staphylococcus aureus) V09.8 ●
Viscera, visceral — *see* condition
Visceroptosis 569.89
Visible peristalsis 787.4
Vision, visual
  binocular, suppression 368.31
  blurred, blurring 368.8
    hysterical 300.11
  defect, defective (*see also* Impaired, vision) 369.9
  disorientation (syndrome) 368.16
  disturbance NEC (*see also* Disturbance, vision) 368.9
    hysterical 300.11
  examination V72.0
  field, limitation 368.40
  fusion, with defective steropsis 368.33
  hallucinations 368.16
  halos 368.16
  loss 369.9
    both eyes (*see also* Blindness, both eyes) 369.3
    complete (*see also* Blindness, both eyes) 369.00
    one eye 369.8
    sudden 368.16
  low (both eyes) 369.20
    one eye (other eye normal) (*see also* Impaired, vision) 369.70
      blindness, other eye 369.10
  perception, simultaneous without fusion 368.32
  tunnel 368.45
Vitality, lack or want of 780.79
  newborn 779.89

Vitamin deficiency NEC (*see also* Deficiency, vitamin) 269.2
Vitelline duct, persistent 751.0
Vitiligo 709.01
  due to pinta (carate) 103.2
  eyelid 374.53
  vulva 624.8
Vitium cordis — *see* Disease, heart
Vitreous — *see also* condition
  touch syndrome 997.99
VLCAD (long chain/very long chain acyl CoA ● dehydrogenase deficiency, LCAD) 277.85 ●
Vocal cord — *see* condition
Vocational rehabilitation V57.22
Vogt's (Cecile) disease or syndrome 333.7
Vogt-Koyanagi syndrome 364.24
Vogt-Spielmeyer disease (amaurotic familial idiocy) 330.1
Voice
  change (*see also* Dysphonia) 784.49
  loss (*see also* Aphonia) 784.41
Volhard-Fahr disease (malignant nephrosclerosis) 403.00
Volhynian fever 083.1
Volkmann's ischemic contracture or paralysis (complicating trauma) 958.6
Voluntary starvation 307.1
Volvulus (bowel) (colon) (intestine) 560.2
  with
    hernia — *see also* Hernia, by site, with obstruction
      gangrenous — *see* Hernia, by site, with gangrene
    perforation 560.2
  congenital 751.5
  duodenum 537.3
  fallopian tube 620.5
  oviduct 620.5
  stomach (due to absence of gastrocolic ligament) 537.89
Vomiting 787.03
  with nausea 787.01
  allergic 535.4 ☑
  asphyxia 933.1
  bilious (cause unknown) 787.0 ☑
    following gastrointestinal surgery 564.3
  blood (*see also* Hematemesis) 578.0
  causing asphyxia, choking, or suffocation (*see also* Asphyxia, food) 933.1
  cyclical 536.2
    psychogenic 306.4
  epidemic 078.82
  fecal matter 569.89
  following gastrointestinal surgery 564.3
  functional 536.8
    psychogenic 306.4
  habit 536.2
  hysterical 300.11
  nervous 306.4
  neurotic 306.4
  newborn 779.3
  of or complicating pregnancy 643.9 ☑
    due to
      organic disease 643.8 ☑
      specific cause NEC 643.8 ☑
    early — *see* Hyperemesis, gravidarum
    late (after 22 completed weeks of gestation) 643.2 ☑
  pernicious or persistent 536.2
    complicating pregnancy — *see* Hyperemesis, gravidarum
    psychogenic 306.4
  physiological 787.0 ☑
  psychic 306.4
  psychogenic 307.54
  stercoral 569.89
  uncontrollable 536.2
    psychogenic 306.4
  uremic — *see* Uremia
  winter 078.82
von Bechterew (-Strumpell) disease or syndrome (ankylosing spondylitis) 720.0
von Bezold's abscess 383.01

☑ Additional Digit Required   ▶◀ Revised Text   ● New Line   ▲ Revised Code

von Economo's disease (encephalitis lethargica) 049.8
von Eulenburg's disease (congenital paramyotonia) 359.2
von Gierke's disease (glycogenosis I) 271.0
von Gies' joint 095.8
von Graefe's disease or syndrome 378.72
von Hippel (-Lindau) disease or syndrome (retinocerebral angiomatosis) 759.6
von Jaksch's anemia or disease (pseudoleukemia infantum) 285.8
von Recklinghausen's
  disease or syndrome (nerves) (skin) (M9540/1) 237.71
    bones (osteitis fibrosa cystica) 252.01 ▲
    tumor (M9540/1) 237.71
von Recklinghausen-Applebaum disease (hemochromatosis) 275.0
von Schroetter's syndrome (intermittent venous claudication) 453.8
von Willebrand (~Jürgens) (-Minot) disease or syndrome (angiohemophilia) 286.4
von Zambusch's disease (lichen sclerosus et atrophicus) 701.0
Voorhoeve's disease or dyschondroplasia 756.4
Vossius' ring 921.3
  late effect 366.21
Voyeurism 302.82
VRE (vancomycin resistant enterococcus) V09.8 ●
Vrolik's disease (osteogenesis imperfecta) 756.51
VRSA (vancomycin resistant staphylococcus aureus) V09.8 ●
Vulva — see condition
Vulvismus 625.1
Vulvitis (acute) (allergic) (aphthous) (chronic) (gangrenous) (hypertrophic) (intertriginous) 616.10
  with
    abortion — see Abortion, by type, with sepsis
    ectopic pregnancy (see also categories 633.0-633.9) 639.0
    molar pregnancy (see also categories 630-632) 639.0
  adhesive, congenital 752.49
  blennorhagic (acute) 098.0
    chronic or duration of 2 months or over 098.2
  chlamydial 099.53
  complicating pregnancy or puerperium 646.6 ✓
  due to Ducrey's bacillus 099.0
  following
    abortion 639.0
    ectopic or molar pregnancy 639.0
  gonococcal (acute) 098.0
    chronic or duration of 2 months or over 098.2
  herpetic 054.11
  leukoplakic 624.0
  monilial 112.1
  puerperal, postpartum, childbirth 646.6 ✓
  syphilitic (early) 091.0
    late 095.8
  trichomonal 131.01
Vulvodynia 625.9
Vulvorectal — see condition
Vulvovaginitis (see also Vulvitis) 616.10
  amebic 006.8
  chlamydial 099.53
  gonococcal (acute) 098.0
    chronic or duration of 2 months or over 098.2
  herpetic 054.11
  monilial 112.1
  trichomonal (Trichomonas vaginalis) 131.01

W

Waardenburg's syndrome 756.89
  meaning ptosis-epicanthus 270.2
Waardenburg-Klein syndrome (ptosis-epicanthus) 270.2
Wagner's disease (colloid milium) 709.3
Wagner (-Unverricht) syndrome (dermatomyositis) 710.3
Waiting list, person on V63.2
  undergoing social agency investigation V63.8
Wakefulness disorder (see also Hypersomnia) 780.54
  nonorganic origin 307.43
Waldenström's
  disease (osteochondrosis, capital femoral) 732.1
  hepatitis (lupoid hepatitis) 571.49
  hypergammaglobulinemia 273.0
  macroglobulinemia 273.3
  purpura, hypergammaglobulinemic 273.0
  syndrome (macroglobulinemia) 273.3
Waldenström-Kjellberg syndrome (sideropenic dysphagia) 280.8
Walking
  difficulty 719.7
    psychogenic 307.9
  sleep 307.46
    hysterical 300.13
Wall, abdominal — see condition
Wallenberg's syndrome (posterior inferior cerebellar artery) (see also Disease, cerebrovascular, acute) 436
Wallgren's
  disease (obstruction of splenic vein with collateral circulation) 459.89
  meningitis (see also Meningitis, aseptic) 047.9
Wandering
  acetabulum 736.39
  gallbladder 751.69
  kidney, congenital 753.3
  organ or site, congenital NEC — see Malposition, congenital
  pacemaker (atrial) (heart) 427.89
  spleen 289.59
Wardrop's disease (with lymphangitis) 681.9
  finger 681.02
  toe 681.11
War neurosis 300.16
Wart (common) (digitate) (filiform) (infectious) (juvenile) (plantar) (viral) 078.10
  external genital organs (venereal) 078.19
  fig 078.19
  Hassall-Henle's (of cornea) 371.41
  Henle's (of cornea) 371.41
  juvenile 078.19
  moist 078.10
  Peruvian 088.0
  plantar 078.19
  prosector (see also Tuberculosis) 017.0 ✓
  seborrheic 702.19
    inflamed 702.11
  senile 702.0
  specified NEC 078.19
  syphilitic 091.3
  tuberculous (see also Tuberculosis) 017.0 ✓
  venereal (female) (male) 078.19
Warthin's tumor (salivary gland) (M8561/0) 210.2
Washerwoman's itch 692.4
Wassilieff's disease (leptospiral jaundice) 100.0
Wasting
  disease 799.4
    due to malnutrition 261
  extreme (due to malnutrition) 261
  muscular NEC 728.2
  palsy, paralysis 335.21
  pelvic muscle 618.83 ●
Water
  clefts 366.12
  deprivation of 994.3
  in joint (see also Effusion, joint) 719.0 ✓
  intoxication 276.6
  itch 120.3
  lack of 994.3

Water — continued
  loading 276.6
  on
    brain — see Hydrocephalus
    chest 511.8
  poisoning 276.6
Waterbrash 787.1
Water-hammer pulse (see also Insufficiency, aortic) 424.1
Waterhouse (-Friderichsen) disease or syndrome 036.3
Water-losing nephritis 588.89 ▲
Wax in ear 380.4
Waxy
  degeneration, any site 277.3
  disease 277.3
  kidney 277.3 [583.81]
  liver (large) 277.3
  spleen 277.3
Weak, weakness (generalized) 780.79
  arches (acquired) 734
    congenital 754.61
  bladder sphincter 596.59
  congenital 779.89
  eye muscle — see Strabismus
  facial 781.94
  foot (double) — see Weak, arches
  heart, cardiac (see also Failure, heart) 428.9
    congenital 746.9
  mind 317
  muscle 728.87
  myocardium (see also Failure, heart) 428.9
  newborn 779.89
  pelvic fundus
    pubocervical tissue 618.81 ●
    rectovaginal tissue 618.82 ●
  pulse 785.9
  senile 797
  valvular — see Endocarditis
Wear, worn, tooth, teeth (approximal) (hard tissues) (interproximal) (occlusal) ▶ (see also Attrition, teeth)◀ 521.10 ▲
Weather, weathered
  effects of
    cold NEC 991.9
      specified effect NEC 991.8
    hot (see also Heat) 992.9
    skin 692.74
Web, webbed (congenital) — see also Anomaly, specified type NEC
  canthus 743.63
  digits (see also Syndactylism) 755.10
  duodenal 751.5
  esophagus 750.3
  fingers (see also Syndactylism, fingers) 755.11
  larynx (glottic) (subglottic) 748.2
  neck (pterygium colli) 744.5
  Paterson-Kelly (sideropenic dysphagia) 280.8
  popliteal syndrome 756.89
  toes (see also Syndactylism, toes) 755.13
Weber's paralysis or syndrome 344.89
Weber-Christian disease or syndrome (nodular nonsuppurative panniculitis) 729.30
Weber-Cockayne syndrome (epidermolysis bullosa) 757.39
Weber-Dimitri syndrome 759.6
Weber-Gubler syndrome 344.89
Weber-Leyden syndrome 344.89
Weber-Osler syndrome (familial hemorrhagic telangiectasia) 448.0
Wedge-shaped or wedging vertebra (see also Osteoporosis) 733.00
Wegener's granulomatosis or syndrome 446.4
Wegner's disease (syphilitic osteochondritis) 090.0
Weight
  gain (abnormal) (excessive) 783.1
    during pregnancy 646.1 ✓
      insufficient 646.8 ✓
  less than 1000 grams at birth 765.0 ✓
  loss (cause unknown) 783.21
Weightlessness 994.9

Wound, open — *continued*

brain — *see* Injury, intracranial, with open intracranial wound
breast 879.0
  complicated 879.1
brow 873.42
  complicated 873.52
buccal mucosa 873.61
  complicated 873.71
buttock 877.0
  complicated 877.1
calf 891.0
  with tendon involvement 891.2
  complicated 891.1
canaliculus lacrimalis 870.8
  with laceration of eyelid 870.2
canthus, eye 870.8
  laceration — *see* Laceration, eyelid
cavernous sinus — *see* Injury, intracranial
cerebellum — *see* Injury, intracranial
cervical esophagus 874.4
  complicated 874.5
cervix — *see* Injury, internal, cervix
cheek(s) (external) 873.41
  complicated 873.51
  internal 873.61
    complicated 873.71
chest (wall) (external) 875.0
  complicated 875.1
chin 873.44
  complicated 873.54
choroid 363.63
ciliary body (eye) (*see also* Wound, open, intraocular) 871.9
clitoris 878.8
  complicated 878.9
cochlea 872.64
  complicated 872.74
complicated 879.9
conjunctiva — *see* Wound, open, intraocular
cornea (nonpenetrating) (*see also* Wound, open, intraocular) 871.9
costal region 875.0
  complicated 875.1
Descemet's membrane (*see also* Wound, open, intraocular) 871.9
digit(s)
  foot 893.0
    with tendon involvement 893.2
    complicated 893.1
  hand 883.0
    with tendon involvement 883.2
    complicated 883.1
drumhead, ear 872.61
  complicated 872.71
ear 872.8
  canal 872.02
    complicated 872.12
  complicated 872.9
  drum 872.61
    complicated 872.71
  external 872.00
    complicated 872.10
  multiple sites 872.69
    complicated 872.79
  ossicles (incus) (malleus) (stapes) 872.62
    complicated 872.72
  specified part NEC 872.69
    complicated 872.79
elbow 881.01
  with tendon involvement 881.21
  complicated 881.11
epididymis 878.2
  complicated 878.3
epigastric region 879.2
  complicated 879.3
epiglottis 874.01
  complicated 874.11
esophagus (cervical) 874.4
  complicated 874.5
  thoracic — *see* Injury, internal, esophagus
Eustachian tube 872.63
  complicated 872.73
extremity
  lower (multiple) NEC 894.0
    with tendon involvement 894.2
    complicated 894.1

Wound, open — *continued*

extremity — *continued*
  upper (multiple) NEC 884.0
    with tendon involvement 884.2
    complicated 884.1
eye(s) (globe) — *see* Wound, open, intraocular
eyeball NEC 871.9
  laceration (*see also* Laceration, eyeball) 871.4
  penetrating (*see also* Penetrating wound, eyeball) 871.7
eyebrow 873.42
  complicated 873.52
eyelid NEC 870.8
  laceration — *see* Laceration, eyelid
face 873.40
  complicated 873.50
  multiple sites 873.49
    complicated 873.59
  specified part NEC 873.49
    complicated 873.59
fallopian tube — *see* Injury, internal, fallopian tube
finger(s) (nail) (subungual) 883.0
  with tendon involvement 883.2
  complicated 883.1
flank 879.4
  complicated 879.5
foot (any part except toe(s) alone) 892.0
  with tendon involvement 892.2
  complicated 892.1
forearm 881.00
  with tendon involvement 881.20
  complicated 881.10
forehead 873.42
  complicated 873.52
genital organs (external) NEC 878.8
  complicated 878.9
  internal — *see* Injury, internal, by site
globe (eye) (*see also* Wound, open, eyeball) 871.9
groin 879.4
  complicated 879.5
gum(s) 873.62
  complicated 873.72
hand (except finger(s) alone) 882.0
  with tendon involvement 882.2
  complicated 882.1
head NEC 873.8
  with intracranial injury — *see* Injury, intracranial
    due to or associated with skull fracture — *see* Fracture, skull
  complicated 873.9
  scalp — *see* Wound, open, scalp
heel 892.0
  with tendon involvement 892.2
  complicated 892.1
high-velocity (grease gun) — *see* Wound, open, complicated, by site
hip 890.0
  with tendon involvement 890.2
  complicated 890.1
hymen 878.6
  complicated 878.7
hypochondrium 879.4
  complicated 879.5
hypogastric region 879.2
  complicated 879.3
iliac (region) 879.4
  complicated 879.5
incidental to
  dislocation — *see* Dislocation, open, by site
  fracture — *see* Fracture, open, by site
  intracranial injury — *see* Injury, intracranial, with open intracranial wound
  nerve injury — *see* Injury, nerve, by site
inguinal region 879.4
  complicated 879.5
instep 892.0
  with tendon involvement 892.2
  complicated 892.1
interscapular region 876.0
  complicated 876.1
intracranial — *see* Injury, intracranial, with open intracranial wound

Wound, open — *continued*

intraocular 871.9
  with
    partial loss (of intraocular tissue) 871.2
    prolapse or exposure (of intraocular tissue) 871.1
  aceration (*see also* Laceration, eyeball) 871.4
  penetrating 871.7
    with foreign body (nonmagnetic) 871.6
      magnetic 871.5
  without prolapse (of intraocular tissue) 871.0
iris (*see also* Wound, open, eyeball) 871.9
jaw (fracture not involved) 873.44
  with fracture — *see* Fracture, jaw
  complicated 873.54
knee 891.0
  with tendon involvement 891.2
  complicated 891.1
labium (majus) (minus) 878.4
  complicated 878.5
lacrimal apparatus, gland, or sac 870.8
  with laceration of eyelid 870.2
larynx 874.01
  with trachea 874.00
    complicated 874.10
  complicated 874.11
leg (multiple) 891.0
  with tendon involvement 891.2
  complicated 891.1
  lower 891.0
    with tendon involvement 891.2
    complicated 891.1
  thigh 890.0
    with tendon involvement 890.2
    complicated 890.1
  upper 890.0
    with tendon involvement 890.2
    complicated 890.1
lens (eye) (alone) (*see also* Cataract, traumatic) 366.20
  with involvement of other eye structures — *see* Wound, open, eyeball
limb
  lower (multiple) NEC 894.0
    with tendon involvement 894.2
    complicated 894.1
  upper (multiple) NEC 884.0
    with tendon involvement 884.2
    complicated 884.1
lip 873.43
  complicated 873.53
loin 876.0
  complicated 876.1
lumbar region 876.0
  complicated 876.1
malar region 873.41
  complicated 873.51
mastoid region 873.49
  complicated 873.59
mediastinum — *see* Injury, internal, mediastinum
midthoracic region 875.0
  complicated 875.1
mouth 873.60
  complicated 873.70
  floor 873.64
    complicated 873.74
  multiple sites 873.69
    complicated 873.79
  specified site NEC 873.69
    complicated 873.79
multiple, unspecified site(s) 879.8

> Note — Multiple open wounds of sites classifiable to the same four-digit category should be classified to that category unless they are in different limbs.
>
> Multiple open wounds of sites classifiable to different four-digit categories, or to different limbs, should be coded separately.

  complicated 879.9
  lower limb(s) (one or both) (sites classifiable to more than one three-digit category in 890 to 893) 894.0

Wound, open — *continued*
  multiple, unspecified site(s) — *continued*
    lower limb(s) — *continued*
      with tendon involvement 894.2
      complicated 894.1
    upper limb(s) (one or both) (sites classifiable to more than one three-digit category in 880 to 883) 884.0
      with tendon involvement 884.2
      complicated 884.1
  muscle — *see* Sprain, by site
  nail
    finger(s) 883.0
      complicated 883.1
    thumb 883.0
      complicated 883.1
    toe(s) 893.0
      complicated 893.1
  nape (neck) 874.8
    complicated 874.9
    specified part NEC 874.8
      complicated 874.9
  nasal — *see also* Wound, open, nose
    cavity 873.22
      complicated 873.32
    septum 873.21
      complicated 873.31
    sinuses 873.23
      complicated 873.33
  nasopharynx 873.22
    complicated 873.32
  neck 874.8
    complicated 874.9
    nape 874.8
      complicated 874.9
    specified part NEC 874.8
      complicated 874.9
  nerve — *see* Injury, nerve, by site
  non-healing surgical 998.83
  nose 873.20
    complicated 873.30
    multiple sites 873.29
      complicated 873.39
    septum 873.21
      complicated 873.31
    sinuses 873.23
      complicated 873.33
  occipital region — *see* Wound, open, scalp
  ocular NEC 871.9
    adnexa 870.9
      specified region NEC 870.8
    laceration (*see also* Laceration, ocular) 871.4
    muscle (extraocular) 870.3
      with foreign body 870.4
      eyelid 870.1
      intraocular — *see* Wound, open, eyeball
    penetrating (*see also* Penetrating wound, ocular) 871.7
  orbit 870.8
    penetrating 870.3
      with foreign body 870.4
  orbital region 870.9
  ovary — *see* Injury, internal, pelvic organs
  palate 873.65
    complicated 873.75
  palm 882.0
    with tendon involvement 882.2
    complicated 882.1
  parathyroid (gland) 874.2
    complicated 874.3
  parietal region — *see* Wound, open, scalp
  pelvic floor or region 879.6
    complicated 879.7
  penis 878.0
    complicated 878.1
  perineum 879.6
    complicated 879.7
  periocular area 870.8
    laceration of skin 870.0
  pharynx 874.4
    complicated 874.5
  pinna 872.01
    complicated 872.11
  popliteal space 891.0
    with tendon involvement 891.2
    complicated 891.1

Wound, open — *continued*
  prepuce 878.0
    complicated 878.1
  pubic region 879.2
    complicated 879.3
  pudenda 878.8
    complicated 878.9
  rectovaginal septum 878.8
    complicated 878.9
  sacral region 877.0
    complicated 877.1
  sacroiliac region 877.0
    complicated 877.1
  salivary (ducts) (glands) 873.69
    complicated 873.79
  scalp 873.0
    complicated 873.1
  scalpel, fetus or newborn 767.8
  scapular region 880.01
    with tendon involvement 880.21
    complicated 880.11
    involving other sites of upper arm 880.09
      with tendon involvement 880.29
      complicated 880.19
  sclera — (*see also* Wound, open, intraocular) 871.9
  scrotum 878.2
    complicated 878.3
  seminal vesicle — *see* Injury, internal, pelvic organs
  shin 891.0
    with tendon involvement 891.2
    complicated 891.1
  shoulder 880.00
    with tendon involvement 880.20
    complicated 880.10
    involving other sites of upper arm 880.09
      with tendon involvement 880.29
      complicated 880.19
  skin NEC 879.8
    complicated 879.9
  skull — *see also* Injury, intracranial, with open intracranial wound
    with skull fracture — *see* Fracture, skull
  spermatic cord (scrotal) 878.2
    complicated 878.3
    pelvic region — *see* Injury, internal, spermatic cord
  spinal cord — *see* Injury, spinal
  sternal region 875.0
    complicated 875.1
  subconjunctival — *see* Wound, open, intraocular
  subcutaneous NEC 879.8
    complicated 879.9
  submaxillary region 873.44
    complicated 873.54
  submental region 873.44
    complicated 873.54
  subungual
    finger(s) (thumb) — *see* Wound, open, finger
    toe(s) — *see* Wound, open, toe
  supraclavicular region 874.8
    complicated 874.9
  supraorbital 873.42
    complicated 873.52
  surgical, non-healing 998.83
  temple 873.49
    complicated 873.59
  temporal region 873.49
    complicated 873.59
  testis 878.2
    complicated 878.3
  thigh 890.0
    with tendon involvement 890.2
    complicated 890.1
  thorax, thoracic (external) 875.0
    complicated 875.1
  throat 874.8
    complicated 874.9
  thumb (nail) (subungual) 883.0
    with tendon involvement 883.2
    complicated 883.1
  thyroid (gland) 874.2
    complicated 874.3

Wound, open — *continued*
  toe(s) (nail) (subungual) 893.0
    with tendon involvement 893.2
    complicated 893.1
  tongue 873.64
    complicated 873.74
  tonsil — *see* Wound, open, neck
  trachea (cervical region) 874.02
    with larynx 874.00
      complicated 874.10
    complicated 874.12
    intrathoracic — *see* Injury, internal, trachea
  trunk (multiple) NEC 879.6
    complicated 879.7
    specified site NEC 879.6
      complicated 879.7
  tunica vaginalis 878.2
    complicated 878.3
  tympanic membrane 872.61
    complicated 872.71
  tympanum 872.61
    complicated 872.71
  umbilical region 879.2
    complicated 879.3
  ureter — *see* Injury, internal, ureter
  urethra — *see* Injury, internal, urethra
  uterus — *see* Injury, internal, uterus
  uvula 873.69
    complicated 873.79
  vagina 878.6
    complicated 878.7
  vas deferens — *see* Injury, internal, vas deferens
  vitreous (humor) 871.2
  vulva 878.4
    complicated 878.5
  wrist 881.02
    with tendon involvement 881.22
    complicated 881.12
Wright's syndrome (hyperabduction) 447.8
  pneumonia 390 [517.1]
Wringer injury — *see* Crush injury, by site
Wrinkling of skin 701.8
Wrist — *see also* condition
  drop (acquired) 736.05
Wrong drug (given in error) NEC 977.9
  specified drug or substance — *see* Table of Drugs and Chemicals
Wry neck — *see also* Torticollis
  congenital 754.1
Wuchereria infestation 125.0
  bancrofti 125.0
  Brugia malayi 125.1
  malayi 125.1
Wuchereriasis 125.0
Wuchereriosis 125.0
Wuchernde struma langhans (M8332/3) 193

X

Xanthelasma 272.2
  eyelid 272.2 [374.51]
  palpebrarum 272.2 [374.51]
Xanthelasmatosis (essential) 272.2
Xanthelasmoidea 757.33
Xanthine stones 277.2
Xanthinuria 277.2
Xanthofibroma (M8831/0) — *see* Neoplasm, connective tissue, benign
Xanthoma(s), xanthomatosis 272.2
  with
    hyperlipoproteinemia
      type I 272.3
      type III 272.2
      type IV 272.1
      type V 272.3
  bone 272.7
  craniohypophyseal 277.89
  cutaneotendinous 272.7
  diabeticorum 250.8 ☑ [272.2]
  disseminatum 272.7
  eruptive 272.2

Xanthoma(s), xanthomatosis — *continued*
eyelid 272.2 *[374.51]*
familial 272.7
hereditary 272.7
hypercholesterinemic 272.0
hypercholesterolemic 272.0
hyperlipemic 272.4
hyperlipidemic 272.4
infantile 272.7
joint 272.7
juvenile 272.7
multiple 272.7
multiplex 272.7
primary familial 272.7
tendon (sheath) 272.7
tuberosum 272.2
tuberous 272.2
tubo-eruptive 272.2
Xanthosis 709.09
surgical 998.81
Xenophobia 300.29
Xeroderma (congenital) 757.39
acquired 701.1
eyelid 373.33
eyelid 373.33
pigmentosum 757.33
vitamin A deficiency 264.8
Xerophthalmia 372.53
vitamin A deficiency 264.7
Xerosis
conjunctiva 372.53
with Bitôt's spot 372.53
vitamin A deficiency 264.1
vitamin A deficiency 264.0
cornea 371.40
with corneal ulceration 370.00
vitamin A deficiency 264.3
vitamin A deficiency 264.2
cutis 706.8
skin 706.8
Xerostomia 527.7
Xiphodynia 733.90
Xiphoidalgia 733.90
Xiphoiditis 733.99
Xiphopagus 759.4
XO syndrome 758.6

X-ray
effects, adverse, NEC 990
of chest
for suspected tuberculosis V71.2
routine V72.5
XXX syndrome 758.81
XXXXY syndrome 758.81
XXY syndrome 758.7
Xyloketosuria 271.8
Xylosuria 271.8
Xylulosuria 271.8
XYY syndrome 758.81

Y

Yawning 786.09
psychogenic 306.1
Yaws 102.9
bone or joint lesions 102.6
butter 102.1
chancre 102.0
cutaneous, less than five years after infection
102.2
early (cutaneous) (macular) (maculopapular)
(micropapular) (papular) 102.2
frambeside 102.2
skin lesions NEC 102.2
eyelid 102.9 *[373.4]*
ganglion 102.6
gangosis, gangosa 102.5
gumma, gummata 102.4
bone 102.6
gummatous
frambeside 102.4
osteitis 102.6
periostitis 102.6
hydrarthrosis 102.6
hyperkeratosis (early) (late) (palmar) (plantar)
102.3
initial lesions 102.0
joint lesions 102.6
juxta-articular nodules 102.7
late nodular (ulcerated) 102.4
latent (without clinical manifestations) (with
positive serology) 102.8
mother 102.0

Yaws — *continued*
mucosal 102.7
multiple papillomata 102.1
nodular, late (ulcerated) 102.4
osteitis 102.6
papilloma, papillomata (palmar) (plantar) 102.1
periostitis (hypertrophic) 102.6
ulcers 102.4
wet crab 102.1
Yeast infection (*see also* Candidiasis) 112.9
Yellow
atrophy (liver) 570
chronic 571.8
resulting from administration of blood,
plasma, serum, or other biological
substance (within 8 months of
administration) — *see* Hepatitis, viral
fever — *see* Fever, yellow
jack (*see also* Fever, yellow) 060.9
jaundice (*see also* Jaundice) 782.4
Yersinia septica 027.8

Z

Zagari's disease (xerostomia) 527.7
Zahorsky's disease (exanthema subitum) 057.8
syndrome (herpangina) 074.0
Zellweger syndrome 277.86 ●
Zenker's diverticulum (esophagus) 530.6
Ziehen-Oppenheim disease 333.6
Zieve's syndrome (jaundice, hyperlipemia, and
hemolytic anemia) 571.1
Zika fever 066.3
Zollinger-Ellison syndrome (gastric
hypersecretion with pancreatic islet cell
tumor) 251.5
Zona (*see also* Herpes, zoster) 053.9
Zoophilia (erotica) 302.1
Zoophobia 300.29
Zoster (herpes) (*see also* Herpes, zoster) 053.9
Zuelzer (-Ogden) anemia or syndrome
(nutritional megaloblastic anemia) 281.2
Zygodactyly (*see also* Syndactylism) 755.10
Zygomycosis 117.7
Zymotic — *see* condition

SECTION 2

Alphabetic Index to Poisoning and External Causes of Adverse Effects of Drugs and Other Chemical Substances
TABLE OF DRUGS AND CHEMICALS

This table contains a classification of drugs and other chemical substances to identify poisoning states and external causes of adverse effects.

Each of the listed substances in the table is assigned a code according to the poisoning classification (960-989). These codes are used when there is a statement of poisoning, overdose, wrong substance given or taken, or intoxication.

The table also contains a listing of external causes of adverse effects. An adverse effect is a pathologic manifestation due to ingestion or exposure to drugs or other chemical substances (e.g., dermatitis, hypersensitivity reaction, aspirin gastritis). The adverse effect is to be identified by the appropriate code found in Section 1, Index to Diseases and Injuries. An external cause code can then be used to identify the circumstances involved. The table headings pertaining to external causes are defined below:

Accidental poisoning (E850-E869) — accidental overdose of drug, wrong substance given or taken, drug taken inadvertently, accidents in the usage of drugs and biologicals in medical and surgical procedures, and to show external causes of poisonings classifiable to 980-989.

Therapeutic use (E930-E949) — a correct substance properly administered in therapeutic or prophylactic dosage as the external cause of adverse effects.

Suicide attempt (E950-E952) — instances in which self-inflicted injuries or poisonings are involved.

Assault (E961-E962) — injury or poisoning inflicted by another person with the intent to injure or kill.

Undetermined (E980-E982) — to be used when the intent of the poisoning or injury cannot be determined whether it was intentional or accidental.

The American Hospital Formulary Service list numbers are included in the table to help classify new drugs not identified in the table by name. The AHFS list numbers are keyed to the continually revised American Hospital Formulary Service (AHFS).* These listings are found in the table under the main term **Drug.**

Excluded from the table are radium and other radioactive substances. The classification of adverse effects and complications pertaining to these substances will be found in Section 1, Index to Diseases and Injuries, and Section 3, Index to External Causes of Injuries.

Although certain substances are indexed with one or more subentries, the majority are listed according to one use or state. It is recognized that many substances may be used in various ways, in medicine and in industry, and may cause adverse effects whatever the state of the agent (solid, liquid, or fumes arising from a liquid). In cases in which the reported data indicates a use or state not in the table, or which is clearly different from the one listed, an attempt should be made to classify the substance in the form which most nearly expresses the reported facts.

*American Hospital Formulary Service, 2 vol. (Washington, D.C.: American Society of Hospital Pharmacists, 1959-)

	Poisoning	Accident	Therapeutic Use	Suicide Attempt	Assault	Undetermined
1-propanol	980.3	E860.4	—	E950.9	E962.1	E980.9
2-propanol	980.2	E860.3	—	E950.9	E962.1	E980.9
2, 4-D (dichlorophenoxyacetic acid)	989.4	E863.5	—	E950.6	E962.1	E980.7
2, 4-toluene diisocyanate	983.0	E864.0	—	E950.7	E962.1	E980.6
2, 4, 5-T (trichlorophenoxyacetic acid)	989.2	E863.5	—	E950.6	E962.1	E980.7
14-hydroxydihydromorph-inone	965.09	E850.2	E935.2	E950.0	E962.0	E980.0
ABOB	961.7	E857	E931.7	E950.4	E962.0	E980.4
Abrus (seed)	988.2	E865.3	—	E950.9	E962.1	E980.9
Absinthe	980.0	E860.1	—	E950.9	E962.1	E980.9
beverage	980.0	E860.0	—	E950.9	E962.1	E980.9
Acenocoumarin, acenocoumarol	964.2	E858.2	E934.2	E950.4	E962.0	E980.4
Acepromazine	969.1	E853.0	E939.1	E950.3	E962.0	E980.3
Acetal	982.8	E862.4	—	E950.9	E962.1	E980.9
Acetaldehyde (vapor)	987.8	E869.8	—	E952.8	E962.2	E982.8
liquid	989.89	E866.8	—	E950.9	E962.1	E980.9
Acetaminophen	965.4	E850.4	E935.4	E950.0	E962.0	E980.0
Acetaminosalol	965.1	E850.3	E935.3	E950.0	E962.0	E980.0
Acetanilid(e)	965.4	E850.4	E935.4	E950.0	E962.0	E980.0
Acetarsol, acetarsone	961.1	E857	E931.1	E950.4	E962.0	E980.4
Acetazolamide	974.2	E858.5	E944.2	E950.4	E962.0	E980.4
Acetic						
acid	983.1	E864.1	—	E950.7	E962.1	E980.6
with sodium acetate (ointment)	976.3	E858.7	E946.3	E950.4	E962.0	E980.4
irrigating solution	974.5	E858.5	E944.5	E950.4	E962.0	E980.4
lotion	976.2	E858.7	E946.2	E950.4	E962.0	E980.4
anhydride	983.1	E864.1	—	E950.7	E962.1	E980.6
ether (vapor)	982.8	E862.4	—	E950.9	E962.1	E980.9
Acetohexamide	962.3	E858.0	E932.3	E950.4	E962.0	E980.4
Acetomenaphthone	964.3	E858.2	E934.3	E950.4	E962.0	E980.4
Acetomorphine	965.01	E850.0	E935.0	E950.0	E962.0	E980.0
Acetone (oils) (vapor)	982.8	E862.4	—	E950.9	E962.1	E980.9
Acetophenazine (maleate)	969.1	E853.0	E939.1	E950.3	E962.0	E980.3
Acetophenetidin	965.4	E850.4	E935.4	E950.0	E962.0	E980.0
Acetophenone	982.0	E862.4	—	E950.9	E962.1	E980.9

	Poisoning	Accident	Therapeutic Use	Suicide Attempt	Assault	Undetermined
Acetorphine	965.09	E850.2	E935.2	E950.0	E962.0	E980.0
Acetosulfone (sodium)	961.8	E857	E931.8	E950.4	E962.0	E980.4
Acetrizoate (sodium)	977.8	E858.8	E947.8	E950.4	E962.0	E980.4
Acetylcarbromal	967.3	E852.2	E937.3	E950.2	E962.0	E980.2
Acetylcholine (chloride)	971.0	E855.3	E941.0	E950.4	E962.0	E980.4
Acetylcysteine	975.5	E858.6	E945.5	E950.4	E962.0	E980.4
Acetyldigitoxin	972.1	E858.3	E942.1	E950.4	E962.0	E980.4
Acetyldihydrocodeine	965.09	E850.2	E935.2	E950.0	E962.0	E980.0
Acetyldihydrocodeinone	965.09	E850.2	E935.2	E950.0	E962.0	E980.0
Acetylene (gas) (industrial)	987.1	E868.1	—	E951.8	E962.2	E981.8
incomplete combustion of — see Carbon monoxide, fuel, utility						
tetrachloride (vapor)	982.3	E862.4	—	E950.9	E962.1	E980.9
Acetyliodosalicylic acid	965.1	E850.3	E935.3	E950.0	E962.0	E980.0
Acetylphenylhydrazine	965.8	E850.8	E935.8	E950.0	E962.0	E980.0
Acetylsalicylic acid	965.1	E850.3	E935.3	E950.0	E962.0	E980.0
Achromycin	960.4	E856	E930.4	E950.4	E962.0	E980.4
ophthalmic preparation	976.5	E858.7	E946.5	E950.4	E962.0	E980.4
topical NEC	976.0	E858.7	E946.0	E950.4	E962.0	E980.4
Acidifying agents	963.2	E858.1	E933.2	E950.4	E962.0	E980.4
Acids (corrosive) NEC	983.1	E864.1	—	E950.7	E962.1	E980.6
Aconite (wild)	988.2	E865.4	—	E950.9	E962.1	E980.9
Aconitine (liniment)	976.8	E858.7	E946.8	E950.4	E962.0	E980.4
Aconitum ferox	988.2	E865.4	—	E950.9	E962.1	E980.9
Acridine	983.0	E864.0	—	E950.7	E962.1	E980.6
vapor	987.8	E869.8	—	E952.8	E962.2	E982.8
Acriflavine	961.9	E857	E931.9	E950.4	E962.0	E980.4
Acrisorcin	976.0	E858.7	E946.0	E950.4	E962.0	E980.4
Acrolein (gas)	987.8	E869.8	—	E952.8	E962.2	E982.8
liquid	989.89	E866.8	—	E950.9	E962.1	E980.9
Actaea spicata	988.2	E865.4	—	E950.9	E962.1	E980.9
Acterol	961.5	E857	E931.5	E950.4	E962.0	E980.4
ACTH	962.4	E858.0	E932.4	E950.4	E962.0	E980.4
Acthar	962.4	E858.0	E932.4	E950.4	E962.0	E980.4
Actinomycin (C)(D)	960.7	E856	E930.7	E950.4	E962.0	E980.4
Adalin (acetyl)	967.3	E852.2	E937.3	E950.2	E962.0	E980.2
Adenosine (phosphate)	977.8	E858.8	E947.8	E950.4	E962.0	E980.4
Adhesives	989.89	E866.6	—	E950.9	E962.1	E980.9

		External Cause (E-Code)				
	Poisoning	Accident	Therapeutic Use	Suicide Attempt	Assault	Undetermined
ADH	962.5	E858.0	E932.5	E950.4	E962.0	E980.4
Adicillin	960.0	E856	E930.0	E950.4	E962.0	E980.4
Adiphenine	975.1	E855.6	E945.1	E950.4	E962.0	E980.4
Adjunct, pharmaceutical	977.4	E858.8	E947.4	E950.4	E962.0	E980.4
Adrenal (extract, cortex or medulla) (glucocorticoids) (hormones) (mineralocorticoids)	962.0	E858.0	E932.0	E950.4	E962.0	E980.4
ENT agent	976.6	E858.7	E946.6	E950.4	E962.0	E980.4
ophthalmic preparation	976.5	E858.7	E946.5	E950.4	E962.0	E980.4
topical NEC	976.0	E858.7	E946.0	E950.4	E962.0	E980.4
Adrenalin	971.2	E855.5	E941.2	E950.4	E962.0	E980.4
Adrenergic blocking agents	971.3	E855.6	E941.3	E950.4	E962.0	E980.4
Adrenergics	971.2	E855.5	E941.2	E950.4	E962.0	E980.4
Adrenochrome (derivatives)	972.8	E858.3	E942.8	E950.4	E962.0	E980.4
Adrenocorticotropic hormone	962.4	E858.0	E932.4	E950.4	E962.0	E980.4
Adrenocorticotropin	962.4	E858.0	E932.4	E950.4	E962.0	E980.4
Adriamycin	960.7	E856	E930.7	E950.4	E962.0	E980.4
Aerosol spray — *see* Sprays						
Aerosporin	960.8	E856	E930.8	E950.4	E962.0	E980.4
ENT agent	976.6	E858.7	E946.6	E950.4	E962.0	E980.4
ophthalmic preparation	976.5	E858.7	E946.5	E950.4	E962.0	E980.4
topical NEC	976.0	E858.7	E946.0	E950.4	E962.0	E980.4
Aethusa cynapium	988.2	E865.4	—	E950.9	E962.1	E980.9
Afghanistan black	969.6	E854.1	E939.6	E950.3	E962.0	E980.3
Aflatoxin	989.7	E865.9	—	E950.9	E962.1	E980.9
African boxwood	988.2	E865.4	—	E950.9	E962.1	E980.9
Agar (-agar)	973.3	E858.4	E943.3	E950.4	E962.0	E980.4
Agricultural agent NEC	989.89	E863.9	—	E950.6	E962.1	E980.7
Agrypnal	967.0	E851	E937.0	E950.1	E962.0	E980.1
Air contaminant(s), source or type not specified	987.9	E869.9	—	E952.9	E962.2	E982.9
specified type — *see* specific substance						
Akee	988.2	E865.4	—	E950.9	E962.1	E980.9
Akrinol	976.0	E858.7	E946.0	E950.4	E962.0	E980.4
Alantolactone	961.6	E857	E931.6	E950.4	E962.0	E980.4
Albamycin	960.8	E856	E930.8	E950.4	E962.0	E980.4
Albumin (normal human serum)	964.7	E858.2	E934.7	E950.4	E962.0	E980.4
Albuterol	975.7	E858.6	E945.7	E950.4	E962.0	E980.4
Alcohol	980.9	E860.9	—	E950.9	E962.1	E980.9
absolute	980.0	E860.1	—	E950.9	E962.1	E980.9
beverage	980.0	E860.0	E947.8	E950.9	E962.1	E980.9
amyl	980.3	E860.4	—	E950.9	E962.1	E980.9
antifreeze	980.1	E860.2	—	E950.9	E962.1	E980.9
butyl	980.3	E860.4	—	E950.9	E962.1	E980.9
dehydrated	980.0	E860.1	—	E950.9	E962.1	E980.9
beverage	980.0	E860.0	E947.8	E950.9	E962.1	E980.9
denatured	980.0	E860.1	—	E950.9	E962.1	E980.9
deterrents	977.3	E858.8	E947.3	E950.4	E962.0	E980.4
diagnostic (gastric function)	977.8	E858.8	E947.8	E950.4	E962.0	E980.4
ethyl	980.0	E860.1	—	E950.9	E962.1	E980.9
beverage	980.0	E860.0	E947.8	E950.9	E962.1	E980.9
grain	980.0	E860.1	—	E950.9	E962.1	E980.9
beverage	980.0	E860.0	E947.8	E950.9	E962.1	E980.9
industrial	980.9	E860.9	—	E950.9	E962.1	E980.9
isopropyl	980.2	E860.3	—	E950.9	E962.1	E980.9
methyl	980.1	E860.2	—	E950.9	E962.1	E980.9
preparation for consumption	980.0	E860.0	E947.8	E950.9	E962.1	E980.9
propyl	980.3	E860.4	—	E950.9	E962.1	E980.9
secondary	980.2	E860.3	—	E950.9	E962.1	E980.9
radiator	980.1	E860.2	—	E950.9	E962.1	E980.9
rubbing	980.2	E860.3	—	E950.9	E962.1	E980.9
specified type NEC	980.8	E860.8	—	E950.9	E962.1	E980.9
surgical	980.9	E860.9	—	E950.9	E962.1	E980.9
vapor (from any type of alcohol)	987.8	E869.8	—	E952.8	E962.2	E982.8
wood	980.1	E860.2	—	E950.9	E962.1	E980.9
Alcuronium chloride	975.2	E858.6	E945.2	E950.4	E962.0	E980.4
Aldactone	974.4	E858.5	E944.4	E950.4	E962.0	E980.4
Aldicarb	989.3	E863.2	—	E950.6	E962.1	E980.7
Aldomet	972.6	E858.3	E942.6	E950.4	E962.0	E980.4
Aldosterone	962.0	E858.0	E932.0	E950.4	E962.0	E980.4
Aldrin (dust)	989.2	E863.0	—	E950.6	E962.1	E980.7
Algeldrate	973.0	E858.4	E943.0	E950.4	E962.0	E980.4
Alidase	963.4	E858.1	E933.4	E950.4	E962.0	E980.4
Aliphatic thiocyanates	989.0	E866.8	—	E950.9	E962.1	E980.9
Alkaline antiseptic solution (aromatic)	976.6	E858.7	E946.6	E950.4	E962.0	E980.4
Alkalinizing agents (medicinal)	963.3	E858.1	E933.3	E950.4	E962.0	E980.4
Alkalis, caustic	983.2	E864.2	—	E950.7	E962.1	E980.6
Alkalizing agents (medicinal)	963.3	E858.1	E933.3	E950.4	E962.0	E980.4
Alka-seltzer	965.1	E850.3	E935.3	E950.0	E962.0	E980.0
Alkavervir	972.6	E858.3	E942.6	E950.4	E962.0	E980.4
Allegron	969.0	E854.0	E939.0	E950.3	E962.0	E980.3
Alleve — Naproxen						
Allobarbital, allobarbitone	967.0	E851	E937.0	E950.1	E962.0	E980.1
Allopurinol	974.7	E858.5	E944.7	E950.4	E962.0	E980.4
Allylestrenol	962.2	E858.0	E932.2	E950.4	E962.0	E980.4
Allylisopropylacetylurea	967.8	E852.8	E937.8	E950.2	E962.0	E980.2
Allylisopropylmalonylurea	967.0	E851	E937.0	E950.1	E962.0	E980.1
Allyltribromide	967.3	E852.2	E937.3	E950.2	E962.0	E980.2
Aloe, aloes, aloin	973.1	E858.4	E943.1	E950.4	E962.0	E980.4
Alosetron	973.8	E858.4	E943.8	E950.4	E962.0	E980.4
Aloxidone	966.0	E855.0	E936.0	E950.4	E962.0	E980.4
Aloxiprin	965.1	E850.3	E935.3	E950.0	E962.0	E980.0
Alpha amylase	963.4	E858.1	E933.4	E950.4	E962.0	E980.4
Alphaprodine (hydrochloride)	965.09	E850.2	E935.2	E950.0	E962.0	E980.0
Alpha tocopherol	963.5	E858.1	E933.5	E950.4	E962.0	E980.4
Alseroxylon	972.6	E858.3	E942.6	E950.4	E962.0	E980.4
Alum (ammonium) (potassium)	983.2	E864.2	—	E950.7	E962.1	E980.6
medicinal (astringent) NEC	976.2	E858.7	E946.2	E950.4	E962.0	E980.4
Aluminium, aluminum (gel) (hydroxide)	973.0	E858.4	E943.0	E950.4	E962.0	E980.4
acetate solution	976.2	E858.7	E946.2	E950.4	E962.0	E980.4
aspirin	965.1	E850.3	E935.3	E950.0	E962.0	E980.0
carbonate	973.0	E858.4	E943.0	E950.4	E962.0	E980.4
glycinate	973.0	E858.4	E943.0	E950.4	E962.0	E980.4
nicotinate	972.2	E858.3	E942.2	E950.4	E962.0	E980.4
ointment (surgical) (topical)	976.3	E858.7	E946.3	E950.4	E962.0	E980.4
phosphate	973.0	E858.4	E943.0	E950.4	E962.0	E980.4
subacetate	976.2	E858.7	E946.2	E950.4	E962.0	E980.4
topical NEC	976.3	E858.7	E946.3	E950.4	E962.0	E980.4
Alurate	967.0	E851	E937.0	E950.1	E962.0	E980.1
Alverine (citrate)	975.1	E858.6	E945.1	E950.4	E962.0	E980.4
Alvodine	965.09	E850.2	E935.2	E950.0	E962.0	E980.0
Amanita phalloides	988.1	E865.5	—	E950.9	E962.1	E980.9
Amantadine (hydrochloride)	966.4	E855.0	E936.4	E950.4	E962.0	E980.4
Ambazone	961.9	E857	E931.9	E950.4	E962.0	E980.4
Ambenonium	971.0	E855.3	E941.0	E950.4	E962.0	E980.4
Ambutonium bromide	971.1	E855.4	E941.1	E950.4	E962.0	E980.4
Ametazole	977.8	E858.8	E947.8	E950.4	E962.0	E980.4
Amethocaine (infiltration) (topical)	968.5	E855.2	E938.5	E950.4	E962.0	E980.4
nerve block (peripheral) (plexus)	968.6	E855.2	E938.6	E950.4	E962.0	E980.4
spinal	968.7	E855.2	E938.7	E950.4	E962.0	E980.4
Amethopterin	963.1	E858.1	E933.1	E950.4	E962.0	E980.4
Amfepramone	977.0	E858.8	E947.0	E950.4	E962.0	E980.4
Amidon	965.02	E850.1	E935.1	E950.0	E962.0	E980.0
Amidopyrine	965.5	E850.5	E935.5	E950.0	E962.0	E980.0
Aminacrine	976.0	E858.7	E946.0	E950.4	E962.0	E980.4
Aminitrozole	961.5	E857	E931.5	E950.4	E962.0	E980.4
Aminoacetic acid	974.5	E858.5	E944.5	E950.4	E962.0	E980.4
Amino acids	974.5	E858.5	E944.5	E950.4	E962.0	E980.4
Aminocaproic acid	964.4	E858.2	E934.4	E950.4	E962.0	E980.4
Aminoethylisothiourium	963.8	E858.1	E933.8	E950.4	E962.0	E980.4
Aminoglutethimide	966.3	E855.0	E936.3	E950.4	E962.0	E980.4
Aminometradine	974.3	E858.5	E944.3	E950.4	E962.0	E980.4
Aminopentamide	971.1	E855.4	E941.1	E950.4	E962.0	E980.4
Aminophenazone	965.5	E850.5	E935.5	E950.0	E962.0	E980.0
Aminophenol	983.0	E864.0	—	E950.7	E962.1	E980.6
Aminophenylpyridone	969.5	E853.8	E939.5	E950.3	E962.0	E980.3
Aminophyllin	975.7	E858.6	E945.7	E950.4	E962.0	E980.4
Aminopterin	963.1	E858.1	E933.1	E950.4	E962.0	E980.4
Aminopyrine	965.5	E850.5	E935.5	E950.0	E962.0	E980.0
Aminosalicylic acid	961.8	E857	E931.8	E950.4	E962.0	E980.4
Amiphenazole	970.1	E854.3	E940.1	E950.4	E962.0	E980.4
Amiquinsin	972.6	E858.3	E942.6	E950.4	E962.0	E980.4
Amisometradine	974.3	E858.5	E944.3	E950.4	E962.0	E980.4
Amitriptyline	969.0	E854.0	E939.0	E950.3	E962.0	E980.3
Ammonia (fumes) (gas) (vapor)	987.8	E869.8	—	E952.8	E962.2	E982.8
liquid (household) NEC	983.2	E861.4	—	E950.7	E962.1	E980.6
spirit, aromatic	970.8	E854.3	E940.8	E950.4	E962.0	E980.4

☑ Additional Digit Required   ▶◀ Revised Text   ● New Line   ▲ Revised Code

	Poisoning	External Cause (E-Code)				
		Accident	Therapeutic Use	Suicide Attempt	Assault	Undetermined
Ammoniated mercury	976.0	E858.7	E946.0	E950.4	E962.0	E980.4
Ammonium						
carbonate	983.2	E864.2	—	E950.7	E962.1	E980.6
chloride (acidifying agent)	963.2	E858.1	E933.2	E950.4	E962.0	E980.4
expectorant	975.5	E858.6	E945.5	E950.4	E962.0	E980.4
compounds (household)						
NEC	983.2	E861.4	—	E950.7	E962.1	E980.6
fumes (any usage)	987.8	E869.8	—	E952.8	E962.2	E982.8
industrial	983.2	E864.2	—	E950.7	E962.1	E980.6
ichthyosulfonate	976.4	E858.7	E946.4	E950.4	E962.0	E980.4
mandelate	961.9	E857	E931.9	E950.4	E962.0	E980.4
Amobarbital	967.0	E851	E937.0	E950.1	E962.0	E980.1
Amodiaquin(e)	961.4	E857	E931.4	E950.4	E962.0	E980.4
Amopyroquin(e)	961.4	E857	E931.4	E950.4	E962.0	E980.4
Amphenidone	969.5	E853.8	E939.5	E950.3	E962.0	E980.3
Amphetamine	969.7	E854.2	E939.7	E950.3	E962.0	E980.3
Amphomycin	960.8	E856	E930.8	E950.4	E962.0	E980.4
Amphotericin B	960.1	E856	E930.1	E950.4	E962.0	E980.4
topical	976.0	E858.7	E946.0	E950.4	E962.0	E980.4
Ampicillin	960.0	E856	E930.0	E950.4	E962.0	E980.4
Amprotropine	971.1	E855.4	E941.1	E950.4	E962.0	E980.4
Amygdalin	977.8	E858.8	E947.8	E950.4	E962.0	E980.4
Amyl						
acetate (vapor)	982.8	E862.4	—	E950.9	E962.1	E980.9
alcohol	980.3	E860.4	—	E950.9	E962.1	E980.9
nitrite (medicinal)	972.4	E858.3	E942.4	E950.4	E962.0	E980.4
Amylase (alpha)	963.4	E858.1	E933.4	E950.4	E962.0	E980.4
Amylene hydrate	980.8	E860.8	—	E950.9	E962.1	E980.9
Amylobarbitone	967.0	E851	E937.0	E950.1	E962.0	E980.1
Amylocaine	968.9	E855.2	E938.9	E950.4	E962.0	E980.4
infiltration (subcutaneous)	968.5	E855.2	E938.5	E950.4	E962.0	E980.4
nerve block (peripheral)						
(plexus)	968.6	E855.2	E938.6	E950.4	E962.0	E980.4
spinal	968.7	E855.2	E938.7	E950.4	E962.0	E980.4
topical (surface)	968.5	E855.2	E938.5	E950.4	E962.0	E980.4
Amytal (sodium)	967.0	E851	E937.0	E950.1	E962.0	E980.1
Analeptics	970.0	E854.3	E940.0	E950.4	E962.0	E980.4
Analgesics	965.9	E850.9	E935.9	E950.0	E962.0	E980.0
aromatic NEC	965.4	E850.4	E935.4	E950.0	E962.0	E980.0
non-narcotic NEC	965.7	E850.7	E935.7	E950.0	E962.0	E980.0
specified NEC	965.8	E850.8	E935.8	E950.0	E962.0	E980.0
Anamirta cocculus	988.2	E865.3	—	E950.9	E962.1	E980.9
Ancillin	960.0	E856	E930.0	E950.4	E962.0	E980.4
Androgens (anabolic congeners)	962.1	E858.0	E932.1	E950.4	E962.0	E980.4
Androstalone	962.1	E858.0	E932.1	E950.4	E962.0	E980.4
Androsterone	962.1	E858.0	E932.1	E950.4	E962.0	E980.4
Anemone pulsatilla	988.2	E865.4	—	E950.9	E962.1	E980.9
Anesthesia, anesthetic						
(general) NEC	968.4	E855.1	E938.4	E950.4	E962.0	E980.4
block (nerve) (plexus)	968.6	E855.2	E938.6	E950.4	E962.0	E980.4
gaseous NEC	968.2	E855.1	E938.2	E950.4	E962.0	E980.4
halogenated hydrocarbon derivatives NEC	968.2	E855.1	E938.2	E950.4	E962.0	E980.4
infiltration (intradermal) (subcutaneous) (submucosal)	968.5	E855.2	E938.5	E950.4	E962.0	E980.4
intravenous	968.3	E855.1	E938.3	E950.4	E962.0	E980.4
local NEC	968.9	E855.2	E938.9	E950.4	E962.0	E980.4
nerve blocking (peripheral) (plexus)	968.6	E855.2	E938.6	E950.4	E962.0	E980.4
rectal NEC	968.3	E855.1	E938.3	E950.4	E962.0	E980.4
spinal	968.7	E855.2	E938.7	E950.4	E962.0	E980.4
surface	968.5	E855.2	E938.5	E950.4	E962.0	E980.4
topical	968.5	E855.2	E938.5	E950.4	E962.0	E980.4
Aneurine	963.5	E858.1	E933.5	E950.4	E962.0	E980.4
Angio-Conray	977.8	E858.8	E947.8	E950.4	E962.0	E980.4
Angiotensin	971.2	E855.5	E941.2	E950.4	E962.0	E980.4
Anhydrohydroxyprogesterone	962.2	E858.0	E932.2	E950.4	E962.0	E980.4
Anhydron	974.3	E858.5	E944.3	E950.4	E962.0	E980.4
Anileridine	965.09	E850.2	E935.2	E950.0	E962.0	E980.0
Aniline (dye) (liquid)	983.0	E864.0	—	E950.7	E962.1	E980.6
analgesic	965.4	E850.4	E935.4	E950.0	E962.0	E980.0
derivatives, therapeutic NEC	965.4	E850.4	E935.4	E950.0	E962.0	E980.0
vapor	987.8	E869.8	—	E952.8	E962.2	E982.8
Anisindione	964.2	E858.2	E934.2	E950.4	E962.0	E980.4
Aniscoropine	971.1	E855.4	E941.1	E950.4	E962.0	E980.4
Anorexic agents	977.0	E858.8	E947.0	E950.4	E962.0	E980.4
Ant (bite) (sting)	989.5	E905.5	—	E950.9	E962.1	E980.9

	Poisoning	External Cause (E-Code)				
		Accident	Therapeutic Use	Suicide Attempt	Assault	Undetermined
Antabuse	977.3	E858.8	E947.3	E950.4	E962.0	E980.4
Antacids	973.0	E858.4	E943.0	E950.4	E962.0	E980.4
Antazoline	963.0	E858.1	E933.0	E950.4	E962.0	E980.4
Anthelmintics	961.6	E857	E931.6	E950.4	E962.0	E980.4
Anthralin	976.4	E858.7	E946.4	E950.4	E962.0	E980.4
Anthramycin	960.7	E856	E930.7	E950.4	E962.0	E980.4
Antiadrenergics	971.3	E855.6	E941.3	E950.4	E962.0	E980.4
Antiallergic agents	963.0	E858.1	E933.0	E950.4	E962.0	E980.4
Antianemic agents NEC	964.1	E858.2	E934.1	E950.4	E962.0	E980.4
Antiaris toxicaria	988.2	E865.4	—	E950.9	E962.1	E980.9
Antiarteriosclerotic agents	972.2	E858.3	E942.2	E950.4	E962.0	E980.4
Antiasthmatics	975.7	E858.6	E945.7	E950.4	E962.0	E980.4
Antibiotics	960.9	E856	E930.9	E950.4	E962.0	E980.4
antifungal	960.1	E856	E930.1	E950.4	E962.0	E980.4
antimycobacterial	960.6	E856	E930.6	E950.4	E962.0	E980.4
antineoplastic	960.7	E856	E930.7	E950.4	E962.0	E980.4
cephalosporin (group)	960.5	E856	E930.5	E950.4	E962.0	E980.4
chloramphenicol (group)	960.2	E856	E930.2	E950.4	E962.0	E980.4
macrolides	960.3	E856	E930.3	E950.4	E962.0	E980.4
specified NEC	960.8	E856	E930.8	E950.4	E962.0	E980.4
tetracycline (group)	960.4	E856	E930.4	E950.4	E962.0	E980.4
Anticancer agents NEC	963.1	E858.1	E933.1	E950.4	E962.0	E980.4
antibiotics	960.7	E856	E930.7	E950.4	E962.0	E980.4
Anticholinergics	971.1	E855.4	E941.1	E950.4	E962.0	E980.4
Anticholinesterase (organophosphorus) (reversible)	971.0	E855.3	E941.0	E950.4	E962.0	E980.4
Anticoagulants	964.2	E858.2	E934.2	E950.4	E962.0	E980.4
antagonists	964.5	E858.2	E934.5	E950.4	E962.0	E980.4
Anti-common cold agents NEC	975.6	E858.6	E945.6	E950.4	E962.0	E980.4
Anticonvulsants NEC	966.3	E855.0	E936.3	E950.4	E962.0	E980.4
Antidepressants	969.0	E854.0	E939.0	E950.3	E962.0	E980.3
Antidiabetic agents	962.3	E858.0	E932.3	E950.4	E962.0	E980.4
Antidiarrheal agents	973.5	E858.4	E943.5	E950.4	E962.0	E980.4
Antidiuretic hormone	962.5	E858.0	E932.5	E950.4	E962.0	E980.4
Antidotes NEC	977.2	E858.8	E947.2	E950.4	E962.0	E980.4
Antiemetic agents	963.0	E858.1	E933.0	E950.4	E962.0	E980.4
Antiepilepsy agent NEC	966.3	E855.0	E936.3	E950.4	E962.0	E980.4
Antifertility pills	962.2	E858.0	E932.2	E950.4	E962.0	E980.4
Antiflatulents	973.8	E858.4	E943.8	E950.4	E962.0	E980.4
Antifreeze	989.89	E866.8	—	E950.9	E962.1	E980.9
alcohol	980.1	E860.2	—	E950.9	E962.1	E980.9
ethylene glycol	982.8	E862.4	—	E950.9	E962.1	E980.9
Antifungals (nonmedicinal) (sprays)	989.4	E863.6	—	E950.6	E962.1	E980.7
medicinal NEC	961.9	E857	E931.9	E950.4	E962.0	E980.4
antibiotic	960.1	E856	E930.1	E950.4	E962.0	E980.4
topical	976.0	E858.7	E946.0	E950.4	E962.0	E980.4
Antigastric secretion agents	973.0	E858.4	E943.0	E950.4	E962.0	E980.4
Anthelmintics	961.6	E857	E931.6	E950.4	E962.0	E980.4
Antihemophilic factor (human)	964.7	E858.2	E934.7	E950.4	E962.0	E980.4
Antihistamine	963.0	E858.1	E933.0	E950.4	E962.0	E980.4
Antihypertensive agents NEC	972.6	E858.3	E942.6	E950.4	E962.0	E980.4
Anti-infectives NEC	961.9	E857	E931.9	E950.4	E962.0	E980.4
antibiotics	960.9	E856	E930.9	E950.4	E962.0	E980.4
specified NEC	960.8	E856	E930.8	E950.4	E962.0	E980.4
anthelmintic	961.6	E857	E931.6	E950.4	E962.0	E980.4
antimalarial	961.4	E857	E931.4	E950.4	E962.0	E980.4
antimycobacterial NEC	961.8	E857	E931.8	E950.4	E962.0	E980.4
antibiotics	960.6	E856	E930.6	E950.4	E962.0	E980.4
antiprotozoal NEC	961.5	E857	E931.5	E950.4	E962.0	E980.4
blood	961.4	E857	E931.4	E950.4	E962.0	E980.4
antiviral	961.7	E857	E931.7	E950.4	E962.0	E980.4
arsenical	961.1	E857	E931.1	E950.4	E962.0	E980.4
ENT agents	976.6	E858.7	E946.6	E950.4	E962.0	E980.4
heavy metals NEC	961.2	E857	E931.2	E950.4	E962.0	E980.4
local	976.0	E858.7	E946.0	E950.4	E962.0	E980.4
ophthalmic preparation	976.5	E858.7	E946.5	E950.4	E962.0	E980.4
topical NEC	976.0	E858.7	E946.0	E950.4	E962.0	E980.4
Anti-inflammatory agents (topical)	976.0	E858.7	E946.0	E950.4	E962.0	E980.4
Antiknock (tetraethyl lead)	984.1	E862.1	—	E950.9	E962.1	E980.9
Antilipemics	972.2	E858.3	E942.2	E950.4	E962.0	E980.4
Antimalarials	961.4	E857	E931.4	E950.4	E962.0	E980.4
Antimony (compounds) (vapor) NEC	985.4	E866.2	—	E950.9	E962.1	E980.9
anti-infectives	961.2	E857	E931.2	E950.4	E962.0	E980.4

☑ Additional Digit Required   ►◄ Revised Text   ● New Line   ▲ Revised Code

		External Cause (E-Code)							External Cause (E-Code)				
	Poisoning	Accident	Therapeutic Use	Suicide Attempt	Assault	Undetermined		Poisoning	Accident	Therapeutic Use	Suicide Attempt	Assault	Undetermined
Antimony — *continued*							**Atophan**	974.7	E858.5	E944.7	E950.4	E962.0	E980.4
pesticides (vapor)	985.4	E863.4	—	E950.6	E962.2	E980.7	**Atropine**	971.1	E855.4	E941.1	E950.4	E962.0	E980.4
potassium tartrate	961.2	E857	E931.2	E950.4	E962.0	E980.4	**Attapulgite**	973.5	E858.4	E943.5	E950.4	E962.0	E980.4
tartrated	961.2	E857	E931.2	E950.4	E962.0	E980.4	**Attenuvax**	979.4	E858.8	E949.4	E950.4	E962.0	E980.4
Antimuscarinic agents	971.1	E855.4	E941.1	E950.4	E962.0	E980.4	**Aureomycin**	960.4	E856	E930.4	E950.4	E962.0	E980.4
Antimycobacterials NEC	961.8	E857	E931.8	E950.4	E962.0	E980.4	ophthalmic preparation	976.5	E858.7	E946.5	E950.4	E962.0	E980.4
antibiotics	960.6	E856	E930.6	E950.4	E962.0	E980.4	topical NEC	976.0	E858.7	E946.0	E950.4	E962.0	E980.4
Antineoplastic agents	963.1	E858.1	E933.1	E950.4	E962.0	E980.4	**Aurothioglucose**	965.69	E850.6	E935.6	E950.0	E962.0	E980.0
antibiotics	960.7	E856	E930.7	E950.4	E962.0	E980.4	**Aurothioglycanide**	965.69	E850.6	E935.6	E950.0	E962.0	E980.0
Anti-Parkinsonism agents	966.4	E855.0	E936.4	E950.4	E962.0	E980.4	**Aurothiomalate**	965.69	E850.6	E935.6	E950.0	E962.0	E980.0
Antiphlogistics	965.69	E850.6	E935.6	E950.0	E962.0	E980.0	**Automobile fuel**	981	E862.1	—	E950.9	E962.1	E980.9
Antiprotozoals NEC	961.5	E857	E931.5	E950.4	E962.0	E980.4	**Autonomic nervous system**						
blood	961.4	E857	E931.4	E950.4	E962.0	E980.4	**agents NEC**	971.9	E855.9	E941.9	E950.4	E962.0	E980.4
Antipruritics (local)	976.1	E858.7	E946.1	E950.4	E962.0	E980.4	**Avlosulfon**	961.8	E857	E931.8	E950.4	E962.0	E980.4
Antipsychotic agents NEC	969.3	E853.8	E939.3	E950.3	E962.0	E980.3	**Avomine**	967.8	E852.8	E937.8	E950.2	E962.0	E980.2
Antipyretics	965.9	E850.9	E935.9	E950.0	E962.0	E980.0	**Azacyclonol**	969.5	E853.8	E939.5	E950.3	E962.0	E980.3
specified NEC	965.8	E850.8	E935.8	E950.0	E962.0	E980.0	**Azapetine**	971.3	E855.6	E941.3	E950.4	E962.0	E980.4
Antipyrine	965.5	E850.5	E935.5	E950.0	E962.0	E980.0	**Azaribine**	963.1	E858.1	E933.1	E950.4	E962.0	E980.4
Antirabies serum (equine)	979.9	E858.8	E949.9	E950.4	E962.0	E980.4	**Azaserine**	960.7	E856	E930.7	E950.4	E962.0	E980.4
Antirheumatics	965.69	E850.6	E935.6	E950.0	E962.0	E980.0	**Azathioprine**	963.1	E858.1	E933.1	E950.4	E962.0	E980.4
Antiseborrheics	976.4	E858.7	E946.4	E950.4	E962.0	E980.4	**Azosulfamide**	961.0	E857	E931.0	E950.4	E962.0	E980.4
Antiseptics (external)							**Azulfidine**	961.0	E857	E931.0	E950.4	E962.0	E980.4
(medicinal)	976.0	E858.7	E946.0	E950.4	E962.0	E980.4	**Azuresin**	977.8	E858.8	E947.8	E950.4	E962.0	E980.4
Antistine	963.0	E858.1	E933.0	E950.4	E962.0	E980.4	**Bacimycin**	976.0	E858.7	E946.0	E950.4	E962.0	E980.4
Antithyroid agents	962.8	E858.0	E932.8	E950.4	E962.0	E980.4	ophthalmic preparation	976.5	E858.7	E946.5	E950.4	E962.0	E980.4
Antitoxin, any	979.9	E858.8	E949.9	E950.4	E962.0	E980.4	**Bacitracin**	960.8	E856	E930.8	E950.4	E962.0	E980.4
Antituberculars	961.8	E857	E931.8	E950.4	E962.0	E980.4	ENT agent	976.6	E858.7	E946.6	E950.4	E962.0	E980.4
antibiotics	960.6	E856	E930.6	E950.4	E962.0	E980.4	ophthalmic preparation	976.5	E858.7	E946.5	E950.4	E962.0	E980.4
Antitussives	975.4	E858.6	E945.4	E950.4	E962.0	E980.4	topical NEC	976.0	E858.7	E946.0	E950.4	E962.0	E980.4
Antivaricose agents							**Baking soda**	963.3	E858.1	E933.3	E950.4	E962.0	E980.4
(sclerosing)	972.7	E858.3	E942.7	E950.4	E962.0	E980.4	**BAL**	963.8	E858.1	E933.8	E950.4	E962.0	E980.4
Antivenin (crotaline)							**Bamethan** (sulfate)	972.5	E858.3	E942.5	E950.4	E962.0	E980.4
(spider-bite)	979.9	E858.8	E949.9	E950.4	E962.0	E980.4	**Bamipine**	963.0	E858.1	E933.0	E950.4	E962.0	E980.4
Antivert	963.0	E858.1	E933.0	E950.4	E962.0	E980.4	**Baneberry**	988.2	E865.4	—	E950.9	E962.1	E980.9
Antivirals NEC	961.7	E857	E931.7	E950.4	E962.0	E980.4	**Banewort**	988.2	E865.4	—	E950.9	E962.1	E980.9
Ant poisons — *see* Pesticides							**Barbenyl**	967.0	E851	E937.0	E950.1	E962.0	E980.1
Antrol	989.4	E863.4	—	E950.6	E962.1	E980.7	**Barbital, barbitone**	967.0	E851	E937.0	E950.1	E962.0	E980.1
fungicide	989.4	E863.6	—	E950.6	E962.1	E980.7	**Barbiturates, barbituric**						
Apomorphine hydrochloride							**acid**	967.0	E851	E937.0	E950.1	E962.0	E980.1
(emetic)	973.6	E858.4	E943.6	E950.4	E962.0	E980.4	anesthetic (intravenous)	968.3	E855.1	E938.3	E950.4	E962.0	E980.4
Appetite depressants,							**Barium** (carbonate) (chloride)						
central	977.0	E858.8	E947.0	E950.4	E962.0	E980.4	(sulfate)	985.8	E866.4	—	E950.9	E962.1	E980.9
Apresoline	972.6	E858.3	E942.6	E950.4	E962.0	E980.4	diagnostic agent	977.8	E858.8	E947.8	E950.4	E962.0	E980.4
Aprobarbital, aprobarbitone	967.0	E851	E937.0	E950.1	E962.0	E980.1	pesticide	985.8	E863.4	—	E950.6	E962.1	E980.7
Apronalide	967.8	E852.8	E937.8	E950.2	E962.0	E980.2	rodenticide	985.8	E863.7	—	E950.6	E962.1	E980.7
Aqua fortis	983.1	E864.1	—	E950.7	E962.1	E980.6	**Barrier cream**	976.3	E858.7	E946.3	E950.4	E962.0	E980.4
Arachis oil (topical)	976.3	E858.7	E946.3	E950.4	E962.0	E980.4	**Battery acid or fluid**	983.1	E864.1	—	E950.7	E962.1	E980.6
cathartic	973.2	E858.4	E943.2	E950.4	E962.0	E980.4	**Bay rum**	980.8	E860.8	—	E950.9	E962.1	E980.9
Aralen	961.4	E857	E931.4	E950.4	E962.0	E980.4	**BCG vaccine**	978.0	E858.8	E948.0	E950.4	E962.0	E980.4
Arginine salts	974.5	E858.5	E944.5	E950.4	E962.0	E980.4	**Bearsfoot**	988.2	E865.4	—	E950.9	E962.1	E980.9
Argyrol	976.0	E858.7	E946.0	E950.4	E962.0	E980.4	**Beclamide**	966.3	E855.0	E936.3	E950.4	E962.0	E980.4
ENT agent	976.6	E858.7	E946.6	E950.4	E962.0	E980.4	**Bee** (sting) (venom)	989.5	E905.3	—	E950.9	E962.1	E980.9
ophthalmic preparation	976.5	E858.7	E946.5	E950.4	E962.0	E980.4	**Belladonna** (alkaloids)	971.1	E855.4	E941.1	E950.4	E962.0	E980.4
Aristocort	962.0	E858.0	E932.0	E950.4	E962.0	E980.4	**Bemegride**	970.0	E854.3	E940.0	E950.4	E962.0	E980.4
ENT agent	976.6	E858.7	E946.6	E950.4	E962.0	E980.4	**Benactyzine**	969.8	E855.8	E939.8	E950.3	E962.0	E980.3
ophthalmic preparation	976.5	E858.7	E946.5	E950.4	E962.0	E980.4	**Benadryl**	963.0	E858.1	E933.0	E950.4	E962.0	E980.4
topical NEC	976.0	E858.7	E946.0	E950.4	E962.0	E980.4	**Bendrofluazide**	974.3	E858.5	E944.3	E950.4	E962.0	E980.4
Aromatics, corrosive	983.0	E864.0	—	E950.7	E962.1	E980.6	**Bendroflumethiazide**	974.3	E858.5	E944.3	E950.4	E962.0	E980.4
disinfectants	983.0	E861.4	—	E950.7	E962.1	E980.6	**Benemid**	974.7	E858.5	E944.7	E950.4	E962.0	E980.4
Arsenate of lead (insecticide)	985.1	E863.4	—	E950.8	E962.1	E980.8	**Benethamine penicillin G**	960.0	E856	E930.0	E950.4	E962.0	E980.4
herbicide	985.1	E863.5	—	E950.8	E962.1	E980.8	**Benisone**	976.0	E858.7	E946.0	E950.4	E962.0	E980.4
Arsenic, arsenicals							**Benoquin**	976.8	E858.7	E946.8	E950.4	E962.0	E980.4
(compounds) (dust)							**Benoxinate**	968.5	E855.2	E938.5	E950.4	E962.0	E980.4
(fumes) (vapor) NEC	985.1	E866.3	—	E950.8	E962.1	E980.8	**Bentonite**	976.3	E858.7	E946.3	E950.4	E962.0	E980.4
anti-infectives	961.1	E857	E931.1	E950.4	E962.0	E980.4	**Benzalkonium** (chloride)	976.0	E858.7	E946.0	E950.4	E962.0	E980.4
pesticide (dust) (fumes)	985.1	E863.4	—	E950.8	E962.1	E980.8	ophthalmic preparation	976.5	E858.7	E946.5	E950.4	E962.0	E980.4
Arsine (gas)	985.1	E866.3	—	E950.8	E962.1	E980.8	**Benzamidosalicylate**						
Arsphenamine (silver)	961.1	E857	E931.1	E950.4	E962.0	E980.4	(calcium)	961.8	E857	E931.8	E950.4	E962.0	E980.4
Arsthinol	961.1	E857	E931.1	E950.4	E962.0	E980.4	**Benzathine penicillin**	960.0	E856	E930.0	E950.4	E962.0	E980.4
Artane	971.1	E855.4	E941.1	E950.4	E962.0	E980.4	**Benzcarbimine**	963.1	E858.1	E933.1	E950.4	E962.0	E980.4
Arthropod (venomous) NEC	989.5	E905.5	—	E950.9	E962.1	E980.9	**Benzedrex**	971.2	E855.5	E941.2	E950.4	E962.0	E980.4
Asbestos	989.81	E866.8	—	E950.9	E962.1	E980.9	**Benzedrine** (amphetamine)	969.7	E854.2	E939.7	E950.3	E962.0	E980.3
Ascaridole	961.6	E857	E931.6	E950.4	E962.0	E980.4	**Benzene** (acetyl) (dimethyl)						
Ascorbic acid	963.5	E858.1	E933.5	E950.4	E962.0	E980.4	(methyl) (solvent)						
Asiaticoside	976.0	E858.7	E946.0	E950.4	E962.0	E980.4	(vapor)	982.0	E862.4	—	E950.9	E962.1	E980.9
Aspidium (oleoresin)	961.6	E857	E931.6	E950.4	E962.0	E980.4	hexachloride (gamma)						
Aspirin	965.1	E850.3	E935.3	E950.0	E962.0	E980.0	(insecticide) (vapor)	989.2	E863.0	—	E950.6	E962.1	E980.7
Astringents (local)	976.2	E858.7	E946.2	E950.4	E962.0	E980.4	**Benzethonium**	976.0	E858.7	E946.0	E950.4	E962.0	E980.4
Atabrine	961.3	E857	E931.3	E950.4	E962.0	E980.4	**Benzhexol** (chloride)	966.4	E855.0	E936.4	E950.4	E962.0	E980.4
Ataractics	969.5	E853.8	E939.5	E950.3	E962.0	E980.3	**Benzilonium**	971.1	E855.4	E941.1	E950.4	E962.0	E980.4
Atonia drug, intestinal	973.3	E858.4	E943.3	E950.4	E962.0	E980.4	**Benzin(e)** — *see* Ligroin						

☑ Additional Digit Required　　　►◄ Revised Text　　　● New Line　　　▲ Revised Code

	Poisoning	External Cause (E-Code)						Poisoning	External Cause (E-Code)				
		Accident	Therapeutic Use	Suicide Attempt	Assault	Undetermined			Accident	Therapeutic Use	Suicide Attempt	Assault	Undetermined
Tessalon	975.4	E858.6	E945.4	E950.4	E962.0	E980.4	Thiouracil	962.8	E858.0	E932.8	E950.4	E962.0	E980.4
Testosterone	962.1	E858.0	E932.1	E950.4	E962.0	E980.4	Thiourea	962.8	E858.0	E932.8	E950.4	E962.0	E980.4
Tetanus (vaccine)	978.4	E858.8	E948.4	E950.4	E962.0	E980.4	Thiphenamil	971.1	E855.4	E941.1	E950.4	E962.0	E980.4
antitoxin	979.9	E858.8	E949.9	E950.4	E962.0	E980.4	Thiram NEC	989.4	E863.6	—	E950.6	E962.1	E980.7
immune globulin (human)	964.6	E858.2	E934.6	E950.4	E962.0	E980.4	medicinal	976.2	E858.7	E946.2	E950.4	E962.0	E980.4
toxoid	978.4	E858.8	E948.4	E950.4	E962.0	E980.4	Thonzylamine	963.0	E858.1	E933.0	E950.4	E962.0	E980.4
with diphtheria toxoid	978.9	E858.8	E948.9	E950.4	E962.0	E980.4	Thorazine	969.1	E853.0	E939.1	E950.3	E962.0	E980.3
with pertussis	978.6	E858.8	E948.6	E950.4	E962.0	E980.4	Thornapple	988.2	E865.4	—	E950.9	E962.1	E980.9
Tetrabenazine	969.5	E853.8	E939.5	E950.3	E962.0	E980.3	Throat preparation						
Tetracaine (infiltration)							(lozenges) NEC	976.6	E858.7	E946.6	E950.4	E962.0	E980.4
(topical)	968.5	E855.2	E938.5	E950.4	E962.0	E980.4	Thrombin	964.5	E858.2	E934.5	E950.4	E962.0	E980.4
nerve block (peripheral)							Thrombolysin	964.4	E858.2	E934.4	E950.4	E962.0	E980.4
(plexus)	968.6	E855.2	E938.6	E950.4	E962.0	E980.4	Thymol	983.0	E864.0	—	E950.7	E962.1	E980.6
spinal	968.7	E855.2	E938.7	E950.4	E962.0	E980.4	Thymus extract	962.9	E858.0	E932.9	E950.4	E962.0	E980.4
Tetrachlorethylene — see Tetrachloroethylene							Thyroglobulin	962.7	E858.0	E932.7	E950.4	E962.0	E980.4
							Thyroid (derivatives) (extract)	962.7	E858.0	E932.7	E950.4	E962.0	E980.4
Tetrachlormethiazide	974.3	E858.5	E944.3	E950.4	E962.0	E980.4	Thyrolar	962.7	E858.0	E932.7	E950.4	E962.0	E980.4
Tetrachloroethane (liquid)							Thyrothrophin, thyrotropin	977.8	E858.8	E947.8	E950.4	E962.0	E980.4
(vapor)	982.3	E862.4	—	E950.9	E962.1	E980.9	Thyroxin(e)	962.7	E858.0	E932.7	E950.4	E962.0	E980.4
paint or varnish	982.3	E861.6	—	E950.9	E962.1	E980.9	Tigan	963.0	E858.1	E933.0	E950.4	E962.0	E980.4
Tetrachloroethylene (liquid)							Tigloidine	968.0	E855.1	E938.0	E950.4	E962.0	E980.4
(vapor)	982.3	E862.4	—	E950.9	E962.1	E980.9	Tin (chloride) (dust) (oxide)						
medicinal	961.6	E857	E931.6	E950.4	E962.0	E980.4	NEC	985.8	E866.4	—	E950.9	E962.1	E980.9
Tetrachloromethane — see Carbon, tetrachloride							anti-infectives	961.2	E857	E931.2	E950.4	E962.0	E980.4
							Tinactin	976.0	E858.7	E946.0	E950.4	E962.0	E980.4
Tetracycline	960.4	E856	E930.4	E950.4	E962.0	E980.4	Tincture, iodine — see Iodine						
ophthalmic preparation	976.5	E858.7	E946.5	E950.4	E962.0	E980.4	Tindal	969.1	E853.0	E939.1	E950.3	E962.0	E980.3
topical NEC	976.0	E858.7	E946.0	E950.4	E962.0	E980.4	Titanium (compounds) (vapor)	985.8	E866.4	—	E950.9	E962.1	E980.9
Tetraethylammonium chloride	972.3	E858.3	E942.3	E950.4	E962.0	E980.4	ointment	976.3	E858.7	E946.3	E950.4	E962.0	E980.4
							Titroid	962.7	E858.0	E932.7	E950.4	E962.0	E980.4
Tetraethyl lead (antiknock compound)	984.1	E862.1	—	E950.9	E962.1	E980.9	TMTD — see Tetramethylthiuram disulfide						
Tetraethyl pyrophosphate	989.3	E863.1	—	E950.6	E962.1	E980.7	TNT	989.89	E866.8	—	E950.9	E962.1	E980.9
Tetraethylthiuram disulfide	977.3	E858.8	E947.3	E950.4	E962.0	E980.4	fumes	987.8	E869.8	—	E952.8	E962.2	E982.8
Tetrahydroaminoacridine	971.0	E855.3	E941.0	E950.4	E962.0	E980.4	Toadstool	988.1	E865.5	—	E950.9	E962.1	E980.9
Tetrahydrocannabinol	969.6	E854.1	E939.6	E950.3	E962.0	E980.3	Tobacco NEC	989.84	E866.8	—	E950.9	E962.1	E980.9
Tetrahydronaphthalene	982.0	E862.4	—	E950.9	E962.1	E980.9	Indian	988.2	E865.4	—	E950.9	E962.1	E980.9
Tetrahydrozoline	971.2	E855.5	E941.2	E950.4	E962.0	E980.4	smoke, second-hand	987.8	E869.4	—	—	—	—
Tetralin	982.0	E862.4	—	E950.9	E962.1	E980.9	Tocopherol	963.5	E858.1	E933.5	E950.4	E962.0	E980.4
Tetramethylthiuram							Tocosamine	975.0	E858.6	E945.0	E950.4	E962.0	E980.4
(disulfide) NEC	989.4	E863.6	—	E950.6	E962.1	E980.7	Tofranil	969.0	E854.0	E939.0	E950.3	E962.0	E980.3
medicinal	976.2	E858.7	E946.2	E950.4	E962.0	E980.4	Toilet deodorizer	989.89	E866.8	—	E950.9	E962.1	E980.9
Tetronal	967.8	E852.8	E937.8	E950.2	E962.0	E980.2	Tolazamide	962.3	E858.0	E932.3	E950.4	E962.0	E980.4
Tetryl	983.0	E864.0	—	E950.7	E962.1	E980.6	Tolazoline	971.3	E855.6	E941.3	E950.4	E962.0	E980.4
Thalidomide	967.8	E852.8	E937.8	E950.2	E962.0	E980.2	Tolbutamide	962.3	E858.0	E932.3	E950.4	E962.0	E980.4
Thallium (compounds) (dust)							sodium	977.8	E858.8	E947.8	E950.4	E962.0	E980.4
NEC	985.8	E866.4	—	E950.9	E962.1	E980.9	Tolmetin	965.69	E850.6	E935.6	E950.0	E962.0	E980.0
pesticide (rodenticide)	985.8	E863.7	—	E950.6	E962.1	E980.7	Tolnaftate	976.0	E858.7	E946.0	E950.4	E962.0	E980.4
THC	969.6	E854.1	E939.6	E950.3	E962.0	E980.3	Tolpropamine	976.1	E858.7	E946.1	E950.4	E962.0	E980.4
Thebacon	965.09	E850.2	E935.2	E950.0	E962.0	E980.0	Tolserol	968.0	E855.1	E938.0	E950.4	E962.0	E980.4
Thebaine	965.09	E850.2	E935.2	E950.0	E962.0	E980.0	Toluene (liquid) (vapor)	982.0	E862.4	—	E950.9	E962.1	E980.9
Theobromine (calcium salicylate)	974.1	E858.5	E944.1	E950.4	E962.0	E980.4	diisocyanate	983.0	E864.0	—	E950.7	E962.1	E980.6
							Toluidine	983.0	E864.0	—	E950.7	E962.1	E980.6
Theophylline (diuretic)	974.1	E858.5	E944.1	E950.4	E962.0	E980.4	vapor	987.8	E869.8	—	E952.8	E962.2	E982.8
ethylenediamine	975.7	E858.6	E945.7	E950.4	E962.0	E980.4	Toluol (liquid) (vapor)	982.0	E862.4	—	E950.9	E962.1	E980.9
Thiabendazole	961.6	E857	E931.6	E950.4	E962.0	E980.4	Tolylene-2, 4-diisocyanate	983.0	E864.0	—	E950.7	E962.1	E980.6
Thialbarbital, thialbarbitone	968.3	E855.1	E938.3	E950.4	E962.0	E980.4	Tonics, cardiac	972.1	E858.3	E942.1	E950.4	E962.0	E980.4
							Toxaphene (dust) (spray)	989.2	E863.0	—	E950.6	E962.1	E980.7
Thiamine	963.5	E858.1	E933.5	E950.4	E962.0	E980.4	Toxoids NEC	978.8	E858.8	E948.8	E950.4	E962.0	E980.4
Thiamylal (sodium)	968.3	E855.1	E938.3	E950.4	E962.0	E980.4	Tractor fuel NEC	981	E862.1	—	E950.9	E962.1	E980.9
Thiazesim	969.0	E854.0	E939.0	E950.3	E962.0	E980.3	Tragacanth	973.3	E858.4	E943.3	E950.4	E962.0	E980.4
Thiazides (diuretics)	974.3	E858.5	E944.3	E950.4	E962.0	E980.4	Tramazoline	971.2	E855.5	E941.2	E950.4	E962.0	E980.4
Thiethylperazine	963.0	E858.1	E933.0	E950.4	E962.0	E980.4	Tranquilizers	969.5	E853.9	E939.5	E950.3	E962.0	E980.3
Thimerosal (topical)	976.0	E858.7	E946.0	E950.4	E962.0	E980.4	benzodiazepine-based	969.4	E853.2	E939.4	E950.3	E962.0	E980.3
ophthalmic preparation	976.5	E858.7	E946.5	E950.4	E962.0	E980.4	butyrophenone-based	969.2	E853.1	E939.2	E950.3	E962.0	E980.3
Thioacetazone	961.8	E857	E931.8	E950.4	E962.0	E980.4	major NEC	969.3	E853.8	E939.3	E950.3	E962.0	E980.3
Thiobarbiturates	968.3	E855.1	E938.3	E950.4	E962.0	E980.4	phenothiazine-based	969.1	E853.0	E939.1	E950.3	E962.0	E980.3
Thiobismol	961.2	E857	E931.2	E950.4	E962.0	E980.4	specified NEC	969.5	E853.8	E939.5	E950.3	E962.0	E980.3
Thiocarbamide	962.8	E858.0	E932.8	E950.4	E962.0	E980.4	Trantoin	961.9	E857	E931.9	E950.4	E962.0	E980.4
Thiocarbarsone	961.1	E857	E931.1	E950.4	E962.0	E980.4	Tranxene	969.4	E853.2	E939.4	E950.3	E962.0	E980.3
Thiocarlide	961.8	E857	E931.8	E950.4	E962.0	E980.4	Tranylcypromine (sulfate)	969.0	E854.0	E939.0	E950.3	E962.0	E980.3
Thioguanine	963.1	E858.1	E933.1	E950.4	E962.0	E980.4	Trasentine	975.1	E858.6	E945.1	E950.4	E962.0	E980.4
Thiomercaptomerin	974.0	E858.5	E944.0	E950.4	E962.0	E980.4	Travert	974.5	E858.5	E944.5	E950.4	E962.0	E980.4
Thiomerin	974.0	E858.5	E944.0	E950.4	E962.0	E980.4	Trecator	961.8	E857	E931.8	E950.4	E962.0	E980.4
Thiopental, thiopentone (sodium)	968.3	E855.1	E938.3	E950.4	E962.0	E980.4	Tretinoin	976.8	E858.7	E946.8	E950.4	E962.0	E980.4
							Triacetin	976.0	E858.7	E946.0	E950.4	E962.0	E980.4
Thiopropazate	969.1	E853.0	E939.1	E950.3	E962.0	E980.3	Triacetyloleandomycin	960.3	E856	E930.3	E950.4	E962.0	E980.4
Thioproperazine	969.1	E853.0	E939.1	E950.3	E962.0	E980.3	Triamcinolone	962.0	E858.0	E932.0	E950.4	E962.0	E980.4
Thioridazine	969.1	E853.0	E939.1	E950.3	E962.0	E980.3	ENT agent	976.6	E858.7	E946.6	E950.4	E962.0	E980.4
Thio-TEPA, thiotepa	963.1	E858.1	E933.1	E950.4	E962.0	E980.4	ophthalmic preparation	976.5	E858.7	E946.5	E950.4	E962.0	E980.4
Thiothixene	969.3	E853.8	E939.3	E950.3	E962.0	E980.3	topical NEC	976.0	E858.7	E946.0	E950.4	E962.0	E980.4

☑ Additional Digit Required ▶◀ Revised Text ● New Line ▲ Revised Code

	Poisoning	External Cause (E-Code)				
		Accident	Therapeutic Use	Suicide Attempt	Assault	Undetermined
Triamterene	974.4	E858.5	E944.4	E950.4	E962.0	E980.4
Triaziquone	963.1	E858.1	E933.1	E950.4	E962.0	E980.4
Tribromacetaldehyde	967.3	E852.2	E937.3	E950.2	E962.0	E980.2
Tribromoethanol	968.2	E855.1	E938.2	E950.4	E962.0	E980.4
Tribromomethane	967.3	E852.2	E937.3	E950.2	E962.0	E980.2
Trichlorethane	982.3	E862.4	—	E950.9	E962.1	E980.9
Trichlormethiazide	974.3	E858.5	E944.3	E950.4	E962.0	E980.4
Trichloroacetic acid	983.1	E864.1	—	E950.7	E962.1	E980.6
medicinal (keratolytic)	976.4	E858.7	E946.4	E950.4	E962.0	E980.4
Trichloroethanol	967.1	E852.0	E937.1	E950.2	E962.0	E980.2
Trichloroethylene (liquid)						
(vapor)	982.3	E862.4	—	E950.9	E962.1	E980.9
anesthetic (gas)	968.2	E855.1	E938.2	E950.4	E962.0	E980.4
Trichloroethyl phosphate	967.1	E852.0	E937.1	E950.2	E962.0	E980.2
Trichlorofluoromethane						
NEC	987.4	E869.2	—	E952.8	E962.2	E982.8
Trichlorotriethylamine	963.1	E858.1	E933.1	E950.4	E962.0	E980.4
Trichomonacides NEC	961.5	E857	E931.5	E950.4	E962.0	E980.4
Trichomycin	960.1	E856	E930.1	E950.4	E962.0	E980.4
Triclofos	967.1	E852.0	E937.1	E950.2	E962.0	E980.2
Tricresyl phosphate	989.89	E866.8	—	E950.9	E962.1	E980.9
solvent	982.8	E862.4	—	E950.9	E962.1	E980.9
Tricyclamol	966.4	E855.0	E936.4	E950.4	E962.0	E980.4
Tridesilon	976.0	E858.7	E946.0	E950.4	E962.0	E980.4
Tridihexethyl	971.1	E855.4	E941.1	E950.4	E962.0	E980.4
Tridione	966.0	E855.0	E936.0	E950.4	E962.0	E980.4
Triethanolamine NEC	983.2	E864.2	—	E950.7	E962.1	E980.6
detergent	983.2	E861.0	—	E950.7	E962.1	E980.6
trinitrate	972.4	E858.3	E942.4	E950.4	E962.0	E980.4
Triethanomelamine	963.1	E858.1	E933.1	E950.4	E962.0	E980.4
Triethylene melamine	963.1	E858.1	E933.1	E950.4	E962.0	E980.4
Triethylenephosphoramide	963.1	E858.1	E933.1	E950.4	E962.0	E980.4
Triethylenethiophospho-ramide	963.1	E858.1	E933.1	E950.4	E962.0	E980.4
Trifluoperazine	969.1	E853.0	E939.1	E950.3	E962.0	E980.3
Trifluperidol	969.2	E853.1	E939.2	E950.3	E962.0	E980.3
Triflupromazine	969.1	E853.0	E939.1	E950.3	E962.0	E980.3
Trihexyphenidyl	971.1	E855.4	E941.1	E950.4	E962.0	E980.4
Triiodothyronine	962.7	E858.0	E932.7	E950.4	E962.0	E980.4
Trilene	968.2	E855.1	E938.2	E950.4	E962.0	E980.4
Trimeprazine	963.0	E858.1	E933.0	E950.4	E962.0	E980.4
Trimetazidine	972.4	E858.3	E942.4	E950.4	E962.0	E980.4
Trimethadione	966.0	E855.0	E936.0	E950.4	E962.0	E980.4
Trimethaphan	972.3	E858.3	E942.3	E950.4	E962.0	E980.4
Trimethidinium	972.3	E858.3	E942.3	E950.4	E962.0	E980.4
Trimethobenzamide	963.0	E858.1	E933.0	E950.4	E962.0	E980.4
Trimethylcarbinol	980.8	E860.8	—	E950.9	E962.1	E980.9
Trimethylpsoralen	976.3	E858.7	E946.3	E950.4	E962.0	E980.4
Trimeton	963.0	E858.1	E933.0	E950.4	E962.0	E980.4
Trimipramine	969.0	E854.0	E939.0	E950.3	E962.0	E980.3
Trimustine	963.1	E858.1	E933.1	E950.4	E962.0	E980.4
Trinitrin	972.4	E858.3	E942.4	E950.4	E962.0	E980.4
Trinitrophenol	983.0	E864.0	—	E950.7	E962.1	E980.6
Trinitrotoluene	989.89	E866.8	—	E950.9	E962.1	E980.9
fumes	987.8	E869.8	—	E952.8	E962.2	E982.8
Trional	967.8	E852.8	E937.8	E950.2	E962.0	E980.2
Trioxide of arsenic — see Arsenic						
Trioxsalen	976.3	E858.7	E946.3	E950.4	E962.0	E980.4
Tripelennamine	963.0	E858.1	E933.0	E950.4	E962.0	E980.4
Triperidol	969.2	E853.1	E939.2	E950.3	E962.0	E980.3
Triprolidine	963.0	E858.1	E933.0	E950.4	E962.0	E980.4
Trisoralen	976.3	E858.7	E946.3	E950.4	E962.0	E980.4
Troleandomycin	960.3	E856	E930.3	E950.4	E962.0	E980.4
Trolnitrate (phosphate)	972.4	E858.3	E942.4	E950.4	E962.0	E980.4
Trometamol	963.3	E858.1	E933.3	E950.4	E962.0	E980.4
Tromethamine	963.3	E858.1	E933.3	E950.4	E962.0	E980.4
Tronothane	968.5	E855.2	E938.5	E950.4	E962.0	E980.4
Tropicamide	971.1	E855.4	E941.1	E950.4	E962.0	E980.4
Troxidone	966.0	E855.0	E936.0	E950.4	E962.0	E980.4
Tryparsamide	961.1	E857	E931.1	E950.4	E962.0	E980.4
Trypsin	963.4	E858.1	E933.4	E950.4	E962.0	E980.4
Tryptizol	969.0	E854.0	E939.0	E950.3	E962.0	E980.3
Tuaminoheptane	971.2	E855.5	E941.2	E950.4	E962.0	E980.4
Tuberculin (old)	977.8	E858.8	E947.8	E950.4	E962.0	E980.4
Tubocurare	975.2	E858.6	E945.2	E950.4	E962.0	E980.4
Tubocurarine	975.2	E858.6	E945.2	E950.4	E962.0	E980.4
Turkish green	969.6	E854.1	E939.6	E950.3	E962.0	E980.3
Turpentine (spirits of) (liquid)						
(vapor)	982.8	E862.4	—	E950.9	E962.1	E980.9
Tybamate	969.5	E853.8	E939.5	E950.3	E962.0	E980.3

	Poisoning	External Cause (E-Code)				
		Accident	Therapeutic Use	Suicide Attempt	Assault	Undetermined
Tyloxapol	975.5	E858.6	E945.5	E950.4	E962.0	E980.4
Tymazoline	971.2	E855.5	E941.2	E950.4	E962.0	E980.4
Typhoid vaccine	978.1	E858.8	E948.1	E950.4	E962.0	E980.4
Typhus vaccine	979.2	E858.8	E949.2	E950.4	E962.0	E980.4
Tyrothricin	976.0	E858.7	E946.0	E950.4	E962.0	E980.4
ENT agent	976.6	E858.7	E946.6	E950.4	E962.0	E980.4
ophthalmic preparation	976.5	E858.7	E946.5	E950.4	E962.0	E980.4
Undecenoic acid	976.0	E858.7	E946.0	E950.4	E962.0	E980.4
Undecylenic acid	976.0	E858.7	E946.0	E950.4	E962.0	E980.4
Unna's boot	976.3	E858.7	E946.3	E950.4	E962.0	E980.4
Uracil mustard	963.1	E858.1	E933.1	E950.4	E962.0	E980.4
Uramustine	963.1	E858.1	E933.1	E950.4	E962.0	E980.4
Urari	975.2	E858.6	E945.2	E950.4	E962.0	E980.4
Urea	974.4	E858.5	E944.4	E950.4	E962.0	E980.4
topical	976.8	E858.7	E946.8	E950.4	E962.0	E980.4
Urethan(e) (antineoplastic)	963.1	E858.1	E933.1	E950.4	E962.0	E980.4
Urginea (maritima) (scilla) — see Squill						
Uric acid metabolism agents NEC	974.7	E858.5	E944.7	E950.4	E962.0	E980.4
Urokinase	964.4	E858.2	E934.4	E950.4	E962.0	E980.4
Urokon	977.8	E858.8	E947.8	E950.4	E962.0	E980.4
Urotropin	961.9	E857	E931.9	E950.4	E962.0	E980.4
Urtica	988.2	E865.4	—	E950.9	E962.1	E980.9
Utility gas — see Gas, utility						
Vaccine NEC	979.9	E858.8	E949.9	E950.4	E962.0	E980.4
bacterial NEC	978.8	E858.8	E948.8	E950.4	E962.0	E980.4
with						
other bacterial component	978.9	E858.8	E948.9	E950.4	E962.0	E980.4
pertussis component	978.6	E858.8	E948.6	E950.4	E962.0	E980.4
viral-rickettsial component	979.7	E858.8	E949.7	E950.4	E962.0	E980.4
mixed NEC	978.9	E858.8	E948.9	E950.4	E962.0	E980.4
BCG	978.0	E858.8	E948.0	E950.4	E962.0	E980.4
cholera	978.2	E858.8	E948.2	E950.4	E962.0	E980.4
diphtheria	978.5	E858.8	E948.5	E950.4	E962.0	E980.4
influenza	979.6	E858.8	E949.6	E950.4	E962.0	E980.4
measles	979.4	E858.8	E949.4	E950.4	E962.0	E980.4
meningococcal	978.8	E858.8	E948.8	E950.4	E962.0	E980.4
mumps	979.6	E858.8	E949.6	E950.4	E962.0	E980.4
paratyphoid	978.1	E858.8	E948.1	E950.4	E962.0	E980.4
pertussis (with diphtheria toxoid) (with tetanus toxoid)	978.6	E858.8	E948.6	E950.4	E962.0	E980.4
plague	978.3	E858.8	E948.3	E950.4	E962.0	E980.4
poliomyelitis	979.5	E858.8	E949.5	E950.4	E962.0	E980.4
poliovirus	979.5	E858.8	E949.5	E950.4	E962.0	E980.4
rabies	979.1	E858.8	E949.1	E950.4	E962.0	E980.4
respiratory syncytial virus	979.6	E858.8	E949.6	E950.4	E962.0	E980.4
rickettsial NEC	979.6	E858.8	E949.6	E950.4	E962.0	E980.4
with						
bacterial component	979.7	E858.8	E949.7	E950.4	E962.0	E980.4
pertussis component	978.6	E858.8	E948.6	E950.4	E962.0	E980.4
viral component	979.7	E858.8	E949.7	E950.4	E962.0	E980.4
Rocky mountain spotted fever	979.6	E858.8	E949.6	E950.4	E962.0	E980.4
rotavirus	979.6	E858.8	E949.6	E950.4	E962.0	E980.4
rubella virus	979.4	E858.8	E949.4	E950.4	E962.0	E980.4
sabin oral	979.5	E858.8	E949.5	E950.4	E962.0	E980.4
smallpox	979.0	E858.8	E949.0	E950.4	E962.0	E980.4
tetanus	978.4	E858.8	E948.4	E950.4	E962.0	E980.4
typhoid	978.1	E858.8	E948.1	E950.4	E962.0	E980.4
typhus	979.2	E858.8	E949.2	E950.4	E962.0	E980.4
viral NEC	979.6	E858.8	E949.6	E950.4	E962.0	E980.4
with						
bacterial component	979.7	E858.8	E949.7	E950.4	E962.0	E980.4
pertussis component	978.6	E858.8	E948.6	E950.4	E962.0	E980.4
rickettsial component	979.7	E858.8	E949.7	E950.4	E962.0	E980.4
yellow fever	979.3	E858.8	E949.3	E950.4	E962.0	E980.4
Vaccinia immune globulin (human)	964.6	E858.2	E934.6	E950.4	E962.0	E980.4
Vaginal contraceptives	976.8	E858.7	E946.8	E950.4	E962.0	E980.4
Valethamate	971.1	E855.4	E941.1	E950.4	E962.0	E980.4

☑ Additional Digit Required   ▶◀ Revised Text   ● New Line   ▲ Revised Code

	Poisoning	External Cause (E-Code)				
		Accident	Therapeutic Use	Suicide Attempt	Assault	Undetermined
Benziodarone	972.4	E858.3	E942.4	E950.4	E962.0	E980.4
Benzocaine	968.5	E855.2	E938.5	E950.4	E962.0	E980.4
Benzodiapin	969.4	E853.2	E939.4	E950.3	E962.0	E980.3
Benzodiazepines						
(tranquilizers) NEC	969.4	E853.2	E939.4	E950.3	E962.0	E980.3
Benzoic acid (with salicylic						
acid) (anti-infective)	976.0	E858.7	E946.0	E950.4	E962.0	E980.4
Benzoin	976.3	E858.7	E946.3	E950.4	E962.0	E980.4
Benzol (vapor)	982.0	E862.4	—	E950.9	E962.1	E980.9
Benzomorphan	965.09	E850.2	E935.2	E950.0	E962.0	E980.0
Benzonatate	975.4	E858.6	E945.4	E950.4	E962.0	E980.4
Benzothiadiazides	974.3	E858.5	E944.3	E950.4	E962.0	E980.4
Benzoylpas	961.8	E857	E931.8	E950.4	E962.0	E980.4
Benzperidol	969.5	E853.8	E939.5	E950.3	E962.0	E980.3
Benzphetamine	977.0	E858.8	E947.0	E950.4	E962.0	E980.4
Benzpyrinium	971.0	E855.3	E941.0	E950.4	E962.0	E980.4
Benzquinamide	963.0	E858.1	E933.0	E950.4	E962.0	E980.4
Benzthiazide	974.3	E858.5	E944.3	E950.4	E962.0	E980.4
Benztropine	971.1	E855.4	E941.1	E950.4	E962.0	E980.4
Benzyl						
acetate	982.8	E862.4	—	E950.9	E962.1	E980.9
benzoate (anti-infective)	976.0	E858.7	E946.0	E950.4	E962.0	E980.4
morphine	965.09	E850.2	E935.2	E950.0	E962.0	E980.0
penicillin	960.0	E856	E930.0	E950.4	E962.0	E980.4
Bephenium						
hydroxynapthoate	961.6	E857	E931.6	E950.4	E962.0	E980.4
Bergamot oil	989.89	E866.8	—	E950.9	E962.1	E980.9
Berries, poisonous	988.2	E865.3	—	E950.9	E962.1	E980.9
Beryllium (compounds)						
(fumes)	985.3	E866.4	—	E950.9	E962.1	E980.9
Beta-carotene	976.3	E858.7	E946.3	E950.4	E962.0	E980.4
Beta-Chlor	967.1	E852.0	E937.1	E950.2	E962.0	E980.2
Betamethasone	962.0	E858.0	E932.0	E950.4	E962.0	E980.4
topical	976.0	E858.7	E946.0	E950.4	E962.0	E980.4
Betazole	977.8	E858.8	E947.8	E950.4	E962.0	E980.4
Bethanechol	971.0	E855.3	E941.0	E950.4	E962.0	E980.4
Bethanidine	972.6	E858.3	E942.6	E950.4	E962.0	E980.4
Betula oil	976.3	E858.7	E946.3	E950.4	E962.0	E980.4
Bhang	969.6	E854.1	E939.6	E950.3	E962.0	E980.3
Bialamicol	961.5	E857	E931.5	E950.4	E962.0	E980.4
Bichloride of mercury —						
see Mercury, chloride						
Bichromates (calcium)						
(crystals) (potassium)						
(sodium)	983.9	E864.3	—	E950.7	E962.1	E980.6
fumes	987.8	E869.8	—	E952.8	E962.2	E982.8
Biguanide derivatives, oral	962.3	E858.0	E932.3	E950.4	E962.0	E980.4
Biligrafin	977.8	E858.8	E947.8	E950.4	E962.0	E980.4
Bilopaque	977.8	E858.8	E947.8	E950.4	E962.0	E980.4
Bioflavonoids	972.8	E858.3	E942.8	E950.4	E962.0	E980.4
Biological substance NEC	979.9	E858.8	E949.9	E950.4	E962.0	E980.4
Biperiden	966.4	E855.0	E936.4	E950.4	E962.0	E980.4
Bisacodyl	973.1	E858.4	E943.1	E950.4	E962.0	E980.4
Bishydroxycoumarin	964.2	E858.2	E934.2	E950.4	E962.0	E980.4
Bismarsen	961.1	E857	E931.1	E950.4	E962.0	E980.4
Bismuth (compounds) NEC	985.8	E866.4	—	E950.9	E962.1	E980.9
anti-infectives	961.2	E857	E931.2	E950.4	E962.0	E980.4
subcarbonate	973.5	E858.4	E943.5	E950.4	E962.0	E980.4
sulfarsphenamine	961.1	E857	E931.1	E950.4	E962.0	E980.4
Bithionol	961.6	E857	E931.6	E950.4	E962.0	E980.4
Bitter almond oil	989.0	E866.8	—	E950.9	E962.1	E980.9
Bittersweet	988.2	E865.4	—	E950.9	E962.1	E930.9
Black						
flag	989.4	E863.4	—	E950.6	E962.1	E980.7
henbane	988.2	E865.4	—	E950.9	E962.1	E980.9
leaf (40)	989.4	E863.4	—	E950.6	E962.1	E980.7
widow spider (bite)	989.5	E905.1	—	E950.9	E962.1	E980.9
antivenin	979.9	E858.8	E949.9	E950.4	E962.0	E980.4
Blast furnace gas (carbon						
monoxide from)	986	E868.8	—	E952.1	E962.2	E982.1
Bleach NEC	983.9	E864.3	—	E950.7	E962.1	E980.6
Bleaching solutions	983.9	E864.3	—	E950.7	E962.1	E980.6
Bleomycin (sulfate)	960.7	E856	E930.7	E950.4	E962.0	E980.4
Blockain	968.9	E855.2	E938.9	E950.4	E962.0	E980.4
infiltration (subcutaneous)	968.5	E855.2	E938.5	E950.4	E962.0	E980.4
nerve block (peripheral)						
(plexus)	968.6	E855.2	E938.6	E950.4	E962.0	E980.4
topical (surface)	968.5	E855.2	E938.5	E950.4	E962.0	E980.4
Blood (derivatives) (natural)						
(plasma) (whole)	964.7	E858.2	E934.7	E950.4	E962.0	E980.4
affecting agent	964.9	E858.2	E934.9	E950.4	E962.0	E980.4
specified NEC	964.8	E858.2	E934.8	E950.4	E962.0	E980.4

	Poisoning	External Cause (E-Code)				
		Accident	Therapeutic Use	Suicide Attempt	Assault	Undetermined
Blood — continued						
substitute (macromolecular)	964.8	E858.2	E934.8	E950.4	E962.0	E980.4
Blue velvet	965.09	E850.2	E935.2	E950.0	E962.0	E980.0
Bone meal	989.89	E866.5	—	E950.9	E962.1	E980.9
Bonine	963.0	E858.1	E933.0	E950.4	E962.0	E980.4
Boracic acid	976.0	E858.7	E946.0	E950.4	E962.0	E980.4
ENT agent	976.6	E858.7	E946.6	E950.4	E962.0	E980.4
ophthalmic preparation	976.5	E858.7	E946.5	E950.4	E962.0	E980.4
Borate (cleanser) (sodium)	989.6	E861.3	—	E950.9	E962.1	E980.9
Borax (cleanser)	989.6	E861.3	—	E950.9	E962.1	E980.9
Boric acid	976.0	E858.7	E946.0	E950.4	E962.0	E980.4
ENT agent	976.6	E858.7	E946.6	E950.4	E962.0	E980.4
ophthalmic preparation	976.5	E858.7	E946.5	E950.4	E962.0	E980.4
Boron hydride NEC	989.89	E866.8	—	E950.9	E962.1	E980.9
fumes or gas	987.8	E869.8	—	E952.8	E962.2	E982.8
Botox	975.3	E858.6	E945.3	E950.4	E962.0	E980.4
Brake fluid vapor	987.8	E869.8	—	E952.8	E962.2	E982.8
Brass (compounds) (fumes)	985.8	E866.4	—	E950.9	E962.1	E980.9
Brasso	981	E861.3	—	E950.9	E962.1	E980.9
Bretylium (tosylate)	972.6	E858.3	E942.6	E950.4	E962.0	E980.4
Brevital (sodium)	968.3	E855.1	E938.3	E950.4	E962.0	E980.4
British antilewisite	963.8	E858.1	E933.8	E950.4	E962.0	E980.4
Bromal (hydrate)	967.3	E852.2	E937.3	E950.2	E962.0	E980.2
Bromelains	963.4	E858.1	E933.4	E950.4	E962.0	E980.4
Bromides NEC	967.3	E852.2	E937.3	E950.2	E962.0	E980.2
Bromine (vapor)	987.8	E869.8	—	E952.8	E962.2	E982.8
compounds (medicinal)	967.3	E852.2	E937.3	E950.2	E962.0	E980.2
Bromisovalum	967.3	E852.2	E937.3	E950.2	E962.0	E980.2
Bromobenzyl cyanide	987.5	E869.3	—	E952.8	E962.2	E982.8
Bromodiphenhydramine	963.0	E858.1	E933.0	E950.4	E962.0	E980.4
Bromoform	967.3	E852.2	E937.3	E950.2	E962.0	E980.2
Bromophenol blue reagent	977.8	E858.8	E947.8	E950.4	E962.0	E980.4
Bromosalicylhydroxamic						
acid	961.8	E857	E931.8	E950.4	E962.0	E980.4
Bromo-seltzer	965.4	E850.4	E935.4	E950.0	E962.0	E980.0
Brompheniramine	963.0	E858.1	E933.0	E950.4	E962.0	E980.4
Bromural	967.3	E852.2	E937.3	E950.2	E962.0	E980.2
Brown spider (bite) (venom)	989.5	E905.1	—	E950.9	E962.1	E980.9
Brucia	988.2	E865.3	—	E950.9	E962.1	E980.9
Brucine	989.1	E863.7	—	E950.6	E962.1	E980.7
Brunswick green — see Copper						
Bruten — see Ibuprofen						
Bryonia (alba) (dioica)	988.2	E865.4	—	E950.9	E962.1	E980.9
Buclizine	969.5	E853.8	E939.5	E950.3	E962.0	E980.3
Bufferin	965.1	E850.3	E935.3	E950.0	E962.0	E980.0
Bufotenine	969.6	E854.1	E939.6	E950.3	E962.0	E980.3
Buphenine	971.2	E855.5	E941.2	E950.4	E962.0	E980.4
Bupivacaine	968.9	E855.2	E938.9	E950.4	E962.0	E980.4
infiltration (subcutaneous)	968.5	E855.2	E938.5	E950.4	E962.0	E980.4
nerve block (peripheral)						
(plexus)	968.6	E855.2	E938.6	E950.4	E962.0	E980.4
Busulfan	963.1	E858.1	E933.1	E950.4	E962.0	E980.4
Butabarbital (sodium)	967.0	E851	E937.0	E950.1	E962.0	E980.1
Butabarbitone	967.0	E851	E937.0	E950.1	E962.0	E980.1
Butabarpal	967.0	E851	E937.0	E950.1	E962.0	E980.1
Butacaine	968.5	E855.2	E938.5	E950.4	E962.0	E980.4
Butallylonal	967.0	E851	E937.0	E950.1	E962.0	E980.1
Butane (distributed in mobile						
container)	987.0	E868.0	—	E951.1	E962.2	E981.1
distributed through pipes	987.0	E867	—	E951.0	E962.2	E981.0
incomplete combustion of						
— see Carbon						
monoxide, butane						
Butanol	980.3	E860.4	—	E950.9	E962.1	E980.9
Butanone	982.8	E862.4	—	E950.9	E962.1	E980.9
Butaperazine	969.1	E853.0	E939.1	E950.3	E962.0	E980.3
Butazolidin	965.5	E850.5	E935.5	E950.0	E962.0	E980.0
Butethal	967.0	E851	E937.0	E950.1	E962.0	E980.1
Butethamate	971.1	E855.4	E941.1	E950.4	E962.0	E980.4
Buthalitone (sodium)	968.3	E855.1	E938.3	E950.4	E962.0	E980.4
Butisol (sodium)	967.0	E851	E937.0	E950.1	E962.0	E980.1
Butobarbital, butobarbitone	967.0	E851	E937.0	E950.1	E962.0	E980.1
Butriptyline	969.0	E854.0	E939.0	E950.3	E962.0	E980.3
Buttercups	988.2	E865.4	—	E950.9	E962.1	E980.9
Butter of antimony — see Antimony						
Butyl						
acetate (secondary)	982.8	E862.4	—	E950.9	E962.1	E980.9
alcohol	980.3	E860.4	—	E950.9	E962.1	E980.9
carbinol	980.8	E860.8	—	E950.9	E962.1	E980.9
carbitol	982.8	E862.4	—	E950.9	E962.1	E980.9
cellosolve	982.8	E862.4	—	E950.9	E962.1	E980.9

		External Cause (E-Code)				
	Poisoning	Accident	Therapeutic Use	Suicide Attempt	Assault	Undetermined
Butyl — *continued*						
chloral (hydrate)	967.1	E852.0	E937.1	E950.2	E962.0	E980.2
formate	982.8	E862.4	—	E950.9	E962.1	E980.9
scopolammonium bromide ...	971.1	E855.4	E941.1	E950.4	E962.0	E980.4
Butyn	968.5	E855.2	E938.5	E950.4	E962.0	E980.4
Butyrophenone (-based tranquilizers)	969.2	E853.1	E939.2	E950.3	E962.0	E980.3
Cacodyl, cacodylic acid — *see* Arsenic						
Cactinomycin	960.7	E856	E930.7	E950.4	E962.0	E980.4
Cade oil	976.4	E858.7	E946.4	E950.4	E962.0	E980.4
Cadmium (chloride) (compounds) (dust) (fumes) (oxide)	985.5	E866.4	—	E950.9	E962.1	E980.9
sulfide (medicinal) NEC	976.4	E858.7	E946.4	E950.4	E962.0	E980.4
Caffeine	969.7	E854.2	E939.7	E950.3	E962.0	E980.3
Calabar bean	988.2	E865.4	—	E950.9	E962.1	E980.9
Caladium seguinium	988.2	E865.4	—	E950.9	E962.1	E980.9
Calamine (liniment) (lotion)	976.3	E858.7	E946.3	E950.4	E962.0	E980.4
Calciferol	963.5	E858.1	E933.5	E950.4	E962.0	E980.4
Calcium (salts) NEC	974.5	E858.5	E944.5	E950.4	E962.0	E980.4
acetylsalicylate	965.1	E850.3	E935.3	E950.0	E962.0	E980.0
benzamidosalicylate	961.8	E857	E931.8	E950.4	E962.0	E980.4
carbaspirin	965.1	E850.3	E935.3	E950.0	E962.0	E980.0
carbimide (citrated)	977.3	E858.8	E947.3	E950.4	E962.0	E980.4
carbonate (antacid)	973.0	E858.4	E943.0	E950.4	E962.0	E980.4
cyanide (citrated)	977.3	E858.8	E947.3	E950.4	E962.0	E980.4
dioctyl sulfosuccinate	973.2	E858.4	E943.2	E950.4	E962.0	E980.4
disodium edathamil	963.8	E858.1	E933.8	E950.4	E962.0	E980.4
disodium edetate	963.8	E858.1	E933.8	E950.4	E962.0	E980.4
EDTA	963.8	E858.1	E933.8	E950.4	E962.0	E980.4
hydrate, hydroxide	983.2	E864.2	—	E950.7	E962.1	E980.6
mandelate	961.9	E857	E931.9	E950.4	E962.0	E980.4
oxide	983.2	E864.2	—	E950.7	E962.1	E980.6
Calomel — *see* Mercury, chloride						
Caloric agents NEC	974.5	E858.5	E944.5	E950.4	E962.0	E980.4
Calusterone	963.1	E858.1	E933.1	E950.4	E962.0	E980.4
Camoquin	961.4	E857	E931.4	E950.4	E962.0	E980.4
Camphor (oil)	976.1	E858.7	E946.1	E950.4	E962.0	E980.4
Candeptin	976.0	E858.7	E946.0	E950.4	E962.0	E980.4
Candicidin	976.0	E858.7	E946.0	E950.4	E962.0	E980.4
Cannabinols	969.6	E854.1	E939.6	E950.3	E962.0	E980.3
Cannabis (derivatives) (indica) (sativa)	969.6	E854.1	E939.6	E950.3	E962.0	E980.3
Canned heat	980.1	E860.2	—	E950.9	E962.1	E980.9
Cantharides, cantharidin, cantharis	976.8	E858.7	E946.8	E950.4	E962.0	E980.4
Capillary agents	972.8	E858.3	E942.8	E950.4	E962.0	E980.4
Capreomycin	960.6	E856	E930.6	E950.4	E962.0	E980.4
Captodiame, captodiamine	969.5	E853.8	E939.5	E950.3	E962.0	E980.3
Caramiphen (hydrochloride)	971.1	E855.4	E941.1	E950.4	E962.0	E980.4
Carbachol	971.0	E855.3	E941.0	E950.4	E962.0	E980.4
Carbacrylamine resins	974.5	E858.5	E944.5	E950.4	E962.0	E980.4
Carbamate (sedative)	967.8	E852.8	E937.8	E950.2	E962.0	E980.2
herbicide	989.3	E863.5	—	E950.6	E962.1	E980.7
insecticide	989.3	E863.2	—	E950.6	E962.1	E980.7
Carbamazepine	966.3	E855.0	E936.3	E950.4	E962.0	E980.4
Carbamic esters	967.8	E852.8	E937.8	E950.2	E962.0	E980.2
Carbamide	974.4	E858.5	E944.4	E950.4	E962.0	E980.4
topical	976.8	E858.7	E946.8	E950.4	E962.0	E980.4
Carbamylcholine chloride	971.0	E855.3	E941.0	E950.4	E962.0	E980.4
Carbarsone	961.1	E857	E931.1	E950.4	E962.0	E980.4
Carbaryl	989.3	E863.2	—	E950.6	E962.1	E980.7
Carbaspirin	965.1	E850.3	E935.3	E950.0	E962.0	E980.0
Carbazochrome	972.8	E858.3	E942.8	E950.4	E962.0	E980.4
Carbenicillin	960.0	E856	E930.0	E950.4	E962.0	E980.4
Carbenoxolone	973.8	E858.4	E943.8	E950.4	E962.0	E980.4
Carbetapentane	975.4	E858.6	E945.4	E950.4	E962.0	E980.4
Carbimazole	962.8	E858.0	E932.8	E950.4	E962.0	E980.4
Carbinol	980.1	E860.2	—	E950.9	E962.1	E980.9
Carbinoxamine	963.0	E858.1	E933.0	E950.4	E962.0	E980.4
Carbitol	982.8	E862.4	—	E950.9	E962.1	E980.9
Carbocaine	968.9	E855.2	E938.9	E950.4	E962.0	E980.4
infiltration (subcutaneous) ...	968.5	E855.2	E938.5	E950.4	E962.0	E980.4
nerve block (peripheral) (plexus)	968.6	E855.2	E938.6	E950.4	E962.0	E980.4
topical (surface)	968.5	E855.2	E938.5	E950.4	E962.0	E980.4
Carbol-fuchsin solution	976.0	E858.7	E946.0	E950.4	E962.0	E980.4
Carbolic acid (*see also* Phenol)	983.0	E864.0	—	E950.7	E962.1	E980.6
Carbomycin	960.8	E856	E930.8	E950.4	E962.0	E980.4
Carbon						
bisulfide (liquid) (vapor)	982.2	E862.4	—	E950.9	E962.1	E980.9
dioxide (gas)	987.8	E869.8	—	E952.8	E962.2	E982.8
disulfide (liquid) (vapor)	982.2	E862.4	—	E950.9	E962.1	E980.9
monoxide (from incomplete combustion of) (in)						
NEC	986	E868.9	—	E952.1	E962.2	E982.1
blast furnace gas	986	E868.8	—	E952.1	E962.2	E982.1
butane (distributed in mobile container)	986	E868.0	—	E951.1	E962.2	E981.1
distributed through pipes	986	E867	—	E951.0	E962.2	E981.0
charcoal fumes	986	E868.3	—	E952.1	E962.2	E982.1
coal						
gas (piped)	986	E867	—	E951.0	E962.2	E981.0
solid (in domestic stoves, fireplaces) ...	986	E868.3	—	E952.1	E962.2	E982.1
coke (in domestic stoves, fireplaces)	986	E868.3	—	E952.1	E962.2	E982.1
exhaust gas (motor) not in transit	986	E868.2	—	E952.0	E962.2	E982.0
combustion engine, any not in watercraft ...	986	E868.2	—	E952.0	E962.2	E982.0
farm tractor, not in transit	986	E868.2	—	E952.0	E962.2	E982.0
gas engine	986	E868.2	—	E952.0	E962.2	E982.0
motor pump	986	E868.2	—	E952.0	E962.2	E982.0
motor vehicle, not in transit	986	E868.2	—	E952.0	E962.2	E982.0
fuel (in domestic use)	986	E868.3	—	E952.1	E962.2	E982.1
gas (piped)	986	E867	—	E951.0	E962.2	E981.0
in mobile con-tainer ...	986	E868.0	—	E951.1	E962.2	E981.1
utility	986	E868.1	—	E951.8	E962.2	E981.1
in mobile con-tainer ...	986	E868.0	—	E951.1	E962.2	E981.1
piped (natural) ..	986	E867	—	E951.0	E962.2	E981.0
illuminating gas	986	E868.1	—	E951.8	E962.2	E981.8
industrial fuels or gases, any	986	E868.8	—	E952.1	E962.2	E982.1
kerosene (in domestic stoves, fireplaces)	986	E868.3	—	E952.1	E962.2	E982.1
kiln gas or vapor	986	E868.8	—	E952.1	E962.2	E982.1
motor exhaust gas, not in transit	986	E868.2	—	E952.0	E962.2	E982.0
piped gas (manufactured) (natural)	986	E867	—	E951.0	E962.2	E981.0
producer gas	986	E868.8	—	E951.8	E962.2	E982.1
propane (distributed in mobile container)	986	E868.0	—	E951.1	E962.2	E981.1
distributed through pipes	986	E867	—	E951.0	E962.2	E981.0
specified source NEC ...	986	E868.8	—	E952.1	E962.2	E982.1
stove gas	986	E868.1	—	E951.8	E962.2	E981.8
piped	986	E867	—	E951.0	E962.2	E981.0
utility gas	986	E868.1	—	E951.8	E962.2	E981.8
piped	986	E867	—	E951.0	E962.2	E981.0
water gas	986	E868.1	—	E951.8	E962.2	E981.8
wood (in domestic stoves, fireplaces)	986	E868.3	—	E952.1	E962.2	E982.1
tetrachloride (vapor) NEC	987.8	E869.8	—	E952.8	E962.2	E982.8
liquid (cleansing agent) NEC	982.1	E861.3	—	E950.9	E962.1	E980.9
solvent	982.1	E862.4	—	E950.9	E962.1	E980.9
Carbonic acid (gas)	987.8	E869.8	—	E952.8	E962.2	E982.8
anhydrase inhibitors	974.2	E858.5	E944.2	E950.4	E962.0	E980.4
Carbowax	976.3	E858.7	E946.3	E950.4	E962.0	E980.4
Carbrital	967.0	E851	E937.0	E950.1	E962.0	E980.1
Carbromal (derivatives)	967.3	E852.2	E937.3	E950.2	E962.0	E980.2
Cardiac						
depressants	972.0	E858.3	E942.0	E950.4	E962.0	E980.4
rhythm regulators	972.0	E858.3	E942.0	E950.4	E962.0	E980.4

☑ Additional Digit Required   ▶◀ Revised Text   ● New Line   ▲ Revised Code

	Poisoning	External Cause (E-Code)						Poisoning	External Cause (E-Code)				
		Accident	Therapeutic Use	Suicide Attempt	Assault	Undetermined			Accident	Therapeutic Use	Suicide Attempt	Assault	Undetermined
Cardiografin	977.8	E858.8	E947.8	E950.4	E962.0	E980.4	Cetrimide	976.2	E858.7	E946.2	E950.4	E962.0	E980.4
Cardio-green	977.8	E858.8	E947.8	E950.4	E962.0	E980.4	Cetylpyridinium	976.0	E858.7	E946.0	E950.4	E962.0	E980.4
Cardiotonic glycosides	972.1	E858.3	E942.1	E950.4	E962.0	E980.4	ENT agent	976.6	E858.7	E946.6	E950.4	E962.0	E980.4
Cardiovascular agents NEC	972.9	E858.3	E942.9	E950.4	E962.0	E980.4	lozenges	976.6	E858.7	E946.6	E950.4	E962.0	E980.4
Cardrase	974.2	E858.5	E944.2	E950.4	E962.0	E980.4	Cevadilla — see Sabadilla						
Carfusin	976.0	E858.7	E946.0	E950.4	E962.0	E980.4	Cevitamic acid	963.5	E858.1	E933.5	E950.4	E962.0	E980.4
Carisoprodol	968.0	E855.1	E938.0	E950.4	E962.0	E980.4	Chalk, precipitated	973.0	E858.4	E943.0	E950.4	E962.0	E980.4
Carmustine	963.1	E858.1	E933.1	E950.4	E962.0	E980.4	Charcoal						
Carotene	963.5	E858.1	E933.5	E950.4	E962.0	E980.4	fumes (carbon monoxide)	986	E868.3	—	E952.1	E962.2	E982.1
Carphenazine (maleate)	969.1	E853.0	E939.1	E950.3	E962.0	E980.3	industrial	986	E868.8	—	E952.1	E962.2	E982.1
Carter's Little Pills	973.1	E858.4	E943.1	E950.4	E962.0	E980.4	medicinal (activated)	973.0	E858.4	E943.0	E950.4	E962.0	E980.4
Cascara (sagrada)	973.1	E858.4	E943.1	E950.4	E962.0	E980.4	Chelating agents NEC	977.2	E858.8	E947.2	E950.4	E962.0	E980.4
Cassava	988.2	E865.4	—	E950.9	E962.1	E980.9	Chelidonium majus	988.2	E865.4	—	E950.9	E962.1	E980.9
Castellani's paint	976.0	E858.7	E946.0	E950.4	E962.0	E980.4	Chemical substance	989.9	E866.9	—	E950.9	E962.1	E980.9
Castor							specified NEC	989.89	E866.8	—	E950.9	E962.1	E980.9
bean	988.2	E865.3	—	E950.9	E962.1	E980.9	Chemotherapy,						
oil	973.1	E858.4	E943.1	E950.4	E962.0	E980.4	antineoplastic	963.1	E858.1	E933.1	E950.4	E962.0	E980.4
Caterpillar (sting)	989.5	E905.5	—	E950.9	E962.1	E980.9	Chenopodium (oil)	961.6	E857	E931.6	E950.4	E962.0	E980.4
Catha (edulis)	970.8	E854.3	E940.8	E950.4	E962.0	E980.4	Cherry laurel	988.2	E865.4	—	E950.9	E962.1	E980.9
Cathartics NEC	973.3	E858.4	E943.3	E950.4	E962.0	E980.4	Chiniofon	961.3	E857	E931.3	E950.4	E962.0	E980.4
contact	973.1	E858.4	E943.1	E950.4	E962.0	E980.4	Chlophedianol	975.4	E858.6	E945.4	E950.4	E962.0	E980.4
emollient	973.2	E858.4	E943.2	E950.4	E962.0	E980.4	Chloral (betaine) (formamide)						
intestinal irritants	973.1	E858.4	E943.1	E950.4	E962.0	E980.4	(hydrate)	967.1	E852.0	E937.1	E950.2	E962.0	E980.2
saline	973.3	E858.4	E943.3	E950.4	E962.0	E980.4	Chloralamide	967.1	E852.0	E937.1	E950.2	E962.0	E980.2
Cathomycin	960.8	E856	E930.8	E950.4	E962.0	E980.4	Chlorambucil	963.1	E858.1	E933.1	E950.4	E962.0	E980.4
Caustic(s)	983.9	E864.4	—	E950.7	E962.1	E980.6	Chloramphenicol	960.2	E856	E930.2	E950.4	E962.0	E980.4
alkali	983.2	E864.2	—	E950.7	E962.1	E980.6	ENT agent	976.6	E858.7	E946.6	E950.4	E962.0	E980.4
hydroxide	983.2	E864.2	—	E950.7	E962.1	E980.6	ophthalmic preparation	976.5	E858.7	E946.5	E950.4	E962.0	E980.4
potash	983.2	E864.2	—	E950.7	E962.1	E980.6	topical NEC	976.0	E858.7	E946.0	E950.4	E962.0	E980.4
soda	983.2	E864.2	—	E950.7	E962.1	E980.6	Chlorate(s) (potassium)						
specified NEC	983.9	E864.3	—	E950.7	E962.1	E980.6	(sodium) NEC	983.9	E864.3	—	E950.7	E962.1	E980.6
Ceepryn	976.0	E858.7	E946.0	E950.4	E962.0	E980.4	herbicides	989.4	E863.5	—	E950.6	E962.1	E980.7
ENT agent	976.6	E858.7	E946.6	E950.4	E962.0	E980.4	Chlorcyclizine	963.0	E858.1	E933.0	E950.4	E962.0	E980.4
lozenges	976.6	E858.7	E946.6	E950.4	E962.0	E980.4	Chlordan(e) (dust)	989.2	E863.0	—	E950.6	E962.1	E980.7
Celestone	962.0	E858.0	E932.0	E950.4	E962.0	E980.4	Chlordantoin	976.0	E858.7	E946.0	E950.4	E962.0	E980.4
topical	976.0	E858.7	E946.0	E950.4	E962.0	E980.4	Chlordiazepoxide	969.4	E853.2	E939.4	E950.3	E962.0	E980.3
Cellosolve	982.8	E862.4	—	E950.9	E962.1	E980.9	Chloresium	976.8	E858.7	E946.8	E950.4	E962.0	E980.4
Cell stimulants and							Chlorethiazol	967.1	E852.0	E937.1	E950.2	E962.0	E980.2
proliferants	976.8	E858.7	E946.8	E950.4	E962.0	E980.4	Chlorethyl — see Ethyl, chloride						
Cellulose derivatives,							Chloretone	967.1	E852.0	E937.1	E950.2	E962.0	E980.2
cathartic	973.3	E858.4	E943.3	E950.4	E962.0	E980.4	Chlorex	982.3	E862.4	—	E950.9	E962.1	E980.9
nitrates (topical)	976.3	E858.7	E946.3	E950.4	E962.0	E980.4	Chlorhexadol	967.1	E852.0	E937.1	E950.2	E962.0	E980.2
Centipede (bite)	989.5	E905.4	—	E950.9	E962.1	E980.9	Chlorhexidine (hydrochloride)	976.0	E858.7	E946.0	E950.4	E962.0	E980.4
Central nervous system							Chlorhydroxyquinolin	976.0	E858.7	E946.0	E950.4	E962.0	E980.4
depressants	968.4	E855.1	E938.4	E950.4	E962.0	E980.4	Chloride of lime (bleach)	983.9	E864.3	—	E950.7	E962.1	E980.6
anesthetic (general) NEC	968.4	E855.1	E938.4	E950.4	E962.0	E980.4	Chlorinated						
gases NEC	968.2	E855.1	E938.2	E950.4	E962.0	E980.4	camphene	989.2	E863.0	—	E950.6	E962.1	E980.7
intravenous	968.3	E855.1	E938.3	E950.4	E962.0	E980.4	diphenyl	989.89	E866.8	—	E950.9	E962.1	E980.9
barbiturates	967.0	E851	E937.0	E950.1	E962.0	E980.1	hydrocarbons NEC	989.2	E863.0	—	E950.6	E962.1	E980.7
bromides	967.3	E852.2	E937.3	E950.2	E962.0	E980.2	solvent	982.3	E862.4	—	E950.9	E962.1	E980.9
cannabis sativa	969.6	E854.1	E939.6	E950.3	E962.0	E980.3	lime (bleach)	983.9	E864.3	—	E950.7	E962.1	E980.6
chloral hydrate	967.1	E852.0	E937.1	E950.2	E962.0	E980.2	naphthalene — see						
hallucinogenics	969.6	E854.1	E939.6	E950.3	E962.0	E980.3	Naphthalene						
hypnotics	967.9	E852.9	E937.9	E950.2	E962.0	E980.2	pesticides NEC	989.2	E863.0	—	E950.6	E962.1	E980.7
specified NEC	967.8	E852.8	E937.8	E950.2	E962.0	E980.2	soda — see Sodium,						
muscle relaxants	968.0	E855.1	E938.0	E950.4	E962.0	E980.4	hypochlorite						
paraldehyde	967.2	E852.1	E937.2	E950.2	E962.0	E980.2	Chlorine (fumes) (gas)	987.6	E869.8	—	E952.8	E962.2	E982.8
sedatives	967.9	E852.9	E937.9	E950.2	E962.0	E980.2	bleach	983.9	E864.3	—	E950.7	E962.1	E980.6
mixed NEC	967.6	E852.5	E937.6	E950.2	E962.0	E980.2	compounds NEC	983.9	E864.3	—	E950.7	E962.1	E980.6
specified NEC	967.8	E852.8	E937.8	E950.2	E962.0	E980.2	disinfectant	983.9	E861.4	—	E950.7	E962.1	E980.6
muscle-tone depressants	968.0	E855.1	E938.0	E950.4	E962.0	E980.4	releasing agents NEC	983.9	E864.3	—	E950.7	E962.1	E980.6
stimulants	970.9	E854.3	E940.9	E950.4	E962.0	E980.4	Chlorisondamine	972.3	E858.3	E942.3	E950.4	E962.0	E980.4
amphetamines	969.7	E854.2	E939.7	E950.3	E962.0	E980.3	Chlormadinone	962.2	E858.0	E932.2	E950.4	E962.0	E980.4
analeptics	970.0	E854.3	E940.0	E950.4	E962.0	E980.4	Chlormerodrin	974.0	E858.5	E944.0	E950.4	E962.0	E980.4
antidepressants	969.0	E854.0	E939.0	E950.3	E962.0	E980.3	Chlormethiazole	967.1	E852.0	E937.1	E950.2	E962.0	E980.2
opiate antagonists	970.1	E854.3	E940.1	E950.4	E962.0	E980.4	Chlormethylenecycline	960.4	E856	E930.4	E950.4	E962.0	E980.4
specified NEC	970.8	E854.3	E940.8	E950.4	E962.0	E980.4	Chlormezanone	969.5	E853.8	E939.5	E950.3	E962.0	E980.3
Cephalexin	960.5	E856	E930.5	E950.4	E962.0	E980.4	Chloroacetophenone	987.5	E869.3	—	E952.8	E962.2	E982.8
Cephaloglycin	960.5	E856	E930.5	E950.4	E962.0	E980.4	Chloroaniline	983.0	E864.0	—	E950.7	E962.1	E980.6
Cephaloridine	960.5	E856	E930.5	E950.4	E962.0	E980.4	Chlorobenzene,						
Cephalosporins NEC	960.5	E856	E930.5	E950.4	E962.0	E980.4	chlorobenzol	982.0	E862.4	—	E950.9	E962.1	E980.9
N (adicillin)	960.0	E856	E930.0	E950.4	E962.0	E980.4	Chlorobutanol	967.1	E852.0	E937.1	E950.2	E962.0	E980.2
Cephalothin (sodium)	960.5	E856	E930.5	E950.4	E962.0	E980.4	Chlorodinitrobenzene	983.0	E864.0	—	E950.7	E962.1	E980.6
Cerbera (odollam)	988.2	E865.4	—	E950.9	E962.1	E980.9	dust or vapor	987.8	E869.8	—	E952.8	E962.2	E982.8
Cerberin	972.1	E858.3	E942.1	E950.4	E962.0	E980.4	Chloroethane — see Ethyl,						
Cerebral stimulants	970.9	E854.3	E940.9	E950.4	E962.0	E980.4	chloride						
psychotherapeutic	969.7	E854.2	E939.7	E950.3	E962.0	E980.3	Chloroform (fumes) (vapor)	987.8	E869.8	—	E952.8	E962.2	E982.8
specified NEC	970.8	E854.3	E940.8	E950.4	E962.0	E980.4	anesthetic (gas)	968.2	E855.1	E938.2	E950.4	E962.0	E980.4
Cetalkonium (chloride)	976.0	E858.7	E946.0	E950.4	E962.0	E980.4	liquid NEC	968.4	E855.1	E938.4	E950.4	E962.0	E980.4
Cetoxime	963.0	E858.1	E933.0	E950.4	E962.0	E980.4	solvent	982.3	E862.4	—	E950.9	E962.1	E980.9
							Chloroguanide	961.4	E857	E931.4	E950.4	E962.0	E980.4

☑ Additional Digit Required   ▶◀ Revised Text   ● New Line   ▲ Revised Code

	Poisoning	External Cause (E-Code)				
	Poisoning	Accident	Therapeutic Use	Suicide Attempt	Assault	Undetermined
Chloromycetin	960.2	E856	E930.2	E950.4	E962.0	E980.4
ENT agent	976.6	E858.7	E946.6	E950.4	E962.0	E980.4
ophthalmic preparation	976.5	E858.7	E946.5	E950.4	E962.0	E980.4
otic solution	976.6	E858.7	E946.6	E950.4	E962.0	E980.4
topical NEC	976.0	E858.7	E946.0	E950.4	E962.0	E980.4
Chloronitrobenzene	983.0	E864.0	—	E950.7	E962.1	E980.6
dust or vapor	987.8	E869.8	—	E952.8	E962.2	E982.8
Chlorophenol	983.0	E864.0	—	E950.7	E962.1	E980.6
Chlorophenothane	989.2	E863.0	—	E950.6	E962.1	E980.7
Chlorophyll (derivatives)	976.8	E858.7	E946.8	E950.4	E962.0	E980.4
Chloropicrin (fumes)	987.8	E869.8	—	E952.8	E962.2	E982.8
fumigant	989.4	E863.8	—	E950.6	E962.1	E980.7
fungicide	989.4	E863.6	—	E950.6	E962.1	E980.7
pesticide (fumes)	989.4	E863.4	—	E950.6	E962.1	E980.7
Chloroprocaine	968.9	E855.2	E938.9	E950.4	E962.0	E980.4
infiltration (subcutaneous)	968.5	E855.2	E938.5	E950.4	E962.0	E980.4
nerve block (peripheral)						
(plexus)	968.6	E855.2	E938.6	E950.4	E962.0	E980.4
Chloroptic	976.5	E858.7	E946.5	E950.4	E962.0	E980.4
Chloropurine	963.1	E858.1	E933.1	E950.4	E962.0	E980.4
Chloroquine (hydrochloride)						
(phosphate)	961.4	E857	E931.4	E950.4	E962.0	E980.4
Chlorothen	963.0	E858.1	E933.0	E950.4	E962.0	E980.4
Chlorothiazide	974.3	E858.5	E944.3	E950.4	E962.0	E980.4
Chlorotrianisene	962.2	E858.0	E932.2	E950.4	E962.0	E980.4
Chlorovinyldichloroarsine	985.1	E866.3	—	E950.8	E962.1	E980.8
Chloroxylenol	976.0	E858.7	E946.0	E950.4	E962.0	E980.4
Chlorphenesin (carbamate)	968.0	E855.1	E938.0	E950.4	E962.0	E980.4
topical (antifungal)	976.0	E858.7	E946.0	E950.4	E962.0	E980.4
Chlorpheniramine	963.0	E858.1	E933.0	E950.4	E962.0	E980.4
Chlorphenoxamine	966.4	E855.0	E936.4	E950.4	E962.0	E980.4
Chlorphentermine	977.0	E858.8	E947.0	E950.4	E962.0	E980.4
Chlorproguanil	961.4	E857	E931.4	E950.4	E962.0	E980.4
Chlorpromazine	969.1	E853.0	E939.1	E950.3	E962.0	E980.3
Chlorpropamide	962.3	E858.0	E932.3	E950.4	E962.0	E980.4
Chlorprothixene	969.3	E853.8	E939.3	E950.3	E962.0	E980.3
Chlorquinaldol	976.0	E858.7	E946.0	E950.4	E962.0	E980.4
Chlortetracycline	960.4	E856	E930.4	E950.4	E962.0	E980.4
Chlorthalidone	974.4	E858.5	E944.4	E950.4	E962.0	E980.4
Chlortrianisene	962.2	E858.0	E932.2	E950.4	E962.0	E980.4
Chlor-Trimeton	963.0	E858.1	E933.0	E950.4	E962.0	E980.4
Chlorzoxazone	968.0	E855.1	E938.0	E950.4	E962.0	E980.4
Choke damp	987.8	E869.8	—	E952.8	E962.2	E982.8
Cholebrine	977.8	E858.8	E947.8	E950.4	E962.0	E980.4
Cholera vaccine	978.2	E858.8	E948.2	E950.4	E962.0	E980.4
Cholesterol-lowering						
agents	972.2	E858.3	E942.2	E950.4	E962.0	E980.4
Cholestyramine (resin)	972.2	E858.3	E942.2	E950.4	E962.0	E980.4
Cholic acid	973.4	E858.4	E943.4	E950.4	E962.0	E980.4
Choline						
dihydrogen citrate	977.1	E858.8	E947.1	E950.4	E962.0	E980.4
salicylate	965.1	E850.3	E935.3	E950.0	E962.0	E980.0
theophyllinate	974.1	E858.5	E944.1	E950.4	E962.0	E980.4
Cholinergics	971.0	E855.3	E941.0	E950.4	E962.0	E980.4
Cholografin	977.8	E858.8	E947.8	E950.4	E962.0	E980.4
Chorionic gonadotropin	962.4	E858.0	E932.4	E950.4	E962.0	E980.4
Chromates	983.9	E864.3	—	E950.7	E962.1	E980.6
dust or mist	987.8	E869.8	—	E952.8	E962.2	E982.8
lead	984.0	E866.0	—	E950.9	E962.1	E980.9
paint	984.0	E861.5	—	E950.9	E962.1	E980.9
Chromic acid	983.9	E864.3	—	E950.7	E962.1	E980.6
dust or mist	987.8	E869.8	—	E952.8	E962.2	E982.8
Chromium	985.6	E866.4	—	E950.9	E962.1	E980.9
compounds — see Chromates						
Chromonar	972.4	E858.3	E942.4	E950.4	E962.0	E980.4
Chromyl chloride	983.9	E864.3	—	E950.7	E962.1	E980.6
Chrysarobin (ointment)	976.4	E858.7	E946.4	E950.4	E962.0	E980.4
Chrysazin	973.1	E858.4	E943.1	E950.4	E962.0	E980.4
Chymar	963.4	E858.1	E933.4	E950.4	E962.0	E980.4
ophthalmic preparation	976.5	E858.7	E946.5	E950.4	E962.0	E980.4
Chymotrypsin	963.4	E858.1	E933.4	E950.4	E962.0	E980.4
ophthalmic preparation	976.5	E858.7	E946.5	E950.4	E962.0	E980.4
Cicuta maculata or virosa	988.2	E865.4	—	E950.9	E962.1	E980.9
Cigarette lighter fluid	981	E862.1	—	E950.9	E962.1	E980.9
Cinchocaine (spinal)	968.7	E855.2	E938.7	E950.4	E962.0	E980.4
topical (surface)	968.5	E855.2	E938.5	E950.4	E962.0	E980.4
Cinchona	961.4	E857	E931.4	E950.4	E962.0	E980.4
Cinchonine alkaloids	961.4	E857	E931.4	E950.4	E962.0	E980.4
Cinchophen	974.7	E858.5	E944.7	E950.4	E962.0	E980.4

	Poisoning	External Cause (E-Code)				
	Poisoning	Accident	Therapeutic Use	Suicide Attempt	Assault	Undetermined
Cinnarizine	963.0	E858.1	E933.0	E950.4	E962.0	E980.4
Citanest	968.9	E855.2	E938.9	E950.4	E962.0	E980.4
infiltration (subcutaneous)	968.5	E855.2	E938.5	E950.4	E962.0	E980.4
nerve block (peripheral)						
(plexus)	968.6	E855.2	E938.6	E950.4	E962.0	E980.4
Citric acid	989.89	E866.8	—	E950.9	E962.1	E980.9
Citrovorum factor	964.1	E858.2	E934.1	E950.4	E962.0	E980.4
Claviceps purpurea	988.2	E865.4	—	E950.9	E962.1	E980.9
Cleaner, cleansing agent						
NEC	989.89	E861.3	—	E950.9	E962.1	E980.9
of paint or varnish	982.8	E862.9	—	E950.9	E962.1	E980.9
Clematis vitalba	988.2	E865.4	—	E950.9	E962.1	E980.9
Clemizole	963.0	E858.1	E933.0	E950.4	E962.0	E980.4
penicillin	960.0	E856	E930.0	E950.4	E962.0	E980.4
Clidinium	971.1	E855.4	E941.1	E950.4	E962.0	E980.4
Clindamycin	960.8	E856	E930.8	E950.4	E962.0	E980.4
Cliradon	965.09	E850.2	E935.2	E950.0	E962.0	E980.0
Clocortolone	962.0	E858.0	E932.0	E950.4	E962.0	E980.4
Clodanol	975.4	E858.6	E945.4	E950.4	E962.0	E980.4
Clofibrate	972.2	E858.3	E942.2	E950.4	E962.0	E980.4
Clomethiazole	967.1	E852.0	E937.1	E950.2	E962.0	E980.2
Clomiphene	977.8	E858.8	E947.8	E950.4	E962.0	E980.4
Clonazepam	969.4	E853.2	E939.4	E950.3	E962.0	E980.3
Clonidine	972.6	E858.3	E942.6	E950.4	E962.0	E980.4
Clopamide	974.3	E858.5	E944.3	E950.4	E962.0	E980.4
Clorazepate	969.4	E853.2	E939.4	E950.3	E962.0	E980.3
Clorexolone	974.4	E858.5	E944.4	E950.4	E962.0	E980.4
Clorox (bleach)	983.9	E864.3	—	E950.7	E962.1	E980.6
Clortermine	977.0	E858.8	E947.0	E950.4	E962.0	E980.4
Clotrimazole	976.0	E858.7	E946.0	E950.4	E962.0	E980.4
Cloxacillin	960.0	E856	E930.0	E950.4	E962.0	E980.4
Coagulants NEC	964.5	E858.2	E934.5	E950.4	E962.0	E980.4
Coal (carbon monoxide from) — see also Carbon, monoxide, coal						
oil — see Kerosene						
tar NEC	983.0	E864.0	—	E950.7	E962.1	E980.6
fumes	987.8	E869.8	—	E952.8	E962.2	E982.8
medicinal (ointment)	976.4	E858.7	E946.4	E950.4	E962.0	E980.4
analgesics NEC	965.5	E850.5	E935.5	E950.0	E962.0	E980.0
naphtha (solvent)	981	E862.0	—	E950.9	E962.1	E980.9
Cobalt (fumes) (industrial)	985.8	E866.4	—	E950.9	E962.1	E980.9
Cobra (venom)	989.5	E905.0	—	E950.9	E962.1	E980.9
Coca (leaf)	970.8	E854.3	E940.8	E950.4	E962.0	E980.4
Cocaine (hydrochloride) (salt)	970.8	E854.3	E940.8	E950.4	E962.0	E980.4
topical anesthetic	968.5	E855.2	E938.5	E950.4	E962.0	E980.4
Coccidioidin	977.8	E858.8	E947.8	E950.4	E962.0	E980.4
Cocculus indicus	988.2	E865.3	—	E950.9	E962.1	E980.9
Cochineal	989.89	E866.8	—	E950.9	E962.1	E980.9
medicinal products	977.4	E858.8	E947.4	E950.4	E962.0	E980.4
Codeine	965.09	E850.2	E935.2	E950.0	E962.0	E980.0
Coffee	989.89	E866.8	—	E950.9	E962.1	E980.9
Cogentin	971.1	E855.4	E941.1	E950.4	E962.0	E980.4
Coke fumes or gas (carbon monoxide)	986	E868.3	—	E952.1	E962.2	E982.1
industrial use	986	E868.8	—	E952.1	E962.2	E982.1
Colace	973.2	E858.4	E943.2	E950.4	E962.0	E980.4
Colchicine	974.7	E858.5	E944.7	E950.4	E962.0	E980.4
Colchicum	988.2	E865.3	—	E950.9	E962.1	E980.9
Cold cream	976.3	E858.7	E946.3	E950.4	E962.0	E980.4
Colestipol	972.2	E858.3	E942.2	E950.4	E962.0	E980.4
Colistimethate	960.8	E856	E930.8	E950.4	E962.0	E980.4
Colistin	960.8	E856	E930.8	E950.4	E962.0	E980.4
Collagenase	976.8	E858.7	E946.8	E950.4	E962.0	E980.4
Collagen	977.8	E866.8	E947.8	E950.9	E962.1	E980.9
Collodion (flexible)	976.3	E858.7	E946.3	E950.4	E962.0	E980.4
Colocynth	973.1	E858.4	E943.1	E950.4	E962.0	E980.4
Coloring matter — see Dye(s)						
Combustion gas — see Carbon, monoxide						
Compazine	969.1	E853.0	E939.1	E950.3	E962.0	E980.3
Compound						
42 (warfarin)	989.4	E863.7	—	E950.6	E962.1	E980.7
269 (endrin)	989.2	E863.0	—	E950.6	E962.1	E980.7
497 (dieldrin)	989.2	E863.0	—	E950.6	E962.1	E980.7
1080 (sodium fluoroacetate)	989.4	E863.7	—	E950.6	E962.1	E980.7
3422 (parathion)	989.3	E863.1	—	E950.6	E962.1	E980.7
3911 (phorate)	989.3	E863.1	—	E950.6	E962.1	E980.7
3956 (toxaphene)	989.2	E863.0	—	E950.6	E962.1	E980.7
4049 (malathion)	989.3	E863.1	—	E950.6	E962.1	E980.7

☑ Additional Digit Required   ►◄ Revised Text   ● New Line   ▲ Revised Code

	External Cause (E-Code)							External Cause (E-Code)				
	Poisoning	Accident	Therapeutic Use	Suicide Attempt	Assault	Undetermined		Poisoning	Accident	Therapeutic Use	Suicide Attempt	Assault	Undetermined
Compound — *continued*							**Cough mixtures**						
4124 (dicapthon)	989.4	E863.4	—	E950.6	E962.1	E980.7	(antitussives)	975.4	E858.6	E945.4	E950.4	E962.0	E980.4
E (cortisone)	962.0	E858.0	E932.0	E950.4	E962.0	E980.4	containing opiates	965.09	E850.2	E935.2	E950.0	E962.0	E980.0
F (hydrocortisone)	962.0	E858.0	E932.0	E950.4	E962.0	E980.4	expectorants	975.5	E858.6	E945.5	E950.4	E962.0	E980.4
Congo red	977.8	E858.8	E947.8	E950.4	E962.0	E980.4	**Coumadin**	964.2	E858.2	E934.2	E950.4	E962.0	E980.4
Coniine, conine	965.7	E850.7	E935.7	E950.0	E962.0	E980.0	rodenticide	989.4	E863.7	—	E950.6	E962.1	E980.7
Conium (maculatum)	988.2	E865.4	—	E950.9	E962.1	E980.9	**Coumarin**	964.2	E858.2	E934.2	E950.4	E962.0	E980.4
Conjugated estrogens							**Coumetarol**	964.2	E858.2	E934.2	E950.4	E962.0	E980.4
(equine)	962.2	E858.0	E932.2	E950.4	E962.0	E980.4	**Cowbane**	988.2	E865.4	—	E950.9	E962.1	E980.9
Contac	975.6	E858.6	E945.6	E950.4	E962.0	E980.4	**Cozyme**	963.5	E858.1	E933.5	E950.4	E962.0	E980.4
Contact lens solution	976.5	E858.7	E946.5	E950.4	E962.0	E980.4	**Crack**	970.8	E854.3	E940.8	E950.4	E962.0	E980.4
Contraceptives (oral)	962.2	E858.0	E932.2	E950.4	E962.0	E980.4	**Creolin**	983.0	E864.0	—	E950.7	E962.1	E980.6
vaginal	976.8	E858.7	E946.8	E950.4	E962.0	E980.4	disinfectant	983.0	E861.4	—	E950.7	E962.1	E980.6
Contrast media							**Creosol** (compound)	983.0	E864.0	—	E950.7	E962.1	E980.6
(roentgenographic)	977.8	E858.8	E947.8	E950.4	E962.0	E980.4	**Creosote** (beechwood)						
Convallaria majalis	988.2	E865.4	—	E950.9	E962.1	E980.9	(coal tar)	983.0	E864.0	—	E950.7	E962.1	E980.6
Copper (dust) (fumes)							medicinal (expectorant)	975.5	E858.6	E945.5	E950.4	E962.0	E980.4
(salts) NEC	985.8	E866.4	—	E950.9	E962.1	E980.9	syrup	975.5	E858.6	E945.5	E950.4	E962.0	E980.4
arsenate, arsenite	985.1	E866.3	—	E950.8	E962.1	E980.8	**Cresol**	983.0	E864.0	—	E950.7	E962.1	E980.6
insecticide	985.1	E863.4	—	E950.8	E962.1	E980.8	disinfectant	983.0	E861.4	—	E950.7	E962.1	E980.6
emetic	973.6	E858.4	E943.6	E950.4	E962.0	E980.4	**Cresylic acid**	983.0	E864.0	—	E950.7	E962.1	E980.6
fungicide	985.8	E863.6	—	E950.6	E962.1	E980.7	**Cropropamide**	965.7	E850.7	E935.7	E950.0	E962.0	E980.0
insecticide	985.8	E863.4	—	E950.6	E962.1	E980.7	with crotethamide	970.0	E854.3	E940.0	E950.4	E962.0	E980.4
oleate	976.0	E858.7	E946.0	E950.4	E962.0	E980.4	**Crotamiton**	976.0	E858.7	E946.0	E950.4	E962.0	E980.4
sulfate	983.9	E864.3	—	E950.7	E962.1	E980.6	**Crotethamide**	965.7	E850.7	E935.7	E950.0	E962.0	E980.0
fungicide	983.9	E863.6	—	E950.7	E962.1	E980.6	with cropropamide	970.0	E854.3	E940.0	E950.4	E962.0	E980.4
cupric	973.6	E858.4	E943.6	E950.4	E962.0	E980.4	**Croton** (oil)	973.1	E858.4	E943.1	E950.4	E962.0	E980.4
cuprous	983.9	E864.3	—	E950.7	E962.1	E980.6	chloral	967.1	E852.0	E937.1	E950.2	E962.0	E980.2
Copperhead snake (bite)							**Crude oil**	981	E862.1	—	E950.9	E962.1	E980.9
(venom)	989.5	E905.0	—	E950.9	E962.1	E980.9	**Cryogenine**	965.8	E850.8	E935.8	E950.0	E962.0	E980.0
Coral (sting)	989.5	E905.6	—	E950.9	E962.1	E980.9	**Cryolite** (pesticide)	989.4	E863.4	—	E950.6	E962.1	E980.7
snake (bite) (venom)	989.5	E905.0	—	E950.9	E962.1	E980.9	**Cryptenamine**	972.6	E858.3	E942.6	E950.4	E962.0	E980.4
Cordran	976.0	E858.7	E946.0	E950.4	E962.0	E980.4	**Crystal violet**	976.0	E858.7	E946.0	E950.4	E962.0	E980.4
Corn cures	976.4	E858.7	E946.4	E950.4	E962.0	E980.4	**Cuckoopint**	988.2	E865.4	—	E950.9	E962.1	E980.9
Cornhusker's lotion	976.3	E858.7	E946.3	E950.4	E962.0	E980.4	**Cumetharol**	964.2	E858.2	E934.2	E950.4	E962.0	E980.4
Corn starch	976.3	E858.7	E946.3	E950.4	E962.0	E980.4	**Cupric sulfate**	973.6	E858.4	E943.6	E950.4	E962.0	E980.4
Corrosive	983.9	E864.4	—	E950.7	E962.1	E980.6	**Cuprous sulfate**	983.9	E864.3	—	E950.7	E962.1	E980.6
acids NEC	983.1	E864.1	—	E950.7	E962.1	E980.6	**Curare, curarine**	975.2	E858.6	E945.2	E950.4	E962.0	E980.4
aromatics	983.0	E864.0	—	E950.7	E962.1	E980.6	**Cyanic acid** — *see* Cyanide(s)						
disinfectant	983.0	E861.4	—	E950.7	E962.1	E980.6	**Cyanide(s)** (compounds)						
fumes NEC	987.9	E869.9	—	E952.9	E962.2	E982.9	(hydrogen) (potassium)						
specified NEC	983.9	E864.3	—	E950.7	E962.1	E980.6	(sodium) NEC	989.0	E866.8	—	E950.9	E962.1	E980.9
sublimate — *see*							dust or gas (inhalation)						
Mercury, chloride							NEC	987.7	E869.8	—	E952.8	E962.2	E982.8
Cortate	962.0	E858.0	E932.0	E950.4	E962.0	E980.4	fumigant	989.0	E863.8	—	E950.6	E962.1	E980.7
Cort-Dome	962.0	E858.0	E932.0	E950.4	E962.0	E980.4	mercuric — *see* Mercury						
ENT agent	976.6	E858.7	E946.6	E950.4	E962.0	E980.4	pesticide (dust) (fumes)	989.0	E863.4	—	E950.6	E962.1	E980.7
ophthalmic preparation	976.5	E858.7	E946.5	E950.4	E962.0	E980.4	**Cyanocobalamin**	964.1	E858.2	E934.1	E950.4	E962.0	E980.4
topical NEC	976.0	E858.7	E946.0	E950.4	E962.0	E980.4	**Cyanogen** (chloride) (gas)						
Cortef	962.0	E858.0	E932.0	E950.4	E962.0	E980.4	NEC	987.8	E869.8	—	E952.8	E962.2	E982.8
ENT agent	976.6	E858.7	E946.6	E950.4	E962.0	E980.4	**Cyclaine**	968.5	E855.2	E938.5	E950.4	E962.0	E980.4
ophthalmic preparation	976.5	E858.7	E946.5	E950.4	E962.0	E980.4	**Cyclamen europaeum**	988.2	E865.4	—	E950.9	E962.1	E980.9
topical NEC	976.0	E858.7	E946.0	E950.4	E962.0	E980.4	**Cyclandelate**	972.5	E858.3	E942.5	E950.4	E962.0	E980.4
Corticosteroids (fluorinated)	962.0	E858.0	E932.0	E950.4	E962.0	E980.4	**Cyclazocine**	965.09	E850.2	E935.2	E950.0	E962.0	E980.0
ENT agent	976.6	E858.7	E946.6	E950.4	E962.0	E980.4	**Cyclizine**	963.0	E858.1	E933.0	E950.4	E962.0	E980.4
ophthalmic preparation	976.5	E858.7	E946.5	E950.4	E962.0	E980.4	**Cyclobarbital,**						
topical NEC	976.0	E858.7	E946.0	E950.4	E962.0	E980.4	**cyclobarbitone**	967.0	E851	E937.0	E950.1	E962.0	E980.1
Corticotropin	962.4	E858.0	E932.4	E950.4	E962.0	E980.4	**Cycloguanil**	961.4	E857	E931.4	E950.4	E962.0	E980.4
Cortisol	962.0	E858.0	E932.0	E950.4	E962.0	E980.4	**Cyclohexane**	982.0	E862.4	—	E950.9	E962.1	E980.9
ENT agent	976.6	E858.7	E946.6	E950.4	E962.0	E980.4	**Cyclohexanol**	980.8	E860.8	—	E950.9	E962.1	E980.9
ophthalmic preparation	976.5	E858.7	E946.5	E950.4	E962.0	E980.4	**Cyclohexanone**	982.8	E862.4	—	E950.9	E962.1	E980.9
topical NEC	976.0	E858.7	E946.0	E950.4	E962.0	E980.4	**Cyclomethycaine**	968.5	E855.2	E938.5	E950.4	E962.0	E980.4
Cortisone derivatives							**Cyclopentamine**	971.2	E855.5	E941.2	E950.4	E962.0	E980.4
(acetate)	962.0	E858.0	E932.0	E950.4	E962.0	E980.4	**Cyclopenthiazide**	974.3	E858.5	E944.3	E950.4	E962.0	E980.4
ENT agent	976.6	E858.7	E946.6	E950.4	E962.0	E980.4	**Cyclopentolate**	971.1	E855.4	E941.1	E950.4	E962.0	E980.4
ophthalmic preparation	976.5	E858.7	E946.5	E950.4	E962.0	E980.4	**Cyclophosphamide**	963.1	E858.1	E933.1	E950.4	E962.0	E980.4
topical NEC	976.0	E858.7	E946.0	E950.4	E962.0	E980.4	**Cyclopropane**	968.2	E855.1	E938.2	E950.4	E962.0	E980.4
Cortogen	962.0	E858.0	E932.0	E950.4	E962.0	E980.4	**Cycloserine**	960.6	E856	E930.6	E950.4	E962.0	E980.4
ENT agent	976.6	E858.7	E946.6	E950.4	E962.0	E980.4	**Cyclothiazide**	974.3	E858.5	E944.3	E950.4	E962.0	E980.4
ophthalmic preparation	976.5	E858.7	E946.5	E950.4	E962.0	E980.4	**Cycrimine**	966.4	E855.0	E936.4	E950.4	E962.0	E980.4
Cortone	962.0	E858.0	E932.0	E950.4	E962.0	E980.4	**Cymarin**	972.1	E858.3	E942.1	E950.4	E962.0	E980.4
ENT agent	976.6	E858.7	E946.6	E950.4	E962.0	E980.4	**Cyproheptadine**	963.0	E858.1	E933.0	E950.4	E962.0	E980.4
ophthalmic preparation	976.5	E858.7	E946.5	E950.4	E962.0	E980.4	**Cyprolidol**	969.0	E854.0	E939.0	E950.3	E962.0	E980.3
Cortril	962.0	E858.0	E932.0	E950.4	E962.0	E980.4	**Cytarabine**	963.1	E858.1	E933.1	E950.4	E962.0	E980.4
ENT agent	976.6	E858.7	E946.6	E950.4	E962.0	E980.4	**Cytisus**						
ophthalmic preparation	976.5	E858.7	E946.5	E950.4	E962.0	E980.4	laburnum	988.2	E865.4	—	E950.9	E962.1	E980.9
topical NEC	976.0	E858.7	E946.0	E950.4	E962.0	E980.4	scoparius	988.2	E865.4	—	E950.9	E962.1	E980.9
Cosmetics	989.89	E866.7	—	E950.9	E962.1	E980.9	**Cytomel**	962.7	E858.0	E932.7	E950.4	E962.0	E980.4
Cosyntropin	977.8	E858.8	E947.8	E950.4	E962.0	E980.4	**Cytosine** (antineoplastic)	963.1	E858.1	E933.1	E950.4	E962.0	E980.4
Cotarnine	964.5	E858.2	E934.5	E950.4	E962.0	E980.4	**Cytoxan**	963.1	E858.1	E933.1	E950.4	E962.0	E980.4
Cottonseed oil	976.3	E858.7	E946.3	E950.4	E962.0	E980.4	**Dacarbazine**	963.1	E858.1	E933.1	E950.4	E962.0	E980.4

		External Cause (E-Code)				
	Poisoning	Accident	Therapeutic Use	Suicide Attempt	Assault	Undetermined
Dactinomycin	960.7	E856	E930.7	E950.4	E962.0	E980.4
DADPS	961.8	E857	E931.8	E950.4	E962.0	E980.4
Dakin's solution (external)	976.0	E858.7	E946.0	E950.4	E962.0	E980.4
Dalmane	969.4	E853.2	E939.4	E950.3	E962.0	E980.3
DAM	977.2	E858.8	E947.2	E950.4	E962.0	E980.4
Danilone	964.2	E858.2	E934.2	E950.4	E962.0	E980.4
Danthron	973.1	E858.4	E943.1	E950.4	E962.0	E980.4
Dantrolene	975.2	E858.6	E945.2	E950.4	E962.0	E980.4
Daphne (gnidium) (mezereum)	988.2	E865.4	—	E950.9	E962.1	E980.9
berry	988.2	E865.3	—	E950.9	E962.1	E980.9
Dapsone	961.8	E857	E931.8	E950.4	E962.0	E980.4
Daraprim	961.4	E857	E931.4	E950.4	E962.0	E980.4
Darnel	988.2	E865.3	—	E950.9	E962.1	E980.9
Darvon	965.8	E850.8	E935.8	E950.0	E962.0	E980.0
Daunorubicin	960.7	E856	E930.7	E950.4	E962.0	E980.4
DBI	962.3	E858.0	E932.3	E950.4	E962.0	E980.4
D-Con (rodenticide)	989.4	E863.7	—	E950.6	E962.1	E980.7
DDS	961.8	E857	E931.8	E950.4	E962.0	E980.4
DDT	989.2	E863.0	—	E950.6	E962.1	E980.7
Deadly nightshade	988.2	E865.4	—	E950.9	E962.1	E980.9
berry	988.2	E865.3	—	E950.9	E962.1	E980.9
Deanol	969.7	E854.2	E939.7	E950.3	E962.0	E980.3
Debrisoquine	972.6	E858.3	E942.6	E950.4	E962.0	E980.4
Decaborane	989.89	E866.8	—	E950.9	E962.1	E980.9
fumes	987.8	E869.8	—	E952.8	E962.2	E982.8
Decadron	962.0	E858.0	E932.0	E950.4	E962.0	E980.4
ENT agent	976.6	E858.7	E946.6	E950.4	E962.0	E980.4
ophthalmic preparation	976.5	E858.7	E946.5	E950.4	E962.0	E980.4
topical NEC	976.0	E858.7	E946.0	E950.4	E962.0	E980.4
Decahydronaphthalene	982.0	E862.4	—	E950.9	E962.1	E980.9
Decalin	982.0	E862.4	—	E950.9	E962.1	E980.9
Decamethonium	975.2	E858.6	E945.2	E950.4	E962.0	E980.4
Decholin	973.4	E858.4	E943.4	E950.4	E962.0	E980.4
sodium (diagnostic)	977.8	E858.8	E947.8	E950.4	E962.0	E980.4
Declomycin	960.4	E856	E930.4	E950.4	E962.0	E980.4
Deferoxamine	963.8	E858.1	E933.8	E950.4	E962.0	E980.4
Dehydrocholic acid	973.4	E858.4	E943.4	E950.4	E962.0	E980.4
DeKalin	982.0	E862.4	—	E950.9	E962.1	E980.9
Delalutin	962.2	E858.0	E932.2	E950.4	E962.0	E980.4
Delphinium	988.2	E865.3	—	E950.9	E962.1	E980.9
Deltasone	962.0	E858.0	E932.0	E950.4	E962.0	E980.4
Delta	962.0	E858.0	E932.0	E950.4	E962.0	E980.4
Delvinal	967.0	E851	E937.0	E950.1	E962.0	E980.1
Demecarium (bromide)	971.0	E855.3	E941.0	E950.4	E962.0	E980.4
Demeclocycline	960.4	E856	E930.4	E950.4	E962.0	E980.4
Demecolcine	963.1	E858.1	E933.1	E950.4	E962.0	E980.4
Demelanizing agents	976.8	E858.7	E946.8	E950.4	E962.0	E980.4
Demerol	965.09	E850.2	E935.2	E950.0	E962.0	E980.0
Demethylchlortetracycline	960.4	E856	E930.4	E950.4	E962.0	E980.4
Demethyltetracycline	960.4	E856	E930.4	E950.4	E962.0	E980.4
Demeton	989.3	E863.1	—	E950.6	E962.1	E980.7
Demulcents	976.3	E858.7	E946.3	E950.4	E962.0	E980.4
Demulen	962.2	E858.0	E932.2	E950.4	E962.0	E980.4
Denatured alcohol	980.0	E860.1	—	E950.9	E962.1	E980.9
Dendrid	976.5	E858.7	E946.5	E950.4	E962.0	E980.4
Dental agents, topical	976.7	E858.7	E946.7	E950.4	E962.0	E980.4
Deodorant spray (feminine hygiene)	976.8	E858.7	E946.8	E950.4	E962.0	E980.4
Deoxyribonuclease	963.4	E858.1	E933.4	E950.4	E962.0	E980.4
Depressants						
appetite, central	977.0	E858.8	E947.0	E950.4	E962.0	E980.4
cardiac	972.0	E858.3	E942.0	E950.4	E962.0	E980.4
central nervous system						
(anesthetic)	968.4	E855.1	E938.4	E950.4	E962.0	E980.4
psychotherapeutic	969.5	E853.9	E939.5	E950.3	E962.0	E980.3
Dequalinium	976.0	E858.7	E946.0	E950.4	E962.0	E980.4
Dermolate	976.2	E858.7	E946.2	E950.4	E962.0	E980.4
DES	962.2	E858.0	E932.2	E950.4	E962.0	E980.4
Desenex	976.0	E858.7	E946.0	E950.4	E962.0	E980.4
Deserpidine	972.6	E858.3	E942.6	E950.4	E962.0	E980.4
Desipramine	969.0	E854.0	E939.0	E950.3	E962.0	E980.3
Deslanoside	972.1	E858.3	E942.1	E950.4	E962.0	E980.4
Desocodeine	965.09	E850.2	E935.2	E950.0	E962.0	E980.0
Desomorphine	965.09	E850.2	E935.2	E950.0	E962.0	E980.0
Desonide	976.0	E858.7	E946.0	E950.4	E962.0	E980.4
Desoxycorticosterone derivatives	962.0	E858.0	E932.0	E950.4	E962.0	E980.4
Desoxyephedrine	969.7	E854.2	E939.7	E950.3	E962.0	E980.3
DET	969.6	E854.1	E939.6	E950.3	E962.0	E980.3
Detergents (ingested) (synthetic)	989.6	E861.0	—	E950.9	E962.1	E980.9
external medication	976.2	E858.7	E946.2	E950.4	E962.0	E980.4

		External Cause (E-Code)				
	Poisoning	Accident	Therapeutic Use	Suicide Attempt	Assault	Undetermined
Deterrent, alcohol	977.3	E858.8	E947.3	E950.4	E962.0	E980.4
Detrothyronine	962.7	E858.0	E932.7	E950.4	E962.0	E980.4
Dettol (external medication)	976.0	E858.7	E946.0	E950.4	E962.0	E980.4
Dexamethasone	962.0	E858.0	E932.0	E950.4	E962.0	E980.4
ENT agent	976.6	E858.7	E946.6	E950.4	E962.0	E980.4
ophthalmic preparation	976.5	E858.7	E946.5	E950.4	E962.0	E980.4
topical NEC	976.0	E858.7	E946.0	E950.4	E962.0	E980.4
Dexamphetamine	969.7	E854.2	E939.7	E950.3	E962.0	E980.3
Dexedrine	969.7	E854.2	E939.7	E950.3	E962.0	E980.3
Dexpanthenol	963.5	E858.1	E933.5	E950.4	E962.0	E980.4
Dextran	964.8	E858.2	E934.8	E950.4	E962.0	E980.4
Dextriferron	964.0	E858.2	E934.0	E950.4	E962.0	E980.4
Dextroamphetamine	969.7	E854.2	E939.7	E950.3	E962.0	E980.3
Dextro calcium pantothenate	963.5	E858.1	E933.5	E950.4	E962.0	E980.4
Dextromethorphan	975.4	E858.6	E945.4	E950.4	E962.0	E980.4
Dextromoramide	965.09	E850.2	E935.2	E950.0	E962.0	E980.0
Dextro pantothenyl alcohol	963.5	E858.1	E933.5	E950.4	E962.0	E980.4
topical	976.8	E858.7	E946.8	E950.4	E962.0	E980.4
Dextropropoxyphene (hydrochloride)	965.8	E850.8	E935.8	E950.0	E962.0	E980.0
Dextrorphan	965.09	E850.2	E935.2	E950.0	E962.0	E980.0
Dextrose NEC	974.5	E858.5	E944.5	E950.4	E962.0	E980.4
Dextrothyroxin	962.7	E858.0	E932.7	E950.4	E962.0	E980.4
DFP	971.0	E855.3	E941.0	E950.4	E962.0	E980.4
DHE-45	972.9	E858.3	E942.9	E950.4	E962.0	E980.4
Diabinese	962.3	E858.0	E932.3	E950.4	E962.0	E980.4
Diacetyl monoxime	977.2	E858.8	E947.2	E950.4	E962.0	E980.4
Diacetylmorphine	965.01	E850.0	E935.0	E950.0	E962.0	E980.0
Diagnostic agents	977.8	E858.8	E947.8	E950.4	E962.0	E980.4
Dial (soap)	976.2	E858.7	E946.2	E950.4	E962.0	E980.4
sedative	967.0	E851	E937.0	E950.1	E962.0	E980.1
Diallylbarbituric acid	967.0	E851	E937.0	E950.1	E962.0	E980.1
Diaminodiphenylsulfone	961.8	E857	E931.8	E950.4	E962.0	E980.4
Diamorphine	965.01	E850.0	E935.0	E950.0	E962.0	E980.0
Diamox	974.2	E858.5	E944.2	E950.4	E962.0	E980.4
Diamthazole	976.0	E858.7	E946.0	E950.4	E962.0	E980.4
Diaphenylsulfone	961.8	E857	E931.8	E950.4	E962.0	E980.4
Diasone (sodium)	961.8	E857	E931.8	E950.4	E962.0	E980.4
Diazepam	969.4	E853.2	E939.4	E950.3	E962.0	E980.3
Diazinon	989.3	E863.1	—	E950.6	E962.1	E980.7
Diazomethane (gas)	987.8	E869.8	—	E952.8	E962.2	E982.8
Diazoxide	972.5	E858.3	E942.5	E950.4	E962.0	E980.4
Dibenamine	971.3	E855.6	E941.3	E950.4	E962.0	E980.4
Dibenzheptropine	963.0	E858.1	E933.0	E950.4	E962.0	E980.4
Dibenzyline	971.3	E855.6	E941.3	E950.4	E962.0	E980.4
Diborane (gas)	987.8	E869.8	—	E952.8	E962.2	E982.8
Dibromomannitol	963.1	E858.1	E933.1	E950.4	E962.0	E980.4
Dibucaine (spinal)	968.7	E855.2	E938.7	E950.4	E962.0	E980.4
topical (surface)	968.5	E855.2	E938.5	E950.4	E962.0	E980.4
Dibunate sodium	975.4	E858.6	E945.4	E950.4	E962.0	E980.4
Dibutoline	971.1	E855.4	E941.1	E950.4	E962.0	E980.4
Dicapthon	989.4	E863.4	—	E950.6	E962.1	E980.7
Dichloralphenazone	967.1	E852.0	E937.1	E950.2	E962.0	E980.2
Dichlorodifluoromethane	987.4	E869.2	—	E952.8	E962.2	E982.8
Dichloroethane	982.3	E862.4	—	E950.9	E962.1	E980.9
Dichloroethylene	982.3	E862.4	—	E950.9	E962.1	E980.9
Dichloroethyl sulfide	987.8	E869.8	—	E952.8	E962.2	E982.8
Dichlorohydrin	982.3	E862.4	—	E950.9	E962.1	E980.9
Dichloromethane (solvent) (vapor)	982.3	E862.4	—	E950.9	E962.1	E980.9
Dichlorophen(e)	961.6	E857	E931.6	E950.4	E962.0	E980.4
Dichlorphenamide	974.2	E858.5	E944.2	E950.4	E962.0	E980.4
Dichlorvos	989.3	E863.1	—	E950.6	E962.1	E980.7
Diclofenac sodium	965.69	E850.6	E935.6	E950.0	E962.0	E980.0
Dicoumarin, dicumarol	964.2	E858.2	E934.2	E950.4	E962.0	E980.4
Dicyanogen (gas)	987.8	E869.8	—	E952.8	E962.2	E982.8
Dicyclomine	971.1	E855.4	E941.1	E950.4	E962.0	E980.4
Dieldrin (vapor)	989.2	E863.0	—	E950.6	E962.1	E980.7
Dienestrol	962.2	E858.0	E932.2	E950.4	E962.0	E980.4
Dietetics	977.0	E858.8	E947.0	E950.4	E962.0	E980.4
Diethazine	966.4	E855.0	E936.4	E950.4	E962.0	E980.4
Diethyl						
barbituric acid	967.0	E851	E937.0	E950.1	E962.0	E980.1
carbamazine	961.6	E857	E931.6	E950.4	E962.0	E980.4
carbinol	980.8	E860.8	—	E950.9	E962.1	E980.9
carbonate	982.8	E862.4	—	E950.9	E962.1	E980.9
ether (vapor) — see ther(s)						
propion	977.0	E858.8	E947.0	E950.4	E962.0	E980.4
stilbestrol	962.2	E858.0	E932.2	E950.4	E962.0	E980.4

☑ Additional Digit Required   ▶◀ Revised Text   ● New Line   ▲ Revised Code

	Poisoning	External Cause (E-Code) Accident	Therapeutic Use	Suicide Attempt	Assault	Undetermined
Diethylene						
dioxide	982.8	E862.4	—	E950.9	E962.1	E980.9
glycol (monoacetate)						
(monoethyl ether)	982.8	E862.4	—	E950.9	E962.1	E980.9
Diethylsulfone-						
diethylmethane	967.8	E852.8	E937.8	E950.2	E962.0	E980.2
Difencloxazine	965.09	E850.2	E935.2	E950.0	E962.0	E980.0
Diffusin	963.4	E858.1	E933.4	E950.4	E962.0	E980.4
Diflos	971.0	E855.3	E941.0	E950.4	E962.0	E980.4
Digestants	973.4	E858.4	E943.4	E950.4	E962.0	E980.4
Digitalin(e)	972.1	E858.3	E942.1	E950.4	E962.0	E980.4
Digitalis glycosides	972.1	E858.3	E942.1	E950.4	E962.0	E980.4
Digitoxin	972.1	E858.3	E942.1	E950.4	E962.0	E980.4
Digoxin	972.1	E858.3	E942.1	E950.4	E962.0	E980.4
Dihydrocodeine	965.09	E850.2	E935.2	E950.0	E962.0	E980.0
Dihydrocodeinone	965.09	E850.2	E935.2	E950.0	E962.0	E980.0
Dihydroergocristine	972.9	E858.3	E942.9	E950.4	E962.0	E980.4
Dihydroergotamine	972.9	E858.3	E942.9	E950.4	E962.0	E980.4
Dihydroergotoxine	972.9	E858.3	E942.9	E950.4	E962.0	E980.4
Dihydrohydroxycodeinone	965.09	E850.2	E935.2	E950.0	E962.0	E980.0
Dihydrohydroxymorphinone	965.09	E850.2	E935.2	E950.0	E962.0	E980.0
Dihydroisocodeine	965.09	E850.2	E935.2	E950.0	E962.0	E980.0
Dihydromorphine	965.09	E850.2	E935.2	E950.0	E962.0	E980.0
Dihydromorphinone	965.09	E850.2	E935.2	E950.0	E962.0	E980.0
Dihydrostreptomycin	960.6	E856	E930.6	E950.4	E962.0	E980.4
Dihydrotachysterol	962.6	E858.0	E932.6	E950.4	E962.0	E980.4
Dihydroxyanthraquinone	973.1	E858.4	E943.1	E950.4	E962.0	E980.4
Dihydroxycodeinone	965.09	E850.2	E935.2	E950.0	E962.0	E980.0
Diiodohydroxyquin	961.3	E857	E931.3	E950.4	E962.0	E980.4
topical	976.0	E858.7	E946.0	E950.4	E962.0	E980.4
Diiodohydroxyquinoline	961.3	E857	E931.3	E950.4	E962.0	E980.4
Dilantin	966.1	E855.0	E936.1	E950.4	E962.0	E980.4
Dilaudid	965.09	E850.2	E935.2	E950.0	E962.0	E980.0
Diloxanide	961.5	E857	E931.5	E950.4	E962.0	E980.4
Dimefline	970.0	E854.3	E940.0	E950.4	E962.0	E980.4
Dimenhydrinate	963.0	E858.1	E933.0	E950.4	E962.0	E980.4
Dimercaprol	963.8	E858.1	E933.8	E950.4	E962.0	E980.4
Dimercaptopropanol	963.8	E858.1	E933.8	E950.4	E962.0	E980.4
Dimetane	963.0	E858.1	E933.0	E950.4	E962.0	E980.4
Dimethicone	976.3	E858.7	E946.3	E950.4	E962.0	E980.4
Dimethindene	963.0	E858.1	E933.0	E950.4	E962.0	E980.4
Dimethisoquin	968.5	E855.2	E938.5	E950.4	E962.0	E980.4
Dimethisterone	962.2	E858.0	E932.2	E950.4	E962.0	E980.4
Dimethoxanate	975.4	E858.6	E945.4	E950.4	E962.0	E980.4
Dimethyl						
arsine, arsinic acid — *see* Arsenic						
carbinol	980.2	E860.3	—	E950.9	E962.1	E980.9
diguanide	962.3	E858.0	E932.3	E950.4	E962.0	E980.4
ketone	982.8	E862.4	—	E950.9	E962.1	E980.9
vapor	987.8	E869.8	—	E952.8	E962.2	E982.8
meperidine	965.09	E850.2	E935.2	E950.0	E962.0	E980.0
parathion	989.3	E863.1	—	E950.6	E962.1	E980.7
polysiloxane	973.8	E858.4	E943.8	E950.4	E962.0	E980.4
sulfate (fumes)	987.8	E869.8	—	E952.8	E962.2	E982.8
liquid	983.9	E864.3	—	E950.7	E962.1	E980.6
sulfoxide NEC	982.8	E862.4	—	E950.9	E962.1	E980.9
medicinal	976.4	E858.7	E946.4	E950.4	E962.0	E980.4
triptamine	969.6	E854.1	E939.6	E950.3	E962.0	E980.3
tubocurarine	975.2	E858.6	E945.2	E950.4	E962.0	E980.4
Dindevan	964.2	E858.2	E934.2	E950.4	E962.0	E980.4
Dinitro (-ortho-) cresol						
(herbicide) (spray)	989.4	E863.5	—	E950.6	E962.1	E980.7
insecticide	989.4	E863.4	—	E950.6	E962.1	E980.7
Dinitrobenzene	983.0	E864.0	—	E950.7	E962.1	E980.6
vapor	987.8	E869.8	—	E952.8	E962.2	E982.8
Dinitro-orthocresol						
(herbicide)	989.4	E863.5	—	E950.6	E962.1	E980.7
insecticide	989.4	E863.4	—	E950.6	E962.1	E980.7
Dinitrophenol (herbicide)						
(spray)	989.4	E863.5	—	E950.6	E962.1	E980.7
insecticide	989.4	E863.4	—	E950.6	E962.1	E980.7
Dinoprost	975.0	E858.6	E945.0	E950.4	E962.0	E980.4
Dioctyl sulfosuccinate						
(calcium) (sodium)	973.2	E858.4	E943.2	E950.4	E962.0	E980.4
Diodoquin	961.3	E857	E931.3	E950.4	E962.0	E980.4
Dione derivatives NEC	966.3	E855.0	E936.3	E950.4	E962.0	E980.4
Dionin	965.09	E850.2	E935.2	E950.0	E962.0	E980.0
Dioxane	982.8	E862.4	—	E950.9	E962.1	E980.9
Dioxin — *see* Herbicide						
Dioxyline	972.5	E858.3	E942.5	E950.4	E962.0	E980.4
Dipentene	982.8	E862.4	—	E950.9	E962.1	E980.9
Diphemanil	971.1	E855.4	E941.1	E950.4	E962.0	E980.4
Diphenadione	964.2	E858.2	E934.2	E950.4	E962.0	E980.4
Diphenhydramine	963.0	E858.1	E933.0	E950.4	E962.0	E980.4
Diphenidol	963.0	E858.1	E933.0	E950.4	E962.0	E980.4
Diphenoxylate	973.5	E858.4	E943.5	E950.4	E962.0	E980.4
Diphenylchloroarsine	985.1	E866.3	—	E950.8	E962.1	E980.8
Diphenylhydantoin (sodium)	966.1	E855.0	E936.1	E950.4	E962.0	E980.4
Diphenylpyraline	963.0	E858.1	E933.0	E950.4	E962.0	E980.4
Diphtheria						
antitoxin	979.9	E858.8	E949.9	E950.4	E962.0	E980.4
toxoid	978.5	E858.8	E948.5	E950.4	E962.0	E980.4
with tetanus toxoid	978.9	E858.8	E948.9	E950.4	E962.0	E980.4
with pertussis component	978.6	E858.8	E948.6	E950.4	E962.0	E980.4
vaccine	978.5	E858.8	E948.5	E950.4	E962.0	E980.4
Dipipanone	965.09	E850.2	E935.2	E950.0	E962.0	E980.0
Diplovax	979.5	E858.8	E949.5	E950.4	E962.0	E980.4
Diprophylline	975.1	E858.6	E945.1	E950.4	E962.0	E980.4
Dipyridamole	972.4	E858.3	E942.4	E950.4	E962.0	E980.4
Dipyrone	965.5	E850.5	E935.5	E950.0	E962.0	E980.0
Diquat	989.4	E863.5	—	E950.6	E962.1	E980.7
Disinfectant NEC	983.9	E861.4	—	E950.7	E962.1	E980.6
alkaline	983.2	E861.4	—	E950.7	E962.1	E980.6
aromatic	983.0	E861.4	—	E950.7	E962.1	E980.6
Disipal	966.4	E855.0	E936.4	E950.4	E962.0	E980.4
Disodium edetate	963.8	E858.1	E933.8	E950.4	E962.0	E980.4
Disulfamide	974.4	E858.5	E944.4	E950.4	E962.0	E980.4
Disulfanilamide	961.0	E857	E931.0	E950.4	E962.0	E980.4
Disulfiram	977.3	E858.8	E947.3	E950.4	E962.0	E980.4
Dithiazanine	961.6	E857	E931.6	E950.4	E962.0	E980.4
Dithioglycerol	963.8	E858.1	E933.8	E950.4	E962.0	E980.4
Dithranol	976.4	E858.7	E946.4	E950.4	E962.0	E980.4
Diucardin	974.3	E858.5	E944.3	E950.4	E962.0	E980.4
Diupres	974.3	E858.5	E944.3	E950.4	E962.0	E980.4
Diuretics NEC	974.4	E858.5	E944.4	E950.4	E962.0	E980.4
carbonic acid anhydrase inhibitors	974.2	E858.5	E944.2	E950.4	E962.0	E980.4
mercurial	974.0	E858.5	E944.0	E950.4	E962.0	E980.4
osmotic	974.4	E858.5	E944.4	E950.4	E962.0	E980.4
purine derivatives	974.1	E858.5	E944.1	E950.4	E962.0	E980.4
saluretic	974.3	E858.5	E944.3	E950.4	E962.0	E980.4
Diuril	974.3	E858.5	E944.3	E950.4	E962.0	E980.4
Divinyl ether	968.2	E855.1	E938.2	E950.4	E962.0	E980.4
D-lysergic acid						
diethylamide	969.6	E854.1	E939.6	E950.3	E962.0	E980.3
DMCT	960.4	E856	E930.4	E950.4	E962.0	E980.4
DMSO	982.8	E862.4	—	E950.9	E962.1	E980.9
DMT	969.6	E854.1	E939.6	E950.3	E962.0	E980.3
DNOC	989.4	E863.5	—	E950.6	E962.1	E980.7
DOCA	962.0	E858.0	E932.0	E950.4	E962.0	E980.4
Dolophine	965.02	E850.1	E935.1	E950.0	E962.0	E980.0
Doloxene	965.8	E850.8	E935.8	E950.0	E962.0	E980.0
DOM	969.6	E854.1	E939.6	E950.3	E962.0	E980.3
Domestic gas — *see* Gas, utility						
Domiphen (bromide)						
(lozenges)	976.6	E858.7	E946.6	E950.4	E962.0	E980.4
Dopa (levo)	966.4	E855.0	E936.4	E950.4	E962.0	E980.4
Dopamine	971.2	E855.5	E941.2	E950.4	E962.0	E980.4
Doriden	967.5	E852.4	E937.5	E950.2	E962.0	E980.2
Dormiral	967.0	E851	E937.0	E950.1	E962.0	E980.1
Dormison	967.8	E852.8	E937.8	E950.2	E962.0	E980.2
Dornase	963.4	E858.1	E933.4	E950.4	E962.0	E980.4
Dorsacaine	968.5	E855.2	E938.5	E950.4	E962.0	E980.4
Dothiepin hydrochloride	969.0	E854.0	E939.0	E950.3	E962.0	E980.3
Doxapram	970.0	E854.3	E940.0	E950.4	E962.0	E980.4
Doxepin	969.0	E854.0	E939.0	E950.3	E962.0	E980.3
Doxorubicin	960.7	E856	E930.7	E950.4	E962.0	E980.4
Doxycycline	960.4	E856	E930.4	E950.4	E962.0	E980.4
Doxylamine	963.0	E858.1	E933.0	E950.4	E962.0	E980.4
Dramamine	963.0	E858.1	E933.0	E950.4	E962.0	E980.4
Drano (drain cleaner)	983.2	E864.2	—	E950.7	E962.1	E980.6
Dromoran	965.09	E850.2	E935.2	E950.0	E962.0	E980.0
Dromostanolone	962.1	E858.0	E932.1	E950.4	E962.0	E980.4
Droperidol	969.2	E853.1	E939.2	E950.3	E962.0	E980.3
Drotrecogin alfa	964.2	E858.2	E934.2	E950.4	E962.0	E980.4
Drug	977.9	E858.9	E947.9	E950.5	E962.0	E980.5
specified NEC	977.8	E858.8	E947.8	E950.4	E962.0	E980.4

☑ Additional Digit Required   ▶◀ Revised Text   ● New Line   ▲ Revised Code

Drug — continued	Poisoning	Accident	Therapeutic Use	Suicide Attempt	Assault	Undetermined
AHFS List						
4:00 antihistamine drugs	963.0	E858.1	E933.0	E950.4	E962.0	E980.4
8:04 amebacides	961.5	E857	E931.5	E950.4	E962.0	E980.4
arsenical anti-infectives	961.1	E857	E931.1	E950.4	E962.0	E980.4
quinoline derivatives	961.3	E857	E931.3	E950.4	E962.0	E980.4
8:08 anthelmintics	961.6	E857	E931.6	E950.4	E962.0	E980.4
quinoline derivatives	961.3	E857	E931.3	E950.4	E962.0	E980.4
8:12.04 antifungal antibiotics	960.1	E856	E930.1	E950.4	E962.0	E980.4
8:12.06 cephalosporins	960.5	E856	E930.5	E950.4	E962.0	E980.4
8:12.08 chloramphenicol	960.2	E856	E930.2	E950.4	E962.0	E980.4
8:12.12 erythromycins	960.3	E856	E930.3	E950.4	E962.0	E980.4
8:12.16 penicillins	960.0	E856	E930.0	E950.4	E962.0	E980.4
8:12.20 streptomycins	960.6	E856	E930.6	E950.4	E962.0	E980.4
8:12.24 tetracyclines	960.4	E856	E930.4	E950.4	E962.0	E980.4
8:12.28 other antibiotics	960.8	E856	E930.8	E950.4	E962.0	E980.4
antimycobacterial	960.6	E856	E930.6	E950.4	E962.0	E980.4
macrolides	960.3	E856	E930.3	E950.4	E962.0	E980.4
8:16 antituberculars	961.8	E857	E931.8	E950.4	E962.0	E980.4
antibiotics	960.6	E856	E930.6	E950.4	E962.0	E980.4
8:18 antivirals	961.7	E857	E931.7	E950.4	E962.0	E980.4
8:20 plasmodicides (antimalarials)	961.4	E857	E931.4	E950.4	E962.0	E980.4
8:24 sulfonamides	961.0	E857	E931.0	E950.4	E962.0	E980.4
8:26 sulfones	961.8	E857	E931.8	E950.4	E962.0	E980.4
8:28 treponemicides	961.2	E857	E931.2	E950.4	E962.0	E980.4
8:32 trichomonacides	961.5	E857	E931.5	E950.4	E962.0	E980.4
quinoline derivatives	961.3	E857	E931.3	E950.4	E962.0	E980.4
nitrofuran derivatives	961.9	E857	E931.9	E950.4	E962.0	E980.4
8:36 urinary germicides	961.9	E857	E931.9	E950.4	E962.0	E980.4
quinoline derivatives	961.3	E857	E931.3	E950.4	E962.0	E980.4
8:40 other anti-infectives	961.9	E857	E931.9	E950.4	E962.0	E980.4
10:00 antineoplastic agents	963.1	E858.1	E933.1	E950.4	E962.0	E980.4
antibiotics	960.7	E856	E930.7	E950.4	E962.0	E980.4
progestogens	962.2	E858.0	E932.2	E950.4	E962.0	E980.4
12:04 parasympathomimetic (cholinergic) agents	971.0	E855.3	E941.0	E950.4	E962.0	E980.4
12:08 parasympatholytic (cholinergic-blocking) agents	971.1	E855.4	E941.1	E950.4	E962.0	E980.4
12:12 Sympathomimetic (adrenergic) agents	971.2	E855.5	E941.2	E950.4	E962.0	E980.4
12:16 sympatholytic (adrenergic-blocking) agents	971.3	E855.6	E941.3	E950.4	E962.0	E980.4
12:20 skeletal muscle relaxants						
central nervous system muscle-tone depressants	968.0	E855.1	E938.0	E950.4	E962.0	E980.4
myoneural blocking agents	975.2	E858.6	E945.2	E950.4	E962.0	E980.4
16:00 blood derivatives	964.7	E858.2	E934.7	E950.4	E962.0	E980.4
20:04 antianemia drugs	964.1	E858.2	E934.1	E950.4	E962.0	E980.4
20:04.04 iron preparations	964.0	E858.2	E934.0	E950.4	E962.0	E980.4
20:04.08 liver and stomach preparations	964.1	E858.2	E934.1	E950.4	E962.0	E980.4
20:12.04 anticoagulants	964.2	E858.2	E934.2	E950.4	E962.0	E980.4
20:12.08 antiheparin agents	964.5	E858.2	E934.5	E950.4	E962.0	E980.4
20:12.12 coagulants	964.5	E858.2	E934.5	E950.4	E962.0	E980.4
20:12.16 hemostatics NEC	964.5	E858.2	E934.5	E950.4	E962.0	E980.4
capillary active drugs	972.8	E858.3	E942.8	E950.4	E962.0	E980.4
24:04 cardiac drugs	972.9	E858.3	E942.9	E950.4	E962.0	E980.4
cardiotonic agents	972.1	E858.3	E942.1	E950.4	E962.0	E980.4
rhythm regulators	972.0	E858.3	E942.0	E950.4	E962.0	E980.4
24:06 antilipemic agents	972.2	E858.3	E942.2	E950.4	E962.0	E980.4
thyroid derivatives	962.7	E858.0	E932.7	E950.4	E962.0	E980.4
24:08 hypotensive agents	972.6	E858.3	E942.6	E950.4	E962.0	E980.4
adrenergic blocking agents	971.3	E855.6	E941.3	E950.4	E962.0	E980.4
ganglion blocking agents	972.3	E858.3	E942.3	E950.4	E962.0	E980.4
vasodilators	972.5	E858.3	E942.5	E950.4	E962.0	E980.4
24:12 vasodilating agents NEC	972.5	E858.3	E942.5	E950.4	E962.0	E980.4
coronary	972.4	E858.3	E942.4	E950.4	E962.0	E980.4
nicotinic acid derivatives	972.2	E858.3	E942.2	E950.4	E962.0	E980.4

Drug — continued	Poisoning	Accident	Therapeutic Use	Suicide Attempt	Assault	Undetermined
24:16 sclerosing agents	972.7	E858.3	E942.7	E950.4	E962.0	E980.4
28:04 general anesthetics	968.4	E855.1	E938.4	E950.4	E962.0	E980.4
gaseous anesthetics	968.2	E855.1	E938.2	E950.4	E962.0	E980.4
halothane	968.1	E855.1	E938.1	E950.4	E962.0	E980.4
intravenous anesthetics	968.3	E855.1	E938.3	E950.4	E962.0	E980.4
28:08 analgesics and antipyretics	965.9	E850.9	E935.9	E950.0	E962.0	E980.0
antirheumatics	965.69	E850.6	E935.6	E950.0	E962.0	E980.0
aromatic analgesics	965.4	E850.4	E935.4	E950.0	E962.0	E980.0
non-narcotic NEC	965.7	E850.7	E935.7	E950.0	E962.0	E980.0
opium alkaloids	965.00	E850.2	E935.2	E950.0	E962.0	E980.0
heroin	965.01	E850.0	E935.0	E950.0	E962.0	E980.0
methadone	965.02	E850.1	E935.1	E950.0	E962.0	E980.0
specified type NEC	965.09	E850.2	E935.2	E950.0	E962.0	E980.0
pyrazole derivatives	965.5	E850.5	E935.5	E950.0	E962.0	E980.0
salicylates	965.1	E850.3	E935.3	E950.0	E962.0	E980.0
specified NEC	965.8	E850.8	E935.8	E950.0	E962.0	E980.0
28:10 narcotic antagonists	970.1	E854.3	E940.1	E950.4	E962.0	E980.4
28:12 anticonvulsants	966.3	E855.0	E936.3	E950.4	E962.0	E980.4
barbiturates	967.0	E851	E937.0	E950.1	E962.0	E980.1
benzodiazepine-based tranquilizers	969.4	E853.2	E939.4	E950.3	E962.0	E980.3
bromides	967.3	E852.2	E937.3	E950.2	E962.0	E980.2
hydantoin derivatives	966.1	E855.0	E936.1	E950.4	E962.0	E980.4
oxazolidine (derivatives)	966.0	E855.0	E936.0	E950.4	E962.0	E980.4
succinimides	966.2	E855.0	E936.2	E950.4	E962.0	E980.4
28:16.04 antidepressants	969.0	E854.0	E939.0	E950.3	E962.0	E980.3
28:16.08 tranquilizers	969.5	E853.9	E939.5	E950.3	E962.0	E980.3
benzodiazepine-based	969.4	E853.2	E939.4	E950.3	E962.0	E980.3
butyrophenone-based	969.2	E853.1	E939.2	E950.3	E962.0	E980.3
major NEC	969.3	E853.8	E939.3	E950.3	E962.0	E980.3
phenothiazine-based	969.1	E853.0	E939.1	E950.3	E962.0	E980.3
28:16.12 other psychotherapeutic agents	969.8	E855.8	E939.8	E950.3	E962.0	E980.3
28:20 respiratory and cerebral stimulants	970.9	E854.3	E940.9	E950.4	E962.0	E980.4
analeptics	970.0	E854.3	E940.0	E950.4	E962.0	E980.4
anorexigenic agents	977.0	E858.8	E947.0	E950.4	E962.0	E980.4
psychostimulants	969.7	E854.2	E939.7	E950.3	E962.0	E980.3
specified NEC	970.8	E854.3	E940.8	E950.4	E962.0	E980.4
28:24 sedatives and hypnotics	967.9	E852.9	E937.9	E950.2	E962.0	E980.2
barbiturates	967.0	E851	E937.0	E950.1	E962.0	E980.1
benzodiazepine-based tranquilizers	969.4	E853.2	E939.4	E950.3	E962.0	E980.3
chloral hydrate (group)	967.1	E852.0	E937.1	E950.2	E962.0	E980.2
glutethamide group	967.5	E852.4	E937.5	E950.2	E962.0	E980.2
intravenous anesthetics	968.3	E855.1	E938.3	E950.4	E962.0	E980.4
methaqualone (compounds)	967.4	E852.3	E937.4	E950.2	E962.0	E980.2
paraldehyde	967.2	E852.1	E937.2	E950.2	E962.0	E980.2
phenothiazine-based tranquilizers	969.1	E853.0	E939.1	E950.3	E962.0	E980.3
specified NEC	967.8	E852.8	E937.8	E950.2	E962.0	E980.2
thiobarbiturates	968.3	E855.1	E938.3	E950.4	E962.0	E980.4
tranquilizer NEC	969.5	E853.9	E939.5	E950.3	E962.0	E980.3
36:04 to 36:88 diagnostic agents	977.8	E858.8	E947.8	E950.4	E962.0	E980.4
40:00 electrolyte, caloric, and water balance agents NEC	974.5	E858.5	E944.5	E950.4	E962.0	E980.4
40:04 acidifying agents	963.2	E858.1	E933.2	E950.4	E962.0	E980.4
40:08 alkalinizing agents	963.3	E858.1	E933.3	E950.4	E962.0	E980.4
40:10 ammonia detoxicants	974.5	E858.5	E944.5	E950.4	E962.0	E980.4
40:12 replacement solutions	974.5	E858.5	E944.5	E950.4	E962.0	E980.4
plasma expanders	964.8	E858.2	E934.8	E950.4	E962.0	E980.4
40:16 sodium-removing resins	974.5	E858.5	E944.5	E950.4	E962.0	E980.4
40:18 potassium-removing resins	974.5	E858.5	E944.5	E950.4	E962.0	E980.4
40:20 caloric agents	974.5	E858.5	E944.5	E950.4	E962.0	E980.4
40:24 salt and sugar substitutes	974.5	E858.5	E944.5	E950.4	E962.0	E980.4

☑ Additional Digit Required   ▶◀ Revised Text   ● New Line   ▲ Revised Code

Drug	Poisoning	External Cause (E-Code)				
		Accident	Therapeutic Use	Suicide Attempt	Assault	Undetermined
Drug — *continued*						
40:28 diuretics NEC	974.4	E858.5	E944.4	E950.4	E962.0	E980.4
carbonic acid anhydrase inhibitors	974.2	E858.5	E944.2	E950.4	E962.0	E980.4
mercurials	974.0	E858.5	E944.0	E950.4	E962.0	E980.4
purine derivatives	974.1	E858.5	E944.1	E950.4	E962.0	E980.4
saluretics	974.3	E858.5	E944.3	E950.4	E962.0	E980.4
thiazides	974.3	E858.5	E944.3	E950.4	E962.0	E980.4
40:36 irrigating solutions	974.5	E858.5	E944.5	E950.4	E962.0	E980.4
40:40 uricosuric agents	974.7	E858.5	E944.7	E950.4	E962.0	E980.4
44:00 enzymes	963.4	E858.1	E933.4	E950.4	E962.0	E980.4
fibrinolysis-affecting agents	964.4	E858.2	E934.4	E950.4	E962.0	E980.4
gastric agents	973.4	E858.4	E943.4	E950.4	E962.0	E980.4
48:00 expectorants and cough preparations						
antihistamine agents	963.0	E858.1	E933.0	E950.4	E962.0	E980.4
antitussives	975.4	E858.6	E945.4	E950.4	E962.0	E980.4
codeine derivatives	965.09	E850.2	E935.2	E950.0	E962.0	E980.0
expectorants	975.5	E858.6	E945.5	E950.4	E962.0	E980.4
narcotic agents NEC	965.09	E850.2	E935.2	E950.0	E962.0	E980.0
52:04 anti-infectives (EENT)						
ENT agent	976.6	E858.7	E946.6	E950.4	E962.0	E980.4
ophthalmic preparation	976.5	E858.7	E946.5	E950.4	E962.0	E980.4
52:04.04 antibiotics (EENT)						
ENT agent	976.6	E858.7	E946.6	E950.4	E962.0	E980.4
ophthalmic preparation	976.5	E858.7	E946.5	E950.4	E962.0	E980.4
52:04.06 antivirals (EENT)						
ENT agent	976.6	E858.7	E946.6	E950.4	E962.0	E980.4
ophthalmic preparation	976.5	E858.7	E946.5	E950.4	E962.0	E980.4
52:04.08 sulfonamides (EENT)						
ENT agent	976.6	E858.7	E946.6	E950.4	E962.0	E980.4
ophthalmic preparation	976.5	E858.7	E946.5	E950.4	E962.0	E980.4
52:04.12 miscellaneous anti-infectives (EENT)						
ENT agent	976.6	E858.7	E946.6	E950.4	E962.0	E980.4
ophthalmic preparation	976.5	E858.7	E946.5	E950.4	E962.0	E980.4
52:08 anti-inflammatory agents (EENT)						
ENT agent	976.6	E858.7	E946.6	E950.4	E962.0	E980.4
ophthalmic preparation	976.5	E858.7	E946.5	E950.4	E962.0	E980.4
52:10 carbonic anhydrase inhibitors	974.2	E858.5	E944.2	E950.4	E962.0	E980.4
52:12 contact lens solutions	976.5	E858.7	E946.5	E950.4	E962.0	E980.4
52:16 local anesthetics (EENT)	968.5	E855.2	E938.5	E950.4	E962.0	E980.4
52:20 miotics	971.0	E855.3	E941.0	E950.4	E962.0	E980.4
52:24 mydriatics						
adrenergics	971.2	E855.5	E941.2	E950.4	E962.0	E980.4
anticholinergics	971.1	E855.4	E941.1	E950.4	E962.0	E980.4
antimuscarinics	971.1	E855.4	E941.1	E950.4	E962.0	E980.4
parasympatholytics	971.1	E855.4	E941.1	E950.4	E962.0	E980.4
spasmolytics	971.1	E855.4	E941.1	E950.4	E962.0	E980.4
sympathomimetics	971.2	E855.5	E941.2	E950.4	E962.0	E980.4
52:28 mouth washes and gargles	976.6	E858.7	E946.6	E950.4	E962.0	E980.4
52:32 vasoconstrictors (EENT)	971.2	E855.5	E941.2	E950.4	E962.0	E980.4
52:36 unclassified agents (EENT)						
ENT agent	976.6	E858.7	E946.6	E950.4	E962.0	E980.4
ophthalmic preparation	976.5	E858.7	E946.5	E950.4	E962.0	E980.4
56:04 antacids and adsorbents	973.0	E858.4	E943.0	E950.4	E962.0	E980.4
56:08 antidiarrhea agents	973.5	E858.4	E943.5	E950.4	E962.0	E980.4
56:10 antiflatulents	973.8	E858.4	E943.8	E950.4	E962.0	E980.4
56:12 cathartics NEC	973.3	E858.4	E943.3	E950.4	E962.0	E980.4
emollients	973.2	E858.4	E943.2	E950.4	E962.0	E980.4
irritants	973.1	E858.4	E943.1	E950.4	E962.0	E980.4
56:16 digestants	973.4	E858.4	E943.4	E950.4	E962.0	E980.4
56:20 emetics and antiemetics						
antiemetics	963.0	E858.1	E933.0	E950.4	E962.0	E980.4
emetics	973.6	E858.4	E943.6	E950.4	E962.0	E980.4
56:24 lipotropic agents	977.1	E858.8	E947.1	E950.4	E962.0	E980.4
56:40 miscellaneous G.I. drugs	973.8	E858.4	E943.8	E950.4	E962.0	E980.4
60:00 gold compounds	965.69	E850.6	E935.6	E950.0	E962.0	E980.0
64:00 heavy metal antagonists	963.8	E858.1	E933.8	E950.4	E962.0	E980.4

Drug	Poisoning	External Cause (E-Code)				
		Accident	Therapeutic Use	Suicide Attempt	Assault	Undetermined
Drug — *continued*						
68:04 adrenals	962.0	E858.0	E932.0	E950.4	E962.0	E980.4
68:08 androgens	962.1	E858.0	E932.1	E950.4	E962.0	E980.4
68:12 contraceptives, oral	962.2	E858.0	E932.2	E950.4	E962.0	E980.4
68:16 estrogens	962.2	E858.0	E932.2	E950.4	E962.0	E980.4
68:18 gonadotropins	962.4	E858.0	E932.4	E950.4	E962.0	E980.4
68:20 insulins and antidiabetic agents	962.3	E858.0	E932.3	E950.4	E962.0	E980.4
68:20.08 insulins	962.3	E858.0	E932.3	E950.4	E962.0	E980.4
68:24 parathyroid	962.6	E858.0	E932.6	E950.4	E962.0	E980.4
68:28 pituitary (posterior)	962.5	E858.0	E932.5	E950.4	E962.0	E980.4
anterior	962.4	E858.0	E932.4	E950.4	E962.0	E980.4
68:32 progestogens	962.2	E858.0	E932.2	E950.4	E962.0	E980.4
68:34 other corpus luteum hormones NEC	962.2	E858.0	E932.2	E950.4	E962.0	E980.4
68:36 thyroid and antithyroid						
antithyroid	962.8	E858.0	E932.8	E950.4	E962.0	E980.4
thyroid (derivatives)	962.7	E858.0	E932.7	E950.4	E962.0	E980.4
72:00 local anesthetics						
NEC	968.9	E855.2	E938.9	E950.4	E962.0	E980.4
topical (surface)	968.5	E855.2	E938.5	E950.4	E962.0	E980.4
infiltration (intradermal) (subcutaneous) (submucosal)	968.5	E855.2	E938.5	E950.4	E962.0	E980.4
nerve blocking (peripheral) (plexus) (regional)	968.6	E855.2	E938.6	E950.4	E962.0	E980.4
spinal	968.7	E855.2	E938.7	E950.4	E962.0	E980.4
76:00 oxytocics	975.0	E858.6	E945.0	E950.4	E962.0	E980.4
78:00 radioactive agents	990	—	—	—	—	—
80:04 serums NEC	979.9	E858.8	E949.9	E950.4	E962.0	E980.4
immune gamma globulin (human)	964.6	E858.2	E934.6	E950.4	E962.0	E980.4
80:08 toxoids NEC	978.8	E858.8	E948.8	E950.4	E962.0	E980.4
diphtheria	978.5	E858.8	E948.5	E950.4	E962.0	E980.4
and tetanus	978.9	E858.8	E948.9	E950.4	E962.0	E980.4
w/pertussis component	978.6	E858.8	E948.6	E950.4	E962.0	E980.4
tetanus	978.4	E858.8	E948.4	E950.4	E962.0	E980.4
and diphtheria	978.9	E858.8	E948.9	E950.4	E962.0	E980.4
with pertussis component	978.6	E858.8	E948.6	E950.4	E962.0	E980.4
80:12 vaccines	979.9	E858.8	E949.9	E950.4	E962.0	E980.4
bacterial NEC	978.8	E858.8	E948.8	E950.4	E962.0	E980.4
with other bacterial components	978.9	E858.8	E948.9	E950.4	E962.0	E980.4
pertussis component	978.6	E858.8	E948.6	E950.4	E962.0	E980.4
viral and rickettsial components	979.7	E858.8	E949.7	E950.4	E962.0	E980.4
rickettsial NEC	979.6	E858.8	E949.6	E950.4	E962.0	E980.4
with bacterial component	979.7	E858.8	E949.7	E950.4	E962.0	E980.4
pertussis component	978.6	E858.8	E948.6	E950.4	E962.0	E980.4
viral component	979.7	E858.8	E949.7	E950.4	E962.0	E980.4
viral NEC	979.6	E858.8	E949.6	E950.4	E962.0	E980.4
with bacterial component	979.7	E858.8	E949.7	E950.4	E962.0	E980.4
pertussis component	978.6	E858.8	E948.6	E950.4	E962.0	E980.4
rickettsial component	979.7	E858.8	E949.7	E950.4	E962.0	E980.4
84:04.04 antibiotics (skin and mucous membrane)	976.0	E858.7	E946.0	E950.4	E962.0	E980.4
84:04.08 fungicides (skin and mucous membrane)	976.0	E858.7	E946.0	E950.4	E962.0	E980.4
84:04.12 scabicides and pediculicides (skin and mucous membrane)	976.0	E858.7	E946.0	E950.4	E962.0	E980.4
84:04.16 miscellaneous local anti-infectives (skin and mucous membrane)	976.0	E858.7	E946.0	E950.4	E962.0	E980.4

	External Cause (E-Code)					
	Poisoning	Accident	Therapeutic Use	Suicide Attempt	Assault	Undetermined
Drug — continued						
84:06 anti-inflammatory agents (skin and mucous membrane)	976.0	E858.7	E946.0	E950.4	E962.0	E980.4
84:08 antipruritics and local anesthetics						
antipruritics	976.1	E858.7	E946.1	E950.4	E962.0	E980.4
local anesthetics	968.5	E855.2	E938.5	E950.4	E962.0	E980.4
84:12 astringents	976.2	E858.7	E946.2	E950.4	E962.0	E980.4
84:16 cell stimulants and proliferants	976.8	E858.7	E946.8	E950.4	E962.0	E980.4
84:20 detergents	976.2	E858.7	E946.2	E950.4	E962.0	E980.4
84:24 emollients, demulcents, and protectants	976.3	E858.7	E946.3	E950.4	E962.0	E980.4
84:28 keratolytic agents	976.4	E858.7	E946.4	E950.4	E962.0	E980.4
84:32 keratoplastic agents	976.4	E858.7	E946.4	E950.4	E962.0	E980.4
84:36 miscellaneous agents (skin and mucous membrane)	976.8	E858.7	E946.8	E950.4	E962.0	E980.4
86:00 spasmolytic agents	975.1	E858.6	E945.1	E950.4	E962.0	E980.4
antiasthmatics	975.7	E858.6	E945.7	E950.4	E962.0	E980.4
papaverine	972.5	E858.3	E942.5	E950.4	E962.0	E980.4
theophylline	974.1	E858.5	E944.1	E950.4	E962.0	E980.4
88:04 vitamin A	963.5	E858.1	E933.5	E950.4	E962.0	E980.4
88:08 vitamin B complex	963.5	E858.1	E933.5	E950.4	E962.0	E980.4
hematopoietic vitamin	964.1	E858.2	E934.1	E950.4	E962.0	E980.4
nicotinic acid derivatives	972.2	E858.3	E942.2	E950.4	E962.0	E980.4
88:12 vitamin C	963.5	E858.1	E933.5	E950.4	E962.0	E980.4
88:16 vitamin D	963.5	E858.1	E933.5	E950.4	E962.0	E980.4
88:20 vitamin E	963.5	E858.1	E933.5	E950.4	E962.0	E980.4
88:24 vitamin K activity	964.3	E858.2	E934.3	E950.4	E962.0	E980.4
88:28 multivitamin preparations	963.5	E858.1	E933.5	E950.4	E962.0	E980.4
92:00 unclassified therapeutic agents	977.8	E858.8	E947.8	E950.4	E962.0	E980.4
Duboisine	971.1	E855.4	E941.1	E950.4	E962.0	E980.4
Dulcolax	973.1	E858.4	E943.1	E950.4	E962.0	E980.4
Duponol (C) (EP)	976.2	E858.7	E946.2	E950.4	E962.0	E980.4
Durabolin	962.1	E858.0	E932.1	E950.4	E962.0	E980.4
Dyclone	968.5	E855.2	E938.5	E950.4	E962.0	E980.4
Dyclonine	968.5	E855.2	E938.5	E950.4	E962.0	E980.4
Dydrogesterone	962.2	E858.0	E932.2	E950.4	E962.0	E980.4
Dyes NEC	989.89	E866.8	—	E950.9	E962.1	E980.9
diagnostic agents	977.8	E858.8	E947.8	E950.4	E962.0	E980.4
pharmaceutical NEC	977.4	E858.8	E947.4	E950.4	E962.0	E980.4
Dyfols	971.0	E855.3	E941.0	E950.4	E962.0	E980.4
Dymelor	962.3	E858.0	E932.3	E950.4	E962.0	E980.4
Dynamite	989.89	E866.8	—	E950.9	E962.1	E980.9
fumes	987.8	E869.8	—	E952.8	E962.2	E982.8
Dyphylline	975.1	E858.6	E945.1	E950.4	E962.0	E980.4
Ear preparations	976.6	E858.7	E946.6	E950.4	E962.0	E980.4
Echothiopate, ecothiopate	971.0	E855.3	E941.0	E950.4	E962.0	E980.4
Ecstasy	969.7	E854.2	E939.7	E950.3	E962.0	E980.3
Ectylurea	967.8	E852.8	E937.8	E950.2	E962.0	E980.2
Edathamil disodium	963.8	E858.1	E933.8	E950.4	E962.0	E980.4
Edecrin	974.4	E858.5	E944.4	E950.4	E962.0	E980.4
Edetate, disodium (calcium)	963.8	E858.1	E933.8	E950.4	E962.0	E980.4
Edrophonium	971.0	E855.3	E941.0	E950.4	E962.0	E980.4
Elase	976.8	E858.7	E946.8	E950.4	E962.0	E980.4
Elaterium	973.1	E858.4	E943.1	E950.4	E962.0	E980.4
Elder	988.2	E865.4	—	E950.9	E962.1	E980.9
berry (unripe)	988.2	E865.3	—	E950.9	E962.1	E980.9
Electrolytes NEC	974.5	E858.5	E944.5	E950.4	E962.0	E980.4
Electrolytic agent NEC	974.5	E858.5	E944.5	E950.4	E962.0	E980.4
Embramine	963.0	E858.1	E933.0	E950.4	E962.0	E980.4
Emetics	973.6	E858.4	E943.6	E950.4	E962.0	E980.4
Emetine (hydrochloride)	961.5	E857	E931.5	E950.4	E962.0	E980.4
Emollients	976.3	E858.7	E946.3	E950.4	E962.0	E980.4
Emylcamate	969.5	E853.8	E939.5	E950.3	E962.0	E980.3
Encyprate	969.0	E854.0	E939.0	E950.3	E962.0	E980.3
Endocaine	968.5	E855.2	E938.5	E950.4	E962.0	E980.4
Endrin	989.2	E863.0	—	E950.6	E962.1	E980.7
Enflurane	968.2	E855.1	E938.2	E950.4	E962.0	E980.4
Enovid	962.2	E858.0	E932.2	E950.4	E962.0	E980.4
ENT preparations (anti-infectives)	976.6	E858.7	E946.6	E950.4	E962.0	E980.4
Enzodase	963.4	E858.1	E933.4	E950.4	E962.0	E980.4
Enzymes NEC	963.4	E858.1	E933.4	E950.4	E962.0	E980.4
Epanutin	966.1	E855.0	E936.1	E950.4	E962.0	E980.4
Ephedra (tincture)	971.2	E855.5	E941.2	E950.4	E962.0	E980.4
Ephedrine	971.2	E855.5	E941.2	E950.4	E962.0	E980.4
Epiestriol	962.2	E858.0	E932.2	E950.4	E962.0	E980.4
Epilim — see Sodium Valproate						
Epinephrine	971.2	E855.5	E941.2	E950.4	E962.0	E980.4
Epsom salt	973.3	E858.4	E943.3	E950.4	E962.0	E980.4
Equanil	969.5	E853.8	E939.5	E950.3	E962.0	E980.3
Equisetum (diuretic)	974.4	E858.5	E944.4	E950.4	E962.0	E980.4
Ergometrine	975.0	E858.6	E945.0	E950.4	E962.0	E980.4
Ergonovine	975.0	E858.6	E945.0	E950.4	E962.0	E980.4
Ergot NEC	988.2	E865.4	—	E950.9	E962.1	E980.9
medicinal (alkaloids)	975.0	E858.6	E945.0	E950.4	E962.0	E980.4
Ergotamine (tartrate) (for migraine) NEC	972.9	E858.3	E942.9	E950.4	E962.0	E980.4
Ergotrate	975.0	E858.6	E945.0	E950.4	E962.0	E980.4
Erythrityl tetranitrate	972.4	E858.3	E942.4	E950.4	E962.0	E980.4
Erythrol tetranitrate	972.4	E858.3	E942.4	E950.4	E962.0	E980.4
Erythromycin	960.3	E856	E930.3	E950.4	E962.0	E980.4
ophthalmic preparation	976.5	E858.7	E946.5	E950.4	E962.0	E980.4
topical NEC	976.0	E858.7	E946.0	E950.4	E962.0	E980.4
Eserine	971.0	E855.3	E941.0	E950.4	E962.0	E980.4
Eskabarb	967.0	E851	E937.0	E950.1	E962.0	E980.1
Eskalith	969.8	E855.8	E939.8	E950.3	E962.0	E980.3
Estradiol (cypionate) (dipropionate) (valerate)	962.2	E858.0	E932.2	E950.4	E962.0	E980.4
Estriol	962.2	E858.0	E932.2	E950.4	E962.0	E980.4
Estrogens (with progestogens)	962.2	E858.0	E932.2	E950.4	E962.0	E980.4
Estrone	962.2	E858.0	E932.2	E950.4	E962.0	E980.4
Etafedrine	971.2	E855.5	E941.2	E950.4	E962.0	E980.4
Ethacrynate sodium	974.4	E858.5	E944.4	E950.4	E962.0	E980.4
Ethacrynic acid	974.4	E858.5	E944.4	E950.4	E962.0	E980.4
Ethambutol	961.8	E857	E931.8	E950.4	E962.0	E980.4
Ethamide	974.2	E858.5	E944.2	E950.4	E962.0	E980.4
Ethamivan	970.0	E854.3	E940.0	E950.4	E962.0	E980.4
Ethamsylate	964.5	E858.2	E934.5	E950.4	E962.0	E980.4
Ethanol	980.0	E860.1	—	E950.9	E962.1	E980.9
beverage	980.0	E860.0	—	E950.9	E962.1	E980.9
Ethchlorvynol	967.8	E852.8	E937.8	E950.2	E962.0	E980.2
Ethebenecid	974.7	E858.5	E944.7	E950.4	E962.0	E980.4
Ether(s) (diethyl) (ethyl) (vapor)	987.8	E869.8	—	E952.8	E962.2	E982.8
anesthetic	968.2	E855.1	E938.2	E950.4	E962.0	E980.4
petroleum — see Ligroin						
solvent	982.8	E862.4	—	E950.9	E962.1	E980.9
Ethidine chloride (vapor)	987.8	E869.8	—	E952.8	E962.2	E982.8
liquid (solvent)	982.3	E862.4	—	E950.9	E962.1	E980.9
Ethinamate	967.8	E852.8	E937.8	E950.2	E962.0	E980.2
Ethinylestradiol	962.2	E858.0	E932.2	E950.4	E962.0	E980.4
Ethionamide	961.8	E857	E931.8	E950.4	E962.0	E980.4
Ethisterone	962.2	E858.0	E932.2	E950.4	E962.0	E980.4
Ethobral	967.0	E851	E937.0	E950.1	E962.0	E980.1
Ethocaine (infiltration) (topical)	968.5	E855.2	E938.5	E950.4	E962.0	E980.4
nerve block (peripheral) (plexus)	968.6	E855.2	E938.6	E950.4	E962.0	E980.4
spinal	968.7	E855.2	E938.7	E950.4	E962.0	E980.4
Ethoheptazine (citrate)	965.7	E850.7	E935.7	E950.0	E962.0	E980.0
Ethopropazine	966.4	E855.0	E936.4	E950.4	E962.0	E980.4
Ethosuximide	966.2	E855.0	E936.2	E950.4	E962.0	E980.4
Ethotoin	966.1	E855.0	E936.1	E950.4	E962.0	E980.4
Ethoxazene	961.9	E857	E931.9	E950.4	E962.0	E980.4
Ethoxzolamide	974.2	E858.5	E944.2	E950.4	E962.0	E980.4
Ethyl						
acetate (vapor)	982.8	E862.4	—	E950.9	E962.1	E980.9
alcohol	980.0	E860.1	—	E950.9	E962.1	E980.9
beverage	980.0	E860.0	—	E950.9	E962.1	E980.9
aldehyde (vapor)	987.8	E869.8	—	E952.8	E962.2	E982.8
liquid	989.89	E866.8	—	E950.9	E962.1	E980.9
aminobenzoate	968.5	E855.2	E938.5	E950.4	E962.0	E980.4
biscoumacetate	964.2	E858.2	E934.2	E950.4	E962.0	E980.4
bromide (anesthetic)	968.2	E855.1	E938.2	E950.4	E962.0	E980.4
carbamate (antineoplastic)	963.1	E858.1	E933.1	E950.4	E962.0	E980.4
carbinol	980.3	E860.4	—	E950.9	E962.1	E980.9
chaulmoograte	961.8	E857	E931.8	E950.4	E962.0	E980.4
chloride (vapor)	987.8	E869.8	—	E952.8	E962.2	E982.8
anesthetic (local)	968.5	E855.2	E938.5	E950.4	E962.0	E980.4
inhaled	968.2	E855.1	E938.2	E950.4	E962.0	E980.4
solvent	982.3	E862.4	—	E950.9	E962.1	E980.9

	Poisoning	External Cause (E-Code)						Poisoning	External Cause (E-Code)				
		Accident	Therapeutic Use	Suicide Attempt	Assault	Undetermined			Accident	Therapeutic Use	Suicide Attempt	Assault	Undetermined
Ethyl — *continued*							**Flavoxate**	975.1	E858.6	E945.1	E950.4	E962.0	E980.4
estranol	962.1	E858.0	E932.1	E950.4	E962.0	E980.4	**Flaxedil**	975.2	E858.6	E945.2	E950.4	E962.0	E980.4
ether — *see* Ether(s)							**Flaxseed** (medicinal)	976.3	E858.7	E946.3	E950.4	E962.0	E980.4
formate (solvent) NEC	982.8	E862.4	—	E950.9	E962.1	E980.9	**Florantyrone**	973.4	E858.4	E943.4	E950.4	E962.0	E980.4
iodoacetate	987.5	E869.3	—	E952.8	E962.2	E982.8	**Floraquin**	961.3	E857	E931.3	E950.4	E962.0	E980.4
lactate (solvent) NEC	982.8	E862.4	—	E950.9	E962.1	E980.9	**Florinef**	962.0	E858.0	E932.0	E950.4	E962.0	E980.4
methylcarbinol	980.8	E860.8	—	E950.9	E962.1	E980.9	ENT agent	976.6	E858.7	E946.6	E950.4	E962.0	E980.4
morphine	965.09	E850.2	E935.2	E950.0	E962.0	E980.0	ophthalmic preparation	976.5	E858.7	E946.5	E950.4	E962.0	E980.4
Ethylene (gas)	987.1	E869.8	—	E952.8	E962.2	E982.8	topical NEC	976.0	E858.7	E946.0	E950.4	E962.0	E980.4
anesthetic (general)	968.2	E855.1	E938.2	E950.4	E962.0	E980.4	**Flowers of sulfur**	976.4	E858.7	E946.4	E950.4	E962.0	E980.4
chlorohydrin (vapor)	982.3	E862.4	—	E950.9	E962.1	E980.9	**Floxuridine**	963.1	E858.1	E933.1	E950.4	E962.0	E980.4
dichloride (vapor)	982.3	E862.4	—	E950.9	E962.1	E980.9	**Flucytosine**	961.9	E857	E931.9	E950.4	E962.0	E980.4
glycol(s) (any) (vapor)	982.8	E862.4	—	E950.9	E962.1	E980.9	**Fludrocortisone**	962.0	E858.0	E932.0	E950.4	E962.0	E980.4
Ethylidene							ENT agent	976.6	E858.7	E946.6	E950.4	E962.0	E980.4
chloride NEC	982.3	E862.4	—	E950.9	E962.1	E980.9	ophthalmic preparation	976.5	E858.7	E946.5	E950.4	E962.0	E980.4
diethyl ether	982.8	E862.4	—	E950.9	E962.1	E980.9	topical NEC	976.0	E858.7	E946.0	E950.4	E962.0	E980.4
Ethynodiol	962.2	E858.0	E932.2	E950.4	E962.0	E980.4	**Flumethasone**	976.0	E858.7	E946.0	E950.4	E962.0	E980.4
Etidocaine	968.9	E855.2	E938.9	E950.4	E962.0	E980.4	**Flumethiazide**	974.3	E858.5	E944.3	E950.4	E962.0	E980.4
infiltration (subcutaneous)	968.5	E855.2	E938.5	E950.4	E962.0	E980.4	**Flumidin**	961.7	E857	E931.7	E950.4	E962.0	E980.4
nerve (peripheral) (plexus)	968.6	E855.2	E938.6	E950.4	E962.0	E980.4	**Flunitrazepam**	969.4	E853.2	E939.4	E950.3	E962.0	E980.3
Etilfen	967.0	E851	E937.0	E950.1	E962.0	E980.1	**Fluocinolone**	976.0	E858.7	E946.0	E950.4	E962.0	E980.4
Etomide	965.7	E850.7	E935.7	E950.0	E962.0	E980.0	**Fluocortolone**	962.0	E858.0	E932.0	E950.4	E962.0	E980.4
Etorphine	965.09	E850.2	E935.2	E950.0	E962.0	E980.0	**Fluohydrocortisone**	962.0	E858.0	E932.0	E950.4	E962.0	E980.4
Etoval	967.0	E851	E937.0	E950.1	E962.0	E980.1	ENT agent	976.6	E858.7	E946.6	E950.4	E962.0	E980.4
Etryptamine	969.0	E854.0	E939.0	E950.3	E962.0	E980.3	ophthalmic preparation	976.5	E858.7	E946.5	E950.4	E962.0	E980.4
Eucaine	968.5	E855.2	E938.5	E950.4	E962.0	E980.4	topical NEC	976.0	E858.7	E946.0	E950.4	E962.0	E980.4
Eucalyptus (oil) NEC	975.5	E858.6	E945.5	E950.4	E962.0	E980.4	**Fluonid**	976.0	E858.7	E946.0	E950.4	E962.0	E980.4
Eucatropine	971.1	E855.4	E941.1	E950.4	E962.0	E980.4	**Fluopromazine**	969.1	E853.0	E939.1	E950.3	E962.0	E980.3
Eucodal	965.09	E850.2	E935.2	E950.0	E962.0	E980.0	**Fluoracetate**	989.4	E863.7	—	E950.6	E962.1	E980.7
Euneryl	967.0	E851	E937.0	E950.1	E962.0	E980.1	**Fluorescein** (sodium)	977.8	E858.8	E947.8	E950.4	E962.0	E980.4
Euphthalmine	971.1	E855.4	E941.1	E950.4	E962.0	E980.4	**Fluoride(s)** (pesticides)						
Eurax	976.0	E858.7	E946.0	E950.4	E962.0	E980.4	(sodium) NEC	989.4	E863.4	—	E950.6	E962.1	E980.7
Euresol	976.4	E858.7	E946.4	E950.4	E962.0	E980.4	hydrogen — *see*						
Euthroid	962.7	E858.0	E932.7	E950.4	E962.0	E980.4	Hydrofluoric acid						
Evans blue	977.8	E858.8	E947.8	E950.4	E962.0	E980.4	medicinal	976.7	E858.7	E946.7	E950.4	E962.0	E980.4
Evipal	967.0	E851	E937.0	E950.1	E962.0	E980.1	not pesticide NEC	983.9	E864.4	—	E950.7	E962.1	E980.6
sodium	968.3	E855.1	E938.3	E950.4	E962.0	E980.4	stannous	976.7	E858.7	E946.7	E950.4	E962.0	E980.4
Evipan	967.0	E851	E937.0	E950.1	E962.0	E980.1	**Fluorinated corticosteroids**	962.0	E858.0	E932.0	E950.4	E962.0	E980.4
sodium	968.3	E855.1	E938.3	E950.4	E962.0	E980.4	**Fluorine** (compounds) (gas)	987.8	E869.8	—	E952.8	E962.2	E982.8
Exalgin	965.4	E850.4	E935.4	E950.0	E962.0	E980.0	salt — *see* Fluoride(s)						
Excipients, pharmaceutical	977.4	E858.8	E947.4	E950.4	E962.0	E980.4	**Fluoristan**	976.7	E858.7	E946.7	E950.4	E962.0	E980.4
Exhaust gas — *see* Carbon,							**Fluoroacetate**	989.4	E863.7	—	E950.6	E962.1	E980.7
monoxide							**Fluorodeoxyuridine**	963.1	E858.1	E933.1	E950.4	E962.0	E980.4
Ex-Lax (phenolphthalein)	973.1	E858.4	E943.1	E950.4	E962.0	E980.4	**Fluorometholone** (topical)						
Expectorants	975.5	E858.6	E945.5	E950.4	E962.0	E980.4	NEC	976.0	E858.7	E946.0	E950.4	E962.0	E980.4
External medications (skin)							ophthalmic preparation	976.5	E858.7	E946.5	E950.4	E962.0	E980.4
(mucous membrane)	976.9	E858.7	E946.9	E950.4	E962.0	E980.4	**Fluorouracil**	963.1	E858.1	E933.1	E950.4	E962.0	E980.4
dental agent	976.7	E858.7	E946.7	E950.4	E962.0	E980.4	**Fluothane**	968.1	E855.1	E938.1	E950.4	E962.0	E980.4
ENT agent	976.6	E858.7	E946.6	E950.4	E962.0	E980.4	**Fluoxetine hydrochloride**	969.0	E854.0	E939.0	E950.3	E962.0	E980.3
ophthalmic preparation	976.5	E858.7	E946.5	E950.4	E962.0	E980.4	**Fluoxymesterone**	962.1	E858.0	E932.1	E950.4	E962.0	E980.4
specified NEC	976.8	E858.7	E946.8	E950.4	E962.0	E980.4	**Fluphenazine**	969.1	E853.0	E939.1	E950.3	E962.0	E980.3
Eye agents (anti-infective)	976.5	E858.7	E946.5	E950.4	E962.0	E980.4	**Fluprednisolone**	962.0	E858.0	E932.0	E950.4	E962.0	E980.4
Factor IX complex (human)	964.5	E858.2	E934.5	E950.4	E962.0	E980.4	**Flurandrenolide**	976.0	E858.7	E946.0	E950.4	E962.0	E980.4
Fecal softeners	973.2	E858.4	E943.2	E950.4	E962.0	E980.4	**Flurazepam** (hydrochloride)	969.4	E853.2	E939.4	E950.3	E962.0	E980.3
Fenbutrazate	977.0	E858.8	E947.0	E950.4	E962.0	E980.4	**Flurbiprofen**	965.61	E850.6	E935.6	E950.0	E962.0	E980.0
Fencamfamin	970.8	E854.3	E940.8	E950.4	E962.0	E980.4	**Flurobate**	976.0	E858.7	E946.0	E950.4	E962.0	E980.4
Fenfluramine	977.0	E858.8	E947.0	E950.4	E962.0	E980.4	**Flurothyl**	969.8	E855.8	E939.8	E950.3	E962.0	E980.3
Fenoprofen	965.61	E850.6	E935.6	E950.0	E962.0	E980.0	**Fluroxene**	968.2	E855.1	E938.2	E950.4	E962.0	E980.4
Fentanyl	965.09	E850.2	E935.2	E950.0	E962.0	E980.0	**Folacin**	964.1	E858.2	E934.1	E950.4	E962.0	E980.4
Fentazin	969.1	E853.0	E939.1	E950.3	E962.0	E980.3	**Folic acid**	964.1	E858.2	E934.1	E950.4	E962.0	E980.4
Fenticlor, fentichlor	976.0	E858.7	E946.0	E950.4	E962.0	E980.4	**Follicle stimulating**						
Fer de lance (bite) (venom)	989.5	E905.0	—	E950.9	E962.1	E980.9	hormone	962.4	E858.0	E932.4	E950.4	E962.0	E980.4
Ferric — *see* Iron							**Food, foodstuffs,**						
Ferrocholinate	964.0	E858.2	E934.0	E950.4	E962.0	E980.4	**nonbacterial or**						
Ferrous fumarate, gluconate,							**noxious**	988.9	E865.9	—	E950.9	E962.1	E980.9
lactate, salt NEC,							berries, seeds	988.2	E865.3	—	E950.9	E962.1	E980.9
sulfate (medicinal)	964.0	E858.2	E934.0	E950.4	E962.0	E980.4	fish	988.0	E865.2	—	E950.9	E962.1	E980.9
Ferrum — *see* Iron							mushrooms	988.1	E865.5	—	E950.9	E962.1	E980.9
Fertilizers NEC	989.89	E866.5	—	E950.9	E962.1	E980.4	plants	988.2	E865.9	—	E950.9	E962.1	E980.9
with herbicide mixture	989.4	E863.5	—	E950.6	E962.1	E980.7	specified type NEC	988.2	E865.4	—	E950.9	E962.1	E980.9
Fibrinogen (human)	964.7	E858.2	E934.7	E950.4	E962.0	E980.4	shellfish	988.0	E865.1	—	E950.9	E962.1	E980.9
Fibrinolysin	964.4	E858.2	E934.4	E950.4	E962.0	E980.4	specified NEC	988.8	E865.8	—	E950.9	E962.1	E980.9
Fibrinolysis-affecting							**Fool's parsley**	988.2	E865.4	—	E950.9	E962.1	E980.9
agents	964.4	E858.2	E934.4	E950.4	E962.0	E980.4	**Formaldehyde** (solution)	989.89	E861.4	—	E950.9	E962.1	E980.9
Filix mas	961.6	E857	E931.6	E950.4	E962.0	E980.4	fungicide	989.4	E863.6	—	E950.6	E962.1	E980.7
Fiorinal	965.1	E850.3	E935.3	E950.0	E962.0	E980.0	gas or vapor	987.8	E869.8	—	E952.8	E962.2	E982.8
Fire damp	987.1	E869.8	—	E952.8	E962.2	E982.8	**Formalin**	989.89	E861.4	—	E950.9	E962.1	E980.9
Fish, nonbacterial or							fungicide	989.4	E863.6	—	E950.6	E962.1	E980.7
noxious	988.0	E865.2	—	E950.9	E962.1	E980.9	vapor	987.8	E869.8	—	E952.8	E962.2	E982.8
shell	988.0	E865.1	—	E950.9	E962.1	E980.9	**Formic acid**	983.1	E864.1	—	E950.7	E962.1	E980.6
Flagyl	961.5	E857	E931.5	E950.4	E962.0	E980.4	vapor	987.8	E869.8	—	E952.8	E962.2	E982.8

	Poisoning	\u00A0	\u00A0	\u00A0	\u00A0	\u00A0

Left table — External Cause (E-Code)

	Poisoning	Accident	Therapeutic Use	Suicide Attempt	Assault	Undetermined
Fowler's solution	985.1	E866.3	—	E950.8	E962.1	E980.8
Foxglove	988.2	E865.4	—	E950.9	E962.1	E980.9
Fox green	977.8	E858.8	E947.8	E950.4	E962.0	E980.4
Framycetin	960.8	E856	E930.8	E950.4	E962.0	E980.4
Frangula (extract)	973.1	E858.4	E943.1	E950.4	E962.0	E980.4
Frei antigen	977.8	E858.8	E947.8	E950.4	E962.0	E980.4
Freons	987.4	E869.2	—	E952.8	E962.2	E982.8
Fructose	974.5	E858.5	E944.5	E950.4	E962.0	E980.4
Frusemide	974.4	E858.5	E944.4	E950.4	E962.0	E980.4
FSH	962.4	E858.0	E932.4	E950.4	E962.0	E980.4
Fuel						
automobile	981	E862.1	—	E950.9	E962.1	E980.9
exhaust gas, not in transit	986	E868.2	—	E952.0	E962.2	E982.0
vapor NEC	987.1	E869.8	—	E952.8	E962.2	E982.8
gas (domestic use) — see also Carbon, monoxide, fuel						
utility	987.1	E868.1	—	E951.8	E962.2	E981.8
incomplete combustion of — see Carbon, monoxide, fuel, utility						
in mobile container	987.0	E868.0	—	E951.1	E962.2	E981.1
piped (natural)	987.1	E867	—	E951.0	E962.2	E981.0
industrial, incomplete combustion	986	E868.3	—	E952.1	E962.2	E982.1
Fugillin	960.8	E856	E930.8	E950.4	E962.0	E980.4
Fulminate of mercury	985.0	E866.1	—	E950.9	E962.1	E980.9
Fulvicin	960.1	E856	E930.1	E950.4	E962.0	E980.4
Fumadil	960.8	E856	E930.8	E950.4	E962.0	E980.4
Fumagillin	960.8	E856	E930.8	E950.4	E962.0	E980.4
Fumes (from)	987.9	E869.9	—	E952.9	E962.2	E982.9
carbon monoxide — see Carbon, monoxide						
charcoal (domestic use)	986	E868.3	—	E952.1	E962.2	E982.1
chloroform — see Chloroform						
coke (in domestic stoves, fireplaces)	986	E868.3	—	E952.1	E962.2	E982.1
corrosive NEC	987.8	E869.8	—	E952.8	E962.2	E982.8
ether — see Ether(s)						
freons	987.4	E869.2	—	E952.8	E962.2	E982.8
hydrocarbons	987.1	E869.8	—	E952.8	E962.2	E982.8
petroleum (liquefied)	987.0	E868.0	—	E951.1	E962.2	E981.1
distributed through pipes (pure or mixed with air)	987.0	E867	—	E951.0	E962.2	E981.0
lead — see Lead						
metals — see specified metal						
nitrogen dioxide	987.2	E869.0	—	E952.8	E962.2	E982.8
pesticides — see Pesticides						
petroleum (liquefied)	987.0	E868.0	—	E951.1	E962.2	E981.1
distributed through pipes (pure or mixed with air)	987.0	E867	—	E951.0	E962.2	E981.0
polyester	987.8	E869.8	—	E952.8	E962.2	E982.8
specified source other (see also substance specified)	987.8	E869.8	—	E952.8	E962.2	E982.8
sulfur dioxide	987.3	E869.1	—	E952.8	E962.2	E982.8
Fumigants	989.4	E863.8	—	E950.6	E962.1	E980.7
Fungi, noxious, used as food	988.1	E865.5	—	E950.9	E962.1	E980.9
Fungicides (see also Antifungals)	989.4	E863.6	—	E950.6	E962.1	E980.7
Fungizone	960.1	E856	E930.1	E950.4	E962.0	E980.4
topical	976.0	E858.7	E946.0	E950.4	E962.0	E980.4
Furacin	976.0	E858.7	E946.0	E950.4	E962.0	E980.4
Furadantin	961.9	E857	E931.9	E950.4	E962.0	E980.4
Furazolidone	961.9	E857	E931.9	E950.4	E962.0	E980.4
Furnace (coal burning) (domestic), gas from	986	E868.3	—	E952.1	E962.2	E982.1
industrial	986	E868.8	—	E952.1	E962.2	E982.1
Furniture polish	989.89	E861.2	—	E950.9	E962.1	E980.9
Furosemide	974.4	E858.5	E944.4	E950.4	E962.0	E980.4
Furoxone	961.9	E857	E931.9	E950.4	E962.0	E980.4
Fusel oil (amyl) (butyl) (propyl)	980.3	E860.4	—	E950.9	E962.1	E980.9
Fusidic acid	960.8	E856	E930.8	E950.4	E962.0	E980.4

Right table — External Cause (E-Code)

	Poisoning	Accident	Therapeutic Use	Suicide Attempt	Assault	Undetermined
Gallamine	975.2	E858.6	E945.2	E950.4	E962.0	E980.4
Gallotannic acid	976.2	E858.7	E946.2	E950.4	E962.0	E980.4
Gamboge	973.1	E858.4	E943.1	E950.4	E962.0	E980.4
Gamimune	964.6	E858.2	E934.6	E950.4	E962.0	E980.4
Gamma-benzene						
hexachloride (vapor)	989.2	E863.0	—	E950.6	E962.1	E980.7
Gamma globulin	964.6	E858.2	E934.6	E950.4	E962.0	E980.4
Gamma hydroxy						
butyrate (GHB)	968.4	E855.1	E938.4	E950.4	E962.0	E980.4
Gamulin	964.6	E858.2	E934.6	E950.4	E962.0	E980.4
Ganglionic blocking agents	972.3	E858.3	E942.3	E950.4	E962.0	E980.4
Ganja	969.6	E854.1	E939.6	E950.3	E962.0	E980.3
Garamycin	960.8	E856	E930.8	E950.4	E962.0	E980.4
ophthalmic preparation	976.5	E858.7	E946.5	E950.4	E962.0	E980.4
topical NEC	976.0	E858.7	E946.0	E950.4	E962.0	E980.4
Gardenal	967.0	E851	E937.0	E950.1	E962.0	E980.1
Gardepanyl	967.0	E851	E937.0	E950.1	E962.0	E980.1
Gas	987.9	E869.9	—	E952.9	E962.2	E982.9
acetylene	987.1	E868.1	—	E951.8	E962.2	E981.8
incomplete combustion of — see Carbon, monoxide, fuel, utility						
air contaminants, source or type not specified	987.9	E869.9	—	E952.9	E962.2	E982.9
anesthetic (general) NEC	968.2	E855.1	E938.2	E950.4	E962.0	E980.4
blast furnace	986	E868.8	—	E952.1	E962.2	E982.1
butane — see Butane						
carbon monoxide — see Carbon, monoxide						
chlorine	987.6	E869.8	—	E952.8	E962.2	E982.8
coal — see Carbon, monoxide, coal						
cyanide	987.7	E869.8	—	E952.8	E962.2	E982.8
dicyanogen	987.8	E869.8	—	E952.8	E962.2	E982.8
domestic — see Gas, utility						
exhaust — see Carbon, monoxide, exhaust gas						
from wood- or coal-burning stove or fireplace	986	E868.3	—	E952.1	E962.2	E982.1
fuel (domestic use) — see also Carbon, monoxide, fuel						
industrial use	986	E868.8	—	E952.1	E962.2	E982.1
utility	987.1	E868.1	—	E951.8	E962.2	E981.8
incomplete combustion of — see Carbon, monoxide, fuel, utility						
in mobile container	987.0	E868.0	—	E951.1	E962.2	E981.1
piped (natural)	987.1	E867	—	E951.0	E962.2	E981.0
garage	986	E868.2	—	E952.0	E962.2	E982.0
hydrocarbon NEC	987.1	E869.8	—	E952.8	E962.2	E982.8
incomplete combustion of — see Carbon, monoxide, fuel, utility						
liquefied (mobile container)	987.0	E868.0	—	E951.1	E962.2	E981.1
piped	987.0	E867	—	E951.0	E962.2	E981.0
hydrocyanic acid	987.7	E869.8	—	E952.8	E962.2	E982.8
illuminating — see Gas, utility						
incomplete combustion, any — see Carbon, monoxide						
kiln	986	E868.8	—	E952.1	E962.2	E982.1
lacrimogenic	987.5	E869.3	—	E952.8	E962.2	E982.8
marsh	987.1	E869.8	—	E952.8	E962.2	E982.8
motor exhaust, not in transit	986	E868.8	—	E952.1	E962.2	E982.1
mustard — see Mustard, gas						
natural	987.1	E867	—	E951.0	E962.2	E981.0
nerve (war)	987.9	E869.9	—	E952.9	E962.2	E982.9
oils	981	E862.1	—	E950.9	E962.1	E980.9
petroleum (liquefied) (distributed in mobile containers)	987.0	E868.0	—	E951.1	E962.2	E981.1
piped (pure or mixed with air)	987.0	E867	—	E951.0	E962.2	E981.1
piped (manufactured) (natural) NEC	987.1	E867	—	E951.0	E962.2	E981.0

	Poisoning	**External Cause (E-Code)**				
		Accident	Therapeutic Use	Suicide Attempt	Assault	Undetermined
Gas — continued						
producer	986	E868.8	—	E952.1	E962.2	E982.1
propane — see Propane						
refrigerant (freon)	987.4	E869.2	—	E952.8	E962.2	E982.8
not freon	987.9	E869.9	—	E952.9	E962.2	E982.9
sewer	987.8	E869.8	—	E952.8	E962.2	E982.8
specified source NEC (*see also* substance specified)	987.8	E869.8	—	E952.8	E962.2	E982.8
stove — *see* Gas, utility						
tear	987.5	E869.3	—	E952.8	E962.2	E982.8
utility (for cooking, heating, or lighting) (piped)						
NEC	987.1	E868.1	—	E951.8	E962.2	E981.8
incomplete combustion of — *see* Carbon, monoxide, fuel, utilty						
in mobile container	987.0	E868.0	—	E951.1	E962.2	E981.1
piped (natural)	987.1	E867	—	E951.0	E962.2	E981.0
water	987.1	E868.1	—	E951.8	E962.2	E981.8
incomplete combustion of — *see* Carbon, monoxide, fuel, utility						
Gaseous substance — *see* Gas						
Gasoline, gasolene	981	E862.1	—	E950.9	E962.1	E980.9
vapor	987.1	E869.8	—	E952.8	E962.2	E982.8
Gastric enzymes	973.4	E858.4	E943.4	E950.4	E962.0	E980.4
Gastrografin	977.8	E858.8	E947.8	E950.4	E962.0	E980.4
Gastrointestinal agents	973.9	E858.4	E943.9	E950.4	E962.0	E980.4
specified NEC	973.8	E858.4	E943.8	E950.4	E962.0	E980.4
Gaultheria procumbens	988.2	E865.4	—	E950.9	E962.1	E980.9
Gelatin (intravenous)	964.8	E858.2	E934.8	E950.4	E962.0	E980.4
absorbable (sponge)	964.5	E858.2	E934.5	E950.4	E962.0	E980.4
Gelfilm	976.8	E858.7	E946.8	E950.4	E962.0	E980.4
Gelfoam	964.5	E858.2	E934.5	E950.4	E962.0	E980.4
Gelsemine	970.8	E854.3	E940.8	E950.4	E962.0	E980.4
Gelsemium (sempervirens)	988.2	E865.4	—	E950.9	E962.1	E980.9
Gemonil	967.0	E851	E937.0	E950.1	E962.0	E980.1
Gentamicin	960.8	E856	E930.8	E950.4	E962.0	E980.4
ophthalmic preparation	976.5	E858.7	E946.5	E950.4	E962.0	E980.4
topical NEC	976.0	E858.7	E946.0	E950.4	E962.0	E980.4
Gentian violet	976.0	E858.7	E946.0	E950.4	E962.0	E980.4
Gexane	976.0	E858.7	E946.0	E950.4	E962.0	E980.4
Gila monster (venom)	989.5	E905.0	—	E950.9	E962.1	E980.9
Ginger, Jamaica	989.89	E866.8	—	E950.9	E962.1	E980.9
Gitalin	972.1	E858.3	E942.1	E950.4	E962.0	E980.4
Gitoxin	972.1	E858.3	E942.1	E950.4	E962.0	E980.4
Glandular extract (medicinal) NEC	977.9	E858.9	E947.9	E950.5	E962.0	E980.5
Glaucarubin	961.5	E857	E931.5	E950.4	E962.0	E980.4
Globin zinc insulin	962.3	E858.0	E932.3	E950.4	E962.0	E980.4
Glucagon	962.3	E858.0	E932.3	E950.4	E962.0	E980.4
Glucochloral	967.1	E852.0	E937.1	E950.2	E962.0	E980.2
Glucocorticoids	962.0	E858.0	E932.0	E950.4	E962.0	E980.4
Glucose	974.5	E858.5	E944.5	E950.4	E962.0	E980.4
oxidase reagent	977.8	E858.8	E947.8	E950.4	E962.0	E980.4
Glucosulfone sodium	961.8	E857	E931.8	E950.4	E962.0	E980.4
Glue(s)	989.89	E866.6	—	E950.9	E962.1	E980.9
Glutamic acid (hydrochloride)	973.4	E858.4	E943.4	E950.4	E962.0	E980.4
Glutaraldehyde	989.89	E861.4	—	E950.9	E962.1	E980.9
Glutathione	963.8	E858.1	E933.8	E950.4	E962.0	E980.4
Glutethimide (group)	967.5	E852.4	E937.5	E950.2	E962.0	E980.2
Glycerin (lotion)	976.3	E858.7	E946.3	E950.4	E962.0	E980.4
Glycerol (topical)	976.3	E858.7	E946.3	E950.4	E962.0	E980.4
Glyceryl						
guaiacolate	975.5	E858.6	E945.5	E950.4	E962.0	E980.4
triacetate (topical)	976.0	E858.7	E946.0	E950.4	E962.0	E980.4
trinitrate	972.4	E858.3	E942.4	E950.4	E962.0	E980.4
Glycine	974.5	E858.5	E944.5	E950.4	E962.0	E980.4
Glycobiarsol	961.1	E857	E931.1	E950.4	E962.0	E980.4
Glycols (ether)	982.8	E862.4	—	E950.9	E962.1	E980.9
Glycopyrrolate	971.1	E855.4	E941.1	E950.4	E962.0	E980.4
Glymidine	962.3	E858.0	E932.3	E950.4	E962.0	E980.4
Gold (compounds) (salts)	965.69	E850.6	E935.6	E950.0	E962.0	E980.0
Golden sulfide of antimony	985.4	E866.2	—	E950.9	E962.1	E980.9
Goldylocks	988.2	E865.4	—	E950.9	E962.1	E980.9
Gonadal tissue extract	962.9	E858.0	E932.9	E950.4	E962.0	E980.4
female	962.2	E858.0	E932.2	E950.4	E962.0	E980.4
male	962.1	E858.0	E932.1	E950.4	E962.0	E980.4

	Poisoning	**External Cause (E-Code)**				
		Accident	Therapeutic Use	Suicide Attempt	Assault	Undetermined
Gonadotropin	962.4	E858.0	E932.4	E950.4	E962.0	E980.4
Grain alcohol	980.0	E860.1	—	E950.9	E962.1	E980.9
beverage	980.0	E860.0	—	E950.9	E962.1	E980.9
Gramicidin	960.8	E856	E930.8	E950.4	E962.0	E980.4
Gratiola officinalis	988.2	E865.4	—	E950.9	E962.1	E980.9
Grease	989.89	E866.8	—	E950.9	E962.1	E980.9
Green hellebore	988.2	E865.4	—	E950.9	E962.1	E980.9
Green soap	976.2	E858.7	E946.2	E950.4	E962.0	E980.4
Grifulvin	960.1	E856	E930.1	E950.4	E962.0	E980.4
Griseofulvin	960.1	E856	E930.1	E950.4	E962.0	E980.4
Growth hormone	962.4	E858.0	E932.4	E950.4	E962.0	E980.4
Guaiacol	975.5	E858.6	E945.5	E950.4	E962.0	E980.4
Guaiac reagent	977.8	E858.8	E947.8	E950.4	E962.0	E980.4
Guaifenesin	975.5	E858.6	E945.5	E950.4	E962.0	E980.4
Guaiphenesin	975.5	E858.6	E945.5	E950.4	E962.0	E980.4
Guanatol	961.4	E857	E931.4	E950.4	E962.0	E980.4
Guanethidine	972.6	E858.3	E942.6	E950.4	E962.0	E980.4
Guano	989.89	E866.5	—	E950.9	E962.1	E980.9
Guanochlor	972.6	E858.3	E942.6	E950.4	E962.0	E980.4
Guanoctine	972.6	E858.3	E942.6	E950.4	E962.0	E980.4
Guanoxan	972.6	E858.3	E942.6	E950.4	E962.0	E980.4
Hair treatment agent NEC	976.4	E858.7	E946.4	E950.4	E962.0	E980.4
Halcinonide	976.0	E858.7	E946.0	E950.4	E962.0	E980.4
Halethazole	976.0	E858.7	E946.0	E950.4	E962.0	E980.4
Hallucinogens	969.6	E854.1	E939.6	E950.3	E962.0	E980.3
Haloperidol	969.2	E853.1	E939.2	E950.3	E962.0	E980.3
Haloprogin	976.0	E858.7	E946.0	E950.4	E962.0	E980.4
Halotex	976.0	E858.7	E946.0	E950.4	E962.0	E980.4
Halothane	968.1	E855.1	E938.1	E950.4	E962.0	E980.4
Halquinols	976.0	E858.7	E946.0	E950.4	E962.0	E980.4
Harmonyl	972.6	E858.3	E942.6	E950.4	E962.0	E980.4
Hartmann's solution	974.5	E858.5	E944.5	E950.4	E962.0	E980.4
Hashish	969.6	E854.1	E939.6	E950.3	E962.0	E980.3
Hawaiian wood rose seeds	969.6	E854.1	E939.6	E950.3	E962.0	E980.3
Headache cures, drugs, powders NEC	977.9	E858.9	E947.9	E950.5	E962.0	E980.9
Heavenly Blue (morning glory)	969.6	E854.1	E939.6	E950.3	E962.0	E980.3
Heavy metal antagonists	963.8	E858.1	E933.8	E950.4	E962.0	E980.4
anti-infectives	961.2	E857	E931.2	E950.4	E962.0	E980.4
Hedaquinium	976.0	E858.7	E946.0	E950.4	E962.0	E980.4
Hedge hyssop	988.2	E865.4	—	E950.9	E962.1	E980.9
Heet	976.8	E858.7	E946.8	E950.4	E962.0	E980.4
Helenin	961.6	E857	E931.6	E950.4	E962.0	E980.4
Hellebore (black) (green) (white)	988.2	E865.4	—	E950.9	E962.1	E980.9
Hemlock	988.2	E865.4	—	E950.9	E962.1	E980.9
Hemostatics	964.5	E858.2	E934.5	E950.4	E962.0	E980.4
capillary active drugs	972.8	E858.3	E942.8	E950.4	E962.0	E980.4
Henbane	988.2	E865.4	—	E950.9	E962.1	E980.9
Heparin (sodium)	964.2	E858.2	E934.2	E950.4	E962.0	E980.4
Heptabarbital, heptabarbitone	967.0	E851	E937.0	E950.1	E962.0	E980.1
Heptachlor	989.2	E863.0	—	E950.6	E962.1	E980.7
Heptalgin	965.09	E850.2	E935.2	E950.0	E962.0	E980.0
Herbicides	989.4	E863.5	—	E950.6	E962.1	E980.7
Heroin	965.01	E850.0	E935.0	E950.0	E962.0	E980.0
Herplex	976.5	E858.7	E946.5	E950.4	E962.0	E980.4
HES	964.8	E858.2	E934.8	E950.4	E962.0	E980.4
Hetastarch	964.8	E858.2	E934.8	E950.4	E962.0	E980.4
Hexachlorocyclohexane	989.2	E863.0	—	E950.6	E962.1	E980.7
Hexachlorophene	976.2	E858.7	E946.2	E950.4	E962.0	E980.4
Hexadimethrine (bromide)	964.5	E858.2	E934.5	E950.4	E962.0	E980.4
Hexafluorenium	975.2	E858.6	E945.2	E950.4	E962.0	E980.4
Hexa-germ	976.2	E858.7	E946.2	E950.4	E962.0	E980.4
Hexahydrophenol	980.8	E860.8	—	E950.9	E962.1	E980.9
Hexalin	980.8	E860.8	—	E950.9	E962.1	E980.9
Hexamethonium	972.3	E858.3	E942.3	E950.4	E962.0	E980.4
Hexamethyleneamine	961.9	E857	E931.9	E950.4	E962.0	E980.4
Hexamine	961.9	E857	E931.9	E950.4	E962.0	E980.4
Hexanone	982.8	E862.4	—	E950.9	E962.1	E980.9
Hexapropymate	967.8	E852.8	E937.8	E950.2	E962.0	E980.2
Hexestrol	962.2	E858.0	E932.2	E950.4	E962.0	E980.4
Hexethal (sodium)	967.0	E851	E937.0	E950.1	E962.0	E980.1
Hexetidine	976.0	E858.7	E946.0	E950.4	E962.0	E980.4
Hexobarbital, hexobarbitone	967.0	E851	E937.0	E950.1	E962.0	E980.1
sodium (anesthetic)	968.3	E855.1	E938.3	E950.4	E962.0	E980.4
soluble	968.3	E855.1	E938.3	E950.4	E962.0	E980.4
Hexocyclium	971.1	E855.4	E941.1	E950.4	E962.0	E980.4
Hexoestrol	962.2	E858.0	E932.2	E950.4	E962.0	E980.4

☑ Additional Digit Required   ▶◀ Revised Text   ● New Line   ▲ Revised Code

	Poisoning	Accident	Therapeutic Use	Suicide Attempt	Assault	Undetermined
External Cause (E-Code)						
Hexone	982.8	E862.4	—	E950.9	E962.1	E980.9
Hexylcaine	968.5	E855.2	E938.5	E950.4	E962.0	E980.4
Hexylresorcinol	961.6	E857	E931.6	E950.4	E962.0	E980.4
Hinkle's pills	973.1	E858.4	E943.1	E950.4	E962.0	E980.4
Histalog	977.8	E858.8	E947.8	E950.4	E962.0	E980.4
Histamine (phosphate)	972.5	E858.3	E942.5	E950.4	E962.0	E980.4
Histoplasmin	977.8	E858.8	E947.8	E950.4	E962.0	E980.4
Holly berries	988.2	E865.3	—	E950.9	E962.1	E980.9
Homatropine	971.1	E855.4	E941.1	E950.4	E962.0	E980.4
Homo-tet	964.6	E858.2	E934.6	E950.4	E962.0	E980.4
Hormones (synthetic						
substitute) NEC	962.9	E858.0	E932.9	E950.4	E962.0	E980.4
adrenal cortical steroids	962.0	E858.0	E932.0	E950.4	E962.0	E980.4
antidiabetic agents	962.3	E858.0	E932.3	E950.4	E962.0	E980.4
follicle stimulating	962.4	E858.0	E932.4	E950.4	E962.0	E980.4
gonadotropic	962.4	E858.0	E932.4	E950.4	E962.0	E980.4
growth	962.4	E858.0	E932.4	E950.4	E962.0	E980.4
ovarian (substitutes)	962.2	E858.0	E932.2	E950.4	E962.0	E980.4
parathyroid (derivatives)	962.6	E858.0	E932.6	E950.4	E962.0	E980.4
pituitary (posterior)	962.5	E858.0	E932.5	E950.4	E962.0	E980.4
anterior	962.4	E858.0	E932.4	E950.4	E962.0	E980.4
thyroid (derivative)	962.7	E858.0	E932.7	E950.4	E962.0	E980.4
Hornet (sting)	989.5	E905.3	—	E950.9	E962.1	E980.9
Horticulture agent NEC	989.4	E863.9	—	E950.6	E962.1	E980.7
Hyaluronidase	963.4	E858.1	E933.4	E950.4	E962.0	E980.4
Hyazyme	963.4	E858.1	E933.4	E950.4	E962.0	E980.4
Hycodan	965.09	E850.2	E935.2	E950.0	E962.0	E980.0
Hydantoin derivatives	966.1	E855.0	E936.1	E950.4	E962.0	E980.4
Hydeltra	962.0	E858.0	E932.0	E950.4	E962.0	E980.4
Hydergine	971.3	E855.6	E941.3	E950.4	E962.0	E980.4
Hydrabamine penicillin	960.0	E856	E930.0	E950.4	E962.0	E980.4
Hydralazine, hydrallazine	972.6	E858.3	E942.6	E950.4	E962.0	E980.4
Hydrargaphen	976.0	E858.7	E946.0	E950.4	E962.0	E980.4
Hydrazine	983.9	E864.3	—	E950.7	E962.1	E980.6
Hydriodic acid	975.5	E858.6	E945.5	E950.4	E962.0	E980.4
Hydrocarbon gas	987.1	E869.8	—	E952.8	E962.2	E982.8
incomplete combustion of — see Carbon, monoxide, fuel, utility						
liquefied (mobile container)	987.0	E868.0	—	E951.1	E962.2	E981.1
piped (natural)	987.0	E867	—	E951.0	E962.2	E981.0
Hydrochloric acid (liquid)	983.1	E864.1	—	E950.7	E962.1	E980.6
medicinal	973.4	E858.4	E943.4	E950.4	E962.0	E980.4
vapor	987.8	E869.8	—	E952.8	E962.2	E982.8
Hydrochlorothiazide	974.3	E858.5	E944.3	E950.4	E962.0	E980.4
Hydrocodone	965.09	E850.2	E935.2	E950.0	E962.0	E980.0
Hydrocortisone	962.0	E858.0	E932.0	E950.4	E962.0	E980.4
ENT agent	976.6	E858.7	E946.6	E950.4	E962.0	E980.4
ophthalmic preparation	976.5	E858.7	E946.5	E950.4	E962.0	E980.4
topical NEC	976.0	E858.7	E946.0	E950.4	E962.0	E980.4
Hydrocortone	962.0	E858.0	E932.0	E950.4	E962.0	E980.4
ENT agent	976.6	E858.7	E946.6	E950.4	E962.0	E980.4
ophthalmic preparation	976.5	E858.7	E946.5	E950.4	E962.0	E980.4
topical NEC	976.0	E858.7	E946.0	E950.4	E962.0	E980.4
Hydrocyanic acid — see Cyanide(s)						
Hydroflumethiazide	974.3	E858.5	E944.3	E950.4	E962.0	E980.4
Hydrofluoric acid (liquid)	983.1	E864.1	—	E950.7	E962.1	E980.6
vapor	987.8	E869.8	—	E952.8	E962.2	E982.8
Hydrogen	987.8	E869.8	—	E952.8	E962.2	E982.8
arsenide	985.1	E866.3	—	E950.8	E962.1	E980.8
arseniureted	985.1	E866.3	—	E950.8	E962.1	E980.8
cyanide (salts)	989.0	E866.8	—	E950.9	E962.1	E980.9
gas	987.7	E869.8	—	E952.8	E962.2	E982.8
fluoride (liquid)	983.1	E864.1	—	E950.7	E962.1	E980.6
vapor	987.8	E869.8	—	E952.8	E962.2	E982.8
peroxide (solution)	976.6	E858.7	E946.6	E950.4	E962.0	E980.4
phosphureted	987.8	E869.8	—	E952.8	E962.2	E982.8
sulfide (gas)	987.8	E869.8	—	E952.8	E962.2	E982.8
arseniureted	985.1	E866.3	—	E950.8	E962.1	E980.8
sulfureted	987.8	E869.8	—	E952.8	E962.2	E982.8
Hydromorphinol	965.09	E850.2	E935.2	E950.0	E962.0	E980.0
Hydromorphinone	965.09	E850.2	E935.2	E950.0	E962.0	E980.0
Hydromorphone	965.09	E850.2	E935.2	E950.0	E962.0	E980.0
Hydromox	974.3	E858.5	E944.3	E950.4	E962.0	E980.4
Hydrophilic lotion	976.3	E858.7	E946.3	E950.4	E962.0	E980.4
Hydroquinone	983.0	E864.0	—	E950.7	E962.1	E980.6
vapor	987.8	E869.8	—	E952.8	E962.2	E982.8
Hydrosulfuric acid (gas)	987.8	E869.8	—	E952.8	E962.2	E982.8
Hydrous wool fat (lotion)	976.3	E858.7	E946.3	E950.4	E962.0	E980.4
Hydroxide, caustic	983.2	E864.2	—	E950.7	E962.1	E980.6

	Poisoning	Accident	Therapeutic Use	Suicide Attempt	Assault	Undetermined
External Cause (E-Code)						
Hydroxocobalamin	964.1	E858.2	E934.1	E950.4	E962.0	E980.4
Hydroxyamphetamine	971.2	E855.5	E941.2	E950.4	E962.0	E980.4
Hydroxychloroquine	961.4	E857	E931.4	E950.4	E962.0	E980.4
Hydroxydihydrocodeinone	965.09	E850.2	E935.2	E950.0	E962.0	E980.0
Hydroxyethyl starch	964.8	E858.2	E934.8	E950.4	E962.0	E980.4
Hydroxyphenamate	969.5	E853.8	E939.5	E950.3	E962.0	E980.3
Hydroxyphenylbutazone	965.5	E850.5	E935.5	E950.0	E962.0	E980.0
Hydroxyprogesterone	962.2	E858.0	E932.2	E950.4	E962.0	E980.4
Hydroxyquinoline derivatives	961.3	E857	E931.3	E950.4	E962.0	E980.4
Hydroxystilbamidine	961.5	E857	E931.5	E950.4	E962.0	E980.4
Hydroxyurea	963.1	E858.1	E933.1	E950.4	E962.0	E980.4
Hydroxyzine	969.5	E853.8	E939.5	E950.3	E962.0	E980.3
Hyoscine (hydrobromide)	971.1	E855.4	E941.1	E950.4	E962.0	E980.4
Hyoscyamine	971.1	E855.4	E941.1	E950.4	E962.0	E980.4
Hyoscyamus (albus) (niger)	988.2	E865.4	—	E950.9	E962.1	E980.9
Hypaque	977.8	E858.8	E947.8	E950.4	E962.0	E980.4
Hypertussis	964.6	E858.2	E934.6	E950.4	E962.0	E980.4
Hypnotics NEC	967.9	E852.9	E937.9	E950.2	E962.0	E980.2
Hypochlorites — see Sodium, hypochlorite						
Hypotensive agents NEC	972.6	E858.3	E942.6	E950.4	E962.0	E980.4
Ibufenac	965.69	E850.6	E935.6	E950.0	E962.0	E980.0
Ibuprofen	965.61	E850.6	E935.6	E950.0	E962.0	E980.0
ICG	977.8	E858.8	E947.8	E950.4	E962.0	E980.4
Ichthammol	976.4	E858.7	E946.4	E950.4	E962.0	E980.4
Ichthyol	976.4	E858.7	E946.4	E950.4	E962.0	E980.4
Idoxuridine	976.5	E858.7	E946.5	E950.4	E962.0	E980.4
IDU	976.5	E858.7	E946.5	E950.4	E962.0	E980.4
Iletin	962.3	E858.0	E932.3	E950.4	E962.0	E980.4
Ilex	988.2	E865.4	—	E950.9	E962.1	E980.9
Illuminating gas — see Gas, utility						
Ilopan	963.5	E858.1	E933.5	E950.4	E962.0	E980.4
Ilotycin	960.3	E856	E930.3	E950.4	E962.0	E980.4
ophthalmic preparation	976.5	E858.7	E946.5	E950.4	E962.0	E980.4
topical NEC	976.0	E858.7	E946.0	E950.4	E962.0	E980.4
Imipramine	969.0	E854.0	E939.0	E950.3	E962.0	E980.3
Immu-G	964.6	E858.2	E934.6	E950.4	E962.0	E980.4
Immuglobin	964.6	E858.2	E934.6	E950.4	E962.0	E980.4
Immune serum globulin	964.6	E858.2	E934.6	E950.4	E962.0	E980.4
Immunosuppressive agents	963.1	E858.1	E933.1	E950.4	E962.0	E980.4
Immu-tetanus	964.6	E858.2	E934.6	E950.4	E962.0	E980.4
Indandione (derivatives)	964.2	E858.2	E934.2	E950.4	E962.0	E980.4
Inderal	972.0	E858.3	E942.0	E950.4	E962.0	E980.4
Indian						
hemp	969.6	E854.1	E939.6	E950.3	E962.0	E980.3
tobacco	988.2	E865.4	—	E950.9	E962.1	E980.9
Indigo carmine	977.8	E858.8	E947.8	E950.4	E962.0	E980.4
Indocin	965.69	E850.6	E935.6	E950.0	E962.0	E980.0
Indocyanine green	977.8	E858.8	E947.8	E950.4	E962.0	E980.4
Indomethacin	965.69	E850.6	E935.6	E950.0	E962.0	E980.0
Industrial						
alcohol	980.9	E860.9	—	E950.9	E962.1	E980.9
fumes	987.8	E869.8	—	E952.8	E962.2	E982.8
solvents (fumes) (vapors)	982.8	E862.9	—	E950.9	E962.1	E980.9
Influenza vaccine	979.6	E858.8	E949.6	E950.4	E962.0	E980.4
Ingested substances NEC	989.9	E866.9	—	E950.9	E962.1	E980.9
INH (isoniazid)	961.8	E857	E931.8	E950.4	E962.0	E980.4
Inhalation, gas (noxious) — see Gas						
Ink	989.89	E866.8	—	E950.9	E962.1	E980.9
Innovar	967.6	E852.5	E937.6	E950.2	E962.0	E980.2
Inositol niacinate	972.2	E858.3	E942.2	E950.4	E962.0	E980.4
Inproquone	963.1	E858.1	E933.1	E950.4	E962.0	E980.4
Insect (sting), venomous	989.5	E905.5	—	E950.9	E962.1	E980.9
Insecticides (see also Pesticides)	989.4	E863.4	—	E950.6	E962.1	E980.7
chlorinated	989.2	E863.0	—	E950.6	E962.1	E980.7
mixtures	989.4	E863.3	—	E950.6	E962.1	E980.7
organochlorine (compounds)	989.2	E863.0	—	E950.6	E962.1	E980.7
organophosphorus (compounds)	989.3	E863.1	—	E950.6	E962.1	E980.7
Insular tissue extract	962.3	E858.0	E932.3	E950.4	E962.0	E980.4
Insulin (amorphous) (globin) (isophane) (Lente) (NPH) (protamine) (Semilente) (Ultralente) (zinc)	962.3	E858.0	E932.3	E950.4	E962.0	E980.4
Intranarcon	968.3	E855.1	E938.3	E950.4	E962.0	E980.4
Inulin	977.8	E858.8	E947.8	E950.4	E962.0	E980.4
Invert sugar	974.5	E858.5	E944.5	E950.4	E962.0	E980.4

☑ Additional Digit Required   ▶◀ Revised Text   ● New Line   ▲ Revised Code

	Poisoning	External Cause (E-Code)						Poisoning	External Cause (E-Code)				
		Accident	Therapeutic Use	Suicide Attempt	Assault	Undeter- mined			Accident	Therapeutic Use	Suicide Attempt	Assault	Undeter- mined
Iodide NEC (*see also* Iodine)	976.0	E858.7	E946.0	E950.4	E962.0	E980.4	**Kenacort**	962.0	E858.0	E932.0	E950.4	E962.0	E980.4
mercury (ointment)	976.0	E858.7	E946.0	E950.4	E962.0	E980.4	**Keratolytics**	976.4	E858.7	E946.4	E950.4	E962.0	E980.4
methylate	976.0	E858.7	E946.0	E950.4	E962.0	E980.4	**Keratoplastics**	976.4	E858.7	E946.4	E950.4	E962.0	E980.4
potassium (expectorant)							**Kerosene, kerosine** (fuel)						
NEC	975.5	E858.6	E945.5	E950.4	E962.0	E980.4	(solvent) NEC	981	E862.1	—	E950.9	E962.1	E980.9
Iodinated glycerol	975.5	E858.6	E945.5	E950.4	E962.0	E980.4	insecticide	981	E863.4	—	E950.6	E962.1	E980.7
Iodine (antiseptic, external)							vapor	987.1	E869.8	—	E952.8	E962.2	E982.8
(tincture) NEC	976.0	E858.7	E946.0	E950.4	E962.0	E980.4	**Ketamine**	968.3	E855.1	E938.3	E950.4	E962.0	E980.4
diagnostic	977.8	E858.8	E947.8	E950.4	E962.0	E980.4	**Ketobemidone**	965.09	E850.2	E935.2	E950.0	E962.0	E980.0
for thyroid conditions							**Ketols**	982.8	E862.4	—	E950.9	E962.1	E980.9
(antithyroid)	962.8	E858.0	E932.8	E950.4	E962.0	E980.4	**Ketone oils**	982.8	E862.4	—	E950.9	E962.1	E980.9
vapor	987.8	E869.8	—	E952.8	E962.2	E982.8	**Ketoprofen**	965.61	E850.6	E935.6	E950.0	E962.0	E980.0
Iodized oil	977.8	E858.8	E947.8	E950.4	E962.0	E980.4	**Kiln gas or vapor** (carbon						
Iodobismitol	961.2	E857	E931.2	E950.4	E962.0	E980.4	monoxide)	986	E868.8	—	E952.1	E962.2	E982.1
Iodochlorhydroxyquin	961.3	E857	E931.3	E950.4	E962.0	E980.4	**Konsyl**	973.3	E858.4	E943.3	E950.4	E962.0	E980.4
topical	976.0	E858.7	E946.0	E950.4	E962.0	E980.4	**Kosam seed**	988.2	E865.3	—	E950.9	E962.1	E980.9
Iodoform	976.0	E858.7	E946.0	E950.4	E962.0	E980.4	**Krait** (venom)	989.5	E905.0	—	E950.9	E962.1	E980.9
Iodopanoic acid	977.8	E858.8	E947.8	E950.4	E962.0	E980.4	**Kwell** (insecticide)	989.2	E863.0	—	E950.6	E962.1	E980.7
Iodophthalein	977.8	E858.8	E947.8	E950.4	E962.0	E980.4	anti-infective (topical)	976.0	E858.7	E946.0	E950.4	E962.0	E980.4
Ion exchange resins	974.5	E858.5	E944.5	E950.4	E962.0	E980.4	**Laburnum** (flowers) (seeds)	988.2	E865.3	—	E950.9	E962.1	E980.9
Iopanoic acid	977.8	E858.8	E947.8	E950.4	E962.0	E980.4	leaves	988.2	E865.4	—	E950.9	E962.1	E980.9
Iophendylate	977.8	E858.8	E947.8	E950.4	E962.0	E980.4	**Lacquers**	989.89	E861.6	—	E950.9	E962.1	E980.9
Iothiouracil	962.8	E858.0	E932.8	E950.4	E962.0	E980.4	**Lacrimogenic gas**	987.5	E869.3	—	E952.8	E962.2	E982.8
Ipecac	973.6	E858.4	E943.6	E950.4	E962.0	E980.4	**Lactic acid**	983.1	E864.1	—	E950.7	E962.1	E980.6
Ipecacuanha	973.6	E858.4	E943.6	E950.4	E962.0	E980.4	**Lactobacillus acidophilus**	973.5	E858.4	E943.5	E950.4	E962.0	E980.4
Ipodate	977.8	E858.8	E947.8	E950.4	E962.0	E980.4	**Lactoflavin**	963.5	E858.1	E933.5	E950.4	E962.0	E980.4
Ipral	967.0	E851	E937.0	E950.1	E962.0	E980.1	**Lactuca** (virosa) (extract)	967.8	E852.8	E937.8	E950.2	E962.0	E980.2
Ipratropium	975.1	E858.6	E945.1	E950.4	E962.0	E980.4	**Lactucarium**	967.8	E852.8	E937.8	E950.2	E962.0	E980.2
Iproniazid	969.0	E854.0	E939.0	E950.3	E962.0	E980.3	**Laevulose**	974.5	E858.5	E944.5	E950.4	E962.0	E980.4
Iron (compounds) (medicinal)							**Lanatoside** (C)	972.1	E858.3	E942.1	E950.4	E962.0	E980.4
(preparations)	964.0	E858.2	E934.0	E950.4	E962.0	E980.4	**Lanolin** (lotion)	976.3	E858.7	E946.3	E950.4	E962.0	E980.4
dextran	964.0	E858.2	E934.0	E950.4	E962.0	E980.4	**Largactil**	969.1	E853.0	E939.1	E950.3	E962.0	E980.3
nonmedicinal (dust)							**Larkspur**	988.2	E865.3	—	E950.9	E962.1	E980.9
(fumes) NEC	985.8	E866.4	—	E950.9	E962.1	E980.9	**Laroxyl**	969.0	E854.0	E939.0	E950.3	E962.0	E980.3
Irritant drug	977.9	E858.9	E947.9	E950.5	E962.0	E980.5	**Lasix**	974.4	E858.5	E944.4	E950.4	E962.0	E980.4
Ismelin	972.6	E858.3	E942.6	E950.4	E962.0	E980.4	**Latex**	989.82	E866.8	—	E950.9	E962.1	E980.9
Isoamyl nitrite	972.4	E858.3	E942.4	E950.4	E962.0	E980.4	**Lathyrus** (seed)	988.2	E865.3	—	E950.9	E962.1	E980.9
Isobutyl acetate	982.8	E862.4	—	E950.9	E962.1	E980.9	**Laudanum**	965.09	E850.2	E935.2	E950.0	E962.0	E980.0
Isocarboxazid	969.0	E854.0	E939.0	E950.3	E962.0	E980.3	**Laudexium**	975.2	E858.6	E945.2	E950.4	E962.0	E980.4
Isoephedrine	971.2	E855.5	E941.2	E950.4	E962.0	E980.4	**Laurel, black or cherry**	988.2	E865.4	—	E950.9	E962.1	E980.9
Isoetharine	971.2	E855.5	E941.2	E950.4	E962.0	E980.4	**Laurolinium**	976.0	E858.7	E946.0	E950.4	E962.0	E980.4
Isofluorophate	971.0	E855.3	E941.0	E950.4	E962.0	E980.4	**Lauryl sulfoacetate**	976.2	E858.7	E946.2	E950.4	E962.0	E980.4
Isoniazid (INH)	961.8	E857	E931.8	E950.4	E962.0	E980.4	**Laxatives NEC**	973.3	E858.4	E943.3	E950.4	E962.0	E980.4
Isopentaquine	961.4	E857	E931.4	E950.4	E962.0	E980.4	emollient	973.2	E858.4	E943.2	E950.4	E962.0	E980.4
Isophane insulin	962.3	E858.0	E932.3	E950.4	E962.0	E980.4	**L-dopa**	966.4	E855.0	E936.4	E950.4	E962.0	E980.4
Isopregnenone	962.2	E858.0	E932.2	E950.4	E962.0	E980.4	**Lead** (dust) (fumes) (vapor)						
Isoprenaline	971.2	E855.5	E941.2	E950.4	E962.0	E980.4	NEC	984.9	E866.0	—	E950.9	E962.1	E980.9
Isopropamide	971.1	E855.4	E941.1	E950.4	E962.0	E980.4	acetate (dust)	984.1	E866.0	—	E950.9	E962.1	E980.9
Isopropanol	980.2	E860.3	—	E950.9	E962.1	E980.9	anti-infectives	961.2	E857	E931.2	E950.4	E962.0	E980.4
topical (germicide)	976.0	E858.7	E946.0	E950.4	E962.0	E980.4	antiknock compound						
Isopropyl							(tetraethyl)	984.1	E862.1		E950.9	E962.1	E980.9
acetate	982.8	E862.4	—	E950.9	E962.1	E980.9	arsenate, arsenite (dust)						
alcohol	980.2	E860.3	—	E950.9	E962.1	E980.9	(insecticide) (vapor)	985.1	E863.4	—	E950.8	E962.1	E980.8
topical (germicide)	976.0	E858.7	E946.0	E950.4	E962.0	E980.4	herbicide	985.1	E863.5	—	E950.8	E962.1	E980.8
ether	982.8	E862.4	—	E950.9	E962.1	E980.9	carbonate	984.0	E866.0	—	E950.9	E962.1	E980.9
Isoproterenol	971.2	E855.5	E941.2	E950.4	E962.0	E980.4	paint	984.0	E861.5	—	E950.9	E962.1	E980.9
Isosorbide dinitrate	972.4	E858.3	E942.4	E950.4	E962.0	E980.4	chromate	984.0	E866.0	—	E950.9	E962.1	E980.9
Isothipendyl	963.0	E858.1	E933.0	E950.4	E962.0	E980.4	paint	984.0	E861.5	—	E950.9	E962.1	E980.9
Isoxazolyl penicillin	960.0	E856	E930.0	E950.4	E962.0	E980.4	dioxide	984.0	E866.0	—	E950.9	E962.1	E980.9
Isoxsuprine hydrochloride	972.5	E858.3	E942.5	E950.4	E962.0	E980.4	inorganic (compound)	984.0	E866.0	—	E950.9	E962.1	E980.9
I-thyroxine sodium	962.7	E858.0	E932.7	E950.4	E962.0	E980.4	paint	984.0	E861.5	—	E950.9	E962.1	E980.9
Jaborandi (pilocarpus)							iodide	984.0	E866.0	—	E950.9	E962.1	E980.9
(extract)	971.0	E855.3	E941.0	E950.4	E962.0	E980.4	pigment (paint)	984.0	E861.5	—	E950.9	E962.1	E980.9
Jalap	973.1	E858.4	E943.1	E950.4	E962.0	E980.4	monoxide (dust)	984.0	E866.0	—	E950.9	E962.1	E980.9
Jamaica							paint	984.0	E861.5	—	E950.9	E962.1	E980.9
dogwood (bark)	965.7	E850.7	E935.7	E950.0	E962.0	E980.0	organic	984.1	E866.0	—	E950.9	E962.1	E980.9
ginger	989.89	E866.8	—	E950.9	E962.1	E980.9	oxide	984.0	E866.0	—	E950.9	E962.1	E980.9
Jatropha	988.2	E865.4	—	E950.9	E962.1	E980.9	paint	984.0	E861.5	—	E950.9	E962.1	E980.9
curcas	988.2	E865.3	—	E950.9	E962.1	E980.9	paint	984.0	E861.5	—	E950.9	E962.1	E980.9
Jectofer	964.0	E858.2	E934.0	E950.4	E962.0	E980.4	salts	984.0	E866.0	—	E950.9	E962.1	E980.9
Jellyfish (sting)	989.5	E905.6	—	E950.9	E962.1	E980.9	specified compound NEC	984.8	E866.0	—	E950.9	E962.1	E980.9
Jequirity (bean)	988.2	E865.3	—	E950.9	E962.1	E980.9	tetra-ethyl	984.1	E862.1	—	E950.9	E962.1	E980.9
Jimson weed	988.2	E865.4	—	E950.9	E962.1	E980.9	**Lebanese red**	969.6	E854.1	E939.6	E950.3	E962.0	E980.3
seeds	988.2	E865.3	—	E950.9	E962.1	E980.9	**Lente Iletin** (insulin)	962.3	E858.0	E932.3	E950.4	E962.0	E980.4
Juniper tar (oil) (ointment)	976.4	E858.7	E946.4	E950.4	E962.0	E980.4	**Leptazol**	970.0	E854.3	E940.0	E950.4	E962.0	E980.4
Kallikrein	972.5	E858.3	E942.5	E950.4	E962.0	E980.4	**Leritine**	965.09	E850.2	E935.2	E950.0	E962.0	E980.0
Kanamycin	960.6	E856	E930.6	E950.4	E962.0	E980.4	**Letter**	962.7	E858.0	E932.7	E950.4	E962.0	E980.4
Kantrex	960.6	E856	E930.6	E950.4	E962.0	E980.4	**Lettuce opium**	967.8	E852.8	E937.8	E950.2	E962.0	E980.2
Kaolin	973.5	E858.4	E943.5	E950.4	E962.0	E980.4	**Leucovorin** (factor)	964.1	E858.2	E934.1	E950.4	E962.0	E980.4
Karaya (gum)	973.3	E858.4	E943.3	E950.4	E962.0	E980.4	**Leukeran**	963.1	E858.1	E933.1	E950.4	E962.0	E980.4
Kemithal	968.3	E855.1	E938.3	E950.4	E962.0	E980.4	**Levalbuterol**	975.7	E858.6	E945.7	E950.4	E962.0	E980.4

☑ Additional Digit Required   ▶◀ Revised Text   ● New Line   ▲ Revised Code

	External Cause (E-Code)					
	Poisoning	Accident	Therapeutic Use	Suicide Attempt	Assault	Undetermined
Levallorphan	970.1	E854.3	E940.1	E950.4	E962.0	E980.4
Levanil	967.8	E852.8	E937.8	E950.2	E962.0	E980.2
Levarterenol	971.2	E855.5	E941.2	E950.4	E962.0	E980.4
Levodopa	966.4	E855.0	E936.4	E950.4	E962.0	E980.4
Levo-dromoran	965.09	E850.2	E935.2	E950.0	E962.0	E980.0
Levoid	962.7	E858.0	E932.7	E950.4	E962.0	E980.4
Levo-iso-methadone	965.02	E850.1	E935.1	E950.0	E962.0	E980.0
Levomepromazine	967.8	E852.8	E937.8	E950.2	E962.0	E980.2
Levoprome	967.8	E852.8	E937.8	E950.2	E962.0	E980.2
Levopropoxyphene	975.4	E858.6	E945.4	E950.4	E962.0	E980.4
Levorphan, levorphanol	965.09	E850.2	E935.2	E950.0	E962.0	E980.0
Levothyroxine (sodium)	962.7	E858.0	E932.7	E950.4	E962.0	E980.4
Levsin	971.1	E855.4	E941.1	E950.4	E962.0	E980.4
Levulose	974.5	E858.5	E944.5	E950.4	E962.0	E980.4
Lewisite (gas)	985.1	E866.3	—	E950.8	E962.1	E980.8
Librium	969.4	E853.2	E939.4	E950.3	E962.0	E980.3
Lidex	976.0	E858.7	E946.0	E950.4	E962.0	E980.4
Lidocaine (infiltration) (topical)	968.5	E855.2	E938.5	E950.4	E962.0	E980.4
nerve block (peripheral) (plexus)	968.6	E855.2	E938.6	E950.4	E962.0	E980.4
spinal	968.7	E855.2	E938.7	E950.4	E962.0	E980.4
Lighter fluid	981	E862.1	—	E950.9	E962.1	E980.9
Lignocaine (infiltration) (topical)	968.5	E855.2	E938.5	E950.4	E962.0	E980.4
nerve block (peripheral) (plexus)	968.6	E855.2	E938.6	E950.4	E962.0	E980.4
spinal	968.7	E855.2	E938.7	E950.4	E962.0	E980.4
Ligroin(e) (solvent)	981	E862.0	—	E950.9	E962.1	E980.9
vapor	987.1	E869.8	—	E952.8	E962.2	E982.8
Ligustrum vulgare	988.2	E865.3	—	E950.9	E962.1	E980.9
Lily of the valley	988.2	E865.4	—	E950.9	E962.1	E980.9
Lime (chloride)	983.2	E864.2	—	E950.7	E962.1	E980.6
solution, sulferated	976.4	E858.7	E946.4	E950.4	E962.0	E980.4
Limonene	982.8	E862.4	—	E950.9	E962.1	E980.9
Lincomycin	960.8	E856	E930.8	E950.4	E962.0	E980.4
Lindane (insecticide) (vapor)	989.2	E863.0	—	E950.6	E962.1	E980.7
anti-infective (topical)	976.0	E858.7	E946.0	E950.4	E962.0	E980.4
Liniments NEC	976.9	E858.7	E946.9	E950.4	E962.0	E980.4
Linoleic acid	972.2	E858.3	E942.2	E950.4	E962.0	E980.4
Liothyronine	962.7	E858.0	E932.7	E950.4	E962.0	E980.4
Liotrix	962.7	E858.0	E932.7	E950.4	E962.0	E980.4
Lipancreatin	973.4	E858.4	E943.4	E950.4	E962.0	E980.4
Lipo-Lutin	962.2	E858.0	E932.2	E950.4	E962.0	E980.4
Lipotropic agents	977.1	E858.8	E947.1	E950.4	E962.0	E980.4
Liquefied petroleum gases	987.0	E868.0	—	E951.1	E962.2	E981.1
piped (pure or mixed with air)	987.0	E867	—	E951.0	E962.2	E981.0
Liquid petrolatum	973.2	E858.4	E943.2	E950.4	E962.0	E980.4
substance	989.9	E866.9	—	E950.9	E962.1	E980.9
specified NEC	989.89	E866.8	—	E950.9	E962.1	E980.9
Lirugen	979.4	E858.8	E949.4	E950.4	E962.0	E980.4
Lithane	969.8	E855.8	E939.8	E950.3	E962.0	E980.3
Lithium	985.8	E866.4	—	E950.9	E962.1	E980.9
carbonate	969.8	E855.8	E939.8	E950.3	E962.0	E980.3
Lithonate	969.8	E855.8	E939.8	E950.3	E962.0	E980.3
Liver (extract) (injection) (preparations)	964.1	E858.2	E934.1	E950.4	E962.0	E980.4
Lizard (bite) (venom)	989.5	E905.0	—	E950.9	E962.1	E980.9
LMD	964.8	E858.2	E934.8	E950.4	E962.0	E980.4
Lobelia	988.2	E865.4	—	E950.9	E962.1	E980.9
Lobeline	970.0	E854.3	E940.0	E950.4	E962.0	E980.4
Locorten	976.0	E858.7	E946.0	E950.4	E962.0	E980.4
Lolium temulentum	988.2	E865.3	—	E950.9	E962.1	E980.9
Lomotil	973.5	E858.4	E943.5	E950.4	E962.0	E980.4
Lomustine	963.1	E858.1	E933.1	E950.4	E962.0	E980.4
Lophophora williamsii	969.6	E854.1	E939.6	E950.3	E962.0	E980.3
Lorazepam	969.4	E853.2	E939.4	E950.3	E962.0	E980.3
Lotions NEC	976.9	E858.7	E946.9	E950.4	E962.0	E980.4
Lotronex	973.8	E858.4	E943.8	E950.4	E962.0	E980.4
Lotusate	967.0	E851	E937.0	E950.1	E962.0	E980.1
Lowila	976.2	E858.7	E946.2	E950.4	E962.0	E980.4
Loxapine	969.3	E853.8	E939.3	E950.3	E962.0	E980.3
Lozenges (throat)	976.6	E858.7	E946.6	E950.4	E962.0	E980.4
LSD (25)	969.6	E854.1	E939.6	E950.3	E962.0	E980.3
Lubricating oil NEC	981	E862.2	—	E950.9	E962.1	E980.9
Lucanthone	961.6	E857	E931.6	E950.4	E962.0	E980.4
Luminal	967.0	E851	E937.0	E950.1	E962.0	E980.1
Lung irritant (gas) NEC	987.9	E869.9	—	E952.9	E962.2	E982.9
Lutocylol	962.2	E858.0	E932.2	E950.4	E962.0	E980.4

	External Cause (E-Code)					
	Poisoning	Accident	Therapeutic Use	Suicide Attempt	Assault	Undetermined
Lutromone	962.2	E858.0	E932.2	E950.4	E962.0	E980.4
Lututrin	975.0	E858.6	E945.0	E950.4	E962.0	E980.4
Lye (concentrated)	983.2	E864.2	—	E950.7	E962.1	E980.6
Lygranum (skin test)	977.8	E858.8	E947.8	E950.4	E962.0	E980.4
Lymecycline	960.4	E856	E930.4	E950.4	E962.0	E980.4
Lymphogranuloma venereum antigen	977.8	E858.8	E947.8	E950.4	E962.0	E980.4
Lynestrenol	962.2	E858.0	E932.2	E950.4	E962.0	E980.4
Lyovac Sodium Edecrin	974.4	E858.5	E944.4	E950.4	E962.0	E980.4
Lypressin	962.5	E858.0	E932.5	E950.4	E962.0	E980.4
Lysergic acid (amide) (diethylamide)	969.6	E854.1	E939.6	E950.3	E962.0	E980.3
Lysergide	969.6	E854.1	E939.6	E950.3	E962.0	E980.3
Lysine vasopressin	962.5	E858.0	E932.5	E950.4	E962.0	E980.4
Lysol	983.0	E864.0	—	E950.7	E962.1	E980.6
Lytta (vitatta)	976.8	E858.7	E946.8	E950.4	E962.0	E980.4
Mace	987.5	E869.3	—	E952.8	E962.2	E982.8
Macrolides (antibiotics)	960.3	E856	E930.3	E950.4	E962.0	E980.4
Mafenide	976.0	E858.7	E946.0	E950.4	E962.0	E980.4
Magaldrate	973.0	E858.4	E943.0	E950.4	E962.0	E980.4
Magic mushroom	969.6	E854.1	E939.6	E950.3	E962.0	E980.3
Magnamycin	960.8	E856	E930.8	E950.4	E962.0	E980.4
Magnesia magma	973.0	E858.4	E943.0	E950.4	E962.0	E980.4
Magnesium (compounds) (fumes) NEC	985.8	E866.4	—	E950.9	E962.1	E980.9
antacid	973.0	E858.4	E943.0	E950.4	E962.0	E980.4
carbonate	973.0	E858.4	E943.0	E950.4	E962.0	E980.4
cathartic	973.3	E858.4	E943.3	E950.4	E962.0	E980.4
citrate	973.3	E858.4	E943.3	E950.4	E962.0	E980.4
hydroxide	973.0	E858.4	E943.0	E950.4	E962.0	E980.4
oxide	973.0	E858.4	E943.0	E950.4	E962.0	E980.4
sulfate (oral)	973.3	E858.4	E943.3	E950.4	E962.0	E980.4
intravenous	966.3	E855.0	E936.3	E950.4	E962.0	E980.4
trisilicate	973.0	E858.4	E943.0	E950.4	E962.0	E980.4
Malathion (insecticide)	989.3	E863.1	—	E950.6	E962.1	E980.7
Male fern (oleoresin)	961.6	E857	E931.6	E950.4	E962.0	E980.4
Mandelic acid	961.9	E857	E931.9	E950.4	E962.0	E980.4
Manganese compounds (fumes) NEC	985.2	E866.4	—	E950.9	E962.1	E980.9
Mannitol (diuretic) (medicinal) NEC	974.4	E858.5	E944.4	E950.4	E962.0	E980.4
hexanitrate	972.4	E858.3	E942.4	E950.4	E962.0	E980.4
mustard	963.1	E858.1	E933.1	E950.4	E962.0	E980.4
Mannomustine	963.1	E858.1	E933.1	E950.4	E962.0	E980.4
MAO inhibitors	969.0	E854.0	E939.0	E950.3	E962.0	E980.3
Mapharsen	961.1	E857	E931.1	E950.4	E962.0	E980.4
Marcaine	968.9	E855.2	E938.9	E950.4	E962.0	E980.4
infiltration (subcutaneous)	968.5	E855.2	E938.5	E950.4	E962.0	E980.4
nerve block (peripheral) (plexus)	968.6	E855.2	E938.6	E950.4	E962.0	E980.4
Marezine	963.0	E858.1	E933.0	E950.4	E962.0	E980.4
Marihuana, marijuana (derivatives)	969.6	E854.1	E939.6	E950.3	E962.0	E980.3
Marine animals or plants (sting)	989.5	E905.6	—	E950.9	E962.1	E980.9
Marplan	969.0	E854.0	E939.0	E950.3	E962.0	E980.3
Marsh gas	987.1	E869.8	—	E952.8	E962.2	E982.8
Marsilid	969.0	E854.0	E939.0	E950.3	E962.0	E980.3
Matulane	963.1	E858.1	E933.1	E950.4	E962.0	E980.4
Mazindol	977.0	E858.8	E947.0	E950.4	E962.0	E980.4
MDMA	969.7	E854.2	E939.7	E950.3	E962.0	E980.3
Meadow saffron	988.2	E865.3	—	E950.9	E962.1	E980.9
Measles vaccine	979.4	E858.8	E949.4	E950.4	E962.0	E980.4
Meat, noxious or nonbacterial	988.8	E865.0	—	E950.9	E962.1	E980.9
Mebanazine	969.0	E854.0	E939.0	E950.3	E962.0	E980.3
Mebaral	967.0	E851	E937.0	E950.1	E962.0	E980.1
Mebendazole	961.6	E857	E931.6	E950.4	E962.0	E980.4
Mebeverine	975.1	E858.6	E945.1	E950.4	E962.0	E980.4
Mebhydroline	963.0	E858.1	E933.0	E950.4	E962.0	E980.4
Mebrophenhydramine	963.0	E858.1	E933.0	E950.4	E962.0	E980.4
Mebutamate	969.5	E853.8	E939.5	E950.3	E962.0	E980.3
Mecamylamine (chloride)	972.3	E858.3	E942.3	E950.4	E962.0	E980.4
Mechlorethamine hydrochloride	963.1	E858.1	E933.1	E950.4	E962.0	E980.4
Meclizene (hydrochloride)	963.0	E858.1	E933.0	E950.4	E962.0	E980.4
Meclofenoxate	970.0	E854.3	E940.0	E950.4	E962.0	E980.4
Meclozine (hydrochloride)	963.0	E858.1	E933.0	E950.4	E962.0	E980.4
Medazepam	969.4	E853.2	E939.4	E950.3	E962.0	E980.3

☑ Additional Digit Required   ▶◀ Revised Text   ● New Line   ▲ Revised Code

	Poisoning	Accident	Therapeutic Use	Suicide Attempt	Assault	Undetermined
Medicine, medicinal substance	977.9	E858.9	E947.9	E950.5	E962.0	E980.5
specified NEC	977.8	E858.8	E947.8	E950.4	E962.0	E980.4
Medinal	967.0	E851	E937.0	E950.1	E962.0	E980.1
Medomin	967.0	E851	E937.0	E950.1	E962.0	E980.1
Medroxyprogesterone	962.2	E858.0	E932.2	E950.4	E962.0	E980.4
Medrysone	976.5	E858.7	E946.5	E950.4	E962.0	E980.4
Mefenamic acid	965.7	E850.7	E935.7	E950.0	E962.0	E980.0
Megahallucinogen	969.6	E854.1	E939.6	E950.3	E962.0	E980.3
Megestrol	962.2	E858.0	E932.2	E950.4	E962.0	E980.4
Meglumine	977.8	E858.8	E947.8	E950.4	E962.0	E980.4
Meladinin	976.3	E858.7	E946.3	E950.4	E962.0	E980.4
Melanizing agents	976.3	E858.7	E946.3	E950.4	E962.0	E980.4
Melarsoprol	961.1	E857	E931.1	E950.4	E962.0	E980.4
Melia azedarach	988.2	E865.3	—	E950.9	E962.1	E980.9
Mellaril	969.1	E853.0	E939.1	E950.3	E962.0	E980.3
Meloxine	976.3	E858.7	E946.3	E950.4	E962.0	E980.4
Melphalan	963.1	E858.1	E933.1	E950.4	E962.0	E980.4
Menadiol sodium diphosphate	964.3	E858.2	E934.3	E950.4	E962.0	E980.4
Menadione (sodium bisulfite)	964.3	E858.2	E934.3	E950.4	E962.0	E980.4
Menaphthone	964.3	E858.2	E934.3	E950.4	E962.0	E980.4
Meningococcal vaccine	978.8	E858.8	E948.8	E950.4	E962.0	E980.4
Menningovax-C	978.8	E858.8	E948.8	E950.4	E962.0	E980.4
Menotropins	962.4	E858.0	E932.4	E950.4	E962.0	E980.4
Menthol NEC	976.1	E858.7	E946.1	E950.4	E962.0	E980.4
Mepacrine	961.3	E857	E931.3	E950.4	E962.0	E980.4
Meparfynol	967.8	E852.8	E937.8	E950.2	E962.0	E980.2
Mepazine	969.1	E853.0	E939.1	E950.3	E962.0	E980.3
Mepenzolate	971.1	E855.4	E941.1	E950.4	E962.0	E980.4
Meperidine	965.09	E850.2	E935.2	E950.0	E962.0	E980.0
Mephenamin(e)	966.4	E855.0	E936.4	E950.4	E962.0	E980.4
Mephenesin (carbamate)	968.0	E855.1	E938.0	E950.4	E962.0	E980.4
Mephenoxalone	969.5	E853.8	E939.5	E950.3	E962.0	E980.3
Mephentermine	971.2	E855.5	E941.2	E950.4	E962.0	E980.4
Mephenytoin	966.1	E855.0	E936.1	E950.4	E962.0	E980.4
Mephobarbital	967.0	E851	E937.0	E950.1	E962.0	E980.1
Mepiperphenidol	971.1	E855.4	E941.1	E950.4	E962.0	E980.4
Mepivacaine	968.9	E855.2	E938.9	E950.4	E962.0	E980.4
infiltration (subcutaneous)	968.5	E855.2	E938.5	E950.4	E962.0	E980.4
nerve block (peripheral) (plexus)	968.6	E855.2	E938.6	E950.4	E962.0	E980.4
topical (surface)	968.5	E855.2	E938.5	E950.4	E962.0	E980.4
Meprednisone	962.0	E858.0	E932.0	E950.4	E962.0	E980.4
Meprobam	969.5	E853.8	E939.5	E950.3	E962.0	E980.3
Meprobamate	969.5	E853.8	E939.5	E950.3	E962.0	E980.3
Mepyramine (maleate)	963.0	E858.1	E933.0	E950.4	E962.0	E980.4
Meralluride	974.0	E858.5	E944.0	E950.4	E962.0	E980.4
Merbaphen	974.0	E858.5	E944.0	E950.4	E962.0	E980.4
Merbromin	976.0	E858.7	E946.0	E950.4	E962.0	E980.4
Mercaptomerin	974.0	E858.5	E944.0	E950.4	E962.0	E980.4
Mercaptopurine	963.1	E858.1	E933.1	E950.4	E962.0	E980.4
Mercumatilin	974.0	E858.5	E944.0	E950.4	E962.0	E980.4
Mercuramide	974.0	E858.5	E944.0	E950.4	E962.0	E980.4
Mercuranin	976.0	E858.7	E946.0	E950.4	E962.0	E980.4
Mercurochrome	976.0	E858.7	E946.0	E950.4	E962.0	E980.4
Mercury, mercuric, mercurous (compounds) (cyanide) (fumes) (nonmedicinal) (vapor) NEC	985.0	E866.1	—	E950.9	E962.1	E980.9
ammoniated	976.0	E858.7	E946.0	E950.4	E962.0	E980.4
anti-infective	961.2	E857	E931.2	E950.4	E962.0	E980.4
topical	976.0	E858.7	E946.0	E950.4	E962.0	E980.4
chloride (antiseptic) NEC	976.0	E858.7	E946.0	E950.4	E962.0	E980.4
fungicide	985.0	E863.6	—	E950.6	E962.1	E980.7
diuretic compounds	974.0	E858.5	E944.0	E950.4	E962.0	E980.4
fungicide	985.0	E863.6	—	E950.6	E962.1	E980.7
organic (fungicide)	985.0	E863.6	—	E950.6	E962.1	E980.7
Merethoxylline	974.0	E858.5	E944.0	E950.4	E962.0	E980.4
Mersalyl	974.0	E858.5	E944.0	E950.4	E962.0	E980.4
Merthiolate (topical)	976.0	E858.7	E946.0	E950.4	E962.0	E980.4
ophthalmic preparation	976.5	E858.7	E946.5	E950.4	E962.0	E980.4
Meruvax	979.4	E858.8	E949.4	E950.4	E962.0	E980.4
Mescal buttons	969.6	E854.1	E939.6	E950.3	E962.0	E980.3
Mescaline (salts)	969.6	E854.1	E939.6	E950.3	E962.0	E980.3
Mesoridazine besylate	969.1	E853.0	E939.1	E950.3	E962.0	E980.3
Mestanolone	962.1	E858.0	E932.1	E950.4	E962.0	E980.4
Mestranol	962.2	E858.0	E932.2	E950.4	E962.0	E980.4
Metacresylacetate	976.0	E858.7	E946.0	E950.4	E962.0	E980.4

	Poisoning	Accident	Therapeutic Use	Suicide Attempt	Assault	Undetermined
Metaldehyde (snail killer) NEC	989.4	E863.4	—	E950.6	E962.1	E980.7
Metals (heavy) (nonmedicinal) NEC	985.9	E866.4	—	E950.9	E962.1	E980.9
dust, fumes, or vapor NEC	985.9	E866.4	—	E950.9	E962.1	E980.9
light NEC	985.9	E866.4	—	E950.9	E962.1	E980.9
dust, fumes, or vapor NEC	985.9	E866.4	—	E950.9	E962.1	E980.9
pesticides (dust) (vapor)	985.9	E863.4	—	E950.6	E962.1	E980.7
Metamucil	973.3	E858.4	E943.3	E950.4	E962.0	E980.4
Metaphen	976.0	E858.7	E946.0	E950.4	E962.0	E980.4
Metaproterenol	975.1	E858.6	E945.1	E950.4	E962.0	E980.4
Metaraminol	972.8	E858.3	E942.8	E950.4	E962.0	E980.4
Metaxalone	968.0	E855.1	E938.0	E950.4	E962.0	E980.4
Metformin	962.3	E858.0	E932.3	E950.4	E962.0	E980.4
Methacycline	960.4	E856	E930.4	E950.4	E962.0	E980.4
Methadone	965.02	E850.1	E935.1	E950.0	E962.0	E980.0
Methallenestril	962.2	E858.0	E932.2	E950.4	E962.0	E980.4
Methamphetamine	969.7	E854.2	E939.7	E950.3	E962.0	E980.3
Methandienone	962.1	E858.0	E932.1	E950.4	E962.0	E980.4
Methandriol	962.1	E858.0	E932.1	E950.4	E962.0	E980.4
Methandrostenolone	962.1	E858.0	E932.1	E950.4	E962.0	E980.4
Methane gas	987.1	E869.8	—	E952.8	E962.2	E982.8
Methanol	980.1	E860.2	—	E950.9	E962.1	E980.9
vapor	987.8	E869.8	—	E952.8	E962.2	E982.8
Methantheline	971.1	E855.4	E941.1	E950.4	E962.0	E980.4
Methaphenilene	963.0	E858.1	E933.0	E950.4	E962.0	E980.4
Methapyrilene	963.0	E858.1	E933.0	E950.4	E962.0	E980.4
Methaqualone (compounds)	967.4	E852.3	E937.4	E950.2	E962.0	E980.2
Metharbital, metharbitone	967.0	E851	E937.0	E950.1	E962.0	E980.1
Methazolamide	974.2	E858.5	E944.2	E950.4	E962.0	E980.4
Methdilazine	963.0	E858.1	E933.0	E950.4	E962.0	E980.4
Methedrine	969.7	E854.2	E939.7	E950.3	E962.0	E980.3
Methenamine (mandelate)	961.9	E857	E931.9	E950.4	E962.0	E980.4
Methenolone	962.1	E858.0	E932.1	E950.4	E962.0	E980.4
Methergine	975.0	E858.6	E945.0	E950.4	E962.0	E980.4
Methiacil	962.8	E858.0	E932.8	E950.4	E962.0	E980.4
Methicillin (sodium)	960.0	E856	E930.0	E950.4	E962.0	E980.4
Methimazole	962.8	E858.0	E932.8	E950.4	E962.0	E980.4
Methionine	977.1	E858.8	E947.1	E950.4	E962.0	E980.4
Methisazone	961.7	E857	E931.7	E950.4	E962.0	E980.4
Methitural	967.0	E851	E937.0	E950.1	E962.0	E980.1
Methixene	971.1	E855.4	E941.1	E950.4	E962.0	E980.4
Methobarbital, methobarbitone	967.0	E851	E937.0	E950.1	E962.0	E980.1
Methocarbamol	968.0	E855.1	E938.0	E950.4	E962.0	E980.4
Methohexital, methohexitone (sodium)	968.3	E855.1	E938.3	E950.4	E962.0	E980.4
Methoin	966.1	E855.0	E936.1	E950.4	E962.0	E980.4
Methopholine	965.7	E850.7	E935.7	E950.0	E962.0	E980.0
Methorate	975.4	E858.6	E945.4	E950.4	E962.0	E980.4
Methoserpidine	972.6	E858.3	E942.6	E950.4	E962.0	E980.4
Methotrexate	963.1	E858.1	E933.1	E950.4	E962.0	E980.4
Methotrimeprazine	967.8	E852.8	E937.8	E950.2	E962.0	E980.2
Methoxa-Dome	976.3	E858.7	E946.3	E950.4	E962.0	E980.4
Methoxamine	971.2	E855.5	E941.2	E950.4	E962.0	E980.4
Methoxsalen	976.3	E858.7	E946.3	E950.4	E962.0	E980.4
Methoxybenzyl penicillin	960.0	E856	E930.0	E950.4	E962.0	E980.4
Methoxychlor	989.2	E863.0	—	E950.6	E962.1	E980.7
Methoxyflurane	968.2	E855.1	E938.2	E950.4	E962.0	E980.4
Methoxyphenamine	971.2	E855.5	E941.2	E950.4	E962.0	E980.4
Methoxypromazine	969.1	E853.0	E939.1	E950.3	E962.0	E980.3
Methoxypsoralen	976.3	E858.7	E946.3	E950.4	E962.0	E980.4
Methscopolamine (bromide)	971.1	E855.4	E941.1	E950.4	E962.0	E980.4
Methsuximide	966.2	E855.0	E936.2	E950.4	E962.0	E980.4
Methyclothiazide	974.3	E858.5	E944.3	E950.4	E962.0	E980.4
Methyl						
acetate	982.8	E862.4	—	E950.9	E962.1	E980.9
acetone	982.8	E862.4	—	E950.9	E962.1	E980.9
alcohol	980.1	E860.2	—	E950.9	E962.1	E980.9
amphetamine	969.7	E854.2	E939.7	E950.3	E962.0	E980.3
androstanolone	962.1	E858.0	E932.1	E950.4	E962.0	E980.4
atropine	971.1	E855.4	E941.1	E950.4	E962.0	E980.4
benzene	982.0	E862.4	—	E950.9	E962.1	E980.9
bromide (gas)	987.8	E869.8	—	E952.8	E962.2	E982.8
fumigant	987.8	E863.8	—	E950.6	E962.2	E980.7
butanol	980.8	E860.8	—	E950.9	E962.1	E980.9
carbinol	980.1	E860.2	—	E950.9	E962.1	E980.9
cellosolve	982.8	E862.4	—	E950.9	E962.1	E980.9
cellulose	973.3	E858.4	E943.3	E950.4	E962.0	E980.4
chloride (gas)	987.8	E869.8	—	E952.8	E962.2	E982.8

		External Cause (E-Code)							External Cause (E-Code)				
	Poisoning	Accident	Therapeutic Use	Suicide Attempt	Assault	Undeter-mined		Poisoning	Accident	Therapeutic Use	Suicide Attempt	Assault	Undeter-mined
Methyl — *continued*							Moroxydine (hydrochloride)	961.7	E857	E931.7	E950.4	E962.0	E980.4
cyclohexane	982.8	E862.4	—	E950.9	E962.1	E980.9	Morphazinamide	961.8	E857	E931.8	E950.4	E962.0	E980.4
cyclohexanone	982.8	E862.4	—	E950.9	E962.1	E980.9	Morphinans	965.09	E850.2	E935.2	E950.0	E962.0	E980.0
dihydromorphinone	965.09	E850.2	E935.2	E950.0	E962.0	E980.0	Morphine NEC	965.09	E850.2	E935.2	E950.0	E962.0	E980.0
ergometrine	975.0	E858.6	E945.0	E950.4	E962.0	E980.4	antagonists	970.1	E854.3	E940.1	E950.4	E962.0	E980.4
ergonovine	975.0	E858.6	E945.0	E950.4	E962.0	E980.4	Morpholinylethylmorphine	965.09	E850.2	E935.2	E950.0	E962.0	E980.0
ethyl ketone	982.8	E862.4	—	E950.9	E962.1	E980.9	Morrhuate sodium	972.7	E858.3	E942.7	E950.4	E962.0	E980.4
hydrazine	983.9	E864.3	—	E950.7	E962.1	E980.6	**Moth balls** (*see also*						
isobutyl ketone	982.8	E862.4	—	E950.9	E962.1	E980.9	Pesticides)	989.4	E863.4	—	E950.6	E962.1	E980.7
morphine NEC	965.09	E850.2	E935.2	E950.0	E962.0	E980.0	naphthalene	983.0	E863.4	—	E950.7	E962.1	E980.6
parafynol	967.8	E852.8	E937.8	E950.2	E962.0	E980.2	**Motor exhaust gas** — *see*						
parathion	989.3	E863.1	—	E950.6	E962.1	E980.7	Carbon, monoxide,						
pentynol NEC	967.8	E852.8	E937.8	E950.2	E962.0	E980.2	exhaust gas						
peridol	969.2	E853.1	E939.2	E950.3	E962.0	E980.3	**Mouth wash**	976.6	E858.7	E946.6	E950.4	E962.0	E980.4
phenidate	969.7	E854.2	E939.7	E950.3	E962.0	E980.3	**Mucolytic agent**	975.5	E858.6	E945.5	E950.4	E962.0	E980.4
prednisolone	962.0	E858.0	E932.0	E950.4	E962.0	E980.4	**Mucomyst**	975.5	E858.6	E945.5	E950.4	E962.0	E980.4
ENT agent	976.6	E858.7	E946.6	E950.4	E962.0	E980.4	**Mucous membrane**						
ophthalmic preparation	976.5	E858.7	E946.5	E950.4	E962.0	E980.4	agents (external)	976.9	E858.7	E946.9	E950.4	E962.0	E980.4
topical NEC	976.0	E858.7	E946.0	E950.4	E962.0	E980.4	specified NEC	976.8	E858.7	E946.8	E950.4	E962.0	E980.4
propylcarbinol	980.8	E860.8	—	E950.9	E962.1	E980.9	**Mumps**						
rosaniline NEC	976.0	E858.7	E946.0	E950.4	E962.0	E980.4	immune globulin (human)	964.6	E858.2	E934.6	E950.4	E962.0	E980.4
salicylate NEC	976.3	E858.7	E946.3	E950.4	E962.0	E980.4	skin test antigen	977.8	E858.8	E947.8	E950.4	E962.0	E980.4
sulfate (fumes)	987.8	E869.8	—	E952.8	E962.2	E982.8	vaccine	979.6	E858.8	E949.6	E950.4	E962.0	E980.4
liquid	983.9	E864.3	—	E950.7	E962.1	E980.6	**Mumpsvax**	979.6	E858.8	E949.6	E950.4	E962.0	E980.4
sulfonal	967.8	E852.8	E937.8	E950.2	E962.0	E980.2	**Muriatic acid** — *see*						
testosterone	962.1	E858.0	E932.1	E950.4	E962.0	E980.4	Hydrochloric acid						
thiouracil	962.8	E858.0	E932.8	E950.4	E962.0	E980.4	**Muscarine**	971.0	E855.3	E941.0	E950.4	E962.0	E980.4
Methylated spirit	980.0	E860.1	—	E950.9	E962.1	E980.9	**Muscle affecting agents**						
Methyldopa	972.6	E858.3	E942.6	E950.4	E962.0	E980.4	NEC	975.3	E858.6	E945.3	E950.4	E962.0	E980.4
Methylene							oxytocic	975.0	E858.6	E945.0	E950.4	E962.0	E980.4
blue	961.9	E857	E931.9	E950.4	E962.0	E980.4	relaxants	975.3	E858.6	E945.3	E950.4	E962.0	E980.4
chloride or dichloride							central nervous system	968.0	E855.1	E938.0	E950.4	E962.0	E980.4
(solvent) NEC	982.3	E862.4	—	E950.9	E962.1	E980.9	skeletal	975.2	E858.6	E945.2	E950.4	E962.0	E980.4
Methylhexabital	967.0	E851	E937.0	E950.1	E962.0	E980.1	smooth	975.1	E858.6	E945.1	E950.4	E962.0	E980.4
Methylparaben (ophthalmic)	976.5	E858.7	E946.5	E950.4	E962.0	E980.4	**Mushrooms, noxious**	988.1	E865.5	—	E950.9	E962.1	E980.9
Methyprylon	967.5	E852.4	E937.5	E950.2	E962.0	E980.2	**Mussel, noxious**	988.0	E865.1	—	E950.9	E962.1	E980.9
Methysergide	971.3	E855.6	E941.3	E950.4	E962.0	E980.4	**Mustard** (emetic)	973.6	E858.4	E943.6	E950.4	E962.0	E980.4
Metoclopramide	963.0	E858.1	E933.0	E950.4	E962.0	E980.4	gas	987.8	E869.8	—	E952.8	E962.2	E982.8
Metofoline	965.7	E850.7	E935.7	E950.0	E962.0	E980.0	nitrogen	963.1	E858.1	E933.1	E950.4	E962.0	E980.4
Metopon	965.09	E850.2	E935.2	E950.0	E962.0	E980.0	**Mustine**	963.1	E858.1	E933.1	E950.4	E962.0	E980.4
Metronidazole	961.5	E857	E931.5	E950.4	E962.0	E980.4	**M-vac**	979.4	E858.8	E949.4	E950.4	E962.0	E980.4
Metycaine	968.9	E855.2	E938.9	E950.4	E962.0	E980.4	**Mycifradin**	960.8	E856	E930.8	E950.4	E962.0	E980.4
infiltration (subcutaneous)	968.5	E855.2	E938.5	E950.4	E962.0	E980.4	topical	976.0	E858.7	E946.0	E950.4	E962.0	E980.4
nerve block (peripheral)							**Mycitracin**	960.8	E856	E930.8	E950.4	E962.0	E980.4
(plexus)	968.6	E855.2	E938.6	E950.4	E962.0	E980.4	ophthalmic preparation	976.5	E858.7	E946.5	E950.4	E962.0	E980.4
topical (surface)	968.5	E855.2	E938.5	E950.4	E962.0	E980.4	**Mycostatin**	960.1	E856	E930.1	E950.4	E962.0	E980.4
Metyrapone	977.8	E858.8	E947.8	E950.4	E962.0	E980.4	topical	976.0	E858.7	E946.0	E950.4	E962.0	E980.4
Mevinphos	989.3	E863.1	—	E950.6	E962.1	E980.7	**Mydriacyl**	971.1	E855.4	E941.1	E950.4	E962.0	E980.4
Mezereon (berries)	988.2	E865.3	—	E950.9	E962.1	E980.9	**Myelobromal**	963.1	E858.1	E933.1	E950.4	E962.0	E980.4
Micatin	976.0	E858.7	E946.0	E950.4	E962.0	E980.4	**Myleran**	963.1	E858.1	E933.1	E950.4	E962.0	E980.4
Miconazole	976.0	E858.7	E946.0	E950.4	E962.0	E980.4	**Myochrysin(e)**	965.69	E850.6	E935.6	E950.0	E962.0	E980.0
Midol	965.1	E850.3	E935.3	E950.0	E962.0	E980.0	**Myoneural blocking agents**	975.2	E858.6	E945.2	E950.4	E962.0	E980.4
Mifepristone	962.9	E858.0	E932.9	E950.4	E962.0	E980.4	**Myristica fragrans**	988.2	E865.3	—	E950.9	E962.1	E980.9
Milk of magnesia	973.0	E858.4	E943.0	E950.4	E962.0	E980.4	**Myristicin**	988.2	E865.3	—	E950.9	E962.1	E980.9
Millipede (tropical)							**Mysoline**	966.3	E855.0	E936.3	E950.4	E962.0	E980.4
(venomous)	989.5	E905.4	—	E950.9	E962.1	E980.9	**Nafcillin** (sodium)	960.0	E856	E930.0	E950.4	E962.0	E980.4
Miltown	969.5	E853.8	E939.5	E950.3	E962.0	E980.3	**Nail polish remover**	982.8	E862.4	—	E950.9	E962.1	E908.9
Mineral							**Nalidixic acid**	961.9	E857	E931.9	E950.4	E962.0	E980.4
oil (medicinal)	973.2	E858.4	E943.2	E950.4	E962.0	E980.4	**Nalorphine**	970.1	E854.3	E940.1	E950.4	E962.0	E980.4
nonmedicinal	981	E862.1	—	E950.9	E962.1	E980.9	**Naloxone**	970.1	E854.3	E940.1	E950.4	E962.0	E980.4
topical	976.3	E858.7	E946.3	E950.4	E962.0	E980.4	**Nandrolone** (decanoate)						
salts NEC	974.6	E858.5	E944.6	E950.4	E962.0	E980.4	(phenproprioate)	962.1	E858.0	E932.1	E950.4	E962.0	E980.4
spirits	981	E862.0	—	E950.9	E962.1	E980.9	**Naphazoline**	971.2	E855.5	E941.2	E950.4	E962.0	E980.4
Minocycline	960.4	E856	E930.4	E950.4	E962.0	E980.4	**Naphtha** (painter's)						
Mithramycin (antineoplastic)	960.7	E856	E930.7	E950.4	E962.0	E980.4	(petroleum)	981	E862.0	—	E950.9	E962.1	E980.9
Mitobronitol	963.1	E858.1	E933.1	E950.4	E962.0	E980.4	solvent	981	E862.0	—	E950.9	E962.1	E980.9
Mitomycin (antineoplastic)	960.7	E856	E930.7	E950.4	E962.0	E980.4	vapor	987.1	E869.8	—	E952.8	E962.2	E982.8
Mitotane	963.1	E858.1	E933.1	E950.4	E962.0	E980.4	**Naphthalene** (chlorinated)	983.0	E864.0	—	E950.7	E962.1	E980.6
Moderil	972.6	E858.3	E942.6	E950.4	E962.0	E980.4	insecticide or moth						
Mogadon — *see Nitrazepam*							repellent	983.0	E863.4	—	E950.7	E962.1	E980.6
Molindone	969.3	E853.8	E939.3	E950.3	E962.0	E980.3	vapor	987.8	E869.8	—	E952.8	E962.2	E982.8
Monistat	976.0	E858.7	E946.0	E950.4	E962.0	E980.4	**Naphthol**	983.0	E864.0	—	E950.7	E962.1	E980.6
Monkshood	988.2	E865.4	—	E950.9	E962.1	E980.9	**Naphthylamine**	983.0	E864.0	—	E950.7	E962.1	E980.6
Monoamine oxidase							**Naprosyn** — *see Naproxen*						
inhibitors	969.0	E854.0	E939.0	E950.3	E962.0	E980.3	**Naproxen**	965.61	E850.6	E935.6	E950.0	E962.0	E980.0
Monochlorobenzene	982.0	E862.4	—	E950.9	E962.1	E980.9	**Narcotic** (drug)	967.9	E852.9	E937.9	E950.2	E962.0	E980.2
Monosodium glutamate	989.89	E866.8	—	E950.9	E962.1	E980.9	analgesic NEC	965.8	E850.8	E935.8	E950.0	E962.0	E980.0
Monoxide, carbon —							antagonist	970.1	E854.3	E940.1	E950.4	E962.0	E980.4
see Carbon, monoxide							specified NEC	967.8	E852.8	E937.8	E950.2	E962.0	E980.2
Moperone	969.2	E853.1	E939.2	E950.3	E962.0	E980.3	**Narcotine**	975.4	E858.6	E945.4	E950.4	E962.0	E980.4
Morning glory seeds	969.6	E854.1	E939.6	E950.3	E962.0	E980.3	**Nardil**	969.0	E854.0	E939.0	E950.3	E962.0	E980.3

☑ Additional Digit Required   ►◄ Revised Text   ● New Line   ▲ Revised Code

		External Cause (E-Code)							External Cause (E-Code)				
	Poisoning	Accident	Therapeutic Use	Suicide Attempt	Assault	Undeter-mined		Poisoning	Accident	Therapeutic Use	Suicide Attempt	Assault	Undeter-mined
Natrium cyanide — *see* Cyanide(s)							Nitroglycerin, nitroglycerol						
Natural							(medicinal)	972.4	E858.3	E942.4	E950.4	E962.0	E980.4
blood (product)	964.7	E858.2	E934.7	E950.4	E962.0	E980.4	nonmedicinal	989.89	E866.8	—	E950.9	E962.1	E980.9
gas (piped)	987.1	E867	—	E951.0	E962.2	E981.0	fumes	987.8	E869.8	—	E952.8	E962.2	E982.8
incomplete combustion	986	E867	—	E951.0	E962.2	E981.0	Nitrohydrochloric acid	983.1	E864.1	—	E950.7	E962.1	E980.6
Nealbarbital, nealbarbitone	967.0	E851	E937.0	E950.1	E962.0	E980.1	Nitromersol	976.0	E858.7	E946.0	E950.4	E962.0	E980.4
Nectadon	975.4	E858.6	E945.4	E950.4	E962.0	E980.4	Nitronaphthalene	983.0	E864.0	—	E950.7	E962.2	E980.6
Nematocyst (sting)	989.5	E905.6	—	E950.9	E962.1	E980.9	Nitrophenol	983.0	E864.0	—	E950.7	E962.2	E980.6
Nembutal	967.0	E851	E937.0	E950.1	E962.0	E980.1	Nitrothiazol	961.6	E857	E931.6	E950.4	E962.0	E980.4
Neoarsphenamine	961.1	E857	E931.1	E950.4	E962.0	E980.4	Nitrotoluene, nitrotoluol	983.0	E864.0	—	E950.7	E962.1	E980.6
Neocinchophen	974.7	E858.5	E944.7	E950.4	E962.0	E980.4	vapor	987.8	E869.8	—	E952.8	E962.2	E982.8
Neomycin	960.8	E856	E930.8	E950.4	E962.0	E980.4	Nitrous	968.2	E855.1	E938.2	E950.4	E962.0	E980.4
ENT agent	976.6	E858.7	E946.6	E950.4	E962.0	E980.4	acid (liquid)	983.1	E864.1	—	E950.7	E962.1	E980.6
ophthalmic preparation	976.5	E858.7	E946.5	E950.4	E962.0	E980.4	fumes	987.2	E869.0	—	E952.8	E962.2	E982.8
topical NEC	976.0	E858.7	E946.0	E950.4	E962.0	E980.4	oxide (anesthetic) NEC	968.2	E855.1	E938.2	E950.4	E962.0	E980.4
Neonal	967.0	E851	E937.0	E950.1	E962.0	E980.1	Nitrozone	976.0	E858.7	E946.0	E950.4	E962.0	E980.4
Neoprontosil	961.0	E857	E931.0	E950.4	E962.0	E980.4	Noctec	967.1	E852.0	E937.1	E950.2	E962.0	E980.2
Neosalvarsan	961.1	E857	E931.1	E950.4	E962.0	E980.4	Noludar	967.5	E852.4	E937.5	E950.2	E962.0	E980.2
Neosilversalvarsan	961.1	E857	E931.1	E950.4	E962.0	E980.4	Noptil	967.0	E851	E937.0	E950.1	E962.0	E980.1
Neosporin	960.8	E856	E930.8	E950.4	E962.0	E980.4	Noradrenalin	971.2	E855.5	E941.2	E950.4	E962.0	E980.4
ENT agent	976.6	E858.7	E946.6	E950.4	E962.0	E980.4	Noramidopyrine	965.5	E850.5	E935.5	E950.0	E962.0	E980.0
opthalmic preparation	976.5	E858.7	E946.5	E950.4	E962.0	E980.4	Norepinephrine	971.2	E855.5	E941.2	E950.4	E962.0	E980.4
topical NEC	976.0	E858.7	E946.0	E950.4	E962.0	E980.4	Norethandrolone	962.1	E858.0	E932.1	E950.4	E962.0	E980.4
Neostigmine	971.0	E855.3	E941.0	E950.4	E962.0	E980.4	Norethindrone	962.2	E858.0	E932.2	E950.4	E962.0	E980.4
Neraval	967.0	E851	E937.0	E950.1	E962.0	E980.1	Norethisterone	962.2	E858.0	E932.2	E950.4	E962.0	E980.4
Neravan	967.0	E851	E937.0	E950.1	E962.0	E980.1	Norethynodrel	962.2	E858.0	E932.2	E950.4	E962.0	E980.4
Nerium oleander	988.2	E865.4	—	E950.9	E962.1	E980.9	Norlestrin	962.2	E858.0	E932.2	E950.4	E962.0	E980.4
Nerve gases (war)	987.9	E869.9	—	E952.9	E962.2	E982.9	Norlutin	962.2	E858.0	E932.2	E950.4	E962.0	E980.4
Nesacaine	968.9	E855.2	E938.9	E950.4	E962.0	E980.4	Normison — *see* Benzodiazepines						
infiltration (subcutaneous)	968.5	E855.2	E938.5	E950.4	E962.0	E980.4	Normorphine	965.09	E850.2	E935.2	E950.0	E962.0	E980.0
nerve block (peripheral) (plexus)	968.6	E855.2	E938.6	E950.4	E962.0	E980.4	Nortriptyline	969.0	E854.0	E939.0	E950.3	E962.0	E980.3
Neurobarb	967.0	E851	E937.0	E950.1	E962.0	E980.1	Noscapine	975.4	E858.6	E945.4	E950.4	E962.0	E980.4
Neuroleptics NEC	969.3	E853.8	E939.3	E950.3	E962.0	E980.3	Nose preparations	976.6	E858.7	E946.6	E950.4	E962.0	E980.4
Neuroprotective agent	977.8	E858.8	E947.8	E950.4	E962.0	E980.4	Novobiocin	960.8	E856	E930.8	E950.4	E962.0	E980.4
Neutral spirits	980.0	E860.1	—	E950.9	E962.1	E980.9	Novocain (infiltration) (topical)	968.5	E855.2	E938.5	E950.4	E962.0	E980.4
beverage	980.0	E860.0	—	E950.9	E962.1	E980.9	nerve block (peripheral) (plexus)	968.6	E855.2	E938.6	E950.4	E962.0	E980.4
Niacin, niacinamide	972.2	E858.3	E942.2	E950.4	E962.0	E980.4	spinal	968.7	E855.2	E938.7	E950.4	E962.0	E980.4
Nialamide	969.0	E854.0	E939.0	E950.3	E962.0	E980.3	Noxythiolin	961.9	E857	E931.9	E950.4	E962.0	E980.4
Nickle (carbonyl) (compounds) (fumes) (tetracarbonyl) (vapor)	985.8	E866.4	—	E950.9	E962.1	E980.9	NPH Iletin (insulin)	962.3	E858.0	E932.3	E950.4	E962.0	E980.4
Niclosamide	961.6	E857	E931.6	E950.4	E962.0	E980.4	Numorphan	965.09	E850.2	E935.2	E950.0	E962.0	E980.0
Nicomorphine	965.09	E850.2	E935.2	E950.0	E962.0	E980.0	Nunol	967.0	E851	E937.0	E950.1	E962.0	E980.1
Nicotinamide	972.2	E858.3	E942.2	E950.4	E962.0	E980.4	Nupercaine (spinal anesthetic)	968.7	E855.2	E938.7	E950.4	E962.0	E980.4
Nicotine (insecticide) (spray) (sulfate) NEC	989.4	E863.4	—	E950.6	E962.1	E980.7	topical (surface)	968.5	E855.2	E938.5	E950.4	E962.0	E980.4
not insecticide	989.89	E866.8	—	E950.9	E962.1	E980.9	Nutmeg oil (liniment)	976.3	E858.7	E946.3	E950.4	E962.0	E980.4
Nicotinic acid (derivatives)	972.2	E858.3	E942.2	E950.4	E962.0	E980.4	Nux vomica	989.1	E863.7	—	E950.6	E962.1	E980.7
Nicotinyl alcohol	972.2	E858.3	E942.2	E950.4	E962.0	E980.4	Nydrazid	961.8	E857	E931.8	E950.4	E962.0	E980.4
Nicoumalone	964.2	E858.2	E934.2	E950.4	E962.0	E980.4	Nylidrin	971.2	E855.5	E941.2	E950.4	E962.0	E980.4
Nifenazone	965.5	E850.5	E935.5	E950.0	E962.0	E980.0	Nystatin	960.1	E856	E930.1	E950.4	E962.0	E980.4
Nifuraldezone	961.9	E857	E931.9	E950.4	E962.0	E980.4	topical	976.0	E858.7	E946.0	E950.4	E962.0	E980.4
Nightshade (deadly)	988.2	E865.4	—	E950.9	E962.1	E980.9	Nytol	963.0	E858.2	E934.2	E950.4	E962.0	E980.4
Nikethamide	970.0	E854.3	E940.0	E950.4	E962.0	E980.4	Oblivion	967.8	E852.8	E937.8	E950.2	E962.0	E980.2
Nilstat	960.1	E856	E930.1	E950.4	E962.0	E980.4	Octyl nitrite	972.4	E858.3	E942.4	E950.4	E962.0	E980.4
topical	976.0	E858.7	E946.0	E950.4	E962.0	E980.4	Oestradiol (cypionate) (dipropionate) (valerate)	962.2	E858.0	E932.2	E950.4	E962.0	E980.4
Nimodipine	977.8	E858.8	E947.8	E950.4	E962.0	E980.4	Oestriol	962.2	E858.0	E932.2	E950.4	E962.0	E980.4
Niridazole	961.6	E857	E931.6	E950.4	E962.0	E980.4	Oestrone	962.2	E858.0	E932.2	E950.4	E962.0	E980.4
Nisentil	965.09	E850.2	E935.2	E950.0	E962.0	E980.0	Oil (of) NEC	989.89	E866.8	—	E950.9	E962.1	E980.9
Nitrates	972.4	E858.3	E942.4	E950.4	E962.0	E980.4	bitter almond	989.0	E866.8	—	E950.9	E962.1	E980.9
Nitrazepam	969.4	E853.2	E939.4	E950.3	E962.0	E980.3	camphor	976.1	E858.7	E946.1	E950.4	E962.0	E980.4
Nitric							colors	989.89	E861.6	—	E950.9	E962.1	E980.9
acid (liquid)	983.1	E864.1	—	E950.7	E962.1	E980.6	fumes	987.8	E869.8	—	E952.8	E962.2	E982.8
vapor	987.8	E869.8	—	E952.8	E962.2	E982.8	lubricating	981	E862.2	—	E950.9	E962.1	E980.9
oxide (gas)	987.2	E869.0	—	E952.8	E962.2	E982.8	specified source, other — *see* substance specified						
Nitrite, amyl (medicinal) (vapor)	972.4	E858.3	E942.4	E950.4	E962.0	E980.4	vitriol (liquid)	983.1	E864.1	—	E950.7	E962.1	E980.6
Nitroaniline	983.0	E864.0	—	E950.7	E962.1	E980.6	fumes	987.8	E869.8	—	E952.8	E962.2	E982.8
vapor	987.8	E869.8	—	E952.8	E962.2	E982.8	wintergreen (bitter) NEC	976.3	E858.7	E946.3	E950.4	E962.0	E980.4
Nitrobenzene, nitrobenzol	983.0	E864.0	—	E950.7	E962.1	E980.6	Ointments NEC	976.9	E858.7	E946.9	E950.4	E962.0	E980.4
vapor	987.8	E869.8	—	E952.8	E962.2	E982.8	Oleander	988.2	E865.4	—	E950.9	E962.1	E980.9
Nitrocellulose	976.3	E858.7	E946.3	E950.4	E962.0	E980.4	Oleandomycin	960.3	E856	E930.3	E950.4	E962.0	E980.4
Nitrofuran derivatives	961.9	E857	E931.9	E950.4	E962.0	E980.4	Oleovitamin A	963.5	E858.1	E933.5	E950.4	E962.0	E980.4
Nitrofurantoin	961.9	E857	E931.9	E950.4	E962.0	E980.4	Oleum ricini	973.1	E858.4	E943.1	E950.4	E962.0	E980.4
Nitrofurazone	976.0	E858.7	E946.0	E950.4	E962.0	E980.4	Olive oil (medicinal) NEC	973.2	E858.4	E943.2	E950.4	E962.0	E980.4
Nitrogen (dioxide) (gas) (oxide)	987.2	E869.0	—	E952.8	E962.2	E982.8	OMPA	989.3	E863.1	—	E950.6	E962.1	E980.7
mustard (antineoplastic)	963.1	E858.1	E933.1	E950.4	E962.0	E980.4							

☑ Additional Digit Required   ▶◀ Revised Text   ● New Line   ▲ Revised Code

	External Cause (E-Code)					
	Poisoning	Accident	Therapeutic Use	Suicide Attempt	Assault	Undetermined
Oncovin	963.1	E858.1	E933.1	E950.4	E962.0	E980.4
Ophthaine	968.5	E855.2	E938.5	E950.4	E962.0	E980.4
Ophthetic	968.5	E855.2	E938.5	E950.4	E962.0	E980.4
Opiates, opioids, opium						
NEC	965.00	E850.2	E935.2	E950.0	E962.0	E980.0
antagonists	970.1	E854.3	E940.1	E950.4	E962.0	E980.4
Oracon	962.2	E858.0	E932.2	E950.4	E962.0	E980.4
Oragrafin	977.8	E858.8	E947.8	E950.4	E962.0	E980.4
Oral contraceptives	962.2	E858.0	E932.2	E950.4	E962.0	E980.4
Orciprenaline	975.1	E858.6	E945.1	E950.4	E962.0	E980.4
Organidin	975.5	E858.6	E945.5	E950.4	E962.0	E980.4
Organophosphates	989.3	E863.1	—	E950.6	E962.1	E980.7
Orimune	979.5	E858.8	E949.5	E950.4	E962.0	E980.4
Orinase	962.3	E858.0	E932.3	E950.4	E962.0	E980.4
Orphenadrine	966.4	E855.0	E936.4	E950.4	E962.0	E980.4
Ortal (sodium)	967.0	E851	E937.0	E950.1	E962.0	E980.1
Orthoboric acid	976.0	E858.7	E946.0	E950.4	E962.0	E980.4
ENT agent	976.6	E858.7	E946.6	E950.4	E962.0	E980.4
ophthalmic preparation	976.5	E858.7	E946.5	E950.4	E962.0	E980.4
Orthocaine	968.5	E855.2	E938.5	E950.4	E962.0	E980.4
Ortho-Novum	962.2	E858.0	E932.2	E950.4	E962.0	E980.4
Orthotolidine (reagent)	977.8	E858.8	E947.8	E950.4	E962.0	E980.4
Osmic acid (liquid)	983.1	E864.1	—	E950.7	E962.1	E980.6
fumes	987.8	E869.8	—	E952.8	E962.2	E982.8
Osmotic diuretics	974.4	E858.5	E944.4	E950.4	E962.0	E980.4
Ouabain	972.1	E858.3	E942.1	E950.4	E962.0	E980.4
Ovarian hormones (synthetic substitutes)	962.2	E858.0	E932.2	E950.4	E962.0	E980.4
Ovral	962.2	E858.0	E932.2	E950.4	E962.0	E980.4
Ovulation suppressants	962.2	E858.0	E932.2	E950.4	E962.0	E980.4
Ovulen	962.2	E858.0	E932.2	E950.4	E962.0	E980.4
Oxacillin (sodium)	960.0	E856	E930.0	E950.4	E962.0	E980.4
Oxalic acid	983.1	E864.1	—	E950.7	E962.1	E980.6
Oxanamide	969.5	E853.8	E939.5	E950.3	E962.0	E980.3
Oxandrolone	962.1	E858.0	E932.1	E950.4	E962.0	E980.4
Oxaprozin	965.61	E850.6	E935.6	E950.0	E962.0	E980.0
Oxazepam	969.4	E853.2	E939.4	E950.3	E962.0	E980.3
Oxazolidine derivatives	966.0	E855.0	E936.0	E950.4	E962.0	E980.4
Ox bile extract	973.4	E858.4	E943.4	E950.4	E962.0	E980.4
Oxedrine	971.2	E855.5	E941.2	E950.4	E962.0	E980.4
Oxeladin	975.4	E858.6	E945.4	E950.4	E962.0	E980.4
Oxethazaine NEC	968.5	E855.2	E938.5	E950.4	E962.0	E980.4
Oxidizing agents NEC	983.9	E864.3	—	E950.7	E962.1	E980.6
Oxolinic acid	961.3	E857	E931.3	E950.4	E962.0	E980.4
Oxophenarsine	961.1	E857	E931.1	E950.4	E962.0	E980.4
Oxsoralen	976.3	E858.7	E946.3	E950.4	E962.0	E980.4
Oxtriphylline	975.7	E858.6	E945.7	E950.4	E962.0	E980.4
Oxybuprocaine	968.5	E855.2	E938.5	E950.4	E962.0	E980.4
Oxybutynin	975.1	E858.6	E945.1	E950.4	E962.0	E980.4
Oxycodone	965.09	E850.2	E935.2	E950.0	E962.0	E980.0
Oxygen	987.8	E869.8	—	E952.8	E962.2	E982.8
Oxylone	976.0	E858.7	E946.0	E950.4	E962.0	E980.4
ophthalmic preparation	976.5	E858.7	E946.5	E950.4	E962.0	E980.4
Oxymesterone	962.1	E858.0	E932.1	E950.4	E962.0	E980.4
Oxymetazoline	971.2	E855.5	E941.2	E950.4	E962.0	E980.4
Oxymetholone	962.1	E858.0	E932.1	E950.4	E962.0	E980.4
Oxymorphone	965.09	E850.2	E935.2	E950.0	E962.0	E980.0
Oxypertine	969.0	E854.0	E939.0	E950.3	E962.0	E980.3
Oxyphenbutazone	965.5	E850.5	E935.5	E950.0	E962.0	E980.0
Oxyphencyclimine	971.1	E855.4	E941.1	E950.4	E962.0	E980.4
Oxyphenisatin	973.1	E858.4	E943.1	E950.4	E962.0	E980.4
Oxyphenonium	971.1	E855.4	E941.1	E950.4	E962.0	E980.4
Oxyquinoline	961.3	E857	E931.3	E950.4	E962.0	E980.4
Oxytetracycline	960.4	E856	E930.4	E950.4	E962.0	E980.4
Oxytocics	975.0	E858.6	E945.0	E950.4	E962.0	E980.4
Oxytocin	975.0	E858.6	E945.0	E950.4	E962.0	E980.4
Ozone	987.8	E869.8	—	E952.8	E962.2	E982.8
PABA	976.3	E858.7	E946.3	E950.4	E962.0	E980.4
Packed red cells	964.7	E858.2	E934.7	E950.4	E962.0	E980.4
Paint NEC	989.89	E861.6	—	E950.9	E962.1	E980.9
cleaner	982.8	E862.9	—	E950.9	E962.1	E980.9
fumes NEC	987.8	E869.8	—	E952.8	E962.1	E982.8
lead (fumes)	984.0	E861.5	—	E950.9	E962.1	E980.9
solvent NEC	982.8	E862.9	—	E950.9	E962.1	E980.9
stripper	982.8	E862.9	—	E950.9	E962.1	E980.9
Palfium	965.09	E850.2	E935.2	E950.0	E962.0	E980.0
Palivizumab	979.9	E858.8	E949.6	E950.4	E962.0	E980.4
Paludrine	961.4	E857	E931.4	E950.4	E962.0	E980.4
PAM	977.2	E855.8	E947.2	E950.4	E962.0	E980.4
Pamaquine (naphthoate)	961.4	E857	E931.4	E950.4	E962.0	E980.4
Pamprin	965.1	E850.3	E935.3	E950.0	E962.0	E980.0

	External Cause (E-Code)					
	Poisoning	Accident	Therapeutic Use	Suicide Attempt	Assault	Undetermined
Panadol	965.4	E850.4	E935.4	E950.0	E962.0	E980.0
Pancreatic dornase (mucolytic)	963.4	E858.1	E933.4	E950.4	E962.0	E980.4
Pancreatin	973.4	E858.4	E943.4	E950.4	E962.0	E980.4
Pancrelipase	973.4	E858.4	E943.4	E950.4	E962.0	E980.4
Pangamic acid	963.5	E858.1	E933.5	E950.4	E962.0	E980.4
Panthenol	963.5	E858.1	E933.5	E950.4	E962.0	E980.4
topical	976.8	E858.7	E946.8	E950.4	E962.0	E980.4
Pantopaque	977.8	E858.8	E947.8	E950.4	E962.0	E980.4
Pantopon	965.00	E850.2	E935.2	E950.0	E962.0	E980.0
Pantothenic acid	963.5	E858.1	E933.5	E950.4	E962.0	E980.4
Panwarfin	964.2	E858.2	E934.2	E950.4	E962.0	E980.4
Papain	973.4	E858.4	E943.4	E950.4	E962.0	E980.4
Papaverine	972.5	E858.3	E942.5	E950.4	E962.0	E980.4
Para-aminobenzoic acid	976.3	E858.7	E946.3	E950.4	E962.0	E980.4
Para-aminophenol derivatives	965.4	E850.4	E935.4	E950.0	E962.0	E980.0
Para-aminosalicylic acid (derivatives)	961.8	E857	E931.8	E950.4	E962.0	E980.4
Paracetaldehyde (medicinal)	967.2	E852.1	E937.2	E950.2	E962.0	E980.2
Paracetamol	965.4	E850.4	E935.4	E950.0	E962.0	E980.0
Paracodin	965.09	E850.2	E935.2	E950.0	E962.0	E980.0
Paradione	966.0	E855.0	E936.0	E950.4	E962.0	E980.4
Paraffin(s) (wax)	981	E862.3	—	E950.9	E962.1	E980.9
liquid (medicinal)	973.2	E858.4	E943.2	E950.4	E962.0	E980.4
nonmedicinal (oil)	981	E862.1	—	E950.9	E962.1	E980.9
Paraldehyde (medicinal)	967.2	E852.1	E937.2	E950.2	E962.0	E980.2
Paramethadione	966.0	E855.0	E936.0	E950.4	E962.0	E980.4
Paramethasone	962.0	E858.0	E932.0	E950.4	E962.0	E980.4
Paraquat	989.4	E863.5	—	E950.6	E962.1	E980.7
Parasympatholytics	971.1	E855.4	E941.1	E950.4	E962.0	E980.4
Parasympathomimetics	971.0	E855.3	E941.0	E950.4	E962.0	E980.4
Parathion	989.3	E863.1	—	E950.6	E962.1	E980.7
Parathormone	962.6	E858.0	E932.6	E950.4	E962.0	E980.4
Parathyroid (derivatives)	962.6	E858.0	E932.6	E950.4	E962.0	E980.4
Paratyphoid vaccine	978.1	E858.8	E948.1	E950.4	E962.0	E980.4
Paredrine	971.2	E855.5	E941.2	E950.4	E962.0	E980.4
Paregoric	965.00	E850.2	E935.2	E950.0	E962.0	E980.0
Pargyline	972.3	E858.3	E942.3	E950.4	E962.0	E980.4
Paris green	985.1	E866.3	—	E950.8	E962.1	E980.8
insecticide	985.1	E863.4	—	E950.8	E962.1	E980.8
Parnate	969.0	E854.0	E939.0	E950.3	E962.0	E980.3
Paromomycin	960.8	E856	E930.8	E950.4	E962.0	E980.4
Paroxypropione	963.1	E858.1	E933.1	E950.4	E962.0	E980.4
Parzone	965.09	E850.2	E935.2	E950.0	E962.0	E980.0
PAS	961.8	E857	E931.8	E950.4	E962.0	E980.4
PCBs	981	E862.3	—	E950.9	E962.1	E980.9
PCP (pentachlorophenol)	989.4	E863.6	—	E950.6	E962.1	E980.7
herbicide	989.4	E863.5	—	E950.6	E962.1	E980.7
insecticide	989.4	E863.4	—	E950.6	E962.1	E980.7
phencyclidine	968.3	E855.1	E938.3	E950.4	E962.0	E980.4
Peach kernel oil (emulsion)	973.2	E858.4	E943.2	E950.4	E962.0	E980.4
Peanut oil (emulsion) NEC	973.2	E858.4	E943.2	E950.4	E962.0	E980.4
topical	976.3	E858.7	E946.3	E950.4	E962.0	E980.4
Pearly Gates (morning glory seeds)	969.6	E854.1	E939.6	E950.3	E962.0	E980.3
Pecazine	969.1	E853.0	E939.1	E950.3	E962.0	E980.3
Pecilocin	960.1	E856	E930.1	E950.4	E962.0	E980.4
Pectin (with kaolin) NEC	973.5	E858.4	E943.5	E950.4	E962.0	E980.4
Pelletierine tannate	961.6	E857	E931.6	E950.4	E962.0	E980.4
Pemoline	969.7	E854.2	E939.7	E950.3	E962.0	E980.3
Pempidine	972.3	E858.3	E942.3	E950.4	E962.0	E980.4
Penamecillin	960.0	E856	E930.0	E950.4	E962.0	E980.4
Penethamate hydriodide	960.0	E856	E930.0	E950.4	E962.0	E980.4
Penicillamine	963.8	E858.1	E933.8	E950.4	E962.0	E980.4
Penicillin (any type)	960.0	E856	E930.0	E950.4	E962.0	E980.4
Penicillinase	963.4	E858.1	E933.4	E950.4	E962.0	E980.4
Pentachlorophenol (fungicide)	989.4	E863.6	—	E950.6	E962.1	E980.7
herbicide	989.4	E863.5	—	E950.6	E962.1	E980.7
insecticide	989.4	E863.4	—	E950.6	E962.1	E980.7
Pentaerythritol	972.4	E858.3	E942.4	E950.4	E962.0	E980.4
chloral	967.1	E852.0	E937.1	E950.2	E962.0	E980.2
tetranitrate NEC	972.4	E858.3	E942.4	E950.4	E962.0	E980.4
Pentagastrin	977.8	E858.8	E947.8	E950.4	E962.0	E980.4
Pentalin	982.3	E862.4	—	E950.9	E962.1	E980.9
Pentamethonium (bromide)	972.3	E858.3	E942.3	E950.4	E962.0	E980.4
Pentamidine	961.5	E857	E931.5	E950.4	E962.0	E980.4
Pentanol	980.8	E860.8	—	E950.9	E962.1	E980.9
Pentaquine	961.4	E857	E931.4	E950.4	E962.0	E980.4
Pentazocine	965.8	E850.8	E935.8	E950.0	E962.0	E980.0

☑ Additional Digit Required   ▶◀ Revised Text   ● New Line   ▲ Revised Code

Substance	Poisoning	External Cause (E-Code) Accident	Therapeutic Use	Suicide Attempt	Assault	Undetermined
Penthienate	971.1	E855.4	E941.1	E950.4	E962.0	E980.4
Pentobarbital, pentobarbitone						
(sodium)	967.0	E851	E937.0	E950.1	E962.0	E980.1
Pentolinium (tartrate)	972.3	E858.3	E942.3	E950.4	E962.0	E980.4
Pentothal	968.3	E855.1	E938.3	E950.4	E962.0	E980.4
Pentylenetetrazol	970.0	E854.3	E940.0	E950.4	E962.0	E980.4
Pentylsalicylamide	961.8	E857	E931.8	E950.4	E962.0	E980.4
Pepsin	973.4	E858.4	E943.4	E950.4	E962.0	E980.4
Peptavlon	977.8	E858.8	E947.8	E950.4	E962.0	E980.4
Percaine (spinal)	968.7	E855.2	E938.7	E950.4	E962.0	E980.4
topical (surface)	968.5	E855.2	E938.5	E950.4	E962.0	E980.4
Perchloroethylene (vapor)	982.3	E862.4	—	E950.9	E962.1	E980.9
medicinal	961.6	E857	E931.6	E950.4	E962.0	E980.4
Percodan	965.09	E850.2	E935.2	E950.0	E962.0	E980.0
Percogesic	965.09	E850.2	E935.2	E950.0	E962.0	E980.0
Percorten	962.0	E858.0	E932.0	E950.4	E962.0	E980.4
Pergonal	962.4	E858.0	E932.4	E950.4	E962.0	E980.4
Perhexiline	972.4	E858.3	E942.4	E950.4	E962.0	E980.4
Periactin	963.0	E858.1	E933.0	E950.4	E962.0	E980.4
Periclor	967.1	E852.0	E937.1	E950.2	E962.0	E980.2
Pericyazine	969.1	E853.0	E939.1	E950.3	E962.0	E980.3
Peritrate	972.4	E858.3	E942.4	E950.4	E962.0	E980.4
Permanganates NEC	983.9	E864.3	—	E950.7	E962.1	E980.6
potassium (topical)	976.0	E858.7	E946.0	E950.4	E962.0	E980.4
Pernocton	967.0	E851	E937.0	E950.1	E962.0	E980.1
Pernoston	967.0	E851	E937.0	E950.1	E962.0	E980.1
Peronin(e)	965.09	E850.2	E935.2	E950.0	E962.0	E980.0
Perphenazine	969.1	E853.0	E939.1	E950.3	E962.0	E980.3
Pertofrane	969.0	E854.0	E939.0	E950.3	E962.0	E980.3
Pertussis						
immune serum (human)	964.6	E858.2	E934.6	E950.4	E962.0	E980.4
vaccine (with diphtheria toxoid) (with tetanus toxoid)	978.6	E858.8	E948.6	E950.4	E962.0	E980.4
Peruvian balsam	976.8	E858.7	E946.8	E950.4	E962.0	E980.4
Pesticides (dust) (fumes)						
(vapor)	989.4	E863.4	—	E950.6	E962.1	E980.7
arsenic	985.1	E863.4	—	E950.8	E962.1	E980.8
chlorinated	989.2	E863.0	—	E950.6	E962.1	E980.7
cyanide	989.0	E863.4	—	E950.6	E962.1	E980.7
kerosene	981	E863.4	—	E950.6	E962.1	E980.7
mixture (of compounds)	989.4	E863.3	—	E950.6	E962.1	E980.7
naphthalene	983.0	E863.4	—	E950.7	E962.1	E980.6
organochlorine (compounds)	989.2	E863.0	—	E950.6	E962.1	E980.7
petroleum (distillate) (products) NEC	981	E863.4	—	E950.6	E962.1	E980.7
specified ingredient NEC	989.4	E863.4	—	E950.6	E962.1	E980.7
strychnine	989.1	E863.4	—	E950.6	E962.1	E980.7
thallium	985.8	E863.7	—	E950.6	E962.1	E980.7
Pethidine (hydrochloride)	965.09	E850.2	E935.2	E950.0	E962.0	E980.0
Petrichloral	967.1	E852.0	E937.1	E950.2	E962.0	E980.2
Petrol	981	E862.1	—	E950.9	E962.1	E980.9
vapor	987.1	E869.8	—	E952.8	E962.2	E982.8
Petrolatum (jelly) (ointment)	976.3	E858.7	E946.3	E950.4	E962.0	E980.4
hydrophilic	976.3	E858.7	E946.3	E950.4	E962.0	E980.4
liquid	973.2	E858.4	E943.2	E950.4	E962.0	E980.4
topical	976.3	E858.7	E946.3	E950.4	E962.0	E980.4
nonmedicinal	981	E862.1	—	E950.9	E962.1	E980.9
Petroleum (cleaners) (fuels) (products) NEC	981	E862.1	—	E950.9	E962.1	E980.9
benzin(e) — see Ligroin						
ether — see Ligroin						
jelly — see Petrolatum						
naphtha — see Ligroin						
pesticide	981	E863.4	—	E950.6	E962.1	E980.7
solids	981	E862.3	—	E950.9	E962.1	E980.9
solvents	981	E862.0	—	E950.9	E962.1	E980.9
vapor	987.1	E869.8	—	E952.8	E962.2	E982.8
Peyote	969.6	E854.1	E939.6	E950.3	E962.0	E980.3
Phanodorm, phanodorn	967.0	E851	E937.0	E950.1	E962.0	E980.1
Phanquinone, phanquone	961.5	E857	E931.5	E950.4	E962.0	E980.4
Pharmaceutical excipient or adjunct	977.4	E858.8	E947.4	E950.4	E962.0	E980.4
Phenacemide	966.3	E855.0	E936.3	E950.4	E962.0	E980.4
Phenacetin	965.4	E850.4	E935.4	E950.0	E962.0	E980.0
Phenadoxone	965.09	E850.2	E935.2	E950.0	E962.0	E980.0
Phenaglycodol	969.5	E853.8	E939.5	E950.3	E962.0	E980.3
Phenantoin	966.1	E855.0	E936.1	E950.4	E962.0	E980.4
Phenaphthazine reagent	977.8	E858.8	E947.8	E950.4	E962.0	E980.4
Phenazocine	965.09	E850.2	E935.2	E950.0	E962.0	E980.0
Phenazone	965.5	E850.5	E935.5	E950.0	E962.0	E980.0
Phenazopyridine	976.1	E858.7	E946.1	E950.4	E962.0	E980.4
Phenbenicillin	960.0	E856	E930.0	E950.4	E962.0	E980.4
Phenbutrazate	977.0	E858.8	E947.0	E950.4	E962.0	E980.4
Phencyclidine	968.3	E855.1	E938.3	E950.4	E962.0	E980.4
Phendimetrazine	977.0	E858.8	E947.0	E950.4	E962.0	E980.4
Phenelzine	969.0	E854.0	E939.0	E950.3	E962.0	E980.3
Phenergan	967.8	E852.8	E937.8	E950.2	E962.0	E980.2
Phenethicillin (potassium)	960.0	E856	E930.0	E950.4	E962.0	E980.4
Phenetsal	965.1	E850.3	E935.3	E950.0	E962.0	E980.0
Pheneturide	966.3	E855.0	E936.3	E950.4	E962.0	E980.4
Phenformin	962.3	E858.0	E932.3	E950.4	E962.0	E980.4
Phenglutarimide	971.1	E855.4	E941.1	E950.4	E962.0	E980.4
Phenicarbazide	965.8	E850.8	E935.8	E950.0	E962.0	E980.0
Phenindamine (tartrate)	963.0	E858.1	E933.0	E950.4	E962.0	E980.4
Phenindione	964.2	E858.2	E934.2	E950.4	E962.0	E980.4
Pheniprazine	969.0	E854.0	E939.0	E950.3	E962.0	E980.3
Pheniramine (maleate)	963.0	E858.1	E933.0	E950.4	E962.0	E980.4
Phenmetrazine	977.0	E858.8	E947.0	E950.4	E962.0	E980.4
Phenobal	967.0	E851	E937.0	E950.1	E962.0	E980.1
Phenobarbital	967.0	E851	E937.0	E950.1	E962.0	E980.1
Phenobarbitone	967.0	E851	E937.0	E950.1	E962.0	E980.1
Phenoctide	976.0	E858.7	E946.0	E950.4	E962.0	E980.4
Phenol (derivatives) NEC	983.0	E864.0	—	E950.7	E962.1	E980.6
disinfectant	983.0	E864.0	—	E950.7	E962.1	E980.6
pesticide	989.4	E863.4	—	E950.6	E962.1	E980.7
red	977.8	E858.8	E947.8	E950.4	E962.0	E980.4
Phenolphthalein	973.1	E858.4	E943.1	E950.4	E962.0	E980.4
Phenolsulfonphthalein	977.8	E858.8	E947.8	E950.4	E962.0	E980.4
Phenomorphan	965.09	E850.2	E935.2	E950.0	E962.0	E980.0
Phenonyl	967.0	E851	E937.0	E950.1	E962.0	E980.1
Phenoperidine	965.09	E850.2	E935.2	E950.0	E962.0	E980.0
Phenoquin	974.7	E858.5	E944.7	E950.4	E962.0	E980.4
Phenothiazines (tranquilizers)						
NEC	969.1	E853.0	E939.1	E950.3	E962.0	E980.3
insecticide	989.3	E863.4	—	E950.6	E962.1	E980.7
Phenoxybenzamine	971.3	E855.6	E941.3	E950.4	E962.0	E980.4
Phenoxymethyl penicillin	960.0	E856	E930.0	E950.4	E962.0	E980.4
Phenprocoumon	964.2	E858.2	E934.2	E950.4	E962.0	E980.4
Phensuximide	966.2	E855.0	E936.2	E950.4	E962.0	E980.4
Phentermine	977.0	E858.8	E947.0	E950.4	E962.0	E980.4
Phentolamine	971.3	E855.6	E941.3	E950.4	E962.0	E980.4
Phenyl						
butazone	965.5	E850.5	E935.5	E950.0	E962.0	E980.0
enediamine	983.0	E864.0	—	E950.7	E962.1	E980.6
hydrazine	983.0	E864.0	—	E950.7	E962.1	E980.6
antineoplastic	963.1	E858.1	E933.1	E950.4	E962.0	E980.4
mercuric compounds — see Mercury						
salicylate	976.3	E858.7	E946.3	E950.4	E962.0	E980.4
Phenylephrin	971.2	E855.5	E941.2	E950.4	E962.0	E980.4
Phenylethylbiguanide	962.3	E858.0	E932.3	E950.4	E962.0	E980.4
Phenylpropanolamine	971.2	E855.5	E941.2	E950.4	E962.0	E980.4
Phenylsulfthion	989.3	E863.1	—	E950.6	E962.1	E980.7
Phenyramidol, phenyramidon	965.7	E850.7	E935.7	E950.0	E962.0	E980.0
Phenytoin	966.1	E855.0	E936.1	E950.4	E962.0	E980.4
pHisoHex	976.2	E858.7	E946.2	E950.4	E962.0	E980.4
Pholcodine	965.09	E850.2	E935.2	E950.0	E962.0	E980.0
Phorate	989.3	E863.1	—	E950.6	E962.1	E980.7
Phosdrin	989.3	E863.1	—	E950.6	E962.1	E980.7
Phosgene (gas)	987.8	E869.8	—	E952.8	E962.2	E982.8
Phosphate (tricresyl)	989.89	E866.8	—	E950.9	E962.1	E980.9
organic	989.3	E863.1	—	E950.6	E962.1	E980.7
solvent	982.8	E862.4	—	E950.9	E926.1	E980.9
Phosphine	987.8	E869.8	—	E952.8	E962.2	E982.8
fumigant	987.8	E863.8	—	E950.6	E962.2	E980.7
Phospholine	971.0	E855.3	E941.0	E950.4	E962.0	E980.4
Phosphoric acid	983.1	E864.1	—	E950.7	E962.1	E980.6
Phosphorus (compounds)						
NEC	983.9	E864.3	—	E950.7	E962.1	E980.6
rodenticide	983.9	E863.7	—	E950.7	E962.1	E980.6
Phthalimidoglutarimide	967.8	E852.8	E937.8	E950.2	E962.0	E980.2
Phthalylsulfathiazole	961.0	E857	E931.0	E950.4	E962.0	E980.4
Phylloquinone	964.3	E858.2	E934.3	E950.4	E962.0	E980.4
Physeptone	965.02	E850.1	E935.1	E950.0	E962.0	E980.0
Physostigma venenosum	988.2	E865.4	—	E950.9	E962.1	E980.9
Physostigmine	971.0	E855.3	E941.0	E950.4	E962.0	E980.4
Phytolacca decandra	988.2	E865.4	—	E950.9	E962.1	E980.9
Phytomenadione	964.3	E858.2	E934.3	E950.4	E962.0	E980.4
Phytonadione	964.3	E858.2	E934.3	E950.4	E962.0	E980.4

☑ Additional Digit Required   ▶◀ Revised Text   ● New Line   ▲ Revised Code

		External Cause (E-Code)								External Cause (E-Code)				
	Poisoning	Accident	Therapeutic Use	Suicide Attempt	Assault	Undetermined		Poisoning	Accident	Therapeutic Use	Suicide Attempt	Assault	Undetermined
Picric (acid)	983.0	E864.0	—	E950.7	E962.1	E980.6	Polythiazide	974.3	E858.5	E944.3	E950.4	E962.0	E980.4
Picrotoxin	970.0	E854.3	E940.0	E950.4	E962.0	E980.4	Polyvinylpyrrolidone	964.8	E858.2	E934.8	E950.4	E962.0	E980.4
Pilocarpine	971.0	E855.3	E941.0	E950.4	E962.0	E980.4	Pontocaine (hydrochloride)						
Pilocarpus (jaborandi)							(infiltration) (topical)	968.5	E855.2	E938.5	E950.4	E962.0	E980.4
extract	971.0	E855.3	E941.0	E950.4	E962.0	E980.4	nerve block (peripheral)						
Pimaricin	960.1	E856	E930.1	E950.4	E962.0	E980.4	(plexus)	968.6	E855.2	E938.6	E950.4	E962.0	E980.4
Piminodine	965.09	E850.2	E935.2	E950.0	E962.0	E980.0	spinal	968.7	E855.2	E938.7	E950.4	E962.0	E980.4
Pine oil, pinesol							Pot	969.6	E854.1	E939.6	E950.3	E962.0	E980.3
(disinfectant)	983.9	E861.4	—	E950.7	E962.1	E980.6	Potash (caustic)	983.2	E864.2	—	E950.7	E962.1	E980.6
Pinkroot	961.6	E857	E931.6	E950.4	E962.0	E980.4	Potassic saline injection						
Pipadone	965.09	E850.2	E935.2	E950.0	E962.0	E980.0	(lactated)	974.5	E858.5	E944.5	E950.4	E962.0	E980.4
Pipamazine	963.0	E858.1	E933.0	E950.4	E962.0	E980.4	Potassium (salts) NEC	974.5	E858.5	E944.5	E950.4	E962.0	E980.4
Pipazethate	975.4	E858.6	E945.4	E950.4	E962.0	E980.4	aminosalicylate	961.8	E857	E931.8	E950.4	E962.0	E980.4
Pipenzolate	971.1	E855.4	E941.1	E950.4	E962.0	E980.4	arsenite (solution)	985.1	E866.3	—	E950.8	E962.1	E980.8
Piperacetazine	969.1	E853.0	E939.1	E950.3	E962.0	E980.3	bichromate	983.9	E864.3	—	E950.7	E962.1	E980.6
Piperazine NEC	961.6	E857	E931.6	E950.4	E962.0	E980.4	bisulfate	983.9	E864.3	—	E950.7	E962.1	E980.6
estrone sulfate	962.2	E858.0	E932.2	E950.4	E962.0	E980.4	bromide (medicinal) NEC	967.3	E852.2	E937.3	E950.2	E962.0	E980.2
Piper cubeba	988.2	E865.4	—	E950.9	E962.1	E980.9	carbonate	983.2	E864.2	—	E950.7	E962.1	E980.6
Piperidione	975.4	E858.6	E945.4	E950.4	E962.0	E980.4	chlorate NEC	983.9	E864.3	—	E950.7	E962.1	E980.6
Piperidolate	971.1	E855.4	E941.1	E950.4	E962.0	E980.4	cyanide — see Cyanide						
Piperocaine	968.9	E855.2	E938.9	E950.4	E962.0	E980.4	hydroxide	983.2	E864.2	—	E950.7	E962.1	E980.6
infiltration (subcutaneous)	968.5	E855.2	E938.5	E950.4	E962.0	E980.4	iodide (expectorant) NEC	975.5	E858.6	E945.5	E950.4	E962.0	E980.4
nerve block (peripheral)							nitrate	989.89	E866.8	—	E950.9	E962.1	E980.9
(plexus)	968.6	E855.2	E938.6	E950.4	E962.0	E980.4	oxalate	983.9	E864.3	—	E950.7	E962.1	E980.6
topical (surface)	968.5	E855.2	E938.5	E950.4	E962.0	E980.4	perchlorate NEC	977.8	E858.8	E947.8	E950.4	E962.0	E980.4
Pipobroman	963.1	E858.1	E933.1	E950.4	E962.0	E980.4	antithyroid	962.8	E858.0	E932.8	E950.4	E962.0	E980.4
Pipradrol	970.8	E854.3	E940.8	E950.4	E962.0	E980.4	permanganate	976.0	E858.7	E946.0	E950.4	E962.0	E980.4
Piscidia (bark) (erythrina)	965.7	E850.7	E935.7	E950.0	E962.0	E980.0	nonmedicinal	983.9	E864.3	—	E950.7	E962.1	E980.6
Pitch	983.0	E864.0	—	E950.7	E962.1	E980.6	Povidone-iodine						
Pitkin's solution	968.7	E855.2	E938.7	E950.4	E962.0	E980.4	(anti-infective) NEC	976.0	E858.7	E946.0	E950.4	E962.0	E980.4
Pitocin	975.0	E858.6	E945.0	E950.4	E962.0	E980.4	Practolol	972.0	E858.3	E942.0	E950.4	E962.0	E980.4
Pitressin (tannate)	962.5	E858.0	E932.5	E950.4	E962.0	E980.4	Pralidoxime (chloride)	977.2	E858.8	E947.2	E950.4	E962.0	E980.4
Pituitary extracts (posterior)	962.5	E858.0	E932.5	E950.4	E962.0	E980.4	Pramoxine	968.5	E855.2	E938.5	E950.4	E962.0	E980.4
anterior	962.4	E858.0	E932.4	E950.4	E962.0	E980.4	Prazosin	972.6	E858.3	E942.6	E950.4	E962.0	E980.4
Pituitrin	962.5	E858.0	E932.5	E950.4	E962.0	E980.4	Prednisolone	962.0	E858.0	E932.0	E950.4	E962.0	E980.4
Placental extract	962.9	E858.0	E932.9	E950.4	E962.0	E980.4	ENT agent	976.6	E858.7	E946.6	E950.4	E962.0	E980.4
Placidyl	967.8	E852.8	E937.8	E950.2	E962.0	E980.2	ophthalmic preparation	976.5	E858.7	E946.5	E950.4	E962.0	E980.4
Plague vaccine	978.3	E858.8	E948.3	E950.4	E962.0	E980.4	topical NEC	976.0	E858.7	E946.0	E950.4	E962.0	E980.4
Plant foods or fertilizers							Prednisone	962.0	E858.0	E932.0	E950.4	E962.0	E980.4
NEC	989.89	E866.5	—	E950.9	E962.1	E980.9	Pregnanediol	962.2	E858.0	E932.2	E950.4	E962.0	E980.4
mixed with herbicides	989.4	E863.5	—	E950.6	E962.1	E980.7	Pregneninolone	962.2	E858.0	E932.2	E950.4	E962.0	E980.4
Plants, noxious, used as							Preludin	977.0	E858.8	E947.0	E950.4	E962.0	E980.4
food	988.2	E865.9	—	E950.9	E962.1	E980.9	Premarin	962.2	E858.0	E932.2	E950.4	E962.0	E980.4
berries and seeds	988.2	E865.3	—	E950.9	E962.1	E980.9	Prenylamine	972.4	E858.3	E942.4	E950.4	E962.0	E980.4
specified type NEC	988.2	E865.4	—	E950.9	E962.1	E980.9	Preparation H	976.8	E858.7	E946.8	E950.4	E962.0	E980.4
Plasma (blood)	964.7	E858.2	E934.7	E950.4	E962.0	E980.4	Preservatives	989.89	E866.8	—	E950.9	E962.1	E980.9
expanders	964.8	E858.2	E934.8	E950.4	E962.0	E980.4	Pride of China	988.2	E865.3	—	E950.9	E962.1	E980.9
Plasmanate	964.7	E858.2	E934.7	E950.4	E962.0	E980.4	Prilocaine	968.9	E855.2	E938.9	E950.4	E962.0	E980.4
Plegicil	969.1	E853.0	E939.1	E950.3	E962.0	E980.3	infiltration (subcutaneous)	968.5	E855.2	E938.5	E950.4	E962.0	E980.4
Podophyllin	976.4	E858.7	E946.4	E950.4	E962.0	E980.4	nerve block (peripheral)						
Podophyllum resin	976.4	E858.7	E946.4	E950.4	E962.0	E980.4	(plexus)	968.6	E855.2	E938.6	E950.4	E962.0	E980.4
Poison NEC	989.9	E866.9	—	E950.9	E962.1	E980.9	Primaquine	961.4	E857	E931.4	E950.4	E962.0	E980.4
Poisonous berries	988.2	E865.3	—	E950.9	E962.1	E980.9	Primidone	966.3	E855.0	E936.3	E950.4	E962.0	E980.4
Pokeweed (any part)	988.2	E865.4	—	E950.9	E962.1	E980.9	Primula (veris)	988.2	E865.4	—	E950.9	E962.1	E980.9
Poldine	971.1	E855.4	E941.1	E950.4	E962.0	E980.4	Prinadol	965.09	E850.2	E935.2	E950.0	E962.0	E980.0
Poliomyelitis vaccine	979.5	E858.8	E949.5	E950.4	E962.0	E980.4	Priscol, Priscoline	971.3	E855.6	E941.3	E950.4	E962.0	E980.4
Poliovirus vaccine	979.5	E858.8	E949.5	E950.4	E962.0	E980.4	Privet	988.2	E865.4	—	E950.9	E962.1	E980.9
Polish (car) (floor) (furniture)							Privine	971.2	E855.5	E941.2	E950.4	E962.0	E980.4
(metal) (silver)	989.89	E861.2	—	E950.9	E962.1	E980.9	Pro-Banthine	971.1	E855.4	E941.1	E950.4	E962.0	E980.4
abrasive	989.89	E861.3	—	E950.9	E962.1	E980.9	Probarbital	967.0	E851	E937.0	E950.1	E962.0	E980.1
porcelain	989.89	E861.3	—	E950.9	E962.1	E980.9	Probenecid	974.7	E858.5	E944.7	E950.4	E962.0	E980.4
Poloxalkol	973.2	E858.4	E943.2	E950.4	E962.0	E980.4	Procainamide (hydrochloride)	972.0	E858.3	E942.0	E950.4	E962.0	E980.4
Polyaminostyrene resins	974.5	E858.5	E944.5	E950.4	E962.0	E980.4	Procaine (hydrochloride)						
Polychlorinated biphenyl							(infiltration) (topical)	968.5	E855.2	E938.5	E950.4	E962.0	E980.4
— see PCBs							nerve block (peripheral)						
Polycycline	960.4	E856	E930.4	E950.4	E962.0	E980.4	(plexus)	968.6	E855.2	E938.6	E950.4	E962.0	E980.4
Polyester resin hardener	982.8	E862.4	—	E950.9	E962.1	E980.9	penicillin G	960.0	E856	E930.0	E950.4	E962.0	E980.4
fumes	987.8	E869.8	—	E952.8	E962.2	E982.8	spinal	968.7	E855.2	E938.7	E950.4	E962.0	E980.4
Polyestradiol (phosphate)	962.2	E858.0	E932.2	E950.4	E962.0	E980.4	Procalmidol	969.5	E853.8	E939.5	E950.3	E962.0	E980.3
Polyethanolamine alkyl							Procarbazine	963.1	E858.1	E933.1	E950.4	E962.0	E980.4
sulfate	976.2	E858.7	E946.2	E950.4	E962.0	E980.4	Prochlorperazine	969.1	E853.0	E939.1	E950.3	E962.0	E980.3
Polyethylene glycol	976.3	E858.7	E946.3	E950.4	E962.0	E980.4	Procyclidine	966.4	E855.0	E936.4	E950.4	E962.0	E980.4
Polyferose	964.0	E858.2	E934.0	E950.4	E962.0	E980.4	Producer gas	986	E868.8	—	E952.1	E962.2	E982.1
Polymyxin B	960.8	E856	E930.8	E950.4	E962.0	E980.4	Profenamine	966.4	E855.0	E936.4	E950.4	E962.0	E980.4
ENT agent	976.6	E858.7	E946.6	E950.4	E962.0	E980.4	Profenil	975.1	E858.6	E945.1	E950.4	E962.0	E980.4
ophthalmic preparation	976.5	E858.7	E946.5	E950.4	E962.0	E980.4	Progesterones	962.2	E858.0	E932.2	E950.4	E962.0	E980.4
topical NEC	976.0	E858.7	E946.0	E950.4	E962.0	E980.4	Progestin	962.2	E858.0	E932.2	E950.4	E962.0	E980.4
Polynoxylin(e)	976.0	E858.7	E946.0	E950.4	E962.0	E980.4	Progestogens (with						
Polyoxymethyleneurea	976.0	E858.7	E946.0	E950.4	E962.0	E980.4	estrogens)	962.2	E858.0	E932.2	E950.4	E962.0	E980.4
Polytetrafluoroethylene							Progestone	962.2	E858.0	E932.2	E950.4	E962.0	E980.4
(inhaled)	987.8	E869.8	—	E952.8	E962.2	E982.8	Proguanil	961.4	E857	E931.4	E950.4	E962.0	E980.4

☑ Additional Digit Required   ▶◀ Revised Text   ● New Line   ▲ Revised Code

	Poisoning	External Cause (E-Code)				
		Accident	Therapeutic Use	Suicide Attempt	Assault	Undetermined
Prolactin	962.4	E858.0	E932.4	E950.4	E962.0	E980.4
Proloid	962.7	E858.0	E932.7	E950.4	E962.0	E980.4
Proluton	962.2	E858.0	E932.2	E950.4	E962.0	E980.4
Promacetin	961.8	E857	E931.8	E950.4	E962.0	E980.4
Promazine	969.1	E853.0	E939.1	E950.3	E962.0	E980.3
Promedol	965.09	E850.2	E935.2	E950.0	E962.0	E980.0
Promethazine	967.8	E852.8	E937.8	E950.2	E962.0	E980.2
Promin	961.8	E857	E931.8	E950.4	E962.0	E980.4
Pronestyl (hydrochloride)	972.0	E858.3	E942.0	E950.4	E962.0	E980.4
Pronetalol, pronethalol	972.0	E858.3	E942.0	E950.4	E962.0	E980.4
Prontosil	961.0	E857	E931.0	E950.4	E962.0	E980.4
Propamidine isethionate	961.5	E857	E931.5	E950.4	E962.0	E980.4
Propanal (medicinal)	967.8	E852.8	E937.8	E950.2	E962.0	E980.2
Propane (gas) (distributed in mobile container)	987.0	E868.0	—	E951.1	E962.2	E981.1
distributed through pipes	987.0	E867	—	E951.0	E962.2	E981.0
incomplete combustion of — see Carbon monoxide, Propane						
Propanidid	968.3	E855.1	E938.3	E950.4	E962.0	E980.4
Propanol	980.3	E860.4	—	E950.9	E962.1	E980.9
Propantheline	971.1	E855.4	E941.1	E950.4	E962.0	E980.4
Proparacaine	968.5	E855.2	E938.5	E950.4	E962.0	E980.4
Propatyl nitrate	972.4	E858.3	E942.4	E950.4	E962.0	E980.4
Propicillin	960.0	E856	E930.0	E950.4	E962.0	E980.4
Propiolactone (vapor)	987.8	E869.8	—	E952.8	E962.2	E982.8
Propiomazine	967.8	E852.8	E937.8	E950.2	E962.0	E980.2
Propionaldehyde (medicinal)	967.8	E852.8	E937.8	E950.2	E962.0	E980.2
Propionate compound	976.0	E858.7	E946.0	E950.4	E962.0	E980.4
Propion gel	976.0	E858.7	E946.0	E950.4	E962.0	E980.4
Propitocaine	968.9	E855.2	E938.9	E950.4	E962.0	E980.4
infiltration (subcutaneous)	968.5	E855.2	E938.5	E950.4	E962.0	E980.4
nerve block (peripheral) (plexus)	968.6	E855.2	E938.6	E950.4	E962.0	E980.4
Propoxur	989.3	E863.2	—	E950.6	E962.1	E980.7
Propoxycaine	968.9	E855.2	E938.9	E950.4	E962.0	E980.4
infiltration (subcutaneous)	968.5	E855.2	E938.5	E950.4	E962.0	E980.4
nerve block (peripheral) (plexus)	968.6	E855.2	E938.6	E950.4	E962.0	E980.4
topical (surface)	968.5	E855.2	E938.5	E950.4	E962.0	E980.4
Propoxyphene (hydrochloride)	965.8	E850.8	E935.8	E950.0	E962.0	E980.0
Propranolol	972.0	E858.3	E942.0	E950.4	E962.0	E980.4
Propyl						
alcohol	980.3	E860.4	—	E950.9	E962.1	E980.9
carbinol	980.3	E860.4	—	E950.9	E962.1	E980.9
hexadrine	971.2	E855.5	E941.2	E950.4	E962.0	E980.4
iodone	977.8	E858.8	E947.8	E950.4	E962.0	E980.4
thiouracil	962.8	E858.0	E932.8	E950.4	E962.0	E980.4
Propylene	987.1	E869.8	—	E952.8	E962.2	E982.8
Propylparaben (ophthalmic)	976.5	E858.7	E946.5	E950.4	E962.0	E980.4
Proscillaridin	972.1	E858.3	E942.1	E950.4	E962.0	E980.4
Prostaglandins	975.0	E858.6	E945.0	E950.4	E962.0	E980.4
Prostigmin	971.0	E855.3	E941.0	E950.4	E962.0	E980.4
Protamine (sulfate)	964.5	E858.2	E934.5	E950.4	E962.0	E980.4
zinc insulin	962.3	E858.0	E932.3	E950.4	E962.0	E980.4
Protectants (topical)	976.3	E858.7	E946.3	E950.4	E962.0	E980.4
Protein hydrolysate	974.5	E858.5	E944.5	E950.4	E962.0	E980.4
Prothiaden — see Dothiepin hydrochloride						
Prothionamide	961.8	E857	E931.8	E950.4	E962.0	E980.4
Prothipendyl	969.5	E853.8	E939.5	E950.3	E962.0	E980.3
Protokylol	971.2	E855.5	E941.2	E950.4	E962.0	E980.4
Protopam	977.2	E858.8	E947.2	E950.4	E962.0	E980.4
Protoveratrine(s) (A) (B)	972.6	E858.3	E942.6	E950.4	E962.0	E980.4
Protriptyline	969.0	E854.0	E939.0	E950.3	E962.0	E980.3
Provera	962.2	E858.0	E932.2	E950.4	E962.0	E980.4
Provitamin A	963.5	E858.1	E933.5	E950.4	E962.0	E980.4
Proxymetacaine	968.5	E855.2	E938.5	E950.4	E962.0	E980.4
Proxyphylline	975.1	E858.6	E945.1	E950.4	E962.0	E980.4
Prozac — see Fluoxetine hydrochloride						
Prunus						
laurocerasus	988.2	E865.4	—	E950.9	E962.1	E980.9
virginiana	988.2	E865.4	—	E950.9	E962.1	E980.9
Prussic acid	989.0	E866.8	—	E950.9	E962.1	E980.9
vapor	987.7	E869.8	—	E952.8	E962.2	E982.8
Pseudoephedrine	971.2	E855.5	E941.2	E950.4	E962.0	E980.4
Psilocin	969.6	E854.1	E939.6	E950.3	E962.0	E980.3
Psilocybin	969.6	E854.1	E939.6	E950.3	E962.0	E980.3
PSP	977.8	E858.8	E947.8	E950.4	E962.0	E980.4
Psychedelic agents	969.6	E854.1	E939.6	E950.3	E962.0	E980.3
Psychodysleptics	969.6	E854.1	E939.6	E950.3	E962.0	E980.3
Psychostimulants	969.7	E854.2	E939.7	E950.3	E962.0	E980.3
Psychotherapeutic agents	969.9	E855.9	E939.9	E950.3	E962.0	E980.3
antidepressants	969.0	E854.0	E939.0	E950.3	E962.0	E980.3
specified NEC	969.8	E855.8	E939.8	E950.3	E962.0	E980.3
tranquilizers NEC	969.5	E853.9	E939.5	E950.3	E962.0	E980.3
Psychotomimetic agents	969.6	E854.1	E939.6	E950.3	E962.0	E980.3
Psychotropic agents	969.9	E854.8	E939.9	E950.3	E962.0	E980.3
specified NEC	969.8	E854.8	E939.8	E950.3	E962.0	E980.3
Psyllium	973.3	E858.4	E943.3	E950.4	E962.0	E980.4
Pteroylglutamic acid	964.1	E858.2	E934.1	E950.4	E962.0	E980.4
Pteroyltriglutamate	963.1	E858.1	E933.1	E950.4	E962.0	E980.4
PTFE	987.8	E869.8	—	E952.8	E962.2	E982.8
Pulsatilla	988.2	E865.4	—	E950.9	E962.1	E980.9
Purex (bleach)	983.9	E864.3	—	E950.7	E962.1	E980.6
Purine diuretics	974.1	E858.5	E944.1	E950.4	E962.0	E980.4
Purinethol	963.1	E858.1	E933.1	E950.4	E962.0	E980.4
PVP	964.8	E858.2	E934.8	E950.4	E962.0	E980.4
Pyrabital	965.7	E850.7	E935.7	E950.0	E962.0	E980.0
Pyramidon	965.5	E850.5	E935.5	E950.0	E962.0	E980.0
Pyrantel (pamoate)	961.6	E857	E931.6	E950.4	E962.0	E980.4
Pyrathiazine	963.0	E858.1	E933.0	E950.4	E962.0	E980.4
Pyrazinamide	961.8	E857	E931.8	E950.4	E962.0	E980.4
Pyrazinoic acid (amide)	961.8	E857	E931.8	E950.4	E962.0	E980.4
Pyrazole (derivatives)	965.5	E850.5	E935.5	E950.0	E962.0	E980.0
Pyrazolone (analgesics)	965.5	E850.5	E935.5	E950.0	E962.0	E980.0
Pyrethrins, pyrethrum	989.4	E863.4	—	E950.6	E962.1	E980.7
Pyribenzamine	963.0	E858.1	E933.0	E950.4	E962.0	E980.4
Pyridine (liquid) (vapor)	982.0	E862.4	—	E950.9	E962.1	E980.9
aldoxime chloride	977.2	E858.8	E947.2	E950.4	E962.0	E980.4
Pyridium	976.1	E858.7	E946.1	E950.4	E962.0	E980.4
Pyridostigmine	971.0	E855.3	E941.0	E950.4	E962.0	E980.4
Pyridoxine	963.5	E858.1	E933.5	E950.4	E962.0	E980.4
Pyrilamine	963.0	E858.1	E933.0	E950.4	E962.0	E980.4
Pyrimethamine	961.4	E857	E931.4	E950.4	E962.0	E980.4
Pyrogallic acid	983.0	E864.0	—	E950.7	E962.1	E980.6
Pyroxylin	976.3	E858.7	E946.3	E950.4	E962.0	E980.4
Pyrrobutamine	963.0	E858.1	E933.0	E950.4	E962.0	E980.4
Pyrrocitine	968.5	E855.2	E938.5	E950.4	E962.0	E980.4
Pyrvinium (pamoate)	961.6	E857	E931.6	E950.4	E962.0	E980.4
PZI	962.3	E858.0	E932.3	E950.4	E962.0	E980.4
Quaalude	967.4	E852.3	E937.4	E950.2	E962.0	E980.2
Quaternary ammonium derivatives	971.1	E855.4	E941.1	E950.4	E962.0	E980.4
Quicklime	983.2	E864.2	—	E950.7	E962.1	E980.6
Quinacrine	961.3	E857	E931.3	E950.4	E962.0	E980.4
Quinaglute	972.0	E858.3	E942.0	E950.4	E962.0	E980.4
Quinalbarbitone	967.0	E851	E937.0	E950.1	E962.0	E980.1
Quinestradiol	962.2	E858.0	E932.2	E950.4	E962.0	E980.4
Quinethazone	974.3	E858.5	E944.3	E950.4	E962.0	E980.4
Quinidine (gluconate) (polygalacturonate) (salts) (sulfate)	972.0	E858.3	E942.0	E950.4	E962.0	E980.4
Quinine	961.4	E857	E931.4	E950.4	E962.0	E980.4
Quiniobine	961.3	E857	E931.3	E950.4	E962.0	E980.4
Quinolines	961.3	E857	E931.3	E950.4	E962.0	E980.4
Quotane	968.5	E855.2	E938.5	E950.4	E962.0	E980.4
Rabies						
immune globulin (human)	964.6	E858.2	E934.6	E950.4	E962.0	E980.4
vaccine	979.1	E858.8	E949.1	E950.4	E962.0	E980.4
Racemoramide	965.09	E850.2	E935.2	E950.0	E962.0	E980.0
Racemorphan	965.09	E850.2	E935.2	E950.0	E962.0	E980.0
Radiator alcohol	980.1	E860.2	—	E950.9	E962.1	E980.9
Radio-opaque (drugs) (materials)	977.8	E858.8	E947.8	E950.4	E962.0	E980.4
Ranunculus	988.2	E865.4	—	E950.9	E962.1	E980.9
Rat poison	989.4	E863.7	—	E950.6	E962.1	E980.7
Rattlesnake (venom)	989.5	E905.0	—	E950.9	E962.1	E980.9
Raudixin	972.6	E858.3	E942.6	E950.4	E962.0	E980.4
Rautensin	972.6	E858.3	E942.6	E950.4	E962.0	E980.4
Rautina	972.6	E858.3	E942.6	E950.4	E962.0	E980.4
Rautotal	972.6	E858.3	E942.6	E950.4	E962.0	E980.4
Rauwiloid	972.6	E858.3	E942.6	E950.4	E962.0	E980.4
Rauwoldin	972.6	E858.3	E942.6	E950.4	E962.0	E980.4
Rauwolfia (alkaloids)	972.6	E858.3	E942.6	E950.4	E962.0	E980.4
Realgar	985.1	E866.3	—	E950.8	E962.1	E980.8
Red cells, packed	964.7	E858.2	E934.7	E950.4	E962.0	E980.4
Reducing agents, industrial NEC	983.9	E864.3	—	E950.7	E962.1	E980.6
Refrigerant gas (freon)	987.4	E869.2	—	E952.8	E962.2	E982.8
not freon	987.9	E869.9	—	E952.9	E962.2	E982.9

☑ Additional Digit Required ◄► Revised Text ● New Line ▲ Revised Code

	Poisoning	External Cause (E-Code)						Poisoning	External Cause (E-Code)				
		Accident	Therapeutic Use	Suicide Attempt	Assault	Undeter-mined			Accident	Therapeutic Use	Suicide Attempt	Assault	Undeter-mined
Regroton	974.4	E858.5	E944.4	E950.4	E962.0	E980.4	Sarkomycin	960.7	E856	E930.7	E950.4	E962.0	E980.4
Rela	968.0	E855.1	E938.0	E950.4	E962.0	E980.4	Saroten	969.0	E854.0	E939.0	E950.3	E962.0	E980.3
Relaxants, skeletal muscle							Saturnine — see Lead						
(autonomic)	975.2	E858.6	E945.2	E950.4	E962.0	E980.4	Savin (oil)	976.4	E858.7	E946.4	E950.4	E962.0	E980.4
central nervous system	968.0	E855.1	E938.0	E950.4	E962.0	E980.4	Scammony	973.1	E858.4	E943.1	E950.4	E962.0	E980.4
Renese	974.3	E858.5	E944.3	E950.4	E962.0	E980.4	Scarlet red	976.8	E858.7	E946.8	E950.4	E962.0	E980.4
Renografin	977.8	E858.8	E947.8	E950.4	E962.0	E980.4	Scheele's green	985.1	E866.3	—	E950.8	E962.1	E980.8
Replacement solutions	974.5	E858.5	E944.5	E950.4	E962.0	E980.4	insecticide	985.1	E863.4	—	E950.8	E962.1	E980.8
Rescinnamine	972.6	E858.3	E942.6	E950.4	E962.0	E980.4	Schradan	989.3	E863.1	—	E950.6	E962.1	E980.7
Reserpine	972.6	E858.3	E942.6	E950.4	E962.0	E980.4	Schweinfurt(h) green	985.1	E866.3	—	E950.8	E962.1	E980.8
Resorcin, resorcinol	976.4	E858.7	E946.4	E950.4	E962.0	E980.4	insecticide	985.1	E863.4	—	E950.8	E962.1	E980.8
Respaire	975.5	E858.6	E945.5	E950.4	E962.0	E980.4	Scilla — see Squill						
Respiratory agents NEC	975.8	E858.6	E945.8	E950.4	E962.0	E980.4	Sclerosing agents	972.7	E858.3	E942.7	E950.4	E962.0	E980.4
Retinoic acid	976.8	E858.7	E946.8	E950.4	E962.0	E980.4	Scopolamine	971.1	E855.4	E941.1	E950.4	E962.0	E980.4
Retinol	963.5	E858.1	E933.5	E950.4	E962.0	E980.4	Scouring powder	989.89	E861.3	—	E950.9	E962.1	E980.9
Rh (D) immune globulin							Sea						
(human)	964.6	E858.2	E934.6	E950.4	E962.0	E980.4	anemone (sting)	989.5	E905.6	—	E950.9	E962.1	E980.9
Rhodine	965.1	E850.3	E935.3	E950.0	E962.0	E980.0	cucumber (sting)	989.5	E905.6	—	E950.9	E962.1	E980.9
RhoGAM	964.6	E858.2	E934.6	E950.4	E962.0	E980.4	snake (bite) (venom)	989.5	E905.0	—	E950.9	E962.1	E980.9
Riboflavin	963.5	E858.1	E933.5	E950.4	E962.0	E980.4	urchin spine (puncture)	989.5	E905.6	—	E950.9	E962.1	E980.9
Ricin	989.89	E866.8	—	E950.9	E962.1	E980.9	Secbutabarbital	967.0	E851	E937.0	E950.1	E962.0	E980.1
Ricinus communis	988.2	E865.3	—	E950.9	E962.1	E980.9	Secbutabarbitone	967.0	E851	E937.0	E950.1	E962.0	E980.1
Rickettsial vaccine NEC	979.6	E858.8	E949.6	E950.4	E962.0	E980.4	Secobarbital	967.0	E851	E937.0	E950.1	E962.0	E980.1
with viral and bacterial							Seconal	967.0	E851	E937.0	E950.1	E962.0	E980.1
vaccine	979.7	E858.8	E949.7	E950.4	E962.0	E980.4	Secretin	977.8	E858.8	E947.8	E950.4	E962.0	E980.4
Rifampin	960.6	E856	E930.6	E950.4	E962.0	E980.4	Sedatives, nonbarbiturate	967.9	E852.9	E937.9	E950.2	E962.0	E980.2
Rimifon	961.8	E857	E931.8	E950.4	E962.0	E980.4	specified NEC	967.8	E852.8	E937.8	E950.2	E962.0	E980.2
Ringer's injection (lactated)	974.5	E858.5	E944.5	E950.4	E962.0	E980.4	Sedormid	967.8	E852.8	E937.8	E950.2	E962.0	E980.2
Ristocetin	960.8	E856	E930.8	E950.4	E962.0	E980.4	Seed (plant)	988.2	E865.3	—	E950.9	E962.1	E980.9
Ritalin	969.7	E854.2	E939.7	E950.3	E962.0	E980.3	disinfectant or dressing	989.89	E866.5	—	E950.9	E962.1	E980.9
Roach killers — see Pesticides							Selenium (fumes) NEC	985.8	E866.4	—	E950.9	E962.1	E980.9
Rocky Mountain spotted							disulfide or sulfide	976.4	E858.7	E946.4	E950.4	E962.0	E980.4
fever vaccine	979.6	E858.8	E949.6	E950.4	E962.0	E980.4	Selsun	976.4	E858.7	E946.4	E950.4	E962.0	E980.4
Rodenticides	989.4	E863.7	—	E950.6	E962.1	E980.7	Senna	973.1	E858.4	E943.1	E950.4	E962.0	E980.4
Rohypnol	969.4	E853.2	E939.4	E950.3	E962.0	E980.3	Septisol	976.2	E858.7	E946.2	E950.4	E962.0	E980.4
Rolaids	973.0	E858.4	E943.0	E950.4	E962.0	E980.4	Serax	969.4	E853.2	E939.4	E950.3	E962.0	E980.3
Rolitetracycline	960.4	E856	E930.4	E950.4	E962.0	E980.4	Serenesil	967.8	E852.8	E937.8	E950.2	E962.0	E980.2
Romilar	975.4	E858.6	E945.4	E950.4	E962.0	E980.4	Serenium (hydrochloride)	961.9	E857	E931.9	E950.4	E962.0	E980.4
Rose water ointment	976.3	E858.7	E946.3	E950.4	E962.0	E980.4	Sernyl	968.3	E855.1	E938.3	E950.4	E962.0	E980.4
Rotenone	989.4	E863.7	—	E950.6	E962.1	E980.7	Serotonin	977.8	E858.8	E947.8	E950.4	E962.0	E980.4
Rotoxamine	963.0	E858.1	E933.0	E950.4	E962.0	E980.4	Serpasil	972.6	E858.3	E942.6	E950.4	E962.0	E980.4
Rough-on-rats	989.4	E863.7	—	E950.6	E962.1	E980.7	Sewer gas	987.8	E869.8	—	E952.8	E962.2	E982.8
RU486	962.9	E858.0	E932.9	E950.4	E962.0	E980.4	Shampoo	989.6	E861.0	—	E950.9	E962.1	E980.9
Rubbing alcohol	980.2	E860.3	—	E950.9	E962.1	E980.9	Shellfish, nonbacterial or						
Rubella virus vaccine	979.4	E858.8	E949.4	E950.4	E962.0	E980.4	noxious	988.0	E865.1	—	E950.9	E962.1	E980.9
Rubelogen	979.4	E858.8	E949.4	E950.4	E962.0	E980.4	Silicones NEC	989.83	E866.8	E947.8	E950.9	E962.1	E980.9
Rubeovax	979.4	E858.8	E949.4	E950.4	E962.0	E980.4	Silvadene	976.0	E858.7	E946.0	E950.4	E962.0	E980.4
Rubidomycin	960.7	E856	E930.7	E950.4	E962.0	E980.4	Silver (compound) (medicinal)						
Rue	988.2	E865.4	—	E950.9	E962.1	E980.9	NEC	976.0	E858.7	E946.0	E950.4	E962.0	E980.4
Ruta	988.2	E865.4	—	E950.9	E962.1	E980.9	anti-infectives	976.0	E858.7	E946.0	E950.4	E962.0	E980.4
Sabadilla (medicinal)	976.0	E858.7	E946.0	E950.4	E962.0	E980.4	arsphenamine	961.1	E857	E931.1	E950.4	E962.0	E980.4
pesticide	989.4	E863.4	—	E950.6	E962.1	E980.7	nitrate	976.0	E858.7	E946.0	E950.4	E962.0	E980.4
Sabin oral vaccine	979.5	E858.8	E949.5	E950.4	E962.0	E980.4	ophthalmic preparation	976.5	E858.7	E946.5	E950.4	E962.0	E980.4
Saccharated iron oxide	964.0	E858.2	E934.0	E950.4	E962.0	E980.4	toughened (keratolytic)	976.4	E858.7	E946.4	E950.4	E962.0	E980.4
Saccharin	974.5	E858.5	E944.5	E950.4	E962.0	E980.4	nonmedicinal (dust)	985.8	E866.4	—	E950.9	E962.1	E980.9
Safflower oil	972.2	E858.3	E942.2	E950.4	E962.0	E980.4	protein (mild) (strong)	976.0	E858.7	E946.0	E950.4	E962.0	E980.4
Salbutamol sulfate	975.7	E858.6	E945.7	E950.4	E962.0	E980.4	salvarsan	961.1	E857	E931.1	E950.4	E962.0	E980.4
Salicylamide	965.1	E850.3	E935.3	E950.0	E962.0	E980.0	Simethicone	973.8	E858.4	E943.8	E950.4	E962.0	E980.4
Salicylate(s)	965.1	E850.3	E935.3	E950.0	E962.0	E980.0	Sinequan	969.0	E854.0	E939.0	E950.3	E962.0	E980.3
methyl	976.3	E858.7	E946.3	E950.4	E962.0	E980.4	Singoserp	972.6	E858.3	E942.6	E950.4	E962.0	E980.4
theobromine calcium	974.1	E858.5	E944.1	E950.4	E962.0	E980.4	Sintrom	964.2	E858.2	E934.2	E950.4	E962.0	E980.4
Salicylazosulfapyridine	961.0	E857	E931.0	E950.4	E962.0	E980.4	Sitosterols	972.2	E858.3	E942.2	E950.4	E962.0	E980.4
Salicylhydroxamic acid	976.0	E858.7	E946.0	E950.4	E962.0	E980.4	Skeletal muscle relaxants	975.2	E858.6	E945.2	E950.4	E962.0	E980.4
Salicylic acid (keratolytic)							Skin						
NEC	976.4	E858.7	E946.4	E950.4	E962.0	E980.4	agents (external)	976.9	E858.7	E946.9	E950.4	E962.0	E980.4
congeners	965.1	E850.3	E935.3	E950.0	E962.0	E980.0	specified NEC	976.8	E858.7	E946.8	E950.4	E962.0	E980.4
salts	965.1	E850.3	E935.3	E950.0	E962.0	E980.0	test antigen	977.8	E858.8	E947.8	E950.4	E962.0	E980.4
Saliniazid	961.8	E857	E931.8	E950.4	E962.0	E980.4	Sleep-eze	963.0	E858.1	E933.0	E950.4	E962.0	E980.4
Salol	976.3	E858.7	E946.3	E950.4	E962.0	E980.4	Sleeping draught (drug) (pill)						
Salt (substitute) NEC	974.5	E858.5	E944.5	E950.4	E962.0	E980.4	(tablet)	967.9	E852.9	E937.9	E950.2	E962.0	E980.2
Saluretics	974.3	E858.5	E944.3	E950.4	E962.0	E980.4	Smallpox vaccine	979.0	E858.8	E949.0	E950.4	E962.0	E980.4
Saluron	974.3	E858.5	E944.3	E950.4	E962.0	E980.4	Smelter fumes NEC	985.9	E866.4	—	E950.9	E962.1	E980.9
Salvarsan 606 (neosilver)							Smog	987.3	E869.1	—	E952.8	E962.2	E982.8
(silver)	961.1	E857	E931.1	E950.4	E962.0	E980.4	Smoke NEC	987.9	E869.9	—	E952.9	E962.2	E982.9
Sambucus canadensis	988.2	E865.4	—	E950.9	E962.1	E980.9	Smooth muscle relaxant	975.1	E858.6	E945.1	E950.4	E962.0	E980.4
berry	988.2	E865.3	—	E950.9	E962.1	E980.9	Snail killer	989.4	E863.4	—	E950.6	E962.1	E980.7
Sandril	972.6	E858.3	E942.6	E950.4	E962.0	E980.4	Snake (bite) (venom)	989.5	E905.0	—	E950.9	E962.1	E980.9
Sanguinaria canadensis	988.2	E865.4	—	E950.9	E962.1	E980.9	Snuff	989.89	E866.8	—	E950.9	E962.1	E980.9
Saniflush (cleaner)	983.9	E861.3	—	E950.7	E962.1	E980.6	Soap (powder) (product)	989.6	E861.1	—	E950.9	E962.1	E980.9
Santonin	961.6	E857	E931.6	E950.4	E962.0	E980.4	medicinal, soft	976.2	E858.7	E946.2	E950.4	E962.0	E980.4
Santyl	976.8	E858.7	E946.8	E950.4	E962.0	E980.4							

		External Cause (E-Code)				
	Poisoning	Accident	Therapeutic Use	Suicide Attempt	Assault	Undetermined
Soda (caustic)	983.2	E864.2	—	E950.7	E962.1	E980.6
bicarb	963.3	E858.1	E933.3	E950.4	E962.0	E980.4
chlorinated — see Sodium, hypochlorite						
Sodium						
acetosulfone	961.8	E857	E931.8	E950.4	E962.0	E980.4
acetrizoate	977.8	E858.8	E947.8	E950.4	E962.0	E980.4
amytal	967.0	E851	E937.0	E950.1	E962.0	E980.1
arsenate — see Arsenic						
bicarbonate	963.3	E858.1	E933.3	E950.4	E962.0	E980.4
bichromate	983.9	E864.3	—	E950.7	E962.1	E980.6
biphosphate	963.2	E858.1	E933.2	E950.4	E962.0	E980.4
bisulfate	983.9	E864.3	—	E950.7	E962.1	E980.6
borate (cleanser)	989.6	E861.3	—	E950.9	E962.1	E980.9
bromide NEC	967.3	E852.2	E937.3	E950.2	E962.0	E980.2
cacodylate (nonmedicinal)						
NEC	978.8	E858.8	E948.8	E950.4	E962.0	E980.4
anti-infective	961.1	E857	E931.1	E950.4	E962.0	E980.4
herbicide	989.4	E863.5	—	E950.6	E962.1	E980.7
calcium edetate	963.8	E858.1	E933.8	E950.4	E962.0	E980.4
carbonate NEC	983.2	E864.2	—	E950.7	E962.1	E980.6
chlorate NEC	983.9	E864.3	—	E950.7	E962.1	E980.6
herbicide	983.9	E863.5	—	E950.7	E962.1	E980.6
chloride NEC	974.5	E858.5	E944.5	E950.4	E962.0	E980.4
chromate	983.9	E864.3	—	E950.7	E962.1	E980.6
citrate	963.3	E858.1	E933.3	E950.4	E962.0	E980.4
cyanide — see Cyanide(s)						
cyclamate	974.5	E858.5	E944.5	E950.4	E962.0	E980.4
diatrizoate	977.8	E858.8	E947.8	E950.4	E962.0	E980.4
dibunate	975.4	E858.6	E945.4	E950.4	E962.0	E980.4
dioctyl sulfosuccinate	973.2	E858.4	E943.2	E950.4	E962.0	E980.4
edetate	963.8	E858.1	E933.8	E950.4	E962.0	E980.4
ethacrynate	974.4	E858.5	E944.4	E950.4	E962.0	E980.4
fluoroacetate (dust) (rodenticide)	989.4	E863.7	—	E950.6	E962.1	E980.7
fluoride — see Fluoride(s)						
free salt	974.5	E858.5	E944.5	E950.4	E962.0	E980.4
glucosulfone	961.8	E857	E931.8	E950.4	E962.0	E980.4
hydroxide	983.2	E864.2	—	E950.7	E962.1	E980.6
hypochlorite (bleach) NEC	983.9	E864.3	—	E950.7	E962.1	E980.6
disinfectant	983.9	E861.4	—	E950.7	E962.1	E980.6
medicinal (anti-infective) (external)	976.0	E858.7	E946.0	E950.4	E962.0	E980.4
vapor	987.8	E869.8	—	E952.8	E962.2	E982.8
hyposulfite	976.0	E858.7	E946.0	E950.4	E962.0	E980.4
indigotindisulfonate	977.8	E858.8	E947.8	E950.4	E962.0	E980.4
iodide	977.8	E858.8	E947.8	E950.4	E962.0	E980.4
iothalamate	977.8	E858.8	E947.8	E950.4	E962.0	E980.4
iron edetate	964.0	E858.2	E934.0	E950.4	E962.0	E980.4
lactate	963.3	E858.1	E933.3	E950.4	E962.0	E980.4
lauryl sulfate	976.2	E858.7	E946.2	E950.4	E962.0	E980.4
L-triiodothyronine	962.7	E858.0	E932.7	E950.4	E962.0	E980.4
metrizoate	977.8	E858.8	E947.8	E950.4	E962.0	E980.4
monofluoroacetate (dust) (rodenticide)	989.4	E863.7	—	E950.6	E962.1	E980.7
morrhuate	972.7	E858.3	E942.7	E950.4	E962.0	E980.4
nafcillin	960.0	E856	E930.0	E950.4	E962.0	E980.4
nitrate (oxidizing agent)	983.9	E864.3	—	E950.7	E962.1	E980.6
nitrite (medicinal)	972.4	E858.3	E942.4	E950.4	E962.0	E980.4
nitroferricyanide	972.6	E858.3	E942.6	E950.4	E962.0	E980.4
nitroprusside	972.6	E858.3	E942.6	E950.4	E962.0	E980.4
para-aminohippurate	977.8	E858.8	E947.8	E950.4	E962.0	E980.4
perborate (nonmedicinal)						
NEC	989.89	E866.8	—	E950.9	E962.1	E980.9
medicinal	976.6	E858.7	E946.6	E950.4	E962.0	E980.4
soap	989.6	E861.1	—	E950.9	E962.1	E980.9
percarbonate — see Sodium, perborate						
phosphate	973.3	E858.4	E943.3	E950.4	E962.0	E980.4
polystyrene sulfonate	974.5	E858.5	E944.5	E950.4	E962.0	E980.4
propionate	976.0	E858.7	E946.0	E950.4	E962.0	E980.4
psylliate	972.7	E858.3	E942.7	E950.4	E962.0	E980.4
removing resins	974.5	E858.5	E944.5	E950.4	E962.0	E980.4
salicylate	965.1	E850.3	E935.3	E950.0	E962.0	E980.0
sulfate	973.3	E858.4	E943.3	E950.4	E962.0	E980.4
sulfoxone	961.8	E857	E931.8	E950.4	E962.0	E980.4
tetradecyl sulfate	972.7	E858.3	E942.7	E950.4	E962.0	E980.4
thiopental	968.3	E855.1	E938.3	E950.4	E962.0	E980.4
thiosalicylate	965.1	E850.3	E935.3	E950.0	E962.0	E980.0
thiosulfate	976.0	E858.7	E946.0	E950.4	E962.0	E980.4
tolbutamide	977.8	E858.8	E947.8	E950.4	E962.0	E980.4
Sodium — continued						
tyropanoate	977.8	E858.8	E947.8	E950.4	E962.0	E980.4
valproate	966.3	E855.0	E936.3	E950.4	E962.0	E980.4
Solanine	977.8	E858.8	E947.8	E950.4	E962.0	E980.4
Solanum dulcamara	988.2	E865.4	—	E950.9	E962.1	E980.9
Solapsone	961.8	E857	E931.8	E950.4	E962.0	E980.4
Solasulfone	961.8	E857	E931.8	E950.4	E962.0	E980.4
Soldering fluid	983.1	E864.1	—	E950.7	E962.1	E980.6
Solid substance	989.9	E866.9	—	E950.9	E962.1	E980.9
specified NEC	989.9	E866.8	—	E950.9	E962.1	E980.9
Solvents, industrial	982.8	E862.9	—	E950.9	E962.1	E980.9
naphtha	981	E862.0	—	E950.9	E962.1	E980.9
petroleum	981	E862.0	—	E950.9	E962.1	E980.9
specified NEC	982.8	E862.4	—	E950.9	E962.1	E980.9
Soma	968.0	E855.1	E938.0	E950.4	E962.0	E980.4
Somatotropin	962.4	E858.0	E932.4	E950.4	E962.0	E980.4
Sominex	963.0	E858.1	E933.0	E950.4	E962.0	E980.4
Somnos	967.1	E852.0	E937.1	E950.2	E962.0	E980.2
Somonal	967.0	E851	E937.0	E950.1	E962.0	E980.1
Soneryl	967.0	E851	E937.0	E950.1	E962.0	E980.1
Soothing syrup	977.9	E858.9	E947.9	E950.5	E962.0	E980.5
Sopor	967.4	E852.3	E937.4	E950.2	E962.0	E980.2
Soporific drug	967.9	E852.9	E937.9	E950.2	E962.0	E980.2
specified type NEC	967.8	E852.8	E937.8	E950.2	E962.0	E980.2
Sorbitol NEC	977.4	E858.8	E947.4	E950.4	E962.0	E980.4
Sotradecol	972.7	E858.3	E942.7	E950.4	E962.0	E980.4
Spacoline	975.1	E858.6	E945.1	E950.4	E962.0	E980.4
Spanish fly	976.8	E858.7	E946.8	E950.4	E962.0	E980.4
Sparine	969.1	E853.0	E939.1	E950.3	E962.0	E980.3
Sparteine	975.0	E858.6	E945.0	E950.4	E962.0	E980.4
Spasmolytics	975.1	E858.6	E945.1	E950.4	E962.0	E980.4
anticholinergics	971.1	E855.4	E941.1	E950.4	E962.0	E980.4
Spectinomycin	960.8	E856	E930.8	E950.4	E962.0	E980.4
Speed	969.7	E854.2	E939.7	E950.3	E962.0	E980.3
Spermicides	976.8	E858.7	E946.8	E950.4	E962.0	E980.4
Spider (bite) (venom)	989.5	E905.1	—	E950.9	E962.1	E980.9
antivenin	979.9	E858.8	E949.9	E950.4	E962.0	E980.4
Spigelia (root)	961.6	E857	E931.6	E950.4	E962.0	E980.4
Spiperone	969.2	E853.1	E939.2	E950.3	E962.0	E980.3
Spiramycin	960.3	E856	E930.3	E950.4	E962.0	E980.4
Spirilene	969.5	E853.8	E939.5	E950.3	E962.0	E980.3
Spirit(s) (neutral) NEC	980.0	E860.1	—	E950.9	E962.1	E980.9
beverage	980.0	E860.0	—	E950.9	E962.1	E980.9
industrial	980.9	E860.9	—	E950.9	E962.1	E980.9
mineral	981	E862.0	—	E950.9	E962.1	E980.9
of salt — see Hydrochloric acid						
surgical	980.9	E860.9	—	E950.9	E962.1	E980.9
Spironolactone	974.4	E858.5	E944.4	E950.4	E962.0	E980.4
Sponge, absorbable (gelatin)	964.5	E858.2	E934.5	E950.4	E962.0	E980.4
Sporostacin	976.0	E858.7	E946.0	E950.4	E962.0	E980.4
Sprays (aerosol)	989.89	E866.8	—	E950.9	E962.1	E980.9
cosmetic	989.89	E866.7	—	E950.9	E962.1	E980.9
medicinal NEC	977.9	E858.9	E947.9	E950.5	E962.0	E980.5
pesticides — see Pesticides						
specified content — see substance specified						
Spurge flax	988.2	E865.4	—	E950.9	E962.1	E980.9
Spurges	988.2	E865.4	—	E950.9	E962.1	E980.9
Squill (expectorant) NEC	975.5	E858.6	E945.5	E950.4	E962.0	E980.4
rat poison	989.4	E863.7	—	E950.6	E962.1	E980.7
Squirting cucumber (cathartic)	973.1	E858.4	E943.1	E950.4	E962.0	E980.4
Stains	989.89	E866.8	—	E950.9	E962.1	E980.9
Stannous — see also Tin						
fluoride	976.7	E858.7	E946.7	E950.4	E962.0	E980.4
Stanolone	962.1	E858.0	E932.1	E950.4	E962.0	E980.4
Stanozolol	962.1	E858.0	E932.1	E950.4	E962.0	E980.4
Staphisagria or stavesacre (pediculicide)	976.0	E858.7	E946.0	E950.4	E962.0	E980.4
Stelazine	969.1	E853.0	E939.1	E950.3	E962.0	E980.3
Stemetil	969.1	E853.0	E939.1	E950.3	E962.0	E980.3
Sterculia (cathartic) (gum)	973.3	E858.4	E943.3	E950.4	E962.0	E980.4
Sternutator gas	987.8	E869.8	—	E952.8	E962.2	E982.8
Steroids NEC	962.0	E858.0	E932.0	E950.4	E962.0	E980.4
ENT agent	976.6	E858.7	E946.6	E950.4	E962.0	E980.4
ophthalmic preparation	976.5	E858.7	E946.5	E950.4	E962.0	E980.4
topical NEC	976.0	E858.7	E946.0	E950.4	E962.0	E980.4
Stibine	985.8	E866.4	—	E950.9	E962.1	E980.9
Stibophen	961.2	E857	E931.2	E950.4	E962.0	E980.4
Stilbamide, stilbamidine	961.5	E857	E931.5	E950.4	E962.0	E980.4

	Poisoning	Accident	Therapeutic Use	Suicide Attempt	Assault	Undetermined
Stilbestrol	962.2	E858.0	E932.2	E950.4	E962.0	E980.4
Stimulants (central nervous system)	970.9	E854.3	E940.9	E950.4	E962.0	E980.4
analeptics	970.0	E854.3	E940.0	E950.4	E962.0	E980.4
opiate antagonist	970.1	E854.3	E940.1	E950.4	E962.0	E980.4
psychotherapeutic NEC	969.0	E854.0	E939.0	E950.3	E962.0	E980.3
specified NEC	970.8	E854.3	E940.8	E950.4	E962.0	E980.4
Storage batteries (acid) (cells)	983.1	E864.1	—	E950.7	E962.1	E980.6
Stovaine	968.9	E855.2	E938.9	E950.4	E962.0	E980.4
infiltration (subcutaneous)	968.5	E855.2	E938.5	E950.4	E962.0	E980.4
nerve block (peripheral) (plexus)	968.6	E855.2	E938.6	E950.4	E962.0	E980.4
spinal	968.7	E855.2	E938.7	E950.4	E962.0	E980.4
topical (surface)	968.5	E855.2	E938.5	E950.4	E962.0	E980.4
Stovarsal	961.1	E857	E931.1	E950.4	E962.0	E980.4
Stove gas — see Gas, utility						
Stoxil	976.5	E858.7	E946.5	E950.4	E962.0	E980.4
STP	969.6	E854.1	E939.6	E950.3	E962.0	E980.3
Stramonium (medicinal) NEC	971.1	E855.4	E941.1	E950.4	E962.0	E980.4
natural state	988.2	E865.4	—	E950.9	E962.1	E980.9
Streptodornase	964.4	E858.2	E934.4	E950.4	E962.0	E980.4
Streptoduocin	960.6	E856	E930.6	E950.4	E962.0	E980.4
Streptokinase	964.4	E858.2	E934.4	E950.4	E962.0	E980.4
Streptomycin	960.6	E856	E930.6	E950.4	E962.0	E980.4
Streptozocin	960.7	E856	E930.7	E950.4	E962.0	E980.4
Stripper (paint) (solvent)	982.8	E862.9	—	E950.9	E962.1	E980.9
Strobane	989.2	E863.0	—	E950.6	E962.1	E980.7
Strophanthin	972.1	E858.3	E942.1	E950.4	E962.0	E980.4
Strophanthus hispidus or kombe	988.2	E865.4	—	E950.9	E962.1	E980.9
Strychnine (rodenticide) (salts)	989.1	E863.7	—	E950.6	E962.1	E980.7
medicinal NEC	970.8	E854.3	E940.8	E950.4	E962.0	E980.4
Strychnos (ignatii) — see Strychnine						
Styramate	968.0	E855.1	E938.0	E950.4	E962.0	E980.4
Styrene	983.0	E864.0	—	E950.7	E962.1	E980.6
Succinimide (anticonvulsant)	966.2	E855.0	E936.2	E950.4	E962.0	E980.4
mercuric — see Mercury						
Succinylcholine	975.2	E858.6	E945.2	E950.4	E962.0	E980.4
Succinylsulfathiazole	961.0	E857	E931.0	E950.4	E962.0	E980.4
Sucrose	974.5	E858.5	E944.5	E950.4	E962.0	E980.4
Sulfacetamide	961.0	E857	E931.0	E950.4	E962.0	E980.4
ophthalmic preparation	976.5	E858.7	E946.5	E950.4	E962.0	E980.4
Sulfachlorpyridazine	961.0	E857	E931.0	E950.4	E962.0	E980.4
Sulfacytine	961.0	E857	E931.0	E950.4	E962.0	E980.4
Sulfadiazine	961.0	E857	E931.0	E950.4	E962.0	E980.4
silver (topical)	976.0	E858.7	E946.0	E950.4	E962.0	E980.4
Sulfadimethoxine	961.0	E857	E931.0	E950.4	E962.0	E980.4
Sulfadimidine	961.0	E857	E931.0	E950.4	E962.0	E980.4
Sulfaethidole	961.0	E857	E931.0	E950.4	E962.0	E980.4
Sulfafurazole	961.0	E857	E931.0	E950.4	E962.0	E980.4
Sulfaguanidine	961.0	E857	E931.0	E950.4	E962.0	E980.4
Sulfamerazine	961.0	E857	E931.0	E950.4	E962.0	E980.4
Sulfameter	961.0	E857	E931.0	E950.4	E962.0	E980.4
Sulfamethizole	961.0	E857	E931.0	E950.4	E962.0	E980.4
Sulfamethoxazole	961.0	E857	E931.0	E950.4	E962.0	E980.4
Sulfamethoxydiazine	961.0	E857	E931.0	E950.4	E962.0	E980.4
Sulfamethoxypyridazine	961.0	E857	E931.0	E950.4	E962.0	E980.4
Sulfamethylthiazole	961.0	E857	E931.0	E950.4	E962.0	E980.4
Sulfamylon	976.0	E858.7	E946.0	E950.4	E962.0	E980.4
Sulfan blue (diagnostic dye)	977.8	E858.8	E947.8	E950.4	E962.0	E980.4
Sulfanilamide	961.0	E857	E931.0	E950.4	E962.0	E980.4
Sulfanilylguanidine	961.0	E857	E931.0	E950.4	E962.0	E980.4
Sulfaphenazole	961.0	E857	E931.0	E950.4	E962.0	E980.4
Sulfaphenylthiazole	961.0	E857	E931.0	E950.4	E962.0	E980.4
Sulfaproxyline	961.0	E857	E931.0	E950.4	E962.0	E980.4
Sulfapyridine	961.0	E857	E931.0	E950.4	E962.0	E980.4
Sulfapyrimidine	961.0	E857	E931.0	E950.4	E962.0	E980.4
Sulfarsphenamine	961.1	E857	E931.1	E950.4	E962.0	E980.4
Sulfasalazine	961.0	E857	E931.0	E950.4	E962.0	E980.4
Sulfasomizole	961.0	E857	E931.0	E950.4	E962.0	E980.4
Sulfasuxidine	961.0	E857	E931.0	E950.4	E962.0	E980.4
Sulfinpyrazone	974.7	E858.5	E944.7	E950.4	E962.0	E980.4
Sulfisoxazole	961.0	E857	E931.0	E950.4	E962.0	E980.4
ophthalmic preparation	976.5	E858.7	E946.5	E950.4	E962.0	E980.4
Sulfomyxin	960.8	E856	E930.8	E950.4	E962.0	E980.4
Sulfonal	967.8	E852.8	E937.8	E950.2	E962.0	E980.2
Sulfonamides (mixtures)	961.0	E857	E931.0	E950.4	E962.0	E980.4
Sulfones	961.8	E857	E931.8	E950.4	E962.0	E980.4
Sulfonethylmethane	967.8	E852.8	E937.8	E950.2	E962.0	E980.2
Sulfonmethane	967.8	E852.8	E937.8	E950.2	E962.0	E980.2
Sulfonphthal, sulfonphthol	977.8	E858.8	E947.8	E950.4	E962.0	E980.4
Sulfonylurea derivatives, oral	962.3	E858.0	E932.3	E950.4	E962.0	E980.4
Sulfoxone	961.8	E857	E931.8	E950.4	E962.0	E980.4
Sulfur, sulfureted, sulfuric, sulfurous, sulfuryl (compounds) NEC	989.89	E866.8	—	E950.9	E962.1	E980.9
acid	983.1	E864.1	—	E950.7	E962.1	E980.6
dioxide	987.3	E869.1	—	E952.8	E962.2	E982.8
ether — see Ether(s)						
hydrogen	987.8	E869.8	—	E952.8	E962.2	E982.8
medicinal (keratolytic) (ointment) NEC	976.4	E858.7	E946.4	E950.4	E962.0	E980.4
pesticide (vapor)	989.4	E863.4	—	E950.6	E962.1	E980.7
vapor NEC	987.8	E869.8	—	E952.8	E962.2	E982.8
Sulkowitch's reagent	977.8	E858.8	E947.8	E950.4	E962.0	E980.4
Sulph — see also Sulf-						
Sulphadione	961.8	E857	E931.8	E950.4	E962.0	E980.4
Sulthiame, sultiame	966.3	E855.0	E936.3	E950.4	E962.0	E980.4
Superinone	975.5	E858.6	E945.5	E950.4	E962.0	E980.4
Suramin	961.5	E857	E931.5	E950.4	E962.0	E980.4
Surfacaine	968.5	E855.2	E938.5	E950.4	E962.0	E980.4
Surital	968.3	E855.1	E938.3	E950.4	E962.0	E980.4
Sutilains	976.8	E858.7	E946.8	E950.4	E962.0	E980.4
Suxamethonium (bromide) (chloride) (iodide)	975.2	E858.6	E945.2	E950.4	E962.0	E980.4
Suxethonium (bromide)	975.2	E858.6	E945.2	E950.4	E962.0	E980.4
Sweet oil (birch)	976.3	E858.7	E946.3	E950.4	E962.0	E980.4
Sym-dichloroethyl ether	982.3	E862.4	—	E950.9	E962.1	E980.9
Sympatholytics	971.3	E855.6	E941.3	E950.4	E962.0	E980.4
Sympathomimetics	971.2	E855.5	E941.2	E950.4	E962.0	E980.4
Synagis	979.6	E858.8	E949.6	E950.4	E962.0	E980.4
Synalar	976.0	E858.7	E946.0	E950.4	E962.0	E980.4
Synthroid	962.7	E858.0	E932.7	E950.4	E962.0	E980.4
Syntocinon	975.0	E858.6	E945.0	E950.4	E962.0	E980.4
Syrosingopine	972.6	E858.3	E942.6	E950.4	E962.0	E980.4
Systemic agents (primarily)	963.9	E858.1	E933.9	E950.4	E962.0	E980.4
specified NEC	963.8	E858.1	E933.8	E950.4	E962.0	E980.4
Tablets (see also specified substance)	977.9	E858.9	E947.9	E950.5	E962.0	E980.5
Tace	962.2	E858.0	E932.2	E950.4	E962.0	E980.4
Tacrine	971.0	E855.3	E941.0	E950.4	E962.0	E980.4
Talbutal	967.0	E851	E937.0	E950.1	E962.0	E980.1
Talc	976.3	E858.7	E946.3	E950.4	E962.0	E980.4
Talcum	976.3	E858.7	E946.3	E950.4	E962.0	E980.4
Tandearil, tanderil	965.5	E850.5	E935.5	E950.0	E962.0	E980.0
Tannic acid	983.1	E864.1	—	E950.7	E962.1	E980.6
medicinal (astringent)	976.2	E858.7	E946.2	E950.4	E962.0	E980.4
Tannin — see Tannic acid						
Tansy	988.2	E865.4	—	E950.9	E962.1	E980.9
TAO	960.3	E856	E930.3	E950.4	E962.0	E980.4
Tapazole	962.8	E858.0	E932.8	E950.4	E962.0	E980.4
Tar NEC	983.0	E864.0	—	E950.7	E962.1	E980.6
camphor — see Naphthalene						
fumes	987.8	E869.8	—	E952.8	E962.2	E982.8
Taractan	969.3	E853.8	E939.3	E950.3	E962.0	E980.3
Tarantula (venomous)	989.5	E905.1	—	E950.9	E962.1	E980.9
Tartar emetic (anti-infective)	961.2	E857	E931.2	E950.4	E962.0	E980.4
Tartaric acid	983.1	E864.1	—	E950.7	E962.1	E980.6
Tartrated antimony (anti-infective)	961.2	E857	E931.2	E950.4	E962.0	E980.4
TCA — see Trichloroacetic acid						
TDI	983.0	E864.0	—	E950.7	E962.1	E980.6
vapor	987.8	E869.8	—	E952.8	E962.2	E982.8
Tear gas	987.5	E869.3	—	E952.8	E962.2	E982.8
Teclothiazide	974.3	E858.5	E944.3	E950.4	E962.0	E980.4
Tegretol	966.3	E855.0	E936.3	E950.4	E962.0	E980.4
Telepaque	977.8	E858.8	E947.8	E950.4	E962.0	E980.4
Tellurium	985.8	E866.4	—	E950.9	E962.1	E980.9
fumes	985.8	E866.4	—	E950.9	E962.1	E980.9
TEM	963.1	E858.1	E933.1	E950.4	E962.0	E980.4
Temazepan — see Benzodiazepines						
TEPA	963.1	E858.1	E933.1	E950.4	E962.0	E980.4
TEPP	989.3	E863.1	—	E950.6	E962.1	E980.7
Terbutaline	971.2	E855.5	E941.2	E950.4	E962.0	E980.4
Teroxalene	961.6	E857	E931.6	E950.4	E962.0	E980.4
Terpin hydrate	975.5	E858.6	E945.5	E950.4	E962.0	E980.4
Terramycin	960.4	E856	E930.4	E950.4	E962.0	E980.4

☑ Additional Digit Required ▶◀ Revised Text ● New Line ▲ Revised Code

	Poisoning	Accident	Therapeutic Use	Suicide Attempt	Assault	Undetermined
External Cause (E-Code)						
Valisone	976.0	E858.7	E946.0	E950.4	E962.0	E980.4
Valium	969.4	E853.2	E939.4	E950.3	E962.0	E980.3
Valmid	967.8	E852.8	E937.8	E950.2	E962.0	E980.2
Vanadium	985.8	E866.4	—	E950.9	E962.1	E980.9
Vancomycin	960.8	E856	E930.8	E950.4	E962.0	E980.4
Vapor (see also Gas)	987.9	E869.9	—	E952.9	E962.2	E982.9
kiln (carbon monoxide)	986	E868.8	—	E952.1	E962.2	E982.1
lead — see Lead						
specified source NEC (see also specific substance)	987.8	E869.8	—	E952.8	E962.2	E982.8
Varidase	964.4	E858.2	E934.4	E950.4	E962.0	E980.4
Varnish	989.89	E861.6	—	E950.9	E962.1	E980.9
cleaner	982.8	E862.9	—	E950.9	E962.1	E980.9
Vaseline	976.3	E858.7	E946.3	E950.4	E962.0	E980.4
Vasodilan	972.5	E858.3	E942.5	E950.4	E962.0	E980.4
Vasodilators NEC	972.5	E858.3	E942.5	E950.4	E962.0	E980.4
coronary	972.4	E858.3	E942.4	E950.4	E962.0	E980.4
Vasopressin	962.5	E858.0	E932.5	E950.4	E962.0	E980.4
Vasopressor drugs	962.5	E858.0	E932.5	E950.4	E962.0	E980.4
Venom, venomous (bite) (sting)	989.5	E905.9	—	E950.9	E962.1	E980.9
arthropod NEC	989.5	E905.5	—	E950.9	E962.1	E980.9
bee	989.5	E905.3	—	E950.9	E962.1	E980.9
centipede	989.5	E905.4	—	E950.9	E962.1	E980.9
hornet	989.5	E905.3	—	E950.9	E962.1	E980.9
lizard	989.5	E905.0	—	E950.9	E962.1	E980.9
marine animals or plants	989.5	E905.6	—	E950.9	E962.1	E980.9
millipede (tropical)	989.5	E905.4	—	E950.9	E962.1	E980.9
plant NEC	989.5	E905.7	—	E950.9	E962.1	E980.9
marine	989.5	E905.6	—	E950.9	E962.1	E980.9
scorpion	989.5	E905.2	—	E950.9	E962.1	E980.9
snake	989.5	E905.0	—	E950.9	E962.1	E980.9
specified NEC	989.5	E905.8	—	E950.9	E962.1	E980.9
spider	989.5	E905.1	—	E950.9	E962.1	E980.9
wasp	989.5	E905.3	—	E950.9	E962.1	E980.9
Veramon	967.0	E851	E937.0	E950.1	E962.0	E980.1
Veratrum						
album	988.2	E865.4	—	E950.9	E962.1	E980.9
alkaloids	972.6	E858.3	E942.6	E950.4	E962.0	E980.4
viride	988.2	E865.4	—	E950.9	E962.1	E980.9
Verdigris (see also Copper)	985.8	E866.4	—	E950.9	E962.1	E980.9
Veronal	967.0	E851	E937.0	E950.1	E962.0	E980.1
Veroxil	961.6	E857	E931.6	E950.4	E962.0	E980.4
Versidyne	965.7	E850.7	E935.7	E950.0	E962.0	E980.0
Viagra	972.5	E858.3	E942.5	E950.4	E962.0	E980.4
Vienna						
green	985.1	E866.3	—	E950.8	E962.1	E980.8
insecticide	985.1	E863.4	—	E950.6	E962.1	E980.7
red	989.89	E866.8	—	E950.9	E962.1	E980.9
pharmaceutical dye	977.4	E858.8	E947.4	E950.4	E962.0	E980.4
Vinbarbital, vinbarbitone	967.0	E851	E937.0	E950.1	E962.0	E980.1
Vinblastine	963.1	E858.1	E933.1	E950.4	E962.0	E980.4
Vincristine	963.1	E858.1	E933.1	E950.4	E962.0	E980.4
Vinesthene, vinethene	968.2	E855.1	E938.2	E950.4	E962.0	E980.4
Vinyl						
bital	967.0	E851	E937.0	E950.1	E962.0	E980.1
ether	968.2	E855.1	E938.2	E950.4	E962.0	E980.4
Vioform	961.3	E857	E931.3	E950.4	E962.0	E980.4
topical	976.0	E858.7	E946.0	E930.4	E962.0	E980.4
Viomycin	960.6	E856	E930.6	E950.4	E962.0	E980.4
Viosterol	963.5	E858.1	E933.5	E950.4	E962.0	E980.4
Viper (venom)	989.5	E905.0	—	E950.9	E962.1	E980.9
Viprynium (embonate)	961.6	E857	E931.6	E950.4	E962.0	E980.4
Virugon	961.7	E857	E931.7	E950.4	E962.0	E980.4
Visine	976.5	E858.7	E946.5	E950.4	E962.0	E980.4
Vitamins NEC	963.5	E858.1	E933.5	E950.4	E962.0	E980.4
B_{12}	964.1	E858.2	E934.1	E950.4	E962.0	E980.4
hematopoietic	964.1	E858.2	E934.1	E950.4	E962.0	E980.4
K	964.3	E858.2	E934.3	E950.4	E962.0	E980.4
Vleminckx's solution	976.4	E858.7	E946.4	E950.4	E962.0	E980.4
Voltaren — see Diclofenac sodium						
Ventolin — see Salbutamol sulfate						
Warfarin (potassium) (sodium)	964.2	E858.2	E934.2	E950.4	E962.0	E980.4
rodenticide	989.4	E863.7	—	E950.6	E962.1	E980.7
Wasp (sting)	989.5	E905.3	—	E950.9	E962.1	E980.9
Water						
balance agents NEC	974.5	E858.5	E944.5	E950.4	E962.0	E980.4
Water — continued						
gas	987.1	E868.1	—	E951.8	E962.2	E981.8
incomplete combustion of — see Carbon, monoxide, fuel, utility						
hemlock	988.2	E865.4	—	E950.9	E962.1	E980.9
moccasin (venom)	989.5	E905.0	—	E950.9	E962.1	E980.9
Wax (paraffin) (petroleum)	981	E862.3	—	E950.9	E962.1	E980.9
automobile	989.89	E861.2	—	E950.9	E962.1	E980.9
floor	981	E862.0	—	E950.9	E962.1	E980.9
Weed killers NEC	989.4	E863.5	—	E950.6	E962.1	E980.7
Welldorm	967.1	E852.0	E937.1	E950.2	E962.0	E980.2
White						
arsenic — see Arsenic						
hellebore	988.2	E865.4	—	E950.9	E962.1	E980.9
lotion (keratolytic)	976.4	E858.7	E946.4	E950.4	E962.0	E980.4
spirit	981	E862.0	—	E950.9	E962.1	E980.9
Whitewashes	989.89	E861.6	—	E950.9	E962.1	E980.9
Whole blood	964.7	E858.2	E934.7	E950.4	E962.0	E980.4
Wild						
black cherry	988.2	E865.4	—	E950.9	E962.1	E980.9
poisonous plants NEC	988.2	E865.4	—	E950.9	E962.1	E980.9
Window cleaning fluid	989.89	E861.3	—	E950.9	E962.1	E980.9
Wintergreen (oil)	976.3	E858.7	E946.3	E950.4	E962.0	E980.4
Witch hazel	976.2	E858.7	E946.2	E950.4	E962.0	E980.4
Wood						
alcohol	980.1	E860.2	—	E950.9	E962.1	E980.9
spirit	980.1	E860.2	—	E950.9	E962.1	E980.9
Woorali	975.2	E858.6	E945.2	E950.4	E962.0	E980.4
Wormseed, American	961.6	E857	E931.6	E950.4	E962.0	E980.4
Xanthine diuretics	974.1	E858.5	E944.1	E950.4	E962.0	E980.4
Xanthocillin	960.0	E856	E930.0	E950.4	E962.0	E980.4
Xanthotoxin	976.3	E858.7	E946.3	E950.4	E962.0	E980.4
Xigris	964.2	E858.2	E934.2	E950.4	E962.0	E980.4
Xylene (liquid) (vapor)	982.0	E862.4	—	E950.9	E962.1	E980.9
Xylocaine (infiltration) (topical)	968.5	E855.2	E938.5	E950.4	E962.0	E980.4
nerve block (peripheral) (plexus)	968.6	E855.2	E938.6	E950.4	E962.0	E980.4
spinal	968.7	E855.2	E938.7	E950.4	E962.0	E980.4
Xylol (liquid) (vapor)	982.0	E862.4	—	E950.9	E962.1	E980.9
Xylometazoline	971.2	E855.5	E941.2	E950.4	E962.0	E980.4
Yellow						
fever vaccine	979.3	E858.8	E949.3	E950.4	E962.0	E980.4
jasmine	988.2	E865.4	—	E950.9	E962.1	E980.9
Yew	988.2	E865.4	—	E950.9	E962.1	E980.9
Zactane	965.7	E850.7	E935.7	E950.0	E962.0	E980.0
Zaroxolyn	974.3	E858.5	E944.3	E950.4	E962.0	E980.4
Zephiran (topical)	976.0	E858.7	E946.0	E950.4	E962.0	E980.4
ophthalmic preparation	976.5	E858.7	E946.5	E950.4	E962.0	E980.4
Zerone	980.1	E860.2	—	E950.9	E962.1	E980.9
Zinc (compounds) (fumes) (salts) (vapor) NEC	985.8	E866.4	—	E950.9	E962.1	E980.9
anti-infectives	976.0	E858.7	E946.0	E950.4	E962.0	E980.4
antivaricose	972.7	E858.3	E942.7	E950.4	E962.0	E980.4
bacitracin	976.0	E858.7	E946.0	E950.4	E962.0	E980.4
chloride	976.2	E858.7	E946.2	E950.4	E962.0	E980.4
gelatin	976.3	E858.7	E946.3	E950.4	E962.0	E980.4
oxide	976.3	E858.7	E946.3	E950.4	E962.0	E980.4
peroxide	976.0	E858.7	E946.0	E950.4	E962.0	E980.4
pesticides	985.8	E863.4	—	E950.6	E962.1	E980.7
phosphide (rodenticide)	985.8	E863.7	—	E950.6	E962.1	E980.7
stearate	976.3	E858.7	E946.3	E950.4	E962.0	E980.4
sulfate (antivaricose)	972.7	E858.3	E942.7	E950.4	E962.0	E980.4
ENT agent	976.6	E858.7	E946.6	E950.4	E962.0	E980.4
ophthalmic solution	976.5	E858.7	E946.5	E950.4	E962.0	E980.4
topical NEC	976.0	E858.7	E946.0	E950.4	E962.0	E980.4
undecylenate	976.0	E858.7	E946.0	E950.4	E962.0	E980.4
Zovant	964.2	E858.2	E934.2	E950.4	E962.0	E980.4
Zoxazolamine	968.0	E855.1	E938.0	E950.4	E962.0	E980.4
Zygadenus (venenosus)	988.2	E865.4	—	E950.9	E962.1	E980.9

☑ Additional Digit Required ▶◀ Revised Text ● New Line ▲ Revised Code

SECTION 3

Alphabetic Index to External Causes of Injury and Poisoning (E Code)

This section contains the index to the codes which classify environmental events, circumstances, and other conditions as the cause of injury and other adverse effects. Where a code from the section Supplementary Classification of External Causes of Injury and Poisoning (E800-E998) is applicable, it is intended that the E code shall be used in addition to a code from the main body of the classification, Chapters 1 to 17.

The alphabetic index to the E codes is organized by main terms which describe the *accident, circumstance, event,* or *specific agent* which caused the injury or other adverse effect.

Note — Transport accidents (E800-E848) include accidents involving:

> *aircraft and spacecraft (E840-E845)*
> *watercraft (E830-E838)*
> *motor vehicle (E810-E825)*
> *railway (E800-E807)*
> *other road vehicles (E826-E829)*

For definitions and examples related to transport accidents — see Volume 1 code categories E800-E848.

The fourth-digit subdivisions for use with categories E800-E848 to identify the injured person are found at the end of this section.

For identifying the place in which an accident or poisoning occurred (circumstances classifiable to categories E850-E869 and E880-E928) — see the listing in this section under "Accident, occurring."

See the Table of Drugs and Chemicals (Section 2 of this volume) for identifying the specific agent involved in drug overdose or a wrong substance given or taken in error, and for intoxication or poisoning by a drug or other chemical substance.

The specific adverse effect, reaction, or localized toxic effect to a correct drug or substance properly administered in therapeutic or prophylactic dosage should be classified according to the nature of the adverse effect (e.g., allergy, dermatitis, tachycardia) listed in Section 1 of this volume.

A

Abandonment
causing exposure to weather conditions — see
    Exposure
child, with intent to injure or kill E968.4
helpless person, infant, newborn E904.0
    with intent to injure or kill E968.4
Abortion, criminal, injury to child E968.8
Abuse (alleged) (suspected)
adult
    by
        child E967.4
        ex-partner E967.3
        ex-spouse E967.3
        father E967.0
        grandchild E967.7
        grandparent E967.6
        mother E967.2
        non-related caregiver E967.8
        other relative E967.7
        other specified person E967.1
        partner E967.3
        sibling E967.5
        spouse E967.3
        stepfather E967.0
        stepmother E967.2
        unspecified person E967.9
child
    by
        boyfriend of parent or guardian E967.0
        child E967.4
        father E967.0
        female partner of parent or guardian
          E967.2
        girlfriend of parent or guardian E967.2
        grandchild E967.7
        grandparent E967.6
        male partner of parent or guardian
          E967.2
        mother E967.2
        non-related caregiver E967.8
        other relative E967.7
        other specified person(s) E967.1
        sibling E967.5
        stepfather E967.0
        stepmother E967.2
        unspecified person E967.9
Accident (to) E928.9
aircraft (in transit) (powered) E841 ☑
    at landing, take-off E840 ☑
    due to, caused by cataclysm — see
        categories E908 ☑, E909 ☑
    late effect of E929.1
    unpowered (see also Collision, aircraft,
        unpowered) E842 ☑
    while alighting, boarding E843 ☑
amphibious vehicle
    on
        land — see Accident, motor vehicle
        water — see Accident, watercraft
animal, ridden NEC E828 ☑
animal-drawn vehicle NEC E827 ☑
balloon (see also Collision, aircraft, unpowered)
    E842 ☑
caused by, due to
    abrasive wheel (metalworking) E919.3
    animal NEC E906.9
        being ridden (in sport or transport)
          E828 ☑
    avalanche NEC E909.2
    band saw E919.4
    bench saw E919.4
    bore, earth-drilling or mining (land) (seabed)
        E919.1
    bulldozer E919.7
    cataclysmic
        earth surface movement or eruption
          E909.9
        storm E908.9
    chain
        hoist E919.2
          agricultural operations E919.0
          mining operations E919.1
        saw E920.1
    circular saw E919.4

Accident (to) — continued
caused by, due to — continued
    cold (excessive) (see also Cold, exposure to)
        E901.9
    combine E919.0
    conflagration — see Conflagration
    corrosive liquid, substance NEC E924.1
    cotton gin E919.8
    crane E919.2
        agricultural operations E919.0
        mining operations E919.1
    cutting or piercing instrument (see also Cut)
        E920.9
    dairy equipment E919.8
    derrick E919.2
        agricultural operations E919.0
        mining operations E919.1
    drill E920.1
        earth (land) (seabed) E919.1
        hand (powered) E920.1
          not powered E920.4
        metalworking E919.3
        woodworking E919.4
    earth(-)
        drilling machine E919.1
        moving machine E919.7
        scraping machine E919.7
    electric
        current (see also Electric shock) E925.9
        motor — see also Accident, machine, by
          type of machine
          current (of) — see Electric shock
    elevator (building) (grain) E919.2
        agricultural operations E919.0
        mining operations E919.1
    environmental factors NEC E928.9
    excavating machine E919.7
    explosive material (see also Explosion)
        E923.9
    farm machine E919.0
    fire, flames — see also Fire
        conflagration — see Conflagration
    firearm missile — see Shooting
    forging (metalworking) machine E919.3
    forklift (truck) E919.2
        agricultural operations E919.0
        mining operations E919.1
    gas turbine E919.5
    harvester E919.0
    hay derrick, mower, or rake E919.0
    heat (excessive) (see also Heat) E900.9
    hoist (see also Accident, caused by, due to,
        lift) E919.2
        chain — see Accident, caused by, due to,
          chain
        shaft E919.1
    hot
        liquid E924.0
          caustic or corrosive E924.1
        object (not producing fire or flames)
          E924.8
        substance E924.9
          caustic or corrosive E924.1
          liquid (metal) NEC E924.0
          specified type NEC E924.8
    human bite E928.3
    ignition — see Ignition
    internal combustion engine E919.5
    landslide NEC E909.2
    lathe (metalworking) E919.3
        turnings E920.8
        woodworking E919.4
    lift, lifting (appliances) E919.2
        agricultural operations E919.0
        mining operations E919.1
        shaft E919.1
    lightning NEC E907
    machine, machinery — see also Accident,
        machine
        drilling, metal E919.3
        manufacturing, for manufacture of
          beverages E919.8
          clothing E919.8
          foodstuffs E919.8
          paper E919.8
          textiles E919.8

Accident (to) — continued
caused by, due to — continued
    machine, machinery — see also Accident,
        machine — continued
        milling, metal E919.3
        moulding E919.4
        power press, metal E919.3
        printing E919.8
        rolling mill, metal E919.3
        sawing, metal E919.3
        specified type NEC E919.8
        spinning E919.8
        weaving E919.8
    natural factor NEC E928.9
    overhead plane E919.4
    plane E920.4
        overhead E919.4
    powered
        hand tool NEC E920.1
        saw E919.4
          hand E920.1
    printing machine E919.8
    pulley (block) E919.2
        agricultural operations E919.0
        mining operations E919.1
        transmission E919.6
    radial saw E919.4
    radiation — see Radiation
    reaper E919.0
    road scraper E919.7
        when in transport under its own power —
          see categories E810-E825 ☑
    roller coaster E919.8
    sander E919.4
    saw E920.4
        band E919.4
        bench E919.4
        chain E920.1
        circular E919.4
        hand E920.4
          powered E920.1
        powered, except hand E919.4
        radial E919.4
    sawing machine, metal E919.3
    shaft
        hoist E919.1
        lift E919.1
        transmission E919.6
    shears E920.4
        hand E920.4
          powered E920.1
        mechanical E919.3
    shovel E920.4
        steam E919.7
    spinning machine E919.8
    steam — see also Burning, steam
        engine E919.5
        shovel E919.7
    thresher E919.0
    thunderbolt NEC E907
    tractor E919.0
        when in transport under its own power —
          see categories E810-E825 ☑
    transmission belt, cable, chain, gear, pinion,
        pulley, shaft E919.6
    turbine (gas) (water driven) E919.5
    under-cutter E919.1
    weaving machine E919.8
    winch E919.2
        agricultural operations E919.0
        mining operations E919.1
diving E883.0
    with insufficient air supply E913.2
glider (hang) (see also Collision, aircraft,
    unpowered) E842 ☑
hovercraft
    on
        land — see Accident, motor vehicle
        water — see Accident, watercraft
ice yacht (see also Accident, vehicle NEC) E848
in
    medical, surgical procedure
        as, or due to misadventure — see
          Misadventure

☑ Additional Digit Required   ▶◀ Revised Text   ● New Line   ▲ Revised Code

Accident (to) — *continued*
  in — *continued*
    medical, surgical procedure — *continued*
      causing an abnormal reaction or later complication without mention of misadventure — *see* Reaction, abnormal
    kite carrying a person (*see also* Collision, aircraft, unpowered) E842 ☑
    land yacht (*see also* Accident, vehicle NEC) E848
    late effect of — *see* Late effect
    launching pad E845 ☑
    machine, machinery (*see also* Accident, caused by, due to, by specific type of machine) E919.9
      agricultural including animal-powered E919.0
      earth-drilling E919.1
      earth moving or scraping E919.7
      excavating E919.7
      involving transport under own power on highway or transport vehicle — *see* categories E810-E825 ☑, E840-E845 ☑
      lifting (appliances) E919.2
      metalworking E919.3
      mining E919.1
      prime movers, except electric motors E919.5
        electric motors — *see* Accident, machine, by specific type of machine
      recreational E919.8
      specified type NEC E919.8
      transmission E919.6
      watercraft (deck) (engine room) (galley) (laundry) (loading) E836 ☑
      woodworking or forming E919.4
    motor vehicle (on public highway) (traffic) E819 ☑
      due to cataclysm — *see* categories E908 ☑, E909 ☑
      involving
        collision (*see also* Collision, motor vehicle) E812 ☑
      nontraffic, not on public highway — *see* categories E820-E825 ☑
      not involving collision — *see* categories E816-E819 ☑
    nonmotor vehicle NEC E829 ☑
      nonroad — *see* Accident, vehicle NEC
      road, except pedal cycle, animal-drawn vehicle, or animal being ridden E829 ☑
    nonroad vehicle NEC — *see* Accident, vehicle NEC
    not elsewhere classifiable involving
      cable car (not on rails) E847
        on rails E829 ☑
      coal car in mine E846
      hand truck — *see* Accident, vehicle NEC
      logging car E846
      sled(ge), meaning snow or ice vehicle E848
      tram, mine or quarry E846
      truck
        mine or quarry E846
        self-propelled, industrial E846
        station baggage E846
      tub, mine or quarry E846
      vehicle NEC E848
        snow and ice E848
        used only on industrial premises E846
      wheelbarrow E848
    occurring (at) (in)
      apartment E849.0
      baseball field, diamond E849.4
      construction site, any E849.3
      dock E849.8
        yard E849.3
      dormitory E849.7
      factory (building) (premises) E849.3
      farm E849.1
        buildings E849.1
        house E849.0
      football field E849.4
      forest E849.8
      garage (place of work) E849.3
        private (home) E849.0

Accident (to) — *continued*
  occurring (at) (in) — *continued*
    gravel pit E849.2
    gymnasium E849.4
    highway E849.5
    home (private) (residential) E849.0
      institutional E849.7
    hospital E849.7
    hotel E849.6
    house (private) (residential) E849.0
      movie E849.6
      public E849.6
    institution, residential E849.7
    jail E849.7
    mine E849.2
    motel E849.6
    movie house E849.6
    office (building) E849.6
    orphanage E849.7
    park (public) E849.4
      mobile home E849.8
      trailer E849.8
    parking lot or place E849.8
    place
      industrial NEC E849.3
      parking E849.8
      public E849.8
        specified place NEC E849.5
      recreational NEC E849.4
      sport NEC E849.4
    playground (park) (school) E849.4
    prison E849.6
    public building NEC E849.6
    quarry E849.2
    railway
      line NEC E849.8
      yard E849.3
    residence
      home (private) E849.0
    resort (beach) (lake) (mountain) (seashore) (vacation) E849.4
    restaurant E849.6
    sand pit E849.2
    school (building) (private) (public) (state) E849.6
      reform E849.7
      riding E849.4
    seashore E849.8
      resort E849.4
    shop (place of work) E849.3
      commercial E849.6
    skating rink E849.4
    sports palace E849.4
    stadium E849.4
    store E849.6
    street E849.5
    swimming pool (public) E849.4
      private home or garden E849.0
    tennis court E849.4
    theatre, theater E849.6
    trailer court E849.8
    tunnel E849.8
      under construction E849.2
    warehouse E849.3
    yard
      dock E849.3
      industrial E849.3
      private (home) E849.0
      railway E849.3
  off-road type motor vehicle (not on public highway) NEC E821 ☑
    on public highway — *see* catagories E810-E819 ☑
  pedal cycle E826 ☑
  railway E807 ☑
    due to cataclysm — *see* categories E908 ☑, E909 ☑
    involving
      avalanche E909.2
      burning by engine, locomotive, train (*see also* Explosion, railway engine) E803 ☑
      collision (*see also* Collision, railway) E800 ☑
      derailment (*see also* Derailment, railway) E802 ☑

Accident (to) — *continued*
  railway — *continued*
    involving — *continued*
      explosion (*see also* Explosion, railway engine) E803 ☑
      fall (*see also* Fall, from, railway rolling stock) E804 ☑
      fire (*see also* Explosion, railway engine) E803 ☑
      hitting by, being struck by
        object falling in, on, from, rolling stock, train, vehicle E806 ☑
        rolling stock, train, vehicle E805 ☑
      overturning, railway rolling stock, train, vehicle (*see also* Derailment, railway) E802 ☑
      running off rails, railway (*see also* Derailment, railway) E802 ☑
      specified circumstances NEC E806 ☑
      train or vehicle hit by
        avalanche E909.2
        falling object (earth, rock, tree) E806 ☑
          due to cataclysm — *see* categories E908 ☑, E909 ☑
        landslide E909.2
  roller skate E885.1
  scooter (nonmotorized) E885.0
  skateboard E885.2
  ski(ing) E885.3
    jump E884.9
    lift or tow (with chair or gondola) E847
  snow vehicle, motor driven (not on public highway) E820 ☑
    on public highway — *see* catagories E810-E819 ☑
  snowboard E885.4
  spacecraft E845 ☑
  specified cause NEC E928.8
  street car E829 ☑
  traffic NEC E819 ☑
  vehicle NEC (with pedestrian) E848
    battery powered
      airport passenger vehicle E846
      truck (baggage) (mail) E846
    powered commercial or industrial (with other vehicle or object within commercial or industrial premises) E846
  watercraft E838 ☑
    with
      drowning or submersion resulting from accident other than to watercraft E832 ☑
        accident to watercraft E830 ☑
      injury, except drowning or submersion, resulting from
        accident other than to watercraft — *see* categories E833-E838 ☑
        accident to watercraft E831 ☑
    due to, caused by cataclysm — *see* categories E908 ☑, E909 ☑
    machinery E836 ☑

Acid throwing E961
Acosta syndrome E902.0
Aeroneurosis E902.1
Aero-otitis media — *see* Effects of, air pressure
Aerosinusitis — *see* Effects of, air pressure
After-effect, late — *see* Late effect
Air
  blast
    in
      terrorism E979.2
      war operations E993
  embolism (traumatic) NEC E928.9
    in
      infusion or transfusion E874.1
      perfusion E874.2
  sickness E903
Alpine sickness E902.0
Altitude sickness — *see* Effects of, air pressure
Anaphylactic shock, anaphylaxis (*see also* Table of Drugs and Chemicals) E947.9
  due to bite or sting (venomous) — *see* Bite, venomous
Andes disease E902.0

Apoplexy
heat — *see* Heat
Arachnidism E905.1
Arson E968.0
Asphyxia, asphyxiation
by
chemical
in
terrorism E979.7
war operations E997.2
explosion — *see* Explosion
food (bone) (regurgitated food) (seed) E911
foreign object, except food E912
fumes
in
terrorism (chemical weapons) E979.7
war operations E997.2
gas — *see also* Table of Drugs and
Chemicals
in
terrorism E979.7
war operations E997.2
legal
execution E978
intervention (tear) E972
tear E972
mechanical means (*see also* Suffocation)
E913.9
from
conflagration — *see* Conflagration
fire — *see also* Fire E899
in
terrorism E979.3
war operations E990.9
ignition — *see* Ignition
Aspiration
foreign body — *see* Foreign body, aspiration
mucus, not of newborn (with asphyxia,
obstruction respiratory passage,
suffocation) E912
phlegm (with asphyxia, obstruction respiratory
passage, suffocation) E912
vomitus (with asphyxia, obstruction respiratory
passage, suffocation) (*see also* Foreign
body, aspiration, food) E911
Assassination (attempt) (*see also* Assault) E968.9
Assault (homicidal) (by) (in) E968.9
acid E961
swallowed E962.1
air gun E968.6
BB gun E968.6
bite NEC E968.8
of human being E968.7
bomb ((placed in) car or house) E965.8
antipersonnel E965.5
letter E965.7
petrol E965.7
brawl (hand) (fists) (foot) E960.0
burning, burns (by fire) E968.0
acid E961
swallowed E962.1
caustic, corrosive substance E961
swallowed E962.1
chemical from swallowing caustic, corrosive
substance NEC E962.1
hot liquid E968.3
scalding E968.3
vitriol E961
swallowed E962.1
caustic, corrosive substance E961
swallowed E962.1
cut, any part of body E966
dagger E966
drowning E964
explosive(s) E965.9
bomb (*see also* Assault, bomb) E965.8
dynamite E965.8
fight (hand) (fists) (foot) E960.0
with weapon E968.9
blunt or thrown E968.2
cutting or piercing E966
firearm — *see* Shooting, homicide
fire E968.0
firearm(s) — *see* Shooting, homicide

Assault — *continued*
garrotting E963
gunshot (wound) — *see* Shooting, homicide
hanging E963
injury NEC E968.9
knife E966
late effect of E969
ligature E963
poisoning E962.9
drugs or medicinals E962.0
gas(es) or vapors, except drugs and
medicinals E962.2
solid or liquid substances, except drugs and
medicinals E962.1
puncture, any part of body E966
pushing
before moving object, train, vehicle E968.5
from high place E968.1
rape E960.1
scalding E968.3
shooting — *see* Shooting, homicide
sodomy E960.1
stab, any part of body E966
strangulation E963
submersion E964
suffocation E963
transport vehicle E968.5
violence NEC E968.9
vitriol E961
swallowed E962.1
weapon E968.9
blunt or thrown E968.2
cutting or piercing E966
firearm — *see* Shooting, homicide
wound E968.9
cutting E966
gunshot — *see* Shooting, homicide
knife E966
piercing E966
puncture E966
stab E966
Attack by animal NEC E906.9
Avalanche E909.2
falling on or hitting
motor vehicle (in motion) (on public
highway) E909.2
railway train E909.2
Aviators' disease E902.1

B

Barotitis, barodontalgia, barosinusitis,
barotrauma (otitic) (sinus) — *see* Effects of,
air pressure
Battered
baby or child (syndrome) — *see* Abuse, child;
category E967 ☑
person other than baby or child — *see* Assault
Bayonet wound (*see also* Cut, by bayonet) E920.3
in
legal intervention E974
terrorism E979.8
war operations E995
Bean in nose E912
Bed set on fire NEC E898.0
Beheading (by guillotine)
homicide E966
legal execution E978
Bending, injury in E927
Bends E902.0
Bite
animal (nonvenomous) NEC E906.5
other specified (except arthropod) E906.3
venomous NEC E905.9
arthropod (nonvenomous) NEC E906.4
venomous — *see* Sting
black widow spider E905.1
cat E906.3
centipede E905.4
cobra E905.0
copperhead snake E905.0
coral snake E905.0
dog E906.0
fer de lance E905.0
gila monster E905.0

Bite — *continued*
human being
accidental E928.3
assault E968.7
insect (nonvenomous) E906.4
venomous — *see* Sting
krait E905.0
late effect of — *see* Late effect
lizard E906.2
venomous E905.0
mamba E905.0
marine animal
nonvenomous E906.3
snake E906.2
venomous E905.6
snake E905.0
millipede E906.4
venomous E905.4
moray eel E906.3
rat E906.1
rattlesnake E905.0
rodent, except rat E906.3
serpent — *see* Bite, snake
shark E906.3
snake (venomous) E905.0
nonvenomous E906.2
sea E905.0
spider E905.1
nonvenomous E906.4
tarantula (venomous) E905.1
venomous NEC E905.9
by specific animal — *see category* E905 ☑
viper E905.0
water moccasin E905.0
Blast (air)
from nuclear explosion E996
in
terrorism E979.2
from nuclear explosion E979.5
underwater E979.0
war operations E993
from nuclear explosion E996
underwater E992
underwater E992
Blizzard E908.3
Blow E928.9
by law-enforcing agent, police (on duty) E975
with blunt object (baton) (nightstick) (stave)
(truncheon) E973
Blowing up (*see also* Explosion) E923.9
Brawl (hand) (fists) (foot) E960.0
Breakage (accidental)
cable of cable car not on rails E847
ladder (causing fall) E881.0
part (any) of
animal-drawn vehicle E827 ☑
ladder (causing fall) E881.0
motor vehicle
in motion (on public highway) E818 ☑
not on public highway E825 ☑
nonmotor road vehicle, except animal-drawn
vehicle or pedal cycle E829 ☑
off-road type motor vehicle (not on public
highway) NEC E821 ☑
on public highway E818 ☑
pedal cycle E826 ☑
scaffolding (causing fall) E881.1
snow vehicle, motor-driven (not on public
highway) E820 ☑
on public highway E818 ☑
vehicle NEC — *see* Accident, vehicle
Broken
glass
fall on E888.0
injury by E920.8
power line (causing electric shock) E925.1
Bumping against, into (accidentally)
object (moving) E917.9
caused by crowd E917.1
with subsequent fall E917.6
furniture E917.3
with subsequent fall E917.7
in
running water E917.2
sports E917.0
with subsequent fall E917.5

☑ Additional Digit Required   ▶◀ Revised Text   ● New Line   ▲ Revised Code

Bumping against, into — *continued*
object — *continued*
stationary E917.4
with subsequent fall E917.8
person(s) E917.9
with fall E886.9
in sports E886.0
as, or caused by, a crowd E917.1
with subsequent fall E917.6
in sports E917.0
with fall E886.0

Burning, burns (accidental) (by) (from) (on) E899
acid (any kind) E924.1
swallowed — *see* Table of Drugs and
Chemicals
bedclothes (*see also* Fire, specified NEC)
E898.0
blowlamp (*see also* Fire, specified NEC) E898.1
blowtorch (*see also* Fire, specified NEC) E898.1
boat, ship, watercraft — *see* categories
E830 ☑, E831 ☑, E837 ☑
bonfire (controlled) E897
uncontrolled E892
candle (*see also* Fire, specified NEC) E898.1
caustic liquid, substance E924.1
swallowed — *see* Table of Drugs and
Chemicals
chemical E924.1
from swallowing caustic, corrosive
substance — *see* Table of Drugs and
Chemicals
in
terrorism E979.7
war operations E997.2
cigar(s) or cigarette(s) (*see also* Fire, specified
NEC) E898.1
clothes, clothing, nightdress — *see* Ignition,
clothes
with conflagration — *see* Conflagration
conflagration — *see* Conflagration
corrosive liquid, substance E924.1
swallowed — *see* Table of Drugs and
Chemicals
electric current (*see also* Electric shock) E925.9
fire, flames (*see also* Fire) E899
flare, Verey pistol E922.8
heat
from appliance (electrical) E924.8
in local application, or packing during
medical or surgical procedure E873.5
homicide (attempt) (*see also* Assault, burning)
E968.0
hot
liquid E924.0
caustic or corrosive E924.1
object (not producing fire or flames) E924.8
substance E924.9
caustic or corrosive E924.1
liquid (metal) NEC E924.0
specified type NEC E924.8
tap water E924.2
ignition — *see* Ignition
clothes, clothing, nightdress — *see also*
Ignition, clothes
with conflagration — *see* Conflagration
highly inflammable material (benzine) (fat)
(gasoline) (kerosene) (paraffin) (petrol)
E894
inflicted by other person
stated as
homicidal, intentional (*see also* Assault,
burning) E968.0
undetermined whether accidental or
intentional (*see also* Burn, stated
as undetermined whether
accidental or intentional) E988.1
internal, from swallowed caustic, corrosive
liquid, substance — *see* Table of Drugs
and Chemicals
in
terrorism E979.3
from nuclear explosion E979.5
petrol bomb E979.3

Burning, burns — *continued*
in — *continued*
war operations (from fire-producing device
or conventional weapon) E990.9
from nuclear explosion E996
petrol bomb E990.0
lamp (*see also* Fire, specified NEC) E898.1
late effect of NEC E929.4
lighter (cigar) (cigarette) (*see also* Fire, specified
NEC) E898.1
lightning E907
liquid (boiling) (hot) (molten) E924.0
caustic, corrosive (external) E924.1
swallowed — *see* Table of Drugs and
Chemicals
local application of externally applied
substance in medical or surgical care
E873.5
machinery — *see* Accident, machine
matches (*see also* Fire, specified NEC) E898.1
medicament, externally applied E873.5
metal, molten E924.0
object (hot) E924.8
producing fire or flames — *see* Fire
oven (electric) (gas) E924.8
pipe (smoking) (*see also* Fire, specified NEC)
E898.1
radiation — *see* Radiation
railway engine, locomotive, train (*see also*
Explosion, railway engine) E803 ☑
self-inflicted (unspecified whether accidental or
intentional) E988.1
caustic or corrosive substance NEC E988.7
stated as intentional, purposeful E958.1
caustic or corrosive substance NEC
E958.7
stated as undetermined whether accidental or
intentional E988.1
caustic or corrosive substance NEC E988.7
steam E924.0
pipe E924.8
substance (hot) E924.9
boiling or molten E924.0
caustic, corrosive (external) E924.1
swallowed — *see* Table of Drugs and
Chemicals
suicidal (attempt) NEC E958.1
caustic substance E958.7
late effect of E959
tanning bed E926.2
therapeutic misadventure
overdose of radiation E873.2
torch, welding (*see also* Fire, specified NEC)
E898.1
trash fire (*see also* Burning, bonfire) E897
vapor E924.0
vitriol E924.1
x-rays E926.3
in medical, surgical procedure — *see*
Misadventure, failure, in dosage,
radiation

Butted by animal E906.8

C

Cachexia, lead or saturnine E866.0
from pesticide NEC (*see also* Table of Drugs
and Chemicals) E863.4

Caisson disease E902.2

Capital punishment (any means) E978

Car sickness E903

Casualty (not due to war) NEC E928.9
terrorism E979.8
war (*see also* War operations) E995

Cat
bite E906.3
scratch E906.8

Cataclysmic (any injury)
earth surface movement or eruption E909.9
specified type NEC E909.8
storm or flood resulting from storm E908.9
specified type NEC E909.8

Catching fire — *see* Ignition

Caught
between
objects (moving) (stationary and moving)
E918
and machinery — *see* Accident, machine
by cable car, not on rails E847
in
machinery (moving parts of) — *see*,
Accident, machine
object E918

Cave-in (causing asphyxia, suffocation (by
pressure)) (*see also* Suffocation, due to,
cave-in) E913.3
with injury other than asphyxia or suffocation
E916
with asphyxia or suffocation (*see also*
Suffocation, due to, cave-in) E913.3
struck or crushed by E916
with asphyxia or suffocation (*see also*
Suffocation, due to, cave-in) E913.3

Change(s) in air pressure — *see also* Effects of,
air pressure
sudden, in aircraft (ascent) (descent) (causing
aeroneurosis or aviators' disease) E902.1

Chilblains E901.0
due to manmade conditions E901.1

Choking (on) (any object except food or vomitus)
E912
apple E911
bone E911
food, any type (regurgitated) E911
mucus or phlegm E912
seed E911

Civil insurrection — *see* War operations

Cloudburst E908.8

Cold, exposure to (accidental) (excessive)
(extreme) (place) E901.9
causing chilblains or immersion foot E901.0
due to
manmade conditions E901.1
specified cause NEC E901.8
weather (conditions) E901.0
late effect of NEC E929.5
self-inflicted (undetermined whether accidental
or intentional) E988.3
suicidal E958.3
suicide E958.3

Colic, lead, painter's, or saturnine — *see*
category E866 ☑

Collapse
building (moveable) E916
burning (uncontrolled fire) E891.8
in terrorism E979.3
private E890.8
dam E909.3
due to heat — *see* Heat
machinery — *see* Accident, machine
man-made structure E909.3
postoperative NEC E878.9
structure, burning NEC E891.8
burning (uncontrolled fire)
in terrorism E979.3

Collision (accidental)

> *Note — In the case of collisions between different types of vehicles, persons and objects, priority in classification is in the following order:*
>
> *Aircraft*
>
> *Watercraft*
>
> *Motor vehicle*
>
> *Railway vehicle*
>
> *Pedal cycle*
>
> *Animal-drawn vehicle*
>
> *Animal being ridden*
>
> *Streetcar or other nonmotor road vehicle*
>
> *Other vehicle*
>
> *Pedestrian or person using pedestrian conveyance*
>
> *Object (except where falling from or set in motion by vehicle etc. listed above)*
>
> *In the listing below, the combinations are listed only under the vehicle etc. having priority. For definitions See Supplementary Classification of External Causes of Injury and Poisoning (E800-E999).*

aircraft (with object or vehicle) (fixed) (movable) (moving) E841 ☑
  with
    person (while landing, taking off) (without accident to aircraft) E844 ☑
    powered (in transit) (with unpowered aircraft) E841 ☑
      while landing, taking off E840 ☑
    unpowered E842 ☑
      while landing, taking off E840 ☑
animal being ridden (in sport or transport) E828 ☑
  and
    animal (being ridden) (herded) (unattended) E828 ☑
    nonmotor road vehicle, except pedal cycle or animal-drawn vehicle E828 ☑
    object (fallen) (fixed) (movable) (moving) not falling from or set in motion by vehicle of higher priority E828 ☑
    pedestrian (conveyance or vehicle) E828 ☑
animal-drawn vehicle E827 ☑
  and
    animal (being ridden) (herded) (unattended) E827 ☑
    nonmotor road vehicle, except pedal cycle E827 ☑
    object (fallen) (fixed) (movable) (moving) not falling from or set in motion by vehicle of higher priority E827 ☑
    pedestrian (conveyance or vehicle) E827 ☑
    streetcar E827 ☑
motor vehicle (on public highway) (traffic accident) E812 ☑
  after leaving, running off, public highway (without antecedent collision) (without re-entry) E816 ☑
  with antecedent collision on public highway — *see* categories E810-E815 ☑
  with re-entrance collision with another motor vehicle E811 ☑
  and
    abutment (bridge) (overpass) E815 ☑
    animal (herded) (unattended) E815 ☑
    carrying person, property E813 ☑
    animal-drawn vehicle E813 ☑
    another motor vehicle (abandoned) (disabled) (parked) (stalled) (stopped) E812 ☑
      with, involving re-entrance (on same roadway) (across median strip) E811 ☑

Collision — *continued*
  motor vehicle — *continued*
    and — *continued*
      any object, person, or vehicle off the public highway resulting from a noncollision motor vehicle nontraffic accident E816 ☑
      avalanche, fallen or not moving E815 ☑
        falling E909.2
      boundary fence E815 ☑
      culvert E815 ☑
      fallen
        stone E815 ☑
        tree E815 ☑
      guard post or guard rail E815 ☑
      inter-highway divider E815 ☑
      landslide, fallen or not moving E815 ☑
        moving E909 ☑
      machinery (road) E815 ☑
      nonmotor road vehicle NEC E813 ☑
      object (any object, person, or vehicle off the public highway resulting from a noncollision motor vehicle nontraffic accident) E815 ☑
        off, normally not on, public highway resulting from a noncollision motor vehicle traffic accident E816 ☑
      pedal cycle E813 ☑
      pedestrian (conveyance) E814 ☑
      person (using pedestrian conveyance) E814 ☑
      post or pole (lamp) (light) (signal) (telephone) (utility) E815 ☑
      railway rolling stock, train, vehicle E810 ☑
      safety island E815 ☑
      street car E813 ☑
      traffic signal, sign, or marker (temporary) E815 ☑
      tree E815 ☑
      tricycle E813 ☑
      wall of cut made for road E815 ☑
    due to cataclysm — *see* categories E908 ☑, E909 ☑
    not on public highway, nontraffic accident E822 ☑
    and
      animal (carrying person, property) (herded) (unattended) E822 ☑
      animal-drawn vehicle E822 ☑
      another motor vehicle (moving), except off-road motor vehicle E822 ☑
        stationary E823 ☑
      avalanche, fallen, not moving E823 ☑
        moving E909.2
      landslide, fallen, not moving E823 ☑
        moving E909.2
      nonmotor vehicle (moving) E822 ☑
        stationary E823 ☑
      object (fallen) (normally) (fixed) (movable but not in motion) (stationary) E823 ☑
        moving, except when falling from, set in motion by, aircraft or cataclysm E822 ☑
      pedal cycle (moving) E822 ☑
        stationary E823 ☑
      pedestrian (conveyance) E822 ☑
      person (using pedestrian conveyance) E822 ☑
      railway rolling stock, train, vehicle (moving) E822 ☑
        stationary E823 ☑
      road vehicle (any) (moving) E822 ☑
        stationary E823 ☑
      tricycle (moving) E822 ☑
        stationary E823 ☑

Collision — *continued*
  off-road type motor vehicle (not on public highway) E821 ☑
  and
    animal (being ridden) (-drawn vehicle) E821 ☑
    another off-road motor vehicle, except snow vehicle E821 ☑
    other motor vehicle, not on public highway E821 ☑
    other object or vehicle NEC, fixed or movable, not set in motion by aircraft, motor vehicle on highway, or snow vehicle, motor driven E821 ☑
    pedal cycle E821 ☑
    pedestrian (conveyance) E821 ☑
    railway train E821 ☑
  on public highway — *see* Collision, motor vehicle
  pedal cycle E826 ☑
  and
    animal (carrying person, property) (herded) (unherded) E826 ☑
    animal-drawn vehicle E826 ☑
    another pedal cycle E826 ☑
    nonmotor road vehicle E826 ☑
    object (fallen) (fixed) (movable) (moving) not falling from or set in motion by aircraft, motor vehicle, or railway train NEC E826 ☑
    pedestrian (conveyance) E826 ☑
    person (using pedestrian conveyance) E826 ☑
    street car E826 ☑
  pedestrian(s) (conveyance) E917.9
  with fall E886.9
    in sports E886.0
  and
    crowd, human stampede E917.1
      with subsequent fall E917.6
    furniture E917.3
      with subsequent fall E917.7
    machinery — *see* Accident, machine
    object (fallen) (moving) not falling from NEC, fixed or set in motion by any vehicle classifiable to E800-E848 E917.9
      with subsequent fall E917.6
      caused by a crowd E917.1
        with subsequent fall E917.6
      furniture E917.3
        with subsequent fall E917.7
      in
        running water E917.2
          with drowning or submersion — *see* Submersion
        sports E917.0
          with subsequent fall E917.5
        stationary E917.4
          with subsequent fall E917.8
    vehicle, nonmotor, nonroad E848
    in
      running water E917.2
        with drowning or submersion — *see* Submersion
      sports E917.0
        with fall E886.0
  person(s) (using pedestrian conveyance) (*see also* Collision, pedestrian) E917.9
  railway (rolling stock) (train) (vehicle) (with (subsequent) derailment, explosion, fall or fire) E800 ☑
  with antecedent derailment E802 ☑
  and
    animal (carrying person) (herded) (unattended) E801 ☑
    another railway train or vehicle E800 ☑
    buffers E801 ☑
    fallen tree on railway E801 ☑
    farm machinery, nonmotor (in transport) (stationary) E801 ☑
    gates E801 ☑
    nonmotor vehicle E801 ☑

Collision — *continued*
  railway — *continued*
    and — *continued*
      object (fallen) (fixed) (movable) (moving)
        not falling from, set in motion by,
        aircraft or motor vehicle NEC
        E801 ☑
      pedal cycle E801 ☑
      pedestrian (conveyance) E805 ☑
      person (using pedestrian conveyance)
        E805 ☑
      platform E801 ☑
      rock on railway E801 ☑
      street car E801 ☑
  snow vehicle, motor-driven (not on public
    highway) E820 ☑
    and
      animal (being ridden) (-drawn vehicle)
        E820 ☑
      another off-road motor vehicle E820 ☑
      other motor vehicle, not on public
        highway E820 ☑
      other object or vehicle NEC, fixed or
        movable, not set in motion by
        aircraft or motor vehicle on highway
        E820 ☑
      pedal cycle E820 ☑
      pedestrian (conveyance) E820 ☑
      railway train E820 ☑
  on public highway — *see* Collision, motor
    vehicle
  street car(s) E829 ☑
  and
    animal, herded, not being ridden,
      unattended E829 ☑
    nonmotor road vehicle NEC E829 ☑
    object (fallen) (fixed) (movable) (moving)
      not falling from or set in motion by
      aircraft, animal-drawn vehicle,
      animal being ridden, motor vehicle,
      pedal cycle, or railway train
      E829 ☑
    pedestrian (conveyance) E829 ☑
    person (using pedestrian conveyance)
      E829 ☑
  vehicle
    animal-drawn — *see* Collision, animal-
      drawn vehicle
    motor — *see* Collision, motor vehicle
    nonmotor
      nonroad E848
      and
        another nonmotor, nonroad vehicle
          E848
        object (fallen) (fixed) (movable)
          (moving) not falling from or
          set in motion by aircraft,
          animal-drawn vehicle, animal
          being ridden, motor vehicle,
          nonmotor road vehicle, pedal
          cycle, railway train, or
          streetcar E848
      road, except animal being ridden, animal-
        drawn vehicle, or pedal cycle
        E829 ☑
      and
        animal, herded, not being ridden,
          unattended E829 ☑
        another nonmotor road vehicle,
          except animal being ridden,
          animal-drawn vehicle, or
          pedal cycle E829 ☑
        object (fallen) (fixed) (movable)
          (moving) not falling from or
          set in motion by, aircraft,
          animal-drawn vehicle, animal
          being ridden, motor vehicle,
          pedal cycle, or railway train
          E829 ☑
        pedestrian (conveyance) E829 ☑
        person (using pedestrian
          conveyance) E829 ☑
        vehicle, nonmotor, nonroad E829 ☑

Collision — *continued*
  watercraft E838 ☑
  and
    person swimming or water skiing E838 ☑
  causing
    drowning, submersion E830 ☑
    injury except drowning, submersion
      E831 ☑
Combustion, spontaneous — *see* Ignition
**Complication of medical or surgical procedure
  or treatment**
  as an abnormal reaction — *see* Reaction,
    abnormal
  delayed, without mention of misadventure —
    see Reaction, abnormal
  due to misadventure — *see* Misadventure
Compression
  divers' squeeze E902.2
  trachea by
    food E911
    foreign body, except food E912
Conflagration
  building or structure, except private dwelling
    (barn) (church) (convalescent or
    residential home) (factory) (farm
    outbuilding) (hospital) (hotel) (institution)
    (educational) (domitory) (residential)
    (school) (shop) (store) (theater) E891.9
    with or causing (injury due to)
      accident or injury NEC E891.9
        specified circumstance NEC E891.8
      burns, burning E891.3
      carbon monoxide E891.2
      fumes E891.2
        polyvinylchloride (PVC) or similar
          material E891.1
      smoke E891.2
      causing explosion E891.0
    in terrorism E979.3
  not in building or structure E892
  private dwelling (apartment) (boarding house)
    (camping place) (caravan) (farmhouse)
    (home (private)) (house) (lodging house)
    (private garage) (rooming house)
    (tenement) E890.9
    with or causing (injury due to)
      accident or injury NEC E890.9
        specified circumstance NEC E890.8
      burns, burning E890.3
      carbon monoxide E890.2
      fumes E890.2
        polyvinylchloride (PVC) or similar
          material E890.1
      smoke E890.2
      causing explosion E890.0
Constriction, external
  caused by
    hair E928.4
    other object E928.5
Contact with
  dry ice E901.1
  liquid air, hydrogen, nitrogen E901.1
Cramp(s)
  Heat — *see* Heat
  swimmers (*see also* category E910 ☑) E910.2
    not in recreation or sport E910.3
Cranking (car) (truck) (bus) (engine), injury by
  E917.9
Crash
  aircraft (in transit) (powered) E841 ☑
    at landing, take-off E840 ☑
    in
      terrorism E979.1
      war operations E994
    on runway NEC E840 ☑
    stated as
      homicidal E968.8
      suicidal E958.6
      undetermined whether accidental or
        intentional E988.6
    unpowered E842 ☑
  glider E842 ☑

Crash — *continued*
  motor vehicle — *see also* Accident, motor
    vehicle
    homicidal E968.5
    suicidal E958.5
    undetermined whether accidental or
      intentional E988.5
Crushed (accidentally) E928.9
  between
    boat(s), ship(s), watercraft (and dock or pier)
      (without accident to watercraft)
      E838 ☑
      after accident to, or collision, watercraft
        E831 ☑
    objects (moving) (stationary and moving)
      E918
  by
    avalanche NEC E909.2
    boat, ship, watercraft after accident to,
      collision, watercraft E831 ☑
    cave-in E916
      with asphyxiation or suffocation (*see also*
        Suffocation, due to, cave-in) E913.3
    crowd, human stampede E917.1
    falling
      aircraft (*see also* Accident, aircraft)
        E841 ☑
        in
          terrorism E979.1
          war operations E994
      earth, material E916
        with asphyxiation or suffocation (*see
          also* Suffocation, due to, cave-in)
          E913.3
      object E916
        on ship, watercraft E838 ☑
        while loading, unloading watercraft
          E838 ☑
    landslide NEC E909.2
    lifeboat after abandoning ship E831 ☑
    machinery — *see* Accident, machine
    railway rolling stock, train, vehicle (part of)
      E805 ☑
    street car E829 ☑
    vehicle NEC — *see* Accident, vehicle NEC
  in
    machinery — *see* Accident, machine
    object E918
    transport accident — *see* categories E800-
      E848 ☑
  late effect of NEC E929.9
Cut, cutting (any part of body) (accidental)
  E920.9
  by
    arrow E920.8
    axe E920.4
    bayonet (*see also* Bayonet wound) E920.3
    blender E920.2
    broken glass E920.8
      following fall E888.0
    can opener E920.4
      powered E920.2
    chisel E920.4
    circular saw E919.4
    cutting or piercing instrument — *see also*
      category E920 ☑
      following fall E888.0
      late effect of E929.8
    dagger E920.3
    dart E920.8
    drill — *see* Accident, caused by drill
    edge of stiff paper E920.8
    electric
      beater E920.2
      fan E920.2
      knife E920.2
      mixer E920.2
    fork E920.4
    garden fork E920.4
    hand saw or tool (not powered) E920.4
      powered E920.1
    hedge clipper E920.4
      powered E920.1
    hoe E920.4
    ice pick E920.4

Collision — Cut, cutting

☑ Additional Digit Required   ▶◀ Revised Text   ● New Line   ▲ Revised Code

Cut, cutting — *continued*
  by — *continued*
    knife E920.3
      electric E920.2
    lathe turnings E920.8
    lawn mower E920.4
      powered E920.0
      riding E919.8
    machine — *see* Accident, machine
    meat
      grinder E919.8
      slicer E919.8
    nails E920.8
    needle E920.4
      hypodermic E920.5
    object, edged, pointed, sharp — *see* category
      E920 ☑
      following fall E888.0
    paper cutter E920.4
    piercing instrument — *see also* category
      E920 ☑
      late effect of E929.8
    pitchfork E920.4
    powered
      can opener E920.2
      garden cultivator E920.1
        riding E919.8
      hand saw E920.1
      hand tool NEC E920.1
      hedge clipper E920.1
      household appliance or implement
        E920.2
      lawn mower (hand) E920.0
        riding E919.8
      rivet gun E920.1
      staple gun E920.1
    rake E920.4
    saw
      circular E919.4
      hand E920.4
    scissors E920.4
    screwdriver E920.4
    sewing machine (electric) (powered) E920.2
      not powered E920.4
    shears E920.4
    shovel E920.4
    spade E920.4
    splinters E920.8
    sword E920.3
    tin can lid E920.8
    wood slivers E920.8
  homicide (attempt) E966
  inflicted by other person
    stated as
      intentional, homicidal E966
      undetermined whether accidental or
        intentional E986
  late effect of NEC E929.8
  legal
    execution E978
    intervention E974
  self-inflicted (unspecified whether accidental or
    intentional) E986
    stated as intentional, purposeful E956
    stated as undetermined whether accidental or
      intentional E986
  suicidal (attempt) E956
  terrorism E979.8
  war operations E995
Cyclone E908.1

D

Death due to injury occurring one year or more previous — *see* Late effect
Decapitation (accidental circumstances) NEC
  E928.9
  homicidal E966
  legal execution (by guillotine) E978
Deprivation — *see also* Privation
  homicidal intent E968.4

Derailment (accidental)
  railway (rolling stock) (train) (vehicle) (with
    subsequent collision) E802 ☑
    with
      collision (antecedent) (*see also* Collision,
        railway) E800 ☑
      explosion (subsequent) (without
        antecedent collision) E802 ☑
      antecedent collision E803 ☑
      fall (without collision (antecedent))
        E802 ☑
      fire (without collision (antecedent))
        E802 ☑
    street car E829 ☑
Descent
  parachute (voluntary) (without accident to
    aircraft) E844 ☑
    due to accident to aircraft — *see* categories
      E840-E842 ☑
Desertion
  child, with intent to injure or kill E968.4
  helpless person, infant, newborn E904.0
    with intent to injure or kill E968.4
Destitution — *see* Privation
Disability, late effect or sequela of injury — *see*
  Late effect
Disease
  Andes E902.0
  aviators' E902.1
  caisson E902.2
  range E902.0
Divers' disease, palsy, paralysis, squeeze
  E902.0
Dog bite E906.0
Dragged by
  cable car (not on rails) E847
    on rails E829 ☑
  motor vehicle (on highway) E814 ☑
    not on highway, nontraffic accident E825 ☑
  street car E829 ☑
Drinking poison (accidental) — *see* Table of
  Drugs and Chemicals
Drowning — *see* Submersion
Dust in eye E914

E

Earth falling (on) (with asphyxia or suffocation
  (by pressure)) (*see also* Suffocation, due to,
  cave-in) E913.3
  as, or due to, a cataclysm (involving any
    transport vehicle) — *see* categories
    E908 ☑, E909 ☑
  not due to cataclysmic action E913.3
    motor vehicle (in motion) (on public
      highway) E810 ☑
      not on public highway E825 ☑
    nonmotor road vehicle NEC E829 ☑
    pedal cycle E826 ☑
    railway rolling stock, train, vehicle E806 ☑
    street car E829 ☑
    struck or crushed by E916
      with asphyxiation or suffocation E913.3
      with injury other than asphyxia,
        suffocation E916
Earthquake (any injury) E909.0
Effect(s) (adverse) of
  air pressure E902.9
    at high altitude E902.9
      in aircraft E902.1
      residence or prolonged visit (causing
        conditions classifiable to E902.0)
        E902.0
    due to
      diving E902.2
      specified cause NEC E902.8
    in aircraft E902.1
  cold, excessive (exposure to) (*see also* Cold,
    exposure to) E901.9
  heat (excessive) (*see also* Heat) E900.9
  hot
    place — *see* Heat
    weather E900.0
  insulation — *see* Heat

Effect(s) (adverse) of — *continued*
  late — *see* Late effect of
  motion E903
  nuclear explosion or weapon
    in
      terrorism E979.5
      war operations (blast) (fireball) (heat)
        (radiation) (direct) (secondary) E996
  radiation — *see* Radiation
  terrorism, secondary E979.9
  travel E903
Electric shock, electrocution (accidental) (from
  exposed wire, faulty appliance, high voltage
  cable, live rail, open socket) (by) (in) E925.9
  appliance or wiring
    domestic E925.0
    factory E925.2
    farm (building) E925.8
      house E925.0
    home E925.0
    industrial (conductor) (control apparatus)
      (transformer) E925.2
    outdoors E925.8
    public building E925.8
    residential institution E925.8
    school E925.8
    specified place NEC E925.8
  caused by other person
    stated as
      intentional, homicidal E968.8
      undetermined whether accidental or
        intentional E988.4
  electric power generating plant, distribution
    station E925.1
  homicidal (attempt) E968.8
  legal execution E978
  lightning E907
  machinery E925.9
    domestic E925.0
    factory E925.2
    farm E925.8
    home E925.0
  misadventure in medical or surgical procedure
    in electroshock therapy E873.4
  self-inflicted (undetermined whether accidental
    or intentional) E988.4
    stated as intentional E958.4
  stated as undetermined whether accidental or
    intentional E988.4
  suicidal (attempt) E958.4
  transmission line E925.1
Electrocution — *see* Electric shock
Embolism
  air (traumatic) NEC — *see* Air, embolism
Encephalitis
  lead or saturnine E866.0
    from pesticide NEC E863.4
Entanglement
  in
    bedclothes, causing suffocation E913.0
    wheel of pedal cycle E826 ☑
Entry of foreign body, material, any — *see*
  Foreign body
Execution, legal (any method) E978
Exhaustion
  cold — *see* Cold, exposure to
  due to excessive exertion E927
  heat — *see* Heat
Explosion (accidental) (in) (of) (on) E923.9
  acetylene E923.2
  aerosol can E921.8
  aircraft (in transit) (powered) E841 ☑
    at landing, take-off E840 ☑
    in
      terrorism E979.1
      war operations E994
    unpowered E842 ☑
  air tank (compressed) (in machinery) E921.1
  anesthetic gas in operating theatre E923.2
  automobile tire NEC E921.8
    causing transport accident — *see* categories
      E810-E825 ☑
  blasting (cap) (materials) E923.1
  boiler (machinery), not on transport vehicle
    E921.0
    steamship — *see* Explosion, watercraft

Explosion — *continued*
  bomb E923.8
    in
      terrorism E979.2
      war operations E993
        after cessation of hostilities E998
        atom, hydrogen or nuclear E996
        injury by fragments from E991.9
          antipersonnel bomb E991.3
  butane E923.2
  caused by
    other person
      stated as
        intentional, homicidal — *see* Assault,
          explosive
        undetermined whether accidental or
          homicidal E985.5
  coal gas E923.2
  detonator E923.1
  dyamite E923.1
  explosive (material) NEC E923.9
    gas(es) E923.2
    missile E923.8
      in
        terrorism E979.2
        war operations E993
          injury by fragments from E991.9
            antipersonnel bomb E991.3
    used in blasting operations E923.1
  fire-damp E923.2
  fireworks E923.0
  gas E923.2
    cylinder (in machinery) E921.1
    pressure tank (in machinery) E921.1
  gasoline (fumes) (tank) not in moving motor
    vehicle E923.2
  grain store (military) (munitions) E923.8
  grenade E923.8
    in
      terrorism E979.2
      war operations E993
        injury by fragments from E991.9
  homicide (attempt) — *see* Assault, explosive
  hot water heater, tank (in machinery) E921.0
  in mine (of explosive gases) NEC E923.2
  late effect of NEC E929.8
  machinery — *see also* Accident, machine
    pressure vessel — *see* Explosion, pressure
      vessel
  methane E923.2
  missile E923.8
    in
      terrorism E979.2
      war operations E993
        injury by fragments from E991.9
  motor vehicle (part of)
    in motion (on public highway) E818 ☑
    not on public highway E825 ☑
  munitions (dump) (factory) E923.8
    in
      terrorism E979.2
      war operations E993
  of mine E923.8
    in
      terrorism
        at sea or in harbor E979.0
        land E979.2
        marine E979.0
      war operations
        after cessation of hostilities E998
        at sea or in harbor E992
        land E993
          after cessation of hostilities E998
          injury by fragments from E991.9
        marine E992
  own weapons
    in
      terrorism (*see also* Suicide) E979.2
      war operations E993
        injury by fragments from E991.9
          antipersonnel bomb E991.3
      injury by fragments from E991.9
        antipersonnel bomb E991.3
  pressure
    cooker E921.8
    gas tank (in machinery) E921.1

Explosion — *continued*
  pressure — *continued*
    vessel (in machinery) E921.9
      on transport vehicle — *see* categories
        E800-E848 ☑
      specified type NEC E921.8
  propane E923.2
  railway engine, locomotive, train (boiler) (with
    subsequent collision, derailment, fall)
    E803 ☑
    with
      collision (antecedent) (*see also* Collision,
        railway) E800 ☑
      derailment (antecedent) E802 ☑
      fire (without antecedent collision or
        derailment) E803 ☑
  secondary fire resulting from — *see* Fire
  self-inflicted (unspecified whether accidental or
    intentional) E985.5
    stated as intentional, purposeful E955.5
  shell (artillery) E923.8
    in
      terrorism E979.2
      war operations E993
        injury by fragments from E991.9
  stated as undetermined whether caused
    accidentally or purposely inflicted E985.5
  steam or water lines (in machinery) E921.0
  suicide (attempted) E955.5
  terrorism — *see* Terrorism, explosion
  torpedo E923.8
    in
      terrorism E979.0
      war operations E992
  transport accident — *see* categories E800-
    E848 ☑
  war operations — *see* War operations,
    explosion
  watercraft (boiler) E837 ☑
    causing drowning, submersion (after
      jumping from watercraft) E830 ☑
Exposure (weather) (conditions) (rain) (wind)
  E904.3
  with homicidal intent E968.4
  excessive E904.3
    cold (*see also* Cold, exposure to) E901.9
      self-inflicted — *see* Cold, exposure to,
        self-inflicted
    heat (*see also* Heat) E900.9
  fire — *see* Fire
  helpless person, infant, newborn due to
    abandonment or neglect E904.0
  noise E928.1
  prolonged in deep-freeze unit or refrigerator
    E901.1
  radiation — *see* Radiation
  resulting from transport accident — *see*
    categories E800-E848 ☑
  smoke from, due to
    fire — *see* Fire
    tobacco, second-hand E869.4
  vibration E928.2

F

Fall, falling (accidental) E888.9
  building E916
    burning E891.8
      private E890.8
  down
    escalator E880.0
    ladder E881.0
      in boat, ship, watercraft E833 ☑
    staircase E880.9
    stairs, steps — *see* Fall, from, stairs
  earth (with asphyxia or suffocation (by
    pressure)) (*see also* Earth, falling) E913.3
  from, off
    aircraft (at landing, take-off) (in-transit)
      (while alighting, boarding) E843 ☑
      resulting from accident to aircraft — *see*
        categories E840-E842 ☑
    animal (in sport or transport) E828 ☑
    animal-drawn vehicle E827 ☑
    balcony E882
    bed E884.4
    bicycle E826 ☑

Fall, falling — *continued*
  from, off — *continued*
    boat, ship, watercraft (into water) E832 ☑
      after accident to, collision, fire on
        E830 ☑
        and subsequently struck by (part of)
          boat E831 ☑
      and subsequently struck by (part of) boat
        E831 ☑
      burning, crushed, sinking E830 ☑
        and subsequently struck by (part of)
          boat E831 ☑
    bridge E882
    building E882
      burning (uncontrolled fire) E891.8
        in terrorism E979.3
      private E890.8
    bunk in boat, ship, watercraft E834 ☑
      due to accident to watercraft E831 ☑
    cable car (not on rails) E847
      on rails E829 ☑
    car — *see* Fall from motor vehicle
    chair E884.2
    cliff E884.1
    commode E884.6
    curb (sidewalk) E880.1
    elevation aboard ship E834 ☑
      due to accident to ship E831 ☑
    embankment E884.9
    escalator E880.0
    fire escape E882
    flagpole E882
    furniture NEC E884.5
    gangplank (into water) (*see also* Fall, from,
      boat) E832 ☑
      to deck, dock E834 ☑
    hammock on ship E834 ☑
      due to accident to watercraft E831 ☑
    haystack E884.9
    high place NEC E884.9
      stated as undetermined whether
        accidental or intentional — *see*
        Jumping, from, high place
    horse (in sport or transport) E828 ☑
    in-line skates E885.1
    ladder E881.0
      in boat, ship, watercraft E833 ☑
        due to accident to watercraft E831 ☑
    machinery — *see also* Accident, machine
      not in operation E884.9
    motor vehicle (in motion) (on public
      highway) E818 ☑
      not on public highway E825 ☑
        stationary, except while alighting,
          boarding, entering, leaving
          E884.9
        while alighting, boarding, entering,
          leaving E824 ☑
      stationary, except while alighting,
        boarding, entering, leaving E884.9
      while alighting, boarding, entering,
        leaving, except off-road type motor
        vehicle E817 ☑
        off-road type — *see* Fall, from, off-road
          type motor vehicle
    nonmotor road vehicle (while alighting,
      boarding) NEC E829 ☑
      stationary, except while alighting,
        boarding, entering, leaving E884.9
    off road type motor vehicle (not on public
      highway) NEC E821 ☑
      on public highway E818 ☑
        while alighting, boarding, entering,
          leaving E817 ☑
    snow vehicle — *see* Fall from snow
      vehicle, motor-driven
    one
      deck to another on ship E834 ☑
        due to accident to ship E831 ☑
      level to another NEC E884.9
        boat, ship, or watercraft E834 ☑
          due to accident to watercraft
            E831 ☑
    pedal cycle E826 ☑
    playground equipment E884.0

(side margin: Explosion — Fall, falling)

Fall, falling — *continued*
  from, off — *continued*
    railway rolling stock, train, vehicle, (while alighting, boarding) E804 ☑
      with
        collision (*see also* Collision, railway) E800 ☑
        derailment (*see also* Derailment, railway) E802 ☑
        explosion (*see also* Explosion, railway engine) E803 ☑
    rigging (aboard ship) E834 ☑
      due to accident to watercraft E831 ☑
    roller skates E885.1
    scaffolding E881.1
    scooter (nonmotorized) E885.0
    sidewalk (curb) E880.1
      moving E885.9
    skateboard E885.2
    skis E885.3
    snow vehicle, motor-driven (not on public highway) E820 ☑
      on public highway E818 ☑
        while alighting, boarding, entering, leaving E817 ☑
    snowboard E885.4
    stairs, step E880.9
      boat, ship, watercraft E833 ☑
        due to accident to watercraft E831 ☑
      motor bus, motor vehicle — *see* Fall, from, motor vehicle, while alighting, boarding
      street car E829 ☑
    stationary vehicle NEC E884.9
    stepladder E881.0
    street car (while boarding, alighting) E829
      stationary, except while boarding or alighting E884.9
    structure NEC E882
      burning (uncontrolled fire) E891.8
        in terrorism E979.3
    table E884.9
    toilet E884.6
    tower E882
    tree E884.9
    turret E882
    vehicle NEC — *see also* Accident, vehicle NEC
      stationary E884.9
    viaduct E882
    wall E882
    wheelchair E884.3
    window E882
  in, on
    aircraft (at landing, take-off) (in-transit) E843 ☑
      resulting from accident to aircraft — *see* categories E840-E842 ☑
    boat, ship, watercraft E835 ☑
      due to accident to watercraft E831 ☑
      one level to another NEC E834 ☑
      on ladder, stairs E833 ☑
    cutting or piercing instrument or machine E888.0
    deck (of boat, ship, watercraft) E835 ☑
      due to accident to watercraft E831 ☑
    escalator E880.0
    gangplank E835 ☑
    glass, broken E888.0
    knife E888.0
    ladder E881.0
      in boat, ship, watercraft E833 ☑
        due to accident to watercraft E831 ☑
    object
      edged, pointed or sharp E888.0
      other E888.1
    pitchfork E888.0
    railway rolling stock, train, vehicle (while alighting, boarding) E804 ☑
      with
        collision (*see also* Collision, railway) E800 ☑
        derailment (*see also* Derailment, railway) E802 ☑
        explosion (see also Explosion, railway engine) E803 ☑

Fall, falling — *continued*
  in, on — *continued*
    scaffolding E881.1
    scissors E888.0
    staircase, stairs, steps (*see also* Fall, from, stairs) E880.9
    street car E829 ☑
    water transport (*see also* Fall, in, boat) E835 ☑
  into
    cavity E883.9
    dock E883.9
      from boat, ship, watercraft (*see also* Fall, from, boat) E832 ☑
    hold (of ship) E834 ☑
      due to accident to watercraft E831 ☑
    hole E883.9
    manhole E883.2
    moving part of machinery — *see* Accident, machine
    opening in surface NEC E883.9
    pit E883.9
    quarry E883.9
    shaft E883.9
    storm drain E883.2
    tank E883.9
    water (with drowning or submersion) E910.9
    well E883.1
  late effect of NEC E929.3
  object (*see also* Hit by, object, falling) E916
  other E888.8
  over
    animal E885.9
    cliff E884.1
    embankment E884.9
    small object E885 ☑
  overboard (*see also* Fall, from, boat) E832 ☑
  resulting in striking against object E888.1
    sharp E888.0
  rock E916
  same level NEC E888.9
    aircraft (any kind) E843 ☑
      resulting from accident to aircraft — *see* categories E840-E842 ☑
    boat, ship, watercraft E835 ☑
      due to accident to, collision, watercraft E831 ☑
    from
      collision, pushing, shoving, by or with other person(s) E886.9
        as, or caused by, a crowd E917.6
        in sports E886.0
      scooter (nonmotorized) E885.0
      slipping stumbling, tripping E885 ☑
  snowslide E916
    as avalanche E909.2
  stone E916
  through
    hatch (on ship) E834 ☑
      due to accident to watercraft E831 ☑
    roof E882
    window E882
  timber E916
  while alighting from, boarding, entering, leaving
    aircraft (any kind) E843 ☑
    motor bus, motor vehicle — *see* Fall, from, motor vehicle, while alighting, boarding
    nonmotor road vehicle NEC E829 ☑
    railway train E804 ☑
    street car E829 ☑

Fallen on by
  animal (horse) (not being ridden) E906.8
    being ridden (in sport or transport) E828 ☑

Fell or jumped from high place, so stated — *see* Jumping, from, high place

Felo-de-se (*see also* Suicide) E958.9

Fever
  heat — *see* Heat
  thermic — *see* Heat

Fight (hand) (fist) (foot) (*see also* Assault, fight) E960.0

Fire (accidental) (caused by great heat from appliance (electrical), hot object or hot substance) (secondary, resulting from explosion) E899

Fire — *continued*
  conflagration — *see* Conflagration
  controlled, normal (in brazier, fireplace, furnace, or stove) (charcoal) (coal) (coke) (electric) (gas) (wood)
    bonfire E897
    brazier, not in building or structure E897
    in building or structure, except private dwelling (barn) (church) (convalescent or residential home) (factory) (farm outbuilding) (hospital) (hotel) (institution (educational) (dormitory) (residential)) (private garage) (school) (shop) (store) (theatre) E896
    in private dwelling (apartment) (boarding house) (camping place) (caravan) (farmhouse) (home (private)) (house) (lodging house) (rooming house) (tenement) E895
    not in building or structure E897
    trash E897
  forest (uncontrolled) E892
  grass (uncontrolled) E892
  hay (uncontrolled) E892
  homicide (attempt) E968.0
    late effect of E969
  in, of, on, starting in E892
    aircraft (in transit) (powered) E841 ☑
      at landing, take-off E840 ☑
      stationary E892
      unpowered (balloon) (glider) E842 ☑
    balloon E842 ☑
    boat, ship, watercraft — *see* categories E830 ☑, E831 ☑, E837 ☑
    building or structure, except private dwelling (barn) (church) (convalescent or residential home) (factory) (farm outbuilding) (hospital) (hotel) (institution (educational) (dormitory) (residential)) (school) (shop) (store) (theatre) (*see also* Conflagration, building or structure, except private dwelling) E891.9
    forest (uncontrolled) E892
    glider E842 ☑
    grass (uncontrolled) E892
    hay (uncontrolled) E892
    lumber (uncontrolled) E892
    machinery — *see* Accident, machine
    mine (uncontrolled) E892
    motor vehicle (in motion) (on public highway) E818 ☑
      not on public highway E825 ☑
      stationary E892
    prairie (uncontrolled) E892
    private dwelling (apartment) (boarding house) (camping place) (caravan) (farmhouse) (home (private)) (house) (lodging house) (private garage) (rooming house) (tenement) (*see also* Conflagration, private dwelling) E890.9
    railway rolling stock, train, vehicle (*see also* Explosion, railway engine) E803 ☑
      stationary E892
    room NEC E898.1
    street car (in motion) E829 ☑
      stationary E892
    terrorism (by fire-producing device) E979.3
      fittings or furniture (burning building) (uncontrolled fire) E979.3
      from nuclear explosion E979.5
    transport vehicle, stationary NEC E892
    tunnel (uncontrolled) E892
    war operations (by fire-producing device or conventional weapon) E990.9
      from nuclear explosion E996
      petrol bomb E990.0
  late effect of NEC E929.4
  lumber (uncontrolled) E892
  mine (uncontrolled) E892
  prairie (uncontrolled) E892
  self-inflicted (unspecified whether accidental or intentional) E988.1
    stated as intentional, purposeful E958.1
  specified NEC E898.1
    with
      conflagration — *see* Conflagration

☑ Additional Digit Required   ▶◀ Revised Text   ● New Line   ▲ Revised Code

Fire — *Hit, hitting*

Fire — *continued*
  specified — *continued*
    with — *continued*
      ignition (of)
        clothing — *see* Ignition, clothes
        highly inflammable material (benzine)
          (fat) (gasoline) (kerosene)
          (paraffin) (petrol) E894
    started by other person
      stated as
        with intent to injure or kill E968.0
        undetermined whether or not with intent
          to injure or kill E988.1
    suicide (attempted) E958.1
      late effect of E959
    tunnel (uncontrolled) E892
Fireball effects from nuclear explosion
  in
    terrorism E979.5
    war operations E996
Fireworks (explosion) E923.0
Flash burns from explosion (*see also* Explosion)
  E923.9
Flood (any injury) (resulting from storm) E908.2
  caused by collapse of dam or manmade
    structure E909.3
Forced landing (aircraft) E840 ☑
Foreign body, object or material (entrance into
  (accidental)
  air passage (causing injury) E915
    with asphyxia, obstruction, suffocation E912
      food or vomitus E911
    nose (with asphyxia, obstruction,
      suffocation) E912
      causing injury without asphyxia,
        obstruction, suffocation E915
  alimentary canal (causing injury) (with
    obstruction) E915
    with asphyxia, obstruction respiratory
      passage, suffocation E912
      food E911
    mouth E915
      with asphyxia, obstruction, suffocation
        E912
      food E911
    pharynx E915
      with asphyxia, obstruction, suffocation
        E912
      food E911
  aspiration (with asphyxia, obstruction
    respiratory passage, suffocation) E912
    causing injury without asphyxia, obstruction
      respiratory passage, suffocation E915
    food (regurgitated) (vomited) E911
      causing injury without asphyxia,
        obstruction respiratory passage,
        suffocation E915
    mucus (not of newborn) E912
    phlegm E912
  bladder (causing injury or obstruction) E915
  bronchus, bronchi — *see* Foreign body, air
    passages
  conjunctival sac E914
  digestive system — *see* Foreign body,
    alimentary canal
  ear (causing injury or obstruction) E915
  esophagus (causing injury or obstruction) (*see
    also* Foreign body, alimentary canal)
    E915
  eye (any part) E914
  eyelid E914
  hairball (stomach) (with obstruction) E915
  ingestion — *see* Foreign body, alimentary canal
  inhalation — *see* Foreign body, aspiration
  intestine (causing injury or obstruction) E915
  iris E914
  lacrimal apparatus E914
  larynx — *see* Foreign body, air passage
  late effect of NEC E929.8
  lung — *see* Foreign body, air passage
  mouth — *see* Foreign body, alimentary canal,
    mouth
  nasal passage — *see* Foreign body, air passage,
    nose
  nose — *see* Foreign body, air passage, nose
  ocular muscle E914

Foreign body, object or material — *continued*
  operation wound (left in) — *see* Misadventure,
    foreign object
  orbit E914
  pharynx — *see* Foreign body, alimentary canal,
    pharynx
  rectum (causing injury or obstruction) E915
  stomach (hairball) (causing injury or
    obstruction) E915
  tear ducts or glands E914
  trachea — *see* Foreign body, air passage
  urethra (causing injury or obstruction) E915
  vagina (causing injury or obstruction) E915
Found dead, injured
  from exposure (to) — *see* Exposure
  on
    public highway E819 ☑
    railway right of way E807 ☑
Fracture (circumstances unknown or unspecified)
  E887
  due to specified external means — *see* manner
    of accident
  late effect of NEC E929.3
  occuring in water transport NEC E835 ☑
Freezing — *see* Cold, exposure to
Frostbite E901.0
  due to manmade conditions E901.1
Frozen — *see* Cold, exposure to

G

Garrotting, homicidal (attempted) E963
Gored E906.8
Gunshot wound (*see also* Shooting) E922.9

H

Hailstones, injury by E904.3
Hairball (stomach) (with obstruction) E915
Hanged himself (*see also* Hanging, self-inflicted)
  E983.0
Hang gliding E842 ☑
Hanging (accidental) E913.8
  caused by other person
    in accidental circumstances E913.8
    stated as
      intentional, homicidal E963
      undetermined whether accidental or
        intentional E983.0
  homicide (attempt) E963
  in bed or cradle E913.0
  legal execution E978
  self-inflicted (unspecified whether accidental or
    intentional) E983.0
    in accidental circumstances E913.8
    stated as intentional, purposeful E953.0
  stated as undetermined whether accidental or
    intentional E983.0
  suicidal (attempt) E953.0
Heat (apoplexy) (collapse) (cramps) (effects of)
  (excessive) (exhaustion) (fever) (prostration)
  (stroke) E900.9
  due to
    manmade conditions (as listed in E900.1,
      except boat, ship, watercraft) E900.1
    weather (conditions) E900.0
  from
    electric heating appartus causing burning
      E924.8
    nuclear explosion
      in
        terrorism E979.5
        war operations E996
  generated in, boiler, engine, evaporator, fire
    room of boat, ship, watercraft E838 ☑
  inappropriate in local application or packing in
    medical or surgical procedure E873.5
  late effect of NEC E989
Hemorrhage
  delayed following medical or surgical treatment
    without mention of misadventure — *see*
    Reaction, abnormal
  during medical or surgical treatment as
    misadventure — *see* Misadventure, cut

High
  altitude, effects E902.9
  level of radioactivity, effects — *see* Radiation
  pressure effects — *see also* Effects of, air
    pressure
    from rapid descent in water (causing caisson
      or divers' disease, palsy, or paralysis)
      E902.2
  temperature, effects — *see* Heat
Hit, hitting (accidental) by
  aircraft (propeller) (without accident to aircraft)
    E844 ☑
    unpowered E842 ☑
  avalanche E909.2
  being thrown against object in or part of
    motor vehicle (in motion) (on public
      highway) E818 ☑
      not on public highway E825 ☑
    nonmotor road vehicle NEC E829 ☑
    street car E829 ☑
  boat, ship, watercraft
    after fall from watercraft E838 ☑
      damaged, involved in accident E831 ☑
    while swimming, water skiing E838 ☑
  bullet (*see also* Shooting) E922.9
    from air gun E922.4
    in
      terrorism E979.4
      war operations E991.2
        rubber E991.0
  flare, Verey pistol (*see also* Shooting) E922.8
  hailstones E904.3
  landslide E909.2
  law-enforcing agent (on duty) E975
    with blunt object (baton) (night stick) (stave)
      (truncheon) E973
  machine — *see* Accident, machine
  missile
    firearm (*see also* Shooting) E922.9
    in
      terrorism — *see* Terrorism, mission
      war operations — *see* War operations,
        missile
  motor vehicle (on public highway) (traffic
    accident) E814 ☑
    not on public highway, nontraffic accident
      E822 ☑
  nonmotor road vehicle NEC E829 ☑
  object
    falling E916
      from, in, on
        aircraft E844 ☑
          due to accident to aircraft — *see*
            categories E840-E842 ☑
          unpowered E842 ☑
        boat, ship, watercraft E838 ☑
          due to accident to watercraft
          E831 ☑
        building E916
          burning (uncontrolled fire) E891.8
            in terrorism E979.3
            private E890.8
        cataclysmic
          earth surface movement or eruption
            E909.9
          storm E908.9
        cave-in E916
          with asphyxiation or suffocation
            (*see also* Suffocation, due to,
            cave-in) E913.3
        earthquake E909.0
        motor vehicle (in motion) (on public
          highway) E818 ☑
          not on public highway E825 ☑
          stationary E916
        nonmotor road vehicle NEC E829 ☑
        pedal cycle E826 ☑
        railway rolling stock, train, vehicle
          E806 ☑
        street car E829 ☑
        structure, burning NEC E891.8
        vehicle, stationary E916
    moving NEC — *see* Striking against, object
    projected NEC — *see* Striking against, object

Hit, hitting by — *continued*
  object — *continued*
    set in motion by
      compressed air or gas, spring, striking,
        throwing — *see* Striking against,
        object
      explosion — *see* Explosion
    thrown into, on, or towards
      motor vehicle (in motion) (on public
        highway) E818 ☑
        not on public highway E825 ☑
      nonmotor road vehicle NEC E829 ☑
      pedal cycle E826 ☑
      strect car E829 ☑
    off-road type motor vehicle (not on public
      highway) E821 ☑
      on public highway E814 ☑
    other person(s) E917.9
      with blunt or thrown object E917.9
        in sports E917.0
          with subsequent fall E917.5
      intentionally, homicidal E968.2
      as, or caused by, a crowd E917.1
        with subsequent fall E917.6
          in sports E917.0
    pedal cycle E826 ☑
    police (on duty) E975
      with blunt object (baton) (nightstick) (stave)
        (truncheon) E973
    railway, rolling stock, train, vehicle (part of)
      E805 ☑
    shot — *see* Shooting
    snow vehicle, motor-driven (not on public
      highway) E820 ☑
      on public highway E814 ☑
    street car E829 ☑
    vehicle NEC — *see* Accident, vehicle NEC
Homicide, homicidal (attempt) (justifiable) (*see
    also* Assault) E968.9
Hot
  liquid, object, substance, accident caused by —
    see also Accident, caused by, hot, by type
    of substance
    late effect of E929.8
  place, effects — *see* Heat
  weather, effects E900.0
Humidity, causing problem E904.3
Hunger E904.1
  resulting from
    abandonment or neglect E904.0
    transport accident — *see* categories E800-
      E848 ☑
Hurricane (any injury) E908.0
Hypobarism, hypobaropathy — *see* Effects of, air
  pressure
Hypothermia — *see* Cold, exposure to

I

Ictus
  caloris — *see* Heat
  solaris E900.0
Ignition (accidental)
  anesthetic gas in operating theatre E923.2
  bedclothes
    with
      conflagration — *see* Conflagration
      ignition (of)
        clothing — *see* Ignition, clothes
        highly inflammable material (benzine)
          (fat) (gasoline) (kerosene)
          (paraffin) (petrol) E894
  benzine E894
  clothes, clothing (from controlled fire) (in
    building) E893.9
    with conflagration — *see* Conflagration
    from
      bonfire E893.2
      highly inflammable material E894
      sources or material as listed in E893.8
      trash fire E893.2
      uncontrolled fire — *see* Conflagration

Ignition — *continued*
  clothes, clothing — *continued*
    in
      private dwelling E893.0
      specified building or structure, except
        private dwelling E893.1
    not in building or structure E893.2
  explosive material — *see* Explosion
  fat E894
  gasoline E894
  kerosene E894
  material
    explosive — *see* Explosion
    highly inflammable E894
      with conflagration — *see* Conflagration
      with explosion E923.2
  nightdress — *see* Ignition, clothes
  paraffin E894
  petrol E894
Immersion — *see* Submersion
Implantation of quills of porcupine E906.8
Inanition (from) E904.9
  hunger — *see* Lack of, food
  resulting from homicidal intent E968.4
  thirst — *see* Lack of, water
Inattention after, at birth E904.0
  homicidal, infanticidal intent E968.4
Infanticide (*see also* Assault)
Ingestion
  foreign body (causing injury) (with obstruction)
    — *see* Foreign body, alimentary canal
  poisonous substance NEC — *see* Table of
    Drugs and Chemicals
Inhalation
  excessively cold substance, manmade E901.1
  foreign body — *see* Foreign body, aspiration
  liquid air, hydrogen, nitrogen E901.1
  mucus, not of newborn (with asphyxia,
    obstruction respiratory passage,
    suffocation) E912
  phlegm (with asphyxia, obstruction respiratory
    passage, suffocation) E912
  poisonous gas — *see* Table of Drugs and
    Chemicals
  smoke from, due to
    fire — *see* Fire
    tobacco, second-hand E869.4
  vomitus (with asphyxia, obstruction respiratory
    passage, suffocation) E911
Injury, injured (accidental(ly)) NEC E928.9
  by, caused by, from
    air rifle (BB gun) E922.4
    animal (not being ridden) NEC E906.9
      being ridden (in sport or transport)
        E828 ☑
    assault (*see also* Assault) E968.9
    avalanche E909.2
    bayonet (*see also* Bayonet wound) E920.3
    being thrown against some part of, or object
      in
        motor vehicle (in motion) (on public
          highway) E818 ☑
          not on public highway E825 ☑
        nonmotor road vehicle NEC E829 ☑
        off-road motor vehicle NEC E821 ☑
        railway train E806 ☑
        snow vehicle, motor-driven E820 ☑
        street car E829 ☑
    bending E927
    broken glass E920.8
    bullet — *see* Shooting
    cave-in (*see also* Suffocation, due to, cave-
      in) E913.3
      earth surface movement or eruption
        E909.9
    earthquake E909.0
    flood E908.2
    hurricane E908.0
    landslide E909.2
    storm E908.9
      without asphyxiation or suffocation E916
    cloudburst E908.8
    cutting or piercing instrument (*see also* Cut)
      E920.9
    cyclone E908.1
    earth surface movement or eruption E909.9

Injury, injured NEC — *continued*
  by, caused by, from — *continued*
    earthquake E909 ☑
    electric current (*see also* Electric shock)
      E925.9
    explosion (*see also* Explosion) E923.9
    fire — *see* Fire
    flare, Verey pistol E922.8
    flood E908 ☑
    foreign body — *see* Foreign body
    hailstones E904.3
    hurricane E908 ☑
    landslide E909 ☑
    law-enforcing agent, police, in course of legal
      intervention — *see* Legal intervention
    lightning E907
    live rail or live wire — *see* Electric shock
    machinery — *see also* Accident, machine
      aircraft, without accident to aircraft
        E844 ☑
      boat, ship, watercraft (deck) (engine
        room) (galley) (laundry) (loading)
        E836 ☑
    missile
      explosive E923.8
      firearm — *see* Shooting
      in
        terrorism — *see* Terrorism, missile
        war operations — *see* War operations,
          missile
    moving part of motor vehicle (in motion) (on
      public highway) E818 ☑
      not on public highway, nontraffic
        accident E825 ☑
      while alighting, boarding, entering,
        leaving — *see* Fall, from, motor
        vehicle, while alighting, boarding
    nail E920.8
    needle (sewing) E920.4
      hypodermic E920.5
    noise E928.1
    object
      fallen on
        motor vehicle (in motion) (on public
          highway) E818 ☑
          not on public highway E825 ☑
      falling — *see* Hit by, object, falling
    paintball gun E922.5
    radiation — *see* Radiation
    railway rolling stock, train, vehicle (part of)
      E805 ☑
      door or window E806 ☑
    rotating propeller, aircraft E844 ☑
    rough landing of off-road type motor vehicle
      (after leaving ground or rough terrain)
      E821 ☑
    snow vehicle E820 ☑
    saber (*see also* Wound, saber) E920.3
    shot — *see* Shooting
    sound waves E928.1
    splinter or sliver, wood E920.8
    straining E927
    street car (door) E829 ☑
    suicide (attempt) E958.9
    sword E920.3
    terrorism — *see* Terrorism
    third rail — *see* Electric shock
    thunderbolt E907
    tidal wave E909.4
      caused by storm E908.0
    tornado E908.1
    torrential rain E908.2
    twisting E927
    vehicle NEC — *see* Accident, vehicle NEC
    vibration E928.2
    volcanic eruption E909.1
    weapon burst, in war operations E993
    weightlessness (in spacecraft, real or
      simulated) E928.0
    wood splinter or sliver E920.8
  due to
    civil insurrection — *see* War operations
      occurring after cessation of hostilities
        E998
    terrorism — *see* Terrorism

☑ Additional Digit Required   ◄► Revised Text   ● New Line   ▲ Revised Code

Injury, injured — Late effect of

Injury, injured NEC — *continued*
  due to — *continued*
    war operations — *see* War operations
      occurring after cessation of hostilities
        E998
    homicidal (*see also* Assault) E968.9
  in, on
    civil insurrection — *see* War operations
    fight E960.0
    parachute descent (voluntary) (without
        accident to aircraft) E844 ☑
      with accident to aircraft — *see* categories
        E840-E842 ☑
    public highway E819 ☑
    railway right of way E807 ☑
    terrorism — *see* Terrorism
    war operations — *see* War operations
  inflicted (by)
    in course of arrest (attempted), suppression
        of disturbance, maintenance of order,
        by law enforcing agents — *see* Legal
        intervention
    law-enforcing agent (on duty) — *see* Legal
        intervention
    other person
      stated as
        accidental E928.9
        homicidal, intentional — *see* Assault
        undetermined whether accidental or
          intentional — *see* Injury, stated
          as undetermined
    police (on duty) — *see* Legal intervention
  late effect of E929.9
  purposely (inflicted) by other person(s) — *see*
    Assault
  self-inflicted (unspecified whether accidental or
      intentional) E988.9
    stated as
      accidental E928.9
      intentionally, purposely E958.9
  specified cause NEC E928.8
  stated as
    undetermined whether accidentally or
        purposely inflicted (by) E988.9
      cut (any part of body) E986
      cutting or piercing instrument
        (classifiable to E920) E986
      drowning E984
      explosive(s) (missile) E985.5
      falling from high place E987.9
        manmade structure, except residential
          E987.1
        natural site E987.2
        residential premises E987.0
      hanging E983.0
      knife E986
      late effect of E989
      puncture (any part of body) E986
      shooting — *see* Shooting, stated as
        undetermined whether accidental or
        intentional
      specified means NEC E988.8
      stab (any part of body) E986
      strangulation — *see* Suffocation, stated as
        undetermined whether accidental or
        intentional
      submersion E984
      suffocation — *see* Suffocation, stated as
        undetermined whether accidental or
        intentional
  to child due to criminal abortion E968.8
Insufficient nourishment — *see also* Lack of,
    food
  homicidal intent E968.4
Insulation, effects — *see* Heat
Interruption of respiration by
  food lodged in esophagus E911
  foreign body, except food, in esophagus E912
Intervention, legal — *see* Legal intervention
Intoxication, drug or poison — *see* Table of
    Drugs and Chemicals
Irradiation — *see* Radiation

J

Jammed (accidentally)
  between objects (moving) (stationary and
      moving) E918
  in object E918
Jumped or fell from high place, so stated — *see*
    Jumping, from, high place, stated as
    in undetermined circumstances
Jumping
  before train, vehicle or other moving object
      (unspecified whether accidental or
      intentional) E988.0
    stated as
      intentional, purposeful E958.0
      suicidal (attempt) E958.0
  from
    aircraft
      by parachute (voluntarily) (without
          accident to aircraft) E844 ☑
      due to accident to aircraft — *see*
          categories E840-E842 ☑
    boat, ship, watercraft (into water)
      after accident to, fire on, watercraft
          E830 ☑
        and subsequently struck by (part of)
          boat E831 ☑
      burning, crushed, sinking E830 ☑
        and subsequently struck by (part of)
          boat E831 ☑
      voluntarily, without accident (to boat)
        with injury other than drowning or
          submersion E883.0
    building — *see also* Jumping, from, high
        place
      burning (uncontrolled fire) E891.8
        in terrorism E979.3
        private E890.8
    cable car (not on rails) E847
      on rails E829 ☑
    high place
      in accidental circumstances or in sport —
          see categories E880-E884 ☑
      stated as
        with intent to injure self E957.9
          man-made structures NEC E957.1
          natural sites E957.2
          residential premises E957.0
        in undetermined circumstances
            E987.9
          man-made structures NEC E987.1
          natural sites E987.2
          residential premises E987.0
        suicidal (attempt) E957.9
          man-made structures NEC E957.1
          natural sites E957.1
          residential premises E957.0
    motor vehicle (in motion) (on public
        highway) — *see* Fall, from, motor
        vehicle
    nonmotor road vehicle NEC E829 ☑
    street car E829 ☑
    structure — *see also* Jumping, from, high
        place
      burning NEC (uncontrolled fire) E891.8
        in terrorism E979.3
  into water
    with injury other than drowning or
        submersion E883.0
      drowning or submersion — *see*
          Submersion
    from, off, watercraft — *see* Jumping, from,
        boat
Justifiable homicide — *see* Assault

K

Kicked by
  animal E906.8
  person(s) (accidentally) E917.9
    with intent to injure or kill E960.0
    as, or caused by a crowd E917.1
      with subsequent fall E917.6
    in fight E960.0

Kicked by — *continued*
  person(s) — *continued*
    in sports E917.0
      with subsequent fall E917.5
Kicking against
  object (moving) E917.9
    in sports E917.0
      with subsequent fall E917.5
    stationary E917.4
      with subsequent fall E917.8
  person — *see* Striking against, person
Killed, killing (accidentally) NEC (*see also* Injury)
    E928.9
  in
    action — *see* War operations
    brawl, fight (hand) (fists) (foot) E960.0
      by weapon — *see also* Assault
        cutting, piercing E966
        firearm — *see* Shooting, homicide
  self
    stated as
      accident E928.9
      suicide — *see* Suicide
    unspecified whether accidental or suicidal
        E988.9
Knocked down (accidentally) (by) NEC E928.9
  animal (not being ridden) E906.8
    being ridden (in sport or transport) E828 ☑
  blast from explosion (*see also* Explosion)
      E923.9
  crowd, human stampede E917.6
  late effect of — *see* Late effect
  person (accidentally) E917.9
    in brawl, fight E960.0
    in sports E917.5
  transport vehicle — *see* vehicle involved under
      Hit by
  while boxing E917.5

L

Laceration NEC E928.9
Lack of
  air (refrigerator or closed place), suffocation by
      E913.2
  care (helpless person) (infant) (newborn) E904.0
    homicidal intent E968.4
  food except as result of transport accident
      E904.1
    helpless person, infant, newborn due to
        abandonment or neglect E904.0
  water except as result of transport accident
      E904.2
    helpless person, infant, newborn due to
        abandonment or neglect E904.0
Landslide E909.2
  falling on, hitting
    motor vehicle (any) (in motion) (on or off
        public highway) E909.2
    railway rolling stock, train, vehicle E909.2
Late effect of
  accident NEC (accident classifiable to E928.9)
      E929.9
    specified NEC (accident classifiable to E910-
        E928.8) E929.8
  assault E969
  fall, accidental (accident classifiable to E880-
      E888) E929.3
  fire, accident caused by (accident classifiable to
      E890-E899) E929.4
  homicide, attempt (any means) E969
  injury due to terrorism E999.1
  injury undetermined whether accidentally or
      purposely inflicted (injury classifiable to
      E980-E988) E989
  legal intervention (injury classifiable to E970-
      E976) E977
  medical or surgical procedure, test or therapy
      as, or resulting in, or from
    abnormal or delayed reaction or
        complication — *see* Reaction,
        abnormal
    misadventure — *see* Misadventure
  motor vehicle accident (accident classifiable to
      E810-E825) E929.0

☑ Additional Digit Required   ▶◀ Revised Text   ● New Line   ▲ Revised Code

Late effect of — *continued*
  natural or environmental factor, accident due to (accident classifiable to E900-E909) E929.5
  poisoning, accidental (accident classifiable to E850-E858, E860-E869) E929.2
  suicide, attempt (any means) E959
  transport accident NEC (accident classifiable to E800-E807, E826-E838, E840-E848) E929.1
  war operations, injury due to (injury classifiable to E990-E998) E999.0
Launching pad accident E845 ☑
Legal
  execution, any method E978
  intervention (by) (injury from) E976
    baton E973
    bayonet E974
    blow E975
    blunt object (baton) (nightstick) (stave) (truncheon) E973
    cutting or piercing instrument E974
    dynamite E971
    execution, any method E973
    explosive(s) (shell) E971
    firearm(s) E970
    gas (asphyxiation) (poisoning) (tear) E972
    grenade E971
    late effect of E977
    machine gun E970
    manhandling E975
    mortar bomb E971
    nightstick E973
    revolver E970
    rifle E970
    specified means NEC E975
    stabbing E974
    stave E973
    truncheon E973
Lifting, injury in E927
Lightning (shock) (stroke) (struck by) E907
Liquid (noncorrosive) in eye E914
  corrosive E924.1
Loss of control
  motor vehicle (on public highway) (without antecedent collision) E816 ☑
    with
      antecedent collision on public highway — *see* Collision, motor vehicle
      involving any object, person or vehicle not on public highway E816 ☑
      on public highway — *see* Collision, motor vehicle
      not on public highway, nontraffic accident E825 ☑
        with antecedent collision — *see* Collision, motor vehicle, not on public highway
  off-road type motor vehicle (not on public highway) E821 ☑
    on public highway — *see* Loss of control, motor vehicle
  snow vehicle, motor-driven (not on public highway) E820 ☑
    on public highway — *see* Loss of control, motor vehicle
Lost at sea E832 ☑
  with accident to watercraft E830 ☑
  in war operations E995
Low
  pressure, effects — *see* Effects of, air pressure
  temperature, effects — *see* Cold, exposure to
Lying before train, vehicle or other moving object (unspecified whether accidental or intentional) E988.0
  stated as intentional, purposeful, suicidal (attempt) E958.0
Lynching (*see also* Assault) E968.9

M

Malfunction, atomic power plant in water transport E838 ☑
Mangled (accidentally) NEC E928.9

Manhandling (in brawl, fight) E960.0
  legal intervention E975
Manslaughter (nonaccidental) — *see* Assault
Marble in nose E912
Mauled by animal E906.8
Medical procedure, complication of
  delayed or as an abnormal reaction
    without mention of misadventure — *see* Reaction, abnormal
  due to or as a result of misadventure — *see* Misadventure
Melting of fittings and furniture in burning
  in terrorism E979.3
Minamata disease E865.2
Misadventure(s) to patient(s) during surgical or medical care E876.9
  contaminated blood, fluid, drug or biological substance (presence of agents and toxins as listed in E875) E875.9
    administered (by) NEC E875.9
      infusion E875.0
      injection E875.1
      specified means NEC E875.2
      transfusion E875.0
      vaccination E875.1
  cut, cutting, puncture, perforation or hemorrhage (accidental) (inadvertent) (inappropriate) (during) E870.9
    aspiration of fluid or tissue (by puncture or catheterization, except heart) E870.5
      biopsy E870.8
        needle (aspirating) E870.5
      blood sampling E870.5
      catheterization E870.5
        heart E870.6
      dialysis (kidney) E870.2
      endoscopic examination E870.4
      enema E870.7
      infusion E870.1
      injection E870.3
      lumbar puncture E870.5
      needle biopsy E870.5
      paracentesis, abdominal E870.5
      perfusion E870.2
      specified procedure NEC E870.8
      surgical operation E870.0
      thoracentesis E870.5
      transfusion E870.1
      vaccination E870.3
  excessive amount of blood or other fluid during transfusion or infusion E873.0
  failure
    in dosage E873.9
      electroshock therapy E873.4
      inappropriate temperature (too hot or too cold) in local application and packing E873.5
      infusion
        excessive amount of fluid E873.0
        incorrect dilution of fluid E873.1
      insulin-shock therapy E873.4
      nonadministration of necessary drug or medicinal E873.6
      overdose — *see also* Overdose
        radiation, in therapy E873.2
      radiation
        inadvertent exposure of patient (receiving radiation for test or therapy) E873.3
        not receiving radiation for test or therapy — *see* Radiation
      overdose E873.2
      specified procedure NEC E873.8
      transfusion
        excessive amount of blood E873.0
    mechanical, of instrument or apparatus (during procedure) E874.9
      aspiration of fluid or tissue (by puncture or catheterization, except of heart) E874.4
      biopsy E874.8
        needle (aspirating) E874.4
      blood sampling E874.4
      catheterization E874.4
        heart E874.5

Misadventure(s) to patient(s) during surgical or medical care — *continued*
  failure — *continued*
    mechanical, of instrument or apparatus — *continued*
      dialysis (kidney) E874.2
      endoscopic examination E874.3
      enema E874.8
      infusion E874.1
      injection E874.8
      lumbar puncture E874.4
      needle biopsy E874.4
      paracentesis, abdominal E874.4
      perfusion E874.2
      specified procedure NEC E874.8
      surgical operation E874.0
      thoracentesis E874.4
      transfusion E874.1
      vaccination E874.8
    sterile precautions (during procedure) E872.9
      aspiration of fluid or tissue (by puncture or catheterization, except heart) E872.5
      biopsy E872.8
        needle (aspirating) E872.5
      blood sampling E872.5
      catheterization E872.5
        heart E872.6
      dialysis (kidney) E872.2
      endoscopic examination E872.4
      enema E872.8
      infusion E872.1
      injection E872.3
      lumbar puncture E872.5
      needle biopsy E872.5
      paracentesis, abdominal E872.5
      perfusion E872.2
      removal of catheter or packing E872.8
      specified procedure NEC E872.8
      surgical operation E872.0
      thoracentesis E872.5
      transfusion E872.1
      vaccination E872.3
    suture or ligature during surgical procedure E876.2
    to introduce or to remove tube or instrument E876.4
      foreign object left in body — *see* Misadventure, foreign object
  foreign object left in body (during procedure) E871.9
    aspiration of fluid or tissue (by puncture or catheterization, except heart) E871.5
    biopsy E871.8
      needle (aspirating) E871.5
    blood sampling E871.5
    catheterization E871.5
      heart E871.6
    dialysis (kidney) E871.2
    endoscopic examination E871.4
    enema E871.8
    infusion E871.1
    injection E871.3
    lumbar puncture E871.5
    needle biopsy E871.5
    paracentesis, abdominal E871.5
    perfusion E871.2
    removal of catheter or packing E871.7
    specified procedure NEC E871.8
    surgical operation E871.0
    thoracentesis E871.5
    transfusion E871.1
    vaccination E871.3
  hemorrhage — *see* Misadventure, cut
  inadvertent exposure of patient to radiation (being received for test or therapy) E873.3
  inappropriate
    operation performed E876.5
    temperature (too hot or too cold) in local application or packing E873.5
  infusion — *see also* Misadventure, by specific type, infusion
    excessive amount of fluid E873.0
    incorrect dilution of fluid E873.1
    wrong fluid E876.1
  mismatched blood in transfusion E876.0

☑ Additional Digit Required   ▶◀ Revised Text   ● New Line   ▲ Revised Code

Misadventure(s) to patient(s) during surgical or medical care — *continued*
　nonadministration of necessary drug or
　　medicinal E873.6
　overdose — *see also* Overdose
　　radiation, in therapy E873.2
　perforation — *see* Misadventure, cut
　performance of inappropriate operation E876.5
　puncture — *see* Misadventure, cut
　specified type NEC E876.8
　　failure
　　　suture or ligature during surgical
　　　　operation E876.2
　　　to introduce or to remove tube or
　　　　instrument E876.4
　　　　foreign object left in body E871.9
　　infusion of wrong fluid E876.1
　　performance of inappropriate operation
　　　E876.5
　　transfusion of mismatched blood E876.0
　　wrong
　　　fluid in infusion E876.1
　　　placement of endotracheal tube during
　　　　anesthetic procedure E876.3
　transfusion — *see also* Misadventure, by
　　specific type, transfusion
　　excessive amount of blood E873.0
　　mismatched blood E876.0
　wrong
　　drug given in error — *see* Table of Drugs
　　　and Chemicals
　　fluid in infusion E876.1
　　placement of endotracheal tube during
　　　anesthetic procedure E876.3
Motion (effects) E903
　sickness E903
Mountain sickness E902.0
Mucus aspiration or inhalation, not of newborn
　(with asphyxia, obstruction respiratory
　passage, suffocation) E912
Mudslide of cataclysmic nature E909.2
Murder (attempt) (*see also* Assault) E968.9

N

Nail, injury by E920.8
Needlestick (sewing needle) E920.4
　hypodermic E920.5
Neglect — *see also* Privation
　criminal E968.4
　homicidal intent E968.4
Noise (causing injury) (pollution) E928.1

O

Object
　falling
　　from, in, on, hitting
　　　aircraft E844 ☑
　　　　due to accident to aircraft — *see*
　　　　　categories E840-E842 ☑
　　　machinery — *see also* Accident, machine
　　　　not in operation E916
　　　motor vehicle (in motion) (on public
　　　　highway) E818 ☑
　　　　not on public highway E825 ☑
　　　　stationary E916
　　　nonmotor road vehicle NEC E829 ☑
　　　pedal cycle E826 ☑
　　　person E916
　　　railway rolling stock, train, vehicle
　　　　E806 ☑
　　　street car E829 ☑
　　　watercraft E838 ☑
　　　　due to accident to watercraft
　　　　　E831 ☑
　　set in motion by
　　　accidental explosion of pressure vessel —
　　　　see category E921 ☑
　　　firearm — *see* category E922 ☑
　　　machine(ry) — *see* Accident, machine
　　　transport vehicle — *see* categories E800-
　　　　E848 ☑

Object — *continued*
　thrown from, in, on, towards
　　aircraft E844 ☑
　　cable car (not on rails) E847
　　　on rails E829 ☑
　　motor vehicle (in motion) (on public
　　　highway) E818 ☑
　　　not on public highway E825 ☑
　　nonmotor road vehicle NEC E829 ☑
　　pedal cycle E826 ☑
　　street car E829 ☑
　　vehicle NEC — *see* Accident, vehicle NEC
Obstruction
　air passages, larynx, respiratory passages
　　by
　　　external means NEC — *see* Suffocation
　　　food, any type (regurgitated) (vomited)
　　　　E911
　　　material or object, except food E912
　　　mucus E912
　　　phlegm E912
　　　vomitus E911
　digestive tract, except mouth or pharynx
　　by
　　　food, any type E915
　　　foreign body (any) E915
　esophagus
　　food E911
　　foreign body, except food E912
　　without asphyxia or obstruction of
　　　respiratory passage E915
　mouth or pharynx
　　by
　　　food, any type E911
　　　material or object, except food E912
　respiration — *see* Obstruction, air passages
Oil in eye E914
Overdose
　anesthetic (drug) — *see* Table of Drugs and
　　Chemicals
　drug — *see* Table of Drugs and Chemicals
Overexertion (lifting) (pulling) (pushing) E927
Overexposure (accidental) (to)
　cold (*see also* Cold, exposure to) E901.9
　　due to manmade conditions E901.1
　heat (*see also* Heat) E900.9
　radiation — *see* Radiation
　radioactivity — *see* Radiation
　sun, except sunburn E900.0
　weather — *see* Exposure
　wind — *see* Exposure
Overheated (*see also* Heat) E900.9
Overlaid E913.0
Overturning (accidental)
　animal-drawn vehicle E827 ☑
　boat, ship, watercraft
　　causing
　　　drowning, submersion E830 ☑
　　　injury except drowning, submersion
　　　　E831 ☑
　machinery — *see* Accident, machine
　motor vehicle (*see also* Loss of control, motor
　　vehicle) E816 ☑
　　with antecedent collision on public highway
　　　— *see* Collision, motor vehicle
　　not on public highway, nontraffic accident
　　　E825 ☑
　　　with antecedent collision — *see* Collision,
　　　　motor vehicle, not on public
　　　　highway
　nonmotor road vehicle NEC E829 ☑
　off-road type motor vehicle — *see* Loss of
　　control, off-road type motor vehicle
　pedal cycle E826 ☑
　railway rolling stock, train, vehicle (*see also*
　　Derailment, railway) E802 ☑
　street car E829 ☑
　vehicle NEC — *see* Accident, vehicle NEC

P

Palsy, divers' E902.2
Parachuting (voluntary) (without accident to
　aircraft) E844 ☑

Parachuting — *continued*
　due to accident to aircraft — *see* categories
　　E840-E842 ☑
Paralysis
　divers' E902.2
　lead or saturnine E866.0
　　from pesticide NEC E863.4
Pecked by bird E906.8
Phlegm aspiration or inhalation (with asphyxia,
　obstruction respiratory passage, suffocation)
　E912
Piercing (*see also* Cut) E920.9
Pinched
　between objects (moving) (stationary and
　　moving) E918
　in object E918
Pinned under
　machine(ry) — *see* Accident, machine
Place of occurrence of accident — *see* Accident
　(to), occurring (at) (in)
Plumbism E866.0
　from insecticide NEC E863.4
Poisoning (accidental) (by) — *see also* Table of
　Drugs and Chemicals
　carbon monoxide
　　generated by
　　　aircraft in transit E844 ☑
　　　motor vehicle
　　　　in motion (on public highway) E818 ☑
　　　　not on public highway E825 ☑
　　　watercraft (in transit) (not in transit)
　　　　E838 ☑
　caused by injection of poisons or toxins into or
　　through skin by plant thorns, spines, or
　　other mechanism E905.7
　　marine or sea plants E905.6
　fumes or smoke due to
　　conflagration — *see* Conflagration
　　explosion or fire — *see* Fire
　　ignition — *see* Ignition
　gas
　　in legal intervention E972
　　legal execution, by E978
　　on watercraft E838 ☑
　　used as anesthetic — *see* Table of Drugs
　　　and Chemicals
　in
　　terrorism (chemical weapons) E979.7
　　war operations E997.2
　late effect of — *see* Late effect
　legal
　　execution E978
　　intervention
　　　by gas E972
Pressure, external, causing asphyxia,
　suffocation (*see also* Suffocation) E913.9
Privation E904.9
　food (*see also* Lack of, food) E904.1
　helpless person, infant, newborn due to
　　abandonment or neglect E904.0
　late effect of NEC E929.5
　resulting from transport accident — *see*
　　categories E800-E848 ☑
　water (*see also* Lack of, water) E904.2
Projected objects, striking against or struck by
　— *see* Striking against, object
Prolonged stay in
　high altitude (causing conditions as listed in
　　E902.0) E902.0
　weightless environment E928.0
Prostration
　heat — *see* Heat
Pulling, injury in E927
Puncture, puncturing (*see also* Cut) E920.9
　by
　　plant thorns or spines E920.8
　　　toxic reaction E905.7
　　　　marine or sea plants E905.6
　　sea-urchin spine E905.6

Pushing (injury in) (overexertion) E927
by other person(s) (accidental) E917.9
as, or caused by, a crowd, human stampede E917.1
with subsequent fall E917.6
before moving vehicle or object
stated as
intentional, homicidal E968.5
undetemined whether accidental or intentional E988.8
from
high place
in accidental circum-stances — see categories E880-E884 ☑
stated as
intentional, homicidal E968.1
undetermined whether accidental or intentional E987.9
man-made structure, except residential E987.1
natural site E987.2
residential E987.0
motor vehicle (see also Fall, from, motor vehicle) E818 ☑
stated as
intentional, homicidal E968.5
undetermined whether accidental or intentional E988.8
in sports E917.0
with fall E886.0
with fall E886.9
in sports E886.0

R

Radiation (exposure to) E926.9
abnormal reaction to medical test or therapy E879.2
arc lamps E926.2
atomic power plant (malfunction) NEC E926.9
in water transport E838 ☑
electromagnetic, ionizing E926.3
gamma rays E926.3
in
terrorism (from or following nuclear explosion) (direct) (secondary) E979.5
laser E979.8
war operations (from or following nuclear explosion) (direct) (secondary) E996
laser(s) E997.0
water transport E838 ☑
inadvertent exposure of patient (receiving test or therapy) E873.3
infrared (heaters and lamps) E926.1
excessive heat E900.1
ionized, ionizing (particles, artificially accelerated) E926.8
electromagnetic E926.3
isotopes, radioactive — see Radiation, radioactive isotopes
laser(s) E926.4
in
terrorism E979.8
war operations E997.0
misadventure in medical care — see Misadventure, failure, in dosage, radiation
late effect of NEC E929.8
excessive heat from — see Heat
light sources (visible) (ultraviolet) E926.2
misadventure in medical or surgical procedure — see Misadventure, failure, in dosage, radiation
overdose (in medical or surgical procedure) E873.2
radar E926.0
radioactive isotopes E926.5
atomic power plant malfunction E926.5
in water transport E838 ☑
misadventure in medical or surgical treatment — see Misadventure, failure, in dosage, radiation
radiobiologicals — see Radiation, radioactive isotopes
radiofrequency E926.0

Radiation — continued
radiopharmaceuticals — see Radiation, radioactive isotopes
radium NEC E926.9
sun E926.2
excessive heat from E900.0
tanning bed E926.2
welding arc or torch E926.2
excessive heat from E900.1
x-rays (hard) (soft) E926.3
misadventure in medical or surgical treatment — see Misadventure, failure, in dosage, radiation

Rape E960.1

Reaction, abnormal to or following (medical or surgical procedure) E879.9
amputation (of limbs) E878.5
anastomosis (arteriovenous) (blood vessel) (gastrojejunal) (skin) (tendon) (natural, artificial material, tissue) E878.2
external stoma, creation of E878.3
aspiration (of fluid) E879.4
tissue E879.8
biopsy E879.8
blood
sampling E879.7
transfusion
procedure E879.8
bypass — see Reaction, abnormal, anastomosis
catheterization
cardiac E879.0
urinary E879.6
colostomy E878.3
cystostomy E878.3
dialysis (kidney) E879.1
drugs or biologicals — see Table of Drugs and Chemicals
duodenostomy E878.3
electroshock therapy E879.3
formation of external stoma E878.3
gastrostomy E878.3
graft — see Reaction, abnormal, anastomosis
hypothermia E879.8
implant, implantation (of)
artificial
internal device (cardiac pacemaker) (electrodes in brain) (heart valve prosthesis) (orthopedic) E878.1
material or tissue (for anastomosis or bypass) E878.2
with creation of external stoma E878.3
natural tissues (for anastomosis or bypass) E878.2
as transplantion — see Reaction, abnormal, transplant
with creation of external stoma E878.3
infusion
procedure E879.8
injection
procedure E879.8
insertion of gastric or duodenal sound E879.5
insulin-shock therapy E879.3
lumbar puncture E879.4
perfusion E879.1
procedures other than surgical operation (see also Reaction, abnormal, by specific type of procedure) E879.9
specified procedure NEC E879.8
radiological procedure or therapy E879.2
removal of organ (partial) (total) NEC E878.6
with
anastomosis, bypass or graft E878.2
formation of external stoma E878.3
implant of artificial internal device E878.1
transplant(ation)
partial organ E878.4
whole organ E878.0
sampling
blood E879.7
fluid NEC E879.4
tissue E879.8
shock therapy E879.3
surgical operation (see also Reaction, abnormal, by specified type of operation) E878.9

Reaction, abnormal to or following — continued
surgical operation (see also Reaction, abnormal, by specified type of operation) — continued
restorative NEC E878.4
with
anastomosis, bypass or graft E878.2
fomation of external stoma E878.3
implant(ation) — see Reaction, abnormal, implant
transplant(ation) — see Reaction, abnormal, transplant
specified operation NEC E878.8
thoracentesis E879.4
transfusion
procedure E879.8
transplant, transplantation (heart) (kidney) (liver) E878.0
partial organ E878.4
ureterostomy E878.3
vaccination E879.8

Reduction in
atmospheric pressure — see also Effects of, air pressure
while surfacing from
deep water diving causing caisson or divers' disease, palsy or paralysis E902.2
underground E902.8

Residual (effect) — see Late effect

Rock falling on or hitting (accidentally)
motor vehicle (in motion) (on public highway) E818 ☑
not on public highway E825 ☑
nonmotor road vehicle NEC E829 ☑
pedal cycle E826 ☑
person E916
railway rolling stock, train, vehicle E806 ☑

Running off, away
animal (being ridden) (in sport or transport) E829 ☑
not being ridden E906.8
animal-drawn vehicle E827 ☑
rails, railway (see also Derailment) E802 ☑
roadway
motor vehicle (without antecedent collision) E816 ☑
nontraffic accident E825 ☑
with antecedent collision — see Collision, motor vehicle, not on public highway
with
antecedent collision — see Collision motor vehicle
subsequent collision
involving any object, person or vehicle not on public highway E816 ☑
on public highway E811 ☑
nonmotor road vehicle NEC E829 ☑
pedal cycle E826 ☑

Run over (accidentally) (by)
animal (not being ridden) E906.8
being ridden (in sport or transport) E828 ☑
animal-drawn vehicle E827 ☑
machinery — see Accident, machine
motor vehicle (on public highway) — see Hit by, motor vehicle
nonmotor road vehicle NEC E829 ☑
railway train E805 ☑
street car E829 ☑
vehicle NEC E848

S

Saturnism E866.0
from insecticide NEC E863.4

Scald, scalding (accidental) (by) (from) (in) E924.0
acid — see Scald, caustic
boiling tap water E924.2
caustic or corrosive liquid, substance E924.1
swallowed — see Table of Drugs and Chemicals
homicide (attempt) — see Assault, burning

Scald, scalding — Sting (side text)

Scald, scalding — *continued*
  inflicted by other person
    stated as
      intentional or homicidal E968.3
      undetermined whether accidental or
          intentional E988.2
  late effect of NEC E929.8
  liquid (boiling) (hot) E924.0
  local application of externally applied
      substance in medical or surgical care
      E873.5
  molten metal E924.0
  self-inflicted (unspecified whether accidental or
      intentional) E988.2
    stated as intentional, purposeful E958.2
    stated as undetermined whether accidental or
        intentional E988.2
  steam E924.0
  tap water (boiling) E924.2
  transport accident — *see* catagories E800-E848
  vapor E924.0
Scratch, cat E906.8
Sea
  sickness E903
Self-mutilation — *see* Suicide
Sequelae (of)
  in
    terrorism E999.1
    war operations E999.0
Shock
  anaphylactic (*see also* Table of Drugs and
      Chemicals) E947.9
    due to
      bite (venomous) — *see* Bite, venomous
          NEC
      sting — *see* Sting
  electric (*see also* Electric shock) E925.9
  from electric appliance or current (*see also*
      Electric shock) E925.9
Shooting, shot (accidental(ly)) E922.9
  air gun E922.4
  BB gun E922.4
  hand gun (pistol) (revolver) E922.0
  himself (*see also* Shooting, self-inflicted)
      E985.4
    hand gun (pistol) (revolver) E985.0
    military firearm, except hand gun E985.3
      hand gun (pistol) (revolver) E985.0
    rifle (hunting) E985.2
      military E985.3
    shotgun (automatic) E985.1
    specified firearm NEC E985.4
    Verey pistol E985.4
  homicide (attempt) E965.4
    air gun E968.6
    BB gun E968.6
    hand gun (pistol) (revolver) E965.0
    military firearm, except hand gun E965.3
      hand gun (pistol) (revolver) E965.0
    paintball gun E965.4
    rifle (hunting) E965.2
      military E965.3
    shotgun (automatic) E965.1
    specified firearm NEC E965.4
    Verey pistol E965.4
  inflicted by other person
    in accidental circumstances E922.9
      hand gun (pistol) (revolver) E922.0
      military firearm, except hand gun E922.3
        hand gun (pistol) (revolver) E922.0
      rifle (hunting) E922.2
        military E922.3
      shotgun (automatic) E922.1
      specified firearm NEC E922.8
      Verey pistol E922.8
    stated as
      intentional, homicidal E965.4
        hand gun (pistol) (revolver) E965.0
        military firearm, except hand gun
            E965.3
          hand gun (pistol) (revolver) E965.0
        paintball gun E965.4
        rifle (hunting) E965.2
          military E965.3
        shotgun (automatic) E965.1
        specified firearm E965.4

Shooting, shot — *continued*
  inflicted by other person — *continued*
    stated as — *continued*
      intentional, homicidal — *continued*
        Verey pistol E965.4
      undetermined whether accidental or
          intentional E985.4
        air gun E985.6
        BB gun E985.6
        hand gun (pistol) (revolver) E985.0
        military firearm, except hand gun
            E985.3
          hand gun (pistol) (revolver) E985.0
        paintball gun E985.7
        rifle (hunting) E985.2
        shotgun (automatic) E985.1
        specified firearm NEC E985.4
        Verey pistol E985.4
  in
    terrorism — *see* Terrorism, shooting
    war operations — *see* War operations,
        shooting
  legal
    execution E978
    intervention E970
  military firearm, except hand gun E922.3
    hand gun (pistol) (revolver) E922.0
  paintball gun E922.5
  rifle (hunting) E922.2
    military E922.3
  self-inflicted (unspecified whether accidental or
      intentional) E985.4
    air gun E985.6
    BB gun E985.6
    hand gun (pistol) (revolver) E985.0
    military firearm, except hand gun E985.3
      hand gun (pistol) (revolver) E985.0
    paintball gun E985.7
    rifle (hunting) E985.2
      military E985.3
    shotgun (automatic) E985.1
    specified firearm NEC E985.4
    stated as
      accidental E922.9
        hand gun (pistol) (revolver) E922.0
        military firearm, except hand gun
            E922.3
          hand gun (pistol) (revolver) E922.0
        paintball gun E922.5
        rifle (hunting) E922.2
          military E922.3
        shotgun (automatic) E922.1
        specified firearm NEC E922.8
        Verey pistol E922.8
      intentional, purposeful E955.4
        hand gun (pistol) (revolver) E955.0
        military firearm, except hand gun
            E955.3
          hand gun (pistol) (revolver) E955.0
        paintball gun E955.7
        rifle (hunting) E955.2
          military E955.3
        shotgun (automatic) E955.1
        specified firearm NEC E955.4
        Verey pistol E955.4
  shotgun (automatic) E922.1
  specified firearm NEC E922.8
  stated as undetermined whether accidental or
      intentional E985.4
    hand gun (pistol) (revolver) E985.0
    military firearm, except hand gun E985.3
      hand gun (pistol) (revolver) E985.0
    paintball gun E985.7
    rifle (hunting) E985.2
      military E985.3
    shotgun (automatic) E985.1
    specified firearm NEC E985.4
    Verey pistol E985.4
  suicidal (attempt) E955.4
    air gun E955.6
    BB gun E955.6
    hand gun (pistol) (revolver) E955.0
    military firearm, except hand gun E955.3
      hand gun (pistol) (revolver) E955.0
    paintball gun E955.7
    rifle (hunting) E955.2
      military E955.3

Shooting, shot — *continued*
  suicidal — *continued*
    shotgun (automatic) E955.1
    specified firearm NEC E955.4
    Verey pistol E955.4
  Verey pistol E922.8
Shoving (accidentally) by other person (*see also*
    Pushing by other person) E917.9
Sickness
  air E903
  alpine E902.0
  car E903
  motion E903
  mountain E902.0
  sea E903
  travel E903
Sinking (accidental)
  boat, ship, watercraft (causing drowning,
      submersion) E830 ☑
  causing injury except drowning, submersion
      E831 ☑
Siriasis E900.0
Skydiving E844 ☑
Slashed wrists (*see also* Cut, self-inflicted) E986
Slipping (accidental)
  on
    deck (of boat, ship, watercraft) (icy) (oily)
        (wet) E835 ☑
    ice E885 ☑
    ladder of ship E833 ☑
      due to accident to watercraft E831 ☑
    mud E885 ☑
    oil E885 ☑
    snow E885 ☑
    stairs of ship E833 ☑
      due to accident to watercraft E831 ☑
    surface
      slippery E885 ☑
      wet E885 ☑
Sliver, wood, injury by E920.8
Smouldering building or structure in terrorism
    E979.3
Smothering, smothered (*see also* Suffocation)
    E913.9
Sodomy (assault) E960.1
Solid substance in eye (any part) or adnexa E914
Sound waves (causing injury) E928.1
Splinter, injury by E920.8
Stab, stabbing E966
  accidental — *see* Cut
Starvation E904.1
  helpless person, infant, newborn — *see* Lack of
      food
  homicidal intent E968.4
  late effect of NEC E929.5
  resulting from accident connected with
      transport — *see* catagories E800-E848
Stepped on
  by
    animal (not being ridden) E906.8
      being ridden (in sport or transport)
          E828 ☑
    crowd E917.1
    person E917.9
      in sports E917.0
  in sports E917.0
Stepping on
  object (moving) E917.9
    in sports E917.0
      with subsequent fall E917.5
    stationary E917.4
      with subsequent fall E917.8
  person E917.9
    as, or caused by a crowd E917.1
      with subsequent fall E917.6
    in sports E917.0
Sting E905.9
  ant E905.5
  bee E905.3
  caterpillar E905.5
  coral E905.6
  hornet E905.3
  insect NEC E905.5
  jellyfish E905.6

☑ Additional Digit Required   ▶◀ Revised Text   ● New Line   ▲ Revised Code

Sting — *continued*
  marine animal or plant E905.6
  nematocysts E905.6
  scorpion E905.2
  sea anemone E905.6
  sea cucumber E905.6
  wasp E905.3
  yellow jacket E905.3
Storm E908.9
  specified type NEC E908.8
Straining, injury in E927
Strangling — *see* Suffocation
Strangulation — *see* Suffocation
Strenuous movements (in recreational or other
    activities) E927
Striking against
  bottom (when jumping or diving into water)
    E883.0
  object (moving) E917.9
    caused by crowd E917.1
      with subsequent fall E917.6
    furniture E917.3
      with subsequent fall E917.7
    in
      running water E917.2
        with drowning or submersion — *see*
          Submersion
      sports E917.0
        with subsequent fall E917.5
    stationary E917.4
      with subsequent fall E917.8
  person(s) E917.9
    with fall E886.9
      in sports E886.0
    as, or caused by, a crowd E917.1
      with subsequent fall E917.6
        in sports E917.0
          with fall E886.0
Stroke
  heat — *see* Heat
  lightning E907
Struck by — *see also* Hit by
  bullet
    in
      terrorism E979.4
      war operations E991.2
        rubber E991.0
  lightning E907
  missile
    in terrorism — *see* Terrorism, missile
  object
    falling
      from, in, on
        building
          burning (uncontrolled fire)
            in terrorism E979.3
  thunderbolt E907
**Stumbling over animal, carpet, curb, rug or
    (small) object (with fall)** E885 ☑
  without fall — *see* Striking against, object
Submersion (accidental) E910.8
  boat, ship, watercraft (causing drowning,
    submersion) E830 ☑
    causing injury except drowning, submersion
      E831 ☑
  by other person
    in accidental circumstances — *see* category
      E910 ☑
    intentional, homicidal E964
    stated as undetermined whether due to
      accidental or intentional E984
  due to
    accident
      machinery — *see* Accident, machine
      to boat, ship, watercraft E830 ☑
      transport — *see* categories E800-E848 ☑
    avalanche E909.2
    cataclysmic
      earth surface movement or eruption E909.9
      storm E908.9
    cloudburst E908.8
    cyclone E908.1

Submersion — *continued*
  due to — *continued*
    fall
      from
        boat, ship, watercraft (not involved in
          accident) E832 ☑
          burning, crushed E830 ☑
          involved in accident, collision
            E830 ☑
        gangplank (into water) E832 ☑
      overboard NEC E832 ☑
    flood E908.2
    hurricane E908.0
    jumping into water E910.8
      from boat, ship, watercraft
        burning, crushed, sinking E830 ☑
        involved in accident, collision E830 ☑
        not involved in accident, for swim
          E910.2
      in recreational activity (without diving
        equipment) E910.2
        with or using diving equipment E910.1
      to rescue another person E910.3
  homicide (attempt) E964
  in
    bathtub E910.4
    specified activity, not sport, transport or
      recreational E910.3
    sport or recreational activity (without diving
      equipment) E910.2
      with or using diving equipment E910.1
      water skiing E910.0
    swimming pool NEC E910.8
    terrorism E979.8
    war operations E995
    water transport E832 ☑
      due to accident to boat, ship, watercraft
        E830 ☑
  landslide E909.2
  overturning boat, ship, watercraft E909.2
  sinking boat, ship, watercraft E909.2
  submersion boat, ship, watercraft E909.2
  tidal wave E909.4
    caused by storm E908.0
  torrential rain E908.2
  late effect of NEC E929.8
  quenching tank E910.8
  self-inflicted (unspecified whether accidental or
    intentional) E984
    in accidental circumstances — *see* category
      E910 ☑
    stated as intentional, purposeful E954
  stated as undetermined whether accidental or
    intentional E984
  suicidal (attempted) E954
  while
    attempting rescue of another person E910.3
    engaged in
      marine salvage E910.3
      underwater construction or repairs
        E910.3
    fishing, not from boat E910.2
    hunting, not from boat E910.2
    ice skating E910.2
    pearl diving E910.3
    placing fishing nets E910.3
    playing in water E910.2
    scuba diving E910.1
      nonrecreational E910.3
    skin diving E910.1
    snorkel diving E910.2
    spear fishing underwater E910.1
    surfboarding E910.2
    swimming (swimming pool) E910.2
    wading (in water) E910.2
    water skiing E910.0
Sucked
  into
    jet (aircraft) E844 ☑
Suffocation (accidental) (by external means) (by
    pressure) (mechanical) E913.9
  caused by other person
    in accidental circumstances — *see category*
      E913 ☑

Suffocation — *continued*
  caused by other person — *continued*
    stated as
      intentional, homicidal E963
      undetermined whether accidental or
        intentional E983.9
      by, in
        hanging E983.0
        plastic bag E983.1
        specified means NEC E983.8
  due to, by
    avalanche E909.2
    bedclothes E913.0
    bib E913.0
    blanket E913.0
    cave-in E913.3
      caused by cataclysmic earth surface
        movement or eruption E909.9
    conflagration — *see* Conflagration
    explosion — *see* Explosion
    falling earth, other substance E913.3
    fire — *see* Fire
    food, any type (ingestion) (inhalation)
      (regurgitated) (vomited) E911
    foreign body, except food (ingestion)
      (inhalation) E912
    ignition — *see* Ignition
    landslide E909.2
    machine(ry) — *see* Accident, machine
    material, object except food entering by nose
      or mouth, ingested, inhaled E912
    mucus (aspiration) (inhalation), not of
      newborn E912
    phlegm (aspiration) (inhalation) E912
    pillow E913.0
    plastic bag — *see* Suffocation, in, plastic bag
    sheet (plastic) E913.0
    specified means NEC E913.8
    vomitus (aspiration) (inhalation) E911
  homicidal (attempt) E963
  in
    airtight enclosed place E913.2
    baby carriage E913.0
    bed E913.0
    closed place E913.2
    cot, cradle E913.0
    perambulator E913.0
    plastic bag (in accidental circumstances)
      E913.1
      homicidal, purposely inflicted by other
        person E963
      self-inflicted (unspecified whether
        accidental or intentional) E983.1
        in accidental circumstances E913.1
        intentional, suicidal E953.1
      stated as undetermined whether
        accidentally or purposely inflicted
        E983.1
      suicidal, purposely self-inflicted E953.1
    refrigerator E913.2
  self-inflicted — *see also* Suffocation, stated as
    undetermined whether accidental or
    intentional E953.9
    in accidental circumstances — *see* category
      E913 ☑
    stated as intentional, purposeful — *see*
      Suicide, suffocation
  stated as undetermined whether accidental or
    intentional E983.9
    by, in
      hanging E983.0
      plastic bag E983.1
      specified means NEC E983.8
  suicidal — *see* Suicide, suffocation
Suicide, suicidal (attempted) (by) E958.9
  burning, burns E958.1
  caustic substance E958.7
    poisoning E950.7
    swallowed E950.7
  cold, extreme E958.3
  cut (any part of body) E956
  cutting or piercing instrument (classifiable to
    E920) E956
  drowning E954
  electrocution E958.4
  explosive(s) (classifiable to E923) E955.5
  fire E958.1

☑ Additional Digit Required   ▶◀ Revised Text   ● New Line   ▲ Revised Code

Suicide, suicidal — *continued*
  firearm (classifiable to E922) — *see* Shooting,
      suicidal
  hanging E953.0
  jumping
      before moving object, train, vehicle E958.0
      from high place — *see* Jumping, from, high
          place, stated as, suicidal
  knife E956
  late effect of E959
  motor vehicle, crashing of E958.5
  poisoning — *see* Table of Drugs and Chemicals
  puncture (any part of body) E956
  scald E958.2
  shooting — *see* Shooting, suicidal
  specified means NEC E958.8
  stab (any part of body) E956
  strangulation — *see* Suicide, suffocation
  submersion E954
  suffocation E953.9
      by, in
          hanging E953.0
          plastic bag E953.1
          specified means NEC E953.8
  wound NEC E958.9
Sunburn E926.2
Sunstroke E900.0
Supersonic waves (causing injury) E928.1
Surgical procedure, complication of
  delayed or as an abnormal reaction without
      mention of misadventure — *see* Reaction,
      abnormal
  due to or as a result of misadventure — *see*
      Misadventure
Swallowed, swallowing
  foreign body — *see* Foreign body, alimentary
      canal
  poison — *see* Table of Drugs and Chemicals
  substance
      caustic — *see* Table of Drugs and Chemicals
      corrosive — *see* Table or drugs and
          chemicals
      poisonous — *see* Table of Drugs and
          Chemicals
Swimmers cramp (*see also* category E910 ☑)
      E910.2
  not in recreation or sport E910.3
Syndrome, battered
  baby or child — *see* Abuse, child
  wife — *see* Assault

T

Tackle in sport E886.0
Terrorism (injury) (by) (in) E979.8
  air blast E979.2
  aircraft burned, destroyed, exploded, shot
      down E979.1
      used as a weapon E979.1
  anthrax E979.6
  asphyxia from
      chemical (weapons) E979.7
      fire, conflagration (caused by fire-producing
          device) E979.3
          from nuclear explosion E979.5
      gas or fumes E979.7
  bayonet E979.8
  biological agents E979.6
  blast (air) (effects) E979.2
      from nuclear explosion E979.5
      underwater E979.0
  bomb (antipersonnel) (mortar) (explosion)
      (fragments) E979.2
  bullet(s) (from carbine, machine gun, pistol,
      rifle, shotgun) E979.4
  burn from
      chemical E979.7
      fire, conflagration (caused by fire-producing
          device) E979.3
          from nuclear explosion E979.5
      gas E979.7
  burning aircraft E979.1
  chemical E979.7
  cholera E979.6
  conflagration E979.3
  crushed by falling aircraft E979.1

Terrorism — *continued*
  depth-charge E979.0
  destruction of aircraft E979.1
  disability, as sequelae one year or more after
      injury E999.1
  drowning E979.8
  effect
      of nuclear weapon (direct) (secondary)
          E979.5
      secondary NEC E979.9
      sequelae E999.1
  explosion (artillery shell) (breech-block) (cannon
      block) E979.2
      aircraft E979.1
      bomb (antipersonnel) (mortar) E979.2
          nuclear (atom) (hydrogen) E979.5
      depth-charge E979.0
      grenade E979.2
      injury by fragments from E979.2
      land-mine E979.2
      marine weapon E979.0
      mine (land) E979.2
          at sea or in harbor E979.0
          marine E979.0
      missile (explosive) NEC E979.2
      munitions (dump) (factory) E979.2
      nuclear (weapon) E979.5
          other direct and secondary effects of
              E979.5
      sea-based artillery shell E979.0
      torpedo E979.0
  exposure to ionizing radiation from nuclear
      explosion E979.5
  falling aircraft E979.1
  fire or fire-producing device E979.3
  firearms E979.4
  fireball effects from nuclear explosion E979.5
  fragments from artillery shell, bomb NEC,
      grenade, guided missile, land-mine,
      rocket, shell, shrapnel E979.2
  gas or fumes E979.7
  grenade (explosion) (fragments) E979.2
  guided missile (explosion) (fragments) E979.2
      nuclear E979.5
  heat from nuclear explosion E979.5
  hot substances E979.3
  hydrogen cyanide E979.7
  land-mine (explosion) (fragments) E979.2
  laser(s) E979.8
  late effect of E999.1
  lewisite E979.7
  lung irritant (chemical) (fumes) (gas) E979.7
  marine mine E979.0
  mine E979.2
      at sea E979.0
      in harbor E979.0
      land (explosion) (fragments) E979.2
      marine E979.0
  missile (explosion) (fragments) (guided) E979.2
      marine E979.0
      nuclear E979.5
  mortar bomb (explosion) (fragments) E979.2
  mustard gas E979.7
  nerve gas E979.7
  nuclear weapons E979.5
  pellets (shotgun) E979.4
  petrol bomb E979.3
  piercing object E979.8
  phosgene E979.7
  poisoning (chemical) (fumes) (gas) E979.7
  radiation, ioninizing from nuclear explosion
      E979.5
  rocket (explosion) (fragments) E979.2
  saber, sabre E979.8
  sarin E979.7
  screening smoke E979.7
  sequelae effect (of) E999.1
  shell (aircraft) (artillery) (cannon) (land-based)
      (explosion) (fragments) E979.2
      sea-based E979.0
  shooting E979.4
      bullet(s) E979.4
      pellet(s) (rifle) (shotgun) E979.4
  shrapnel E979.2

Terrorism — *continued*
  smallpox E979.7
  stabbing object(s) E979.8
  submersion E979.8
  torpedo E979.0
  underwater blast E979.0
  vesicant (chemical) (fumes) (gas) E979.7
  weapon burst E979.2
Thermic fever E900.9
Thermoplegia E900.9
Thirst — *see also* Lack of water
  resulting from accident connected with
      transport — *see* categories E800-E848 ☑
Thrown (accidently)
  against object in or part of vehicle
      by motion of vehicle
          aircraft E844 ☑
          boat, ship, watercraft E838 ☑
          motor vehicle (on public highway)
              E818 ☑
              not on public highway E825 ☑
              off-road type (not on public highway)
                  E821 ☑
                  on public highway E818 ☑
                  snow vehicle E820 ☑
                      on public high-way E818 ☑
          nonmotor road vehicle NEC E829 ☑
          railway rolling stock, train, vehicle E806 ☑
          street car E829 ☑
  from
      animal (being ridden) (in sport or transport)
          E828 ☑
      high place, homicide (attempt) E968.1
      machinery — *see* Accident, machine
      vehicle NEC — *see* Accident, vehicle NEC
  off — *see* Thrown, from
  overboard (by motion of boat, ship, watercraft)
      E832 ☑
      by accident to boat, ship, watercraft E830 ☑
Thunderbolt NEC E907
Tidal wave (any injury) E909.4
  caused by storm E908.0
Took
  overdose of drug — *see* Table of Drugs and
      Chemicals
  poison — *see* Table of Drugs and Chemicals
Tornado (any injury) E908.1
Torrential rain (any injury) E908.2
Traffic accident NEC E819 ☑
Trampled by animal E906.8
  being ridden (in sport or transport) E828 ☑
Trapped (accidently)
  between
      objects (moving) (stationary and moving)
          E918
  by
      door of
          elevator E918
          motor vehicle (on public highway) (while
              alighting, boarding) — *see* Fall,
              from, motor vehicle, while alighting
          railway train (underground) E806 ☑
          street car E829 ☑
          subway train E806 ☑
      in object E918
Travel (effects) E903
  sickness E903
Tree
  falling on or hitting E916
      motor vehicle (in motion) (on public
          highway) E818 ☑
          not on public highway E825 ☑
      nonmotor road vehicle NEC E829 ☑
      pedal cycle E826 ☑
      person E916
      railway rolling stock, train, vehicle E806 ☑
      street car E829 ☑
Trench foot E901.0
**Tripping over animal, carpet, curb, rug, or
  small object** (with fall) E885 ☑
  without fall — *see* Striking against, object

☑ Additional Digit Required   ▶◀ Revised Text   ● New Line   ▲ Revised Code

Tsunami E909.4
Twisting, injury in E927

V

Violence, nonaccidental (*see also* Assault) E968.9
Volcanic eruption (any injury) E909.1
Vomitus in air passages (with asphyxia, obstruction or suffocation) E911

W

War operations (during hostilities) (injury) (by) (in) E995
after cessation of hostilities, injury due to E998
air blast E993
aircraft burned, destroyed, exploded, shot down E994
asphyxia from
chemical E997.2
fire, conflagration (caused by fire producing device or conventional weapon) E990.9
from nuclear explosion E996
petrol bomb E990.0
fumes E997.2
gas E997.2
battle wound NEC E995
bayonet E995
biological warfare agents E997.1
blast (air) (effects) E993
from nuclear explosion E996
underwater E992
bomb (mortar) (explosion) E993
after cessation of hostilities E998
fragments, injury by E991.9
antipersonnel E991.3
bullet(s) (from carbine, machine gun, pistol, rifle, shotgun) E991.2
rubber E991.0
burn from
chemical E997.2
fire, conflagration (caused by fire-producing device or conventional weapon) E990.9
from nuclear explosion E996
petrol bomb E990.0
gas E997.2
burning aircraft E994
chemical E997.2
chlorine E997.2
conventional warfare, specified from NEC E995
crushing by falling aircraft E994
depth charge E992
destruction of aircraft E994
disability as sequela one year or more after injury E999.0
drowning E995
effect (direct) (secondary) nuclear weapon E996
explosion (artillery shell) (breech block) (cannon shell) E993
after cessation of hostilities of bomb, mine placed in war E998
aircraft E994
bomb (mortar) E993
atom E996
hydrogen E996
injury by fragments from E991.9
antipersonnel E991.3
nuclear E996
depth charge E992
injury by fragments from E991.9
antipersonnel E991.3
marine weapon E992
mine
at sea or in harbor E992
land E993
injury by fragments from E991.9
marine E992
munitions (accidental) (being used in war) (dump) (factory) E993
nuclear (weapon) E996
own weapons (accidental) E993
injury by fragments from E991.9
antipersonnel E991.3
sea-based artillery shell E992
torpedo E992

War operations — *continued*
exposure to ionizing radiation from nuclear explosion E996
falling aircraft E994
fire or fire-producing device E990.9
petrol bomb E990.0
fireball effects from nuclear explosion E996
fragments from
antipersonnel bomb E991.3
artillery shell, bomb NEC, grenade, guided missile, land mine, rocket, shell, shrapnel E991.9
fumes E997.2
gas E997.2
grenade (explosion) E993
fragments, injury by E991.9
guided missile (explosion) E993
fragments, injury by E991.9
nuclear E996
heat from nuclear explosion E996
injury due to, but occurring after cessation of hostilities E998
lacrimator (gas) (chemical) E997.2
land mine (explosion) E993
after cessation of hostilities E998
fragments, injury by E991.9
laser(s) E997.0
late effect of E999.0
lewisite E997.2
lung irritant (chemical) (fumes) (gas) E997.2
marine mine E992
mine
after cessation of hostilities E998
at sea E992
in harbor E992
land (explosion) E993
fragments, injury by E991.9
marine E992
missile (guided) (explosion) E993
fragments, injury by E991.9
marine E992
nuclear E996
mortar bomb (explosion) E993
fragments, injury by E991.9
mustard gas E997.2
nerve gas E997.2
phosgene E997.2
poisoning (chemical) (fumes) (gas) E997.2
radiation, ionizing from nuclear explosion E996
rocket (explosion) E993
fragments, injury by E991.9
saber, sabre E995
screening smoke E997.8
shell (aircraft) (artillery) (cannon) (land based) (explosion) E993
fragments, injury by E991.9
sea-based E992
shooting E991.2
after cessation of hostilities E998
bullet(s) E991.2
rubber E991.0
pellet(s) (rifle) E991.1
shrapnel E991.9
submersion E995
torpedo E992
unconventional warfare, except by nuclear weapon E997.9
biological (warfare) E997.1
gas, fumes, chemicals E997.2
laser(s) E997.0
specified type NEC E997.8
underwater blast E992
vesicant (chemical) (fumes) (gas) E997.2
weapon burst E993

Washed
away by flood — *see* Flood
away by tidal wave — *see* Tidal wave
off road by storm (transport vehicle) E908.9
overboard E832 ☑

Weather exposure — *see also* Exposure
cold E901.0
hot E900.0

Weightlessness (causing injury) (effects of) (in spacecraft, real or simulated) E928.0

Wound (accidental) NEC (*see also* Injury) E928.9
battle (*see also* War operations) E995
bayonet E920.3
in
legal intervention E974
war operations E995
gunshot — *see* Shooting
incised — *see* Cut
saber, sabre E920.3
in war operations E995

☑ Additional Digit Required   ►◄ Revised Text   ● New Line   ▲ Revised Code

Railway Accidents (E800-E807)

The following fourth-digit subdivisions are for use with categories E800-E807 to identify the injured person:

.0 Railway employee
Any person who by virtue of his employment in connection with a railway, whether by the railway company or not, is at increased risk of involvement in a railway accident, such as:
　　catering staff on train
　　postal staff on train
　　driver
　　railway fireman
　　guard
　　shunter
　　porter
　　sleeping car attendant

.1 Passenger on railway
Any authorized person traveling on a train, except a railway employee
　　EXCLUDES intending passenger waiting at station (.8)
　　　　　　　unauthorized rider on railway vehicle (.8)

.2 Pedestrian See definition (r), E-Codes-2

.3 Pedal cyclist See definition (p), E-Codes-2

.8 Other specified person Intending passenger waiting at station
Unauthorized rider on railway vehicle

.9 Unspecified person

Motor Vehicle Traffic and Nontraffic Accidents (E810-E825)

The following fourth-digit subdivisions are for use with categories E810-E819 and E820-E825 to identify the injured person:

.0 Driver of motor vehicle other than motorcycle See definition (1), E-Codes-2

.1 Passenger in motor vehicle other than motorcycle See definition (1), E-Codes-2

.2 Motorcyclist See definition (1), E-Codes-2

.3 Passenger on motorcycle See definition (1), E-Codes-2

.4 Occupant of streetcar

.5 Rider of animal; occupant of animal-drawn vehicle

.6 Pedal cyclist See definition (p), E-Codes-2

.7 Pedestrian See definition (r), E-Codes-2

.8 Other specified person
Occupant of vehicle other than above
Person in railway train involved in accident
Unauthorized rider of motor vehicle

.9 Unspecified person

Other Road Vehicle Accidents (E826-E829)

(animal-drawn vehicle, streetcar, pedal cycle, and other nonmotor road vehicle accidents)

The following fourth-digit subdivisions are for use with categories E826-E829 to identify the injured person:

.0 Pedestrian See definition (r), E-Codes-2

.1 Pedal cyclist (does not apply to codes E827, E828, E829) See definition (p), E-Codes-2

.2 Rider of animal (does not apply to code E829)

.3 Occupant of animal-drawn vehicle (does not apply to codes E828, E829)

.4 Occupant of streetcar

.8 Other specified person

.9 Unspecified person

Water Transport Accidents (E830-E838)

The following fourth-digit subdivisions are for use with categories E830-E838 to identify the injured person:

.0 Occupant of small boat, unpowered

.1 Occupant of small boat, powered See definition (t), E-Codes-2
　　EXCLUDES water skier (.4)

.2 Occupant of other watercraft — crew
Persons:
　　engaged in operation of watercraft
　　providing passenger services [cabin attendants, ship's physician, catering personnel]
　　working on ship during voyage in other capacity [musician in band, operators of shops and beauty parlors]

.3 Occupant of other watercraft — other than crew
Passenger
Occupant of lifeboat, other than crew, after abandoning ship

.4 Water skier

.5 Swimmer

.6 Dockers, stevedores
Longshoreman employed on the dock in loading and unloading ships

.8 Other specified person
Immigration and custom officials on board ship
Persons:
　　accompanying passenger or member of crew visiting boat
Pilot (guiding ship into port)

.9 Unspecified person

Air and Space Transport Accidents (E840-E845)

The following fourth-digit subdivisions are for use with categories E840-E845 to identify the injured person:

.0 Occupant of spacecraft

```
Crew
Passenger (civilian)  }  in military aircraft [air force]
(military)                [army] [national guard] [navy]
Troops
```

.1 Occupant of military aircraft, any
　　EXCLUDES occupants of aircraft operated under jurisdiction of police departments (.5) parachutist (.7)

.2 Crew of commercial aircraft (powered) in surface to surface transport

.3 Other occupant of commercial aircraft (powered) in surface to surface transport
Flight personnel:
　　not part of crew
　　on familiarization flight
Passenger on aircraft

.4 Occupant of commercial aircraft (powered) in surface to air transport
Occupant [crew] [passenger] of aircraft (powered) engaged in activities, such as:
　　air drops of emergency supplies
　　air drops of parachutists, except from military craft
　　crop dusting
　　lowering of construction material [bridge or telephone pole]
　　sky writing

.5 Occupant of other powered aircraft
Occupant [crew] [passenger] of aircraft (powered) engaged in activities, such as:
　　aerial spraying (crops) (fire retardants)
　　aerobatic flying
　　aircraft racing
　　rescue operation
　　storm surveillance
　　traffic suveillance
Occupant of private plane NOS

.6 Occupant of unpowered aircraft, except parachutist
Occupant of aircraft classifiable to E842

.7 Parachutist (military) (other)
Person making voluntary descent
　　person making descent after accident to aircraft (.1-.6)

.8 Ground crew, airline employee
Persons employed at airfields (civil) (military) or launching pads, not occupants of aircraft

.9 Other person

☑ Additional Digit Required　　　◄► Revised Text　　　● New Line　　　▲ Revised Code

1. INFECTIOUS AND PARASITIC DISEASES (001-139)

Note: Categories for "late effects" of infectious and parasitic diseases are to be found at 137-139.

INCLUDES   diseases generally recognized as communicable or transmissible as well as a few diseases of unknown but possibly infectious origin

EXCLUDES   *acute respiratory infections (460-466)*
carrier or suspected carrier of infectious organism (V02.0-V02.9)
certain localized infections
influenza (487.0-487.8)

INTESTINAL INFECTIOUS DISEASES (001-009)

EXCLUDES   *helminthiases (120.0-129)*

√4ᵗʰ 001 Cholera

DEF: An acute infectious enteritis caused by a potent enterotoxin elaborated by *Vibrio cholerae*; the vibrio produces a toxin in the intestinal tract that changes the permeability of the mucosa leading to diarrhea and dehydration.

001.0   Due to Vibrio cholerae
001.1   Due to Vibrio cholerae el tor
001.9   Cholera, unspecified

√4ᵗʰ 002 Typhoid and paratyphoid fevers

DEF: Typhoid fever: an acute generalized illness caused by *Salmonella typhi*; notable clinical features are fever, headache, abdominal pain, cough, toxemia, leukopenia, abnormal pulse, rose spots on the skin, bacteremia, hyperplasia of intestinal lymph nodes, mesenteric lymphadenopathy, and Peyer's patches in the intestines.

DEF: Paratyphoid fever: a prolonged febrile illness, much like typhoid but usually less severe; caused by salmonella serotypes other than *S. typhi*, especially *S. enteritidis* serotypes paratyphi A and B and S. *choleraesuis*.

002.0   Typhoid fever
Typhoid (fever) (infection) [any site]
002.1   Paratyphoid fever A
002.2   Paratyphoid fever B
002.3   Paratyphoid fever C
002.9   Paratyphoid fever, unspecified

√4ᵗʰ 003 Other salmonella infections

INCLUDES   infection or food poisoning by Salmonella [any serotype]

DEF: Infections caused by a genus of gram-negative, anaerobic bacteria of the family *Enterobacteriaceae*; affecting warm-blooded animals, like humans; major symptoms are enteric fevers, acute gastroenteritis and septicemia.

003.0   Salmonella gastroenteritis
Salmonellosis
003.1   Salmonella septicemia
√5ᵗʰ 003.2   Localized salmonella infections
    003.20 Localized salmonella infection, unspecified
    003.21 Salmonella meningitis
    003.22 Salmonella pneumonia
    003.23 Salmonella arthritis
    003.24 Salmonella osteomyelitis
    003.29 Other
003.8   Other specified salmonella infections
003.9   Salmonella infection, unspecified

√4ᵗʰ 004 Shigellosis

INCLUDES   bacillary dysentery

DEF: Acute infectious dysentery caused by the genus *Shigella*, of the family *Enterobacteriaceae*; affecting the colon causing the release of blood-stained stools with accompanying tenesmus, abdominal cramps and fever.

004.0   Shigella dysenteriae
Infection by group A Shigella (Schmitz) (Shiga)
004.1   Shigella flexneri
Infection by group B Shigella
004.2   Shigella boydii
Infection by group C Shigella

004.3   Shigella sonnei
Infection by group D Shigella
004.8   Other specified Shigella infections
004.9   Shigellosis, unspecified

√4ᵗʰ 005 Other food poisoning (bacterial)

EXCLUDES   *salmonella infections (003.0-003.9)*
toxic effect of:
food contaminants (989.7)
noxious foodstuffs (988.0-988.9)

DEF: Enteritis caused by ingesting contaminated foods and characterized by diarrhea, abdominal pain, vomiting; symptoms may be mild or life threatening.

005.0   Staphylococcal food poisoning
Staphylococcal toxemia specified as due to food
005.1   Botulism
Food poisoning due to Clostridium botulinum
005.2   Food poisoning due to Clostridium perfringens [C. welchii]
Enteritis necroticans
005.3   Food poisoning due to other Clostridia
005.4   Food poisoning due to Vibrio parahaemolyticus
√5ᵗʰ 005.8   Other bacterial food poisoning
    EXCLUDES   *salmonella food poisoning (003.0-003.9)*
    005.81 Food poisoning due to Vibrio vulnificus
    005.89 Other bacterial food poisoning
        Food poisoning due to Bacillus cereus
005.9   Food poisoning, unspecified

√4ᵗʰ 006 Amebiasis

INCLUDES   infection due to Entamoeba histolytica
EXCLUDES   *amebiasis due to organisms other than Entamoeba histolytica (007.8)*

DEF: Infection of the large intestine caused by *Entamoeba histolytica*; usually asymptomatic but symptoms may range from mild diarrhea to profound life-threatening dysentery. Extraintestinal complications include hepatic abscess, which may rupture into the lung, pericardium or abdomen, causing life-threatening infections.

006.0   Acute amebic dysentery without mention of abscess
Acute amebiasis
006.1   Chronic intestinal amebiasis without mention of abscess
    Chronic: Chronic:
        amebiasis   amebic dysentery
006.2   Amebic nondysenteric colitis
    DEF: *Entamoeba histolytica* infection with inflamed colon but no dysentery.
006.3   Amebic liver abscess
    Hepatic amebiasis
006.4   Amebic lung abscess
    Amebic abscess of lung (and liver)
006.5   Amebic brain abscess
    Amebic abscess of brain (and liver) (and lung)
006.6   Amebic skin ulceration
    Cutaneous amebiasis
006.8   Amebic infection of other sites
    Amebic: Ameboma
        appendicitis
        balanitis
    EXCLUDES   *specific infections by free-living amebae (136.2)*
006.9   Amebiasis, unspecified
    Amebiasis NOS

√4ᵗʰ 007 Other protozoal intestinal diseases

INCLUDES   protozoal: protozoal:
            colitis   dysentery
            diarrhea

007.0   Balantidiasis
    Infection by Balantidium coli
007.1   Giardiasis
    Infection by Giardia lamblia   Lambliasis

√4ᵗʰ
√5ᵗʰ Additional Digit Required   Unspecified Code   Other Specified Code   Manifestation Code   ►◄ Revised Text   ● New Code   ▲ Revised Code Title

007.2 Coccidiosis
Infection by Isospora belli and Isospora hominis
Isosporiasis

007.3 Intestinal trichomoniasis
DEF: Colitis, diarrhea, or dysentery caused by the protozoa *Trichomonas.*

007.4 Cryptosporidiosis
AHA: 4Q, '97, 30

DEF: An intestinal infection by protozoan parasites causing intractable diarrhea in patients with AIDS and other immunosuppressed individuals.

007.5 Cyclosporiasis
AHA: 4Q, '00, 38

DEF: An infection of the small intestine by the protozoal organism, *Cyclospora caytenanesis,* spread to humans though ingestion of contaminated water or food. Symptoms include watery diarrhea with frequent explosive bowel movements, loss of appetite, loss of weight, bloating, increased gas, stomach cramps, nausea, vomiting, muscle aches, low grade fever, and fatigue.

007.8 Other specified protozoal intestinal diseases
Amebiasis due to organisms other than Entamoeba histolytica

007.9 Unspecified protozoal intestinal disease
Flagellate diarrhea
Protozoal dysentery NOS

√4ᵗʰ 008 Intestinal infections due to other organisms
INCLUDES   any condition classifiable to 009.0-009.3 with mention of the responsible organisms
EXCLUDES   *food poisoning by these organisms (005.0-005.9)*

√5ᵗʰ 008.0 Escherichia coli [E. coli]
AHA: 4Q, '92, 17

008.00 E. coli, unspecified
E. coli enteritis NOS

008.01 Enteropathogenic E. coli
DEF: E. coli causing inflammation of intestines.

008.02 Enterotoxigenic E. coli
DEF: A toxic reaction to E. coli of the intestinal mucosa, causing voluminous watery secretions.

008.03 Enteroinvasive E. coli
DEF: E. coli infection penetrating intestinal mucosa.

008.04 Enterohemorrhagic E. coli
DEF: E. coli infection penetrating the intestinal mucosa, producing microscopic ulceration and bleeding.

008.09 Other intestinal E. coli infections

008.1 Arizona group of paracolon bacilli

008.2 Aerobacter aerogenes
Enterobacter aeogenes

008.3 Proteus (mirabilis) (morganii)

√5ᵗʰ 008.4 Other specified bacteria
AHA: 4Q, '92, 18

008.41 Staphylococcus
Staphylococcal enterocolitis

008.42 Pseudomonas
AHA: 2Q, '89, 10

008.43 Campylobacter

008.44 Yersinia enterocolitica

008.45 Clostridium difficile
Pseudomembranous colitis
DEF: An overgrowth of a species of bacterium that is a part of the normal colon flora in human infants and sometimes in adults; produces a toxin that causes pseudomembranous enterocolitis; typically is seen in patients undergoing antibiotic therapy.

008.46 Other anaerobes
Anaerobic enteritis NOS
Bacteroides (fragilis)
Gram-negative anaerobes

008.47 Other gram-negative bacteria
Gram-negative enteritis NOS
EXCLUDES   *gram-negative anaerobes (008.46)*

008.49 Other
AHA: 2Q, '89, 10; 1Q, '88, 6

008.5 Bacterial enteritis, unspecified

√5ᵗʰ 008.6 Enteritis due to specified virus
AHA: 4Q, '92, 18

008.61 Rotavirus

008.62 Adenovirus

008.63 Norwalk virus
Norwalk-like agent

008.64 Other small round viruses [SRVs]
Small round virus NOS

008.65 Calicivirus
DEF: Enteritis due to a subgroup of *Picornaviruses.*

008.66 Astrovirus

008.67 Enterovirus NEC
Coxsackie virus Echovirus
EXCLUDES   *poliovirus (045.0-045.9)*

008.69 Other viral enteritis
Torovirus
AHA: 1Q, '03,10

008.8 Other organism, not elsewhere classified
Viral:
  enteritis NOS
  gastroenteritis
EXCLUDES   *influenza with involvement of gastrointestinal tract (487.8)*

√4ᵗʰ 009 Ill-defined intestinal infections
EXCLUDES   *diarrheal disease or intestinal infection due to specified organism (001.0-008.8)*
diarrhea following gastrointestinal surgery (564.4)
intestinal malabsorption (579.0-579.9)
ischemic enteritis (557.0-557.9)
other noninfectious gastroenteritis and colitis (558.1-558.9)
regional enteritis (555.0-555.9)
ulcerative colitis (556)

009.0 Infectious colitis, enteritis, and gastroenteritis
Colitis ⎫
Enteritis ⎬ septic
Gastroenteritis ⎭

Dysentery:
  NOS
  catarrhal
  hemorrhagic
AHA: 3Q, '99, 4

DEF: Colitis: An inflammation of mucous membranes of the colon.

DEF: Enteritis: An inflammation of mucous membranes of the small intestine.

DEF: Gastroenteritis: An inflammation of mucous membranes of stomach and intestines.

009.1 Colitis, enteritis, and gastroenteritis of presumed infectious origin
EXCLUDES   *colitis NOS (558.9)*
enteritis NOS (558.9)
gastroenteritis NOS (558.9)
AHA: 3Q, '99, 6

009.2 Infectious diarrhea
Diarrhea:
dysenteric
epidemic
Infectious diarrheal disease NOS

009.3 Diarrhea of presumed infectious origin
EXCLUDES   diarrhea NOS (787.91)

AHA: N-D, '87, 7

TUBERCULOSIS (010-018)

INCLUDES   infection by Mycobacterium tuberculosis
(human) (bovine)

EXCLUDES   congenital tuberculosis (771.2)
late effects of tuberculosis (137.0-137.4)

The following fifth-digit subclassification is for use with
categories 010-018:

  0   **unspecified**
  1   **bacteriological or histological examination not
done**
  2   **bacteriological or histological examination
unknown (at present)**
  3   **tubercle bacilli found (in sputum) by
microscopy**
  4   **tubercle bacilli not found (in sputum) by
microscopy, but found by bacterial culture**
  5   **tubercle bacilli not found by bacteriological
examination, but tuberculosis confirmed
histologically**
  6   **tubercle bacilli not found by bacteriological or
histological examination but tuberculosis
confirmed by other methods [inoculation of
animals]**

DEF: An infection by *Mycobacterium tuberculosis* causing the formation of
small, rounded nodules, called tubercles, that can disseminate throughout the
body via lymph and blood vessels. Localized tuberculosis is most often seen
in the lungs.

✓4th **010 Primary tuberculous infection**
DEF: Tuberculosis of the lungs occurring when the patient is first infected.

✓5th **010.0 Primary tuberculous infection**
EXCLUDES   nonspecific reaction to tuberculin skin
test without active tuberculosis
(795.5)
positive PPD (795.5)
positive tuberculin skin test without
active tuberculosis (795.5)

DEF: Hilar or paratracheal lymph node enlargement in pulmonary
tuberculosis.

✓5th **010.1 Tuberculous pleurisy in primary progressive
tuberculosis**
DEF: Inflammation and exudation in the lining of the tubercular
lung.

✓5th **010.8 Other primary progressive tuberculosis**
EXCLUDES   tuberculous erythema nodosum (017.1)

✓5th **010.9 Primary tuberculous infection, unspecified**

✓4th **011 Pulmonary tuberculosis**
Use additional code to identify any associated silicosis (502)

✓5th **011.0 Tuberculosis of lung, infiltrative**

✓5th **011.1 Tuberculosis of lung, nodular**

✓5th **011.2 Tuberculosis of lung with cavitation**

✓5th **011.3 Tuberculosis of bronchus**
EXCLUDES   isolated bronchial tuberculosis (012.2)

✓5th **011.4 Tuberculous fibrosis of lung**

✓5th **011.5 Tuberculous bronchiectasis**

✓5th **011.6 Tuberculous pneumonia [any form]**
DEF: Inflammatory pulmonary reaction to tuberculous cells.

✓5th **011.7 Tuberculous pneumothorax**
DEF: Spontaneous rupture of damaged tuberculous pulmonary
tissue.

✓5th **011.8 Other specified pulmonary tuberculosis**

✓5th **011.9 Pulmonary tuberculosis, unspecified**
Respiratory tuberculosis NOS
Tuberculosis of lung NOS

✓4th **012 Other respiratory tuberculosis**
EXCLUDES   respiratory tuberculosis, unspecified (011.9)

✓5th **012.0 Tuberculous pleurisy**
Tuberculosis of pleura
Tuberculous empyema
Tuberculous hydrothorax
EXCLUDES   pleurisy with effusion without mention
of cause (511.9)
tuberculous pleurisy in primary
progressive tuberculosis (010.1)

DEF: Inflammation and exudation in the lining of the tubercular
lung.

✓5th **012.1 Tuberculosis of intrathoracic lymph nodes**
Tuberculosis of lymph nodes:
hilar
mediastinal
tracheobronchial
Tuberculous tracheobronchial adenopathy
EXCLUDES   that specified as primary (010.0-010.9)

✓5th **012.2 Isolated tracheal or bronchial tuberculosis**

✓5th **012.3 Tuberculous laryngitis**
Tuberculosis of glottis

✓5th **012.8 Other specified respiratory tuberculosis**
Tuberculosis of: Tuberculosis of:
mediastinum   nose (septum)
nasopharynx   sinus [any nasal]

✓4th **013 Tuberculosis of meninges and central nervous system**

✓5th **013.0 Tuberculous meningitis**
Tuberculosis of meninges (cerebral) (spinal)
Tuberculous:
leptomeningitis
meningoencephalitis
EXCLUDES   tuberculoma of meninges (013.1)

✓5th **013.1 Tuberculoma of meninges**

✓5th **013.2 Tuberculoma of brain**
Tuberculosis of brain (current disease)

✓5th **013.3 Tuberculous abscess of brain**

✓5th **013.4 Tuberculoma of spinal cord**

✓5th **013.5 Tuberculous abscess of spinal cord**

✓5th **013.6 Tuberculous encephalitis or myelitis**

✓5th **013.8 Other specified tuberculosis of central nervous
system**

✓5th **013.9 Unspecified tuberculosis of central nervous
system**
Tuberculosis of central nervous system NOS

✓4th **014 Tuberculosis of intestines, peritoneum, and mesenteric
glands**

✓5th **014.0 Tuberculous peritonitis**
Tuberculous ascites
DEF: Tuberculous inflammation of the membrane lining the
abdomen.

✓5th **014.8 Other**
Tuberculosis (of):
anus
intestine (large) (small)
mesenteric glands
rectum
retroperitoneal (lymph nodes)
Tuberculous enteritis

✓4th
✓5th   Additional Digit Required   Unspecified Code   Other Specified Code   Manifestation Code   ▶◀ Revised Text   ● New Code   ▲ Revised Code Title

2005 ICD•9•CM   **Volume 1 — 3**

✓4ᵗʰ **015 Tuberculosis of bones and joints**
Use additional code to identify manifestation, as:
tuberculous:
arthropathy (711.4)
necrosis of bone (730.8)
osteitis (730.8)
osteomyelitis (730.8)
synovitis (727.01)
tenosynovitis (727.01)

§ ✓5ᵗʰ **015.0 Vertebral column**
Pott's disease
Use additional code to identify manifestation, as:
curvature of spine [Pott's] (737.4)
kyphosis (737.4)
spondylitis (720.81)

§ ✓5ᵗʰ **015.1 Hip**

§ ✓5ᵗʰ **015.2 Knee**

§ ✓5ᵗʰ **015.5 Limb bones**
Tuberculous dactylitis

§ ✓5ᵗʰ **015.6 Mastoid**
Tuberculous mastoiditis

§ ✓5ᵗʰ **015.7 Other specified bone**

§ ✓5ᵗʰ **015.8 Other specified joint**

§ ✓5ᵗʰ **015.9 Tuberculosis of unspecified bones and joints**

✓4ᵗʰ **016 Tuberculosis of genitourinary system**

§ ✓5ᵗʰ **016.0 Kidney**
Renal tuberculosis
Use additional code to identify manifestation, as:
tuberculous:
nephropathy (583.81)
pyelitis (590.81)
pyelonephritis (590.81)

§ ✓5ᵗʰ **016.1 Bladder**

§ ✓5ᵗʰ **016.2 Ureter**

§ ✓5ᵗʰ **016.3 Other urinary organs**

§ ✓5ᵗʰ **016.4 Epididymis**   ♂

§ ✓5ᵗʰ **016.5 Other male genital organs**   ♂
Use additional code to identify manifestation, as:
tuberculosis of:
prostate (601.4)
seminal vesicle (608.81)
testis (608.81)

§ ✓5ᵗʰ **016.6 Tuberculous oophoritis and salpingitis**   ♀

§ ✓5ᵗʰ **016.7 Other female genital organs**   ♀
Tuberculous:
cervicitis
endometritis

§ ✓5ᵗʰ **016.9 Genitourinary tuberculosis, unspecified**

✓4ᵗʰ **017 Tuberculosis of other organs**

§ ✓5ᵗʰ **017.0 Skin and subcutaneous cellular tissue**

Lupus:	Tuberculosis:
exedens	cutis
vulgaris	lichenoides
Scrofuloderma	papulonecrotica
Tuberculosis:	verrucosa cutis
colliquativa	

EXCLUDES   *lupus erythematosus (695.4)*
disseminated (710.0)
lupus NOS (710.0)
nonspecific reaction to tuberculin skin
test without active tuberculosis
(795.5)
positive PPD (795.5)
positive tuberculin skin test without
active tuberculosis (795.5)

§ ✓5ᵗʰ **017.1 Erythema nodosum with hypersensitivity reaction in tuberculosis**

Bazin's disease	Erythema:
Erythema:	nodosum, tuberculous
induratum	Tuberculosis indurativa

EXCLUDES   *erythema nodosum NOS (695.2)*

DEF: Tender, inflammatory, bilateral nodules appearing on the shins and thought to be an allergic reaction to tuberculotoxin.

§ ✓5ᵗʰ **017.2 Peripheral lymph nodes**
Scrofula
Scrofulous abscess
Tuberculous adenitis
EXCLUDES   *tuberculosis of lymph nodes:*
bronchial and mediastinal (012.1)
mesenteric and retroperitoneal
(014.8)
tuberculous tracheobronchial
adenopathy (012.1)

DEF: Scrofula: Old name for tuberculous cervical lymphadenitis.

§ ✓5ᵗʰ **017.3 Eye**
Use additional code to identify manifestation, as:
tuberculous:
chorioretinitis, disseminated (363.13)
episcleritis (379.09)
interstitial keratitis (370.59)
iridocyclitis, chronic (364.11)
keratoconjunctivitis (phlyctenular) (370.31)

§ ✓5ᵗʰ **017.4 Ear**
Tuberculosis of ear
Tuberculous otitis media
EXCLUDES   *tuberculous mastoiditis (015.6)*

§ ✓5ᵗʰ **017.5 Thyroid gland**

§ ✓5ᵗʰ **017.6 Adrenal glands**
Addison's disease, tuberculous

§ ✓5ᵗʰ **017.7 Spleen**

§ ✓5ᵗʰ **017.8 Esophagus**

§ ✓5ᵗʰ **017.9 Other specified organs**
Use additional code to identify manifestation, as:
tuberculosis of:
endocardium [any valve] (424.91)
myocardium (422.0)
pericardium (420.0)

✓4ᵗʰ **018 Miliary tuberculosis**
INCLUDES   tuberculosis:
disseminated
generalized
miliary, whether of a single specified site,
multiple sites, or unspecified site
polyserositis

DEF: A form of tuberculosis caused by caseous material carried through the bloodstream planting seedlike tubercles in various body organs.

§ ✓5ᵗʰ **018.0 Acute miliary tuberculosis**

§ ✓5ᵗʰ **018.8 Other specified miliary tuberculosis**

§ ✓5ᵗʰ **018.9 Miliary tuberculosis, unspecified**

ZOONOTIC BACTERIAL DISEASES (020–027)

✓4ᵗʰ **020 Plague**
INCLUDES   infection by Yersinia [Pasteurella] pestis

020.0 Bubonic
DEF: Most common acute and severe form of plague characterized by lymphadenopathy (buboes), chills, fever and headache.

020.1 Cellulocutaneous
DEF: Plague characterized by inflammation and necrosis of skin.

020.2 Septicemic
DEF: Plague characterized by massive infection in the bloodstream.

---

§ Requires fifth-digit. See beginning of section 010–018 for codes and definitions.

N Newborn Age: 0   P Pediatric Age: 0-17   M Maternity Age: 12-55   A Adult Age: 15-124   MSP Medicare Secondary Payer

020.3 Primary pneumonic
DEF: Plague characterized by massive pulmonary infection.

020.4 Secondary pneumonic
DEF: Lung infection as a secondary complication of plague.

020.5 Pneumonic, unspecified

020.8 Other specified types of plague
Abortive plague   Pestis minor
Ambulatory plague

020.9 Plague, unspecified

✓4ᵗʰ **021 Tularemia**
INCLUDES   deerfly fever
infection by Francisella [Pasteurella] tularensis
rabbit fever

DEF: A febrile disease transmitted by the bites of deer flies, fleas and ticks, by inhalations of aerosolized *F. tuarensis* or by ingestion of contaminated food or water; patients quickly develop fever, chills, weakness, headache, backache and malaise.

021.0 Ulceroglandular tularemia
DEF: Lesions occur at the site *Francisella tularensis;* organism enters body, usually the fingers or hands.

021.1 Enteric tularemia
Tularemia: Tularemia:
cryptogenic   typhoidal
intestinal

021.2 Pulmonary tularemia
Bronchopneumonic tularemia

021.3 Oculoglandular tularemia
DEF: Painful conjunctival infection by *Francisella tularensis* organism with possible corneal, preauricular lymph, or lacrimal involvement.

021.8 Other specified tularemia
Tularemia:
generalized or disseminated
glandular

021.9 Unspecified tularemia

✓4ᵗʰ **022 Anthrax**
AHA: 4Q '02, 70

DEF: An infectious bacterial disease usually transmitted by contact with infected animals or their discharges or products; it is classified by primary routes of inoculation as cutaneous, gastrointestinal and by inhalation.

022.0 Cutaneous anthrax
Malignant pustule

022.1 Pulmonary anthrax
Respiratory anthrax   Wool-sorters' disease

022.2 Gastrointestinal anthrax

022.3 Anthrax septicemia

022.8 Other specified manifestations of anthrax

022.9 Anthrax, unspecified

✓4ᵗʰ **023 Brucellosis**
INCLUDES   fever:
Malta
Mediterranean
undulant

DEF: An infectious disease caused by gram-negative, *aerobic coccobacilli* organisms; it is transmitted to humans through contact with infected tissue or dairy products; fever, sweating, weakness and aching are symptoms of the disease.

023.0 Brucella melitensis
DEF: Infection from direct or indirect contact with infected sheep or goats.

023.1 Brucella abortus
DEF: Infection from direct or indirect contact with infected cattle.

023.2 Brucella suis
DEF: Infection from direct or indirect contact with infected swine.

023.3 Brucella canis
DEF: Infection from direct or indirect contact with infected dogs.

023.8 Other brucellosis
Infection by more than one organism

023.9 Brucellosis, unspecified

024 Glanders
Infection by:
Actinobacillus mallei
Malleomyces mallei
Pseudomonas mallei
Farcy
Malleus

DEF: Equine infection causing mucosal inflammation and skin ulcers in humans.

025 Melioidosis
Infection by:
Malleomyces pseudomallei
Pseudomonas pseudomallei
Whitmore's bacillus
Pseudoglanders

DEF: Rare infection caused by *Pseudomonas pseudomallei;* clinical symptoms range from localized infection to fatal septicemia.

✓4ᵗʰ **026 Rat-bite fever**

026.0 Spirillary fever
Rat-bite fever due to Spirillum minor [S. minus]
Sodoku

026.1 Streptobacillary fever
Epidemic arthritic erythema
Haverhill fever
Rat-bite fever due to Streptobacillus moniliformis

026.9 Unspecified rat-bite fever

✓4ᵗʰ **027 Other zoonotic bacterial diseases**

027.0 Listeriosis
Infection }
Septicemia } by Listeria monocytogenes

Use additional code to identify manifestation, as meningitis (320.7)
EXCLUDES   congenital listeriosis (771.2)

027.1 Erysipelothrix infection
Erysipeloid (of Rosenbach)
Infection } by Erysipelothrix insidiosa
Septicemia } [E. rhusiopathiae]

DEF: Usually associated with handling of fish, meat, or poultry; symptoms range from localized inflammation to septicemia.

027.2 Pasteurellosis
Pasteurella pseudotuberculosis infection
Mesenteric adenitis } by Pasteurella
Septic infection (cat bite) } multocida [P.
(dog bite) } septica]

EXCLUDES   infection by:
Francisella [Pasteurella] tularensis (021.0-021.9)
Yersinia [Pasteurella] pestis (020.0-020.9)

DEF: Swelling, abscesses, or septicemia from *Pasteurella multocida,* commonly transmitted to humans by a dog or cat scratch.

027.8 Other specified zoonotic bacterial diseases
027.9 Unspecified zoonotic bacterial disease

OTHER BACTERIAL DISEASES (030-041)
EXCLUDES   bacterial venereal diseases (098.0-099.9)
bartonellosis (088.0)

✓4ᵗʰ **030 Leprosy**
INCLUDES   Hansen's disease
infection by Mycobacterium leprae

Additional Digit Required | Unspecified Code | Other Specified Code | Manifestation Code | ▶◀ Revised Text | ● New Code | ▲ Revised Code Title

2005 ICD•9•CM | Volume 1 — 5

030.0 Lepromatous [type L]
Lepromatous leprosy (macular) (diffuse) (infiltrated) (nodular) (neuritic)

DEF: Infectious disseminated leprosy bacilli with lesions and deformities.

030.1 Tuberculoid [type T]
Tuberculoid leprosy (macular) (maculoanesthetic) (major) (minor) (neuritic)

DEF: Relatively benign, self-limiting leprosy with neuralgia and scales.

030.2 Indeterminate [group I]
Indeterminate [uncharacteristic] leprosy (macular) (neuritic)

DEF: Uncharacteristic leprosy, frequently an early manifestation.

030.3 Borderline [group B]
Borderline or dimorphous leprosy (infiltrated) (neuritic)

DEF: Transitional form of leprosy, neither lepromatous nor tuberculoid.

030.8 Other specified leprosy
030.9 Leprosy, unspecified

✓4ᵗʰ **031 Diseases due to other mycobacteria**

031.0 Pulmonary
Battey disease
Infection by Mycobacterium:
avium
intracellulare [Battey bacillus]
kansasii

031.1 Cutaneous
Buruli ulcer
Infection by Mycobacterium:
marinum [M. balnei]
ulcerans

031.2 Disseminated
Disseminated mycobacterium avium-intracellulare complex (DMAC)
Mycobacterium avium-intracellulare complex (MAC) bacteremia

AHA: 4Q, '97, 31

DEF: Disseminated mycobacterium avium-intracellulare complex (DMAC): A serious systemic form of MAC commonly observed in patients in the late course of AIDS.

DEF: Mycobacterium avium-intracellulare complex (MAC) bacterium: Human pulmonary disease, lymphadenitis in children and systemic disease in immunocompromised individuals caused by a slow growing, gram-positive, aerobic organism.

031.8 Other specified mycobacterial diseases
031.9 Unspecified diseases due to mycobacteria
Atypical mycobacterium infection NOS

✓4ᵗʰ **032 Diphtheria**
INCLUDES infection by Corynebacterium diphtheriae

032.0 Faucial diphtheria
Membranous angina, diphtheritic
DEF: Diphtheria of the throat.

032.1 Nasopharyngeal diphtheria
032.2 Anterior nasal diphtheria
032.3 Laryngeal diphtheria
Laryngotracheitis, diphtheritic

✓5ᵗʰ **032.8 Other specified diphtheria**
032.81 Conjunctival diphtheria
Pseudomembranous diphtheritic conjunctivitis
032.82 Diphtheritic myocarditis
032.83 Diphtheritic peritonitis
032.84 Diphtheritic cystitis
032.85 Cutaneous diphtheria
032.89 Other

032.9 Diphtheria, unspecified

✓4ᵗʰ **033 Whooping cough**
INCLUDES pertussis
Use additional code to identify any associated pneumonia (484.3)

DEF: An acute, highly contagious respiratory tract infection caused by *Bordetella pertussis* and *B. bronchiseptica*; characteristic paroxysmal cough.

033.0 Bordetella pertussis [B. pertussis]
033.1 Bordetella parapertussis [B. parapertussis]
033.8 Whooping cough due to other specified organism
Bordetella bronchiseptica [B. bronchiseptica]
033.9 Whooping cough, unspecified organism

✓4ᵗʰ **034 Streptococcal sore throat and scarlet fever**
034.0 Streptococcal sore throat
Septic:
angina
sore throat
Streptococcal:
angina
Streptococcal:
laryngitis
pharyngitis
tonsillitis

034.1 Scarlet fever
Scarlatina
EXCLUDES parascarlatina (057.8)
DEF: Streptococcal infection and fever with red rash spreading from trunk.

035 Erysipelas
EXCLUDES postpartum or puerperal erysipelas (670)
DEF: An acute superficial cellulitis involving the dermal lymphatics; it is often caused by group A streptococci.

✓4ᵗʰ **036 Meningococcal infection**
036.0 Meningococcal meningitis
Cerebrospinal fever (meningococcal)
Meningitis:
cerebrospinal
epidemic

036.1 Meningococcal encephalitis
036.2 Meningococcemia
Meningococcal septicemia
036.3 Waterhouse-Friderichsen syndrome, meningococcal
Meningococcal hemorrhagic adrenalitis
Meningococcic adrenal syndrome
Waterhouse-Friderichsen syndrome NOS

✓5ᵗʰ **036.4 Meningococcal carditis**
036.40 Meningococcal carditis, unspecified
036.41 Meningococcal pericarditis
DEF: Meningococcal infection of the outer membrane of the heart.
036.42 Meningococcal endocarditis
DEF: Meningococcal infection of the membranes lining the cavities of the heart.
036.43 Meningococcal myocarditis
DEF: Meningococcal infection of the muscle of the heart.

✓5ᵗʰ **036.8 Other specified meningococcal infections**
036.81 Meningococcal optic neuritis
036.82 Meningococcal arthropathy
036.89 Other
036.9 Meningococcal infection, unspecified
Meningococcal infection NOS

037 Tetanus

> **EXCLUDES**   tetanus:
> > complicating:
> > > abortion (634-638 with .0, 639.0)
> > > ectopic or molar pregnancy (639.0)
> >
> > neonatorum (771.3)
> > puerperal (670)

DEF: An acute, often fatal, infectious disease caused by the anaerobic, spore-forming bacillus *Clostridium tetani*; the bacillus most often enters the body through a contaminated wound, burns, surgical wounds, or cutaneous ulcers. Symptoms include lockjaw, spasms, seizures, and paralysis.

√4ᵗʰ 038 Septicemia

Use additional code for systemic inflammatory response syndrome (SIRS) (995.91-995.92)

> **EXCLUDES**   bacteremia (790.7)
> > during labor (659.3)
> > following ectopic or molar pregnancy (639.0)
> > following infusion, injection, transfusion, or vaccination (999.3)
> > postpartum, puerperal (670)
> > septicemia (sepsis) of newborn (771.81)
> > that complicating abortion (634-638 with .0, 639.0)

AHA: 4Q, '88, 10; 3Q, '88, 12

DEF: A systemic disease associated with the presence and persistence of pathogenic microorganisms or their toxins in the blood.

038.0 Streptococcal septicemia
    AHA: ▶4Q, '03, 79;◀ 2Q, '96. 5

√5ᵗʰ 038.1 Staphylococcal septicemia
    AHA: 4Q, '97, 32

     038.10 Staphylococcal septicemia, unspecified
     038.11 Staphylococcus aureus septicemia
        AHA: 2Q, '00, 5; 4Q, '98, 42

     038.19 Other staphylococcal septicemia
        AHA: 2Q, '00, 5

038.2 Pneumococcal septicemia [Streptococcus pneumoniae septicemia]
    AHA: 2Q, '96, 5; 1Q, '91, 13

038.3 Septicemia due to anaerobes
    Septicemia due to bacteroides
> **EXCLUDES**   gas gangrene (040.0)
> > that due to anaerobic streptococci (038.0)

DEF: Infection of blood by microorganisms that thrive without oxygen.

√5ᵗʰ 038.4 Septicemia due to other gram-negative organisms
DEF: Infection of blood by microorganisms categorized as gram-negative by Gram's method of staining for identification of bacteria.

     038.40 Gram-negative organism, unspecified
        Gram-negative septicemia NOS
     038.41 Hemophilus influenzae [H. influenzae]
     038.42 Escherichia coli [E. coli]
        AHA: ▶4Q, '03, 73◀
     038.43 Pseudomonas
     038.44 Serratia
     038.49 Other

038.8 Other specified septicemias
> **EXCLUDES**   septicemia (due to):
> > anthrax (022.3)
> > gonococcal (098.89)
> > herpetic (054.5)
> > meningococcal (036.2)
> > septicemic plague (020.2)

038.9 Unspecified septicemia
    Septicemia NOS
> **EXCLUDES**   bacteremia NOS (790.7)

AHA: ▶4Q, '03, 79;◀ 2Q, '00, 3; 3Q, '99. 5. 9; 1Q, '98, 5; 3Q, '96, 16; 2Q, '96, 6

√4ᵗʰ 039 Actinomycotic infections

> **INCLUDES**   actinomycotic mycetoma
> > infection by Actinomycetales, such as species of Actinomyces, Actinomadura, Nocardia, Streptomyces
> > maduromycosis (actinomycotic)
> > schizomycetoma (actinomycotic)

DEF: Inflammatory lesions and abscesses at site of infection by *Actinomyces israelii.*

039.0 Cutaneous
    Erythrasma   Trichomycosis axillaris
039.1 Pulmonary
    Thoracic actinomycosis
039.2 Abdominal
039.3 Cervicofacial
039.4 Madura foot
> **EXCLUDES**   madura foot due to mycotic infection (117.4)

039.8 Of other specified sites
039.9 Of unspecified site
    Actinomycosis NOS   Nocardiosis NOS
    Maduromycosis NOS

√4ᵗʰ 040 Other bacterial diseases

> **EXCLUDES**   bacteremia NOS (790.7)
> > bacterial infection NOS (041.9)

040.0 Gas gangrene
    Gas bacillus infection or gangrene
    Infection by Clostridium:
      histolyticum
      oedematiens
      perfringens [welchii]
      septicum
      sordellii
    Malignant edema
    Myonecrosis, clostridial
    Myositis, clostridial
    AHA: 1Q, '95, 11

040.1 Rhinoscleroma
DEF: Growths on the nose and nasopharynx caused by *Klebsiella rhinoscleromatis.*

040.2 Whipple's disease
    Intestinal lipodystrophy
040.3 Necrobacillosis
DEF: Infection with *Fusobacterium necrophorum* causing abscess or necrosis.

√5ᵗʰ 040.8 Other specified bacterial diseases
     040.81 Tropical pyomyositis
     040.82 Toxic shock syndrome
        Use additional code to identify the organism
        AHA: 4Q, '02, 44

        DEF: Syndrome caused by staphylococcal exotoxin that may rapidly progress to severe and intractable shock; symptoms include characteristic sunburn-like rash with peeling of skin on palms and soles, sudden onset high fever, vomiting, diarrhea, malagia, and hypotension.

     040.89 Other
        AHA: N-D, '86, 7

√4ᵗʰ 041 Bacterial infection in conditions classified elsewhere and of unspecified site

Note: This category is provided to be used as an additional code to identify the bacterial agent in diseases classified elsewhere. This category will also be used to classify bacterial infections of unspecified nature or site.

> **EXCLUDES**   bacteremia NOS (790.7)
> > septicemia (038.0-038.9)

AHA: 2Q, '01, 12; J-A, '84, 19

√4ᵗʰ / √5ᵗʰ Additional Digit Required   Unspecified Code   Other Specified Code   Manifestation Code   ▶◀ Revised Text   ● New Code   ▲ Revised Code Title

2005 ICD•9•CM   **February 2004 • Volume 1 — 7**

√5ᵗʰ **041.0** Streptococcus
    041.00 Streptococcus, unspecified
    041.01 Group A
        AHA: 1Q, '02, 3
    041.02 Group B
    041.03 Group C
    041.04 Group D [Enterococcus]
    041.05 Group G
    041.09 Other Streptococcus

√5ᵗʰ **041.1** Staphylococcus
    041.10 Staphylococcus, unspecified
    041.11 Staphylococcus aureus
        AHA: 4Q, '03, 104, 106; 2Q, '01, 11; 4Q, '98, 42, 54; 4Q, '97, 32
    041.19 Other Staphylococcus

    041.2 Pneumococcus
    041.3 Friedländer's bacillus
        Infection by Klebsiella pneumoniae
    041.4 Escherichia coli [E. coli]
    041.5 Hemophilus influenzae [H. influenzae]
    041.6 Proteus (mirabilis) (morganii)
    041.7 Pseudomonas
        AHA: 4Q, '02, 45

√5ᵗʰ **041.8** Other specified bacterial infections
    041.81 Mycoplasma
        Eaton's agent
        Pleuropneumonia-like organisms [PPLO]
▲   **041.82** Bacteroides fragilis
    041.83 Clostridium perfringens
    041.84 Other anaerobes
        Gram-negative anaerobes
        EXCLUDES   Helicobacter pylori (041.86)
    041.85 Other gram-negative organisms
        Aerobacter aerogenes
        Gram-negative bacteria NOS
        Mima polymorpha
        Serratia
        EXCLUDES   gram-negative anaerobes
                   (041.84)
        AHA: 1Q, 95, 18
    041.86 Helicobacter pylori (H. pylori)
        AHA: 4Q, '95, 60
    041.89 Other specified bacteria
        AHA: 2Q, '03, 7

    041.9 Bacterial infection, unspecified
        AHA: 2Q, '91, 9

HUMAN IMMUNODEFICIENCY VIRUS (HIV) INFECTION (042)

042 Human immunodeficiency virus [HIV] disease
    Acquired immune deficiency syndrome
    Acquired immunodeficiency syndrome
    AIDS
    AIDS-like syndrome
    AIDS-related complex
    ARC
    HIV infection, symptomatic
    Use additional code(s) to identify all manifestations of HIV.
    Use additional code to identify HIV-2 infection (079.53)
    EXCLUDES   asymptomatic HIV infection status (V08)
                 exposure to HIV virus ▶(V01.79)◀
                 nonspecific serologic evidence of HIV (795.71)
    AHA: ▶1Q, '04, 5;◀ 1Q, '03, 15; 1Q, '99, 14, 4Q, '97, 30, 31; 1Q, '93, 21; 2Q, '92, 11;
        3Q, '90, 17; J-A, '87, 8

POLIOMYELITIS AND OTHER NON-ARTHROPOD-BORNE VIRAL DISEASES OF CENTRAL NERVOUS SYSTEM (045-049)

√4ᵗʰ **045** Acute poliomyelitis
    EXCLUDES   late effects of acute poliomyelitis (138)
    The following fifth-digit subclassification is for use with category 045:
        0 poliovirus, unspecified type
        1 poliovirus type I
        2 poliovirus type II
        3 poliovirus type III

√5ᵗʰ **045.0** Acute paralytic poliomyelitis specified as bulbar
    Infantile paralysis (acute) ⎫
    Poliomyelitis (acute)   ⎬ specified as bulbar
      (anterior)   ⎭
    Polioencephalitis (acute) (bulbar)
    Polioencephalomyelitis (acute) (anterior) (bulbar)
    DEF: Acute paralytic infection occurring where the brain merges with the spinal cord; affecting breathing, swallowing, and heart rate.

√5ᵗʰ **045.1** Acute poliomyelitis with other paralysis
    Paralysis:
      acute atrophic, spinal
      infantile, paralytic
    Poliomyelitis (acute) ⎫
      anterior   ⎬ with paralysis except
      epidemic   ⎭   bulbar
    DEF: Paralytic infection affecting peripheral or spinal nerves.

√5ᵗʰ **045.2** Acute nonparalytic poliomyelitis
    Poliomyelitis (acute) ⎫
      anterior   ⎬ specified as
      epidemic   ⎭   nonparalytic
    DEF: Nonparalytic infection causing pain, stiffness, and paresthesias.

√5ᵗʰ **045.9** Acute poliomyelitis, unspecified
    Infantile paralysis   ⎫ unspecified whether
    Poliomyelitis (acute) ⎬   paralytic or
      anterior   ⎪   nonparalytic
      epidemic   ⎭

√4ᵗʰ **046** Slow virus infection of central nervous system
    046.0 Kuru
        DEF: A chronic, progressive, fatal nervous system disorder; clinical symptoms include cerebellar ataxia, trembling, spasticity and progressive dementia.
    046.1 Jakob-Creutzfeldt disease
        Subacute spongiform encephalopathy
        DEF: Communicable, progressive spongiform encephalopathy thought to be caused by an infectious particle known as a "prion" (proteinaceous infection particle). This is a progressive, fatal disease manifested principally by mental deterioration.
    046.2 Subacute sclerosing panencephalitis
        Dawson's inclusion body encephalitis
        Van Bogaert's sclerosing leukoencephalitis
        DEF: Progressive viral infection causing cerebral dysfunction, blindness, dementia, and death (SSPE).
    046.3 Progressive multifocal leukoencephalopathy
        Multifocal leukoencephalopathy NOS
        DEF: Infection affecting cerebral cortex in patients with weakened immune systems.
    046.8 Other specified slow virus infection of central nervous system
    046.9 Unspecified slow virus infection of central nervous system

---

✓4ᵗʰ **047 Meningitis due to enterovirus**
    INCLUDES   meningitis:
                  abacterial
                  aseptic
                  viral
    EXCLUDES   *meningitis due to:*
            adenovirus (049.1)
            arthropod-borne virus (060.0-066.9)
            leptospira (100.81)
            virus of:
                herpes simplex (054.72)
                herpes zoster (053.0)
                lymphocytic choriomeningitis (049.0)
                mumps (072.1)
                poliomyelitis (045.0-045.9)
            any other infection specifically classified
              elsewhere

    AHA: J-F, '87, 6

    047.0 Coxsackie virus
    047.1 ECHO virus
        Meningo-eruptive syndrome
    047.8 Other specified viral meningitis
    047.9 Unspecified viral meningitis
        Viral meningitis NOS

048 Other enterovirus diseases of central nervous system
    Boston exanthem

✓4ᵗʰ **049 Other non-arthropod-borne viral diseases of central nervous system**
    EXCLUDES   *late effects of viral encephalitis (139.0)*

    049.0 Lymphocytic choriomeningitis
        Lymphocytic:
            meningitis (serous) (benign)
            meningoencephalitis (serous) (benign)
    049.1 Meningitis due to adenovirus
        DEF: Inflammation of lining of brain caused by Arenaviruses and usually occurring in adults in fall and winter months.
    049.8 Other specified non-arthropod-borne viral diseases of central nervous system
        Encephalitis:
            acute:
                inclusion body
                necrotizing
            epidemic
            lethargica
            Rio Bravo
            von Economo's disease
    049.9 Unspecified non-arthropod-borne viral diseases of central nervous system
        Viral encephalitis NOS

VIRAL DISEASES ACCOMPANIED BY EXANTHEM (050-057)
    EXCLUDES   *arthropod-borne viral diseases (060.0-066.9)*
                Boston exanthem (048)

✓4ᵗʰ **050 Smallpox**
    050.0 Variola major
        Hemorrhagic (pustular) smallpox
        Malignant smallpox
        Purpura variolosa
        DEF: Form of smallpox known for its high mortality; exists only in laboratories.
    050.1 Alastrim
        Variola minor
        DEF: Mild form of smallpox known for its low mortality rate.
    050.2 Modified smallpox
        Varioloid
        DEF: Mild form occurring in patients with history of infection or vaccination.
    050.9 Smallpox, unspecified

✓4ᵗʰ **051 Cowpox and paravaccinia**
    051.0 Cowpox
        Vaccinia not from vaccination
        EXCLUDES   *vaccinia (generalized) (from vaccination) (999.0)*
        DEF: A disease contracted by milking infected cows; vesicles usually appear on the fingers, may spread to hands and adjacent areas and usually disappear without scarring; other associated features of the disease may include local edema, lymphangitis and regional lymphadenitis with or without fever.
    051.1 Pseudocowpox
        Milkers' node
        DEF: Hand lesions and mild fever in dairy workers caused by exposure to paravaccinia.
    051.2 Contagious pustular dermatitis
        Ecthyma contagiosum
        Orf
        DEF: Skin eruptions caused by exposure to poxvirus-infected sheep or goats.
    051.9 Paravaccinia, unspecified

✓4ᵗʰ **052 Chickenpox**
    DEF: Contagious infection by varicella-zoster virus causing rash with pustules and fever.
    052.0 Postvaricella encephalitis
        Postchickenpox encephalitis
    052.1 Varicella (hemorrhagic) pneumonitis
    052.7 With other specified complications
        AHA: 1Q, '02, 3
    052.8 With unspecified complication
    052.9 Varicella without mention of complication
        Chickenpox NOS
        Varicella NOS

✓4ᵗʰ **053 Herpes zoster**
    INCLUDES   shingles
                  zona
    DEF: Self-limiting infection by varicella-zoster virus causing unilateral eruptions and neuralgia along affected nerves.
    053.0 With meningitis
        DEF: Varicella-zoster virus infection causing inflammation of the lining of the brain and/or spinal cord.
    ✓5ᵗʰ **053.1 With other nervous system complications**
        053.10 With unspecified nervous system complication
        053.11 Geniculate herpes zoster
            Herpetic geniculate ganglionitis
            DEF: Unilateral eruptions and neuralgia along the facial nerve geniculum affecting face and outer and middle ear.
        053.12 Postherpetic trigeminal neuralgia
            DEF: Severe oral or nasal pain following a herpes zoster infection.
        053.13 Postherpetic polyneuropathy
            DEF: Multiple areas of pain following a herpes zoster infection.
        053.19 Other
    ✓5ᵗʰ **053.2 With ophthalmic complications**
        053.20 Herpes zoster dermatitis of eyelid
            Herpes zoster ophthalmicus
        053.21 Herpes zoster keratoconjunctivitis
        053.22 Herpes zoster iridocyclitis
        053.29 Other
    ✓5ᵗʰ **053.7 With other specified complications**
        053.71 Otitis externa due to herpes zoster
        053.79 Other
    053.8 With unspecified complication

✓4ᵗʰ
✓5ᵗʰ Additional Digit Required   Unspecified Code   Other Specified Code   Manifestation Code   ►◄ Revised Text   ● New Code   ▲ Revised Code Title

2005 ICD•9•CM   Volume 1 — 9

053.9   **Herpes zoster without mention of complication**
Herpes zoster NOS

☑4th **054 Herpes simplex**
EXCLUDES   *congenital herpes simplex (771.2)*

054.0   **Eczema herpeticum**
Kaposi's varicelliform eruption
DEF: Herpes simplex virus invading site of preexisting skin inflammation.

☑5th **054.1**   **Genital herpes**
AHA: J-F, '87, 15, 16

054.10 Genital herpes, unspecified
Herpes progenitalis
054.11 Herpetic vulvovaginitis   ♀
054.12 Herpetic ulceration of vulva   ♀
054.13 Herpetic infection of penis   ♂
054.19 Other

054.2   **Herpetic gingivostomatitis**
054.3   **Herpetic meningoencephalitis**
Herpes encephalitis
Simian B disease
DEF: Inflammation of the brain and its lining; caused by infection of herpes simplex 1 in adults and simplex 2 in newborns.

☑5th **054.4**   **With ophthalmic complications**
054.40 With unspecified ophthalmic complication
054.41 Herpes simplex dermatitis of eyelid
054.42 Dendritic keratitis
054.43 Herpes simplex disciform keratitis
054.44 Herpes simplex iridocyclitis
054.49 Other

054.5   **Herpetic septicemia**
AHA: 2Q, '00, 5

054.6   **Herpetic whitlow**
Herpetic felon
DEF: A primary infection of the terminal segment of a finger by herpes simplex; intense itching and pain start the disease, vesicles form, and tissue ultimately is destroyed.

☑5th **054.7**   **With other specified complications**
054.71 Visceral herpes simplex
054.72 Herpes simplex meningitis
054.73 Herpes simplex otitis externa
054.79 Other
054.8   **With unspecified complication**
054.9   **Herpes simplex without mention of complication**

☑4th **055 Measles**
INCLUDES   morbilli
rubeola
055.0   **Postmeasles encephalitis**
055.1   **Postmeasles pneumonia**
055.2   **Postmeasles otitis media**
☑5th **055.7**   **With other specified complications**
055.71 Measles keratoconjunctivitis
Measles keratitis
055.79 Other
055.8   **With unspecified complication**
055.9   **Measles without mention of complication**
☑4th **056 Rubella**
INCLUDES   German measles
EXCLUDES   *congenital rubella (771.0)*
DEF: Acute but usually benign togavirus infection causing fever, sore throat, and rash; associated with complications to fetus as a result of maternal infection.

☑5th **056.0**   **With neurological complications**
056.00 With unspecified neurological complication
056.01 Encephalomyelitis due to rubella
Encephalitis   } due to
Meningoencephalitis }   rubella
056.09 Other
☑5th **056.7**   **With other specified complications**
056.71 Arthritis due to rubella
056.79 Other
056.8   **With unspecified complications**
056.9   **Rubella without mention of complication**
☑4th **057 Other viral exanthemata**
DEF: Skin eruptions or rashes and fever caused by viruses, including poxviruses.

057.0   **Erythema infectiosum [fifth disease]**
DEF: A moderately contagious, benign, epidemic disease, usually seen in children, and of probable viral etiology; a red macular rash appears on the face and may spread to the limbs and trunk.

057.8   **Other specified viral exanthemata**
Dukes (-Filatow) disease
Exanthema subitum [sixth disease]
Fourth disease
Parascarlatina
Pseudoscarlatina
Roseola infantum
057.9   **Viral exanthem, unspecified**

ARTHROPOD-BORNE VIRAL DISEASES (060-066)

Use additional code to identify any associated meningitis (321.2)
EXCLUDES   *late effects of viral encephalitis (139.0)*

☑4th **060 Yellow fever**
DEF: Fever and jaundice from infection by mosquito-borne virus of genus Flavivirus.

060.0   **Sylvatic**
Yellow fever:
jungle
sylvan
DEF: Yellow fever transmitted from animal to man, via mosquito.

060.1   **Urban**
DEF: Yellow fever transmitted from man to man, via mosquito.

060.9   **Yellow fever, unspecified**
061 Dengue
Breakbone fever
EXCLUDES   *hemorrhagic fever caused by dengue virus (065.4)*
DEF: Acute, self-limiting infection by mosquito-borne virus characterized by fever and generalized aches

☑4th **062 Mosquito-borne viral encephalitis**
062.0   **Japanese encephalitis**
Japanese B encephalitis
DEF: Flavivirus causing inflammation of the brain, and Russia, with a wide range of clinical manifestations

062.1   **Western equine encephalitis**
DEF: Alphavirus WEE infection causing inflammation of the brain, found in areas west of the Mississippi; transmitted horse to mosquito to man.

062.2   **Eastern equine encephalitis**
EXCLUDES   *Venezuelan equine encephalitis (066.2)*
DEF: Alphavirus EEE causing inflammation of the brain and spinal cord, found as far north as Canada and south into South America and Mexico; transmitted horse to mosquito to man.

N Newborn Age: 0   P Pediatric Age: 0-17   M Maternity Age: 12-55   A Adult Age: 15-124   MSP Medicare Secondary Payer

062.3   **St. Louis encephalitis**
DEF: Epidemic form caused by Flavivirus and transmitted by mosquito, and characterized by fever, difficulty in speech, and headache.

062.4   **Australian encephalitis**
Australian arboencephalitis
Australian X disease
Murray Valley encephalitis
DEF: Flavivirus causing inflammation of the brain, occurring in Australia and New Guinea.

062.5   **California virus encephalitis**
Encephalitis: Tahyna fever
    California
    La Crosse
DEF: Bunya virus causing inflammation of the brain.

062.8   **Other specified mosquito-borne viral encephalitis**
Encephalitis by Ilheus virus
   EXCLUDES   West Nile virus ▶(066.40-066.49)◀

062.9   **Mosquito-borne viral encephalitis, unspecified**

✓4th **063**   **Tick-borne viral encephalitis**
   INCLUDES   diphasic meningoencephalitis

063.0   **Russian spring-summer [taiga] encephalitis**

063.1   **Louping ill**
DEF: Inflammation of brain caused by virus transmitted sheep to tick to man; incidence usually limited to British Isles.

063.2   **Central European encephalitis**
DEF: Inflammation of brain caused by virus transmitted by tick; limited to central Europe and presenting with two distinct phases.

063.8   **Other specified tick-borne viral encephalitis**
Langat encephalitis   Powassan encephalitis

063.9   **Tick-borne viral encephalitis, unspecified**

064   **Viral encephalitis transmitted by other and unspecified arthropods**
Arthropod-borne viral encephalitis, vector unknown
Negishi virus encephalitis
   EXCLUDES   viral encephalitis NOS (049.9)

✓4th **065**   **Arthropod-borne hemorrhagic fever**

065.0   **Crimean hemorrhagic fever [CHF Congo virus]**
Central Asian hemorrhagic fever

065.1   **Omsk hemorrhagic fever**

065.2   **Kyasanur Forest disease**

065.3   **Other tick-borne hemorrhagic fever**

065.4   **Mosquito-borne hemorrhagic fever**
Chikungunya hemorrhagic fever
Dengue hemorrhagic fever
   EXCLUDES   Chikungunya fever (066.3)
                dengue (061)
                yellow fever (060.0-060.9)

065.8   **Other specified arthropod-borne hemorrhagic fever**
Mite-borne hemorrhagic fever

065.9   **Arthropod-borne hemorrhagic fever, unspecified**
Arbovirus hemorrhagic fever NOS

✓4th **066**   **Other arthropod-borne viral diseases**

066.0   **Phlebotomus fever**
Changuinola fever   Sandfly fever
DEF: Sandfly-borne viral infection occurring in Asia, Middle East and South America.

066.1   **Tick-borne fever**
Nairobi sheep disease   Tick fever:
Tick fever: Kemerovo
    American mountain   Quaranfil
    Colorado

066.2   **Venezuelan equine fever**
Venezuelan equine encephalitis
DEF: Alphavirus VEE infection causing inflammation of the brain, usually limited to South America, Mexico, and Florida; transmitted horse to mosquito to man.

066.3   **Other mosquito-borne fever**
Fever (viral):   Fever (viral):
   Bunyamwera   Oropouche
   Bwamba   Pixuna
   Chikungunya   Rift valley
   Guama   Ross river
   Mayaro   Wesselsbron
   Mucambo   Zika
   O'Nyong-Nyong
   EXCLUDES   dengue (061)
                yellow fever (060.0-060.9)

✓5th **066.4**   **West Nile fever**
AHA: 4Q, '02, 44
DEF: Mosquito-borne fever causing fatal inflammation of the brain, the lining of the brain, or of the lining of the brain and spinal cord.

   ●   **066.40**   **West Nile fever, unspecified**
West Nile fever NOS
West Nile fever without complications
West Nile virus NOS

   ●   **066.41**   **West Nile fever with encephalitis**
West Nile encephalitis
West Nile encephalomyelitis

   ●   **066.42**   **West Nile fever with other neurologic manifestation**
Use additional code to specify the neurologic manifestation

   ●   **066.49**   **West Nile fever with other complications**
Use additional code to specify the other conditions

066.8   **Other specified arthropod-borne viral diseases**
Chandipura fever   Piry fever

066.9   **Arthropod-borne viral disease, unspecified**
Arbovirus infection NOS

OTHER DISEASES DUE TO VIRUSES AND CHLAMYDIAE (070-079)

✓4th **070**   **Viral hepatitis**
   INCLUDES   viral hepatitis (acute) (chronic)
   EXCLUDES   cytomegalic inclusion virus hepatitis (078.5)

The following fifth-digit subclassification is for use with categories 070.2 and 070.3:
   0   **acute or unspecified, without mention of hepatitis delta**
   1   **acute or unspecified, with hepatitis delta**
   2   **chronic, without mention of hepatitis delta**
   3   **chronic, with hepatitis delta**

DEF: Hepatitis A: HAV infection is self-limiting with flu like symptoms; transmission, fecal-oral.
DEF: Hepatitis B: HBV infection can be chronic and systemic; transmission, bodily fluids.
DEF: Hepatitis C: HCV infection can be chronic and systemic; transmission, blood transfusion and unidentified agents.
DEF: Hepatitis D (delta): HDV occurs only in the presence of hepatitis B virus.
DEF: Hepatitis E: HEV is epidemic form; transmission and nature under investigation.

070.0   **Viral hepatitis A with hepatic coma**

070.1   **Viral hepatitis A without mention of hepatic coma**
Infectious hepatitis

✓5th **070.2**   **Viral hepatitis B with hepatic coma**
AHA: 4Q, '91, 28

✓5th **070.3**   **Viral hepatitis B without mention of hepatic coma**
Serum hepatitis
AHA: 1Q, '93, 28; 4Q, '91, 28

✓5th **070.4**   **Other specified viral hepatitis with hepatic coma**
AHA: 4Q, '91, 28

   ▲   **070.41**   **Acute hepatitis C with hepatic coma**

       070.42   **Hepatitis delta without mention of active hepatitis B disease with hepatic coma**
Hepatitis delta with hepatitis B carrier state

✓4th ✓5th   Additional Digit Required   Unspecified Code   Other Specified Code   Manifestation Code   ▶◀ Revised Text   ● New Code   ▲ Revised Code Title

2005 ICD•9•CM   **October 2004 • Volume 1 — 11**

070.43 Hepatitis E with hepatic coma

070.44 Chronic hepatitis C with hepatic coma

070.49 Other specified viral hepatitis with hepatic coma

√5th **070.5** Other specified viral hepatitis without mention of hepatic coma

AHA: 4Q, '91, 28

070.51 Acute hepatitis C without mention of hepatic coma

070.52 Hepatitis delta without mention of active hepatitits B disease or hepatic coma

070.53 Hepatitis E without mention of hepatic coma

070.54 Chronic hepatitis C without mention of hepatic coma

070.59 Other specified viral hepatitis without mention of hepatic coma

070.6 Unspecified viral hepatitis with hepatic coma

> EXCLUDES ▶ unspecified viral hepatitis C with hepatic coma (070.71)◀

√5th **070.7** Unspecified viral hepatitis C

070.70 Unspecified viral hepatitis C without hepatic coma

Unspecified viral hepatitis C NOS

070.71 Unspecified viral hepatitis C with hepatic coma

070.9 Unspecified viral hepatitis without mention of hepatic coma

Viral hepatitis NOS

> EXCLUDES ▶ unspecified viral hepatitis C without hepatic coma (070.70)◀

071 Rabies

Hydrophobia   Lyssa

DEF: Acute infectious disease of the CNS caused by a rhabdovirus; usually spread by virus-laden saliva from bites by infected animals; it progresses from fever, restlessness, and extreme excitability, to hydrophobia, seizures, confusion and death.

√4th **072 Mumps**

DEF: Acute infectious disease caused by paramyxovirus; usually seen in children less than 15 years of age; salivary glands are typically enlarged, and other organs, such as testes, pancreas and meninges, are often involved.

072.0 Mumps orchitis ♂

072.1 Mumps meningitis

072.2 Mumps encephalitis

Mumps meningoencephalitis

072.3 Mumps pancreatitis

√5th 072.7 Mumps with other specified complications

072.71 Mumps hepatitis

072.72 Mumps polyneuropathy

072.79 Other

072.8 Mumps with unspecified complication

072.9 Mumps without mention of complication

Epidemic parotitis   Infectious parotitis

√4th **073 Ornithosis**

INCLUDES parrot fever
psittacosis

DEF: *Chlamydia psittaci* infection often transmitted from birds to humans.

073.0 With pneumonia

Lobular pneumonitis due to ornithosis

073.7 With other specified complications

073.8 With unspecified complication

073.9 Ornithosis, unspecified

√4th **074 Specific diseases due to Coxsackie virus**

EXCLUDES Coxsackie virus:
infection NOS (079.2)
meningitis (047.O)

074.0 Herpangina

Vesicular pharyngitis

DEF: Acute infectious coxsackie virus infection causing throat lesions, fever, and vomiting; generally affects children in summer.

074.1 Epidemic pleurodynia

Bornholm disease   Epidemic:
Devil's grip   myalgia
myositis

DEF: Paroxysmal pain in chest, accompanied by fever and usually limited to children and young adults; caused by coxsackie virus.

√5th 074.2 Coxsackie carditis

074.20 Coxsackie carditis, unspecified

074.21 Coxsackie pericarditis

DEF: Coxsackie infection of the outer lining of the heart.

074.22 Coxsackie endocarditis

DEF: Coxsackie infection within the heart's cavities.

074.23 Coxsackie myocarditis

Aseptic myocarditis of newborn

DEF: Coxsackie infection of the muscle of the heart.

074.3 Hand, foot, and mouth disease

Vesicular stomatitis and exanthem

DEF: Mild coxsackie infection causing lesions on hands, feet and oral mucosa; most commonly seen in preschool children.

074.8 Other specified diseases due to Coxsackie virus

Acute lymphonodular pharyngitis

075 Infectious mononucleosis

Glandular fever   Pfeiffer's disease
Monocytic angina

AHA: 3Q, '01, 13; M-A, '87, 8

DEF: Acute infection by Epstein-Barr virus causing fever, sore throat, enlarged lymph glands and spleen, and fatigue; usually seen in teens and young adults.

√4th **076 Trachoma**

EXCLUDES late effect of trachoma (139.1)

DEF: A chronic infectious disease of the cornea and conjunctiva caused by a strain of the bacteria *Chlamydia trachomatis*; the infection can cause photophobia, pain, excessive tearing and sometimes blindness.

076.0 Initial stage

Trachoma dubium

076.1 Active stage

Granular conjunctivitis (trachomatous)
Trachomatous
follicular conjunctivitis
pannus

076.9 Trachoma, unspecified

Trachoma NOS

√4th **077 Other diseases of conjunctiva due to viruses and Chlamydiae**

EXCLUDES ophthalmic complications of viral diseases classified elsewhere

077.0 Inclusion conjunctivitis

Paratrachoma
Swimming pool conjunctivitis

EXCLUDES inclusion blennorrhea (neonatal) (771.6)

DEF: Pus in conjunctiva caused by *Chlamydiae trachomatis* infection.

077.1 Epidemic keratoconjunctivitis

Shipyard eye

DEF: Highly contagious corneal or conjunctival infection caused by adenovirus type 8; symptoms include inflammation and corneal infiltrates.

077.2 Pharyngoconjunctival fever

Viral pharyngoconjunctivitis

077.3 Other adenoviral conjunctivitis

Acute adenoviral follicular conjunctivitis

077.4 Epidemic hemorrhagic conjunctivitis

Apollo:
conjunctivitis
disease

Conjunctivitis due to enterovirus type 70
Hemorrhagic conjunctivitis (acute) (epidemic)

077.8   Other viral conjunctivitis
Newcastle conjunctivitis

✓5ᵗʰ **077.9   Unspecified diseases of conjunctiva due to viruses and Chlamydiae**

077.98 Due to Chlamydiae

077.99 Due to viruses
Viral conjunctivitis NOS

✓4ᵗʰ **078 Other diseases due to viruses and Chlamydiae**
> **EXCLUDES**   *viral infection NOS (079.0-079.9)*
> *viremia NOS (790.8)*

078.0   Molluscum contagiosum
DEF: Benign poxvirus infection causing small bumps on the skin or conjunctiva; transmitted by close contact.

✓5ᵗʰ **078.1   Viral warts**
Viral warts due to human papilloma virus
AHA: 2Q, '97, 9; 4Q, '93, 22

DEF: A keratotic papilloma of the epidermis caused by the human papilloma virus; the superficial vegetative lesions last for varying durations and eventually regress spontaneously.

078.10 Viral warts, unspecified
Condyloma NOS
Verruca:
  NOS
  Vulgaris
Warts (infectious)

078.11 Condyloma acuminatum
DEF: Clusters of mucosa or epidermal lesions on external genitalia; viral infection is sexually transmitted.

078.19 Other specified viral warts
Genital warts NOS
Verruca:
  plana
  plantaris

078.2   Sweating fever
Miliary fever
Sweating disease
DEF: A viral infection characterized by profuse sweating; various papular, vesicular and other eruptions cause the blockage of sweat glands.

078.3   Cat-scratch disease
Benign lymphoreticulosis (of inoculation)
Cat-scratch fever

078.4   Foot and mouth disease
Aphthous fever
Epizootic:
  aphthae
  stomatitis
DEF: Ulcers on oral mucosa, legs, and feet after exposure to infected animal.

078.5   Cytomegaloviral disease
Cytomegalic inclusion disease
Salivary gland virus disease
Use additional code to identify manifestation, as:
  cytomegalic inclusion virus:
    hepatitis (573.1)
    pneumonia (484.1)
> **EXCLUDES**   *congenital cytomegalovirus infection (771.1)*

AHA: 1Q, '03 ,10; 3Q, '98, 4; 2Q, '93, 11; 1Q, '89, 9

DEF: A herpes virus inclusion associated with serious disease morbidity including fever, leukopenia, pneumonia, retinitis, hepatitis and organ transplant; often leads to syndromes such as hepatomegaly, splenomegaly and thrombocytopenia; a common post-transplant complication for organ transplant recipients.

078.6   Hemorrhagic nephrosonephritis
Hemorrhagic fever:
  epidemic
  Korean
  Russian
  with renal syndrome
DEF: Viral infection causing kidney dysfunction and bleeding disorders.

078.7   Arenaviral hemorrhagic fever
Hemorrhagic fever:
  Argentine
  Bolivian
  Junin virus
  Machupo virus

✓5ᵗʰ **078.8   Other specified diseases due to viruses and Chlamydiae**
> **EXCLUDES**   *epidemic diarrhea (009.2)*
> *lymphogranuloma venereum (099.1)*

078.81 Epidemic vertigo

078.82 Epidemic vomiting syndrome
Winter vomiting disease

078.88 Other specified diseases due to Chlamydiae
AHA: 4Q, '96, 22

078.89 Other specified diseases due to viruses
Epidemic cervical myalgia
Marburg disease
Tanapox

✓4ᵗʰ **079 Viral and chlamydial infection in conditions classified elsewhere and of unspecified site**
Note: This category is provided to be used as an additional code to identify the viral agent in diseases classifiable elsewhere. This category will also be used to classify virus infection of unspecified nature or site.

079.0   Adenovirus

079.1   ECHO virus
DEF: An "orphan" enteric RNA virus, certain serotypes of which are associated with human disease, especially aseptic meningitis.

079.2   Coxsackie virus
DEF: A heterogenous group of viruses associated with aseptic meningitis, myocarditis, pericarditis, and acute onset juvenile diabetes.

079.3   Rhinovirus
DEF: Rhinoviruses affect primarily the upper respiratory tract. Over 100 distinct types infect humans.

079.4   Human papillomavirus
AHA: 2Q, '97, 9; 4Q, '93, 22

DEF: Viral infection caused by the genus *Papillomavirus* causing cutaneous and genital warts, including verruca vulgaris and condyloma acuminatum; certain types are associated with cervical dysplasia, cancer and other genital malignances.

✓5ᵗʰ **079.5   Retrovirus**
> **EXCLUDES**   *human immunodeficiency virus, type 1 [HIV-1] (042)*
> *human T-cell lymphotrophic virus, type III [HTLV-III] (042)*
> *lymphadenopathy-associated virus [LAV] (042)*

AHA: 4Q, '93, 22, 23

DEF: A large group of RNA viruses that carry reverse transcriptase and include the leukoviruses and lentiviruses.

079.50 Retrovirus, unspecified

079.51 Human T-cell lymphotrophic virus, type I [HTLV-I]

079.52 Human T-cell lymphotrophic virus, type II [HTLV-II]

✓4ᵗʰ
✓5ᵗʰ Additional Digit Required   Unspecified Code   Other Specified Code   Manifestation Code   ►◄ Revised Text   ● New Code   ▲ Revised Code Title

2005 ICD•9•CM   Volume 1 — 13

079.53 Human immunodeficiency virus, type 2 [HIV-2]

079.59 Other specified retrovirus

079.6 Respiratory syncytial virus (RSV)
AHA: 4Q, '96, 27, 28

DEF: The major respiratory pathogen of young children, causing severe bronchitis and bronchopneumonia, and minor infection in adults.

√5ᵗʰ **079.8 Other specified viral and chlamydial infections**
AHA: 1Q, '88, 12

079.81 Hantavirus
AHA: 4Q, '95, 60

DEF: An infection caused by the Muerto Canyon virus whose primary rodent reservoir is the deer mouse Peromyscus maniculatus; commonly characterized by fever, myalgias, headache, cough and rapid respiratory failure.

079.82 SARS-associated coronavirus
AHA:▶ 4Q, '03, 46◀

DEF: ▶ A life-threatening respiratory disease described as severe acute respiratory syndrome (SARS); etiology coronavirus; most common presenting symptoms may range from mild to more severe forms of flu-like conditions; fever, chills, cough, headache, myalgia; diagnosis of SARS is based upon clinical, laboratory, and epidemiological criteria.◀

079.88 Other specified chlamydial infection

079.89 Other specified viral infection

√5ᵗʰ **079.9 Unspecified viral and chlamydial infections**
EXCLUDES   viremia NOS (790.8)

AHA: 2Q, '91, 8

079.98 Unspecified chlamydial infection
Chlamydial infections NOS

079.99 Unspecified viral infection
Viral infections NOS

RICKETTSIOSES AND OTHER ARTHROPOD-BORNE DISEASES (080-088)

EXCLUDES   arthropod-borne viral diseases (060.0-066.9)

080 Louse-borne [epidemic] typhus

Typhus (fever):   Typhus (fever):
  classical   exanthematic NOS
  epidemic   louse-borne

DEF: Rickettsia prowazekii; causes severe headache, rash, high fever.

√4ᵗʰ **081 Other typhus**

081.0 Murine [endemic] typhus
Typhus (fever):   Typhus (fever):
  endemic   flea-borne
DEF: Milder typhus caused by Rickettsia typhi (mooseri); transmitted by rat flea.

081.1 Brill's disease
Brill-Zinsser disease
Recrudescent typhus (fever)

081.2 Scrub typhus
Japanese river fever   Mite-borne typhus
Kedani fever   Tsutsugamushi
DEF: Typhus caused by Rickettsia tsutsugamushi transmitted by chigger.

081.9 Typhus, unspecified
Typhus (fever) NOS

√4ᵗʰ **082 Tick-borne rickettsioses**

082.0 Spotted fevers
Rocky mountain spotted fever
Sao Paulo fever

082.1 Boutonneuse fever
African tick typhus   Marseilles fever
India tick typhus   Mediterranean tick fever
Kenya tick typhus

082.2 North Asian tick fever
Siberian tick typhus

082.3 Queensland tick typhus

√5ᵗʰ **082.4 Ehrlichiosis**
AHA: 4Q, '00, 38

082.40 Ehrlichiosis, unspecified

082.41 Ehrlichiosis chaffeensis [E. chaffeensis]
DEF: A febrile illness caused by bacterial infection, also called human monocytic ehrlichiosis (HME). Causal organism is Ehrlichia chaffeensis, transmitted by the Lone Star tick, Amblyomma americanum. Symptoms include fever, chills, myalgia, nausea, vomiting, diarrhea, confusion, and severe headache occurring one week after a tick bite. Clinical findings are lymphadenopathy, rash, thrombocytopenia, leukopenia, and abnormal liver function tests

082.49 Other ehrlichiosis

082.8 Other specified tick-borne rickettsioses
Lone star fever
AHA: 4Q, '99, 19

082.9 Tick-borne rickettsiosis, unspecified
Tick-borne typhus NOS

√4ᵗʰ **083 Other rickettsioses**

083.0 Q fever
DEF: Infection of Coxiella burnetii usually acquired through airborne organisms.

083.1 Trench fever
Quintan fever   Wolhynian fever

083.2 Rickettsialpox
Vesicular rickettsiosis
DEF: Infection of Rickettsia akari usually acquired through a mite bite.

083.8 Other specified rickettsioses

083.9 Rickettsiosis, unspecified

√4ᵗʰ **084 Malaria**
Note: Subcategories 084.0-084.6 exclude the listed conditions with mention of pernicious complications (084.8-084.9).
EXCLUDES   congenital malaria (771.2)

DEF: Mosquito-borne disease causing high fever and prostration and cataloged by species of Plasmodium: P. falciparum, P. malariae, P. ovale, and P. vivax.

084.0 Falciparum malaria [malignant tertian]
Malaria (fever):
  by Plasmodium falciparum
  subtertian

084.1 Vivax malaria [benign tertian]
Malaria (fever) by Plasmodium vivax

084.2 Quartan malaria
Malaria (fever) by Plasmodium malariae
Malariae malaria

084.3 Ovale malaria
Malaria (fever) by Plasmodium ovale

084.4 Other malaria
Monkey malaria

084.5 Mixed malaria
Malaria (fever) by more than one parasite

084.6 Malaria, unspecified
Malaria (fever) NOS

084.7 Induced malaria
Therapeutically induced malaria
EXCLUDES   accidental infection from syringe, blood transfusion, etc. (084.0-084.6, above, according to parasite species)
transmission from mother to child during delivery (771.2)

N Newborn Age: 0   P Pediatric Age: 0-17   M Maternity Age: 12-55   A Adult Age: 15-124   MSP Medicare Secondary Payer

084.8 Blackwater fever

Hemoglobinuric: Malarial hemoglobinuria
  fever (bilious)
  malaria

DEF: Severe hemic and renal complication of *Plasmodium falciparum* infection.

084.9 Other pernicious complications of malaria

Algid malaria
Cerebral malaria
Use additional code to identify complication, as:
  malarial:
    hepatitis (573.2)
    nephrosis (581.81)

✓4ᵗʰ 085 Leishmaniasis

085.0 Visceral [kala-azar]

Dumdum fever
Infection by Leishmania:
  donovani
  infantum
Leishmaniasis:
  dermal, post-kala-azar
  Mediterranean
  visceral (Indian)

085.1 Cutaneous, urban

Aleppo boil   Leishmaniasis, cutaneous:
Baghdad boil   dry form
Delhi boil   late
Infection by Leishmania   recurrent
  tropica (minor)   ulcerating
                      Oriental sore

085.2 Cutaneous, Asian desert

Infection by Leishmania tropica major
Leishmaniasis, cutaneous:
  acute necrotizing
  rural
  wet form
  zoonotic form

085.3 Cutaneous, Ethiopian

Infection by Leishmania ethiopica
Leishmaniasis, cutaneous:
  diffuse
  lepromatous

085.4 Cutaneous, American

Chiclero ulcer
Infection by Leishmania mexicana
Leishmaniasis tegumentaria diffusa

085.5 Mucocutaneous (American)

Espundia
Infection by Leishmania braziliensis
Uta

085.9 Leishmaniasis, unspecified

✓4ᵗʰ 086 Trypanosomiasis

Use additional code to identify manifestations, as:
  trypanosomiasis:
    encephalitis (323.2)
    meningitis (321.3)

086.0 Chagas' disease with heart involvement

American trypanosomiasis } with heart
Infection by Trypanosoma   involvement
  cruzi

Any condition classifiable to 086.2 with heart involvement

086.1 Chagas' disease with other organ involvement

American
  trypanosomiasis   } with involvement of
Infection by   organ other
  Trypanosoma cruzi   than heart

Any condition classifiable to 086.2 with involvement of organ other than heart

086.2 Chagas' disease without mention of organ involvement

American trypanosomiasis
Infection by Trypanosoma cruzi

086.3 Gambian trypanosomiasis

Gambian sleeping sickness
Infection by Trypanosoma gambiense

086.4 Rhodesian trypanosomiasis

Infection by Trypanosoma rhodesiense
Rhodesian sleeping sickness

086.5 African trypanosomiasis, unspecified

Sleeping sickness NOS

086.9 Trypanosomiasis, unspecified

✓4ᵗʰ 087 Relapsing fever

INCLUDES recurrent fever

DEF: Infection by *Borrelia*; symptoms are episodic and include fever and arthralgia.

087.0 Louse-borne

087.1 Tick-borne

087.9 Relapsing fever, unspecified

✓4ᵗʰ 088 Other arthropod-borne diseases

088.0 Bartonellosis

Carrión's disease   Verruga peruana
Oroya fever

✓5ᵗʰ 088.8 Other specified arthropod-borne diseases

088.81 Lyme disease

Erythema chronicum migrans
AHA: 4Q, '91, 15; 3Q, '90, 14; 2Q, '89, 10

DEF: A recurrent multisystem disorder caused by the spirochete *Borrelia burgdorferi* with the carrier being the tick *Ixodes damminii*; the disease begins with lesions of erythema chronicum migrans; it is followed by arthritis of the large joints, myalgia, malaise, and neurological and cardiac manifestations.

088.82 Babesiosis

Babesiasis
AHA: 4Q, '93, 23

DEF: A tick-borne disease caused by infection of *Babesia*, characterized by fever, malaise, listlessness, severe anemia and hemoglobinuria.

088.89 Other

088.9 Arthropod-borne disease, unspecified

SYPHILIS AND OTHER VENEREAL DISEASES (090-099)

EXCLUDES nonvenereal endemic syphilis (104.0)
          urogenital trichomoniasis (131.0)

✓4ᵗʰ 090 Congenital syphilis

DEF: Infection by spirochete *Treponema pallidum* acquired in utero from the infected mother.

090.0 Early congenital syphilis, symptomatic

Congenital syphilitic: Congenital syphilitic:
  choroiditis   splenomegaly
  coryza (chronic)   Syphilitic (congenital):
  hepatomegaly   epiphysitis
  mucous patches   osteochondritis
  periostitis   pemphigus
Any congenital syphilitic condition specified as early or manifest less than two years after birth

090.1 Early congenital syphilis, latent

Congenital syphilis without clinical manifestations, with positive serological reaction and negative spinal fluid test, less than two years after birth

090.2 Early congenital syphilis, unspecified

Congenital syphilis NOS, less than two years after birth

✓4ᵗʰ
✓5ᵗʰ Additional Digit Required   Unspecified Code   Other Specified Code   Manifestation Code   ▶◀ Revised Text   ● New Code   ▲ Revised Code Title

2005 ICD•9•CM   Volume 1 — 15

090.3 **Syphilitic interstitial keratitis**
Syphilitic keratitis:
parenchymatous
punctata profunda
EXCLUDES interstitial keratitis NOS (370.50)

√5ᵗʰ **090.4** **Juvenile neurosyphilis**
Use additional code to identify any associated
mental disorder
DEF: *Treponema pallidum* infection involving the nervous system.

090.40 **Juvenile neurosyphilis, unspecified**
Congenital neurosyphilis
Dementia paralytica juvenilis
Juvenile:
general paresis
tabes
taboparesis

090.41 **Congenital syphilitic encephalitis**
DEF: Congenital *Treponema pallidum* infection involving the brain.

090.42 **Congenital syphilitic meningitis**
DEF: Congenital *Treponema pallidum* infection involving the lining of the brain and/or spinal cord.

090.49 **Other**

090.5 **Other late congenital syphilis, symptomatic**
Gumma due to congenital syphilis
Hutchinson's teeth
Syphilitic saddle nose
Any congenital syphilitic condition specified as late
or manifest two years or more after birth

090.6 **Late congenital syphilis, latent**
Congenital syphilis without clinical manifestations,
with positive serological reaction and negative
spinal fluid test, two years or more after birth

090.7 **Late congenital syphilis, unspecified**
Congenital syphilis NOS, two years or more after birth

090.9 **Congenital syphilis, unspecified**

√4ᵗʰ **091** **Early syphilis, symptomatic**
EXCLUDES early cardiovascular syphilis (093.0-093.9)
early neurosyphilis (094.0-094.9)

091.0 **Genital syphilis (primary)**
Genital chancre
DEF: Genital lesion at the site of initial infection by *Treponema pallidum*.

091.1 **Primary anal syphilis**
DEF: Anal lesion at the site of initial infection by *Treponema pallidum*.

091.2 **Other primary syphilis**
Primary syphilis of: Primary syphilis of:
breast   lip
fingers   tonsils
DEF: Lesion at the site of initial infection by *Treponema pallidum*.

091.3 **Secondary syphilis of skin or mucous membranes**
Condyloma latum   Secondary syphilis of:
Secondary syphilis of: skin
anus   tonsils
mouth   vulva
pharynx
DEF: Transitory or chronic lesions following initial syphilis infection.

091.4 **Adenopathy due to secondary syphilis**
Syphilitic adenopathy (secondary)
Syphilitic lymphadenitis (secondary)

√5ᵗʰ **091.5** **Uveitis due to secondary syphilis**
091.50 **Syphilitic uveitis, unspecified**
091.51 **Syphilitic chorioretinitis (secondary)**
DEF: Inflammation of choroid and retina as a secondary infection.

091.52 **Syphilitic iridocyclitis (secondary)**
DEF: Inflammation of iris and ciliary body as a secondary infection.

√5ᵗʰ **091.6** **Secondary syphilis of viscera and bone**
091.61 **Secondary syphilitic periostitis**
DEF: Inflammation of outer layers of bone as a secondary infection.

091.62 **Secondary syphilitic hepatitis**
Secondary syphilis of liver

091.69 **Other viscera**

091.7 **Secondary syphilis, relapse**
Secondary syphilis, relapse (treated) (untreated)

√5ᵗʰ **091.8** **Other forms of secondary syphilis**
091.81 **Acute syphilitic meningitis (secondary)**
DEF: Sudden, severe inflammation of the lining of the brain and/or spinal cord as a secondary infection.

091.82 **Syphilitic alopecia**
DEF: Hair loss following initial syphilis infection.

091.89 **Other**

091.9 **Unspecified secondary syphilis**

√4ᵗʰ **092** **Early syphilis, latent**
INCLUDES syphilis (acquired) without clinical
manifestations, with positive serological
reaction and negative spinal fluid test,
less than two years after infection

092.0 **Early syphilis, latent, serological relapse after treatment**

092.9 **Early syphilis, latent, unspecified**

√4ᵗʰ **093** **Cardiovascular syphilis**
093.0 **Aneurysm of aorta, specified as syphilitic**
Dilatation of aorta, specified as syphilitic

093.1 **Syphilitic aortitis**
DEF: Inflammation of the aorta - the main artery leading from the heart.

√5ᵗʰ **093.2** **Syphilitic endocarditis**
DEF: Inflammation of the tissues lining the cavities of the heart.

093.20 **Valve, unspecified**
Syphilitic ostial coronary disease
093.21 **Mitral valve**
093.22 **Aortic valve**
Syphilitic aortic incompetence or stenosis
093.23 **Tricuspid valve**
093.24 **Pulmonary valve**

√5ᵗʰ **093.8** **Other specified cardiovascular syphilis**
093.81 **Syphilitic pericarditis**
DEF: Inflammation of the outer lining of the heart.

093.82 **Syphilitic myocarditis**
DEF: Inflammation of the muscle of the heart.

093.89 **Other**

093.9 **Cardiovascular syphilis, unspecified**

√4ᵗʰ **094** **Neurosyphilis**
Use additional code to identify any associated mental disorder
094.0 **Tabes dorsalis**
Locomotor ataxia (progressive)
Posterior spinal sclerosis (syphilitic)
Tabetic neurosyphilis
Use additional code to identify manifestation, as:
neurogenic arthropathy [Charcot's joint disease] (713.5)
DEF: Progressive degeneration of nerves associated with long-term syphilis; causing pain, wasting away, incontinence, and ataxia.

094.1 **General paresis**
     Dementia paralytica
     General paralysis (of the insane) (progressive)
     Paretic neurosyphilis
     Taboparesis
     DEF: Degeneration of brain associated with long-term syphilis, causing loss of brain function, progressive dementia, and paralysis.

094.2 **Syphilitic meningitis**
     Meningovascular syphilis
        EXCLUDES   acute syphilitic meningitis (secondary) (091.81)
     DEF: Inflammation of the lining of the brain and/or spinal cord.

094.3 **Asymptomatic neurosyphilis**

✓5ᵗʰ **094.8** **Other specified neurosyphilis**
     094.81 Syphilitic encephalitis
     094.82 Syphilitic Parkinsonism
        DEF: Decreased motor function, tremors, and muscular rigidity.
     094.83 Syphilitic disseminated retinochoroiditis
        DEF: Inflammation of retina and choroid due to neurosyphilis.
     094.84 Syphilitic optic atrophy
        DEF: Degeneration of the eye and its nerves due to neurosyphilis.
     094.85 Syphilitic retrobulbar neuritis
        DEF: Inflammation of the posterior optic nerve due to neurosyphilis.
     094.86 Syphilitic acoustic neuritis
        DEF: Inflammation of acoustic nerve due to neurosyphilis.
     094.87 Syphilitic ruptured cerebral aneurysm
     094.89 Other

094.9 **Neurosyphilis, unspecified**
     Gumma (syphilitic)
     Syphilis (early) (late) } of central nervous
     Syphiloma   system NOS

✓4ᵗʰ **095 Other forms of late syphilis, with symptoms**
        INCLUDES   gumma (syphilitic)
                 syphilis, late, tertiary, or unspecified stage

     095.0 **Syphilitic episcleritis**
     095.1 **Syphilis of lung**
     095.2 **Syphilitic peritonitis**
     095.3 **Syphilis of liver**
     095.4 **Syphilis of kidney**
     095.5 **Syphilis of bone**
     095.6 **Syphilis of muscle**
        Syphilitic myositis
     095.7 **Syphilis of synovium, tendon, and bursa**
        Syphilitic: Syphilitic:
        bursitis   synovitis
     095.8 **Other specified forms of late symptomatic syphilis**
        EXCLUDES   cardiovascular syphilis (093.0-093.9)
                 neurosyphilis (094.0-094.9)
     095.9 **Late symptomatic syphilis, unspecified**

096 Late syphilis, latent
     Syphilis (acquired) without clinical manifestations, with positive serological reaction and negative spinal fluid test, two years or more after infection

✓4ᵗʰ **097 Other and unspecified syphilis**
     097.0 **Late syphilis, unspecified**
     097.1 **Latent syphilis, unspecified**
        Positive serological reaction for syphilis
     097.9 **Syphilis, unspecified**
        Syphilis (acquired) NOS
        EXCLUDES   syphilis NOS causing death under two years of age (090.9)

✓4ᵗʰ **098 Gonococcal infections**
     DEF: *Neisseria gonorrhoeae* infection generally acquired in utero or in sexual congress.

     098.0 **Acute, of lower genitourinary tract**
        Gonococcal: Gonorrhea (acute):
        Bartholinitis (acute)   NOS
        urethritis (acute)   genitourinary (tract) NOS
        vulvovaginitis (acute)

✓5ᵗʰ **098.1** **Acute, of upper genitourinary tract**
     098.10 Gonococcal infection (acute) of upper genitourinary tract, site unspecified
     098.11 Gonococcal cystitis (acute)
        Gonorrhea (acute) of bladder
     098.12 Gonococcal prostatitis (acute)   ♂
     098.13 Gonococcal epididymo-orchitis (acute)   ♂
        Gonococcal orchitis (acute)
        DEF: Acute inflammation of the testes.
     098.14 Gonococcal seminal vesiculitis (acute)   ♂
        Gonorrhea (acute) of seminal vesicle
     098.15 Gonococcal cervicitis (acute)   ♀
        Gonorrhea (acute) of cervix
     098.16 Gonococcal endometritis (acute)   ♀
        Gonorrhea (acute) of uterus
     098.17 Gonococcal salpingitis, specified as acute ♀
        DEF: Acute inflammation of the fallopian tubes.
     098.19 Other

     098.2 **Chronic, of lower genitourinary tract**
        Gonococcal:
        Bartholinitis
        urethritis   } specified as chronic or
        vulvovaginitis   with duration of
        Gonorrhea: two months or
        NOS   more
        genitourinary (tract) }

        Any condition classifiable to 098.0 specified as chronic or with duration of two months or more

✓5ᵗʰ **098.3** **Chronic, of upper genitourinary tract**
        INCLUDES   any condition classifiable to 098.1 stated as chronic or with a duration of two months or more
     098.30 Chronic gonococcal infection of upper genitourinary tract, site unspecified
     098.31 Gonococcal cystitis, chronic
        Any condition classifiable to 098.11, specified as chronic
        Gonorrhea of bladder, chronic
     098.32 Gonococcal prostatitis, chronic   ♂
        Any condition classifiable to 098.12, specified as chronic
     098.33 Gonococcal epididymo-orchitis, chronic ♂
        Any condition classifiable to 098.13, specified as chronic
        Chronic gonococcal orchitis
        DEF: Chronic inflammation of the testes.
     098.34 Gonococcal seminal vesiculitis, chronic ♂
        Any condition classifiable to 098.14, specified as chronic
        Gonorrhea of seminal vesicle, chronic
     098.35 Gonococcal cervicitis, chronic   ♀
        Any condition classifiable to 098.15, specified as chronic
        Gonorrhea of cervix, chronic
     098.36 Gonococcal endometritis, chronic   ♀
        Any condition classifiable to 098.16, specified as chronic
        DEF: Chronic inflammation of the uterus.

✓4ᵗʰ
✓5ᵗʰ   Additional Digit Required   Unspecified Code   Other Specified Code   Manifestation Code   ►◄ Revised Text   ● New Code   ▲ Revised Code Title

2005 ICD•9•CM   **Volume 1 — 17**

098.37 Gonococcal salpingitis (chronic) ♀
DEF: Chronic inflammation of the fallopian tubes.

098.39 Other

√5ᵗʰ **098.4 Gonococcal infection of eye**
098.40 Gonococcal conjunctivitis (neonatorum)
Gonococcal ophthalmia (neonatorum)
DEF: Inflammation and infection of conjunctiva present at birth.

098.41 Gonococcal iridocyclitis
DEF: Inflammation and infection of iris and ciliary body.

098.42 Gonococcal endophthalmia
DEF: Inflammation and infection of the contents of the eyeball.

098.43 Gonococcal keratitis
DEF: Inflammation and infection of the cornea.

098.49 Other

√5ᵗʰ **098.5 Gonococcal infection of joint**
098.50 Gonococcal arthritis
Gonococcal infection of joint NOS
098.51 Gonococcal synovitis and tenosynovitis
098.52 Gonococcal bursitis
DEF: Inflammation of the sac-like cavities in a joint.

098.53 Gonococcal spondylitis
098.59 Other
Gonococcal rheumatism

098.6 Gonococcal infection of pharynx
098.7 Gonococcal infection of anus and rectum
Gonococcal proctitis

√5ᵗʰ **098.8 Gonococcal infection of other specified sites**
098.81 Gonococcal keratosis (blennorrhagica)
DEF: Pustular skin lesions caused by *Neisseria gonorrhoeae*.

098.82 Gonococcal meningitis
DEF: Inflammation of the lining of the brain and/or spinal cord.

098.83 Gonococcal pericarditis
DEF: Inflammation of the outer lining of the heart.

098.84 Gonococcal endocarditis
DEF: Inflammation of the tissues lining the cavities of the heart.

098.85 Other gonococcal heart disease
098.86 Gonococcal peritonitis
DEF: Inflammation of the membrane lining the abdomen.

098.89 Other
Gonococcemia

√4ᵗʰ **099 Other venereal diseases**
099.0 Chancroid

Bubo (inguinal):	Chancre:
chancroidal	Ducrey's
due to Hemophilus	simple
ducreyi	soft
	Ulcus molle (cutis) (skin)

DEF: A sexually transmitted disease caused by *Haemophilus ducreyi*; it is identified by a painful primary ulcer at the site of inoculation (usually on the external genitalia) with related lymphadenitis.

099.1 Lymphogranuloma venereum
Climatic or tropical bubo
(Durand-) Nicolas-Favre disease
Esthiomene
Lymphogranuloma inguinale
DEF: Sexually transmitted infection of *Chlamydia trachomatis* causing skin lesions.

099.2 Granuloma inguinale

Donovanosis	Granuloma venereum
Granuloma pudendi	Pudendal ulcer
(ulcerating)	

DEF: Chronic, sexually transmitted infection of *Calymmatobacterium granulomatis*, resulting in progressive, anogenital skin ulcers.

099.3 Reiter's disease
Reiter's syndrome
Use additional code for associated:
arthropathy (711.1)
conjunctivitis (372.33)
DEF: A symptom complex of unknown etiology consisting of urethritis, conjunctivitis, arthritis and myocutaneous lesions. It occurs most commonly in young men and patients with HIV and may precede or follow AIDS. Also a form of reactive arthritis.

√5ᵗʰ **099.4 Other nongonococcal urethritis [NGU]**
099.40 Unspecified
Nonspecific urethritis
099.41 Chlamydia trachomatis
099.49 Other specified organism

√5ᵗʰ **099.5 Other venereal diseases due to Chlamydia trachomatis**
    EXCLUDES   *Chlamydia trachomatis infection of conjunctiva (076.0-076.9, 077.0, 077.9)*
    Lymphogranuloma venereum (099.1)
DEF: Venereal diseases caused by *Chlamydia trachomatis* at other sites besides the urethra (e.g., pharynx, anus and rectum, conjunctiva and peritoneum).

099.50 Unspecified site
099.51 Pharynx
099.52 Anus and rectum
099.53 Lower genitourinary sites
    EXCLUDES   *urethra (099.41)*
Use additional code to specify site of infection, such as:
bladder (595.4)
cervix (616.0)
vagina and vulva (616.11)
099.54 Other genitourinary sites
Use additional code to specify site of infection, such as:
pelvic inflammatory disease NOS (614.9)
testis and epididymis (604.91)
099.55 Unspecified genitourinary site
099.56 Peritoneum
Perihepatitis
099.59 Other specified site
099.8 Other specified venereal diseases
099.9 Venereal disease, unspecified

OTHER SPIROCHETAL DISEASES (100-104)

√4ᵗʰ **100 Leptospirosis**
DEF: An infection of any spirochete of the genus Leptospire in blood. This zoonosis is transmitted to humans most often by exposure with contaminated animal tissues or water and less often by contact with urine. Patients present with flulike symptoms, the most common being muscle aches involving the thighs and low back. Treatment is with hydration and antibiotics.

100.0 Leptospirosis icterohemorrhagica
Leptospiral or spirochetal jaundice (hemorrhagic)
Weil's disease

√5ᵗʰ **100.8 Other specified leptospiral infections**
100.81 Leptospiral meningitis (aseptic)
100.89 Other

Fever:	Infection by Leptospira:
Fort Bragg	australis
pretibial	bataviae
swamp	pyrogenes

100.9 Leptospirosis, unspecified

101 Vincent's angina

Acute necrotizing ulcerative: Trench mouth
   gingivitis   Vincent's:
   stomatitis   gingivitis
Fusospirochetal pharyngitis   infection [any site]
Spirochetal stomatitis

DEF: Painful ulceration with edema and hypermic patches of the oropharyngeal and throat membranes; it is caused by spreading of acute ulcerative gingivitis.

✓4ᵗʰ 102 Yaws

   INCLUDES   frambesia
              pian

DEF: An infectious, endemic, tropical disease caused by *Treponema pertenue*; it usually affects persons 15 years old or younger; a primary cutaneous lesion develops, then a granulomatous skin eruption, and occasionally lesions that destroy skin and bone.

102.0 Initial lesions

Chancre of yaws
Frambesia, initial or primary
Initial frambesial ulcer
Mother yaw

102.1 Multiple papillomata and wet crab yaws

Butter yaws   Plantar or palmar
Frambesioma   papilloma of yaws
Pianoma

102.2 Other early skin lesions

Cutaneous yaws, less than five years after infection
Early yaws (cutaneous) (macular) (papular)
   (maculopapular) (micropapular)
Frambeside of early yaws

102.3 Hyperkeratosis

Ghoul hand
Hyperkeratosis, palmar or plantar (early) (late) due
   to yaws
Worm-eaten soles

DEF: Overgrowth of the skin of the palms or bottoms of the feet, due to yaws.

102.4 Gummata and ulcers

Gummatous frambeside
Nodular late yaws (ulcerated)

DEF: Rubbery lesions and areas of dead skin caused by yaws.

102.5 Gangosa

Rhinopharyngitis mutilans

DEF: Massive, mutilating lesions of the nose and oral cavity caused by yaws.

102.6 Bone and joint lesions

Goundou
Gumma, bone   } of yaws (late)
Gummatous osteitis or
   periostitis

Hydrarthrosis
Osteitis   } of yaws (early) (late)
Periostitis (hypertrophic)

102.7 Other manifestations

Juxta-articular nodules of yaws
Mucosal yaws

102.8 Latent yaws

Yaws without clinical manifestations, with positive
   serology

102.9 Yaws, unspecified

✓4ᵗʰ 103 Pinta

DEF: A chronic form of treponematosis, endemic in areas of tropical America; it is identified by the presence of red, violet, blue, coffee-colored or white spots on the skin.

103.0 Primary lesions

Chancre (primary)
Papule (primary)   } of pinta [carate]
Pintid

103.1 Intermediate lesions

Erythematous plaques
Hyperchromic lesions   } of pinta [carate]
Hyperkeratosis

103.2 Late lesions

Cardiovascular lesions
Skin lesions:
   achromic   } of pinta [carate]
   cicatricial
   dyschromic
Vitiligo

103.3 Mixed lesions

Achromic and hyperchromic skin lesions of pinta
   [carate]

103.9 Pinta, unspecified

✓4ᵗʰ 104 Other spirochetal infection

104.0 Nonvenereal endemic syphilis

Bejel
Njovera

DEF: *Treponema pallidum, T. pertenue*, or *T. carateum* infection transmitted non-sexually, causing lesions on mucosa and skin.

104.8 Other specified spirochetal infections

   EXCLUDES   relapsing fever (087.0-087.9)
              syphilis (090.0-097.9)

104.9 Spirochetal infection, unspecified

MYCOSES (110-118)

Use additional code to identify manifestation as:
   arthropathy (711.6)
   meningitis (321.0-321.1)
   otitis externa (380.15)

   EXCLUDES   infection by Actinomycetales, such as species of
              Actinomyces, Actinomadura, Nocardia,
              Streptomyces (039.0-039.9)

✓4ᵗʰ 110 Dermatophytosis

   INCLUDES   infection by species of Epidermophyton,
              Microsporum, and Trichophyton
              tinea, any type except those in 111

DEF: Superficial infection of the skin caused by a parasitic fungus.

110.0 Of scalp and beard

Kerion   Trichophytic tinea
Sycosis, mycotic   [black dot tinea], scalp

110.1 Of nail

Dermatophytic onychia   Tinea unguium
Onychomycosis

110.2 Of hand

Tinea manuum

110.3 Of groin and perianal area

Dhobie itch   Tinea cruris
Eczema marginatum

110.4 Of foot

Athlete's foot   Tinea pedis

110.5 Of the body

Herpes circinatus   Tinea imbricata [Tokelau]

110.6 Deep seated dermatophytosis

Granuloma trichophyticum
Majocchi's granuloma

110.8 Of other specified sites

110.9 Of unspecified site

Favus NOS   Ringworm NOS
Microsporic tinea NOS

✓4ᵗʰ
✓5ᵗʰ Additional Digit Required   Unspecified Code   Other Specified Code   Manifestation Code   ►◄ Revised Text   ● New Code   ▲ Revised Code Title

2005 ICD•9•CM   **Volume 1 — 19**

√4ᵗʰ **111 Dermatomycosis, other and unspecified**

111.0 Pityriasis versicolor
Infection by Malassezia [Pityrosporum] furfur
Tinea flava
Tinea versicolor

111.1 Tinea nigra
Infection by Cladosporium species
Keratomycosis nigricans
Microsporosis nigra
Pityriasis nigra
Tinea palmaris nigra

111.2 Tinea blanca
Infection by Trichosporon (beigelii) cutaneum
White piedra

111.3 Black piedra
Infection by Piedraia hortai

111.8 Other specified dermatomycoses

111.9 Dermatomycosis, unspecified

√4ᵗʰ **112 Candidiasis**

INCLUDES   infection by Candida species
moniliasis

EXCLUDES   neonatal monilial infection (771.7)

DEF: Fungal infection caused by *Candida*; usually seen in mucous membranes or skin.

112.0 Of mouth
Thrush (oral)

112.1 Of vulva and vagina   ♀
Candidal vulvovaginitis   Monilial vulvovaginitis

112.2 Of other urogenital sites
Candidal balanitis

AHA: ▶4Q, '03, 105;◀ 4Q, '96, 33

112.3 Of skin and nails
Candidal intertrigo   Candidal perionyxis
Candidal onychia   [paronychia]

112.4 Of lung
Candidal pneumonia

AHA: 2Q, '98, 7

112.5 Disseminated
Systemic candidiasis

AHA: 2Q, '00, 5; 2Q, '89, 10

√5ᵗʰ **112.8 Of other specified sites**

112.81 Candidal endocarditis

112.82 Candidal otitis externa
Otomycosis in moniliasis

112.83 Candidal meningitis

112.84 Candidal esophagitis
AHA: 4Q, '92, 19

112.85 Candidal enteritis
AHA: 4Q, '92, 19

112.89 Other
AHA: 1Q, '92, 17; 3Q, '91, 20

112.9 Of unspecified site

√4ᵗʰ **114 Coccidioidomycosis**

INCLUDES   infection by Coccidioides (immitis)
Posada-Wernicke disease

AHA: 4Q, '93, 23

DEF: A fungal disease caused by inhalation of dust particles containing arthrospores of *Coccidiodes immitis*; a self-limited respiratory infection; the primary form is known as San Joaquin fever, desert fever or valley fever.

114.0 Primary coccidioidomycosis (pulmonary)
Acute pulmonary coccidioidomycosis
Coccidioidomycotic pneumonitis
Desert rheumatism
Pulmonary coccidioidomycosis
San Joaquin Valley fever

DEF: Acute, self-limiting *Coccidioides immitis* infection of the lung.

114.1 Primary extrapulmonary coccidioidomycosis
Chancriform syndrome
Primary cutaneous coccidioidomycosis

DEF: Acute, self-limiting *Coccidioides immitis* infection in non-pulmonary site.

114.2 Coccidioidal meningitis

DEF: *Coccidioides immitis* infection of the lining of the brain and/or spinal cord.

114.3 Other forms of progressive coccidioidomycosis
Coccidioidal granuloma
Disseminated coccidioidomycosis

114.4 Chronic pulmonary coccidioidomycosis

114.5 Pulmonary coccidioidomycosis, unspecified

114.9 Coccidioidomycosis, unspecified

√4ᵗʰ **115 Histoplasmosis**

The following fifth-digit subclassification is for use with category 115:
 0 **without mention of manifestation**
 1 **meningitis**
 2 **retinitis**
 3 **pericarditis**
 4 **endocarditis**
 5 **pneumonia**
 9 **other**

√5ᵗʰ **115.0 Infection by Histoplasma capsulatum**
American histoplasmosis
Darling's disease
Reticuloendothelial cytomycosis
Small form histoplasmosis

DEF: Infection resulting from inhalation of fungal spores, causing acute pneumonia, an influenza-like illness, or a disseminated disease of the reticuloendothelial system. In immunocompromised patients it can reactivate, affecting lungs, meninges, heart, peritoneum and adrenals.

√5ᵗʰ **115.1 Infection by Histoplasma duboisii**
African histoplasmosis
Large form histoplasmosis

√5ᵗʰ **115.9 Histoplasmosis, unspecified**
Histoplasmosis NOS

√4ᵗʰ **116 Blastomycotic infection**

116.0 Blastomycosis
Blastomycotic dermatitis
Chicago disease
Cutaneous blastomycosis
Disseminated blastomycosis
Gilchrist's disease
Infection by Blastomyces [Ajellomyces] dermatitidis
North American blastomycosis
Primary pulmonary blastomycosis

116.1 Paracoccidioidomycosis
Brazilian blastomycosis
Infection by Paracoccidioides [Blastomyces]
    brasiliensis
Lutz-Splendore-Almeida disease
Mucocutaneous-lymphangitic
    paracoccidioidomycosis
Pulmonary paracoccidioidomycosis
South American blastomycosis
Visceral paracoccidioidomycosis

116.2 Lobomycosis
Infections by Loboa [Blastomyces] loboi
Keloidal blastomycosis
Lobo's disease

√4ᵗʰ **117 Other mycoses**

117.0 Rhinosporidiosis
Infection by Rhinosporidium seeberi

N Newborn Age: 0   P Pediatric Age: 0-17   M Maternity Age: 12-55   A Adult Age: 15-124   MSP Medicare Secondary Payer

117.1 Sporotrichosis
Cutaneous sporotrichosis
Disseminated sporotrichosis
Infection by Sporothrix [Sporotrichum] schenckii
Lymphocutaneous sporotrichosis
Pulmonary sporotrichosis
Sporotrichosis of the bones

117.2 Chromoblastomycosis
Chromomycosis
Infection by Cladosporidium carrionii, Fonsecaea
compactum, Fonsecaea pedrosoi, Phialophora
verrucosa

117.3 Aspergillosis
Infection by Aspergillus species, mainly A.
fumigatus, A. flavus group, A. terreus group
AHA: 4Q, '97, 40

117.4 Mycotic mycetomas
Infection by various genera and species of
Ascomycetes and Deuteromycetes, such as
Acremonium [Cephalosporium] falciforme,
Neotestudina rosatii, Madurella grisea,
Madurella mycetomii, Pyrenochaeta romeroi,
Zopfia [Leptosphaeria] senegalensis
Madura foot, mycotic
Maduromycosis, mycotic
EXCLUDES *actinomycotic mycetomas (039.0-039.9)*

117.5 Cryptococcosis
Busse-Buschke's disease
European cryptococcosis
Infection by Cryptococcus neoformans
Pulmonary cryptococcosis
Systemic cryptococcosis
Torula

117.6 Allescheriosis [Petriellidosis]
Infections by Allescheria [Petriellidium] boydii
[Monosporium apiospermum]
EXCLUDES *mycotic mycetoma (117.4)*

117.7 Zygomycosis [Phycomycosis or Mucormycosis]
Infection by species of Absidia, Basidiobolus,
Conidiobolus, Cunninghamella,
Entomophthora, Mucor, Rhizopus, Saksenaea

**117.8 Infection by dematiacious fungi,
[Phaehyphomycosis]**
Infection by dematiacious fungi, such as
Cladosporium trichoides [bantianum],
Dreschlera hawaiiensis, Phialophora
gougerotii, Phialophora jeanselmi

117.9 Other and unspecified mycoses

118 Opportunistic mycoses
Infection of skin, subcutaneous tissues, and/or organs by a
wide variety of fungi generally considered to be
pathogenic to compromised hosts only (e.g., infection
by species of Alternaria, Dreschlera, Fusarium)

HELMINTHIASES (120-129)

✓4th 120 Schistosomiasis [bilharziasis]
DEF: Infection caused by *Schistosoma*, a genus of flukes or trematode
parasites.

120.0 Schistosoma haematobium
Vesical schistosomiasis NOS

120.1 Schistosoma mansoni
Intestinal schistosomiasis NOS

120.2 Schistosoma japonicum
Asiatic schistosomiasis NOS
Katayama disease or fever

120.3 Cutaneous
Cercarial dermatitis
Infection by cercariae of Schistosoma
Schistosome dermatitis
Swimmers' itch

120.8 Other specified schistosomiasis
Infection by Schistosoma:
bovis
intercalatum
mattheii
spindale
Schistosomiasis chestermani

120.9 Schistosomiasis, unspecified
Blood flukes NOS
Hemic distomiasis

✓4th 121 Other trematode infections
121.0 Opisthorchiasis
Infection by:
cat liver fluke
Opisthorchis (felineus) (tenuicollis) (viverrini)

121.1 Clonorchiasis
Biliary cirrhosis due to clonorchiasis
Chinese liver fluke disease
Hepatic distomiasis due to Clonorchis sinensis
Oriental liver fluke disease

121.2 Paragonimiasis
Infection by Paragonimus
Lung fluke disease (oriental)
Pulmonary distomiasis

121.3 Fascioliasis
Infection by Fasciola:
gigantica
hepatica
Liver flukes NOS
Sheep liver fluke infection

121.4 Fasciolopsiasis
Infection by Fasciolopsis (buski)
Intestinal distomiasis

121.5 Metagonimiasis
Infection by Metagonimus yokogawai

121.6 Heterophyiasis
Infection by:
Heterophyes heterophyes
Stellantchasmus falcatus

121.8 Other specified trematode infections
Infection by:
Dicrocoelium dendriticum
Echinostoma ilocanum
Gastrodiscoides hominis

121.9 Trematode infection, unspecified
Distomiasis NOS
Fluke disease NOS

✓4th 122 Echinococcosis
INCLUDES echinococciasis
hydatid disease
hydatidosis

DEF: Infection caused by larval forms of tapeworms of the genus
Echinococcus.

122.0 Echinococcus granulosus infection of liver
122.1 Echinococcus granulosus infection of lung
122.2 Echinococcus granulosus infection of thyroid
122.3 Echinococcus granulosus infection, other
122.4 Echinococcus granulosus infection, unspecified
122.5 Echinococcus multilocularis infection of liver
122.6 Echinococcus multilocularis infection, other
122.7 Echinococcus multilocularis infection, unspecified
122.8 Echinococcosis, unspecified, of liver
122.9 Echinococcosis, other and unspecified

✓4th 123 Other cestode infection
123.0 Taenia solium infection, intestinal form
Pork tapeworm (adult) (infection)

123.1 Cysticercosis
Cysticerciasis
Infection by Cysticercus cellulosae [larval form of
Taenia solium]
AHA: 2Q, '97, 8

✓4th ✓5th Additional Digit Required   Unspecified Code   Other Specified Code   Manifestation Code   ▶◀ Revised Text   ● New Code   ▲ Revised Code Title

2005 ICD•9•CM   **Volume 1 — 21**

123.2　Taenia saginata infection
　Beef tapeworm (infection)
　Infection by Taeniarhynchus saginatus

123.3　Taeniasis, unspecified

123.4　Diphyllobothriasis, intestinal
　Diphyllobothrium (adult) (latum) (pacificum) infection
　Fish tapeworm (infection)

123.5　Sparganosis [larval diphyllobothriasis]
　Infection by:
　　Diphyllobothrium larvae
　　Sparganum (mansoni) (proliferum)
　　Spirometra larvae

123.6　Hymenolepiasis
　Dwarf tapeworm (infection)
　Hymenolepis (diminuta) (nana) infection
　Rat tapeworm (infection)

123.8　Other specified cestode infection
　Diplogonoporus (grandis)　⎱
　Dipylidium (caninum)　　　⎬ infection
　Dog tapeworm (infection)　⎰

123.9　Cestode infection, unspecified
　Tapeworm (infection) NOS

124　Trichinosis
　Trichinella spiralis infection
　Trichinellosis
　Trichiniasis
　DEF: Infection by *Trichinella spiralis*, the smallest of the parasitic nematodes.

✓4ᵗʰ　125　Filarial infection and dracontiasis

125.0　Bancroftian filariasis
　Chyluria　　　　⎱
　Elephantiasis　 ⎮
　Infection　　　 ⎬ due to Wuchereria bancrofti
　Lymphadenitis　 ⎮
　Lymphangitis　　⎰
　Wuchereriasis

125.1　Malayan filariasis
　Brugia filariasis　⎱
　Chyluria　　　　　⎮
　Elephantiasis　　 ⎬ due to Brugia [Wuchereria]
　Infection　　　　 ⎮　　malayi
　Lymphadenitis　　⎮
　Lymphangitis　　 ⎰

125.2　Loiasis
　Eyeworm disease of Africa　Loa loa infection

125.3　Onchocerciasis
　Onchocerca volvulus infection
　Onchocercais

125.4　Dipetalonemiasis
　Infection by:
　　Acanthocheilonema perstans
　　Dipetalonema perstans

125.5　Mansonella ozzardi infection
　Filariasis ozzardi

125.6　Other specified filariasis
　Dirofilaria infection
　Infection by:
　　Acanthocheilonema streptocerca
　　Dipetalonema streptocerca

125.7　Dracontiasis
　Guinea-worm infection
　Infection by Dracunculus medinensis

125.9　Unspecified filariasis

✓4ᵗʰ　126　Ancylostomiasis and necatoriasis
　INCLUDES　cutaneous larva migrans due to Ancylostoma
　　hookworm (disease) (infection)
　　uncinariasis

126.0　Ancylostoma duodenale
126.1　Necator americanus
126.2　Ancylostoma braziliense

126.3　Ancylostoma ceylanicum
126.8　Other specified Ancylostoma
126.9　Ancylostomiasis and necatoriasis, unspecified
　Creeping eruption NOS
　Cutaneous larva migrans NOS

✓4ᵗʰ　127　Other intestinal helminthiases

127.0　Ascariasis
　Ascaridiasis
　Infection by Ascaris lumbricoides
　Roundworm infection

127.1　Anisakiasis
　Infection by Anisakis larva

127.2　Strongyloidiasis
　Infection by Strongyloides stercoralis
　EXCLUDES　trichostrongyliasis (127.6)

127.3　Trichuriasis
　Infection by Trichuris trichiuria
　Trichocephaliasis
　Whipworm (disease) (infection)

127.4　Enterobiasis
　Infection by Enterobius vermicularis
　Oxyuriasis
　Oxyuris vermicularis infection
　Pinworm (disease) (infection)
　Threadworm infection

127.5　Capillariasis
　Infection by Capillaria philippinensis
　EXCLUDES　infection by Capillaria hepatica (128.8)

127.6　Trichostrongyliasis
　Infection by Trichostrongylus species

127.7　Other specified intestinal helminthiasis
　Infection by:
　　Oesophagostomum apiostomum and related species
　　Ternidens diminutus
　　other specified intestinal helminth
　Physalopteriasis

127.8　Mixed intestinal helminthiasis
　Infection by intestinal helminths classified to more than one of the categories 120.0-127.7
　Mixed helminthiasis NOS

127.9　Intestinal helminthiasis, unspecified

✓4ᵗʰ　128　Other and unspecified helminthiases

128.0　Toxocariasis
　Larva migrans visceralis
　Toxocara (canis) (cati) infection
　Visceral larva migrans syndrome

128.1　Gnathostomiasis
　Infection by Gnathostoma spinigerum and related species

128.8　Other specified helminthiasis
　Infection by:
　　Angiostrongylus cantonensis
　　Capillaria hepatica
　　other specified helminth

128.9　Helminth infection, unspecified
　Helminthiasis NOS
　Worms NOS

129　Intestinal parasitism, unspecified

OTHER INFECTIOUS AND PARASITIC DISEASES (130–136)

✓4ᵗʰ　130　Toxoplasmosis
　INCLUDES　infection by toxoplasma gondii
　　toxoplasmosis (acquired)
　EXCLUDES　congenital toxoplasmosis (771.2)

130.0　Meningoencephalitis due to toxoplasmosis
　Encephalitis due to acquired toxoplasmosis

130.1　Conjunctivitis due to toxoplasmosis

130.2　Chorioretinitis due to toxoplasmosis
　Focal retinochoroiditis due to acquired toxoplasmosis

N　Newborn Age: 0　　P　Pediatric Age: 0-17　　M　Maternity Age: 12-55　　A　Adult Age: 15-124　　MSP　Medicare Secondary Payer

130.3   **Myocarditis due to toxoplasmosis**
130.4   **Pneumonitis due to toxoplasmosis**
130.5   **Hepatitis due to toxoplasmosis**
130.7   **Toxoplasmosis of other specified sites**
130.8   **Multisystemic disseminated toxoplasmosis**
     Toxoplasmosis of multiple sites
130.9   **Toxoplasmosis, unspecified**

√4th **131 Trichomoniasis**
     INCLUDES   infection due to Trichomonas (vaginalis)

√5th **131.0   Urogenital trichomoniasis**
131.00   **Urogenital trichomoniasis, unspecified**

     Fluor (vaginalis) ⎫ trichomonal or due
     Leukorrhea ⎬ to Trichomonas
       (vaginalis) ⎭ (vaginalis)

     DEF: *Trichomonas vaginalis* infection of reproductive and urinary organs, transmitted through coitus.

131.01   **Trichomonal vulvovaginitis**   ♀
     Vaginitis, trichomonal or due to Trichomonas (vaginalis)
     DEF: *Trichomonas vaginalis* infection of vulva and vagina; often asymptomatic, transmitted through coitus.

131.02   **Trichomonal urethritis**
     DEF: *Trichomonas vaginalis* infection of the urethra.

131.03   **Trichomonal prostatitis**   ♂
     DEF: *Trichomonas vaginalis* infection of the prostate.

131.09   **Other**
131.8   **Other specified sites**
     EXCLUDES   intestinal (007.3)
131.9   **Trichomoniasis, unspecified**

√4th **132 Pediculosis and phthirus infestation**
132.0   **Pediculus capitis [head louse]**
132.1   **Pediculus corporis [body louse]**
132.2   **Phthirus pubis [pubic louse]**
     Pediculus pubis
132.3   **Mixed infestation**
     Infestation classifiable to more than one of the categories 132.0-132.2
132.9   **Pediculosis, unspecified**

√4th **133 Acariasis**
133.0   **Scabies**
     Infestation by Sarcoptes scabiei
     Norwegian scabies
     Sarcoptic itch
133.8   **Other acariasis**
     Chiggers
     Infestation by:
       Demodex folliculorum
       Trombicula
133.9   **Acariasis, unspecified**
     Infestation by mites NOS

√4th **134 Other infestation**
134.0   **Myiasis**
     Infestation by:
       Dermatobia (hominis)
       fly larvae
       Gasterophilus (intestinalis)
       maggots
       Oestrus ovis
134.1   **Other arthropod infestation**
     Infestation by:
       chigoe
       sand flea
     Tunga penetrans
     Jigger disease
     Tungiasis
     Scarabiasis

134.2   **Hirudiniasis**
     Hirudiniasis (external) (internal)
     Leeches (aquatic) (land)
134.8   **Other specified infestations**
134.9   **Infestation, unspecified**
     Infestation (skin) NOS
     Skin parasites NOS

135 Sarcoidosis
     Besnier-Boeck-Schaumann disease
     Lupoid (miliary) of Boeck
     Lupus pernio (Besnier)
     Lymphogranulomatosis, benign (Schaumann's)
     Sarcoid (any site):
       NOS
       Boeck
       Darier-Roussy
     Uveoparotid fever
     DEF: A chronic, granulomatous reticulosis (abnormal increase in cells), affecting any organ or tissue; acute form has high rate of remission; chronic form is progressive.

√4th **136 Other and unspecified infectious and parasitic diseases**
136.0   **Ainhum**
     Dactylolysis spontanea
     DEF: A disease affecting the toes, especially the fifth digit, and sometimes the fingers, especially seen in black adult males; it is characterized by a linear constriction around the affected digit leading to spontaneous amputation of the distal part of the digit.
136.1   **Behçet's syndrome**
     DEF: A chronic inflammatory disorder of unknown etiology involving the small blood vessels; it is characterized by recurrent aphthous ulceration of the oral and pharyngeal mucous membranes and the genitalia, skin lesions, severe uvetis, retinal vascularitis and optic atrophy.
136.2   **Specific infections by free-living amebae**
     Meningoencephalitis due to Naegleria
136.3   **Pneumocystosis**
     Pneumonia due to Pneumocystis carinii
     AHA: 1Q, '03, 15; N-D, '87, 5, 6
     DEF: *Pneumocystis carinii* fungus causing pneumonia in immunocompromised patients; a leading cause of death among AIDS patients.
136.4   **Psorospermiasis**
136.5   **Sarcosporidiosis**
     Infection by Sarcocystis lindemanni
     DEF: Sarcocystis infection causing muscle cysts of intestinal inflammation.
136.8   **Other specified infectious and parasitic diseases**
     Candiru infestation
136.9   **Unspecified infectious and parasitic diseases**
     Infectious disease NOS
     Parasitic disease NOS
     AHA: 2Q, '91, 8

LATE EFFECTS OF INFECTIOUS AND PARASITIC DISEASES (137-139)

√4th **137 Late effects of tuberculosis**
     Note: This category is to be used to indicate conditions classifiable to 010-018 as the cause of late effects, which are themselves classified elsewhere. The "late effects" include those specified as such, as sequelae, or as due to old or inactive tuberculosis, without evidence of active disease.
137.0   **Late effects of respiratory or unspecified tuberculosis**
137.1   **Late effects of central nervous system tuberculosis**
137.2   **Late effects of genitourinary tuberculosis**
137.3   **Late effects of tuberculosis of bones and joints**
137.4   **Late effects of tuberculosis of other specified organs**

√4th √5th Additional Digit Required   Unspecified Code   Other Specified Code   Manifestation Code   ►◄ Revised Text   ● New Code   ▲ Revised Code Title

2005 ICD•9•CM   Volume 1 — 23

138 Late effects of acute poliomyelitis

> Note: This category is to be used to indicate conditions
> classifiable to 045 as the cause of late effects, which
> are themselves classified elsewhere. The "late effects"
> include conditions specified as such, or as sequelae, or
> as due to old or inactive poliomyelitis, without evidence
> of active disease.

✓4ᵗʰ 139 Late effects of other infectious and parasitic diseases

> Note: This category is to be used to indicate conditions
> classifiable to categories 001-009, 020-041, 046-136 as
> the cause of late effects, which are themselves
> classified elsewhere. The "late effects" include
> conditions specified as such; they also include sequela
> of diseases classifiable to the above categories if there
> is evidence that the disease itself is no longer present.

139.0 Late effects of viral encephalitis

> Late effects of conditions classifiable to 049.8-049.9,
> 062-064

139.1 Late effects of trachoma

> Late effects of conditions classifiable to 076

139.8 Late effects of other and unspecified infectious and parasitic diseases

> AHA: 4Q, '91, 15; 3Q, '90, 14; M-A, '87, 8

2. NEOPLASMS (140-239)

Notes:

1. Content

This chapter contains the following broad groups:

140-195   Malignant neoplasms, stated or presumed to be primary, of specified sites, except of lymphatic and hematopoietic tissue

196-198   Malignant neoplasms, stated or presumed to be secondary, of specified sites

199   Malignant neoplasms, without specification of site

200-208   Malignant neoplasms, stated or presumed to be primary, of lymphatic and hematopoietic tissue

210-229   Benign neoplasms

230-234   Carcinoma in situ

235-238   Neoplasms of uncertain behavior [see Note at beginning of section]

239   Neoplasms of unspecified nature

2. Functional activity

All neoplasms are classified in this chapter, whether or not functionally active. An additional code from Chapter 3 may be used to identify such functional activity associated with any neoplasm, e.g.:

catecholamine-producing malignant pheochromocytoma of adrenal:

code 194.0, additional code 255.6

basophil adenoma of pituitary with Cushing's syndrome:

code 227.3, additional code 255.0

3. Morphology [Histology]

For those wishing to identify the histological type of neoplasms, a comprehensive coded nomenclature, which comprises the morphology rubrics of the ICD-Oncology, is given in Appendix A.

4. Malignant neoplasms overlapping site boundaries

Categories 140-195 are for the classification of primary malignant neoplasms according to their point of origin. A malignant neoplasm that overlaps two or more subcategories within a three-digit rubric and whose point of origin cannot be determined should be classified to the subcategory .8 "Other."

For example, "carcinoma involving tip and ventral surface of tongue" should be assigned to 141.8. On the other hand, "carcinoma of tip of tongue, extending to involve the ventral surface" should be coded to 141.2, as the point of origin, the tip, is known. Three subcategories (149.8, 159.8, 165.8) have been provided for malignant neoplasms that overlap the boundaries of three-digit rubrics within certain systems.

Overlapping malignant neoplasms that cannot be classified as indicated above should be assigned to the appropriate subdivision of category 195 (Malignant neoplasm of other and ill-defined sites).

AHA: 2Q, '90, 7

DEF: An abnormal growth, such as a tumor. Morphology determines behavior, i.e., whether it will remain intact (benign) or spread to adjacent tissue (malignant). The term mass is not synonymous with neoplasm, as it is often used to describe cysts and thickenings such as those occurring with hematoma or infection.

MALIGNANT NEOPLASM OF LIP, ORAL CAVITY, AND PHARYNX (140-149)

EXCLUDES   carcinoma in situ (230.0)

✓4ᵗʰ 140   Malignant neoplasm of lip

EXCLUDES   skin of lip (173.0)

140.0   Upper lip, vermilion border

Upper lip: Upper lip:
NOS   lipstick area
external

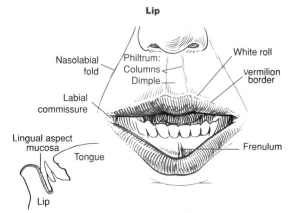

Lip

140.1   Lower lip, vermilion border

Lower lip: Lower lip:
NOS   lipstick area
external

140.3   Upper lip, inner aspect

Upper lip: Upper lip:
buccal aspect   mucosa
frenulum   oral aspect

140.4   Lower lip, inner aspect

Lower lip: Lower lip:
buccal aspect   mucosa
frenulum   oral aspect

140.5   Lip, unspecified, inner aspect

Lip, not specified whether upper or lower:
buccal aspect
frenulum
mucosa
oral aspect

140.6   Commissure of lip

Labial commissure

140.8   Other sites of lip

Malignant neoplasm of contiguous or overlapping sites of lip whose point of origin cannot be determined

140.9   Lip, unspecified, vermilion border

Lip, not specified as upper or lower:
NOS
external
lipstick area

✓4ᵗʰ 141   Malignant neoplasm of tongue

141.0   Base of tongue

Dorsal surface of base of tongue
Fixed part of tongue NOS

141.1   Dorsal surface of tongue

Anterior two-thirds of tongue, dorsal surface
Dorsal tongue NOS
Midline of tongue

EXCLUDES   dorsal surface of base of tongue (141.0)

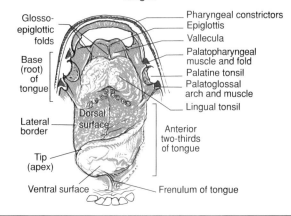

Tongue

✓4ᵗʰ
✓5ᵗʰ   Additional Digit Required   Unspecified Code   Other Specified Code   Manifestation Code   ▶◀ Revised Text   ● New Code   ▲ Revised Code Title

2005 ICD•9•CM   **Volume 1 — 25**

141.2   **Tip and lateral border of tongue**

141.3   **Ventral surface of tongue**
Anterior two-thirds of tongue, ventral surface
Frenulum linguae

141.4   **Anterior two-thirds of tongue, part unspecified**
Mobile part of tongue NOS

141.5   **Junctional zone**
Border of tongue at junction of fixed and mobile
parts at insertion of anterior tonsillar pillar

141.6   **Lingual tonsil**

141.8   **Other sites of tongue**
Malignant neoplasm of contiguous or overlapping
sites of tongue whose point of origin cannot be
determined

141.9   **Tongue, unspecified**
Tongue NOS

✓4ᵗʰ **142 Malignant neoplasm of major salivary glands**
> INCLUDES   salivary ducts
> EXCLUDES   *malignant neoplasm of minor salivary glands:*
> *NOS (145.9)*
> *buccal mucosa (145.0)*
> *soft palate (145.3)*
> *tongue (141.0-141.9)*
> *tonsil, palatine (146.0)*

142.0   **Parotid gland**

142.1   **Submandibular gland**
Submaxillary gland

142.2   **Sublingual gland**

142.8   **Other major salivary glands**
Malignant neoplasm of contiguous or overlapping
sites of salivary glands and ducts whose point
of origin cannot be determined

142.9   **Salivary gland, unspecified**
Salivary gland (major) NOS

✓4ᵗʰ **143 Malignant neoplasm of gum**
> INCLUDES   alveolar (ridge) mucosa
> gingiva (alveolar) (marginal)
> interdental papillae
> EXCLUDES   *malignant odontogenic neoplasms (170.0-170.1)*

143.0   **Upper gum**

143.1   **Lower gum**

143.8   **Other sites of gum**
Malignant neoplasm of contiguous or overlapping
sites of gum whose point of origin cannot be
determined

143.9   **Gum, unspecified**

✓4ᵗʰ **144 Malignant neoplasm of floor of mouth**

144.0   **Anterior portion**
Anterior to the premolar-canine junction

144.1   **Lateral portion**

Main Salivary Glands

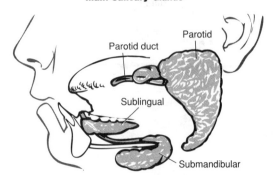

Parotid
Parotid duct
Sublingual
Submandibular

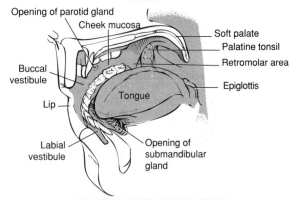

Mouth

Opening of parotid gland
Cheek mucosa
Soft palate
Palatine tonsil
Retromolar area
Buccal vestibule
Epiglottis
Lip
Tongue
Labial vestibule
Opening of submandibular gland

144.8   **Other sites of floor of mouth**
Malignant neoplasm of contiguous or overlapping
sites of floor of mouth whose point of origin
cannot be determined

144.9   **Floor of mouth, part unspecified**

✓4ᵗʰ **145 Malignant neoplasm of other and unspecified parts of mouth**
> EXCLUDES   *mucosa of lips (140.0-140.9)*

145.0   **Cheek mucosa**
Buccal mucosa
Cheek, inner aspect

145.1   **Vestibule of mouth**
Buccal sulcus (upper) (lower)
Labial sulcus (upper) (lower)

145.2   **Hard palate**

145.3   **Soft palate**
> EXCLUDES   *nasopharyngeal [posterior] [superior]*
> *surface of soft palate (147.3)*

145.4   **Uvula**

145.5   **Palate, unspecified**
Junction of hard and soft palate
Roof of mouth

145.6   **Retromolar area**

145.8   **Other specified parts of mouth**
Malignant neoplasm of contiguous or overlapping
sites of mouth whose point of origin cannot be
determined

145.9   **Mouth, unspecified**
Buccal cavity NOS
Minor salivary gland, unspecified site
Oral cavity NOS

✓4ᵗʰ **146 Malignant neoplasm of oropharynx**

146.0   **Tonsil**
Tonsil: Tonsil:
NOS   palatine
faucial
> EXCLUDES   *lingual tonsil (141.6)*
> *pharyngeal tonsil (147.1)*

AHA: S-O, '87, 8

146.1   **Tonsillar fossa**

146.2   **Tonsillar pillars (anterior) (posterior)**
Faucial pillar   Palatoglossal arch
Glossopalatine fold   Palatopharyngeal arch

146.3   **Vallecula**
Anterior and medial surface of the
pharyngoepiglottic fold

146.4   **Anterior aspect of epiglottis**
Epiglottis, free border [margin]
Glossoepiglottic fold(s)
> EXCLUDES   *epiglottis:*
> *NOS (161.1)*
> *suprahyoid portion (161.1)*

N   Newborn Age: 0   **P**   Pediatric Age: 0-17   **M**   Maternity Age: 12-55   **A**   Adult Age: 15-124   **MSP**   Medicare Secondary Payer

26 — Volume 1   *2005 ICD•9•CM*

Oropharynx

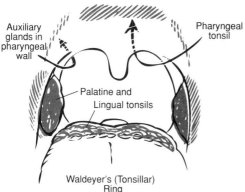

Auxiliary glands in pharyngeal wall

Pharyngeal tonsil

Palatine and Lingual tonsils

Waldeyer's (Tonsillar) Ring

146.5 Junctional region

Junction of the free margin of the epiglottis, the aryepiglottic fold, and the pharyngoepiglottic fold

146.6 Lateral wall of oropharynx

146.7 Posterior wall of oropharynx

146.8 Other specified sites of oropharynx

Branchial cleft

Malignant neoplasm of contiguous or overlapping sites of oropharynx whose point of origin cannot be determined

146.9 Oropharynx, unspecified

AHA: 2Q, '02, 6

✓4th **147 Malignant neoplasm of nasopharynx**

147.0 Superior wall

Roof of nasopharynx

147.1 Posterior wall

Adenoid

Pharyngeal tonsil

147.2 Lateral wall

Fossa of Rosenmüller

Opening of auditory tube

Pharyngeal recess

147.3 Anterior wall

Floor of nasopharynx

Nasopharyngeal [posterior] [superior] surface of soft palate

Posterior margin of nasal septum and choanae

147.8 Other specified sites of nasopharynx

Malignant neoplasm of contiguous or overlapping sites of nasopharynx whose point of origin cannot be determined

147.9 Nasopharynx, unspecified

Nasopharyngeal wall NOS

✓4th **148 Malignant neoplasm of hypopharynx**

148.0 Postcricoid region

148.1 Pyriform sinus

Pyriform fossa

Nasopharynx

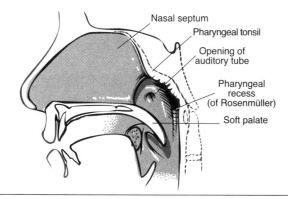

Nasal septum

Pharyngeal tonsil

Opening of auditory tube

Pharyngeal recess (of Rosenmüller)

Soft palate

Hypopharynx

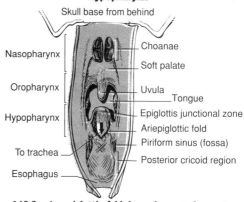

Skull base from behind

Nasopharynx — Choanae

Soft palate

Oropharynx — Uvula

Tongue

Hypopharynx — Epiglottis junctional zone

Ariepiglottic fold

Piriform sinus (fossa)

To trachea — Posterior cricoid region

Esophagus

148.2 Aryepiglottic fold, hypopharyngeal aspect

Aryepiglottic fold or interarytenoid fold:

NOS

marginal zone

EXCLUDES *aryepiglottic fold or interarytenoid fold, laryngeal aspect (161.1)*

148.3 Posterior hypopharyngeal wall

148.8 Other specified sites of hypopharynx

Malignant neoplasm of contiguous or overlapping sites of hypopharynx whose point of origin cannot be determined

148.9 Hypopharynx, unspecified

Hypopharyngeal wall NOS

Hypopharynx NOS

✓4th **149 Malignant neoplasm of other and ill-defined sites within the lip, oral cavity, and pharynx**

149.0 Pharynx, unspecified

149.1 Waldeyer's ring

149.8 Other

Malignant neoplasms of lip, oral cavity, and pharynx whose point of origin cannot be assigned to any one of the categories 140-148

EXCLUDES *"book leaf" neoplasm [ventral surface of tongue and floor of mouth] (145.8)*

149.9 Ill-defined

MALIGNANT NEOPLASM OF DIGESTIVE ORGANS AND PERITONEUM (150-159)

EXCLUDES *carcinoma in situ (230.1-230.9)*

✓4th **150 Malignant neoplasm of esophagus**

150.0 Cervical esophagus

150.1 Thoracic esophagus

150.2 Abdominal esophagus

EXCLUDES *adenocarcinoma (151.0)*
cardio-esophageal junction (151.0)

150.3 Upper third of esophagus

Proximal third of esophagus

150.4 Middle third of esophagus

150.5 Lower third of esophagus

Distal third of esophagus

EXCLUDES *adenocarcinoma (151.0)*
cardio-esophageal junction (151.0)

150.8 Other specified part

Malignant neoplasm of contiguous or overlapping sites of esophagus whose point of origin cannot be determined

150.9 Esophagus, unspecified

✓4th **151 Malignant neoplasm of stomach**

151.0 Cardia

Cardiac orifice   Cardio-esophageal junction

EXCLUDES *squamous cell carcinoma (150.2, 150.5)*

✓4th / ✓5th Additional Digit Required | Unspecified Code | Other Specified Code | Manifestation Code | ▶◀ Revised Text | ● New Code | ▲ Revised Code Title

2005 ICD•9•CM

Volume 1 — 27

Colon

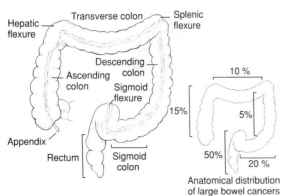

Anatomical distribution of large bowel cancers

151.1 Pylorus
Prepylorus   Pyloric canal

151.2 Pyloric antrum
Antrum of stomach NOS

151.3 Fundus of stomach

151.4 Body of stomach

151.5 Lesser curvature, unspecified
Lesser curvature, not classifiable to 151.1-151.4

151.6 Greater curvature, unspecified
Greater curvature, not classifiable to 151.0-151.4

151.8 Other specified sites of stomach
Anterior wall, not classifiable to 151.0-151.4
Posterior wall, not classifiable to 151.0-151.4
Malignant neoplasm of contiguous or overlapping
sites of stomach whose point of origin cannot
be determined

151.9 Stomach, unspecified
Carcinoma ventriculi   Gastric cancer
AHA: 2Q, '01, 17

✓4ᵗʰ **152 Malignant neoplasm of small intestine, including duodenum**

152.0 Duodenum

152.1 Jejunum

152.2 Ileum
EXCLUDES   ileocecal valve (153.4)

152.3 Meckel's diverticulum

152.8 Other specified sites of small intestine
Duodenojejunal junction
Malignant neoplasm of contiguous or overlapping
sites of small intestine whose point of origin
cannot be determined

152.9 Small intestine, unspecified

✓4ᵗʰ **153 Malignant neoplasm of colon**

153.0 Hepatic flexure

153.1 Transverse colon

153.2 Descending colon
Left colon

153.3 Sigmoid colon
Sigmoid (flexure)
EXCLUDES   rectosigmoid junction (154.0)

153.4 Cecum
Ileocecal valve

153.5 Appendix

153.6 Ascending colon
Right colon

153.7 Splenic flexure

153.8 Other specified sites of large intestine
Malignant neoplasm of contiguous or overlapping
sites of colon whose point of origin cannot be
determined
EXCLUDES   ileocecal valve (153.4)
                rectosigmoid junction (154.0)

153.9 Colon, unspecified
Large intestine NOS

✓4ᵗʰ **154 Malignant neoplasm of rectum, rectosigmoid junction, and anus**

154.0 Rectosigmoid junction
Colon with rectum
Rectosigmoid (colon)

154.1 Rectum
Rectal ampulla

154.2 Anal canal
Anal sphincter
EXCLUDES   skin of anus (172.5, 173.5)
AHA: 1Q, '01, 8

154.3 Anus, unspecified
EXCLUDES   anus:
            margin (172.5, 173.5)
            skin (172.5, 173.5)
            perianal skin (172.5, 173.5)

154.8 Other
Anorectum
Cloacogenic zone
Malignant neoplasm of contiguous or overlapping
sites of rectum, rectosigmoid junction, and
anus whose point of origin cannot be
determined

✓4ᵗʰ **155 Malignant neoplasm of liver and intrahepatic bile ducts**

155.0 Liver, primary
Carcinoma:
   hepatocellular
   liver cell
   liver, specified as primary
Hepatoblastoma

155.1 Intrahepatic bile ducts
Canaliculi biliferi   Intrahepatic:
Interlobular: biliary passages
   bile ducts   canaliculi
   biliary canals   gall duct
EXCLUDES   hepatic duct (156.1)

155.2 Liver, not specified as primary or secondary

✓4ᵗʰ **156 Malignant neoplasm of gallbladder and extrahepatic bile ducts**

156.0 Gallbladder

156.1 Extrahepatic bile ducts
Biliary duct or passage NOS
Common bile duct
Cystic duct
Hepatic duct
Sphincter of Oddi

156.2 Ampulla of Vater
DEF: Malignant neoplasm in the area of dilation at the juncture of
the common bile and pancreatic ducts near the opening into the
lumen of the duodenum.

**156.8 Other specified sites of gallbladder and
extrahepatic bile ducts**
Malignant neoplasm of contiguous or overlapping
sites of gallbladder and extrahepatic bile ducts
whose point of origin cannot be determined

156.9 Biliary tract, part unspecified
Malignant neoplasm involving both intrahepatic and
extrahepatic bile ducts

✓4ᵗʰ **157 Malignant neoplasm of pancreas**

157.0 Head of pancreas
AHA: 4Q, '00, 40

157.1 Body of pancreas

157.2 Tail of pancreas

157.3 Pancreatic duct
Duct of:
   Santorini
   Wirsung

N Newborn Age: 0   **P** Pediatric Age: 0-17   **M** Maternity Age: 12-55   **A** Adult Age: 15-124   **MSP** Medicare Secondary Payer

28 — Volume 1   ***2005 ICD•9•CM***

Retroperitoneum and Peritoneum

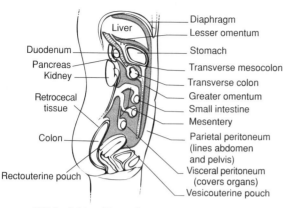

157.4 Islets of Langerhans
Islets of Langerhans, any part of pancreas
Use additional code to identify any functional
activity
DEF: Malignant neoplasm within the structures of the pancreas that
produce insulin, somatostatin and glucagon.

157.8 Other specified sites of pancreas
Ectopic pancreatic tissue
Malignant neoplasm of contiguous or overlapping
sites of pancreas whose point of origin cannot
be determined

157.9 Pancreas, part unspecified
AHA: 4Q, '89, 11

✓4ᵗʰ **158 Malignant neoplasm of retroperitoneum and peritoneum**
158.0 Retroperitoneum
Periadrenal tissue
Perinephric tissue
Perirenal tissue
Retrocecal tissue

158.8 Specified parts of peritoneum
Cul-de-sac (of Douglas)
Mesentery
Mesocolon
Omentum
Peritoneum:
  parietal
  pelvic
Rectouterine pouch
Malignant neoplasm of contiguous or overlapping
sites of retroperitoneum and peritoneum whose
point of origin cannot be determined

158.9 Peritoneum, unspecified

✓4ᵗʰ **159 Malignant neoplasm of other and ill-defined sites within the
digestive organs and peritoneum**
159.0 Intestinal tract, part unspecified
Intestine NOS

159.1 Spleen, not elsewhere classified
Angiosarcoma }
Fibrosarcoma } of spleen
    EXCLUDES Hodgkin's disease (201.0-201.9)
              lymphosarcoma (200.1)
              reticulosarcoma (200.0)

**159.8 Other sites of digestive system and
intra-abdominal organs**
Malignant neoplasm of digestive organs and
peritoneum whose point of origin cannot be
assigned to any one of the categories 150-158
    EXCLUDES anus and rectum (154.8)
              cardio-esophageal junction (151.0)
              colon and rectum (154.0)

159.9 Ill-defined
Alimentary canal or tract NOS
Gastrointestinal tract NOS
    EXCLUDES abdominal NOS (195.2)
              intra-abdominal NOS (195.2)

MALIGNANT NEOPLASM OF RESPIRATORY AND INTRATHORACIC ORGANS (160-165)
    EXCLUDES carcinoma in situ (231.0-231.9)

✓4ᵗʰ **160 Malignant neoplasm of nasal cavities, middle ear, and
accessory sinuses**
160.0 Nasal cavities
Cartilage of nose   Septum of nose
Conchae, nasal   Vestibule of nose
Internal nose
    EXCLUDES nasal bone (170.0)
              nose NOS (195.0)
              olfactory bulb (192.0)
              posterior margin of septum and
                  choanae (147.3)
              skin of nose (172.3, 173.3)
              turbinates (170.0)

160.1 Auditory tube, middle ear, and mastoid air cells
Antrum tympanicum Tympanic cavity
Eustachian tube
    EXCLUDES auditory canal (external) (172.2, 173.2)
              bone of ear (meatus) (170.0)
              cartilage of ear (171.0)
              ear (external) (skin) (172.2, 173.2)

160.2 Maxillary sinus
Antrum (Highmore) (maxillary)

160.3 Ethmoidal sinus

160.4 Frontal sinus

160.5 Sphenoidal sinus

160.8 Other
Malignant neoplasm of contiguous or overlapping
sites of nasal cavities, middle ear, and
accessory sinuses whose point of origin cannot
be determined

160.9 Accessory sinus, unspecified

✓4ᵗʰ **161 Malignant neoplasm of larynx**
161.0 Glottis
Intrinsic larynx
Laryngeal commissure (anterior) (posterior)
True vocal cord
Vocal cord NOS

161.1 Supraglottis
Aryepiglottic fold or interarytenoid fold, laryngeal
aspect
Epiglottis (suprahyoid portion) NOS
Extrinsic larynx
False vocal cords
Posterior (laryngeal) surface of epiglottis
Ventricular bands
    EXCLUDES anterior aspect of epiglottis (146.4)
              aryepiglottic fold or interarytenoid fold:
                  NOS (148.2)
                  hypopharyngeal aspect (148.2)
                  marginal zone (148.2)

161.2 Subglottis

161.3 Laryngeal cartilages
Cartilage: Cartilage:
  arytenoid   cuneiform
  cricoid   thyroid

161.8 Other specified sites of larynx
Malignant neoplasm of contiguous or overlapping
sites of larynx whose point of origin cannot be
determined

161.9 Larynx, unspecified

✓4ᵗʰ ✓5ᵗʰ Additional Digit Required   Unspecified Code   Other Specified Code   Manifestation Code   ▶◀ Revised Text   ● New Code   ▲ Revised Code Title

☑4ᵗʰ **162 Malignant neoplasm of trachea, bronchus, and lung**

     162.0 **Trachea**
         Cartilage ⎫
         Mucosa ⎬ of trachea

     162.2 **Main bronchus**
         Carina
         Hilus of lung

     162.3 **Upper lobe, bronchus or lung**
         AHA: ▶1Q, '04, 4◀

     162.4 **Middle lobe, bronchus or lung**

     162.5 **Lower lobe, bronchus or lung**

     162.8 **Other parts of bronchus or lung**
         Malignant neoplasm of contiguous or overlapping sites of bronchus or lung whose point of origin cannot be determined

     162.9 **Bronchus and lung, unspecified**
         AHA: 2Q, '97, 3; 4Q, '96, 48

☑4ᵗʰ **163 Malignant neoplasm of pleura**

     163.0 **Parietal pleura**

     163.1 **Visceral pleura**

     163.8 **Other specified sites of pleura**
         Malignant neoplasm of contiguous or overlapping sites of pleura whose point of origin cannot be determined

     163.9 **Pleura, unspecified**

☑4ᵗʰ **164 Malignant neoplasm of thymus, heart, and mediastinum**

     164.0 **Thymus**

     164.1 **Heart**
         Endocardium
         Epicardium
         Myocardium
         Pericardium
         EXCLUDES *great vessels (171.4)*

     164.2 **Anterior mediastinum**

     164.3 **Posterior mediastinum**

     164.8 **Other**
         Malignant neoplasm of contiguous or overlapping sites of thymus, heart, and mediastinum whose point of origin cannot be determined

     164.9 **Mediastinum, part unspecified**

☑4ᵗʰ **165 Malignant neoplasm of other and ill-defined sites within the respiratory system and intrathoracic organs**

     165.0 **Upper respiratory tract, part unspecified**

     165.8 **Other**
         Malignant neoplasm of respiratory and intrathoracic organs whose point of origin cannot be assigned to any one of the categories 160-164

     165.9 **Ill-defined sites within the respiratory system**
         Respiratory tract NOS
         EXCLUDES *intrathoracic NOS (195.1)*
                          thoracic NOS (195.1)

Skull

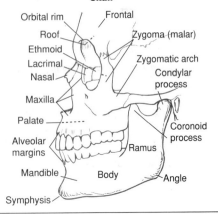

MALIGNANT NEOPLASM OF BONE, CONNECTIVE TISSUE, SKIN, AND BREAST (170-176)

     EXCLUDES *carcinoma in situ:*
                 breast (233.0)
                 skin (232.0-232.9)

☑4ᵗʰ **170 Malignant neoplasm of bone and articular cartilage**

     INCLUDES cartilage (articular) (joint)
                 periosteum

     EXCLUDES *bone marrow NOS (202.9)*
                 cartilage:
                     ear (171.0)
                     eyelid (171.0)
                     larynx (161.3)
                     nose (160.0)
                 synovia (171.0-171.9)

     170.0 **Bones of skull and face, except mandible**
         Bone: Bone:
            ethmoid   sphenoid
            frontal   temporal
            malar   zygomatic
            nasal   Maxilla (superior)
            occipital   Turbinate
            orbital   Upper jaw bone
            parietal   Vomer
         EXCLUDES *carcinoma, any type except intraosseous or odontogenic:*
                 maxilla, maxillary (sinus) (160.2)
                 upper jaw bone (143.0)
                 jaw bone (lower) (170.1)

     170.1 **Mandible**
         Inferior maxilla
         Jaw bone NOS
         Lower jaw bone
         EXCLUDES *carcinoma, any type except intraosseous or odontogenic:*
                 jaw bone NOS (143.9)
                 lower (143.1)
                 upper jaw bone (170.0)

     170.2 **Vertebral column, excluding sacrum and coccyx**
         Spinal column   Vertebra
         Spine
         EXCLUDES *sacrum and coccyx (170.6)*

     170.3 **Ribs, sternum, and clavicle**
         Costal cartilage
         Costovertebral joint
         Xiphoid process

     170.4 **Scapula and long bones of upper limb**
         Acromion
         Bones NOS of upper limb
         Humerus
         Radius
         Ulna
         AHA: 2Q, '99, 9

     170.5 **Short bones of upper limb**
         Carpal   Scaphoid (of hand)
         Cuneiform, wrist   Semilunar or lunate
         Metacarpal   Trapezium
         Navicular, of hand   Trapezoid
         Phalanges of hand   Unciform
         Pisiform

     170.6 **Pelvic bones, sacrum, and coccyx**
         Coccygeal vertebra   Pubic bone
         Ilium   Sacral vertebra
         Ischium

     170.7 **Long bones of lower limb**
         Bones NOS of lower limb
         Femur
         Fibula
         Tibia

Ⓝ Newborn Age: 0   Ⓟ Pediatric Age: 0-17   Ⓜ Maternity Age: 12-55   Ⓐ Adult Age: 15-124   MSP Medicare Secondary Payer

170.8   Short bones of lower limb
  Astragalus [talus]   Navicular (of ankle)
  Calcaneus   Patella
  Cuboid   Phalanges of foot
  Cuneiform, ankle   Tarsal
  Metatarsal

170.9   Bone and articular cartilage, site unspecified

✓4ᵗʰ **171 Malignant neoplasm of connective and other soft tissue**

INCLUDES   blood vessel
           bursa
           fascia
           fat
           ligament, except uterine
           muscle
           peripheral, sympathetic, and parasympathetic
               nerves and ganglia
           synovia
           tendon (sheath)

EXCLUDES   *cartilage (of):*
               articular (170.0-170.9)
               larynx (161.3)
               nose (160.0)
           connective tissue:
               breast (174.0-175.9)
               internal organs—code to malignant neoplasm
                   of the site [e.g., leiomyosarcoma of
                   stomach, 151.9]
           heart (164.1)
           uterine ligament (183.4)

171.0   Head, face, and neck
  Cartilage of: Cartilage of:
     ear   eyelid
  AHA: 2Q, '99, 6

171.2   Upper limb, including shoulder
  Arm   Forearm
  Finger   Hand

171.3   Lower limb, including hip
  Foot   Thigh
  Leg   Toe
  Popliteal space

171.4   Thorax
  Axilla   Great vessels
  Diaphragm
  EXCLUDES   *heart (164.1)*
             mediastinum (164.2-164.9)
             thymus (164.0)

171.5   Abdomen
  Abdominal wall
  Hypochondrium
  EXCLUDES   *peritoneum (158.8)*
             retroperitoneum (158.0)

171.6   Pelvis
  Buttock   Inguinal region
  Groin   Perineum
  EXCLUDES   *pelvic peritoneum (158.8)*
             retroperitoneum (158.0)
             uterine ligament, any (183.3-183.5)

171.7   Trunk, unspecified
  Back NOS
  Flank NOS

**171.8   Other specified sites of connective and other
          soft tissue**
  Malignant neoplasm of contiguous or overlapping
      sites of connective tissue whose point of origin
      cannot be determined

**171.9   Connective and other soft tissue, site
          unspecified**

✓4ᵗʰ **172 Malignant melanoma of skin**

INCLUDES   melanocarcinoma
           melanoma (skin) NOS

EXCLUDES   *skin of genital organs (184.0-184.9, 187.1-*
               187.9)
           sites other than skin—code to malignant
               neoplasm of the site

DEF: Malignant neoplasm of melanocytes; most common in skin, may involve
oral cavity, esophagus, anal canal, vagina, leptomeninges or conjunctiva.

172.0   Lip
  EXCLUDES   *vermilion border of lip (140.0-140.1,*
               140.9)

172.1   Eyelid, including canthus

172.2   Ear and external auditory canal
  Auricle (ear)
  Auricular canal, external
  External [acoustic] meatus
  Pinna

172.3   Other and unspecified parts of face
  Cheek (external)   Forehead
  Chin   Nose, external
  Eyebrow   Temple

172.4   Scalp and neck

172.5   Trunk, except scrotum
  Axilla   Perianal skin
  Breast   Perineum
  Buttock   Umbilicus
  Groin
  EXCLUDES   *anal canal (154.2)*
             anus NOS (154.3)
             scrotum (187.7)

172.6   Upper limb, including shoulder
  Arm   Forearm
  Finger   Hand

172.7   Lower limb, including hip
  Ankle   Leg
  Foot   Popliteal area
  Heel   Thigh
  Knee   Toe

172.8   Other specified sites of skin
  Malignant melanoma of contiguous or overlapping
      sites of skin whose point of origin cannot be
      determined

172.9   Melanoma of skin, site unspecified

✓4ᵗʰ **173 Other malignant neoplasm of skin**

INCLUDES   malignant neoplasm of:
               sebaceous glands
               sudoriferous, sudoriparous glands
               sweat glands

EXCLUDES   *Kaposi's sarcoma (176.0-176.9)*
           malignant melanoma of skin (172.0-172.9)
           skin of genital organs (184.0-184.9, 187.1-
               187.9)

AHA: 1Q, '00, 18; 2Q, '96, 12

173.0   Skin of lip
  EXCLUDES   *vermilion border of lip (140.0-140.1,*
               140.9)

173.1   Eyelid, including canthus
  EXCLUDES   *cartilage of eyelid (171.0)*

173.2   Skin of ear and external auditory canal
  Auricle (ear)
  Auricular canal, external
  External meatus
  Pinna
  EXCLUDES   *cartilage of ear (171.0)*

173.3   Skin of other and unspecified parts of face
  Cheek, external   Forehead
  Chin   Nose, external
  Eyebrow   Temple
  AHA: 1Q, '00, 3

| ✓4ᵗʰ ✓5ᵗʰ Additional Digit Required | Unspecified Code | Other Specified Code | Manifestation Code | ►◄ Revised Text | ● New Code | ▲ Revised Code Title |

2005 ICD•9•CM   Volume 1 — 31

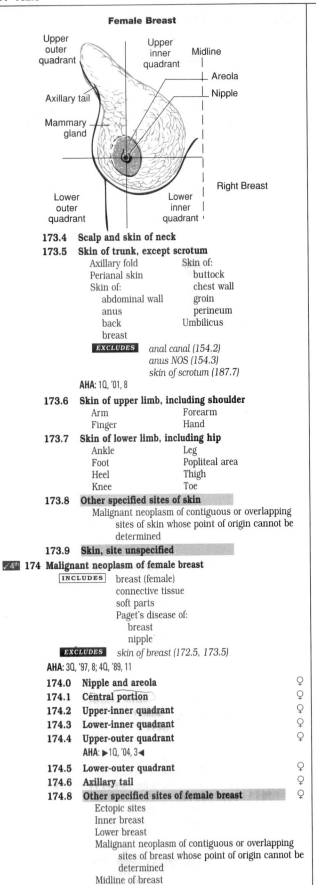

Female Breast

173.4 **Scalp and skin of neck**

173.5 **Skin of trunk, except scrotum**
Axillary fold
Perianal skin
Skin of:
  abdominal wall
  anus
  back
  breast
Skin of:
  buttock
  chest wall
  groin
  perineum
  Umbilicus

EXCLUDES anal canal (154.2)
  anus NOS (154.3)
  skin of scrotum (187.7)

AHA: 1Q, '01, 8

173.6 **Skin of upper limb, including shoulder**
Arm Forearm
Finger Hand

173.7 **Skin of lower limb, including hip**
Ankle Leg
Foot Popliteal area
Heel Thigh
Knee Toe

173.8 **Other specified sites of skin**
Malignant neoplasm of contiguous or overlapping sites of skin whose point of origin cannot be determined

173.9 **Skin, site unspecified**

✓4ᵗʰ 174 **Malignant neoplasm of female breast**
INCLUDES breast (female)
  connective tissue
  soft parts
  Paget's disease of:
    breast
    nipple
EXCLUDES skin of breast (172.5, 173.5)

AHA: 3Q, '97, 8; 4Q, '89, 11

174.0 **Nipple and areola** ♀
174.1 **Central portion** ♀
174.2 **Upper-inner quadrant** ♀
174.3 **Lower-inner quadrant** ♀
174.4 **Upper-outer quadrant** ♀
  AHA: ▶1Q, '04, 3◀
174.5 **Lower-outer quadrant** ♀
174.6 **Axillary tail** ♀
174.8 **Other specified sites of female breast** ♀
Ectopic sites
Inner breast
Lower breast
Malignant neoplasm of contiguous or overlapping sites of breast whose point of origin cannot be determined
Midline of breast
Outer breast
Upper breast
174.9 **Breast (female), unspecified** ♀

✓4ᵗʰ 175 **Malignant neoplasm of male breast**
EXCLUDES skin of breast (172.5, 173.5)
175.0 **Nipple and areola** ♂
175.9 **Other and unspecified sites of male breast** ♂
Ectopic breast tissue, male

✓4ᵗʰ 176 **Kaposi's sarcoma**
AHA: 4Q, '91, 24

176.0 **Skin**
176.1 **Soft tissue**
▶Blood vessel
Connective tissue
Fascia
Ligament
Lymphatic(s) NEC
Muscle◀
EXCLUDES lymph glands and nodes (176.5)
176.2 **Palate**
176.3 **Gastrointestinal sites**
176.4 **Lung**
176.5 **Lymph nodes**
176.8 **Other specified sites**
▶Oral cavity NEC◀
176.9 **Unspecified**
Viscera NOS

MALIGNANT NEOPLASM OF GENITOURINARY ORGANS (179-189)
EXCLUDES carcinoma in situ (233.1-233.9)

179 **Malignant neoplasm of uterus, part unspecified** ♀

✓4ᵗʰ 180 **Malignant neoplasm of cervix uteri**
INCLUDES invasive malignancy [carcinoma]
EXCLUDES carcinoma in situ (233.1)
180.0 **Endocervix** ♀
Cervical canal NOS Endocervical gland
Endocervical canal
180.1 **Exocervix** ♀
180.8 **Other specified sites of cervix** ♀
Cervical stump
Squamocolumnar junction of cervix
Malignant neoplasm of contiguous or overlapping sites of cervix uteri whose point of origin cannot be determined
180.9 **Cervix uteri, unspecified** ♀

181 **Malignant neoplasm of placenta** ♀
Choriocarcinoma NOS
Chorioepithelioma NOS
EXCLUDES chorioadenoma (destruens) (236.1)
  hydatidiform mole (630)
    malignant (236.1)
  invasive mole (236.1)
  male choriocarcinoma NOS (186.0-186.9)

✓4ᵗʰ 182 **Malignant neoplasm of body of uterus**
EXCLUDES carcinoma in situ (233.2)
182.0 **Corpus uteri, except isthmus** ♀
Cornu Fundus
Endometrium Myometrium
182.1 **Isthmus** ♀
Lower uterine segment
182.8 **Other specified sites of body of uterus** ♀
Malignant neoplasm of contiguous or overlapping sites of body of uterus whose point of origin cannot be determined
EXCLUDES uterus NOS (179)

N Newborn Age: 0 P Pediatric Age: 0-17 M Maternity Age: 12-55 A Adult Age: 15-124 MSP Medicare Secondary Payer

✓4ᵗʰ 183 Malignant neoplasm of ovary and other uterine adnexa
     EXCLUDES   *Douglas' cul-de-sac (158.8)*

183.0 Ovary   ♀
     Use additional code to identify any functional activity

183.2 Fallopian tube   ♀
     Oviduct   Uterine tube

183.3 Broad ligament   ♀
     Mesovarium   Parovarian region

183.4 Parametrium   ♀
     Uterine ligament NOS Uterosacral ligament

183.5 Round ligament   ♀
     AHA: 3Q, '99, 5

183.8 Other specified sites of uterine adnexa   ♀
     Tubo-ovarian
     Utero-ovarian
     Malignant neoplasm of contiguous or overlapping sites of ovary and other uterine adnexa whose point of origin cannot be determined

183.9 Uterine adnexa, unspecified   ♀

✓4ᵗʰ 184 Malignant neoplasm of other and unspecified female genital organs
     EXCLUDES   *carcinoma in situ (233.3)*

184.0 Vagina   ♀
     Gartner's duct   Vaginal vault

184.1 Labia majora   ♀
     Greater vestibular [Bartholin's] gland

184.2 Labia minora   ♀

184.3 Clitoris   ♀

184.4 Vulva, unspecified   ♀
     External female genitalia NOS
     Pudendum

184.8 Other specified sites of female genital organs   ♀
     Malignant neoplasm of contiguous or overlapping sites of female genital organs whose point of origin cannot be determined

184.9 Female genital organ, site unspecified   ♀
     Female genitourinary tract NOS

185 Malignant neoplasm of prostate   ♂
     EXCLUDES   *seminal vesicles (187.8)*
     AHA: ▶ 3Q, '03, 13; ◀, 3Q, '99, 5; 3Q, '92, 7

✓4ᵗʰ 186 Malignant neoplasm of testis
     Use additional code to identify any functional activity

186.0 Undescended testis   ♂
     Ectopic testis   Retained testis

186.9 Other and unspecified testis   ♂
     Testis: Testis:
     NOS   scrotal
     descended

✓4ᵗʰ 187 Malignant neoplasm of penis and other male genital organs

187.1 Prepuce   ♂
     Foreskin

187.2 Glans penis   ♂

187.3 Body of penis   ♂
     Corpus cavernosum

187.4 Penis, part unspecified   ♂
     Skin of penis NOS

187.5 Epididymis   ♂

187.6 Spermatic cord   ♂
     Vas deferens

187.7 Scrotum   ♂
     Skin of scrotum

187.8 Other specified sites of male genital organs   ♂
     Seminal vesicle
     Tunica vaginalis
     Malignant neoplasm of contiguous or overlapping sites of penis and other male genital organs whose point of origin cannot be determined

187.9 Male genital organ, site unspecified   ♂
     Male genital organ or tract NOS

✓4ᵗʰ 188 Malignant neoplasm of bladder
     EXCLUDES   *carcinoma in situ (233.7)*

188.0 Trigone of urinary bladder

188.1 Dome of urinary bladder

188.2 Lateral wall of urinary bladder

188.3 Anterior wall of urinary bladder

188.4 Posterior wall of urinary bladder

188.5 Bladder neck
     Internal urethral orifice

188.6 Ureteric orifice

188.7 Urachus

188.8 Other specified sites of bladder
     Malignant neoplasm of contiguous or overlapping sites of bladder whose point of origin cannot be determined

188.9 Bladder, part unspecified
     Bladder wall NOS
     AHA: 1Q, '00, 5

✓4ᵗʰ 189 Malignant neoplasm of kidney and other and unspecified urinary organs

189.0 Kidney, except pelvis
     Kidney NOS   Kidney parenchyma

189.1 Renal pelvis
     Renal calyces   Ureteropelvic junction

189.2 Ureter
     EXCLUDES   *ureteric orifice of bladder (188.6)*

189.3 Urethra
     EXCLUDES   *urethral orifice of bladder (188.5)*

189.4 Paraurethral glands

189.8 Other specified sites of urinary organs
     Malignant neoplasm of contiguous or overlapping sites of kidney and other urinary organs whose point of origin cannot be determined

189.9 Urinary organ, site unspecified
     Urinary system NOS

MALIGNANT NEOPLASM OF OTHER AND UNSPECIFIED SITES (190-199)

     EXCLUDES   *carcinoma in situ (234.0-234.9)*

✓4ᵗʰ 190 Malignant neoplasm of eye
     EXCLUDES   *carcinoma in situ (234.0)*
         eyelid (skin) (172.1, 173.1)
            cartilage (171.0)
         optic nerve (192.0)
         orbital bone (170.0)

190.0 Eyeball, except conjunctiva, cornea, retina, and choroid
     Ciliary body   Sclera
     Crystalline lens   Uveal tract
     Iris

190.1 Orbit
     Connective tissue of orbit Retrobulbar
     Extraocular muscle
     EXCLUDES   *bone of orbit (170.0)*

190.2 Lacrimal gland

190.3 Conjunctiva

190.4 Cornea

190.5 Retina

190.6 Choroid

✓4ᵗʰ
✓5ᵗʰ Additional Digit Required   Unspecified Code   Other Specified Code   Manifestation Code   ▶◀ Revised Text   ● New Code   ▲ Revised Code Title

2005 ICD•9•CM   **February 2004 • Volume 1 — 33**

Brain

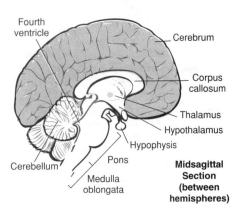

Fourth ventricle

Cerebrum

Corpus callosum

Thalamus

Hypothalamus

Hypophysis

Pons

Cerebellum

Medulla oblongata

Midsagittal Section (between hemispheres)

190.7　Lacrimal duct
　　　Lacrimal sac　　　　Nasolacrimal duct

190.8　Other specified sites of eye
　　　Malignant neoplasm of contiguous or overlapping sites of eye whose point of origin cannot be determined

190.9　Eye, part unspecified

✓4th **191　Malignant neoplasm of brain**
　　　EXCLUDES　cranial nerves (192.0)
　　　　　　　　retrobulbar area (190.1)

191.0　Cerebrum, except lobes and ventricles
　　　Basal ganglia　　　　Globus pallidus
　　　Cerebral cortex　　　Hypothalamus
　　　Corpus striatum　　　Thalamus

191.1　Frontal lobe

191.2　Temporal lobe
　　　Hippocampus　　　　Uncus

191.3　Parietal lobe

191.4　Occipital lobe

191.5　Ventricles
　　　Choroid plexus　　　Floor of ventricle

191.6　Cerebellum NOS
　　　Cerebellopontine angle

191.7　Brain stem
　　　Cerebral peduncle　　Midbrain
　　　Medulla oblongata　　Pons

191.8　Other parts of brain
　　　Corpus callosum
　　　Tapetum
　　　Malignant neoplasm of contiguous or overlapping sites of brain whose point of origin cannot be determined

191.9　Brain, unspecified
　　　Cranial fossa NOS

✓4th **192　Malignant neoplasm of other and unspecified parts of nervous system**
　　　EXCLUDES　peripheral, sympathetic, and parasympathetic nerves and ganglia (171.0-171.9)

192.0　Cranial nerves
　　　Olfactory bulb

192.1　Cerebral meninges
　　　Dura (mater)　　　　Meninges NOS
　　　Falx (cerebelli) (cerebri)　Tentorium

192.2　Spinal cord
　　　Cauda equina

192.3　Spinal meninges

192.8　Other specified sites of nervous system
　　　Malignant neoplasm of contiguous or overlapping sites of other parts of nervous system whose point of origin cannot be determined

192.9　Nervous system, part unspecified
　　　Nervous system (central) NOS
　　　EXCLUDES　meninges NOS (192.1)

193　Malignant neoplasm of thyroid gland
　　　Sipple's syndrome
　　　Thyroglossal duct
　　　Use additional code to identify any functional activity

✓4th **194　Malignant neoplasm of other endocrine glands and related structures**
　　　Use additional code to identify any functional activity
　　　EXCLUDES　islets of Langerhans (157.4)
　　　　　　　　ovary (183.0)
　　　　　　　　testis (186.0-186.9)
　　　　　　　　thymus (164.0)

194.0　Adrenal gland
　　　Adrenal cortex　　　Suprarenal gland
　　　Adrenal medulla

194.1　Parathyroid gland

194.3　Pituitary gland and craniopharyngeal duct
　　　Craniobuccal pouch　Rathke's pouch
　　　Hypophysis　　　　　Sella turcica
　　　AHA: J-A, '85, 9

194.4　Pineal gland

194.5　Carotid body

194.6　Aortic body and other paraganglia
　　　Coccygeal body　　　Para-aortic body
　　　Glomus jugulare

194.8　Other
　　　Pluriglandular involvement NOS
　　　Note: If the sites of multiple involvements are known, they should be coded separately.

194.9　Endocrine gland, site unspecified

✓4th **195　Malignant neoplasm of other and ill-defined sites**
　　　INCLUDES　malignant neoplasms of contiguous sites, not elsewhere classified, whose point of origin cannot be determined
　　　EXCLUDES　malignant neoplasm:
　　　　　　　　lymphatic and hematopoietic tissue (200.0-208.9)
　　　　　　　　secondary sites (196.0-198.8)
　　　　　　　　unspecified site (199.0-199.1)

195.0　Head, face, and neck
　　　Cheek NOS　　　　　Nose NOS
　　　Jaw NOS　　　　　　Supraclavicular region NOS
　　　AHA: ▶4Q, '03, 107◀

195.1　Thorax
　　　Axilla　　　　　　　Intrathoracic NOS
　　　Chest (wall) NOS

195.2　Abdomen
　　　Intra-abdominal NOS
　　　AHA: 2Q, '97, 3

195.3　Pelvis
　　　Groin
　　　Inguinal region NOS
　　　Presacral region
　　　Sacrococcygeal region
　　　Sites overlapping systems within pelvis, as:
　　　　rectovaginal (septum)
　　　　rectovesical (septum)

195.4　Upper limb

195.5　Lower limb

195.8　Other specified sites
　　　Back NOS　　　　　　Trunk NOS
　　　Flank NOS

✓4th **196　Secondary and unspecified malignant neoplasm of lymph nodes**
　　　EXCLUDES　any malignant neoplasm of lymph nodes, specified as primary (200.0-202.9)
　　　　　　　　Hodgkin's disease (201.0-201.9)
　　　　　　　　lymphosarcoma (200.1)
　　　　　　　　reticulosarcoma (200.0)
　　　　　　　　other forms of lymphoma (202.0-202.9)
　　　AHA: 2Q, '92, 3; M-J, '85, 3

N Newborn Age: 0　　　　P Pediatric Age: 0-17　　　　M Maternity Age: 12-55　　　　A Adult Age: 15-124　　　　MSP Medicare Secondary Payer

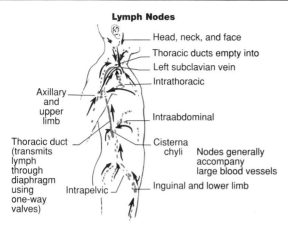

Lymph Nodes

- Head, neck, and face
- Thoracic ducts empty into
- Left subclavian vein
- Intrathoracic
- Axillary and upper limb
- Intraabdominal
- Thoracic duct (transmits lymph through diaphragm using one-way valves)
- Cisterna chyli
- Nodes generally accompany large blood vessels
- Intrapelvic
- Inguinal and lower limb

196.0 Lymph nodes of head, face, and neck
Cervical   Scalene
Cervicofacial   Supraclavicular

196.1 Intrathoracic lymph nodes
Bronchopulmonary   Mediastinal
Intercostal   Tracheobronchial

196.2 Intra-abdominal lymph nodes
Intestinal   Retroperitoneal
Mesenteric
AHA: ▶4Q, '03, 111◀

196.3 Lymph nodes of axilla and upper limb
Brachial   Infraclavicular
Epitrochlear   Pectoral

196.5 Lymph nodes of inguinal region and lower limb
Femoral   Popliteal
Groin   Tibial

196.6 Intrapelvic lymph nodes
Hypogastric   Obturator
Iliac   Parametrial

196.8 Lymph nodes of multiple sites

196.9 Site unspecified
Lymph nodes NOS

✓4ᵗʰ 197 Secondary malignant neoplasm of respiratory and digestive systems
> **EXCLUDES**   lymph node metastasis (196.0-196.9)

AHA: M-J, '85, 3

197.0 Lung
Bronchus
AHA: 2Q, '99, 9

197.1 Mediastinum

197.2 Pleura
AHA: ▶4Q, '03, 110;◀ 4Q, '89, 11

197.3 Other respiratory organs
Trachea

197.4 Small intestine, including duodenum

197.5 Large intestine and rectum

197.6 Retroperitoneum and peritoneum
AHA: 4Q, '89, 11

197.7 Liver, specified as secondary

197.8 Other digestive organs and spleen
AHA: 2Q, '97, 3; 2Q, '92, 3

✓4ᵗʰ 198 Secondary malignant neoplasm of other specified sites
> **EXCLUDES**   lymph node metastasis (196.0-196.9)

AHA: M-J, '85, 3

198.0 Kidney

198.1 Other urinary organs

198.2 Skin
Skin of breast

198.3 Brain and spinal cord
AHA: 3Q, '99, 7

198.4 Other parts of nervous system
Meninges (cerebral) (spinal)
AHA: J-F, '87, 7

198.5 Bone and bone marrow
AHA: ▶4Q, '03, 110;◀ 3Q, '99, 5; 2Q, '92, 3; 1Q, '91, 16; 4Q, '89, 10

198.6 Ovary   ♀

198.7 Adrenal gland
Suprarenal gland

✓5ᵗʰ 198.8 Other specified sites

198.81 Breast
> **EXCLUDES**   skin of breast (198.2)

198.82 Genital organs

198.89 Other
> **EXCLUDES**   retroperitoneal lymph nodes (196.2)

AHA: 2Q, '97, 4

✓4ᵗʰ 199 Malignant neoplasm without specification of site

199.0 Disseminated
Carcinomatosis
Generalized: unspecified site
  cancer   (primary)
  malignancy   (secondary)
Multiple cancer

AHA: 4Q, '89, 10

199.1 Other
Cancer   unspecified site
Carcinoma   (primary)
Malignancy   (secondary)

MALIGNANT NEOPLASM OF LYMPHATIC AND HEMATOPOIETIC TISSUE (200-208)

> **EXCLUDES**   secondary neoplasm of:
>   bone marrow (198.5)
>   spleen (197.8)
>   secondary and unspecified neoplasm of lymph nodes (196.0-196.9)

The following fifth-digit subclassification is for use with categories 200-202:

0 unspecified site, extranodal and solid organ sites
1 lymph nodes of head, face, and neck
2 intrathoracic lymph nodes
3 intra-abdominal lymph nodes
4 lymph nodes of axilla and upper limb
5 lymph nodes of inguinal region and lower limb
6 intrapelvic lymph nodes
7 spleen
8 lymph nodes of multiple sites

✓4ᵗʰ 200 Lymphosarcoma and reticulosarcoma
AHA: 2Q, '92, 3; N-D, '86, 5

✓5ᵗʰ 200.0 Reticulosarcoma
Lymphoma (malignant):
  histiocytic (diffuse):
    nodular
    pleomorphic cell type
  reticulum cell type
Reticulum cell sarcoma:
  NOS
  pleomorphic cell type
AHA: For Code 200.03: 3Q, '01, 12

DEF: Malignant lymphoma of primarily histolytic cells; commonly originates in reticuloendothelium of lymph nodes.

✓4ᵗʰ ✓5ᵗʰ Additional Digit Required   Unspecified Code   Other Specified Code   Manifestation Code   ▶◀ Revised Text   ● New Code   ▲ Revised Code Title

2005 ICD•9•CM   **February 2004 • Volume 1 — 35**

§ ✓5ᵗʰ **200.1 Lymphosarcoma**
Lymphoblastoma (diffuse)
Lymphoma (malignant):
lymphoblastic (diffuse)
lymphocytic (cell type) (diffuse)
lymphosarcoma type
Lymphosarcoma:
NOS
diffuse NOS
lymphoblastic (diffuse)
lymphocytic (diffuse)
prolymphocytic
EXCLUDES *lymphosarcoma:*
follicular or nodular (202.0)
mixed cell type (200.8)
lymphosarcoma cell leukemia (207.8)
DEF: Malignant lymphoma created from anaplastic lymphoid cells resembling lymphocytes or lymphoblasts.

§ ✓5ᵗʰ **200.2 Burkitt's tumor or lymphoma**
Malignant lymphoma, Burkitt's type
DEF: Large osteolytic lesion most common in jaw or as abdominal mass; usually found in central Africa but reported elsewhere.

§ ✓5ᵗʰ **200.8 Other named variants**
Lymphoma (malignant):
lymphoplasmacytoid type
mixed lymphocytic-histiocytic (diffuse)
Lymphosarcoma, mixed cell type (diffuse)
Reticulolymphosarcoma (diffuse)

✓4ᵗʰ **201 Hodgkin's disease**
AHA: 2Q, '92, 3; N-D, '86, 5
DEF: Painless, progressive enlargement of lymph nodes, spleen and general lymph tissue; symptoms include anorexia, lassitude, weight loss, fever, pruritis, night sweats, anemia.

§ ✓5ᵗʰ **201.0 Hodgkin's paragranuloma**
§ ✓5ᵗʰ **201.1 Hodgkin's granuloma**
AHA: 2Q, '99, 7
§ ✓5ᵗʰ **201.2 Hodgkin's sarcoma**
§ ✓5ᵗʰ **201.4 Lymphocytic-histiocytic predominance**
§ ✓5ᵗʰ **201.5 Nodular sclerosis**
Hodgkin's disease, nodular sclerosis:
NOS
cellular phase
§ ✓5ᵗʰ **201.6 Mixed cellularity**
§ ✓5ᵗʰ **201.7 Lymphocytic depletion**
Hodgkin's disease, lymphocytic depletion:
NOS
diffuse fibrosis
reticular type
§ ✓5ᵗʰ **201.9 Hodgkin's disease, unspecified**
Hodgkin's: Malignant:
disease NOS   lymphogranuloma
lymphoma NOS   lymphogranulomatosis

✓4ᵗʰ **202 Other malignant neoplasms of lymphoid and histiocytic tissue**
AHA: 2Q, '92, 3; N-D, '86, 5

§ ✓5ᵗʰ **202.0 Nodular lymphoma**
Brill-Symmers disease
Lymphoma:
follicular (giant)
lymphocytic, nodular
Lymphosarcoma:
follicular (giant)
nodular
Reticulosarcoma, follicular or nodular
DEF: Lymphomatous cells clustered into nodules within the lymph node; usually occurs in older adults and may involve all nodes and possibly extranodal sites.

§ ✓5ᵗʰ **202.1 Mycosis fungoides**
AHA: 2Q, '92, 4
DEF: Type of cutaneous T-cell lymphoma; may evolve into generalized lymphoma; formerly thought to be of fungoid origin.

§ ✓5ᵗʰ **202.2 Sézary's disease**
AHA: 2Q, '99, 7
DEF: Type of cutaneous T-cell lymphoma with erythroderma, intense pruritus, peripheral lymphadenopathy, abnormal hyperchromatic mononuclear cells in skin, lymph nodes and peripheral blood.

§ ✓5ᵗʰ **202.3 Malignant histiocytosis**
Histiocytic medullary reticulosis
Malignant:
reticuloendotheliosis
reticulosis
§ ✓5ᵗʰ **202.4 Leukemic reticuloendotheliosis**
Hairy-cell leukemia
DEF: Chronic leukemia with large, mononuclear cells with "hairy" appearance in marrow, spleen, liver, blood.

§ ✓5ᵗʰ **202.5 Letterer-Siwe disease**
Acute:
differentiated progressive histiocytosis
histiocytosis X (progressive)
infantile reticuloendotheliosis
reticulosis of infancy
EXCLUDES *Hand-Schüller-Christian disease (277.89)*
histiocytosis (acute) (chronic) (277.89)
histiocytosis X (chronic) (277.89)
DEF: A recessive reticuloendotheliosis of early childhood, with a hemorrhagic tendency, eczema-like skin eruption, hepato-splenomegaly, including lymph node enlargement, and progressive anemia; it is often a fatal disease with no established cause.

§ ✓5ᵗʰ **202.6 Malignant mast cell tumors**
Malignant: Mast cell sarcoma
mastocytoma   Systemic tissue mast
mastocytosis   cell disease
EXCLUDES *mast cell leukemia (207.8)*

§ ✓5ᵗʰ **202.8 Other lymphomas**
Lymphoma (malignant):
NOS
diffuse
EXCLUDES *benign lymphoma (229.0)*
AHA: 2Q, '92, 4

§ ✓5ᵗʰ **202.9 Other and unspecified malignant neoplasms of lymphoid and histiocytic tissue**
Follicular dendritic cell sarcoma
Interdigitating dendritic cell sarcoma
Langerhans cell sarcom
Malignant neoplasm of bone marrow NOS

§ Requires fifth-digit. See beginning of section 200–208 for codes and definitions.

√4ᵗʰ 203 Multiple myeloma and immunoproliferative neoplasms

The following fifth-digit subclassification is for use with category 203:

    0 **without mention of remission**
    1 **in remission**

√5ᵗʰ 203.0 Multiple myeloma
    Kahler's disease   Myelomatosis
    EXCLUDES *solitary myeloma (238.6)*
    AHA: 1Q, '96, 16; 4Q, '91, 26

√5ᵗʰ 203.1 Plasma cell leukemia
    Plasmacytic leukemia
    AHA: 4Q, '90, 26; S-O, '86, 12

√5ᵗʰ 203.8 Other immunoproliferative neoplasms
    AHA: 4Q, '90, 26; S-O, '86, 12

√4ᵗʰ 204 Lymphoid leukemia
    INCLUDES leukemia:
        lymphatic
        lymphoblastic
        lymphocytic
        lymphogenous

    AHA: 3Q, '93, 4

The following fifth-digit subclassification is for use with category 204:

    0 **without mention of remission**
    1 **in remission**

√5ᵗʰ 204.0 Acute
    EXCLUDES *acute exacerbation of chronic lymphoid leukemia (204.1)*
    AHA: 3Q, '99, 6

√5ᵗʰ 204.1 Chronic

√5ᵗʰ 204.2 Subacute

√5ᵗʰ 204.8 Other lymphoid leukemia
    Aleukemic leukemia: Aleukemic leukemia:
      lymphatic   lymphoid
      lymphocytic

√5ᵗʰ 204.9 Unspecified lymphoid leukemia

√4ᵗʰ 205 Myeloid leukemia
    INCLUDES leukemia:
        granulocytic
        myeloblastic
        myelocytic
        myelogenous
        myelomonocytic
        myelosclerotic
        myelosis

    AHA: 3Q, '93, 3; 4Q, '91, 26; 4Q, '90, 3; M-J, '85, 18

The following fifth-digit subclassification is for use with category 205:

    0 **without mention of remission**
    1 **in remission**

√5ᵗʰ 205.0 Acute
    Acute promyelocytic leukemia
    EXCLUDES *acute exacerbation of chronic myeloid leukemia (205.1)*

√5ᵗʰ 205.1 Chronic
    Eosinophilic leukemia
    Neutrophilic leukemia
    AHA: 1Q, 00, 6; J-A, '85, 13

√5ᵗʰ 205.2 Subacute

√5ᵗʰ 205.3 Myeloid sarcoma
    Chloroma
    Granulocytic sarcoma

√5ᵗʰ 205.8 Other myeloid leukemia
    Aleukemic leukemia: Aleukemic leukemia:
      granulocytic   myeloid
      myelogenous   Aleukemic myelosis

√5ᵗʰ 205.9 Unspecified myeloid leukemia

√4ᵗʰ 206 Monocytic leukemia
    INCLUDES leukemia:
        histiocytic
        monoblastic
        monocytoid

The following fifth-digit subclassification is for use with category 206:

    0 **without mention of remission**
    1 **in remission**

√5ᵗʰ 206.0 Acute
    EXCLUDES *acute exacerbation of chronic monocytic leukemia (206.1)*

√5ᵗʰ 206.1 Chronic

√5ᵗʰ 206.2 Subacute

√5ᵗʰ 206.8 Other monocytic leukemia
    Aleukemic: Aleukemic:
      monocytic leukemia   monocytoid leukemia

√5ᵗʰ 206.9 Unspecified monocytic leukemia

√4ᵗʰ 207 Other specified leukemia
    EXCLUDES *leukemic reticuloendotheliosis (202.4)*
                plasma cell leukemia (203.1)

The following fifth-digit subclassification is for use with category 207:

    0 **without mention of remission**
    1 **in remission**

√5ᵗʰ 207.0 Acute erythremia and erythroleukemia
    Acute erythremic myelosis   Erythremic myelosis
    Di Guglielmo's disease
    DEF: Erythremia: polycythemia vera.
    DEF: Erythroleukemia: a malignant blood dyscrasia (a myeloproliferative disorder).

√5ᵗʰ 207.1 Chronic erythremia
    Heilmeyer-Schöner disease

√5ᵗʰ 207.2 Megakaryocytic leukemia
    Megakaryocytic myelosis   Thrombocytic leukemia

√5ᵗʰ 207.8 Other specified leukemia
    Lymphosarcoma cell leukemia

√4ᵗʰ 208 Leukemia of unspecified cell type

The following fifth-digit subclassification is for use with category 208:

    0 **without mention of remission**
    1 **in remission**

√5ᵗʰ 208.0 Acute
    Acute leukemia NOS   Stem cell leukemia
    Blast cell leukemia
    EXCLUDES *acute exacerbation of chronic unspecified leukemia (208.1)*

√5ᵗʰ 208.1 Chronic
    Chronic leukemia NOS

√5ᵗʰ 208.2 Subacute
    Subacute leukemia NOS

√5ᵗʰ 208.8 Other leukemia of unspecified cell type

√5ᵗʰ 208.9 Unspecified leukemia
    Leukemia NOS

√4ᵗʰ / √5ᵗʰ Additional Digit Required   Unspecified Code   Other Specified Code   Manifestation Code   ►◄ Revised Text   ● New Code   ▲ Revised Code Title

BENIGN NEOPLASMS (210-229)

☑4ᵗʰ **210 Benign neoplasm of lip, oral cavity, and pharynx**

EXCLUDES   cyst (of):
jaw (526.0-526.2,526.89)
oral soft tissue (528.4)
radicular (522.8)

210.0 Lip
Frenulum labii
Lip (inner aspect) (mucosa) (vermilion border)
EXCLUDES   labial commissure (210.4)
skin of lip (216.0)

210.1 Tongue
Lingual tonsil

210.2 Major salivary glands
Gland:
parotid
sublingual
submandibular
EXCLUDES   benign neoplasms of minor salivary
glands:
NOS (210.4)
buccal mucosa (210.4)
lips (210.0)
palate (hard) (soft) (210.4)
tongue (210.1)
tonsil, palatine (210.5)

210.3 Floor of mouth

210.4 Other and unspecified parts of mouth
Gingiva   Oral mucosa
Gum (upper) (lower)   Palate (hard) (soft)
Labial commissure   Uvula
Oral cavity NOS
EXCLUDES   benign odontogenic neoplasms of bone
(213.0-213.1)
developmental odontogenic cysts
(526.0)
mucosa of lips (210.0)
nasopharyngeal [posterior] [superior]
surface of soft palate (210.7)

210.5 Tonsil
Tonsil (faucial) (palatine)
EXCLUDES   lingual tonsil (210.1)
pharyngeal tonsil (210.7)
tonsillar:
fossa (210.6)
pillars (210.6)

210.6 Other parts of oropharynx
Branchial cleft or vestiges   Tonsillar:
Epiglottis, anterior aspect   fossa
Fauces NOS   pillars
Mesopharynx NOS   Vallecula
EXCLUDES   epiglottis:
NOS (212.1)
suprahyoid portion (212.1)

210.7 Nasopharynx
Adenoid tissue   Pharyngeal tonsil
Lymphadenoid tissue Posterior nasal septum

210.8 Hypopharynx
Arytenoid fold   Postcricoidregion
Laryngopharynx   Pyriform fossa

210.9 Pharynx, unspecified
Throat NOS

☑4ᵗʰ **211 Benign neoplasm of other parts of digestive system**

211.0 Esophagus

211.1 Stomach
Body ⎫
Cardia ⎬ of stomach
Fundus ⎭

Cardiac orifice
Pylorus

211.2 Duodenum, jejunum, and ileum
Small intestine NOS
EXCLUDES   ampulla of Vater (211.5)
ileocecal valve (211.3)

211.3 Colon
Appendix   Ileocecal valve
Cecum   Large intestine NOS
EXCLUDES   rectosigmoid junction (211.4)

AHA: 4Q, '01, 56

211.4 Rectum and anal canal
Anal canal or sphincter   Rectosigmoid junction
Anus NOS
EXCLUDES   anus:
margin (216.5)
skin (216.5)
perianal skin (216.5)

211.5 Liver and biliary passages
Ampulla of Vater   Gallbladder
Common bile duct   Hepatic duct
Cystic duct   Sphincter of Oddi

211.6 Pancreas, except islets of Langerhans

211.7 Islets of Langerhans
Islet cell tumor
Use additional code to identify any functional
activity

211.8 Retroperitoneum and peritoneum
Mesentery   Omentum
Mesocolon   Retroperitoneal tissue

211.9 Other and unspecified site
Alimentary tract NOS
Digestive system NOS
Gastrointestinal tract NOS
Intestinal tract NOS
Intestine NOS
Spleen, not elsewhere classified

☑4ᵗʰ **212 Benign neoplasm of respiratory and intrathoracic organs**

212.0 Nasal cavities, middle ear, and accessory sinuses
Cartilage of nose   Sinus:
Eustachian tube   ethomoidal
Nares   frontal
Septum of nose   maxillary
sphenoidal
EXCLUDES   auditory canal (external) (216.2)
bone of:
ear (213.0)
nose [turbinates] (213.0)
cartilage of ear (215.0)
ear (external) (skin) (216.2)
nose NOS (229.8)
skin (216.3)
olfactory bulb (225.1)
polyp of:
accessory sinus (471.8)
ear (385.30-385.35)
nasal cavity (471.0)
posterior margin of septum and
choanae (210.7)

212.1 Larynx
Cartilage:
arytenoid
cricoid
cuneiform
thyroid
Epiglottis (suprahyoid portion) NOS
Glottis
Vocal cords (false) (true)
EXCLUDES   epiglottis, anterior aspect (210.6)
polyp of vocal cord or larynx (478.4)

212.2 Trachea

212.3 Bronchus and lung
Carina   Hilus of lung

212.4 Pleura

212.5 **Mediastinum**

212.6 **Thymus**

212.7 **Heart**
> EXCLUDES *great vessels (215.4)*

212.8 **Other specified sites**

212.9 **Site unspecified**
Respiratory organ NOS
Upper respiratory tract NOS
> EXCLUDES *intrathoracic NOS (229.8)*
> *thoracic NOS (229.8)*

√4ᵗʰ **213 Benign neoplasm of bone and articular cartilage**
> INCLUDES cartilage (articular) (joint)
> periosteum
> EXCLUDES *cartilage of:*
> *ear (215.0)*
> *eyelid (215.0)*
> *larynx (212.1)*
> *nose (212.0)*
> *exostosis NOS (726.91)*
> *synovia (215.0-215.9)*

213.0 **Bones of skull and face**
> EXCLUDES *lower jaw bone (213.1)*

213.1 **Lower jaw bone**

213.2 **Vertebral column, excluding sacrum and coccyx**

213.3 **Ribs, sternum, and clavicle**

213.4 **Scapula and long bones of upper limb**

213.5 **Short bones of upper limb**

213.6 **Pelvic bones, sacrum, and coccyx**

213.7 **Long bones of lower limb**

213.8 **Short bones of lower limb**

213.9 **Bone and articular cartilage, site unspecified**

√4ᵗʰ **214 Lipoma**
> INCLUDES angiolipoma
> fibrolipoma
> hibernoma
> lipoma (fetal) (infiltrating) (intramuscular)
> myelolipoma
> myxolipoma

DEF: Benign tumor frequently composed of mature fat cells; may occasionally be composed of fetal fat cells.

214.0 **Skin and subcutaneous tissue of face**

214.1 **Other skin and subcutaneous tissue**

214.2 **Intrathoracic organs**

214.3 **Intra-abdominal organs**

214.4 **Spermatic cord**   ♂

214.8 **Other specified sites**
AHA: 3Q, '94, 7

214.9 **Lipoma, unspecified site**

√4ᵗʰ **215 Other benign neoplasm of connective and other soft tissue**
> INCLUDES blood vessel
> bursa
> fascia
> ligament
> muscle
> peripheral, sympathetic, and parasympathetic
> nerves and ganglia
> synovia
> tendon (sheath)
> EXCLUDES *cartilage:*
> *articular (213.0-213.9)*
> *larynx (212.1)*
> *nose (212.0)*
> *connective tissue of:*
> *breast (217)*
> *internal organ, except lipoma and*
> *hemangioma—code to benign neoplasm*
> *of the site*
> *lipoma (214.0-214.9)*

215.0 **Head, face, and neck**

215.2 **Upper limb, including shoulder**

215.3 **Lower limb, including hip**

215.4 **Thorax**
> EXCLUDES *heart (212.7)*
> *mediastinum (212.5)*
> *thymus (212.6)*

215.5 **Abdomen**
Abdominal wall   Hypochondrium

215.6 **Pelvis**
Buttock   Inguinal region
Groin   Perineum
> EXCLUDES *uterine:*
> *leiomyoma (218.0-218.9)*
> *ligament, any (221.0)*

215.7 **Trunk, unspecified**
Back NOS   Flank NOS

215.8 **Other specified sites**

215.9 **Site unspecified**

√4ᵗʰ **216 Benign neoplasm of skin**
> INCLUDES blue nevus
> dermatofibroma
> hydrocystoma
> pigmented nevus
> syringoadenoma
> syringoma
> EXCLUDES *skin of genital organs (221.0-222.9)*

AHA: 1Q, '00, 21

216.0 **Skin of lip**
> EXCLUDES *vermilion border of lip (210.0)*

216.1 **Eyelid, including canthus**
> EXCLUDES *cartilage of eyelid (215.0)*

216.2 **Ear and external auditory canal**
Auricle (ear)
Auricular canal, external
External meatus
Pinna
> EXCLUDES *cartilage of ear (215.0)*

216.3 **Skin of other and unspecified parts of face**
Cheek, external   Nose, external
Eyebrow   Temple

216.4 **Scalp and skin of neck**
AHA: 3Q, '91, 12

216.5 **Skin of trunk, except scrotum**
Axillary fold   Skin of:
Perianal skin   buttock
Skin of: chest wall
abdominal wall   groin
anus   perineum
back   Umbilicus
breast
> EXCLUDES *anal canal (211.4)*
> *anus NOS (211.4)*
> *skin of scrotum (222.4)*

216.6 **Skin of upper limb, including shoulder**

216.7 **Skin of lower limb, including hip**

216.8 **Other specified sites of skin**

216.9 **Skin, site unspecified**

217 Benign neoplasm of breast
Breast (male) (female):   Breast (male) (female):
connective tissue   soft parts
glandular tissue
> EXCLUDES *adenofibrosis (610.2)*
> *benign cyst of breast (610.0)*
> *fibrocystic disease (610.1)*
> *skin of breast (216.5)*

AHA: 1Q, '00, 4

√4ᵗʰ **218 Uterine leiomyoma**

     INCLUDES   fibroid (bleeding) (uterine)
                   uterine:
                      fibromyoma
                      myoma

DEF: Benign tumor primarily derived from uterine smooth muscle tissue; may contain fibrous, fatty, or epithelial tissue; also called uterine fibroid or myoma.

   218.0 Submucous leiomyoma of uterus ♀
   218.1 Intramural leiomyoma of uterus ♀
          Interstitial leiomyoma of uterus
   218.2 Subserous leiomyoma of uterus ♀
   218.9 Leiomyoma of uterus, unspecified ♀
          AHA: 1Q, '03, 4

√4ᵗʰ **219 Other benign neoplasm of uterus**

   219.0 Cervix uteri ♀
   219.1 Corpus uteri ♀
          Endometrium   Myometrium
          Fundus
   219.8 Other specified parts of uterus ♀
   219.9 Uterus, part unspecified ♀
   220 Benign neoplasm of ovary ♀
          Use additional code to identify any functional activity (256.0-256.1)
          EXCLUDES   cyst:
                  corpus albicans (620.2)
                  corpus luteum (620.1)
                  endometrial (617.1)
                  follicular (atretic) (620.0)
                  graafian follicle (620.0)
                  ovarian NOS (620.2)
                  retention (620.2)

√4ᵗʰ **221 Benign neoplasm of other female genital organs**

     INCLUDES   adenomatous polyp
                   benign teratoma
     EXCLUDES   cyst:
                  epoophoron (752.11)
                  fimbrial (752.11)
                  Gartner's duct (752.11)
                  parovarian (752.11)

   221.0 Fallopian tube and uterine ligaments ♀
          Oviduct
          Parametruim
          Uterine ligament (broad) (round) (uterosacral)
          Uterine tube
   221.1 Vagina ♀
   221.2 Vulva ♀
          Clitoris
          External female genitalia NOS
          Greater vestibular [Bartholin's] gland
          Labia (majora) (minora)
          Pudendum
          EXCLUDES   Bartholin's (duct) (gland) cyst (616.2)

Eyeball

√4ᵗʰ **222 Benign neoplasm of male genital organs**

   221.8 Other specified sites of female genital organs ♀
   221.9 Female genital organ, site unspecified ♀
          Female genitourinary tract NOS

   222.0 Testis ♂
          Use additional code to identify any functional activity
   222.1 Penis ♂
          Corpus cavernosum   Prepuce
          Glans penis
   222.2 Prostate ♂
          EXCLUDES   adenomatous hyperplasia of prostate (600.20-600.21)
                       prostatic:
                         adenoma (600.20-600.21)
                         enlargement (600.00-600.01)
                         hypertrophy (600.00-600.01)
   222.3 Epididymis ♂
   222.4 Scrotum ♂
          Skin of scrotum
   222.8 Other specified sites of male genital organs ♂
          Seminal vesicle
          Spermatic cord
   222.9 Male genital organ, site unspecified ♂
          Male genitourinary tract NOS

√4ᵗʰ **223 Benign neoplasm of kidney and other urinary organs**

   223.0 Kidney, except pelvis
          Kidney NOS
          EXCLUDES   renal:
                    calyces (223.1)
                    pelvis (223.1)
   223.1 Renal pelvis
   223.2 Ureter
          EXCLUDES   ureteric orifice of bladder (223.3)
   223.3 Bladder

√5ᵗʰ **223.8 Other specified sites of urinary organs**
      223.81 Urethra
          EXCLUDES   urethral orifice of bladder (223.3)
      223.89 Other
          Paraurethral glands
   223.9 Urinary organ, site unspecified
          Urinary system NOS

√4ᵗʰ **224 Benign neoplasm of eye**

     EXCLUDES   cartilage of eyelid (215.0)
               eyelid (skin) (216.1)
               optic nerve (225.1)
               orbital bone (213.0)
   224.0 Eyeball, except conjunctiva, cornea, retina, and choroid
          Ciliary body   Sclera
          Iris   Uveal tract
   224.1 Orbit
          EXCLUDES   bone of orbit (213.0)
   224.2 Lacrimal gland
   224.3 Conjunctiva
   224.4 Cornea
   224.5 Retina
          EXCLUDES   hemangioma of retina (228.03)
   224.6 Choroid
   224.7 Lacrimal duct
          Lacrimal sac
          Nasolacrimal duct
   224.8 Other specified parts of eye
   224.9 Eye, part unspecified

N Newborn Age: 0   P Pediatric Age: 0-17   M Maternity Age: 12-55   A Adult Age: 15-124   MSP Medicare Secondary Payer

☑4th **225 Benign neoplasm of brain and other parts of nervous system**

> EXCLUDES   *hemangioma (228.02)*
> *neurofibromatosis (237.7)*
> *peripheral, sympathetic, and parasympathetic*
> *nerves and ganglia (215.0-215.9)*
> *retrobulbar (224.1)*

225.0 Brain

225.1 Cranial nerves

225.2 Cerebral meninges
Meninges NOS   Meningioma (cerebral)

225.3 Spinal cord
Cauda equina

225.4 Spinal meninges
Spinal meningioma

225.8 Other specified sites of nervous system

225.9 Nervous system, part unspecified
Nervous system (central) NOS
> EXCLUDES   *meninges NOS (225.2)*

226 Benign neoplasm of thyroid glands
Use additional code to identify any functional activity

☑4th **227 Benign neoplasm of other endocrine glands and related structures**
Use additional code to identify any functional activity
> EXCLUDES   *ovary (220)*
> *pancreas (211.6)*
> *testis (222.0)*

227.0 Adrenal gland
Suprarenal gland

227.1 Parathyroid gland

227.3 Pituitary gland and craniopharyngeal duct (pouch)
Craniobuccal pouch   Rathke's pouch
Hypophysis   Sella turcica

227.4 Pineal gland
Pineal body

227.5 Carotid body

227.6 Aortic body and other paraganglia
Coccygeal body   Para-aortic body
Glomus jugulare
AHA: N-D, '84, 17

227.8 Other

227.9 Endocrine gland, site unspecified

☑4th **228 Hemangioma and lymphangioma, any site**
> INCLUDES   angioma (benign) (cavernous) (congenital) NOS
> cavernous nevus
> glomus tumor
> hemangioma (benign) (congenital)
> EXCLUDES   *benign neoplasm of spleen, except hemangioma*
> *and lymphangioma (211.9)*
> *glomus jugulare (227.6)*
> *nevus:*
> *NOS (216.0-216.9)*
> *blue or pigmented (216.0-216.9)*
> *vascular (757.32)*

AHA: 1Q, '00, 21

☑5th **228.0 Hemangioma, any site**
AHA: J-F, '85, 19

DEF: A common benign tumor usually occurring in infancy; composed of newly formed blood vessels due to malformation of angioblastic tissue.

228.00 Of unspecified site

228.01 Of skin and subcutaneous tissue

228.02 Of intracranial structures

228.03 Of retina

228.04 Of intra-abdominal structures
Peritoneum   Retroperitoneal tissue

228.09 Of other sites
Systemic angiomatosis
AHA: 3Q, '91, 20

228.1 Lymphangioma, any site
Congenital lymphangioma
Lymphatic nevus

☑4th **229 Benign neoplasm of other and unspecified sites**

229.0 Lymph nodes
> EXCLUDES   *lymphangioma (228.1)*

229.8 Other specified sites
Intrathoracic NOS   Thoracic NOS

229.9 Site unspecified

CARCINOMA IN SITU (230-234)

> INCLUDES   Bowen's disease
> erythroplasia
> Queyrat's erythroplasia
> EXCLUDES   *leukoplakia—see Alphabetic Index*

DEF: A neoplastic type; with tumor cells confined to epithelium of origin; without further invasion.

☑4th **230 Carcinoma in situ of digestive organs**

230.0 Lip, oral cavity, and pharynx
Gingiva   Oropharynx
Hypopharynx   Salivary gland or duct
Mouth [any part]   Tongue
Nasopharynx
> EXCLUDES   *aryepiglottic fold or interarytenoid fold,*
> *laryngeal aspect (231.0)*
> *epiglottis:*
> *NOS (231.0)*
> *suprahyoid portion (231.0)*
> *skin of lip (232.0)*

230.1 Esophagus

230.2 Stomach
Body
Cardia   } of stomach
Fundus

Cardiac orifice
Pylorus

230.3 Colon
Appendix   Ileocecal valve
Cecum   Large intestine NOS
> EXCLUDES   *rectosigmoid junction (230.4)*

230.4 Rectum
Rectosigmoid junction

230.5 Anal canal
Anal sphincter

230.6 Anus, unspecified
> EXCLUDES   *anus:*
> *margin (232.5)*
> *skin (232.5)*
> *perianal skin (232.5)*

230.7 Other and unspecified parts of intestine
Duodenum   Jejunum
Ileum   Small intestine NOS
> EXCLUDES   *ampulla of Vater (230.8)*

230.8 Liver and biliary system
Ampulla of Vater   Gallbladder
Common bile duct   Hepatic duct
Cystic duct   Sphincter of Oddi

230.9 Other and unspecified digestive organs
Digestive organ NOS
Gastrointestinal tract NOS
Pancreas
Spleen

☑4th ☑5th Additional Digit Required   Unspecified Code   Other Specified Code   Manifestation Code   ▶◀ Revised Text   ● New Code   ▲ Revised Code Title

2005 ICD•9•CM   **Volume 1 — 41**

✓4ᵗʰ **231 Carcinoma in situ of respiratory system**

231.0 **Larynx**

Cartilage: Epiglottis:
arytenoid NOS
cricoid posterior surface
cuneiform suprahyoid portion
thyroid Vocal cords (false) (true)

EXCLUDES *aryepiglottic fold or interarytenoid fold:*
NOS (230.0)
hypopharyngeal aspect (230.0)
marginal zone (230.0)

231.1 **Trachea**

231.2 **Bronchus and lung**

Carina Hilus of lung

231.8 **Other specified parts of respiratory system**

Accessory sinuses Nasal cavities
Middle ear Pleura

EXCLUDES *ear (external) (skin) (232.2)*
nose NOS (234.8)
skin (232.3)

231.9 **Respiratory system, part unspecified**

Respiratory organ NOS

✓4ᵗʰ **232 Carcinoma in situ of skin**

INCLUDES pigment cells

232.0 **Skin of lip**

EXCLUDES *vermilion border of lip (230.0)*

232.1 **Eyelid, including canthus**

232.2 **Ear and external auditory canal**

232.3 **Skin of other and unspecified parts of face**

232.4 **Scalp and skin of neck**

232.5 **Skin of trunk, except scrotum**

Anus, margin Skin of:
Axillary fold breast
Perianal skin buttock
Skin of: chest wall
abdominal wall groin
anus perineum
back Umbilicus

EXCLUDES *anal canal (230.5)*
anus NOS (230.6)
skin of genital organs (233.3, 233.5-233.6)

232.6 **Skin of upper limb, including shoulder**

232.7 **Skin of lower limb, including hip**

232.8 **Other specified sites of skin**

232.9 **Skin, site unspecified**

✓4ᵗʰ **233 Carcinoma in situ of breast and genitourinary system**

233.0 **Breast**

EXCLUDES *Paget's disease (174.0-174.9)*
skin of breast (232.5)

233.1 **Cervix uteri** ♀
▶Cervical intraepithelial neoplasia III [CIN III]
Severe dysplasia of cervix◀

EXCLUDES ▶*cervical intraepithelial neoplasia II [CIN II] (622.12)*
cytologic evidence of malignancy without histologic confirmation (795.04)
high grade squamous intraepithelial lesion (HGSIL) (795.04)
moderate dysplasia of cervix (622.12)◀

AHA: 3Q, '92, 7; 3Q, '92, 8; 1Q, '91, 11

233.2 **Other and unspecified parts of uterus** ♀

233.3 **Other and unspecified female genital organs** ♀

233.4 **Prostate** ♂

233.5 **Penis** ♂

233.6 **Other and unspecified male genital organs** ♂

233.7 **Bladder**

233.9 **Other and unspecified urinary organs**

✓4ᵗʰ **234 Carcinoma in situ of other and unspecified sites**

234.0 **Eye**

EXCLUDES *cartilage of eyelid (234.8)*
eyelid (skin) (232.1)
optic nerve (234.8)
orbital bone (234.8)

234.8 **Other specified sites**
Endocrine gland [any]

234.9 **Site unspecified**
Carcinoma in situ NOS

NEOPLASMS OF UNCERTAIN BEHAVIOR (235-238)

Note: Categories 235–238 classify by site certain histomorphologically well-defined neoplasms, the subsequent behavior of which cannot be predicted from the present appearance.

✓4ᵗʰ **235 Neoplasm of uncertain behavior of digestive and respiratory systems**

235.0 **Major salivary glands**

Gland: Gland:
parotid submandibular
sublingual

EXCLUDES *minor salivary glands (235.1)*

235.1 **Lip, oral cavity, and pharynx**

Gingiva Nasopharynx
Hypopharynx Oropharynx
Minor salivary glands Tongue
Mouth

EXCLUDES *aryepiglottic fold or interarytenoid fold, laryngeal aspect (235.6)*
epiglottis:
NOS (235.6)
suprahyoid portion (235.6)
skin of lip (238.2)

235.2 **Stomach, intestines, and rectum**

235.3 **Liver and biliary passages**

Ampulla of Vater Gallbladder
Bile ducts [any] Liver

235.4 **Retroperitoneum and peritoneum**

235.5 **Other and unspecified digestive organs**

Anal: Esophagus
canal Pancreas
sphincter Spleen
Anus NOS

EXCLUDES *anus:*
margin (238.2)
skin (238.2)
perianal skin (238.2)

235.6 **Larynx**

EXCLUDES *aryepiglottic fold or interarytenoid fold:*
NOS (235.1)
hypopharyngeal aspect (235.1)
marginal zone (235.1)

235.7 **Trachea, bronchus, and lung**

235.8 **Pleura, thymus, and mediastinum**

235.9 **Other and unspecified respiratory organs**

Accessory sinuses Nasal cavities
Middle ear Respiratory organ NOS

EXCLUDES *ear (external) (skin) (238.2)*
nose (238.8)
skin (238.2)

✓4ᵗʰ **236 Neoplasm of uncertain behavior of genitourinary organs**

236.0 **Uterus** ♀

236.1 **Placenta** ♀
Chorioadenoma (destruens)
Invasive mole
Malignant hydatid(iform) mole

236.2 **Ovary** ♀
Use additional code to identify any functional activity

236.3 **Other and unspecified female genital organs** ♀

236.4 Testis ♂
Use additional code to identify any functional activity

236.5 Prostate ♂

236.6 Other and unspecified male genital organs ♂

236.7 Bladder

✓5th **236.9 Other and unspecified urinary organs**

236.90 Urinary organ, unspecified

236.91 Kidney and ureter

236.99 Other

✓4th **237 Neoplasm of uncertain behavior of endocrine glands and nervous system**

237.0 Pituitary gland and craniopharyngeal duct
Use additional code to identify any functional activity

237.1 Pineal gland

237.2 Adrenal gland
Suprarenal gland
Use additional code to identify any functional activity

237.3 Paraganglia
Aortic body   Coccygeal body
Carotid body   Glomus jugulare
AHA: N-D, '84, 17

237.4 Other and unspecified endocrine glands
Parathyroid gland   Thyroid gland

237.5 Brain and spinal cord

237.6 Meninges
Meninges: Meninges:
NOS   spinal
cerebral

✓5th **237.7 Neurofibromatosis**
von Recklinghausen's disease
DEF: An inherited condition with developmental changes in the nervous system, muscles, bones and skin; multiple soft tumors (neurofibromas) distributed over the entire body.

237.70 Neurofibromatosis, unspecified

237.71 Neurofibromatosis, type 1 [von Recklinghausen's disease]

237.72 Neurofibromatosis, type 2 [acoustic neurofibromatosis]
DEF: Inherited condition with cutaneous lesions, benign tumors of peripheral nerves and bilateral 8th nerve masses.

237.9 Other and unspecified parts of nervous system
Cranial nerves
EXCLUDES peripheral, sympathetic, and parasympathetic nerves and ganglia (238.1)

✓4th **238 Neoplasm of uncertain behavior of other and unspecified sites and tissues**

238.0 Bone and articular cartilage
EXCLUDES cartilage:
ear (238.1)
eyelid (238.1)
larynx (235.6)
nose (235.9)
synovia (238.1)

238.1 Connective and other soft tissue
Peripheral, sympathetic, and parasympathetic nerves and ganglia
EXCLUDES cartilage (of):
articular (238.0)
larynx (235.6)
nose (235.9)
connective tissue of breast (238.3)

238.2 Skin
EXCLUDES anus NOS (235.5)
skin of genital organs (236.3, 236.6)
vermilion border of lip (235.1)

238.3 Breast
EXCLUDES skin of breast (238.2)

238.4 Polycythemia vera
DEF: Abnormal proliferation of all bone marrow elements, increased red cell mass and total blood volume; unknown etiology, frequently associated with splenomegaly, leukocytosis, and thrombocythemia.

238.5 Histiocytic and mast cells
Mast cell tumor NOS
Mastocytoma NOS

238.6 Plasma cells
Plasmacytoma NOS
Solitary myeloma

238.7 Other lymphatic and hematopoietic tissues
Disease:
lymphoproliferative (chronic) NOS
myeloproliferative (chronic) NOS
Idiopathic thrombocythemia
Megakaryocytic myelosclerosis
Myelodysplastic syndrome
Myelosclerosis with myeloid metaplasia
Panmyelosis (acute)
EXCLUDES myelofibrosis (289.89)
myelosclerosis NOS (289.89)
myelosis:
NOS (205.9)
megakaryocytic (207.2)
AHA: 3Q, '01, 13; 1Q, '97, 5; 2Q, '89, 8

238.8 Other specified sites
Eye
Heart
EXCLUDES eyelid (skin) (238.2)
cartilage (238.1)

238.9 Site unspecified

NEOPLASMS OF UNSPECIFIED NATURE (239)

✓4th **239 Neoplasms of unspecified nature**
Note: Category 239 classifies by site neoplasms of unspecified morphology and behavior. The term "mass,"unless otherwise stated, is not to be regarded as a neoplastic growth.
INCLUDES "growth" NOS
neoplasm NOS
new growth NOS
tumor NOS

239.0 Digestive system
EXCLUDES anus:
margin (239.2)
skin (239.2)
perianal skin (239.2)

239.1 Respiratory system

239.2 Bone, soft tissue, and skin
EXCLUDES anal canal (239.0)
anus NOS (239.0)
bone marrow (202.9)
cartilage:
larynx (239.1)
nose (239.1)
connective tissue of breast (239.3)
skin of genital organs (239.5)
vermilion border of lip (239.0)

239.3 Breast
EXCLUDES skin of breast (239.2)

239.4 Bladder

239.5 Other genitourinary organs

✓4th ✓5th Additional Digit Required   Unspecified Code   Other Specified Code   Manifestation Code   ▶◀ Revised Text   ● New Code   ▲ Revised Code Title

2005 ICD•9•CM   **Volume 1 — 43**

Neoplasms

239.6   **Brain**
      EXCLUDES   *cerebral meninges (239.7)*
                     cranial nerves (239.7)

239.7   **Endocrine glands and other parts of nervous system**
      EXCLUDES   *peripheral, sympathetic, and parasympathetic nerves and ganglia (239.2)*

239.8   **Other specified sites**
      EXCLUDES   *eyelid (skin) (239.2)*
                     cartilage (239.2)
                     great vessels (239.2)
                     optic nerve (239.7)

239.9   **Site unspecified**

Endocrine System

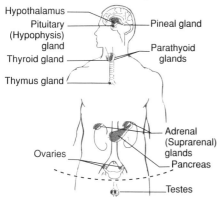

Hypothalamus
Pituitary (Hypophysis) gland
Thyroid gland
Thymus gland
Pineal gland
Parathyroid glands
Adrenal (Suprarenal) glands
Ovaries
Pancreas
Testes

3. ENDOCRINE, NUTRITIONAL AND METABOLIC DISEASES, AND IMMUNITY DISORDERS (240-279)

EXCLUDES *endocrine and metabolic disturbances specific to the fetus and newborn (775.0-775.9)*

Note: All neoplasms, whether functionally active or not, are classified in Chapter 2. Codes in Chapter 3 (i.e., 242.8, 246.0, 251-253, 255-259) may be used to identify such functional activity associated with any neoplasm, or by ectopic endocrine tissue.

DISORDERS OF THYROID GLAND (240-246)

✓4ᵗʰ 240 Simple and unspecified goiter

DEF: An enlarged thyroid gland often caused by an inadequate dietary intake of iodine.

240.0 Goiter, specified as simple

Any condition classifiable to 240.9, specified as simple

240.9 Goiter, unspecified

Enlargement of thyroid
Goiter or struma:
   NOS
   diffuse colloid
   endemic
Goiter or struma:
   hyperplastic
   nontoxic (diffuse)
   parenchymatous
   sporadic
   EXCLUDES *congenital (dyshormonogenic) goiter (246.1)*

✓4ᵗʰ 241 Nontoxic nodular goiter

EXCLUDES *adenoma of thyroid (226)*
cystadenoma of thyroid (226)

241.0 Nontoxic uninodular goiter

Thyroid nodule   Uninodular goiter (nontoxic)

DEF: Enlarged thyroid, commonly due to decreased thyroid production, with single nodule; no clinical hypothyroidism.

241.1 Nontoxic multinodular goiter

Multinodular goiter (nontoxic)

DEF: Enlarged thyroid, commonly due to decreased thyroid production with multiple nodules; no clinical hypothyroidism.

241.9 Unspecified nontoxic nodular goiter

Adenomatous goiter
Nodular goiter (nontoxic) NOS
Struma nodosa (simplex)

✓4ᵗʰ 242 Thyrotoxicosis with or without goiter

EXCLUDES *neonatal thyrotoxicosis (775.3)*

The following fifth-digit subclassification is for use with category 242:

  0 without mention of thyrotoxic crisis or storm
  1 with mention of thyrotoxic crisis or storm

DEF: A condition caused by excess quantities of thyroid hormones being introduced into the tissues.

✓5ᵗʰ 242.0 Toxic diffuse goiter

Basedow's disease
Exophthalmic or toxic goiter NOS
Graves' disease
Primary thyroid hyperplasia

DEF: Diffuse thyroid enlargement accompanied by hyperthyroidism, bulging eyes, and dermopathy.

✓5ᵗʰ 242.1 Toxic uninodular goiter

Thyroid nodule   } toxic or with
Uninodular goiter   }   hyperthyroidism

DEF: Symptomatic hyperthyroidism with a single nodule on the enlarged thyroid gland. Abrupt onset of symptoms; including extreme nervousness, insomnia, weight loss, tremors, and psychosis or coma.

✓5ᵗʰ 242.2 Toxic multinodular goiter

Secondary thyroid hyperplasia

DEF: Symptomatic hyperthyroidism with multiple nodules on the enlarged thyroid gland. Abrupt onset of symptoms; including extreme nervousness, insomnia, weight loss, tremors, and psychosis or coma.

✓5ᵗʰ 242.3 Toxic nodular goiter, unspecified

Adenomatous goiter   }
Nodular goiter   } toxic or with
Struma nodosa   }   hyperthyroidism

Any condition classifiable to 241.9 specified as toxic or with hyperthyroidism

✓5ᵗʰ 242.4 Thyrotoxicosis from ectopic thyroid nodule

✓5ᵗʰ 242.8 Thyrotoxicosis of other specified origin

Overproduction of thyroid-stimulating hormone [TSH]
Thyrotoxicosis:
  factitia from ingestion of excessive thyroid material
Use additional E code to identify cause, if drug-induced

✓5ᵗʰ 242.9 Thyrotoxicosis without mention of goiter or other cause

Hyperthyroidism NOS
Thyrotoxicosis NOS

243 Congenital hypothyroidism

Congenital thyroid insufficiency
Cretinism (athyrotic) (endemic)
Use additional code to identify associated mental retardation
EXCLUDES *congenital (dyshormonogenic) goiter (246.1)*

DEF: Underproduction of thyroid hormone present from birth.

✓4ᵗʰ 244 Acquired hypothyroidism

INCLUDES athyroidism (acquired)
hypothyroidism (acquired)
myxedema (adult) (juvenile)
thyroid (gland) insufficiency (acquired)

244.0 Postsurgical hypothyroidism

DEF: Underproduction of thyroid hormone due to surgical removal of all or part of the thyroid gland.

244.1 Other postablative hypothyroidism

Hypothyroidism following therapy, such as irradiation

244.2 Iodine hypothyroidism

Hypothyroidism resulting from administration or ingestion of iodide
Use additional E code to identify drug

244.3 Other iatrogenic hypothyroidism

Hypothyroidism resulting from:
  P-aminosalicylic acid [PAS]
  Phenylbutazone
  Resorcinol
Iatrogenic hypothyroidism NOS
Use additional E code to identify drug

✓4ᵗʰ
✓5ᵗʰ Additional Digit Required   Unspecified Code   Other Specified Code   Manifestation Code   ►◄ Revised Text   ● New Code   ▲ Revised Code Title

Endocrine, Nutritional, Metabolic, Immunity

244.8–250.4

244.8   Other specified acquired hypothyroidism
Secondary hypothyroidism NEC

AHA: J-A, '85, 9

244.9   Unspecified hypothyroidism

Hypothyroidism
Myxedema   } primary or NOS

AHA: 3Q, '99, 19; 4Q, '96, 29

√4ᵗʰ 245 Thyroiditis

245.0   Acute thyroiditis
Abscess of thyroid
Thyroiditis:
  nonsuppurative, acute
  pyogenic
  suppurative
Use additional code to identify organism

DEF: Inflamed thyroid caused by infection, with abscess and liquid puris.

245.1   Subacute thyroiditis
Thyroiditis:
  de Quervain's
  giant cell
  granulomatous
  viral

DEF: Inflammation of the thyroid, characterized by fever and painful enlargement of the thyroid gland, with granulomas in the gland.

245.2   Chronic lymphocytic thyroiditis
Hashimoto's disease
Struma lymphomatosa
Thyroiditis:
  autoimmune
  lymphocytic (chronic)

DEF: Autoimmune disease of thyroid; lymphocytes infiltrate the gland and thyroid antibodies are produced; women more often affected.

245.3   Chronic fibrous thyroiditis
Struma fibrosa
Thyroiditis:
  invasive (fibrous)
  ligneous
  Riedel's

DEF: Persistent fibrosing inflammation of thyroid with adhesions to nearby structures; rare condition.

245.4   Iatrogenic thyroiditis
Use additional code to identify cause

DEF: Thyroiditis resulting from treatment or intervention by physician or in a patient intervention setting.

245.8   Other and unspecified chronic thyroiditis
Chronic thyroiditis: Chronic thyroiditis:
  NOS   nonspecific

245.9   Thyroiditis, unspecified
Thyroiditis NOS

√4ᵗʰ 246 Other disorders of thyroid

246.0   Disorders of thyrocalcitonin secretion
Hypersecretion of calcitonin or thyrocalcitonin

246.1   Dyshormonogenic goiter
Congenital (dyshormonogenic) goiter
Goiter due to enzyme defect in synthesis of thyroid
  hormone
Goitrous cretinism (sporadic)

246.2   Cyst of thyroid
EXCLUDES   cystadenoma of thyroid (226)

246.3   Hemorrhage and infarction of thyroid

246.8   Other specified disorders of thyroid
Abnormality of thyroid-binding globulin
Atrophy of thyroid
Hyper-TBG-nemia
Hypo-TBG-nemia

246.9   Unspecified disorder of thyroid

DISEASES OF OTHER ENDOCRINE GLANDS (250-259)

√4ᵗʰ 250 Diabetes mellitus
EXCLUDES   gestational diabetes (648.8)
hyperglycemia NOS (790.6)
neonatal diabetes mellitus (775.1)
nonclinical diabetes (790.29

The following fifth-digit subclassification is for use with category 250:

▲ **0   type II or unspecified type, not stated as uncontrolled**
Fifth-digit 0 is for use for type II patients, even if the patient requires insulin
▶Use additional code, if applicable, for associated long-term (current) insulin use V58.67◀

▲ **1   type I [juvenile type], not stated as uncontrolled**

▲ **2   type II or unspecified type, uncontrolled**
Fifth-digit 2 is for use for type II patients, even if the patient requires insulin
▶Use additional code, if applicable, for associated long-term (current) insulin use V58.67◀

▲ **3   type I [juvenile type], uncontrolled**

AHA: 2Q, '02, 13; 2Q, '01, 16; 2Q, '98, 15; 4Q, '97, 32; 2Q, '97, 14; 3Q, '96, 5; 4Q, '93, 19; 2Q, '92, 5; 3Q, '91, 3; 2Q, '90, 22; N-D, '85, 11

DEF: Diabetes mellitus: Inability to metabolize carbohydrates, proteins, and fats with insufficient secretion of insulin. Symptoms may be unremarkable, with long-term complications, involving kidneys, nerves, blood vessels, and eyes.

DEF: Uncontrolled diabetes: A nonspecific term indicating that the current treatment regimen does not keep the blood sugar level of a patient within acceptable levels.

√5ᵗʰ 250.0   Diabetes mellitus without mention of complication
Diabetes mellitus without mention of complication or manifestation classifiable to 250.1-250.9
Diabetes (mellitus) NOS

AHA: 4Q, '97, 32; 3Q, '91, 3, 12; N-D, '85, 11; **For code 250.00:** 4Q, '03, 105, 108; 2Q, '03, 16; 1Q, '02, 7, 11; **For code: 250.01:** 4Q, '03, 110; 2Q, '03, 6; **For code: 250.02:** 1Q, '03, 5

√5ᵗʰ 250.1   Diabetes with ketoacidosis
Diabetic:
  acidosis   } without mention of coma
  ketosis

AHA: 3Q, '91, 6; **For code 250.11:** 4Q, '03, 82

DEF: Diabetic hyperglycemic crisis causing ketone presence in body fluids.

√5ᵗʰ 250.2   Diabetes with hyperosmolarity
Hyperosmolar (nonketotic) coma

AHA: 4Q, '93, 19; 3Q, '91, 7

√5ᵗʰ 250.3   Diabetes with other coma
Diabetic coma (with ketoacidosis)
Diabetic hypoglycemic coma
Insulin coma NOS
EXCLUDES   diabetes with hyperosmolar coma (250.2)

AHA: 3Q, '91, 7,12

DEF: Coma (not hyperosmolar) caused by hyperglycemia or hypoglycemia as complication of diabetes.

√5ᵗʰ 250.4   Diabetes with renal manifestations
Use additional code to identify manifestation, as:
diabetic:
  nephropathy NOS (583.81)
  nephrosis (581.81)
  intercapillary glomerulosclerosis (581.81)
  Kimmelstiel-Wilson syndrome (581.81)

AHA: 3Q, '91, 8,12; S-O, '87, 9; S-O, '84, 3; **For code: 250.40:** 1Q, '03, 20

N Newborn Age: 0   P Pediatric Age: 0-17   M Maternity Age: 12-55   A Adult Age: 15-124   MSP Medicare Secondary Payer

250.5 **Diabetes with ophthalmic manifestations**
Use additional code to identify manifestation, as:
diabetic:
blindness (369.00-369.9)
cataract (366.41)
glaucoma (365.44)
retinal edema (362.01)
retinopathy (362.01-362.02)

AHA: 3Q, '91, 8; S-O, '85, 11

250.6 **Diabetes with neurological manifestations**
Use additional code to identify manifestation, as:
diabetic:
amyotrophy (358.1)
▶gastroparalysis (536.3)
gastroparesis (536.3)◀
mononeuropathy (354.0-355.9)
neurogenic arthropathy (713.5)
peripheral autonomic neuropathy (337.1)
polyneuropathy (357.2)

AHA: 2Q, '93, 6; 2Q, '92, 15; 3Q, '91, 9; N-D, '84, 9; **For code 250.60:** 4Q, '03, 105

250.7 **Diabetes with peripheral circulatory disorders**
Use additional code to identify manifestation, as:
diabetic:
gangrene (785.4)
peripheral angiopathy (443.81)

DEF: Blood vessel damage or disease, usually in the feet, legs, or hands, as a complication of diabetes.

AHA: 1Q, '96, 10; 3Q, '94, 5; 2Q, '94, 17; 3Q, '91, 10, 12; 3Q, '90, 15; **For code 250.70:** ▶1Q, '04, 14◀

250.8 **Diabetes with other specified manifestations**
Diabetic hypoglycemia
Hypoglycemic shock
Use additional code to identify manifestation, as:
any associated ulceration (707.10-707.9)
diabetic bone changes (731.8)
Use additional E code to identify cause, if drug-induced

AHA: 4Q, '00, 44; 4Q, '97, 43; 2Q, '97, 16; 4Q, '93, 20; 3Q, '91, 10; **For code 250.80:** ▶1Q, '04, 14◀

250.9 **Diabetes with unspecified complication**
AHA: 2Q, '92, 15; 3Q, '91, 7, 12

251 Other disorders of pancreatic internal secretion

251.0 **Hypoglycemic coma**
Iatrogenic hyperinsulinism
Non-diabetic insulin coma
Use additional E code to identify cause, if drug-induced

EXCLUDES   *hypoglycemic coma in diabetes mellitus (250.3)*

AHA: M-A, '85, 8

DEF: Coma induced by low blood sugar in non-diabetic patient.

251.1 **Other specified hypoglycemia**
Hyperinsulinism:
NOS
ectopic
functional
Hyperplasia of pancreatic
islet beta cells NOS

EXCLUDES   *hypoglycemia:*
in diabetes mellitus (250.8)
in infant of diabetic mother (775.0)
neonatal hypoglycemia (775.6)
hypoglycemic coma (251.0)
Use additional E code to identify cause, if drug-induced.

DEF: Excessive production of insulin by the pancreas; associated with obesity and insulin-producing tumors.

AHA: 1Q, '03, 10

Dorsal View of Parathyroid Glands

Pharynx — Thyroid gland
Parathyroid glands — Parathyroid glands
Parathyroid glands
Trachea — Esophagus

Parathyroid glands
↓
Parathyroid hormone (PTH)
↓
Calcium in bones ⟶ Calcium in blood

251.2 **Hypoglycemia, unspecified**
Hypoglycemia:
NOS
reactive
spontaneous

EXCLUDES   *hypoglycemia:*
with coma (251.0)
in diabetes mellitus (250.8)
leucine-induced (270.3)

AHA: M-A, '85, 8

251.3 **Postsurgical hypoinsulinemia**
Hypoinsulinemia following complete or partial pancreatectomy
Postpancreatectomy hyperglycemia

AHA: 3Q, '91, 6

251.4 **Abnormality of secretion of glucagon**
Hyperplasia of pancreatic islet alpha cells with glucagon excess

DEF: Production malfunction of a pancreatic hormone secreted by cells of the islets of Langerhans

251.5 **Abnormality of secretion of gastrin**
Hyperplasia of pancreatic alpha cells with gastrin excess
Zollinger-Ellison syndrome

251.8 **Other specified disorders of pancreatic internal secretion**
AHA: 2Q, '98, 15; 3Q, '91, 6

251.9 **Unspecified disorder of pancreatic internal secretion**
Islet cell hyperplasia NOS

252 Disorders of parathyroid gland

252.0 **Hyperparathyroidism**
EXCLUDES   *ectopic hyperparathyroidism (259.3)*

DEF: Abnormally high secretion of parathyroid hormones causing bone deterioration, reduced renal function, kidney stones.

●   **252.00** **Hyperparathyroidism, unspecified**
●   **252.01** **Primary hyperparathyroidism**
Hyperplasia of parathyroid

     252.02 **Secondary hyperparathyroidism, non-renal**
EXCLUDES   *secondary hyperparathyroidism (of renal origin) (588.81)*

●   **252.08** **Other hyperparathyroidism**
Tertiary hyperparathyroidism

✓4ᵗʰ ✓5ᵗʰ Additional Digit Required   Unspecified Code   Other Specified Code   Manifestation Code   ▶◀ Revised Text   ● New Code   ▲ Revised Code Title

2005 ICD•9•CM   **October 2004 • Volume 1 — 47**

252.1 Hypoparathyroidism
Parathyroiditis (autoimmune)
Tetany:
   parathyroid
   parathyroprival
    EXCLUDES   *pseudohypoparathyroidism (275.4)*
           pseudopseudohypoparathyroidism
             (275.4)
           tetany NOS (781.7)
           transitory neonatal
             hypoparathyroidism (775.4)

DEF: Abnormally low secretion of parathyroid hormones which causes decreased calcium and increased phosphorus in the blood. Resulting in muscle cramps, tetany, urinary frequency and cataracts.

252.8 Other specified disorders of parathyroid gland
Cyst
Hemorrhage } of parathyroid gland

252.9 Unspecified disorder of parathyroid gland

√4ᵗʰ **253 Disorders of the pituitary gland and its hypothalamic control**
    INCLUDES   the listed conditions whether the disorder is in
            the pituitary or the hypothalamus
    EXCLUDES   *Cushing's syndrome (255.0)*

253.0 Acromegaly and gigantism
Overproduction of growth hormone
DEF: Acromegaly: chronic, beginning in middle age; caused by hypersecretion of the pituitary growth hormone; produces enlarged parts of skeleton, especially the nose, ears, jaws, fingers and toes.

DEF: Gigantism: pituitary gigantism caused by excess growth of short flat bones; men may grow 78 to 80 inches tall.

253.1 Other and unspecified anterior pituitary hyperfunction
Forbes-Albright syndrome
    EXCLUDES   *overproduction of:*
           ACTH (255.3)
           thyroid-stimulating hormone [TSH]
             (242.8)

AHA: J-A, '85, 9

DEF: Spontaneous galactorrhea-amenorrhea syndrome unrelated to pregnancy; usually related to presence of pituitary tumor.

253.2 Panhypopituitarism
Cachexia, pituitary
Necrosis of pituitary (postpartum)
Pituitary insufficiency NOS
Sheehan's syndrome
Simmonds' disease
    EXCLUDES   *iatrogenic hypopituitarism (253.7)*

DEF: Damage to or absence of pituitary gland leading to impaired sexual function, weight loss, fatigue, bradycardia, hypotension, pallor, depression, and impaired growth in children; called Simmonds' disease if cachexia is prominent.

253.3 Pituitary dwarfism
Isolated deficiency of (human) growth hormone [HGH]
Lorain-Levi dwarfism
DEF: Dwarfism with infantile physical characteristics due to abnormally low secretion of growth hormone and gonadotropin deficiency.

253.4 Other anterior pituitary disorders
Isolated or partial deficiency of an anterior pituitary
      hormone, other than growth hormone
Prolactin deficiency
AHA: J-A, '85, 9

253.5 Diabetes insipidus
Vasopressin deficiency
    EXCLUDES   *nephrogenic diabetes insipidus (588.1)*
DEF: Metabolic disorder causing insufficient antidiuretic hormone release; symptoms include frequent urination, thirst, ravenous hunger, loss of weight, fatigue.

253.6 Other disorders of neurohypophysis
Syndrome of inappropriate secretion of antidiuretic
      hormone [ADH]
    EXCLUDES   *ectopic antidiuretic hormone secretion*
            (259.3)

253.7 Iatrogenic pituitary disorders
Hypopituitarism: Hypopituitarism:
   hormone-induced   postablative
   hypophysectomy-induced   radiotherapy-induced
Use additional E code to identify cause
DEF: Pituitary dysfunction that results from drug therapy, radiation therapy, or surgery, causing mild to severe symptoms.

253.8 Other disorders of the pituitary and other syndromes of diencephalohypophyseal origin
Abscess of pituitary   Cyst of Rathke's pouch
Adiposogenital dystrophy   Fröhlich's syndrome
    EXCLUDES   *craniopharyngioma (237.0)*

253.9 Unspecified
Dyspituitarism

√4ᵗʰ **254 Diseases of thymus gland**
    EXCLUDES   *aplasia or dysplasia with immunodeficiency*
            (279.2)
           hypoplasia with immunodeficiency (279.2)
           myasthenia gravis (358.00-358.01)

254.0 Persistent hyperplasia of thymus
Hypertrophy of thymus
DEF: Continued abnormal growth of the twin lymphoid lobes that produce T lymphocytes.

254.1 Abscess of thymus

254.8 Other specified diseases of thymus gland
Atrophy
Cyst } of thymus
    EXCLUDES   *thymoma (212.6)*

254.9 Unspecified disease of thymus gland

√4ᵗʰ **255 Disorders of adrenal glands**
    INCLUDES   the listed conditions whether the basic
            disorder is in the adrenals or is pituitary-
            induced

255.0 Cushing's syndrome
Adrenal hyperplasia due to excess ACTH
Cushing's syndrome:
   NOS
   iatrogenic
   idiopathic
   pituitary-dependent
Ectopic ACTH syndrome
Iatrogenic syndrome of excess cortisol
Overproduction of cortisol
Use additional E code to identify cause, if drug-
     induced
    EXCLUDES   *congenital adrenal hyperplasia (255.2)*

DEF: Due to adrenal cortisol oversecretion or glucocorticoid medications; may cause fatty tissue of the face, neck and body, osteoporosis and curvature of spine, hypertension, diabetes mellitus, female genitourinary problems, male impotence, degeneration of muscle tissues, weakness.

√5ᵗʰ **255.1 Hyperaldosteronism**
AHA: 4Q, '03, 48

DEF: Oversecretion of aldosterone causing fluid retention, hypertension.

255.10 Primary aldosteronism
Aldosteronism NOS
Hyperaldosteronism, unspecified
    EXCLUDES ► *Conn's syndrome (255.12)*◄

N Newborn Age: 0   P Pediatric Age: 0-17   M Maternity Age: 12-55   A Adult Age: 15-124   MSP Medicare Secondary Payer

255.11 Glucocorticoid-remediable aldosteronism

Familial aldosteronism type I

> **EXCLUDES** ▶ *Conn's syndrome (255.12)*◄

DEF: A rare autosomal dominant familial form of primary aldosteronism in which the secretion of aldosterone is under the influence of adrenocorticotrophic hormone (ACTH) rather than the renin-angiotensin mechanism; characterized by moderate hypersecretion of aldosterone and suppressed plasma renin activity rapidly reversed by administration of glucosteroids; symptoms include hypertension and mild hypokalemia.

255.12 Conn's syndrome

DEF: A type of primary aldosteronism caused by an adenoma of the glomerulosa cells in the adrenal cortex; there is an absence of hypertension.

255.13 Bartter's syndrome

DEF: A cluster of symptoms caused by a defect in the ability of the kidney to reabsorb potassium; signs include alkalosis (hypokalemic alkalosis), increased aldosterone, increased plasma renin, and normal blood pressure; symptoms include muscle cramping, weakness, constipation, frequency of urination, and failure to grow; also known as urinary potassium wasting or juxtaglomerular cell hyperplasia.

255.14 Other secondary aldosteronism

255.2 Adrenogenital disorders

Achard-Thiers syndrome

Adrenogenital syndromes, virilizing or feminizing, whether acquired or associated with congenital adrenal hyperplasia consequent on inborn enzyme defects in hormone synthesis

Congenital adrenal hyperplasia

Female adrenal pseudohermaphroditism

Male:
macrogenitosomia praecox
sexual precocity with adrenal hyperplasia

Virilization (female) (suprarenal)

> **EXCLUDES** *adrenal hyperplasia due to excess ACTH (255.0)*
> *isosexual virilization (256.4)*

255.3 Other corticoadrenal overactivity

Acquired benign adrenal androgenic overactivity

Overproduction of ACTH

255.4 Corticoadrenal insufficiency

Addisonian crisis

Addison's disease NOS

Adrenal:
atrophy (autoimmune)
calcification
crisis
hemorrhage
infarction
insufficiency NOS

> **EXCLUDES** *tuberculous Addison's disease (017.6)*

DEF: Underproduction of adrenal hormones causing low blood pressure.

255.5 Other adrenal hypofunction

Adrenal medullary insufficiency

> **EXCLUDES** *Waterhouse-Friderichsen syndrome (meningococcal) (036.3)*

255.6 Medulloadrenal hyperfunction

Catecholamine secretion by pheochromocytoma

255.8 Other specified disorders of adrenal glands

Abnormality of cortisol-binding globulin

255.9 Unspecified disorder of adrenal glands

✓4ᵗʰ **256 Ovarian dysfunction**

AHA: 4Q, '00, 51

256.0 Hyperestrogenism   ♀

DEF: Excess secretion of estrogen by the ovaries; characterized by ovaries containing multiple follicular cysts filled with serous fluid.

256.1 Other ovarian hyperfunction   ♀

Hypersecretion of ovarian androgens

AHA: 3Q, '95, 15

256.2 Postablative ovarian failure   ♀

Ovarian failure: Ovarian failure:
iatrogenic   postsurgical
postirradiation

Use additional code for states associated with artificial menopause (627.4)

> **EXCLUDES** *acquired absence of ovary (V45.77)*
> *asymptomatic age-related (natural) postmenopausal status (V49.81)*

AHA: 2Q, '02, 12

DEF: Failed ovarian function after medical or surgical intervention.

✓5ᵗʰ **256.3 Other ovarian failure**

Use additional code for states associated with natural menopause (627.2)

> **EXCLUDES** *asymptomatic age-related (natural) postmenopausal status (V49.81)*

AHA: 4Q, '01, 41

256.31 Premature menopause   ▲ ♀

DEF: Permanent cessation of ovarian function before the age of 40 occurring naturally of unknown cause.

256.39 Other ovarian failure   ♀

Delayed menarche
Ovarian hypofunction
Primary ovarian failure NOS

256.4 Polycystic ovaries   ♀

Isosexual virilization   Stein-Leventhal syndrome

DEF: Multiple serous filled cysts of ovary; symptoms of infertility, hirsutism, oligomenorrhea or amenorrhea.

256.8 Other ovarian dysfunction   ♀

256.9 Unspecified ovarian dysfunction   ♀

✓4ᵗʰ **257 Testicular dysfunction**

257.0 Testicular hyperfunction   ♂

Hypersecretion of testicular hormones

257.1 Postablative testicular hypofunction   ♂

Testicular hypofunction: Testicular hypofunction:
iatrogenic   postsurgical
postirradiation

257.2 Other testicular hypofunction   ♂

Defective biosynthesis of testicular androgen

Eunuchoidism:
NOS
hypogonadotropic

Failure:
Leydig's cell, adult
seminiferous tubule, adult

Testicular hypogonadism

> **EXCLUDES** *azoospermia (606.0)*

257.8 Other testicular dysfunction   ♂

Goldberg-Maxwell syndrome

Male pseudohermaphroditism with testicular feminization

Testicular feminization

257.9 Unspecified testicular dysfunction   ♂

✓4ᵗʰ **258 Polyglandular dysfunction and related disorders**

258.0 Polyglandular activity in multiple endocrine adenomatosis

Wermer's syndrome

DEF: Wermer's syndrome: A rare hereditary condition characterized by the presence of adenomas or hyperplasia in more than one endocrine gland causing premature aging.

258.1 Other combinations of endocrine dysfunction

Lloyd's syndrome
Schmidt's syndrome

258.8 Other specified polyglandular dysfunction

258.9 Polyglandular dysfunction, unspecified

✓4ᵗʰ ✓5ᵗʰ Additional Digit Required   Unspecified Code   Other Specified Code   Manifestation Code   ▶◄ Revised Text   ● New Code   ▲ Revised Code Title

2005 ICD•9•CM   **October 2004 • Volume 1 — 49**

Endocrine, Nutritional, Metabolic, Immunity

259–266.0

✓4ᵗʰ 259 Other endocrine disorders

259.0 Delay in sexual development and puberty, not elsewhere classified
Delayed puberty

259.1 Precocious sexual development and puberty, not elsewhere classified   P
Sexual precocity: Sexual precocity:
    NOS   cryptogenic
    constitutional   idiopathic

259.2 Carcinoid syndrome
Hormone secretion by carcinoid tumors
DEF: Presence of carcinoid tumors that spread to liver; characterized by cyanotic flushing of skin, diarrhea, bronchospasm, acquired tricuspid and pulmonary stenosis, sudden drops in blood pressure, edema, ascites.

259.3 Ectopic hormone secretion, not elsewhere classified
Ectopic:
    antidiuretic hormone secretion [ADH]
    hyperparathyroidism
    EXCLUDES   *ectopic ACTH syndrome (255.0)*
AHA: N-D, '85, 4

259.4 Dwarfism, not elsewhere classified
Dwarfism:
    NOS
    constitutional
    EXCLUDES   *dwarfism:*
          achondroplastic (756.4)
          intrauterine (759.7)
          nutritional (263.2)
          pituitary (253.3)
          renal (588.0)
          progeria (259.8)

259.8 Other specified endocrine disorders
Pineal gland dysfunction   Werner's syndrome
Progeria

259.9 Unspecified endocrine disorder
Disturbance: Infantilism NOS
    endocrine NOS
    hormone NOS

NUTRITIONAL DEFICIENCIES (260-269)

EXCLUDES   *deficiency anemias (280.0-281.9)*

260 Kwashiorkor
Nutritional edema with dyspigmentation of skin and hair
DEF: Syndrome, particularly of children; excessive carbohydrate with inadequate protein intake, inhibited growth potential, anomalies in skin and hair pigmentation, edema and liver disease.

261 Nutritional marasmus
Nutritional atrophy
Severe calorie deficiency
Severe malnutrition NOS
DEF: Protein-calorie malabsorption or malnutrition of children; characterized by tissue wasting, dehydration, and subcutaneous fat depletion; may occur with infectious disease; also called infantile atrophy.

262 Other severe, protein-calorie malnutrition
Nutritional edema without mention of dyspigmentation of skin and hair
AHA: 4Q, '92, 24; J-A, '85, 12

✓4ᵗʰ 263 Other and unspecified protein-calorie malnutrition
AHA: 4Q, '92, 24

263.0 Malnutrition of moderate degree
AHA: J-A, '85, 1
DEF: Malnutrition characterized by biochemical changes in electrolytes, lipids, blood plasma.

263.1 Malnutrition of mild degree
AHA: J-A, '85, 1

263.2 Arrested development following protein-calorie malnutrition
Nutritional dwarfism
Physical retardation due to malnutrition

263.8 Other protein-calorie malnutrition

263.9 Unspecified protein-calorie malnutrition
Dystrophy due to malnutrition
Malnutrition (calorie) NOS
    EXCLUDES   *nutritional deficiency NOS (269.9)*
AHA: ▶4Q, '03, 109;◄ N-D, '84, 19

✓4ᵗʰ 264 Vitamin A deficiency

264.0 With conjunctival xerosis
DEF: Vitamin A deficiency with conjunctival dryness.

264.1 With conjunctival xerosis and Bitot's spot
Bitot's spot in the young child
DEF: Vitamin A deficiency with conjunctival dryness, superficial spots of keratinized epithelium.

264.2 With corneal xerosis
DEF: Vitamin A deficiency with corneal dryness.

264.3 With corneal ulceration and xerosis
DEF: Vitamin A deficiency with corneal dryness, epithelial ulceration.

264.4 With keratomalacia
DEF: Vitamin A deficiency creating corneal dryness; progresses to corneal insensitivity, softness, necrosis; usually bilateral.

264.5 With night blindness
DEF: Vitamin A deficiency causing vision failure in dim light.

264.6 With xerophthalmic scars of cornea
DEF: Vitamin A deficiency with corneal scars from dryness.

264.7 Other ocular manifestations of vitamin A deficiency
Xerophthalmia due to vitamin A deficiency

264.8 Other manifestations of vitamin A deficiency
Follicular keratosis ⎤ due to vitamin A
Xeroderma   ⎦   deficiency

264.9 Unspecified vitamin A deficiency
Hypovitaminosis A NOS

✓4ᵗʰ 265 Thiamine and niacin deficiency states

265.0 Beriberi
DEF: Inadequate vitamin B_1 (thiamine) intake, affects heart and peripheral nerves; individual may become edematous and develop cardiac disease due to the excess fluid; alcoholics and people with a diet of excessive polished rice prone to the disease.

265.1 Other and unspecified manifestations of thiamine deficiency
Other vitamin B_1 deficiency states

265.2 Pellagra
Deficiency: Deficiency:
    niacin (-tryptophan)   vitamin PP
    nicotinamide   Pellagra (alcoholic)
    nicotinic acid
DEF: Niacin deficiency causing dermatitis, inflammation of mucous membranes, diarrhea, and psychic disturbances.

✓4ᵗʰ 266 Deficiency of B-complex components

266.0 Ariboflavinosis
Riboflavin [vitamin B_2] deficiency
DEF: Vitamin B_2 (riboflavin) deficiency marked by swollen lips and tongue fissures, corneal vascularization, scaling lesions, and anemia.
AHA: S-O, '86, 10

N Newborn Age: 0   **P** Pediatric Age: 0-17   **M** Maternity Age: 12-55   **A** Adult Age: 15-124   **MSP** Medicare Secondary Payer

266.1   Vitamin B₆ deficiency

Deficiency: Deficiency:

   pyridoxal   pyridoxine

   pyridoxamine   Vitamin B₆ deficiency

                    syndrome

   EXCLUDES   *vitamin B₆-responsive sideroblastic anemia (285.0)*

DEF: Vitamin B₆ deficiency causing skin, lip, and tongue disturbances, peripheral neuropathy; and convulsions in infants.

266.2   Other B-complex deficiencies

Deficiency: Deficiency:

   cyanocobalamin   vitamin B₁₂

   folic acid

   EXCLUDES   *combined system disease with anemia (281.0-281.1)*
deficiency anemias (281.0-281.9)
subacute degeneration of spinal cord with anemia (281.0-281.1)

266.9   Unspecified vitamin B deficiency

267 Ascorbic acid deficiency

Deficiency of vitamin C

Scurvy

   EXCLUDES   *scorbutic anemia (281.8)*

DEF: Vitamin C deficiency causing swollen gums, myalgia, weight loss, and weakness.

√4ᵗʰ 268 Vitamin D deficiency

   EXCLUDES   *vitamin D-resistant:*
osteomalacia (275.3)
rickets (275.3)

268.0   Rickets, active

   EXCLUDES   *celiac rickets (579.0)*
renal rickets (588.0)

DEF: Inadequate vitamin D intake, usually in pediatrics, that affects bones most involved with muscular action; may cause nodules on ends and sides of bones; delayed closure of fontanels in infants; symptoms may include muscle soreness, and profuse sweating.

268.1   Rickets, late effect

Any condition specified as due to rickets and stated to be a late effect or sequela of rickets

Use additional code to identify the nature of late effect

DEF: Distorted or demineralized bones as a result of vitamin D deficiency.

268.2   Osteomalacia, unspecified

DEF: Softening of bones due to decrease in calcium; marked by pain, tenderness, muscular weakness, anorexia, and weight loss.

268.9   Unspecified vitamin D deficiency

Avitaminosis D

√4ᵗʰ 269 Other nutritional deficiencies

269.0   Deficiency of vitamin K

   EXCLUDES   *deficiency of coagulation factor due to vitamin K deficiency (286.7)*
vitamin K deficiency of newborn (776.0)

269.1   Deficiency of other vitamins

Deficiency: Deficiency:

   vitamin E   vitamin P

269.2   Unspecified vitamin deficiency

Multiple vitamin deficiency NOS

269.3   Mineral deficiency, not elsewhere classified

Deficiency: Deficiency:

   calcium, dietary   iodine

   EXCLUDES   *deficiency:*
calcium NOS (275.4)
potassium (276.8)
sodium (276.1)

269.8   Other nutritional deficiency

   EXCLUDES   *adult failure to thrive (783.7)*
failure to thrive in childhood (783.41)
feeding problems (783.3)
newborn (779.3)

269.9   Unspecified nutritional deficiency

OTHER METABOLIC AND IMMUNITY DISORDERS (270-279)

Use additional code to identify any associated mental retardation

√4ᵗʰ 270 Disorders of amino-acid transport and metabolism

   EXCLUDES   *abnormal findings without manifest disease (790.0-796.9)*
disorders of purine and pyrimidine metabolism (277.1-277.2)
gout (274.0-274.9)

270.0   Disturbances of amino-acid transport

Cystinosis

Cystinuria

Fanconi (-de Toni) (-Debré) syndrome

Glycinuria (renal)

Hartnup disease

270.1   Phenylketonuria [PKU]

Hyperphenylalaninemia

DEF: Inherited metabolic condition causing excess phenylpyruvic and other acids in urine; results in mental retardation, neurological manifestations, including spasticity and tremors, light pigmentation, eczema, and mousy odor.

270.2   Other disturbances of aromatic amino-acid metabolism

Albinism

Alkaptonuria

Alkaptonuric ochronosis

Disturbances of metabolism of tyrosine and tryptophan

Homogentisic acid defects

Hydroxykynureninuria

Hypertyrosinemia

Indicanuria

Kynureninase defects

Oasthouse urine disease

Ochronosis

Tyrosinosis

Tyrosinuria

Waardenburg syndrome

   EXCLUDES   *vitamin B₆-deficiency syndrome (266.1)*

AHA: 3Q, '99, 20

270.3   Disturbances of branched-chain amino-acid metabolism

Disturbances of metabolism of leucine, isoleucine, and valine

Hypervalinemia

Intermittent branched-chain ketonuria

Leucine-induced hypoglycemia

Leucinosis

Maple syrup urine disease

AHA: 3Q, '00, 8

270.4   Disturbances of sulphur-bearing amino-acid metabolism

Cystathioninemia

Cystathioninuria

Disturbances of metabolism of methionine, homocystine, and cystathionine

Homocystinuria

Hypermethioninemia

Methioninemia

AHA: ▶1Q, '04, 6◀

270.5   Disturbances of histidine metabolism

Carnosinemia   Hyperhistidinemia

Histidinemia   Imidazole aminoaciduria

√4ᵗʰ √5ᵗʰ Additional Digit Required   Unspecified Code   Other Specified Code   Manifestation Code   ▶◀ Revised Text   ● New Code   ▲ Revised Code Title

Endocrine, Nutritional, Metabolic, Immunity

270.6–272.4

Lipid Metabolism

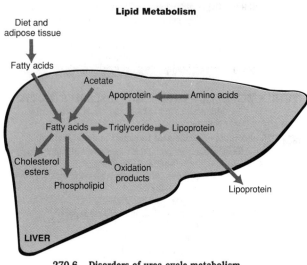

270.6   Disorders of urea cycle metabolism
Argininosuccinic aciduria
Citrullinemia
Disorders of metabolism of ornithine, citrulline,
     argininosuccinic acid, arginine, and ammonia
Hyperammonemia
Hyperornithinemia

270.7   Other disturbances of straight-chain amino-acid metabolism
Glucoglycinuria
Glycinemia (with methyl-malonic acidemia)
Hyperglycinemia
Hyperlysinemia
Other disturbances of metabolism of glycine,
     threonine, serine, glutamine, and lysine
Pipecolic acidemia
Saccharopinuria

AHA: 3Q, '00, 8

270.8   Other specified disorders of amino-acid metabolism
Alaninemia   Iminoacidopathy
Ethanolaminuria   Prolinemia
Glycoprolinuria   Prolinuria
Hydroxyprolinemia   Sarcosinemia
Hyperprolinemia

270.9   Unspecified disorder of amino-acid metabolism

✓4ᵗʰ 271   Disorders of carbohydrate transport and metabolism
     EXCLUDES   abnormality of secretion of glucagon (251.4)
                 diabetes mellitus (250.0-250.9)
                  hypoglycemia NOS (251.2)
                  mucopolysaccharidosis (277.5)

271.0   Glycogenosis
Amylopectinosis
Glucose-6-phosphatase deficiency
Glycogen storage disease
McArdle's disease
Pompe's disease
von Gierke's disease

AHA: 1Q, '98, 5

DEF: Excess glycogen storage; rare inherited trait affects liver, kidneys; causes various symptoms depending on type, though often weakness, and muscle cramps.

271.1   Galactosemia
Galactose-1-phosphate uridyl transferase deficiency
Galactosuria

DEF: Any of three genetic disorders due to defective galactose metabolism; symptoms include failure to thrive in infancy, jaundice, liver and spleen damage, cataracts, and mental retardation.

271.2   Hereditary fructose intolerance
Essential benign fructosuria   Fructosemia

DEF: Chromosome recessive disorder of carbohydrate metabolism; in infants, occurs after dietary sugar introduced; characterized by enlarged spleen, yellowish cast to skin, and progressive inability to thrive.

271.3   Intestinal disaccharidase deficiencies and disaccharide malabsorption
Intolerance or malabsorption (congenital) (of):
     glucose-galactose
     lactose
     sucrose-isomaltose

271.4   Renal glycosuria
Renal diabetes

DEF: Persistent abnormal levels of glucose in urine, with normal blood glucose levels; caused by failure of the renal tubules to reabsorb glucose.

271.8   Other specified disorders of carbohydrate transport and metabolism
Essential benign pentosuria   Mannosidosis
Fucosidosis   Oxalosis
Glycolic aciduria   Xylosuria
Hyperoxaluria (primary)   Xylulosuria

271.9   Unspecified disorder of carbohydrate transport and metabolism

✓4ᵗʰ 272   Disorders of lipoid metabolism
     EXCLUDES   localized cerebral lipidoses (330.1)

272.0   Pure hypercholesterolemia
Familial hypercholesterolemia
Fredrickson Type IIa hyperlipoproteinemia
Hyperbetalipoproteinemia
Hyperlipidemia, Group A
Low-density-lipoid-type [LDL] hyperlipoproteinemia

272.1   Pure hyperglyceridemia
Endogenous hyperglyceridemia
Fredrickson Type IV hyperlipoproteinemia
Hyperlipidemia, Group B
Hyperprebetalipoproteinemia
Hypertriglyceridemia, essential
Very-low-density-lipoid-type [VLDL]
     hyperlipoproteinemia

272.2   Mixed hyperlipidemia
Broad- or floating-betalipoproteinemia
Fredrickson Type IIb or III hyperlipoproteinemia
Hypercholesterolemia with endogenous
     hyperglyceridemia
Hyperbetalipoproteinemia with
     prebetalipoproteinemia
Tubo-eruptive xanthoma
Xanthoma tuberosum

DEF: Elevated levels of lipoprotein, a complex of fats and proteins, in blood due to inherited metabolic disorder.

272.3   Hyperchylomicronemia
Bürger-Grütz syndrome
Fredrickson type I or V hyperlipoproteinemia
Hyperlipidemia, Group D
Mixed hyperglyceridemia

272.4   Other and unspecified hyperlipidemia
Alpha-lipoproteinemia
Combined hyperlipidemia
Hyperlipidemia NOS
Hyperlipoproteinemia NOS

DEF: Hyperlipoproteinemia: elevated levels of transient chylomicrons in the blood which are a form of lipoproteins which transport dietary cholesterol and triglycerides from the small intestine to the blood.

272.5   **Lipoprotein deficiencies**
Abetalipoproteinemia
Bassen-Kornzweig syndrome
High-density lipoid deficiency (familial)
Hypoalphalipoproteinemia
Hypobetalipoproteinemia
DEF: Abnormally low levels of lipoprotein, a complex of fats and protein, in the blood.

272.6   **Lipodystrophy**
Barraquer-Simons disease
Progressive lipodystrophy
Use additional E code to identify cause, if iatrogenic
EXCLUDES   *intestinal lipodystrophy (040.2)*
DEF: Disturbance of fat metabolism resulting in loss of fatty tissue in some areas of the body.

272.7   **Lipidoses**
Chemically-induced lipidosis
Disease:
    Anderson's
    Fabry's
    Gaucher's
    I cell [mucolipidosis I]
    lipoid storage NOS
    Niemann-Pick
    pseudo-Hurler's or mucolipidosis III
    triglyceride storage, Type I or II
    Wolman's or triglyceride storage, Type III
Mucolipidosis II
Primary familial xanthomatosis
EXCLUDES   *cerebral lipidoses (330.1)*
               Tay-Sachs disease (330.1)
DEF: Lysosomal storage diseases marked by an abnormal amount of lipids in reticuloendothelial cells.

272.8   **Other disorders of lipoid metabolism**
Hoffa's disease or liposynovitis prepatellaris
Launois-Bensaude's lipomatosis
Lipoid dermatoarthritis

272.9   **Unspecified disorder of lipoid metabolism**

√4ᵗʰ **273 Disorders of plasma protein metabolism**
EXCLUDES   *agammaglobulinemia and*
             hypogammaglobulinemia (279.0-279.2)
             coagulation defects (286.0-286.9)
             hereditary hemolytic anemias (282.0-282.9)

273.0   **Polyclonal hypergammaglobulinemia**
Hypergammaglobulinemic purpura:
    benign primary
    Waldenström's
DEF: Elevated blood levels of gamma globulins, frequently found in patients with chronic infectious diseases.

273.1   **Monoclonal paraproteinemia**
Benign monoclonal hypergammaglobulinemia [BMH]
Monoclonal gammopathy:
    NOS
    associated with lymphoplasmacytic dyscrasias
    benign
Paraproteinemia:
    benign (familial)
    secondary to malignant or inflammatory disease
DEF: Elevated blood levels of macroglobulins (plasma globulins of high weight); characterized by malignant neoplasms of bone marrow, spleen, liver, or lymph nodes; symptoms include weakness, fatigue, bleeding disorders, and vision problems.

273.2   **Other paraproteinemias**
Cryoglobulinemic: Mixed cryoglobulinemia
    purpura
    vasculitis

273.3   **Macroglobulinemia**
Macroglobulinemia (idiopathic) (primary)
Waldenström's macroglobulinemia

● **273.4**   **Alpha-1-antitrypsin deficiency**
AAT deficiency

273.8   **Other disorders of plasma protein metabolism**
Abnormality of transport protein
Bisalbuminemia
AHA: 2Q, '98, 11

273.9   **Unspecified disorder of plasma protein metabolism**

√4ᵗʰ **274 Gout**
EXCLUDES   *lead gout (984.0-984.9)*
AHA: 2Q, '95, 4
DEF: Purine and pyrimidine metabolic disorders; manifested by hyperuricemia and recurrent acute inflammatory arthritis; monosodium urate or monohydrate crystals may be deposited in and around the joints, leading to joint destruction, and severe crippling.

274.0   **Gouty arthropathy**

√5ᵗʰ **274.1**   **Gouty nephropathy**
274.10 Gouty nephropathy, unspecified
AHA: N-D, '85, 15

274.11 Uric acid nephrolithiasis
DEF: Sodium urate stones in the kidney.

274.19 Other

√5ᵗʰ **274.8**   **Gout with other specified manifestations**
274.81 Gouty tophi of ear
DEF: Chalky sodium urate deposit in the ear due to gout; produces chronic inflammation of external ear.

274.82 Gouty tophi of other sites
Gouty tophi of heart
274.89 Other
Use additional code to identify manifestations, as:
    gouty:
       iritis (364.11)
       neuritis (357.4)

274.9   **Gout, unspecified**

√4ᵗʰ **275 Disorders of mineral metabolism**
EXCLUDES   *abnormal findings without manifest disease (790.0-796.9)*

275.0   **Disorders of iron metabolism**
Bronzed diabetes
Hemochromatosis
Pigmentary cirrhosis (of liver)
EXCLUDES   *anemia:*
          iron deficiency (280.0-280.9)
          sideroblastic (285.0)
AHA: 2Q, '97, 11

275.1   **Disorders of copper metabolism**
Hepatolenticular degeneration
Wilson's disease

275.2   **Disorders of magnesium metabolism**
Hypermagnesemia
Hypomagnesemia

275.3   **Disorders of phosphorus metabolism**
Familial hypophosphatemia
Hypophosphatasia
Vitamin D-resistant:
    osteomalacia
    rickets

√5ᵗʰ **275.4**   **Disorders of calcium metabolism**
EXCLUDES   *parathyroid disorders* ▶*(252.00-252.9)*◀
          vitamin D deficiency (268.0-268.9)
AHA: 4Q, '97, 33

275.40 Unspecified disorder of calcium metabolism

275.41 Hypocalcemia
DEF: Abnormally decreased blood calcium level; symptoms include hyperactive deep tendon reflexes, muscle, abdominal cramps, and carpopedal spasm.

√4ᵗʰ √5ᵗʰ Additional Digit Required   Unspecified Code   Other Specified Code   Manifestation Code   ▶◀ Revised Text   ● New Code   ▲ Revised Code Title

Endocrine, Nutritional, Metabolic, Immunity

275.42–277.2

275.42 Hypercalcemia

AHA: ▶4Q, '03, 110◀

DEF: Abnormally increased blood calcium level; symptoms include muscle weakness, fatigue, nausea, depression, and constipation.

275.49 Other disorders of calcium metabolism

Nephrocalcinosis
Pseudohypoparathyroidism
Pseudopseudohypoparathryoidism

DEF: Nephrocalcinosis: calcium phosphate deposits in the tubules of the kidney with resultant renal insufficiency.

DEF: Pseudohypoparathyroidism: inherited disorder with signs and symptoms of hypoparathyroidism; caused by inadequate response to parathyroid hormone, not hormonal deficiency. Symptoms include muscle cramps, tetany, urinary frequency, blurred vision due to cataracts, and dry scaly skin.

DEF: Pseudopseudohypoparathyroidism: clinical manifestations of hypoparathyroidism without affecting blood calcium levels.

275.8 Other specified disorders of mineral metabolism

275.9 Unspecified disorder of mineral metabolism

√4ᵗʰ **276 Disorders of fluid, electrolyte, and acid-base balance**

EXCLUDES   *diabetes insipidus (253.5)*
familial periodic paralysis (359.3)

276.0 Hyperosmolality and/or hypernatremia

Sodium [Na] excess   Sodium [Na] overload

276.1 Hyposmolality and/or hyponatremia

Sodium [Na] deficiency

276.2 Acidosis

Acidosis: Acidosis:
   NOS   metabolic
   lactic   respiratory

EXCLUDES   *diabetic acidosis (250.1)*

AHA: J-F, '87, 15

DEF: Disorder involves decrease of pH (hydrogen ion) concentration in blood and cellular tissues; caused by increase in acid and decrease in bicarbonate.

276.3 Alkalosis

Alkalosis: Alkalosis:
   NOS   respiratory
   metabolic

DEF: Accumulation of base (non-acid part of salt), or loss of acid without relative loss of base in body fluids; caused by increased arterial plasma bicarbonate concentration or loss of carbon dioxide due to hyperventilation.

276.4 Mixed acid-base balance disorder

Hypercapnia with mixed acid-base disorder

276.5 Volume depletion

Dehydration
Depletion of volume of plasma or extracellular fluid
Hypovolemia

EXCLUDES   *hypovolemic shock:*
postoperative (998.0)
traumatic (958.4)

AHA: 3Q, '02, 21; 4Q, '97, 30; 2Q, '88, 9

276.6 Fluid overload

Fluid retention

EXCLUDES   *ascites (789.5)*
localized edema (782.3)

276.7 Hyperpotassemia

Hyperkalemia   Potassium [K]:
Potassium [K]:   intoxication
   excess   overload

AHA: 2Q, '01, 12

DEF: Elevated blood levels of potassium; symptoms include abnormal EKG readings, weakness; related to defective renal excretion.

276.8 Hypopotassemia

Hypokalemia   Potassium [K] deficiency

DEF: Decreased blood levels of potassium; symptoms include neuromuscular disorders.

276.9 Electrolyte and fluid disorders not elsewhere classified

Electrolyte imbalance   Hypochloremia
Hyperchloremia

EXCLUDES   *electrolyte imbalance:*
associated with hyperemesis gravidarum (643.1)
complicating labor and delivery (669.0)
following abortion and ectopic or molar pregnancy (634-638 with .4, 639.4)

AHA: J-F, '87, 15

√4ᵗʰ **277 Other and unspecified disorders of metabolism**

√5ᵗʰ **277.0 Cystic fibrosis**

Fibrocystic disease of the pancreas
Mucoviscidosis

DEF: Generalized, genetic disorder of infants, children, and young adults marked by exocrine gland dysfunction; characterized by chronic pulmonary disease with excess mucus production, pancreatic deficiency, high levels of electrolytes in the sweat.

AHA: 4Q, '90, 16; 3Q, '90, 18

277.00 Without mention of meconium ileus

Cystic fibrosis NOS

AHA: ▶2Q, '03, 12◀

277.01 With meconium ileus   N

Meconium:
   ileus (of newborn)
   obstruction of intestine in mucoviscidosis

277.02 With pulmonary manifestations

Cystic fibrosis with pulmonary exacerbation
Use additional code to identify any infectious organism present, such as: pseudomonas (041.7)

AHA: 4Q, '02, 45, 46

277.03 With gastrointestinal manifestations

EXCLUDES   *with meconium ileus (277.01)*

AHA: 4Q, '02, 45

277.09 With other manifestations

277.1 Disorders of porphyrin metabolism

Hematoporphyria
Hematoporphyrinuria
Hereditary coproporphyria
Porphyria
Porphyrinuria
Protocoproporphyria
Protoporphyria
Pyrroloporphyria

277.2 Other disorders of purine and pyrimidine metabolism

Hypoxanthine-guanine-phosphoribosyltransferase deficiency [HG-PRT deficiency]
Lesch-Nyhan syndrome
Xanthinuria

EXCLUDES   *gout (274.0-274.9)*
orotic aciduric anemia (281.4)

N   Newborn Age: 0   P   Pediatric Age: 0-17   M   Maternity Age: 12-55   A   Adult Age: 15-124   MSP   Medicare Secondary Payer

277.3 Amyloidosis
Amyloidosis:
NOS
inherited systemic
nephropathic
neuropathic (Portuguese) (Swiss)
secondary
Benign paroxysmal peritonitis
Familial Mediterranean fever
Hereditary cardiac amyloidosis
AHA: 1Q, '96, 16

DEF: Conditions of diverse etiologies characterized by the accumulation of insoluble fibrillar proteins (amyloid) in various organs and tissues of the body, compromising vital functions.

277.4 Disorders of bilirubin excretion
Hyperbilirubinemia: Syndrome:
  congenital   Dubin-Johnson
  constitutional   Gilbert's
Syndrome: Rotor's
  Crigler-Najjar
     EXCLUDES   *hyperbilirubinemias specific to the perinatal period (774.0-774.7)*

277.5 Mucopolysaccharidosis
Gargoylism   Morquio-Brailsford disease
Hunter's syndrome   Osteochondrodystrophy
Hurler's syndrome   Sanfilippo's syndrome
Lipochondrodystrophy   Scheie's syndrome
Maroteaux-Lamy
  syndrome

DEF: Metabolism disorders evidenced by excretion of various mucopolysaccharides in urine and infiltration of these substances into connective tissue, with resulting various defects of bone, cartilage and connective tissue.

277.6 Other deficiencies of circulating enzymes
Hereditary angioedema

277.7 Dysmetabolic syndrome X   [A]
Use additional code for associated manifestation,
  such as:
  cardiovascular disease (414.00-414.07)
  obesity (278.00-278.01)
AHA: 4Q, '01, 42

DEF: A specific group of metabolic disorders that are related to the state of insulin resistance (decreased cellular response to insulin) without elevated blood sugars; often related to elevated cholesterol and triglycerides, obesity, cardiovascular disease, and high blood pressure.

√5ᵗʰ 277.8 Other specified disorders of metabolism
AHA: 4Q, '03, 50; 2Q, '01, 18; S-O, '87, 9

277.81 Primary carnitine deficiency

277.82 Carnitine deficiency due to inborn errors of metabolism

277.83 Iatrogenic carnitine deficiency
Carnitine deficiency due to:
  hemodialysis
  valproic acid therapy

277.84 Other secondary carnitine deficiency

277.85 Disorders of fatty acid oxidation
Carnitine palmitoyltransferase deficiencies
  (CPT1, CPT2)
Glutaric aciduria type II (type IIA, IIB, IIC)
Long chain 3-hydroxyacyl CoA
  dehydrogenase deficiency (LCHAD)
Long chain/very long chain acyl CoA dehy-
  drogenase deficiency (LCAD, VLCAD)
Medium chain acyl CoA dehydrogenase
  deficiency (MCAD)
Short chain acyl CoA dehydrogenase
  deficiency (SCAD)
     EXCLUDES   *primary carnitine deficiency (277.81)*

277.86 Peroxisomal disorders
Adrenomyeloneuropathy
Neonatal adrenoleukodystrophy
Rhizomelic chrondrodysplasia punctata
X-linked adrenoleukodystrophy
Zellweger syndrome
     EXCLUDES   *infantile Refsum disease (356.3)*

277.87 Disorders of mitochondrial metabolism
Kearns-Sayre syndrome
Mitochondrial Encephalopathy, Lactic
  Acidosis and Stroke-like episodes
  (MELAS syndrome)
Mitochondrial Neurogastrointestinal
  Encephalopathy syndrome (MNGIE)
Myoclonus with Epilepsy and with Ragged
  Red Fibers (MERRF syndrome)
Neuropathy, Ataxia and Retinitis
  Pigmentosa (NARP syndrome)
Use additional code for associated
  conditions
     EXCLUDES   *disorders of pyruvate metabolism (271.8)*
                   Leber's optic atrophy (377.16)
                   Leigh's subacute necrotizing encephalopathy (330.8)
                   Reye's syndrome (331.81)

277.89 Other specified disorders of metabolism
Hand-Schüller-Christian disease
Histiocytosis (acute) (chronic)
Histiocytosis X (chronic)
     EXCLUDES   *histiocytosis:*
                   acute differentiated progressive (202.5)
                   X, acute (progressive) (202.5)

277.9 Unspecified disorder of metabolism
Enzymopathy NOS

√4ᵗʰ 278 Obesity and other hyperalimentation
     EXCLUDES   *hyperalimentation NOS (783.6)*
                   poisoning by vitamins NOS (963.5)
                   polyphagia (783.6)

√5ᵗʰ 278.0 Obesity
     EXCLUDES   *adiposogenital dystrophy (253.8)*
                   obesity of endocrine origin NOS (259.9)

278.00 Obesity, unspecified
Obesity NOS
AHA: 4Q, '01, 42;1Q, '99, 5, 6

278.01 Morbid obesity
Severe obesity
AHA: 3Q, '03, 6-8

DEF: Increased weight beyond limits of skeletal and physical requirements (125 percent or more over ideal body weight), as a result of excess fat in subcutaneous connective tissues.

278.1 Localized adiposity
Fat pad

278.2 Hypervitaminosis A

278.3 Hypercarotinemia
DEF: Elevated blood carotene level due to ingesting excess carotenoids or the inability to convert carotenoids to vitamin A.

278.4 Hypervitaminosis D
DEF: Weakness, fatigue, loss of weight, and other symptoms resulting from ingesting excessive amounts of vitamin D.

278.8 Other hyperalimentation

√4ᵗʰ 279 Disorders involving the immune mechanism

√5ᵗʰ 279.0 Deficiency of humoral immunity
DEF: Inadequate immune response to bacterial infections with potential reinfection by viruses due to lack of circulating immunoglobulins (acquired antibodies).

√4ᵗʰ / √5ᵗʰ Additional Digit Required   Unspecified Code   Other Specified Code   Manifestation Code   ►◄ Revised Text   ● New Code   ▲ Revised Code Title

Endocrine, Nutritional, Metabolic, Immunity

277.3–279.0

Endocrine, Nutritional, Metabolic, Immunity

279.00–279.9

279.00 Hypogammaglobulinemia, unspecified
Agammaglobulinemia NOS

279.01 Selective IgA immunodeficiency

279.02 Selective IgM immunodeficiency

279.03 Other selective immunoglobulin deficiencies
Selective deficiency of IgG

279.04 Congenital hypogammaglobulinemia
Agammaglobulinemia:
    Bruton's type
    X-linked

279.05 Immunodeficiency with increased IgM
Immunodeficiency with hyper-IgM:
    autosomal recessive
    X-linked

279.06 Common variable immunodeficiency
Dysgammaglobulinemia (acquired)
    (congenital) (primary)
Hypogammaglobulinemia:
    acquired primary
    congenital non-sex-linked
    sporadic

279.09 Other
Transient hypogammaglobulinemia of infancy

√5ᵗʰ   **279.1 Deficiency of cell-mediated immunity**

279.10 Immunodeficiency with predominant T-cell defect, unspecified
AHA: S-O, '87, 10

279.11 DiGeorge's syndrome
Pharyngeal pouch syndrome
Thymic hypoplasia
DEF: Congenital disorder due to defective development of the third and fourth pharyngeal pouches; results in hypoplasia or aplasia of the thymus, parathyroid glands; related to congenital heart defects, anomalies of the great vessels, esophageal atresia, and abnormalities of facial structures.

279.12 Wiskott-Aldrich syndrome
DEF: A disease characterized by chronic conditions, such as eczema, suppurative otitis media and anemia; it results from an X-linked recessive gene and is classified as an immune deficiency syndrome.

279.13 Nezelof's syndrome
Cellular immunodeficiency with abnormal immunoglobulin deficiency
DEF: Immune system disorder characterized by a pathological deficiency in cellular immunity and humoral antibodies resulting in inability to fight infectious diseases.

279.19 Other
EXCLUDES   *ataxia-telangiectasia (334.8)*

279.2 Combined immunity deficiency
Agammaglobulinemia:
    autosomal recessive
    Swiss-type
    x-linked recessive
Severe combined immunodeficiency [SCID]
Thymic:
    alymophoplasia
    aplasia or dysplasia with immunodeficiency
EXCLUDES   *thymic hypoplasia (279.11)*
DEF: Agammaglobulinemia: no immunoglobulins in the blood.

DEF: Thymic alymphoplasia: severe combined immunodeficiency; result of failed lymphoid tissue development.

279.3 Unspecified immunity deficiency

279.4 Autoimmune disease, not elsewhere classified
Autoimmune disease NOS
EXCLUDES   *transplant failure or rejection (996.80-996.89)*

279.8 Other specified disorders involving the immune mechanism
Single complement [C1-C9] deficiency or dysfunction

279.9 Unspecified disorder of immune mechanism
AHA: 3Q, '92, 13

---

4. DISEASES OF THE BLOOD AND BLOOD-FORMING ORGANS (280-289)

EXCLUDES *anemia complicating pregnancy or the puerperium (648.2)*

✓4ᵗʰ 280 Iron deficiency anemias

INCLUDES anemia:
asiderotic
hypochromic-microcytic
sideropenic

EXCLUDES *familial microcytic anemia (282.49)*

280.0 Secondary to blood loss (chronic)
Normocytic anemia due to blood loss
EXCLUDES *acute posthemorrhagic anemia (285.1)*

AHA: 4Q, '93, 34

280.1 Secondary to inadequate dietary iron intake

280.8 Other specified iron deficiency anemias
Paterson-Kelly syndrome
Plummer-Vinson syndrome
Sideropenic dysphagia

280.9 Iron deficiency anemia, unspecified
Anemia:
achlorhydric
chlorotic
idiopathic hypochromic
iron [Fe] deficiency NOS

✓4ᵗʰ 281 Other deficiency anemias

281.0 Pernicious anemia
Anemia:
Addison's
Biermer's
congenital pernicious
Congenital intrinsic factor [Castle's] deficiency
EXCLUDES *combined system disease without mention of anemia (266.2)*
subacute degeneration of spinal cord without mention of anemia (266.2)

AHA: N-D, '84, 1; S-O, '84, 16

DEF: Chronic progressive anemia due to Vitamin B_{12} malabsorption; caused by lack of a secretion known as intrinsic factor, which is produced by the gastric mucosa of the stomach.

281.1 Other vitamin B_{12} deficiency anemia
Anemia:
vegan's
vitamin B_{12} deficiency (dietary)
due to selective vitamin B_{12} malabsorption with proteinuria
Syndrome:
Imerslund's
Imerslund-Gräsbeck
EXCLUDES *combined system disease without mention of anemia (266.2)*
subacute degeneration of spinal cord without mention of anemia (266.2)

281.2 Folate-deficiency anemia
Congenital folate malabsorption
Folate or folic acid deficiency anemia:
NOS
dietary
drug-induced
Goat's milk anemia
Nutritional megaloblastic anemia (of infancy)
Use additional E code to identify drug
DEF: Macrocytic anemia resembles pernicious anemia but without absence of hydrochloric acid secretions; responsive to folic acid therapy.

281.3 Other specified megaloblastic anemias not elsewhere classified
Combined B_{12} and folate-deficiency anemia
Refractory megaloblastic anemia
DEF: Megaloblasts predominant in bone marrow with few normoblasts; rare familial type associated with proteinuria and genitourinary tract anomalies.

281.4 Protein-deficiency anemia
Amino-acid-deficiency anemia

281.8 Anemia associated with other specified nutritional deficiency
Scorbutic anemia

281.9 Unspecified deficiency anemia
Anemia:
dimorphic
macrocytic
megaloblastic NOS
nutritional NOS
simple chronic

✓4ᵗʰ 282 Hereditary hemolytic anemias

DEF: Escalated rate of erythrocyte destruction; similar to all anemias, occurs when imbalance exists between blood loss and blood production.

282.0 Hereditary spherocytosis
Acholuric (familial) jaundice
Congenital hemolytic anemia (spherocytic)
Congenital spherocytosis
Minkowski-Chauffard syndrome
Spherocytosis (familial)
EXCLUDES *hemolytic anemia of newborn (773.0-773.5)*
DEF: Hereditary, chronic illness marked by abnormal red blood cell membrane; symptoms include enlarged spleen, jaundice; and anemia in severe cases.

282.1 Hereditary elliptocytosis
Elliptocytosis (congenital)
Ovalocytosis (congenital) (hereditary)
DEF: Genetic hemolytic anemia characterized by malformed, elliptical erythrocytes; there is increased destruction of red cells with resulting anemia.

282.2 Anemias due to disorders of glutathione metabolism
Anemia:
6-phosphogluconic dehydrogenase deficiency
enzyme deficiency, drug-induced
erythrocytic glutathione deficiency
glucose-6-phosphate dehydrogenase [G-6-PD] deficiency
glutathione-reductase deficiency
hemolytic nonspherocytic (hereditary), type I
Disorder of pentose phosphate pathway
Favism

282.3 Other hemolytic anemias due to enzyme deficiency
Anemia:
hemolytic nonspherocytic (hereditary), type II
hexokinase deficiency
pyruvate kinase [PK] deficiency
triosephosphate isomerase deficiency

✓5ᵗʰ 282.4 Thalassemias
EXCLUDES *sickle-cell:*
disease (282.60-282.69)
trait (282.5)

AHA: ▶4Q, '03, 51◀

DEF: ▶A group of inherited hemolytic disorders characterized by decreased production of at least one of the four polypeptide globin chains which results in defective hemoglobin synthesis; symptoms include severe anemia, expanded marrow spaces, transfusional and absorptive iron overload, impaired growth rate, thickened cranial bones, and pathologic fractures.◀

✓4ᵗʰ / ✓5ᵗʰ Additional Digit Required   Unspecified Code   Other Specified Code   Manifestation Code   ▶◀ Revised Text   ● New Code   ▲ Revised Code Title

Blood and Blood-Forming Organs

282.41–283.19

282.41 Sickle-cell thalassemia without crisis
Sickle-cell thalassemia NOS
Thalassemia Hb-S disease without crisis

282.42 Sickle-cell thalassemia with crisis
Sickle-cell thalassemia with vaso-occlusive
pain
Thalassemia Hb-S disease with crisis
Use additional code for type of crisis, such as:
acute chest syndrome (517.3)
splenic sequestration (289.52)

282.49 Other thalassemia
Cooley's anemia
Hereditary leptocytosis
Mediterranean anemia (with other
hemoglobinopathy)
Microdrepanocytosis
Thalassemia (alpha) (beta) (intermedia)
(major) (minima) (minor) (mixed) (trait)
(with other hemoglobinopathy)
Thalassemia NOS

282.5 Sickle-cell trait
Hb-AS genotype
Hemoglobin S [Hb-S] trait
Heterozygous:
hemoglobin S
Hb-S

> **EXCLUDES**   *that with other hemoglobinopathy*
> *(282.60-282.69)*
> *that with thalassemia (282.49)*

DEF: Heterozygous genetic makeup characterized by one gene for
normal hemoglobin and one for sickle-cell hemoglobin; clinical
disease rarely present.

√5ᵗʰ 282.6 Sickle-cell disease
Sickle-cell anemia

> **EXCLUDES**   *sickle-cell thalassemia (282.41-282.42)*
> *sickle-cell trait (282.5)*

DEF: Inherited blood disorder; sickle-shaped red blood cells are
hard and pointed, clogging blood flow; anemia characterized by,
periodic episodes of pain, acute abdominal discomfort, skin
ulcerations of the legs, increased infections; occurs primarily in
persons of African descent.

282.60 Sickle-cell disease, unspecified
Sickle-cell anemia NOS
AHA: 2Q, '97, 11

282.61 Hb-SS disease without crisis

282.62 Hb-SS disease with crisis
Hb-SS disease with vaso-occlusive pain
Sickle-cell crisis NOS
Use additional code for type of crisis, such as:
acute chest syndrome (517.3)
splenic sequestration (289.52)
AHA: ▶4Q, '03, 56;◀ 2Q, '98, 8; 2Q, '91, 15

282.63 Sickle-cell/Hb-C disease without crisis
Hb-S/Hb-C disease without crisis

282.64 Sickle-cell/Hb-C disease with crisis
Hb-S/Hb-C disease with crisis
Sickle-cell/Hb-C disease with vaso-occlusive
pain
Use additional code for type of crisis, such as:
acute chest syndrome (517.3)
splenic sequestration (289.52)
AHA: ▶4Q, '03, 51◀

282.68 Other sickle-cell disease without crisis
Hb-S/Hb-D ⎫
Hb-S/Hb-E ⎬ disease without
Sickle-cell/Hb-D ⎮ crisis
Sickle-cell/Hb-E ⎭
AHA: ▶4Q, '03, 51◀

282.69 Other sickle-cell disease with crisis
Hb-S/Hb-D ⎫
Hb-S/Hb-E ⎬ disease with crisis
Sickle-cell/Hb-D ⎮
Sickle-cell/Hb-E ⎭
Other sickle-cell disease with vaso-occlusive
pain
Use additional code for type of crisis, such as:
acute chest syndrome (517.3)
splenic sequestration (289.52)

282.7 Other hemoglobinopathies
Abnormal hemoglobin NOS
Congenital Heinz-body anemia
Disease:
Hb-Bart's
hemoglobin C [Hb-C]
hemoglobin D [Hb-D]
hemoglobin E [Hb-E]
hemoglobin Zurich [Hb-Zurich]
Hemoglobinopathy NOS
Hereditary persistence of fetal hemoglobin [HPFH]
Unstable hemoglobin hemolytic disease

> **EXCLUDES**   *familial polycythemia (289.6)*
> *hemoglobin M [Hb-M] disease (289.7)*
> *high-oxygen-affinity hemoglobin (289.0)*

DEF: Any disorder of hemoglobin due to alteration of molecular
structure; may include overt anemia.

282.8 Other specified hereditary hemolytic anemias
Stomatocytosis

282.9 Hereditary hemolytic anemia, unspecified
Hereditary hemolytic anemia NOS

√4ᵗʰ 283 Acquired hemolytic anemias
AHA: N-D, '84, 1

DEF: Non-heriditary anemia characterized by premature destruction of red
blood cells; caused by infectious organisms, poisons, and physical agents.

283.0 Autoimmune hemolytic anemias
Autoimmune hemolytic disease (cold type) (warm
type)
Chronic cold hemagglutinin disease
Cold agglutinin disease or hemoglobinuria
Hemolytic anemia:
cold type (secondary) (symptomatic)
drug-induced
warm type (secondary) (symptomatic)
Use additional E code to identify cause, if drug-
induced

> **EXCLUDES**   *Evans' syndrome (287.3)*
> *hemolytic disease of newborn (773.0-*
> *773.5)*

√5ᵗʰ 283.1 Non-autoimmune hemolytic anemias
Use additional E code to identify cause
AHA: 4Q, '93, 25

DEF: Hemolytic anemia and thrombocytopenia with acute renal
failure; relatively rare condition; 50 percent of patients require
renal dialysis.

**283.10 Non-autoimmune hemolytic anemia,
unspecified**

283.11 Hemolytic-uremic syndrome

**283.19 Other non-autoimmune hemolytic
anemias**
Hemolytic anemia:
mechanical
microangiopathic
toxic

Ⓝ Newborn Age: 0   Ⓟ Pediatric Age: 0-17   Ⓜ Maternity Age: 12-55   Ⓐ Adult Age: 15-124   **MSP** Medicare Secondary Payer

283.2 Hemoglobinuria due to hemolysis from external causes
Acute intravascular hemolysis
Hemoglobinuria:
  from exertion
  march
  paroxysmal (cold) (nocturnal)
  due to other hemolysis
Marchiafava-Micheli syndrome
Use additional E code to identify cause

283.9 Acquired hemolytic anemia, unspecified
Acquired hemolytic anemia NOS
Chronic idiopathic hemolytic anemia

✓4ᵗʰ 284 Aplastic anemia
AHA: 1Q, '91, 14; N-D, '84, 1; S-O, '84, 16

DEF: Bone marrow failure to produce the normal amount of blood components; generally non-responsive to usual therapy.

284.0 Constitutional aplastic anemia
Aplasia, (pure) red cell:
  congenital
  of infants
  primary
Blackfan-Diamond syndrome
Familial hypoplastic anemia
Fanconi's anemia
Pancytopenia with malformations
AHA: 1Q, '91, 14

284.8 Other specified aplastic anemias
Aplastic anemia (due to):
  chronic systemic disease
  drugs
  infection
  radiation
  toxic (paralytic)
Pancytopenia (acquired)
Red cell aplasia (acquired) (adult) (pure) (with thymoma)
Use additional E code to identify cause
AHA: 1Q, '97, 5; 1Q, '92, 15; 1Q, '91, 14

284.9 Aplastic anemia, unspecified
Anemia:
  aplastic (idiopathic) NOS
  aregenerative
  hypoplastic NOS
  nonregenerative
  refractory
Medullary hypoplasia

✓4ᵗʰ 285 Other and unspecified anemias
AHA: 1Q, '91, 14; N-D, '84, 1

285.0 Sideroblastic anemia
Anemia:
  hypochromic with iron loading
  sideroachrestic
  sideroblastic
    acquired
    congenital
    hereditary
    primary
    refractory
    secondary (drug-induced) (due to disease)
    sex-linked hypochromic
    vitamin B_6-responsive
Pyridoxine-responsive (hypochromic) anemia
Use additional E code to identify cause, if drug induced

DEF: Characterized by a disruption of final heme synthesis; results in iron overload of reticuloendothelial tissues.

285.1 Acute posthemorrhagic anemia
Anemia due to acute blood loss
EXCLUDES   anemia due to chronic blood loss (280.0)
    blood loss anemia NOS (280.0)
AHA: 2Q, '92, 15

✓5ᵗʰ 285.2 Anemia in chronic illness
AHA: 4Q, '00, 39

285.21 Anemia in end-stage renal disease
Erythropoietin-resistant anemia (EPO resistant anemia)

285.22 Anemia in neoplastic disease

285.29 Anemia of other chronic illness

285.8 Other specified anemias
Anemia:
  dyserythropoietic (congenital)
  dyshematopoietic (congenital)
  leukoerythroblastic
  von Jaksch's
Infantile pseudoleukemia
AHA: 21Q, '91, 16

285.9 Anemia, unspecified
Anemia:
  NOS
  essential
  normocytic, not due to blood loss
  profound
  progressive
  secondary
Oligocythemia
EXCLUDES   anemia (due to):
    blood loss:
      acute (285.1)
      chronic or unspecified (280.0)
    iron deficiency (280.0-280.9)
AHA: 1Q, '02, 14; 2Q, '92, 16; M-A, '85, 13; ND, '84, 1

✓4ᵗʰ 286 Coagulation defects
286.0 Congenital factor VIII disorder
Antihemophilic globulin [AHG] deficiency
Factor VIII (functional) deficiency
Hemophilia:
  NOS
  A
  classical
  familial
  hereditary
Subhemophilia
EXCLUDES   factor VIII deficiency with vascular defect (286.4)

DEF: Hereditary, sex-linked, results in missing antihemophilic globulin (AHG) (factor VIII); causes abnormal coagulation characterized by increased tendency to bleeding, large bruises of skin, soft tissue; may also be bleeding in mouth, nose, gastrointestinal tract; after childhood, hemorrhages in joints, resulting in swelling and impaired function.

286.1 Congenital factor IX disorder
Christmas disease
Deficiency:
  factor IX (functional)
  plasma thromboplastin component [PTC]
Hemophilia B
DEF: Deficiency of plasma thromboplastin component (PTC) (factor IX) and plasma thromboplastin antecedent (PTA); PTC deficiency clinically indistinguishable from classical hemophilia; PTA deficiency found in both sexes.

286.2 Congenital factor XI deficiency
Hemophilia C
Plasma thromboplastin antecedent [PTA] deficiency
Rosenthal's disease

✓4ᵗʰ / ✓5ᵗʰ Additional Digit Required   Unspecified Code   Other Specified Code   Manifestation Code   ▶◀ Revised Text   ● New Code   ▲ Revised Code Title

2005 ICD•9•CM   **Volume 1 — 59**

Blood and Blood-Forming Organs

286.3–287.3

286.3 **Congenital deficiency of other clotting factors**
Congenital afibrinogenemia
Deficiency:
  AC globulin factor:
    I [fibrinogen]
    II [prothrombin]
    V [labile]
    VII [stable]
    X [Stuart-Prower]
    XII [Hageman]
    XIII [fibrin stabilizing]
  Laki-Lorand factor
  proaccelerin
Disease
  Owren's
  Stuart-Prower
Dysfibrinogenemia (congenital)
Dysprothrombinemia (constitutional)
Hypoproconvertinemia
Hypoprothrmbinemia (hereditary)
Parahemophilia

286.4 **von Willebrand's disease**
Angiohemophilia (A) (B)
Constitutional thrombopathy
Factor VIII deficiency with vascular defect
Pseudohemophilia type B
Vascular hemophilia
von Willebrand's (-Jürgens') disease
> **EXCLUDES** *factor VIII deficiency:*
>   *NOS (286.0)*
>   *with functional defect (286.0)*
>   *hereditary capillary fragility (287.8)*

DEF: Abnormal blood coagulation caused by deficient blood Factor VII; congenital; symptoms include excess or prolonged bleeding, such as hemorrhage during menstruation, following birthing, or after surgical procedure.

▲   **286.5** **Hemorrhagic disorder due to intrinsic circulating anticoagulants**
Antithrombinemia
Antithromboplastinemia
Antithromboplastino-genemia
Hyperheparinemia
Increase in:
  anti-VIIIa
  anti-IXa
  anti-Xa
  anti-XIa
  antithrombin
▶Secondary hemophilia◀
Systemic lupus erythematosus [SLE] inhibitor
AHA: 3Q, '92, 15; 3Q, '90, 14

286.6 **Defibrination syndrome**
Afibrinogenemia, acquired
Consumption coagulopathy
Diffuse or disseminated intravascular coagulation
  [DIC syndrome]
Fibrinolytic hemorrhage, acquired
Hemorrhagic fibrinogenolysis
Pathologic fibrinolysis
Purpura:
  fibrinolytic
  fulminans
> **EXCLUDES** *that complicating:*
>   *abortion (634-638 with .1, 639.1)*
>   *pregnancy or the puerperium (641.3,*
>   *666.3)*
>   *disseminated intravascular coagulation*
>   *in newborn (776.2)*

AHA: 4Q, '93, 29

DEF: Characterized by destruction of circulating fibrinogen; often precipitated by other conditions, such as injury, causing release of thromboplastic particles in blood stream.

286.7 **Acquired coagulation factor deficiency**
Deficiency of coagulation factor due to:
  liver disease
  vitamin K deficiency
Hypoprothrombinemia, acquired
Use additional E code to identify cause, if drug
  induced
> **EXCLUDES** *vitamin K deficiency of newborn*
>   *(776.0)*

AHA: 4Q, '93, 29

286.9 **Other and unspecified coagulation defects**
Defective coagulation NOS
Deficiency, coagulation factor NOS
Delay, coagulation
Disorder:
  coagulation
  hemostasis
> **EXCLUDES** *abnormal coagulation profile (790.92)*
>   *hemorrhagic disease of newborn*
>   *(776.0)*
>   *that complicating:*
>   *abortion (634-638 with .1, 639.1)*
>   *pregnancy or the puerperium (641.3,*
>   *666.3)*

✓4ᵗʰ **287** **Purpura and other hemorrhagic conditions**
> **EXCLUDES** *hemorrhagic thrombocythemia (238.7)*
>   *purpura fulminans (286.6)*

AHA: 1Q, '91, 14

287.0 **Allergic purpura**
Peliosis rheumatica   Purpura:
Purpura: rheumatica
  anaphylactoid   Schönlein-Henoch
  autoimmune   vascular
  Henoch's   Vasculitis, allergic
  nonthrombocytopenic:
    hemorrhagic
    idiopathic
> **EXCLUDES** *hemorrhagic purpura (287.3)*
>   *purpura annularis telangiectodes*
>   *(709.1)*

DEF: Any hemorrhagic condition, thrombocytic or nonthrombocytopenic in origin, caused by a presumed allergic reaction.

287.1 **Qualitative platelet defects**
Thrombasthenia (hemorrhagic) (hereditary)
Thrombocytasthenia
Thrombocytopathy (dystrophic)
Thrombopathy (Bernard-Soulier)
> **EXCLUDES** *von Willebrand's disease (286.4)*

287.2 **Other nonthrombocytopenic purpuras**
Purpura: Purpura:
  NOS   simplex
  senile

287.3 **Primary thrombocytopenia**
Evans' syndrome
Megakaryocytic hypoplasia
Purpura, thrombocytopenic
  congenital
  hereditary
  idiopathic
Thrombocytopenia:
  congenital
  hereditary
  primary
Tidal platelet dysgenesis
> **EXCLUDES** *thrombotic thrombocytopenic purpura*
>   *(446.6)*
>   *transient thrombocytopenia of newborn*
>   *(776.1)*

AHA: M-A, '85, 14

DEF: Decrease in number of blood platelets in circulating blood and purpural skin hemorrhages.

Ⓝ Newborn Age: 0   Ⓟ Pediatric Age: 0-17   Ⓜ Maternity Age: 12-55   Ⓐ Adult Age: 15-124   **MSP** Medicare Secondary Payer

287.4 Secondary thrombocytopenia
Posttransfusion purpura
Thrombocytopenia (due to):
  dilutional
  drugs
  extracorporeal circulation of blood
  platelet alloimmunization
Use additional E code to identify cause
  EXCLUDES transient thrombocytopenia of newborn
  (776.1)

AHA: 4Q, '99, 22; 4Q, '93, 29

DEF: Reduced number of platelets in circulating blood as consequence of an underlying disease or condition.

287.5 Thrombocytopenia, unspecified

287.8 Other specified hemorrhagic conditions
Capillary fragility (hereditary)
Vascular pseudohemophilia

287.9 Unspecified hemorrhagic conditions
Hemorrhagic diathesis (familial)

✓4ᵗʰ 288 Diseases of white blood cells
  EXCLUDES leukemia (204.0-208.9)

AHA: 1Q, '91, 14

288.0 Agranulocytosis
Infantile genetic agranulocytosis
Kostmann's syndrome
Neutropenia:
  NOS
  cyclic
  drug-induced
  immune
  periodic
  toxic
Neutropenic splenomegaly
Use additional E code to identify drug or other cause
  EXCLUDES transitory neonatal neutropenia (776.7)

AHA: 3Q, '99, 6; 2Q, '99, 9; 3Q, '96, 16; 2Q, '96, 6

DEF: Sudden, severe condition characterized by reduced number of white blood cells; results in sores in the throat, stomach or skin; symptoms include chills, fever; some drugs can bring on condition.

288.1 Functional disorders of polymorphonuclear neutrophils
Chronic (childhood) granulomatous disease
Congenital dysphagocytosis
Job's syndrome
Lipochrome histiocytosis (familial)
Progressive septic granulomatosis

288.2 Genetic anomalies of leukocytes
Anomaly (granulation) (granulocyte) or syndrome:
  Alder's (-Reilly)
  Chédiak-Steinbrinck (-Higashi)
  Jordan's
  May-Hegglin
  Pelger-Huet
Hereditary:
  hypersegmentation
  hyposegmentation
  leukomelanopathy

288.3 Eosinophilia
Eosinophilia:
  allergic
  hereditary
  idiopathic
  secondary
Eosinophilic leukocytosis
  EXCLUDES Löffler's syndrome (518.3)
  pulmonary eosinophilia (518.3)

AHA: 3Q, '00, 11

DEF: Elevated number of eosinophils in the blood; characteristic of allergic states and various parasitic infections.

288.8 Other specified disease of white blood cells
Leukemoid reaction:
  lymphocytic
  monocytic
  myelocytic
Leukocytosis
Lymphocytopenia
Lymphocytosis (symptomatic)
Lymphopenia
Monocytosis (symptomatic)
Plasmacytosis
  EXCLUDES immunity disorders (279.0-279.9)

AHA: M-A, '87, 12

288.9 Unspecified disease of white blood cells

✓4ᵗʰ 289 Other diseases of blood and blood-forming organs

289.0 Polycythemia, secondary
High-oxygen-affinity hemoglobin
Polycythemia:
  acquired
  benign
  due to:
    fall in plasma volume
    high altitude
  emotional
  erythropoietin
  hypoxemic
  nephrogenous
  relative
  spurious
  stress
  EXCLUDES polycythemia:
    neonatal (776.4)
    primary (238.4)
    vera (238.4)

DEF: Elevated number of red blood cells in circulating blood as result of reduced oxygen supply to the tissues.

289.1 Chronic lymphadenitis
Chronic:
  adenitis   } any lymph node, except
  lymphadenitis }   mesenteric
  EXCLUDES acute lymphadenitis (683)
    mesenteric (289.2)
    enlarged glands NOS (785.6)

DEF: Persistent inflammation of lymph node tissue; origin of infection is usually elsewhere.

289.2 Nonspecific mesenteric lymphadenitis
Mesenteric lymphadenitis (acute) (chronic)

DEF: Inflammation of the lymph nodes in peritoneal fold that encases abdominal organs; disease resembles acute appendicitis; unknown etiology.

289.3 Lymphadenitis, unspecified, except mesenteric
AHA: 2Q, '92, 8

289.4 Hypersplenism
"Big spleen" syndrome   Hypersplenia
Dyssplenism
  EXCLUDES primary splenic neutropenia (288.0)
DEF: An overactive spleen; it causes a deficiency of the peripheral blood components, an increase in bone marrow cells and sometimes a notable increase in the size of the spleen.

✓5ᵗʰ 289.5 Other diseases of spleen
  289.50 Disease of spleen, unspecified
  289.51 Chronic congestive splenomegaly
  289.52 Splenic sequestration
Code first sickle-cell disease in crisis
  (282.42, 282.62, 282.64, 282.69)

AHA: ▶4Q, '03, 51◄

DEF: ▶Blood is entrapped in the spleen due to vessel occlusion; most often associated with sickle-cell disease; spleen becomes enlarged and there is a sharp drop in hemoglobin.◄

✓4ᵗʰ / ✓5ᵗʰ Additional Digit Required   Unspecified Code   Other Specified Code   Manifestation Code   ▶◄ Revised Text   ● New Code   ▲ Revised Code Title

Blood and Blood-Forming Organs

289.59–289.9

289.59 Other

Lien migrans	Splenic:
Perisplenitis	fibrosis
Splenic:	infarction
abscess	rupture, nontraumatic
atrophy	Splenitis
cyst	Wandering spleen

    EXCLUDES *bilharzial splenic fibrosis*
                      (120.0-120.9)
              hepatolienal fibrosis (571.5)
              splenomegaly NOS (789.2)

289.6 Familial polycythemia

Familial:
    benign polycythemia
    erythrocytosis

DEF: Elevated number of red blood cells.

289.7 Methemoglobinemia

Congenital NADH [DPNH]-methemoglobin-reductase
    deficiency
Hemoglobin M [Hb-M] disease
Methemoglobinemia:
    NOS
    acquired (with sulfhemoglobinemia)
    hereditary
    toxic
Stokvis' disease
Sulfhemoglobinemia
Use additional E code to identify cause

DEF: Presence in the blood of methemoglobin, a chemically altered form of hemoglobin; causes cyanosis, headache, dizziness, ataxia dyspnea, tachycardia, nausea, stupor, coma, and, rarely, death.

✓5ᵗʰ 289.8 Other specified diseases of blood and blood-forming organs

AHA: ▶4Q, '03, 56;◄ 1Q, '02, 16; 2Q, '89, 8; M-A, '87, 12

DEF: ▶Hypercoagulable states: a group of inherited or acquired abnormalities of specific proteins and anticoagulant factors; also called thromboembolic states or thrombotic disorders, these disorders result in the abnormal development of blood clots.◄

289.81 Primary hypercoagulable state

Activated protein C resistance
Antithrombin III deficiency
Factor V Leiden mutation
Lupus anticoagulant
Protein C deficiency
Protein S deficiency
Prothrombin gene mutation

DEF: ▶Activated protein C resistance: decreased effectiveness of protein C to degrade factor V, necessary to inhibit clotting cascade; also called Factor V Leiden mutation.◄

DEF: ▶Antithrombin III deficiency: deficiency in plasma antithrombin III one of six naturally occurring antithrombins that limit coagulation.◄

DEF: ▶Factor V Leiden mutation: also called activated protein C resistance.◄

DEF: ▶Lupus anticoagulant: deficiency in a circulating anticoagulant that inhibits the conversion of prothrombin into thrombin; autoimmune antibodies induce procoagulant surfaces in platelets; also called anti-phospholipid syndrome.◄

DEF: ▶Protein C deficiency: deficiency of activated protein C which functions to bring the blood-clotting process into balance; same outcome as factor V Leiden mutation.◄

DEF: ▶Protein S deficiency: similar to protein C deficiency; protein S is a vitamin K dependent cofactor in the activation of protein C.◄

DEF: ▶Prothrombin gene mutation: increased levels of prothrombin, or factor II, a plasma protein that is converted to thrombin, which acts upon fibrinogen to form the fibrin.◄

289.82 Secondary hypercoagulable state

289.89 Other specified diseases of blood and blood-forming organs

Hypergammaglobulinemia
Myelofibrosis
Pseudocholinesterase deficiency

289.9 Unspecified diseases of blood and blood-forming organs

Blood dyscrasia NOS
Erythroid hyperplasia

AHA: M-A, '85, 14

5. MENTAL DISORDERS (290-319)

In the *International Classification of Diseases, 9th Revision* (ICD-9), the corresponding Chapter V, "Mental Disorders," includes a glossary which defines the contents of each category. The introduction to Chapter V in ICD-9 indicates that the glossary is intended so that psychiatrists can make the diagnosis based on the descriptions provided rather than from the category titles. Lay coders are instructed to code whatever diagnosis the physician records.

Chapter 5, "Mental Disorders," in ICD-9-CM uses the standard classification format with inclusion and exclusion terms, omitting the glossary as part of the main text.

The mental disorders section of ICD-9-CM has been expanded to incorporate additional psychiatric disorders not listed in ICD-9. The glossary from ICD-9 does not contain all these terms. It now appears in Appendix B, which also contains descriptions and definitions for the terms added in ICD-9-CM. Some of these were provided by the American Psychiatric Association's Task Force on Nomenclature and Statistics who are preparing the Diagnostic and Statistical Manual, Third Edition (DSM-III), and others from A Psychiatric Glossary.

The American Psychiatric Association provided invaluable assistance in modifying Chapter 5 of ICD-9-CM to incorporate detail useful to American clinicians and gave permission to use material from the aforementioned sources.

1. Manual of the *International Statistical Classification of Diseases, Injuries, and Causes of Death, 9th Revision*, World Health Organization, Geneva, Switzerland, 1975.

2. American Psychiatric Association, Task Force on Nomenclature and Statistics, Robert L. Spitzer, M.D., Chairman.

3. *A Psychiatric Glossary*, Fourth Edition, American Psychiatric Association, Washington, D.C., 1975.

PSYCHOSES (290-299)

EXCLUDES   *mental retardation (317-319)*

ORGANIC PSYCHOTIC CONDITIONS (290-294)

INCLUDES   psychotic organic brain syndrome
EXCLUDES   *nonpsychotic syndromes of organic etiology (310.0-310.9)*
            psychoses classifiable to 295-298 and without impairment of orientation, comprehension, calculation, learning capacity, and judgment, but associated with physical disease, injury, or condition affecting the brain [eg., following childbirth] (295.0-298.8)

▲ ✓4ᵗʰ **290 Dementias**
        Code first the associated neurological condition
        EXCLUDES ▶ *dementia due to alcohol (291.0-291.2)*
        dementia due to drugs (292.82)◀
        dementia not classified as senile, presenile, or arteriosclerotic (294.10-294.11)
        psychoses classifiable to 295-298 occurring in the senium without dementia or delirium (295.0-298.8)
        senility with mental changes of nonpsychotic severity (310.1)
        transient organic psychotic conditions (293.0-293.9)

    290.0 Senile dementia, uncomplicated   Ⓐ
        Senile dementia:
            NOS
            simple type
        EXCLUDES *mild memory disturbances, not amounting to dementia, associated with senile brain disease (310.1)*
        senile dementia with:
            delirium or confusion (290.3)
            delusional [paranoid] features (290.20)
            depressive features (290.21)

        AHA: 4Q, '99, 4

✓5ᵗʰ **290.1 Presenile dementia**
        Brain syndrome with presenile brain disease
        EXCLUDES *arteriosclerotic dementia (290.40-290.43)*
        dementia associated with other cerebral conditions (294.10-294.11)

    AHA: N-D, '84, 20

    290.10 Presenile dementia, uncomplicated   Ⓐ
            Presenile dementia: Presenile dementia:
                NOS   simple type
    290.11 Presenile dementia with delirium   Ⓐ
            Presenile dementia with acute confusional state

        AHA: 1Q, '88, 3

    290.12 Presenile dementia with delusional features   Ⓐ
            Presenile dementia, paranoid type
    290.13 Presenile dementia with depressive features   Ⓐ
            Presenile dementia, depressed type

✓5ᵗʰ **290.2 Senile dementia with delusional or depressive features**
        EXCLUDES *senile dementia:*
            NOS (290.0)
            with delirium and/or confusion (290.3)

    290.20 Senile dementia with delusional features   Ⓐ
            Senile dementia, paranoid type
            Senile psychosis NOS
    290.21 Senile dementia with depressive features   Ⓐ

    290.3 Senile dementia with delirium   Ⓐ
            Senile dementia with acute confusional state
        EXCLUDES *senile:*
            dementia NOS (290.0)
            psychosis NOS (290.20)

▲ ✓5ᵗʰ **290.4 Vascular dementia**
        Multi-infarct dementia or psychosis
        Use additional code to identify cerebral atherosclerosis (437.0)
        EXCLUDES *suspected cases with no clear evidence of arteriosclerosis (290.9)*

    AHA: 1Q, '88, 3

▲   **290.40 Vascular dementia, uncomplicated**   Ⓐ
            Arteriosclerotic dementia:
                NOS
                simple type
▲   **290.41 Vascular dementia with delirium**   Ⓐ
            Arteriosclerotic dementia with acute confusional state
▲   **290.42 Vascular dementia with delusions**   Ⓐ
            Arteriosclerotic dementia, paranoid type
▲   **290.43 Vascular dementia with depressed mood**   Ⓐ
            Arteriosclerotic dementia, depressed type
    290.8 Other specified senile psychotic conditions
            Presbyophrenic psychosis
    290.9 Unspecified senile psychotic condition   Ⓐ

▲ ✓4ᵗʰ **291 Alcohol-induced mental disorders**
        EXCLUDES *alcoholism without psychosis (303.0-303.9)*
    AHA: 1Q, '88, 3; S-O, '86, 3

    291.0 Alcohol withdrawal delirium
            Alcoholic delirium
            Delirium tremens
        EXCLUDES *alcohol withdrawal (291.81)*
        AHA: 2Q, '91, 11

✓4ᵗʰ
✓5ᵗʰ Additional Digit Required   Unspecified Code   Other Specified Code   Manifestation Code   ▶◀ Revised Text   ● New Code   ▲ Revised Code Title

2005 ICD•9•CM   October 2004 • Volume 1 — 63

Mental Disorders

291.1–293.0

▲   **291.1 Alcohol-induced persisting amnestic disorder**
Alcoholic polyneuritic psychosis
Korsakoff's psychosis, alcoholic
Wernicke-Korsakoff syndrome (alcoholic)

DEF: Prominent and lasting reduced memory span, disordered time appreciation and confabulation, occurring in alcoholics, as sequel to acute alcoholic psychosis.

▲   **291.2 Alcohol-induced persisting dementia**
Alcoholic dementia NOS
Alcoholism associated with dementia NOS
Chronic alcoholic brain syndrome

▲   **291.3 Alcohol-induced psychotic disorder with hallucinations**
Alcoholic:
hallucinosis (acute)
psychosis with hallucinosis
   EXCLUDES   *alcohol withdrawal with delirium (291.0)*
schizophrenia (295.0-295.9) and paranoid states (297.0-297.9) taking the form of chronic hallucinosis with clear consciousness in an alcoholic

AHA: 2Q, '91, 11

DEF: Psychosis lasting less than six months with slight or no clouding of consciousness in which auditory hallucinations predominate.

▲   **291.4 Idiosyncratic alcohol intoxication**
Pathologic:
alcohol intoxication
drunkenness
   EXCLUDES   *acute alcohol intoxication (305.0) in alcoholism (303.0) simple drunkenness (305.0)*

DEF: Unique behavioral patterns, like belligerence, after intake of relatively small amounts of alcohol; behavior not due to excess consumption.

▲   **291.5 Alcohol-induced psychotic disorder with delusions**
Alcoholic: Alcoholic:
paranoia   psychosis, paranoid type
   EXCLUDES   *nonalcoholic paranoid states (297.0-297.9)*
schizophrenia, paranoid type (295.3)

▲ ✓5th **291.8 Other specified alcohol-induced mental disorders**
AHA: 3Q, '94, 13; J-A, '85, 10

   291.81 Alcohol withdrawal
Alcohol:
abstinence syndrome or symptoms
withdrawal syndrome or symptoms
   EXCLUDES   *alcohol withdrawal: delirium (291.0) hallucinosis (291.3) delirium tremens (291.0)*

AHA: 4Q, '96, 28; 2Q, '91, 11

▲   **291.89 Other**
▶Alcohol-induced anxiety disorder◀
Alcohol-induced mood disorder
Alcohol-induced sexual dysfunction
Alcohol-induced sleep disorder◀

▲   **291.9 Unspecified alcohol-induced mental disorders**
Alcoholic:
mania NOS
psychosis NOS
Alcoholism (chronic) with psychosis
▶Alcohol-related disorder NOS◀

▲ ✓4th **292 Drug-induced mental disorders**
INCLUDES   organic brain syndrome associated with consumption of drugs
Use additional code for any associated drug dependence (304.0-304.9)
Use additional E code to identify drug
AHA: 2Q, '91, 11; S-O, '86, 3

▲   **292.0 Drug withdrawal**
Drug:
abstinence syndrome or symptoms
withdrawal syndrome or symptoms
AHA: 1Q, '97, 12; 1Q, '88, 3

▲ ✓5th **292.1 Drug-induced psychotic disorders**
▲   **292.11 Drug-induced psychotic disorder with delusions**
Paranoid state induced by drugs

▲   **292.12 Drug-induced psychotic disorder with hallucinations**
Hallucinatory state induced by drugs
   EXCLUDES   *states following LSD or other hallucinogens, lasting only a few days or less ["bad trips"] (305.3)*

   292.2 Pathological drug intoxication
Drug reaction:
NOS
idiosyncratic   } resulting in brief psychotic states
pathologic
   EXCLUDES   *expected brief psychotic reactions to hallucinogens ["bad trips"] (305.3)*
physiological side-effects of drugs (e.g., dystonias)

✓5th **292.8 Other specified drug-induced mental disorders**
   292.81 Drug-induced delirium
AHA: 1Q, '88, 3

▲   **292.82 Drug-induced persisting dementia**
▲   **292.83 Drug-induced persisting amnestic disorder**
▲   **292.84 Drug-induced mood disorder**
Depressive state induced by drugs

   292.89 Other
▶Drug-induced anxiety disorder◀
Drug-induced organic personality syndrome
▶Drug-induced sexual dysfunction
Drug-induced sleep disorder
Drug intoxication◀

   292.9 Unspecified drug-induced mental disorder
▶Drug-related disorder NOS◀
Organic psychosis NOS due to or associated with drugs

▲ ✓4th **293 Transient mental disorders due to conditions classified elsewhere**
INCLUDES   transient organic mental disorders not associated with alcohol or drugs
Code first the associated physical or neurological condition
   EXCLUDES   *confusional state or delirium superimposed on senile dementia (290.3)*
dementia due to: alcohol (291.0-291.9) arteriosclerosis (290.40-290.43) drugs (292.82) senility (290.0)

▲   **293.0 Delirium due to conditions classified elsewhere**
Acute:
confusional state
infective psychosis
organic reaction
posttraumatic organic psychosis
psycho-organic syndrome
Acute psychosis associated with endocrine, metabolic, or cerebrovascular disorder
Epileptic:
confusional state
twilight state
AHA: 1Q, '88, 3

N Newborn Age: 0   P Pediatric Age: 0-17   M Maternity Age: 12-55   A Adult Age: 15-124   MSP Medicare Secondary Payer

Mental Disorders

293.1 Subacute delirium
Subacute:
confusional state
infective psychosis
organic reaction
posttraumatic organic psychosis
psycho-organic syndrome
psychosis associated with endocrine or metabolic
disorder

▲ √5ᵗʰ **293.8 Other specified transient mental disorders due to conditions classified elsewhere**

▲ **293.81 Psychotic disorder with delusions in conditions classified elsewhere**
Transient organic psychotic condition, paranoid type

▲ **293.82 Psychotic disorder with hallucinations in conditions classified elsewhere**
Transient organic psychotic condition, hallucinatory type

▲ **293.83 Mood disorder in conditions classified elsewhere**
Transient organic psychotic condition, depressive type

▲ **293.84 Anxiety disorder in conditions classified elsewhere**
AHA: 4Q, '96, 29

▲ **293.89 Other**
▶Catatonic disorder in conditions classified elsewhere◀

▲ **293.9 Unspecified transient mental disorder in conditions classified elsewhere**
Organic psychosis:
infective NOS
posttraumatic NOS
transient NOS
Psycho-organic syndrome

▲ √4ᵗʰ **294 Persistent mental disorders due to conditions classified elsewhere**
INCLUDES organic psychotic brain syndromes (chronic), not elsewhere classified

AHA: M-A, '85, 12

▲ **294.0 Amnestic disorder in conditions classified elsewhere**
Korsakoff's psychosis or syndrome (nonalcoholic)
▶Code first underlying condition◀
EXCLUDES alcoholic:
amnestic syndrome (291.1)
Korsakoff's psychosis (291.1)

√5ᵗʰ **294.1 Dementia in conditions classified elsewhere**
▶Dementia of the Alzheimer's type◀
Code first any underlying physical condition, as:
dementia in:
Alzheimer's disease (331.0)
cerebral lipidoses (330.1)
dementia with Lewy bodies (331.82)
dementia with Parkinsonism (331.82)
epilepsy (345.0-345.9)
frontal dementia (331.19)
frontotemporal dementia (331.19)
general paresis [syphilis] (094.1)
hepatolenticular degeneration (275.1)
Huntington's chorea (333.4)
Jakob-Creutzfeldt disease (046.1)
multiple sclerosis (340)
Pick's disease of the brain (331.11)
polyarteritis nodosa (446.0)
syphilis (094.1)
EXCLUDES dementia:
arteriosclerotic (290.40-290.43)
presenile (290.10-290.13)
senile (290.0)
epileptic psychosis NOS (294.8)

AHA: 4Q, '00, 40; 1Q, '99, 14; N-D, '85, 5

294.10 Dementia in conditions classified elsewhere without behavioral disturbance
Dementia in conditions classified elsewhere NOS

294.11 Dementia in conditions classified elsewhere with behavioral disturbance
Aggressive behavior   Violent behavior
Combative behavior   Wandering off
AHA: 4Q, '00, 41

▲ **294.8 Other persistent mental disorders due to conditions classified elsewhere**
▶Amnestic disorder NOS
Dementia NOS◀
Epileptic psychosis NOS
Mixed paranoid and affective organic psychotic states
Use additional code for associated epilepsy (345.0-345.9)
EXCLUDES mild memory disturbances, not amounting to dementia (310.1)

AHA: 3Q, '03, 14; 1Q, '88, 5

▲ **294.9 Unspecified persistent mental disorders due to conditions classified elsewhere**
▶Cognitive disorder NOS◀
Organic psychosis (chronic)

OTHER PSYCHOSES (295-299)
Use additional code to identify any associated physical disease, injury, or condition affecting the brain with psychoses classifiable to 295-298

√4ᵗʰ **295 Schizophrenic disorders**
INCLUDES schizophrenia of the types described in 295.0-295.9 occurring in children
EXCLUDES childhood type schizophrenia (299.9)
infantile autism (299.0)

The following fifth-digit subclassification is for use with category 295:

0 **unspecified**
1 **subchronic**
2 **chronic**
3 **subchronic with acute exacerbation**
4 **chronic with acute exacerbation**
5 **in remission**

DEF: Group of disorders with disturbances in thought (delusions, hallucinations), mood (blunted, flattened, inappropriate affect), sense of self, relationship to world; also bizarre, purposeless behavior, repetitious activity, or inactivity.

√5ᵗʰ **295.0 Simple type**
Schizophrenia simplex
EXCLUDES latent schizophrenia (295.5)

√5ᵗʰ **295.1 Disorganized type**
Hebephrenia   Hebephrenic type schizophrenia
DEF: Inappropriate behavior; results in extreme incoherence and disorganization of time, place and sense of social appropriateness; withdrawal from routine social interaction may occur.

√5ᵗʰ **295.2 Catatonic type**
Catatonic (schizophrenia):   Schizophrenic:
agitation   catalepsy
excitation   catatonia
excited type   flexibilitas cerea
stupor
withdrawn type
DEF: Extreme changes in motor activity; one extreme is decreased response or reaction to the environment and the other is spontaneous activity.

√4ᵗʰ
√5ᵗʰ Additional Digit Required   Unspecified Code   Other Specified Code   Manifestation Code   ▶◀ Revised Text   ● New Code   ▲ Revised Code Title

2005 ICD•9•CM   October 2004 • Volume 1 — 65

Mental Disorders

295.3–296.7

§ ✓5ᵗʰ **295.3** **Paranoid type**
Paraphrenic schizophrenia
EXCLUDES   *involutional paranoid state (297.2)*
paranoia (297.1)
paraphrenia (297.2)

DEF: Preoccupied with delusional suspicions and auditory hallucinations related to single theme; usually hostile, grandiose, overly religious, occasionally hypochondriacal.

▲ § ✓5ᵗʰ **295.4** **Schizophreniform disorder**
Oneirophrenia   Schizophreniform:
Schizophreniform: psychosis, confusional type
attack
EXCLUDES   *acute forms of schizophrenia of:*
catatonic type (295.2)
hebephrenic type (295.1)
paranoid type (295.3)
simple type (295.0)
undifferentiated type (295.8)

§ ✓5ᵗʰ **295.5** **Latent schizophrenia**
Latent schizophrenic reaction
Schizophrenia:
borderline
incipient
prepsychotic
prodromal
pseudoneurotic
pseudopsychopathic
EXCLUDES   *schizoid personality (301.20-301.22)*

▲ § ✓5ᵗʰ **295.6** **Residual type**
Chronic undifferentiated schizophrenia
Restzustand (schizophrenic)
Schizophrenic residual state

▲ § ✓5ᵗʰ **295.7** **Schizoaffective disorder**
Cyclic schizophrenia
Mixed schizophrenic and affective psychosis
Schizo-affective psychosis
Schizophreniform psychosis, affective type

§ ✓5ᵗʰ **295.8** **Other specified types of schizophrenia**
Acute (undifferentiated) schizophrenia
Atypical schizophrenia
Cenesthopathic schizophrenia
EXCLUDES   *infantile autism (299.0)*

§ ✓5ᵗʰ **295.9** **Unspecified schizophrenia**
Schizophrenia:
NOS
mixed NOS
undifferentiated NOS
►undifferentiated type◄
Schizophrenic reaction NOS
Schizophreniform psychosis NOS
AHA: 3Q, '95, 6

▲ ✓4ᵗʰ **296** **Episodic mood disorders**
INCLUDES   episodic affective disorders
EXCLUDES   *neurotic depression (300.4)*
reactive depressive psychosis (298.0)
reactive excitation (298.1)

The following fifth-digit subclassification is for use with categories 296.0-296.6:
0   unspecified
1   mild
2   moderate
3   severe, without mention of psychotic behavior
4   severe, specified as with psychotic behavior
5   in partial or unspecified remission
6   in full remission

AHA: M-A, '85, 14

▲ ✓5ᵗʰ **296.0** **Bipolar I disorder, single manic episode**
Hypomania (mild) NOS ⎫
Hypomanic psychosis ⎪
Mania (monopolar) NOS ⎬ single episode or
Manic-depressive psychosis ⎪ unspecified
   or reaction: ⎪
    hypomanic ⎪
    manic ⎭
EXCLUDES   *circular type, if there was a previous attack of depression (296.4)*

DEF: Mood disorder identified by hyperactivity; may show extreme agitation or exaggerated excitability; speech and thought processes may be accelerated.

✓5ᵗʰ **296.1** **Manic disorder, recurrent episode**
Any condition classifiable to 296.0, stated to be recurrent
EXCLUDES   *circular type, if there was a previous attack of depression (296.4)*

✓5ᵗʰ **296.2** **Major depressive disorder, single episode**
Depressive psychosis ⎫
Endogenous depression ⎪
Involutional melancholia ⎪
Manic-depressive psychosis ⎬ single episode or
   or reaction, ⎪ unspecified
    depressed type ⎪
Monopolar depression ⎪
Psychotic depression ⎭
EXCLUDES   *circular type, if previous attack was of manic type (296.5)*
depression NOS (311)
reactive depression (neurotic) (300.4)
psychotic (298.0)

DEF: Mood disorder that produces depression; may exhibit as sadness, low self-esteem, or guilt feelings; other manifestations may be withdrawal from friends and family; interrupted normal sleep.

✓5ᵗʰ **296.3** **Major depressive disorder, recurrent episode**
Any condition classifiable to 296.2, stated to be recurrent
EXCLUDES   *circular type, if previous attack was of manic type (296.5)*
depression NOS (311)
reactive depression (neurotic) (300.4)
psychotic (298.0)

▲ ✓5ᵗʰ **296.4** **Bipolar I disorder, most recent episode (or current) manic**
Bipolar disorder, now manic
Manic-depressive psychosis, circular type but currently manic
EXCLUDES   *brief compensatory or rebound mood swings (296.99)*

▲ ✓5ᵗʰ **296.5** **Bipolar I disorder, most recent episode (or current) depressed**
Bipolar disorder, now depressed
Manic-depressive psychosis, circular type but currently depressed
EXCLUDES   *brief compensatory or rebound mood swings (296.99)*

▲ ✓5ᵗʰ **296.6** **Bipolar I disorder, most recent episode (or current) mixed**
Manic-depressive psychosis, circular type, mixed

▲ **296.7** **Bipolar I disorder, most recent episode (or current) unspecified**
Atypical bipolar affective disorder NOS
Manic-depressive psychosis, circular type, current condition not specified as either manic or depressive

DEF: Manic-depressive disorder referred to as bipolar because of the mood range from manic to depressive.

---

§ Requres fifth-digit. See category 295 for codes and definitions.

N Newborn Age: 0   P Pediatric Age: 0-17   M Maternity Age: 12-55   A Adult Age: 15-124   MSP Medicare Secondary Payer

▲　✓5ᵗʰ **296.8　Other and unspecified bipolar disorders**
▲　　　　　**296.80　Bipolar disorder, unspecified**
　　　　　　　　▶Bipolar disorder NOS◀
　　　　　　　Manic-depressive:
　　　　　　　　　reaction NOS
　　　　　　　　　syndrome NOS
　　　　　　296.81　Atypical manic disorder
　　　　　　296.82　Atypical depressive disorder
▲　　　　　**296.89　Other**
　　　　　　　　▶Bipolar II disorder◀
　　　　　　　Manic-depressive psychosis, mixed type
▲　✓5ᵗʰ **296.9　Other and unspecified episodic mood disorder**
　　　　　　EXCLUDES　*psychogenic affective psychoses
　　　　　　　　　　　(298.0-298.8)*
▲　　　　　**296.90　Unspecified episodic mood disorder**
　　　　　　　Affective psychosis NOS
　　　　　　　Melancholia NOS
　　　　　　　▶Mood disorder NOS◀
　　　　　　AHA: M-A, '85, 14

▲　　　　　**296.99　Other specified episodic mood disorder**
　　　　　　　Mood swings:
　　　　　　　　brief compensatory
　　　　　　　　rebound
▲　✓4ᵗʰ **297　Delusional disorders**
　　　　INCLUDES　paranoid disorders
　　　　EXCLUDES　*acute paranoid reaction (298.3)
　　　　　　　　alcoholic jealousy or paranoid state (291.5)
　　　　　　　　paranoid schizophrenia (295.3)*
　　　297.0　Paranoid state, simple
▲　　**297.1　Delusional disorder**
　　　　　Chronic paranoid psychosis
　　　　　Sander's disease
　　　　　Systematized delusions
　　　　　EXCLUDES　*paranoid personality disorder (301.0)*
　　　297.2　Paraphrenia
　　　　　Involutional paranoid state　Paraphrenia
　　　　　　　　(involutional)
　　　　　Late paraphrenia
　　　　　DEF: Paranoid schizophrenic disorder that persists over a
　　　　　prolonged period but does not distort personality despite persistent
　　　　　delusions.

▲　　**297.3　Shared psychotic disorder**
　　　　　Folie à deux
　　　　　Induced psychosis or paranoid disorder
　　　　　DEF: Mental disorder two people share; first person with the
　　　　　delusional disorder convinces second person because of a close
　　　　　relationship and shared experiences to accept the delusions.

　　　297.8　Other specified paranoid states
　　　　　Paranoia querulans　　Sensitiver Beziehungswahn
　　　　　EXCLUDES　*acute paranoid reaction or state (298.3)
　　　　　　　　senile paranoid state (290.20)*
　　　297.9　Unspecified paranoid state
　　　　　Paranoid:　　　　　Paranoid:
　　　　　　disorder NOS　　　　reaction NOS
　　　　　　psychosis NOS　　　state NOS
　　　　　AHA: J-A, '85, 9

✓4ᵗʰ **298　Other nonorganic psychoses**
　　　INCLUDES　psychotic conditions due to or provoked by:
　　　　　　　emotional stress
　　　　　　　environmental factors as major part of
　　　　　　　　etiology
　　298.0　Depressive type psychosis
　　　　Psychogenic depressive psychosis
　　　　Psychotic reactive depression
　　　　Reactive depressive psychosis
　　　　EXCLUDES　*manic-depressive psychosis, depressed
　　　　　　　type (296.2-296.3)
　　　　　　　neurotic depression (300.4)
　　　　　　　reactive depression NOS (300.4)*

298.1　Excitative type psychosis
　　　Acute hysterical psychosis　Reactive excitation
　　　Psychogenic excitation
　　　EXCLUDES　*manic-depressive psychosis, manic
　　　　　　　type (296.0-296.1)*
　　　DEF: Affective disorder similar to manic-depressive psychosis, in
　　　the manic phase, seemingly brought on by stress.

298.2　Reactive confusion
　　　Psychogenic confusion
　　　Psychogenic twilight state
　　　EXCLUDES　*acute confusional state (293.0)*
　　　DEF: Confusion, disorientation, cloudiness in consciousness;
　　　brought on by severe emotional upheaval.

298.3　Acute paranoid reaction
　　　Acute psychogenic paranoid psychosis
　　　Bouffée délirante
　　　EXCLUDES　*paranoid states (297.0-297.9)*

298.4　Psychogenic paranoid psychosis
　　　Protracted reactive paranoid psychosis

298.8　Other and unspecified reactive psychosis
　　　▶Brief psychotic disorder◀
　　　Brief reactive psychosis NOS
　　　Hysterical psychosis
　　　Psychogenic psychosis NOS
　　　Psychogenic stupor
　　　EXCLUDES　*acute hysterical psychosis (298.1)*

298.9　Unspecified psychosis
　　　Atypical psychosis
　　　Psychosis NOS
　　　▶Psychotic disorder NOS◀

▲　✓4ᵗʰ **299　Pervasive developmental disorders**
　　　EXCLUDES　*adult type psychoses occurring in childhood, as:
　　　　　　affective disorders (296.0-296.9)
　　　　　　manic-depressive disorders (296.0-296.9)
　　　　　　schizophrenia (295.0-295.9)*

The following fifth-digit subclassification is for use with
category 299:
　　　0　current or active state
　　　1　residual state

▲　✓5ᵗʰ **299.0　Autistic disorder**
　　　Childhood autism
　　　Infantile psychosis
　　　Kanner's syndrome
　　　EXCLUDES　*disintegrative psychosis (299.1)
　　　　　　Heller's syndrome (299.1)
　　　　　　schizophrenic syndrome of childhood
　　　　　　　(299.9)*

　　　DEF: Severe mental disorder of children, results in impaired social
　　　behavior; abnormal development of communicative skills, appears
　　　to be unaware of the need for emotional support and offers little
　　　emotional response to family members.

▲　✓5ᵗʰ **299.1　Childhood disintegrative disorder**
　　　Heller's syndrome
　　　Use additional code to identify any associated
　　　　neurological disorder
　　　EXCLUDES　*infantile autism (299.0)
　　　　　　schizophrenic syndrome of childhood
　　　　　　　(299.9)*

　　　DEF: Mental disease of children identified by impaired development
　　　of reciprocal social skills, verbal and nonverbal communication
　　　skills, imaginative play.

✓5ᵗʰ **299.8　Other specified pervasive developmental
disorders**
　　　▶Asperger's disorder◀
　　　Atypical childhood psychosis
　　　Borderline psychosis of childhood
　　　EXCLUDES　*simple stereotypes without psychotic
　　　　　　disturbance (307.3)*

✓4ᵗʰ
✓5ᵗʰ　Additional Digit Required　　Unspecified Code　　Other Specified Code　　Manifestation Code　　▶◀ Revised Text　　● New Code　　▲ Revised Code Title

§ ✓5ᵗʰ **299.9 Unspecified pervasive developmental disorder**
  Child psychosis NOS
  Schizophrenia, childhood type NOS
  Schizophrenic syndrome of childhood NOS
  EXCLUDES *schizophrenia of adult type occurring in childhood (295.0-295.9)*

NEUROTIC DISORDERS, PERSONALITY DISORDERS, AND OTHER NONPSYCHOTIC MENTAL DISORDERS (300-316)

▲ ✓4ᵗʰ **300 Anxiety, dissociative and somatoform disorders**

✓5ᵗʰ **300.0 Anxiety states**
  EXCLUDES *anxiety in:*
      acute stress reaction (308.0)
      transient adjustment reaction (309.24)
    neurasthenia (300.5)
    psychophysiological disorders (306.0-306.9)
    separation anxiety (309.21)

  DEF: Mental disorder characterized by anxiety and avoidance behavior not particularly related to any specific situation or stimulus; symptoms include emotional instability, apprehension, fatigue.

300.00 Anxiety state, unspecified
  Anxiety: Anxiety:
    neurosis   state (neurotic)
    reaction   Atypical anxiety disorder
  AHA: 1Q, '02, 6

300.01 Panic disorder without agoraphobia
  Panic: Panic:
    attack   state
  EXCLUDES ▶ *panic disorder with agoraphobia (300.21)*◀

  DEF: Neurotic disorder characterized by recurrent panic or anxiety, apprehension, fear or terror; symptoms include shortness of breath, palpitations, dizziness, faintness or shakiness; fear of dying may persist or fear of other morbid consequences.

300.02 Generalized anxiety disorder
300.09 Other

▲ ✓5ᵗʰ **300.1 Dissociative, conversion and factitious disorders**
  EXCLUDES *adjustment reaction (309.0-309.9)*
    anorexia nervosa (307.1)
    gross stress reaction (308.0-308.9)
    hysterical personality (301.50-301.59)
    psychophysiologic disorders (306.0-306.9)

300.10 Hysteria, unspecified
300.11 Conversion disorder
  Astasia-abasia, hysterical
  Conversion hysteria or reaction
  Hysterical
    blindness
    deafness
    paralysis
  AHA: N-D, '85, 15

  DEF: Mental disorder that impairs physical functions with no physiological basis; sensory motor symptoms include seizures, paralysis, temporary blindness; increase in stress or avoidance of unpleasant responsibilities may precipitate.

300.12 Dissociative amnesia
  Hysterical amnesia
300.13 Dissociative fugue
  Hysterical fugue
  DEF: Dissociative hysteria; identified by loss of memory, flight from familiar surroundings; conscious activity is not associated with perception of surroundings, no later memory of episode.

300.14 Dissociative identity disorder
  Dissociative identity disorder
300.15 Dissociative disorder or reaction, unspecified
  DEF: Hysterical neurotic episode; sudden but temporary changes in perceived identity, memory, consciousness, segregated memory patterns exist separate from dominant personality.
300.16 Factitious disorder with predominantly psychological signs and symptoms
  Compensation neurosis
  Ganser's syndrome, hysterical
  DEF: A disorder characterized by the purposeful assumption of mental illness symptoms; the symptoms are not real, possibly representing what the patient imagines mental illness to be like, and are acted out more often when another person is present.
300.19 Other and unspecified factitious illness
  ▶Factitious disorder (with combined psychological and physical signs and symptoms) (with predominantly physical signs and symptoms) NOS◀
  EXCLUDES *multiple operations or hospital addiction syndrome (301.51)*

✓5ᵗʰ **300.2 Phobic disorders**
  EXCLUDES *anxiety state not associated with a specific situation or object (300.00-300.09)*
    obsessional phobias (300.3)
300.20 Phobia, unspecified
  Anxiety-hysteria NOS
  Phobia NOS
300.21 Agoraphobia with panic disorder
  Fear of:
    open spaces ⎤
    streets   ⎬ with panic attacks
    travel   ⎦
  ▶Panic disorder with agoraphobia◀
  EXCLUDES ▶ *agoraphobia without panic disorder (300.22)*
    panic disorder without agoraphobia (300.01)◀
300.22 Agoraphobia without mention of panic attacks
  Any condition classifiable to 300.21 without mention of panic attacks
300.23 Social phobia
  Fear of: Fear of:
    eating in public   washing in public
    public speaking
300.29 Other isolated or specific phobias
  Acrophobia   Claustrophobia
  Animal phobias   Fear of crowds
300.3 Obsessive-compulsive disorders
  Anancastic neurosis   Obsessional phobia [any]
  Compulsive neurosis
  EXCLUDES *obsessive-compulsive symptoms occurring in:*
    endogenous depression (296.2-296.3)
    organic states (eg., encephalitis)
    schizophrenia (295.0-295.9)

§ Requires fifth-digit. See category 299 for codes and definitions.

Mental Disorders

300.4–301.59

▲ **300.4 Dysthymic disorder**
Anxiety depression
Depression with anxiety
Depressive reaction
Neurotic depressive state
Reactive depression

> **EXCLUDES**   adjustment reaction with depressive symptoms (309.0-309.1)
> depression NOS (311)
> manic-depressive psychosis, depressed type (296.2-296.3)
> reactive depressive psychosis (298.0)

DEF: Depression without psychosis; less severe depression related to personal change or unexpected circumstances; also referred to as "reactional depression."

300.5 Neurasthenia
Fatigue neurosis
Nervous debility
Psychogenic:
    asthenia
    general fatigue
Use additional code to identify any associated physical disorder

> **EXCLUDES**   anxiety state (300.00-300.09)
> neurotic depression (300.4)
> psychophysiological disorders (306.0-306.9)
> specific nonpsychotic mental disorders following organic brain damage (310.0-310.9)

DEF: Physical and mental symptoms caused primarily by what is known as mental exhaustion; symptoms include chronic weakness, fatigue.

▲ **300.6 Depersonalization disorder**
Derealization (neurotic)
Neurotic state with depersonalization episode

> **EXCLUDES**   depersonalization associated with:
> anxiety (300.00-300.09)
> depression (300.4)
> manic-depressive disorder or psychosis (296.0-296.9)
> schizophrenia (295.0-295.9)

DEF: Dissociative disorder characterized by feelings of strangeness about self or body image; symptoms include dizziness, anxiety, fear of insanity, loss of reality of surroundings.

300.7 Hypochondriasis
Body dysmorphic disorder

> **EXCLUDES**   hypochondriasis in:
> hysteria (300.10-300.19)
> manic-depressive psychosis, depressed type (296.2-296.3)
> neurasthenia (300.5)
> obsessional disorder (300.3)
> schizophrenia (295.0-295.9)

▲ ✓5ᵗʰ **300.8 Somatoform disorders**

300.81 Somatization disorder
Briquet's disorder
Severe somatoform disorder

300.82 Undifferentiated somatoform disorder
Atypical somatoform disorder
Somatoform disorder NOS

AHA: 4Q, '96, 29

DEF: Disorders in which patients have symptoms that suggest an organic disease but no evidence of physical disorder after repeated testing.

▲ **300.89 Other somatoform disorders**
Occupational neurosis, including writers' cramp
Psychasthenia
Psychasthenic neurosis

300.9 Unspecified nonpsychotic mental disorder
Psychoneurosis NOS

✓4ᵗʰ **301 Personality disorders**
> **INCLUDES**   character neurosis
Use additional code to identify any associated neurosis or psychosis, or physical condition

> **EXCLUDES**   nonpsychotic personality disorder associated with organic brain syndromes (310.0-310.9)

301.0 Paranoid personality disorder
Fanatic personality
Paranoid personality (disorder)
Paranoid traits

> **EXCLUDES**   acute paranoid reaction (298.3)
> alcoholic paranoia (291.5)
> paranoid schizophrenia (295.3)
> paranoid states (297.0-297.9)

AHA: J-A, '85, 9

✓5ᵗʰ **301.1 Affective personality disorder**
> **EXCLUDES**   affective psychotic disorders (296.0-296.9)
> neurasthenia (300.5)
> neurotic depression (300.4)

301.10 Affective personality disorder, unspecified

301.11 Chronic hypomanic personality disorder
Chronic hypomanic disorder
Hypomanic personality

301.12 Chronic depressive personality disorder
Chronic depressive disorder
Depressive character or personality

301.13 Cyclothymic disorder
Cycloid personality
Cyclothymia
Cyclothymic personality

✓5ᵗʰ **301.2 Schizoid personality disorder**
> **EXCLUDES**   schizophrenia (295.0-295.9)

301.20 Schizoid personality disorder, unspecified

301.21 Introverted personality

301.22 Schizotypal personality disorder

▲ **301.3 Explosive personality disorder**
Aggressive:
    personality
    reaction
Aggressiveness
Emotional instability (excessive)
Pathological emotionality
Quarrelsomeness

> **EXCLUDES**   dyssocial personality (301.7)
> hysterical neurosis (300.10-300.19)

▲ **301.4 Obsessive-compulsive personality disorder**
Anancastic personality
Obsessional personality

> **EXCLUDES**   obsessive-compulsive disorder (300.3)
> phobic state (300.20-300.29)

✓5ᵗʰ **301.5 Histrionic personality disorder**
> **EXCLUDES**   hysterical neurosis (300.10-300.19)

DEF: Extreme emotional behavior, often theatrical; often concerned about own appeal; may demand attention, exhibit seductive behavior.

301.50 Histrionic personality disorder, unspecified
Hysterical personality NOS

301.51 Chronic factitious illness with physical symptoms
Hospital addiction syndrome
Multiple operations syndrome
Munchausen syndrome

301.59 Other histrionic personality disorder
Personality:
    emotionally unstable
    labile
Personality:
    psychoinfantile

✓4ᵗʰ ✓5ᵗʰ Additional Digit Required   Unspecified Code   Other Specified Code   Manifestation Code   ▶◀ Revised Text   ● New Code   ▲ Revised Code Title

2005 ICD•9•CM   **October 2004 • Volume 1 — 69**

Mental Disorders

301.6–302.84

301.6 Dependent personality disorder
Asthenic personality   Passive personality
Inadequate personality
> **EXCLUDES**   *neurasthenia (300.5)*
> *passive-aggressive personality (301.84)*

DEF: Overwhelming feeling of helplessness; fears of abandonment may persist; difficulty in making personal decisions without confirmation by others; low self-esteem due to irrational sensitivity to criticism.

301.7 Antisocial personality disorder
Amoral personality
Asocial personality
Dyssocial personality
Personality disorder with predominantly sociopathic or asocial manifestation
> **EXCLUDES**   *disturbance of conduct without specifiable personality disorder (312.0-312.9)*
> *explosive personality (301.3)*

AHA: S-0, '84, 16

DEF: Continuous antisocial behavior that violates rights of others; social traits include extreme aggression, total disregard for traditional social rules.

✓5ᵗʰ **301.8 Other personality disorders**
▲   **301.81 Narcissistic personality disorder**
DEF: Grandiose fantasy or behavior, lack of social empathy, hypersensitive to the lack of others' judgment, exploits others; also sense of entitlement to have expectations met, need for continual admiration.

▲   **301.82 Avoidant personality disorder**
DEF: Personality disorder marked by feelings of social inferiority; sensitivity to criticism, emotionally restrained due to fear of rejection.

▲   **301.83 Borderline personality disorder**
DEF: Personality disorder characterized by unstable moods, self-image, and interpersonal relationships; uncontrolled anger, impulsive and self-destructive acts, fears of abandonment, feelings of emptiness and boredom, recurrent suicide threats or self-mutilation.

   301.84 Passive-aggressive personality
DEF: Pattern of procrastination and refusal to meet standards; introduce own obstacles to success and exploit failure.

   301.89 Other
Personality: Personality:
   eccentric   masochistic
   "haltlose" type   psychoneurotic
   immature
> **EXCLUDES**   *psychoinfantile personality (301.59)*

301.9 Unspecified personality disorder
Pathological personality NOS
Personality disorder NOS
Psychopathic:
   constitutional state
   personality (disorder)

▲ ✓4ᵗʰ **302 Sexual and gender identity disorders**
> **EXCLUDES**   *sexual disorder manifest in:*
> *organic brain syndrome (290.0-294.9, 310.0-310.9)*
> *psychosis (295.0-298.9)*

▲   **302.0 Ego-dystonic sexual orientation**
Ego-dystonic lesbianism
▶Sexual orientation conflict disorder◀
> **EXCLUDES**   *homosexual pedophilia (302.2)*

   302.1 Zoophilia
Bestiality
DEF: A sociodeviant disorder marked by engaging in sexual intercourse with animals.

   302.2 Pedophilia
DEF: A sociodeviant condition of adults characterized by sexual activity with children.

▲   **302.3 Transvestic fetishism**
> **EXCLUDES**   *trans-sexualism (302.5)*

DEF: The desire to dress in clothing of opposite sex.

   302.4 Exhibitionism
DEF: Sexual deviant behavior; exposure of genitals to strangers; behavior prompted by intense sexual urges and fantasies.

✓5ᵗʰ **302.5 Trans-sexualism**
> **EXCLUDES**   *transvestism (302.3)*

DEF: Gender identity disturbance; overwhelming desire to change anatomic sex, due to belief that individual is a member of the opposite sex.

   302.50 With unspecified sexual history
   302.51 With asexual history
   302.52 With homosexual history
   302.53 With heterosexual history

▲   **302.6 Gender identity disorder in children**
Feminism in boys
▶Gender identity disorder NOS◀
> **EXCLUDES**   *gender identity disorder in adult (302.85)*
> *trans-sexualism (302.50-302.53)*
> *transvestism (302.3)*

✓5ᵗʰ **302.7 Psychosexual dysfunction**
> **EXCLUDES**   *impotence of organic origin (607.84)*
> *normal transient symptoms from ruptured hymen*
> *transient or occasional failures of erection due to fatigue, anxiety, alcohol, or drugs*

   302.70 Psychosexual dysfunction, unspecified
▶Sexual dysfunction NOS◀

   302.71 Hypoactive sexual desire disorder
> **EXCLUDES**   *decreased sexual desire NOS (799.81)*

   302.72 With inhibited sexual excitement
▶Female sexual arousal disorder◀
Frigidity
Impotence
▶Male erectile disorder◀

▲   **302.73 Female orgasmic disorder**   ♀
▲   **302.74 Male orgasmic disorder**   ♂
▲   **302.75 Premature ejaculation**   ♂
▲   **302.76 Dyspareunia, psychogenic**   ♀
Dyspareunia, psychogenic
DEF: Difficult or painful sex due to psychosomatic state.

▲   **302.79 With other specified psychosexual dysfunctions**
▶Sexual aversion disorder◀

✓5ᵗʰ **302.8 Other specified psychosexual disorders**
   302.81 Fetishism
DEF: Psychosexual disorder noted for intense sexual urges and arousal precipitated by fantasies; use of inanimate objects, such as clothing, to stimulate sexual arousal, orgasm.

   302.82 Voyeurism
DEF: Psychosexual disorder characterized by uncontrollable impulse to observe others, without their knowledge, who are nude or engaged in sexual activity.

   302.83 Sexual masochism
DEF: Psychosexual disorder noted for need to achieve sexual gratification through humiliating or hurtful acts inflicted on self.

   302.84 Sexual sadism
DEF: Psychosexual disorder noted for need to achieve sexual gratification through humiliating or hurtful acts inflicted on someone else.

▲   **302.85 Gender identity disorder in adolescents or adults**
EXCLUDES ▶ *gender identity disorder NOS (302.6)*
gender identity disorder in children (302.6)◀

302.89 Other
▶Frotteurism◀
Nymphomania
Satyriasis

302.9 Unspecified psychosexual disorder
▶Paraphilia NOS◀
Pathologic sexuality NOS
Sexual deviation NOS
▶Sexual disorder NOS◀

✓4th **303 Alcohol dependence syndrome**
Use additional code to identify any associated condition, as:
alcoholic psychoses (291.0-291.9)
drug dependence (304.0-304.9)
physical complications of alcohol, such as:
cerebral degeneration (331.7)
cirrhosis of liver (571.2)
epilepsy (345.0-345.9)
gastritis (535.3)
hepatitis (571.1)
liver damage NOS (571.3)
EXCLUDES *drunkenness NOS (305.0)*

The following fifth-digit subclassification is for use with category 303:
0 unspecified
1 continuous
2 episodic
3 in remission

AHA: 3Q, '95, 6; 2Q, '91, 9; 4Q, '88, 8; S-O, '86, 3

✓5th **303.0 Acute alcoholic intoxication**
Acute drunkenness in alcoholism

✓5th **303.9 Other and unspecified alcohol dependence**
Chronic alcoholism
Dipsomania
AHA: 2Q, '02, 4; 2Q, '89, 9

✓4th **304 Drug dependence**
EXCLUDES *nondependent abuse of drugs (305.1-305.9)*

The following fifth-digit subclassification is for use with category 304:
0 unspecified
1 continuous
2 episodic
3 in remission

AHA: 2Q, '91, 10; 4Q, '88, 8; S-O, '86, 3

✓5th **304.0 Opioid type dependence**
Heroin   Opium alkaloids and their
Meperidine   derivatives
Methadone   Synthetics with morphine-like
Morphine   effects
Opium

▲ ✓5th **304.1 Sedative, hypnotic or anxiolytic dependence**
Barbiturates
Nonbarbiturate sedatives and tranquilizers with a similar effect:
chlordiazepoxide   meprobamate
diazepam   methaqualone
glutethimide

✓5th **304.2 Cocaine dependence**
Coca leaves and derivatives

✓5th **304.3 Cannabis dependence**
Hashish   Marihuana
Hemp

✓5th **304.4 Amphetamine and other psychostimulant dependence**
Methylphenidate   Phenmetrazine

✓5th **304.5 Hallucinogen dependence**
Dimethyltryptamine [DMT]   Mescaline
Lysergic acid diethylamide   Psilocybin
[LSD] and derivatives

✓5th **304.6 Other specified drug dependence**
Absinthe addiction
Glue sniffing
▶Inhalant dependence
Phencyclidine dependence◀
EXCLUDES *tobacco dependence (305.1)*

✓5th **304.7 Combinations of opioid type drug with any other**
AHA: M-A, '86, 12

✓5th **304.8 Combinations of drug dependence excluding opioid type drug**
AHA: M-A, '86, 12

✓5th **304.9 Unspecified drug dependence**
Drug addiction NOS   Drug dependence NOS
AHA: For code 304.90: 4Q, '03, 103

✓4th **305 Nondependent abuse of drugs**
Note: Includes cases where a person, for whom no other diagnosis is possible, has come under medical care because of the maladaptive effect of a drug on which he is not dependent and that he has taken on his own initiative to the detriment of his health or social functioning.
EXCLUDES *alcohol dependence syndrome (303.0-303.9)*
drug dependence (304.0-304.9)
drug withdrawal syndrome (292.0)
poisoning by drugs or medicinal substances (960.0-979.9)

The following fifth-digit subclassification is for use with codes 305.0, 305.2-305.9:
0 unspecified
1 continuous
2 episodic
3 in remission

AHA: 2Q, '91, 10; 4Q, '88, 8; S-O, '86, 3

✓5th **305.0 Alcohol abuse**
Drunkenness NOS   "Hangover" (alcohol)
Excessive drinking   Inebriety NOS
of alcohol NOS
EXCLUDES *acute alcohol intoxication in alcoholism (303.0)*
alcoholic psychoses (291.0-291.9)
AHA: 3Q, '96, 16

305.1 Tobacco use disorder
Tobacco dependence
EXCLUDES *history of tobacco use (V15.82)*
AHA: 2Q, '96, 10; N-D, '84, 12

✓5th **305.2 Cannabis abuse**

✓5th **305.3 Hallucinogen abuse**
Acute intoxication from hallucinogens ["bad trips"]
LSD reaction

▲ ✓5th **305.4 Sedative, hypnotic or anxiolytic abuse**

✓5th **305.5 Opioid abuse**

✓5th **305.6 Cocaine abuse**
AHA: 1Q, '93, 25

✓5th **305.7 Amphetamine or related acting sympathomimetic abuse**
AHA: For code 305.70: 2Q, '03, 10-11

✓5th **305.8 Antidepressant type abuse**

✓5th **305.9 Other, mixed, or unspecified drug abuse**
▶Caffeine intoxication
Inhalant abuse◀
"Laxative habit"
Misuse of drugs NOS
Nonprescribed use of drugs or patent medicinals
▶Phencyclidine abuse◀
AHA: 3Q, '99, 20

✓4th ✓5th Additional Digit Required   Unspecified Code   Other Specified Code   Manifestation Code   ▶◀ Revised Text   ● New Code   ▲ Revised Code Title

Mental Disorders

306–307.23

✓4ᵗʰ **306 Physiological malfunction arising from mental factors**

INCLUDES   psychogenic:

physical symptoms ⎫ not involving
physiological   ⎬ tissue
manifestations   ⎭ damage

EXCLUDES   *hysteria (300.11-300.19)*
physical symptoms secondary to a psychiatric
    disorder classified elsewhere
psychic factors associated with physical
    conditions involving tissue damage
    classified elsewhere (316)
specific nonpsychotic mental disorders following
    organic brain damage (310.0-310.9)

DEF: Functional disturbances or interruptions due to mental or psychological causes; no tissue damage sustained in these conditions.

306.0   Musculoskeletal

Psychogenic paralysis   Psychogenic torticollis

EXCLUDES   *Gilles de la Tourette's syndrome*
    (307.23)
paralysis as hysterical or conversion
    reaction (300.11)
tics (307.20-307.22)

306.1   Respiratory

Psychogenic: Psychogenic:
air hunger   hyperventilation
cough   yawning
hiccough

EXCLUDES   *psychogenic asthma (316 and 493.9)*

306.2   Cardiovascular

Cardiac neurosis
Cardiovascular neurosis
Neurocirculatory asthenia
Psychogenic cardiovascular disorder

EXCLUDES   *psychogenic paroxysmal tachycardia*
    (316 and 427.2)

AHA: J-A, '85, 14

DEF: Neurocirculatory asthenia: functional nervous and circulatory irregularities with palpitations, dyspnea, fatigue, rapid pulse, precordial pain, fear of effort, discomfort during exercise, anxiety; also called DaCosta's syndrome, Effort syndrome, Irritable or Soldier's Heart.

306.3   Skin

Psychogenic pruritus

EXCLUDES   *psychogenic:*
    alopecia (316 and 704.00)
    dermatitis (316 and 692.9)
    eczema (316 and 691.8 or 692.9)
    urticaria (316 and 708.0-708.9)

306.4   Gastrointestinal

Aerophagy
Cyclical vomiting, psychogenic
Diarrhea, psychogenic
Nervous gastritis
Psychogenic dyspepsia

EXCLUDES   *cyclical vomiting NOS (536.2)*
globus hystericus (300.11)
mucous colitis (316 and 564.9)
psychogenic:
    cardiospasm (316 and 530.0)
    duodenal ulcer (316 and 532.0-
        532.9)
    gastric ulcer (316 and 531.0-531.9)
    peptic ulcer NOS (316 and 533.0-
        533.9)
    vomiting NOS (307.54)

AHA: 2Q, '89, 11

DEF: Aerophagy: excess swallowing of air, usually unconscious; related to anxiety; results in distended abdomen or belching, often interpreted by the patient as a physical disorder.

✓5ᵗʰ **306.5   Genitourinary**

EXCLUDES   *enuresis, psychogenic (307.6)*
frigidity (302.72)
impotence (302.72)
psychogenic dyspareunia (302.76)

306.50 Psychogenic genitourinary malfunction, unspecified

306.51 Psychogenic vaginismus   ♀

Functional vaginismus

DEF: Psychogenic response resulting in painful contractions of vaginal canal muscles; can be severe enough to prevent sexual intercourse.

306.52 Psychogenic dysmenorrhea   ♀

306.53 Psychogenic dysuria

306.59 Other

AHA: M-A, '87, 11

306.6   Endocrine

306.7   Organs of special sense

EXCLUDES   *hysterical blindness or deafness*
    (300.11)
psychophysical visual disturbances
    (368.16)

306.8   Other specified psychophysiological malfunction

Bruxism   Teeth grinding

306.9   Unspecified psychophysiological malfunction

Psychophysiologic disorder NOS
Psychosomatic disorder NOS

✓4ᵗʰ **307 Special symptoms or syndromes, not elsewhere classified**

Note: This category is intended for use if the psychopathology is manifested by a single specific symptom or group of symptoms which is not part of an organic illness or other mental disorder classifiable elsewhere.

EXCLUDES   *those due to mental disorders classified*
    elsewhere
those of organic origin

▲   **307.0   Stuttering**

EXCLUDES   *dysphasia (784.5)*
lisping or lalling (307.9)
retarded development of speech
    (315.31-315.39)

307.1   Anorexia nervosa

EXCLUDES   *eating disturbance NOS (307.50)*
feeding problem (783.3)
    of nonorganic origin (307.59)
loss of appetite (783.0)
    of nonorganic origin (307.59)

AHA: 4Q, '89, 11

✓5ᵗʰ **307.2   Tics**

EXCLUDES   *nail-biting or thumb-sucking (307.9)*
stereotypes occurring in isolation
    (307.3)
tics of organic origin (333.3)

DEF: Involuntary muscle response usually confined to the face, shoulders.

307.20 Tic disorder, unspecified

▶Tic disorder NOS◀

▲   **307.21 Transient tic disorder**
▲   **307.22 Chronic motor or vocal tic disorder**
▲   **307.23 Tourette's disorder**

Motor-verbal tic disorder

DEF: Syndrome of facial and vocal tics in childhood; progresses to spontaneous or involuntary jerking, obscene utterances, other uncontrollable actions considered inappropriate.

▲   **307.3 Stereotypic movement disorder**
Body-rocking   Spasmus nutans
Head banging   Stereotypes NOS
EXCLUDES   tics (307.20-307.23)
     of organic origin (333.3)

√5ᵗʰ **307.4 Specific disorders of sleep of nonorganic origin**
EXCLUDES   narcolepsy ▶(347.00-347.11)◀
     those of unspecified cause (780.50-780.59)

307.40 Nonorganic sleep disorder, unspecified

307.41 Transient disorder of initiating or maintaining sleep
Hyposomnia ⎱ associated with inter-
Insomnia   ⎰ mittent emotional
Sleeplessness   reactions or conflicts

307.42 Persistent disorder of initiating or maintaining sleep
Hyposomnia, insomnia, or sleeplessness associated with:
anxiety
conditioned arousal
depression (major) (minor)
psychosis

307.43 Transient disorder of initiating or maintaining wakefulness
Hypersomnia associated with acute or intermittent emotional reactions or conflicts

307.44 Persistent disorder of initiating or maintaining wakefulness
Hypersomnia associated with depression (major) (minor)

▲   **307.45 Circadian rhythm sleep disorder**
Irregular sleep-wake rhythm, nonorganic origin
Jet lag syndrome
Rapid time-zone change
Shifting sleep-work schedule

▲   **307.46 Sleep arousal disorder**
▶Night terror disorder
Night terrors
Sleep terror disorder
Sleepwalking
Somnambulism◀
DEF: Sleepwalking marked by extreme terror, panic, screaming, confusion; no recall of event upon arousal; term may refer to simply the act of sleepwalking.

307.47 Other dysfunctions of sleep stages or arousal from sleep
▶Dyssomnia NOS
Nightmare disorder◀
Nightmares:
NOS
REM-sleep type
Sleep drunkenness
▶Parasomnia NOS◀

307.48 Repetitive intrusions of sleep
Repetitive intrusion of sleep with:
atypical polysomnographic features
environmental disturbances
repeated REM-sleep interruptions

307.49 Other
"Short-sleeper"
Subjective insomnia complaint

√5ᵗʰ **307.5 Other and unspecified disorders of eating**
EXCLUDES   anorexia:
     nervosa (307.1)
     of unspecified cause (783.0)
     overeating, of unspecified cause (783.6)
     vomiting:
       NOS (787.0)
       cyclical (536.2)
       psychogenic (306.4)

307.50 Eating disorder, unspecified
▶Eating disorder NOS◀

▲   **307.51 Bulimia nervosa**
Overeating of nonorganic origin
DEF: Mental disorder commonly characterized by binge eating followed by self-induced vomiting; perceptions of being fat; and fear the inability to stop eating voluntarily.

307.52 Pica
Perverted appetite of nonorganic origin
DEF: Compulsive eating disorder characterized by craving for substances, other than food; such as paint chips or dirt.

▲   **307.53 Rumination disorder**
Regurgitation, of nonorganic origin, of food with reswallowing
EXCLUDES   obsessional rumination (300.3)

307.54 Psychogenic vomiting

307.59 Other
▶Feeding disorder of infancy or early childhood◀
Infantile feeding ⎱ of nonorganic
   disturbances   ⎰ origin
Loss of appetite

307.6 Enuresis
Enuresis (primary) (secondary) of nonorganic origin
EXCLUDES   enuresis of unspecified cause (788.3)
DEF: Involuntary urination past age of normal control; also called bedwetting; no trace to biological problem; focus on psychological issues.

307.7 Encopresis
Encopresis (continuous) (discontinuous) of nonorganic origin
EXCLUDES   encopresis of unspecified cause (787.6)
DEF: Inability to control bowel movements; cause traced to psychological, not biological, problems.

▲ √5ᵗʰ **307.8 Pain disorders related to psychological factors**
307.80 Psychogenic pain, site unspecified

307.81 Tension headache
EXCLUDES   headache:
     NOS (784.0)
     migraine (346.0-346.9)
AHA: N-D, '85, 16

▲   **307.89 Other**
▶Code first to site of pain◀
EXCLUDES ▶ pain disorder exclusively attributed to psychological factors (307.80)
     psychogenic pain (307.80)◀

307.9 Other and unspecified special symptoms or syndromes, not elsewhere classified
▶Communication   Lisping
   disorder NOS◀   Masturbation
Hair plucking   Nail-biting
Lalling   Thumb-sucking

√4ᵗʰ **308 Acute reaction to stress**
INCLUDES   catastrophic stress
     combat fatigue
     gross stress reaction (acute)
     transient disorders in response to exceptional physical or mental stress which usually subside within hours or days
EXCLUDES   adjustment reaction or disorder (309.0-309.9)
     chronic stress reaction (309.1-309.9)

308.0 Predominant disturbance of emotions
Anxiety   ⎱ as acute reaction to
Emotional crisis ⎰ exceptional
Panic state   [gross] stress

√4ᵗʰ √5ᵗʰ Additional Digit Required   Unspecified Code   Other Specified Code   Manifestation Code   ▶◀ Revised Text   ● New Code   ▲ Revised Code Title

Mental Disorders

308.1–310.9

308.1 Predominant disturbance of consciousness
Fugues as acute reaction to exceptional [gross] stress

308.2 Predominant psychomotor disturbance
Agitation states ⎱ as acute reaction to
Stupor   ⎰ exceptional [gross] stress

308.3 Other acute reactions to stress
Acute situational disturbance
▶Acute stress disorder◀
EXCLUDES   *prolonged posttraumatic emotional disturbance (309.81)*

308.4 Mixed disorders as reaction to stress

308.9 Unspecified acute reaction to stress

✓4ᵗʰ **309 Adjustment reaction**
INCLUDES   adjustment disorders
reaction (adjustment) to chronic stress
EXCLUDES   *acute reaction to major stress (308.0-308.9)*
neurotic disorders (300.0-300.9)

▲ **309.0 Adjustment disorder with depressed mood**
Grief reaction
EXCLUDES   *affective psychoses (296.0-296.9)*
neurotic depression (300.4)
prolonged depressive reaction (309.1)
psychogenic depressive psychosis (298.0)

309.1 Prolonged depressive reaction
EXCLUDES   *affective psychoses (296.0-296.9)*
brief depressive reaction (309.0)
neurotic depression (300.4)
psychogenic depressive psychosis (298.0)

✓5ᵗʰ **309.2 With predominant disturbance of other emotions**

309.21 Separation anxiety disorder
DEF: Abnormal apprehension by a child when physically separated from support environment; byproduct of abnormal symbiotic child-parent relationship.

309.22 Emancipation disorder of adolescence and early adult life
DEF: Adjustment reaction of late adolescence; conflict over independence from parental supervision; symptoms include difficulty in making decisions, increased reliance on parental advice, deliberate adoption of values in opposition of parents.

309.23 Specific academic or work inhibition

▲ **309.24 Adjustment disorder with anxiety**

▲ **309.28 Adjustment disorder with mixed anxiety and depressed mood**
Adjustment reaction with anxiety and depression

309.29 Other
Culture shock

▲ **309.3 Adjustment disorder with disturbance of conduct**
Conduct disturbance ⎱ as adjustment reaction
Destructiveness   ⎰
EXCLUDES   *destructiveness in child (312.9)*
disturbance of conduct NOS (312.9)
dyssocial behavior without manifest psychiatric disorder (V71.01-V71.02)
personality disorder with predominantly sociopathic or asocial manifestations (301.7)

▲ **309.4 Adjustment disorder with mixed disturbance of emotions and conduct**

✓5ᵗʰ **309.8 Other specified adjustment reactions**

▲ **309.81 Posttraumatic stress disorder**
Chronic posttraumatic stress disorder
Concentration camp syndrome
▶Posttraumatic stress disorder NOS◀
EXCLUDES   ▶*acute stress disorder (308.3)*◀
posttraumatic brain syndrome:
nonpsychotic (310.2)
psychotic (293.0-293.9)

DEF: Preoccupation with traumatic events beyond normal experience; events such as rape, personal assault, combat, natural disasters, accidents, torture precipitate disorder; also recurring flashbacks of trauma; symptoms include difficulty remembering, sleeping, or concentrating, and guilt feelings for surviving.

309.82 Adjustment reaction with physical symptoms

309.83 Adjustment reaction with withdrawal
Elective mutism as adjustment reaction
Hospitalism (in children) NOS

309.89 Other

309.9 Unspecified adjustment reaction
Adaptation reaction NOS
Adjustment reaction NOS

▲ ✓4ᵗʰ **310 Specific nonpsychotic mental disorders due to brain damage**
EXCLUDES   *neuroses, personality disorders, or other nonpsychotic conditions occurring in a form similar to that seen with functional disorders but in association with a physical condition (300.0-300.9, 301.0-301.9)*

310.0 Frontal lobe syndrome
Lobotomy syndrome
Postleucotomy syndrome [state]
EXCLUDES   *postcontusion syndrome (310.2)*

▲ **310.1 Personality change due to conditions classified elsewhere**
Cognitive or personality change of other type, of nonpsychotic severity
Organic psychosyndrome of nonpsychotic severity
Presbyophrenia NOS
Senility with mental changes of nonpsychotic severity
EXCLUDES   *memory loss of unknown cause (780.93)*

DEF: Personality disorder caused by organic factors, such as brain lesions, head trauma, or cerebrovascular accident (CVA).

310.2 Postconcussion syndrome
Postcontusion syndrome or encephalopathy
Posttraumatic brain syndrome, nonpsychotic
Status postcommotio cerebri
EXCLUDES   *frontal lobe syndrome (310.0)*
postencephalitic syndrome (310.8)
any organic psychotic conditions following head injury (293.0-294.0)

AHA: 4Q, '90, 24

DEF: Nonpsychotic disorder due to brain trauma, causes symptoms unrelated to any disease process; symptoms include amnesia, serial headaches, rapid heartbeat, fatigue, disrupted sleep patterns, inability to concentrate.

310.8 Other specified nonpsychotic mental disorders following organic brain damage
▶Mild memory disturbance◀
Postencephalitic syndrome
Other focal (partial) organic psychosyndromes

310.9 Unspecified nonpsychotic mental disorder following organic brain damage
AHA: 4Q, '03, 103

N Newborn Age: 0   P Pediatric Age: 0-17   M Maternity Age: 12-55   A Adult Age: 15-124   MSP Medicare Secondary Payer

311 Depressive disorder, not elsewhere classified

Depressive disorder NOS   Depression NOS
Depressive state NOS

> **EXCLUDES**   *acute reaction to major stress with depressive symptoms (308.0)*
> *affective personality disorder (301.10-301.13)*
> *affective psychoses (296.0-296.9)*
> *brief depressive reaction (309.0)*
> *depressive states associated with stressful events (309.0-309.1)*
> *disturbance of emotions specific to childhood and adolescence, with misery and unhappiness (313.1)*
> *mixed adjustment reaction with depressive symptoms (309.4)*
> *neurotic depression (300.4)*
> *prolonged depressive adjustment reaction (309.1)*
> *psychogenic depressive psychosis (298.0)*

AHA: 4Q, '03, 75

✓4ᵗʰ 312 Disturbance of conduct, not elsewhere classified

> **EXCLUDES**   *adjustment reaction with disturbance of conduct (309.3)*
> *drug dependence (304.0-304.9)*
> *dyssocial behavior without manifest psychiatric disorder (V71.01-V71.02)*
> *personality disorder with predominantly sociopathic or asocial manifestations (301.7)*
> *sexual deviations (302.0-302.9)*

The following fifth-digit subclassification is for use with categories 312.0-312.2:

     0   unspecified
     1   mild
     2   moderate
     3   severe

✓5ᵗʰ 312.0 Undersocialized conduct disorder, aggressive type

Aggressive outburst   Unsocialized aggressive
Anger reaction   disorder

DEF: Mental condition identified by behaviors disrespectful of others' rights and of age-appropriate social norms or rules; symptoms include bullying, vandalism, verbal and physical abusiveness, lying, stealing, defiance.

✓5ᵗʰ 312.1 Undersocialized conduct disorder, unaggressive type

Childhood truancy, unsocialized
Solitary stealing
Tantrums

✓5ᵗʰ 312.2 Socialized conduct disorder

Childhood truancy, socialized   Group delinquency
> **EXCLUDES**   *gang activity without manifest psychiatric disorder (V71.01)*

✓5ᵗʰ 312.3 Disorders of impulse control, not elsewhere classified

     312.30 Impulse control disorder, unspecified
     312.31 Pathological gambling
     312.32 Kleptomania
     312.33 Pyromania
     312.34 Intermittent explosive disorder
     312.35 Isolated explosive disorder
     312.39 Other
         ▶Trichotillomania◀

312.4 Mixed disturbance of conduct and emotions

Neurotic delinquency
> **EXCLUDES**   *compulsive conduct disorder (312.3)*

✓5ᵗʰ 312.8 Other specified disturbances of conduct, not elsewhere classified

     312.81 Conduct disorder, childhood onset type
     312.82 Conduct disorder, adolescent onset type
     312.89 Other conduct disorder
         ▶Conduct disorder of unspecified onset◀

312.9 Unspecified disturbance of conduct

Delinquency (juvenile)
▶Disruptive behavior disorder NOS◀

✓4ᵗʰ 313 Disturbance of emotions specific to childhood and adolescence

> **EXCLUDES**   *adjustment reaction (309.0-309.9)*
> *emotional disorder of neurotic type (300.0-300.9)*
> *masturbation, nail-biting, thumbsucking, and other isolated symptoms (307.0-307.9)*

313.0 Overanxious disorder

Anxiety and fearfulness   } of childhood and
Overanxious disorder   } adolescence

> **EXCLUDES**   *abnormal separation anxiety (309.21)*
> *anxiety states (300.00-300.09)*
> *hospitalism in children (309.83)*
> *phobic state (300.20-300.29)*

313.1 Misery and unhappiness disorder

> **EXCLUDES**   *depressive neurosis (300.4)*

✓5ᵗʰ 313.2 Sensitivity, shyness, and social withdrawal disorder

> **EXCLUDES**   *infantile autism (299.0)*
> *schizoid personality (301.20-301.22)*
> *schizophrenia (295.0-295.9)*

     313.21 Shyness disorder of childhood

Sensitivity reaction of childhood or adolescence

     313.22 Introverted disorder of childhood

Social withdrawal   } of childhood or
Withdrawal reaction } adolescence

     313.23 Selective mutism

> **EXCLUDES**   *elective mutism as adjustment reaction (309.83)*

313.3 Relationship problems

Sibling jealousy
> **EXCLUDES**   *relationship problems associated with aggression, destruction, or other forms of conduct disturbance (312.0-312.9)*

✓5ᵗʰ 313.8 Other or mixed emotional disturbances of childhood or adolescence

     313.81 Oppositional defiant disorder

DEF: Mental disorder of children noted for pervasive opposition, defiance of authority.

     313.82 Identity disorder

▶Identity problem◀
DEF: Distress of adolescents caused by inability to form acceptable self-identity; uncertainty about career choice, sexual orientation, moral values.

     313.83 Academic underachievement disorder
     313.89 Other   P

▶Reactive attachment disorder of infancy or early childhood◀

313.9 Unspecified emotional disturbance of childhood or adolescence   P

▶Mental disorder of infancy, childhood or adolescence NOS◀

✓4ᵗʰ 314 Hyperkinetic syndrome of childhood

> **EXCLUDES**   *hyperkinesis as symptom of underlying disorder—code the underlying disorder*

DEF: A behavioral disorder usually diagnosed at an early age; characterized by the inability to focus attention for a normal period of time.

✓5ᵗʰ 314.0 Attention deficit disorder

Adult   Child

     314.00 Without mention of hyperactivity

Predominantly inattentive type
AHA: 1Q, '97, 8

✓4ᵗʰ
✓5ᵗʰ Additional Digit Required   Unspecified Code   Other Specified Code   Manifestation Code   ▶◀ Revised Text   ● New Code   ▲ Revised Code Title

2005 ICD•9•CM   **October 2004 • Volume 1 — 75**

Mental Disorders

314.01–319

314.01 With hyperactivity
Combined type
Overactivity NOS
Predominantly hyperactive/impulsive type
Simple disturbance of attention with
overactivity
AHA: 1Q, '97, 8

314.1 Hyperkinesis with developmental delay
Developmental disorder of hyperkinesis
Use additional code to identify any associated
neurological disorder

314.2 Hyperkinetic conduct disorder
Hyperkinetic conduct disorder without
developmental delay
EXCLUDES *hyperkinesis with significant delays in
specific skills (314.1)*

**314.8 Other specified manifestations of hyperkinetic
syndrome**

314.9 Unspecified hyperkinetic syndrome
Hyperkinetic reaction of childhood or adolescence
NOS
Hyperkinetic syndrome NOS

✓4ᵗʰ **315 Specific delays in development**
EXCLUDES *that due to a neurological disorder (320.0-389.9)*

✓5ᵗʰ **315.0 Specific reading disorder**

315.00 Reading disorder, unspecified

315.01 Alexia
DEF: Lack of ability to understand written language;
manifestation of aphasia.

315.02 Developmental dyslexia
DEF: Serious impairment of reading skills unexplained in
relation to general intelligence and teaching processes;
it can be inherited or congenital.

315.09 Other
Specific spelling difficulty

▲ **315.1 Mathematics disorder**
Dyscalculia

315.2 Other specific learning difficulties
▶Disorder of written expression◀
EXCLUDES *specific arithmetical disorder (315.1)
specific reading disorder (315.00-
315.09)*

✓5ᵗʰ **315.3 Developmental speech or language disorder**
▲ **315.31 Expressive language disorder**
Developmental aphasia
Word deafness
EXCLUDES *acquired aphasia (784.3)
elective mutism (309.83,
313.0, 313.23)*

▲ **315.32 Mixed receptive-expressive language
disorder**
AHA: 4Q, '96, 30

315.39 Other
Developmental articulation disorder
Dyslalia
▶Phonological disorder◀
EXCLUDES *lisping and lalling (307.9)
stammering and stuttering
(307.0)*

▲ **315.4 Developmental coordination disorder**
Clumsiness syndrome   Specific motor development
Dyspraxia syndrome   disorder

315.5 Mixed development disorder
AHA: 2Q, '02, 11

315.8 Other specified delays in development
315.9 Unspecified delay in development
Developmental disorder NOS
▶Learning disorder NOS◀

**316 Psychic factors associated with diseases classified
elsewhere**
Psychologic factors in physical conditions classified elsewhere
Use additional code to identify the associated physical
condition, as:
psychogenic:
asthma (493.9)
dermatitis (692.9)
duodenal ulcer (532.0-532.9)
eczema (691.8, 692.9)
gastric ulcer (531.0-531.9)
mucous colitis (564.9)
paroxysmal tachycardia (427.2)
ulcerative colitis (556)
urticaria (708.0-708.9)
psychosocial dwarfism (259.4)
EXCLUDES *physical symptoms and physiological
malfunctions, not involving tissue damage,
of mental origin (306.0-306.9)*

MENTAL RETARDATION (317-319)
Use additional code(s) to identify any associated psychiatric
or physical condition(s)

317 Mild mental retardation
High-grade defect
IQ 50-70
Mild mental subnormality

✓4ᵗʰ **318 Other specified mental retardation**
318.0 Moderate mental retardation
IQ 35-49
Moderate mental subnormality

318.1 Severe mental retardation
IQ 20-34
Severe mental subnormality

318.2 Profound mental retardation
IQ under 20
Profound mental subnormality

319 Unspecified mental retardation
Mental deficiency NOS
Mental subnormality NOS

6. NERVOUS SYSTEM AND SENSE ORGANS (320-389)

INFLAMMATORY DISEASES OF THE CENTRAL NERVOUS SYSTEM
(320-326)

√4ᵗʰ **320 Bacterial meningitis**

INCLUDES
arachnoiditis ⎫
leptomeningitis ⎪
meningitis ⎬ bacterial
meningoencephalitis ⎪
meningomyelitis ⎪
pachymeningitis ⎭

AHA: J-F, '87, 6

DEF: Bacterial infection causing inflammation of the lining of the brain and/or spinal cord.

320.0 Hemophilus meningitis
Meningitis due to Hemophilus influenzae [H. influenzae]

320.1 Pneumococcal meningitis

320.2 Streptococcal meningitis

320.3 Staphylococcal meningitis

320.7 Meningitis in other bacterial diseases classified elsewhere
Code first underlying disease, as:
actinomycosis (039.8)
listeriosis (027.0)
typhoid fever (002.0)
whooping cough (033.0-033.9)
EXCLUDES meningitis (in):
epidemic (036.0)
gonococcal (098.82)
meningococcal (036.0)
salmonellosis (003.21)
syphilis:
NOS (094.2)
congenital (090.42)
meningovascular (094.2)
secondary (091.81)
tuberculous (013.0)

√5ᵗʰ **320.8 Meningitis due to other specified bacteria**
320.81 Anaerobic meningitis
Bacteroides (fragilis)
Gram-negative anaerobes

320.82 Meningitis due to gram-negative bacteria, not elsewhere classified
Aerobacter aerogenes
Escherichia coli [E. coli]
Friedländer bacillus
Klebsiella pneumoniae
Proteus morganii
Pseudomonas
EXCLUDES gram-negative anaerobes (320.81)

320.89 Meningitis due to other specified bacteria
Bacillus pyocyaneus

320.9 Meningitis due to unspecified bacterium
Meningitis:
bacterial NOS
purulent NOS
pyogenic NOS
suppurative NOS

√4ᵗʰ **321 Meningitis due to other organisms**

INCLUDES
arachnoiditis ⎫
leptomeningitis ⎪ due to organisms
meningitis ⎬ other than
pachymeningitis ⎭ bacteria

AHA: J-F, '87, 6

DEF: Infection causing inflammation of the lining of the brain and/or spinal cord, due to organisms other than bacteria.

321.0 Cryptococcal meningitis
Code first underlying disease (117.5)

321.1 Meningitis in other fungal diseases
Code first underlying disease (110.0-118)
EXCLUDES meningitis in:
candidiasis (112.83)
coccidioidomycosis (114.2)
histoplasmosis (115.01, 115.11, 115.91)

321.2 Meningitis due to viruses not elsewhere classified
Code first underlying disease, as:
meningitis due to arbovirus (060.0-066.9)
EXCLUDES meningitis (due to):
abacterial (047.0-047.9)
adenovirus (049.1)
aseptic NOS (047.9)
Coxsackie (virus)(047.0)
ECHO virus (047.1)
enterovirus (047.0-047.9)
herpes simplex virus (054.72)
herpes zoster virus (053.0)
lymphocytic choriomeningitis virus (049.0)
mumps (072.1)
viral NOS (047.9)
meningo-eruptive syndrome (047.1)

321.3 Meningitis due to trypanosomiasis
Code first underlying disease (086.0-086.9)

321.4 Meningitis in sarcoidosis
Code first underlying disease (135)

321.8 Meningitis due to other nonbacterial organisms classified elsewhere
Code first underlying disease
EXCLUDES leptospiral meningitis (100.81)

√4ᵗʰ **322 Meningitis of unspecified cause**

INCLUDES
arachnoiditis ⎫
leptomeningitis ⎪ with no organism
meningitis ⎬ specified as
pachymeningitis ⎭ cause

AHA: J-F, '87, 6

DEF: Infection causing inflammation of the lining of the brain and/or spinal cord, due to unspecified cause.

322.0 Nonpyogenic meningitis
Meningitis with clear cerebrospinal fluid

322.1 Eosinophilic meningitis

322.2 Chronic meningitis

322.9 Meningitis, unspecified

√4ᵗʰ **323 Encephalitis, myelitis, and encephalomyelitis**

INCLUDES
acute disseminated encephalomyelitis
meningoencephalitis, except bacterial
meningomyelitis, except bacterial
myelitis (acute):
ascending
transverse
EXCLUDES bacterial:
meningoencephalitis (320.0-320.9)
meningomyelitis (320.0-320.9)

DEF: Encephalitis: inflammation of brain tissues.

DEF: Myelitis: inflammation of the spinal cord.

DEF: Encephalomyelitis: inflammation of brain and spinal cord.

√4ᵗʰ
√5ᵗʰ Additional Digit Required   Unspecified Code   Other Specified Code   Manifestation Code   ▶◀ Revised Text   ● New Code   ▲ Revised Code Title

Nervous System and Sense Organs

323.0–330.2

323.0 *Encephalitis in viral diseases classified elsewhere*

Code first underlying disease, as:
cat-scratch disease (078.3)
infectious mononucleosis (075)
ornithosis (073.7)

EXCLUDES   encephalitis (in):
arthropod-borne viral (062.0-064)
herpes simplex (054.3)
mumps (072.2)
other viral diseases of central
nervous system (049.8-049.9)
poliomyelitis (045.0-045.9)
rubella (056.01)
slow virus infections of central
nervous system (046.0-046.9)
viral NOS (049.9)

323.1 *Encephalitis in rickettsial diseases classified elsewhere*

Code first underlying disease (080-083.9)

DEF: Inflammation of the brain caused by rickettsial disease carried by louse, tick, or mite.

323.2 *Encephalitis in protozoal diseases classified elsewhere*

Code first underlying disease, as:
malaria (084.0-084.9)
trypanosomiasis (086.0-086.9)

DEF: Inflammation of the brain caused by protozoal disease carried by mosquitoes and flies.

323.4 *Other encephalitis due to infection classified elsewhere*

Code first underlying disease

EXCLUDES   encephalitis (in):
meningococcal (036.1)
syphilis:
NOS (094.81)
congenital (090.41)
toxoplasmosis (130.0)
tuberculosis (013.6)
meningoencephalitis due to free-living
ameba [Naegleria] (136.2)

323.5 **Encephalitis following immunization procedures**

Encephalitis   } postimmunization or
Encephalomyelitis }   postvaccinal

Use additional E code to identify vaccine

323.6 *Postinfectious encephalitis*

Code first underlying disease

EXCLUDES   encephalitis:
postchickenpox (052.0)
postmeasles (055.0)

DEF: Infection, inflammation of brain several weeks following the outbreak of a systemic infection.

323.7 *Toxic encephalitis*

Code first underlying cause, as:
carbon tetrachloride (982.1)
hydroxyquinoline derivatives (961.3)
lead (984.0-984.9)
mercury (985.0)
thallium (985.8)

AHA: 2Q, '97, 8

323.8 **Other causes of encephalitis**

323.9 **Unspecified cause of encephalitis**

✓4ᵗʰ **324 Intracranial and intraspinal abscess**

324.0 **Intracranial abscess**

Abscess (embolic):   Abscess (embolic) of brain
cerebellar   [any part]:
cerebral   epidural
                           extradural
                           otogenic
                           subdural

EXCLUDES   tuberculous (013.3)

324.1 **Intraspinal abscess**

Abscess (embolic) of spinal cord [any part]:
epidural
extradural
subdural

EXCLUDES   tuberculous (013.5)

324.9 **Of unspecified site**

Extradural or subdural abscess NOS

325 Phlebitis and thrombophlebitis of intracranial venous sinuses

Embolism   } of cavernous, lateral, or
Endophlebitis   }   other intracranial
Phlebitis, septic or   }   or unspecified
    suppurative   }   intracranial
Thrombophlebitis   }   venous sinus
Thrombosis   }

EXCLUDES   that specified as:
complicating pregnancy, childbirth, or the
puerperium (671.5)
of nonpyogenic origin (437.6)

DEF: Inflammation and formation of blood clot in a vein within the brain or its lining.

326 Late effects of intracranial abscess or pyogenic infection

Note: This category is to be used to indicate conditions whose primary classification is to 320-325 [excluding 320.7, 321.0-321.8, 323.0-323.4, 323.6-323.7] as the cause of late effects, themselves classifiable elsewhere. The "late effects" include conditions specified as such, or as sequelae, which may occur at any time after the resolution of the causal condition.
Use additional code to identify condition, as:
hydrocephalus (331.4)
paralysis (342.0-342.9, 344.0-344.9)

HEREDITARY AND DEGENERATIVE DISEASES OF THE CENTRAL NERVOUS SYSTEM (330-337)

EXCLUDES   hepatolenticular degeneration (275.1)
multiple sclerosis (340)
other demyelinating diseases of central nervous
system (341.0-341.9)

✓4ᵗʰ **330 Cerebral degenerations usually manifest in childhood**

Use additional code to identify associated mental retardation

330.0 **Leukodystrophy**

Krabbe's disease   Pelizaeus-Merzbacher
Leukodystrophy   disease
   NOS   Sulfatide lipidosis
   globoid cell
   metachromatic
   sudanophilic

DEF: Hereditary disease of arylsulfatase or cerebroside sulfatase; characterized by a diffuse loss of myelin in CNS; infantile form causes blindness, motor disturbances, rigidity, mental deterioration and, occasionally, convulsions.

330.1 **Cerebral lipidoses**

Amaurotic (familial) idiocy   Disease:
Disease: Spielmeyer-Vogt
   Batten   Tay-Sachs
   Jansky-Bielschowsky   Gangliosidosis
   Kufs'

DEF: Genetic disorder causing abnormal lipid accumulation in the reticuloendothelial cells of the brain.

330.2 *Cerebral degeneration in generalized lipidoses*

Code first underlying disease, as:
Fabry's disease (272.7)
Gaucher's disease (272.7)
Niemann-Pick disease (272.7)
sphingolipidosis (272.7)

330.3   *Cerebral degeneration of childhood in other diseases classified elsewhere*

     Code first underlying disease, as:
        Hunter's disease (277.5)
        mucopolysaccharidosis (277.5)

330.8   **Other specified cerebral degenerations in childhood**

     Alpers' disease or gray-matter degeneration
     Infantile necrotizing encephalomyelopathy
     Leigh's disease
     Subacute necrotizing encephalopathy or encephalomyelopathy

     AHA: N-D, '85, 5

330.9   **Unspecified cerebral degeneration in childhood**

✓4th **331**   **Other cerebral degenerations**

331.0   **Alzheimer's disease**

     AHA: 4Q, '00, 41; 4Q, '99, 7; N-D, '84, 20

     DEF: Diffuse atrophy of cerebral cortex; causing a progressive decline in intellectual and physical functions, including memory loss, personality changes and profound dementia.

✓5th **331.1**   **Frontotemporal dementia**
     Use additional code for associated behavioral disturbance (294.10-294.11)

     AHA: ▶4Q, '03, 57◀

     DEF: Rare, progressive degenerative brain disease, similar to Alzheimer's; cortical atrophy affects the frontal and temporal lobes.

     331.11   **Pick's disease**

        DEF: ▶ A less common form of progressive frontotemporal dementia with asymmetrical atrophy of the frontal and temporal regions of the cerebral cortex including abnormal rounded brain cells called Pick cells together with the presence of abnormal staining of protein (called tau) within the cells, called Pick bodies; symptoms include prominent apathy, deterioration of social skills, behavioral changes such as disinhibition and restlessness, echolalia, impairment of language, memory, and intellect, increased carelessness, poor personal hygiene, and decreased attention span. ◀

     331.19   **Other frontotemporal dementia**
        Frontal dementia

331.2   **Senile degeneration of brain**
     EXCLUDES   senility NOS (797)

331.3   **Communicating hydrocephalus**
     EXCLUDES   congenital hydrocephalus (741.0, 742.3)

     AHA: S-O, '85, 12

     DEF: Subarachnoid hemorrhage and meningitis causing excess buildup of cerebrospinal fluid in cavities due to nonabsorption of fluid back through fluid pathways.

331.4   **Obstructive hydrocephalus**
     Acquired hydrocephalus NOS
     EXCLUDES   congenital hydrocephalus (741.0, 742.3)

     AHA: ▶4Q, '03, 106;◀ 1Q, '99, 9

     DEF: Obstruction of cerebrospinal fluid passage from brain into spinal canal.

331.7   *Cerebral degeneration in diseases classified elsewhere*

     Code first underlying disease, as:
        alcoholism (303.0-303.9)
        beriberi (265.0)
        cerebrovascular disease (430-438)
        congenital hydrocephalus (741.0, 742.3)
        neoplastic disease (140.0-239.9)
        myxedema (244.0-244.9)
        vitamin B_{12} deficiency (266.2)

     EXCLUDES   cerebral degeneration in:
        Jakob-Creutzfeldt disease (046.1)
        progressive multifocal leukoencephalopathy (046.3)
        subacute spongiform encephalopathy (046.1)

✓5th **331.8**   **Other cerebral degeneration**

331.81   **Reye's syndrome**   P

     DEF: Rare childhood illness, often developed after a bout of viral upper respiratory infection; characterized by vomiting, elevated serum transaminase, changes in liver and other viscera; symptoms may be followed by an encephalopathic phase with brain swelling, disturbances of consciousness and seizures; can be fatal.

331.82   **Dementia with Lewy bodies**
     Dementia with Parkinsonism
     Lewy body dementia
     Lewy body disease
     Use additional code for associated behavioral disturbance (294.10-294.11)

     AHA: ▶4Q, '03, 57◀

     DEF: ▶A cerebral dementia with neurophysiologic changes including increased hippocampal volume, hypoperfusion in the occipital lobes, and beta amyloid deposits with neurofibrillarity tangles, atrophy of cortex and brainstem, hallmark neuropsychologic characteristics are fluctuating cognition with pronounced variation in attention and alertness; recurrent hallucinations; and parkinsonism. ◀

331.89   **Other**
     Cerebral ataxia

331.9   **Cerebral degeneration, unspecified**

✓4th **332**   **Parkinson's disease**
     EXCLUDES   dementia with Parkinsonism (331.82)

332.0   **Paralysis agitans**
     Parkinsonism or Parkinson's disease:
        NOS
        idiopathic
        primary

     AHA: M-A, '87, 7

     DEF: Form of parkinsonism; progressive, occurs in senior years; characterized by masklike facial expression; condition affects ability to stand erect, walk smoothly; weakened muscles, also tremble and involuntarily movement.

332.1   **Secondary Parkinsonism**
     Parkinsonism due to drugs
     Use additional E code to identify drug, if drug-induced

     EXCLUDES   Parkinsonism (in):
        Huntington's disease (333.4)
        progressive supranuclear palsy (333.0)
        Shy-Drager syndrome (333.0)
        syphilitic (094.82)

Nervous System and Sense Organs

330.3–332.1

✓4th ✓5th   Additional Digit Required   Unspecified Code   Other Specified Code   Manifestation Code   ▶◀ Revised Text   ● New Code   ▲ Revised Code Title

2005 ICD•9•CM   **February 2004 • Volume 1 — 79**

Nervous System and Sense Organs

333–335.19

✓4ᵗʰ **333 Other extrapyramidal disease and abnormal movement disorders**

> INCLUDES   other forms of extrapyramidal, basal ganglia, or striatopallidal disease
>
> EXCLUDES   *abnormal movements of head NOS (781.0)*

333.0 Other degenerative diseases of the basal ganglia

> Atrophy or degeneration:
>> olivopontocerebellar [Déjérine-Thomas syndrome]
>> pigmentary pallidal [Hallervorden-Spatz disease]
>> striatonigral
>
> Parkinsonian syndrome associated with:
>> idiopathic orthostatic hypotension
>> symptomatic orthostatic hypotension
>
> Progressive supranuclear ophthalmoplegia
> Shy-Drager syndrome
>
> **AHA:** 3Q, '96, 8

333.1 Essential and other specified forms of tremor

> Benign essential tremor
> Familial tremor
> Use additional E code to identify drug, if drug-induced
>
> EXCLUDES   *tremor NOS (781.0)*

333.2 Myoclonus

> Familial essential myoclonus
> Progressive myoclonic epilepsy
> Unverricht-Lundborg disease
> Use additional E code to identify drug, if drug-induced
>
> **AHA:** 3Q, '97, 4; M-A, '87, 12
>
> **DEF:** Spontaneous movements or contractions of muscles.

333.3 Tics of organic origin

> Use additional E code to identify drug, if drug-induced
>
> EXCLUDES   *Gilles de la Tourette's syndrome (307.23)*
>   *habit spasm (307.22)*
>   *tic NOS (307.20)*

333.4 Huntington's chorea

> **DEF:** Genetic disease; characterized by chronic progressive mental deterioration; dementia and death within 15 years of onset.

333.5 Other choreas

> Hemiballism(us)
> Paroxysmal choreo-athetosis
> Use additional E code to identify drug, if drug-induced
>
> EXCLUDES   *Sydenham's or rheumatic chorea (392.0-392.9)*

333.6 Idiopathic torsion dystonia

> Dystonia:
>> deformans progressiva
>> musculorum deformans
>> (Schwalbe-) Ziehen-Oppenheim disease
>
> **DEF:** Sustained muscular contractions, causing twisting and repetitive movements that result in abnormal postures of trunk and limbs; etiology unknown.

333.7 Symptomatic torsion dystonia

> Athetoid cerebral palsy [Vogt's disease]
> Double athetosis (syndrome)
> Use additional E code to identify drug, if drug-induced

✓5ᵗʰ **333.8 Fragments of torsion dystonia**

> Use additional E code to identify drug, if drug-induced

333.81 Blepharospasm

> **DEF:** Uncontrolled winking or blinking due to orbicularis oculi muscle spasm.

333.82 Orofacial dyskinesia

> **DEF:** Uncontrolled movement of mouth or facial muscles.

333.83 Spasmodic torticollis

> EXCLUDES   *torticollis:*
>   *NOS (723.5)*
>   *hysterical (300.11)*
>   *psychogenic (306.0)*
>
> **DEF:** Uncontrolled movement of head due to spasms of neck muscle.

333.84 Organic writers' cramp

> EXCLUDES   *pychogenic (300.89)*

333.89 Other

✓5ᵗʰ **333.9 Other and unspecified extrapyramidal diseases and abnormal movement disorders**

333.90 Unspecified extrapyramidal disease and abnormal movement disorder

333.91 Stiff-man syndrome

333.92 Neuroleptic malignant syndrome

> Use additional E code to identify drug
>
> **AHA:** 4Q, '94, 37

333.93 Benign shuddering attacks

> **AHA:** 4Q, '94, 37

333.99 Other

> Restless legs
>
> **AHA:** 4Q, '94, 37

✓4ᵗʰ **334 Spinocerebellar disease**

> EXCLUDES   *olivopontocerebellar degeneration (333.0)*
>   *peroneal muscular atrophy (356.1)*

334.0 Friedreich's ataxia

> **DEF:** Genetic recessive disease of children; sclerosis of dorsal, lateral spinal cord columns; characterized by ataxia, speech impairment, swaying and irregular movements, with muscle paralysis, especially of lower limbs.

334.1 Hereditary spastic paraplegia

334.2 Primary cerebellar degeneration

> Cerebellar ataxia: Primary cerebellar
>   Marie's   degeneration:
>   Sanger-Brown   NOS
>   Dyssynergia cerebellaris   hereditary
>   myoclonica   sporadic
>
> **AHA:** M-A, '87, 9

334.3 Other cerebellar ataxia

> Cerebellar ataxia NOS
> Use additional E code to identify drug, if drug-induced

334.4 *Cerebellar ataxia in diseases classified elsewhere*

> *Code first underlying disease, as:*
>> alcoholism (303.0-303.9)
>> myxedema (244.0-244.9)
>> neoplastic disease (140.0-239.9)

334.8 Other spinocerebellar diseases

> Ataxia-telangiectasia [Louis-Bar syndrome]
> Corticostriatal-spinal degeneration

334.9 Spinocerebellar disease, unspecified

✓4ᵗʰ **335 Anterior horn cell disease**

335.0 Werdnig-Hoffmann disease

> Infantile spinal muscular atrophy
> Progressive muscular atrophy of infancy
>
> **DEF:** Spinal muscle atrophy manifested in prenatal period or shortly after birth; symptoms include hypotonia, atrophy of skeletal muscle; death occurs in infancy.

✓5ᵗʰ **335.1 Spinal muscular atrophy**

335.10 Spinal muscular atrophy, unspecified

335.11 Kugelberg-Welander disease

> Spinal muscular atrophy:
>> familial
>> juvenile
>
> **DEF:** Hereditary; juvenile muscle atrophy; appears during first two decades of life; due to lesions of anterior horns of spinal cord; includes wasting, diminution of lower body muscles and twitching.

335.19 Other

> Adult spinal muscular atrophy

N   Newborn Age: 0   P   Pediatric Age: 0-17   M   Maternity Age: 12-55   A   Adult Age: 15-124   MSP   Medicare Secondary Payer

✓5th **335.2　Motor neuron disease**

　　335.20　**Amyotrophic lateral sclerosis**　　▲
　　　　　Motor neuron disease (bulbar) (mixed type)
　　　　AHA: 4Q, '95, 81

　　335.21　**Progressive muscular atrophy**
　　　　　Duchenne-Aran muscular atrophy
　　　　　Progressive muscular atrophy (pure)
　　335.22　**Progressive bulbar palsy**
　　335.23　**Pseudobulbar palsy**
　　335.24　**Primary lateral sclerosis**
　　335.29　**Other**

335.8　**Other anterior horn cell diseases**
335.9　**Anterior horn cell disease, unspecified**

✓4th **336　Other diseases of spinal cord**

336.0　**Syringomyelia and syringobulbia**
　　AHA: 1Q, '89, 10

336.1　**Vascular myelopathies**
　　Acute infarction of spinal cord (embolic)
　　　(nonembolic)
　　Arterial thrombosis of spinal cord
　　Edema of spinal cord
　　Hematomyelia
　　Subacute necrotic myelopathy

336.2　***Subacute combined degeneration of spinal
　　　cord in diseases classified elsewhere***
　　Code first underlying disease, as:
　　　pernicious anemia (281.0)
　　　other vitamin B$_{12}$ deficiency anemia (281.1)
　　　vitamin B$_{12}$ deficiency (266.2)

336.3　***Myelopathy in other diseases classified elsewhere***
　　Code first underlying disease, as:
　　　myelopathy in neoplastic disease (140.0-239.9)
　　　EXCLUDES *myelopathy in:*
　　　　　intervertebral disc disorder (722.70-
　　　　　722.73)
　　　　　spondylosis (721.1, 721.41-721.42,
　　　　　721.91)
　　AHA: 3Q, '99, 5

336.8　**Other myelopathy**
　　Myelopathy:　　　　Myelopathy:
　　　drug-induced　　　　radiation-induced
　　Use additonal E code to identify cause

336.9　**Unspecified disease of spinal cord**
　　Cord compression NOS　　Myelopathy NOS
　　　EXCLUDES *myelitis (323.0-323.9)*
　　　　　spinal (canal) stenosis (723.0, 724.00-
　　　　　724.09)

✓4th **337　Disorders of the autonomic nervous system**
　　INCLUDES　disorders of peripheral autonomic,
　　　　sympathetic, parasympathetic, or
　　　　vegetative system
　　EXCLUDES　*familial dysautonomia [Riley-Day syndrome]*
　　　　(742.8)

337.0　**Idiopathic peripheral autonomic neuropathy**
　　Carotid sinus syncope or syndrome
　　Cervical sympathetic dystrophy or paralysis

337.1　***Peripheral autonomic neuropathy in disorders
　　　classified elsewhere***
　　Code first underlying disease, as:
　　　amyloidosis (277.3)
　　　diabetes (250.6)
　　AHA: 2Q, '93, 6; 3Q, '91, 9; N-D, '84, 9

✓5th 337.2　**Reflex sympathetic dystrophy**
　　AHA: 4Q, '93, 24

　　DEF: Disturbance of the sympathetic nervous system evidenced by
　　sweating, pain, pallor and edema following injury to nerves or
　　blood vessels.

　　337.20　**Reflex sympathetic dystrophy,unspecified**
　　337.21　**Reflex sympathetic dystrophy of the upper
　　　　limb**
　　337.22　**Reflex sympathetic dystrophy of the lower
　　　　limb**
　　337.29　**Reflex sympathetic dystrophy of other
　　　　specified site**

337.3　**Autonomic dysreflexia**
　　Use additional code to identify the cause, such as:
　　　decubitus ulcer ▶(707.00-707.09)◀
　　　fecal impaction (560.39)
　　　urinary tract infection (599.0)
　　AHA: 4Q, '98, 37

　　DEF: Noxious stimuli evokes paroxysmal hypertension,
　　bradycardia, excess sweating, headache, pilomotor responses,
　　facial flushing, and nasal congestion due to uncontrolled
　　parasympathetic nerve response; usually occurs in patients with
　　spinal cord injury above major sympathetic outflow tract (T$_6$).

337.9　**Unspecified disorder of autonomic nervous system**

OTHER DISORDERS OF THE CENTRAL NERVOUS SYSTEM (340-349)

340　Multiple sclerosis　　▲
　　Disseminated or multiple sclerosis:
　　　NOS
　　　brain stem
　　　cord
　　　generalized

✓4th **341　Other demyelinating diseases of central nervous system**

341.0　**Neuromyelitis optica**
341.1　**Schilder's disease**
　　Baló's concentric sclerosis
　　Encephalitis periaxialis:
　　　concentrica [Baló's]
　　　diffusa [Schilder's]
　　DEF: Chronic leukoencephalopathy of children and adolescents;
　　symptoms include blindness, deafness, bilateral spasticity and
　　progressive mental deterioration.

341.8　**Other demyelinating diseases of central
　　　nervous system**
　　Central demyelination of corpus callosum
　　Central pontine myelinosis
　　Marchiafava (-Bignami) disease
　　AHA: N-D, '87, 6

341.9　**Demyelinating disease of central nervous
　　　system, unspecified**

✓4th **342　Hemiplegia and hemiparesis**
　　Note: This category is to be used when hemiplegia (complete)
　　　(incomplete) is reported without further specification, or
　　　is stated to be old or long-standing but of unspecified
　　　cause. The category is also for use in multiple coding to
　　　identify these types of hemiplegia resulting from any
　　　cause.
　　EXCLUDES　*congenital (343.1)*
　　　　hemiplegia due to late effect of cerebrovascular
　　　　accident (438.20-438.22)
　　　　infantile NOS (343.4)

　　The following fifth-digits are for use with codes 342.0-342.9:
　　　0　**affecting unspecified side**
　　　1　**affecting dominant side**
　　　2　**affecting nondominant side**
　　AHA: 4Q, '94, 38

✓5th 342.0　**Flaccid hemiplegia**
✓5th 342.1　**Spastic hemiplegia**
✓5th 342.8　**Other specified hemiplegia**
✓5th 342.9　**Hemiplegia, unspecified**
　　AHA: 4Q, '98, 87

✓4th
✓5th Additional Digit Required　　　Unspecified Code　　　Other Specified Code　　　Manifestation Code　　　▶◀ Revised Text　　　● New Code　　　▲ Revised Code Title

Nervous System and Sense Organs

335.2–342.9

Nervous System and Sense Organs

343–345.3

√4th **343 Infantile cerebral palsy**
INCLUDES   cerebral:
palsy NOS
spastic infantile paralysis
congenital spastic paralysis (cerebral)
Little's disease
paralysis (spastic) due to birth injury:
intracranial
spinal
EXCLUDES   *hereditary cerebral paralysis, such as:*
hereditary spastic paraplegia (334.1)
Vogt's disease (333.7)
spastic paralysis specified as noncongenital or
noninfantile (344.0-344.9)

343.0   Diplegic
Congenital diplegia   Congenital paraplegia
DEF: Paralysis affecting both sides of the body simultaneously.

343.1   Hemiplegic
Congenital hemiplegia
EXCLUDES   *infantile hemiplegia NOS (343.4)*

343.2   Quadriplegic
Tetraplegic

343.3   Monoplegic

343.4   Infantile hemiplegia
Infantile hemiplegia (postnatal) NOS

343.8   Other specified infantile cerebral palsy

343.9   Infantile cerebral palsy, unspecified
Cerebral palsy NOS

√4th **344 Other paralytic syndromes**
Note: This category is to be used when the listed conditions
are reported without further specification or are stated
to be old or long-standing but of unspecified cause. The
category is also for use in multiple coding to identify
these conditions resulting from any cause.
INCLUDES   paralysis (complete) (incomplete), except as
classifiable to 342 and 343
EXCLUDES   *congenital or infantile cerebral palsy (343.0-*
343.9)
hemiplegia (342.0-342.9)
congenital or infantile (343.1, 343.4)

√5th **344.0   Quadriplegia and quadriparesis**
344.00   Quadriplegia unspecified
AHA: 4Q, '03, 103; 4Q, '98, 38

344.01   C$_1$-C$_4$ complete
344.02   C$_1$-C$_4$ incomplete
344.03   C$_5$-C$_7$ complete
344.04   C$_5$-C$_7$ incomplete
344.09   Other
AHA: 1Q, '01, 12; 4Q, '98, 39

344.1   Paraplegia
Paralysis of both lower limbs
Paraplegia (lower)
AHA: 4Q, '03, 110; M-A, '87, 10

344.2   Diplegia of upper limbs
Diplegia (upper)   Paralysis of both upper limbs

√5th **344.3   Monoplegia of lower limb**
Paralysis of lower limb
EXCLUDES   *monoplegia of lower limb due to late*
effect of cerebrovascular accident
(438.40-438.42)

344.30   Affecting unspecified side
344.31   Affecting dominant side
344.32   Affecting nondominant side

√5th **344.4   Monoplegia of upper limb**
Paralysis of upper limb
EXCLUDES   *monoplegia of upper limb due to late*
effect of cerebrovascular accident
(438.30-438.32)

344.40   Affecting unspecified side
344.41   Affecting dominant side
344.42   Affecting nondominant side

344.5   Unspecified monoplegia

√5th **344.6   Cauda equina syndrome**
DEF: Dull pain and paresthesias in sacrum, perineum and bladder
due to compression of spinal nerve roots; pain radiates down
buttocks, back of thigh, calf of leg and into foot with prickling,
burning sensations.

344.60   Without mention of neurogenic bladder
344.61   With neurogenic bladder
Acontractile bladder
Autonomic hyperreflexia of bladder
Cord bladder
Detrusor hyperreflexia
AHA: M-J, '87, 12; M-A, '87, 10

√5th **344.8   Other specified paralytic syndromes**
344.81   Locked-in state
AHA: 4Q, '93, 24
DEF: State of consciousness where patients are
paralyzed and unable to respond to environmental
stimuli; patients have eye movements, and stimuli can
enter the brain but patients cannot respond to stimuli.

344.89   Other specified paralytic syndrome
AHA: 2Q, '99, 4

344.9   Paralysis, unspecified

√4th **345 Epilepsy**
EXCLUDES   *progressive myoclonic epilepsy (333.2)*
The following fifth-digit subclassification is for use with
categories 345.0, .1, .4–.9:
0   without mention of intractable epilepsy
1   with intractable epilepsy
AHA: 1Q, '93, 24; 2Q, '92, 8 4Q, '92, 23
DEF: Brain disorder characterized by electrical-like disturbances; may
include occasional impairment or loss of consciousness, abnormal motor
phenomena and psychic or sensory disturbances.

√5th **345.0   Generalized nonconvulsive epilepsy**
Absences: Pykno-epilepsy
atonic   Seizures:
typical   akinetic
Minor epilepsy   atonic
Petit mal
AHA: For code 345.00: ▶1Q, '04, 18◀

√5th **345.1   Generalized convulsive epilepsy**
Epileptic seizures: Epileptic seizures:
clonic   tonic-clonic
myoclonic   Grand mal
tonic   Major epilepsy
EXCLUDES   *convulsions:*
NOS (780.3)
infantile (780.3)
newborn (779.0)
infantile spasms (345.6)
AHA: 3Q, '97, 4
DEF: Convulsive seizures with tension of limbs (tonic) or rhythmic
contractions (clonic).

345.2   Petit mal status
Epileptic absence status
DEF: Minor myoclonic spasms and sudden momentary loss of
consciousness in epilepsy.

345.3   Grand mal status
Status epilepticus NOS
EXCLUDES   *epilepsia partialis continua (345.7)*
status:
psychomotor (345.7)
temporal lobe (345.7)
DEF: Sudden loss of consciousness followed by generalized
convulsions in epilepsy.

N Newborn Age: 0   P Pediatric Age: 0-17   M Maternity Age: 12-55   A Adult Age: 15-124   MSP Medicare Secondary Payer

√5ᵗʰ **345.4 Partial epilepsy, with impairment of consciousness**
Epilepsy:
  limbic system
  partial:
    secondarily generalized
    with memory and ideational disturbances
  psychomotor
  psychosensory
  temporal lobe
Epileptic automatism

√5ᵗʰ **345.5 Partial epilepsy, without mention of impairment of consciousness**
Epilepsy: Epilepsy:
  Bravais-Jacksonian NOS   sensory-induced
  focal (motor) NOS   somatomotor
  Jacksonian NOS   somatosensory
  motor partial   visceral
  partial NOS   visual

√5ᵗʰ **345.6 Infantile spasms**
Hypsarrhythmia   Salaam attacks
Lightning spasms
EXCLUDES salaam tic (781.0)
AHA: N-D, '84, 12

√5ᵗʰ **345.7 Epilepsia partialis continua**
Kojevnikov's epilepsy
DEF: Continuous muscle contractions and relaxation; result of abnormal neural discharge.

√5ᵗʰ **345.8 Other forms of epilepsy**
Epilepsy: Epilepsy:
  cursive [running]   gelastic

√5ᵗʰ **345.9 Epilepsy, unspecified**
Epileptic convulsions, fits, or seizures NOS
EXCLUDES convulsive seizure or fit NOS (780.3)
AHA: N-D, '87, 12

√4ᵗʰ **346 Migraine**
DEF: Benign vascular headache of extreme pain; commonly associated with irritability, nausea, vomiting and often photophobia; premonitory visual hallucination of a crescent in the visual field (scotoma).

The following fifth-digit subclassification is for use with category 346:
  0   without mention of intractable migraine
  1   with intractable migraine, so stated

√5ᵗʰ **346.0 Classical migraine**
Migraine preceded or accompanied by transient focal neurological phenomena
Migraine with aura

√5ᵗʰ **346.1 Common migraine**
Atypical migraine   Sick headache

√5ᵗʰ **346.2 Variants of migraine**
Cluster headache   Migraine:
Histamine cephalgia   lower half
Horton's neuralgia   retinal
Migraine: Neuralgia:
  abdominal   ciliary
  basilar   migrainous

√5ᵗʰ **346.8 Other forms of migraine**
Migraine: Migraine:
  hemiplegic   ophthalmoplegic

√5ᵗʰ **346.9 Migraine, unspecified**
AHA: N-D, '85, 16

√4ᵗʰ **347 Cataplexy and narcolepsy**
DEF: Cataplexy: sudden onset of muscle weakness with loss of tone and strength; caused by aggressive or spontaneous emotions.
DEF: Narcolepsy: brief, recurrent, uncontrollable episodes of sound sleep.

√5ᵗʰ **347.0 Narcolepsy**
  347.00 Without cataplexy
    Narcolepsy NOS
  347.01 With cataplexy

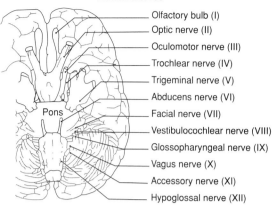
Cranial Nerves
Olfactory bulb (I)
Optic nerve (II)
Oculomotor nerve (III)
Trochlear nerve (IV)
Trigeminal nerve (V)
Abducens nerve (VI)
Facial nerve (VII)
Vestibulocochlear nerve (VIII)
Glossopharyngeal nerve (IX)
Vagus nerve (X)
Accessory nerve (XI)
Hypoglossal nerve (XII)
Pons

√5ᵗʰ **347.1 Narcolepsy in conditions classified elsewhere**
Code first underlying condition
  347.10 Without cataplexy
  347.11 With cataplexy

√4ᵗʰ **348 Other conditions of brain**
348.0 Cerebral cysts
Arachnoid cyst   Porencephaly, acquired
Porencephalic cyst   Pseudoporencephaly
EXCLUDES porencephaly (congenital) (742.4)

348.1 Anoxic brain damage
EXCLUDES that occurring in:
  abortion (634-638 with .7, 639.8)
  ectopic or molar pregnancy (639.8)
  labor or delivery (668.2, 669.4)
  that of newborn (767.0, 768.0-768.9, 772.1-772.2)
Use additional E code to identify cause
DEF: Brain injury due to lack of oxygen, other than birth trauma.

348.2 Benign intracranial hypertension
Pseudotumor cerebri
EXCLUDES hypertensive encephalopathy (437.2)
DEF: Elevated pressure in brain due to fluid retention in brain cavities.

√5ᵗʰ **348.3 Encephalopathy, not elsewhere classified**
AHA: 4Q, '03, 58; 3Q, '97, 4
  348.30 Encephalopathy, unspecified
  348.31 Metabolic encephalopathy
    Septic encephalopathy
  348.39 Other encephalopathy
    EXCLUDES encephalopathy:
     alcoholic (291.2)
     hepatic (572.2)
     hypertensive (437.2)
     toxic (349.82)

348.4 Compression of brain
Compression } brain (stem)
Herniation
Posterior fossa compression syndrome
AHA: 4Q, '94, 37
DEF: Elevated pressure in brain due to blood clot, tumor, fracture, abscess, other condition.

348.5 Cerebral edema
DEF: Elevated pressure in the brain due to fluid retention in brain tissues.

348.8 Other conditions of brain
Cerebral: Cerebral:
  calcification   fungus
AHA: S-O, '87, 9

348.9 Unspecified condition of brain

Nervous System and Sense Organs

349–353

✓4ᵗʰ **349 Other and unspecified disorders of the nervous system**

349.0 Reaction to spinal or lumbar puncture
Headache following lumbar puncture
AHA: 2Q, '99, 9; 3Q, '90, 18

349.1 Nervous system complications from surgically implanted device
EXCLUDES   *immediate postoperative complications (997.00-997.09)*
mechanical complications of nervous system device (996.2)

349.2 Disorders of meninges, not elsewhere classified
Adhesions, meningeal (cerebral) (spinal)
Cyst, spinal meninges
Meningocele, acquired
Pseudomeningocele, acquired
AHA: 2Q, '98, 18; 3Q, '94, 4

✓5ᵗʰ **349.8 Other specified disorders of nervous system**
349.81 Cerebrospinal fluid rhinorrhea
EXCLUDES   *cerebrospinal fluid otorrhea (388.61)*

DEF: Cerebrospinal fluid discharging from the nose; caused by fracture of frontal bone with tearing of dura mater and arachnoid.

349.82 Toxic encephalopathy
Use additional E code, if desired, to identify cause
AHA: 4Q, '93, 29

DEF: Brain tissue degeneration due to toxic substance.

349.89 Other
349.9 Unspecified disorders of nervous system
Disorder of nervous system (central) NOS

DISORDERS OF THE PERIPHERAL NERVOUS SYSTEM (350-359)

EXCLUDES   *diseases of:*
acoustic [8th] nerve (388.5)
oculomotor [3rd, 4th, 6th] nerves (378.0-378.9)
optic [2nd] nerve (377.0-377.9)
peripheral autonomic nerves (337.0-337.9)
neuralgia
neuritis } *NOS or "rheumatic" (729.2)*
radiculitis
peripheral neuritis in pregnancy (646.4)

✓4ᵗʰ **350 Trigeminal nerve disorders**
INCLUDES   disorders of 5th cranial nerve

350.1 Trigeminal neuralgia
Tic douloureux   Trigeminal neuralgia NOS
Trifacial neuralgia
EXCLUDES   *postherpetic (053.12)*

350.2 Atypical face pain
350.8 Other specified trigeminal nerve disorders
350.9 Trigeminal nerve disorder, unspecified

✓4ᵗʰ **351 Facial nerve disorders**
INCLUDES   disorders of 7th cranial nerve
EXCLUDES   *that in newborn (767.5)*

351.0 Bell's palsy
Facial palsy

DEF: Unilateral paralysis of face due to lesion on facial nerve; produces facial distortion.

351.1 Geniculate ganglionitis
Geniculate ganglionitis NOS
EXCLUDES   *herpetic (053.11)*

DEF: Inflammation of tissue at bend in facial nerve.

351.8 Other facial nerve disorders
Facial myokymia   Melkersson's syndrome
AHA: 3Q, '02, 13

351.9 Facial nerve disorder, unspecified

Peripheral Nervous System

✓4ᵗʰ **352 Disorders of other cranial nerves**
352.0 Disorders of olfactory [1st] nerve
352.1 Glossopharyngeal neuralgia
AHA: 2Q, '02, 8

DEF: Pain between throat and ear along petrosal and jugular ganglia.

352.2 Other disorders of glossopharyngeal [9th] nerve
352.3 Disorders of pneumogastric [10th] nerve
Disorders of vagal nerve
EXCLUDES   *paralysis of vocal cords or larynx (478.30-478.34)*

DEF: Nerve disorder affecting ear, tongue, pharynx, larynx, esophagus, viscera and thorax.

352.4 Disorders of accessory [11th] nerve
DEF: Nerve disorder affecting palate, pharynx, larynx, thoracic viscera, sternocleidomastoid and trapezius muscles.

352.5 Disorders of hypoglossal [12th] nerve
DEF: Nerve disorder affecting tongue muscles.

352.6 Multiple cranial nerve palsies
Collet-Sicard syndrome   Polyneuritis cranialis

352.9 Unspecified disorder of cranial nerves

✓4ᵗʰ **353 Nerve root and plexus disorders**
EXCLUDES   *conditions due to:*
intervertebral disc disorders (722.0-722.9)
spondylosis (720.0-721.9)
vertebrogenic disorders (723.0-724.9)

N   Newborn Age: 0   P   Pediatric Age: 0-17   M   Maternity Age: 12-55   A   Adult Age: 15-124   MSP   Medicare Secondary Payer

Trigeminal and Facial Nerve Branches

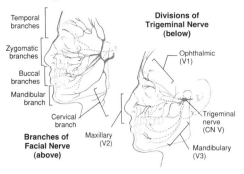

353.0 **Brachial plexus lesions**
Cervical rib syndrome
Costoclavicular syndrome
Scalenus anticus syndrome
Thoracic outlet syndrome

EXCLUDES *brachial neuritis or radiculitis NOS (723.4)*
that in newborn (767.6)

DEF: Acquired disorder in tissue along nerves in shoulder; causes corresponding motor and sensory dysfunction.

353.1 **Lumbosacral plexus lesions**
DEF: Acquired disorder in tissue along nerves in lower back; causes corresponding motor and sensory dysfunction.

353.2 **Cervical root lesions, not elsewhere classified**
353.3 **Thoracic root lesions, not elsewhere classified**
353.4 **Lumbosacral root lesions, not elsewhere classified**
353.5 **Neuralgic amyotrophy**
Parsonage-Aldren-Turner syndrome
353.6 **Phantom limb (syndrome)**
DEF: Abnormal tingling or a burning sensation, transient aches, and intermittent or continuous pain perceived as originating in the absent limb.

353.8 **Other nerve root and plexus disorders**
353.9 **Unspecified nerve root and plexus disorder**

√4ᵗʰ **354 Mononeuritis of upper limb and mononeuritis multiplex**
DEF: Inflammation of a single nerve; known as mononeuritis multiplex when several nerves in unrelated body areas are affected.

354.0 **Carpal tunnel syndrome**
Median nerve entrapment   Partial thenar atrophy
DEF: Compression of median nerve by tendons; causes pain, tingling, numbness and burning sensation in hand.

354.1 **Other lesion of median nerve**
Median nerve neuritis

354.2 **Lesion of ulnar nerve**
Cubital tunnel syndrome
Tardy ulnar nerve palsy

354.3 **Lesion of radial nerve**
Acute radial nerve palsy
AHA: N-D, '87, 6

354.4 **Causalgia of upper limb**
EXCLUDES *causalgia:*
NOS (355.9)
lower limb (355.71)
DEF: Peripheral nerve damage, upper limb; usually due to injury; causes burning sensation and trophic skin changes.

354.5 **Mononeuritis multiplex**
Combinations of single conditions classifiable to 354 or 355

354.8 **Other mononeuritis of upper limb**
354.9 **Mononeuritis of upper limb, unspecified**

√4ᵗʰ **355 Mononeuritis of lower limb**
355.0 **Lesion of sciatic nerve**
EXCLUDES *sciatica NOS (724.3)*
AHA: 2Q, '89, 12
DEF: Acquired disorder of sciatic nerve; causes motor and sensory dysfunction in back, buttock and leg.

355.1 **Meralgia paresthetica**
Lateral cutaneous femoral nerve of thigh compression or syndrome
DEF: Inguinal ligament entraps lateral femoral cutaneous nerve; causes tingling, pain and numbness along outer thigh.

355.2 **Other lesion of femoral nerve**
355.3 **Lesion of lateral popliteal nerve**
Lesion of common peroneal nerve
355.4 **Lesion of medial popliteal nerve**
355.5 **Tarsal tunnel syndrome**
DEF: Compressed, entrapped posterior tibial nerve; causes tingling, pain and numbness in sole of foot.

355.6 **Lesion of plantar nerve**
Morton's metatarsalgia, neuralgia, or neuroma

√5ᵗʰ **355.7** **Other mononeuritis of lower limb**
355.71 **Causalgia of lower limb**
EXCLUDES *causalgia:*
NOS (355.9)
upper limb (354.4)
DEF: Dysfunction of lower limb peripheral nerve, usually due to injury; causes burning pain and trophic skin changes.

355.79 **Other mononeuritis of lower limb**
355.8 **Mononeuritis of lower limb, unspecified**
355.9 **Mononeuritis of unspecified site**
Causalgia NOS
EXCLUDES *causalgia:*
lower limb (355.71)
upper limb (354.4)

√4ᵗʰ **356 Hereditary and idiopathic peripheral neuropathy**
356.0 **Hereditary peripheral neuropathy**
Déjérine-Sottas disease
356.1 **Peroneal muscular atrophy**
Charcôt-Marie-Tooth disease
Neuropathic muscular atrophy
DEF: Genetic disorder, in muscles innervated by peroneal nerves; symptoms include muscle wasting in lower limbs and locomotor difficulties.

356.2 **Hereditary sensory neuropathy**
DEF: Inherited disorder in dorsal root ganglia, optic nerve, and cerebellum, causing sensory losses, shooting pains, and foot ulcers.

356.3 **Refsum's disease**
Heredopathia atactica polyneuritiformis
DEF: Genetic disorder of lipid metabolism; causes persistent, painful inflammation of nerves and retinitis pigmentosa.

356.4 **Idiopathic progressive polyneuropathy**
356.8 **Other specified idiopathic peripheral neuropathy**
Supranuclear paralysis
356.9 **Unspecified**

√4ᵗʰ **357 Inflammatory and toxic neuropathy**
357.0 **Acute infective polyneuritis**
Guillain-Barré syndrome Postinfectious polyneuritis
AHA: 2Q, '98, 12
DEF: Guillain-Barré syndrome: acute demyelinatry polyneuropathy preceded by viral illness (i.e., herpes, cytomegalovirus [CMV], Epstein-Barr virus [EBV]) or a bacterial illness; areflexic motor paralysis with mild sensory disturbance and acellular rise in spinal fluid protein.

√4ᵗʰ √5ᵗʰ Additional Digit Required   Unspecified Code   Other Specified Code   Manifestation Code   ►◄ Revised Text   ● New Code   ▲ Revised Code Title

2005 ICD•9•CM   **Volume 1 — 85**

Nervous System and Sense Organs

357.1–359.81

357.1 Polyneuropathy in collagen vascular disease
Code first underlying disease, as:
disseminated lupus erythematosus (710.0)
polyarteritis nodosa (446.0)
rheumatoid arthritis (714.0)

357.2 Polyneuropathy in diabetes
Code first underlying disease (250.6)
AHA: ▶4Q, '03, 105;◀ 2Q, '92, 15; 3Q, '91, 9

357.3 Polyneuropathy in malignant disease
Code first underlying disease (140.0-208.9)

357.4 Polyneuropathy in other diseases classified elsewhere
Code first underlying disease, as:
amyloidosis (277.3)
beriberi (265.0)
deficiency of B vitamins (266.0-266.9)
diphtheria (032.0-032.9)
hypoglycemia (251.2)
pellagra (265.2)
porphyria (277.1)
sarcoidosis (135)
uremia (585)
EXCLUDES   polyneuropathy in:
herpes zoster (053.13)
mumps (072.72)
AHA: 2Q, '98, 15

357.5 Alcoholic polyneuropathy

357.6 Polyneuropathy due to drugs
Use additional E code to identify drug

357.7 Polyneuropathy due to other toxic agents
Use additional E code to identify toxic agent

✓5th **357.8 Other**
AHA: 4Q, '02, 47; 2Q, '98, 12

357.81 Chronic inflammatory demyelinating polyneuritis
DEF: Chronic inflammatory demyelinating polyneuritis: inflammation of peripheral nerves resulting in destruction of myelin sheath; associated with diabetes mellitus, dysproteinemias, renal failure and malnutrition; symptoms include tingling, numbness, burning pain, diminished tendon reflexes, weakness, and atrophy in lower extremities.

357.82 Critical illness polyneuropathy
Acute motor neuropathy
AHA: ▶4Q, '03, 111◀
DEF: An acute axonal neuropathy, both sensory and motor, that is associated with Systemic Inflammatory Response Syndrome (SIRS).

357.89 Other inflammatory and toxicneuropathy

357.9 Unspecified

✓4th **358 Myoneural disorders**

✓5th **358.0 Myasthenia gravis**
AHA: ▶4Q, '03, 59◀
DEF: Autoimmune disorder of acetylcholine at neuromuscular junction; causing fatigue of voluntary muscles.

358.00 Myasthenia gravis without (acute) exacerbation
Myasthenia gravis NOS

358.01 Myasthenia gravis with (acute) exacerbation
Myasthenia gravis in crisis

358.1 Myasthenic syndromes in diseases classified elsewhere
Amyotrophy ⎫ from stated cause clas-
Eaton-Lambert syndrome ⎭ sified elsewhere
Code first underlying disease, as:
botulism (005.1)
diabetes mellitus (250.6)
hypothyroidism (244.0-244.9)
malignant neoplasm (140.0-208.9)
pernicious anemia (281.0)
thyrotoxicosis (242.0-242.9)

358.2 Toxic myoneural disorders
Use additional E code to identify toxic agent

358.8 Other specified myoneural disorders

358.9 Myoneural disorders, unspecified
AHA: 2Q, '02, 16

✓4th **359 Muscular dystrophies and other myopathies**
EXCLUDES   idiopathic polymyositis (710.4)

359.0 Congenital hereditary muscular dystrophy
Benign congenital myopathy
Central core disease
Centronuclear myopathy
Myotubular myopathy
Nemaline body disease
EXCLUDES   arthrogryposis multiplex congenita (754.89)
DEF: Genetic disorder; causing progressive or nonprogressive muscle weakness.

359.1 Hereditary progressive muscular dystrophy
Muscular dystrophy: Muscular dystrophy:
NOS   Gower's
distal   Landouzy-Déjérine
Duchenne   limb-girdle
Erb's   ocular
fascioscapulohumeral   oculopharyngeal
DEF: Genetic degenerative, muscle disease; causes progressive weakness, wasting of muscle with no nerve involvement.

359.2 Myotonic disorders
Dystrophia myotonica Paramyotonia congenita
Eulenburg's disease   Steinert's disease
Myotonia congenita   Thomsen's disease
DEF: Impaired movement due to spasmatic, rigid muscles.

359.3 Familial periodic paralysis
Hypokalemic familial periodic paralysis
DEF: Genetic disorder; characterized by rapidly progressive flaccid paralysis; attacks often occur after exercise or exposure to cold or dietary changes.

359.4 Toxic myopathy
Use additional E code to identify toxic agent
AHA: 1Q, '88, 5
DEF: Muscle disorder caused by toxic agent.

359.5 Myopathy in endocrine diseases classified elsewhere
Code first underlying disease, as:
Addison's disease (255.4)
Cushing's syndrome (255.0)
hypopituitarism (253.2)
myxedema (244.0-244.9)
thyrotoxicosis (242.0-242.9)
DEF: Muscle disorder secondary to dysfunction in hormone secretion.

359.6 Symptomatic inflammatory myopathy in diseases classified elsewhere
Code first underlying disease, as:
amyloidosis (277.3)
disseminated lupus erythematosus (710.0)
malignant neoplasm (140.0-208.9)
polyarteritis nodosa (446.0)
rheumatoid arthritis (714.0)
sarcoidosis (135)
scleroderma (710.1)
Sjögren's disease (710.2)

✓5th **359.8 Other myopathies**
AHA: 4Q, '02, 47; 3Q, '90, 17

359.81 Critical illness myopathy
Acute necrotizing myopathy
Acute quadriplegic myopathy
Intensive care (ICU) myopathy
Myopathy of critical illness

N Newborn Age: 0   P Pediatric Age: 0-17   M Maternity Age: 12-55   A Adult Age: 15-124   MSP Medicare Secondary Payer

359.89 Other myopathies

359.9 Myopathy, unspecified

DISORDERS OF THE EYE AND ADNEXA (360-379)

☑4ᵗʰ **360 Disorders of the globe**

> INCLUDES   disorders affecting multiple structures of eye

☑5ᵗʰ **360.0 Purulent endophthalmitis**

360.00 Purulent endophthalmitis, unspecified

360.01 Acute endophthalmitis

360.02 Panophthalmitis

360.03 Chronic endophthalmitis

360.04 Vitreous abscess

☑5ᵗʰ **360.1 Other endophthalmitis**

360.11 Sympathetic uveitis

> DEF: Inflammation of vascular layer of uninjured eye; follows injury to other eye.

360.12 Panuveitis

> DEF: Inflammation of entire vascular layer of eye, including choroid, iris and ciliary body.

360.13 Parasitic endophthalmitis NOS

> DEF: Parasitic infection causing inflammation of the entire eye.

360.14 Ophthalmia nodosa

> DEF: Conjunctival inflammation caused by embedded hairs.

360.19 Other

> Phacoanaphylactic endophthalmitis

☑5ᵗʰ **360.2 Degenerative disorders of globe**

> AHA: 3Q, '91, 3

360.20 Degenerative disorder of globe, unspecified

360.21 Progressive high (degenerative) myopia

> Malignant myopia
>
> DEF: Severe, progressive nearsightedness in adults, complicated by serious disease of the choroid; leads to retinal detachment and blindness.

360.23 Siderosis

> DEF: Iron pigment deposits within tissue of eyeball; caused by high iron content of blood.

360.24 Other metallosis

> Chalcosis
>
> DEF: Metal deposits, other than iron, within eyeball tissues.

360.29 Other

> EXCLUDES   xerophthalmia (264.7)

☑5ᵗʰ **360.3 Hypotony of eye**

360.30 Hypotony, unspecified

> DEF: Low osmotic pressure causing lack of tone, tension and strength.

360.31 Primary hypotony

360.32 Ocular fistula causing hypotony

> DEF: Low intraocular pressure due to leak through abnormal passage.

360.33 Hypotony associated with other ocular disorders

360.34 Flat anterior chamber

> DEF: Low pressure behind cornea, causing compression.

☑5ᵗʰ **360.4 Degenerated conditions of globe**

360.40 Degenerated globe or eye, unspecified

360.41 Blind hypotensive eye

> Atrophy of globe
> Phthisis bulbi
>
> DEF: Vision loss due to extremely low intraocular pressure.

Eye

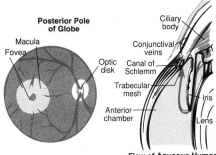

Posterior Pole of Globe

Flow of Aqueous Humor

360.42 Blind hypertensive eye

> Absolute glaucoma
>
> DEF: Vision loss due to painful, high intraocular pressure.

360.43 Hemophthalmos, except current injury

> EXCLUDES   traumatic (871.0-871.9, 921.0-921.9)
>
> DEF: Pool of blood within eyeball, not from current injury.

360.44 Leucocoria

> DEF: Whitish mass or reflex in the pupil behind lens; also called cat's eye reflex; often indicative of retinoblastoma.

☑5ᵗʰ **360.5 Retained (old) intraocular foreign body, magnetic**

> EXCLUDES   current penetrating injury with magnetic foreign body (871.5) retained (old) foreign body of orbit (376.6)

360.50 Foreign body, magnetic, intraocular, unspecified

360.51 Foreign body, magnetic, in anterior chamber

360.52 Foreign body, magnetic, in iris or ciliary body

360.53 Foreign body, magnetic, in lens

360.54 Foreign body, magnetic, in vitreous

360.55 Foreign body, magnetic, in posterior wall

360.59 Foreign body, magnetic, in other or multiple sites

☑5ᵗʰ **360.6 Retained (old) intraocular foreign body, nonmagnetic**

> Retained (old) foreign body:
>   NOS
>   nonmagnetic
> EXCLUDES   current penetrating injury with (nonmagnetic) foreign body (871.6) retained (old) foreign body in orbit (376.6)

360.60 Foreign body, intraocular, unspecified

360.61 Foreign body in anterior chamber

360.62 Foreign body in iris or ciliary body

360.63 Foreign body in lens

360.64 Foreign body in vitreous

☑4ᵗʰ
☑5ᵗʰ Additional Digit Required   Unspecified Code   Other Specified Code   Manifestation Code   ▶◀ Revised Text   ● New Code   ▲ Revised Code Title

2005 ICD•9•CM   Volume 1 — 87

Nervous System and Sense Organs

360.65–362.17

Adnexa

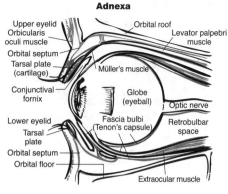

360.65 **Foreign body in posterior wall**

360.69 **Foreign body in other or multiple sites**

√5ᵗʰ 360.8 **Other disorders of globe**

360.81 **Luxation of globe**

> DEF: Displacement of eyeball.

360.89 **Other**

360.9 **Unspecified disorder of globe**

√4ᵗʰ 361 **Retinal detachments and defects**

> DEF: Light-sensitive layer at back of eye, separates from blood supply; disrupting vision.

√5ᵗʰ 361.0 **Retinal detachment with retinal defect**

> Rhegmatogenous retinal detachment
>
> EXCLUDES   *detachment of retinal pigment epithelium (362.42-362.43)*
> *retinal detachment (serous) (without defect) (361.2)*

361.00 **Retinal detachment with retinal defect, unspecified**

361.01 **Recent detachment, partial, with single defect**

361.02 **Recent detachment, partial, with multiple defects**

361.03 **Recent detachment, partial, with giant tear**

361.04 **Recent detachment, partial, with retinal dialysis**

> Dialysis (juvenile) of retina (with detachment)

361.05 **Recent detachment, total or subtotal**

361.06 **Old detachment, partial**

> Delimited old retinal detachment

361.07 **Old detachment, total or subtotal**

√5ᵗʰ 361.1 **Retinoschisis and retinal cysts**

> EXCLUDES   *juvenile retinoschisis (362.73)*
> *microcystoid degeneration of retina (362.62)*
> *parasitic cyst of retina (360.13)*

361.10 **Retinoschisis, unspecified**

> DEF: Separation of retina due to degenerative process of aging; should not be confused with acute retinal detachment.

361.11 **Flat retinoschisis**

> DEF: Slow, progressive split of retinal sensory layers.

361.12 **Bullous retinoschisis**

> DEF: Fluid retention between split retinal sensory layers.

361.13 **Primary retinal cysts**

361.14 **Secondary retinal cysts**

361.19 **Other**

> Pseudocyst of retina

361.2 **Serous retinal detachment**

> Retinal detachment without retinal defect
>
> EXCLUDES   *central serous retinopathy (362.41)*
> *retinal pigment epithelium detachment (362.42-362.43)*

√5ᵗʰ 361.3 **Retinal defects without detachment**

> EXCLUDES   *chorioretinal scars after surgery for detachment (363.30-363.35)*
> *peripheral retinal degeneration without defect (362.60-362.66)*

361.30 **Retinal defect, unspecified**

> Retinal break(s) NOS

361.31 **Round hole of retina without detachment**

361.32 **Horseshoe tear of retina without detachment**

> Operculum of retina without mention of detachment

361.33 **Multiple defects of retina without detachment**

√5ᵗʰ 361.8 **Other forms of retinal detachment**

361.81 **Traction detachment of retina**

> Traction detachment with vitreoretinal organization

361.89 **Other**

> AHA: 3Q, '99, 12

361.9 **Unspecified retinal detachment**

> AHA: N-D, '87, 10

√4ᵗʰ 362 **Other retinal disorders**

> EXCLUDES   *chorioretinal scars (363.30-363.35)*
> *chorioretinitis (363.0-363.2)*

√5ᵗʰ 362.0 **Diabetic retinopathy**

> *Code first diabetes (250.5)*
>
> AHA: 3Q, '91, 8
>
> DEF: Retinal changes in diabetes of long duration; causes hemorrhages, microaneurysms, waxy deposits and proliferative noninflammatory degenerative disease of retina.

362.01 *Background diabetic retinopathy*

> Diabetic macular edema
> Diabetic retinal edema
> Diabetic retinal microaneurysms
> Diabetic retinopathy NOS

362.02 *Proliferative diabetic retinopathy*

> AHA: 3Q, '96, 5

√5ᵗʰ 362.1 **Other background retinopathy and retinal vascular changes**

362.10 **Background retinopathy, unspecified**

362.11 **Hypertensive retinopathy**

> AHA: 3Q, '90, 3
>
> DEF: Retinal irregularities caused by systemic hypertension.

362.12 **Exudative retinopathy**

> Coats' syndrome
>
> AHA: 3Q, '99, 12

362.13 **Changes in vascular appearance**

> Vascular sheathing of retina
> Use additional code for any associated atherosclerosis (440.8)

362.14 **Retinal microaneurysms NOS**

> DEF: Microscopic dilation of retinal vessels in nondiabetic.

362.15 **Retinal telangiectasia**

> DEF: Dilation of blood vessels of the retina.

362.16 **Retinal neovascularization NOS**

> Neovascularization:
> choroidal
> subretinal
>
> DEF: New and abnormal vascular growth in the retina.

362.17 **Other intraretinal microvascular abnormalities**

> Retinal varices

362.18 **Retinal vasculitis**
   Eales' disease   Retinal:
   Retinal: perivasculitis
      arteritis   phlebitis
      endarteritis
   DEF: Inflammation of retinal blood vessels.

√5ᵗʰ 362.2 **Other proliferative retinopathy**

362.21 **Retrolental fibroplasia**
   DEF: Fibrous tissue in vitreous, from retina to lens, causing blindness; associated with premature infants requiring high amounts of oxygen.

362.29 **Other nondiabetic proliferative retinopathy**
   AHA: 3Q, '96, 5

√5ᵗʰ 362.3 **Retinal vascular occlusion**
   DEF: Obstructed blood flow to and from retina.

362.30 **Retinal vascular occlusion, unspecified**
362.31 **Central retinal artery occlusion**
362.32 **Arterial branch occlusion**
362.33 **Partial arterial occlusion**
   Hollenhorst plaque
   Retinal microembolism

362.34 **Transient arterial occlusion**
   Amaurosis fugax
   AHA: 1Q, '00, 16

362.35 **Central retinal vein occlusion**
   AHA: 2Q, '93, 6

362.36 **Venous tributary (branch) occlusion**
362.37 **Venous engorgement**
   Occlusion:
      incipient } of retinal vein
      partial

√5ᵗʰ 362.4 **Separation of retinal layers**
   EXCLUDES   retinal detachment (serous) (361.2)
                    rhegmatogenous (361.00-361.07)

362.40 **Retinal layer separation, unspecified**
362.41 **Central serous retinopathy**
   DEF: Serous-filled blister causing detachment of retina from pigment epithelium.

362.42 **Serous detachment of retinal pigment epithelium**
   Exudative detachment of retinal pigment epithelium
   DEF: Blister of fatty fluid causing detachment of retina from pigment epithelium.

362.43 **Hemorrhagic detachment of retinal pigment epithelium**
   DEF: Blood-filled blister causing detachment of retina from pigment epithelium.

√5ᵗʰ 362.5 **Degeneration of macula and posterior pole**
   EXCLUDES   degeneration of optic disc (377.21-377.24)
                    hereditary retinal degeneration [dystrophy] (362.70-362.77)

362.50 **Macular degeneration (senile), unspecified**
362.51 **Nonexudative senile macular degeneration**
   Senile macular degeneration:
      atrophic
      dry

362.52 **Exudative senile macular degeneration**
   Kuhnt-Junius degeneration
   Senile macular degeneration:
      disciform
      wet
   DEF: Leakage in macular blood vessels with loss of visual acuity.

362.53 **Cystoid macular degeneration**
   Cystoid macular edema
   DEF: Retinal swelling and cyst formation in macula.

362.54 **Macular cyst, hole, or pseudohole**
362.55 **Toxic maculopathy**
   Use additional E code to identify drug, if drug induced

362.56 **Macular puckering**
   Preretinal fibrosis

362.57 **Drusen (degenerative)**
   DEF: White, hyaline deposits on Bruch's membrane (lamina basalis choroideae).

√5ᵗʰ 362.6 **Peripheral retinal degenerations**
   EXCLUDES   hereditary retinal degeneration [dystrophy] (362.70-362.77)
                    retinal degeneration with retinal defect (361.00-361.07)

362.60 **Peripheral retinal degeneration, unspecified**
362.61 **Paving stone degeneration**
   DEF: Degeneration of peripheral retina; causes thinning through which choroid is visible.

362.62 **Microcystoid degeneration**
   Blessig's cysts   Iwanoff's cysts

362.63 **Lattice degeneration**
   Palisade degeneration of retina
   DEF: Degeneration of retina; often bilateral, usually benign; characterized by lines intersecting at irregular intervals in peripheral retina; retinal thinning and retinal holes may occur.

362.64 **Senile reticular degeneration**
   DEF: Net-like appearance of retina; sign of degeneration.

362.65 **Secondary pigmentary degeneration**
   Pseudoretinitis pigmentosa

362.66 **Secondary vitreoretinal degenerations**

√5ᵗʰ 362.7 **Hereditary retinal dystrophies**
   DEF: Genetically induced progressive changes in retina.

362.70 **Hereditary retinal dystrophy, unspecified**
362.71 *Retinal dystrophy in systemic or cerebroretinal lipidoses*
   Code first underlying disease, as:
      cerebroretinal lipidoses (330.1)
      systemic lipidoses (272.7)

362.72 *Retinal dystrophy in other systemic disorders and syndromes*
   Code first underlying disease, as:
      Bassen-Kornzweig syndrome (272.5)
      Refsum's disease (356.3)

362.73 **Vitreoretinal dystrophies**
   Juvenile retinoschisis

362.74 **Pigmentary retinal dystrophy**
   Retinal dystrophy, albipunctate
   Retinitis pigmentosa

362.75 **Other dystrophies primarily involving the sensory retina**
   Progressive cone(-rod) dystrophy
   Stargardt's disease

362.76 **Dystrophies primarily involving the retinal pigment epithelium**
   Fundus flavimaculatus
   Vitelliform dystrophy

362.77 **Dystrophies primarily involving Bruch's membrane**
   Dystrophy:
      hyaline
      pseudoinflammatory foveal
   Hereditary drusen

√5ᵗʰ 362.8 **Other retinal disorders**
   EXCLUDES   chorioretinal inflammations (363.0-363.2)
                    chorioretinal scars (363.30-363.35)

√4ᵗʰ √5ᵗʰ Additional Digit Required   Unspecified Code   Other Specified Code   Manifestation Code   ►◄ Revised Text   ● New Code   ▲ Revised Code Title

Nervous System and Sense Organs

362.81–363.55

362.81 Retinal hemorrhage
Hemorrhage:
preretinal
retinal (deep) (superficial)
subretinal
AHA: 4Q, '96, 43

362.82 Retinal exudates and deposits

362.83 Retinal edema
Retinal:
cotton wool spots
edema (localized) (macular) (peripheral)
DEF: Retinal swelling due to fluid accumulation.

362.84 Retinal ischemia
DEF: Reduced retinal blood supply.

362.85 Retinal nerve fiber bundle defects

362.89 Other retinal disorders

362.9 Unspecified retinal disorder

√4th **363 Chorioretinal inflammations, scars, and other disorders of choroid**

√5th **363.0 Focal chorioretinitis and focal retinochoroiditis**
EXCLUDES *focal chorioretinitis or retinochoroiditis in:*
histoplasmosis (115.02, 115.12, 115.92)
toxoplasmosis (130.2)
congenital infection (771.2)

363.00 Focal chorioretinitis, unspecified
Focal:
choroiditis or chorioretinitis NOS
retinitis or retinochoroiditis NOS

363.01 Focal choroiditis and chorioretinitis, juxtapapillary

363.03 Focal choroiditis and chorioretinitis of other posterior pole

363.04 Focal choroiditis and chorioretinitis, peripheral

363.05 Focal retinitis and retinochoroiditis, juxtapapillary
Neuroretinitis

363.06 Focal retinitis and retinochoroiditis, macular or paramacular

363.07 Focal retinitis and retinochoroiditis of other posterior pole

363.08 Focal retinitis and retinochoroiditis, peripheral

√5th **363.1 Disseminated chorioretinitis and disseminated retinochoroiditis**
EXCLUDES *disseminated choroiditis or chorioretinitis in secondary syphilis (091.51)*
neurosyphilitic disseminated retinitis or retinochoroiditis (094.83)
retinal (peri)vasculitis (362.18)

363.10 Disseminated chorioretinitis, unspecified
Disseminated:
choroiditis or chorioretinitis NOS
retinitis or retinochoroiditis NOS

363.11 Disseminated choroiditis and chorioretinitis, posterior pole

363.12 Disseminated choroiditis and chorioretinitis, peripheral

363.13 Disseminated choroiditis and chorioretinitis, generalized
Code first any underlying disease, as:
tuberculosis (017.3)

363.14 Disseminated retinitis and retinochoroiditis, metastatic

363.15 Disseminated retinitis and retinochoroiditis, pigment epitheliopathy
Acute posterior multifocal placoid pigment epitheliopathy
DEF: Widespread inflammation of retina and choroid; characterized by pigmented epithelium involvement.

√5th **363.2 Other and unspecified forms of chorioretinitis and retinochoroiditis**
EXCLUDES *panophthalmitis (360.02)*
sympathetic uveitis (360.11)
uveitis NOS (364.3)

363.20 Chorioretinitis, unspecified
Choroiditis NOS   Uveitis, posterior NOS
Retinitis NOS

363.21 Pars planitis
Posterior cyclitis
DEF: Inflammation of peripheral retina and ciliary body; characterized by bands of white cells.

363.22 Harada's disease
DEF: Retinal detachment and bilateral widespread exudative choroiditis; symptoms include headache, vomiting, increased lymphocytes in cerebrospinal fluid; and temporary or permanent deafness may occur.

√5th **363.3 Chorioretinal scars**
Scar (postinflammatory) (postsurgical) (posttraumatic):
choroid
retina

363.30 Chorioretinal scar, unspecified

363.31 Solar retinopathy
DEF: Retinal scarring caused by solar radiation.

363.32 Other macular scars

363.33 Other scars of posterior pole

363.34 Peripheral scars

363.35 Disseminated scars

√5th **363.4 Choroidal degenerations**

363.40 Choroidal degeneration, unspecified
Choroidal sclerosis NOS

363.41 Senile atrophy of choroid
DEF: Wasting away of choroid; due to aging.

363.42 Diffuse secondary atrophy of choroid
DEF: Wasting away of choroid in systemic disease.

363.43 Angioid streaks of choroid
DEF: Degeneration of choroid; characterized by dark brown steaks radiating from optic disk; occurs with pseudoxanthoma, elasticum or Paget's disease.

√5th **363.5 Hereditary choroidal dystrophies**
Hereditary choroidal atrophy:
partial [choriocapillaris]
total [all vessels]

363.50 Hereditary choroidal dystrophy or atrophy, unspecified

363.51 Circumpapillary dystrophy of choroid, partial

363.52 Circumpapillary dystrophy of choroid, total
Helicoid dystrophy of choroid

363.53 Central dystrophy of choroid, partial
Dystrophy, choroidal: Dystrophy, choroidal:
central areolar   circinate

363.54 Central choroidal atrophy, total
Dystrophy, choroidal: Dystrophy, choroidal:
central gyrate   serpiginous

363.55 Choroideremia
DEF: Hereditary choroid degeneration, occurs in first decade; characterized by constricted visual field and ultimately blindness in males; less debilitating in females.

363.56 **Other diffuse or generalized dystrophy, partial**
Diffuse choroidal sclerosis

363.57 **Other diffuse or generalized dystrophy, total**
Generalized gyrate atrophy, choroid

✓5th 363.6 **Choroidal hemorrhage and rupture**

363.61 **Choroidal hemorrhage, unspecified**

363.62 **Expulsive choroidal hemorrhage**

363.63 **Choroidal rupture**

✓5th 363.7 **Choroidal detachment**

363.70 **Choroidal detachment, unspecified**

363.71 **Serous choroidal detachment**
DEF: Detachment of choroid from sclera; due to blister of serous fluid.

363.72 **Hemorrhagic choroidal detachment**
DEF: Detachment of choroid from sclera; due to blood-filled blister.

363.8 **Other disorders of choroid**

363.9 **Unspecified disorder of choroid**

✓4th 364 **Disorders of iris and ciliary body**

✓5th 364.0 **Acute and subacute iridocyclitis**
Anterior uveitis ⎫
Cyclitis ⎪
Iridocyclitis ⎬ acute, subacute
Iritis ⎭

EXCLUDES gonococcal (098.41)
herpes simplex (054.44)
herpes zoster (053.22)

364.00 **Acute and subacute iridocyclitis, unspecified**

364.01 **Primary iridocyclitis**

364.02 **Recurrent iridocyclitis**

364.03 **Secondary iridocyclitis, infectious**

364.04 **Secondary iridocyclitis, noninfectious**
Aqueous: Aqueous:
cells   flare
fibrin

364.05 **Hypopyon**
DEF: Accumulation of white blood cells between cornea and lens.

✓5th 364.1 **Chronic iridocyclitis**
EXCLUDES posterior cyclitis (363.21)

364.10 **Chronic iridocyclitis, unspecified**

364.11 *Chronic iridocyclitis in diseases classified elsewhere*
Code first underlying disease, as:
sarcoidosis (135)
tuberculosis (017.3)
EXCLUDES syphilitic iridocyclitis (091.52)
DEF: Persistent inflammation of iris and ciliary body; due to underlying disease or condition.

✓5th 364.2 **Certain types of iridocyclitis**
EXCLUDES posterior cyclitis (363.21)
sympathetic uveitis (360.11)

364.21 **Fuchs' heterochromic cyclitis**
DEF: Chronic cyclitis characterized by differences in the color of the two irises; the lighter iris appears in the inflamed eye.

364.22 **Glaucomatocyclitic crises**
DEF: One-sided form of secondary open angle glaucoma; recurrent, uncommon and of short duration; causes high intraocular pressure, rarely damage.

364.23 **Lens-induced iridocyclitis**
DEF: Inflammation of iris; due to immune reaction to proteins in lens following trauma or other lens abnormality.

364.24 **Vogt-Koyanagi syndrome**
DEF: Uveomeningitis with exudative iridocyclitis and choroiditis; causes depigmentation of hair and skin, detached retina; tinnitus and loss of hearing may occur.

364.3 **Unspecified iridocyclitis**
Uveitis NOS

✓5th 364.4 **Vascular disorders of iris and ciliary body**

364.41 **Hyphema**
Hemorrhage of iris or ciliary body
DEF: Hemorrhage in anterior chamber; also called hyphemia or "blood shot" eyes.

364.42 **Rubeosis iridis**
Neovascularization of iris or ciliary body
DEF: Blood vessel and connective tissue formation on surface of iris; symptomatic of diabetic retinopathy, central retinal vein occlusion and retinal detachment.

✓5th 364.5 **Degenerations of iris and ciliary body**

364.51 **Essential or progressive iris atrophy**

364.52 **Iridoschisis**
DEF: Splitting of iris into two layers.

364.53 **Pigmentary iris degeneration**
Acquired heterochromia ⎫
Pigment dispersion ⎪
syndrome ⎬ of iris
Translucency ⎭

364.54 **Degeneration of pupillary margin**
Atrophy of sphincter ⎫
Ectropion of pigment ⎬ of iris
epithelium ⎭

364.55 **Miotic cysts of pupillary margin**
DEF: Serous-filled sacs in pupillary margin of iris.

364.56 **Degenerative changes of chamber angle**

364.57 **Degenerative changes of ciliary body**

364.59 **Other iris atrophy**
Iris atrophy (generalized) (sector shaped)

✓5th 364.6 **Cysts of iris, ciliary body, and anterior chamber**
EXCLUDES miotic pupillary cyst (364.55)
parasitic cyst (360.13)

364.60 **Idiopathic cysts**
DEF: Fluid-filled sacs in iris or ciliary body; unknown etiology.

364.61 **Implantation cysts**
Epithelial down-growth, anterior chamber
Implantation cysts (surgical) (traumatic)

364.62 **Exudative cysts of iris or anterior chamber**

364.63 **Primary cyst of pars plana**
DEF: Fluid-filled sacs of outermost ciliary ring.

364.64 **Exudative cyst of pars plana**
DEF: Protein, fatty-filled sacs of outermost ciliary ring; due to fluid lead from blood vessels.

✓5th 364.7 **Adhesions and disruptions of iris and ciliary body**
EXCLUDES flat anterior chamber (360.34)

364.70 **Adhesions of iris, unspecified**
Synechiae (iris) NOS

364.71 **Posterior synechiae**
DEF: Adhesion binding iris to lens.

364.72 **Anterior synechiae**
DEF: Adhesion binding the iris to cornea.

✓4th
✓5th Additional Digit Required   Unspecified Code   Other Specified Code   Manifestation Code   ▶◀ Revised Text   ● New Code   ▲ Revised Code Title

2005 ICD•9•CM   Volume 1 — 91

Nervous System and Sense Organs

364.73–365.63

364.73 Goniosynechiae
Peripheral anterior synechiae
DEF: Adhesion binding the iris to cornea at the angle of the anterior chamber.

364.74 Pupillary membranes
Iris bombé　　　　Pupillary:
Pupillary:　　　　　seclusion
　occlusion
DEF: Membrane traversing the pupil and blocking vision.

364.75 Pupillary abnormalities
Deformed pupil　Rupture of sphincter, pupil
Ectopic pupil

364.76 Iridodialysis
DEF: Separation of the iris from the ciliary body base; due to trauma or surgical accident.

364.77 Recession of chamber angle
DEF: Receding of anterior chamber angle of the eye; restricts vision.

364.8　Other disorders of iris and ciliary body
Prolapse of iris NOS
EXCLUDES prolapse of iris in recent wound (871.1)

364.9　Unspecified disorder of iris and ciliary body

✓4ᵗʰ **365 Glaucoma**
EXCLUDES blind hypertensive eye [absolute glaucoma] (360.42)
congenital glaucoma (743.20-743.22)
DEF: Rise in intraocular pressure which restricts blood flow; multiple causes.

✓5ᵗʰ **365.0　Borderline glaucoma [glaucoma suspect]**
AHA: 1Q, '90, 8

365.00 Preglaucoma, unspecified
365.01 Open angle with borderline findings
Open angle with:
　borderline intraocular pressure
　cupping of optic discs
DEF: Minor block of aqueous outflow from eye.

365.02 Anatomical narrow angle
365.03 Steroid responders
365.04 Ocular hypertension
DEF: High fluid pressure within eye; no apparent cause.

✓5ᵗʰ **365.1　Open-angle glaucoma**
365.10 Open-angle glaucoma, unspecified
Wide-angle glaucoma NOS
365.11 Primary open angle glaucoma
Chronic simple glaucoma
DEF: High intraocular pressure, despite free flow of aqueous.

365.12 Low tension glaucoma
365.13 Pigmentary glaucoma
DEF: High intraocular pressure; due to iris pigment granules blocking aqueous flow.

365.14 Glaucoma of childhood
Infantile or juvenile glaucoma
365.15 Residual stage of open angle glaucoma

✓5ᵗʰ **365.2　Primary angle-closure glaucoma**
365.20 Primary angle-closure glaucoma, unspecified
365.21 Intermittent angle-closure glaucoma
Angle-closure glaucoma:
　interval
　subacute
DEF: Recurring attacks of high intraocular pressure; due to blocked aqueous flow.

365.22 Acute angle-closure glaucoma
DEF: Sudden, severe rise in intraocular pressure due to blockage in aqueous drainage.

365.23 Chronic angle-closure glaucoma
AHA: 2Q, '98, 16

365.24 Residual stage of angle-closure glaucoma•

✓5ᵗʰ **365.3　Corticosteroid-induced glaucoma**
DEF: Elevated intraocular pressure; due to long-term corticosteroid therapy.

365.31 Glaucomatous stage
365.32 Residual stage

✓5ᵗʰ **365.4　Glaucoma associated with congenital anomalies, dystrophies, and systemic syndromes**
365.41 Glaucoma associated with chamber angle anomalies
Code first associated disorder, as:
　Axenfeld's anomaly (743.44)
　Rieger's anomaly or syndrome (743.44)

365.42 Glaucoma associated with anomalies of iris
Code first associated disorder, as:
　aniridia (743.45)
　essential iris atrophy (364.51)

365.43 Glaucoma associated with other anterior segment anomalies
Code first associated disorder, as:
　microcornea (743.41)

365.44 Glaucoma associated with systemic syndromes
Code first associated disease, as
　neurofibromatosis (237.7)
　Sturge-Weber (-Dimitri) syndrome (759.6)

✓5ᵗʰ **365.5　Glaucoma associated with disorders of the lens**
365.51 Phacolytic glaucoma
Use additional code for associated
　hypermature cataract (366.18)
DEF: Elevated intraocular pressure; due to lens protein blocking aqueous flow.

365.52 Pseudoexfoliation glaucoma
Use additional code for associated
　pseudoexfoliation of capsule (366.11)
DEF: Glaucoma characterized by small grayish particles deposited on the lens.

365.59 Glaucoma associated with other lens disorders
Use additional code for associated disorder, as:
　dislocation of lens (379.33-379.34)
　spherophakia (743.36)

✓5ᵗʰ **365.6　Glaucoma associated with other ocular disorders**
365.60 Glaucoma associated with unspecified ocular disorder
365.61 Glaucoma associated with pupillary block
Use additional code for associated disorder, as:
　seclusion of pupil [iris bombé] (364.74)
DEF: Acute, open-angle glaucoma caused by mature cataract; aqueous flow is blocked by lens material and macrophages.

365.62 Glaucoma associated with ocular inflammations
Use additional code for associated disorder, as:
　glaucomatocyclitic crises (364.22)
　iridocyclitis (364.0-364.3)

365.63 Glaucoma associated with vascular disorders
Use additional code for associated disorder, as:
　central retinal vein occlusion (362.35)
　hyphema (364.41)

Aqueous Misdirection Syndrome

Cornea — Anterior chamber — Filtration angle (open)   **Normal aqueous flow**

Iris — Canal of Schlemm (open)

Lens

Posterior chamber — Filtration angle (obstructed)

Aqueous misdirection syndrome — Canal of Schlemm (obstructed)

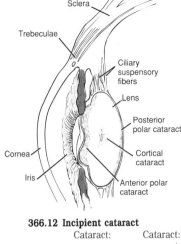

Cataract

Sclera

Trebeculae

Ciliary suspensory fibers

Lens

Posterior polar cataract

Cornea

Cortical cataract

Iris

Anterior polar cataract

365.64 Glaucoma associated with tumors or cysts
Use additional code for associated disorder, as:
benign neoplasm (224.0-224.9)
epithelial down-growth (364.61)
malignant neoplasm (190.0-190.9)

365.65 Glaucoma associated with ocular trauma
Use additional code for associated condition, as:
contusion of globe (921.3)
recession of chamber angle (364.77)

√5ᵗʰ **365.8 Other specified forms of glaucoma**

365.81 Hypersecretion glaucoma

365.82 Glaucoma with increased episcleral venous pressure

365.83 Aqueous misdirection
Malignant glaucoma
AHA: 4Q, '02, 48

DEF: A form of glaucoma that occurs when aqueous humor flows into the posterior chamber of the eye (vitreous) rather than through the normal recycling channels into the anterior chamber.

365.89 Other specified glaucoma
AHA: 2Q, '98, 16

365.9 Unspecified glaucoma
AHA: ▶3Q, '03, 14;◀ 2Q, '01, 16

√4ᵗʰ **366 Cataract**
EXCLUDES congenital cataract (743.30-743.34)

DEF: A variety of conditions that create a cloudy, or calcified lens that obstructs vision.

√5ᵗʰ **366.0 Infantile, juvenile, and presenile cataract**

366.00 Nonsenile cataract, unspecified

366.01 Anterior subcapsular polar cataract
DEF: Defect within the front, center lens surface.

366.02 Posterior subcapsular polar cataract
DEF: Defect within the rear, center lens surface.

366.03 Cortical, lamellar, or zonular cataract
DEF: Opacities radiating from center to edge of lens; appear as thin, concentric layers of lens.

366.04 Nuclear cataract

366.09 Other and combined forms of nonsenile cataract

√5ᵗʰ **366.1 Senile cataract**
AHA: 3Q, '91, 9; S-O, '85, 10

366.10 Senile cataract, unspecified   A
AHA: 1Q, '03, 5

366.11 Pseudoexfoliation of lens capsule   A

366.12 Incipient cataract   A
Cataract: Cataract:
coronary   punctate
immature NOS   Water clefts
DEF: Minor disorders of lens not affecting vision; due to aging.

366.13 Anterior subcapsular polar senile cataract   A

366.14 Posterior subcapsular polar senile cataract   A

366.15 Cortical senile cataract   A

366.16 Nuclear sclerosis   A
Cataracta brunescens
Nuclear cataract

366.17 Total or mature cataract   A

366.18 Hypermature cataract   A
Morgagni cataract

366.19 Other and combined forms of senile cataract   A

√5ᵗʰ **366.2 Traumatic cataract**

366.20 Traumatic cataract, unspecified

366.21 Localized traumatic opacities
Vossius' ring

366.22 Total traumatic cataract

366.23 Partially resolved traumatic cataract

√5ᵗʰ **366.3 Cataract secondary to ocular disorders**

366.30 Cataracta complicata, unspecified

366.31 Glaucomatous flecks (subcapsular)
Code first underlying glaucoma (365.0-365.9)

366.32 Cataract in inflammatory disorders
Code first underlying condition, as:
chronic choroiditis (363.0-363.2)

366.33 Cataract with neovascularization
Code first underlying condition, as:
chronic iridocyclitis (364.10)

366.34 Cataract in degenerative disorders
Sunflower cataract
Code first underlying condition, as:
chalcosis (360.24)
degenerative myopia (360.21)
pigmentary retinal dystrophy (362.74)

√5ᵗʰ **366.4 Cataract associated with other disorders**

366.41 Diabetic cataract
Code first diabetes (250.5)
AHA: 3Q, '91, 9; S-O, '85, 11

366.42 Tetanic cataract
Code first underlying disease, as:
calcinosis (275.4)
hypoparathyroidism (252.1)

366.43 Myotonic cataract
Code first underlying disorder (359.2)

√4ᵗʰ Additional Digit Required   Unspecified Code   Other Specified Code   Manifestation Code   ▶◀ Revised Text   ● New Code   ▲ Revised Code Title

Nervous System and Sense Organs

366.44–368.13

366.44 Cataract associated with other syndromes
Code first underlying condition, as:
craniofacial dysostosis (756.0)
galactosemia (271.1)

366.45 Toxic cataract
Drug-induced cataract
Use additional E code to identify drug or
other toxic substance

**366.46 Cataract associated with radiation and
other physical influences**
Use additional E code to identify cause

√5ᵗʰ **366.5 After-cataract**

366.50 After-cataract, unspecified
Secondary cataract NOS

366.51 Soemmering's ring
DEF: A donut-shaped lens remnant and a capsule behind
the pupil as a result of cataract surgery or trauma.

**366.52 Other after-cataract, not obscuring
vision**

366.53 After-cataract, obscuring vision

366.8 Other cataract
Calcification of lens

366.9 Unspecified cataract

Classification		LEVELS OF VISUAL IMPAIRMENT	Additional descriptors which may be encountered
"legal"	WHO	Visual acuity and/or visual field limitation (whichever is worse)	
LEGAL BLINDNESS (U.S.A.) both eyes	(NEAR-) NORMAL VISION	RANGE OF NORMAL VISION 20/10 20/13 20/16 20/20 20/25 2.0 1.6 1.25 1.0 0.8	
		NEAR-NORMAL VISION 20/30 20/40 20/50 20/60 0.7 0.6 0.5 0.4 0.3	
	LOW VISION	MODERATE VISUAL IMPAIRMENT 20/70 20/80 20/100 20/125 20/160 0.25 0.20 0.16 0.12	Moderate low vision
		SEVERE VISUAL IMPAIRMENT 20/200 20/250 20/320 20/400 0.10 0.08 0.06 0.05 Visual field: 20 degrees or less	Severe low vision, "Legal" blindness
	BLINDNESS (WHO) one or both eyes	PROFOUND VISUAL IMPAIRMENT 20/500 20/630 20/800 20/1000 0.04 0.03 0.025 0.02 Count fingers at: less than 3m (10 ft.) Visual field: 10 degrees or less	Profound low vision, Moderate blindness
		NEAR-TOTAL VISUAL IMPAIRMENT Visual acuity: less than 0.02 (20/1000) Count fingers at: 1m (3 ft.) or less Hand movements: 5m (15 ft.) or less Light projection, light perception Visual field: 5 degrees or less	Severe blindness, Near-total blindness
		TOTAL VISUAL IMPAIRMENT No light perception (NLP)	Total blindness

Visual acuity refers to best achievable acuity with correction.
Non-listed Snellen fractions may be classified by converting to the nearest decimal equivalent, e.g. 10/200 = 0.05, 6/30 = 0.20.
CF (count fingers) without designation of distance, may be classified to profound impairment.
HM (hand motion) without designation of distance, may be classified to near-total impairment.
Visual field measurements refer to the largest field diameter for a 1/100 white test object.

√4ᵗʰ **367 Disorders of refraction and accommodation**

367.0 Hypermetropia
Far-sightedness   Hyperopia
DEF: Refraction error, called also hyperopia, focal point is posterior
to retina; abnormally short anteroposterior diameter or subnormal
refractive power; causes farsightedness.

367.1 Myopia
Near-sightedness
DEF: Refraction error, focal point is anterior to retina; causes near-
sightedness.

√5ᵗʰ **367.2 Astigmatism**

367.20 Astigmatism, unspecified

367.21 Regular astigmatism

367.22 Irregular astigmatism

√5ᵗʰ **367.3 Anisometropia and aniseikonia**

367.31 Anisometropia
DEF: Eyes with refractive powers that differ by at least
one diopter.

367.32 Aniseikonia
DEF: Eyes with unequal retinal imaging; usually due to
refractive error.

367.4 Presbyopia
DEF: Loss of crystalline lens elasticity; causes errors of
accommodation; due to aging.

√5ᵗʰ **367.5 Disorders of accommodation**

367.51 Paresis of accommodation
Cycloplegia
DEF: Partial paralysis of ciliary muscle; causing focus
problems.

367.52 Total or complete internal ophthalmoplegia
DEF: Total paralysis of ciliary muscle; large pupil
incapable of focus.

367.53 Spasm of accommodation
DEF: Abnormal contraction of ciliary muscle; causes
focus problems.

√5ᵗʰ **367.8 Other disorders of refraction and accommodation**

367.81 Transient refractive change

367.89 Other
Drug-induced   } disorders of refraction
Toxic   & accommodation

**367.9 Unspecified disorder of refraction and
accommodation**

√4ᵗʰ **368 Visual disturbances**
EXCLUDES   electrophysiological disturbances (794.11-
794.14)

√5ᵗʰ **368.0 Amblyopia ex anopsia**
DEF: Vision impaired due to disuse; esotropia often cause.

368.00 Amblyopia, unspecified

368.01 Strabismic amblyopia
Suppression amblyopia

368.02 Deprivation amblyopia
DEF: Decreased vision associated with suppressed
retinal image of one eye.

368.03 Refractive amblyopia

√5ᵗʰ **368.1 Subjective visual disturbances**

368.10 Subjective visual disturbance, unspecified

368.11 Sudden visual loss

368.12 Transient visual loss
Concentric fading   Scintillating scotoma

368.13 Visual discomfort
Asthenopia   Photophobia
Eye strain

Ⓝ Newborn Age: 0   Ⓟ Pediatric Age: 0-17   Ⓜ Maternity Age: 12-55   Ⓐ Adult Age: 15-124   **MSP** Medicare Secondary Payer

368.14 Visual distortions of shape and size
Macropsia   Micropsia
Metamorphopsia

368.15 Other visual distortions and entoptic phenomena
Photopsia   Refractive:
Refractive: polyopia
   diplopia   Visual halos

368.16 Psychophysical visual disturbances
Visual: Visual:
   agnosia   hallucinations
   disorientation syndrome

368.2   Diplopia
Double vision

√5ᵗʰ 368.3   Other disorders of binocular vision

368.30 Binocular vision disorder, unspecified

368.31 Suppression of binocular vision

368.32 Simultaneous visual perception without fusion

368.33 Fusion with defective stereopsis

DEF: Faulty depth perception though normal ability to focus.

368.34 Abnormal retinal correspondence

√5ᵗʰ 368.4   Visual field defects

368.40 Visual field defect, unspecified

368.41 Scotoma involving central area
Scotoma: Scotoma:
   central   paracentral
   centrocecal

DEF: Vision loss (blind spot) in central five degrees of visual field.

368.42 Scotoma of blind spot area
Enlarged: Paracecal scotoma
   angioscotoma
   blind spot

368.43 Sector or arcuate defects
Scotoma:
   arcuate
   Bjerrum
   Seidel

DEF: Arc-shaped blind spot caused by retinal nerve damage.

368.44 Other localized visual field defect
Scotoma: Visual field defect:
   NOS   nasal step
   ring   peripheral

368.45 Generalized contraction or constriction

368.46 Homonymous bilateral field defects
Hemianopsia (altitudinal) (homonymous)
Quadrant anopia

DEF: Disorders found in the corresponding vertical halves of the visual fields of both eyes .

368.47 Heteronymous bilateral field defects
Hemianopsia: Hemianopsia:
   binasal   bitemporal

DEF: Disorders in the opposite halves of the visual fields of both eyes.

√5ᵗʰ 368.5   Color vision deficiencies
Color blindness

368.51 Protan defect
Protanomaly   Protanopia

DEF: Mild difficulty distinguishing green and red hues with shortened spectrum; sex-linked affecting one percent of males.

368.52 Deutan defect
Deuteranomaly   Deuteranopia

DEF: Male-only disorder; difficulty in distinguishing green and red, no shortened spectrum.

368.53 Tritan defect
Tritanomaly   Tritanopia

DEF: Difficulty in distinguishing blue and yellow; occurs often due to drugs, retinal detachment and central nervous system diseases.

368.54 Achromatopsia
Monochromatism (cone) (rod)

DEF: Complete color blindness; caused by disease, injury to retina, optic nerve or pathway.

368.55 Acquired color vision deficiencies

368.59 Other color vision deficiencies

√5ᵗʰ 368.6   Night blindness
Nyctalopia

DEF: Nyctalopia: disorder of vision in dim light or night blindness.

368.60 Night blindness, unspecified

368.61 Congenital night blindness
Hereditary night blindness
Oguchi's disease

368.62 Acquired night blindness
EXCLUDES   *that due to vitamin A deficiency (264.5)*

368.63 Abnormal dark adaptation curve
Abnormal threshold   } of cones or rods
Delayed adaptation

368.69 Other night blindness

368.8   Other specified visual disturbances
Blurred vision NOS

AHA: 4Q, '02, 56

368.9   Unspecified visual disturbance

AHA: ▶1Q, '04, 15◀

√4ᵗʰ 369   Blindness and low vision

Note: Visual impairment refers to a functional limitation of the eye (e.g., limited visual acuity or visual field). It should be distinguished from visual disability, indicating a limitation of the abilities of the individual (e.g., limited reading skills, vocational skills), and from visual handicap, indicating a limitation of personal and socioeconomic independence (e.g., limited mobility, limited employability).

The levels of impairment defined in the table on page 94 are based on the recommendations of the WHO Study Group on Prevention of Blindness (Geneva, November 6–10, 1972; WHO Technical Report Series 518), and of the International Council of Ophthalmology (1976).

Note that definitions of blindness vary in different settings.

For international reporting WHO defines blindness as profound impairment. This definition can be applied to blindness of one eye (369.1, 369.6) and to blindness of the individual (369.0).

For determination of benefits in the U.S.A., the definition of legal blindness as severe impairment is often used. This definition applies to blindness of the individual only.

EXCLUDES   *correctable impaired vision due to refractive errors (367.0-367.9)*

√5ᵗʰ 369.0   Profound impairment, both eyes

369.00 Impairment level not further specified
Blindness:
   NOS according to WHO definition
   both eyes

369.01 Better eye: total impairment; lesser eye: total impairment

369.02 Better eye: near-total impairment; lesser eye: not further specified

---

◢4ᵗʰ◣ Additional Digit Required   Unspecified Code   Other Specified Code   Manifestation Code   ►◄ Revised Text   ● New Code   ▲ Revised Code Title
◢5ᵗʰ◣

2005 ICD•9•CM   **October 2004 • Volume 1 — 95**

Nervous System and Sense Organs

369.03–370.24

369.03 Better eye: near-total impairment; lesser eye: total impairment

369.04 Better eye: near-total impairment; lesser eye: near-total impairment

369.05 Better eye: profound impairment; lesser eye: not further specified

369.06 Better eye: profound impairment; lesser eye: total impairment

369.07 Better eye: profound impairment; lesser eye: near-total impairment

369.08 Better eye: profound impairment; lesser eye: profound impairment

√5th 369.1 Moderate or severe impairment, better eye, profound impairment lesser eye

369.10 Impairment level not further specified
    Blindness, one eye, low vision other eye

369.11 Better eye: severe impairment; lesser eye: blind, not further specified

369.12 Better eye: severe impairment; lesser eye: total impairment

369.13 Better eye: severe impairment; lesser eye: near-total impairment

369.14 Better eye: severe impairment; lesser eye: profound impairment

369.15 Better eye: moderate impairment; lesser eye: blind, not further specified

369.16 Better eye: moderate impairment; lesser eye: total impairment

369.17 Better eye: moderate impairment; lesser eye: near-total impairment

369.18 Better eye: moderate impairment; lesser eye: profound impairment

√5th 369.2 Moderate or severe impairment, both eyes

369.20 Impairment level not further specified
    Low vision, both eyes NOS

369.21 Better eye: severe impairment; lesser eye: not further specified

369.22 Better eye: severe impairment; lesser eye: severe impairment

369.23 Better eye: moderate impairment; lesser eye: not further specified

369.24 Better eye: moderate impairment; lesser eye: severe impairment

369.25 Better eye: moderate impairment; lesser eye: moderate impairment

369.3 Unqualified visual loss, both eyes
    EXCLUDES   blindness NOS:
        legal [U.S.A. definition] (369.4)
        WHO definition (369.00)

369.4 Legal blindness, as defined in U.S.A.
    Blindness NOS according to U.S.A. definition
    EXCLUDES   legal blindness with specification of
        impairment level (369.01-369.08,
        369.11-369.14, 369.21-369.22)

√5th 369.6 Profound impairment, one eye

369.60 Impairment level not further specified
    Blindness, one eye

369.61 One eye: total impairment; other eye: not specified

369.62 One eye: total impairment; other eye: near-normal vision

369.63 One eye: total impairment; other eye: normal vision

369.64 One eye: near-total impairment; other eye: not specified

369.65 One eye: near-total impairment; other eye: near-normal vision

369.66 One eye: near-total impairment; other eye: normal vision

369.67 One eye: profound impairment; other eye: not specified

369.68 One eye: profound impairment; other eye: near-normal vision

369.69 One eye: profound impairment; other eye: normal vision

√5th 369.7 Moderate or severe impairment, one eye

369.70 Impairment level not further specified
    Low vision, one eye

369.71 One eye: severe impairment; other eye: not specified

369.72 One eye: severe impairment; other eye: near-normal vision

369.73 One eye: severe impairment; other eye: normal vision

369.74 One eye: moderate impairment; other eye: not specified

369.75 One eye: moderate impairment; other eye: near-normal vision

369.76 One eye: moderate impairment; other eye: normal vision

369.8 Unqualified visual loss, one eye

369.9 Unspecified visual loss
    AHA: 4Q, '02, 114; 3Q, '02, 20

√4th 370 Keratitis

√5th 370.0 Corneal ulcer
    EXCLUDES   that due to vitamin A deficiency (264.3)

369.00 Corneal ulcer, unspecified

370.01 Marginal corneal ulcer

370.02 Ring corneal ulcer

370.03 Central corneal ulcer

370.04 Hypopyon ulcer
    Serpiginous ulcer
    DEF: Corneal ulcer with an accumulation of pus in the eye's anterior chamber.

370.05 Mycotic corneal ulcer
    DEF: Fungal infection causing corneal tissue loss.

370.06 Perforated corneal ulcer
    DEF: Tissue loss through all layers of cornea.

370.07 Mooren's ulcer
    DEF: Tissue loss, with chronic inflammation, at junction of cornea and sclera; seen in elderly.

√5th 370.2 Superficial keratitis without conjunctivitis
    EXCLUDES   dendritic [herpes simplex] keratitis (054.42)

370.20 Superficial keratitis, unspecified

370.21 Punctate keratitis
    Thygeson's superficial punctate keratitis
    DEF: Formation of cellular and fibrinous deposits (keratic precipitates) on posterior surface; deposits develop after injury or iridocyclitis.

370.22 Macular keratitis
    Keratitis: Keratitis:
      areolar   stellate
      nummular   striate

370.23 Filamentary keratitis
    DEF: Keratitis characterized by twisted filaments of mucoid material on the cornea's surface.

370.24 Photokeratitis
    Snow blindness
    Welders' keratitis
    AHA: 3Q, '96, 6
    DEF: Painful, inflamed cornea; due to extended exposure to ultraviolet light.

✓5ᵗʰ **370.3   Certain types of keratoconjunctivitis**

370.31 Phlyctenular keratoconjunctivitis
Phlyctenulosis
Use additional code for any associated tuberculosis (017.3)
DEF: Miniature blister on conjunctiva or cornea; associated with tuberculosis and malnutrition disorders.

370.32 Limbar and corneal involvement in vernal conjunctivitis
Use additional code for vernal conjunctivitis (372.13)
DEF: Corneal itching and inflammation in conjunctivitis; often limited to lining of eyelids.

370.33 Keratoconjunctivitis sicca, not specified as Sjögren's
EXCLUDES   Sjögren's syndrome (710.2)
DEF: Inflammation of conjunctiva and cornea; characterized by "horny" looking tissue and excess blood in these areas; decreased flow of lacrimal (tear) is a contributing factor.

370.34 Exposure keratoconjunctivitis
AHA: 3Q, '96, 6
DEF: Incomplete closure of eyelid causing dry, inflamed eye.

370.35 Neurotrophic keratoconjunctivitis

✓5ᵗʰ **370.4   Other and unspecified keratoconjunctivitis**

370.40 Keratoconjunctivitis, unspecified
Superficial keratitis with conjunctivitis NOS

370.44 Keratitis or keratoconjunctivitis in exanthema
Code first underlying condition (050.0-052.9)
EXCLUDES   herpes simplex (054.43)
herpes zoster (053.21)
measles (055.71)

370.49 Other
EXCLUDES   epidemic keratoconjunctivitis (077.1)

✓5ᵗʰ **370.5   Interstitial and deep keratitis**

370.50 Interstitial keratitis, unspecified

370.52 Diffuse interstitial keratitis
Cogan's syndrome
DEF: Inflammation of cornea; with deposits in middle corneal layers; may obscure vision.

370.54 Sclerosing keratitis
DEF: Chronic corneal inflammation leading to opaque scarring.

370.55 Corneal abscess
DEF: Pocket of pus and inflammation on the cornea.

370.59 Other
EXCLUDES   disciform herpes simplex keratitis (054.43)
syphilitic keratitis (090.3)

✓5ᵗʰ **370.6   Corneal neovascularization**

370.60 Corneal neovascularization, unspecified

370.61 Localized vascularization of cornea
DEF: Limited infiltration of cornea by new blood vessels.

370.62 Pannus (corneal)
AHA: 3Q, '02, 20
DEF: Buildup of superficial vascularization and granulated tissue under epithelium of cornea.

370.63 Deep vascularization of cornea
DEF: Deep infiltration of cornea by new blood vessels.

370.64 Ghost vessels (corneal)

370.8   Other forms of keratitis
AHA: 3Q, '94, 5

370.9   Unspecified keratitis

✓4ᵗʰ **371   Corneal opacity and other disorders of cornea**

✓5ᵗʰ **371.0   Corneal scars and opacities**
EXCLUDES   that due to vitamin A deficiency (264.6)

371.00 Corneal opacity, unspecified
Corneal scar NOS

371.01 Minor opacity of cornea
Corneal nebula

371.02 Peripheral opacity of cornea
Corneal macula not interfering with central vision

371.03 Central opacity of cornea
Corneal:
leucoma ⎫ interfering with central
macula ⎭ vision

371.04 Adherent leucoma
DEF: Dense, opaque corneal growth adhering to the iris; also spelled as leukoma.

371.05 Phthisical cornea
Code first underlying tuberculosis (017.3)

✓5ᵗʰ **371.1   Corneal pigmentations and deposits**

371.10 Corneal deposit, unspecified

371.11 Anterior pigmentations
Stähli's lines

371.12 Stromal pigmentations
Hematocornea

371.13 Posterior pigmentations
Krukenberg spindle

371.14 Kayser-Fleischer ring
DEF: Copper deposits forming ring at outer edge of cornea; seen in Wilson's disease and other liver disorders.

371.15 Other deposits associated with metabolic disorders

371.16 Argentous deposits
DEF: Silver deposits in cornea.

✓5ᵗʰ **371.2   Corneal edema**

371.20 Corneal edema, unspecified

371.21 Idiopathic corneal edema
DEF: Corneal swelling and fluid retention of unknown cause.

371.22 Secondary corneal edema
DEF: Corneal swelling and fluid retention caused by an underlying disease, injury, or condition.

371.23 Bullous keratopathy
DEF: Corneal degeneration; characterized by recurring, rupturing epithelial "blisters;" ruptured blebs expose corneal nerves, cause great pain; occurs in glaucoma, iridocyclitis and Fuchs' epithelial dystrophy.

371.24 Corneal edema due to wearing of contact lenses

✓5ᵗʰ **371.3   Changes of corneal membranes**

371.30 Corneal membrane change, unspecified

371.31 Folds and rupture of Bowman's membrane

371.32 Folds in Descemet's membrane

371.33 Rupture in Descemet's membrane

✓5ᵗʰ **371.4   Corneal degenerations**

371.40 Corneal degeneration, unspecified

371.41 Senile corneal changes
Arcus senilis   Hassall-Henle bodies

371.42 Recurrent erosion of cornea
EXCLUDES   Mooren's ulcer (370.07)

✓4ᵗʰ / ✓5ᵗʰ Additional Digit Required | Unspecified Code | | Other Specified Code | | Manifestation Code | ▶◄ Revised Text   ● New Code   ▲ Revised Code Title

371.43 Band-shaped keratopathy
DEF: Horizontal bands of superficial corneal calcium deposits.

371.44 Other calcerous degenerations of cornea

371.45 Keratomalacia NOS
    EXCLUDES   *that due to vitamin A deficiency (264.4)*
DEF: Destruction of the cornea by keratinization of the epithelium with ulceration and perforation of the cornea; seen in cases of vitamin A deficiency.

371.46 Nodular degeneration of cornea
Salzmann's nodular dystrophy

371.48 Peripheral degenerations of cornea
Marginal degeneration of cornea [Terrien's]

371.49 Other
Discrete colliquative keratopathy

√5ᵗʰ **371.5 Hereditary corneal dystrophies**
DEF: Genetic disorder; leads to opacities, edema or lesions of cornea.

371.50 Corneal dystrophy, unspecified

371.51 Juvenile epithelial corneal dystrophy

371.52 Other anterior corneal dystrophies
Corneal dystrophy:
    microscopic cystic
    ring-like

371.53 Granular corneal dystrophy

371.54 Lattice corneal dystrophy

371.55 Macular corneal dystrophy

371.56 Other stromal corneal dystrophies
Crystalline corneal dystrophy

371.57 Endothelial corneal dystrophy
Combined corneal dystrophy
Cornea guttata
Fuchs' endothelial dystrophy

371.58 Other posterior corneal dystrophies
Polymorphous corneal dystrophy

√5ᵗʰ **371.6 Keratoconus**
DEF: Bilateral bulging protrusion of anterior cornea; often due to noninflammatory thinning.

371.60 Keratoconus, unspecified

371.61 Keratoconus, stable condition

371.62 Keratoconus, acute hydrops

√5ᵗʰ **371.7 Other corneal deformities**

371.70 Corneal deformity, unspecified

371.71 Corneal ectasia
DEF: Bulging protrusion of thinned, scarred cornea.

371.72 Descemetocele
DEF: Protrusion of Descemet's membrane into cornea.

371.73 Corneal staphyloma
DEF: Protrusion of cornea into adjacent tissue.

√5ᵗʰ **371.8 Other corneal disorders**

371.81 Corneal anesthesia and hypoesthesia
DEF: Decreased or absent sensitivity of cornea.

371.82 Corneal disorder due to contact lens
    EXCLUDES   *corneal edema due to contact lens (371.24)*
DEF: Contact lens wear causing cornea disorder, excluding swelling.

371.89 Other
AHA: 3Q, '99, 12

371.9 Unspecified corneal disorder

√4ᵗʰ **372 Disorders of conjunctiva**
    EXCLUDES   *keratoconjunctivitis (370.3-370.4)*

√5ᵗʰ **372.0 Acute conjunctivitis**

372.00 Acute conjunctivitis, unspecified

372.01 Serous conjunctivitis, except viral
    EXCLUDES   *viral conjunctivitis NOS (077.9)*

372.02 Acute follicular conjunctivitis
Conjunctival folliculosis NOS
    EXCLUDES   *conjunctivitis:*
      adenoviral (acute follicular) (077.3)
      epidemic hemorrhagic (077.4)
      inclusion (077.0)
      Newcastle (077.8)
      epidemic keratoconjunctivitis (077.1)
      pharyngoconjunctival fever (077.2)
DEF: Severe conjunctival inflammation with dense infiltrations of lymphoid tissues of inner eyelids; may be traced to a viral or chlamydial etiology.

372.03 Other mucopurulent conjunctivitis
Catarrhal conjunctivitis
    EXCLUDES   *blennorrhea neonatorum (gonococcal) (098.40)*
      neonatal conjunctivitis(771.6)
      ophthalmia neonatorum NOS (771.6)

372.04 Pseudomembranous conjunctivitis
Membranous conjunctivitis
    EXCLUDES   *diphtheritic conjunctivitis (032.81)*
DEF: Severe inflammation of conjunctiva; false membrane develops on inner surface of eyelid; membrane can be removed without harming epithelium, due to bacterial infections, toxic and allergic factors, and viral infections.

372.05 Acute atopic conjunctivitis
DEF: Sudden, severe conjunctivitis due to allergens.

√5ᵗʰ **372.1 Chronic conjunctivitis**

372.10 Chronic conjunctivitis, unspecified

372.11 Simple chronic conjunctivitis

372.12 Chronic follicular conjunctivitis
DEF: Persistent inflammation of conjunctiva; with infiltration of lymphoid tissue of inner eyelids.

372.13 Vernal conjunctivitis
AHA: 3Q, '96, 8

372.14 Other chronic allergic conjunctivitis
AHA: 3Q, '96, 8

372.15 *Parasitic conjunctivitis*
Code first underlying disease, as:
    filariasis (125.0-125.9)
    mucocutaneous leishmaniasis (085.5)

√5ᵗʰ **372.2 Blepharoconjunctivitis**

372.20 Blepharoconjunctivitis, unspecified

372.21 Angular blepharoconjunctivitis
DEF: Inflammation at junction of upper and lower eyelids; may block lacrimal secretions.

372.22 Contact blepharoconjunctivitis

√5ᵗʰ **372.3 Other and unspecified conjunctivitis**

372.30 Conjunctivitis, unspecified

372.31 *Rosacea conjunctivitis*
Code first underlying rosacea dermatitis (695.3)

N Newborn Age: 0   P Pediatric Age: 0-17   M Maternity Age: 12-55   A Adult Age: 15-124   MSP Medicare Secondary Payer

372.33 Conjunctivitis in mucocutaneous disease

Code first underlying disease, as:
erythema multiforme (695.1)
Reiter's disease (099.3)

EXCLUDES   ocular pemphigoid (694.61)

372.39 Other

√5ᵗʰ **372.4 Pterygium**

EXCLUDES   pseudopterygium (372.52)

DEF: Wedge-shaped, conjunctival thickening that advances from the inner corner of the eye toward the cornea.

372.40 Pterygium, unspecified

372.41 Peripheral pterygium, stationary

372.42 Peripheral pterygium, progressive

372.43 Central pterygium

372.44 Double pterygium

372.45 Recurrent pterygium

√5ᵗʰ **372.5 Conjunctival degenerations and deposits**

372.50 Conjunctival degeneration, unspecified

372.51 Pinguecula

DEF: Proliferative spot on the bulbar conjunctiva located near the sclerocorneal junction, usually on the nasal side; it is seen in elderly people.

372.52 Pseudopterygium

DEF: Conjunctival scar joined to the cornea; it looks like a pterygium but is not attached to the tissue.

372.53 Conjunctival xerosis

EXCLUDES   conjunctival xerosis due to vitamin A deficiency (264.0, 264.1, 264.7)

DEF: Dry conjunctiva due to vitamin A deficiency; related to Bitot's spots; may develop into xerophthalmia and keratomalacia.

372.54 Conjunctival concretions

DEF: Calculus or deposit on conjunctiva.

372.55 Conjunctival pigmentations

Conjunctival argyrosis

DEF: Color deposits in conjunctiva.

372.56 Conjunctival deposits

√5ᵗʰ **372.6 Conjunctival scars**

372.61 Granuloma of conjunctiva

372.62 Localized adhesions and strands of conjunctiva

DEF: Abnormal fibrous connections in conjunctiva.

372.63 Symblepharon

Extensive adhesions of conjunctiva

DEF: Adhesion of the eyelids to the eyeball.

372.64 Scarring of conjunctiva

Contraction of eye socket (after enucleation)

√5ᵗʰ **372.7 Conjunctival vascular disorders and cysts**

372.71 Hyperemia of conjunctiva

DEF: Conjunctival blood vessel congestion causing eye redness.

372.72 Conjunctival hemorrhage

Hyposphagma
Subconjunctival hemorrhage

372.73 Conjunctival edema

Chemosis of conjunctiva
Subconjunctival edema

DEF: Fluid retention and swelling in conjunctival tissue.

372.74 Vascular abnormalities of conjunctiva

Aneurysm(ata) of conjunctiva

372.75 Conjunctival cysts

DEF: Abnormal sacs of fluid in conjunctiva.

√5ᵗʰ **372.8 Other disorders of conjunctiva**

372.81 Conjunctivochalasis

AHA: 4Q, '00, 41

DEF: Bilateral condition of redundant conjunctival tissue between globe and lower eyelid margin; may cover lower punctum, interferring with normal tearing.

372.89 Other disorders of conjunctiva

372.9 Unspecified disorder of conjunctiva

√4ᵗʰ **373 Inflammation of eyelids**

√5ᵗʰ **373.0 Blepharitis**

EXCLUDES   blepharoconjunctivitis (372.20-372.22)

373.00 Blepharitis, unspecified

373.01 Ulcerative blepharitis

373.02 Squamous blepharitis

√5ᵗʰ **373.1 Hordeolum and other deep inflammation of eyelid**

DEF: Purulent, localized, staphylococcal infection in sebaceous glands of eyelids.

373.11 Hordeolum externum

Hordeolum NOS
Stye

DEF: Infection of oil gland in eyelash follicles.

373.12 Hordeolum internum

Infection of meibomian gland

DEF: Infection of oil gland of eyelid margin.

373.13 Abscess of eyelid

Furuncle of eyelid

DEF: Inflamed pocket of pus on eyelid.

373.2 Chalazion

Meibomian (gland) cyst

EXCLUDES   infected meibomian gland (373.12)

DEF: Chronic inflammation of the meibomian gland, causing an eyelid mass.

√5ᵗʰ **373.3 Noninfectious dermatoses of eyelid**

373.31 Eczematous dermatitis of eyelid

373.32 Contact and allergic dermatitis of eyelid

373.33 Xeroderma of eyelid

373.34 Discoid lupus erythematosus of eyelid

373.4 Infective dermatitis of eyelid of types resulting in deformity

Code first underlying disease, as:
leprosy (030.0-030.9)
lupus vulgaris (tuberculous) (017.0)
yaws (102.0-102.9)

373.5 Other infective dermatitis of eyelid

Code first underlying disease, as:
actinomycosis (039.3)
impetigo (684)
mycotic dermatitis (110.0-111.9)
vaccinia (051.0)
postvaccination (999.0)

EXCLUDES   herpes:
simplex (054.41)
zoster (053.20)

373.6 Parasitic infestation of eyelid

Code first underlying disease, as:
leishmaniasis (085.0-085.9)
loiasis (125.2)
onchocerciasis (125.3)
pediculosis (132.0)

373.8 Other inflammations of eyelids

373.9 Unspecified inflammation of eyelid

√4ᵗʰ **374 Other disorders of eyelids**

√5ᵗʰ **374.0 Entropion and trichiasis of eyelid**

DEF: Entropion: turning inward of eyelid edge toward eyeball.

DEF: Trichiasis: ingrowing eyelashes marked by irritation with possible distortion of sight.

√4ᵗʰ
√5ᵗʰ Additional Digit Required   Unspecified Code   Other Specified Code   Manifestation Code   ▶◀ Revised Text   ● New Code   ▲ Revised Code Title

2005 ICD•9•CM   **Volume 1 — 99**

Nervous System and Sense Organs

374.00–375.14

Entropion and Ectropion

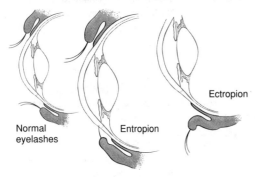

Normal eyelashes   Entropion   Ectropion

374.00 **Entropion, unspecified**   A

374.01 **Senile entropion**

374.02 **Mechanical entropion**

374.03 **Spastic entropion**

374.04 **Cicatricial entropion**

374.05 **Trichiasis without entropion**

√5ᵗʰ 374.1 **Ectropion**

DEF: Turning outward (eversion) of eyelid edge; exposes palpebral conjunctiva; dryness, irritation result.

374.10 **Ectropion, unspecified**   A

374.11 **Senile ectropion**

374.12 **Mechanical ectropion**

374.13 **Spastic ectropion**

374.14 **Cicatricial ectropion**

√5ᵗʰ 374.2 **Lagophthalmos**

DEF: Incomplete closure of eyes; causes dry eye and other complications.

374.20 **Lagophthalmos, unspecified**

374.21 **Paralytic lagophthalmos**

374.22 **Mechanical lagophthalmos**

374.23 **Cicatricial lagophthalmos**

√5ᵗʰ 374.3 **Ptosis of eyelid**

374.30 **Ptosis of eyelid, unspecified**

AHA: 2Q, '96, 11

374.31 **Paralytic ptosis**

DEF: Drooping of upper eyelid due to nerve disorder.

374.32 **Myogenic ptosis**

DEF: Drooping of upper eyelid due to muscle disorder.

374.33 **Mechanical ptosis**

DEF: Outside force causes drooping of upper eyelid.

374.34 **Blepharochalasis**

Pseudoptosis

DEF: Loss of elasticity, thickened or indurated skin of eyelids associated with recurrent episodes of idiopathic edema causing intracellular tissue atrophy.

√5ᵗʰ 374.4 **Other disorders affecting eyelid function**

EXCLUDES   blepharoclonus (333.81)
blepharospasm (333.81)
facial nerve palsy (351.0)
third nerve palsy or paralysis (378.51-378.52)
tic (psychogenic) (307.20-307.23)
organic (333.3)

374.41 **Lid retraction or lag**

374.43 **Abnormal innervation syndrome**

Jaw-blinking
Paradoxical facial movements

374.44 **Sensory disorders**

374.45 **Other sensorimotor disorders**

Deficient blink reflex

374.46 **Blepharophimosis**

Ankyloblepharon

DEF: Narrowing of palpebral fissure horizontally; caused by laterally displaced inner canthi; either acquired or congenital.

√5ᵗʰ 374.5 **Degenerative disorders of eyelid and periocular area**

374.50 **Degenerative disorder of eyelid, unspecified**

374.51 *Xanthelasma*

Xanthoma (planum) (tuberosum) of eyelid
Code first underlying condition (272.0-272.9)

DEF: Fatty tumors of eyelid linked to high fat content of blood.

374.52 **Hyperpigmentation of eyelid**

Chloasma   Dyspigmentation

DEF: Excess pigment of eyelid.

374.53 **Hypopigmentation of eyelid**

Vitiligo of eyelid

DEF: Lack of color pigment of the eyelid.

374.54 **Hypertrichosis of eyelid**

DEF: Excess eyelash growth.

374.55 **Hypotrichosis of eyelid**

Madarosis of eyelid

DEF: Less than normal, or .absent, eyelashes.

374.56 **Other degenerative disorders of skin affecting eyelid**

√5ᵗʰ 374.8 **Other disorders of eyelid**

374.81 **Hemorrhage of eyelid**

EXCLUDES   black eye (921.0)

374.82 **Edema of eyelid**

Hyperemia of eyelid

DEF: Swelling and fluid retention in eyelid.

374.83 **Elephantiasis of eyelid**

DEF: Filarial disease causing dermatitis and enlarged eyelid.

374.84 **Cysts of eyelids**

Sebaceous cyst of eyelid

374.85 **Vascular anomalies of eyelid**

374.86 **Retained foreign body of eyelid**

374.87 **Dermatochalasis**

DEF: Acquired form of connective tissue disorder associated with decreased elastic tissue and abnormal elastin formation resulting in loss of elasticity of the skin of the eyelid, generally associated with aging.

374.89 **Other disorders of eyelid**

374.9 **Unspecified disorder of eyelid**

√4ᵗʰ 375 **Disorders of lacrimal system**

√5ᵗʰ 375.0 **Dacryoadenitis**

375.00 **Dacryoadenitis, unspecified**

375.01 **Acute dacryoadenitis**

DEF: Severe, sudden inflammation of lacrimal gland.

375.02 **Chronic dacryoadenitis**

DEF: Persistent inflammation of lacrimal gland.

375.03 **Chronic enlargement of lacrimal gland**

√5ᵗʰ 375.1 **Other disorders of lacrimal gland**

375.11 **Dacryops**

DEF: Overproduction and constant flow of tears; may cause distended lacrimal duct.

375.12 **Other lacrimal cysts and cystic degeneration**

375.13 **Primary lacrimal atrophy**

375.14 **Secondary lacrimal atrophy**

DEF: Wasting away of lacrimal gland due to another disease.

375.15 Tear film insufficiency, unspecified
Dry eye syndrome
AHA: 3Q, '96, 6

DEF: Eye dryness and irritation due to insufficient tear production.

375.16 Dislocation of lacrimal gland

√5th **375.2 Epiphora**
DEF: Abnormal development of tears due to stricture of lacrimal passages.

375.20 Epiphora, unspecified as to cause
375.21 Epiphora due to excess lacrimation
DEF: Tear overflow due to overproduction.

375.22 Epiphora due to insufficient drainage
DEF: Tear overflow due to blocked drainage.

√5th **375.3 Acute and unspecified inflammation of lacrimal passages**
EXCLUDES *neonatal dacryocystitis (771.6)*
375.30 Dacryocystitis, unspecified
375.31 Acute canaliculitis, lacrimal
375.32 Acute dacryocystitis
Acute peridacryocystitis
375.33 Phlegmonous dacryocystitis
DEF: Infection of tear sac with pockets of pus.

√5th **375.4 Chronic inflammation of lacrimal passages**
375.41 Chronic canaliculitis
375.42 Chronic dacryocystitis
375.43 Lacrimal mucocele

√5th **375.5 Stenosis and insufficiency of lacrimal passages**
375.51 Eversion of lacrimal punctum
DEF: Abnormal turning outward of tear duct.
375.52 Stenosis of lacrimal punctum
DEF: Abnormal narrowing of tear duct.
375.53 Stenosis of lacrimal canaliculi
375.54 Stenosis of lacrimal sac
DEF: Abnormal narrowing of tear sac.
375.55 Obstruction of nasolacrimal duct, neonatal
EXCLUDES *congenital anomaly of nasolacrimal duct (743.65)*
DEF: Acquired, abnormal obstruction of lacrimal system, from eye to nose; in an infant.
375.56 Stenosis of nasolacrimal duct, acquired
375.57 Dacryolith
DEF: Concretion or stone in lacrimal system.

√5th **375.6 Other changes of lacrimal passages**
375.61 Lacrimal fistula
DEF: Abnormal communication from lacrimal system.
375.69 Other

√5th **375.8 Other disorders of lacrimal system**
375.81 Granuloma of lacrimal passages
DEF: Abnormal nodules within lacrimal system.
375.89 Other

375.9 Unspecified disorder of lacrimal system

√4th **376 Disorders of the orbit**
√5th **376.0 Acute inflammation of orbit**
376.00 Acute inflammation of orbit, unspecified
376.01 Orbital cellulitis
Abscess of orbit
DEF: Infection of tissue between orbital bone and eyeball.
376.02 Orbital periostitis
DEF: Inflammation of connective tissue covering orbital bone.

Lacrimal System

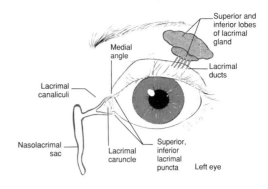

376.03 Orbital osteomyelitis
DEF: Inflammation of orbital bone.

376.04 Tenonitis
√5th **376.1 Chronic inflammatory disorders of orbit**
376.10 Chronic inflammation of orbit, unspecified
376.11 Orbital granuloma
Pseudotumor (inflammatory) of orbit
DEF: Abnormal nodule between orbital bone and eyeball.
376.12 Orbital myositis
DEF: Painful inflammation of eye muscles.
376.13 *Parasitic infestation of orbit*
Code first underlying disease, as:
hydatid infestation of orbit (122.3, 122.6, 122.9)
myiasis of orbit (134.0)

√5th **376.2 Endocrine exophthalmos**
Code first underlying thyroid disorder (242.0-242.9)
376.21 *Thyrotoxic exophthalmos*
DEF: Bulging eyes due to hyperthyroidism.
376.22 *Exophthalmic ophthalmoplegia*
DEF: Inability to rotate eye due to bulging eyes.

√5th **376.3 Other exophthalmic conditions**
376.30 Exophthalmos, unspecified
DEF: Abnormal protrusion of eyeball.
376.31 Constant exophthalmos
DEF: Continuous, abnormal protrusion or bulging of eyeball.
376.32 Orbital hemorrhage
DEF: Bleeding behind the eyeball, causing forward bulge.
376.33 Orbital edema or congestion
DEF: Fluid retention behind eyeball, causing forward bulge.
376.34 Intermittent exophthalmos
376.35 Pulsating exophthalmos
DEF: Bulge or protrusion; associated with a carotid-cavernous fistula.
376.36 Lateral displacement of globe
DEF: Abnormal displacement of the eyeball away from nose, toward temple.

√5th **376.4 Deformity of orbit**
376.40 Deformity of orbit, unspecified
376.41 Hypertelorism of orbit
DEF: Abnormal increase in interorbital distance; associated with congenital facial deformities; may be accompanied by mental deficiency.

√4th Additional Digit Required   Unspecified Code   Other Specified Code   Manifestation Code   ▶◀ Revised Text   ● New Code   ▲ Revised Code Title

2005 ICD•9•CM   **Volume 1 — 101**

Nervous System and Sense Organs

376.42–377.9

376.42 Exostosis of orbit
DEF: Abnormal bony growth of orbit.

376.43 Local deformities due to bone disease
DEF: Acquired abnormalities of orbit; due to bone disease.

376.44 Orbital deformities associated with craniofacial deformities

376.45 Atrophy of orbit
DEF: Wasting away of bone tissue of orbit.

376.46 Enlargement of orbit

376.47 Deformity due to trauma or surgery

√5ᵗʰ **376.5 Enophthalmos**
DEF: Recession of eyeball deep into eye socket.

376.50 Enophthalmos, unspecified as to cause

376.51 Enophthalmos due to atrophy of orbital tissue

376.52 Enophthalmos due to trauma or surgery

376.6 Retained (old) foreign body following penetrating wound of orbit
Retrobulbar foreign body

√5ᵗʰ **376.8 Other orbital disorders**
376.81 Orbital cysts
Encephalocele of orbit
AHA: 3Q, '99, 13

376.82 Myopathy of extraocular muscles
DEF: Disease in the muscles that control eyeball movement.

376.89 Other

376.9 Unspecified disorder of orbit

√4ᵗʰ **377 Disorders of optic nerve and visual pathways**

√5ᵗʰ **377.0 Papilledema**
377.00 Papilledema, unspecified

377.01 Papilledema associated with increased intracranial pressure

377.02 Papilledema associated with decreased ocular pressure

377.03 Papilledema associated with retinal disorder

377.04 Foster-Kennedy syndrome
DEF: Retrobulbar optic neuritis, central scotoma and optic atrophy; caused by tumors in frontal lobe of brain that press downward.

√5ᵗʰ **377.1 Optic atrophy**
377.10 Optic atrophy, unspecified

377.11 Primary optic atrophy
EXCLUDES   neurosyphilitic optic atrophy (094.84)

377.12 Postinflammatory optic atrophy
DEF: Adverse effect of inflammation causing wasting away of eye.

377.13 Optic atrophy associated with retinal dystrophies
DEF: Progressive changes in retinal tissue due to metabolic disorder causing wasting away of eye.

377.14 Glaucomatous atrophy [cupping] of optic disc

377.15 Partial optic atrophy
Temporal pallor of optic disc

377.16 Hereditary optic atrophy
Optic atrophy:
    dominant hereditary
    Leber's

√5ᵗʰ **377.2 Other disorders of optic disc**
377.21 Drusen of optic disc
377.22 Crater-like holes of optic disc

377.23 Coloboma of optic disc
DEF: Ocular malformation caused by the failure of fetal fissure of optic stalk to close.

377.24 Pseudopapilledema

√5ᵗʰ **377.3 Optic neuritis**
EXCLUDES   meningococcal optic neuritis (036.81)

377.30 Optic neuritis, unspecified

377.31 Optic papillitis
DEF: Swelling and inflammation of optic disc.

377.32 Retrobulbar neuritis (acute)
EXCLUDES   syphilitic retrobulbar neuritis (094.85)
DEF: Inflammation of optic nerve immediately behind the eyeball.

377.33 Nutritional optic neuropathy
DEF: Malnutrition causing optic nerve disorder.

377.34 Toxic optic neuropathy
Toxic amblyopia
DEF: Toxic substance causing optic nerve disorder.

377.39 Other
EXCLUDES   ischemic optic neuropathy (377.41)

√5ᵗʰ **377.4 Other disorders of optic nerve**
377.41 Ischemic optic neuropathy
DEF: Decreased blood flow affecting optic nerve.

377.42 Hemorrhage in optic nerve sheaths
DEF: Bleeding in meningeal lining of optic nerve.

377.49 Other
Compression of optic nerve

√5ᵗʰ **377.5 Disorders of optic chiasm**
377.51 Associated with pituitary neoplasms and disorders
DEF: Abnormal pituitary growth causing disruption in nerve chain from retina to brain.

377.52 Associated with other neoplasms
DEF: Abnormal growth, other than pituitary, causing disruption in nerve chain from retina to brain.

377.53 Associated with vascular disorders
DEF: Vascular disorder causing disruption in nerve chain from retina to brain.

377.54 Associated with inflammatory disorders
DEF: Inflammatory disease causing disruption in nerve chain from retina to brain.

√5ᵗʰ **377.6 Disorders of other visual pathways**
377.61 Associated with neoplasms
377.62 Associated with vascular disorders
377.63 Associated with inflammatory disorders

√5ᵗʰ **377.7 Disorders of visual cortex**
EXCLUDES   visual:
    agnosia (368.16)
    hallucinations (368.16)
    halos (368.15)

377.71 Associated with neoplasms
377.72 Associated with vascular disorders
377.73 Associated with inflammatory disorders
377.75 Cortical blindness
DEF: Blindness due to brain disorder, rather than eye disorder.

377.9 Unspecified disorder of optic nerve and visual pathways

---

√4ᵗʰ **378 Strabismus and other disorders of binocular eye movements**

> **EXCLUDES** *nystagmus and other irregular eye movements (379.50-379.59)*

DEF: Misalignment of the eyes due to imbalance in extraocular muscles.

√5ᵗʰ **378.0 Esotropia**

Convergent concomitant strabismus

> **EXCLUDES** *intermittent esotropia (378.20-378.22)*

DEF: Visual axis deviation created by one eye fixing upon an image and the other eye deviating inward.

378.00 Esotropia, unspecified

378.01 Monocular esotropia

378.02 Monocular esotropia with A pattern

378.03 Monocular esotropia with V pattern

378.04 Monocular esotropia with other noncomitancies

Monocular esotropia with X or Y pattern

378.05 Alternating esotropia

378.06 Alternating esotropia with A pattern

378.07 Alternating esotropia with V pattern

378.08 Alternating esotropia with other noncomitancies

Alternating esotropia with X or Y pattern

√5ᵗʰ **378.1 Exotropia**

Divergent concomitant strabismus

> **EXCLUDES** *intermittent exotropia (378.20, 378.23-378.24)*

DEF: Visual axis deviation created by one eye fixing upon an image and the other eye deviating outward.

378.10 Exotropia, unspecified

378.11 Monocular exotropia

378.12 Monocular exotropia with A pattern

378.13 Monocular exotropia with V pattern

378.14 Monocular exotropia with other noncomitancies

Monocular exotropia with X or Y pattern

378.15 Alternating exotropia

378.16 Alternating exotropia with A pattern

378.17 Alternating exotropia with V pattern

378.18 Alternating exotropia with other noncomitancies

Alternating exotropia with X or Y pattern

√5ᵗʰ **378.2 Intermittent heterotropia**

> **EXCLUDES** *vertical heterotropia (intermittent) (378.31)*

DEF: Deviation of eyes seen only at intervals; it is also called strabismus.

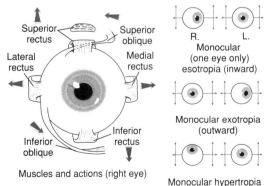

Eye Musculature

Superior rectus — Superior oblique — Lateral rectus — Medial rectus — Inferior oblique — Inferior rectus

Muscles and actions (right eye)

R.   L.
Monocular (one eye only) esotropia (inward)

Monocular exotropia (outward)

Monocular hypertropia (upward)

√5ᵗʰ **378.20 Intermittent heterotropia, unspecified**

Intermittent:
esotropia NOS
exotropia NOS

378.21 Intermittent esotropia, monocular

378.22 Intermittent esotropia, alternating

378.23 Intermittent exotropia, monocular

378.24 Intermittent exotropia, alternating

√5ᵗʰ **378.3 Other and unspecified heterotropia**

378.30 Heterotropia, unspecified

378.31 Hypertropia

Vertical heterotropia (constant)
(intermittent)

378.32 Hypotropia

378.33 Cyclotropia

378.34 Monofixation syndrome

Microtropia

378.35 Accommodative component in esotropia

√5ᵗʰ **378.4 Heterophoria**

DEF: Deviation occurring only when the other eye is covered.

378.40 Heterophoria, unspecified

378.41 Esophoria

378.42 Exophoria

378.43 Vertical heterophoria

378.44 Cyclophoria

378.45 Alternating hyperphoria

√5ᵗʰ **378.5 Paralytic strabismus**

DEF: Deviation of the eye due to nerve paralysis affecting muscle.

378.50 Paralytic strabismus, unspecified

378.51 Third or oculomotor nerve palsy, partial

AHA: 3Q, '91, 9

378.52 Third or oculomotor nerve palsy, total

AHA: 2Q, '89, 12

378.53 Fourth or trochlear nerve palsy

AHA: 2Q, '01, 21

378.54 Sixth or abducens nerve palsy

AHA: 2Q, '89, 12

378.55 External ophthalmoplegia

378.56 Total ophthalmoplegia

√5ᵗʰ **378.6 Mechanical strabismus**

DEF: Deviation of the eye due to an outside force on extraocular muscle.

378.60 Mechanical strabismus, unspecified

378.61 Brown's (tendon) sheath syndrome

DEF: Congenital or acquired shortening of the anterior sheath of the superior oblique muscle; the eye is unable to move upward and inward; it is usually unilateral.

378.62 Mechanical strabismus from other musculofascial disorders

378.63 Limited duction associated with other conditions

√5ᵗʰ **378.7 Other specified strabismus**

378.71 Duane's syndrome

DEF: Congenital, affects one eye; due to abnormal fibrous bands attached to rectus muscle; inability to abduct affected eye with retraction of globe.

378.72 Progressive external ophthalmoplegia

DEF: Paralysis progressing from one eye muscle to another.

378.73 Strabismus in other neuromuscular disorders

√5ᵗʰ **378.8 Other disorders of binocular eye movements**

> **EXCLUDES** *nystagmus (379.50-379.56)*

√4ᵗʰ
√5ᵗʰ Additional Digit Required   Unspecified Code   Other Specified Code   Manifestation Code   ►◄ Revised Text   ● New Code   ▲ Revised Code Title

2005 ICD•9•CM   **Volume 1 — 103**

Nervous System and Sense Organs

378–378.8

Nervous System and Sense Organs

378.81 Palsy of conjugate gaze
DEF: Muscle dysfunction impairing parallel movement of the eye.

378.82 Spasm of conjugate gaze
DEF: Muscle contractions impairing parallel movement of eye.

378.83 Convergence insufficiency or palsy

378.84 Convergence excess or spasm

378.85 Anomalies of divergence

378.86 Internuclear ophthalmoplegia
DEF: Eye movement anomaly due to brainstem lesion.

378.87 Other dissociated deviation of eye movements
Skew deviation

378.9 Unspecified disorder of eye movements
Ophthalmoplegia NOS Strabismus NOS
AHA: 2Q, '01, 21

✓4ᵗʰ **379 Other disorders of eye**

✓5ᵗʰ **379.0 Scleritis and episcleritis**
EXCLUDES syphilitic episcleritis (095.0)

379.00 Scleritis, unspecified
Episcleritis NOS

379.01 Episcleritis periodica fugax
DEF: Hyperemia (engorgement) of the sclera and overlying conjunctiva characterized by a sudden onset and short duration.

379.02 Nodular episcleritis
DEF: Inflammation of the outermost layer of the sclera, with formation of nodules.

379.03 Anterior scleritis

379.04 Scleromalacia perforans
DEF: Scleral thinning, softening and degeneration; seen with rheumatoid arthritis.

379.05 Scleritis with corneal involvement
Scleroperikeratitis

379.06 Brawny scleritis
DEF: Severe inflammation of the sclera; with thickened corneal margins.

379.07 Posterior scleritis
Sclerotenonitis

379.09 Other
Scleral abscess

✓5ᵗʰ **379.1 Other disorders of sclera**
EXCLUDES blue sclera (743.47)

379.11 Scleral ectasia
Scleral staphyloma NOS
DEF: Protrusion of the contents of the eyeball where the sclera has thinned.

379.12 Staphyloma posticum
DEF: Ring-shaped protrusion or bulging of sclera and uveal tissue at posterior pole of eye.

379.13 Equatorial staphyloma
DEF: Ring-shaped protrusion or bulging of sclera and uveal tissue midway between front and back of eye.

379.14 Anterior staphyloma, localized

379.15 Ring staphyloma

379.16 Other degenerative disorders of sclera

379.19 Other

✓5ᵗʰ **379.2 Disorders of vitreous body**
DEF: Disorder of clear gel that fills space between retina and lens.

379.21 Vitreous degeneration
Vitreous: Vitreous:
  cavitation   liquefaction
  detachment

379.22 Crystalline deposits in vitreous
Asteroid hyalitis
Synchysis scintillans

379.23 Vitreous hemorrhage
AHA: 3Q, '91, 15

379.24 Other vitreous opacities
Vitreous floaters

379.25 Vitreous membranes and strands

379.26 Vitreous prolapse
DEF: Slipping of vitreous from normal position.

379.29 Other disorders of vitreous
EXCLUDES vitreous abscess (360.04)
AHA: 1Q, '99, 11

✓5ᵗʰ **379.3 Aphakia and other disorders of lens**
EXCLUDES after-cataract (366.50-366.53)

379.31 Aphakia
EXCLUDES cataract extraction status (V45.61)
DEF: Absence of eye's crystalline lens.

379.32 Subluxation of lens

379.33 Anterior dislocation of lens
DEF: Lens displaced toward iris.

379.34 Posterior dislocation of lens
DEF: Lens displaced backward toward vitreous.

379.39 Other disorders of lens

✓5ᵗʰ **379.4 Anomalies of pupillary function**

379.40 Abnormal pupillary function, unspecified

379.41 Anisocoria
DEF: Unequal pupil diameter.

379.42 Miosis (persistent), not due to miotics
DEF: Abnormal contraction of pupil less than 2 millimeters.

379.43 Mydriasis (persistent), not due to mydriatics
DEF: Morbid dilation of pupil.

379.45 Argyll Robertson pupil, atypical
Argyll Robertson phenomenon or pupil, nonsyphilitic
EXCLUDES Argyll Robertson pupil (syphilitic) (094.89)
DEF: Failure of pupil to respond to light; affects both eyes; may be caused by diseases such as syphilis of the central nervous system or miosis.

379.46 Tonic pupillary reaction
Adie's pupil or syndrome

379.49 Other
Hippus
Pupillary paralysis

✓5ᵗʰ **379.5 Nystagmus and other irregular eye movements**

379.50 Nystagmus, unspecified
AHA: 4Q, '02, 68; 2Q, '01, 21
DEF: Involuntary, rapid, rhythmic movement of eyeball; vertical, horizontal, rotatory or mixed; cause may be congenital, acquired, physiological, neurological, myopathic, or due to ocular diseases.

379.51 Congenital nystagmus

379.52 Latent nystagmus

379.53 Visual deprivation nystagmus

379.54 Nystagmus associated with disorders of the vestibular system

379.55 Dissociated nystagmus

379.56 Other forms of nystagmus

N   Newborn Age: 0   P   Pediatric Age: 0-17   M   Maternity Age: 12-55   A   Adult Age: 15-124   MSP   Medicare Secondary Payer

Ear and Mastoid Process

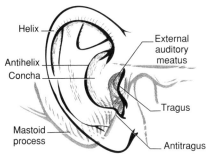

379.57 Deficiencies of saccadic eye movements
Abnormal optokinetic response

DEF: Saccadic eye movements; small, rapid, involuntary movements by both eyes simultaneously, due to changing point of fixation on visualized object.

379.58 Deficiencies of smooth pursuit movements
379.59 Other irregularities of eye movements
Opsoclonus

379.8 Other specified disorders of eye and adnexa
✓5ᵗʰ **379.9 Unspecified disorder of eye and adnexa**
379.90 Disorder of eye, unspecified
379.91 Pain in or around eye
379.92 Swelling or mass of eye
379.93 Redness or discharge of eye
379.99 Other ill-defined disorders of eye
EXCLUDES *blurred vision NOS (368.8)*

DISEASES OF THE EAR AND MASTOID PROCESS (380-389)

✓4ᵗʰ **380 Disorders of external ear**
▲ ✓5ᵗʰ **380.0 Perichondritis and chondritis of pinna**
▶Chondritis of auricle◀
Perichondritis of auricle
380.00 Perichondritis of pinna, unspecified
380.01 Acute perichondritis of pinna
380.02 Chronic perichondritis of pinna
● **380.03 Chondritis of pinna**
✓5ᵗʰ **380.1 Infective otitis externa**
380.10 Infective otitis externa, unspecified

Otitis externa (acute):	Otitis externa (acute):
NOS	hemorrhagica
circumscribed	infective NOS
diffuse	

380.11 Acute infection of pinna
EXCLUDES *furuncular otitis externa (680.0)*

380.12 Acute swimmers' ear
Beach ear   Tank ear
DEF: Otitis externa due to swimming.

380.13 Other acute infections of external ear
Code first underlying disease, as:
erysipelas (035)
impetigo (684)
seborrheic dermatitis (690.10-690.18)
EXCLUDES *herpes simplex (054.73)*
herpes zoster (053.71)

380.14 Malignant otitis externa
DEF: Severe necrotic otitis externa; due to bacteria.

380.15 Chronic mycotic otitis externa
Code first underlying disease, as:
aspergillosis (117.3)
otomycosis NOS (111.9)
EXCLUDES *candidal otitis externa (112.82)*

380.16 Other chronic infective otitis externa
Chronic infective otitis externa NOS

✓5ᵗʰ **380.2 Other otitis externa**
380.21 Cholesteatoma of external ear
Keratosis obturans of external ear (canal)
EXCLUDES *cholesteatoma NOS (385.30-385.35)*
postmastoidectomy (383.32)

DEF: Cystlike mass filled with debris, including cholesterol; rare, congenital condition.

380.22 Other acute otitis externa

Acute otitis externa:	Acute otitis externa:
actinic	eczematoid
chemical	reactive
contact	

380.23 Other chronic otitis externa
Chronic otitis externa NOS

✓5ᵗʰ **380.3 Noninfectious disorders of pinna**
380.30 Disorder of pinna, unspecified
380.31 Hematoma of auricle or pinna
380.32 Acquired deformities of auricle or pinna
EXCLUDES *cauliflower ear (738.7)*
AHA: 3Q, '03, 12

380.39 Other
EXCLUDES *gouty tophi of ear (274.81)*

380.4 Impacted cerumen
Wax in ear

✓5ᵗʰ **380.5 Acquired stenosis of external ear canal**
Collapse of external ear canal
380.50 Acquired stenosis of external ear canal, unspecified as to cause
380.51 Secondary to trauma
DEF: Narrowing of external ear canal; due to trauma.

380.52 Secondary to surgery
DEF: Postsurgical narrowing of external ear canal.

380.53 Secondary to inflammation
DEF: Narrowing, external ear canal; due to chronic inflammation.

✓5ᵗʰ **380.8 Other disorders of external ear**
380.81 Exostosis of external ear canal
380.89 Other
380.9 Unspecified disorder of external ear

✓4ᵗʰ **381 Nonsuppurative otitis media and Eustachian tube disorders**
✓5ᵗʰ **381.0 Acute nonsuppurative otitis media**
Acute tubotympanic catarrh
Otitis media, acute or subacute:
catarrhal
exudative
transudative
with effusion
EXCLUDES *otitic barotrauma (993.0)*

381.00 Acute nonsuppurative otitis media, unspecified
381.01 Acute serous otitis media
Acute or subacute secretory otitis media
DEF: Sudden, severe infection of middle ear.

381.02 Acute mucoid otitis media
Acute or subacute seromucinous otitis media
Blue drum syndrome
DEF: Sudden, severe infection of middle ear, with mucous.

381.03 Acute sanguinous otitis media
DEF: Sudden, severe infection of middle ear, with blood.

381.04 Acute allergic serous otitis media
381.05 Acute allergic mucoid otitis media
381.06 Acute allergic sanguinous otitis media

✓4ᵗʰ ✓5ᵗʰ Additional Digit Required   Unspecified Code   Other Specified Code   Manifestation Code   ▶◀ Revised Text   ● New Code   ▲ Revised Code Title

2005 ICD•9•CM   October 2004 • Volume 1 — 105

Nervous System and Sense Organs

381.1–383.1

√5ᵗʰ **381.1 Chronic serous otitis media**
Chronic tubotympanic catarrh

381.10 Chronic serous otitis media, simple or unspecified
DEF: Persistent infection of middle ear, without pus.

381.19 Other
Serosanguinous chronic otitis media

√5ᵗʰ **381.2 Chronic mucoid otitis media**
Glue ear
EXCLUDES   *adhesive middle ear disease (385.10-385.19)*
DEF: Chronic condition; characterized by viscous fluid in middle ear; due to obstructed Eustachian tube.

381.20 Chronic mucoid otitis media, simple or unspecified

381.29 Other
Mucosanguinous chronic otitis media

381.3 Other and unspecified chronic nonsuppurative otitis media

Otitis media, chronic:	Otitis media, chronic:
allergic	seromucinous
exudative	transudative
secretory	with effusion

381.4 Nonsuppurative otitis media, not specified as acute or chronic

Otitis media:	Otitis media:
allergic	seromucinous
catarrhal	serous
exudative	transudative
mucoid	with effusion
secretory	

√5ᵗʰ **381.5 Eustachian salpingitis**

381.50 Eustachian salpingitis, unspecified

381.51 Acute Eustachian salpingitis
DEF: Sudden, severe inflammation of Eustachian tube.

381.52 Chronic Eustachian salpingitis
DEF: Persistent inflammation of Eustachian tube.

√5ᵗʰ **381.6 Obstruction of Eustachian tube**
Stenosis ⎫
Stricture ⎬ of Eustachian tube

381.60 Obstruction of Eustachian tube, unspecified

381.61 Osseous obstruction of Eustachian tube
Obstruction of Eustachian tube from cholesteatoma, polyp, or other osseous lesion

381.62 Intrinsic cartilagenous obstruction of Eustachian tube
DEF: Blockage of Eustachian tube; due to cartilage overgrowth.

381.63 Extrinsic cartilagenous obstruction of Eustachian tube
Compression of Eustachian tube

381.7 Patulous Eustachian tube
DEF: Distended, oversized Eustachian tube.

√5ᵗʰ **381.8 Other disorders of Eustachian tube**
381.81 Dysfunction of Eustachian tube
381.89 Other

381.9 Unspecified Eustachian tube disorder

√4ᵗʰ **382 Suppurative and unspecified otitis media**
√5ᵗʰ **382.0 Acute suppurative otitis media**

Otitis media, acute:	Otitis media, acute:
necrotizing NOS	purulent

382.00 Acute suppurative otitis media without spontaneous rupture of ear drum
DEF: Sudden, severe inflammation of middle ear, with pus.

382.01 Acute suppurative otitis media with spontaneous rupture of ear drum
DEF: Sudden, severe inflammation of middle ear, with pressure tearing ear drum tissue.

382.02 Acute suppurative otitis media in diseases classified elsewhere
Code first underlying disease, as:
influenza (487.8)
scarlet fever (034.1)
EXCLUDES   *postmeasles otitis (055.2)*

382.1 Chronic tubotympanic suppurative otitis media
Benign chronic suppurative otitis media ⎫
Chronic tubotympanic disease ⎬ (with anterior perforation of ear drum)
DEF: Inflammation of tympanic cavity and auditory tube; with pus formation.

382.2 Chronic atticoantral suppurative otitis media
Chronic atticoantral disease ⎫
Persistent mucosal disease ⎬ (with posterior or superior marginal perforation of ear drum)
DEF: Inflammation of upper tympanic membrane and mastoid antrum; with pus formation.

382.3 Unspecified chronic suppurative otitis media
Chronic purulent otitis media
EXCLUDES   *tuberculous otitis media (017.4)*

382.4 Unspecified suppurative otitis media
Purulent otitis media NOS

382.9 Unspecified otitis media

Otitis media:	Otitis media:
NOS	chronic NOS
acute NOS	

AHA: N-D, '84, 16

√4ᵗʰ **383 Mastoiditis and related conditions**
√5ᵗʰ **383.0 Acute mastoiditis**
Abscess of mastoid   Empyema of mastoid

383.00 Acute mastoiditis without complications
DEF: Sudden, severe inflammation of mastoid air cells.

383.01 Subperiosteal abscess of mastoid
DEF: Pocket of pus within mastoid bone.

383.02 Acute mastoiditis with other complications
Gradenigo's syndrome

383.1 Chronic mastoiditis
Caries of mastoid
Fistula of mastoid
EXCLUDES   *tuberculous mastoiditis (015.6)*
DEF: Persistent inflammation of mastoid air cells.

Middle and Inner Ear

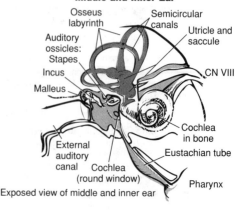

Exposed view of middle and inner ear

√5ᵗʰ **383.2　Petrositis**

Coalescing osteitis
Inflammation　　} of petrous bone
Osteomyelitis

383.20 Petrositis, unspecified

383.21 Acute petrositis

DEF: Sudden, severe inflammation of dense bone behind ear.

383.22 Chronic petrositis

DEF: Persistent inflammation of dense bone behind ear.

√5ᵗʰ **383.3　Complications following mastoidectomy**

383.30 Postmastoidectomy complication, unspecified

383.31 Mucosal cyst of postmastoidectomy cavity

DEF: Mucous-lined cyst cavity following removal of mastoid bone.

383.32 Recurrent cholesteatoma of postmastoidectomy cavity

DEF: Cystlike mass of cell debris in cavity following removal of mastoid bone.

383.33 Granulations of postmastoidectomy cavity

Chronic inflammation of postmastoidectomy cavity

DEF: Granular tissue in cavity following removal of mastoid bone.

√5ᵗʰ **383.8　Other disorders of mastoid**

383.81 Postauricular fistula

DEF: Abnormal passage behind mastoid cavity.

383.89 Other

383.9　Unspecified mastoiditis

√4ᵗʰ **384　Other disorders of tympanic membrane**

√5ᵗʰ **384.0　Acute myringitis without mention of otitis media**

384.00 Acute myringitis, unspecified

Acute tympanitis NOS

DEF: Sudden, severe inflammation of ear drum.

384.01 Bullous myringitis

Myringitis bullosa hemorrhagica

DEF: Type of viral otitis media characterized by the appearance of serous or hemorrhagic blebs on the tympanic membrane.

384.09 Other

384.1　Chronic myringitis without mention of otitis media

Chronic tympanitis

DEF: Persistent inflammation of ear drum; with no evidence of middle ear infection.

√5ᵗʰ **384.2　Perforation of tympanic membrane**

Perforation of ear drum:　Perforation of ear drum:
　NOS　　　　　　　　　　postinflammatory
　persistent　　　　　　　posttraumatic

EXCLUDES　*otitis media with perforation of tympanic membrane (382.00-382.9)*

traumatic perforation [current injury] (872.61)

384.20 Perforation of tympanic membrane, unspecified

384.21 Central perforation of tympanic membrane

384.22 Attic perforation of tympanic membrane

Pars flaccida

384.23 Other marginal perforation of tympanic membrane

384.24 Multiple perforations of tympanic membrane

384.25 Total perforation of tympanic membrane

√5ᵗʰ **384.8　Other specified disorders of tympanic membrane**

384.81 Atrophic flaccid tympanic membrane

Healed perforation of ear drum

384.82 Atrophic nonflaccid tympanic membrane

384.9　Unspecified disorder of tympanic membrane

√4ᵗʰ **385　Other disorders of middle ear and mastoid**

EXCLUDES　*mastoiditis (383.0-383.9)*

√5ᵗʰ **385.0　Tympanosclerosis**

385.00 Tympanosclerosis, unspecified as to involvement

385.01 Tympanosclerosis involving tympanic membrane only

DEF: Tough, fibrous tissue impeding functions of ear drum.

385.02 Tympanosclerosis involving tympanic membrane and ear ossicles

DEF: Tough, fibrous tissue impeding functions of middle ear bones (stapes, malleus, incus).

385.03 Tympanosclerosis involving tympanic membrane, ear ossicles, and middle ear

DEF: Tough, fibrous tissue impeding functions of ear drum, middle ear bones and middle ear canal.

385.09 Tympanosclerosis involving other combination of structures

√5ᵗʰ **385.1　Adhesive middle ear disease**

Adhesive otitis　　　Otitis media:
Otitis media:　　　　　fibrotic
　chronic adhesive

EXCLUDES　*glue ear (381.20-381.29)*

DEF: Adhesions of middle ear structures.

385.10 Adhesive middle ear disease, unspecified as to involvement

385.11 Adhesions of drum head to incus

385.12 Adhesions of drum head to stapes

385.13 Adhesions of drum head to promontorium

385.19 Other adhesions and combinations

√5ᵗʰ **385.2　Other acquired abnormality of ear ossicles**

385.21 Impaired mobility of malleus

Ankylosis of malleus

385.22 Impaired mobility of other ear ossicles

Ankylosis of ear ossicles, except malleus

385.23 Discontinuity or dislocation of ear ossicles

DEF: Disruption in auditory chain; created by malleus, incus and stapes.

385.24 Partial loss or necrosis of ear ossicles

DEF: Tissue loss in malleus, incus and stapes.

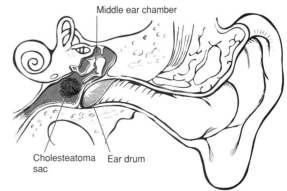

Cholesteatoma

Middle ear chamber

Cholesteatoma sac　　Ear drum

√4ᵗʰ
√5ᵗʰ　Additional Digit Required　　Unspecified Code　　Other Specified Code　　Manifestation Code　　►◄ Revised Text　　● New Code　　▲ Revised Code Title

2005 ICD•9•CM　　　　　　　　　　　　　　　　　　　　　　　　　　　　　　　　　　**Volume 1 — 107**

Nervous System and Sense Organs

383.2–385.24

Nervous System and Sense Organs

385.3–388.00

✓5ᵗʰ **385.3 Cholesteatoma of middle ear and mastoid**

Cholesterosis ⎫
Epidermosis ⎬ of (middle) ear
Keratosis ⎪
Polyp ⎭

> **EXCLUDES**   cholesteatoma:
> external ear canal (380.21)
> recurrent of postmastoidectomy
> cavity (383.32)

DEF: Cystlike mass of middle ear and mastoid antrum filled with debris, including cholesterol.

385.30 Cholesteatoma, unspecified

385.31 Cholesteatoma of attic

385.32 Cholesteatoma of middle ear

385.33 Cholesteatoma of middle ear and mastoid
AHA: 3Q, '00, 10

DEF: Cystlike mass of cell debris in middle ear and mastoid air cells behind ear.

385.35 Diffuse cholesteatosis

✓5ᵗʰ **385.8 Other disorders of middle ear and mastoid**

385.82 Cholesterin granuloma
DEF: Granuloma formed of fibrotic tissue; contains cholesterol crystals surrounded by foreign-body cells; found in the middle ear and mastoid area.

385.83 Retained foreign body of middle ear
AHA: 3Q, '94, 7; N-D, '87, 9

385.89 Other

385.9 Unspecified disorder of middle ear and mastoid

✓4ᵗʰ **386 Vertiginous syndromes and other disorders of vestibular system**
> **EXCLUDES**   vertigo NOS (780.4)

AHA: M-A, '85, 12

✓5ᵗʰ **386.0 Ménière's disease**
Endolymphatic hydrops
Lermoyez's syndrome
Ménière's syndrome or vertigo

DEF: Distended membranous labyrinth of middle ear from endolymphatic hydrops; causes ischemia, failure of nerve function; hearing and balance dysfunction; symptoms include fluctuating deafness, ringing in ears and dizziness.

386.00 Ménière's disease, unspecified
Ménière's disease (active)

386.01 Active Ménière's disease, cochleovestibular

386.02 Active Ménière's disease, cochlear

386.03 Active Ménière's disease, vestibular

386.04 Inactive Ménière's disease
Ménière's disease in remission

✓5ᵗʰ **386.1 Other and unspecified peripheral vertigo**
> **EXCLUDES**   epidemic vertigo (078.81)

386.10 Peripheral vertigo, unspecified

386.11 Benign paroxysmal positional vertigo
Benign paroxysmal positional nystagmus

386.12 Vestibular neuronitis
Acute (and recurrent) peripheral vestibulopathy
DEF: Transient benign vertigo, unknown cause; characterized by response to caloric stimulation on one side, nystagmus with rhythmic movement of eyes; normal auditory function present; occurs in young adults.

386.19 Other
Aural vertigo
Otogenic vertigo

386.2 Vertigo of central origin
Central positional nystagmus
Malignant positional vertigo

✓5ᵗʰ **386.3 Labyrinthitis**

386.30 Labyrinthitis, unspecified

386.31 Serous labyrinthitis
Diffuse labyrinthitis
DEF: Inflammation of labyrinth; with fluid buildup.

386.32 Circumscribed labyrinthitis
Focal labyrinthitis

386.33 Suppurative labyrinthitis
Purulent labyrinthitis
DEF: Inflammation of labyrinth; with pus.

386.34 Toxic labyrinthitis
DEF: Inflammation of labyrinth; due to toxic reaction.

386.35 Viral labyrinthitis

✓5ᵗʰ **386.4 Labyrinthine fistula**

386.40 Labyrinthine fistula, unspecified

386.41 Round window fistula

386.42 Oval window fistula

386.43 Semicircular canal fistula

386.48 Labyrinthine fistula of combined sites

✓5ᵗʰ **386.5 Labyrinthine dysfunction**

386.50 Labyrinthine dysfunction, unspecified

386.51 Hyperactive labyrinth, unilateral
DEF: Oversensitivity of labyrinth to auditory signals; affecting one ear.

386.52 Hyperactive labyrinth, bilateral
DEF: Oversensitivity of labyrinth to auditory signals; affecting both ears.

386.53 Hypoactive labyrinth, unilateral
DEF: Reduced sensitivity of labyrinth to auditory signals; affecting one ear.

386.54 Hypoactive labyrinth, bilateral
DEF: Reduced sensitivity of labyrinth to auditory signals; affecting both ears.

386.55 Loss of labyrinthine reactivity, unilateral
DEF: Reduced reaction of labyrinth to auditory signals, affecting one ear.

386.56 Loss of labyrinthine reactivity, bilateral
DEF: Reduced reaction of labyrinth to auditory signals; affecting both ears.

386.58 Other forms and combinations

386.8 Other disorders of labyrinth

386.9 Unspecified vertiginous syndromes and labyrinthine disorders

✓4ᵗʰ **387 Otosclerosis**
> **INCLUDES**   otospongiosis

DEF: Synonym for otospongiosis, spongy bone formation in the labyrinth bones of the ear; it causes progressive hearing impairment.

387.0 Otosclerosis involving oval window, nonobliterative
DEF: Tough, fibrous tissue impeding functions of oval window.

387.1 Otosclerosis involving oval window, obliterative
DEF: Tough, fibrous tissue blocking oval window.

387.2 Cochlear otosclerosis
Otosclerosis involving: Otosclerosis involving:
otic capsule   round window
DEF: Tough, fibrous tissue impeding functions of cochlea.

387.8 Other otosclerosis

387.9 Otosclerosis, unspecified

✓4ᵗʰ **388 Other disorders of ear**

✓5ᵗʰ **388.0 Degenerative and vascular disorders of ear**

388.00 Degenerative and vascular disorders, unspecified

N Newborn Age: 0	P Pediatric Age: 0-17	M Maternity Age: 12-55	A Adult Age: 15-124	MSP Medicare Secondary Payer

388.01 **Presbyacusis**
> DEF: Progressive, bilateral perceptive hearing loss caused by advancing age; it is also known as presbycusis.

388.02 **Transient ischemic deafness**
> DEF: Restricted blood flow to auditory organs causing temporary hearing loss.

√5ᵗʰ 388.1 **Noise effects on inner ear**
388.10 Noise effects on inner ear, unspecified
388.11 **Acoustic trauma (explosive) to ear**
> Otitic blast injury

388.12 **Noise-induced hearing loss**

388.2 Sudden hearing loss, unspecified

√5ᵗʰ 388.3 **Tinnitus**
> DEF: Abnormal noises in ear; may be heard by others beside the affected individual; noises include ringing, clicking, roaring and buzzing.

388.30 Tinnitus, unspecified
388.31 **Subjective tinnitus**
388.32 **Objective tinnitus**

√5ᵗʰ 388.4 **Other abnormal auditory perception**
388.40 Abnormal auditory perception, unspecified
388.41 **Diplacusis**
> DEF: Perception of a single auditory sound as two sounds at two different levels of intensity.

388.42 **Hyperacusis**
> DEF: Exceptionally acute sense of hearing caused by such conditions as Bell's palsy; this term may also refer to painful sensitivity to sounds.

388.43 **Impairment of auditory discrimination**
> DEF: Impaired ability to distinguish tone of sound.

388.44 **Recruitment**
> DEF: Perception of abnormally increased loudness caused by a slight increase in sound intensity; it is a term used in audiology.

388.5 **Disorders of acoustic nerve**
> Acoustic neuritis
> Degeneration ⎱ of acoustic or eighth nerve
> Disorder ⎰
>
> **EXCLUDES** acoustic neuroma (225.1)
> syphilitic acoustic neuritis (094.86)

AHA: M-A, '87, 8

√5ᵗʰ 388.6 **Otorrhea**
388.60 Otorrhea, unspecified
> Discharging ear NOS

388.61 **Cerebrospinal fluid otorrhea**
> **EXCLUDES** cerebrospinal fluid rhinorrhea (349.81)
>
> DEF: Spinal fluid leakage from ear.

388.69 Other
> Otorrhagia

√5ᵗʰ 388.7 **Otalgia**
388.70 Otalgia, unspecified
> Earache NOS

388.71 **Otogenic pain**
388.72 **Referred pain**

388.8 Other disorders of ear
388.9 Unspecified disorder of ear

√4ᵗʰ 389 **Hearing loss**

√5ᵗʰ 389.0 **Conductive hearing loss**
> Conductive deafness

AHA: 4Q, '89, 5

> DEF: Dysfunction in sound-conducting structures of external or middle ear causing hearing loss.

389.00 Conductive hearing loss, unspecified
389.01 **Conductive hearing loss, external ear**
389.02 **Conductive hearing loss, tympanic membrane**
389.03 **Conductive hearing loss, middle ear**
389.04 **Conductive hearing loss, inner ear**
389.08 **Conductive hearing loss of combined types**

√5ᵗʰ 389.1 **Sensorineural hearing loss**
> Perceptive hearing loss or deafness
> **EXCLUDES** abnormal auditory perception (388.40-388.44)
> psychogenic deafness (306.7)

AHA: 4Q, '89, 5

> DEF: Nerve conduction causing hearing loss.

389.10 Sensorineural hearing loss, unspecified
> **AHA:** 1Q, '93, 29

389.11 **Sensory hearing loss**
389.12 **Neural hearing loss**
389.14 **Central hearing loss**
389.18 **Sensorineural hearing loss of combined types**

389.2 **Mixed conductive and sensorineural hearing loss**
> Deafness or hearing loss of type classifiable to 389.0 with type classifiable to 389.1

389.7 **Deaf mutism, not elsewhere classifiable**
> Deaf, nonspeaking

389.8 Other specified forms of hearing loss
389.9 Unspecified hearing loss
> Deafness NOS

AHA: ▶1Q, '04, 15◀

√4ᵗʰ
√5ᵗʰ Additional Digit Required   Unspecified Code   Other Specified Code   Manifestation Code   ▶◀ Revised Text   ● New Code   ▲ Revised Code Title

2005 ICD•9•CM   October 2004 • Volume 1 — 109

Nervous System and Sense Organs

388.01–389.9

7. DISEASES OF THE CIRCULATORY SYSTEM (390-459)

ACUTE RHEUMATIC FEVER (390-392)

DEF: Febrile disease occurs mainly in children or young adults following throat infection by group A streptococci; symptoms include fever, joint pain, lesions of heart, blood vessels and joint connective tissue, abdominal pain, skin changes, and chorea.

390 Rheumatic fever without mention of heart involvement
Arthritis, rheumatic, acute or subacute
Rheumatic fever (active) (acute)
Rheumatism, articular, acute or subacute
EXCLUDES *that with heart involvement (391.0-391.9)*

√4ᵗʰ **391 Rheumatic fever with heart involvement**
EXCLUDES *chronic heart diseases of rheumatic origin (393.0-398.9) unless rheumatic fever is also present or there is evidence of recrudescence or activity of the rheumatic process*

391.0 Acute rheumatic pericarditis
Rheumatic:
fever (active) (acute) with pericarditis
pericarditis (acute)
Any condition classifiable to 390 with pericarditis
EXCLUDES *that not specified as rheumatic (420.0-420.9)*
DEF: Sudden, severe inflammation of heart lining due to rheumatic fever.

391.1 Acute rheumatic endocarditis
Rheumatic:
endocarditis, acute
fever (active) (acute) with endocarditis or valvulitis
valvulitis acute
Any condition classifiable to 390 with endocarditis or valvulitis
DEF: Sudden, severe inflammation of heart cavities due to rheumatic fever.

391.2 Acute rheumatic myocarditis
Rheumatic fever (active) (acute) with myocarditis
Any condition classifiable to 390 with myocarditis
DEF: Sudden, severe inflammation of heart muscles due to rheumatic fever.

391.8 Other acute rheumatic heart disease
Rheumatic:
fever (active) (acute) with other or multiple types of heart involvement
pancarditis, acute
Any condition classifiable to 390 with other or multiple types of heart involvement

391.9 Acute rheumatic heart disease, unspecified
Rheumatic:
carditis, acute
fever (active) (acute) with unspecified type of heart involvement
heart disease, active or acute
Any condition classifiable to 390 with unspecified type of heart involvement

√4ᵗʰ **392 Rheumatic chorea**
INCLUDES Sydenham's chorea
EXCLUDES *chorea:*
NOS (333.5)
Huntington's (333.4)
DEF: Childhood disease linked with rheumatic fever and streptococcal infections; symptoms include spasmodic, involuntary movements of limbs or facial muscles, psychic symptoms, and irritability.

392.0 With heart involvement
Rheumatic chorea with heart involvement of any type classifiable to 391

392.9 Without mention of heart involvement

CHRONIC RHEUMATIC HEART DISEASE (393-398)

393 Chronic rheumatic pericarditis
Adherent pericardium, rheumatic
Chronic rheumatic:
mediastinopericarditis
myopericarditis
EXCLUDES *pericarditis NOS or not specified as rheumatic (423.0-423.9)*
DEF: Persistent inflammation of heart lining due to rheumatic heart disease.

√4ᵗʰ **394 Diseases of mitral valve**
EXCLUDES *that with aortic valve involvement (396.0-396.9)*

394.0 Mitral stenosis
Mitral (valve):
obstruction (rheumatic)
stenosis NOS
DEF: Narrowing, of mitral valve between left atrium and left ventricle due to rheumatic heart disease.

394.1 Rheumatic mitral insufficiency
Rheumatic mitral: Rheumatic mitral:
incompetence   regurgitation
EXCLUDES *that not specified as rheumatic (424.0)*
DEF: Malfunction of mitral valve between left atrium and left ventricle due to rheumatic heart disease.

394.2 Mitral stenosis with insufficiency
Mitral stenosis with incompetence or regurgitation
DEF: A narrowing or stricture of the mitral valve situated between the left atrium and left ventricle. The stenosis interferes with blood flow from the atrium into the ventricle. If the valve does not completely close, it becomes insufficient (inadequate) and cannot prevent regurgitation (abnormal backward flow) into the atrium when the left ventricle contracts. This abnormal function is also called incompetence.

394.9 Other and unspecified mitral valve diseases
Mitral (valve):   Mitral (valve):
disease (chronic)   failure

√4ᵗʰ **395 Diseases of aortic valve**
EXCLUDES *that not specified as rheumatic (424.1)*
that with mitral valve involvement (396.0-396.9)

395.0 Rheumatic aortic stenosis
Rheumatic aortic (valve) obstruction
AHA: 4Q, '88, 8
DEF: Narrowing of the aortic valve; results in backflow into ventricle due to rheumatic heart disease.

395.1 Rheumatic aortic insufficiency
Rheumatic aortic: Rheumatic aortic:
incompetence   regurgitation
DEF: Malfunction of the aortic valve; results in backflow into left ventricle due to rheumatic heart disease.

395.2 Rheumatic aortic stenosis with insufficiency
Rheumatic aortic stenosis with incompetence or regurgitation
DEF: Malfunction and narrowing, of the aortic valve; results in backflow into left ventricle due to rheumatic heart disease.

395.9 Other and unspecified rheumatic aortic diseases
Rheumatic aortic (valve) disease

√4ᵗʰ **396 Diseases of mitral and aortic valves**
INCLUDES involvement of both mitral and aortic valves, whether specified as rheumatic or not
AHA: N-D, '87, 8

396.0 Mitral valve stenosis and aortic valve stenosis
Atypical aortic (valve) stenosis
Mitral and aortic (valve) obstruction (rheumatic)

396.1 Mitral valve stenosis and aortic valve insufficiency

396.2 Mitral valve insufficiency and aortic valve stenosis
AHA: 2Q, '00, 16

√4ᵗʰ
√5ᵗʰ Additional Digit Required   Unspecified Code   Other Specified Code   Manifestation Code   ▶◀ Revised Text   ● New Code   ▲ Revised Code Title

Circulatory System

396.3–402.91

396.3 Mitral valve insufficiency and aortic valve insufficiency
Mitral and aortic (valve):   Mitral and aortic (valve):
   incompetence   regurgitation

396.8 Multiple involvement of mitral and aortic valves
Stenosis and insufficiency of mitral or aortic valve
with stenosis or insufficiency, or both, of the
other valve

396.9 Mitral and aortic valve diseases, unspecified

✓4ᵗʰ 397 Diseases of other endocardial structures

397.0 Diseases of tricuspid valve
Tricuspid (valve) (rheumatic):
disease
insufficiency
obstruction
regurgitation
stenosis

AHA: 2Q, '00, 16

DEF: Malfunction of the valve between right atrium and right
ventricle due to rheumatic heart disease.

397.1 Rheumatic diseases of pulmonary valve
EXCLUDES   *that not specified as rheumatic (424.3)*

397.9 Rheumatic diseases of endocardium, valve unspecified
Rheumatic:
endocarditis (chronic)
valvulitis (chronic)
EXCLUDES   *that not specified as rheumatic
(424.90-424.99)*

✓4ᵗʰ 398 Other rheumatic heart disease

398.0 Rheumatic myocarditis
Rheumatic degeneration of myocardium
EXCLUDES   *myocarditis not specified as rheumatic
(429.0)*

DEF: Chronic inflammation of heart muscle due to rheumatic heart
disease.

✓5ᵗʰ 398.9 Other and unspecified rheumatic heart diseases

398.90 Rheumatic heart disease, unspecified
Rheumatic: Rheumatic:
carditis   heart disease NOS
EXCLUDES   *carditis not specified as
rheumatic (429.89)*
*heart disease NOS not
specified as rheumatic
(429.9)*

398.91 Rheumatic heart failure (congestive)
Rheumatic left ventricular failure
AHA: 1Q, '95, 6; 3Q, '88, 3

DEF: Decreased cardiac output, edema and hypertension
due to rheumatic heart disease.

398.99 Other

HYPERTENSIVE DISEASE (401-405)

EXCLUDES   *that complicating pregnancy, childbirth, or the
puerperium (642.0-642.9)*
that involving coronary vessels (410.00-414.9)
AHA: 3Q, '90, 3; 2Q, '89, 12; S-O, '87, 9; J-A, '84, 11

✓4ᵗʰ 401 Essential hypertension
INCLUDES   high blood pressure
hyperpiesia
hyperpiesis
hypertension (arterial) (essential) (primary)
(systemic)
hypertensive vascular:
degeneration
disease
EXCLUDES   *elevated blood pressure without diagnosis of
hypertension (796.2)*
pulmonary hypertension (416.0-416.9)
*that involving vessels of:
brain (430-438)
eye (362.11)*

AHA: 2Q, '92, 5

DEF: Hypertension that occurs without apparent organic cause; idiopathic.

401.0 Malignant
AHA: M-J, '85, 19

DEF: Severe high arterial blood pressure; results in necrosis in
kidney, retina, etc.; hemorrhages occur and death commonly due to
uremia or rupture of cerebral vessel.

401.1 Benign
DEF: Mildly elevated arterial blood pressure.

401.9 Unspecified
AHA: 4Q, '03, 105, 108, 111; 3Q, '03, 14; 2Q, '03, 16; 4Q, '97, 37

✓4ᵗʰ 402 Hypertensive heart disease
INCLUDES   hypertensive:
cardiomegaly
cardiopathy
cardiovascular disease
heart (disease) (failure)
►any condition classifiable to 429.0-429.3,
429.8, 429.9 due to hypertension◄
Use additional code to specify type of heart failure (428.0,
428.20-428.23, 428.30-428.33, 428.40-428.43)
AHA: 4Q, '02, 49; 2Q, '93, 9; N-D, '84, 18

✓5ᵗʰ 402.0 Malignant
402.00 Without heart failure
402.01 With heart failure

✓5ᵗʰ 402.1 Benign
402.10 Without heart failure
402.11 With heart failure

✓5ᵗʰ 402.9 Unspecified
402.90 Without heart failure
402.91 With heart failure
AHA: 4Q, '02, 52; 1Q, '93, 19; 2Q, '89, 12

Sections of Heart Muscle

Pericardial layers:
- Pleural
- Fibrous
- Parietal
- Epicardium
- Serous (fluid)
- Pericardial cavity
- Endocardium
- Myocardium (muscular)
- Endocardial cavity

Sectional Schematic

Pericardial sac

Pericardial reflection (layers fused)

Septum:
- Membranous
- Muscular

Pericardial sinus

✓4th **403 Hypertensive renal disease**

INCLUDES
arteriolar nephritis
arteriosclerosis of:
    kidney
    renal arterioles
arteriosclerotic nephritis (chronic) (interstitial)
hypertensive:
    nephropathy
    renal failure
    uremia (chronic)
nephrosclerosis
renal sclerosis with hypertension
any condition classifiable to 585, 586, or 587
    with any condition classifiable to 401

EXCLUDES
acute renal failure (584.5-584.9)
renal disease stated as not due to hypertension
renovascular hypertension (405.0-405.9 with
    fifth-digit 1)

The following fifth-digit subclassification is for use with category 403:

    0 without mention of renal failure
    1 with renal failure

AHA: 4Q, '92, 22; 2Q, '92, 5

✓5th **403.0 Malignant**
✓5th **403.1 Benign**
✓5th **403.9 Unspecified**

AHA: For code 403.91: ▶1Q, '04, 14;◀ 1Q, '03, 20; 2Q, '01, 11; 3Q, '91, 8

✓4th **404 Hypertensive heart and renal disease**

INCLUDES
disease:
    cardiorenal
    cardiovascular renal
    any condition classifiable to 402 with any
        condition classifiable to 403

Use additional code to specify type of heart failure (428.0, 428.20-428.23, 428.30-428.33, 428.40-428.43)

The following fifth-digit subclassification is for use with category 404:

    0 without mention of heart failure or renal failure
    1 with heart failure
    2 with renal failure
    3 with heart failure and renal failure

AHA: 4Q, '02, 49; 3Q, '90, 3; J-A, '84, 14

✓5th **404.0 Malignant**
✓5th **404.1 Benign**
✓5th **404.9 Unspecified**

✓4th **405 Secondary hypertension**

AHA: 3Q, '90, 3; S-O, '87, 9, 11; J-A, '84, 14

DEF: High arterial blood pressure due to or with a variety of primary diseases, such as renal disorders, CNS disorders, endocrine, and vascular diseases.

✓5th **405.0 Malignant**

    405.01 Renovascular
    405.09 Other

✓5th **405.1 Benign**

    405.11 Renovascular
    405.19 Other

✓5th **405.9 Unspecified**

    405.91 Renovascular
    405.99 Other

AHA: 3Q, '00, 4

ISCHEMIC HEART DISEASE (410-414)

INCLUDES that with mention of hypertension

Use additional code to identify presence of hypertension (401.0-405.9)

AHA: 3Q, '91, 10; J-A, '84, 5

✓4th **410 Acute myocardial infarction**

INCLUDES
cardiac infarction
coronary (artery):
    embolism
    occlusion
    rupture
    thrombosis
infarction of heart, myocardium, or ventricle
rupture of heart, myocardium, or ventricle
any condition classifiable to 414.1-414.9
    specified as acute or with a stated
    duration of 8 weeks or less

The following fifth-digit subclassification is for use with category 410:

    0 episode of care unspecified
        Use when the source document does not
        contain sufficient information for the
        assignment of fifth digit 1 or 2.

    1 initial episode of care
        Use fifth-digit 1 to designate the first episode
        of care (regardless of facility site) for a
        newly diagnosed myocardial infarction.
        The fifth-digit 1 is assigned regardless of
        the number of times a patient may be
        transferred during the initial episode of
        care.

    2 subsequent episode of care
        Use fifth-digit 2 to designate an episode of care
        following the initial episode when the
        patient is admitted for further
        observation, evaluation or treatment for a
        myocardial infarction that has received
        initial treatment, but is still less than 8
        weeks old.

AHA: 3Q, '01, 21; 3Q, '98, 15; 4Q, '97, 37; 3Q, '95, 9; 4Q, '92, 24; 1Q, '92,10; 3Q, '91, 18; 1Q, '91, 14; 3Q, '89, 3

DEF: A sudden insufficiency of blood supply to an area of the heart muscle; usually due to a coronary artery occlusion.

Acute Myocardial Infarction

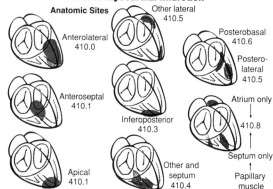

Anatomic Sites
- Anterolateral 410.0
- Other lateral 410.5
- Posterobasal 410.6
- Postero-lateral 410.5
- Anteroseptal 410.1
- Inferoposterior 410.3
- Atrium only 410.8
- Septum only
- Papillary muscle
- Apical 410.1
- Other and septum 410.4

Additional Digit Required | Unspecified Code | Other Specified Code | Manifestation Code | ▶◀ Revised Text | ● New Code | ▲ Revised Code Title

2005 ICD•9•CM

October 2004 • Volume 1 — 113

Circulatory System

410.0–413.9

§ ✓5th **410.0** **Of anterolateral wall** A

§ ✓5th **410.1** **Of other anterior wall** A
Infarction:
anterior (wall) ⎫
NOS ⎬ (with contiguous portion of
anteroapical ⎬ intraventricular septum)
anteroseptal ⎭

AHA: For code 410.11: ▶3Q, '03, 10◄

§ ✓5th **410.2** **Of inferolateral wall** A
§ ✓5th **410.3** **Of inferoposterior wall** A
§ ✓5th **410.4** **Of other inferior wall** A
Infarction:
diaphragmatic ⎫ (with contiguous portion
wall NOS ⎬ of intraventricular
inferior (wall) NOS ⎭ septum)

AHA: 1Q, '00, 7, 26; 4Q, '99, 9; 3Q, '97, 10

AHA: For code 410.41: 2Q, '01, 8, 9

§ ✓5th **410.5** **Of other lateral wall** A
Infarction: Infarction:
apical-lateral   high lateral
basal-lateral   posterolateral

§ ✓5th **410.6** **True posterior wall infarction** A
Infarction: Infarction:
posterobasal   strictly posterior

§ ✓5th **410.7** **Subendocardial infarction** A
Nontransmural infarction
AHA: 1Q, '00, 7

§ ✓5th **410.8** **Of other specified sites** A
Infarction of: Infarction of:
atrium   septum alone
papillary muscle

§ ✓5th **410.9** **Unspecified site** A
Acute myocardial infarction NOS
Coronary occlusion NOS
AHA: 1Q, '96, 17; 1Q, '92, 9; **For code 410.91:** 3Q,'02, 5

✓4th **411** **Other acute and subacute forms of ischemic heart disease**
AHA: 4Q, '94, 55; 3Q, '91, 24

411.0 **Postmyocardial infarction syndrome** A
Dressler's syndrome

DEF: Complication developing several days/weeks after myocardial infarction; symptoms include fever, leukocytosis, chest pain, evidence of pericarditis, pleurisy, and pneumonitis; tendency to recur.

411.1 **Intermediate coronary syndrome** A
Impending infarction   Preinfarction syndrome
Preinfarction angina   Unstable angina
EXCLUDES   angina (pectoris) (413.9)
decubitus (413.0)

AHA: 1Q, '03, 12; 3Q, '01, 15; 2Q, '01, 7, 9; 4Q, '98, 86; 2Q, '96, 10; 3Q, '91, 24; 1Q, '91, 14; 3Q, '90, 6; 4Q, '89, 10

DEF: A condition representing an intermediate stage between angina of effort and acute myocardial infarction. It is often documented by the physician as "unstable angina."

✓5th **411.8** **Other**
AHA: 3Q, '91, 18; 3Q, '89, 4

Arteries of the Heart

411.81 → Left coronary artery / Circumflex branch; Aortic valve; Right coronary artery; Marginal branches; Descending branch (posterior interventricular artery); Descending branch (anterior interventricular artery)

411.81 **Acute coronary occlusion without** A
myocardial infarction
Acute coronary (artery):
embolism ⎫ without or not
obstruction ⎬ resulting in
occlusion ⎬ myocardial
thrombosis ⎭ infarction

EXCLUDES   obstruction without infarction
due to atherosclerosis
(414.00-414.0)
occlusion without infarction
due to atherosclerosis
(414.00-414.07)

AHA: 3Q, '91, 24; 1Q, '91, 14

DEF: Interrupted blood flow to a portion of the heart; without tissue death.

411.89 **Other** A
Coronary insufficiency (acute)
Subendocardial ischemia
AHA: 3Q, '01, 14; 1Q, '92, 9

412 **Old myocardial infarction** A
Healed myocardial infarction
Past myocardial infarction diagnosed on ECG [EKG] or other special investigation, but currently presenting no symptoms
AHA: ▶2Q, '03, 10;◄ 2Q, '01, 9; 3Q, '98, 15; 2Q, '91, 22; 3Q, '90, 7

✓4th **413** **Angina pectoris**
DEF: Severe constricting pain in the chest, often radiating from the precordium to the left shoulder and down the arm, due to ischemia of the heart muscle; usually caused by coronary disease; pain is often precipitated by effort or excitement.

413.0 **Angina decubitus** A
Nocturnal angina
DEF: Angina occurring only in the recumbent position.

413.1 **Prinzmetal angina** A
Variant angina pectoris
DEF: Angina occurring when patient is recumbent; associated with ST-segment elevations.

413.9 **Other and unspecified angina pectoris** A
Angina: Anginal syndrome
NOS   Status anginosus
cardiac   Stenocardia
of effort   Syncope anginosa
EXCLUDES   preinfarction angina (411.1)
AHA: 3Q, '02, 4; 3Q, '91, 16; 3Q, '90, 6

§ Requires fifth-digit. See category 410 for codes and definitions.

√4th **414 Other forms of chronic ischemic heart disease**
　　EXCLUDES *arteriosclerotic cardiovascular disease [ASCVD] (429.2)*
　　cardiovascular:
　　　arteriosclerosis or sclerosis (429.2)
　　　degeneration or disease (429.2)

√5th **414.0 Coronary atherosclerosis**
Arteriosclerotic heart disease [ASHD]
Atherosclerotic heart disease
Coronary (artery):
　arteriosclerosis
　arteritis or endarteritis
　atheroma
　sclerosis
　stricture
　　EXCLUDES *embolism of graft (996.72)*
　　occlusion NOS of graft (996.72)
　　thrombus of graft (996.72)
AHA: 2Q, '97, 13; 2Q, '95, 17; 4Q, '94, 49; 2Q, '94, 13; 1Q, '94, 6; 3Q, '90, 7

DEF: A chronic condition marked by thickening and loss of elasticity of the coronary artery; caused by deposits of plaque containing cholesterol, lipoid material and lipophages.

414.00 Of unspecified type of vessel, native or graft A
AHA: ▶1Q, '04, 24;◀ 2Q, '03, 16; 3Q, '01, 15; 4Q, '99, 4; 3Q, '97, 15; 4Q, '96, 31

414.01 Of native coronary artery A
AHA: 4Q, '03, 108; 3Q, '03, 9, 14; 3Q, '02, 4-9; 3Q, '01, 15; 2Q, '01, 8, 9; 3Q, '97, 15; 2Q, '96, 10; 4Q, '96, 31

DEF: Plaque deposits in natural heart vessels.

414.02 Of autologous vein bypass graft A
DEF: Plaque deposit in grafted vein originating within patient.

414.03 Of nonautologous biological bypass graft A
DEF: Plaque deposits in grafted vessel originating outside patient.

414.04 Of artery bypass graft A
Internal mammary artery
AHA: 4Q, '96, 31
DEF: Plaque deposits in grafted artery originating within patient.

414.05 Of unspecified type of bypass graft A
Bypass graft NOS
AHA: 3Q, '97, 15; 4Q, '96, 31

414.06 Of native coronary artery of transplanted heart
AHA: 4Q, '03, 60

414.07 Of bypass graft (artery) (vein) of transplanted heart A

√5th **414.1 Aneurysm and dissection of heart**
AHA: 4Q, '02, 54

414.10 Aneurysm of heart (wall)
Aneurysm (arteriovenous):
　mural
　ventricular

414.11 Aneurysm of coronary vessels
Aneurysm (arteriovenous) of coronary vessels
AHA: 3Q, '03, 10; 1Q, '99, 17
DEF: Dilatation of all three-vessel wall layers forming a sac filled with blood.

414.12 Dissection of coronary artery
DEF: A tear in the intimal arterial wall of a coronary artery resulting in the sudden intrusion of blood within the layers of the wall.

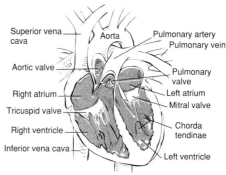

Anatomy

Superior vena cava — Aorta — Pulmonary artery — Pulmonary vein — Aortic valve — Pulmonary valve — Right atrium — Left atrium — Mitral valve — Tricuspid valve — Chorda tendinae — Right ventricle — Inferior vena cava — Left ventricle

Blood Flow

414.19 Other aneurysm of heart
Arteriovenous fistula, acquired, of heart

414.8 Other specified forms of chronic ischemic heart disease
Chronic coronary insufficiency
Ischemia, myocardial (chronic)
Any condition classifiable to 410 specified as chronic, or presenting with symptoms after 8 weeks from date of infarction
　EXCLUDES *coronary insufficiency (acute) (411.89)*
AHA: 3Q, '01, 15; 1Q, '92, 10; 3Q, '90, 7, 15; 2Q, '90, 19

414.9 Chronic ischemic heart disease, unspecified
Ischemic heart disease NOS

DISEASES OF PULMONARY CIRCULATION (415–417)

√4th **415 Acute pulmonary heart disease**

415.0 Acute cor pulmonale
　　EXCLUDES *cor pulmonale NOS (416.9)*
DEF: A heart-lung disease marked by dilation and failure of the right side of heart; due to pulmonary embolism; ventilatory function is impaired and pulmonary hypertension results within hours.

√5th **415.1 Pulmonary embolism and infarction**
Pulmonary (artery) (vein):
　apoplexy
　embolism
　infarction (hemorrhagic)
　thrombosis
　　EXCLUDES *that complicating:*
　　abortion (634-638 with .6, 639.6)
　　ectopic or molar pregnancy (639.6)
　　pregnancy, childbirth, or the puerperium (673.0-673.8)
AHA: 4Q, '90, 25

DEF: Embolism: closure of the pulmonary artery or branch; due to thrombosis (blood clot).

DEF: Infarction: necrosis of lung tissue; due to obstructed arterial blood supply, most often by pulmonary embolism.

√4th √5th Additional Digit Required　　Unspecified Code　　Other Specified Code　　Manifestation Code　　▶◀ Revised Text　　● New Code　　▲ Revised Code Title

Circulatory System

415.11–422.90

415.11 Iatrogenic pulmonary embolism and infarction
AHA: 4Q, '95, 58

415.19 Other

✓4ᵗʰ **416 Chronic pulmonary heart disease**

416.0 Primary pulmonary hypertension
Idiopathic pulmonary arteriosclerosis
Pulmonary hypertension (essential) (idiopathic) (primary)

DEF: A rare increase in pulmonary circulation, often resulting in right ventricular failure or fatal syncope.

416.1 Kyphoscoliotic heart disease

DEF: High blood pressure within the lungs as a result of curvature of the spine.

416.8 Other chronic pulmonary heart diseases
Pulmonary hypertension, secondary

416.9 Chronic pulmonary heart disease, unspecified
Chronic cardiopulmonary disease
Cor pulmonale (chronic) NOS

✓4ᵗʰ **417 Other diseases of pulmonary circulation**

417.0 Arteriovenous fistula of pulmonary vessels
EXCLUDES   *congenital arteriovenous fistula (747.3)*

DEF: Abnormal communication between blood vessels within lung.

417.1 Aneurysm of pulmonary artery
EXCLUDES   *congenital aneurysm (747.3)*

417.8 Other specified diseases of pulmonary circulation

Pulmonary: Pulmonary:
   arteritis   endarteritis
Rupture ⎱
Stricture ⎰ of pulmonary vessel

417.9 Unspecified disease of pulmonary circulation

OTHER FORMS OF HEART DISEASE (420-429)

✓4ᵗʰ **420 Acute pericarditis**
INCLUDES   acute:
      mediastinopericarditis
      myopericarditis
      pericardial effusion
      pleuropericarditis
      pneumopericarditis
EXCLUDES   *acute rheumatic pericarditis (391.0)*
      postmyocardial infarction syndrome [Dressler's] (411.0)

DEF: Inflammation of the pericardium (heart sac); pericardial friction rub results from this inflammation and is heard as a scratchy or leathery sound.

420.0 Acute pericarditis in diseases classified elsewhere
Code first underlying disease, as:
     actinomycosis (039.8)
     amebiasis (006.8)
     nocardiosis (039.8)
     tuberculosis (017.9)
     uremia (585)
EXCLUDES   *pericarditis (acute) (in):*
     Coxsackie (virus) (074.21)
     gonococcal (098.83)
     histoplasmosis (115.0-115.9 with fifth-digit 3)
     meningococcal infection (036.41)
     syphilitic (093.81)

✓5ᵗʰ **420.9 Other and unspecified acute pericarditis**
420.90 Acute pericarditis, unspecified
Pericarditis (acute):   Pericarditis (acute):
   NOS   sicca
   infective NOS
AHA: 2Q, '89, 12

420.91 Acute idiopathic pericarditis
Pericarditis, acute: Pericarditis, acute:
   benign   viral
   nonspecific

420.99 Other
Pericarditis (acute):
   pneumococcal
   purulent
   staphylococcal
   streptococcal
   suppurative
Pneumopyopericardium
Pyopericardium
EXCLUDES   *pericarditis in diseases classified elsewhere (420.0)*

✓4ᵗʰ **421 Acute and subacute endocarditis**

DEF: Bacterial inflammation of the endocardium (intracardiac area); major symptoms include fever, fatigue, heart murmurs, splenomegaly, embolic episodes and areas of infarction.

421.0 Acute and subacute bacterial endocarditis
Endocarditis (acute)   Endocarditis (acute)
   (chronic) (subacute):   (chronic) (subacute):
   bacterial   ulcerative
   infective NOS   vegetative
   lenta   Infective aneurysm
   malignant   Subacute bacterial
   purulent   endocarditis [SBE]
   septic
Use additional code to identify infectious organism [e.g., Streptococcus 041.0, Staphylococcus 041.1]
AHA: 1Q, '99, 12; 1Q, '91, 15

421.1 Acute and subacute infective endocarditis in diseases classified elsewhere
Code first underlying disease, as:
   blastomycosis (116.0)
   Q fever (083.0)
   typhoid (fever) (002.0)
EXCLUDES   *endocarditis (in):*
     Coxsackie (virus) (074.22)
     gonococcal (098.84)
     histoplasmosis (115.0-115.9 with fifth-digit 4)
     meningococcal infection (036.42)
     monilial (112.81)

421.9 Acute endocarditis, unspecified
Endocarditis ⎱
Myoendocarditis ⎰ acute or subacute
Periendocarditis
EXCLUDES   *acute rheumatic endocarditis (391.1)*

✓4ᵗʰ **422 Acute myocarditis**
EXCLUDES   *acute rheumatic myocarditis (391.2)*

DEF: Acute inflammation of the muscular walls of the heart (myocardium).

422.0 Acute myocarditis in diseases classified elsewhere
Code first underlying disease, as:
   myocarditis (acute):
     influenzal (487.8)
     tuberculous (017.9)
EXCLUDES   *myocarditis (acute) (due to):*
     aseptic, of newborn (074.23)
     Coxsackie (virus) (074.23)
     diphtheritic (032.82)
     meningococcal infection (036.43)
     syphilitic (093.82)
     toxoplasmosis (130.3)

✓5ᵗʰ **422.9 Other and unspecified acute myocarditis**
422.90 Acute myocarditis, unspecified
Acute or subacute (interstitial) myocarditis

422.91 Idiopathic myocarditis

Myocarditis (acute or subacute):
    Fiedler's
    giant cell
    isolated (diffuse) (granulomatous)
    nonspecific granulomatous

422.92 Septic myocarditis

Myocarditis, acute or subacute:
    pneumococcal
    staphylococcal
Use additional code to identify infectious
    organism [e.g., Staphylococcus 041.1]

> **EXCLUDES** *myocarditis, acute or*
> *subacute:*
> *in bacterial diseases*
> *classified elsewhere*
> *(422.0)*
> *streptococcal (391.2)*

422.93 Toxic myocarditis

DEF: Inflammation of the heart muscle due to an adverse
reaction to certain drugs or chemicals reaching the heart
through the bloodstream.

422.99 Other

✓4ᵗʰ **423 Other diseases of pericardium**

> **EXCLUDES** *that specified as rheumatic (393)*

423.0 Hemopericardium

DEF: Blood in the pericardial sac (pericardium).

423.1 Adhesive pericarditis

Adherent pericardium
Fibrosis of pericardium
Milk spots
Pericarditis:
    adhesive
    obliterative
Soldiers' patches

DEF: Two layers of serous pericardium adhere to each other by
fibrous adhesions.

Normal Heart Valve Function

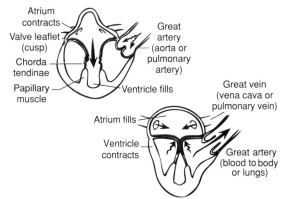

Atrium contracts
Valve leaflet (cusp)
Chorda tendinae
Papillary muscle
Great artery (aorta or pulmonary artery)
Ventricle fills
Atrium fills
Ventricle contracts
Great vein (vena cava or pulmonary vein)
Great artery (blood to body or lungs)

Heart Valve Disorders

Valve stenosis (trouble opening)
Incompetent valve (trouble closing) causes regurgitation (backflow of blood)
Insuficient valve (unable to close completely)
Shortened, fused chorda tendinae
Ventricular hypertrophy

423.2 Constrictive pericarditis

Concato's disease
Pick's disease of heart (and liver)

DEF: Inflammation identified by a rigid, thickened and sometimes
calcified pericardium; ventricles of the heart cannot be adequately
filled and congestive heart failure may result.

423.8 Other specified diseases of pericardium

Calcification ⎤
Fistula   ⎦ of pericardium

AHA: 2Q, '89, 12

423.9 Unspecified disease of pericardium

✓4ᵗʰ **424 Other diseases of endocardium**

> **EXCLUDES** *bacterial endocarditis (421.0-421.9)*
> *rheumatic endocarditis (391.1, 394.0-397.9)*
> *syphilitic endocarditis (093.20-093.24)*

424.0 Mitral valve disorders

Mitral (valve):
    incompetence ⎤
    insufficiency ⎬ NOS of specified cause,
    regurgitation ⎦   except rheumatic

> **EXCLUDES** *mitral (valve):*
> *disease (394.9)*
> *failure (394.9)*
> *stenosis (394.0)*
> *the listed conditions:*
> *specified as rheumatic (394.1)*
> *unspecified as to cause but with*
> *mention of:*
> *diseases of aortic valve (396.0-*
> *396.9)*
> *mitral stenosis or obstruction*
> *(394.2)*

AHA: 2Q, '00, 16; 3Q, '98, 11; N-D, '87, 8; N-D, '84, 8

424.1 Aortic valve disorders

Aortic (valve):
    incompetence ⎤
    insufficiency ⎬ NOS of specified
    regurgitation ⎪   cause, except
    stenosis   ⎦   rheumatic

> **EXCLUDES** *hypertrophic subaortic stenosis (425.1)*
> *that specified as rheumatic (395.0-*
> *395.9)*
> *that of unspecified cause but with*
> *mention of diseases of mitral*
> *valve (396.0-396.9)*

AHA: 4Q, '88, 8; N-D, '87, 8

Nerve Conduction of the Heart

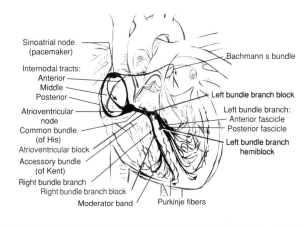

Sinoatrial node (pacemaker)
Internodal tracts:
    Anterior
    Middle
    Posterior
Atrioventricular node
Common bundle (of His)
Atrioventricular block
Accessory bundle (of Kent)
Right bundle branch
Right bundle branch block
Moderator band
Bachmann s bundle
Left bundle branch block
Left bundle branch: Anterior fascicle Posterior fascicle
Left bundle branch hemiblock
Purkinje fibers

✓4ᵗʰ
✓5ᵗʰ
Additional Digit Required   Unspecified Code   Other Specified Code   Manifestation Code   ►◄ Revised Text   ● New Code   ▲ Revised Code Title

2005 ICD•9•CM   **Volume 1 — 117**

424.2　Tricuspid valve disorders, specified as nonrheumatic

Tricuspid valve:
incompetence
insufficiency
regurgitation
stenosis
} of specified cause, except rheumatic

EXCLUDES　rheumatic or of unspecified cause (397.0)

424.3　Pulmonary valve disorders

Pulmonic:　　　　　　Pulmonic:
incompetence NOS　　regurgitation NOS
insufficiency NOS　　stenosis NOS

EXCLUDES　that specified as rheumatic (397.1)

✓5th 424.9　Endocarditis, valve unspecified

424.90　Endocarditis, valve unspecified, unspecified cause

Endocarditis (chronic):
NOS
nonbacterial thrombotic
Valvular:
incompetence
insufficiency
regurgitation
stenosis
} of unspecified valve, unspecified cause
Valvulitis (chronic)

424.91　Endocarditis in diseases classified elsewhere

Code first underlying disease as:
atypical verrucous endocarditis [Libman-Sacks] (710.0)
disseminated lupus erythematosus (710.0)
tuberculosis (017.9)

EXCLUDES　syphilitic (093.20-093.24)

424.99　Other

Any condition classifiable to 424.90 with specified cause, except rheumatic

EXCLUDES　endocardial fibroelastosis (425.3)
that specified as rheumatic (397.9)

✓4th 425　Cardiomyopathy

INCLUDES　myocardiopathy

AHA: J-A, '85, 15

425.0　Endomyocardial fibrosis

425.1　Hypertrophic obstructive cardiomyopathy

Hypertrophic subaortic stenosis (idiopathic)

DEF: Cardiomyopathy marked by left ventricle hypertrophy, enlarged septum; results in obstructed blood flow.

425.2　Obscure cardiomyopathy of Africa

Becker's disease
Idiopathic mural endomyocardial disease

425.3　Endocardial fibroelastosis

Elastomyofibrosis

DEF: A condition marked by left ventricle hypertrophy and conversion of the endocardium into a thick fibroelastic coat; capacity of the ventricle may be reduced, but is often increased.

425.4　Other primary cardiomyopathies

Cardiomyopathy:　　　Cardiomyopathy:
NOS　　　　　　　　idiopathic
congestive　　　　　nonobstructive
constrictive　　　　　obstructive
familial　　　　　　　restrictive
hypertrophic　　　　　Cardiovascular collagenosis

AHA: 1Q, '00, 22; 4Q, '97, 55; 2Q, '90, 19

425.5　Alcoholic cardiomyopathy

AHA: S-O, '85, 15

DEF: Heart disease as result of excess alcohol consumption.

425.7　Nutritional and metabolic cardiomyopathy

Code first underlying disease, as:
amyloidosis (277.3)
beriberi (265.0)
cardiac glycogenosis (271.0)
mucopolysaccharidosis (277.5)
thyrotoxicosis (242.0-242.9)

EXCLUDES　gouty tophi of heart (274.82)

425.8　Cardiomyopathy in other diseases classified elsewhere

Code first underlying disease, as:
Friedreich's ataxia (334.0)
myotonia atrophica (359.2)
progressive muscular dystrophy (359.1)
sarcoidosis (135)

EXCLUDES　cardiomyopathy in Chagas' disease (086.0)

AHA: 2Q, '93, 9

425.9　Secondary cardiomyopathy, unspecified

✓4th 426　Conduction disorders

DEF: Disruption or disturbance in the electrical impulses that regulate heartbeats.

426.0　Atrioventricular block, complete

Third degree atrioventricular block

✓5th 426.1　Atrioventricular block, other and unspecified

426.10　Atrioventricular block, unspecified

Atrioventricular [AV] block (incomplete) (partial)

426.11　First degree atrioventricular block

Incomplete atrioventricular block, first degree
Prolonged P-R interval NOS

426.12　Mobitz (type) II atrioventricular block

Incomplete atrioventricular block:
Mobitz (type) II
second degree, Mobitz (type) II

DEF: Impaired conduction of excitatory impulse from cardiac atrium to ventricle through AV node.

426.13　Other second degree atrioventricular block

Incomplete atrioventricular block:
Mobitz (type) I [Wenckebach's]
second degree:
NOS
Mobitz (type) I
with 2:1 atrioventricular response [block]
Wenckebach's phenomenon

DEF: Wenckebach's phenomenon: impulses generated at constant rate to sinus node, P-R interval lengthens; results in cycle of ventricular inadequacy and shortened P-R interval; second-degree A-V block commonly called "Mobitz type 1."

426.2　Left bundle branch hemiblock

Block:
left anterior fascicular
left posterior fascicular

426.3　Other left bundle branch block

Left bundle branch block:
NOS
anterior fascicular with posterior fascicular
complete
main stem

426.4　Right bundle branch block

AHA: 3Q, '00, 3

✓5th 426.5　Bundle branch block, other and unspecified

426.50　Bundle branch block, unspecified

426.51　Right bundle branch block and left posterior fascicular block

426.52　Right bundle branch block and left anterior fascicular block

426.53 Other bilateral bundle branch block
Bifascicular block NOS
Bilateral bundle branch block NOS
Right bundle branch with left bundle
branch block (incomplete) (main stem)

426.54 Trifascicular block

426.6 Other heart block
Intraventricular block:　Sinoatrial block
NOS　　　　　　　　Sinoauricular block
diffuse
myofibrillar

426.7 Anomalous atrioventricular excitation
Atrioventricular conduction:
accelerated
accessory
pre-excitation
Ventricular pre-excitation
Wolff-Parkinson-White syndrome

DEF: Wolff-Parkinson-White: normal conduction pathway is bypassed; results in short P-R interval on EKG; tendency to supraventricular tachycardia.

√5ᵗʰ 426.8 Other specified conduction disorders
426.81 Lown-Ganong-Levine syndrome
Syndrome of short P-R interval, normal QRS complexes, and supraventricular tachycardias

426.89 Other
Dissociation:
atrioventricular [AV]
interference
isorhythmic
Nonparoxysmal AV nodal tachycardia

426.9 Conduction disorder, unspecified
Heart block NOS
Stokes-Adams syndrome

√4ᵗʰ 427 Cardiac dysrhythmias
EXCLUDES　that complicating:
abortion (634-638 with .7, 639.8)
ectopic or molar pregnancy (639.8)
labor or delivery (668.1, 669.4)

AHA: J-A, '85, 15

DEF: Disruption or disturbance in the rhythm of heartbeats.

427.0 Paroxysmal supraventricular tachycardia
Paroxysmal tachycardia:　Paroxysmal tachycardia:
atrial [PAT]　　　　　junctional
atrioventricular [AV]　nodal

DEF: Rapid atrial rhythm.

427.1 Paroxysmal ventricular tachycardia
Ventricular tachycardia (paroxysmal)
AHA: 3Q, '95, 9; M-A, '86, 11

DEF: Rapid ventricular rhythm.

427.2 Paroxysmal tachycardia, unspecified
Bouveret-Hoffmann syndrome
Paroxysmal tachycardia:
NOS
essential

√5ᵗʰ 427.3 Atrial fibrillation and flutter
427.31 Atrial fibrillation
AHA: ▶4Q, '03, 95, 105;◀ 1Q, '03, 8; 2Q, '99, 17; 3Q, '95, 8
DEF: Irregular, rapid atrial contractions.

427.32 Atrial flutter
AHA: ▶4Q, '03, 94◀
DEF: Regular, rapid atrial contractions.

√5ᵗʰ 427.4 Ventricular fibrillation and flutter
427.41 Ventricular fibrillation
AHA: 3Q, '02, 5
DEF: Irregular, rapid ventricular contractions.

427.42 Ventricular flutter
DEF: Regular, rapid, ventricular contractions.

427.5 Cardiac arrest
Cardiorespiratory arrest
AHA: 3Q,'02, 5; 2Q, '00, 12; 3Q, '95, 8; 2Q, '88, 8

√5ᵗʰ 427.6 Premature beats
427.60 Premature beats, unspecified
Ectopic beats　　Premature contractions
Extrasystoles　　　or systoles NOS
Extrasystolic arrhythmia

427.61 Supraventricular premature beats
Atrial premature beats, contractions, or systoles

427.69 Other
Ventricular premature beats, contractions, or systoles
AHA: 4Q, '93, 42

√5ᵗʰ 427.8 Other specified cardiac dysrhythmias
427.81 Sinoatrial node dysfunction
Sinus bradycardia:
persistent
severe
Syndrome:
sick sinus
tachycardia-bradycardia
EXCLUDES　sinus bradycardia NOS (427.89)
AHA: 3Q, '00, 8
DEF: Complex cardiac arrhythmia; appears as severe sinus bradycardia, sinus bradycardia with tachycardia, or sinus bradycardia with atrioventricular block.

427.89 Other
Rhythm disorder:　Rhythm disorder:
coronary sinus　　nodal
ectopic　　　　　Wandering (atrial)
　　　　　　　　　　pacemaker
EXCLUDES　carotid sinus syncope (337.0)
neonatal bradycardia (779.81)
neonatal tachycardia (779.82)
reflex bradycardia (337.0)
tachycardia NOS (785.0)

427.9 Cardiac dysrhythmia, unspecified
Arrhythmia (cardiac) NOS
AHA: 2Q, '89, 10

√4ᵗʰ 428 Heart failure
EXCLUDES　following cardiac surgery (429.4)
rheumatic (398.91)
that complicating:
abortion (634-638 with .7, 639.8)
ectopic or molar pregnancy (639.8)
labor or delivery (668.1, 669.4)
Code, if applicable, heart failure due to hypertension first (402.0-402.9, with fifth-digit 1 or 404.0-404.9 with fifth-digit 1 or 3)
AHA: 4Q, '02, 49; 3Q, '98, 5; 2Q, '90, 16; 2Q, '90, 19; 2Q, '89, 10; 3Q, '88, 3

428.0 Congestive heart failure, unspecified
Congestive heart disease
Right heart failure (secondary to left heart failure)
EXCLUDES　fluid overload NOS (276.6)
AHA: ▶4Q, '03, 109;◀ 1Q, '03, 9; 4Q, '02, 52; 2Q, '01, 13; 4Q, '00, 48; 2Q, '00, 16; 1Q, '00, 22; 4Q, '99, 4; 1Q, '99, 11; 4Q, '97, 55; 3Q, '97, 10; 3Q, '96, 9; 3Q, '91, 18; 3Q, '91, 19; 2Q, '89, 12
DEF: Mechanical inadequacy; caused by inability of heart to pump and circulate blood; results in fluid collection in lungs, hypertension, congestion and edema of tissue.

428.1 Left heart failure
Acute edema of lung　} with heart disease NOS
Acute pulmonary edema } or heart failure
Cardiac asthma
Left ventricular failure
DEF: Mechanical inadequacy of left ventricle; causing fluid in lungs.

√4ᵗʰ/√5ᵗʰ Additional Digit Required　　Unspecified Code　　Other Specified Code　　Manifestation Code　　▶◀ Revised Text　　● New Code　　▲ Revised Code Title

2005 ICD•9•CM　　　　　　　　　　　　　　　　　　　　February 2004 • Volume 1 — 119

Circulatory System

428.2–429.71

√5ᵗʰ **428.2 Systolic heart failure**
    EXCLUDES   *combined systolic and diastolic heart failure (428.40-428.43)*
    DEF: Heart failure due to a defect in expulsion of blood caused by an abnormality in systolic function, or ventricular contractile dysfunction.

    428.20 Unspecified
    428.21 Acute
    428.22 Chronic
    428.23 Acute on chronic
       AHA: 1Q, '03, 9

√5ᵗʰ **428.3 Diastolic heart failure**
    EXCLUDES   *combined systolic and diastolic heart failure (428.40-428.43)*
    DEF: Heart failure due to resistance to ventricular filling caused by an abnormality in the diastolic function.

    428.30 Unspecified
       AHA: 4Q, '02, 52
    428.31 Acute
    428.32 Chronic
    428.33 Acute on chronic

√5ᵗʰ **428.4 Combined systolic and diastolic heart failure**
    428.40 Unspecified
    428.41 Acute
    428.42 Chronic
    428.43 Acute on chronic
       AHA: 4Q, '02, 52

    428.9 Heart failure, unspecified
    Cardiac failure NOS   Myocardial failure NOS
    Heart failure NOS   Weak heart
       AHA: 2Q, '89, 10; N-D, '85, 14

√4ᵗʰ **429 Ill-defined descriptions and complications of heart disease**
    429.0 Myocarditis, unspecified

    Myocarditis:
      NOS
      chronic (interstitial) } (with mention of
      fibroid   arteriosclerosis)
      senile

    Use additional code to identify presence of arteriosclerosis
    EXCLUDES   *acute or subacute (422.0-422.9)*
                rheumatic (398.0)
                acute (391.2)
                that due to hypertension (402.0-402.9)

    429.1 Myocardial degeneration
    Degeneration of heart or
      myocardium:
      fatty
      mural
      muscular } (with mention of
    Myocardial: arteriosclerosis)
      degeneration
      disease

    Use additional code to identify presence of arteriosclerosis
    EXCLUDES   *that due to hypertension (402.0-402.9)*

    429.2 Cardiovascular disease, unspecified   A
    Arteriosclerotic cardiovascular disease [ASCVD]
    Cardiovascular arteriosclerosis
    Cardiovascular:
      degeneration
      disease } (with mention of
      sclerosis   arteriosclerosis)
    Use additional code to identify presence of arteriosclerosis
    EXCLUDES   *that due to hypertension (402.0-402.9)*

Cerebrovascular Arteries

Echocardiography of Heart Failure

Four-chamber echocardiograms, two-dimensional views.
LV: Left ventricle
RV: Right ventricle
RA: Right atrium
LA: Left atrium

Systolic dysfunction with dilated LV

Diastolic dysfunction with LV hypertrophy

    429.3 Cardiomegaly
    Cardiac: Ventricular dilatation
      dilatation
      hypertrophy
    EXCLUDES   *that due to hypertension (402.0-402.9)*

    429.4 Functional disturbances following cardiac surgery
    Cardiac insufficiency } following cardiac surgery
    Heart failure   or due to prosthesis

    Postcardiotomy syndrome
    Postvalvulotomy syndrome
    EXCLUDES   *cardiac failure in the immediate postoperative period (997.1)*
       AHA: 2Q, '02, 12; N-D, '85, 6

    429.5 Rupture of chordae tendineae
    DEF: Torn tissue, between heart valves and papillary muscles.

    429.6 Rupture of papillary muscle
    DEF: Torn muscle, between chordae tendineae and heart wall.

√5ᵗʰ **429.7 Certain sequelae of myocardial infarction, not elsewhere classified**
    Use additional code to identify the associated myocardial infarction:
      with onset of 8 weeks or less (410.00-410.92)
      with onset of more than 8 weeks (414.8)
    EXCLUDES   *congenital defects of heart (745, 746)*
             coronary aneurysm (414.11)
             disorders of papillary muscle (429.6, 429.81)
             postmyocardial infarction syndrome (411.0)
             rupture of chordae tendineae (429.5)
       AHA: 3Q, '89, 5

    429.71 Acquired cardiac septal defect   A
    EXCLUDES   *acute septal infarction (410.00-410.92)*
    DEF: Abnormal communication, between opposite heart chambers; due to defect of septum; not present at birth.

N   Newborn Age: 0   P   Pediatric Age: 0-17   M   Maternity Age: 12-55   A   Adult Age: 15-124   MSP   Medicare Secondary Payer

429.79 Other   A
     Mural thrombus (atrial) (ventricular),
       acquired, following myocardial
       infarction
     AHA: 1Q, '92, 10

√5th **429.8 Other ill-defined heart diseases**
     429.81 Other disorders of papillary muscle

Papillary muscle:	Papillary muscle:
atrophy	incompetence
degeneration	incoordination
dysfunction	scarring

     429.82 Hyperkinetic heart disease
       DEF: Condition of unknown origin in young adults;
       marked by increased cardiac output at rest, increased
       rate of ventricular ejection; may lead to heart failure.

     429.89 Other
       Carditis
       EXCLUDES   *that due to hypertension*
         (402.0-402.9)
       AHA: 1Q, '92, 10

429.9 Heart disease, unspecified
     Heart disease (organic) NOS   Morbus cordis NOS
     EXCLUDES   *that due to hypertension (402.0-402.9)*
     AHA: 1Q, '93, 19

CEREBROVASCULAR DISEASE (430-438)
   INCLUDES   with mention of hypertension (conditions
       classifiable to 401-405)
   Use additional code to identify presence of hypertension
   EXCLUDES   *any condition classifiable to 430-434, 436, 437*
       occurring during pregnancy, childbirth, or
       the puerperium, or specified as puerperal
       (674.0)
       iatrogenic cerebrovascular infarction or
       hemorrhage (997.02)
   AHA: 1Q, '93, 27; 3Q, '91, 10; 3Q, '90, 3; 2Q, '89, 8; M-A, '85, 6

430 Subarachnoid hemorrhage
   Meningeal hemorrhage
   Ruptured:
     berry aneurysm
     (congenital) cerebral aneurysm NOS
     EXCLUDES   *syphilitic ruptured cerebral aneurysm (094.87)*
   DEF: Bleeding in space between brain and lining.

431 Intracerebral hemorrhage

Hemorrhage (of):	Hemorrhage (of):
basilar	internal capsule
bulbar	intrapontine
cerebellar	pontine
cerebral	subcortical
cerebromeningeal	ventricular
cortical	Rupture of blood vessel in brain

   DEF: Bleeding within the brain.

Berry Aneurysm

√4th **432 Other and unspecified intracranial hemorrhage**
     432.0 Nontraumatic extradural hemorrhage
       Nontraumatic epidural hemorrhage
       DEF: Bleeding, nontraumatic, between skull and brain lining.

     432.1 Subdural hemorrhage
       Subdural hematoma, nontraumatic
       DEF: Bleeding, between outermost and other layers of brain lining.

     432.9 Unspecified intracranial hemorrhage
       Intracranial hemorrhage NOS

√4th **433 Occlusion and stenosis of precerebral arteries**
     INCLUDES   embolism
       narrowing   } of basilar, carotid, and
       obstruction   vertebral arteries
       thrombosis

     EXCLUDES   *insufficiency NOS of precerebral arteries (435.0-*
       435.9)

   The following fifth-digit subclassification is for use with
   category 433:
       0 without mention of cerebral infarction   A
       1 with cerebral infarction

   AHA: 2Q, '95, 14; 3Q, '90, 16

   DEF: Blockage, stricture, arteries branching into brain.

√5th **433.0 Basilar artery**
√5th **433.1 Carotid artery**
     AHA: 1Q, '00, 16; For code 433.10: 1Q, '02, 7, 10
√5th **433.2 Vertebral artery**
√5th **433.3 Multiple and bilateral**
     AHA: 2Q, '02, 19
√5th **433.8 Other specified precerebral artery**
√5th **433.9 Unspecified precerebral artery**
     Precerebral artery NOS

√4th **434 Occlusion of cerebral arteries**
   The following fifth-digit subclassification is for use with
   category 434:
       0 without mention of cerebral infarction
       1 with cerebral infarction

   AHA: 2Q, '95, 14

√5th **434.0 Cerebral thrombosis**   A
     Thrombosis of cerebral arteries
√5th **434.1 Cerebral embolism**   A
     AHA: 3Q, '97, 11
√5th **434.9 Cerebral artery occlusion, unspecified**   A
     AHA: 4Q, '98, 87

√4th **435 Transient cerebral ischemia**
     INCLUDES   cerebrovascular insufficiency (acute) with
       transient focal neurological signs and
       symptoms
       insufficiency of basilar, carotid, and vertebral
       arteries
       spasm of cerebral arteries
     EXCLUDES   *acute cerebrovascular insufficiency NOS (437.1)*
       that due to any condition classifiable to 433
       (433.0-433.9)
   DEF: Temporary restriction of blood flow, to arteries branching into brain.

     435.0 Basilar artery syndrome
     435.1 Vertebral artery syndrome
     435.2 Subclavian steal syndrome
       DEF: Cerebrovascular insufficiency, due to occluded subclavian
       artery; symptoms include pain in mastoid and posterior head
       regions, flaccid paralysis of arm and diminished or absent radical
       pulse on affected side.

     435.3 Vertebrobasilar artery syndrome
       AHA: 4Q, '95, 60
       DEF: Transient ischemic attack; due to brainstem dysfunction;
       symptoms include confusion, vertigo, binocular blindness, diplopia,
       unilateral or bilateral weakness and paresthesis of extremities.

√4th √5th Additional Digit Required   Unspecified Code   Other Specified Code   Manifestation Code   ►◄ Revised Text   ● New Code   ▲ Revised Code Title

Map of Major Arteries

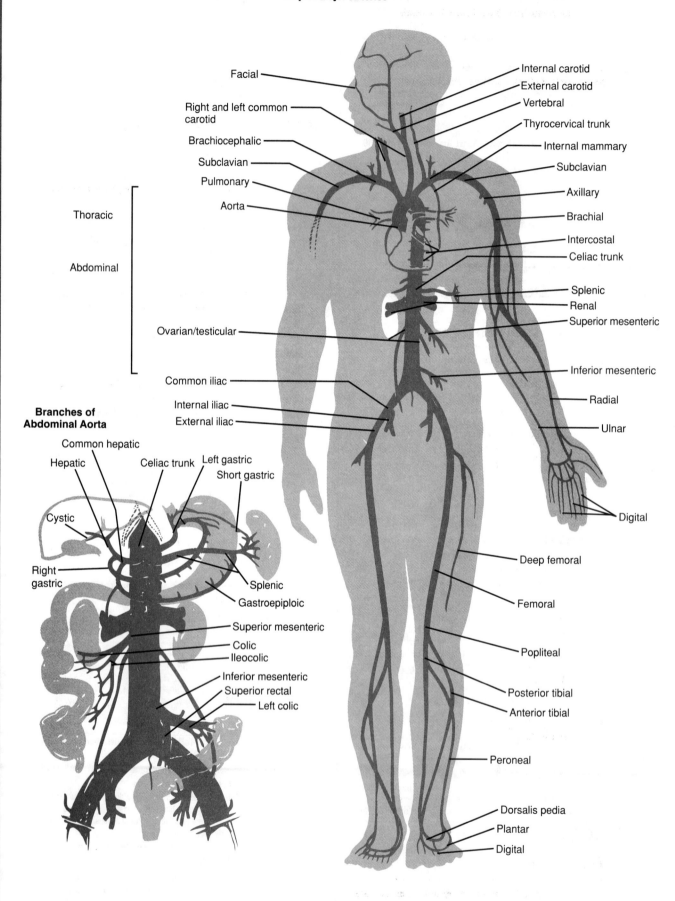

Facial

Right and left common carotid

Brachiocephalic

Subclavian

Pulmonary

Aorta

Thoracic

Abdominal

Ovarian/testicular

Common iliac

Internal iliac

External iliac

Internal carotid

External carotid

Vertebral

Thyrocervical trunk

Internal mammary

Subclavian

Axillary

Brachial

Intercostal

Celiac trunk

Splenic

Renal

Superior mesenteric

Inferior mesenteric

Radial

Ulnar

Digital

Deep femoral

Femoral

Popliteal

Posterior tibial

Anterior tibial

Peroneal

Dorsalis pedia

Plantar

Digital

Branches of Abdominal Aorta

Common hepatic

Hepatic

Celiac trunk

Left gastric

Short gastric

Cystic

Right gastric

Splenic

Gastroepiploic

Superior mesenteric

Colic

Ileocolic

Inferior mesenteric

Superior rectal

Left colic

435.8 Other specified transient cerebral ischemias   A

435.9 Unspecified transient cerebral ischemia   A

    Impending cerebrovascular accident

    Intermittent cerebral ischemia

    Transient ischemic attack [TIA]

    AHA: N-D, '85, 12

436 Acute, but ill-defined, cerebrovascular disease

    Apoplexy, apoplectic: Apoplexy, apoplectic:

      NOS   seizure

      attack   Cerebral seizure

      cerebral

      EXCLUDES   *any condition classifiable to categories 430-435*

           ▶*cerebrovascular accident (434.91)*

           CVA (ischemic) (434.91)

             embolic (434.11)

             hemorrhagic (430, 431, 432.0-432.9)

             thrombotic (434.01)◀

           postoperative cerebrovascular accident (997.02)

           ▶*stroke (ischemic) (434.91)*

             embolic (434.11)

             hemorrhagic (430, 431, 432.0-432.9)

             thrombotic (434.01)◀

   AHA: 4Q, '99, 3

✓4th **437** Other and ill-defined cerebrovascular disease

437.0 Cerebral atherosclerosis   A

    Atheroma of cerebral arteries

    Cerebral arteriosclerosis

437.1 Other generalized ischemic cerebrovascular disease

    Acute cerebrovascular insufficiency NOS

    Cerebral ischemia (chronic)

437.2 Hypertensive encephalopathy

    AHA: J-A, '84, 14

    DEF: Cerebral manifestations (such as visual disturbances and headache) due to high blood pressure.

437.3 Cerebral aneurysm, nonruptured

    Internal carotid artery, intracranial portion

    Internal carotid artery NOS

      EXCLUDES   *congenital cerebral aneurysm, nonruptured (747.81)*

                   internal carotid artery, extracranial portion (442.81)

437.4 Cerebral arteritis

    AHA: 4Q, '99, 21

    DEF: Inflammation of a cerebral artery or arteries.

437.5 Moyamoya disease

    DEF: Cerebrovascular ischemia; vessels occlude and rupture causing tiny hemorrhages at base of brain; predominantly affects Japanese.

437.6 Nonpyogenic thrombosis of intracranial venous sinus

      EXCLUDES   *pyogenic (325)*

437.7 Transient global amnesia

    AHA: 4Q, '92, 20

    DEF: Episode of short-term memory loss, not often recurrent; pathogenesis unknown; with no signs or symptoms of neurological disorder.

437.8 Other

437.9 Unspecified

    Cerebrovascular disease or lesion NOS

✓4th **438** Late effects of cerebrovascular disease

    Note: This category is to be used to indicate conditions in 430-437 as the cause of late effects. The "late effects" include conditions specified as such, as sequelae, which may occur at any time after the onset of the causal condition.

    AHA: 4Q, '99, 4, 6, 7; 4Q, '98, 39, 88; 4Q, '97, 35, 37; 4Q, '92, 21;N-D,'86, 12; M-A, '86, 7

438.0 Cognitive deficits

✓5th **438.1** Speech and language deficits

    438.10 Speech and language deficit, unspecified

438.11 Aphasia

    AHA: 4Q, '03, 105; 4Q, '97, 36

    DEF: Impairment or absence of the ability to communicate by speech, writing or signs or to comprehend the spoken or written language due to disease or injury to the brain. Total aphasia is the loss of function of both sensory and motor areas of the brain.

438.12 Dysphasia

    AHA: 4Q, '99, 3, 9

    DEF: Impaired speech; marked by inability to sequence language.

438.19 Other speech and language deficits

✓5th **438.2** Hemiplegia/hemiparesis

    DEF: Paralysis of one side of the body.

    438.20 Hemiplegia affecting unspecified side

      AHA: 4Q, '03, 105; 4Q, '99, 3, 9

    438.21 Hemiplegia affecting dominant side

    438.22 Hemiplegia affecting nondominant side

      AHA: 4Q, '03, 105; 1Q, '02, 16

✓5th **438.3** Monoplegia of upper limb

    DEF: Paralysis of one limb or one muscle group.

    438.30 Monoplegia of upper limb affecting unspecified side

    438.31 Monoplegia of upper limb affecting dominant side

    438.32 Monoplegia of upper limb affecing nondominant side

✓5th **438.4** Monoplegia of lower limb

    438.40 Monoplegia of lower limb affecting unspecified side

    438.41 Monoplegia of lower limb affecting dominant side

    438.42 Monoplegia of lower limb affecting nondominant side

✓5th **438.5** Other paralytic syndrome

    Use additional code to identify type of paralytic syndrome, such as:

    locked-in state (344.81)

    quadriplegia (344.00-344.09)

      EXCLUDES   *late effects of cerebrovascular accident with:*

           hemiplegia/hemiparesis (438.20-438.22)

           monoplegia of lower limb (438.40-438.42)

           monoplegia of upper limb (438.30-438.32)

    438.50 Other paralytic syndrome affecting unspecified side

    438.51 Other paralytic syndrome affecting dominant side

    438.52 Other paralytic syndrome affecting nondominant side

    438.53 Other paralytic syndrome, bilateral

      AHA: 4Q, '98, 39

438.6 Alterations of sensations

    Use additional code to identify the altered sensation

438.7 Disturbances of vision

    Use additional code to identify the visual disturbance

    AHA: 4Q, '02, 56

✓5th **438.8** Other late effects of cerebrovascular disease

    438.81 Apraxia

      DEF: Inability to activate learned movements; no known sensory or motor impairment.

    438.82 Dysphagia

      DEF: Inability or difficulty in swallowing.

    438.83 Facial weakness

      Facial droop

✓4th ✓5th   Additional Digit Required   Unspecified Code   Other Specified Code   Manifestation Code   ▶◀ Revised Text   ● New Code   ▲ Revised Code Title

2005 ICD•9•CM   **October 2004 • Volume 1 — 123**

Circulatory System

438.84 Ataxia
> AHA: 4Q, '02, 56

438.85 Vertigo

438.89 Other late effects of cerebrovascular disease
> Use additional code to identify the late effect
>
> AHA: 4Q, '98, 39

438.9 Unspecified late effects of cerebrovascular disease

DISEASES OF ARTERIES, ARTERIOLES, AND CAPILLARIES (440-448)

✓4ᵗʰ 440 Atherosclerosis

> INCLUDES   arteriolosclerosis
> arteriosclerosis (obliterans) (senile)
> arteriosclerotic vascular disease
> atheroma
> degeneration:
>> arterial   vascular
>> arteriovascular
> endarteritis deformans or obliterans
> senile:
>> arteritis   endarteritis

> EXCLUDES   *atheroembolism (445.01-445.89)*
> *atherosclerosis of bypass graft of the extremities (403.30-403.32)*

> DEF: Stricture and reduced elasticity of an artery; due to plaque deposits.

440.0 Of aorta   A
> AHA: 2Q, '93, 7; 2Q, '93, 8; 4Q, '88, 8

440.1 Of renal artery   A
> EXCLUDES   *atherosclerosis of renal arterioles (403.00-403.91)*

✓5ᵗʰ 440.2 Of native arteries of the extremities
> EXCLUDES   *atherosclerosis of bypass graft of the extremities (440.30-440.32)*
>
> AHA: 4Q, '94, 49; 4Q, '93, 27; 4Q, '92, 25; 3Q, '90, 15; M-A, '87, 6

440.20 Atherosclerosis of the extremities, unspecified   A

440.21 Atherosclerosis of the extremities with intermittent claudication   A
> DEF: Atherosclerosis; marked by pain, tension and weakness after walking; no symptoms while at rest.

440.22 Atherosclerosis of the extremities with rest pain   A
> INCLUDES   any condition classifiable to 440.21
>
> DEF: Atherosclerosis, marked by pain, tension and weakness while at rest.

Thoracic, Abdominal and Aortic Aneurysm

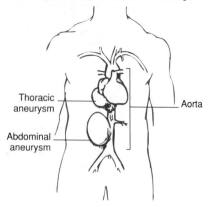

Thoracic aneurysm — Aorta
Abdominal aneurysm

Arterial Diseases and Disorders

Lipids — Calcium deposits

Intimal proliferation   Atherosclerosis narrowing lumen   Thrombus (clot) forming in lumen   Organization of thrombus and recanalization

Embolus (from elsewhere) occluding lumen   Aneurysm bypasses lumen or...   ...bulges from arterial wall   Arteriovenous fistula

440.23 Atherosclerosis of the extremities with ulceration   A
> Use additional code for any associated ulceration (707.10-707.9)
>
> INCLUDES   any condition classifiable to 440.21 and 440.22
>
> AHA: 4Q, '00, 44

440.24 Atherosclerosis of the extremities with gangrene
> INCLUDES   any condition classifiable to 440.21, 440.22, and 440.23 with ischemic gangrene 785.4
>
> EXCLUDES   *gas gangrene (040.0)*
>
> AHA: ▶4Q, '03, 109; 3Q. '03, 14;◀ 4Q, '95, 54; 1Q, '95, 11

440.29 Other   A

✓5ᵗʰ 440.3 Of bypass graft of extremities
> EXCLUDES   *atherosclerosis of native arteries of the extremities (440.21-440.24)*
> *embolism [occlusion NOS] [thrombus] of graft (996.74)*
>
> AHA: 4Q, '94, 49

440.30 Of unspecified graft   A

440.31 Of autologous vein bypass graft   A

440.32 Of nonautologous biological bypass graft   A

440.8 Of other specified arteries   A
> EXCLUDES   *basilar (433.0)*
> *carotid (433.1)*
> *cerebral (437.0)*
> *coronary (414.00-414.07)*
> *mesenteric (557.1)*
> *precerebral (433.0-433.9)*
> *pulmonary (416.0)*
> *vertebral (433.2)*

440.9 Generalized and unspecified atherosclerosis   A
> Arteriosclerotic vascular disease NOS
>
> EXCLUDES   *arteriosclerotic cardiovascular disease [ASCVD] (429.2)*

✓4ᵗʰ 441 Aortic aneurysm and dissection
> EXCLUDES   *syphilitic aortic aneurysm (093.0)*
> *traumatic aortic aneurysm (901.0, 902.0)*

✓5ᵗʰ 441.0 Dissection of aorta
> AHA: 4Q, '89, 10
>
> DEF: Dissection or splitting of wall of the aorta; due to blood entering through intimal tear or interstitial hemorrhage.

441.00 Unspecified site   A

441.01 Thoracic   A

441.02 Abdominal   A

441.03 Thoracoabdominal   A

441.1 Thoracic aneurysm, ruptured `A`

441.2 Thoracic aneurysm without mention of rupture `A`
AHA: 3Q, '92, 10

441.3 Abdominal aneurysm, ruptured `A`

441.4 Abdominal aneurysm without mention of rupture `A`
AHA: 4Q, '00, 64; 1Q, '99, 15, 16, 17; 3Q, '92, 10

441.5 Aortic aneurysm of unspecified site, ruptured `A`
Rupture of aorta NOS

441.6 Thoracoabdominal aneurysm, ruptured `A`

441.7 Thoracoabdominal aneurysm, without mention of rupture `A`

441.9 Aortic aneurysm of unspecified site without mention of rupture `A`
Aneurysm
Dilatation   } of aorta
Hyaline necrosis

√4ᵗʰ 442 Other aneurysm
INCLUDES   aneurysm (ruptured) (cirsoid) (false) (varicose)
aneurysmal varix
EXCLUDES   arteriovenous aneurysm or fistula:
acquired (447.0)
congenital (747.60-747.69)
traumatic (900.0-904.9)

DEF: Dissection or splitting of arterial wall; due to blood entering through intimal tear or interstitial hemorrhage.

442.0 Of artery of upper extremity `A`

442.1 Of renal artery `A`

442.2 Of iliac artery `A`
AHA: 1Q, '99, 16, 17

442.3 Of artery of lower extremity `A`
Aneurysm:
femoral   }
popliteal } artery

AHA: 3Q, '02, 24-26; 1Q, '99, 16

√5ᵗʰ 442.8 Of other specified artery
442.81 Artery of neck
Aneurysm of carotid artery (common) (external) (internal, extracranial portion)
EXCLUDES   internal carotid artery, intracranial portion (437.3)

442.82 Subclavian artery `A`
442.83 Splenic artery `A`
442.84 Other visceral artery `A`
Aneurysm:
celiac
gastroduodenal
gastroepiploic
hepatic   } artery
pancreaticoduodenal
superior mesenteric

442.89 Other `A`
Aneurysm:
mediastinal }
spinal   } artery
EXCLUDES   cerebral (nonruptured) (437.3)
congenital (747.81)
ruptured (430)
coronary (414.11)
heart (414.10)
pulmonary (417.1)

442.9 Of unspecified site `A`

√4ᵗʰ 443 Other peripheral vascular disease
443.0 Raynaud's syndrome
Raynaud's:
disease
phenomenon (secondary)
Use additional code to identify gangrene (785.4)

DEF: Constriction of the arteries, due to cold or stress; bilateral ischemic attacks of fingers, toes, nose or ears; symptoms include pallor, paresthesia and pain; more common in females.

443.1 Thromboangiitis obliterans [Buerger's disease]
Presenile gangrene

DEF: Inflammatory disease of extremity blood vessels, mainly the lower; occurs primarily in young men and leads to tissue ischemia and gangrene.

√5ᵗʰ 443.2 Other arterial dissection
EXCLUDES   dissection of aorta (441.00-441.03)
dissection of coronary arteries (414.12)
AHA: 4Q, '02, 54

443.21 Dissection of carotid artery
443.22 Dissection of iliac artery
443.23 Dissection of renal artery
443.24 Dissection of vertebral artery
443.29 Dissection of other artery

√5ᵗʰ 443.8 Other specified peripheral vascular diseases
443.81 *Peripheral angiopathy in diseases classified elsewhere*
Code first underlying disease, as:
diabetes mellitus (250.7)
AHA: ▶1Q, '04, 14;◀ 3Q, '91, 10

443.89 Other
Acrocyanosis   Erythrocyanosis
Acroparesthesia: Erythromelalgia
simple [Schultze's type]
vasomotor [Nothnagel's type]
EXCLUDES   chilblains (991.5)
frostbite (991.0-991.3)
immersion foot (991.4)

443.9 Peripheral vascular disease, unspecified
Intermittent claudication NOS
Peripheral:
angiopathy NOS
vascular disease NOS
Spasm of artery
EXCLUDES   atherosclerosis of the arteries of the extremities (440.20-440.22)
spasm of cerebral artery (435.0-435.9)
AHA: 4Q, '92, 25; 3Q, '91, 10

√4ᵗʰ 444 Arterial embolism and thrombosis
INCLUDES   infarction:
embolic
thrombotic
occlusion
EXCLUDES   atheroembolism (445.01-445.89)
that complicating:
abortion (634-638 with .6, 639.6)
ectopic or molar pregnancy (639.6)
pregnancy, childbirth, or the pueperium (673.0-673.8)
AHA: 2Q, '92, 11; 4Q, '90, 27

444.0 Of abdominal aorta
Aortic bifurcation syndrome
Aortoiliac obstruction
Leriche's syndrome
Saddle embolus
AHA: 2Q, '93, 7; 4Q, '90, 27

444.1 Of thoracic aorta
Embolism or thrombosis of aorta (thoracic)

√4ᵗʰ √5ᵗʰ Additional Digit Required   Unspecified Code   Other Specified Code   Manifestation Code   ▶◀ Revised Text   ● New Code   ▲ Revised Code Title

2005 ICD•9•CM   October 2004 • Volume 1 — 125

Map of Major Veins

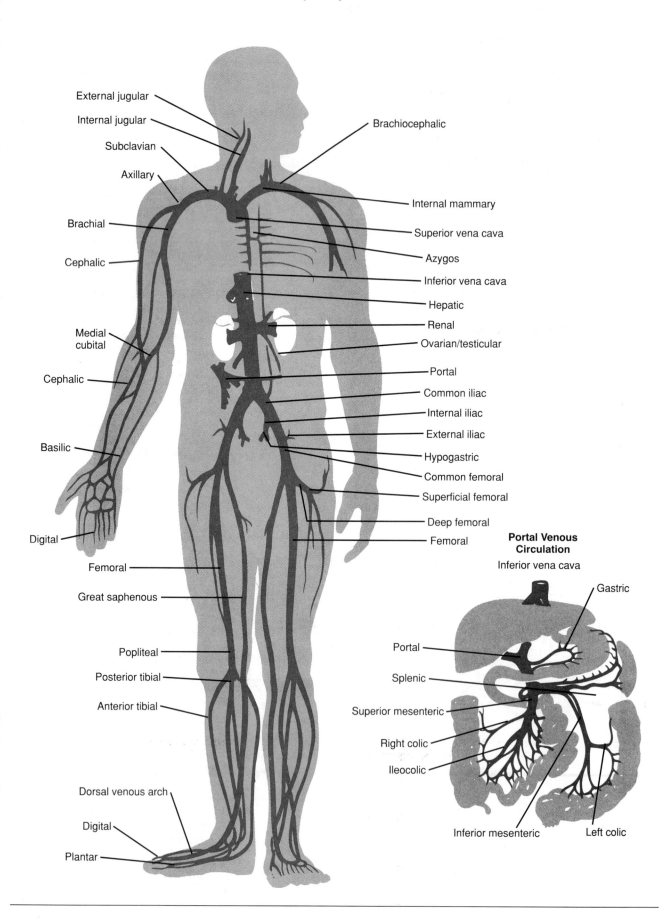

External jugular

Internal jugular

Subclavian

Axillary

Brachial

Cephalic

Medial cubital

Cephalic

Basilic

Digital

Femoral

Great saphenous

Popliteal

Posterior tibial

Anterior tibial

Dorsal venous arch

Digital

Plantar

Brachiocephalic

Internal mammary

Superior vena cava

Azygos

Inferior vena cava

Hepatic

Renal

Ovarian/testicular

Portal

Common iliac

Internal iliac

External iliac

Hypogastric

Common femoral

Superficial femoral

Deep femoral

Femoral

Portal Venous Circulation

Inferior vena cava

Gastric

Portal

Splenic

Superior mesenteric

Right colic

Ileocolic

Inferior mesenteric

Left colic

| N Newborn Age: 0 | P Pediatric Age: 0-17 | M Maternity Age: 12-55 | A Adult Age: 15-124 | MSP Medicare Secondary Payer |

√5th 444.2　Of arteries of the extremities
　　　AHA: M-A, '87, 6

444.21　Upper extremity

444.22　Lower extremity
　　　Arterial embolism or thrombosis:
　　　　femoral
　　　　peripheral NOS
　　　　popliteal
　　　　　EXCLUDES　　*iliofemoral (444.81)*
　　　AHA: ▶3Q, '03, 10;◀ 1Q, '03, 17; 3Q, '90, 16

√5th 444.8　Of other specified artery

444.81　Iliac artery
　　　AHA: 1Q, '03, 16

444.89　Other
　　　　　EXCLUDES　　*basilar (433.0)*
　　　　　　　　　　carotid (433.1)
　　　　　　　　　　cerebral (434.0-434.9)
　　　　　　　　　　coronary (410.00-410.92)
　　　　　　　　　　mesenteric (557.0)
　　　　　　　　　　ophthalmic (362.30-362.34)
　　　　　　　　　　precerebral (433.0-433.9)
　　　　　　　　　　pulmonary (415.19)
　　　　　　　　　　renal (593.81)
　　　　　　　　　　retinal (362.30-362.34)
　　　　　　　　　　vertebral (433.2)

444.9　Of unspecified artery

√4th 445　Atheroembolism
　　　INCLUDES　　atherothrombotic microembolism
　　　　　　　　　cholesterol embolism

　　　AHA: 4Q, '02, 57

√5th 445.0　Of extremities

445.01　Upper extremity

445.02　Lower extremity

√5th 445.8　Of other sites

445.81　Kidney
　　　Use additional code for any associated
　　　　kidney failure (584, 585)

445.89　Other site

√4th 446　Polyarteritis nodosa and allied conditions

446.0　Polyarteritis nodosa
　　　Disseminated necrotizing periarteritis
　　　Necrotizing angiitis
　　　Panarteritis (nodosa)
　　　Periarteritis (nodosa)
　　　DEF: Inflammation of small and mid-size arteries; symptoms related
　　　to involved arteries in kidneys, muscles, gastrointestinal tract and
　　　heart; results in tissue death.

446.1　Acute febrile mucocutaneous lymph node syndrome [MCLS]
　　　Kawasaki disease
　　　DEF: Acute febrile disease of children; marked by erythema of
　　　conjunctiva and mucous membranes of upper respiratory tract, skin
　　　eruptions and edema.

√5th 446.2　Hypersensitivity angiitis
　　　　　EXCLUDES　　*antiglomerular basement membrane*
　　　　　　　　　　　disease without pulmonary
　　　　　　　　　　　hemorrhage (583.89)

446.20　Hypersensitivity angiitis, unspecified

446.21　Goodpasture's syndrome
　　　Antiglomerular basement membrane
　　　　antibody-mediated nephritis with
　　　　pulmonary hemorrhage
　　　Use additional code to identify renal disease
　　　　(583.81)
　　　DEF: Glomerulonephritis associated with hematuria,
　　　progresses rapidly; results in death from renal failure.

446.29　Other specified hypersensitivity angiitis
　　　AHA: 1Q, '95, 3

446.3　Lethal midline granuloma
　　　Malignant granuloma of face
　　　DEF: Granulomatous lesion; in nose or paranasal sinuses; often
　　　fatal; occurs chiefly in males.
　　　AHA: 3Q, '00, 11

446.4　Wegener's granulomatosis
　　　Necrotizing respiratory granulomatosis
　　　Wegener's syndrome
　　　DEF: A disease occurring mainly in men; marked by necrotizing
　　　granulomas and ulceration of the upper respiratory tract;
　　　underlying condition is a vasculitis affecting small vessels and is
　　　possibly due to an immune disorder.
　　　AHA: 3Q, '00, 11

446.5　Giant cell arteritis
　　　Cranial arteritis　　　Temporal arteritis
　　　Horton's disease
　　　DEF: Inflammation of arteries; due to giant cells affecting carotid
　　　artery branches, resulting in occlusion; symptoms include fever,
　　　headache and neurological problems; occurs in elderly.

446.6　Thrombotic microangiopathy
　　　Moschcowitz's syndrome
　　　Thrombotic thrombocytopenic purpura
　　　DEF: Blockage of small blood vessels; due to hyaline deposits;
　　　symptoms include purpura, CNS disorders; results in protracted
　　　disease or rapid death.

446.7　Takayasu's disease
　　　Aortic arch arteritis　　Pulseless disease
　　　DEF: Progressive obliterative arteritis of brachiocephalic trunk, left
　　　subclavian, and left common carotid arteries above aortic arch;
　　　results in ischemia in brain, heart and arm; pulses impalpable in
　　　head, neck and arms; more common in young adult females.

√4th 447　Other disorders of arteries and arterioles

447.0　Arteriovenous fistula, acquired
　　　Arteriovenous aneurysm, acquired
　　　　EXCLUDES　　*cerebrovascular (437.3)*
　　　　　　　　　　coronary (414.19)
　　　　　　　　　　pulmonary (417.0)
　　　　　　　　　　surgically created arteriovenous shunt
　　　　　　　　　　　or fistula:
　　　　　　　　　　　complication (996.1, 996.61-996.62)
　　　　　　　　　　　status or presence (V45.1)
　　　　　　　　　　traumatic (900.0-904.9)
　　　DEF: Communication between an artery and vein caused by error in
　　　healing.

447.1　Stricture of artery
　　　AHA: 2Q, '93, 8; M-A, '87, 6

447.2　Rupture of artery
　　　Erosion
　　　Fistula, except arteriovenous　}　of artery
　　　Ulcer
　　　　　EXCLUDES　　*traumatic rupture of artery (900.0-904.9)*

447.3　Hyperplasia of renal artery
　　　Fibromuscular hyperplasia of renal artery
　　　DEF: Overgrowth of cells in muscular lining of renal artery.

447.4　Celiac artery compression syndrome
　　　Celiac axis syndrome　Marable's syndrome

447.5　Necrosis of artery

447.6　Arteritis, unspecified
　　　Aortitis NOS　　　　　Endarteritis NOS
　　　　EXCLUDES　　*arteritis, endarteritis:*
　　　　　　　　　　aortic arch (446.7)
　　　　　　　　　　cerebral (437.4)
　　　　　　　　　　coronary (414.00-414.07)
　　　　　　　　　　deformans (440.0-440.9)
　　　　　　　　　　obliterans (440.0-440.9)
　　　　　　　　　　pulmonary (417.8)
　　　　　　　　　　senile (440.0-440.9)
　　　　　　　　　polyarteritis NOS (446.0)
　　　　　　　　　syphilitic aortitis (093.1)
　　　AHA: 1Q, '95, 3

√4th　Additional Digit Required　　**Unspecified Code**　　　**Other Specified Code**　　　**Manifestation Code**　　　▶◀ Revised Text　　　● New Code　　　▲ Revised Code Title
√5th

Circulatory System

447.8 Other specified disorders of arteries and arterioles
Fibromuscular hyperplasia of arteries, except renal

447.9 Unspecified disorders of arteries and arterioles

√4ᵗʰ 448 Disease of capillaries

448.0 Hereditary hemorrhagic telangiectasia
Rendu-Osler-Weber disease

DEF: Genetic disease with onset after puberty; results in multiple telangiectases, dilated venules on skin and mucous membranes; recurrent bleeding may occur.

448.1 Nevus, non-neoplastic
Nevus: Nevus:
 araneus   spider
 senile   stellar
EXCLUDES neoplastic (216.0-216.9)
 port wine (757.32)
 strawberry (757.32)

DEF: Enlarged or malformed blood vessels of skin; results in reddish swelling, skin patch, or birthmark.

448.9 Other and unspecified capillary diseases
Capillary: Capillary:
 hemorrhage   thrombosis
 hyperpermeability
EXCLUDES capillary fragility (hereditary) (287.8)

DISEASES OF VEINS AND LYMPHATICS, AND OTHER DISEASES OF CIRCULATORY SYSTEM (451-459)

√4ᵗʰ 451 Phlebitis and thrombophlebitis
INCLUDES endophlebitis
 inflammation, vein
 periphlebitis
 suppurative phlebitis
Use additional E code to identify drug, if drug-induced
EXCLUDES that complicating:
 abortion (634-638 with .7, 639.8)
 ectopic or molar pregnancy (639.8)
 pregnancy, childbirth, or the puerperium (671.0-671.9)
 that due to or following:
 implant or catheter device (996.61-996.62)
 infusion, perfusion, or transfusion (999.2)

AHA: 1Q, '92, 16

DEF: Inflammation of a vein (phlebitis) with formation of a thrombus (thrombophlebitis).

451.0 Of superficial vessels of lower extremities
AHA: 3Q, '91, 16
Saphenous vein (greater) (lesser)

√5ᵗʰ 451.1 Of deep vessels of lower extremities
AHA: 3Q, '91, 16
451.11 Femoral vein (deep) (superficial)
451.19 Other
Femoropopliteal vein   Tibial vein
Popliteal vein

451.2 Of lower extremities, unspecified

√5ᵗʰ 451.8 Of other sites
EXCLUDES intracranial venous sinus (325)
 nonpyogenic (437.6)
 portal (vein) (572.1)
451.81 Iliac vein
451.82 Of superficial veins of upper extremities
Antecubital vein   Cephalic vein
Basilic vein
451.83 Of deep veins of upper extremities
Brachial vein   Ulnar vein
Radial vein
451.84 Of upper extremities, unspecified

451.89 Other
Axillary vein   Thrombophlebitis of
Jugular vein   breast (Mondor's
Subclavian vein   disease)

451.9 Of unspecified site

452 Portal vein thrombosis
Portal (vein) obstruction
EXCLUDES hepatic vein thrombosis (453.0)
 phlebitis of portal vein (572.1)
DEF: Formation of a blood clot in main vein of liver.

√4ᵗʰ 453 Other venous embolism and thrombosis
EXCLUDES that complicating:
 abortion (634-638 with .7, 639.8)
 ectopic or molar pregnancy (639.8)
 pregnancy, childbirth, or the puerperium (671.0-671.9)
 that with inflammation, phlebitis, and thrombophlebitis (451.0-451.9)
AHA: 1Q, '92, 16

453.0 Budd-Chiari syndrome
Hepatic vein thrombosis
DEF: Thrombosis or other obstruction of hepatic vein; symptoms include enlarged liver, extensive collateral vessels, intractable ascites and severe portal hypertension.

453.1 Thrombophlebitis migrans
DEF: Slow, advancing thrombophlebitis; appearing first in one vein then another.

453.2 Of vena cava
453.3 Of renal vein
√5ᵗʰ 453.4 Venous embolism and thrombosis of deep vessels of lower extremity
453.40 Venous embolism and thrombosis of unspecified deep vessels of lower extremity
Deep vein thrombosis NOS
DVT NOS
453.41 Venous embolism and thrombosis of deep vessels of proximal lower extremity
Femoral   Thigh
Iliac   Upper leg NOS
Popliteal
453.42 Venous embolism and thrombosis of deep vessels of distal lower extremity
Calf   Peroneal
Lower leg NOS Tibial

453.8 Of other specified veins
EXCLUDES cerebral (434.0-434.9)
 coronary (410.00-410.92)
 intracranial venous sinus (325)
 nonpyogenic (437.6)
 mesenteric (557.0)
 portal (452)
 precerebral (433.0-433.9)
 pulmonary (415.19)
AHA: 3Q, '91, 16; M-A, '87, 6

453.9 Of unspecified site
Embolism of vein   Thrombosis (vein)

√4ᵗʰ 454 Varicose veins of lower extremities
EXCLUDES that complicating pregnancy, childbirth, or the puerperium (671.0)
AHA: 2Q, '91, 20
DEF: Dilated leg veins; due to incompetent vein valves that allow reversed blood flow and cause tissue erosion or weakness of wall; may be painful.

454.0 With ulcer   A
Varicose ulcer (lower extremity, any part)
Varicose veins with ulcer of lower extremity [any part] or of unspecified site
Any condition classifiable to 454.9 with ulcer or specified as ulcerated
AHA: 4Q, '99, 18

454.1 With inflammation   `A`
Stasis dermatitis
Varicose veins with inflammation of lower extremity [any part] or of unspecified site
Any condition classifiable to 454.9 with inflammation or specified as inflamed

454.2 With ulcer and inflammation   `A`
Varicose veins with ulcer and inflammation of lower extremity [any part] or of unspecified site
Any condition classifiable to 454.9 with ulcer and inflammation

454.8 With other complications
Edema
Pain
Swelling
AHA: 4Q, '02, 58

454.9 Asymptomatic varicose veins   `A`
Phlebectasia
Varicose veins } of lower extremity [any part] or of unspecified site
Varix

Varicose veins NOS
AHA: 4Q, '02, 58

√4ᵗʰ 455 Hemorrhoids
> `INCLUDES`   hemorrhoids (anus) (rectum)
> piles
> varicose veins, anus or rectum
>
> `EXCLUDES`   that complicating pregnancy, childbirth, or the puerperium (671.8)

DEF: Varicose condition of external hemorrhoidal veins causing painful swellings at the anus.

455.0 Internal hemorrhoids without mention of complication

455.1 Internal thrombosed hemorrhoids

455.2 Internal hemorrhoids with other complication
Internal hemorrhoids: Internal hemorrhoids:
  bleeding   strangulated
  prolapsed   ulcerated
AHA: 1Q, '03, 8

455.3 External hemorrhoids without mention of complication

455.4 External thrombosed hemorrhoids

455.5 External hemorrhoids with other complication
External hemorrhoids: External hemorrhoids:
  bleeding   strangulated
  prolapsed   ulcerated
AHA: 1Q, '03, 8

455.6 Unspecified hemorrhoids without mention of complication
Hemorrhoids NOS

455.7 Unspecified thrombosed hemorrhoids
Thrombosed hemorrhoids, unspecified whether internal or external

455.8 Unspecified hemorrhoids with other complication
Hemorrhoids, unspecified whether internal or external:
  bleeding
  prolapsed
  strangulated
  ulcerated

455.9 Residual hemorrhoidal skin tags
Skin tags, anus or rectum

√4ᵗʰ 456 Varicose veins of other sites

456.0 Esophageal varices with bleeding
DEF: Distended, tortuous, veins of lower esophagus, usually due to portal hypertension.

456.1 Esophageal varices without mention of bleeding

√5ᵗʰ 456.2 Esophageal varices in diseases classified elsewhere
Code first underlying disease, as:
  cirrhosis of liver (571.0-571.9)
  portal hypertension (572.3)

456.20 With bleeding
AHA: N-D, '85, 14

456.21 Without mention of bleeding
AHA: 2Q, '02, 4

456.3 Sublingual varices
DEF: Distended, tortuous veins beneath tongue.

456.4 Scrotal varices   ♂
Varicocele

456.5 Pelvic varices
Varices of broad ligament

456.6 Vulval varices   ♀
Varices of perineum
> `EXCLUDES`   that complicating pregnancy, childbirth, or the puerperium (671.1)

456.8 Varices of other sites
Varicose veins of nasal septum (with ulcer)
> `EXCLUDES`   placental varices (656.7)
> retinal varices (362.17)
> varicose ulcer of unspecified site (454.0)
> varicose veins of unspecified site (454.9)

AHA: 2Q, '02, 4

√4ᵗʰ 457 Noninfectious disorders of lymphatic channels

457.0 Postmastectomy lymphedema syndrome   `A`
Elephantiasis
Obliteration of lymphatic vessel } due to mastectomy

DEF: Reduced lymphatic circulation following mastectomy; symptoms include swelling of the arm on the operative side.

AHA: 2Q, '02, 12

457.1 Other lymphedema
Elephantiasis   Lymphedema:
  (nonfilarial) NOS   praecox
Lymphangiectasis   secondary
Lymphedema: Obliteration, lymphatic vessel
  acquired (chronic)
> `EXCLUDES`   elephantiasis (nonfilarial):
>   congenital (757.0)
>   eyelid (374.83)
>   vulva (624.8)

DEF: Fluid retention due to reduced lymphatic circulation; due to other than mastectomy.

457.2 Lymphangitis
Lymphangitis: Lymphangitis:
  NOS   subacute
  chronic
> `EXCLUDES`   acute lymphangitis (682.0-682.9)

457.8 Other noninfectious disorders of lymphatic channels
Chylocele (nonfilarial)   Lymph node or vessel:
Chylous: fistula
  ascites   infarction
  cyst   rupture
> `EXCLUDES`   chylocele:
>   filarial (125.0-125.9)
>   tunica vaginalis (nonfilarial) (608.84)

AHA: ▶1Q, '04, 5;◀ 3Q, '03, 17

457.9 Unspecified noninfectious disorder of lymphatic channels

---

`√4ᵗʰ` `√5ᵗʰ` Additional Digit Required   Unspecified Code   Other Specified Code   Manifestation Code   ▶◀ Revised Text   ● New Code   ▲ Revised Code Title

2005 ICD•9•CM   **October 2004 • Volume 1 — 129**

Circulatory System

458–459.9

✓4ᵗʰ **458 Hypotension**
     INCLUDES   hypopiesis
     EXCLUDES   *cardiovascular collapse (785.50)*
                maternal hypotension syndrome (669.2)
                shock (785.50-785.59)
                Shy-Drager syndrome (333.0)

     458.0 Orthostatic hypotension
         Hypotension: Hypotension:
           orthostatic (chronic)   postural
         AHA: 3Q, '00, 8; 3Q, '91, 9

         DEF: Low blood pressure; occurs when standing.

     458.1 Chronic hypotension
         Permanent idiopathic hypotension
         DEF: Persistent low blood pressure.

     ✓5ᵗʰ **458.2 Iatrogenic hypotension**
         AHA: ▶4Q, '03, 60;◀ 3Q, '02, 12; 4Q, '95, 57
         DEF: Abnormally low blood pressure; due to medical treatment.

         458.21 Hypotension of hemodialysis
             Intra-dialytic hypotension
             AHA: ▶ 4Q, '03, 61◀

         458.29 Other iatrogenic hypotension
             Postoperative hypotension

     458.8 Other specified hypotension
         AHA: 4Q, '97, 37

     458.9 Hypotension, unspecified
         Hypotension (arterial) NOS

✓4ᵗʰ **459 Other disorders of circulatory system**
     459.0 Hemorrhage, unspecified
         Rupture of blood vessel NOS
         Spontaneous hemorrhage NEC
         EXCLUDES   *hemorrhage:*
                 gastrointestinal NOS (578.9)
                 in newborn NOS (772.9)
                 secondary or recurrent following
                     trauma (958.2)
                 traumatic rupture of blood vessel
                     (900.0-904.9)
         AHA: 4Q, '90, 26

     ✓5ᵗʰ **459.1 Postphlebitic syndrome**
         Chronic venous hypertension due to deep vein
             thrombosis
         EXCLUDES   *chronic venous hypertension without*
                 deep vein thrombosis (459.30-
                 459.39)
         AHA: 4Q, '02, 58; 2Q, '91, 20

         DEF: Various conditions following deep vein thrombosis; including
         edema, pain, stasis dermatitis, cellulitis, varicose veins and
         ulceration of the lower leg.

     459.10 Postphlebitic syndrome without
               complications
             Asymptomatic postphlebitic syndrome
             Postphlebitic syndrome NOS

     459.11 Postphlebitic syndrome with ulcer

     459.12 Postphlebitic syndrome with inflammation

     459.13 Postphlebitic syndrome with ulcer and
               inflammation

     459.19 Postphlebitic syndrome with other
               complication

     459.2 Compression of vein
         Stricture of vein
         Vena cava syndrome (inferior) (superior)

✓5ᵗʰ **459.3 Chronic venous hypertension (idiopathic)**
         Stasis edema
         EXCLUDES   *chronic venous hypertension due to*
                 deep vein thrombosis (459.10-
                 459.19)
                 varicose veins (454.0-454.9)

         AHA: 4Q, '02, 59

     459.30 Chronic venous hypertension without
               complications
             Asymptomatic chronic venous hypertension
             Chronic venous hypertension NOS

     459.31 Chronic venous hypertension with ulcer
             AHA: 4Q, '02, 43

     459.32 Chronic venous hypertension with
               inflammation

     459.33 Chronic venous hypertension with ulcer and
               inflammation

     459.39 Chronic venous hypertension with
               other complication

✓5ᵗʰ **459.8 Other specified disorders of circulatory system**
     459.81 Venous (peripheral) insufficiency,
               unspecified
             Chronic venous insufficiency NOS
             Use additional code for any associated
                 ulceration (707.10-707.9)
             AHA: 2Q, '91, 20; M-A, '87, 6

             DEF: Insufficient drainage, venous blood, any part of
             body, results in edema or dermatosis.

     459.89 Other
             Collateral circulation (venous), any site
             Phlebosclerosis
             Venofibrosis

     459.9 Unspecified circulatory system disorder

N Newborn Age: 0   P Pediatric Age: 0-17   M Maternity Age: 12-55   A Adult Age: 15-124   MSP Medicare Secondary Payer

8. DISEASES OF THE RESPIRATORY SYSTEM (460-519)

Use additional code to identify infectious organism

ACUTE RESPIRATORY INFECTIONS (460-466)

> **EXCLUDES**   *pneumonia and influenza (480.0-487.8)*

460 Acute nasopharyngitis [common cold]

Coryza (acute)	Nasopharyngitis:
Nasal catarrh, acute	infective NOS
Nasopharyngitis:	Rhinitis:
NOS	acute
acute	infective

> **EXCLUDES**   *nasopharyngitis, chronic (472.2)*
> *pharyngitis:*
>   *acute or unspecified (462)*
>   *chronic (472.1)*
> *rhinitis:*
>   *allergic (477.0-477.9)*
>   *chronic or unspecified (472.0)*
> *sore throat:*
>   *acute or unspecified (462)*
>   *chronic (472.1)*

AHA: 1Q, '88, 12

DEF: Acute inflammation of mucous membranes; extends from nares to pharynx.

✓4ᵗʰ 461 Acute sinusitis

> **INCLUDES**   abscess   }
>   empyema   } acute, of sinus (accessory)
>   infection   } (nasal)
>   inflammation   }
>   suppuration   }

> **EXCLUDES**   *chronic or unspecified sinusitis (473.0-473.9)*

461.0 Maxillary
     Acute antritis

461.1 Frontal

461.2 Ethmoidal

461.3 Sphenoidal

461.8 Other acute sinusitis
     Acute pansinusitis

461.9 Acute sinusitis, unspecified
     Acute sinusitis NOS

462 Acute pharyngitis

Acute sore throat NOS	Pharyngitis (acute):
Pharyngitis (acute):	staphylococcal
NOS	suppurative
gangrenous	ulcerative
infective	Sore throat (viral) NOS
phlegmonous	Viral pharyngitis
pneumococcal	

> **EXCLUDES**   *abscess:*
>   *peritonsillar [quinsy] (475)*
>   *pharyngeal NOS (478.29)*
>   *retropharyngeal (478.24)*
> *chronic pharyngitis (472.1)*
> *infectious mononucleosis (075)*
> *that specified as (due to):*
>   *Coxsackie (virus) (074.0)*
>   *gonococcus (098.6)*
>   *herpes simplex (054.79)*
>   *influenza (487.1)*
>   *septic (034.0)*
>   *streptococcal (034.0)*

AHA: 4Q, '99, 26; S-O, '85, 8

463 Acute tonsillitis

Tonsillitis (acute):	Tonsillitis (acute):
NOS	septic
follicular	staphylococcal
gangrenous	suppurative
infective	ulcerative
pneumococcal	viral

> **EXCLUDES**   *chronic tonsillitis (474.0)*
> *hypertrophy of tonsils (474.1)*
> *peritonsillar abscess [quinsy] (475)*
> *sore throat:*
>   *acute or NOS (462)*
>   *septic (034.0)*
> *streptococcal tonsillitis (034.0)*

AHA: N-D, '84, 16

✓4ᵗʰ 464 Acute laryngitis and tracheitis

> **EXCLUDES**   *that associated with influenza (487.1)*
> *that due to Streptococcus (034.0)*

✓5ᵗʰ 464.0 Acute laryngitis

Laryngitis (acute):
   NOS
   edematous
   Hemophilus influenzae [H. influenzae]
   pneumococcal
   septic
   suppurative
   ulcerative

> **EXCLUDES**   *chronic laryngitis (476.0-476.1)*
> *influenzal laryngitis (487.1)*

AHA: 4Q, '01, 42

464.00 Without mention of obstruction

464.01 With obstruction

✓5ᵗʰ 464.1 Acute tracheitis

Tracheitis (acute):	Tracheitis (acute):
NOS	viral
catarrhal	

> **EXCLUDES**   *chronic tracheitis (491.8)*

464.10 Without mention of obstruction

464.11 With obstruction

✓5ᵗʰ 464.2 Acute laryngotracheitis

Laryngotracheitis (acute)
Tracheitis (acute) with laryngitis (acute)

> **EXCLUDES**   *chronic laryngotracheitis (476.1)*

464.20 Without mention of obstruction

464.21 With obstruction

✓5ᵗʰ 464.3 Acute epiglottitis

Viral epiglottitis

> **EXCLUDES**   *epiglottitis, chronic (476.1)*

464.30 Without mention of obstruction

464.31 With obstruction

464.4 Croup
Croup syndrome

DEF: Acute laryngeal obstruction due to allergy, foreign body or infection; symptoms include barking cough, hoarseness and harsh, persistent high-pitched respiratory sound.

✓5ᵗʰ 464.5 Supraglottitis, unspecified

AHA: 4Q, '01, 42

DEF: A rapidly advancing generalized upper respiratory infection of the lingual tonsillar area, epiglottic folds, false vocal cords, and the epiglottis; seen most commonly in children, but can affect people of any age.

464.50 Without mention of obstruction
     AHA: 4Q, '01, 43

464.51 With obstruction

✓4ᵗʰ ✓5ᵗʰ Additional Digit Required   Unspecified Code   Other Specified Code   Manifestation Code   ▶◀ Revised Text   ● New Code   ▲ Revised Code Title

2005 ICD•9•CM   **Volume 1 — 131**

Respiratory System

Respiratory System

Upper Respiratory System

√4ᵗʰ **465 Acute upper respiratory infections of multiple or unspecified sites**

EXCLUDES   *upper respiratory infection due to:*
     influenza (487.1)
     Streptococcus (034.0)

465.0 Acute laryngopharyngitis

DEF: Acute infection of the vocal cords and pharynx.

465.8 Other multiple sites

Multiple URI

465.9 Unspecified site

Acute URI NOS
Upper respiratory infection (acute)

√4ᵗʰ **466 Acute bronchitis and bronchiolitis**

INCLUDES   that with:
     bronchospasm
     obstruction

466.0 Acute bronchitis

Bronchitis, acute or subacute:	Bronchitis, acute or subacute:
fibrinous	viral
membranous	with tracheitis
pneumococcal	Croupous bronchitis
purulent	Tracheobronchitis, acute
septic	

EXCLUDES ▶ *acute bronchitis with chronic obstructive pulmonary disease (491.22)*◀

AHA: ▶1Q, '04, 3;◀ 4Q, '02, 46; 4Q, '96, 28; 4Q, '91, 24; 1Q, '88, 12

DEF: Acute inflammation of main branches of bronchial tree due to infectious or irritant agents; symptoms include cough with a varied production of sputum, fever, substernal soreness, and lung rales.

√5ᵗʰ **466.1 Acute bronchiolitis**

Bronchiolitis (acute)   Capillary pneumonia

DEF: Acute inflammation of finer subdivisions of bronchial tree due to infectious or irritant agents; symptoms include cough with a varied production of sputum, fever, substernal soreness, and lung rales.

466.11 Acute bronchiolitis due to respiratory syncytial virus (RSV)

AHA: 4Q, '96, 27

466.19 Acute bronchiolitis due to other infectious organisms

Use additional code to identify organism

OTHER DISEASES OF THE UPPER RESPIRATORY TRACT (470-478)

470 Deviated nasal septum

Deflected septum (nasal) (acquired)

EXCLUDES   *congenital (754.0)*

√4ᵗʰ **471 Nasal polyps**

EXCLUDES   *adenomatous polyps (212.0)*

471.0 Polyp of nasal cavity

Polyp:
   choanal
   nasopharyngeal

471.1 Polypoid sinus degeneration

Woakes' syndrome or ethmoiditis

471.8 Other polyp of sinus

Polyp of sinus:	Polyp of sinus:
accessory	maxillary
ethmoidal	sphenoidal

471.9 Unspecified nasal polyp

Nasal polyp NOS

√4ᵗʰ **472 Chronic pharyngitis and nasopharyngitis**

472.0 Chronic rhinitis

Ozena	Rhinitis:
Rhinitis:	hypertrophic
NOS	obstructive
atrophic	purulent
granulomatous	ulcerative

EXCLUDES   *allergic rhinitis (477.0-477.9)*

DEF: Persistent inflammation of mucous membranes of nose.

472.1 Chronic pharyngitis

Chronic sore throat	Pharyngitis:
Pharyngitis:	granular (chronic)
atrophic	hypertrophic

472.2 Chronic nasopharyngitis

EXCLUDES   *acute or unspecified nasopharyngitis (460)*

DEF: Persistent inflammation of mucous membranes extending from nares to pharynx.

Paranasal Sinuses

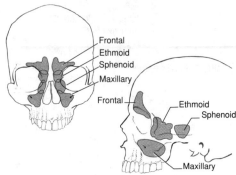

N Newborn Age: 0	P Pediatric Age: 0-17	M Maternity Age: 12-55	A Adult Age: 15-124	MSP Medicare Secondary Payer

√4th **473 Chronic sinusitis**

INCLUDES
abscess
empyema
infection
suppuration
(chronic) of sinus (accessory) (nasal)

EXCLUDES *acute sinusitis (461.0-461.9)*

473.0 Maxillary
Antritis (chronic)

473.1 Frontal

473.2 Ethmoidal
EXCLUDES *Woakes' ethmoiditis (471.1)*

473.3 Sphenoidal

473.8 Other chronic sinusitis
Pansinusitis (chronic)

473.9 Unspecified sinusitis (chronic)
Sinusitis (chronic) NOS

√4th **474 Chronic disease of tonsils and adenoids**

√5th **474.0 Chronic tonsillitis and adenoiditis**
EXCLUDES *acute or unspecified tonsillitis (463)*

AHA: 4Q, '97, 38

474.00 Chronic tonsillitis
474.01 Chronic adenoiditis
474.02 Chronic tonsillitis and adenoiditis

√5th **474.1 Hypertrophy of tonsils and adenoids**
Enlargement
Hyperplasia
Hypertrophy
of tonsils or adenoids

EXCLUDES *that with:*
adenoiditis (474.01)
adenoiditis and tonsillitis (474.02)
tonsillitis (474.00)

474.10 Tonsils with adenoids
474.11 Tonsils alone
474.12 Adenoids alone

474.2 Adenoid vegetations
DEF: Fungus-like growth of lymph tissue between the nares and pharynx.

474.8 Other chronic disease of tonsils and adenoids
Amygdalolith   Tonsillar tag
Calculus, tonsil   Ulcer, tonsil
Cicatrix of tonsil (and adenoid)

474.9 Unspecified chronic disease of tonsils and adenoids
Disease (chronic) of tonsils (and adenoids)

475 Peritonsillar abscess
Abscess of tonsil   Quinsy
Peritonsillar cellulitis
EXCLUDES *tonsillitis:*
acute or NOS (463)
chronic (474.0)

√4th **476 Chronic laryngitis and laryngotracheitis**

476.0 Chronic laryngitis
Laryngitis: Laryngitis:
catarrhal   sicca
hypertrophic

476.1 Chronic laryngotracheitis
Laryngitis, chronic, with tracheitis (chronic)
Tracheitis, chronic, with laryngitis
EXCLUDES *chronic tracheitis (491.8)*
laryngitis and tracheitis, acute or
unspecified (464.00-464.51)

√4th **477 Allergic rhinitis**

INCLUDES
allergic rhinitis (nonseasonal) (seasonal)
hay fever
spasmodic rhinorrhea

EXCLUDES *allergic rhinitis with asthma (bronchial) (493.0)*

DEF: True immunoglobulin E (IgE)-mediated allergic reaction of nasal mucosa; seasonal (typical hay fever) or perennial (year-round allergens: dust, food, dander).

477.0 Due to pollen
Pollinosis

477.1 Due to food
AHA: 4Q, '00, 42

● **477.2 Due to animal (cat) (dog) hair and dander**

477.8 Due to other allergen

477.9 Cause unspecified
AHA: 2Q, '97, 9

√4th **478 Other diseases of upper respiratory tract**

478.0 Hypertrophy of nasal turbinates
DEF: Overgrowth, enlargement of shell-shaped bones, in nasal cavity.

478.1 Other diseases of nasal cavity and sinuses
Abscess
Necrosis
Ulcer
of nose (septum)

Cyst or mucocele of sinus (nasal)
Rhinolith
EXCLUDES *varicose ulcer of nasal septum (456.8)*

√5th **478.2 Other diseases of pharynx, not elsewhere classified**
478.20 Unspecified disease of pharynx
478.21 Cellulitis of pharynx or nasopharynx
478.22 Parapharyngeal abscess
478.24 Retropharyngeal abscess
DEF: Purulent infection, behind pharynx and front of precerebral fascia.

478.25 Edema of pharynx or nasopharynx
478.26 Cyst of pharynx or nasopharynx
478.29 Other
Abscess of pharynx or nasopharynx
EXCLUDES *ulcerative pharyngitis (462)*

√5th **478.3 Paralysis of vocal cords or larynx**
DEF: Loss of motor ability of vocal cords or larynx; due to nerve or muscle damage.

478.30 Paralysis, unspecified
Laryngoplegia   Paralysis of glottis
478.31 Unilateral, partial
478.32 Unilateral, complete
478.33 Bilateral, partial
478.34 Bilateral, complete

478.4 Polyp of vocal cord or larynx
EXCLUDES *adenomatous polyps (212.1)*

478.5 Other diseases of vocal cords
Abscess
Cellulitis
Granuloma
Leukoplakia
of vocal cords

Chorditis (fibrinous) (nodosa) (tuberosa)
Singers' nodes

478.6 Edema of larynx
Edema (of):   Edema (of):
glottis   supraglottic
subglottic

√5th **478.7 Other diseases of larynx, not elsewhere classified**
478.70 Unspecified disease of larynx
478.71 Cellulitis and perichondritis of larynx
DEF: Inflammation of deep soft tissues or lining of bone of the larynx.

√4th √5th Additional Digit Required · Unspecified Code · Other Specified Code · Manifestation Code · ►◄ Revised Text · ● New Code · ▲ Revised Code Title

Respiratory System

478.74–483.8

Lungs

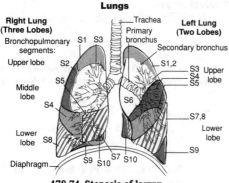

Right Lung (Three Lobes)
Bronchopulmonary segments:
Upper lobe — S1 S3
S2
S5
Middle lobe
S4
Lower lobe — S8
Diaphragm — S9 S10 S7 S10

Trachea
Primary bronchus
Secondary bronchus

Left Lung (Two Lobes)
S1,2 — Upper lobe
S3
S4
S5
S6
S7,8 — Lower lobe
S9

478.74 Stenosis of larynx

478.75 Laryngeal spasm
Laryngismus (stridulus)
DEF: Involuntary muscle contraction of the larynx.

478.79 Other
Abscess
Necrosis
Obstruction } of larynx
Pachyderma
Ulcer

EXCLUDES　ulcerative laryngitis
(464.00-464.01)

AHA: 3Q, '91, 20

478.8 Upper respiratory tract hypersensitivity reaction, site unspecified
EXCLUDES　hypersensitivity reaction of lower respiratory tract, as:
extrinsic allergic alveolitis (495.0-495.9)
pneumoconiosis (500-505)

478.9 Other and unspecified diseases of upper respiratory tract
Abscess } of trachea
Cicatrix

PNEUMONIA AND INFLUENZA (480-487)
EXCLUDES　pneumonia:
allergic or eosinophilic (518.3)
aspiration:
NOS (507.0)
newborn (770.1)
solids and liquids (507.0-507.8)
congenital (770.0)
lipoid (507.1)
passive (514)
rheumatic (390)

✓4ᵗʰ **480 Viral pneumonia**

480.0 Pneumonia due to adenovirus

480.1 Pneumonia due to respiratory syncytial virus
AHA: 4Q, '96, 28; 1Q, '88, 12

480.2 Pneumonia due to parainfluenza virus

480.3 Pneumonia due to SARS-associated coronavirus
AHA: ►4Q, '03, 46-47◄

DEF: ►A severe adult respiratory syndrome caused by the coronavirus, specified as inflammation of the lungs with consolidation.◄

480.8 Pneumonia due to other virus not elsewhere classified
EXCLUDES　congenital rubella pneumonitis (771.0)
influenza with pneumonia, any form (487.0)
pneumonia complicating viral diseases classified elsewhere (484.1-484.8)

480.9 Viral pneumonia, unspecified
AHA: 3Q, '98, 5

481 Pneumococcal pneumonia [Streptococcus pneumoniae pneumonia]
Lobar pneumonia, organism unspecified
AHA: 2Q, '98, 7; 4Q, '92, 19; 1Q, '92, 18; 1Q, '91, 13; 1Q, '88, 13; M-A, '85, 6

✓4ᵗʰ **482 Other bacterial pneumonia**
AHA: 4Q, '93, 39

482.0 Pneumonia due to Klebsiella pneumoniae

482.1 Pneumonia due to Pseudomonas

482.2 Pneumonia due to Hemophilus influenzae [H. influenzae]

✓5ᵗʰ **482.3 Pneumonia due to Streptococcus**
EXCLUDES　Streptococcus pneumoniae (481)
AHA: 1Q, '88, 13

482.30 Streptococcus, unspecified
482.31 Group A
482.32 Group B
482.39 Other Streptococcus

✓5ᵗʰ **482.4 Pneumonia due to Staphylococcus**
AHA: 3Q, '91, 16

482.40 Pneumonia due to Staphylococcus, unspecified
482.41 Pneumonia due to Staphylococcus aureus
482.49 Other Staphylococcus pneumonia

✓5ᵗʰ **482.8 Pneumonia due to other specified bacteria**
EXCLUDES　pneumonia, complicating infectious disease classified elsewhere (484.1-484.8)
AHA: 3Q, '88, 11

482.81 Anaerobes
Bacteroides (melaninogenicus)
Gram-negative anaerobes

482.82 Escherichia coli [E. coli]

482.83 Other gram-negative bacteria
Gram-negative pneumonia NOS
Proteus
Serratia marcescens
EXCLUDES　gram-negative anaerobes (482.81)
Legionnaires' disease (482.84)
AHA: 2Q, '98, 5; 3Q, '94, 9

482.84 Legionnaires' disease
AHA: 4Q, '97, 38

DEF: Severe and often fatal infection by *Legionella pneumophilia;* symptoms include high fever, gastrointestinal pain, headache, myalgia, dry cough, and pneumonia; transmitted airborne via air conditioning systems, humidifiers, water faucets, shower heads; not person-to-person contact.

482.89 Other specified bacteria
AHA: 2Q, '97, 6

482.9 Bacterial pneumonia unspecified
AHA: 2Q, '98, 6; 2Q, '97, 6; 1Q, '94, 17

✓4ᵗʰ **483 Pneumonia due to other specified organism**
AHA: N-D, '87, 5

483.0 Mycoplasma pneumoniae
Eaton's agent
Pleuropneumonia-like organism [PPLO]

483.1 Chlamydia
AHA: 4Q, '96, 31

483.8 Other specified organism

N　Newborn Age: 0　　P　Pediatric Age: 0-17　　M　Maternity Age: 12-55　　A　Adult Age: 15-124　　MSP　Medicare Secondary Payer

√4th **484 Pneumonia in infectious diseases classified elsewhere**

> EXCLUDES   *influenza with pneumonia, any form (487.0)*

484.1   **Pneumonia in cytomegalic inclusion disease**
> *Code first underlying disease, as (078.5)*

484.3   **Pneumonia in whooping cough**
> *Code first underlying disease, as (033.0-033.9)*

484.5   **Pneumonia in anthrax**
> *Code first underlying disease (022.1)*

484.6   **Pneumonia in aspergillosis**
> *Code first underlying disease (117.3)*

> **AHA:** 4Q, '97, 40

484.7   **Pneumonia in other systemic mycoses**
> *Code first underlying disease*
> EXCLUDES   *pneumonia in:*
> *candidiasis (112.4)*
> *coccidioidomycosis (114.0)*
> *histoplasmosis (115.0-115.9 with fifth-digit 5)*

484.8   **Pneumonia in other infectious diseases classified elsewhere**
> *Code first underlying disease, as:*
> Q fever (083.0)
> typhoid fever (002.0)
> EXCLUDES   *pneumonia in:*
> *actinomycosis (039.1)*
> *measles (055.1)*
> *nocardiosis (039.1)*
> *ornithosis (073.0)*
> *Pneumocystis carinii (136.3)*
> *salmonellosis (003.22)*
> *toxoplasmosis (130.4)*
> *tuberculosis (011.6)*
> *tularemia (021.2)*
> *varicella (052.1)*

485 Bronchopneumonia, organism unspecified

Bronchopneumonia: Pneumonia:
    hemorrhagic   lobular
    terminal   segmental
Pleurobronchopneumonia
> EXCLUDES   *bronchiolitis (acute) (466.11-466.19)*
> *chronic (491.8)*
> *lipoid pneumonia (507.1)*

486 Pneumonia, organism unspecified
> EXCLUDES   *hypostatic or passive pneumonia (514)*
> *influenza with pneumonia, any form (487.0)*
> *inhalation or aspiration pneumonia due to foreign materials (507.0-507.8)*
> *pneumonitis due to fumes and vapors (506.0)*

AHA: 4Q, '99, 6; 3Q, '99, 9; 3Q, '98, 7; 2Q, '98, 4, 5; 1Q, '98, 8; 3Q, '97, 9; 3Q, '94, 10; 3Q, '88, 11

Bronchioli and Alveoli

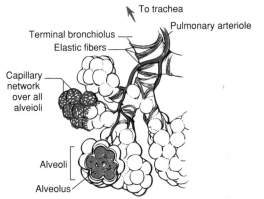

√4th **487 Influenza**

> EXCLUDES   *Hemophilus influenzae [H. influenzae]:*
> *infection NOS (041.5)*
> *laryngitis (464.00-464.01)*
> *meningitis (320.0)*
> *pneumonia (482.2)*

487.0   **With pneumonia**
> Influenza with pneumonia, any form
> Influenzal:
>   bronchopneumonia
>   pneumonia

487.1   **With other respiratory manifestations**
> Influenza NOS
> Influenzal:
>   laryngitis
>   pharyngitis
>   respiratory infection (upper) (acute)

> **AHA:** 4Q, '99, 26

487.8   **With other manifestations**
> Encephalopathy due to influenza
> Influenza with involvement of gastrointestinal tract
> EXCLUDES   *"intestinal flu" [viral gastroenteritis] (008.8)*

CHRONIC OBSTRUCTIVE PULMONARY DISEASE AND ALLIED CONDITIONS (490-496)

> **AHA:** 3Q, '88, 5

490 Bronchitis, not specified as acute or chronic
> Bronchitis NOS:
>   catarrhal
>   with tracheitis NOS
> Tracheobronchitis NOS
> EXCLUDES   *bronchitis:*
> *allergic NOS (493.9)*
> *asthmatic NOS (493.9)*
> *due to fumes and vapors (506.0)*

√4th **491 Chronic bronchitis**
> EXCLUDES   *chronic obstructive asthma (493.2)*

491.0   **Simple chronic bronchitis**
> Catarrhal bronchitis, chronic
> Smokers' cough

491.1   **Mucopurulent chronic bronchitis**
> Bronchitis (chronic) (recurrent):
>   fetid
>   mucopurulent
>   purulent

> **AHA:** 3Q, '88, 12

> **DEF:** Chronic bronchial infection characterized by both mucus and pus secretions in the bronchial tree; recurs after asymptomatic periods; signs are coughing, expectoration and secondary changes in the lung.

√5th **491.2**   **Obstructive chronic bronchitis**
> Bronchitis:
>   emphysematous
>   obstructive (chronic) (diffuse)
> Bronchitis with:
>   chronic airway obstruction
>   emphysema
> EXCLUDES   *asthmatic bronchitis (acute) NOS (493.9)*
> *chronic obstructive asthma (493.2)*

> **AHA:** 3Q, '97, 9; 4Q, '91, 25; 2Q, '91, 21

491.20   **Without exacerbation**
> Emphysema with chronic bronchitis
> **AHA:** 3Q, '97, 9

√4th / √5th Additional Digit Required   Unspecified Code   Other Specified Code   Manifestation Code   ▶◀ Revised Text   ● New Code   ▲ Revised Code Title

2005 ICD•9•CM   Volume 1 — 135

Respiratory System

491.21–494.1

Interrelationship Between Chronic Airway Obstruction, Chronic Bronchitis and Emphysema

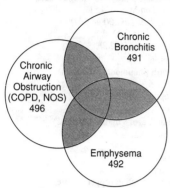

Shaded area:
Obstructive Chronic
Bronchitis (Chronic Bronchitis
with COPD) 491.20-491.21

491.21 With (acute) exacerbation
Acute exacerbation of chronic obstructive
pulmonary disease [COPD]
Decompensated chronic obstructive
pulmonary disease [COPD]
Decompensated chronic obstructive
pulmonary disease [COPD] with
exacerbation
> **EXCLUDES** *chronic obstructive asthma*
> *with acute exacerbation*
> *(493.22)*

AHA: ▶1Q, '04, 3;◀3Q, '02, 18, 19; 4Q, '01, 43; 2Q, '96, 10

491.22 With acute bronchitis

491.8 Other chronic bronchitis
Chronic: Chronic:
   tracheitis   tracheobronchitis

491.9 Unspecified chronic bronchitis

✓4ᵗʰ 492 Emphysema
AHA: 2Q, '91, 21

492.0 Emphysematous bleb
Giant bullous emphysema
Ruptured emphysematous bleb
Tension pneumatocele
Vanishing lung
AHA: 2Q, '93, 3

DEF: Formation of vesicle or bulla in emphysematous lung, more
than one millimeter; contains serum or blood.

492.8 Other emphysema
Emphysema (lung or   Emphysema (lung or
  pulmonary):   pulmonary):
  NOS   unilateral
  centriacinar   vesicular
  centrilobular   MacLeod's syndrome
  obstructive   Swyer-James syndrome
  panacinar   Unilateral hyperlucent lung
  panlobular
> **EXCLUDES** *emphysema:*
> *with chronic bronchitis* ▶*(491.20-*
> *491.22)*◀
> *compensatory (518.2)*
> *due to fumes and vapors (506.4)*
> *interstitial (518.1)*
>   *newborn (770.2)*
> *mediastinal (518.1)*
> *surgical (subcutaneous) (998.81)*
> *traumatic (958.7)*

AHA: 4Q, '93, 41; J-A, '84, 17

✓4ᵗʰ 493 Asthma
> **EXCLUDES** *wheezing NOS (786.07)*

The following fifth-digit subclassification is for use with
codes 493.0-493.2, 493.9:
   0   unspecified
   1   with status asthmaticus
   2   with (acute) exacerbation

AHA: 4Q, '03, 62; 4Q, '01, 43; 4Q, '00, 42; 1Q, '91, 13; 3Q, '88, 9; J-A, '85, 8;
N-D, '84, 17

DEF: Status asthmaticus: Severe, intractable episode of asthma unresponsive
to normal therapeutic measures.

✓5ᵗʰ 493.0 Extrinsic asthma
Asthma: Asthma:
  allergic with   hay
     stated cause   platinum
  atopic   Hay fever with asthma
  childhood
> **EXCLUDES** *asthma:*
> *allergic NOS (493.9)*
> *detergent (507.8)*
> *miners' (500)*
> *wood (495.8)*

DEF: Transient stricture of airway diameters of bronchi; due to
environmental factor; also called allergic (bronchial) asthma.

✓5ᵗʰ 493.1 Intrinsic asthma
Late-onset asthma
AHA: 3Q, '88, 9; M-A, '85, 7

DEF: Transient stricture, of airway diameters of bronchi; due to
pathophysiological disturbances.

✓5ᵗʰ 493.2 Chronic obstructive asthma
Asthma with chronic obstructive pulmonary disease
[COPD]
Chronic asthmatic bronchitis
> **EXCLUDES** *acute bronchitis (466.0)*
> *chronic obstructive bronchitis* ▶*(491.20-*
> *491.22)*◀

AHA: 4Q, '03, 108; 2Q, '91, 21; 2Q, '90, 20

DEF: Persistent narrowing of airway diameters in the bronchial
tree, restricting airflow and causing constant labored breathing.

✓5ᵗʰ 493.8 Other forms of asthma
AHA: 4Q, '03, 62

493.81 Exercise induced bronchospasm
493.82 Cough variant asthma

✓5ᵗʰ 493.9 Asthma, unspecified
Asthma (bronchial) (allergic NOS)
Bronchitis:
  allergic
  asthmatic
AHA: 4Q, '97, 40; **For code 493.90:** 4Q, '03, 108; 4Q, '99, 25; 1Q, '97, 7;
For code 493.92: 1Q, '03, 9

✓4ᵗʰ 494 Bronchiectasis
Bronchiectasis (fusiform) (postinfectious) (recurrent)
Bronchiolectasis
> **EXCLUDES** *congenital (748.61)*
> *tuberculous bronchiectasis (current disease)*
> *(011.5)*

AHA: 4Q, '00, 42

DEF: Dilation of bronchi; due to infection or chronic conditions; causes
decreased lung capacity and recurrent infections of lungs.

494.0 Bronchiectasis without acute exacerbation
494.1 Bronchiectasis with acute exacerbation

√4th **495 Extrinsic allergic alveolitis**

INCLUDES allergic alveolitis and pneumonitis due to inhaled organic dust particles of fungal, thermophilic actinomycete, or other origin

DEF: Pneumonitis due to particles inhaled into lung, often at workplace; symptoms include cough, chills, fever, increased heart and respiratory rates; develops within hours of exposure.

495.0 Farmers' lung

495.1 Bagassosis

495.2 Bird-fanciers' lung
Budgerigar-fanciers' disease or lung
Pigeon-fanciers' disease or lung

495.3 Suberosis
Cork-handlers' disease or lung

495.4 Malt workers' lung
Alveolitis due to Aspergillus clavatus

495.5 Mushroom workers' lung

495.6 Maple bark-strippers' lung
Alveolitis due to Cryptostroma corticale

495.7 "Ventilation" pneumonitis
Allergic alveolitis due to fungal, thermophilic actinomycete, and other organisms growing in ventilation [air conditioning] systems

495.8 Other specified allergic alveolitis and pneumonitis
Cheese-washers' lung
Coffee workers' lung
Fish-meal workers' lung
Furriers' lung
Grain-handlers' disease or lung
Pituitary snuff-takers' disease
Sequoiosis or red-cedar asthma
Wood asthma

495.9 Unspecified allergic alveolitis and pneumonitis
Alveolitis, allergic (extrinsic)
Hypersensitivity pneumonitis

496 Chronic airway obstruction, not elsewhere classified A

Note: This code is not to be used with any code from categories 491-493
Chronic:
nonspecific lung disease
obstructive lung disease
obstructive pulmonary disease [COPD] NOS

EXCLUDES chronic obstructive lung disease [COPD] specified (as) (with):
allergic alveolitis (495.0-495.9)
asthma (493.2)
bronchiectasis (494.0-494.1)
bronchitis ▶(491.20-491.22)◄
with emphysema ▶(491.20-491.22)◄
emphysema (492.0-492.8)

AHA: 4Q, '03, 109; 2Q, '00, 15; 2Q, '92, 16; 2Q, '91, 21; 3Q, '88, 56

PNEUMOCONIOSES AND OTHER LUNG DISEASES DUE TO EXTERNAL AGENTS (500-508)

DEF: Permanent deposits of particulate matter, within lungs; due to occupational or environmental exposure; results in chronic induration and fibrosis. (See specific listings in 500-508 code range)

500 Coal workers' pneumoconiosis A
Anthracosilicosis   Coal workers' lung
Anthracosis   Miner's asthma
Black lung disease

501 Asbestosis A

502 Pneumoconiosis due to other silica or silicates
Pneumoconiosis due to talc
Silicotic fibrosis (massive) of lung
Silicosis (simple) (complicated)

503 Pneumoconiosis due to other inorganic dust
Aluminosis (of lung)   Graphite fibrosis (of lung)
Bauxite fibrosis (of lung)   Siderosis
Berylliosis   Stannosis

504 Pneumonopathy due to inhalation of other dust
Byssinosis   Flax-dressers' disease
Cannabinosis

EXCLUDES allergic alveolitis (495.0-495.9)
asbestosis (501)
bagassosis (495.1)
farmers' lung (495.0)

505 Pneumoconiosis, unspecified

√4th **506 Respiratory conditions due to chemical fumes and vapors**
Use additional E code to identify cause

506.0 Bronchitis and pneumonitis due to fumes and vapors
Chemical bronchitis (acute)

506.1 Acute pulmonary edema due to fumes and vapors
Chemical pulmonary edema (acute)

EXCLUDES acute pulmonary edema NOS (518.4)
chronic or unspecified pulmonary edema (514)

AHA: 3Q, '88, 4

506.2 Upper respiratory inflammation due to fumes and vapors

506.3 Other acute and subacute respiratory conditions due to fumes and vapors

506.4 Chronic respiratory conditions due to fumes and vapors
Emphysema (diffuse) (chronic)
Obliterative bronchiolitis (chronic) (subacute)
Pulmonary fibrosis (chronic)
} due to inhalation of chemical fumes and vapors

506.9 Unspecified respiratory conditions due to fumes and vapors
Silo-fillers' disease

√4th **507 Pneumonitis due to solids and liquids**
EXCLUDES fetal aspiration pneumonitis (770.1)

AHA: 3Q, '91, 16

507.0 Due to inhalation of food or vomitus
Aspiration pneumonia (due to):   Aspiration pneumonia (due to):
NOS   milk
food (regurgitated)   saliva
gastric secretions   vomitus

AHA: 1Q, '89, 10

507.1 Due to inhalation of oils and essences
Lipoid pneumonia (exogenous)

EXCLUDES endogenous lipoid pneumonia (516.8)

507.8 Due to other solids and liquids
Detergent asthma

√4th **508 Respiratory conditions due to other and unspecified external agents**
Use additional E code to identify cause

508.0 Acute pulmonary manifestations due to radiation
Radiation pneumonitis

AHA: 2Q, '88, 4

508.1 Chronic and other pulmonary manifestations due to radiation
Fibrosis of lung following radiation

508.8 Respiratory conditions due to other specified external agents

508.9 Respiratory conditions due to unspecified external agent

OTHER DISEASES OF RESPIRATORY SYSTEM (510-519)

√4th **510 Empyema**
Use additional code to identify infectious organism (041.0-041.9)

EXCLUDES abscess of lung (513.0)

DEF: Purulent infection, within pleural space.

√4th Additional Digit Required   Unspecified Code   Other Specified Code   Manifestation Code   ▶◄ Revised Text   ● New Code   ▲ Revised Code Title

510.0   With fistula

Fistula: Fistula:
   bronchocutaneous   mediastinal
   bronchopleural   pleural
   hepatopleural   thoracic
Any condition classifiable to 510.9 with fistula

DEF: Purulent infection of respiratory cavity; with communication
from cavity to another structure.

510.9   Without mention of fistula

Abscess: Pleurisy:
   pleura   septic
   thorax   seropurulent
Empyema (chest) (lung)   suppurative
   (pleura)   Pyopneumothorax
Fibrinopurulent pleurisy Pyothorax
Pleurisy:
   purulent

AHA: 3Q, '94, 6

✓4ᵗʰ 511 Pleurisy

EXCLUDES   malignant pleural effusion (197.2)
           pleurisy with mention of tuberculosis, current
              disease (012.0)

DEF: Inflammation of serous membrane of lungs and lining of thoracic cavity;
causes exudation in cavity or membrane surface.

511.0   Without mention of effusion or current tuberculosis

Adhesion, lung or pleura   Pleurisy:
Calcification of pleura   NOS
Pleurisy (acute) (sterile):   pneumococcal
   diaphragmatic   staphylococcal
   fibrinous   streptococcal
   interlobar   Thickening of pleura

AHA: 3Q, '94, 5

511.1   With effusion, with mention of a bacterial cause other than tuberculosis

Pleurisy with effusion (exudative) (serous):
   pneumococcal
   staphylococcal
   streptococcal
   other specified nontuberculous bacterial cause

511.8   Other specified forms of effusion, except tuberculous

Encysted pleurisy   Hydropneumothorax
Hemopneumothorax   Hydrothorax
Hemothorax
   EXCLUDES   traumatic (860.2-860.5, 862.29,
                 862.39)

AHA: 1Q, '97, 10

511.9   Unspecified pleural effusion

Pleural effusion NOS   Pleurisy:
Pleurisy: serous
   exudative   with effusion NOS
   serofibrinous

AHA: ▶2Q, '03, 7;◄ 3Q, '91, 19; 4Q, '89, 11

✓4ᵗʰ 512 Pneumothorax

DEF: Collapsed lung; due to gas or air in pleural space.

512.0   Spontaneous tension pneumothorax

AHA: 3Q, '94, 5

DEF: Leaking air from lung into lining causing collapse.

512.1   Iatrogenic pneumothorax

Postoperative pneumothorax

AHA: 4Q, '94, 40

DEF: Air trapped in the lining of the lung following surgery.

512.8   Other spontaneous pneumothorax

Pneumothorax: Pneumothorax:
   NOS   chronic
   acute
   EXCLUDES   pneumothorax:
                 congenital (770.2)
                 traumatic (860.0-860.1, 860.4-
                    860.5)
                 tuberculous, current disease (011.7)

AHA: 2Q, '93, 3

✓4ᵗʰ 513 Abscess of lung and mediastinum

513.0   Abscess of lung

Abscess (multiple) of lung
Gangrenous or necrotic pneumonia
Pulmonary gangrene or necrosis

AHA: 2Q, '98, 7

513.1   Abscess of mediastinum

514 Pulmonary congestion and hypostasis

Hypostatic: Pulmonary edema:
   bronchopneumonia   NOS
   pneumonia   chronic
Passive pneumonia
Pulmonary congestion
   (chronic) (passive)
   EXCLUDES   acute pulmonary edema:
                 NOS (518.4)
                 with mention of heart disease or failure
                    (428.1)

AHA: 2Q, '98, 6; 3Q, '88, 5

DEF: Excessive retention of interstitial fluid in the lungs and pulmonary
vessels; due to poor circulation.

515 Postinflammatory pulmonary fibrosis

Cirrhosis of lung   ⎫
Fibrosis of lung (atrophic) ⎪
   (confluent) (massive)   ⎬ chronic or unspecified
   (perialveolar)   ⎪
   (peribronchial)   ⎪
Induration of lung   ⎭

DEF: Fibrosis and scarring of the lungs due to inflammatory reaction.

✓4ᵗʰ 516 Other alveolar and parietoalveolar pneumonopathy

516.0   Pulmonary alveolar proteinosis

DEF: Reduced ventilation; due to proteinaceous deposits on alveoli;
symptoms include dyspnea, cough, chest pain, weakness, weight
loss, and hemoptysis.

516.1   Idiopathic pulmonary hemosiderosis

Essential brown induration of lung
Code first underlying disease (275.0)

DEF: Fibrosis of alveolar walls; marked by abnormal amounts
hemosiderin in lungs; primarily affects children; symptoms include
anemia, fluid in lungs, and blood in sputum; etiology unknown.

516.2   Pulmonary alveolar microlithiasis

DEF: Small calculi in pulmonary alveoli resembling sand-like
particles on x-ray.

516.3   Idiopathic fibrosing alveolitis

Alveolar capillary block
Diffuse (idiopathic) (interstitial) pulmonary fibrosis
Hamman-Rich syndrome

516.8   Other specified alveolar and parietoalveolar pneumonopathies

Endogenous lipoid pneumonia
Interstitial pneumonia (desquamative) (lymphoid)
   EXCLUDES   lipoid pneumonia, exogenous or
                 unspecified (507.1)

AHA: 1Q, '92, 12

516.9   Unspecified alveolar and parietoalveolar pneumonopathy

---

☑4ᵗʰ **517 Lung involvement in conditions classified elsewhere**

EXCLUDES *rheumatoid lung (714.81)*

517.1 Rheumatic pneumonia

Code first underlying disease (390)

517.2 Lung involvement in systemic sclerosis

Code first underlying disease (710.1)

517.3 Acute chest syndrome

Code first sickle-cell disease in crisis (282.42, 282.62, 282.64, 282.69)

AHA: ▶4Q, '03, 51, 56◀

517.8 Lung involvement in other diseases classified elsewhere

Code first underlying disease, as:
amyloidosis (277.3)
polymyositis (710.4)
sarcoidosis (135)
Sjögren's disease (710.2)
systemic lupus erythematosus (710.0)

EXCLUDES *syphilis (095.1)*

AHA: ▶2Q, '03, 7◀

☑4ᵗʰ **518 Other diseases of lung**

518.0 Pulmonary collapse

Atelectasis　　　　　Middle lobe syndrome
Collapse of lung

EXCLUDES *atelectasis:*
congenital (partial) (770.5)
primary (770.4)
tuberculous, current disease (011.8)

AHA: 4Q, '90, 25

518.1 Interstitial emphysema

Mediastinal emphysema

EXCLUDES *surgical (subcutaneous) emphysema (998.81)*
that in fetus or newborn (770.2)
traumatic emphysema (958.7)

DEF: Escaped air from the alveoli trapped in the interstices of the lung; trauma or cough may cause the disease.

518.2 Compensatory emphysema

DEF: Distention of all or part of the lung caused by disease processes or surgical intervention that decreased volume in another part of the lung; overcompensation reaction to the loss of capacity in another part of the lung.

518.3 Pulmonary eosinophilia

Eosinophilic asthma　　Pneumonia:
Löffler's syndrome　　　eosinophilic
Pneumonia:　　　　　　Tropical eosinophilia
allergic

DEF: Infiltration, into pulmonary parenchyma of eosinophilia; results in cough, fever, and dyspnea.

518.4 Acute edema of lung, unspecified

Acute pulmonary edema NOS
Pulmonary edema, postoperative

EXCLUDES *pulmonary edema:*
acute, with mention of heart disease or failure (428.1)
chronic or unspecified (514)
due to external agents (506.0-508.9)

DEF: Severe, sudden fluid retention within lung tissues.

518.5 Pulmonary insufficiency following trauma and surgery

Adult respiratory distress syndrome
Pulmonary insufficiency following:
shock
surgery
trauma
Shock lung

EXCLUDES *adult respiratory distress syndrome associated with other conditions (518.82)*
pneumonia:
aspiration (507.0)
hypostatic (514)
respiratory failure in other conditions (518.81, 518.83-518.84)

AHA: 3Q, '88, 3; 3Q, '88, 7; S-O, '87, 1

518.6 Allergic bronchopulmonary aspergillosis

AHA: 4Q, '97, 39

DEF: Noninvasive hypersensitive reaction; due to allergic reaction to *Aspergillus fumigatus* (mold).

☑5ᵗʰ **518.8 Other diseases of lung**

518.81 Acute respiratory failure

Respiratory failure NOS

EXCLUDES *acute and chronic respiratory failure (518.84)*
acute respiratory distress (518.82)
chronic respiratory failure (518.83)
respiratory arrest (799.1)
respiratory failure, newborn (770.84)

AHA: 1Q, '03, 15; 4Q, '98, 41; 3Q, '91, 14; 2Q, '91, 3; 4Q, '90, 25; 2Q, '90, 20; 3Q, '88, 7; 3Q, '88, 10; S-O, '87, 1

518.82 Other pulmonary insufficiency, not elsewhere classified

Acute respiratory distress
Acute respiratory insufficiency
Adult respiratory distress syndrome NEC

EXCLUDES *adult respiratory distress syndrome associated with trauma and surgery (518.5)*
pulmonary insufficiency following trauma and surgery (518.5)
respiratory distress:
NOS (786.09)
newborn (770.89)
syndrome, newborn (769)
shock lung (518.5)

AHA: ▶4Q, '03, 105;◀ 2Q, '91, 21; 3Q, '88, 7

518.83 Chronic respiratory failure

AHA: ▶4Q, '03, 103, 111◀

518.84 Acute and chronic respiratory failure

Acute on chronic respiratory failure

518.89 Other diseases of lung, not elsewhere classified

Broncholithiasis　　　Lung disease NOS
Calcification of lung　　Pulmolithiasis

AHA: 3Q, '90, 18; 4Q, '88, 6

DEF: Broncholithiasis: calculi in lumen of transbronchial tree.

DEF: Pulmolithiasis: calculi in lung.

☑4ᵗʰ
☑5ᵗʰ Additional Digit Required　　Unspecified Code　　Other Specified Code　　Manifestation Code　　▶◀ Revised Text　　● New Code　　▲ Revised Code Title

2005 ICD•9•CM　　　　　　　　　　　　　　　　　　　　　　　　**February 2004 • Volume 1 — 139**

Respiratory System

517–518.89

Respiratory System

519–519.9

✓4ᵗʰ **519 Other diseases of respiratory system**

    ✓5ᵗʰ **519.0 Tracheostomy complications**

        519.00 Tracheostomy complication, unspecified

        519.01 Infection of tracheostomy

            Use additional code to identify type of infection, such as:

                abscess or cellulitis of neck (682.1)

                septicemia (038.0-038.9)

            Use additional code to identify organism (041.00-041.9)

            AHA: 4Q, '98, 41

        519.02 Mechanical complication of tracheostomy

            Tracheal stenosis due to tracheostomy

        519.09 Other tracheostomy complications

            Hemorrhage due to tracheostomy

            Tracheoesophageal fistula due to tracheostomy

    519.1 Other diseases of trachea and bronchus, not elsewhere classified

        Calcification ⎱
        Stenosis   ⎰ of bronchus or trachea
        Ulcer

        AHA: 3Q, '02, 18; 3Q, '88, 6

519.2 Mediastinitis

    DEF: Inflammation of tissue between organs behind sternum.

519.3 Other diseases of mediastinum, not elsewhere classified

    Fibrosis ⎱
    Hernia   ⎰ of mediastinum
    Retraction

519.4 Disorders of diaphragm

    Diaphragmitis   Relaxation of diaphragm

    Paralysis of diaphragm

      EXCLUDES   *congenital defect of diaphragm (756.6)*

              diaphragmatic hernia (551-553 with .3)

              congenital (756.6)

519.8 Other diseases of respiratory system, not elsewhere classified

    AHA: 4Q, '89, 12

519.9 Unspecified disease of respiratory system

    Respiratory disease (chronic) NOS

Ⓝ Newborn Age: 0   Ⓟ Pediatric Age: 0-17   Ⓜ Maternity Age: 12-55   Ⓐ Adult Age: 15-124   MSP Medicare Secondary Payer

9. DISEASES OF THE DIGESTIVE SYSTEM (520-579)

DISEASES OF ORAL CAVITY, SALIVARY GLANDS, AND JAWS (520-529)

☑4th 520 Disorders of tooth development and eruption

520.0 Anodontia
Absence of teeth (complete) (congenital) (partial)
Hypodontia
Oligodontia
> **EXCLUDES** *acquired absence of teeth (525.10-525.19)*

520.1 Supernumerary teeth
Distomolar	Paramolar
Fourth molar	Supplemental teeth
Mesiodens	
> **EXCLUDES** *supernumerary roots (520.2)*

520.2 Abnormalities of size and form
Concrescence ⎫
Fusion   ⎬ of teeth
Gemination ⎭

Dens evaginatus	Microdontia
Dens in dente	Peg-shaped [conical] teeth
Dens invaginatus	Supernumerary roots
Enamel pearls	Taurodontism
Macrodontia	Tuberculum paramolare
> **EXCLUDES** *that due to congenital syphilis (090.5)*
> *tuberculum Carabelli, which is regarded as a normal variation*

520.3 Mottled teeth
Dental fluorosis
Mottling of enamel
Nonfluoride enamel opacities

Digestive System

The Oral Cavity

Teeth

Maxillary view

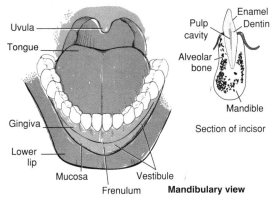

Mandibulary view

520.4 Disturbances of tooth formation
Aplasia and hypoplasia of cementum
Dilaceration of tooth
Enamel hypoplasia (neonatal) (postnatal) (prenatal)
Horner's teeth
Hypocalcification of teeth
Regional odontodysplasia
Turner's tooth
> **EXCLUDES** *Hutchinson's teeth and mulberry molars in congenital syphilis (090.5)*
> *mottled teeth (520.3)*

520.5 Hereditary disturbances in tooth structure, not elsewhere classified
Amelogenesis   ⎫
Dentinogenesis ⎬ imperfecta
Odontogenesis ⎭

Dentinal dysplasia   Shell teeth

520.6 Disturbances in tooth eruption
Teeth:	Tooth eruption:
embedded	late
impacted	obstructed
natal	premature
neonatal	
primary [deciduous]:	
persistent	
shedding, premature	
> **EXCLUDES** *exfoliation of teeth (attributable to disease of surrounding tissues) (525.0-525.19)*

520.7 Teething syndrome

520.8 Other specified disorders of tooth development and eruption
Color changes during tooth formation
Pre-eruptive color changes
> **EXCLUDES** *posteruptive color changes (521.7)*

520.9 Unspecified disorder of tooth development and eruption

☑4th ☑5th Additional Digit Required   `Unspecified Code`   `Other Specified Code`   `Manifestation Code`   ►◄ Revised Text   ● New Code   ▲ Revised Code Title

2005 ICD•9•CM   **Volume 1 — 141**

✓4ᵗʰ **521 Diseases of hard tissues of teeth**

    ✓5ᵗʰ **521.0 Dental caries**
        AHA: 4Q, '01, 44

        521.00 Dental caries, unspecified

        521.01 Dental caries limited to enamel
            Initial caries   White spot lesion

        521.02 Dental caries extending into dentine

        521.03 Dental caries extending into pulp

        521.04 Arrested dental caries

        521.05 Odontoclasia
            Infantile melanodontia
            Melanodontoclasia
            EXCLUDES *internal and external*
                        resorption of teeth
                        ►*(521.40-521.49)*◄

            DEF: A pathological dental condition described as stained areas, loss of tooth substance, and hypoplasia linked to nutritional deficiencies during tooth development and to cariogenic oral conditions; synonyms are melanodontoclasia and infantile melanodontia.

        ● **521.06 Dental caries pit and fissure**

        ● **521.07 Dental caries of smooth surface**

        ● **521.08 Dental caries of root surface**

        521.09 Other dental caries
            AHA: 3Q, '02, 14

▲ ✓5ᵗʰ **521.1 Excessive attrition (approximal wear) (occlusal wear)**
        ● **521.10 Excessive attrition, unspecified**
        521.11 Excessive attrition, limited to enamel
        521.12 Excessive attrition, extending into dentine
        521.13 Excessive attrition, extending into pulp
        521.14 Excessive attrition, localized
        521.15 Excessive attrition, generalized

    ✓5ᵗʰ **521.2 Abrasion**
        Abrasion:
          dentifrice
          habitual
          occupational   } of teeth
          ritual
          traditional
        Wedge defect NOS

        ● **521.20 Abrasion, unspecified**
        ● **521.21 Abrasion, limited to enamel**
        ● **521.22 Abrasion, extending into dentine**
        ● **521.23 Abrasion, extending into pulp**
        ● **521.24 Abrasion, localized**
        ● **521.25 Abrasion, generalized**

    ✓5ᵗʰ **521.3 Erosion**
        Erosion of teeth: Erosion of teeth:
          NOS   idiopathic
          due to: occupational
            medicine
            persistent vomiting

        ● **521.30 Erosion, unspecified**
        521.31 Erosion, limited to enamel
        521.32 Erosion, extending into dentine
        521.33 Erosion, extending into pulp
        521.34 Erosion, localized
        521.35 Erosion, generalized

    ✓5ᵗʰ **521.4 Pathological resorption**
        DEF: Loss of dentin and cementum due to disease process.

        ● **521.40 Pathological resorption, unspecified**
        ● **521.41 Pathological resorption, internal**
        ● **521.42 Pathological resorption, external**
        ● **521.49 Other pathological resorption**
            Internal granuloma of pulp

    521.5 Hypercementosis
        Cementation hyperplasia
        DEF: Excess deposits of cementum, on tooth root.

521.6 Ankylosis of teeth
    DEF: Adhesion of tooth to surrounding bone.

▲ **521.7 Intrinsic posteruptive color changes**
    Staining [discoloration] of teeth:
      NOS
      due to:
        drugs
        metals
        pulpal bleeding
      EXCLUDES *accretions [deposits] on teeth (523.6)*
                  ►*extrinsic color changes (523.6)*◄
                  pre-eruptive color changes (520.8)

521.8 Other specified diseases of hard tissues of teeth
    Irradiated enamel   Sensitive dentin

521.9 Unspecified disease of hard tissues of teeth

✓4ᵗʰ **522 Diseases of pulp and periapical tissues**

    522.0 Pulpitis
        Pulpal: Pulpitis:
          abscess   chronic (hyperplastic)
          polyp   (ulcerative)
        Pulpitis: suppurative
          acute

    522.1 Necrosis of the pulp
        Pulp gangrene
        DEF: Death of pulp tissue.

    522.2 Pulp degeneration
        Denticles   Pulp stones
        Pulp calcifications

    522.3 Abnormal hard tissue formation in pulp
        Secondary or irregular dentin

    522.4 Acute apical periodontitis of pulpal origin
        DEF: Severe inflammation of periodontal ligament due to pulpal inflammation or necrosis.

    522.5 Periapical abscess without sinus
        Abscess: Abscess:
          dental   dentoalveolar
      EXCLUDES *periapical abscess with sinus (522.7)*

    522.6 Chronic apical periodontitis
        Apical or periapical granuloma
        Apical periodontitis NOS

    522.7 Periapical abscess with sinus
        Fistula: Fistula:
          alveolar process   dental

    522.8 Radicular cyst
        Cyst: Cyst:
          apical (periodontal)   radiculodental
          periapical   residual radicular
      EXCLUDES *lateral developmental or lateral periodontal cyst (526.0)*
        DEF: Cyst in tissue around tooth apex due to chronic infection of granuloma around root.

    522.9 Other and unspecified diseases of pulp and periapical tissues

✓4ᵗʰ **523 Gingival and periodontal diseases**

    523.0 Acute gingivitis
      EXCLUDES *acute necrotizing ulcerative gingivitis (101)*
                  herpetic gingivostomatitis (054.2)

    523.1 Chronic gingivitis
        Gingivitis (chronic):   Gingivitis (chronic):
          NOS   simple marginal
          desquamative   ulcerative
          hyperplastic   Gingivostomatitis
      EXCLUDES *herpetic gingivostomatitis (054.2)*

    ✓5ᵗʰ **523.2 Gingival recession**
        ►Gingival recession (postinfective) (postoperative)◄
        ● **523.20 Gingival recession, unspecified**
        ● **523.21 Gingival recession, minimal**
        ● **523.22 Gingival recession, moderate**

● **523.23 Gingival recession, severe**
● **523.24 Gingival recession, localized**
● **523.25 Gingival recession, generalized**

523.3 Acute periodontitis
Acute:
  pericementitis
  pericoronitis
  Paradontal abscess
  Periodontal abscess
> EXCLUDES   acute apical periodontitis (522.4)
>   periapical abscess (522.5, 522.7)

DEF: Severe inflammation, of tissues supporting teeth.

523.4 Chronic periodontitis
Alveolar pyorrhea   Periodontitis:
Chronic pericoronitis   NOS
Pericementitis (chronic)   complex
     simplex
> EXCLUDES   chronic apical periodontitis (522.6)

523.5 Periodontosis

523.6 Accretions on teeth
Dental calculus:
  subgingival
  supragingival
Deposits on teeth:
  betel
  materia alba
  soft
  tartar
  tobacco
▶Extrinsic discoloration of teeth◀
> EXCLUDES ▶ intrinsic discoloration of teeth (521.7)◀

DEF: Foreign material on tooth surface, usually plaque or calculus.

523.8 Other specified periodontal diseases
Giant cell:
  epulis
  peripheral granuloma
Gingival:
  cysts
  enlargement NOS
  fibromatosis
Gingival polyp
Periodontal lesions due to traumatic occlusion
Peripheral giant cell granuloma
> EXCLUDES   leukoplakia of gingiva (528.6)

523.9 Unspecified gingival and periodontal disease
AHA: 3Q, '02, 14

✓4th **524 Dentofacial anomalies, including malocclusion**
✓5th **524.0 Major anomalies of jaw size**
> EXCLUDES   hemifacial atrophy or hypertrophy (754.0)
>   unilateral condylar hyperplasia or hypoplasia of mandible (526.89)

524.00 Unspecified anomaly
DEF: Unspecified deformity of jaw size.

524.01 Maxillary hyperplasia
DEF: Overgrowth or overdevelopment of upper jaw bone.

524.02 Mandibular hyperplasia
DEF: Overgrowth or overdevelopment of lower jaw bone.

524.03 Maxillary hypoplasia
DEF: Incomplete or underdeveloped, upper jaw bone.

524.04 Mandibular hypoplasia
DEF: Incomplete or underdeveloped, lower jaw bone.

524.05 Macrogenia
DEF: Enlarged, jaw, especially chin; affects bone, soft tissue, or both.

524.06 Microgenia
DEF: Underdeveloped mandible, characterized by an extremely small chin.

● **524.07 Excessive tuberosity of jaw**

524.09 Other specified anomaly
✓5th **524.1 Anomalies of relationship of jaw to cranial base**
524.10 Unspecified anomaly
Prognathism   Retrognathism
DEF: Prognathism: protrusion of lower jaw.

DEF: Retrognathism: jaw is located posteriorly to a normally positioned jaw; backward position of mandible.

524.11 Maxillary asymmetry
DEF: Absence of symmetry of maxilla.

524.12 Other jaw asymmetry
524.19 Other specified anomaly
✓5th **524.2 Anomalies of dental arch relationship**
> EXCLUDES   hemifacial atrophy or hypertrophy (754.0)
>   ▶soft tissue impingement (524.81-524.82)◀
>   unilateral condylar hyperplasia or hypoplasia of mandible (526.89)

● **524.20 Unspecified anomaly of dental arch relationship**
● **524.21 Angle's class I**
Neutro-occlusion
● **524.22 Angle's class II**
Disto-occlusion Division I
Disto-occlusion Division II
● **524.23 Angle's class III**
Mesio-occlusion
● **524.24 Open anterior occlusal relationship**
● **524.25 Open posterior occlusal relationship**
● **524.26 Excessive horizontal overlap**
● **524.27 Reverse articulation**
Anterior articulation
Posterior articulation
● **524.28 Anomalies of interarch distance**
Excessive interarch distance
Inadequate interarch distance
● **524.29 Other anomalies of dental arch relationship**
▲ ✓5th **524.3 Anomalies of tooth position of fully erupted teeth**
> EXCLUDES ▶ impacted or embedded teeth with abnormal position of such teeth or adjacent teeth (520.6)◀

● **524.30 Unspecified anomaly of tooth position**
Diastema of teeth NOS
Displacement of teeth NOS
Transposition of teeth NOS
● **524.31 Crowding of teeth**
● **524.32 Excessive spacing of teeth**
● **524.33 Horizontal displacement of teeth**
Tipping of teeth
● **524.34 Vertical displacement of teeth**
Infraeruption of teeth
Supraeruption of teeth
● **524.35 Rotation of teeth**
● **524.36 Insufficient interocclusal distance of teeth (ridge)**
● **524.37 Excessive interocclusal distance of teeth**
Loss of occlusal vertical dimension
● **524.39 Other anomalies of tooth position**
524.4 Malocclusion, unspecified
DEF: Malposition of top and bottom teeth; interferes with chewing.
✓5th **524.5 Dentofacial functional abnormalities**
● **524.50 Dentofacial functional abnormality, unspecified**
● **524.51 Abnormal jaw closure**
Dyskinesia
● **524.52 Limited mandibular range of motion**
● **524.53 Deviation in opening and closing of the mandible**

✓4th / ✓5th Additional Digit Required   Unspecified Code   Other Specified Code   Manifestation Code   ▶◀ Revised Text   ● New Code   ▲ Revised Code Title

Digestive System

524.54–527.1

● 524.54 Insufficient anterior guidance
● 524.55 Centric occlusion maximum intercuspation discrepancy
● 524.56 Non-working side interference
● 524.57 Lack of posterior occlusal support
● 524.59 Other dentofacial functional abnormalities
Abnormal swallowing
Mouth breathing
Sleep postures
Tongue, lip, or finger habits

√5ᵗʰ 524.6 Temporomandibular joint disorders
EXCLUDES current temporomandibular joint:
dislocation (830.0-830.1)
strain (848.1)

524.60 Temporomandibular joint disorders, unspecified
Temporomandibular joint-pain-dysfunction syndrome [TMJ]

524.61 Adhesions and ankylosis (bony or fibrous)
DEF: Stiffening or union of temporomandibular joint due to bony or fibrous union across joint.

524.62 Arthralgia of temporomandibular joint
DEF: Pain in temporomandibular joint; not inflammatory in nature.

524.63 Articular disc disorder (reducing or non-reducing)

● 524.64 Temporomandibular joint sounds on opening and/or closing the jaw

524.69 Other specified temporomandibular joint disorders

√5ᵗʰ 524.7 Dental alveolar anomalies
524.70 Unspecified alveolar anomaly
524.71 Alveolar maxillary hyperplasia
DEF: Excessive tissue formation in the dental alveoli of upper jaw.

524.72 Alveolar mandibular hyperplasia
DEF: Excessive tissue formation in the dental alveoli of lower jaw.

524.73 Alveolar maxillary hypoplasia
DEF: Incomplete or underdeveloped, alveolar tissue of upper jaw.

524.74 Alveolar mandibular hypoplasia
DEF: Incomplete or underdeveloped, alveolar tissue of lower jaw.

● 524.75 Vertical displacement of alveolus and teeth
Extrusion of alveolus and teeth

● 524.76 Occlusal plane deviation
524.79 Other specified alveolar anomaly

√4ᵗʰ 524.8 Other specified dentofacial anomalies
● 524.81 Anterior soft tissue impingement
● 524.82 Posterior soft tissue impingement
● 524.89 Other specified dentofacial anomalies

524.9 Unspecified dentofacial anomalies

√4ᵗʰ 525 Other diseases and conditions of the teeth and supporting structures
525.0 Exfoliation of teeth due to systemic causes
DEF: Deterioration of teeth and surrounding structures due to systemic disease.

√5ᵗʰ 525.1 Loss of teeth due to trauma, extraction, or periodontal disease
AHA: 4Q, '01, 44

525.10 Acquired absence of teeth, unspecified
Edentulism
Tooth extraction status, NOS

525.11 Loss of teeth due to trauma
525.12 Loss of teeth due to periodontal disease

525.13 Loss of teeth due to caries
525.19 Other loss of teeth

√5ᵗʰ 525.2 Atrophy of edentulous alveolar ridge
● 525.20 Unspecified atrophy of edentulous alveolar ridge
Atrophy of the mandible NOS
Atrophy of the maxilla NOS

● 525.21 Minimal atrophy of the mandible
● 525.22 Moderate atrophy of the mandible
● 525.23 Severe atrophy of the mandible
● 525.24 Minimal atrophy of the maxilla
● 525.25 Moderate atrophy of the maxilla
● 525.26 Severe atrophy of the maxilla

525.3 Retained dental root
525.8 Other specified disorders of the teeth and supporting structures
Enlargement of alveolar ridge NOS
Irregular alveolar process

525.9 Unspecified disorder of the teeth and supporting structures

√4ᵗʰ 526 Diseases of the jaws
526.0 Developmental odontogenic cysts
Cyst: Cyst:
dentigerous   lateral periodontal
eruption   primordial
follicular   Keratocyst
lateral developmental
EXCLUDES radicular cyst (522.8)

526.1 Fissural cysts of jaw
Cyst: Cyst:
globulomaxillary   median palatal
incisor canal   nasopalatine
median anterior   palatine of papilla
maxillary
EXCLUDES cysts of oral soft tissues (528.4)

526.2 Other cysts of jaws
Cyst of jaw: Cyst of jaw:
NOS   hemorrhagic
aneurysmal   traumatic

526.3 Central giant cell (reparative) granuloma
EXCLUDES peripheral giant cell granuloma (523.8)

526.4 Inflammatory conditions
Abscess
Osteitis   } of jaw (acute) (chronic)
Osteomyelitis (neonatal)   (suppurative)
Periostitis
Sequestrum of jaw bone
EXCLUDES alveolar osteitis (526.5)

526.5 Alveolitis of jaw
Alveolar osteitis   Dry socket
DEF: Inflammation, of alveoli or tooth socket.

√5ᵗʰ 526.8 Other specified diseases of the jaws
526.81 Exostosis of jaw
Torus mandibularis
Torus palatinus
DEF: Spur or bony outgrowth on the jaw.

526.89 Other
Cherubism
Fibrous dysplasia   } of jaw(s)
Latent bone cyst
Osteoradionecrosis
Unilateral condylar hyperplasia or hypoplasia of mandible

526.9 Unspecified disease of the jaws

√4ᵗʰ 527 Diseases of the salivary glands
527.0 Atrophy
DEF: Wasting away, necrosis of salivary gland tissue.

527.1 Hypertrophy
DEF: Overgrowth or overdeveloped salivary gland tissue.

N Newborn Age: 0   P Pediatric Age: 0-17   M Maternity Age: 12-55   A Adult Age: 15-124   MSP Medicare Secondary Payer

527.2 Sialoadenitis
Parotitis: Sialoangitis
NOS Sialodochitis
allergic
toxic

EXCLUDES *epidemic or infectious parotitis (072.0-072.9)*
uveoparotid fever (135)

DEF: Inflammation of salivary gland.

527.3 Abscess
527.4 Fistula
EXCLUDES *congenital fistula of salivary gland (750.24)*

527.5 Sialolithiasis
Calculus ⎫ of salivary gland or duct
Stone ⎭
Sialodocholithiasis

527.6 Mucocele
Mucous:
extravasation cyst of salivary gland
retention cyst of salivary gland
Ranula

DEF: Dilated salivary gland cavity filled with mucous.

527.7 Disturbance of salivary secretion
Hyposecretion Sialorrhea
Ptyalism Xerostomia

527.8 Other specified diseases of the salivary glands
Benign lymphoepithelial lesion of salivary gland
Sialectasia
Sialosis
Stenosis ⎫ of salivary duct
Stricture ⎭

527.9 Unspecified disease of the salivary glands

✓4ᵗʰ 528 Diseases of the oral soft tissues, excluding lesions specific for gingiva and tongue

528.0 Stomatitis
Stomatitis: Vesicular stomatitis
NOS
ulcerative

EXCLUDES *stomatitis:*
acute necrotizing ulcerative (101)
aphthous (528.2)
gangrenous (528.1)
herpetic (054.2)
Vincent's (101)

AHA: 2Q, '99, 9

DEF: Inflammation of oral mucosa; labial and buccal mucosa, tongue, plate, floor of the mouth, and gingivae.

528.1 Cancrum oris
Gangrenous stomatitis Noma

DEF: A severely gangrenous lesion of mouth due to fusospirochetal infection; destroys buccal, labial and facial tissues; can be fatal; found primarily in debilitated and malnourished children.

528.2 Oral aphthae
Aphthous stomatitis
Canker sore
Periadenitis mucosa necrotica recurrens
Recurrent aphthous ulcer
Stomatitis herpetiformis

EXCLUDES *herpetic stomatitis (054.2)*

DEF: Small oval or round ulcers of the mouth marked by a grayish exudate and a red halo effect.

528.3 Cellulitis and abscess
Cellulitis of mouth (floor) Oral fistula
Ludwig's angina

EXCLUDES *abscess of tongue (529.0)*
cellulitis or abscess of lip (528.5)
fistula (of):
dental (522.7)
lip (528.5)
gingivitis (523.0-523.1)

528.4 Cysts
Dermoid cyst ⎫
Epidermoid cyst ⎪
Epstein's pearl ⎪ of mouth
Lymphoepithelial cyst ⎬
Nasoalveolar cyst ⎪
Nasolabial cyst ⎭

EXCLUDES *cyst:*
gingiva (523.8)
tongue (529.8)

528.5 Diseases of lips
Abscess ⎫
Cellulitis ⎪ of lip(s)
Fistula ⎬
Hypertrophy ⎭

Cheilitis: Cheilodynia
NOS Cheilosis
angular

EXCLUDES *actinic cheilitis (692.79)*
congenital fistula of lip (750.25)
leukoplakia of lips (528.6)

AHA: S-O, '86, 10

528.6 Leukoplakia of oral mucosa, including tongue
Leukokeratosis of Leukoplakia of:
oral mucosa lips
Leukoplakia of: tongue
gingiva

EXCLUDES *carcinoma in situ (230.0, 232.0)*
leukokeratosis nicotina palati
▶*(528.79)*◀

DEF: Thickened white patches of epithelium on mucous membranes of mouth.

✓5ᵗʰ 528.7 Other disturbances of oral epithelium, including tongue

EXCLUDES *carcinoma in situ (230.0, 232.0)*
leukokeratosis NOS (702)

● **528.71 Minimal keratinized residual ridge mucosa**
● **528.72 Excessive keratinized residual ridge mucosa**
● **528.79 Other disturbances of oral epithelium, including tongue**
Erythroplakia of mouth or tongue
Focal epithelial hyperplasia of mouth or tongue
Leukoedema of mouth or tongue
Leukokeratosis nicotina palate

528.8 Oral submucosal fibrosis, including of tongue
528.9 Other and unspecified diseases of the oral soft tissues
Cheek and lip biting
Denture sore mouth
Denture stomatitis
Melanoplakia
Papillary hyperplasia of palate
Eosinophilic granuloma ⎫
Irritative hyperplasia ⎪ of oral mucosa
Pyogenic granuloma ⎬
Ulcer (traumatic) ⎭

Digestive System

529–530.6

✓4ᵗʰ **529 Diseases and other conditions of the tongue**

529.0 Glossitis

Abscess
Ulceration (traumatic) } of tongue

> EXCLUDES   glossitis:
>   benign migratory (529.1)
>   Hunter's (529.4)
>   median rhomboid (529.2)
>   Moeller's (529.4)

529.1 Geographic tongue

Benign migratory glossitis
Glossitis areata exfoliativa

DEF: Chronic glossitis; marked by filiform papillae atrophy and inflammation; no known etiology.

529.2 Median rhomboid glossitis

DEF: A noninflammatory, congenital disease characterized by rhomboid-like lesions at the middle third of the tongue's dorsal surface.

529.3 Hypertrophy of tongue papillae

Black hairy tongue   Hypertrophy of foliate papillae
Coated tongue   Lingua villosa nigra

529.4 Atrophy of tongue papillae

Bald tongue   Glossitis:
Glazed tongue   Moeller's
Glossitis: Glossodynia exfoliativa
   Hunter's   Smooth atrophic tongue

529.5 Plicated tongue

Fissured
Furrowed } tongue
Scrotal

> EXCLUDES   fissure of tongue, congenital (750.13)

DEF: Cracks, fissures or furrows, on dorsal surface of tongue.

529.6 Glossodynia

Glossopyrosis   Painful tongue

> EXCLUDES   glossodynia exfoliativa (529.4)

529.8 Other specified conditions of the tongue

Atrophy
Crenated
Enlargement } (of) tongue
Hypertrophy

Glossocele
Glossoptosis

> EXCLUDES   erythroplasia of tongue ▶(528.79)◀
>   leukoplakia of tongue (528.6)
>   macroglossia (congenital) (750.15)
>   microglossia (congenital) (750.16)
>   oral submucosal fibrosis (528.8)

529.9 Unspecified condition of the tongue

DISEASES OF ESOPHAGUS, STOMACH, AND DUODENUM (530-537)

✓4ᵗʰ **530 Diseases of esophagus**

> EXCLUDES   esophageal varices (456.0-456.2)

530.0 Achalasia and cardiospasm

Achalasia (of cardia)   Megaesophagus
Aperistalsis of esophagus

> EXCLUDES   congenital cardiospasm (750.7)

DEF: Failure of smooth muscle fibers to relax, at gastrointestinal junctures; such as esophagogastric sphincter when swallowing.

✓5ᵗʰ **530.1 Esophagitis**

Abscess of esophagus   Esophagitis:
Esophagitis: peptic
   NOS   postoperative
   chemical   regurgitant
Use additional E code to identify cause, if induced by chemical

> EXCLUDES   tuberculous esophagitis (017.8)

AHA: 4Q, '93, 27; 1Q, '92, 17; 3Q, '91, 20

Esophagus

Pharyngeal constrictors

Front view

Epiglottis

Cricoid cartilage

C6

Trachea

Pharyngoesophageal sphincter

Gastroesophageal sphincter

Diaphragm

Side view

Stomach

530.10 Esophagitis, unspecified

530.11 Reflux esophagitis

AHA: 4Q, '95, 82

DEF: Inflammation of lower esophagus; due to regurgitated gastric acid from malfunctioning lower esophageal sphincter; causes heartburn and substernal pain.

530.12 Acute esophagitis

AHA: 4Q, '01, 45

DEF: An acute inflammation of the mucous lining or submucosal coat of the esophagus.

530.19 Other esophagitis

AHA: 3Q, '01, 10

✓5ᵗʰ **530.2 Ulcer of esophagus**

Ulcer of esophagus
  fungal
  peptic
Ulcer of esophagus due to ingestion of:
  aspirin
  chemicals
  medicines
Use additional E code to identify cause, if induced by chemical or drug

AHA: 4Q, '03, 63

530.20 Ulcer of esophagus without bleeding

Ulcer of esophagus NOS

530.21 Ulcer of esophagus with bleeding

> EXCLUDES   bleeding esophageal varices (456.0, 456.20)

530.3 Stricture and stenosis of esophagus

Compression of esophagus
Obstruction of esophagus

> EXCLUDES   congenital stricture of esophagus (750.3)

AHA: 2Q, '01, 4; 2Q, '97, 3; 1Q, '88, 13

530.4 Perforation of esophagus

Rupture of esophagus

> EXCLUDES   traumatic perforation of esophagus (862.22, 862.32, 874.4-874.5)

530.5 Dyskinesia of esophagus

Corkscrew esophagus   Esophagospasm
Curling esophagus   Spasm of esophagus

> EXCLUDES   cardiospasm (530.0)

AHA: 1Q, '88, 13; N-D, '84, 19

DEF: Difficulty performing voluntary esophageal movements.

530.6 Diverticulum of esophagus, acquired

Diverticulum, acquired:
  epiphrenic
  pharyngoesophageal
  pulsion
  subdiaphragmatic
  traction
  Zenker's (hypopharyngeal)
Esophageal pouch, acquired
Esophagocele, acquired

> EXCLUDES   congenital diverticulum of esophagus (750.4)

AHA: J-F, '85, 3

N Newborn Age: 0	P Pediatric Age: 0-17	M Maternity Age: 12-55	A Adult Age: 15-124	MSP Medicare Secondary Payer

530.7 Gastroesophageal laceration-hemorrhage syndrome
Mallory-Weiss syndrome
DEF: Laceration of distal esophagus and proximal stomach due to vomiting, hiccups or other sustained activity.

√5ᵗʰ 530.8 Other specified disorders of esophagus

530.81 Esophageal reflux
Gastroesophageal reflux
EXCLUDES *reflux esophagitis (530.11)*
AHA: 2Q, '01, 4; 1Q, '95, 7; 4Q, '92, 27

DEF: Regurgitation of the gastric contents into esophagus and possibly pharynx; where aspiration may occur between the vocal cords and down into the trachea.

530.82 Esophageal hemorrhage
EXCLUDES *hemorrhage due to esophageal varices (456.0-456.2)*

530.83 Esophageal leukoplakia

530.84 Tracheoesophageal fistula
EXCLUDES *congenital tracheoesophageal fistula (750.3)*

530.85 Barrett's esophagus
AHA: 4Q, '03, 63

DEF: A metaplastic disorder in which specialized columnar epithelial cells replace the normal squamous epithelial cells; an acquired condition secondary to chronic gastroesophageal reflux damage to the mucosa; associated with increased risk of developing adenocarcinoma.

● **530.86 Infection of esophagostomy**
Use additional code to specify infection

● **530.87 Mechanical complication of esophagostomy**
Malfunction of esophagostomy

530.89 Other
EXCLUDES *Paterson-Kelly syndrome (280.8)*

530.9 Unspecified disorder of esophagus

√4ᵗʰ 531 Gastric ulcer
INCLUDES ulcer (peptic):
prepyloric
pylorus
stomach
Use additional E code to identify drug, if drug-induced
EXCLUDES *peptic ulcer NOS (533.0-533.9)*

The following fifth-digit subclassification is for use with category 531:
0 without mention of obstruction
1 with obstruction

AHA: 1Q, '91, 15; 4Q, '90, 27

DEF: Destruction of tissue in lumen of stomach due to action of gastric acid and pepsin on gastric mucosa decreasing resistance to ulcers.

√5ᵗʰ 531.0 Acute with hemorrhage
AHA: N-D, '84, 15

√5ᵗʰ 531.1 Acute with perforation

Stomach

√5ᵗʰ 531.2 Acute with hemorrhage and perforation

√5ᵗʰ 531.3 Acute without mention of hemorrhage or perforation

√5ᵗʰ 531.4 Chronic or unspecified with hemorrhage
AHA: 4Q, '90, 22

√5ᵗʰ 531.5 Chronic or unspecified with perforation

√5ᵗʰ 531.6 Chronic or unspecified with hemorrhage and perforation

√5ᵗʰ 531.7 Chronic without mention of hemorrhage or perforation

√5ᵗʰ 531.9 Unspecified as acute or chronic, without mention of hemorrhage or perforation

√4ᵗʰ 532 Duodenal ulcer
INCLUDES erosion (acute) of duodenum
ulcer (peptic):
duodenum
postpyloric
Use additional E code to identify drug, if drug-induced
EXCLUDES *peptic ulcer NOS (533.0-533.9)*

The following fifth-digit subclassification is for use with category 532:
0 without mention of obstruction
1 with obstruction

AHA: 4Q, '90, 27, 1Q, '91, 15
DEF: Ulcers in duodenum due to action of gastric acid and pepsin on mucosa decreasing resistance to ulcers.

√5ᵗʰ 532.0 Acute with hemorrhage
AHA: 4Q, '90, 22

√5ᵗʰ 532.1 Acute with perforation

√5ᵗʰ 532.2 Acute with hemorrhage and perforation

√5ᵗʰ 532.3 Acute without mention of hemorrhage or perforation

√5ᵗʰ 532.4 Chronic or unspecified with hemorrhage

√5ᵗʰ 532.5 Chronic or unspecified with perforation

√5ᵗʰ 532.6 Chronic or unspecified with hemorrhage and perforation

√5ᵗʰ 532.7 Chronic without mention of hemorrhage or perforation

√5ᵗʰ 532.9 Unspecified as acute or chronic, without mention of hemorrhage or perforation

√4ᵗʰ 533 Peptic ulcer, site unspecified
INCLUDES gastroduodenal ulcer NOS
peptic ulcer NOS
stress ulcer NOS
Use additional E code to identify drug, if drug-induced
EXCLUDES *peptic ulcer:*
duodenal (532.0-532.9)
gastric (531.0-531.9)

The following fifth-digit subclassification is for use with category 533:
0 without mention of obstruction
1 with obstruction

AHA: 1Q, '91, 15; 4Q, '90, 27

√5ᵗʰ 533.0 Acute with hemorrhage

√5ᵗʰ 533.1 Acute with perforation

√5ᵗʰ 533.2 Acute with hemorrhage and perforation

√5ᵗʰ 533.3 Acute without mention of hemorrhage and perforation

√5ᵗʰ 533.4 Chronic or unspecified with hemorrhage

√5ᵗʰ 533.5 Chronic or unspecified with perforation

√5ᵗʰ 533.6 Chronic or unspecified with hemorrhage and perforation

√5ᵗʰ 533.7 Chronic without mention of hemorrhage or perforation
AHA: 2Q, '89, 16

√5ᵗʰ 533.9 Unspecified as acute or chronic, without mention of hemorrhage or perforation

√4ᵗʰ / √5ᵗʰ Additional Digit Required   Unspecified Code   Other Specified Code   Manifestation Code   ▶◀ Revised Text   ● New Code   ▲ Revised Code Title

2005 ICD•9•CM   October 2004 • Volume 1 — 147

Digestive System

534–537.2

✓4ᵗʰ **534 Gastrojejunal ulcer**

INCLUDES   ulcer (peptic) or erosion:
- anastomotic
- gastrocolic
- gastrointestinal
- gastrojejunal
- jejunal
- marginal
- stomal

EXCLUDES   *primary ulcer of small intestine (569.82)*

The following fifth-digit subclassification is for use with category 534:

    0   without mention of obstruction
    1   with obstruction

AHA: 1Q, '91, 15; 4Q, '90, 27

✓5ᵗʰ **534.0   Acute with hemorrhage**
✓5ᵗʰ **534.1   Acute with perforation**
✓5ᵗʰ **534.2   Acute with hemorrhage and perforation**
✓5ᵗʰ **534.3   Acute without mention of hemorrhage or perforation**
✓5ᵗʰ **534.4   Chronic or unspecified with hemorrhage**
✓5ᵗʰ **534.5   Chronic or unspecified with perforation**
✓5ᵗʰ **534.6   Chronic or unspecified with hemorrhage and perforation**
✓5ᵗʰ **534.7   Chronic without mention of hemorrhage or perforation**
✓5ᵗʰ **534.9   Unspecified as acute or chronic, without mention of hemorrhage or perforation**

✓4ᵗʰ **535 Gastritis and duodenitis**

The following fifth-digit subclassification is for use with category 535:

    0   without mention of hemorrhage
    1   with hemorrhage

AHA: 2Q, '92, 9; 4Q, '91, 25

✓5ᵗʰ **535.0   Acute gastritis**
    AHA: 2Q, '92, 8; N-D, '86, 9

✓5ᵗʰ **535.1   Atrophic gastritis**
    Gastritis: Gastritis:
      atrophic-hyperplastic   chronic (atrophic)
    AHA: 1Q, '94, 18

    DEF: Inflammation of stomach, with mucous membrane atrophy and peptic gland destruction.

✓5ᵗʰ **535.2   Gastric mucosal hypertrophy**
    Hypertrophic gastritis

✓5ᵗʰ **535.3   Alcoholic gastritis**

✓5ᵗʰ **535.4   Other specified gastritis**
    Gastritis: Gastritis:
      allergic   superficial
      bile induced   toxic
      irritant
    AHA: 4Q, '90, 27

✓5ᵗʰ **535.5   Unspecified gastritis and gastroduodenitis**
    AHA: For code 535.50: 4Q, '99, 25

✓5ᵗʰ **535.6   Duodenitis**
    DEF: Inflammation of intestine, between pylorus and jejunum.

✓4ᵗʰ **536 Disorders of function of stomach**
    EXCLUDES   *functional disorders of stomach specified as psychogenic (306.4)*

536.0   Achlorhydria
    DEF: Absence of gastric acid due to gastric mucosa atrophy; unresponsive to histamines; also known as gastric anacidity.

536.1   Acute dilatation of stomach
    Acute distention of stomach

536.2   Persistent vomiting
- Habit vomiting
- Persistent vomiting [not of pregnancy]
- Uncontrollable vomiting

    EXCLUDES   *excessive vomiting in pregnancy (643.0-643.9)*
                        vomiting NOS (787.0)

536.3   Gastroparesis
    ▶Gastroparalysis◀
    AHA: 2Q, '01, 4; 4Q, '94, 42

    DEF: Slight degree of paralysis within muscular coat of stomach.

✓5ᵗʰ **536.4   Gastrostomy complications**
    AHA: 4Q, '98, 42

    536.40 Gastrostomy complication, unspecified
    536.41 Infection of gastrostomy
         Use additional code to specify type of infection, such as:
         abscess or cellulitis of abdomen (682.2)
         septicemia (038.0-038.9)
         Use additional code to identify organism (041.00-041.9)
         AHA: 4Q, '98, 42

    536.42 Mechanical complication of gastrostomy
    536.49 Other gastrostomy complications
         AHA: 4Q, '98, 42

536.8   Dyspepsia and other specified disorders of function of stomach
    Achylia gastrica   Hyperchlorhydria
    Hourglass contraction   Hypochlorhydria
      of stomach   Indigestion
    Hyperacidity

    EXCLUDES   *achlorhydria (536.0)*
                        heartburn (787.1)
    AHA: 2Q, '93, 6; 2Q, '89, 16; N-D, '84, 9

536.9   Unspecified functional disorder of stomach
    Functional gastrointestinal:
      disorder
      disturbance
      irritation

✓4ᵗʰ **537 Other disorders of stomach and duodenum**
    537.0   Acquired hypertrophic pyloric stenosis
       Constriction
       Obstruction } of pylorus, acquired or adult
       Stricture

       EXCLUDES   *congenital or infantile pyloric stenosis (750.5)*
       AHA: 2Q, '01, 4; J-F, '85, 14

    537.1   Gastric diverticulum
       EXCLUDES   *congenital diverticulum of stomach (750.7)*
       AHA: J-F, '85, 4

       DEF: Herniated sac or pouch, within stomach or duodenum.

    537.2   Chronic duodenal ileus
       DEF: Persistent obstruction between pylorus and jejunum.

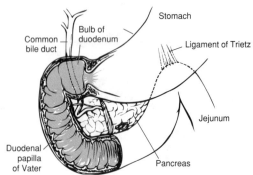

Duodenum

Stomach

Bulb of duodenum

Common bile duct

Ligament of Trietz

Duodenal papilla of Vater

Jejunum

Pancreas

N   Newborn Age: 0   P   Pediatric Age: 0-17   M   Maternity Age: 12-55   A   Adult Age: 15-124   MSP   Medicare Secondary Payer

537.3 Other obstruction of duodenum

Cicatrix
Stenosis } of duodenum
Stricture
Volvulus

> **EXCLUDES** *congenital obstruction of duodenum (751.1)*

537.4 Fistula of stomach or duodenum

Gastrocolic fistula   Gastrojejunocolic fistula

537.5 Gastroptosis

DEF: Downward displacement of stomach.

537.6 Hourglass stricture or stenosis of stomach

Cascade stomach

> **EXCLUDES** *congenital hourglass stomach (750.7)*
> *hourglass contraction of stomach (536.8)*

√5ᵗʰ **537.8 Other specified disorders of stomach and duodenum**

AHA: 4Q, '91, 25

537.81 Pylorospasm

> **EXCLUDES** *congenital pylorospasm (750.5)*

DEF: Spasm of the pyloric sphincter.

537.82 Angiodysplasia of stomach and duodenum (without mention of hemorrhage)

AHA: 3Q, '96, 10; 4Q, '90, 4

537.83 Angiodysplasia of stomach and duodenum with hemorrhage

DEF: Bleeding of stomach and duodenum due to vascular abnormalities.

537.84 Dieulafoy lesion (hemorrhagic) of stomach and duodenum

AHA: 4Q, '02, 60

DEF: An abnormally large and convoluted submucosal artery protruding through a defect in the mucosa in the stomach or intestines that can erode the epithelium causing hemorrhaging; also called Dieulafoy's vascular malformation.

537.89 Other

Gastric or duodenal:
  prolapse
  rupture
Intestinal metaplasia of gastric mucosa
Passive congestion of stomach

> **EXCLUDES** *diverticula of duodenum (562.00-562.01)*
> *gastrointestinal hemorrhage (578.0-578.9)*

AHA: N-D, '84, 7

537.9 Unspecified disorder of stomach and duodenum

APPENDICITIS (540-543)

√4ᵗʰ **540 Acute appendicitis**

AHA: N-D, '84, 19

DEF: Inflammation of vermiform appendix due to fecal obstruction, neoplasm or foreign body of appendiceal lumen; causes infection, edema and infarction of appendiceal wall; may result in mural necrosis, and perforation.

540.0 With generalized peritonitis

Appendicitis (acute):
  fulminating   with:
  gangrenous   perforation
  obstructive   peritonitis (generalized)
  Cecitis (acute)   rupture

Rupture of appendix

> **EXCLUDES** *acute appendicitis with peritoneal abscess (540.1)*

540.1 With peritoneal abscess

With generalized peritonitis
Abscess of appendix

AHA: N-D, '84, 19

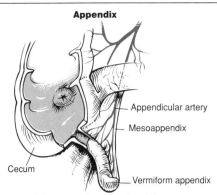

Appendix

Appendicular artery — Mesoappendix — Cecum — Vermiform appendix

540.9 Without mention of peritonitis

Acute:
  appendicitis:
   fulminating   without mention of
   gangrenous   perforation, peritonitis,
   inflamed   or rupture
   obstructive
   cecitis

AHA: 1Q, '01, 15; 4Q, '97, 52

541 Appendicitis, unqualified

AHA: 2Q, '90, 26

542 Other appendicitis

Appendicitis: Appendicitis:
  chronic   relapsing
  recurrent   subacute

> **EXCLUDES** *hyperplasia (lymphoid) of appendix (543.0)*

AHA: 1Q, '01, 15

√4ᵗʰ **543 Other diseases of appendix**

543.0 Hyperplasia of appendix (lymphoid)

DEF: Proliferation of cells in appendix tissue.

543.9 Other and unspecified diseases of appendix

Appendicular or appendiceal:
  colic
  concretion
  fistula
Diverticulum
Fecalith
Intussusception } of appendix
Mucocele
Stercolith

HERNIA OF ABDOMINAL CAVITY (550-553)

> **INCLUDES** hernia:
>   acquired
>   congenital, except diaphragmatic or hiatal

√4ᵗʰ **550 Inguinal hernia**

> **INCLUDES** bubonocele
>   inguinal hernia (direct) (double) (indirect)
>   (oblique) (sliding)
>   scrotal hernia

The following fifth-digit subclassification is for use with category 550:

  0 unilateral or unspecified (not specified as recurrent)
    Unilateral NOS
  1 unilateral or unspecified, recurrent
  2 bilateral (not specified as recurrent)
    Bilateral NOS
  3 bilateral, recurrent

AHA: N-D, '85, 12

DEF: Hernia: protrusion of an abdominal organ or tissue through inguinal canal.

DEF: Indirect inguinal hernia: (external or oblique) leaves abdomen through deep inguinal ring, passes through inguinal canal lateral to the inferior epigastric artery.

DEF: Direct inguinal hernia: (internal) emerges between inferior epigastric artery and rectus muscle edge.

√4ᵗʰ Additional Digit Required   √5ᵗʰ
Unspecified Code   Other Specified Code   Manifestation Code   ▶◀ Revised Text   ● New Code   ▲ Revised Code Title

Digestive System

550.0–552.20

Inguinal Hernia

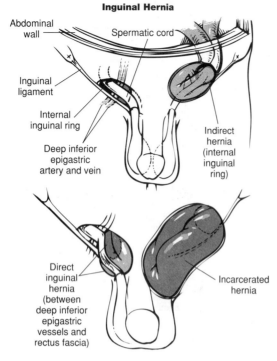

551.21 Incisional, with gangrene
Hernia:
postoperative
recurrent, ventral } specified as gangrenous

551.29 Other
Epigastric hernia specified as gangrenous

551.3 Diaphragmatic hernia with gangrene
Hernia:
hiatal (esophageal)
(sliding)
paraesophageal } specified as gangrenous
Thoracic stomach

EXCLUDES *congenital diaphragmatic hernia (756.6)*

551.8 Hernia of other specified sites, with gangrene
Any condition classifiable to 553.8 if specified as gangrenous

551.9 Hernia of unspecified site, with gangrene
Any condition classifiable to 553.9 if specified as gangrenous

✓4th **552 Other hernia of abdominal cavity, with obstruction, but without mention of gangrene**
EXCLUDES *that with mention of gangrene (551.0-551.9)*

✓5th **552.0 Femoral hernia with obstruction**
Femoral hernia specified as incarcerated, irreducible, strangulated, or causing obstruction

552.00 Unilateral or unspecified (not specified as recurrent)

552.01 Unilateral or unspecified, recurrent

552.02 Bilateral (not specified as recurrent)

552.03 Bilateral, recurrent

552.1 Umbilical hernia with obstruction
Parumbilical hernia specified as incarcerated, irreducible, strangulated, or causing obstruction

✓5th **552.2 Ventral hernia with obstruction**
Ventral hernia specified as incarcerated, irreducible, strangulated, or causing obstruction

552.20 Ventral, unspecified, with obstruction

§ ✓5th **550.0 Inguinal hernia, with gangrene**
Inguinal hernia with gangrene (and obstruction)

§ ✓5th **550.1 Inguinal hernia, with obstruction, without mention of gangrene**
Inguinal hernia with mention of incarceration, irreducibility, or strangulation

§ ✓5th **550.9 Inguinal hernia, without mention of obstruction or gangrene**
Inguinal hernia NOS
AHA: For code 550.91: ▶3Q, '03, 10;◀ 1Q, '03, 4

✓4th **551 Other hernia of abdominal cavity, with gangrene**
INCLUDES that with gangrene (and obstruction)

✓5th **551.0 Femoral hernia with gangrene**

551.00 Unilateral or unspecified (not specified as recurrent)
Femoral hernia NOS with gangrene

551.01 Unilateral or unspecified, recurrent

551.02 Bilateral (not specified as recurrent)

551.03 Bilateral, recurrent

551.1 Umbilical hernia with gangrene
Parumbilical hernia specified as gangrenous

✓5th **551.2 Ventral hernia with gangrene**

551.20 Ventral, unspecified, with gangrene

Femoral Hernia

Diaphragmatic Hernia

§ Requires fifth-digit. See category 550 for codes and definitions.

552.21 Incisional, with obstruction

Hernia:

postoperative ⎫
recurrent, ⎬ specified as incarcerated,
ventral ⎭ irreducible, strangulated, or causing obstruction

AHA: 3Q, '03, 11

552.29 Other

Epigastric hernia specified as incarcerated, irreducible, strangulated, or causing obstruction

552.3 Diaphragmatic hernia with obstruction

Hernia:

hiatal (esophageal) ⎫
(sliding) ⎬ specified as incarcerated,
paraesophageal ⎬ irreducible,
Thoracic stomach ⎭ strangulated, or causing obstruction

EXCLUDES congenital diaphragmatic hernia (756.6)

552.8 Hernia of other specified sites, with obstruction

Any condition classifiable to 553.8 if specified as incarcerated, irreducible, strangulated, or causing obstruction

AHA: ▶1Q, '04, 10◀

552.9 Hernia of unspecified site, with obstruction

Any condition classifiable to 553.9 if specified as incarcerated, irreducible, strangulated, or causing obstruction

✓4ᵗʰ **553 Other hernia of abdominal cavity without mention of obstruction or gangrene**

EXCLUDES the listed conditions with mention of:
gangrene (and obstruction) (551.0-551.9)
obstruction (552.0-552.9)

✓5ᵗʰ **553.0 Femoral hernia**

553.00 Unilateral or unspecified (not specified as recurrent)

Femoral hernia NOS

553.01 Unilateral or unspecified, recurrent

553.02 Bilateral (not specified as recurrent)

553.03 Bilateral, recurrent

553.1 Umbilical hernia

Parumbilical hernia

✓5ᵗʰ **553.2 Ventral hernia**

553.20 Ventral, unspecified

AHA: 3Q, '03, 6

553.21 Incisional

Hernia: Hernia:
postoperative recurrent, ventral

AHA: 3Q, '03, 6

553.29 Other

Hernia: Hernia:
epigastric spigelian

553.3 Diaphragmatic hernia

Hernia:
hiatal (esophageal) (sliding)
paraesophageal
Thoracic stomach

EXCLUDES congenital:
diaphragmatic hernia (756.6)
hiatal hernia (750.6)
esophagocele (530.6)

AHA: 2Q, '01, 6; 1Q, '00, 6

553.8 Hernia of other specified sites

Hernia: Hernia:
ischiatic retroperitoneal
ischiorectal sciatic
lumbar Other abdominal
obturator hernia of specified
pudendal site

EXCLUDES vaginal enterocele (618.6)

553.9 Hernia of unspecified site

Enterocele Hernia:
Epiplocele intestinal
Hernia: intra-abdominal
NOS Rupture (nontraumatic)
interstitial Sarcoepiplocele

NONINFECTIOUS ENTERITIS AND COLITIS (555-558)

✓4ᵗʰ **555 Regional enteritis**

INCLUDES Crohn's disease
Granulomatous enteritis

EXCLUDES ulcerative colitis (556)

DEF: Inflammation of intestine; classified to site.

555.0 Small intestine

Ileitis: Regional enteritis or
regional Crohn's disease of:
segmental duodenum
terminal ileum
jejunum

555.1 Large intestine

Colitis: Regional enteritis or
granulmatous Crohn's disease of:
regional colon
transmural large bowel
rectum

AHA: 3Q, '99, 8

555.2 Small intestine with large intestine

Regional ileocolitis

AHA: 1Q, '03, 18

555.9 Unspecified site

Crohn's disease NOS Regional enteritis NOS

AHA: 3Q, '99, 8; 4Q, '97, 42; 2Q, '97, 3

✓4ᵗʰ **556 Ulcerative colitis**

AHA: 3Q, '99, 8

DEF: Chronic inflammation of mucosal lining of intestinal tract; may be single area or entire colon.

556.0 Ulcerative (chronic) enterocolitis

556.1 Ulcerative (chronic) ileocolitis

556.2 Ulcerative (chronic) proctitis

556.3 Ulcerative (chronic) proctosigmoiditis

556.4 Pseudopolyposis of colon

556.5 Left-sided ulcerative (chronic) colitis

556.6 Universal ulcerative (chronic) colitis

Pancolitis

556.8 Other ulcerative colitis

556.9 Ulcerative colitis, unspecified

Ulcerative enteritis NOS

AHA: 1Q, '03, 10

✓4ᵗʰ **557 Vascular insufficiency of intestine**

EXCLUDES necrotizing enterocolitis of the newborn (777.5)

DEF: Inadequacy of intestinal vessels.

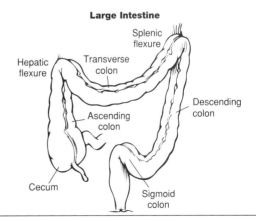

Large Intestine

Splenic flexure
Hepatic flexure
Transverse colon
Descending colon
Ascending colon
Cecum
Sigmoid colon

✓4ᵗʰ Additional Digit Required | Unspecified Code | Other Specified Code | Manifestation Code | ▶◀ Revised Text | ● New Code | ▲ Revised Code Title
✓5ᵗʰ

2005 ICD•9•CM | October 2004 • Volume 1 — 151

Digestive System

557.0–560.9

557.0   **Acute vascular insufficiency of intestine**
Acute:
     hemorrhagic enterocolitis
     ischemic colitis, enteritis, or enterocolitis
     massive necrosis of intestine
Bowel infarction
Embolism of mesenteric artery
Fulminant enterocolitis
Hemorrhagic necrosis of intestine
Infarction of appendices epiploicae
Intestinal gangrene
Intestinal infarction (acute) (agnogenic)
     (hemorrhagic) (nonocclusive)
Mesenteric infarction (embolic) (thrombotic)
Necrosis of intestine
Terminal hemorrhagic enteropathy
Thrombosis of mesenteric artery
AHA: 4Q, '01, 53

557.1   **Chronic vascular insufficiency of intestine**
Angina, abdominal
Chronic ischemic colitis, enteritis, or enterocolitis
Ischemic stricture of intestine
Mesenteric:
     angina
     artery syndrome (superior)
     vascular insufficiency
AHA: 3Q, '96, 9; 4Q, '90, 4; N-D, '86, 11; N-D, '84, 7

557.9   **Unspecified vascular insufficiency of intestine**
Alimentary pain due to vascular insufficiency
Ischemic colitis, enteritis, or enterocolitis NOS

√4ᵗʰ **558**   **Other and unspecified noninfectious gastroenteritis and colitis**
     EXCLUDES   *infectious:*
         colitis, enteritis, or gastroenteritis (009.0-009.1)
         diarrhea (009.2-009.3)

558.1   **Gastroenteritis and colitis due to radiation**
Radiation enterocolitis

558.2   **Toxic gastroenteritis and colitis**
Use additional E code, if desired, to identify cause

558.3   **Allergic gastroenteritis and colitis**
Use additional code to identify type of food allergy (V15.01-V15.05)
AHA: 1Q, '03, 12; 4Q, '00, 42

DEF: True immunoglobulin E (IgE)-mediated allergic reaction of the lining of the stomach, intestines, or colon to food proteins; causes nausea, vomiting, diarrhea, and abdominal cramping.

558.9   **Other and unspecified noninfectious gastroenteritis and colitis**

Colitis ⎫
Enteritis ⎪
Gastroenteritis ⎬ NOS, dietetic, or
Ileitis ⎪ noninfectious
Jejunitis ⎪
Sigmoiditis ⎭

AHA: 3Q, '99, 4, 6; N-D, '87, 7

Volvulus, Diverticulitis

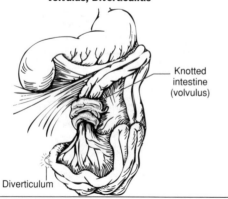

Knotted intestine (volvulus)

Diverticulum

OTHER DISEASES OF INTESTINES AND PERITONEUM (560-569)

√4ᵗʰ **560**   **Intestinal obstruction without mention of hernia**
     EXCLUDES   *duodenum (537.2-537.3)*
         inguinal hernia with obstruction (550.1)
         intestinal obstruction complicating hernia
            (552.0-552.9)
         mesenteric:
            embolism (557.0)
            infarction (557.0)
            thrombosis (557.0)
         neonatal intestinal obstruction (277.01, 777.1-
            777.2, 777.4)

560.0   **Intussusception**
Intussusception (colon) (intestine) (rectum)
Invagination of intestine or colon
     EXCLUDES   *intussusception of appendix (543.9)*
AHA: 4Q, '98, 82

DEF: Prolapse of a bowel section into adjacent section; occurs primarily in children; symptoms include paroxysmal pain, vomiting, presence of lower abdominal tumor and blood, and mucous passage from rectum.

560.1   **Paralytic ileus**
Adynamic ileus
Ileus (of intestine) (of bowel) (of colon)
Paralysis of intestine or colon
     EXCLUDES   *gallstone ileus (560.31)*
AHA: J-F, '87, 13

DEF: Obstruction of ileus due to inhibited bowel motility.

560.2   **Volvulus**
Knotting ⎫
Strangulation ⎪
Torsion ⎬ of intestine, bowel, or colon
Twist ⎭

DEF: Entanglement of bowel; causes obstruction; may compromise bowel circulation.

√5ᵗʰ **560.3**   **Impaction of intestine**
     560.30 Impaction of intestine, unspecified
         Impaction of colon
     560.31 Gallstone ileus
         Obstruction of intestine by gallstone
     560.39 Other
         Concretion of intestine   Fecal impaction
         Enterolith
         AHA: 4Q, '98, 38

√5ᵗʰ **560.8**   **Other specified intestinal obstruction**
     560.81 Intestinal or peritoneal adhesions with obstruction (postoperative) (postinfection)
         EXCLUDES   *adhesions without obstruction (568.0)*
         AHA: 4Q, '95, 55; 3Q, '95, 6; N-D, '87, 9

         DEF: Obstruction of peritoneum or intestine due to abnormal union of tissues.

     560.89 Other
         ▶Acute pseudo-obstruction of intestine◀
         Mural thickening causing obstruction
         EXCLUDES   *ischemic stricture of intestine (557.1)*
         AHA: 2Q, '97, 3; 1Q, '88, 6

560.9   **Unspecified intestinal obstruction**
Enterostenosis
Obstruction ⎫
Occlusion ⎪
Stenosis ⎬ of intestine or colon
Stricture ⎭
     EXCLUDES   *congenital stricture or stenosis of intestine (751.1-751.2)*

N Newborn Age: 0   P Pediatric Age: 0-17   M Maternity Age: 12-55   A Adult Age: 15-124   MSP Medicare Secondary Payer

Digestive System

✓4th 562 Diverticula of intestine

Use additional code to identify any associated:
peritonitis (567.0-567.9)

> **EXCLUDES**   congenital diverticulum of colon (751.5)
> diverticulum of appendix (543.9)
> Meckel's diverticulum (751.0)

AHA: 4Q, '91, 25; J-F, '85, 1

✓5th 562.0 Small intestine

562.00 Diverticulosis of small intestine (without mention of hemorrhage)

Diverticulosis:
duodenum ⎫
ileum   ⎬ without mention of
jejunum ⎭ diverticulitis

DEF: Saclike herniations of mucous lining of small intestine.

562.01 Diverticulitis of small intestine (without mention of hemorrhage)

Diverticulitis (with diverticulosis):
duodenum
ileum
jejunum
small intestine

DEF: Inflamed saclike herniations of mucous lining of small intestine.

562.02 Diverticulosis of small intestine with hemorrhage

562.03 Diverticulitis of small intestine with hemorrhage

✓5th 562.1 Colon

562.10 Diverticulosis of colon (without mention of hemorrhage)

Diverticulosis:
  NOS   ⎫ without mention
  intestine (large) ⎬ of
Diverticular disease ⎭ diverticulitis
  (colon)

AHA: 3Q, '02, 15; 4Q, '90, 21; J-F, '85, 5

DEF: Saclike herniations of mucous lining of large intestine

562.11 Diverticulitis of colon (without mention of hemorrhage)

Diverticulitis (with diverticulosis):
  NOS   intestine (large)
  colon

AHA: 1Q, '96, 14; J-F, '85, 5

DEF: Inflamed saclike herniations of mucosal lining of large intestine.

562.12 Diverticulosis of colon with hemorrhage

562.13 Diverticulitis of colon with hemorrhage

✓4th 564 Functional digestive disorders, not elsewhere classified

> **EXCLUDES**   functional disorders of stomach (536.0-536.9)
> those specified as psychogenic (306.4)

✓5th 564.0 Constipation

AHA: 4Q, '01, 45

564.00 Constipation, unspecified

564.01 Slow transit constipation

DEF: Delay in the transit of fecal material through the colon secondary to smooth muscle dysfunction or decreased peristaltic contractions along the colon: also called colonic inertia or delayed transit.

564.02 Outlet dysfunction constipation

DEF: Failure to relax the paradoxical contractions of the striated pelvic floor muscles during the attempted defecation.

564.09 Other constipation

564.1 Irritable bowel syndrome

Irritable colon   Spastic colon

AHA: 1Q, '88, 6

DEF: Functional gastrointestinal disorder (FGID); symptoms following meals include diarrhea, constipation, abdominal pain; other symptoms include bloating, gas, distended abdomen, nausea, vomiting, appetite loss, emotional distress, and depression.

564.2 Postgastric surgery syndromes

Dumping syndrome   Postgastrectomy syndrome
Jejunal syndrome   Postvagotomy syndrome

> **EXCLUDES**   malnutrition following gastrointestinal surgery (579.3)
> postgastrojejunostomy ulcer (534.0-534.9)

AHA: 1Q, '95, 11

564.3 Vomiting following gastrointestinal surgery

Vomiting (bilious) following gastrointestinal surgery

564.4 Other postoperative functional disorders

Diarrhea following gastrointestinal surgery

> **EXCLUDES**   colostomy and enterostomy complications (569.60-569.69)

564.5 Functional diarrhea

> **EXCLUDES**   diarrhea:
> NOS (787.91)
> psychogenic (306.4)

DEF: Diarrhea with no detectable organic cause.

564.6 Anal spasm

Proctalgia fugax

564.7 Megacolon, other than Hirschsprung's

Dilatation of colon

> **EXCLUDES**   megacolon:
> congenital [Hirschsprung's] (751.3)
> toxic (556)

DEF: Enlarged colon; congenital or acquired; can occur acutely or become chronic.

✓5th 564.8 Other specified functional disorders of intestine

> **EXCLUDES**   malabsorption (579.0-579.9)

AHA: 1Q, '88, 6

Anal Fistula and Abscess

Rectum and Anus

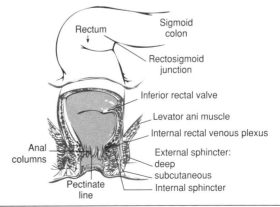

✓4th ✓5th Additional Digit Required   Unspecified Code   Other Specified Code   Manifestation Code   ▶◀ Revised Text   ● New Code   ▲ Revised Code Title

2005 ICD•9•CM   Volume 1 — 153

Digestive System

564.81–569.60

564.81 Neurogenic bowel

AHA: 1Q, '01, 12; 4Q, '98, 45

DEF: Disorder of bowel due to spinal cord lesion above conus medullaris; symptoms include precipitous micturition, nocturia, catheter intolerance, headache, sweating, nasal obstruction and spastic contractions.

564.89 Other functional disorders of intestine

Atony of colon

DEF: Absence of normal bowel tone or strength.

564.9 Unspecified functional disorder of intestine

√4th **565 Anal fissure and fistula**

565.0 Anal fissure

Tear of anus, nontraumatic

EXCLUDES   traumatic (863.89, 863.99)

DEF: Ulceration of cleft at anal mucosa; causes pain, itching, bleeding, infection, and sphincter spasm; may occur with hemorrhoids.

565.1 Anal fistula

Fistula: Fistula:

anorectal   rectum to skin

rectal

EXCLUDES   fistula of rectum to internal organs—
see Alphabetic Index
ischiorectal fistula (566)
rectovaginal fistula (619.1)

DEF: Abnormal opening on cutaneous surface near anus; may lack connection with rectum.

566 Abscess of anal and rectal regions

Abscess: Cellulitis:

ischiorectal   anal

perianal   perirectal

perirectal   rectal

           Ischiorectal fistula

√4th **567 Peritonitis**

EXCLUDES   peritonitis:
benign paroxysmal (277.3)
pelvic, female (614.5, 614.7)
periodic familial (277.3)
puerperal (670)
with or following:
abortion (634-638 with .0, 639.0)
appendicitis (540.0-540.1)
ectopic or molar pregnancy (639.0)

DEF: Inflammation of the peritoneal cavity.

567.0 Peritonitis in infectious diseases classified elsewhere

Code first underlying disease

EXCLUDES   peritonitis:
gonococcal (098.86)
syphilitic (095.2)
tuberculous (014.0)

567.1 Pneumococcal peritonitis

567.2 Other suppurative peritonitis

Abscess (of):   Abscess (of):

abdominopelvic   subhepatic

mesenteric   subphrenic

omentum   Peritonitis (acute):

peritoneum   general

retrocecal   pelvic, male

retroperitoneal   subphrenic

subdiaphragmatic   suppurative

AHA: 2Q, '01, 11, 12; 3Q, '99, 9; 2Q, '98, 19

567.8 Other specified peritonitis

Chronic proliferative   Peritonitis due to:

peritonitis   bile

Fat necrosis of peritoneum   urine

Mesenteric saponification

567.9 Unspecified peritonitis

Peritonitis: Peritonitis:

NOS   of unspecified cause

AHA: ▶1Q, '04, 10◀

√4th **568 Other disorders of peritoneum**

568.0 Peritoneal adhesions (postoperative) (postinfection)

Adhesions (of):   Adhesions (of):

abdominal (wall)   mesenteric

diaphragm   omentum

intestine   stomach

male pelvis   Adhesive bands

EXCLUDES   adhesions:
pelvic, female (614.6)
with obstruction:
duodenum (537.3)
intestine (560.81)

AHA: 3Q, '03, 7, 11; 4Q, '95, 55; 3Q, '95, 7; S-O, '85, 11

DEF: Abnormal union of tissues in peritoneum.

√5th **568.8 Other specified disorders of peritoneum**

568.81 Hemoperitoneum (nontraumatic)

568.82 Peritoneal effusion (chronic)

EXCLUDES   ascites NOS (789.5)

DEF: Persistent leakage of fluid within peritoneal cavity.

568.89 Other

Peritoneal: Peritoneal:

cyst   granuloma

568.9 Unspecified disorder of peritoneum

√4th **569 Other disorders of intestine**

569.0 Anal and rectal polyp

Anal and rectal polyp NOS

EXCLUDES   adenomatous anal and rectal polyp (211.4)

569.1 Rectal prolapse

Procidentia:

anus (sphincter)

rectum (sphincter)

Proctoptosis

Prolapse:

anal canal

rectal mucosa

EXCLUDES   prolapsed hemorrhoids (455.2, 455.5)

569.2 Stenosis of rectum and anus

Stricture of anus (sphincter)

569.3 Hemorrhage of rectum and anus

EXCLUDES   gastrointestinal bleeding NOS (578.9)
melena (578.1)

√5th **569.4 Other specified disorders of rectum and anus**

569.41 Ulcer of anus and rectum

Solitary ulcer ⎫ of anus (sphincter) or

Stercoral ulcer ⎬ rectum (sphincter)

569.42 Anal or rectal pain

AHA: 1Q, '03, 8; 1Q, '96, 13

569.49 Other

Granuloma ⎫ of rectum (sphincter)

Rupture ⎬

Hypertrophy of anal papillae

Proctitis NOS

EXCLUDES   fistula of rectum to:
internal organs—see
Alphabetic Index
skin (565.1)
hemorrhoids (455.0-455.9)
incontinence of sphincter ani (787.6)

569.5 Abscess of intestine

EXCLUDES   appendiceal abscess (540.1)

√5th **569.6 Colostomy and enterostomy complications**

AHA: 4Q, '95, 58

DEF: Complication in a surgically created opening, from intestine to surface skin.

569.60 Colostomy and enterostomy complication, unspecified

569.61 Infection of colostomy or enterostomy
Use additional code to identify organism
(041.00-041.9)
Use additional code to specify type of
infection, such as:
abscess or cellulitis of abdomen (682.2)
septicemia (038.0-038.9)

569.62 Mechanical complication of colostomy and enterostomy
Malfunction of colostomy and enterostomy
AHA: 1Q, '03, 10; 4Q, '98, 44

569.69 Other complication
Fistula
Hernia
Prolapse
AHA: 3Q, '98, 16

√5ᵗʰ **569.8 Other specified disorder of intestine**
AHA: 4Q, '91, 25

569.81 Fistula of intestine, excluding rectum and anus
Fistula: Fistula:
abdominal wall   enteroenteric
enterocolic   ileorectal
EXCLUDES *fistula of intestine to internal organs—see Alphabetic Index*
persistent postoperative fistula (998.6)
AHA: 3Q, '99, 8

569.82 Ulceration of intestine
Primary ulcer of intestine
Ulceration of colon
EXCLUDES *that with perforation (569.83)*

569.83 Perforation of intestine

569.84 Angiodysplasia of intestine (without mention of hemorrhage)
AHA: 3Q, '96, 10; 4Q, '90, 4; 4Q, '90, 21
DEF: Small vascular abnormalities of the intestinal tract without bleeding problems.

569.85 Angiodysplasia of intestine with hemorrhage
AHA: 3Q, '96, 9
DEF: Small vascular abnormalities of the intestinal tract with bleeding problems.

569.86 Dieulafoy lesion (hemorrhagic) of intestine
AHA: 4Q, '02, 60-61

569.89 Other
Enteroptosis
Granuloma } of intestine
Prolapse
Pericolitis
Perisigmoiditis
Visceroptosis
EXCLUDES *gangrene of intestine, mesentery, or omentum (557.0)*
hemorrhage of intestine NOS (578.9)
obstruction of intestine (560.0-560.9)
AHA: 3Q, '96, 9

569.9 Unspecified disorder of intestine

OTHER DISEASES OF DIGESTIVE SYSTEM (570-579)

570 Acute and subacute necrosis of liver
Acute hepatic failure
Acute or subacute hepatitis, not specified as infective
Necrosis of liver (acute) (diffuse) (massive) (subacute)
Parenchymatous degeneration of liver
Yellow atrophy (liver) (acute) (subacute)
EXCLUDES *icterus gravis of newborn (773.0-773.2)*
serum hepatitis (070.2-070.3)
that with:
abortion (634-638 with .7, 639.8)
ectopic or molar pregnancy (639.8)
pregnancy, childbirth, or the puerperium (646.7)
viral hepatitis (070.0-070.9)
AHA: 1Q, '00, 22

√4ᵗʰ **571 Chronic liver disease and cirrhosis**

571.0 Alcoholic fatty liver 🄰

571.1 Acute alcoholic hepatitis 🄰
Acute alcoholic liver disease
AHA: 2Q, '02, 4

571.2 Alcoholic cirrhosis of liver 🄰
Florid cirrhosis   Laennec's cirrhosis (alcoholic)
AHA: 2Q, '02, 4; 1Q, '02, 3; N-D, '85, 14
DEF: Fibrosis and dysfunction, of liver; due to alcoholic liver disease.

571.3 Alcoholic liver damage, unspecified 🄰

√5ᵗʰ **571.4 Chronic hepatitis**
EXCLUDES *viral hepatitis (acute) (chronic) (070.0-070.9)*

571.40 Chronic hepatitis, unspecified
571.41 Chronic persistent hepatitis
571.49 Other
Chronic hepatitis: Recurrent hepatitis
active
aggressive
AHA: 3Q, '99, 19; N-D, '85, 14

571.5 Cirrhosis of liver without mention of alcohol
Cirrhosis of liver: Cirrhosis of liver:
NOS   postnecrotic
cryptogenic   Healed yellow atrophy
macronodular   (liver)
micronodular   Portal cirrhosis
posthepatitic
DEF: Fibrosis and dysfunction of liver; not alcohol related.

571.6 Biliary cirrhosis
Chronic nonsuppurative destructive cholangitis
Cirrhosis:
cholangitic
cholestatic

571.8 Other chronic nonalcoholic liver disease
Chronic yellow atrophy (liver)
Fatty liver, without mention of alcohol
AHA: 2Q, '96, 12

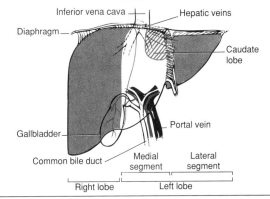

Liver

Inferior vena cava
Hepatic veins
Diaphragm
Caudate lobe
Portal vein
Gallbladder
Common bile duct
Medial segment
Lateral segment
Right lobe
Left lobe

▨4ᵗʰ Additional Digit Required   Unspecified Code   Other Specified Code   Manifestation Code   ▶◀ Revised Text   ● New Code   ▲ Revised Code Title

2005 ICD•9•CM   **Volume 1 — 155**

Digestive System

571.9–574.8

571.9 Unspecified chronic liver disease without mention of alcohol

✓4ᵗʰ 572 Liver abscess and sequelae of chronic liver disease

572.0 Abscess of liver

> **EXCLUDES** amebic liver abscess (006.3)

572.1 Portal pyemia

Phlebitis of portal vein   Pylephlebitis
Portal thrombophlebitis   Pylethrombophlebitis
DEF: Inflammation of portal vein or branches; may be due to intestinal disease; symptoms include fever, chills, jaundice, sweating, and abscess in various body parts.

572.2 Hepatic coma

Hepatic encephalopathy
Hepatocerebral intoxication
Portal-systemic encephalopathy
AHA: 1Q, '02, 3; 3Q, '95, 14

572.3 Portal hypertension

DEF: Abnormally high blood pressure in the portal vein.

572.4 Hepatorenal syndrome

> **EXCLUDES** that following delivery (674.8)

AHA: 3Q, '93, 15

DEF: Hepatic and renal failure characterized by cirrhosis with ascites or obstructive jaundice, oliguria, and low sodium concentration.

572.8 Other sequelae of chronic liver disease

✓4ᵗʰ 573 Other disorders of liver

> **EXCLUDES** amyloid or lardaceous degeneration of liver (277.3)
> congenital cystic disease of liver (751.62)
> glycogen infiltration of liver (271.0)
> hepatomegaly NOS (789.1)
> portal vein obstruction (452)

573.0 Chronic passive congestion of liver

DEF: Blood accumulation in liver tissue.

573.1 Hepatitis in viral diseases classified elsewhere

Code first underlying disease as:
Coxsackie virus disease (074.8)
cytomegalic inclusion virus disease (078.5)
infectious mononucleosis (075)

> **EXCLUDES** hepatitis (in):
> mumps (072.71)
> viral (070.0-070.9)
> yellow fever (060.0-060.9)

573.2 Hepatitis in other infectious diseases classified elsewhere

Code first underlying disease, as:
malaria (084.9)

> **EXCLUDES** hepatitis in:
> late syphilis (095.3)
> secondary syphilis (091.62)
> toxoplasmosis (130.5)

Gallbladder and Bile Ducts

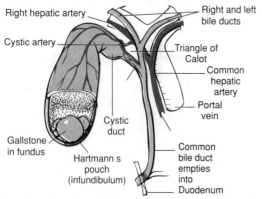

Right hepatic artery
Cystic artery
Gallstone in fundus
Cystic duct
Hartmann's pouch (infundibulum)
Right and left bile ducts
Triangle of Calot
Common hepatic artery
Portal vein
Common bile duct empties into Duodenum

573.3 Hepatitis, unspecified

Toxic (noninfectious) hepatitis
Use additional E code to identify cause
AHA: 3Q, '98, 3, 4; 4Q, '90, 26

573.4 Hepatic infarction

573.8 Other specified disorders of liver

Hepatoptosis

573.9 Unspecified disorder of liver

✓4ᵗʰ 574 Cholelithiasis

The following fifth-digit subclassification is for use with category 574:

0 without mention of obstruction
1 with obstruction

✓5ᵗʰ 574.0 Calculus of gallbladder with acute cholecystitis

Biliary calculus
Calculus of cystic duct   } with acute cholecystitis
Cholelithiasis

Any condition classifiable to 574.2 with acute cholecystitis
AHA: 4Q, '96, 32

✓5ᵗʰ 574.1 Calculus of gallbladder with other cholecystitis

Biliary calculus
Calculus of cystic duct   } with cholecystitis
Cholelithiasis

Cholecystitis with cholelithiasis NOS
Any condition classifiable to 574.2 with cholecystitis (chronic)
AHA: 3Q, '99, 9; 4Q, '96, 32, 69; 2Q, '96, 13; For code 574.10: 1Q, '03, 5

✓5ᵗʰ 574.2 Calculus of gallbladder without mention of cholecystitis

Biliary: Cholelithiasis NOS
calculus NOS   Colic (recurrent) of
colic NOS   gallbladder
Calculus of cystic duct Gallstone (impacted)
AHA: For code 574.20: 1Q, '88, 14

✓5ᵗʰ 574.3 Calculus of bile duct with acute cholecystitis

Calculus of bile duct [any] } with acute cholecystitis
Choledocholithiasis

Any condition classifiable to 574.5 with acute cholecystitis

✓5ᵗʰ 574.4 Calculus of bile duct with other cholecystitis

Calculus of bile duct [any] } with cholecystitis (chronic)
Choledocholithiasis

Any condition classifiable to 574.5 with cholecystitis (chronic)

✓5ᵗʰ 574.5 Calculus of bile duct without mention of cholecystitis

Calculus of: Choledocholithiasis
bile duct [any]   Hepatic:
common duct   colic (recurrent)
hepatic duct   lithiasis
AHA: 3Q, '94, 11

✓5ᵗʰ 574.6 Calculus of gallbladder and bile duct with acute cholecystitis

Any condition classifiable to 574.0 and 574.3
AHA: 4Q, '96, 32

✓5ᵗʰ 574.7 Calculus of gallbladder and bile duct with other cholecystitis

Any condition classifiable to 574.1 and 574.4
AHA: 4Q, '96, 32

✓5ᵗʰ 574.8 Calculus of gallbladder and bile duct with acute and chronic cholecystitis

Any condition classifiable to 574.6 and 574.7
AHA: 4Q, '96, 32

N Newborn Age: 0   P Pediatric Age: 0-17   M Maternity Age: 12-55   A Adult Age: 15-124   MSP Medicare Secondary Payer

√5ᵗʰ **574.9 Calculus of gallbladder and bile duct without cholecystitis**
> Any condition classifiable to 574.2 and 574.5
> **AHA:** 4Q, '96, 32

√4ᵗʰ **575 Other disorders of gallbladder**

575.0 Acute cholecystitis
> Abscess of gallbladder
> Angiocholecystitis
> Cholecystitis:
>> emphysematous (acute)
>> gangrenous   } without mention of calculus
>> suppurative
> Empyema of gallbladder
> Gangrene of gallbladder

> **EXCLUDES**   *that with:*
>> *acute and chronic cholecystitis (575.12)*
>> *choledocholithiasis (574.3)*
>> *choledocholithiasis and cholelithiasis (574.6)*
>> *cholelithiasis (574.0)*

> **AHA:** 3Q, '91, 17

√5ᵗʰ **575.1 Other cholecystitis**
> Cholecystitis:
>> NOS   } without mention of calculus
>> chronic

> **EXCLUDES**   *that with:*
>> *choledocholithiasis (574.4)*
>> *choledocholithiasis and cholelithiasis (574.8)*
>> *cholelithiasis (574.1)*

> **AHA:** 4Q, '96, 32

575.10 Cholecystitis, unspecified
> Cholecystitis NOS

575.11 Chronic cholecystitis

575.12 Acute and chronic cholecystitis
> **AHA:** 4Q, '97, 52; 4Q, '96, 32

575.2 Obstruction of gallbladder
> Occlusion
> Stenosis   } of cystic duct or gallbladder without mention of calculus
> Stricture

> **EXCLUDES**   *that with calculus (574.0-574.2 with fifth-digit 1)*

575.3 Hydrops of gallbladder
> Mucocele of gallbladder
> **AHA:** 2Q, '89, 13

> DEF: Serous fluid accumulation in bladder.

575.4 Perforation of gallbladder
> Rupture of cystic duct or gallbladder

575.5 Fistula of gallbladder
> Fistula: Fistula:
>> cholecystoduodenal   cholecystoenteric

575.6 Cholesterolosis of gallbladder
> Strawberry gallbladder
> **AHA:** 4Q, '90, 17

> DEF: Cholesterol deposits in gallbladder tissue.

575.8 Other specified disorders of gallbladder
> Adhesions
> Atrophy
> Cyst
> Hypertrophy   } (of) cystic duct or gallbladder
> Nonfunctioning
> Ulcer
>
> Biliary dyskinesia

> **EXCLUDES**   *Hartmann's pouch of intestine (V44.3)*
>> *nonvisualization of gallbladder (793.3)*

> **AHA:** 4Q, '90, 26; 2Q, '89, 13

575.9 Unspecified disorder of gallbladder

√4ᵗʰ **576 Other disorders of biliary tract**
> **EXCLUDES**   *that involving the:*
>> *cystic duct (575.0-575.9)*
>> *gallbladder (575.0-575.9)*

576.0 Postcholecystectomy syndrome
> **AHA:** 1Q, '88, 10

> DEF: Jaundice or abdominal pain following cholecystectomy.

576.1 Cholangitis
> Cholangitis: Cholangitis:
>> NOS   recurrent
>> acute   sclerosing
>> ascending   secondary
>> chronic   stenosing
>> primary   suppurative

> **AHA:** 2Q, '99, 13

576.2 Obstruction of bile duct
> Occlusion   } of bile duct, except cystic
> Stenosis   duct, without mention
> Stricture   of calculus

> **EXCLUDES**   *congenital (751.61)*
>> *that with calculus (574.3-574.5 with fifth-digit 1)*

> **AHA:** ▶3Q, '03. 17-18;◄ 1Q, '01, 8; 2Q, '99, 13

576.3 Perforation of bile duct
> Rupture of bile duct, except cystic duct

576.4 Fistula of bile duct
> Choledochoduodenal fistula

576.5 Spasm of sphincter of Oddi

576.8 Other specified disorders of biliary tract
> Adhesions
> Atrophy
> Cyst
> Hypertrophy   } of bile duct [any]
> Stasis
> Ulcer

> **EXCLUDES**   *congenital choledochal cyst (751.69)*
> **AHA:** ▶3Q, '03, 17;◄ 2Q, '99, 14

576.9 Unspecified disorder of biliary tract

√4ᵗʰ **577 Diseases of pancreas**

577.0 Acute pancreatitis
> Abscess of pancreas   Pancreatitis:
> Necrosis of pancreas: acute (recurrent)
>> acute   apoplectic
>> infective   hemorrhagic
> Pancreatitis: subacute
>> NOS   suppurative

> **EXCLUDES**   *mumps pancreatitis (072.3)*
> **AHA:** 3Q, '99, 9; 2Q, '98, 19; 2Q, '96, 13; 2Q, '89, 9

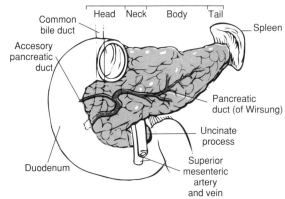

Pancreas

Common bile duct — Head | Neck | Body | Tail — Spleen
Accesory pancreatic duct
Duodenum
Pancreatic duct (of Wirsung)
Uncinate process
Superior mesenteric artery and vein

√4ᵗʰ √5ᵗʰ Additional Digit Required   Unspecified Code   Other Specified Code   Manifestation Code   ▶◀ Revised Text   ● New Code   ▲ Revised Code Title

2005 ICD•9•CM   **February 2004 • Volume 1 — 157**

Digestive System

577.1 Chronic pancreatitis

Chronic pancreatitis: Pancreatitis:
  NOS   painless
  infectious   recurrent
  interstitial   relapsing

AHA: 1Q, '01, 8; 2Q, '96, 13; 3Q, '94, 11

577.2 Cyst and pseudocyst of pancreas

577.8 Other specified diseases of pancreas

Atrophy ⎫
Calculus ⎪
Cirrhosis ⎬ of pancreas
Fibrosis ⎭

Pancreatic: Pancreatic:
  infantilism   necrosis:
  necrosis: fat
    NOS   Pancreatolithiasis
    aseptic

EXCLUDES   fibrocystic disease of pancreas (277.00-
           277.09)
           islet cell tumor of pancreas (211.7)
           pancreatic steatorrhea (579.4)

AHA: 1Q, '01, 8

577.9 Unspecified disease of pancreas

✓4ᵗʰ **578 Gastrointestinal hemorrhage**

EXCLUDES   that with mention of:
           angiodysplasia of stomach and duodenum
             (537.83)
           angiodysplasia of intestine (569.85)
           diverticulitis, intestine:
             large (562.13)
             small (562.03)
           diverticulosis, intestine:
             large (562.12)
             small (562.02)
           gastritis and duodenitis (535.0-535.6)
           ulcer:
             duodenal, gastric, gastrojejuunal or peptic
               (531.00-534.91)

AHA: 2Q, '92, 9; 4Q, '90, 20

578.0 Hematemesis
Vomiting of blood
AHA: 2Q, '02, 4

578.1 Blood in stool
Melena
EXCLUDES   melena of the newborn (772.4, 777.3)
           occult blood (792.1)

AHA: 2Q, '92, 8

578.9 Hemorrhage of gastrointestinal tract, unspecified
Gastric hemorrhage
Intestinal hemorrhage
AHA: N-D, '86, 9

✓4ᵗʰ **579 Intestinal malabsorption**

579.0 Celiac disease

Celiac: Gee (-Herter) disease
  crisis   Gluten enteropathy
  infantilism   Idiopathic steatorrhea
  rickets   Nontropical sprue

DEF: Malabsorption syndrome due to gluten consumption;
symptoms include fetid, bulky, frothy, oily stools; distended
abdomen, gas, weight loss, asthenia, electrolyte depletion and
vitamin B, D and K deficiency.

579.1 Tropical sprue
Sprue: Tropical steatorrhea
  NOS
  tropical

DEF: Diarrhea, occurs in tropics; may be due to enteric infection
and malnutrition.

579.2 Blind loop syndrome
Postoperative blind loop syndrome

DEF: Obstruction or impaired passage in small intestine due to
alterations, from strictures or surgery; causes stasis, abnormal
bacterial flora, diarrhea, weight loss, multiple vitamin deficiency,
and megaloblastic anemia.

579.3 Other and unspecified postsurgical nonabsorption

Hypoglycemia ⎫ following gastrointestinal
Malnutrition ⎭ surgery

AHA: ►4Q, '03, 104◄

579.4 Pancreatic steatorrhea
DEF: Excess fat in feces due to absence of pancreatic juice in
intestine.

579.8 Other specified intestinal malabsorption
Enteropathy: Steatorrhea (chronic)
  exudative
  protein-losing
AHA: 1Q, '88, 6

579.9 Unspecified intestinal malabsorption
Malabsorption syndrome NOS

Kidney

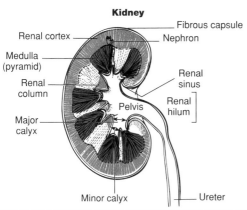

10. DISEASES OF THE GENITOURINARY SYSTEM (580-629)

NEPHRITIS, NEPHROTIC SYNDROME, AND NEPHROSIS (580-589)

EXCLUDES hypertensive renal disease (403.00-403.91)

√4ᵗʰ 580 Acute glomerulonephritis

INCLUDES acute nephritis

DEF: Acute, severe inflammation in tuft of capillaries that filter the kidneys.

580.0 With lesion of proliferative glomerulonephritis
Acute (diffuse) proliferative glomerulonephritis
Acute poststreptococcal glomerulonephritis

580.4 With lesion of rapidly progressive glomerulonephritis
Acute nephritis with lesion of necrotizing glomerulitis

DEF: Acute glomerulonephritis; progresses to ESRD with diffuse epithelial proliferation.

√5ᵗʰ 580.8 With other specified pathological lesion in kidney

580.81 Acute glomerulonephritis in diseases classified elsewhere
Code first underlying disease, as:
infectious hepatitis (070.0-070.9)
mumps (072.79)
subacute bacterial endocarditis (421.0)
typhoid fever (002.0)

580.89 Other
Glomerulonephritis, acute, with lesion of:
exudative nephritis
interstitial (diffuse) (focal) nephritis

580.9 Acute glomerulonephritis with unspecified pathological lesion in kidney
Glomerulonephritis:
NOS
hemorrhagic   } specified as acute
Nephritis
Nephropathy

Nephron

Nephron diagram labels

√4ᵗʰ 581 Nephrotic syndrome

DEF: Disease process marked by symptoms such as; extensive edema, notable proteinuria, hypoalbuminemia, and susceptibility to intercurrent infections.

581.0 With lesion of proliferative glomerulonephritis

581.1 With lesion of membranous glomerulonephritis
Epimembranous nephritis
Idiopathic membranous glomerular disease
Nephrotic syndrome with lesion of:
focal glomerulosclerosis
sclerosing membranous glomerulonephritis
segmental hyalinosis

581.2 With lesion of membranoproliferative glomerulonephritis
Nephrotic syndrome with lesion (of):
endothelial
hypocomplementemic
persistent
lobular   } glomerulonephritis
mesangiocapillary
mixed membranous
and proliferative

DEF: Glomerulonephritis combined with clinical features of nephrotic syndrome; characterized by uneven thickening of glomerular capillary walls and mesangial cell increase; slowly progresses to ESRD.

581.3 With lesion of minimal change glomerulonephritis
Foot process disease   Minimal change:
Lipoid nephrosis   glomerulitis
Minimal change: nephrotic syndrome
glomerular disease

√5ᵗʰ 581.8 With other specified pathological lesion in kidney

581.81 Nephrotic syndrome in diseases classified elsewhere
Code first underlying disease, as:
amyloidosis (277.3)
diabetes mellitus (250.4)
malaria (084.9)
polyarteritis (446.0)
systemic lupus erythematosus (710.0)
EXCLUDES nephrosis in epidemic hemorrhagic fever (078.6)

AHA: 3Q, '91, 8,12; S-O, '85, 3

581.89 Other
Glomerulonephritis with edema and lesion of:
exudative nephritis
interstitial (diffuse) (focal) nephritis

581.9 Nephrotic syndrome with unspecified pathological lesion in kidney
Glomerulonephritis with edema NOS
Nephritis:
nephrotic NOS
with edema NOS
Nephrosis NOS
Renal disease with edema NOS

√4ᵗʰ 582 Chronic glomerulonephritis

INCLUDES chronic nephritis

DEF: Slow progressive type of nephritis characterized by inflammation of the capillary loops in the glomeruli of the kidney, which leads to renal failure.

582.0 With lesion of proliferative glomerulonephritis
Chronic (diffuse) proliferative glomerulonephritis

582.1 With lesion of membranous glomerulonephritis
Chronic glomerulonephritis:
membranous
sclerosing
Focal glomerulosclerosis
Segmental hyalinosis

AHA: S-O, '84, 16

√4ᵗʰ
√5ᵗʰ Additional Digit Required   Unspecified Code   Other Specified Code   Manifestation Code   ►◄ Revised Text   ● New Code   ▲ Revised Code Title

Genitourinary System

580–582.1

Genitourinary System

582.2–584.6

582.2 With lesion of membranoproliferative glomerulonephritis
Chronic glomerulonephritis:
endothelial
hypocomplementemic persistent
lobular
membranoproliferative
mesangiocapillary
mixed membranous and proliferative

DEF: Chronic glomerulonephritis with mesangial cell proliferation.

582.4 With lesion of rapidly progressive glomerulonephritis
Chronic nephritis with lesion of necrotizing glomerulitis

DEF: Chronic glomerulonephritisrapidly progresses to ESRD; marked by diffuse epithelial proliferation.

√5th 582.8 With other specified pathological lesion in kidney

582.81 Chronic glomerulonephritis in diseases classified elsewhere
Code first underlying disease, as:
amyloidosis (277.3)
systemic lupus erythematosus (710.0)

582.89 Other
Chronic glomerulonephritis with lesion of:
exudative nephritis
interstitial (diffuse) (focal) nephritis

582.9 Chronic glomerulonephritis with unspecified pathological lesion in kidney

Glomerulonephritis: ⎫
NOS ⎪
hemorrhagic ⎬ specified as chronic
Nephritis ⎪
Nephropathy ⎭

AHA: 2Q, '01, 12

√4th 583 Nephritis and nephropathy, not specified as acute or chronic
INCLUDES "renal disease" so stated, not specified as acute or chronic but with stated pathology or cause

583.0 With lesion of proliferative glomerulonephritis
Proliferative: Proliferative
glomerulonephritis   nephritis NOS
(diffuse) NOS   nephropathy NOS

583.1 With lesion of membranous glomerulonephritis
Membranous:
glomerulonephritis NOS
nephritis NOS
Membranous nephropathy:
NOS

DEF: Kidney inflammation or dysfunction with deposits on glomerular capillary basement membranes.

583.2 With lesion of membranoproliferative glomerulonephritis
Membranoproliferative:
glomerulonephritis NOS
nephritis NOS
nephropathy NOS
Nephritis NOS, with lesion of:
hypocomplementemic ⎫
persistent ⎪
lobular ⎬ glomerulonephritis
mesangiocapillary ⎪
mixed membranous ⎪
and proliferative ⎭

DEF: Kidney inflammation or dysfunction with mesangial cell proliferation.

583.4 With lesion of rapidly progressive glomerulonephritis
Necrotizing or rapidly progressive:
glomerulitis NOS
glomerulonephritis NOS
nephritis NOS
nephropathy NOS
Nephritis, unspecified, with lesion of necrotizing glomerulitis

DEF: Kidney inflammation or dysfunction; rapidly progresses to ESRD marked by diffuse epithelial proliferation.

583.6 With lesion of renal cortical necrosis
Nephritis NOS ⎫ with (renal) cortical
Nephropathy NOS ⎭ necrosis

Renal cortical necrosis NOS

583.7 With lesion of renal medullary necrosis
Nephritis NOS ⎫ with (renal) medullary
Nephropathy NOS ⎭ [papillary] necrosis

√5th 583.8 With other specified pathological lesion in kidney

583.81 Nephritis and nephropathy, not specified as acute or chronic, in diseases classified elsewhere
Code first underlying disease, as:
amyloidosis (277.3)
diabetes mellitus (250.4)
gonococcal infection (098.19)
Goodpasture's syndrome (446.21)
systemic lupus erythematosus (710.0)
tuberculosis (016.0)
EXCLUDES gouty nephropathy (274.10)
syphilitic nephritis (095.4)

AHA: ▶2Q, '03, 7;◀ 3Q, '91, 8; S-0, '85, 3

583.89 Other
Glomerulitis ⎫ with lesion of:
Glomerulonephritis ⎪ exudative
Nephritis ⎬ nephritis
Nephropathy ⎪ interstitial
Renal disease ⎭ nephritis

583.9 With unspecified pathological lesion in kidney
Glomerulitis NOS   Nephritis NOS
Glomerulonephritis NOS   Nephropathy NOS
EXCLUDES nephropathy complicating pregnancy, labor, or the puerperium (642.0-642.9, 646.2)
renal disease NOS with no stated cause (593.9)

√4th 584 Acute renal failure
EXCLUDES following labor and delivery (669.3)
posttraumatic (958.5)
that complicating:
abortion (634-638 with .3, 639.3)
ectopic or molar pregnancy (639.3)

AHA: 1Q, '93, 18; 2Q, '92, 5; 4Q, '92, 22

DEF: State resulting from increasing urea and related substances from the blood (azotemia), often with urine output of less than 500 ml per day.

584.5 With lesion of tubular necrosis
Lower nephron nephrosis
Renal failure with (acute) tubular necrosis
Tubular necrosis:
NOS
acute

DEF: Acute decline in kidney efficiency with destruction of tubules.

584.6 With lesion of renal cortical necrosis
DEF: Acute decline in kidney efficiency with destruction of renal tissues that filter blood.

N Newborn Age: 0   P Pediatric Age: 0-17   M Maternity Age: 12-55   A Adult Age: 15-124   MSP Medicare Secondary Payer

584.7 With lesion of renal medullary [papillary] necrosis
Necrotizing renal papillitis
DEF: Acute decline in kidney efficiency with destruction of renal tissues that collect urine.

584.8 With other specified pathological lesion in kidney
AHA: N-D, '85, 1

584.9 Acute renal failure, unspecified
AHA: 2Q, '03, 7; 1Q, 03, 22; 3Q, '02, 21, 28; 2Q, '01, 14; 1Q, '00, 22; 3Q, '96, 9; 4Q, '88, 1

585 Chronic renal failure
Chronic uremia
Use additional code to identify manifestation as:
uremic:
neuropathy (357.4)
pericarditis (420.0)
> **EXCLUDES** *that with any condition classifiable to 401 (403.0-403.9 with fifth-digit 1)*

AHA: ▶1Q, '04, 5;◀ 4Q, '03, 61, 111; 2Q, '03, 7; 2Q, '01, 12, 13; 1Q, '01, 3; 4Q, '98, 55; 3Q, '98, 6, 7; 2Q, '98, 20; 3Q, '96, 9; 1Q, '93, 18; 3Q, '91, 8; 4Q, '89, 1; N-D, '85, 15; S-O, '84, 3

586 Renal failure, unspecified
Uremia NOS
> **EXCLUDES** *following labor and delivery (669.3)*
> *posttraumatic renal failure (958.5)*
> *that complicating:*
>   *abortion (634-638 with .3, 639.3)*
>   *ectopic or molar pregnancy (639.3)*
> *uremia:*
>   *extrarenal (788.9)*
>   *prerenal (788.9)*
> *with any condition classifiable to 401 (403.0-403.9 with fifth-digit 1)*

AHA: 3Q, '98, 6; 1Q, '93, 18
DEF: Renal failure: kidney functions cease; malfunction may be due to inability to excrete metabolized substances or retain level of electrolytes.
DEF: Uremia: excess urea, creatinine and other nitrogenous products of protein and amino acid metabolism in blood due to reduced excretory function in bilateral kidney disease; also called azotemia.

587 Renal sclerosis, unspecified
Atrophy of kidney
Contracted kidney
Renal:
cirrhosis
fibrosis
> **EXCLUDES** *nephrosclerosis (arteriolar) (arteriosclerotic) (403.00-403.92)*
> *with hypertension (403.00-403.91)*

√4ᵗʰ 588 Disorders resulting from impaired renal function

588.0 Renal osteodystrophy
Azotemic osteodystrophy
Phosphate-losing tubular disorders
Renal:
dwarfism
infantilism
rickets
DEF: Bone disorder that results in various bone diseases such as osteomalacia, osteoporosis or osteosclerosis; caused by impaired renal function, an abnormal level of phosphorus in the blood and impaired stimulation of the parathyroid.

588.1 Nephrogenic diabetes insipidus
> **EXCLUDES** *diabetes insipidus NOS (253.5)*

DEF: Type of diabetes due to renal tubules inability to reabsorb water; not responsive to vasopressin; may develop into chronic renal insufficiency.

√5ᵗʰ 588.8 Other specified disorders resulting from impaired renal function
> **EXCLUDES** *secondary hypertension (405.0-405.9)*

588.81 Secondary hyperparathyroidism (of renal origin)
Secondary hyperparathyroidism NOS

Genitourinary System

Inferior vena cava — Aorta — Right kidney — Left kidney — Anterior division of internal iliac artery — Ureter — Superior and Inferior vesicular arteries — Ovarian or testicular artery and vein — Ureteral orifice — Urinary bladder — Urethra — Urogenital diaphragm

588.89 Other specified disorders resulting from impaired renal function
Hypokalemic nephropathy

588.9 Unspecified disorder resulting from impaired renal function

√4ᵗʰ 589 Small kidney of unknown cause

589.0 Unilateral small kidney

589.1 Bilateral small kidneys

589.9 Small kidney, unspecified

OTHER DISEASES OF URINARY SYSTEM (590-599)

√4ᵗʰ 590 Infections of kidney
Use additional code to identify organism, such as Escherichia coli [E. coli] (041.4)

√5ᵗʰ 590.0 Chronic pyelonephritis
Chronic pyelitis
Chronic pyonephrosis
Code, if applicable, any causal condition first

590.00 Without lesion of renal medullary necrosis

590.01 With lesion of renal medullary necrosis

√5ᵗʰ 590.1 Acute pyelonephritis
Acute pyelitis   Acute pyonephrosis

590.10 Without lesion of renal medullary necrosis

590.11 With lesion of renal medullary necrosis

590.2 Renal and perinephric abscess
Abscess: Abscess:
kidney   perirenal
nephritic   Carbuncle of kidney

590.3 Pyeloureteritis cystica
Infection of renal pelvis and ureter
Ureteritis cystica
DEF: Inflammation and formation of submucosal cysts in the kidney, pelvis, and ureter.

√5ᵗʰ 590.8 Other pyelonephritis or pyonephrosis, not specified as acute or chronic

590.80 Pyelonephritis, unspecified
Pyelitis NOS   Pyelonephritis NOS
AHA: 1Q, '98, 10; 4Q, '97, 40

590.81 Pyelitis or pyelonephritis in diseases classified elsewhere
Code first underlying disease, as:
tuberculosis (016.0)

590.9 Infection of kidney, unspecified
> **EXCLUDES** *urinary tract infection NOS (599.0)*

591 Hydronephrosis
Hydrocalycosis   Hydroureteronephrosis
Hydronephrosis
> **EXCLUDES** *congenital hydronephrosis (753.29)*
> *hydroureter (593.5)*

AHA: 2Q, '98, 9
DEF: Distention of kidney and pelvis, with urine build-up due to ureteral obstruction; pyonephrosis may result.

√4ᵗʰ / √5ᵗʰ Additional Digit Required   Unspecified Code   Other Specified Code   Manifestation Code   ▶◀ Revised Text   ● New Code   ▲ Revised Code Title

2005 ICD•9•CM   October 2004 • Volume 1 — 161

Genitourinary System

592–595.3

√4th **592 Calculus of kidney and ureter**
> EXCLUDES   nephrocalcinosis (275.4)

592.0 Calculus of kidney
> Nephrolithiasis NOS   Staghorn calculus
> Renal calculus or stone   Stone in kidney
> > EXCLUDES   uric acid nephrolithiasis (274.11)

AHA: 1Q, '00, 4

592.1 Calculus of ureter
> Ureteric stone   Ureterolithiasis

AHA: 2Q, '98, 9; 1Q, '98, 10; 1Q, '91, 11

592.9 Urinary calculus, unspecified

AHA: 1Q, '98, 10; 4Q, '97, 40

√4th **593 Other disorders of kidney and ureter**

593.0 Nephroptosis
> Floating kidney   Mobile kidney

593.1 Hypertrophy of kidney

593.2 Cyst of kidney, acquired
> Cyst (multiple) (solitary) of kidney, not congenital
> Peripelvic (lymphatic) cyst
> > EXCLUDES   calyceal or pyelogenic cyst of kidney
> >   (591)
> >   congenital cyst of kidney (753.1)
> >   polycystic (disease of) kidney (753.1)

AHA: 4Q, '90, 3

DEF: Abnormal, fluid-filled sac in the kidney, not present at birth.

593.3 Stricture or kinking of ureter
> Angulation ⎫
> Constriction ⎬ of ureter (post-operative)
>   ⎭
> Stricture of pelviureteric junction

AHA: 2Q, '98, 9

DEF: Stricture or knot in tube connecting kidney to bladder.

593.4 Other ureteric obstruction
> Idiopathic retroperitoneal fibrosis
> Occlusion NOS of ureter
> > EXCLUDES   that due to calculus (592.1)

AHA: 2Q, '97, 4

593.5 Hydroureter
> > EXCLUDES   congenital hydroureter (753.22)
> >   hydroureteronephrosis (591)

593.6 Postural proteinuria
> Benign postural proteinuria
> Orthostatic proteinuria
> > EXCLUDES   proteinuria NOS (791.0)

DEF: Excessive amounts of serum protein in the urine caused by the body position, e.g., orthostatic and lordotic.

√5th **593.7 Vesicoureteral reflux**

AHA: 4Q, '94, 42

DEF: Backflow of urine, from bladder into ureter due to obstructed bladder neck.

593.70 Unspecified or without reflux nephropathy
593.71 With reflux nephropathy, unilateral
593.72 With reflux nephropathy, bilateral
593.73 With reflux nephropathy NOS

√5th **593.8 Other specified disorders of kidney and ureter**
> **593.81 Vascular disorders of kidney**
> > Renal (artery):   Renal (artery):
> >   embolism   thrombosis
> >   hemorrhage   Renal infarction

593.82 Ureteral fistula
> Intestinoureteral fistula
> > EXCLUDES   fistula between ureter and
> >   female genital tract
> >   (619.0)

DEF: Abnormal communication, between tube connecting kidney to bladder and another structure.

593.89 Other
> Adhesions, kidney   Polyp of ureter
>   or ureter   Pyelectasia
> Periureteritis   Ureterocele
> > EXCLUDES   tuberculosis of ureter (016.2)
> >   ureteritis cystica (590.3)

593.9 Unspecified disorder of kidney and ureter
> Renal disease (chronic) NOS
> Renal insufficiency (acute) (chronic)
> Salt-losing nephritis or syndrome
> > EXCLUDES   cystic kidney disease (753.1)
> >   nephropathy, so stated (583.0-583.9)
> >   renal disease:
> >   acute (580.0-580.9)
> >   arising in pregnancy or the
> >   puerperium (642.1-642.2,
> >   642.4-642.7, 646.2)
> >   chronic (582.0-582.9)
> >   not specified as acute or chronic, but
> >   with stated pathology or cause
> >   (583.0-583.9)

AHA: 1Q, '93, 17

√4th **594 Calculus of lower urinary tract**
594.0 Calculus in diverticulum of bladder
> DEF: Stone or mineral deposit in abnormal sac on the bladder wall.

594.1 Other calculus in bladder
> Urinary bladder stone
> > EXCLUDES   staghorn calculus (592.0)

DEF: Stone or mineral deposit in bladder.

594.2 Calculus in urethra
> DEF: Stone or mineral deposit in tube that empties urine from bladder.

594.8 Other lower urinary tract calculus

AHA: J-F, '85, 16

594.9 Calculus of lower urinary tract, unspecified
> > EXCLUDES   calculus of urinary tract NOS (592.9)

√4th **595 Cystitis**
> > EXCLUDES   prostatocystitis (601.3)
> Use additional code to identify organism, such as Escherichia coli [E. coli] (041.4)

595.0 Acute cystitis
> > EXCLUDES   trigonitis (595.3)

AHA: 2Q, '99, 15

DEF: Acute inflammation of bladder.

595.1 Chronic interstitial cystitis
> Hunner's ulcer   Submucous cystitis
> Panmural fibrosis of bladder

DEF: Inflamed lesion affecting bladder wall; symptoms include urinary frequency, pain on bladder filling, nocturia, and distended bladder.

595.2 Other chronic cystitis
> Chronic cystitis NOS   Subacute cystitis
> > EXCLUDES   trigonitis (595.3)

DEF: Persistent inflammation of bladder.

595.3 Trigonitis
> Follicular cystitis   Urethrotrigonitis
> Trigonitis (acute) (chronic)

DEF: Inflammation of the triangular area of the bladder called the trigonum vesicae.

N Newborn Age: 0   P Pediatric Age: 0-17   M Maternity Age: 12-55   A Adult Age: 15-124   MSP Medicare Secondary Payer

595.4 Cystitis in diseases classified elsewhere

Code first underlying disease, as:
actinomycosis (039.8)
amebiasis (006.8)
bilharziasis (120.0-120.9)
Echinococcus infestation (122.3, 122.6)

EXCLUDES cystitis:
diphtheritic (032.84)
gonococcal (098.11, 098.31)
monilial (112.2)
trichomonal (131.09)
tuberculous (016.1)

√5ᵗʰ **595.8 Other specified types of cystitis**

595.81 Cystitis cystica

DEF: Inflammation of the bladder characterized by formation of multiple cysts.

595.82 Irradiation cystitis

Use additional E code to identify cause

DEF: Inflammation of the bladder due to effects of radiation.

595.89 Other

Abscess of bladder	Cystitis:
Cystitis:	emphysematous
bullous	glandularis

595.9 Cystitis, unspecified

√4ᵗʰ **596 Other disorders of bladder**

Use additional code to identify urinary incontinence (625.6, 788.30-788.39)

AHA: M-A, '87, 10

596.0 Bladder neck obstruction

Contracture (acquired) ⎫
Obstruction (acquired) ⎬ of bladder neck or
Stenosis (acquired) ⎭ vesicourethral orifice

EXCLUDES congenital (753.6)

AHA: 3Q '02, 28; 2Q, '01, 14; N-D, '86, 10

DEF: Bladder outlet and vesicourethral obstruction; occurs more often in males as a consequence of benign prostatic hypertrophy or prostatic cancer; may also occur in either sex due to strictures, following radiation, cystoscopy, catheterization, injury, infection, blood clots, bladder cancer, impaction or disease compressing bladder neck.

596.1 Intestinovesical fistula

Fistula:	Fistula:
enterovesical	vesicoenteric
vesicocolic	vesicorectal

DEF: Abnormal communication, between intestine and bladder.

596.2 Vesical fistula, not elsewhere classified

Fistula:	Fistula:
bladder NOS	vesicocutaneous
urethrovesical	vesicoperineal

EXCLUDES fistula between bladder and female genital tract (619.0)

DEF: Abnormal communication between bladder and another structure.

596.3 Diverticulum of bladder

Diverticulitis ⎫
Diverticulum (acquired) (false) ⎬ of bladder

EXCLUDES that with calculus in diverticulum of bladder (594.0)

DEF: Abnormal pouch in bladder wall.

596.4 Atony of bladder

High compliance bladder
Hypotonicity ⎫
Inertia ⎬ of bladder

EXCLUDES neurogenic bladder (596.54)

DEF: Distended, bladder with loss of expulsive force; linked to CNS disease.

√5ᵗʰ **596.5 Other functional disorders of bladder**

EXCLUDES cauda equina syndrome with neurogenic bladder (344.61)

596.51 Hypertonicity of bladder

Hyperactivity
Overactive bladder

DEF: Abnormal tension of muscular wall of bladder; may appear after surgery of voluntary nerve.

596.52 Low bladder compliance

DEF: Low bladder capacity; causes increased pressure and frequent urination.

596.53 Paralysis of bladder

DEF: Impaired bladder motor function due to nerve or muscle damage.

596.54 Neurogenic bladder NOS

AHA: 1Q, '01, 12

DEF: Unspecified dysfunctional bladder due to lesion of central, peripheral nervous system; may result in incontinence, residual urine retention, urinary infection, stones and renal failure.

596.55 Detrusor sphincter dyssynergia

DEF: Instability of the urinary bladder sphincter muscle associated with urinary incontinence.

596.59 Other functional disorder of bladder

Detrusor instability

DEF: Detrusor instability: instability of bladder; marked by uninhibited contractions often leading to incontinence.

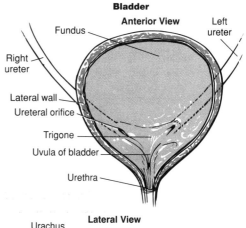

Bladder
Anterior View

Fundus — Left ureter
Right ureter
Lateral wall
Ureteral orifice
Trigone
Uvula of bladder
Urethra

Lateral View

Urachus
Left ureter
Peritoneum
Pubic bone
Urogenital diaphragm

√4ᵗʰ
√5ᵗʰ Additional Digit Required   Unspecified Code   Other Specified Code   Manifestation Code   ▶◀ Revised Text   ● New Code   ▲ Revised Code Title

2005 ICD•9•CM   **Volume 1 — 163**

Genitourinary System

596.6–599.84

596.6　Rupture of bladder, nontraumatic

596.7　Hemorrhage into bladder wall
Hyperemia of bladder
> EXCLUDES　*acute hemorrhagic cystitis (595.0)*

596.8　Other specified disorders of bladder
Bladder:　　　　　　　　Bladder:
　calcified　　　　　　　　hemorrhage
　contracted　　　　　　　hypertrophy
> EXCLUDES　*cystocele, female ▶(618.01-618.02,*
> *618.09, 618.2-618.4)◀*
> *hernia or prolapse of bladder,*
> *female ▶(618.01-618.02, 618.09,*
> *618.2-618.4)◀*

AHA: J-F, '85, 8

596.9　Unspecified disorder of bladder
AHA: J-F, '85, 8

✓4ᵗʰ **597　Urethritis, not sexually transmitted, and urethral syndrome**
> EXCLUDES　*nonspecific urethritis, so stated (099.4)*

597.0　Urethral abscess
Abscess:　　　　　　　　Abscess of:
　periurethral　　　　　　Cowper's gland
　urethral (gland)　　　　Littré's gland
Abscess of:　　　　　　　Periurethral cellulitis
　bulbourethral gland
> EXCLUDES　*urethral caruncle (599.3)*

DEF: Pocket of pus in tube that empties urine from the bladder.

✓5ᵗʰ **597.8　Other urethritis**

597.80　Urethritis, unspecified

597.81　Urethral syndrome NOS

597.89　Other
Adenitis, Skene's glands
Cowperitis
Meatitis, urethral
Ulcer, urethra (meatus)
Verumontanitis
> EXCLUDES　*trichomonal (131.02)*

✓4ᵗʰ **598　Urethral stricture**
Use additional code to identify urinary incontinence (625.6, 788.30-788.39)
> INCLUDES　pinhole meatus
> stricture of urinary meatus
> EXCLUDES　*congenital stricture of urethra and urinary*
> *meatus (753.6)*

DEF: Narrowing of tube that empties urine from bladder.

✓5ᵗʰ **598.0　Urethral stricture due to infection**

598.00　Due to unspecified infection

598.01　Due to infective diseases classified elsewhere
Code first underlying disease, as:
　gonococcal infection (098.2)
　schistosomiasis (120.0-120.9)
　syphilis (095.8)

598.1　Traumatic urethral stricture
Stricture of urethra:　　Stricture of urethra:
　late effect of injury　　postobstetric
> EXCLUDES　*postoperative following surgery on*
> *genitourinary tract (598.2)*

598.2　Postoperative urethral stricture
Postcatheterization stricture of urethra
AHA: 3Q, '97, 6

598.8　Other specified causes of urethral stricture
AHA: N-D, '84, 9

598.9　Urethral stricture, unspecified

✓4ᵗʰ **599　Other disorders of urethra and urinary tract**

599.0　Urinary tract infection, site not specified
> EXCLUDES　*candidiasis of urinary tract (112.2)*
> *urinary tract infection of newborn*
> *(771.82)*
Use additional code to identify organism, such as Escherichia coli [E. coli] (041.4)

AHA: 4Q, '03, 79; 4Q, '99, 6; 2Q, '99, 15; 1Q, '98, 5; 2Q, '96, 7; 4Q, '96, 33; 2Q, '95, 7; 1Q, '92, 13

599.1　Urethral fistula
Fistula:　　　　　　　　Urinary fistula NOS
　urethroperineal
　urethrorectal
> EXCLUDES　*fistula:*
> *urethroscrotal (608.89)*
> *urethrovaginal (619.0)*
> *urethrovesicovaginal (619.0)*

AHA: 3Q, '97, 6

599.2　Urethral diverticulum
DEF: Abnormal pouch in urethral wall.

599.3　Urethral caruncle
Polyp of urethra

599.4　Urethral false passage
DEF: Abnormal opening in urethra due to surgery, trauma or disease.

599.5　Prolapsed urethral mucosa
Prolapse of urethra　　Urethrocele
> EXCLUDES　*urethrocele, female ▶(618.03, 618.09,*
> *618.2-618.4)◀*

599.6　Urinary obstruction, unspecified
Obstructive uropathy NOS
Urinary (tract) obstruction NOS
Use additional code to identify urinary incontinence (625.6, 788.30-788.39)
> EXCLUDES　*obstructive nephropathy NOS (593.89)*

599.7　Hematuria
Hematuria (benign) (essential)
> EXCLUDES　*hemoglobinuria (791.2)*

AHA: 1Q, '00, 5; 3Q, '95, 8

DEF: Blood in urine.

✓5ᵗʰ **599.8　Other specified disorders of urethra and urinary tract**
Use additional code to identify urinary incontinence (625.6, 788.30-788.39)
> EXCLUDES　*symptoms and other conditions*
> *classifiable to 788.0-788.2,*
> *788.4-788.9, 791.0-791.9*

599.81　Urethral hypermobility
DEF: Hyperactive urethra.

599.82　Intrinsic (urethral) spincter deficiency [ISD]
AHA: 2Q, '96, 15
DEF: Malfunctioning urethral sphincter.

599.83　Urethral instability
DEF: Inconsistent functioning of urethra.

599.84　Other specified disorders of urethra
Rupture of urethra (nontraumatic)
Urethral:
　cyst
　granuloma
DEF: Rupture of urethra; due to herniation or breaking down of tissue; not due to trauma.
DEF: Urethral cyst: abnormal sac in urethra; usually fluid filled.
DEF: Granuloma: inflammatory cells forming small nodules in urethra.

N　Newborn Age: 0　　　P　Pediatric Age: 0-17　　　M　Maternity Age: 12-55　　　A　Adult Age: 15-124　　　MSP　Medicare Secondary Payer

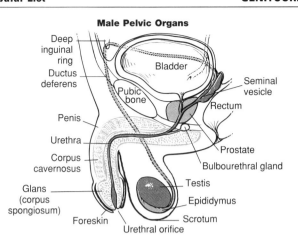

Male Pelvic Organs

599.89 **Other specified disorders of urinary tract**

599.9 **Unspecified disorder of urethra and urinary tract**

DISEASES OF MALE GENITAL ORGANS (600-608)

✓4th **600 Hyperplasia of prostate**

Use additional code to identify urinary incontinence (788.30-788.39)

AHA: 4Q, '00, 43; 3Q, '94, 12; 3Q, '92, 7; N-D, '86, 10

DEF: Fibrostromal proliferation in periurethral glands, causes blood in urine; etiology unknown.

✓5th **600.0 Hypertrophy (benign) of prostate**

Benign prostatic hypertrophy
Enlargement of prostate
Smooth enlarged prostate
Soft enlarged prostate

AHA: ▶4Q, '03, 63;◀ 1Q, '03, 6; 3Q '02, 28; 2Q, '01, 14

600.00 Hypertrophy (benign) of prostate without urinary obstruction   A ♂

Hypertrophy (benign) of prostate NOS

600.01 Hypertrophy (benign) of prostate with urinary obstruction   A ♂

Hypertrophy (benign) of prostate with urinary retention

AHA: ▶4Q, '03, 64◀

✓5th **600.1 Nodular prostate**

Hard, firm prostate   Multinodular prostate

EXCLUDES *malignant neoplasm of prostate (185)*

AHA: ▶4Q, '03, 63◀

DEF: Hard, firm nodule in prostate.

Common Inguinal Canal Anomalies

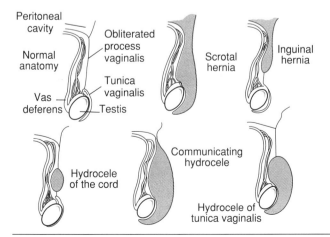

600.10 Nodular prostate without urinary obstruction   A ♂

Nodular prostate NOS

600.11 Nodular prostate with urinary obstruction   A ♂

Nodular prostate with urinary retention

✓5th **600.2 Benign localized hyperplasia of prostate**

Adenofibromatous hypertrophy of prostate
Adenoma of prostate
Fibroadenoma of prostate
Fibroma of prostate
Myoma of prostate
Polyp of prostate

EXCLUDES *benign neoplasms of prostate (222.2)
hypertrophy of prostate (600.00-600.01)
malignant neoplasm of prostate (185)*

AHA: ▶4Q, '03, 63◀

DEF: Benign localized hyperplasia is a clearly defined epithelial tumor. Other terms used for this condition are adenofibromatous hypertrophy of prostate, adenoma of prostate, fibroadenoma of prostate, fibroma of prostate, myoma of prostate, and polyp of prostate.

600.20 Benign localized hyperplasia of prostate without urinary obstruction   A ♂

Benign localized hyperplasia of prostate NOS

600.21 Benign localized hyperplasia of prostate with urinary obstruction   A ♂

Benign localized hyperplasia of prostate with urinary retention

600.3 Cyst of prostate   A ♂

DEF: Sacs of fluid, which differentiate this from either nodular or adenomatous tumors.

✓5th **600.9 Hyperplasia of prostate, unspecified**

Median bar
Prostatic obstruction NOS

AHA: ▶4Q, '03, 63◀

600.90 Hyperplasia of prostate, unspecified, without urinary obstruction   A ♂

Hyperplasia of prostate NOS

600.91 Hyperplasia of prostate, unspecified, with urinary obstruction   A ♂

Hyperplasia of prostate, unspecified, with urinary obstruction

✓4th **601 Inflammatory diseases of prostate**

Use additional code to identify organism, such as Staphylococcus (041.1), or Streptococcus (041.0)

601.0 Acute prostatitis   A ♂

601.1 Chronic prostatitis   A ♂

601.2 Abscess of prostate   A ♂

601.3 Prostatocystitis   A ♂

601.4 *Prostatitis in diseases classified elsewhere*   A ♂

Code first underlying disease, as:
actinomycosis (039.8)
blastomycosis (116.0)
syphilis (095.8)
tuberculosis (016.5)

EXCLUDES *prostatitis:
gonococcal (098.12, 098.32)
monilial (112.2)
trichomonal (131.03)*

601.8 Other specified inflammatory diseases of prostate   A ♂

Prostatitis: Prostatitis:
cavitary   granulomatous
diverticular

601.9 Prostatitis, unspecified   A ♂

Prostatitis NOS

✓4th Additional Digit Required   Unspecified Code   Other Specified Code   Manifestation Code   ▶◀ Revised Text   ● New Code   ▲ Revised Code Title

Genitourinary System

602–607.85

✓4ᵗʰ **602 Other disorders of prostate**

602.0 Calculus of prostate   Ⓐ♂
    Prostatic stone
    DEF: Stone or mineral deposit in prostate.

602.1 Congestion or hemorrhage of prostate   Ⓐ♂
    DEF: Bleeding or fluid collection in prostate.

602.2 Atrophy of prostate   Ⓐ♂
602.3 Dysplasia of prostate   ♂
    Prostatic intraepithelial neoplasia I (PIN I)
    Prostatic intraepithelial neoplasia II (PIN II)
      EXCLUDES *prostatic intraepithelial neoplasia III (PIN III) (233.4)*

    AHA: 4Q, '01, 46

    DEF: Abnormality of shape and size of the intraepithelial tissues of the prostate; pre-malignant condition characterized by stalks and absence of a basilar cell layer; synonyms are intraductal dysplasia, large acinar atypical hyperplasia, atypical primary hyperplasia, hyperplasia with malignant changes, marked atypia, or duct-acinar dysplasia.

602.8 Other specified disorders of prostate   Ⓐ♂
    Fistula ⎫
    Infarction ⎬ of prostate
    Stricture ⎭

    Periprostatic adhesions

602.9 Unspecified disorder of prostate   Ⓐ♂

✓4ᵗʰ **603 Hydrocele**
    INCLUDES hydrocele of spermatic cord, testis, or tunica vaginalis
    EXCLUDES *congenital (778.6)*

    DEF: Circumscribed collection of fluid in tunica vaginalis, spermatic cord or testis.

603.0 Encysted hydrocele
603.1 Infected hydrocele
    Use additional code to identify organism
603.8 Other specified types of hydrocele
603.9 Hydrocele, unspecified

✓4ᵗʰ **604 Orchitis and epididymitis**
    Use additional code to identify organism, such as Escherichia coli [E. coli] (041.4), Staphylococcus (041.1), or Streptococcus (041.0)

604.0 Orchitis, epididymitis, and epididymo-orchitis, with abscess   ♂
    Abscess of epididymis or testis

✓5ᵗʰ **604.9 Other orchitis, epididymitis, and epididymo-orchitis, without mention of abscess**
    604.90 Orchitis and epididymitis, unspecified   ♂
    604.91 Orchitis and epididymitis in diseases classified elsewhere   ♂
        Code first underlying disease, as:
          diphtheria (032.89)
          filariasis (125.0-125.9)
          syphilis (095.8)
        EXCLUDES *orchitis:*
           gonococcal (098.13, 098.33)
           mumps (072.0)
           tuberculous (016.5)
           tuberculous epididymitis (016.4)   ♂
        604.99 Other   ♂

605 Redundant prepuce and phimosis   ♂
    Adherent prepuce   Phimosis (congenital)
    Paraphimosis   Tight foreskin
    DEF: Constriction of preputial orifice causing inability of the prepuce to be drawn back over the glans; it may be congenital or caused by infection.

✓4ᵗʰ **606 Infertility, male**
    AHA: 2Q, '96, 9

606.0 Azoospermia   Ⓐ♂
    Absolute infertility
    Infertility due to:
      germinal (cell) aplasia
      spermatogenic arrest (complete)
    DEF: Absence of spermatozoa in the semen or inability to produce spermatozoa.

606.1 Oligospermia   Ⓐ♂
    Infertility due to:
      germinal cell desquamation
      hypospermatogenesis
      incomplete spermatogenic arrest
    DEF: Insufficient number of sperm in semen.

606.8 Infertility due to extratesticular causes   Ⓐ♂
    Infertility due to: Infertility due to:
      drug therapy   radiation
      infection   systemic disease
      obstruction of efferent
        ducts

606.9 Male infertility, unspecified   Ⓐ♂

✓4ᵗʰ **607 Disorders of penis**
    EXCLUDES *phimosis (605)*

607.0 Leukoplakia of penis   ♂
    Kraurosis of penis
      EXCLUDES *carcinoma in situ of penis (233.5)*
               erythroplasia of Queyrat (233.5)
    DEF: White, thickened patches on glans penis.

607.1 Balanoposthitis   ♂
    Balanitis
    Use additional code to identify organism
    DEF: Inflammation of glans penis and prepuce.

607.2 Other inflammatory disorders of penis   ♂
    Abscess ⎫
    Boil   ⎬ of corpus cavernosum or penis
    Carbuncle ⎪
    Cellulitis ⎭

    Cavernitis (penis)
    Use additional code to identify organism
      EXCLUDES *herpetic infection (054.13)*

607.3 Priapism   ♂
    Painful erection
    DEF: Prolonged penile erection without sexual stimulation.

✓5ᵗʰ **607.8 Other specified disorders of penis**
    607.81 Balanitis xerotica obliterans   ♂
        Induratio penis plastica
        DEF: Inflammation of the glans penis, caused by stricture of the opening of the prepuce.

    607.82 Vascular disorders of penis   ♂
        Embolism   ⎫
        Hematoma   ⎪ of corpus
          (nontraumatic) ⎬ cavernosum
        Hemorrhage   ⎪ or penis
        Thrombosis   ⎭

    607.83 Edema of penis   ♂
        DEF: Fluid retention within penile tissues.

    607.84 Impotence of organic origin   Ⓐ♂
        EXCLUDES *nonorganic or unspecified (302.72)*

        AHA: 3Q, '91, 11

        DEF: Physiological cause interfering with erection.

    607.85 Peyronie's disease   ♂
        AHA: ▶4Q, '03, 64◀

        DEF: ▶A severe curvature of the erect penis due to fibrosis of the cavernous sheaths.◀

Ⓝ Newborn Age: 0   Ⓟ Pediatric Age: 0-17   Ⓜ Maternity Age: 12-55   Ⓐ Adult Age: 15-124   MSP Medicare Secondary Payer

Torsion of Testis

Torsion of testis

Testes after correction showing bilateral fixation

607.89 Other ♂

Atrophy
Fibrosis
Hypertrophy
Ulcer (chronic)
} of corpus cavernosum or penis

607.9 Unspecified disorder of penis ♂

√4ᵗʰ **608 Other disorders of male genital organs**

608.0 Seminal vesiculitis ♂

Abscess
Cellulitis
} of seminal vesicle

Vesiculitis (seminal)
Use additional code to identify organism
EXCLUDES *gonococcal infection (098.14, 098.34)*
DEF: Inflammation of seminal vesicle.

608.1 Spermatocele ♂
DEF: Cystic enlargement of the epididymis or the testis; the cysts contain spermatozoa.

608.2 Torsion of testis ♂
Torsion of: Torsion of:
   epididymis   testicle
   spermatic cord
DEF: Twisted or rotated testis; may compromise blood flow.

608.3 Atrophy of testis ♂

608.4 Other inflammatory disorders of male genital organs ♂

Abscess
Boil
Carbuncle
Cellulitis
} of scrotum, spermatic cord, testis [except abscess], tunica vaginalis, or vas deferens

Vasitis
Use additional code to identify organism
EXCLUDES *abscess of testis (604.0)*

√5ᵗʰ **608.8 Other specified disorders of male genital organs**

608.81 Disorders of male genital organs in diseases classified elsewhere ♂
Code first underlying disease, as:
   filariasis (125.0-125.9)
   tuberculosis (016.5)

608.82 Hematospermia ♂
AHA: 4Q, '01, 46

DEF: Presence of blood in the ejaculate; relatively common, affecting men of any age after puberty; cause is often difficult to determine since the semen originates in several organs, often the result of a viral bacterial infection and inflammation.

608.83 Vascular disorders ♂
Hematoma
(non-traumatic)
Hemorrhage
Thrombosis
} of seminal vesicle, spermatic cord, testis, scrotum, tunica vaginalis, or vas deferens

Hematocele NOS, male
AHA: ►4Q, '03, 110◄

608.84 Chylocele of tunica vaginalis ♂
DEF: Chylous effusion into tunica vaginalis; due to infusion of lymphatic fluids.

608.85 Stricture ♂
Stricture of: Stricture of:
   spermatic cord   vas deferens
   tunica vaginalis

608.86 Edema ♂

608.87 Retrograde ejaculation ♂
AHA: 4Q, '01, 46

DEF: Condition where the semen travels to the bladder rather than out through the urethra due to damaged nerves causing the bladder neck to remain open during ejaculation.

608.89 Other ♂

Atrophy
Fibrosis
Hypertrophy
Ulcer
} of seminal vesicle, spermatic cord, testis, scrotum, tunica vaginalis, or vas deferens

EXCLUDES *atrophy of testis (608.3)*

608.9 Unspecified disorder of male genital organs ♂

DISORDERS OF BREAST (610-611)

√4ᵗʰ **610 Benign mammary dysplasias**

610.0 Solitary cyst of breast
Cyst (solitary) of breast

610.1 Diffuse cystic mastopathy Ⓐ
Chronic cystic mastitis   Fibrocystic disease of
Cystic breast   breast
DEF: Extensive formation of nodular cysts in breast tissue; symptoms include tenderness, change in size and hyperplasia of ductal epithelium.

610.2 Fibroadenosis of breast
Fibroadenosis of breast: Fibroadenosis of breast:
   NOS   diffuse
   chronic   periodic
   cystic   segmental
DEF: Non-neoplastic nodular condition of breast.

610.3 Fibrosclerosis of breast
DEF: Fibrous tissue in breast.

610.4 Mammary duct ectasia
Comedomastitis   Mastitis:
Duct ectasia   periductal
                        plasma cell

DEF: Atrophy of duct epithelium; causes distended collecting ducts of mammary gland; drying up of breast secretion, intraductal inflammation and periductal and interstitial chronic inflammatory reaction.

610.8 Other specified benign mammary dysplasias
Mazoplasia   Sebaceous cyst of breast

610.9 Benign mammary dysplasia, unspecified

√4ᵗʰ **611 Other disorders of breast**
EXCLUDES *that associated with lactation or the puerperium (675.0-676.9)*

611.0 Inflammatory disease of breast
Abscess (acute) (chronic) Mastitis (acute) (subacute)
   (nonpuerperal) of: (nonpuerperal):
   areola   NOS
   breast   infective
   Mammillary fistula   retromammary
                            submammary

EXCLUDES *carbuncle of breast (680.2)*
chronic cystic mastitis (610.1)
neonatal infective mastitis (771.5)
thrombophlebitis of breast [Mondor's disease] (451.89)

√4ᵗʰ √5ᵗʰ Additional Digit Required   Unspecified Code   Other Specified Code   Manifestation Code   ►◄ Revised Text   ● New Code   ▲ Revised Code Title

Genitourinary System

611.1–615.9

611.1   **Hypertrophy of breast**
Gynecomastia
Hypertrophy of breast:
  NOS
  massive pubertal

611.2   **Fissure of nipple**

611.3   **Fat necrosis of breast**
Fat necrosis (segmental) of breast

DEF: Splitting of neutral fats in adipose tissue cells as a result of trauma; a firm circumscribed mass is then formed in the breast.

611.4   **Atrophy of breast**

611.5   **Galactocele**

DEF: Milk-filled cyst in breast; due to blocked duct.

611.6   **Galactorrhea not associated with childbirth**

DEF: Flow of milk not associated with childbirth or pregnancy.

√5ᵗʰ **611.7**   **Signs and symptoms in breast**

    611.71 Mastodynia
        Pain in breast

    611.72 Lump or mass in breast
        AHA: 2Q, '03, 4-5

    611.79 Other
        Induration of breast   Nipple discharge
        Inversion of nipple   Retraction of nipple

611.8   **Other specified disorders of breast**
Hematoma (nontraumatic) ⎫
Infarction   ⎬ of breast
Occlusion of breast duct
Subinvolution of breast (postlactational)
  (postpartum)

611.9   **Unspecified breast disorder**

INFLAMMATORY DISEASE OF FEMALE PELVIC ORGANS (614-616)

Use additional code to identify organism, such as Staphylococcus (041.1), or Streptococcus (041.0)

EXCLUDES   *that associated with pregnancy, abortion, childbirth, or the puerperium (630-676.9)*

√4ᵗʰ **614**   **Inflammatory disease of ovary, fallopian tube, pelvic cellular tissue, and peritoneum**

EXCLUDES   *endometritis (615.0-615.9)*
major infection following delivery (670)
that complicating:
  abortion (634-638 with .0, 639.0)
  ectopic or molar pregnancy (639.0)
  pregnancy or labor (646.6)

614.0   **Acute salpingitis and oophoritis**   ♀
Any condition classifiable to 614.2, specified as acute or subacute

DEF: Acute inflammation, of ovary and fallopian tube.

614.1   **Chronic salpingitis and oophoritis**   ♀
Hydrosalpinx
Salpingitis:
  follicularis
  isthmica nodosa
Any condition classifiable to 614.2, specified as chronic

DEF: Persistent inflammation of ovary and fallopian tube.

614.2   **Salpingitis and oophoritis not specified as acute, subacute, or chronic**   ♀
Abscess (of):   Pyosalpinx
  fallopian tube   Perisalpingitis
  ovary   Salpingitis
  tubo-ovarian   Salpingo-oophoritis
Oophoritis   Tubo-ovarian inflammatory
Perioophoritis   disease
    EXCLUDES   *gonococcal infection (chronic) (098.37)*
                acute (098.17)
                tuberculous (016.6)

AHA: 2Q, '91, 5

614.3   **Acute parametritis and pelvic cellulitis**   ♀
Acute inflammatory pelvic disease
Any condition classifiable to 614.4, specified as acute

DEF: Parametritis: inflammation of the parametrium; pelvic cellulitis is a synonym for parametritis.

614.4   **Chronic or unspecified parametritis and pelvic cellulitis**   ♀
Abscess (of):
  broad ligament   ⎫
  parametrium   ⎬ chronic or NOS
  pelvis, female   ⎪
  pouch of Douglas   ⎭
Chronic inflammatory pelvic disease
Pelvic cellulitis, female
    EXCLUDES   *tuberculous (016.7)*

614.5   **Acute or unspecified pelvic peritonitis, female**   ♀

614.6   **Pelvic peritoneal adhesions, female (postoperative) (postinfection)**   ♀
Adhesions:
  peritubal
  tubo-ovarian
Use additional code to identify any associated infertility (628.2)

AHA: 3Q, '03, 6; 1Q, '03, 4; 3Q, '95, 7; 3Q, '94, 12

DEF: Fibrous scarring abnormally joining structures within abdomen.

614.7   **Other chronic pelvic peritonitis, female**   ♀
    EXCLUDES   *tuberculous (016.7)*

614.8   **Other specified inflammatory disease of female pelvic organs and tissues**   ♀

614.9   **Unspecified inflammatory disease of female pelvic organs and tissues**   ♀
Pelvic infection or inflammation, female NOS
Pelvic inflammatory disease [PID]

√4ᵗʰ **615**   **Inflammatory diseases of uterus, except cervix**
    EXCLUDES   *following delivery (670)*
hyperplastic endometritis ▶*(621.30-621.33)*◀
that complicating:
  abortion (634-638 with .0, 639.0)
  ectopic or molar pregnancy (639.0)
  pregnancy or labor (646.6)

615.0   **Acute**   ♀
Any condition classifiable to 615.9, specified as acute or subacute

615.1   **Chronic**   ♀
Any condition classifiable to 615.9, specified as chronic

615.9   **Unspecified inflammatory disease of uterus**   ♀
Endometritis   Perimetritis
Endomyometritis   Pyometra
Metritis   Uterine abscess
Myometritis

Female Genitourinary System

N Newborn Age: 0   **P** Pediatric Age: 0-17   **M** Maternity Age: 12-55   **A** Adult Age: 15-124   **MSP** Medicare Secondary Payer

Common Sites of Endometriosis

Common sites of endometriosis, in descending order of frequency:
(1) ovary
(2) cul de sac
(3) utersacral ligaments
(4) broad ligaments
(5) fallopian tube
(6) uterovesical fold
(7) round ligament
(8) vermiform appendix
(9) vagina
(10) rectovaginal septum

√4ᵗʰ **616 Inflammatory disease of cervix, vagina, and vulva**

    EXCLUDES *that complicating:*
        abortion (634-638 with .0, 639.0)
        ectopic or molar pregnancy (639.0)
        pregnancy, childbirth, or the puerperium
        (646.6)

616.0 Cervicitis and endocervicitis ♀

    Cervicitis } with or without mention of
    Endocervicitis } erosion or ectropion

    Nabothian (gland) cyst or follicle
    EXCLUDES *erosion or ectropion without mention*
        of cervicitis (622.0)

√5ᵗʰ **616.1 Vaginitis and vulvovaginitis**

    DEF: Inflammation or infection of vagina or external female genitalia.

    616.10 Vaginitis and vulvovaginitis, unspecified ♀
        Vaginitis:
          NOS
          postirradiation
        Vulvitis NOS
        Vulvovaginitis NOS
        Use additional code to identify organism, such as Escherichia coli [E. coli] (041.4), Staphylococcus (041.1), or Streptococcus (041.0)
        EXCLUDES *noninfective leukorrhea (623.5)*
            postmenopausal or senile
            vaginitis (627.3)

    616.11 Vaginitis and vulvovaginitis in diseases classified elsewhere ♀
        Code first underlying disease, as:
        pinworm vaginitis (127.4)
        EXCLUDES *herpetic vulvovaginitis*
            (054.11)
            monilial vulvotaginitis (112.1)
            trichomonal vaginitis or
            vulvovaginitis (131.01)

616.2 Cyst of Bartholin's gland ♀
    Bartholin's duct cyst
    DEF: Fluid-filled sac within gland of vaginal orifice.

616.3 Abscess of Bartholin's gland ♀
    Vulvovaginal gland abscess

616.4 Other abscess of vulva ♀
    Abscess
    Carbuncle } of vulva
    Furuncle

√5ᵗʰ **616.5 Ulceration of vulva**
    616.50 Ulceration of vulva, unspecified ♀
        Ulcer NOS of vulva

    616.51 **Ulceration of vulva in diseases classified elsewhere** ♀
        Code first underlying disease, as:
        Behçet's syndrome (136.1)
        tuberculosis (016.7)
        EXCLUDES *vulvar ulcer (in):*
            gonococcal (098.0)
            herpes simplex (054.12)
            syphilitic (091.0)

616.8 Other specified inflammatory diseases of cervix, vagina, and vulva ♀
    Caruncle, vagina or labium
    Ulcer, vagina
    EXCLUDES *noninflammatory disorders of:*
        cervix (622.0-622.9)
        vagina (623.0-623.9)
        vulva (624.0-624.9)

616.9 Unspecified inflammatory disease of cervix, vagina, and vulva ♀

OTHER DISORDERS OF FEMALE GENITAL TRACT (617-629)

√4ᵗʰ **617 Endometriosis**

617.0 Endometriosis of uterus ♀
    Adenomyosis   Endometriosis:
    Endometriosis: internal
      cervix   myometrium
    EXCLUDES *stromal endometriosis (236.0)*
    AHA: 3Q, '92, 7
    DEF: Aberrant uterine mucosal tissue; creating products of menses and inflamed uterine tissues.

617.1 Endometriosis of ovary ♀
    Chocolate cyst of ovary
    Endometrial cystoma of ovary
    DEF: Aberrant uterine tissue; creating products of menses and inflamed ovarian tissues.

617.2 Endometriosis of fallopian tube ♀
    DEF: Aberrant uterine tissue; creating products of menses and inflamed tissues of fallopian tubes.

617.3 Endometriosis of pelvic peritoneum ♀
    Endometriosis: Endometriosis:
      broad ligament   parametrium
      cul-de-sac (Douglas')   round ligament
    DEF: Aberrant uterine tissue; creating products of menses and inflamed peritoneum tissues.

617.4 Endometriosis of rectovaginal septum and vagina ♀
    DEF: Aberrant uterine tissue; creating products of menses and inflamed tissues in and behind vagina.

617.5 Endometriosis of intestine ♀
    Endometriosis: Endometriosis:
      appendix   rectum
      colon
    DEF: Aberrant uterine tissue; creating products of menses and inflamed intestinal tissues.

Types of Vaginal Hernias

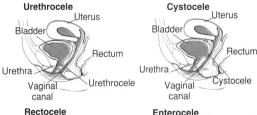

Urethrocele — Uterus, Bladder, Rectum, Urethra, Vaginal canal, Urethrocele

Cystocele — Uterus, Bladder, Rectum, Urethra, Vaginal canal, Cystocele

Rectocele — Uterus, Bladder, Rectum, Urethra, Vaginal canal, Rectocele

Enterocele — Uterus, Bladder, Rectum, Urethra, Vaginal canal, Terminal ileum

√4ᵗʰ √5ᵗʰ Additional Digit Required   Unspecified Code   Other Specified Code   Manifestation Code   ►◄ Revised Text   ● New Code   ▲ Revised Code Title

2005 ICD•9•CM   **Volume 1 — 169**

617.6   **Endometriosis in scar of skin** ♀

617.8   **Endometriosis of other specified sites** ♀
> Endometriosis: Endometriosis:
>   bladder   umbilicus
>   lung   vulva

617.9   **Endometriosis, site unspecified** ♀

✓4th **618 Genital prolapse**
> Use additional code to identify urinary incontinence (625.6, 788.31, 788.33-788.39)
> **EXCLUDES**   *that complicating pregnancy, labor, or delivery (654.4)*

✓5th **618.0**   **Prolapse of vaginal walls without mention of uterine prolapse**
> **EXCLUDES**   *that with uterine prolapse (618.2-618.4)*
>   *enterocele (618.6)*
>   *vaginal vault prolapse following hysterectomy (618.5)*

●   **618.00** **Unspecified prolapse of vaginal walls** ♀
> Vaginal prolapse NOS

●   **618.01** **Cystocele, midline** ♀
> Cystocele NOS

●   **618.02** **Cystocele, lateral** ♀
> Paravaginal

●   **618.03** **Urethrocele** ♀

●   **618.04** **Rectocele** ♀
> Proctocele

●   **618.05** **Perineocele** ♀

●   **618.09** **Other prolapse of vaginal walls without mention of uterine prolapse** ♀
> Cystourethrocele

618.1   **Uterine prolapse without mention of vaginal wall prolapse** ♀
> Descensus uteri   Uterine prolapse:
> Uterine prolapse: first degree
>   NOS   second degree
>   complete   third degree
> **EXCLUDES**   *that with mention of cystocele, urethrocele, or rectocele (618.2-618.4)*

618.2   **Uterovaginal prolapse, incomplete** ♀
> DEF: Downward displacement of uterus downward into vagina.

618.3   **Uterovaginal prolapse, complete** ♀
> DEF: Downward displacement of uterus exposed within external genitalia.

618.4   **Uterovaginal prolapse, unspecified** ♀

618.5   **Prolapse of vaginal vault after hysterectomy** ♀

618.6   **Vaginal enterocele, congenital or acquired** ♀
> Pelvic enterocele, congenital or acquired
> DEF: Vaginal vault hernia formed by the loop of the small intestine protruding into the rectal vaginal pouch; can also accompany uterine prolapse or follow hysterectomy.

618.7   **Old laceration of muscles of pelvic floor** ♀

✓5th **618.8**   **Other specified genital prolapse**

●   **618.81** **Incompetence or weakening of pubocervical tissue** ♀

●   **618.82** **Incompetence or weakening of rectovaginal tissue** ♀

●   **618.83** **Pelvic muscle wasting** ♀
> Disuse atrophy of pelvic muscles and anal sphincter

●   **618.89** **Other specified genital prolapse** ♀
> Incompetence or weakening of pelvic fundus
> Relaxation of vaginal outlet or pelvis

618.9   **Unspecified genital prolapse** ♀

Uterus and Ovaries

✓4th **619 Fistula involving female genital tract**
> **EXCLUDES**   *vesicorectal and intestinovesical fistula (596.1)*

619.0   **Urinary-genital tract fistula, female** ♀
> Fistula: Fistula:
>   cervicovesical   uteroureteric
>   ureterovaginal   uterovesical
>   urethrovaginal   vesicocervicovaginal
>   urethrovesicovaginal   vesicovaginal

619.1   **Digestive-genital tract fistula, female** ♀
> Fistula: Fistula:
>   intestinouterine   rectovulval
>   intestinovaginal   sigmoidovaginal
>   rectovaginal   uterorectal

619.2   **Genital tract-skin fistula, female** ♀
> Fistula:
>   uterus to abdominal wall
>   vaginoperineal

619.8   **Other specified fistulas involving female genital tract** ♀
> Fistula: Fistula:
>   cervix   uterus
>   cul-de-sac (Douglas')   vagina
> DEF: Abnormal communication between female reproductive tract and skin.

619.9   **Unspecified fistula involving female genital tract** ♀

✓4th **620 Noninflammatory disorders of ovary, fallopian tube, and broad ligament**
> **EXCLUDES**   *hydrosalpinx (614.1)*

620.0   **Follicular cyst of ovary** ♀
> Cyst of graafian follicle
> DEF: Fluid-filled, encapsulated cyst due to occluded follicle duct that secretes hormones into ovaries.

620.1   **Corpus luteum cyst or hematoma** ♀
> Corpus luteum hemorrhage or rupture
> Lutein cyst
> DEF: Fluid-filled cyst due to serous developing from corpus luteum or clotted blood.

620.2   **Other and unspecified ovarian cyst** ♀
> Cyst:
>   NOS
>   corpus albicans
>   retention NOS   } of ovary
>   serous
>   theca-lutein
> Simple cystoma of ovary
> **EXCLUDES**   *cystadenoma (benign) (serous) (220)*
>   *developmental cysts (752.0)*
>   *neoplastic cysts (220)*
>   *polycystic ovaries (256.4)*
>   *Stein-Leventhal syndrome (256.4)*

620.3   **Acquired atrophy of ovary and fallopian tube** ♀
> Senile involution of ovary

620.4   **Prolapse or hernia of ovary and fallopian tube**   ♀
Displacement of ovary and fallopian tube
Salpingocele

620.5   **Torsion of ovary, ovarian pedicle, or fallopian tube**   ♀
Torsion: Torsion:
   accessory tube   hydatid of Morgagni

620.6   **Broad ligament laceration syndrome**   ♀
Masters-Allen syndrome

620.7   **Hematoma of broad ligament**   ♀
Hematocele, broad ligament
DEF: Blood within peritoneal fold that supports uterus.

620.8   **Other noninflammatory disorders of ovary, fallopian tube, and broad ligament**   ♀

Cyst } of broad ligament or fallopian tube
Polyp

Infarction } of ovary or fallopian tube
Rupture

Hematosalpinx
   EXCLUDES   *hematosalpinx in ectopic pregnancy (639.2)*
            peritubal adhesions (614.6)
            torsion of ovary, ovarian pedicle, or fallopian tube (620.5)

620.9   **Unspecified noninflammatory disorder of ovary, fallopian tube, and broad ligament**   ♀

√4ᵗʰ **621 Disorders of uterus, not elsewhere classified**

621.0   **Polyp of corpus uteri**   ♀
Polyp: Polyp:
   endometrium   uterus NOS
   EXCLUDES   *cervical polyp NOS (622.7)*

621.1   **Chronic subinvolution of uterus**   ♀
   EXCLUDES   *puerperal (674.8)*
AHA: 1Q, '91, 11
DEF: Abnormal size of uterus after delivery; the uterus does not return to its normal size after the birth of a child.

621.2   **Hypertrophy of uterus**   ♀
Bulky or enlarged uterus
   EXCLUDES   *puerperal (674.8)*

▲ √5ᵗʰ **621.3**   **Endometrial hyperplasia**
Hyperplasia (adenomatous) (cystic) (glandular) of endometrium
DEF: Abnormal cystic overgrowth of endometrial tissue.

●   **621.30**   **Endometrial hyperplasia, unspecified**   ♀
Endometrial hyperplasia NOS

●   **621.31**   **Simple endometrial hyperplasia without atypia**   ♀

●   **621.32**   **Complex endometrial hyperplasia without atypia**   ♀

●   **621.33**   **Endometrial hyperplasia with atypia**   ♀

621.4   **Hematometra**   ♀
Hemometra
   EXCLUDES   *that in congenital anomaly (752.2-752.3)*
DEF: Accumulated blood in uterus.

621.5   **Intrauterine synechiae**   ♀
Adhesions of uterus
Band(s) of uterus

621.6   **Malposition of uterus**   ♀
Anteversion
Retroflexion } of uterus
Retroversion
   EXCLUDES   *malposition complicating pregnancy, labor, or delivery (654.3-654.4)*
            prolapse of uterus (618.1-618.4)

621.7   **Chronic inversion of uterus**   ♀
   EXCLUDES   *current obstetrical trauma (665.2)*
            prolapse of uterus (618.1-618.4)

621.8   **Other specified disorders of uterus, not elsewhere classified**   ♀
Atrophy, acquired
Cyst
Fibrosis NOS } of uterus
Old laceration (postpartum)
Ulcer
   EXCLUDES   *bilharzial fibrosis (120.0-120.9)*
            endometriosis (617.0)
            fistulas (619.0-619.8)
            inflammatory diseases (615.0-615.9)

621.9   **Unspecified disorder of uterus**   ♀

√4ᵗʰ **622 Noninflammatory disorders of cervix**
   EXCLUDES   *abnormality of cervix complicating pregnancy, labor, or delivery (654.5-654.6)*
            fistula (619.0-619.8)

622.0   **Erosion and ectropion of cervix**   ♀
Eversion } of cervix
Ulcer
   EXCLUDES   *that in chronic cervicitis (616.0)*
DEF: Ulceration or turning outward of uterine cervix.

√5ᵗʰ **622.1**   **Dysplasia of cervix (uteri)**
   EXCLUDES   ► *abnormal results from cervical cytologic examination without histologic confirmation (795.00-795.09)* ◄
            carcinoma in situ of cervix (233.1)
            cervical intraepithelial neoplasia III [CIN III] (233.1)
AHA: 1Q, '91, 11
DEF: Abnormal cell structures in portal between uterus and vagina.

●   **622.10**   **Dysplasia of cervix, unspecified**   ♀
Anaplasia of cervix
Cervical atypism
Cervical dysplasia NOS

●   **622.11**   **Mild dysplasia of cervix**   ♀
Cervical intraepithelial neoplasia I [CIN I]

●   **622.12**   **Moderate dysplasia of cervix**   ♀
Cervical intraepithelial neoplasia II [CIN II]
   EXCLUDES   *carcinoma in situ of cervix (233.1)*
            cervical intraepithelial neoplasia III [CIN III] (233.1)
            severe dysplasia (233.1)

622.2   **Leukoplakia of cervix (uteri)**   ♀
DEF: Abnormal cell structures in portal between uterus and vagina.
   EXCLUDES   *carcinoma in situ of cervix (233.1)*
DEF: Thickened, white patches on portal between uterus and vagina.

622.3   **Old laceration of cervix**   ♀
Adhesions
Band(s) } of cervix
Cicatrix (postpartum)
   EXCLUDES   *current obstetrical trauma (665.3)*
DEF: Scarring or other evidence of old wound on cervix.

622.4   **Stricture and stenosis of cervix**   ♀
Atresia (acquired)
Contracture } of cervix
Occlusion
Pinpoint os uteri
   EXCLUDES   *congenital (752.49)*
            that complicating labor (654.6)

622.5   **Incompetence of cervix**   ♀
   EXCLUDES   *complicating pregnancy (654.5)*
            that affecting fetus or newborn (761.0)
DEF: Inadequate functioning of cervix; marked by abnormal widening during pregnancy; causing miscarriage.

√4ᵗʰ √5ᵗʰ Additional Digit Required   Unspecified Code   Other Specified Code   Manifestation Code   ►◄ Revised Text   ● New Code   ▲ Revised Code Title

Genitourinary System

620.4–622.5

Genitourinary System

622.6–625.9

622.6   Hypertrophic elongation of cervix ♀
DEF: Overgrowth of cervix tissues extending down into vagina.

622.7   Mucous polyp of cervix ♀
Polyp NOS of cervix
EXCLUDES   adenomatous polyp of cervix (219.0)

622.8   Other specified noninflammatory disorders of cervix ♀
Atrophy (senile) ⎤
Cyst   ⎬ of cervix
Fibrosis   ⎪
Hemorrhage ⎦
EXCLUDES   endometriosis (617.0)
            fistula (619.0-619.8)
            inflammatory diseases (616.0)

622.9   Unspecified noninflammatory disorder of cervix ♀

✓4ᵗʰ **623   Noninflammatory disorders of vagina**
EXCLUDES   abnormality of vagina complicating pregnancy, labor, or delivery (654.7)
            congenital absence of vagina (752.49)
            congenital diaphragm or bands (752.49)
            fistulas involving vagina (619.0-619.8)

623.0   Dysplasia of vagina ♀
EXCLUDES   carcinoma in situ of vagina (233.3)

623.1   Leukoplakia of vagina ♀
DEF: Thickened white patches on vaginal canal.

623.2   Stricture or atresia of vagina ♀
Adhesions (postoperative) (postradiation) of vagina
Occlusion of vagina
Stenosis, vagina
Use additional E code to identify any external cause
EXCLUDES   congenital atresia or stricture (752.49)

623.3   Tight hymenal ring ♀
Rigid hymen   ⎤
Tight hymenal ring ⎬ acquired or congenital
Tight introitus   ⎦
EXCLUDES   imperforate hymen (752.42)

623.4   Old vaginal laceration ♀
EXCLUDES   old laceration involving muscles of pelvic floor (618.7)
DEF: Scarring or other evidence of old wound on vagina.

623.5   Leukorrhea, not specified as infective ♀
Leukorrhea NOS of vagina
Vaginal discharge NOS
EXCLUDES   trichomonal (131.00)
DEF: Viscid whitish discharge, from vagina.

623.6   Vaginal hematoma ♀
EXCLUDES   current obstetrical trauma (665.7)

623.7   Polyp of vagina

623.8   Other specified noninflammatory disorders of vagina ♀
Cyst   ⎤
Hemorrhage ⎦ of vagina

623.9   Unspecified noninflammatory disorder of vagina ♀

✓4ᵗʰ **624   Noninflammatory disorders of vulva and perineum**
EXCLUDES   abnormality of vulva and perineum complicating pregnancy, labor, or delivery (654.8)
            condyloma acuminatum (078.1)
            fistulas involving:
               perineum — see Alphabetic Index
               vulva (619.0-619.8)
            vulval varices (456.6)
            vulvar involvement in skin conditions (690-709.9)

624.0   Dystrophy of vulva ♀
Kraurosis   ⎤
Leukoplakia ⎦ of vulva
EXCLUDES   carcinoma in situ of vulva (233.3)

624.1   Atrophy of vulva ♀

624.2   Hypertrophy of clitoris ♀
EXCLUDES   that in endocrine disorders (255.2, 256.1)

624.3   Hypertrophy of labia ♀
Hypertrophy of vulva NOS
DEF: Overgrowth of fleshy folds on either side of vagina.

624.4   Old laceration or scarring of vulva ♀
DEF: Scarring or other evidence of old wound on external female genitalia.

624.5   Hematoma of vulva ♀
EXCLUDES   that complicating delivery (664.5)
DEF: Blood in tissue of external genitalia.

624.6   Polyp of labia and vulva ♀

624.8   Other specified noninflammatory disorders of vulva and perineum ♀
Cyst   ⎤
Edema   ⎬ of vulva
Stricture ⎦
AHA: ▶1Q, '03, 13; ◀ 1Q, '95, 8

624.9   Unspecified noninflammatory disorder of vulva and perineum ♀

✓4ᵗʰ **625   Pain and other symptoms associated with female genital organs**

625.0   Dyspareunia ♀
EXCLUDES   psychogenic dyspareunia (302.76)
DEF: Difficult or painful sexual intercourse.

625.1   Vaginismus ♀
Colpospasm   Vulvismus
EXCLUDES   psychogenic vaginismus (306.51)
DEF: Vaginal spasms; due to involuntary contraction of musculature; prevents intercourse.

625.2   Mittelschmerz ♀
Intermenstrual pain   Ovulation pain
DEF: Pain occurring between menstrual periods.

625.3   Dysmenorrhea ♀
Painful menstruation
EXCLUDES   psychogenic dysmenorrhea (306.52)
AHA: 2Q, '94, 12

625.4   Premenstrual tension syndromes ♀
Menstrual:
   migraine
   molimen
Premenstrual dysphoric disorder
Premenstrual syndrome
Premenstrual tension NOS
AHA: ▶4Q, '03, 116◀

625.5   Pelvic congestion syndrome ♀
Congestion-fibrosis syndrome   Taylor's syndrome
DEF: Excessive accumulated of blood in vessels of pelvis; may occur after orgasm; causes abnormal menstruation, lower back pain and vaginal discharge.

625.6   Stress incontinence, female ♀
EXCLUDES   mixed incontinence (788.33)
            stress incontinence, male (788.32)
DEF: Involuntary leakage of urine due to insufficient sphincter control; occurs upon sneezing, laughing, coughing, sudden movement or lifting.

625.8   Other specified symptoms associated with female genital organs ♀
AHA: N-D, '85, 16

625.9   Unspecified symptom associated with female genital organs ♀

Ⓝ Newborn Age: 0   Ⓟ Pediatric Age: 0-17   Ⓜ Maternity Age: 12-55   Ⓐ Adult Age: 15-124   ⓂⓈⓅ Medicare Secondary Payer

✓4ᵗʰ 626 Disorders of menstruation and other abnormal bleeding from female genital tract

> **EXCLUDES** menopausal and premenopausal bleeding (627.0)
> pain and other symptoms associated with menstrual cycle (625.2-625.4)
> postmenopausal bleeding (627.1)

626.0 Absence of menstruation ♀
Amenorrhea (primary) (secondary)

626.1 Scanty or infrequent menstruation ♀
Hypomenorrhea   Oligomenorrhea

626.2 Excessive or frequent menstruation ♀
Heavy periods   Menorrhagia
Menometrorrhagia   Plymenorrhea
> **EXCLUDES** premenopausal(627.0)
> that in puberty (626.3)

626.3 Puberty bleeding ♀
Excessive bleeding associated with onset of menstrual periods
Pubertal menorrhagia

626.4 Irregular menstrual cycle ♀
Irregular: Irregular:
  bleeding NOS   periods
  menstruation

626.5 Ovulation bleeding ♀
Regular intermenstrual bleeding

626.6 Metrorrhagia ♀
Bleeding unrelated to menstrual cycle
Irregular intermenstrual bleeding

626.7 Postcoital bleeding ♀
DEF: Bleeding from vagina after sexual intercourse.

626.8 Other ♀
Dysfunctional or functional uterine hemorrhage NOS
Menstruation:
  retained
  suppression of

626.9 Unspecified ♀

✓4ᵗʰ 627 Menopausal and postmenopausal disorders
> **EXCLUDES** asymptomatic age-related (natural) postmenopausal status (V49.81)

627.0 Premenopausal menorrhagia ♀
Excessive bleeding associated with onset of menopause
Menorrhagia:
  climacteric
  menopausal
  preclimacteric

627.1 Postmenopausal bleeding ♀

627.2 Symptomatic menopausal or female climacteric states ♀
Symptoms, such as flushing, sleeplessness, headache, lack of concentration, associated with the menopause

627.3 Postmenopausal atrophic vaginitis ♀
Senile (atrophic) vaginitis

627.4 Symptomatic states associated with artificial menopause ♀
Postartificial menopause syndromes
Any condition classifiable to 627.1, 627.2, or 627.3 which follows induced menopause
DEF: Conditions arising after hysterectomy.

627.8 Other specified menopausal and postmenopausal disorders ♀
> **EXCLUDES** premature menopause NOS (256.31)

627.9 Unspecified menopausal and postmenopausal disorder ♀

✓4ᵗʰ 628 Infertility, female
> **INCLUDES** primary and secondary sterility

AHA: 2Q, '96, 9; 1Q, '95, 7

DEF: Infertility: inability to conceive for at least one year with regular intercourse.

DEF: Primary infertility: occurring in patients who have never conceived.

DEF: Secondary infertility; occurring in patients who have previously conceived.

628.0 Associated with anovulation ♀
Anovulatory cycle
Use additional code for any associated Stein-Leventhal syndrome (256.4)

628.1 Of pituitary-hypothalamic origin ♀
Code first underlying cause, as:
  adiposogenital dystrophy (253.8)
  anterior pituitary disorder (253.0-253.4)

628.2 Of tubal origin ♀
Infertility associated with congenital anomaly of tube
Tubal:
  block
  occlusion
  stenosis
Use additional code for any associated peritubal adhesions (614.6)

628.3 Of uterine origin ♀
Infertility associated with congenital anomaly of uterus
Nonimplantation
Use additional code for any associated tuberculous endometritis (016.7)

628.4 Of cervical or vaginal origin ♀
Infertility associated with:
  anomaly of cervical mucus
  congenital structural anomaly
  dysmucorrhea

628.8 Of other specified origin ♀

628.9 Of unspecified origin ♀

✓4ᵗʰ 629 Other disorders of female genital organs

629.0 Hematocele, female, not elsewhere classified ♀
> **EXCLUDES** hematocele or hematoma:
> broad ligament (620.7)
> fallopian tube (620.8)
> that associated with ectopic pregnancy (633.00-633.91)
> uterus (621.4)
> vagina (623.6)
> vulva (624.5)

629.1 Hydrocele, canal of Nuck ♀
Cyst of canal of Nuck (acquired)
> **EXCLUDES** congenital (752.41)

● **✓5ᵗʰ 629.2 Female genital mutilation status**
Female circumcision status

● **629.20 Female genital mutilation status, unspecified** ♀
Female genital mutilation status NOS

● **629.21 Female genital mutilation Type I status** ♀
Clitorectomy status

● **629.22 Female genital mutilation Type II status** ♀
Clitorectomy with excision of labia minora status

● **629.23 Female genital mutilation Type III status** ♀
Infibulation status

629.8 Other specified disorders of female genital organs ♀

629.9 Unspecified disorder of female genital organs ♀
Habitual aborter without current pregnancy

✓4ᵗʰ / ✓5ᵗʰ Additional Digit Required   Unspecified Code   Other Specified Code   Manifestation Code   ▶◀ Revised Text   ● New Code   ▲ Revised Code Title

2005 ICD•9•CM   **October 2004 • Volume 1 — 173**

11. COMPLICATIONS OF PREGNANCY, CHILDBIRTH AND THE PUERPERIUM (630-677)

ECTOPIC AND MOLAR PREGNANCY (630-633)

Use additional code from category 639 to identify any complications

630 Hydatidiform mole   Ⓜ ♀

Trophoblastic disease NOS   Vesicularmole

> **EXCLUDES**   *chorioadenoma (destruens) (236.1)*
> *chorionepithelioma (181)*
> *malignant hydatidiform mole (236.1)*

DEF: Abnormal product of pregnancy; marked by mass of cysts resembling bunch of grapes due to chorionic villi proliferation, and dissolution; must be surgically removed.

631 Other abnormal product of conception   Ⓜ ♀

Blighted ovum   Mole:
Mole: fleshy
    NOS   stone
    carneous

632 Missed abortion   Ⓜ ♀

Early fetal death before completion of 22 weeks' gestation with retention of dead fetus

Retained products of conception, not following spontaneous or induced abortion or delivery

> **EXCLUDES**   *failed induced abortion (638.0-638.9)*
> *fetal death (intrauterine) (late) (656.4)*
> *missed delivery (656.4)*
> *that with abnormal product of conception (630, 631)*

AHA: 1Q, '01, 5

√4ᵗʰ 633 Ectopic pregnancy

> **INCLUDES**   ruptured ectopic pregnancy

AHA: 4Q, '02, 61

DEF: Fertilized egg develops outside uterus.

√5ᵗʰ 633.0 Abdominal pregnancy

Intraperitoneal pregnancy

    633.00 Abdominal pregnancy without intrauterine pregnancy   Ⓜ ♀

    633.01 Abdominal pregnancy with intrauterine pregnancy   Ⓜ ♀

√5ᵗʰ 633.1 Tubal pregnancy

Fallopian pregnancy
Rupture of (fallopian) tube due to pregnancy
Tubal abortion

AHA: 2Q, '90, 27

    633.10 Tubal pregnancy without intrauterine pregnancy   Ⓜ ♀

    633.11 Tubal pregnancy with intrauterine pregnancy   Ⓜ ♀

√5ᵗʰ 633.2 Ovarian pregnancy

    633.20 Ovarian pregnancy without intrauterine pregnancy   Ⓜ ♀

    633.21 Ovarian pregnancy with intrauterine pregnancy   Ⓜ ♀

√5ᵗʰ 633.8 Other ectopic pregnancy

Pregnancy: Pregnancy:
   cervical   intraligamentous
   combined   mesometric
   cornual   mural

    633.80 Other ectopic pregnancy without intrauterine pregnancy   Ⓜ ♀

    633.81 Other ectopic pregnancy with intrauterine pregnancy   Ⓜ ♀

√5ᵗʰ 633.9 Unspecified ectopic pregnancy

    633.90 Unspecified ectopic pregnancy without intrauterine pregnancy   Ⓜ ♀

    633.91 Unspecified ectopic pregnancy with intrauterine pregnancy   Ⓜ ♀

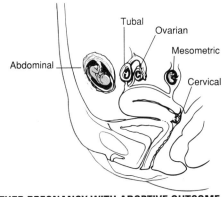

Ectopic Pregnancy Sites

Tubal — Ovarian — Mesometric — Cervical — Abdominal

OTHER PREGNANCY WITH ABORTIVE OUTCOME (634-639)

The following fourth-digit subdivisions are for use with categories 634-638:

.0 Complicated by genital tract and pelvic infection

Endometritis
Salpingo-oophoritis
Sepsis NOS
Septicemia NOS
Any condition classifiable to 639.0, with condition classifiable to 634-638

> **EXCLUDES**   *urinary tract infection (634-638 with .7)*

.1 Complicated by delayed or excessive hemorrhage

Afibrinogenemia
Defibrination syndrome
Intravascular hemolysis
Any condition classifiable to 639.1, with condition classifiable to 634-638

.2 Complicated by damage to pelvic organs and tissues

Laceration, perforation, or tear of:
   bladder
   uterus
Any condition classifiable to 639.2, with condition classifiable to 634-638

.3 Complicated by renal failure

Oliguria
Uremia
Any condition classifiable to 639.3, with condition classifiable to 634-638

.4 Complicated by metabolic disorder

Electrolyte imbalance with conditions classifiable to 634-638

.5 Complicated by shock

Circulatory collapse
Shock (postoperative) (septic)
Any condition classifiable to 639.5, with condition classifiable to 634-638

.6 Complicated by embolism

Embolism:
   NOS
   amniotic fluid
   pulmonary
Any condition classifiable to 639.6, with condition classifiable to 634-638

.7 With other specified complications

Cardiac arrest or failure
Urinary tract infection
Any condition classifiable to 639.8, with condition classifiable to 634-638

.8 With unspecified complication

.9 Without mention of complication

√4ᵗʰ / **√5ᵗʰ** Additional Digit Required   Unspecified Code   Other Specified Code   Manifestation Code   ▶◀ Revised Text   ● New Code   ▲ Revised Code Title

2005 ICD•9•CM   **Volume 1 — 175**

Complications of Pregnancy, Childbirth & Puerperium

634–639

§ ✓4th **634 Spontaneous abortion**
     INCLUDES   miscarriage
                     spontaneous abortion

     Requires fifth-digit to identify stage:
         0   unspecified
         1   incomplete
         2   complete

     AHA: 2Q, '91, 16

     DEF: Spontaneous premature expulsion of the products of conception from the uterus.

✓5th **634.0 Complicated by genital tract and pelvic infection**   M♀
✓5th **634.1 Complicated by delayed or excessive hemorrhage**   M♀
     AHA: For code 634.11: 1Q, '03, 6
✓5th **634.2 Complicated by damage to pelvic organs or tissues**   M♀
✓5th **634.3 Complicated by renal failure**   M♀
✓5th **634.4 Complicated by metabolic disorder**   M♀
✓5th **634.5 Complicated by shock**   M♀
✓5th **634.6 Complicated by embolism**   M♀
✓5th **634.7 With other specified complications**   M♀
✓5th **634.8 With unspecified complication**   M♀
✓5th **634.9 Without mention of complication**   M♀

§ ✓4th **635 Legally induced abortion**
     INCLUDES   abortion or termination of pregnancy:
                     elective
                     legal
                     therapeutic
     EXCLUDES   *menstrual extraction or regulation (V25.3)*

     Requires fifth-digit to identify stage:
         0   unspecified
         1   incomplete
         2   complete

     AHA: 2Q, '94, 14

     DEF: Intentional expulsion of products of conception from uterus performed by medical professionals inside boundaries of law.

✓5th **635.0 Complicated by genital tract and pelvic infection**   M♀
✓5th **635.1 Complicated by delayed or excessive hemorrhage**   M♀
✓5th **635.2 Complicated by damage to pelvic organs or tissues**   M♀
✓5th **635.3 Complicated by renal failure**   M♀
✓5th **635.4 Complicated by metabolic disorder**   M♀
✓5th **635.5 Complicated by shock**   M♀
✓5th **635.6 Complicated by embolism**   M♀
✓5th **635.7 With other specified complications**   M♀
✓5th **635.8 With unspecified complication**   M♀
✓5th **635.9 Without mention of complication**   M♀

§ ✓4th **636 Illegally induced abortion**
     INCLUDES   abortion: abortion:
                     criminal   self-induced
                     illegal

     Requires fifth-digit to identify stage:
         0   unspecified
         1   incomplete
         2   complete

     DEF: Intentional expulsion of products of conception from uterus; outside boundaries of law.

✓5th **636.0 Complicated by genital tract and pelvic infection**   M♀
✓5th **636.1 Complicated by delayed or excessive hemorrhage**   M♀
✓5th **636.2 Complicated by damage to pelvic organs or tissues**   M♀
✓5th **636.3 Complicated by renal failure**   M♀
✓5th **636.4 Complicated by metabolic disorder**   M♀
✓5th **636.5 Complicated by shock**   M♀
✓5th **636.6 Complicated by embolism**   M♀
✓5th **636.7 With other specified complications**   M♀
✓5th **636.8 With unspecified complication**   M♀
✓5th **636.9 Without mention of complication**   M♀

§ ✓4th **637 Unspecified abortion**
     INCLUDES   abortion NOS
                     retained products of conception following abortion, not classifiable elsewhere

     Requires fifth-digit to identify stage:
         0   unspecified
         1   incomplete
         2   complete

✓5th **637.0 Complicated by genital tract and pelvic infection**   M♀
✓5th **637.1 Complicated by delayed or excessive hemorrhage**   M♀
✓5th **637.2 Complicated by damage to pelvic organs or tissues**   M♀
✓5th **637.3 Complicated by renal failure**   M♀
✓5th **637.4 Complicated by metabolic disorder**   M♀
✓5th **637.5 Complicated by shock**   M♀
✓5th **637.6 Complicated by embolism**   M♀
✓5th **637.7 With other specified complications**   M♀
✓5th **637.8 With unspecified complication**   M♀
✓5th **637.9 Without mention of complication**   M♀

§ ✓4th **638 Failed attempted abortion**
     INCLUDES   failure of attempted induction of (legal) abortion
     EXCLUDES   *incomplete abortion (634.0-637.9)*
     DEF: Continued pregnancy despite an attempted legal abortion.

638.0 Complicated by genital tract and pelvic infection   M♀
638.1 Complicated by delayed or excessive hemorrhage   M♀
638.2 Complicated by damage to pelvic organs or tissues   M♀
638.3 Complicated by renal failure   M♀
638.4 Complicated by metabolic disorder   M♀
638.5 Complicated by shock   M♀
638.6 Complicated by embolism   M♀
638.7 With other specified complications   M♀
638.8 With unspecified complication   M♀
638.9 Without mention of complication   M♀

✓4th **639 Complications following abortion and ectopic and molar pregnancies**
     Note: This category is provided for use when it is required to classify separately the complications classifiable to the fourth-digit level in categories 634-638; for example:
     a) when the complication itself was responsible for an episode of medical care, the abortion, ectopic or molar pregnancy itself having been dealt with at a previous episode
     b) when these conditions are immediate complications of ectopic or molar pregnancies classifiable to 630-633 where they cannot be identified at fourth-digit level.

§ See beginning of section 634–639 for fourth-digit definitions.

639.0   **Genital tract and pelvic infection**   Ⓜ ♀

Endometritis
Parametritis
Pelvic peritonitis
Salpingitis   } following conditions classifiable to 630-638
Salpingo-oophoritis
Sepsis NOS
Septicemia NOS

> **EXCLUDES**   *urinary tract infection (639.8)*

639.1   **Delayed or excessive hemorrhage**   Ⓜ ♀

Afibrinogenemia
Defibrination syndrome   } following conditions classifiable to 630-638
Intravascular hemolysis

639.2   **Damage to pelvic organs and tissues**   Ⓜ ♀

Laceration, perforation, or tear of:
   bladder
   bowel
   broad ligament   } following conditions classifiable to 630-638
   cervix
   periurethral tissue
   uterus
   vagina

639.3   **Renal failure**   Ⓜ ♀

Oliguria
Renal:
   failure (acute)
   shutdown   } following conditions classifiable to 630-638
   tubular necrosis
Uremia

639.4   **Metabolic disorders**   Ⓜ ♀

Electrolyte imbalance following conditions classifiable to 630-638

639.5   **Shock**   Ⓜ ♀

Circulatory collapse
Shock (postoperative)   } following conditions classifiable to 630-638
   (septic)

639.6   **Embolism**   Ⓜ ♀

Embolism:
   NOS
   air
   amniotic fluid
   blood-clot   } following conditions classifiable to 630-638
   fat
   pulmonary
   pyemic
   septic
   soap

639.8   **Other specified complications following abortion or ectopic and molar pregnancy**   Ⓜ ♀

Acute yellow atrophy or necrosis of liver
Cardiac arrest or failure   } following conditions classifiable to 630-638
Cerebral anoxia
Urinary tract infection

639.9   **Unspecified complication following abortion or ectopic and molar pregnancy**   Ⓜ ♀

Complication(s) not further specified following conditions classifiable to 630-638

COMPLICATIONS MAINLY RELATED TO PREGNANCY (640-648)

> **INCLUDES**   the listed conditions even if they arose or were present during labor, delivery, or the puerperium

The following fifth-digit subclassification is for use with categories 640-648 to denote the current episode of care. Valid fifth-digits are in [brackets] under each code.

   0   **unspecified as to episode of care or not applicable**

   1   **delivered, with or without mention of antepartum condition**

     Antepartum condition with delivery
     Delivery NOS (with mention of antepartum complication during current episode of care)
     Intrapartum obstetric condition (with mention of antepartum complication during current episode of care)
     Pregnancy, delivered (with mention of antepartum complication during current episode of care)

   2   **delivered, with mention of postpartum complication**

     Delivery with mention of puerperal complication during current episode of care

   3   **antepartum condition or complication**

     Antepartum obstetric condition, not delivered during the current episode of care

   4   **postpartum condition or complication**

     Postpartum or puerperal obstetric condition or complication following delivery that occurred:
      during previous episode of care
      outside hospital, with subsequent admission for observation or care

AHA: 2Q, '90, 11

√4ᵗʰ **640**   **Hemorrhage in early pregnancy**

> **INCLUDES**   hemorrhage before completion of 22 weeks' gestation

√5ᵗʰ **640.0**   **Threatened abortion**   Ⓜ ♀
[0,1,3]   DEF: Bloody discharge during pregnancy; cervix may be dilated and pregnancy is threatened, but the pregnancy is not terminated.

√5ᵗʰ **640.8**   **Other specified hemorrhage in early pregnancy**   Ⓜ ♀
[0,1,3]

√5ᵗʰ **640.9**   **Unspecified hemorrhage in early pregnancy**   Ⓜ ♀
[0,1,3]

√4ᵗʰ **641**   **Antepartum hemorrhage, abruptio placentae, and placenta previa**

√5ᵗʰ **641.0**   **Placenta previa without hemorrhage**   Ⓜ ♀
[0,1,3]

Low implantation of placenta
Placenta previa noted: } without hemorrhage
   during pregnancy
   before labor (and delivered by cesarean delivery)

DEF: Placenta implanted in lower segment of uterus; commonly causes hemorrhage in the last trimester of pregnancy.

√5ᵗʰ **641.1**   **Hemorrhage from placenta previa**   Ⓜ ♀
[0,1,3]

Low-lying placenta
Placenta previa: } NOS or with hemorrhage (intrapartum)
   incomplete
   marginal
   partial
   total

> **EXCLUDES**   *hemorrhage from vasa previa (663.5)*

✓4ᵗʰ ✓5ᵗʰ Additional Digit Required   Unspecified Code   Other Specified Code   Manifestation Code   ▶◀ Revised Text   ● New Code   ▲ Revised Code Title

2005 ICD•9•CM   **Volume 1 — 177**

Complications of Pregnancy, Childbirth & Puerperium

641.2–643

Placenta Previa

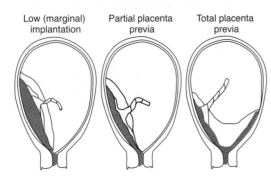

Low (marginal) implantation   Partial placenta previa   Total placenta previa

§ ✓5ᵗʰ 641.2   **Premature separation of placenta**   Ⓜ ♀
[0,1,3]
     Ablatio placentae
     Abruptio placentae
     Accidental antepartum hemorrhage
     Couvelaire uterus
     Detachment of placenta (premature)
     Premature separation of normally implanted
       placenta

     DEF: Abruptio placentae: premature detachment of the placenta, characterized by shock, oliguria and decreased fibrinogen.

§ ✓5ᵗʰ 641.3   **Antepartum hemorrhage associated with**   Ⓜ ♀
[0,1,3]   **coagulation defects**
     Antepartum or intrapartum hemorrhage associated
       with:
       afibrinogenemia
       hyperfibrinolysis
       hypofibrinogenemia

     DEF: Uterine hemorrhage prior to delivery.

§ ✓5ᵗʰ 641.8   **Other antepartum hemorrhage**   Ⓜ ♀
[0,1,3]
     Antepartum or intrapartum hemorrhage associated
       with:
       trauma
       uterine leiomyoma

§ ✓5ᵗʰ 641.9   **Unspecified antepartum hemorrhage**   Ⓜ ♀
[0,1,3]   Hemorrhage: Hemorrhage:
       antepartum NOS   of pregnancy NOS
       intrapartum NOS

✓4ᵗʰ 642   **Hypertension complicating pregnancy, childbirth and the**
puerperium

Abruptio Placentae

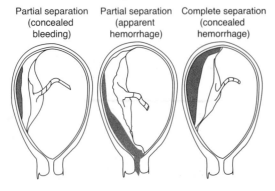

Partial separation (concealed bleeding)   Partial separation (apparent hemorrhage)   Complete separation (concealed hemorrhage)

§ ✓5ᵗʰ 642.0   **Benign essential hypertension complicating**   Ⓜ ♀
[0-4]   **pregnancy, childbirth and the puerperium**
     Hypertension:
       benign essential   } specified as complicating,
       chronic NOS   or as a reason for
       essential   obstetric care during
       pre-existing NOS   pregnancy, childbirth
                               or the puerperium

§ ✓5ᵗʰ 642.1   **Hypertension secondary to renal disease,**   Ⓜ ♀
[0-4]   **complicating pregnancy, childbirth and the**
   puerperium
     Hypertension secondary to renal disease, specified
       as complicating, or as a reason for obstetric
       care during pregnancy, childbirth or the
       puerperium

§ ✓5ᵗʰ 642.2   **Other pre-existing hypertension complicating** Ⓜ ♀
[0-4]   **pregnancy, childbirth and the puerperium**
     Hypertensive:
       heart and renal   } specified as complicating,
         disease   or as a reason for
       heart disease   obstetric care
       renal disease   during pregnancy,
       Malignant   childbirth or the
         hypertension   puerperium

§ ✓5ᵗʰ 642.3   **Transient hypertension of pregnancy**   Ⓜ ♀
[0-4]   Gestational hypertension
     Transient hypertension, so described, in pregnancy,
       childbirth or the puerperium

     AHA: 3Q, '90, 4

§ ✓5ᵗʰ 642.4   **Mild or unspecified pre-eclampsia**   Ⓜ ♀
[0-4]   Hypertension in pregnancy, childbirth or the
       puerperium, not specified as pre-existing, with
       either albuminuria or edema, or both; mild or
       unspecified
     Pre-eclampsia: Toxemia (pre-eclamptic):
       NOS   NOS
       mild   mild

     EXCLUDES   albuminuria in pregnancy, without
                   mention of hypertension (646.2)
                  edema in pregnancy, without mention
                   of hypertension (646.1)

§ ✓5ᵗʰ 642.5   **Severe pre-eclampsia**   Ⓜ ♀
[0-4]   Hypertension in pregnancy, childbirth or the
       puerperium, not specified as pre-existing, with
       either albuminuria or edema, or both; specified
       as severe
     Pre-eclampsia, severe
     Toxemia (pre-eclamptic), severe

     AHA: N-D, '85, 3

§ ✓5ᵗʰ 642.6   **Eclampsia**   Ⓜ ♀
[0-4]   Toxemia: Toxemia:
       eclamptic   with convulsions

§ ✓5ᵗʰ 642.7   **Pre-eclampsia or eclampsia superimposed on** Ⓜ ♀
[0-4]   **pre existing hypertension**
     Conditions classifiable to 642.4-642.6, with
       conditions classifiable to 642.0-642.2

§ ✓5ᵗʰ 642.9   **Unspecified hypertension complicating** Ⓜ ♀
[0-4]   **pregnancy, childbirth or the puerperium**
     Hypertension NOS, without mention of albuminuria
       or edema, complicating pregnancy, childbirth
       or the puerperium

✓4ᵗʰ 643   **Excessive vomiting in pregnancy**
     INCLUDES   hyperemesis   }
              vomiting: } arising during pregnancy
                persistent   }
                vicious

     hyperemesis gravidarum

---

§ Requires fifth digit. Valid digits are in [brackets] under each code. See beginning of section 640–648 for codes and definitions.

Ⓝ Newborn Age: 0   Ⓟ Pediatric Age: 0-17   Ⓜ Maternity Age: 12-55   Ⓐ Adult Age: 15-124   MSP Medicare Secondary Payer

§ ✓5ᵗʰ **643.0** **Mild hyperemesis gravidarum** Ⓜ♀
[0,1,3]
Hyperemesis gravidarum, mild or unspecified, starting before the end of the 22nd week of gestation
DEF: Detrimental vomiting and nausea.

§ ✓5ᵗʰ **643.1** **Hyperemesis gravidarum with metabolic** Ⓜ♀
[0,1,3] **disturbance**
Hyperemesis gravidarum, starting before the end of the 22nd week of gestation, with metabolic disturbance, such as:
carbohydrate depletion
dehydration
electrolyte imbalance

§ ✓5ᵗʰ **643.2** **Late vomiting of pregnancy** Ⓜ♀
[0,1,3]
Excessive vomiting starting after 22 completed weeks of gestation

§ ✓5ᵗʰ **643.8** **Other vomiting complicating pregnancy** Ⓜ♀
[0,1,3]
Vomiting due to organic disease or other cause, specified as complicating pregnancy, or as a reason for obstetric care during pregnancy
Use additional code to specify cause

§ ✓5ᵗʰ **643.9** **Unspecified vomiting of pregnancy** Ⓜ♀
[0,1,3]
Vomiting as a reason for care during pregnancy, length of gestation unspecified

✓4ᵗʰ **644 Early or threatened labor**

§ ✓5ᵗʰ **644.0** **Threatened premature labor** Ⓜ♀
[0,3]
Premature labor after 22 weeks, but before 37 completed weeks of gestation without delivery
EXCLUDES *that occurring before 22 completed weeks of gestation (640.0)*

§ ✓5ᵗʰ **644.1** **Other threatened labor** Ⓜ♀
[0,3]
False labor:
NOS
after 37 completed
  weeks of gestation } without delivery
Threatened labor NOS

§ ✓5ᵗʰ **644.2** **Early onset of delivery** Ⓜ♀
[0,1]
Onset (spontaneous) of
  delivery
Premature labor with
  onset of delivery } before 37 completed weeks of gestation
AHA: 2Q, '91, 16

✓4ᵗʰ **645 Late pregnancy**
AHA: 4Q. '00, 43; 4Q, '91, 26

§ ✓5ᵗʰ **645.1** **Post term pregnancy** Ⓜ♀
[0,1,3]
Pregnancy over 40 completed weeks to 42 completed weeks gestation

§ ✓5ᵗʰ **645.2** **Prolonged pregnancy** Ⓜ♀
[0,1,3]
Pregnancy which has advanced beyond 42 completed weeks of gestation

✓4ᵗʰ **646 Other complications of pregnancy, not elsewhere classified**
Use additional code(s) to further specify complication
AHA: 4Q, '95, 59

§ ✓5ᵗʰ **646.0** **Papyraceous fetus** Ⓜ♀
[0,1,3] DEF: Fetus retained in the uterus beyond natural term, exhibits parchment-like skin.

§ ✓5ᵗʰ **646.1** **Edema or excessive weight gain in pregnancy,** Ⓜ♀
[0-4] **without mention of hypertension**
Gestational edema   Maternal obesity syndrome
EXCLUDES *that with mention of hypertension (642.0-642.)*

§ ✓5ᵗʰ **646.2** **Unspecified renal disease in pregnancy,** Ⓜ♀
[0-4] **without mention of hypertension**
Albuminuria
Nephropathy NOS } in pregnancy or the puerperium, without mention of hypertension
Renal disease NOS
Uremia

Gestational proteinuria
EXCLUDES *that with mention of hypertension (642.0-642.9)*

§ ✓5ᵗʰ **646.3** **Habitual aborter** Ⓜ♀
[0,1,3] EXCLUDES *with current abortion (634.0-634.9)*
without current pregnancy (629.9)
DEF: Three or more consecutive spontaneous abortions.

§ ✓5ᵗʰ **646.4** **Peripheral neuritis in pregnancy** Ⓜ♀
[0-4]

§ ✓5ᵗʰ **646.5** **Asymptomatic bacteriuria in pregnancy** Ⓜ♀
[0-4]

§ ✓5ᵗʰ **646.6** **Infections of genitourinary tract in pregnancy** Ⓜ♀
[0-4]
Conditions classifiable to 590, 595, 597, 599.0, 616 complicating pregnancy, childbirth or the puerperium
Conditions classifiable to (614.0-614.5, 614.7-614.9, 615) complicating pregnancy or labor
EXCLUDES *major puerperal infection (670)*

§ ✓5ᵗʰ **646.7** **Liver disorders in pregnancy** Ⓜ♀
[0,1,3]
Acute yellow atrophy of liver
  (obstetric) (true)
Icterus gravis } of pregnancy
Necrosis of liver

EXCLUDES *hepatorenal syndrome following delivery (674.8)*
viral hepatitis (647.6)

§ ✓5ᵗʰ **646.8** **Other specified complications of pregnancy** Ⓜ♀
[0-4]
Fatigue during pregnancy
Herpes gestationis
Insufficient weight gain of pregnancy
Uterine size-date discrepancy
AHA: 3Q, '98, 16, J-F, '85, 15

§ ✓5ᵗʰ **646.9** **Unspecified complication of pregnancy** Ⓜ♀
[0,1,3]

✓4ᵗʰ **647 Infectious and parasitic conditions in the mother classifiable elsewhere, but complicating pregnancy, childbirth or the puerperium**
INCLUDES the listed conditions when complicating the pregnant state, aggravated by the pregnancy, or when a main reason for obstetric care
EXCLUDES *those conditions in the mother known or suspected to have affected the fetus (655.0-655.9)*
Use additional code(s) to further specify complication

§ ✓5ᵗʰ **647.0** **Syphilis** Ⓜ♀
[0-4] Conditions classifiable to 090-097

§ ✓5ᵗʰ **647.1** **Gonorrhea** Ⓜ♀
[0-4] Conditions classifiable to 098

§ ✓5ᵗʰ **647.2** **Other venereal diseases** Ⓜ♀
[0-4] Conditions classifiable to 099

§ ✓5ᵗʰ **647.3** **Tuberculosis** Ⓜ♀
[0-4] Conditions classifiable to 010-018

§ ✓5ᵗʰ **647.4** **Malaria** Ⓜ♀
[0-4] Conditions classifiable to 084

§ ✓5ᵗʰ **647.5** **Rubella** Ⓜ♀
[0-4] Conditions classifiable to 056

§ Requires fifth digit. Valid digits are in [brackets] under each code. See beginning of section 640–648 for codes and definitions.

✓4ᵗʰ / ✓5ᵗʰ Additional Digit Required   Unspecified Code   Other Specified Code   Manifestation Code   ▶◀ Revised Text   ● New Code   ▲ Revised Code Title

Complications of Pregnancy, Childbirth & Puerperium

647.6–652.2

§ ✓5ᵗʰ **647.6** **Other viral diseases** Ⓜ ♀
[0-4]   Conditions classifiable to 042 and 050-079, except 056
     AHA: J-F, '85, 15

§ ✓5ᵗʰ **647.8** **Other specified infectious and parasitic diseases** Ⓜ ♀
[0-4]

§ ✓5ᵗʰ **647.9** **Unspecified infection or infestation** Ⓜ ♀
[0-4]

✓4ᵗʰ **648** **Other current conditions in the mother classifiable elsewhere, but complicating pregnancy, childbirth or the puerperium**

     INCLUDES   the listed conditions when complicating the pregnant state, aggravated by the pregnancy, or when a main reason for obstetric care

     EXCLUDES   *those conditions in the mother known or suspected to have affected the fetus (655.0-665.9)*

     Use additional code(s) to identify the condition

§ ✓5ᵗʰ **648.0** **Diabetes mellitus** Ⓜ ♀
[0-4]   Conditions classifiable to 250
     EXCLUDES   *gestational diabetes (648.8)*
     AHA: 3Q, '91, 5, 11

§ ✓5ᵗʰ **648.1** **Thyroid dysfunction** Ⓜ ♀
[0-4]   Conditions classifiable to 240-246

§ ✓5ᵗʰ **648.2** **Anemia** Ⓜ ♀
[0-4]   Conditions classifiable to 280-285
     AHA: For Code 648.22: 1Q, '02, 14

§ ✓5ᵗʰ **648.3** **Drug dependence** Ⓜ ♀
[0-4]   Conditions classifiable to 304
     AHA: 2Q, '98, 13; 4Q, '88, 8

§ ✓5ᵗʰ **648.4** **Mental disorders** Ⓜ ♀
[0-4]   Conditions classifiable to 290-303, 305-316, 317-319
     AHA: 2Q, '98, 13; 4Q, '95, 63

§ ✓5ᵗʰ **648.5** **Congenital cardiovascular disorders** Ⓜ ♀
[0-4]   Conditions classifiable to 745-747

§ ✓5ᵗʰ **648.6** **Other cardiovascular diseases** Ⓜ ♀
[0-4]   Conditions classifiable to 390-398, 410-429
     EXCLUDES   *cerebrovascular disorders in the puerperium (674.0)*
       ▶*peripartum cardiomyopathy (674.5)*◀
       venous complications (671.0-671.9)
     AHA: 3Q, '98, 11

§ ✓5ᵗʰ **648.7** **Bone and joint disorders of back, pelvis, and lower limbs** Ⓜ ♀
[0-4]   Conditions classifiable to 720-724, and those classifiable to 711-719 or 725-738, specified as affecting the lower limbs

§ ✓5ᵗʰ **648.8** **Abnormal glucose tolerance** Ⓜ ♀
[0-4]   Conditions classifiable to 790.2
     Gestational diabetes
     AHA: 3Q, '91, 5

     DEF: Glucose intolerance arising in pregnancy, resolving at end of pregnancy.

§ ✓5ᵗʰ **648.9** **Other current conditions classifiable elsewhere** Ⓜ ♀
[0-4]   Conditions classifiable to 440-459
     Nutritional deficiencies [conditions classifiable to 260-269]
     AHA: N-D, '87, 10; **For code 648.91:** 1Q, '02, 14

NORMAL DELIVERY, AND OTHER INDICATIONS FOR CARE IN PREGNANCY, LABOR, AND DELIVERY (650-659)

The following fifth-digit subclassification is for use with categories 651-659 to denote the current episode of care. Valid fifth-digits are in [brackets] under each code.

   0   **unspecified as to episode of care or not applicable**
   1   delivered, with or without mention of antepartum condition
   2   delivered, with mention of postpartum complication
   3   antepartum condition or complication
   4   postpartum condition or complication

650 **Normal delivery** Ⓜ ♀
Delivery requiring minimal or no assistance, with or without episiotomy, without fetal manipulation [e.g., rotation version] or instrumentation [forceps] of spontaneous, cephalic, vaginal, full-term, single, live-born infant. This code is for use as a single diagnosis code and is not to be used with any other code in the range 630-676.

     EXCLUDES   *breech delivery (assisted) (spontaneous) NOS (652.2)*
       delivery by vacuum extractor, forceps, cesarean section, or breech extraction, without specified complication (669.5-669.7)

     Use additional code to indicate outcome of delivery (V27.0)

     AHA: 2Q, '02, 10; 3Q, '01, 12; 3Q, '00, 5; 4Q, '95, 28, 59

✓4ᵗʰ **651** **Multiple gestation**

§ ✓5ᵗʰ **651.0** **Twin pregnancy** Ⓜ ♀
[0,1,3]

§ ✓5ᵗʰ **651.1** **Triplet pregnancy** Ⓜ ♀
[0,1,3]

§ ✓5ᵗʰ **651.2** **Quadruplet pregnancy** Ⓜ ♀
[0,1,3]

§ ✓5ᵗʰ **651.3** **Twin pregnancy with fetal loss and retention of one fetus** Ⓜ ♀
[0,1,3]   Vanishing twin syndrome (651.33)

§ ✓5ᵗʰ **651.4** **Triplet pregnancy with fetal loss and retention of one or more fetus(es)** Ⓜ ♀
[0,1,3]

§ ✓5ᵗʰ **651.5** **Quadruplet pregnancy with fetal loss and retention of one or more fetus(es)** Ⓜ ♀
[0,1,3]

§ ✓5ᵗʰ **651.6** **Other multiple pregnancy with fetal loss and retention of one or more fetus(es)** Ⓜ ♀
[0,1,3]

§ ✓5ᵗʰ **651.8** **Other specified multiple gestation** Ⓜ ♀
[0,1,3]

§ ✓5ᵗʰ **651.9** **Unspecified multiple gestation** Ⓜ ♀
[0,1,3]

✓4ᵗʰ **652** **Malposition and malpresentation of fetus**
     Code first any associated obstructed labor (660.0)

§ ✓5ᵗʰ **652.0** **Unstable lie** Ⓜ ♀
[0,1,3]   DEF: Changing fetal position.

§ ✓5ᵗʰ **652.1** **Breech or other malpresentation successfully converted to cephalic presentation** Ⓜ ♀
[0,1,3]   Cephalic version NOS

§ ✓5ᵗʰ **652.2** **Breech presentation without mention of version** Ⓜ ♀
[0,1,3]
     Breech delivery (assisted) (spontaneous) NOS
     Buttocks presentation
     Complete breech
     Frank breech
     EXCLUDES   *footling presentation (652.8)*
       incomplete breech (652.8)

     DEF: Fetal presentation of buttocks or feet at birth canal.

---

§ Requires fifth digit. Valid digits are in [brackets] under each code. See beginning of section 640–648 for codes and definitions.

Ⓝ Newborn Age: 0   Ⓟ Pediatric Age: 0-17   Ⓜ Maternity Age: 12-55   Ⓐ Adult Age: 15-124   MSP Medicare Secondary Payer

Malposition and Malpresentation

Breech

Shoulder (arm prolapse)

Mother's pelvis

Face (mentum)

Compound (extremity together with head)

Oblique

Cephalopelvic Disproportion

Pubic symphysis

Cephalopelvic disproportion due to: Contraction of pelvic inlet, or large fetus, or hydrocephalus

Ischial tuberosity

Contraction of pelvic outlet (from below)

Pubic symphysis

Pelvic inlet from above

§ ✓5th **652.3** **Transverse or oblique presentation**   M♀
[0,1,3]   Oblique lie   Transverse lie
EXCLUDES   *transverse arrest of fetal head (660.3)*
DEF: Delivery of fetus, shoulder first.

§ ✓5th **652.4** **Face or brow presentation**   M♀
[0,1,3]   Mentum presentation

§ ✓5th **652.5** **High head at term**   M♀
[0,1,3]   Failure of head to enter pelvic brim

§ ✓5th **652.6** **Multiple gestation with malpresentation**   M♀
[0,1,3]   **of one fetus or more**

§ ✓5th **652.7** **Prolapsed arm**   M♀
[0,1,3]

§ ✓5th **652.8** **Other specified malposition or**   M♀
[0,1,3]   **malpresentation**
    Compound presentation

§ ✓5th **652.9** **Unspecified malposition or malpresentation**   M♀
[0,1,3]

✓4th **653** **Disproportion**
    Code first any associated obstructed labor (660.1)

§ ✓5th **653.0** **Major abnormality of bony pelvis, not further**   M♀
[0,1,3]   **specified**
    Pelvic deformity NOS

§ ✓5th **653.1** **Generally contracted pelvis**   M♀
[0,1,3]   Contracted pelvis NOS

§ ✓5th **653.2** **Inlet contraction of pelvis**   M♀
[0,1,3]   Inlet contraction (pelvis)

§ ✓5th **653.3** **Outlet contraction of pelvis**   M♀
[0,1,3]   Outlet contraction (pelvis)

§ ✓5th **653.4** **Fetopelvic disproportion**   M♀
[0,1,3]   Cephalopelvic disproportion NOS
    Disproportion of mixed maternal and fetal origin, with normally formed fetus

§ ✓5th **653.5** **Unusually large fetus causing disproportion**   M♀
[0,1,3]   Disproportion of fetal origin with normally formed fetus
    Fetal disproportion NOS
    EXCLUDES   *that when the reason for medical care was concern for the fetus (656.6)*

§ ✓5th **653.6** **Hydrocephalic fetus causing disproportion**   M♀
[0,1,3]   *EXCLUDES*   *that when the reason for medical care was concern for the fetus (655.0)*

§ ✓5th **653.7** **Other fetal abnormality causing disproportion**   M♀
[0,1,3]   Conjoined twins   Fetal:
    Fetal: myelomeningocele
    ascites   sacral teratoma
    hydrops   tumor

§ ✓5th **653.8** **Disproportion of other origin**   M♀
[0,1,3]   *EXCLUDES*   *shoulder (girdle) dystocia (660.4)*

§ ✓5th **653.9** **Unspecified disproportion**   M♀
[0,1,3]

✓4th **654** **Abnormality of organs and soft tissues of pelvis**
    INCLUDES   the listed conditions during pregnancy, childbirth or the puerperium
    Code first any associated obstructed labor (660.2)

§ ✓5th **654.0** **Congenital abnormalities of uterus**   M♀
[0-4]   Double uterus   Uterus bicornis

§ ✓5th **654.1** **Tumors of body of uterus**   M♀
[0-4]   Uterine fibroids

§ ✓5th **654.2** **Previous cesarean delivery**   M♀
[0,1,3]   Uterine scar from previous cesarean delivery
    AHA: 1Q, '92, 8

§ ✓5th **654.3** **Retroverted and incarcerated gravid uterus**   M♀
[0-4]   DEF: Retroverted: tilted back uterus; no change in angle of longitudinal axis.
    DEF: Incarcerated: immobile, fixed uterus.

§ ✓5th **654.4** **Other abnormalities in shape or position of**   M♀
[0-4]   **gravid uterus and of neighboring structures**
    Cystocele   Prolapse of gravid uterus
    Pelvic floor repair   Rectocele
    Pendulous abdomen   Rigid pelvic floor

§ ✓5th **654.5** **Cervical incompetence**   M♀
[0-4]   Presence of Shirodkar suture with or without mention of cervical incompetence
    DEF: Abnormal cervix; tendency to dilate in second trimester; causes premature fetal expulsion.
    DEF: Shirodkar suture: purse-string suture used to artificially close incompetent cervix.

§ ✓5th **654.6** **Other congenital or acquired abnormality of**   ♀
[0-4]   **cervix**
    Cicatricial cervix   Rigid cervix (uteri)
    Polyp of cervix   Stenosis or stricture of cervix
    Previous surgery to cervix   Tumor of cervix

§ ✓5th **654.7** **Congenital or acquired abnormality of vagina**   M♀
[0-4]   Previous surgery to vagina   Stricture of vagina
    Septate vagina   Tumor of vagina
    Stenosis of vagina (acquired) (congenital)

§ ✓5th **654.8** **Congenital or acquired abnormality of vulva**   M♀
[0-4]   Fibrosis of perineum   Rigid perineum
    Persistent hymen   Tumor of vulva
    Previous surgery to perineum or vulva
    EXCLUDES   *varicose veins of vulva (671.1)*
    AHA: 1Q, '03, 14

§ ✓5th **654.9** **Other and unspecified**   M♀
[0-4]   Uterine scar NEC

§ Requires fifth digit. Valid digits are in [brackets] under each code. See beginning of section 640–648 for codes and definitions.

✓4th **Additional Digit Required**   **Unspecified Code**   **Other Specified Code**   **Manifestation Code**   ►◄ Revised Text   ● New Code   ▲ Revised Code Title

√4th **655 Known or suspected fetal abnormality affecting management of mother**

INCLUDES the listed conditions in the fetus as a reason for observation or obstetrical care of the mother, or for termination of pregnancy

AHA: 3Q, '90, 4

§ √5th **655.0 Central nervous system malformation in fetus** M♀
[0,1,3]   Fetal or suspected fetal:
         anencephaly
         hydrocephalus
         spina bifida (with myelomeningocele)

§ √5th **655.1 Chromosomal abnormality in fetus** M♀
[0,1,3]

§ √5th **655.2 Hereditary disease in family possibly** M♀
[0,1,3] **affecting fetus**

§ √5th **655.3 Suspected damage to fetus from viral disease** M♀
[0,1,3] **in the mother**
     Suspected damage to fetus from maternal rubella

§ √5th **655.4 Suspected damage to fetus from other** M♀
[0,1,3] **disease in the mother**
     Suspected damage to fetus from maternal:
         alcohol addiction
         listeriosis
         toxoplasmosis

§ √5th **655.5 Suspected damage to fetus from drugs** M♀
[0,1,3]

§ √5th **655.6 Suspected damage to fetus from radiation** M♀
[0,1,3]

§ √5th **655.7 Decreased fetal movements** M♀
[0,1,3] AHA: 4Q, '97, 41

§ √5th **655.8 Other known or suspected fetal abnormality,** M♀
[0,1,3] **not elsewhere classified**
     Suspected damage to fetus from:
         environmental toxins
         intrauterine contraceptive device

§ √5th **655.9 Unspecified** M♀
[0,1,3]

√4th **656 Other fetal and placental problems affecting management of mother**

§ √5th **656.0 Fetal-maternal hemorrhage** M♀
[0,1,3]   Leakage (microscopic) of fetal blood into maternal circulation

§ √5th **656.1 Rhesus isoimmunization** M♀
[0,1,3]   Anti-D [Rh] antibodies
         Rh incompatibility
     DEF: Antibodies developing against Rh factor; mother with Rh negative develops antibodies against Rh positive fetus.

§ √5th **656.2 Isoimmunization from other and unspecified** M♀
[0,1,3] **blood-group incompatibility**
     ABO isoimmunization

§ √5th **656.3 Fetal distress** M♀
[0,1,3]   Fetal metabolic acidemia
         EXCLUDES   abnormal fetal acid-base balance (656.8)
                     abnormality in fetal heart rate or rhythm (659.7)
                     fetal bradycardia (659.7)
                     fetal tachycardia (659.7)
                     meconium in liquor (656.8)
     AHA: N-D, '86, 4
     DEF: Life-threatening disorder; fetal anoxia, hemolytic disease and other miscellaneous diseases cause fetal distress.

§ √5th **656.4 Intrauterine death** M♀
[0,1,3]   Fetal death:
         NOS
         after completion of 22 weeks' gestation
         late
     Missed delivery
         EXCLUDES   missed abortion (632)

§ √5th **656.5 Poor fetal growth** M♀
[0,1,3]   "Light-for-dates"   "Small-for-dates"
     "Placental insufficiency"

§ √5th **656.6 Excessive fetal growth** M♀
[0,1,3]   "Large-for-dates"

§ √5th **656.7 Other placental conditions** M♀
[0,1,3]   Abnormal placenta   Placental infarct
         EXCLUDES   placental polyp (674.4)
                     placentitis (658.4)

§ √5th **656.8 Other specified fetal and placental problems** M♀
[0,1,3]   Abnormal acid-base balance
     Intrauterine acidosis
     Lithopedian
     Meconium in liquor
     DEF: Lithopedion: Calcified fetus; not expelled by mother.

§ √5th **656.9 Unspecified fetal and placental problem** M♀
[0,1,3]

√4th **657 Polyhydramnios** M♀
[0,1,3]
§ √5th   Use 0 as fourth-digit for this category
     Hydramnios
AHA: 4Q, '91, 26

DEF: Excess amniotic fluid.

√4th **658 Other problems associated with amniotic cavity and membranes**
     EXCLUDES   amniotic fluid embolism (673.1)

§ √5th **658.0 Oligohydramnios** M♀
[0,1,3]   Oligohydramnios without mention of rupture of membranes
     DEF: Deficient amount of amniotic fluid.

§ √5th **658.1 Premature rupture of membranes** M♀
[0,1,3]   Rupture of amniotic sac less than 24 hours prior to the onset of labor
     AHA: For code 658.13: 1Q, '01, 5; 4Q, '98, 77

§ √5th **658.2 Delayed delivery after spontaneous or** M♀
[0,1,3] **unspecified rupture of membranes**
     Prolonged rupture of membranes NOS
     Rupture of amniotic sac 24 hours or more prior to the onset of labor

§ √5th **658.3 Delayed delivery after artificial rupture of** M♀
[0,1,3] **membranes**

§ √5th **658.4 Infection of amniotic cavity** M♀
[0,1,3]   Amnionitis   Membranitis
     Chorioamnionitis   Placentitis

§ √5th **658.8 Other** M♀
[0,1,3]   Amnion nodosum   Amniotic cyst

§ √5th **658.9 Unspecified** M♀
[0,1,3]

√4th **659 Other indications for care or intervention related to labor and delivery, not elsewhere classified**

§ √5th **659.0 Failed mechanical induction** M♀
[0,1,3]   Failure of induction of labor by surgical or other instrumental methods

§ √5th **659.1 Failed medical or unspecified induction** M♀
[0,1,3]   Failed induction NOS
     Failure of induction of labor by medical methods, such as oxytocic drugs

---

§ Requires fifth digit. Valid digits are in [brackets] under each code. See beginning of section 640–648 for codes and definitions.

N Newborn Age: 0   P Pediatric Age: 0-17   M Maternity Age: 12-55   A Adult Age: 15-124   MSP Medicare Secondary Payer

§ ✓5ᵗʰ **659.2** **Maternal pyrexia during labor, unspecified** Ⓜ♀
[0,1,3]   DEF: Fever during labor.

§ ✓5ᵗʰ **659.3** **Generalized infection during labor** Ⓜ♀
[0,1,3]   Septicemia during labor

§ ✓5ᵗʰ **659.4** **Grand multiparity** Ⓜ♀
[0,1,3]   **EXCLUDES**   *supervision only, in pregnancy (V23.3)*
     without current pregnancy (V61.5)

     DEF: Having borne six or more children previously.

§ ✓5ᵗʰ **659.5** **Elderly primigravida** Ⓜ♀
[0,1,3]   First pregnancy in a woman who will be 35 years of
     age or older at expected date of delivery
     EXCLUDES   *supervision only, in pregnancy (V23.81)*

     AHA: 3Q, '01, 12

§ ✓5ᵗʰ **659.6** **Elderly multigravida** Ⓜ♀
[0,1,3]   Second or more pregnancy in a woman who will be
     35 years of age or older at expected date of
     delivery
     EXCLUDES   *elderly primigravida 659.5*
     supervision only, in pregnancy (V23.82)

     AHA: 3Q, '01, 12

§ ✓5ᵗʰ **659.7** **Abnormality in fetal heart rate or rhythm** Ⓜ♀
[0,1,3]   Depressed fetal heart tones
     Fetal:
       bradycardia
       tachycardia
     Fetal heart rate decelerations
     Non-reassuring fetal heart rate or rhythm

     AHA: 4Q, '98, 48

§ ✓5ᵗʰ **659.8** **Other specified indications for care or** Ⓜ♀
[0,1,3] **intervention related to labor and delivery**
     Pregnancy in a female less than 16 years old at
     expected date of delivery
     Very young maternal age

     AHA: 3Q, '01, 12

§ ✓5ᵗʰ **659.9** **Unspecified indication for care or** Ⓜ♀
[0,1,3] **intervention related to labor and delivery**

COMPLICATIONS OCCURRING MAINLY IN THE COURSE OF LABOR AND DELIVERY (660-669)

The following fifth-digit subclassification is for use with
categories 660-669 to denote the current episode of care.
Valid fifth-digits are in [brackets] under each code.

   0   **unspecified as to episode of care or not applicable**

   1   **delivered, with or without mention of antepartum condition**

   2   **delivered, with mention of postpartum complication**

   3   **antepartum condition or complication**

   4   **postpartum condition or complication**

✓4ᵗʰ **660 Obstructed labor**
     AHA: 3Q, '95, 10

§ ✓5ᵗʰ **660.0** **Obstruction caused by malposition of fetus** Ⓜ♀
[0,1,3] **at onset of labor**
     Any condition classifiable to 652, causing
     obstruction during labor
     Use additional code from 652.0-652.9 to identify
     condition

§ ✓5ᵗʰ **660.1** **Obstruction by bony pelvis** Ⓜ♀
[0,1,3]   Any condition classifiable to 653, causing
     obstruction during labor
     Use additional code from 653.0-653.9 to identify
     condition

§ ✓5ᵗʰ **660.2** **Obstruction by abnormal pelvic soft tissues** Ⓜ♀
[0,1,3]   Prolapse of anterior lip of cervix
     Any condition classifiable to 654, causing
     obstruction during labor
     Use additional code from 654.0-654.9 to identify
     condition

§ ✓5ᵗʰ **660.3** **Deep transverse arrest and persistent** Ⓜ♀
[0,1,3] **occipitoposterior position**

§ ✓5ᵗʰ **660.4** **Shoulder (girdle) dystocia** Ⓜ♀
[0,1,3]   Impacted shoulders

     DEF: Obstructed labor due to impacted fetal shoulders.

§ ✓5ᵗʰ **660.5** **Locked twins** Ⓜ♀
[0,1,3]

§ ✓5ᵗʰ **660.6** **Failed trial of labor, unspecified** Ⓜ♀
[0,1,3]   Failed trial of labor, without mention of
     condition or suspected condition

§ ✓5ᵗʰ **660.7** **Failed forceps or vacuum extractor,** Ⓜ♀
[0,1,3] **unspecified**
     Application of ventouse or forceps, without
     mention of condition

§ ✓5ᵗʰ **660.8** **Other causes of obstructed labor** Ⓜ♀
[0,1,3]

§ ✓5ᵗʰ **660.9** **Unspecified obstructed labor** Ⓜ♀
[0,1,3]   Dystocia: Dystocia:
     NOS   maternal NOS
     fetal NOS

✓4ᵗʰ **661 Abnormality of forces of labor**

§ ✓5ᵗʰ **661.0** **Primary uterine inertia** Ⓜ♀
[0,1,3]   Failure of cervical dilation
     Hypotonic uterine dysfunction, primary
     Prolonged latent phase of labor

     DEF: Lack of efficient contractions during labor causing
     prolonged labor.

§ ✓5ᵗʰ **661.1** **Secondary uterine inertia** Ⓜ♀
[0,1,3]   Arrested active phase of labor
     Hypotonic uterine dysfunction, secondary

§ ✓5ᵗʰ **661.2** **Other and unspecified uterine inertia** Ⓜ♀
[0,1,3]   Desultory labor   Poor contractions
     Irregular labor   Slow slope active phase
         of labor

§ ✓5ᵗʰ **661.3** **Precipitate labor** Ⓜ♀
[0,1,3]   DEF: Rapid labor and delivery.

§ ✓5ᵗʰ **661.4** **Hypertonic, incoordinate, or prolonged** Ⓜ♀
[0,1,3] **uterine contractions**
     Cervical spasm
     Contraction ring (dystocia)
     Dyscoordinate labor
     Hourglass contraction of uterus
     Hypertonic uterine dysfunction
     Incoordinate uterine action
     Retraction ring (Bandl's) (pathological)
     Tetanic contractions
     Uterine dystocia NOS
     Uterine spasm

§ ✓5ᵗʰ **661.9** **Unspecified abnormality of labor** Ⓜ♀
[0,1,3]

✓4ᵗʰ **662 Long labor**

§ ✓5ᵗʰ **662.0** **Prolonged first stage** Ⓜ♀
[0,1,3]

§ ✓5ᵗʰ **662.1** **Prolonged labor, unspecified** Ⓜ♀
[0,1,3]

§ ✓5ᵗʰ **662.2** **Prolonged second stage** Ⓜ♀
[0,1,3]

§ ✓5ᵗʰ **662.3** **Delayed delivery of second twin, triplet, etc.** Ⓜ♀
[0,1,3]

§ Requires fifth digit. Valid digits are in [brackets] under each code. See beginning of section 640–648 for codes and definitions.

✓4ᵗʰ Additional Digit Required   **Unspecified Code**   **Other Specified Code**   **Manifestation Code**   ►◄ Revised Text   ● New Code   ▲ Revised Code Title

√4ᵗʰ **663 Umbilical cord complications**

§ √5ᵗʰ **663.0 Prolapse of cord**   M♀
[0,1,3]   Presentation of cord

DEF: Abnormal presentation of fetus; marked by protruding umbilical cord during labor; can cause fetal death.

§ √5ᵗʰ **663.1 Cord around neck, with compression**   M♀
[0,1,3]   Cord tightly around neck

§ √5ᵗʰ **663.2 Other and unspecified cord entanglement, with compression**   M♀
[0,1,3]   Entanglement of cords of twins in mono-amniotic sac
Knot in cord (with compression)

§ √5ᵗʰ **663.3 Other and unspecified cord entanglement, without mention of compression**   M♀
[0,1,3]

AHA: For code 663.31: ▶2Q, '03, 9◀

§ √5ᵗʰ **663.4 Short cord**   M♀
[0,1,3]

§ √5ᵗʰ **663.5 Vasa previa**   M♀
[0,1,3]

DEF: Abnormal presentation of fetus marked by blood vessels of umbilical cord in front of fetal head.

§ √5ᵗʰ **663.6 Vascular lesions of cord**   M♀
[0,1,3]   Bruising of cord   Thrombosis of vessels of
Hematoma of cord   cord

§ √5ᵗʰ **663.8 Other umbilical cord complications**   M♀
[0,1,3]   Velamentous insertion of umbilical cord

§ √5ᵗʰ **663.9 Unspecified umbilical cord complication**   M♀
[0,1,3]

√4ᵗʰ **664 Trauma to perineum and vulva during delivery**

INCLUDES   damage from instruments
that from extension of episiotomy

AHA: 1Q, '92, 11; N-D, '84, 10

§ √5ᵗʰ **664.0 First-degree perineal laceration**   M♀
[0,1,4]   Perineal laceration, rupture, or tear involving:
fourchette   skin
hymen   vagina
labia   vulva

§ √5ᵗʰ **664.1 Second-degree perineal laceration**   M♀
[0,1,4]   Perineal laceration, rupture, or tear (following episiotomy) involving:
pelvic floor
perineal muscles
vaginal muscles

EXCLUDES   that involving anal sphincter (664.2)

§ √5ᵗʰ **664.2 Third-degree perineal laceration**   M♀
[0,1,4]   Perineal laceration, rupture, or tear (following episiotomy) involving:
anal sphincter
rectovaginal septum
sphincter NOS

EXCLUDES   that with anal or rectal mucosal laceration (664.3)

§ √5ᵗʰ **664.3 Fourth-degree perineal laceration**   M♀
[0,1,4]   Perineal laceration, rupture, or tear as classifiable to 664.2 and involving also:
anal mucosa
rectal mucosa

§ √5ᵗʰ **664.4 Unspecified perineal laceration**   M♀
[0,1,4]   Central laceration

AHA: 1Q, '92, 8

§ √5ᵗʰ **664.5 Vulval and perineal hematoma**   M♀
[0,1,4]   AHA: N-D, '84, 10

§ √5ᵗʰ **664.8 Other specified trauma to perineum and vulva**   M♀
[0,1,4]

§ √5ᵗʰ **664.9 Unspecified trauma to perineum and vulva**   M♀
[0,1,4]

√4ᵗʰ **665 Other obstetrical trauma**

INCLUDES   damage from instruments

§ √5ᵗʰ **665.0 Rupture of uterus before onset of labor**   M♀
[0,1,3]

§ √5ᵗʰ **665.1 Rupture of uterus during labor**   M♀
[0,1]   Rupture of uterus NOS

§ √5ᵗʰ **665.2 Inversion of uterus**   M♀
[0,2,4]

§ √5ᵗʰ **665.3 Laceration of cervix**   M♀
[0,1,4]

§ √5ᵗʰ **665.4 High vaginal laceration**   M♀
[0,1,4]   Laceration of vaginal wall or sulcus without mention of perineal laceration

§ √5ᵗʰ **665.5 Other injury to pelvic organs**   M♀
[0,1,4]   Injury to:
bladder
urethra

AHA: M-A, '87, 10

§ √5ᵗʰ **665.6 Damage to pelvic joints and ligaments**   M♀
[0,1,4]   Avulsion of inner symphyseal cartilage
Damage to coccyx
Separation of symphysis (pubis)

AHA: N-D, '84, 12

§ √5ᵗʰ **665.7 Pelvic hematoma**   M♀
[0,1,2,4]   Hematoma of vagina

§ √5ᵗʰ **665.8 Other specified obstetrical trauma**   M♀
[0-4]

§ √5ᵗʰ **665.9 Unspecified obstetrical trauma**   M♀
[0-4]

√4ᵗʰ **666 Postpartum hemorrhage**

AHA: 1Q, '88, 14

§ √5ᵗʰ **666.0 Third-stage hemorrhage**   M♀
[0,2,4]   Hemorrhage associated with retained, trapped, or adherent placenta
Retained placenta NOS

§ √5ᵗʰ **666.1 Other immediate postpartum hemorrhage**   M♀
[0,2,4]   Atony of uterus
Hemorrhage within the first 24 hours following delivery of placenta
Postpartum hemorrhage (atonic) NOS

Perineal Lacerations

First degree

Anus

Second degree

Third degree

Fourth degree

---

§ Requires fifth digit. Valid digits are in [brackets] under each code. See beginning of section 640–648 for codes and definitions.

N Newborn Age: 0   P Pediatric Age: 0-17   M Maternity Age: 12-55   A Adult Age: 15-124   MSP Medicare Secondary Payer

§ ✓5ᵗʰ **666.2 Delayed and secondary postpartum hemorrhage** M ♀
[0,2,4]
    Hemorrhage:
        after the first 24 hours following delivery
        associated with retained portions of placenta or
          membranes
    Postpartum hemorrhage specified as delayed or
        secondary
    Retained products of conception NOS, following
        delivery

§ ✓5ᵗʰ **666.3 Postpartum coagulation defects** M ♀
[0,2,4]
  Postpartum: Postpartum:
    afibrinogenemia   fibrinolysis

✓4ᵗʰ **667 Retained placenta or membranes, without hemorrhage**
    Requires fifth-digit; valid digits are in [brackets] under each
        code. See beginning of section 660-669 for definitions.
AHA: 1Q, '88, 14

DEF: Postpartum condition resulting from failure to expel placental membrane
tissues due to failed contractions of uterine wall.

§ ✓5ᵗʰ **667.0 Retained placenta without hemorrhage** M ♀
[0,2,4]
    Placenta accreta
    Retained placenta:
      NOS   } without hemorrhage
      total

§ ✓5ᵗʰ **667.1 Retained portions of placenta or membranes,** M ♀
[0,2,4] **without hemorrhage**
    Retained products of conception following delivery,
        without hemorrhage

✓4ᵗʰ **668 Complications of the administration of anesthetic or other**
sedation in labor and delivery
  INCLUDES complications arising from the administration
        of a general or local anesthetic, analgesic,
        or other sedation in labor and delivery
  EXCLUDES *reaction to spinal or lumbar puncture (349.0)*
        spinal headache (349.0)
  Use additional code(s) to further specify complication

§ ✓5ᵗʰ **668.0 Pulmonary complications** M ♀
[0-4]
    Inhalation [aspiration] of   } following anesthesia
      stomach contents   or other
      or secretions   sedation in
    Mendelson's syndrome   labor or
    Pressure collapse of lung delivery

§ ✓5ᵗʰ **668.1 Cardiac complications** M ♀
[0-4]
    Cardiac arrest or failure following anesthesia or
        other sedation in labor and delivery

§ ✓5ᵗʰ **668.2 Central nervous system complications** M ♀
[0-4]
    Cerebral anoxia following anesthesia or other
        sedation in labor and delivery

§ ✓5ᵗʰ **668.8 Other complications of anesthesia or other** M ♀
[0-4] **sedation in labor and delivery**
  AHA: 2Q, '99, 9

§ ✓5ᵗʰ **668.9 Unspecified complication of anesthesia and** M ♀
[0-4] **other sedation**

✓4ᵗʰ **669 Other complications of labor and delivery, not elsewhere**
classified

§ ✓5ᵗʰ **669.0 Maternal distress** M ♀
[0-4]
    Metabolic disturbance in labor and delivery

§ ✓5ᵗʰ **669.1 Shock during or following labor and delivery** M ♀
[0-4]
    Obstetric shock

§ ✓5ᵗʰ **669.2 Maternal hypotension syndrome** M ♀
[0-4]
  DEF: Low arterial blood pressure, in mother, during labor and
  delivery.

§ ✓5ᵗʰ **669.3 Acute renal failure following labor and delivery** M ♀
[0,2,4]

§ ✓5ᵗʰ **669.4 Other complications of obstetrical surgery** M ♀
[0-4] **and procedures**
    Cardiac: } following cesarean or other
      arrest   obstetrical surgery or
      failure   procedure, including
    Cerebral anoxia } delivery NOS
  EXCLUDES *complications of obstetrical surgical*
        wounds (674.1-674.3)

§ ✓5ᵗʰ **669.5 Forceps or vacuum extractor delivery** M ♀
[0,1] **without mention of indication**
    Delivery by ventouse, without mention of indication

§ ✓5ᵗʰ **669.6 Breech extraction, without mention of** M ♀
[0,1] **indication**
  EXCLUDES *breech delivery NOS (652.2)*

§ ✓5ᵗʰ **669.7 Cesarean delivery, without mention of** M ♀
[0,1] **indication**
  AHA: For code 658.71: 1Q, '01, 11

§ ✓5ᵗʰ **669.8 Other complications of labor and delivery** M ♀
[0-4]

§ ✓5ᵗʰ **669.9 Unspecified complication of labor and delivery** M ♀
[0-4]

COMPLICATIONS OF THE PUERPERIUM (670-677)

Note: Categories 671 and 673-676 include the listed
conditions even if they occur during pregnancy or
childbirth.

The following fifth-digit subclassification is for use with
categories 670-676 to denote the current episode of care.
Valid fifth-digits are in [brackets] under each code.
    0 unspecified as to episode of care or not
      applicable
    1 delivered, with or without mention of
      antepartum condition
    2 delivered, with mention of postpartum
      complication
    3 antepartum condition or complication
    4 postpartum condition or complication

✓4ᵗʰ **670 Major puerperal infection** M ♀
[0,2,4]
§ ✓5ᵗʰ   Use 0 as fourth-digit for this category
    Puerperal:
      endometritis
      fever (septic)
      pelvic:
        cellulitis
        sepsis
      peritonitis
      pyemia
      salpingitis
      septicemia
  EXCLUDES *infection following abortion (639.0)*
        minor genital tract infection following delivery
        (646.6)
        puerperal pyrexia NOS (672)
        puerperal fever NOS (672)
        puerperal pyrexia of unknown origin (672)
        urinary tract infection following delivery (646.6)
  AHA: 4Q, '91, 26; 2Q, '91, 7

DEF: Infection and inflammation, following childbirth.

✓4ᵗʰ **671 Venous complications in pregnancy and the puerperium**
§ ✓5ᵗʰ **671.0 Varicose veins of legs** M ♀
[0-4]
    Varicose veins NOS
  DEF: Distended, tortuous veins on legs associated with pregnancy.

---

§ Requires fifth digit. Valid digits are in [brackets] under each code. See beginning of section 640–648 for codes and definitions.

✓4ᵗʰ ✓5ᵗʰ Additional Digit Required   Unspecified Code   Other Specified Code   Manifestation Code   ▶◀ Revised Text   ● New Code   ▲ Revised Code Title

Complications of Pregnancy, Childbirth & Puerperium

671.1–675.9

§ ✓5ᵗʰ **671.1**   **Varicose veins of vulva and perineum**   Ⓜ♀
[0-4]   DEF: Distended, tortuous veins on external female genitalia associated with pregnancy.

§ ✓5ᵗʰ **671.2**   **Superficial thrombophlebitis**   Ⓜ♀
[0-4]   Thrombophlebitis (superficial)

§ ✓5ᵗʰ **671.3**   **Deep phlebothrombosis, antepartum**   Ⓜ♀
[0,1,3]   Deep-vein thrombosis, antepartum

§ ✓5ᵗʰ **671.4**   **Deep phlebothrombosis, postpartum**   Ⓜ♀
[0,2,4]   Deep-vein thrombosis, postpartum
     Pelvic thrombophlebitis, postpartum
     Phlegmasia alba dolens (puerperal)

§ ✓5ᵗʰ **671.5**   **Other phlebitis and thrombosis**   Ⓜ♀
[0-4]   Cerebral venous thrombosis
     Thrombosis of intracranial venous sinus

§ ✓5ᵗʰ **671.8**   **Other venous complications**   Ⓜ♀
[0-4]   Hemorrhoids

§ ✓5ᵗʰ **671.9**   **Unspecified venous complication**   Ⓜ♀
[0-4]   Phlebitis NOS   Thrombosis NOS

✓4ᵗʰ **672**   **Pyrexia of unknown origin during the puerperium**   Ⓜ♀
[0,2,4]

§ ✓5ᵗʰ   Use 0 as fourth-digit for this category
    Postpartum fever NOS   Puerperal pyrexia NOS
    Puerperal fever NOS

AHA: 4Q, '91, 26

DEF: Fever of unknown origin experienced by the mother after childbirth.

✓4ᵗʰ **673**   **Obstetrical pulmonary embolism**
    Requires fifth-digit; valid digits are in [brackets] under each code. See beginning of section 670-676 for definitions.
    INCLUDES   pulmonary emboli in pregnancy, childbirth or the puerperium, or specified as puerperal
    EXCLUDES   embolism following abortion (639.6)

§ ✓5ᵗʰ **673.0**   **Obstetrical air embolism**   Ⓜ♀
[0-4]   DEF: Sudden blocking of pulmonary artery with air or nitrogen bubbles during puerperium..

§ ✓5ᵗʰ **673.1**   **Amniotic fluid embolism**   Ⓜ♀
[0-4]   DEF: Sudden onset of pulmonary artery blockage from amniotic fluid entering the mother's circulation near the end of pregnancy due to strong uterine contractions.

§ ✓5ᵗʰ **673.2**   **Obstetrical blood-clot embolism**   Ⓜ♀
[0-4]   Puerperal pulmonary embolism NOS
   DEF: Blood clot blocking artery in the lung; associated with pregnancy.

§ ✓5ᵗʰ **673.3**   **Obstetrical pyemic and septic embolism**   Ⓜ♀
[0-4]

§ ✓5ᵗʰ **673.8**   **Other pulmonary embolism**   Ⓜ♀
[0-4]   Fat embolism

✓4ᵗʰ **674**   **Other and unspecified complications of the puerperium, not elsewhere classified**

§ ✓5ᵗʰ **674.0**   **Cerebrovascular disorders in the puerperium**   Ⓜ♀
[0-4]   Any condition classifiable to 430-434, 436-437 occurring during pregnancy, childbirth or the puerperium, or specified as puerperal
    EXCLUDES   intracranial venous sinus thrombosis (671.5)

§ ✓5ᵗʰ **674.1**   **Disruption of cesarean wound**   Ⓜ♀
[0,2,4]   Dehiscence or disruption of uterine wound
    EXCLUDES   uterine rupture before onset of labor (665.0)
            uterine rupture during labor (665.1)

§ ✓5ᵗʰ **674.2**   **Disruption of perineal wound**   Ⓜ♀
[0,2,4]   Breakdown of perineum   Disruption of wound of:
    Disruption of wound of: perineal laceration
      episiotomy   Secondary perineal tear
    AHA: For code 674.24: 1Q, '97, 9

§ ✓5ᵗʰ **674.3**   **Other complications of obstetrical surgical**   Ⓜ♀
[0,2,4]   **wounds**

    Hematoma
    Hemorrhage } of cesarean section or perineal wound
    Infection

    EXCLUDES   damage from instruments in delivery (664.0-665.9)

AHA: 2Q, '91, 7

§ ✓5ᵗʰ **674.4**   **Placental polyp**   Ⓜ♀
[0,2,4]

§ ✓5ᵗʰ **674.5**   **Peripartum cardiomyopathy**   Ⓜ♀
[0-4]   Postpartum cardiomyopathy

AHA: ▶4Q, '03, 65◀

DEF: ▶Any structural or functional abnormality of the ventricular myocardium, non-inflammatory disease of obscure or unknown etiology with onset during the postpartum period.◀

§ ✓5ᵗʰ **674.8**   **Other**   Ⓜ♀
[0,2,4]   Hepatorenal syndrome, following delivery
    Postpartum:
      subinvolution of uterus
      uterine hypertrophy

AHA: 3Q, '98, 16

§ ✓5ᵗʰ **674.9**   **Unspecified**   Ⓜ♀
[0,2,4]   Sudden death of unknown cause during the puerperium

✓4ᵗʰ **675**   **Infections of the breast and nipple associated with childbirth**
    INCLUDES   the listed conditions during pregnancy, childbirth or the puerperium

§ ✓5ᵗʰ **675.0**   **Infections of nipple**   Ⓜ♀
[0-4]   Abscess of nipple

§ ✓5ᵗʰ **675.1**   **Abscess of breast**   Ⓜ♀
[0-4]   Abscess: Mastitis:
      mammary   purulent
      subareolar   retromammary
      submammary   submammary

§ ✓5ᵗʰ **675.2**   **Nonpurulent mastitis**   Ⓜ♀
[0-4]   Lymphangitis of breast   Mastitis:
    Mastitis: interstitial
     NOS   parenchymatous

§ ✓5ᵗʰ **675.8**   **Other specified infections of the breast and nipple**   Ⓜ♀
[0-4]

§ ✓5ᵗʰ **675.9**   **Unspecified infection of the breast and nipple**   Ⓜ♀
[0-4]

Lactation Process: Ejection Reflex Arc

§ Requires fifth digit. Valid digits are in [brackets] under each code. See beginning of section 640-648 for codes and definitions.

Ⓝ Newborn Age: 0   Ⓟ Pediatric Age: 0-17   Ⓜ Maternity Age: 12-55   Ⓐ Adult Age: 15-124   MSP Medicare Secondary Payer

√4ᵗʰ **676 Other disorders of the breast associated with childbirth and disorders of lactation**
     INCLUDES   the listed conditions during pregnancy, the puerperium, or lactation

§ √5ᵗʰ **676.0 Retracted nipple**   Ⓜ ♀
   [0-4]

§ √5ᵗʰ **676.1 Cracked nipple**   Ⓜ ♀
   [0-4]   Fissure of nipple

§ √5ᵗʰ **676.2 Engorgement of breasts**   Ⓜ ♀
   [0-4]   DEF: Abnormal accumulation of milk in ducts of breast.

§ √5ᵗʰ **676.3 Other and unspecified disorder of breast**   Ⓜ ♀
   [0-4]

§ √5ᵗʰ **676.4 Failure of lactation**   Ⓜ ♀
   [0-4]   Agalactia
       DEF: Abrupt ceasing of milk secretion by breast.

§ √5ᵗʰ **676.5 Suppressed lactation**   Ⓜ ♀
   [0-4]

§ √5ᵗʰ **676.6 Galactorrhea**   Ⓜ ♀
   [0-4]   EXCLUDES   *galactorrhea not associated with childbirth (611.6)*
       DEF: Excessive or persistent milk secretion by breast; may be in absence of nursing.

§ √5ᵗʰ **676.8 Other disorders of lactation**   Ⓜ ♀
   [0-4]   Galactocele
       DEF: Galactocele: obstructed mammary gland, creating retention cyst, results in milk-filled cysts enlarging mammary gland.

§ √5ᵗʰ **676.9 Unspecified disorder of lactation**   Ⓜ ♀
   [0-4]

677 Late effect of complication of pregnancy, childbirth and the puerperium   ♀
    Note: This category is to be used to indicate conditions in 632-648.9 and 651-676.9 as the cause of the late effect, themselves classifiable elsewhere. The "late effects" include conditions specified as such, or as sequelae, which may occur at any time after puerperium.
    Code first any sequelae
    AHA: 1Q, '97, 9; 4Q, '94, 42

---

§ Requires fifth digit. Valid digits are in [brackets] under each code. See beginning of section 640-648 for codes and definitions.

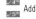
√4ᵗʰ √5ᵗʰ Additional Digit Required   Unspecified Code   Other Specified Code   Manifestation Code   ▶◀ Revised Text   ● New Code   ▲ Revised Code Title

12. DISEASES OF THE SKIN AND SUBCUTANEOUS TISSUE
(680-709)

INFECTIONS OF SKIN AND SUBCUTANEOUS TISSUE (680-686)

EXCLUDES *certain infections of skin classified under "Infectious and Parasitic Diseases," such as:*
erysipelas (035)
erysipeloid of Rosenbach (027.1)
herpes:
  simplex (054.0-054.9)
  zoster (053.0-053.9)
molluscum contagiosum (078.0)
viral warts (078.1)

✓4ᵗʰ **680 Carbuncle and furuncle**

INCLUDES boil
furunculosis

DEF: Carbuncle: necrotic boils in skin and subcutaneous tissue of neck or back mainly due to staphylococcal infection.

DEF: Furuncle: circumscribed inflammation of corium and subcutaneous tissue due to staphylococcal infection.

680.0   Face
Ear [any part]   Nose (septum)
Face [any part, except eye]   Temple (region)
EXCLUDES *eyelid (373.13)*
lacrimal apparatus (375.31)
orbit (376.01)

680.1   Neck

680.2   Trunk
Abdominal wall   Flank
Back [any part, except   Groin
  buttocks]   Pectoral region
Breast   Perineum
Chest wall   Umbilicus
EXCLUDES *buttocks (680.5)*
external genital organs:
  female (616.4)
  male (607.2, 608.4)

680.3   Upper arm and forearm
Arm [any part, except hand]
Axilla
Shoulder

680.4   Hand
Finger [any]   Wrist
Thumb

680.5   Buttock
Anus   Gluteal region

680.6   Leg, except foot
Ankle   Knee
Hip   Thigh

680.7   Foot
Heel
Toe

680.8   Other specified sites
Head [any part, except face]
Scalp
EXCLUDES *external genital organs:*
  female (616.4)
  male (607.2, 608.4)

680.9   Unspecified site
Boil NOS   Furuncle NOS
Carbuncle NOS

✓4ᵗʰ **681 Cellulitis and abscess of finger and toe**
INCLUDES   that with lymphangitis
Use additional code to identify organism, such as Staphylococcus (041.1)
AHA: 2Q, '91, 5; J-F, '87, 12

DEF: Acute suppurative inflammation and edema in subcutaneous tissue or muscle of finger or toe.

✓5ᵗʰ **681.0   Finger**
681.00 Cellulitis and abscess, unspecified
681.01 Felon
Pulp abscess
Whitlow
EXCLUDES *herpetic whitlow (054.6)*

DEF: Painful abscess of fingertips caused by infection in the closed space of terminal phalanx.

681.02 Onychia and paronychia of finger
Panaritium ⎫
Perionychia ⎬ of finger

DEF: Onychia: inflammation of nail matrix; causes nail loss.

DEF: Paronychia: inflammation of tissue folds around nail.

✓5ᵗʰ **681.1   Toe**
681.10 Cellulitis and abscess, unspecified
681.11 Onychia and paronychia of toe
Panaritium ⎫
Perionychia ⎬ of toe

681.9   Cellulitis and abscess of unspecified digit
Infection of nail NOS

✓4ᵗʰ **682 Other cellulitis and abscess**
INCLUDES   abscess (acute)   ⎫ (with lymphangitis)
cellulitis (diffuse)   ⎬ except of finger
lymphangitis, acute   ⎭ or toe

Use additional code to identify organism, such as Staphylococcus (041.1)
EXCLUDES *lymphangitis (chronic) (subacute) (457.2)*
AHA: 2Q, '91, 5; J-F, '87, 12; S-O, '85, 10

DEF: Cellulitis: Acute suppurative inflammation of deep subcutaneous tissue and sometimes muscle due to infection of wound, burn or other lesion.

682.0   Face
Cheek, external   Nose, external
Chin   Submandibular
Forehead   Temple (region)
EXCLUDES *ear [any part] (380.10-380.16)*
eyelid (373.13)
lacrimal apparatus (375.31)
lip (528.5)
mouth (528.3)
nose (internal) (478.1)
orbit (376.01)

682.1   Neck

Skin and Subcutaneous Layer

Hair follicle
Epidermis
Dermis
Hypodermis (subcutaneous layer)
Bulb

Sebaceous gland
Arrector pili muscle
Thick-skin epidermis
Hair shaft
Pacinian corpuscle
Hair matrix
Sweat (eccrine gland)
Sensory nerve
Blood vessels

✓4ᵗʰ
✓5ᵗʰ Additional Digit Required   Unspecified Code   Other Specified Code   Manifestation Code   ▶◀ Revised Text   ● New Code   ▲ Revised Code Title

682.2   Trunk
Abdominal wall   Groin
Back [any part, except   Pectoral region
    buttock]   Perineum
Chest wall   Umbilicus, except newborn
Flank

EXCLUDES   *anal and rectal regions (566)*
breast:
    NOS (611.0)
    puerperal (675.1)
external genital organs:
    female (616.3-616.4)
    male (604.0, 607.2, 608.4)
umbilicus, newborn (771.4)

AHA: 4Q, '98, 42

682.3   Upper arm and forearm
Arm [any part, except hand]
Axilla
Shoulder

EXCLUDES   *hand (682.4)*

AHA: ▶2Q, '03, 7◀

682.4   Hand, except fingers and thumb
Wrist

EXCLUDES   *finger and thumb (681.00-681.02)*

682.5   Buttock
Gluteal region

EXCLUDES   *anal and rectal regions (566)*

682.6   Leg, except foot
Ankle   Knee
Hip   Thigh

AHA: ▶4Q, '03, 108◀

682.7   Foot, except toes
Heel

EXCLUDES   *toe (681.10-681.11)*

682.8   Other specified sites
Head [except face]
Scalp

EXCLUDES   *face (682.0)*

682.9   Unspecified site
Abscess NOS   Lymphangitis, acute NOS
Cellulitis NOS

EXCLUDES   *lymphangitis NOS (457.2)*

683 Acute lymphadenitis
Abscess (acute)
Adenitis, acute   } lymph gland or node,
Lymphadenitis, acute   except mesenteric

Use additional code to identify organism, such as
Staphylococcus (041.1)

EXCLUDES   *enlarged glands NOS (785.6)*
lymphadenitis:
    chronic or subacute, except mesenteric
      (289.1)
    mesenteric (acute) (chronic) (subacute) (289.2)
    unspecified (289.3)

DEF: Acute inflammation of lymph nodes due to primary infection located elsewhere in the body.

684 Impetigo
Impetiginization of other dermatoses
Impetigo (contagiosa) [any site] [any organism]:
    bullous   neonatorum
    circinate   simplex
Pemphigus neonatorum

EXCLUDES   *impetigo herpetiformis (694.3)*

DEF: Infectious skin disease commonly occurring in children; caused by group A streptococci or *Staphylococcus aureus*; skin lesions usually appear on the face and consist of subcorneal vesicles and bullae that burst and form yellow crusts.

Lymphatic System of Head and Neck

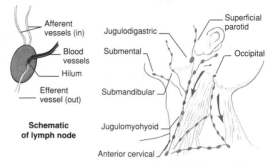

Lymphatic drainage of the
head, neck, and face

✓4th **685 Pilonidal cyst**

INCLUDES   fistula   } coccygeal or pilonidal
          sinus

DEF: Hair-containing cyst or sinus in the tissues of the sacrococcygeal area; often drains through opening at the postanal dimple.

685.0   With abscess
685.1   Without mention of abscess

✓4th **686 Other local infections of skin and subcutaneous tissue**
Use additional code to identify any infectious organism
(041.0-041.8)

✓5th **686.0   Pyoderma**
Dermatitis: Dermatitis:
    purulent   suppurative
    septic

DEF: Nonspecific purulent skin disease related most to furuncles, pustules, or possibly carbuncles.

686.00   Pyoderma, unspecified

686.01   Pyoderma gangrenosum
AHA: 4Q, '97, 42

DEF: Persistent debilitating skin disease, characterized by irregular, boggy, blue-red ulcerations, with central healing and undermined edges.

686.09   Other pyoderma

686.1   Pyogenic granuloma
Granuloma: Granuloma:
    septic   telangiectaticum
    suppurative

EXCLUDES   *pyogenic granuloma of oral mucosa*
    (528.9)

DEF: Solitary polypoid capillary hemangioma often asociated with local irritation, trauma, and superimposed inflammation; located on the skin and gingival or oral mucosa.

Stages of Pilonidal Disease

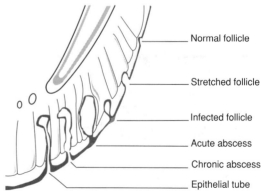

686.8 Other specified local infections of skin and subcutaneous tissue

Bacterid (pustular) Ecthyma
Dermatitis vegetans Perlèche

EXCLUDES *dermatitis infectiosa eczematoides (690.8)*
panniculitis (729.30-729.39)

686.9 Unspecified local infection of skin and subcutaneous tissue

Fistula of skin NOS
Skin infection NOS

EXCLUDES *fistula to skin from internal organs — see Alphabetic Index*

OTHER INFLAMMATORY CONDITIONS OF SKIN AND SUBCUTANEOUS TISSUE (690-698)

EXCLUDES *panniculitis (729.30-729.39)*

√4ᵗʰ **690 Erythematosquamous dermatosis**

EXCLUDES *eczematous dermatitis of eyelid (373.31)*
parakeratosis variegata (696.2)
psoriasis (696.0-696.1)
seborrheic keratosis (702.11-702.19)

DEF: Dry material desquamated from the scalp, associated with disease.

√5ᵗʰ **690.1 Seborrheic dermatitis**

AHA: 4Q, '95, 58

690.10 Seborrheic dermatitis, unspecified
Seborrheic dermatitis NOS

690.11 Seborrhea capitis P
Cradle cap

690.12 Seborrheic infantile dermatitis P

690.18 Other seborrheic dermatitis

690.8 Other erythematosquamous dermatosis

√4ᵗʰ **691 Atopic dermatitis and related conditions**

DEF: Atopic dermatitis: chronic, pruritic, inflammatory skin disorder found on the face and antecubital and popliteal fossae; noted in persons with a hereditary predisposition to pruritus, and often accompanied by allergic rhinitis, hay fever, asthma, and extreme itching; also called allergic dermatitis, allergic or atopic eczema, or disseminated neurodermatitis.

691.0 Diaper or napkin rash

Ammonia dermatitis Diaper or napkin:
Diaper or napkin: rash
  dermatitis   Psoriasiform napkin eruption
  erythema

691.8 Other atopic dermatitis and related conditions

Atopic dermatitis   Neurodermatitis:
Besnier's prurigo   atopic
Eczema: diffuse (of Brocq)
  atopic
  flexural
  intrinsic (allergic)

√4ᵗʰ **692 Contact dermatitis and other eczema**

INCLUDES dermatitis:
  NOS
  contact
  occupational
  venenata
eczema (acute) (chronic):
  NOS
  allergic
  erythematous
  occupational

EXCLUDES *allergy NOS (995.3)*
contact dermatitis of eyelids (373.32)
dermatitis due to substances taken internally (693.0-693.9)
eczema of external ear (380.22)
perioral dermatitis (695.3)
urticarial reactions (708.0-708.9, 995.1)

DEF: Contact dermatitis: acute or chronic dermatitis caused by initial irritant effect of a substance, or by prior sensitization to a substance coming once again in contact with skin.

692.0 Due to detergents

692.1 Due to oils and greases

692.2 Due to solvents

Dermatitis due to solvents of:
  chlorocompound
  cyclohexane
  ester
  glycol   } group
  hydrocarbon
  ketone

692.3 Due to drugs and medicines in contact with skin

Dermatitis (allergic)   Dermatitis (allergic)
(contact) due to: (contact) due to:
  arnica   neomycin
  fungicides   pediculocides
  iodine   phenols
  keratolytics   scabicides
  mercurials   any drug applied to skin
Dermatitis medicamentosa due to drug applied to skin
Use additional E code to identify drug

EXCLUDES *allergy NOS due to drugs (995.2)*
dermatitis due to ingested drugs (693.0)
dermatitis medicamentosa NOS (693.0)

692.4 Due to other chemical products

Dermatitis due to: Dermatitis due to:
  acids   insecticide
  adhesive plaster   nylon
  alkalis   plastic
  caustics   rubber
  dichromate

AHA: 2Q, '89, 16

692.5 Due to food in contact with skin

Dermatitis, contact,   Dermatitis, contact,
  due to: due to:
  cereals   fruit
  fish   meat
  flour   milk

EXCLUDES *dermatitis due to:*
dyes (692.89)
ingested foods (693.1)
preservatives (692.89)

692.6 Due to plants [except food]

Dermatitis due to:
  lacquer tree [Rhus verniciflua]
  poison:
    ivy [Rhus toxicodendron]
    oak [Rhus diversiloba]
    sumac [Rhus venenata]
    vine [Rhus radicans]
  primrose [Primula]
  ragweed [Senecio jacobae]
  other plants in contact with the skin

EXCLUDES *allergy NOS due to pollen (477.0)*
nettle rash (708.8)

√5ᵗʰ **692.7 Due to solar radiation**

EXCLUDES *sunburn due to other ultraviolet radiation exposure (692.82)*

692.70 Unspecified dermatitis due to sun

692.71 Sunburn
First degree sunburn
Sunburn NOS

AHA: 4Q, '01, 47

√4ᵗʰ √5ᵗʰ Additional Digit Required   Unspecified Code   Other Specified Code   Manifestation Code   ►◄ Revised Text   ● New Code   ▲ Revised Code Title

Skin and Subcutaneous Tissue

692.72–694.3

692.72 Acute dermatitis due to solar radiation
Acute solar skin damage NOS
Berlogue dermatitis
Photoallergic response
Phototoxic response
Polymorphus light eruption
> **EXCLUDES**   sunburn (692.71, 692.76-692.77)

Use additional E code to identify drug, if drug induced

DEF: Berloque dermatitis: phytophotodermatitis due to sun exposure after use of a product containing bergamot oil; causes red patches, which may turn brown.

DEF: Photoallergic response: dermatitis due to hypersensitivity to the sun; causes papulovesicular, eczematous or exudative eruptions.

DEF: Phototoxic response: chemically induced sensitivity to sun causes burn-like reaction, occasionally vesiculation and subsequent hyperpigmentation.

DEF: Polymorphous light eruption: inflammatory skin eruptions due to sunlight exposure; eruptions differ in size and shape.

DEF: Acute solar skin damage (NOS): rapid, unspecified injury to skin from sun.

692.73 Actinic reticuloid and actinic granuloma
DEF: Actinic reticuloid: dermatosis aggravated by light, causes chronic eczema-like eruption on exposed skin which extends to other unexposed surfaces; occurs in the eldery.

DEF: Actinic granuloma: inflammatory response of skin to sun causing small nodule of microphages.

692.74 Other chronic dermatitis due to solar radiation
Solar elastosis
Chronic solar skin damage NOS
> **EXCLUDES**   actinic [solar] keratosis (702.0)

DEF: Solar elastosis: premature aging of skin of light-skinned people; causes inelasticity, thinning or thickening, wrinkling, dryness, scaling and hyperpigmentation.

DEF: Chronic solar skin damage (NOS): chronic skin impairment due to exposure to the sun, not otherwise specified.

692.75 Disseminated superficial actinic porokeratosis (DSAP)
AHA: 4Q, '00, 43

DEF: Autosomal dominant skin condition occurring in skin that has been overexposed to the sun. Primarily affects women over the age of 16; characterized by numerous superficial annular, keratotic, brownish-red spots or thickenings with depressed centers and sharp, ridged borders. High risk that condition will evolve into squamous cell carcinoma.

692.76 Sunburn of second degree
AHA: 4Q, '01, 47

692.77 Sunburn of third degree
AHA: 4Q, '01, 47

692.79 Other dermatitis due to solar radiation
Hydroa aestivale
Photodermatitis
Photosensitiveness } (due to sun)

Solar skin damage NOS

√5th **692.8 Due to other specified agents**

692.81 Dermatitis due to cosmetics

692.82 Dermatitis due to other radiation
Infrared rays   Tanning bed
Light   Ultraviolet rays
Radiation NOS   X-rays
> **EXCLUDES**   solar radiation (692.70-692.79)

AHA: 4Q, '01, 47; 3Q, '00, 5

692.83 Dermatitis due to metals
Jewelry

692.84 Due to animal (cat) (dog) dander
Due to animal (cat) (dog) hair

692.89 Other
Dermatitis due to: Dermatitis due to:
   cold weather   hot weather
   dyes   preservatives
> **EXCLUDES** ▶ allergy (NOS) (rhinitis) due to animal hair or dander (477.2)
> allergy to dust (477.8)◀
> sunburn (692.71, 692.76-692.77)

692.9 Unspecified cause
Dermatitis: Dermatitis:
   NOS   venenata NOS
   contact NOS   Eczema NOS

√4th **693 Dermatitis due to substances taken internally**
> **EXCLUDES**   adverse effect NOS of drugs and medicines (995.2)
> allergy NOS (995.3)
> contact dermatitis (692.0-692.9)
> urticarial reactions (708.0-708.9, 995.1)

DEF: Inflammation of skin due to ingested substance.

693.0 Due to drugs and medicines
Dermatitis medicamentosa NOS
Use additional E code to identify drug
> **EXCLUDES**   that due to drugs in contact with skin (692.3)

693.1 Due to food

693.8 Due to other specified substances taken internally

693.9 Due to unspecified substance taken internally
> **EXCLUDES**   dermatitis NOS (692.9)

√4th **694 Bullous dermatoses**

694.0 Dermatitis herpetiformis
Dermatosis herpetiformis   Hydroa herpetiformis
Duhring's disease
> **EXCLUDES**   herpes gestationis (646.8)
> dermatitis herpetiformis:
>   juvenile (694.2)
>   senile (694.5)

DEF: Chronic, relapsing multisystem disease manifested most in the cutaneous system; seen as an extremely pruritic eruption of various combinations of lesions that frequently heal leaving hyperpigmentation or hypopigmentation and occasionally scarring; usually associated with an asymptomatic gluten-sensitive enteropathy, and immunogenic factors are believed to play a role in its origin.

694.1 Subcorneal pustular dermatosis
Sneddon-Wilkinson disease or syndrome

DEF: Chronic relapses of sterile pustular blebs beneath the horny skin layer of the trunk and skin folds; resembles dermatitis herpetiformis.

694.2 Juvenile dermatitis herpetiformis
Juvenile pemphigoid

694.3 Impetigo herpetiformis
DEF: Rare dermatosis associated with pregnancy; marked by itching pustules in third trimester, hypocalcemia, tetany, fever and lethargy; may result in maternal or fetal death.

694.4 Pemphigus

Pemphigus: Pemphigus:
    NOS   malignant
    erythematosus   vegetans
    foliaceus   vulgaris

> EXCLUDES   pemphigus neonatorum (684)

DEF: Chronic, relapsing, sometimes fatal skin diseases; causes vesicles, bullae; autoantibodies against intracellular connections cause acantholysis.

694.5 Pemphigoid

Benign pemphigus NOS
Bullous pemphigoid
Herpes circinatus bullosus
Senile dermatitis herpetiformis

√5ᵗʰ 694.6 Benign mucous membrane pemphigoid

Cicatricial pemphigoid
Mucosynechial atrophic bullous dermatitis

694.60 Without mention of ocular involvement

694.61 With ocular involvement

Ocular pemphigus

694.8 Other specified bullous dermatoses

> EXCLUDES   herpes gestationis (646.8)

694.9 Unspecified bullous dermatoses

√4ᵗʰ 695 Erythematous conditions

695.0 Toxic erythema

Erythema venenatum

695.1 Erythema multiforme

Erythema iris   Scalded skin syndrome
Herpes iris   Stevens-Johnson syndrome
Lyell's syndrome   Toxic epidermal necrolysis

DEF: Symptom complex with a varied skin eruption pattern of macular, bullous, papular, nodose, or vesicular lesions on the neck, face, and legs; gastritis and rheumatic pains are also noticeable, first-seen symptoms; complex is secondary to a number of factors, including infections, ingestants, physical agents, malignancy and pregnancy.

695.2 Erythema nodosum

> EXCLUDES   tuberculous erythema nodosum (017.1)

DEF: Panniculitis (an inflammatory reaction of the subcutaneous fat) of women, usually seen as a hypersensitivity reaction to various infections, drugs, sarcoidosis, and specific enteropathies; the acute stage is often associated with other symptoms, including fever, malaise, and arthralgia; the lesions are pink to blue in color, appear in crops as tender nodules and are found on the front of the legs below the knees.

695.3 Rosacea

Acne: Perioral dermatitis
    erythematosa   Rhinophyma
    rosacea

DEF: Chronic skin disease, usually of the face, characterized by persistent erythema and sometimes by telangiectasis with acute episodes of edema, engorgement papules, and pustules.

695.4 Lupus erythematosus

Lupus:
    erythematodes (discoid)
    erythematosus (discoid), not disseminated

> EXCLUDES   lupus (vulgaris) NOS (017.0)
>   systemic [disseminated] lupus
>   erythematosus (710.0)

DEF: Group of connective tissue disorders occurring as various cutaneous diseases of unknown origin; it primarily affects women between the ages of 20 and 40.

√5ᵗʰ 695.8 Other specified erythematous conditions

695.81 Ritter's disease

Dermatitis exfoliativa neonatorum

DEF: Infectious skin disease of infants and young children marked by eruptions ranging from a localized bullous type to widespread development of easily ruptured fine vesicles and bullae; results in exfoliation of large planes of skin and leaves raw areas; also called staphylococcal scalded skin syndrome.

695.89 Other

Erythema intertrigo
Intertrigo
Pityriasis rubra (Hebra)

> EXCLUDES   mycotic intertrigo (111.0-
>   111.9)

AHA:: S-O, '86, 10

695.9 Unspecified erythematous condition

Erythema NOS   Erythroderma (secondary)

√4ᵗʰ 696 Psoriasis and similar disorders

696.0 Psoriatic arthropathy

DEF: Psoriasis associated with inflammatory arthritis; often involves interphalangeal joints.

696.1 Other psoriasis

Acrodermatitis continua
Dermatitis repens
Psoriasis:
    NOS
    any type, except arthropathic

> EXCLUDES   psoriatic arthropathy (696.0)

696.2 Parapsoriasis

Parakeratosis variegata
Parapsoriasis lichenoides chronica
Pityriasis lichenoides et varioliformis

DEF: Erythrodermas similar to lichen, planus and psoriasis; symptoms include redness and itching; resistant to treatment.

696.3 Pityriasis rosea

Pityriasis circinata (et maculata)

DEF: Common, self-limited rash of unknown etiology marked by a solitary erythematous, salmon or fawn-colored herald plaque on the trunk, arms or thighs; followed by development of papular or macular lesions that tend to peel and form a scaly collarette.

696.4 Pityriasis rubra pilaris

Devergie's disease   Lichen ruber acuminatus

> EXCLUDES   pityriasis rubra (Hebra) (695.89)

DEF: Inflammatory disease of hair follicles; marked by firm, red lesions topped by horny plugs; may form patches; occurs on fingers elbows, knees.

696.5 Other and unspecified pityriasis

Pityriasis: Pityriasis:
    NOS   streptogenes
    alba

> EXCLUDES   pityriasis:
>   simplex (690.18)
>   versicolor (111.0)

696.8 Other

√4ᵗʰ 697 Lichen

> EXCLUDES   lichen:
>   obtusus corneus (698.3)
>   pilaris (congenital) (757.39)
>   ruber acuminatus (696.4)
>   sclerosus et atrophicus (701.0)
>   scrofulosus (017.0)
>   simplex chronicus (698.3)
>   spinulosus (congenital) (757.39)
>   urticatus (698.2)

√4ᵗʰ √5ᵗʰ Additional Digit Required   Unspecified Code   Other Specified Code   Manifestation Code   ►◄ Revised Text   ● New Code   ▲ Revised Code Title

2005 ICD•9•CM   **Volume 1 — 193**

Skin and Subcutaneous Tissue

697.0–701.9

697.0   Lichen planus
     Lichen: Lichen:
       planopilaris   ruber planus
     DEF: Inflammatory, pruritic skin disease; marked by angular, flat-top, violet-colored papules; may be acute and widespread or chronic and localized.

697.1   Lichen nitidus
     Pinkus' disease
     DEF: Chronic, inflammatory, usually asymptomatic skin disorder, characterized by numerous glistening, flat-topped, discrete, smooth, skin-colored micropapules most often on penis, lower abdomen, inner thighs, wrists, forearms, breasts and buttocks.

697.8   Other lichen, not elsewhere classified
     Lichen: Lichen:
       ruber moniliforme   striata

697.9   Lichen, unspecified

✓4ᵗʰ 698   Pruritus and related conditions
     EXCLUDES   *pruritus specified as psychogenic (306.3)*
     DEF: Pruritus: Intense, persistent itching due to irritation of sensory nerve endings from organic or psychogenic causes.

698.0   Pruritus ani
     Perianal itch

698.1   Pruritus of genital organs

698.2   Prurigo
     Lichen urticatus   Prurigo:
     Prurigo: mitis
       NOS   simplex
       Hebra's   Urticaria papulosa (Hebra)
     EXCLUDES   *prurigo nodularis (698.3)*

698.3   Lichenification and lichen simplex chronicus
     Hyde's disease
     Neurodermatitis (circumscripta) (local)
     Prurigo nodularis
     EXCLUDES   *neurodermatitis, diffuse (of Brocq) (691.8)*
     DEF: Lichenification: thickening of skin due to prolonged rubbing or scratching.

     DEF: Lichen simplex chronicus: eczematous dermatitis, of face, neck, extremities, scrotum, vulva, and perianal region due to repeated itching, rubbing and scratching; spontaneous or evolves with other dermatoses.

698.4   Dermatitis factitia [artefacta]
     Dermatitis ficta
     Neurotic excoriation
     Use additional code to identify any associated mental disorder
     DEF: Various types of self-inflicted skin lesions characterized in appearance as an erythema to a gangrene.

698.8   Other specified pruritic conditions
     Pruritus: Winter itch
       hiemalis
       senilis

698.9   Unspecified pruritic disorder
     Itch NOS
     Pruritus NOS

OTHER DISEASES OF SKIN AND SUBCUTANEOUS TISSUE (700-709)
     EXCLUDES   *conditions confined to eyelids (373.0-374.9)*
                     congenital conditions of skin, hair, and nails (757.0-757.9)

700   Corns and callosities
     Callus
     Clavus
     DEF: Corns: conical or horny thickening of skin on toes, due to friction, pressure from shoes and hosiery; pain and inflammation may develop.

     DEF: Callosities: localized overgrowth (hyperplasia) of the horny epidermal layer due to pressure or friction.

✓4ᵗʰ 701   Other hypertrophic and atrophic conditions of skin
     EXCLUDES   *dermatomyositis (710.3)*
                     hereditary edema of legs (757.0)
                     scleroderma (generalized) (710.1)

701.0   Circumscribed scleroderma
     Addison's keloid
     Dermatosclerosis, localized
     Lichen sclerosus et atrophicus
     Morphea
     Scleroderma, circumscribed or localized
     DEF: Thickened, hardened, skin and subcutaneous tissue; may involve musculoskeletal system.

701.1   Keratoderma, acquired
     Acquired:
       ichthyosis
       keratoderma palmaris et plantaris
     Elastosis perforans serpiginosa
     Hyperkeratosis:
       NOS
       follicularis in cutem penetrans
       palmoplantaris climacterica
     Keratoderma:
       climactericum
       tylodes, progressive
     Keratosis (blennorrhagica)
     EXCLUDES   *Darier's disease [keratosis follicularis] (congenital) (757.39)*
                    keratosis:
                      arsenical (692.4)
                      gonococcal (098.81)

     AHA: 4Q, '94, 48

701.2   Acquired acanthosis nigricans
     Keratosis nigricans
     DEF: Diffuse velvety hyperplasia of the spinous skin layer of the axilla and other body folds marked by gray, brown, or black pigmentation; in adult form it is often associated with an internal carcinoma (malignant acanthosis nigricans) in a benign, nevoid form it is relatively generalized; benign juvenile form with obesity is sometimes caused by an endocrine disturbance.

701.3   Striae atrophicae
     Atrophic spots of skin
     Atrophoderma maculatum
     Atrophy blanche (of Milian)
     Degenerative colloid atrophy
     Senile degenerative atrophy
     Striae distensae
     DEF: Bands of atrophic, depressed, wrinkled skin associated with stretching of skin from pregnancy, obesity, or rapid growth during puberty.

701.4   Keloid scar
     Cheloid   Keloid
     Hypertrophic scar
     DEF: Overgrowth of scar tissue due to excess amounts of collagen during connective tissue repair; occurs mainly on upper trunk, face.

701.5   Other abnormal granulation tissue
     Excessive granulation

701.8   Other specified hypertrophic and atrophic conditions of skin
     Acrodermatitis atrophicans chronica
     Atrophia cutis senilis
     Atrophoderma neuriticum
     Confluent and reticulate papillomatosis
     Cutis laxa senilis
     Elastosis senilis
     Folliculitis ulerythematosa reticulata
     Gougerot-Carteaud syndrome or disease

701.9   Unspecified hypertrophic and atrophic conditions of skin
     Atrophoderma

√4ᵗʰ **702 Other dermatoses**

> EXCLUDES   carcinoma in situ (232.0-232.9)

702.0 Actinic keratosis

AHA: 1Q, '92, 18

DEF: Wart-like growth, red or skin-colored; may form a cutaneous horn.

√5ᵗʰ **702.1 Seborrheic keratosis**

DEF: Common, benign, lightly pigmented, warty growth composed of basaloid cells.

702.11 Inflamed seborrheic keratosis

AHA: 4Q, '94, 48

702.19 Other seborrheic keratosis

Seborrheic keratosis NOS

702.8 Other specified dermatoses

√4ᵗʰ **703 Diseases of nail**

> EXCLUDES   congenital anomalies (757.5)
> onychia and paronychia (681.02, 681.11)

703.0 Ingrowing nail

Ingrowing nail with infection   Unguis incarnatus

> EXCLUDES   infection, nail NOS (681.9)

703.8 Other specified diseases of nail

Dystrophia unguium   Onychauxis
Hypertrophy of nail   Onychogryposis
Koilonychia   Onycholysis
Leukonychia (punctata) (striata)

703.9 Unspecified disease of nail

√4ᵗʰ **704 Diseases of hair and hair follicles**

> EXCLUDES   congenital anomalies (757.4)

√5ᵗʰ **704.0 Alopecia**

> EXCLUDES   madarosis (374.55)
> syphilitic alopecia (091.82)

DEF: Lack of hair, especially on scalp; often called baldness; may be partial or total; occurs at any age.

704.00 Alopecia, unspecified

Baldness   Loss of hair

704.01 Alopecia areata

Ophiasis

DEF: Alopecia areata: usually reversible, inflammatory, patchy hair loss found in beard or scalp.

DEF: Ophiasis: alopecia areata of children; marked by band around temporal and occipital scalp margins.

704.02 Telogen effluvium

DEF: Shedding of hair from premature telogen development in follicles due to stress, including shock, childbirth, surgery, drugs or weight loss.

704.09 Other

Folliculitis decalvans
Hypotrichosis:
    NOS
    postinfectional NOS
Pseudopelade

704.1 Hirsutism

Hypertrichosis: Polytrichia
    NOS
    lanuginosa, acquired

> EXCLUDES   hypertrichosis of eyelid (374.54)

DEF: Excess hair growth; often in unexpected places and amounts.

704.2 Abnormalities of the hair

Atrophic hair   Trichiasis:
Clastothrix   NOS
Fragilitas crinium   cicatrical
    Trichorrhexis (nodosa)

> EXCLUDES   trichiasis of eyelid (374.05)

704.3 Variations in hair color

Canities (premature)
Grayness, hair (premature)
Heterochromia of hair
Poliosis:
    NOS
    circumscripta, acquired

704.8 Other specified diseases of hair and hair follicles

Folliculitis: Sycosis:
    NOS   NOS
    abscedens et suffodiens   barbae [not parasitic]
    pustular   lupoid
Perifolliculitis: vulgaris
    NOS
    capitis abscedens et suffodiens
    scalp

704.9 Unspecified disease of hair and hair follicles

√4ᵗʰ **705 Disorders of sweat glands**

705.0 Anhidrosis

Hypohidrosis   Oligohidrosis

DEF: Lack or deficiency of ability to sweat.

● √5ᵗʰ **705.2 Focal hyperhidrosis**

> EXCLUDES   generalized (secondary) hyperhidrosis (780.8)

● **705.21 Primary focal hyperhidrosis**

Focal hyperhidrosis NOS
Hyperhidrosis NOS
Hyperhidrosis of:
    axilla
    face
    palms
    soles

● **705.22 Secondary focal hyperhidrosis**

Frey's syndrome

705.1 Prickly heat

Heat rash   Sudamina
Miliaria rubra (tropicalis)

√5ᵗʰ **705.8 Other specified disorders of sweat glands**

705.81 Dyshidrosis

Cheiropompholyx   Pompholyx

DEF: Vesicular eruption, on hands, feet causing itching and burning.

705.82 Fox-Fordyce disease

DEF: Chronic, usually pruritic disease chiefly of women evidenced by small follicular papular eruptions, especially in the axillary and pubic areas; develops from the closure and rupture of the affected apocrine glands' intraepidermal portion of the ducts.

705.83 Hidradenitis

Hidradenitis suppurativa

DEF: Inflamed sweat glands.

705.89 Other

Bromhidrosis   Granulosis rubra nasi
Chromhidrosis   Urhidrosis

> EXCLUDES   ▶ generalized hyperhidrosis (780.8)◀
> hidrocystoma (216.0-216.9)

DEF: Bromhidrosis: foul-smelling axillary sweat due to decomposed bacteria.

DEF: Chromhidrosis: secretion of colored sweat.

DEF: Granulosis rubra nasi: ideopathic condition of children; causes redness, sweating around nose, face and chin; tends to end by puberty.

DEF: Urhidrosis: urinous substance, such as uric acid, in sweat; occurs in uremia.

705.9 Unspecified disorder of sweat glands

Disorder of sweat glands NOS

√4ᵗʰ √5ᵗʰ Additional Digit Required   Unspecified Code   Other Specified Code   Manifestation Code   ▶◀ Revised Text   ● New Code   ▲ Revised Code Title

✓4ᵗʰ 706 Diseases of sebaceous glands

706.0 Acne varioliformis

Acne: Acne:
frontalis   necrotica

DEF: Rare form of acne characterized by persistent brown papulopustules usually on the brow and temporoparietal part of the scalp.

706.1 Other acne

Acne: Acne:
NOS   vulgaris
conglobata   Blackhead
cystic   Comedo
pustular

EXCLUDES   acne rosacea (695.3)

706.2 Sebaceous cyst

Atheroma, skin   Wen
Keratin cyst

DEF: Benign epidermal cyst, contains sebum and keratin; presents as firm, circumscribed nodule.

706.3 Seborrhea

EXCLUDES   seborrhea:
     capitis (690.11)
     sicca (690.18)
   seborrheic:
     dermatitis (690.10)
     keratosis (702.11-702.19)

DEF: Seborrheic dermatitis marked by excessive secretion of sebum; the sebum forms an oily coating, crusts, or scales on the skin; it is also called hypersteatosis.

706.8 Other specified diseases of sebaceous glands

Asteatosis (cutis)   Xerosis cutis

706.9 Unspecified disease of sebaceous glands

✓4ᵗʰ 707 Chronic ulcer of skin

INCLUDES   non-infected sinus of skin
     non-healing ulcer

EXCLUDES   specific infections classified under "Infectious and Parasitic Diseases" (001.0-136.9)
     varicose ulcer (454.0, 454.2)

✓5ᵗʰ 707.0 Decubitus ulcer

Bed sore
Decubitus ulcer [any site]
Plaster ulcer
Pressure ulcer

AHA: ▶1Q, '04, 14;◀ 4Q, '03, 110; 4Q, '99, 20; 1Q, '96, 15; 3Q, '90, 15; N-D, '87, 9

● **707.00 Unspecified site**

● **707.01 Elbow**

● **707.02 Upper back**
Shoulder blades

● **707.03 Lower back**
Sacrum

● **707.04 Hip**

● **707.05 Buttock**

Six Stages of Decubitus Ulcers

Skin is warm, firm, or stretched   Bacteria enter   Fat layer exposed

First Stage   Second Stage   Third Stage

Muscle necrosis   Advanced muscle necrosis   Bone necrosis

Fourth Stage   Fifth Stage   Sixth Stage

● **707.06 Ankle**

● **707.07 Heel**

● **707.09 Other site**
Head

✓5ᵗʰ 707.1 Ulcer of lower limbs, except decubitus

Ulcer, chronic:
   neurogenic }
   trophic   } of lower limb

Code, if applicable, any casual condition first:
atherosclerosis of the extremities with ulceration (440.23)
chronic venous hypertension with ulcer (459.31)
chronic venous hypertension with ulcer and inflammation (459.33)
diabetes mellitus (250.80-250.83)
postphlebitic syndrome with ulcer (459.11)
postphlebitic syndrome with ulcer and inflammation (459.13)

AHA: 4Q, '00, 44; 4Q, '99, 15

707.10 Ulcer of lower limb, unspecified

AHA: 4Q, '02, 43

707.11 Ulcer of thigh

707.12 Ulcer of calf

707.13 Ulcer of ankle

707.14 Ulcer of heel and midfoot
Plantar surface of midfoot

707.15 Ulcer of other part of foot
Toes

707.19 Ulcer of other part of lower limb

707.8 Chronic ulcer of other specified sites

Ulcer, chronic:
   neurogenic }
   trophic   } of other specified sites

707.9 Chronic ulcer of unspecified site

Chronic ulcer NOS   Tropical ulcer NOS
Trophic ulcer NOS   Ulcer of skin NOS

✓4ᵗʰ 708 Urticaria

EXCLUDES   edema:
     angioneurotic (995.1)
     Quincke's (995.1)
   hereditary angioedema (277.6)
   urticaria:
     giant (995.1)
     papulosa (Hebra) (698.2)
     pigmentosa (juvenile) (congenital) (757.33)

DEF: Skin disorder marked by raised edematous patches of skin or mucous membrane with intense itching; also called hives.

708.0 Allergic urticaria

708.1 Idiopathic urticaria

708.2 Urticaria due to cold and heat
Thermal urticaria

Cutaneous Lesions
Surface Lesions

Fissure   Polyp growth   Ulcer

Solid Lesions

Flat macule   Slightly elevated wheal   Solid papule

Sac Lesions

Cyst   Clear fluid vesicle   Pustule

N Newborn Age: 0   **P** Pediatric Age: 0-17   **M** Maternity Age: 12-55   **A** Adult Age: 15-124   **MSP** Medicare Secondary Payer

708.3 Dermatographic urticaria
  Dermatographia   Factitial urticaria

708.4 Vibratory urticaria

708.5 Cholinergic urticaria

708.8 Other specified urticaria
  Nettle rash   Urticaria:
  Urticaria: recurrent periodic
    chronic

708.9 Urticaria, unspecified
  Hives NOS

✓4ᵗʰ **709 Other disorders of skin and subcutaneous tissue**

  ✓5ᵗʰ **709.0 Dyschromia**
       EXCLUDES *albinism (270.2)*
                     pigmented nevus (216.0-216.9)
                     that of eyelid (374.52-374.53)

       DEF: Pigment disorder of skin or hair.

    709.00 Dyschromia, unspecified

    709.01 Vitiligo
         DEF: Persistent, progressive development of
         nonpigmented white patches on otherwise normal skin.

    709.09 Other

  709.1 Vascular disorders of skin
    Angioma serpiginosum
    Purpura (primary)annularis telangiectodes

709.2 Scar conditions and fibrosis of skin
  Adherent scar (skin)   Fibrosis, skin NOS
  Cicatrix   Scar NOS
  Disfigurement (due to scar)
       EXCLUDES *keloid scar (701.4)*

  AHA: N-D, '84, 19

709.3 Degenerative skin disorders
  Calcinosis: Degeneration, skin
    circumscripta   Deposits, skin
    cutis   Senile dermatosis NOS
  Colloid milium   Subcutaneous calcification

**709.4 Foreign body granuloma of skin and subcutaneous
         tissue**
       EXCLUDES *residual foreign body without*
                     granuloma of skin and
                     subcutaneous tissue (729.6)
                     that of muscle (728.82)

709.8 Other specified disorders of skin
  Epithelial hyperplasia Vesicular eruption
  Menstrual dermatosis

  AHA: N-D, '87, 6

  DEF: Epithelial hyperplasia: increased number of epitheleal cells.

  DEF: Vesicular eruption: liquid-filled structures appearing through
  skin.

**709.9 Unspecified disorder of skin and subcutaneous
         tissue**
  Dermatosis NOS

✓4ᵗʰ
✓5ᵗʰ Additional Digit Required   Unspecified Code   Other Specified Code   Manifestation Code   ►◄ Revised Text   ● New Code   ▲ Revised Code Title

2005 ICD•9•CM   **Volume 1 — 197**

13. DISEASES OF THE MUSCULOSKELETAL SYSTEM AND CONNECTIVE TISSUE (710-739)

The following fifth-digit subclassification is for use with categories 711-712, 715-716, 718-719, and 730:

0 site unspecified

1 shoulder region
Acromioclavicular joint(s)
Clavicle
Glenohumeral joint(s)
Scapula
Sternoclavicular joint(s)

2 upper arm
Elbow joint   Humerus

3 forearm
Radius   Wrist joint
Ulna

4 hand
Carpus   Phalanges [fingers]
Metacarpus

5 pelvic region and thigh
Buttock   Hip (joint)
Femur

6 lower leg
Fibula   Patella
Knee joint   Tibia

7 ankle and foot
Ankle joint   Phalanges, foot
Digits [toes]   Tarsus
Metatarsus   Other joints in foot

8 other specified sites
Head   Skull
Neck   Trunk
Ribs   Vertebral column

9 multiple sites

ARTHROPATHIES AND RELATED DISORDERS (710-719)

EXCLUDES   disorders of spine (720.0-724.9)

✓4ᵗʰ **710 Diffuse diseases of connective tissue**

INCLUDES   all collagen diseases whose effects are not mainly confined to a single system

EXCLUDES   those affecting mainly the cardiovascular system, i.e., polyarteritis nodosa and allied conditions (446.0-446.7)

710.0 Systemic lupus erythematosus
Disseminated lupus erythematosus
Libman-Sacks disease
Use additional code to identify manifestation, as:
   endocarditis (424.91)
   nephritis (583.81)
      chronic (582.81)
   nephrotic syndrome (581.81)
    EXCLUDES   lupus erythematosus (discoid) NOS (695.4)

AHA: ▶2Q, '03, 7-8;◀ 2Q, '97, 8

DEF: A chronic multisystemic inflammatory disease affecting connective tissue; marked by anemia, leukopenia, muscle and joint pains, fever, rash of a butterfly pattern around cheeks and forehead area; of unknown etiology.

710.1 Systemic sclerosis
Acrosclerosis   Progressive systemic sclerosis
CRST syndrome   Scleroderma
   EXCLUDES   circumscribed scleroderma (701.0)
Use additional code to identify manifestation, as:
   lung involvement (517.2)
   myopathy (359.6)

AHA: 1Q, '88, 6

DEF: Systemic disease, involving excess fibrotic collagen build-up; symptoms include thickened skin; fibrotic degenerative changes in various organs; and vascular abnormalities; condition occurs more often in females.

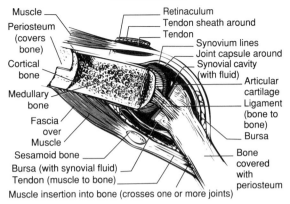

Joint Structures

710.2 Sicca syndrome
Keratoconjunctivitis sicca
Sjögren's disease

DEF: Autoimmune disease; associated with keratoconjunctivitis, laryngopharyngitis, rhinitis, dry mouth, enlarged parotid gland, and chronic polyarthritis.

710.3 Dermatomyositis
Poikilodermatomyositis
Polymyositis with skin involvement

DEF: Polymyositis associated with flat-top purple papules on knuckles; marked by upper eyelid rash, edema of eyelids and orbit area, red rash on forehead, neck, shoulders, trunk and arms; symptoms include fever, weight loss aching muscles; visceral cancer (in individuals older than 40).

710.4 Polymyositis

DEF: Chronic, progressive, inflammatory skeletal muscle disease; causes weakness of limb girdles, neck, pharynx; may precede or follow scleroderma, Sjogren's disease, systemic lupus erythematosus, arthritis, or malignancy.

710.5 Eosinophilia myalgia syndrome
Toxic oil syndrome
Use additional E code to identify drug, if drug induced

AHA: 4Q, '92, 21

DEF: Eosinophilia myalgia syndrome (EMS): inflammatory, multisystem fibrosis; associated with ingesting elemetary L-tryptophan; symptoms include myalgia, weak limbs and bulbar muscles, distal sensory loss, areflexia, arthralgia, cough, fever, fatigue, skin rashes myopathy, and eosinophil counts greater than 1000/microliter.

DEF: Toxic oil syndrome: syndrome similar to EMS due to ingesting contaminated cooking oil.

710.8 Other specified diffuse diseases of connective tissue
Multifocal fibrosclerosis (idiopathic) NEC
Systemic fibrosclerosing syndrome

AHA: M-A, '87, 12

710.9 Unspecified diffuse connective tissue disease
Collagen disease NOS

✓4ᵗʰ / ✓5ᵗʰ Additional Digit Required   Unspecified Code   Other Specified Code   Manifestation Code   ▶◀ Revised Text   ● New Code   ▲ Revised Code Title

2005 ICD•9•CM   **February 2004 • Volume 1 — 199**

Musculoskeletal System and Connective Tissue

711–713

√4ᵗʰ **711 Arthropathy associated with infections**

INCLUDES

arthritis
arthropathy
polyarthritis
polyarthropathy
} associated with conditions classifiable below

EXCLUDES   rheumatic fever (390)

The following fifth-digit subclassification is for use with category 711; valid digits are in [brackets] under each code. See list at beginning of chapter for definitions.

0 site unspecified
1 shoulder region
2 upper arm
3 forearm
4 hand
5 pelvic region and thigh
6 lower leg
7 ankle and foot
8 other specified sites
9 multiple sites

AHA: 1Q, '92, 17

§ √5ᵗʰ **711.0 Pyogenic arthritis**
[0-9]   Arthritis or polyarthritis (due to):
     coliform [Escherichia coli]
     Hemophilus influenzae [H. influenzae]
     pneumococcal
     Pseudomonas
     staphylococcal
     streptococcal
    Pyarthrosis
    Use additional code to identify infectious organism
     (041.0-041.8)

AHA: 1Q, '92, 16; 1Q, '91, 15

DEF: Infectious arthritis caused by various bacteria; marked by inflamed synovial membranes, and purulent effusion in joints.

§ √5ᵗʰ **711.1 Arthropathy associated with Reiter's disease and nonspecific urethritis**
[0-9]   Code first underlying disease as:
     nonspecific urethritis (099.4)
     Reiter's disease (099.3)

DEF: Reiter's disease: joint disease marked by diarrhea, urethritis, conjunctivitis, keratosis and arthritis; of unknown etiology; affects young males.

DEF: Urethritis: inflamed urethra.

§ √5ᵗʰ **711.2 Arthropathy in Behçet's syndrome**
[0-9]   Code first underlying disease (136.1)

DEF: Behçet's syndrome: chronic inflammatory disorder, of unknown etiology; affects small blood vessels; causes ulcers of oral and pharyngeal mucous membranes and genitalia, skin lesions, retinal vasculitis, optic atrophy and severe uveitis.

§ √5ᵗʰ **711.3 Postdysenteric arthropathy**
[0-9]   Code first underlying disease as:
     dysentery (009.0)
     enteritis, infectious (008.0-009.3)
     paratyphoid fever (002.1-002.9)
     typhoid fever (002.0)
     EXCLUDES   salmonella arthritis (003.23)

§ √5ᵗʰ **711.4 Arthropathy associated with other bacterial diseases**
[0-9]   Code first underlying disease as:
     diseases classifiable to 010-040, 090-099, except as in 711.1, 711.3, and 713.5
     leprosy (030.0-030.9)
     tuberculosis (015.0-015.9)
     EXCLUDES   gonococcal arthritis (098.50)
                 meningococcal arthritis (036.82)

§ √5ᵗʰ **711.5 Arthropathy associated with other viral diseases**
[0-9]   Code first underlying disease as:
     diseases classifiable to 045-049, 050-079, 480, 487
    O'nyong nyong (066.3)
     EXCLUDES   that due to rubella (056.71)

§ √5ᵗʰ **711.6 Arthropathy associated with mycoses**
[0-9]   Code first underlying disease (110.0-118)

§ √5ᵗʰ **711.7 Arthropathy associated with helminthiasis**
[0-9]   Code first underlying disease as:
     filariasis (125.0-125.9)

§ √5ᵗʰ **711.8 Arthropathy associated with other infectious and parasitic diseases**
[0-9]   Code first underlying disease as:
     diseases classifiable to 080-088, 100-104, 130-136
     EXCLUDES   arthropathy associated with sarcoidosis (713.7)

AHA: 4Q, '91, 15; 3Q, '90, 14

§ √5ᵗʰ **711.9 Unspecified infective arthritis**
[0-9]   Infective arthritis or polyarthritis (acute) (chronic) (subacute) NOS

√4ᵗʰ **712 Crystal arthropathies**

INCLUDES   crystal-induced arthritis and synovitis
EXCLUDES   gouty arthropathy (274.0)

DEF: Joint disease due to urate crystal deposit in joints or synovial membranes.

The following fifth-digit subclassification is for use with category 712; valid digits are in [brackets] under each code. See list at beginning of chapter for definitions.

0 site unspecified
1 shoulder region
2 upper arm
3 forearm
4 hand
5 pelvic region and thigh
6 lower leg
7 ankle and foot
8 other specified sites
9 multiple sites

§ √5ᵗʰ **712.1 Chondrocalcinosis due to dicalcium phosphate crystals**
[0-9]   Chondrocalcinosis due to dicalcium phosphate crystals (with other crystals)
    Code first underlying disease (275.4)

§ √5ᵗʰ **712.2 Chondrocalcinosis due to pyrophosphate crystals**
[0-9]   Code first underlying disease (275.4)

§ √5ᵗʰ **712.3 Chondrocalcinosis, unspecified**
[0-9]   Code first underlying disease (275.4)

§ √5ᵗʰ **712.8 Other specified crystal arthropathies**
[0-9]

§ √5ᵗʰ **712.9 Unspecified crystal arthropathy**
[0-9]

√4ᵗʰ **713 Arthropathy associated with other disorders classified elsewhere**

INCLUDES

arthritis
arthropathy
polyarthritis
polyarthropathy
} associated with conditions classifiable below

§ Requires fifth digit. Valid digits are in [brackets] under each code. See beginning of section 710–739 for codes and definitions.

N Newborn Age: 0   P Pediatric Age: 0-17   M Maternity Age: 12-55   A Adult Age: 15-124   MSP Medicare Secondary Payer

713.0   *Arthropathy associated with other endocrine and metabolic disorders*
  Code first underlying disease as:
    acromegaly (253.0)
    hemochromatosis (275.0)
    hyperparathyroidism ▶(252.00-252.08)◀
    hypogammaglobulinemia (279.00-279.09)
    hypothyroidism (243-244.9)
    lipoid metabolism disorder (272.0-272.9)
    ochronosis (270.2)
    EXCLUDES arthropathy associated with:
        amyloidosis (713.7)
        crystal deposition disorders, except gout (712.1-712.9)
        diabetic neuropathy (713.5)
        gouty arthropathy (274.0)

713.1   *Arthropathy associated with gastrointestinal conditions other than infections*
  Code first underlying disease as:
    regional enteritis (555.0-555.9)
    ulcerative colitis (556)

713.2   *Arthropathy associated with hematological disorders*
  Code first underlying disease as:
    hemoglobinopathy (282.4-282.7)
    hemophilia (286.0-286.2)
    leukemia (204.0-208.9)
    malignant reticulosis (202.3)
    multiple myelomatosis (203.0)
    EXCLUDES arthropathy associated with Henoch-Schönlein purpura (713.6)

713.3   *Arthropathy associated with dermatological disorders*
  Code first underlying disease as:
    erythema multiforme (695.1)
    erythema nodosum (695.2)
    EXCLUDES psoriatic arthropathy (696.0)

713.4   *Arthropathy associated with respiratory disorders*
  Code first underlying disease as:
    diseases classifiable to 490-519
    EXCLUDES arthropathy associated with respiratory infections (711.0, 711.4-711.8)

713.5   *Arthropathy associated with neurological disorders*

    Charcôt's arthropathy ⎫ associated with
    Neuropathic arthritis ⎬ diseases classifiable elsewhere ⎭

  Code first underlying disease as:
    neuropathic joint disease [Charcôt's joints]:
      NOS (094.0)
      diabetic (250.6)
      syringomyelic (336.0)
      tabetic [syphilitic] (094.0)

713.6   *Arthropathy associated with hypersensitivity reaction*
  Code first underlying disease as:
    Henoch (-Schönlein) purpura (287.0)
    serum sickness (999.5)
    EXCLUDES allergic arthritis NOS (716.2)

713.7   *Other general diseases with articular involvement*
  Code first underlying disease as:
    amyloidosis (277.3)
    familial Mediterranean fever (277.3)
    sarcoidosis (135)
  AHA: 2Q, '97, 12

713.8   *Arthropathy associated with other conditions classifiable elsewhere*
  Code first underlying disease as:
    conditions classifiable elsewhere except as in 711.1-711.8, 712, and 713.0-713.7

✓4ᵗʰ **714 Rheumatoid arthritis and other inflammatory polyarthropathies**
    EXCLUDES rheumatic fever (390)
        rheumatoid arthritis of spine NOS (720.0)

AHA: 2Q, '95, 3

714.0   Rheumatoid arthritis
    Arthritis or polyarthritis:
      atrophic
      rheumatic (chronic)
    Use additional code to identify manifestation, as:
      myopathy (359.6)
      polyneuropathy (357.1)
      EXCLUDES juvenile rheumatoid arthritis NOS (714.30)

AHA: 1Q, '90, 5

DEF: Chronic systemic disease principally of joints, manifested by inflammatory changes in articular structures and synovial membranes, atrophy, and loss in bone density.

714.1   Felty's syndrome
    Rheumatoid arthritis with splenoadenomegaly and leukopenia
DEF: Syndrome marked by rheumatoid arthritis, splenomegaly, leukopenia, pigmented spots on lower extremity skin, anemia, and thrombocytopenia.

714.2   Other rheumatoid arthritis with visceral or systemic involvement
    Rheumatoid carditis

✓5ᵗʰ **714.3   Juvenile chronic polyarthritis**
    DEF: Rheumatoid arthritis of more than one joint; lasts longer than six weeks in age 17 or younger; symptoms include fever, erythematous rash, weight loss, lymphadenopathy, hepatosplenomegaly and pericarditis.

    714.30 Polyarticular juvenile rheumatoid arthritis, chronic or unspecified
        Juvenile rheumatoid arthritis NOS
        Still's disease

    714.31 Polyarticular juvenile rheumatoid arthritis, acute

    714.32 Pauciarticular juvenile rheumatoid arthritis

    714.33 Monoarticular juvenile rheumatoid arthritis

714.4   Chronic postrheumatic arthropathy
    Chronic rheumatoid nodular fibrositis
    Jaccoud's syndrome
    DEF: Persistent joint disorder; follows previous rheumatic infection.

✓5ᵗʰ **714.8   Other specified inflammatory polyarthropathies**
    714.81 Rheumatoid lung
        Caplan's syndrome
        Diffuse interstitial rheumatoid disease of lung
        Fibrosing alveolitis, rheumatoid
        DEF: Lung disorders associated with rheumatoid arthritis.

    714.89 Other

714.9   Unspecified inflammatory polyarthropathy
    Inflammatory polyarthropathy or polyarthritis NOS
    EXCLUDES polyarthropathy NOS (716.5)

✓4ᵗʰ ✓5ᵗʰ Additional Digit Required   Unspecified Code   Other Specified Code   Manifestation Code   ▶◀ Revised Text   ● New Code   ▲ Revised Code Title

2005 ICD•9•CM   **October 2004 • Volume 1 — 201**

Musculoskeletal System and Connective Tissue

715–717.3

√4ᵗʰ **715 Osteoarthrosis and allied disorders**

Note: Localized, in the subcategories below, includes bilateral involvement of the same site.

INCLUDES   arthritis or polyarthritis:
degenerative
hypertrophic
degenerative joint disease
osteoarthritis

EXCLUDES   *Marie-Strümpell spondylitis (720.0)*
osteoarthrosis [osteoarthritis] of spine (721.0-721.9)

The following fifth-digit subclassification is for use with category 715; valid digits are in [brackets] under each code. See list at beginning of chapter for definitions.

0   site unspecified
1   shoulder region
2   upper arm
3   forearm
4   hand
5   pelvic region and thigh
6   lower leg
7   ankle and foot
8   other specified sites
9   multiple sites

§ √5ᵗʰ **715.0 Osteoarthrosis, generalized**
[0,4,9]   Degenerative joint disease, involving multiple joints
Primary generalized hypertrophic osteoarthrosis
DEF: Chronic noninflammatory arthritis; marked by degenerated articular cartilage and enlarged bone; symptoms include pain and stiffness with activity; occurs among elderly.

§ √5ᵗʰ **715.1 Osteoarthrosis, localized, primary**
[0-8]   Localized osteoarthropathy, idiopathic

§ √5ᵗʰ **715.2 Osteoarthrosis, localized, secondary**
[0-8]   Coxae malum senilis

§ √5ᵗʰ **715.3 Osteoarthrosis, localized, not specified whether primary or secondary**
[0-8]   Otto's pelvis
AHA: For code 715.36: ▶4Q, '03, 118;◀ 2Q, '95, 5

§ √5ᵗʰ **715.8 Osteoarthrosis involving, or with mention of more than one site, but not specified as generalized**
[0,9]

§ √5ᵗʰ **715.9 Osteoarthrosis, unspecified whether generalized or localized**
[0-8]
AHA: For code 715.90: 2Q, '97, 12

√4ᵗʰ **716 Other and unspecified arthropathies**
EXCLUDES   *cricoarytenoid arthropathy (478.79)*

The following fifth-digit subclassification is for use with category 716; valid digits are in [brackets] under each code. See list at beginning of chapter for definitions.

0   site unspecified
1   shoulder region
2   upper arm
3   forearm
4   hand
5   pelvic region and thigh
6   lower leg
7   ankle and foot
8   other specified sites
9   multiple sites

AHA: 2Q, '95, 3

§ √5ᵗʰ **716.0 Kaschin-Beck disease**
[0-9]   Endemic polyarthritis
DEF: Chronic degenerative disease of spine and peripheral joints; occurs in eastern Siberian, northern Chinese, and Korean youth; may a mycotoxicosis caused by eating cereals infected with fungus.

§ √5ᵗʰ **716.1 Traumatic arthropathy**
[0-9]   AHA: For Code 716.11: 1Q, '02, 9

§ √5ᵗʰ **716.2 Allergic arthritis**
[0-9]   EXCLUDES   *arthritis associated with Henoch-Schönlein purpura or serum sickness (713.6)*

§ √5ᵗʰ **716.3 Climacteric arthritis**   ♀
[0-9]   Menopausal arthritis
DEF: Ovarian hormone deficiency; causes pain in small joints, shoulders, elbows or knees; affects females at menopause; also called arthropathia ovaripriva.

§ √5ᵗʰ **716.4 Transient arthropathy**
[0-9]   EXCLUDES   *palindromic rheumatism (719.3)*

§ √5ᵗʰ **716.5 Unspecified polyarthropathy or polyarthritis**
[0-9]

§ √5ᵗʰ **716.6 Unspecified monoarthritis**
[0-8]   Coxitis

§ √5ᵗʰ **716.8 Other specified arthropathy**
[0-9]

§ √5ᵗʰ **716.9 Arthropathy, unspecified**
[0-9]   Arthritis
Arthropathy } (acute) (chronic) (subacute)

Articular rheumatism (chronic)
Inflammation of joint NOS

√4ᵗʰ **717 Internal derangement of knee**
INCLUDES   degeneration
rupture, old } of articular cartilage or meniscus of knee
tear, old

EXCLUDES   *acute derangement of knee (836.0-836.6)*
ankylosis (718.5)
contracture (718.4)
current injury (836.0-836.6)
deformity (736.4-736.6)
recurrent dislocation (718.3)

717.0 Old bucket handle tear of medial meniscus
Old bucket handle tear of unspecified cartilage

717.1 Derangement of anterior horn of medial meniscus

717.2 Derangement of posterior horn of medial meniscus

717.3 Other and unspecified derangement of medial meniscus
Degeneration of internal semilunar cartilage

Disruption and Tears of Meniscus

Bucket-handle

Flap-type

Radial
Peripheral

Horizontal cleavage

Vertical

Congenital discoid meniscus

§ Requires fifth digit. Valid digits are in [brackets] under each code. See beginning of section 710–739 for codes and definitions.

N Newborn Age: 0   P Pediatric Age: 0-17   M Maternity Age: 12-55   A Adult Age: 15-124   MSP Medicare Secondary Payer

Internal Derangements of Knee

Disruptions of Cruciate Ligament

Anterior

Posterior

Chondromalacia of Patella

"Kissing" lesion of fermur

✓5th **717.4 Derangement of lateral meniscus**

717.40 Derangement of lateral meniscus, unspecified

717.41 Bucket handle tear of lateral meniscus

717.42 Derangement of anterior horn of lateral meniscus

717.43 Derangement of posterior horn of lateral meniscus

717.49 Other

717.5 Derangement of meniscus, not elsewhere classified
Congenital discoid meniscus
Cyst of semilunar cartilage
Derangement of semilunar cartilage NOS

717.6 Loose body in knee
Joint mice, knee
Rice bodies, knee (joint)

DEF: The presence in the joint synovial area of a small, frequently calcified, loose body created from synovial membrane, organized fibrin fragments of articular cartilage or arthritis osteophytes.

717.7 Chondromalacia of patella
Chondromalacia patellae
Degeneration [softening] of articular cartilage of patella

AHA: M-A, '85, 14; N-D, '84, 9

DEF: Softened patella cartilage.

✓5th **717.8 Other internal derangement of knee**

717.81 Old disruption of lateral collateral ligament

717.82 Old disruption of medial collateral ligament

717.83 Old disruption of anterior cruciate ligament

717.84 Old disruption of posterior cruciate ligament

717.85 Old disruption of other ligaments of knee
Capsular ligament of knee

717.89 Other
Old disruption of ligaments of knee NOS

717.9 Unspecified internal derangement of knee
Derangement NOS of knee

✓4th **718 Other derangement of joint**
    EXCLUDES current injury (830.0-848.9)
                jaw ▶(524.60-524.69)◀

The following fifth-digit subclassification is for use with category 718; valid digits are in [brackets] under each code. See list at beginning of chapter for definitions.
    0 site unspecified
    1 shoulder region
    2 upper arm
    3 forearm
    4 hand
    5 pelvic region and thigh
    6 lower leg
    7 ankle and foot
    8 other specified sites
    9 multiple sites

§ ✓5th **718.0 Articular cartilage disorder**
[0-5,7-9]   Meniscus: Meniscus:
                disorder   tear, old
                rupture, old   Old rupture of ligament(s) of
                                                  joint NOS
            EXCLUDES articular cartilage disorder:
                        in ochronosis (270.2)
                        knee (717.0-717.9)
                      chondrocalcinosis (275.4)
                      metastatic calcification (275.4)

§ ✓5th **718.1 Loose body in joint**
[0-5,7-9]   Joint mice
            EXCLUDES knee (717.6)

AHA: For code 718.17: 2Q, '01, 15

DEF: Calcified loose bodies in synovial fluid; due to arthritic osteophytes.

§ ✓5th **718.2 Pathological dislocation**
[0-9]   Dislocation or displacement of joint, not recurrent
                and not current injury
            Spontaneous dislocation (joint)

§ ✓5th **718.3 Recurrent dislocation of joint**
[0-9]   AHA: N-D, '87, 7

§ ✓5th **718.4 Contracture of joint**
[0-9]   AHA: 4Q, '98, 40

§ ✓5th **718.5 Ankylosis of joint**
[0-9]   Ankylosis of joint (fibrous) (osseous)
            EXCLUDES spine (724.9)
                        stiffness of joint without mention of
                          ankylosis (719.5)

DEF: Immobility and solidification, of joint; due to disease, injury or surgical procedure.

§ ✓5th **718.6 Unspecified intrapelvic protrusion of acetabulum**
[0,5]   Protrusio acetabuli, unspecified

DEF: Sinking of the floor of acetabulum; causing femoral head to protrude, limits hip movement; of unknown etiology.

§ ✓5th **718.7 Developmental dislocation of joint**
[0-9]   EXCLUDES congenital dislocation of joint (754.0-
                          755.8)
                      traumatic dislocation of joint (830-839)

AHA: 4Q, '01, 48

§ ✓5th **718.8 Other joint derangement, not elsewhere classified**
[0-9]   Flail joint (paralytic)
            Instability of joint
            EXCLUDES deformities classifiable to 736 (736.0-
                          736.9)

AHA: For code 718.81: 2Q, '00, 14

Musculoskeletal System and Connective Tissue

717.4–718.8

Musculoskeletal System and Connective Tissue

718.9–721.1

Joint Derangements and Disorders

Loose body in joint

Dislocation of joint

Joint contracture

Ankylosis of joint

Synovial effusion (fluid)

Hemarthrosis (blood)

§ ✓5ᵗʰ **718.9** **Unspecified derangement of joint**
[0-5,7-9]   **EXCLUDES**   *knee (717.9)*

✓4ᵗʰ **719 Other and unspecified disorders of joint**
     EXCLUDES   *jaw ▶(524.60-524.69)◀*

> The following fifth-digit subclassification is for use with codes 719.0-719.6, 719.8-719.9; valid digits are in [brackets] under each code. See list at beginning of chapter for definitions.
>
> 0 site unspecified
> 1 shoulder region
> 2 upper arm
> 3 forearm
> 4 hand
> 5 pelvic region and thigh
> 6 lower leg
> 7 ankle and foot
> 8 other specified sites
> 9 multiple sites

§ ✓5ᵗʰ **719.0** **Effusion of joint**
[0-9]   Hydrarthrosis
        Swelling of joint, with or without pain
        EXCLUDES   *intermittent hydrarthrosis (719.3)*

§ ✓5ᵗʰ **719.1** **Hemarthrosis**
[0-9]   **EXCLUDES**   *current injury (840.0-848.9)*

§ ✓5ᵗʰ **719.2** **Villonodular synovitis**
[0-9]   DEF: Overgrowth of synovial tissue, especially at knee joint; due to macrophage infiltration of giant cells in synovial villi and fibrous nodules.

§ ✓5ᵗʰ **719.3** **Palindromic rheumatism**
[0-9]   Hench-Rosenberg syndrome
        Intermittent hydrarthrosis
     DEF: Recurrent episodes of afebrile arthritis and periarthritis marked by their complete disappearance after a few days or hours; causes swelling, redness, and disability usually affecting only one joint; no known cause; affects adults of either sex.

§ ✓5ᵗʰ **719.4** **Pain in joint**
[0-9]   Arthralgia
     AHA: For code 719.46: 1Q, '01, 3

§ ✓5ᵗʰ **719.5** **Stiffness of joint, not elsewhere classified**
[0-9]

§ ✓5ᵗʰ **719.6** **Other symptoms referable to joint**
[0-9]   Joint crepitus   Snapping hip
     AHA: 1Q, '94, 15

     719.7 **Difficulty in walking**
        EXCLUDES   *abnormality of gait (781.2)*
     AHA: 4Q, '03, 66

§ ✓5ᵗʰ **719.8** **Other specified disorders of joint**
[0-9]   Calcification of joint   Fistula of joint
        EXCLUDES   *temporomandibular joint-pain-dysfunction syndrome [Costen's syndrome] ▶(524.60)◀*

§ ✓5ᵗʰ **719.9** **Unspecified disorder of joint**
[0-9]

DORSOPATHIES (720-724)

     EXCLUDES   *curvature of spine (737.0-737.9)*
                   osteochondrosis of spine (juvenile) (732.0)
                   adult (732.8)

✓4ᵗʰ **720 Ankylosing spondylitis and other inflammatory spondylopathies**

     720.0 **Ankylosing spondylitis**
        Rheumatoid arthritis of spine NOS
        Spondylitis:
           Marie-Strümpell
           rheumatoid
     DEF: Rheumatoid arthritis of spine and sacroiliac joints; fusion and deformity in spine follows; affects mainly males; cause unknown.

     720.1 **Spinal enthesopathy**
        Disorder of peripheral ligamentous or muscular attachments of spine
        Romanus lesion
     DEF: Tendinous or muscular vertebral bone attachment abnormality.

     720.2 **Sacroiliitis, not elsewhere classified**
        Inflammation of sacroiliac joint NOS
     DEF: Pain due to inflammation in joint, at juncture of sacrum and hip.

✓5ᵗʰ   **720.8** **Other inflammatory spondylopathies**
     720.81 *Inflammatory spondylopathies in diseases classified elsewhere*
        Code first underlying disease as:
           tuberculosis (015.0)
     720.89 **Other**
     720.9 **Unspecified inflammatory spondylopathy**
        Spondylitis NOS

✓4ᵗʰ **721 Spondylosis and allied disorders**
     AHA: 2Q, '89, 14

     DEF: Degenerative changes in spinal joint.

     721.0 **Cervical spondylosis without myelopathy**
        Cervical or cervicodorsal: Cervical or cervicodorsal:
           arthritis   spondylarthritis
           osteoarthritis

     721.1 **Cervical spondylosis with myelopathy**
        Anterior spinal artery compression syndrome
        Spondylogenic compression of cervical spinal cord
        Vertebral artery compression syndrome

Normal Anatomy of Vertebral Disc

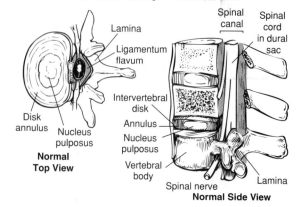

Lamina

Spinal canal

Spinal cord in dural sac

Ligamentum flavum

Intervertebral disk

Annulus

Nucleus pulposus

Vertebral body

Disk annulus

Nucleus pulposus

Spinal nerve

Lamina

Normal Top View

Normal Side View

---

§ Requires fifth digit. Valid digits are in [brackets] under each code. See beginning of section 710–739 for codes and definitions.

Ⓝ Newborn Age: 0   Ⓟ Pediatric Age: 0-17   Ⓜ Maternity Age: 12-55   Ⓐ Adult Age: 15-124   MSP Medicare Secondary Payer

721.2 Thoracic spondylosis without myelopathy
Thoracic: Thoracic:
  arthritis   spondylarthritis
  osteoarthritis

721.3 Lumbosacral spondylosis without myelopathy
Lumbar or lumbosacral: Lumbar or lumbosacral:
  arthritis   spondylarthritis
  osteoarthritis
AHA: 4Q, '02, 107

√5th **721.4 Thoracic or lumbar spondylosis with myelopathy**
  721.41 Thoracic region
    Spondylogenic compression of thoracic spinal cord
  721.42 Lumbar region
    Spondylogenic compression of lumbar spinal cord

721.5 Kissing spine
Baastrup's syndrome
DEF: Compression of spinous processes of adjacent vertebrae; due to mutual contact.

721.6 Ankylosing vertebral hyperostosis
721.7 Traumatic spondylopathy
Kümmell's disease or spondylitis
721.8 Other allied disorders of spine
√5th **721.9 Spondylosis of unspecified site**
  721.90 Without mention of myelopathy
    Spinal:
      arthritis (deformans) (degenerative) (hypertrophic)
      osteoarthritis NOS
    Spondylarthrosis NOS
  721.91 With myelopathy
    Spondylogenic compression of spinal cord NOS

√4th **722 Intervertebral disc disorders**
AHA: 1Q, '88. 10

  722.0 Displacement of cervical intervertebral disc without myelopathy
    Neuritis (brachial) or radiculitis due to displacement or rupture of cervical intervertebral disc
    Any condition classifiable to 722.2 of the cervical or cervicothoracic intervertebral disc

√5th **722.1 Displacement of thoracic or lumbar intervertebral disc without myelopathy**
  722.10 Lumbar intervertebral disc without myelopathy
    Lumbago or sciatica due to displacement of intervertebral disc
    Neuritis or radiculitis due to displacement or rupture of lumbar intervertebral disc
    Any condition classifiable to 722.2 of the lumbar or lumbosacral intervertebral disc
AHA: ▶3Q, '03, 12;◀ 1Q, '03, 7; 4Q, '02, 107

  722.11 Thoracic intervertebral disc without myelopathy
    Any condition classifiable to 722.2 of thoracic intervertebral disc

722.2 Displacement of intervertebral disc, site unspecified, without myelopathy
Discogenic syndrome NOS
Herniation of nucleus pulposus NOS
Intervertebral disc NOS:
  extrusion
  prolapse
  protrusion
  rupture
Neuritis or radiculitis due to displacement or rupture of intervertebral disc

√5th **722.3 Schmorl's nodes**
DEF: Irregular bone defect in the margin of the vertebral body; causes herniation into end plate of vertebral body.
  722.30 Unspecified region
  722.31 Thoracic region
  722.32 Lumbar region
  722.39 Other

722.4 Degeneration of cervical intervertebral disc
Degeneration of cervicothoracic intervertebral disc

√5th **722.5 Degeneration of thoracic or lumbar intervertebral disc**
  722.51 Thoracic or thoracolumbar intervertebral disc
  722.52 Lumbar or lumbosacral intervertebral disc

722.6 Degeneration of intervertebral disc, site unspecified
Degenerative disc disease NOS
Narrowing of intervertebral disc or space NOS

√5th **722.7 Intervertebral disc disorder with myelopathy**
  722.70 Unspecified region
  722.71 Cervical region
  722.72 Thoracic region
  722.73 Lumbar region

√5th **722.8 Postlaminectomy syndrome**
AHA: J-F, '87, 7
DEF: Spinal disorder due to spinal laminectomy surgery.
  722.80 Unspecified region
  722.81 Cervical region
  722.82 Thoracic region
  722.83 Lumbar region
  AHA: 2Q, '97, 15

√5th **722.9 Other and unspecified disc disorder**
Calcification of intervertebral cartilage or disc
Discitis

Derangement of Vertebral Disc

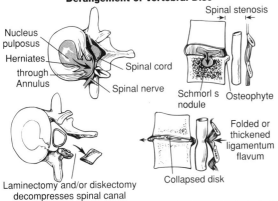

Spinal Stenosis in Cervical Region

√4th √5th Additional Digit Required | Unspecified Code | Other Specified Code | Manifestation Code | ▶◀ Revised Text | ● New Code | ▲ Revised Code Title

Musculoskeletal System and Connective Tissue

722.90–726.33

722.90 Unspecified region   A
> AHA: N-D, '84, 19

722.91 Cervical region   A
722.92 Thoracic region   A
722.93 Lumbar region   A

√4ᵗʰ **723 Other disorders of cervical region**
> EXCLUDES   conditions due to:
>> intervertebral disc disorders (722.0-722.9)
>> spondylosis (721.0-721.9)

AHA: 3Q, '94, 14; 2Q, '89, 14

723.0 Spinal stenosis in cervical region
> AHA: ▶4Q, '03, 101◀

723.1 Cervicalgia
> Pain in neck
> DEF: Pain in cervical spine or neck region.

723.2 Cervicocranial syndrome
> Barré-Liéou syndrome
> Posterior cervical sympathetic syndrome
> DEF: Neurologic disorder of upper cervical spine and nerve roots.

723.3 Cervicobrachial syndrome (diffuse)
> AHA: N-D, '85, 12
>
> DEF: Complex of symptoms due to scalenus anterior muscle compressing the brachial plexus; pain radiates from shoulder to arm or back of neck.

723.4 Brachial neuritis or radiculitis NOS
> Cervical radiculitis
> Radicular syndrome of upper limbs

723.5 Torticollis, unspecified
> Contracture of neck
>> EXCLUDES   congenital (754.1)
>>> due to birth injury (767.8)
>>> hysterical (300.11)
>>> ocular torticollis (781.93)
>>> psychogenic (306.0)
>>> spasmodic (333.83)
>>> traumatic, current (847.0)
>
> AHA: 2Q, '01, 21; 1Q, '95, 7
>
> DEF: Abnormally positioned neck relative to head; due to cervical muscle or fascia contractions; also called wryneck.

723.6 Panniculitis specified as affecting neck
> DEF: Inflammation of the panniculus adiposus (subcutaneous fat) in the neck.

723.7 Ossification of posterior longitudinal ligament in cervical region

723.8 Other syndromes affecting cervical region
> Cervical syndrome NEC
> Klippel's disease
> Occipital neuralgia
> AHA: 1Q, '00, 7

723.9 Unspecified musculoskeletal disorders and symptoms referable to neck
> Cervical (region) disorder NOS

√4ᵗʰ **724 Other and unspecified disorders of back**
> EXCLUDES   collapsed vertebra (code to cause, e.g.,
>> osteoporosis, 733.00-733.09)
>> conditions due to:
>>> intervertebral disc disorders (722.0-722.9)
>>> spondylosis (721.0-721.9)

AHA: 2Q, '89, 14

√5ᵗʰ **724.0 Spinal stenosis, other than cervical**
> **724.00 Spinal stenosis, unspecified region**   A
> **724.01 Thoracic region**   A
> **724.02 Lumbar region**   A
>> AHA: 4Q, '99, 13
>
> **724.09 Other**   A

724.1 Pain in thoracic spine

724.2 Lumbago
> Low back pain   Lumbalgia
> Low back syndrome
> AHA: N-D, '85, 12

724.3 Sciatica
> Neuralgia or neuritis of sciatic nerve
>> EXCLUDES   specified lesion of sciatic nerve (355.0)
> AHA: 2Q, '89, 12

724.4 Thoracic or lumbosacral neuritis or radiculitis, unspecified
> Radicular syndrome of lower limbs
> AHA: 2Q, '99, 3

724.5 Backache, unspecified
> Vertebrogenic (pain) syndrome NOS

724.6 Disorders of sacrum
> Ankylosis � lumbosacral or sacroiliac (joint)
> Instability

√5ᵗʰ **724.7 Disorders of coccyx**
> **724.70 Unspecified disorder of coccyx**
> **724.71 Hypermobility of coccyx**
> **724.79 Other**
>> Coccygodynia

724.8 Other symptoms referable to back
> Ossification of posterior longitudinal ligament NOS
> Panniculitis specified as sacral or affecting back

724.9 Other unspecified back disorders
> Ankylosis of spine NOS
> Compression of spinal nerve root NEC
> Spinal disorder NOS
>> EXCLUDES   sacroiliitis (720.2)

RHEUMATISM, EXCLUDING THE BACK (725-729)
> INCLUDES   disorders of muscles and tendons and their attachments, and of other soft tissues

725 Polymyalgia rheumatica
> DEF: Joint and muscle pain, pelvis, and shoulder girdle stiffness, high sedimentation rate and temporal arteritis; occurs in elderly.

√4ᵗʰ **726 Peripheral enthesopathies and allied syndromes**
> Note: Enthesopathies are disorders of peripheral ligamentous or muscular attachments.
>> EXCLUDES   spinal enthesopathy (720.1)

726.0 Adhesive capsulitis of shoulder

√5ᵗʰ **726.1 Rotator cuff syndrome of shoulder and allied disorders**
> **726.10 Disorders of bursae and tendons in shoulder region, unspecified**
>> Rotator cuff syndrome NOS
>> Supraspinatus syndrome NOS
>> AHA: 2Q, '01, 11
>
> **726.11 Calcifying tendinitis of shoulder**
> **726.12 Bicipital tenosynovitis**
> **726.19 Other specified disorders**
>> EXCLUDES   complete rupture of rotator cuff, nontraumatic (727.61)

726.2 Other affections of shoulder region, not elsewhere classified
> Periarthritis of shoulder   Scapulohumeral fibrositis

√5ᵗʰ **726.3 Enthesopathy of elbow region**
> **726.30 Enthesopathy of elbow, unspecified**
> **726.31 Medial epicondylitis**
> **726.32 Lateral epicondylitis**
>> Epicondylitis NOS   Tennis elbow
>> Golfers' elbow
> **726.33 Olecranon bursitis**
>> Bursitis of elbow

N Newborn Age: 0   P Pediatric Age: 0-17   M Maternity Age: 12-55   A Adult Age: 15-124   MSP Medicare Secondary Payer

Bunion

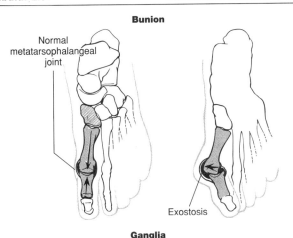

Normal metatarsophalangeal joint

Exostosis

Ganglia

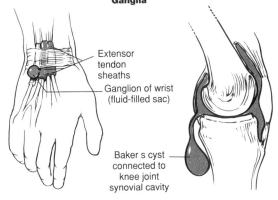

Extensor tendon sheaths

Ganglion of wrist (fluid-filled sac)

Baker s cyst connected to knee joint synovial cavity

726.39 Other

726.4 Enthesopathy of wrist and carpus
Bursitis of hand or wrist
Periarthritis of wrist

726.5 Enthesopathy of hip region
Bursitis of hip
Gluteal tendinitis
Iliac crest spur
Psoas tendinitis
Trochanteric tendinitis

✓5ᵗʰ 726.6 Enthesopathy of knee
726.60 Enthesopathy of knee, unspecified
Bursitis of knee NOS

726.61 Pes anserinus tendinitis or bursitis
DEF: Inflamed tendons of sartorius, gracilis and semitendinosus muscles of medial aspect of knee.

726.62 Tibial collateral ligament bursitis
Pellegrini-Stieda syndrome

726.63 Fibular collateral ligament bursitis

726.64 Patellar tendinitis

726.65 Prepatellar bursitis

726.69 Other
Bursitis:
infrapatellar
Bursitis:
subpatellar

✓5ᵗʰ 726.7 Enthesopathy of ankle and tarsus
726.70 Enthesopathy of ankle and tarsus, unspecified
Metatarsalgia NOS
EXCLUDES Morton's metatarsalgia (355.6)

726.71 Achilles bursitis or tendinitis

726.72 Tibialis tendinitis
Tibialis (anterior) (posterior) tendinitis

726.73 Calcaneal spur
DEF: Overgrowth of calcaneous bone; causes pain on walking; due to chronic avulsion injury of plantar fascia from calcaneus.

726.79 Other
Peroneal tendinitis

726.8 Other peripheral enthesopathies

✓5ᵗʰ 726.9 Unspecified enthesopathy
726.90 Enthesopathy of unspecified site
Capsulitis NOS
Periarthritis NOS
Tendinitis NOS

726.91 Exostosis of unspecified site
Bone spur NOS
AHA: 2Q, '01, 15

✓4ᵗʰ 727 Other disorders of synovium, tendon, and bursa
✓5ᵗʰ 727.0 Synovitis and tenosynovitis
727.00 Synovitis and tenosynovitis, unspecified
Synovitis NOS
Tenosynovitis NOS

727.01 Synovitis and tenosynovitis in diseases classified elsewhere
Code first underlying disease as:
tuberculosis (015.0-015.9)
EXCLUDES crystal-induced (275.4)
gonococcal (098.51)
gouty (274.0)
syphilitic (095.7)

727.02 Giant cell tumor of tendon sheath

727.03 Trigger finger (acquired)
DEF: Stenosing tenosynovitis or nodule in flexor tendon; cessation of flexion or extension movement in finger, followed by snapping into place.

727.04 Radial styloid tenosynovitis
de Quervain's disease

727.05 Other tenosynovitis of hand and wrist

727.06 Tenosynovitis of foot and ankle

727.09 Other

727.1 Bunion
DEF: Enlarged first metatarsal head due to inflamed bursa; results in laterally displaced great toe.

727.2 Specific bursitides often of occupational origin
Beat:
elbow
hand
knee
Miners':
elbow
knee
Chronic crepitant synovitis of wrist

727.3 Other bursitis
Bursitis NOS
EXCLUDES bursitis:
gonococcal (098.52)
subacromial (726.19)
subcoracoid (726.19)
subdeltoid (726.19)
syphilitic (095.7)
"frozen shoulder" (726.0)

✓5ᵗʰ 727.4 Ganglion and cyst of synovium, tendon, and bursa
727.40 Synovial cyst, unspecified
EXCLUDES that of popliteal space (727.51)
AHA: 2Q, '97, 6

727.41 Ganglion of joint

727.42 Ganglion of tendon sheath

727.43 Ganglion, unspecified

727.49 Other
Cyst of bursa

✓5ᵗʰ 727.5 Rupture of synovium
727.50 Rupture of synovium, unspecified
727.51 Synovial cyst of popliteal space
Baker's cyst (knee)
727.59 Other

✓5ᵗʰ 727.6 Rupture of tendon, nontraumatic
727.60 Nontraumatic rupture of unspecified tendon

✓4ᵗʰ
✓5ᵗʰ Additional Digit Required   Unspecified Code   Other Specified Code   Manifestation Code   ▶◀ Revised Text   ● New Code   ▲ Revised Code Title

2005 ICD•9•CM

Musculoskeletal System and Connective Tissue

727.61–728.88

727.61   Complete rupture of rotator cuff
727.62   Tendons of biceps (long head)
727.63   Extensor tendons of hand and wrist
727.64   Flexor tendons of hand and wrist
727.65   Quadriceps tendon
727.66   Patellar tendon
727.67   Achilles tendon
727.68   Other tendons of foot and ankle
727.69   Other

√5th **727.8   Other disorders of synovium, tendon, and bursa**

727.81   **Contracture of tendon (sheath)**
    Short Achilles tendon (acquired)

727.82   **Calcium deposits in tendon and bursa**
    Calcification of tendon NOS
    Calcific tendinitis NOS
    EXCLUDES   peripheral ligamentous or muscular attachments (726.0-726.9)

727.83   **Plica syndrome**
    Plica knee
    AHA: 4Q, '00, 44
    DEF: A fold in the synovial tissue that begins to form before birth, creating a septum between two pockets of synovial tissue; two most common plicae are the medial patellar plica and the suprapatellar plica. Plica syndrome, or plica knee, refers to symptomatic plica. Experienced by females more commonly than males.

727.89   **Other**
    Abscess of bursa or tendon
    EXCLUDES   xanthomatosis localized to tendons (272.7)
    AHA: 2Q, '89, 15

727.9   **Unspecified disorder of synovium, tendon, and bursa**

√4th **728   Disorders of muscle, ligament, and fascia**
    EXCLUDES   enthesopathies (726.0-726.9)
       muscular dystrophies (359.0-359.1)
       myoneural disorders (358.00-358.9)
       myopathies (359.2-359.9)
       old disruption of ligaments of knee (717.81-717.89)

728.0   **Infective myositis**
    Myositis:
      purulent
      suppurative
    EXCLUDES   myositis:
        epidemic (074.1)
        interstitial (728.81)
        syphilitic (095.6)
        tropical (040.81)
    DEF: Inflamed connective septal tissue of muscle.

√5th **728.1   Muscular calcification and ossification**

728.10   **Calcification and ossification, unspecified**
    Massive calcification (paraplegic)

728.11   **Progressive myositis ossificans**
    DEF: Progressive myositic disease; marked by bony tissue formed by voluntary muscle; occurs among very young.

728.12   **Traumatic myositis ossificans**
    Myositis ossificans (circumscripta)

728.13   **Postoperative heterotopic calcification**
    DEF: Abnormal formation of calcium deposits in muscular tissue after surgery, marked by a corresponding loss of muscle tone and tension.

728.19   **Other**
    Polymyositis ossificans

728.2   **Muscular wasting and disuse atrophy, not elsewhere classified**
    Amyotrophia NOS   Myofibrosis
    EXCLUDES   neuralgic amyotrophy (353.5)
       ▶pelvic muscle wasting and disuse atrophy (618.83)◀
       progressive muscular atrophy (335.0-335.9)

728.3   **Other specific muscle disorders**
    Arthrogryposis
    Immobility syndrome (paraplegic)
    EXCLUDES   arthrogryposis multiplex congenita (754.89)
       stiff-man syndrome (333.91)

728.4   **Laxity of ligament**

728.5   **Hypermobility syndrome**

728.6   **Contracture of palmar fascia**   A
    Dupuytren's contracture
    DEF: Dupuytren's contracture: flexion deformity of finger, due to shortened, thickened fibrosing of palmar fascia; cause unknown; associated with long-standing epilepsy; occurs more often in males.

√5th **728.7   Other fibromatoses**

728.71   **Plantar fascial fibromatosis**
    Contracture of plantar fascia
    Plantar fasciitis (traumatic)
    DEF: Plantar fascia fibromatosis; causes nodular swelling and pain; not associated with contractures.

728.79   **Other**
    Garrod's or knuckle pads
    Nodular fasciitis
    Pseudosarcomatous fibromatosis (proliferative) (subcutaneous)
    DEF: Knuckle pads: pea-size nodules on dorsal surface of interphalangeal joints; new growth of fibrous tissue with thickened dermis and epidermis.

√5th **728.8   Other disorders of muscle, ligament, and fascia**

728.81   **Interstitial myositis**
    DEF: Inflammation of septal connective parts of muscle tissue.

728.82   **Foreign body granuloma of muscle**
    Talc granuloma of muscle

728.83   **Rupture of muscle, nontraumatic**

728.84   **Diastasis of muscle**
    Diastasis recti (abdomen)
    EXCLUDES   diastasis recti complicating pregnancy, labor, and delivery (665.8)
    DEF: Muscle separation, such as recti abdominis after repeated pregnancies.

728.85   **Spasm of muscle**

728.86   **Necrotizing fasciitis**
    Use additional code to identify:
      infectious organism (041.00-041.89)
      gangrene (785.4), if applicable
    AHA: 4Q, '95, 54
    DEF: Fulminating infection begins with extensive cellulitis, spreads to superficial and deep fascia; causes thrombosis of subcutaneous vessels, and gangrene of underlying tissue.

728.87   **Muscle weakness**
    EXCLUDES   generalized weakness (780.79)
    AHA: 4Q, '03, 66

728.88   **Rhabdomyolysis**
    AHA: 4Q, '03, 66
    DEF: A disintegration or destruction of muscle; an acute disease characterized by the excretion of myoglobin into the urine.

P Pediatric Age: 0-17   M Maternity Age: 12-55   A Adult Age: 15-124   MSP Medicare Secondary Payer

2005 ICD•9•CM

728.89 Other
Eosinophilic fasciitis
Use additional E code to identify drug, if
drug induced
AHA: 3Q, '02, 28; 2Q, '01, 14, 15

DEF: Eosinophilic fasciitis: inflammation of fascia of
extremities associated with eosinophilia, edema, and
swelling; occurs alone or as part of myalgia syndrome.

**728.9 Unspecified disorder of muscle, ligament, and
fascia**
AHA: 4Q, '88, 11

✓4ᵗʰ 729 Other disorders of soft tissues
    EXCLUDES *acroparesthesia (443.89)*
carpal tunnel syndrome (354.0)
disorders of the back (720.0-724.9)
entrapment syndromes (354.0-355.9)
palindromic rheumatism (719.3)
periarthritis (726.0-726.9)
psychogenic rheumatism (306.0)

729.0 Rheumatism, unspecified and fibrositis
DEF: General term describes diseases of muscle, tendon, nerve,
joint, or bone; symptoms include pain and stiffness.

729.1 Myalgia and myositis, unspecified
Fibromyositis NOS
DEF: Myalgia: muscle pain.

DEF: Myositis: inflamed voluntary muscle.

DEF: Fibromyositis: inflamed fibromuscular tissue.

729.2 Neuralgia, neuritis, and radiculitis, unspecified
    EXCLUDES *brachial radiculitis (723.4)*
cervical radiculitis (723.4)
lumbosacral radiculitis (724.4)
mononeuritis (354.0-355.9)
*radiculitis due to intervertebral disc
involvement (722.0-722.2, 722.7)*
sciatica (724.3)

DEF: Neuralgia: paroxysmal pain along nerve symptoms include
brief pain and tenderness at point nerve exits.

DEF: Neuritis: inflamed nerve, symptoms include paresthesia,
paralysis and loss of reflexes at nerve site.

DEF: Radiculitis: inflamed nerve root.

✓5ᵗʰ 729.3 Panniculitis, unspecified
DEF: Inflammatory reaction of subcutaneous fat; causes nodules;
often develops in abdominal region.

729.30 Panniculitis, unspecified site
Weber-Christian disease
DEF: Febrile, nodular, nonsuppurative, relapsing
inflammation of subcutaneous fat.

729.31 Hypertrophy of fat pad, knee
Hypertrophy of infrapatellar fat pad
729.39 Other site
    EXCLUDES *panniculitis specified as
(affecting):
back (724.8)
neck (723.6)
sacral (724.8)*

729.4 Fasciitis, unspecified
    EXCLUDES *necrotizing fasciitis (728.86)*
nodular fasciitis (728.79)

AHA: 2Q, '94, 13

729.5 Pain in limb

729.6 Residual foreign body in soft tissue
    EXCLUDES *foreign body granuloma:
muscle (728.82)
skin and subcutaneous tissue
(709.4)*

✓5ᵗʰ 729.8 Other musculoskeletal symptoms referable to limbs
729.81 Swelling of limb
AHA: 4Q, '88, 6

729.82 Cramp
729.89 Other
    EXCLUDES *abnormality of gait (781.2)*
tetany (781.7)
*transient paralysis of limb
(781.4)*

AHA: 4Q, '88, 12

729.9 Other and unspecified disorders of soft tissue
Polyalgia

OSTEOPATHIES, CHONDROPATHIES, AND ACQUIRED
MUSCULOSKELETAL DEFORMITIES (730-739)

**✓4ᵗʰ 730 Osteomyelitis, periostitis, and other infections involving
bone**
    EXCLUDES *jaw (526.4-526.5)*
petrous bone (383.2)
Use additional code to identify organism, such as
Staphylococcus (041.1)

The following fifth-digit subclassification is for use with
category 730; valid digits are in [brackets] under each
code. See list at beginning of chapter for definitions.
0   site unspecified
1   shoulder region
2   upper arm
3   forearm
4   hand
5   pelvic region and thigh
6   lower leg
7   ankle and foot
8   other specified sites
9   multiple sites

AHA: 4Q, '97, 43

DEF: Osteomyelitis: bacterial inflammation of bone tissue and marrow.

DEF: Periostitis: inflammation of specialized connective tissue; causes
swelling of bone and aching pain.

§ **✓5ᵗʰ 730.0 Acute osteomyelitis**
[0-9]   Abscess of any bone except accessory sinus, jaw, or
mastoid
Acute or subacute osteomyelitis, with or without
mention of periostitis
AHA: For code 730.06: 1Q, '02, 4; **For code 730.07:** ▶1Q, '04, 14◀

§ **✓5ᵗʰ 730.1 Chronic osteomyelitis**
[0-9]   Brodie's abscess
Chronic or old osteomyelitis, with or without
mention of periostitis
Sequestrum of bone
Sclerosing osteomyelitis of Garré
    EXCLUDES *aseptic necrosis of bone (733.40-733.49)*
AHA: For code 730.17: 3Q, '00, 4

§ **✓5ᵗʰ 730.2 Unspecified osteomyelitis**
[0-9]   Osteitis or osteomyelitis NOS, with or without
mention of periostitis

§ **✓5ᵗʰ 730.3 Periostitis without mention of osteomyelitis**
[0-9]   Abscess of periosteum ⎱ without mention of
Periostosis ⎰ osteomyelitis

    EXCLUDES *that in secondary syphilis (091.61)*

---

§ Requires fifth digit. Valid digits are in [brackets] under each code. See beginning of section 710–739 for codes and definitions.

✓4ᵗʰ / ✓5ᵗʰ Additional Digit Required   Unspecified Code   Other Specified Code   Manifestation Code   ▶◀ Revised Text   ● New Code   ▲ Revised Code Title

2005 ICD•9•CM   October 2004 • Volume 1 — 209

Musculoskeletal System and Connective Tissue

730.7–733.11

§ ✓5ᵗʰ **730.7 Osteopathy resulting from poliomyelitis**
[0-9]
  Code first underlying disease (045.0-045.9)

§ ✓5ᵗʰ **730.8 Other infections involving bone in diseases classified elsewhere**
[0-9]
  Code first underlying disease as:
    tuberculosis (015.0-015.9)
    typhoid fever (002.0)
  EXCLUDES   syphilis of bone NOS (095.5)
  AHA: 2Q, '97, 16; 3Q, '91, 10

§ ✓5ᵗʰ **730.9 Unspecified infection of bone**
[0-9]

✓4ᵗʰ **731 Osteitis deformans and osteopathies associated with other disorders classified elsewhere**
  DEF: Osteitis deformans: Bone disease marked by episodes of increased bone loss, excessive repair attempts follow; causes weakened, deformed bones with increased mass, bowed long bones, deformed flat bones, pain and pathological fractures; may be fatal if associated with congestive heart failure, giant cell tumors or bone sarcoma; also called Paget's disease.

731.0 Osteitis deformans without mention of bone tumor
  Paget's disease of bone

731.1 Osteitis deformans in diseases classified elsewhere
  Code first underlying disease as:
    malignant neoplasm of bone (170.0-170.9)

731.2 Hypertrophic pulmonary osteoarthropathy
  Bamberger-Marie disease
  DEF: Clubbing, of fingers and toes; related to enlarged ends of long bones; due to chronic lung and heart disease.

731.8 Other bone involvement in diseases classified elsewhere
  Code first underlying disease as:
    diabetes mellitus (250.8)
  Use additional code to specify bone condition, such as:
    acute osteomyelitis (730.00-730.09)
  AHA: 1Q, '04, 14; 4Q, '97, 43; 2Q, '97, 16

✓4ᵗʰ **732 Osteochondropathies**
  DEF: Conditions related to both bone and cartilage, or conditions in which cartilage is converted to bone (enchondral ossification).

732.0 Juvenile osteochondrosis of spine
  Juvenile osteochondrosis (of):
    marginal or vertebral epiphysis (of Scheuermann)
    spine NOS
  Vertebral epiphysitis
  EXCLUDES   adolescent postural kyphosis (737.0)

732.1 Juvenile osteochondrosis of hip and pelvis
  Coxa plana
  Ischiopubic synchondrosis (of van Neck)
  Osteochondrosis (juvenile) of:
    acetabulum
    head of femur (of Legg-Calvé-Perthes)
    iliac crest (of Buchanan)
    symphysis pubis (of Pierson)
  Pseudocoxalgia

732.2 Nontraumatic slipped upper femoral epiphysis
  Slipped upper femoral epiphysis NOS

732.3 Juvenile osteochondrosis of upper extremity
  Osteochondrosis (juvenile) of:
    capitulum of humerus (of Panner)
    carpal lunate (of Kienbock)
    hand NOS
    head of humerus (of Haas)
    heads of metacarpals (of Mauclaire)
    lower ulna (of Burns)
    radial head (of Brailsford)
    upper extremity NOS

732.4 Juvenile osteochondrosis of lower extremity, excluding foot
  Osteochondrosis (juvenile) of:
    lower extremity NOS
    primary patellar center (of Köhler)
    proximal tibia (of Blount)
    secondary patellar center (of Sinding-Larsen)
    tibial tubercle (of Osgood-Schlatter)
  Tibia vara

732.5 Juvenile osteochondrosis of foot
  Calcaneal apophysitis
  Epiphysitis, os calcis
  Osteochondrosis (juvenile) of:
    astragalus (of Diaz)
    calcaneum (of Sever)
    foot NOS
    metatarsal:
      second (of Freiberg)
      fifth (of Iselin)
    os tibiale externum (of Haglund)
    tarsal navicular (of Köhler)

732.6 Other juvenile osteochondrosis
  Apophysitis
  Epiphysitis   }   specified as juvenile, of other
  Osteochondritis   }   site, or site NOS
  Osteochondrosis }

732.7 Osteochondritis dissecans

732.8 Other specified forms of osteochondropathy
  Adult osteochondrosis of spine

732.9 Unspecified osteochondropathy
  Apophysitis
  Epiphysitis   }   NOS
  Osteochondritis   }   not specified as adult or juve-
  Osteochondrosis }   nile, of unspecified site

✓4ᵗʰ **733 Other disorders of bone and cartilage**
  EXCLUDES   bone spur (726.91)
    cartilage of, or loose body in, joint (717.0-717.9, 718.0-718.9)
    giant cell granuloma of jaw (526.3)
    osteitis fibrosa cystica generalisata ▶(252.01)◀
    osteomalacia (268.2)
    polyostotic fibrous dysplasia of bone (756.54)
    prognathism, retrognathism (524.1)
    xanthomatosis localized to bone (272.7)

✓5ᵗʰ **733.0 Osteoporosis**
  DEF: Bone mass reduction that ultimately results in fractures after minimal trauma; dorsal kyphosis or loss of height often occur.

  733.00 Osteoporosis, unspecified
    Wedging of vertebra NOS
    AHA: 3Q, '01, 19; 2Q, '98, 12

  733.01 Senile osteoporosis
    Postmenopausal osteoporosis

  733.02 Idiopathic osteoporosis

  733.03 Disuse osteoporosis

  733.09 Other
    Drug-induced osteoporosis
    Use additional E code to identify drug
    AHA: 4Q, '03, 108

✓5ᵗʰ **733.1 Pathologic fracture**
    Spontaneous fracture
    EXCLUDES   stress fracture (733.93-733.95)
      traumatic fracture (800-829)
    AHA: 4Q, '93, 25; N-D, '86, 10; N-D, '85, 16
    DEF: Fracture due to bone structure weakening by pathological processes (e.g., osteoporosis, neoplasms and osteomalacia).

  733.10 Pathologic fracture, unspecified site
  733.11 Pathologic fracture of humerus

---

§ Requires fifth digit. Valid digits are in [brackets] under each code. See beginning of section 710–739 for codes and definitions.

N Newborn Age: 0   P Pediatric Age: 0-17   M Maternity Age: 12-55   A Adult Age: 15-124   MSP Medicare Secondary Payer

Acquired Deformities of Toe

Hallux valgus

Hallux varus

Hallux malleus
(hammer of big toe)

Hammertoe

Acquired Deformities of Forearm

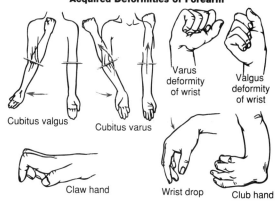

Cubitus valgus

Cubitus varus

Varus deformity of wrist

Valgus deformity of wrist

Claw hand

Wrist drop

Club hand

733.12 Pathologic fracture of distal radius and ulna
Wrist NOS

733.13 Pathologic fracture of vertebrae
Collapse of vertebra NOS
AHA: 3Q, '99, 5

733.14 Pathologic fracture of neck of femur
Femur NOS   Hip NOS
AHA: 1Q, '01, 1; 1Q, '96, 16

733.15 Pathologic fracture of other specified part of femur
AHA: 2Q, '98, 12

733.16 Pathologic fracture of tibia or fibula
Ankle NOS

733.19 Pathologic fracture of other specified site

✓5ᵗʰ **733.2 Cyst of bone**

733.20 Cyst of bone (localized), unspecified

733.21 Solitary bone cyst
Unicameral bone cyst

733.22 Aneurysmal bone cyst
DEF: Solitary bone lesion, bulges into periosteum; marked by calcified rim.

733.29 Other
Fibrous dysplasia (monostotic)
EXCLUDES   cyst of jaw (526.0-526.2, 526.89)
osteitis fibrosa cystica
▶(252.01)◀
polyostotic fibrousdyplasia of bone (756.54)

733.3 Hyperostosis of skull
Hyperostosis interna frontalis
Leontiasis ossium
DEF: Abnormal bone growth on inner aspect of cranial bones.

✓5ᵗʰ **733.4 Aseptic necrosis of bone**
EXCLUDES   osteochondropathies (732.0-732.9)
DEF: Infarction of bone tissue due to a nonfectious etiology, such as a fracture, ischemic disorder or administration of immunosuppressive drugs; leads to degenerative joint disease or nonunion of fractures.

733.40 Aseptic necrosis of bone, site unspecified

733.41 Head of humerus

733.42 Head and neck of femur
Femur NOS
EXCLUDES   Legg-Calvé-Perthes disease (732.1)

733.43 Medial femoral condyle

733.44 Talus

733.49 Other

733.5 Osteitis condensans
Piriform sclerosis of ilium
DEF: Idiopathic condition marked by low back pain; associated with oval or triangular sclerotic, opaque bone next to sacroiliac joints in the ileum.

733.6 Tietze's disease
Costochondral junction syndrome
Costochondritis
DEF: Painful, idiopathic, nonsuppurative, swollen costal cartilage sometimes confused with cardiac symptoms because the anterior chest pain resembles that of coronary artery disease.

733.7 Algoneurodystrophy
Disuse atrophy of bone
Sudeck's atrophy
DEF: Painful, idiopathic.

✓5ᵗʰ **733.8 Malunion and nonunion of fracture**
AHA: 2Q, '94, 5

733.81 Malunion of fracture

733.82 Nonunion of fracture
Pseudoarthrosis (bone)

✓5ᵗʰ **733.9 Other and unspecified disorders of bone and cartilage**

733.90 Disorder of bone and cartilage, unspecified

733.91 Arrest of bone development or growth
Epiphyseal arrest

733.92 Chondromalacia
Chondromalacia:
  NOS
  localized, except patella
  systemic
  tibial plateau
EXCLUDES   chondromalacia of patella (717.7)
DEF: Articular cartilage softening.

733.93 Stress fracture of tibia or fibula
Stress reaction of tibia or fibula
AHA: 4Q, '01, 48

733.94 Stress fracture of the metatarsals
Stress reaction of metatarsals
AHA: 4Q, '01, 48

733.95 Stress fracture of other bone
Stress reaction of other bone
AHA: 4Q, '01, 48

733.99 Other
Diaphysitis
Hypertrophy of bone
Relapsing polychondritis
AHA: J-F, '87, 14

✓4ᵗʰ
✓5ᵗʰ Additional Digit Required   Unspecified Code   Other Specified Code   Manifestation Code   ▶◀ Revised Text   ● New Code   ▲ Revised Code Title

734   Flat foot
> Pes planus (acquired)
> Talipes planus (acquired)
>> **EXCLUDES**   *congenital (754.61)*
>> *rigid flat foot (754.61)*
>> *spastic (everted) flat foot (754.61)*

✓4ᵗʰ   735   Acquired deformities of toe
> **EXCLUDES**   *congenital (754.60-754.69, 755.65-755.66)*

> **735.0   Hallux valgus (acquired)**
>> DEF: Angled displacement of the great toe, causing it to ride over or under other toes.

> **735.1   Hallux varus (acquired)**
>> DEF: Angled displacement of the great toe toward the body midline, away from the other toes.

> **735.2   Hallux rigidus**
>> DEF: Limited flexion movement at metatarsophalangeal joint of great toe; due to degenerative joint disease.

> **735.3   Hallux malleus**
>> DEF: Extended proximal phalanx, flexed distal phalanges, of great toe; foot resembles claw or hammer.

> **735.4   Other hammer toe (acquired)**
> **735.5   Claw toe (acquired)**
>> DEF: Hyperextended proximal phalanges, flexed middle and distal phalanges.

> **735.8   Other acquired deformities of toe**
> **735.9   Unspecified acquired deformity of toe**

✓4ᵗʰ   736   Other acquired deformities of limbs
> **EXCLUDES**   *congenital (754.3-755.9)*

> **✓5ᵗʰ   736.0   Acquired deformities of forearm, excluding fingers**
>> **736.00   Unspecified deformity**
>>> Deformity of elbow, forearm, hand, or wrist (acquired) NOS

Acquired Deformities of Hip

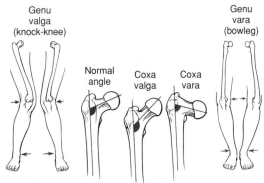

Genu valga (knock-knee)   Normal angle   Coxa valga   Coxa vara   Genu vara (bowleg)

Acquired Deformities of Lower Limb

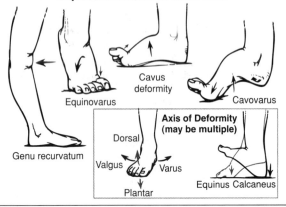

Equinovarus   Cavus deformity   Cavovarus
Genu recurvatum
Axis of Deformity (may be multiple)   Dorsal   Valgus   Varus   Plantar   Equinus Calcaneus

---

> **736.01   Cubitus valgus (acquired)**
>> DEF: Deviation of the elbow away from the body midline upon extension; it occurs when the palm is turning outward.

> **736.02   Cubitus varus (acquired)**
>> DEF: Elbow joint displacement angled laterally; when the forearm is extended, it is deviated toward the midline of the body; also called "gun stock" deformity.

> **736.03   Valgus deformity of wrist (acquired)**
>> DEF: Abnormal angulation away from the body midline.

> **736.04   Varus deformity of wrist (acquired)**
>> DEF: Abnormal angulation toward the body midline.

> **736.05   Wrist drop (acquired)**
>> DEF: Inability to extend the hand at the wrist due to extensor muscle paralysis.

> **736.06   Claw hand (acquired)**
>> DEF: Flexion and atrophy of the hand and fingers; found in ulnar nerve lesions, syringomyelia, and leprosy.

> **736.07   Club hand, acquired**
>> DEF: Twisting of the hand out of shape or position; caused by the congenital absence of the ulna or radius.

> **736.09   Other**

736.1   Mallet finger
> DEF: Permanently flexed distal phalanx.

✓5ᵗʰ   736.2   Other acquired deformities of finger
> **736.20   Unspecified deformity**
>> Deformity of finger (acquired) NOS

> **736.21   Boutonniere deformity**
>> DEF: A deformity of the finger caused by flexion of the proximal interphalangeal joint and hyperextension of the distal joint; also called buttonhole deformity.

> **736.22   Swan-neck deformity**
>> DEF: Flexed distal and hyperextended proximal interphalangeal joint.

> **736.29   Other**
>> **EXCLUDES**   *trigger finger (727.03)*
>> **AHA:** 2Q, '89, 13

✓5ᵗʰ   736.3   Acquired deformities of hip
> **736.30   Unspecified deformity**
>> Deformity of hip (acquired) NOS

> **736.31   Coxa valga (acquired)**
>> DEF: Increase of at least 140 degrees in the angle formed by the axis of the head and the neck of the femur, and the axis of its shaft.

Kyphosis and Lordosis

Kyphosis (hump)
Lordosis (concave)

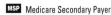

N   Newborn Age: 0   P   Pediatric Age: 0-17   M   Maternity Age: 12-55   A   Adult Age: 15-124   MSP   Medicare Secondary Payer

Scoliosis and Kyphoscoliosis

Scoliosis

Kyphoscoliosis

736.32 Coxa vara (acquired)
DEF: The bending downward of the neck of the femur: causing difficulty in movement; a right angle or less may be formed by the axis of the head and neck of the femur, and the axis of its shaft.

736.39 Other
AHA: 2Q, '91, 18

√5th **736.4 Genu valgum or varum (acquired)**

736.41 Genu valgum (acquired)
DEF: Abnormally close together and an abnormally large space between the ankles; also called "knock-knees."

736.42 Genu varum (acquired)
DEF: Abnormally separated knees and the inward bowing of the legs; it is also called "bowlegs."

736.5 Genu recurvatum (acquired)
DEF: Hyperextended knees; also called "backknee."

736.6 Other acquired deformities of knee
Deformity of knee (acquired) NOS

√5th **736.7 Other acquired deformities of ankle and foot**
EXCLUDES   deformities of toe (acquired) (735.0-735.9)
pes planus (acquired) (734)

736.70 Unspecified deformity of ankle and foot, acquired

736.71 Acquired equinovarus deformity
Clubfoot, acquired
EXCLUDES   clubfoot not specified as acquired (754.5-754.7)

736.72 Equinus deformity of foot, acquired
DEF: A plantar flexion deformity that forces people to walk on their toes.

736.73 Cavus deformity of foot
EXCLUDES   that with claw foot (736.74)
DEF: Abnormally high longitudinal arch of the foot.

736.74 Claw foot, acquired
DEF: High foot arch with hyperextended toes at metatarsophalangeal joint and flexed toes at distal joints; also called "main en griffe."

736.75 Cavovarus deformity of foot, acquired
DEF: Inward turning of the heel from the midline of the leg and an abnormally high longitudinal arch.

736.76 Other calcaneus deformity
736.79 Other
Acquired:
pes
talipes } not elsewhere classified

√5th **736.8 Acquired deformities of other parts of limbs**
736.81 Unequal leg length (acquired)
736.89 Other
Deformity (acquired):
arm or leg, not elsewhere classified
shoulder

736.9 Acquired deformity of limb, site unspecified

√4th **737 Curvature of spine**
EXCLUDES   congenital (754.2)

737.0 Adolescent postural kyphosis
EXCLUDES   osteochondrosis of spine (juvenile) (732.0)
adult (732.8)

√5th **737.1 Kyphosis (acquired)**
737.10 Kyphosis (acquired) (postural)
737.11 Kyphosis due to radiation
737.12 Kyphosis, postlaminectomy
AHA: J-F, '87, 7

737.19 Other
EXCLUDES   that associated with conditions classifiable elsewhere (737.41)

√5th **737.2 Lordosis (acquired)**
DEF: Swayback appearance created by an abnormally increased spinal curvature; it is also referred to as "hollow back" or "saddle back."

737.20 Lordosis (acquired) (postural)
737.21 Lordosis, postlaminectomy
737.22 Other postsurgical lordosis
737.29 Other
EXCLUDES   that associated with conditions classifiable elsewhere (737.42)

√5th **737.3 Kyphoscoliosis and scoliosis**
DEF: Kyphoscoliosis: backward and lateral curvature of the spinal column; it is found in vertebral osteochondrosis.
DEF: Scoliosis: an abnormal deviation of the spine to the left or right of the midline

737.30 Scoliosis [and kyphoscoliosis], idiopathic
AHA: 3Q, '03, 19

737.31 Resolving infantile idiopathic scoliosis
737.32 Progressive infantile idiopathic scoliosis
AHA: 3Q, '02, 12

737.33 Scoliosis due to radiation
737.34 Thoracogenic scoliosis
737.39 Other
EXCLUDES   that associated with conditions classifiable elsewhere (737.43)
that in kyphoscoliotic heart disease (416.1)
AHA: 2Q, '02, 16

√5th **737.4 Curvature of spine associated with other conditions**
Code first associated condition as:
Charcôt-Marie-Tooth disease (356.1)
mucopolysaccharidosis (277.5)
neurofibromatosis (237.7)
osteitis deformans (731.0)
osteitis fibrosa cystica ▶(252.01)◀
osteoporosis (733.00-733.09)
poliomyelitis (138)
tuberculosis [Pott's curvature] (015.0)
737.40 Curvature of spine, unspecified
737.41 Kyphosis
737.42 Lordosis
737.43 Scoliosis

√4th Additional Digit Required   Unspecified Code   Other Specified Code   Manifestation Code   ▶◀ Revised Text   ● New Code   ▲ Revised Code Title

737.8   Other curvatures of spine

737.9   Unspecified curvature of spine
Curvature of spine (acquired) (idiopathic) NOS
Hunchback, acquired
> **EXCLUDES**   *deformity of spine NOS (738.5)*

✓4ᵗʰ **738   Other acquired deformity**
> **EXCLUDES**   *congenital (754.0-756.9, 758.0-759.9)*
> *dentofacial anomalies (524.0-524.9)*

738.0   Acquired deformity of nose
Deformity of nose (acquired)
Overdevelopment of nasal bones
> **EXCLUDES**   *deflected or deviated nasal septum*
> *(470)*

✓5ᵗʰ **738.1   Other acquired deformity of head**

738.10   Unspecified deformity

738.11   Zygomatic hyperplasia
DEF: Abnormal enlargement of the zygoma (processus zygomaticus temporalis).

738.12   Zygomatic hypoplasia
DEF: Underdevelopment of the zygoma (processus zygomaticus temporalis).

738.19   Other specified deformity
AHA: ▶2Q, '03, 13◀

738.2   Acquired deformity of neck

738.3   Acquired deformity of chest and rib

Deformity:	Pectus:
chest (acquired)	carinatum, acquired
rib (acquired)	excavatum, acquired

738.4   Acquired spondylolisthesis
Degenerative spondylolisthesis
Spondylolysis, acquired
> **EXCLUDES**   *congenital (756.12)*

DEF: Vertebra displaced forward over another; due to bilateral defect in vertebral arch, eroded articular surface of posterior facts and elongated pedicle between fifth lumbar vertebra and sacrum.

738.5   Other acquired deformity of back or spine
Deformity of spine NOS
> **EXCLUDES**   *curvature of spine (737.0-737.9)*

738.6   Acquired deformity of pelvis
Pelvic obliquity
> **EXCLUDES**   *intrapelvic protrusion of acetabulum*
> *(718.6)*
> *that in relation to labor and delivery*
> *(653.0-653.4, 653.8-653.9)*

DEF: Pelvic obliquity: slanting or inclination of the pelvis at an angle between 55 and 60 degrees between the plane of the pelvis and the horizontal plane.

738.7   Cauliflower ear
DEF: Abnormal external ear; due to injury, subsequent perichondritis.

738.8   Acquired deformity of other specified site
Deformity of clavicle
AHA: 2Q, '01, 15

738.9   Acquired deformity of unspecified site

✓4ᵗʰ **739   Nonallopathic lesions, not elsewhere classified**
> **INCLUDES**   segmental dysfunction
> somatic dysfunction

DEF: Disability, loss of function or abnormality of a body part that is neither classifiable to a particular system nor brought about therapeutically to counteract another disease.

739.0   Head region
Occipitocervical region

739.1   Cervical region
Cervicothoracic region

739.2   Thoracic region
Thoracolumbar region

739.3   Lumbar region
Lumbosacral region

739.4   Sacral region
Sacrococcygeal region   Sacroiliac region

739.5   Pelvic region
Hip region
Pubic region

739.6   Lower extremities

739.7   Upper extremities
Acromioclavicular region
Sternoclavicular region

739.8   Rib cage
Costochondral region   Sternochondral region
Costovertebral region

739.9   Abdomen and other
AHA: 2Q, '89, 14

N Newborn Age: 0   P Pediatric Age: 0-17   M Maternity Age: 12-55   A Adult Age: 15-124   MSP Medicare Secondary Payer

14. CONGENITAL ANOMALIES (740-759)

✓4ᵗʰ 740 Anencephalus and similar anomalies

740.0 Anencephalus

Acrania   Hemicephaly
Amyelencephalus   Hemianencephaly

DEF: Fetus without cerebrum, cerebellum and flat bones of skull.

740.1 Craniorachischisis

DEF: Congenital slit in cranium and vertebral column.

740.2 Iniencephaly

DEF: Spinal cord passes through enlarged occipital bone (foramen magnum); absent vertebral bone layer and spinal processes; resulting in both reduction in number and proper fusion of the vertebrae.

✓4ᵗʰ 741 Spina bifida

EXCLUDES spina bifida occulta (756.17)

The following fifth-digit subclassification is for use with category 741:

    0   unspecified region
    1   cervical region
    2   dorsal [thoracic] region
    3   lumbar region

AHA: 3Q, '94, 7

DEF: Lack of closure of spinal cord's bony encasement; marked by cord protrusion into lumbosacral area; evident by elevated alpha-fetoprotein of amniotic fluid.

✓5ᵗʰ 741.0 With hydrocephalus

Arnold-Chiari syndrome, type II
Any condition classifiable to 741.9 with any condition classifiable to 742.3
Chiari malformation, type II

AHA: 4Q, '97, 51; 4Q, '94, 37; S-O, '87, 10

✓5ᵗʰ 741.9 Without mention of hydrocephalus

Hydromeningocele (spinal)   Myelocystocele
Hydromyelocele   Rachischisis
Meningocele (spinal)   Spina bifida (aperta)
Meningomyelocele   Syringomyelocele
Myelocele

✓4ᵗʰ 742 Other congenital anomalies of nervous system

742.0 Encephalocele

Encephalocystocele   Hydromeningocele, cranial
Encephalomyelocele   Meningocele, cerebral
Hydroencephalocele   Meningoencephalocele

AHA: 4Q, '94, 37

DEF: Brain tissue protrudes through skull defect.

742.1 Microcephalus

Hydromicrocephaly
Micrencephaly

DEF: Extremely small head or brain.

742.2 Reduction deformities of brain

Absence ⎤
Agenesis ⎥ of part of brain
Aplasia ⎥
Hypoplasia ⎦

Agyria   Holoprosencephaly
Arhinencephaly   Microgyria

AHA: ▶3Q, '03, 15;◀ 4Q, '94, 37

742.3 Congenital hydrocephalus

Aqueduct of Sylvius:
    anomaly
    obstruction, congenital
    stenosis
Atresia of foramina of Magendie and Luschka
Hydrocephalus in newborn

EXCLUDES hydrocephalus:
    acquired (331.3-331.4)
    due to congenital toxoplasmosis
      (771.2)
    with any condition classifiable to
      741.9 (741.0)

DEF: Fluid accumulation within the skull; involves subarachnoid (external) or ventricular (internal) brain spaces.

742.4 Other specified anomalies of brain

Congenital cerebral cyst   Multiple anomalies of brain
Macroencephaly   NOS
Macrogyria   Porencephaly
Megalencephaly   Ulegyria

AHA: 1Q, '99, 9; 3Q, '92, 12

✓5ᵗʰ 742.5 Other specified anomalies of spinal cord

742.51 Diastematomyelia

DEF: Congenital anomaly often associated with spina bifida; the spinal cord is separated into halves by bony tissue resembling a "spike" (spicule), each half surrounded by a dural sac.

742.53 Hydromyelia

Hydrorhachis

DEF: Dilated central spinal cord canal; characterized by increased fluid accumulation.

Normal Ventricles and Hydrocephalus

Cerebrospinal fluid in ventricles   **Normal Ventricles**

Third ventricle (III)

Choroid plexus produces Cerebrospinal fluid (CSF)

Lateral ventricles (I and II)

Foramen of Monro

Cerebral aqueduct (Sylvius)

Fourth ventricle (IV)

Foramen of Luschka

Foramen of Magendie

Hydrocephalus

Blockage of any CSF passage increases pressure in skull, which may push tissue through the Incisura tentorii or through the Foramen magnum

Enlarged ventricles

Spina Bifida

Normal spinal cord

Skin

Cerebrospinal fluid space

Spinal cord (placode) in section

Cerebrospinal fluid

Skin

Unfused posterior vertebral bone

✓4ᵗʰ / ✓5ᵗʰ Additional Digit Required   Unspecified Code   Other Specified Code   Manifestation Code   ▶◀ Revised Text   ● New Code   ▲ Revised Code Title

Congenital Anomalies

742.59–743.62

742.59 Other
Amyelia
Atelomyelia
Congenital anomaly of spinal meninges
Defective development of cauda equina
Hypoplasia of spinal cord
Myelatelia
Myelodysplasia
AHA: 2Q, '91, 14; 1Q, '89, 10

742.8 Other specified anomalies of nervous system
Agenesis of nerve
Displacement of brachial plexus
Familial dysautonomia
Jaw-winking syndrome
Marcus-Gunn syndrome
Riley-Day syndrome
EXCLUDES *neurofibromatosis (237.7)*

742.9 Unspecified anomaly of brain, spinal cord, and nervous system
Anomaly
Congenital:
  disease
  lesion
  Deformity
} of:
  brain
  nervous system
  spinal cord

✓4ᵗʰ 743 Congenital anomalies of eye

✓5ᵗʰ 743.0 Anophthalmos
DEF: Complete absence of the eyes or the presence of vestigial eyes.

743.00 Clinical anophthalmos, unspecified
Agenesis
Congenital absence
} of eye

Anophthalmos NOS

743.03 Cystic eyeball, congenital
743.06 Cryptophthalmos
DEF: Eyelids continue over eyeball, results in apparent absence of eyelids.

✓5ᵗʰ 743.1 Microphthalmos
Dysplasia
Hypoplasia
} of eye

Rudimentary eye
DEF: Abnormally small eyeballs, may be opacities of cornea and lens, scarring of choroid and retina.

743.10 Microphthalmos, unspecified
743.11 Simple microphthalmos
743.12 Microphthalmos associated with other anomalies of eye and adnexa

✓5ᵗʰ 743.2 Buphthalmos
Glaucoma: Hydrophthalmos
  congenital
  newborn
EXCLUDES *glaucoma of childhood (365.14)*
traumatic glaucoma due to birth injury (767.8)
DEF: Distended, enlarged fibrous coats of eye; due to intraocular pressure of congenital glaucoma.

743.20 Buphthalmos, unspecified
743.21 Simple buphthalmos
743.22 Buphthalmos associated with other ocular anomalies
Keratoglobus,
  congenital
Megalocornea
} associated with buphthalmos

✓5ᵗʰ 743.3 Congenital cataract and lens anomalies
EXCLUDES *infantile cataract (366.00-366.09)*
DEF: Opaque eye lens.

743.30 Congenital cataract, unspecified
743.31 Capsular and subcapsular cataract
743.32 Cortical and zonular cataract
743.33 Nuclear cataract
743.34 Total and subtotal cataract, congenital
743.35 Congenital aphakia
Congenital absence of lens
743.36 Anomalies of lens shape
Microphakia   Spherophakia
743.37 Congenital ectopic lens
743.39 Other

✓5ᵗʰ 743.4 Coloboma and other anomalies of anterior segment
DEF: Coloboma: ocular tissue defect associated with defect of ocular fetal intraocular fissure; may cause small pit on optic disk, major defects of iris, ciliary body, choroid, and retina.

743.41 Anomalies of corneal size and shape
Microcornea
EXCLUDES *that associated with buphthalmos (743.22)*
743.42 Corneal opacities, interfering with vision, congenital
743.43 Other corneal opacities, congenital
743.44 Specified anomalies of anterior chamber, chamber angle, and related structures
Anomaly: Anomaly:
  Axenfeld's   Rieger's
  Peters'
743.45 Aniridia
AHA: 3Q, '02, 20
DEF: Incompletely formed or absent iris; affects both eyes; dominant trait; also called congenital hyperplasia of iris.
743.46 Other specified anomalies of iris and ciliary body
Anisocoria, congenital   Coloboma of iris
Atresia of pupil   Corectopia
743.47 Specified anomalies of sclera
743.48 Multiple and combined anomalies of anterior segment
743.49 Other

✓5ᵗʰ 743.5 Congenital anomalies of posterior segment
743.51 Vitreous anomalies
Congenital vitreous opacity
743.52 Fundus coloboma
DEF: Absent retinal and choroidal tissue; occurs in lower fundus; a bright white ectatic zone of exposed sclera extends into and changes the optic disk.
743.53 Chorioretinal degeneration, congenital
743.54 Congenital folds and cysts of posterior segment
743.55 Congenital macular changes
743.56 Other retinal changes, congenital
AHA: 3Q, '99, 12
743.57 Specified anomalies of optic disc
Coloboma of optic disc (congenital)
743.58 Vascular anomalies
Congenital retinal aneurysm
743.59 Other

✓5ᵗʰ 743.6 Congenital anomalies of eyelids, lacrimal system, and orbit
743.61 Congenital ptosis
DEF: Drooping of eyelid.
743.62 Congenital deformities of eyelids
Ablepharon   Congenital:
Absence of eyelid   ectropion
Accessory eyelid   entropion
AHA: 1Q, '00, 22

743.63 Other specified congenital anomalies of eyelid
Absence, agenesis, of cilia

743.64 Specified congenital anomalies of lacrimal gland

743.65 Specified congenital anomalies of lacrimal passages
Absence, agenesis of:
    lacrimal apparatus
    punctum lacrimale
Accessory lacrimal canal

743.66 Specified congenital anomalies of orbit

743.69 Other
Accessory eye muscles

743.8 Other specified anomalies of eye
> EXCLUDES   *congenital nystagmus (379.51)*
> *ocular albinism (270.2)*
> *retinitis pigmentosa (362.74)*

743.9 Unspecified anomaly of eye
Congenital:
anomaly NOS } of eye [any part]
deformity NOS

✓4th **744 Congenital anomalies of ear, face, and neck**
> EXCLUDES   *anomaly of:*
> *cervical spine (754.2, 756.10-756.19)*
> *larynx (748.2-748.3)*
> *nose (748.0-748.1)*
> *parathyroid gland (759.2)*
> *thyroid gland (759.2)*
> *cleft lip (749.10-749.25)*

✓5th **744.0 Anomalies of ear causing impairment of hearing**
> EXCLUDES   *congenital deafness without mention of cause (389.0-389.9)*

744.00 Unspecified anomaly of ear with impairment of hearing

744.01 Absence of external ear
Absence of:
    auditory canal (external)
    auricle (ear) (with stenosis or atresia of auditory canal)

744.02 Other anomalies of external ear with impairment of hearing
Atresia or stricture of auditory canal (external)

744.03 Anomaly of middle ear, except ossicles
Atresia or stricture of osseous meatus (ear)

744.04 Anomalies of ear ossicles
Fusion of ear ossicles

744.05 Anomalies of inner ear
Congenital anomaly of:
    membranous labyrinth
    organ of Corti

744.09 Other
Absence of ear, congenital

744.1 Accessory auricle
Accessory tragus   Supernumerary:
Polyotia   ear
Preauricular appendage   lobule
DEF: Redundant tissue or structures of ear.

✓5th **744.2 Other specified anomalies of ear**
> EXCLUDES   *that with impairment of hearing (744.00-744.09)*

744.21 Absence of ear lobe, congenital

744.22 Macrotia
DEF: Abnormally large pinna of ear.

744.23 Microtia
DEF: Hypoplasia of pinna; associated with absent or closed auditory canal.

744.24 Specified anomalies of Eustachian tube
Absence of Eustachian tube

744.29 Other
Bat ear   Prominence of auricle
Darwin's tubercle   Ridge ear
Pointed ear
> EXCLUDES   *preauricular sinus (744.46)*

744.3 Unspecified anomaly of ear
Congenital:
anomaly NOS } of ear, not elsewhere
deformity NOS   classified

✓5th **744.4 Branchial cleft cyst or fistula; preauricular sinus**

744.41 Branchial cleft sinus or fistula
Branchial:
    sinus (external) (internal)
    vestige
DEF: Cyst due to failed closure of embryonic branchial cleft.

744.42 Branchial cleft cyst

744.43 Cervical auricle

744.46 Preauricular sinus or fistula

744.47 Preauricular cyst

744.49 Other
Fistula (of):   Fistula (of):
    auricle, congenital   cervicoaural

744.5 Webbing of neck
Pterygium colli
DEF: Thick, triangular skinfold, stretches from lateral side of neck across shoulder; associated with Turner's and Noonan's syndromes.

✓5th **744.8 Other specified anomalies of face and neck**

744.81 Macrocheilia
Hypertrophy of lip, congenital
DEF: Abnormally large lips.

744.82 Microcheilia
DEF: Abnormally small lips.

744.83 Macrostomia
DEF: Bilateral or unilateral anomaly, of mouth due to malformed maxillary and mandibular processes; results in mouth extending toward ear.

744.84 Microstomia
DEF: Abnormally small mouth.

744.89 Other
> EXCLUDES   *congenital fistula of lip (750.25)*
> *musculoskeletal anomalies (754.0-754.1, 756.0)*

744.9 Unspecified anomalies of face and neck
Congenital:
anomaly NOS } of face [any part] or
deformity NOS   neck [any part]

✓4th **745 Bulbus cordis anomalies and anomalies of cardiac septal closure**

745.0 Common truncus
Absent septum } between aorta and
Communication   pulmonary artery
(abnormal)

Aortic septal defect
Common aortopulmonary trunk
Persistent truncus arteriosus

✓4th Additional Digit Required   Unspecified Code   Other Specified Code   Manifestation Code   ▶◀ Revised Text   ● New Code   ▲ Revised Code Title
✓5th

2005 ICD•9•CM   **Volume 1 — 217**

Congenital Anomalies

745.1–746.7

Heart Defects

Atrial septal defect

Ventricular septal defect

Aortic stenosis

Patent ductus arteriosus

Pulmonary stenosis

Transposition of the great vessels

Tetralogy of Fallot

√5ᵗʰ **745.1 Transposition of great vessels**

745.10 Complete transposition of great vessels
Transposition of great vessels:
NOS
classical

745.11 Double outlet right ventricle
Dextratransposition of aorta
Incomplete transposition of great vessels
Origin of both great vessels from right ventricle
Taussig-Bing syndrome or defect

745.12 Corrected transposition of great vessels

745.19 Other

745.2 Tetralogy of Fallot
Fallot's pentalogy
Ventricular septal defect with pulmonary stenosis or atresia, dextraposition of aorta, and hypertrophy of right ventricle
  EXCLUDES   *Fallot's triad (746.09)*
DEF: Obstructed cardiac outflow causes pulmonary stenosis, interventricular septal defect and right ventricular hypertrophy.

745.3 Common ventricle
Cor triloculare biatriatum
Single ventricle

745.4 Ventricular septal defect
Eisenmenger's defect or complex
Gerbo dedefect
Interventricular septal defect
Left ventricular-right atrial communication
Roger's disease
  EXCLUDES   *common atrioventricular canal type (745.69)*
  single ventricle (745.3)

745.5 Ostium secundum type atrial septal defect
Defect: Patent or persistent:
  atrium secundum   foramen ovale
  fossa ovalis   ostium secundum
Lutembacher's syndrome
DEF: Opening in atrial septum due to failure of the septum secundum and the endocardial cushions to fuse; there is a rim of septum surrounding the defect.

√5ᵗʰ **745.6 Endocardial cushion defects**
DEF: Atrial and/or ventricular septal defects causing abnormal fusion of cushions in atrioventricular canal.

745.60 Endocardial cushion defect, unspecified type
DEF: Septal defect due to imperfect fusion of endocardial cushions.

745.61 Ostium primum defect
Persistent ostium primum
DEF: Opening in low, posterior septum primum; causes cleft in basal portion of atrial septum; associated with cleft mitral valve.

745.69 Other
Absence of atrial septum
Atrioventricular canal type ventricular septal defect
Common atrioventricular canal
Common atrium

745.7 Cor biloculare
Absence of atrial and ventricular septa
DEF: Atrial and ventricular septal defect; marked by heart with two cardiac chambers (one atrium, one ventricle), and one atrioventricular valve.

745.8 Other

745.9 Unspecified defect of septal closure
Septal defect NOS

√4ᵗʰ **746 Other congenital anomalies of heart**
  EXCLUDES   *endocardial fibroelastosis (425.3)*

√5ᵗʰ **746.0 Anomalies of pulmonary valve**
  EXCLUDES   *infundibular or subvalvular pulmonic stenosis (746.83)*
  tetralogy of Fallot (745.2)

746.00 Pulmonary valve anomaly, unspecified

746.01 Atresia, congenital
Congenital absence of pulmonary valve

746.02 Stenosis, congenital
DEF: Stenosis of opening between pulmonary artery and right ventricle; causes obstructed blood outflow from right ventricle.

746.09 Other
Congenital insufficiency of pulmonary valve
Fallot's triad or trilogy

746.1 Tricuspid atresia and stenosis, congenital
Absence of tricuspid valve

746.2 Ebstein's anomaly
DEF: Malformation of the tricuspid valve characterized by septal and posterior leaflets attaching to the wall of the right ventricle; causing the right ventricle to fuse with the atrium producing a large right atrium and a small ventricle; causes a malfunction of the right ventricle with accompanying complications such as heart failure and abnormal cardiac rhythm.

746.3 Congenital stenosis of aortic valve
Congenital aortic stenosis
  EXCLUDES   *congenital:*
  subaortic stenosis (746.81)
  supravalvular aortic stenosis (747.22)

AHA: 4Q, '88, 8

DEF: Stenosis of orifice of aortic valve; obstructs blood outflow from left ventricle.

746.4 Congenital insufficiency of aortic valve
Bicuspid aortic valve
Congenital aortic insufficiency
DEF: Impaired functioning of aortic valve due to incomplete closure; causes backflow (regurgitation) of blood from aorta to left ventricle.

746.5 Congenital mitral stenosis
Fused commissure
Parachute deformity   } of mitral valve
Supernumerary cusps
DEF: Stenosis of left atrioventricular orifice.

746.6 Congenital mitral insufficiency
DEF: Impaired functioning of mitral valve due to incomplete closure; causes backflow of blood from left ventricle to left atrium.

746.7 Hypoplastic left heart syndrome
Atresia, or marked hypoplasia, of aortic orifice or valve, with hypoplasia of ascending aorta and defective development of left ventricle (with mitral valve atresia)

☑5th **746.8 Other specified anomalies of heart**

746.81 Subaortic stenosis

DEF: Stenosis, of left ventricular outflow tract due to fibrous tissue ring or septal hypertrophy below aortic valve.

746.82 Cor triatriatum

DEF: Transverse septum divides left atrium due to failed resorption of embryonic common pulmonary vein; results in three atrial chambers.

746.83 Infundibular pulmonic stenosis

Subvalvular pulmonic stenosis

DEF: Stenosis of right ventricle outflow tract within infundibulum due to fibrous diaphragm below valve or long, narrow fibromuscular channel.

746.84 Obstructive anomalies of heart, not elsewhere classified

Uhl's disease

746.85 Coronary artery anomaly

Anomalous origin or communication of coronary artery

Arteriovenous malformation of coronary artery

Coronary artery:
absence
arising from aorta or pulmonary trunk
single

AHA: N-D, '85, 3

746.86 Congenital heart block

Complete or incomplete atrioventricular [AV] block

DEF: Impaired conduction of electrical impulses; due to maldeveloped junctional tissue.

746.87 Malposition of heart and cardiac apex

Abdominal heart   Levocardia (isolated)
Dextrocardia   Mesocardia
Ectopia cordis

EXCLUDES   dextrocardia with complete transposition of viscera (759.3)

746.89 Other

Atresia   }
Hypoplasia } of cardiac vein

Congenital:
cardiomegaly
diverticulum, left ventricle
pericardial defect

AHA: 3Q, '00, 3; 1Q, '99, 11; J-F, '85, 3

746.9 Unspecified anomaly of heart

Congenital:
anomaly of heart NOS
heart disease NOS

☑4th **747 Other congenital anomalies of circulatory system**

747.0 Patent ductus arteriosus

Patent ductus Botalli Persistent ductus arteriosus

DEF: Open lumen in ductus arteriosus causes arterial blood recirculation in lungs; inhibits blood supply to aorta; symptoms such as shortness of breath more noticeable upon activity.

☑5th **747.1 Coarctation of aorta**

DEF: Localized deformity of aortic media seen as a severe constriction of the vessel lumen; major symptom is high blood pressure in the arms and low pressure in the legs; a CVA, rupture of the aorta, bacterial endocarditis or congestive heart failure can follow if left untreated.

747.10 Coarctation of aorta (preductal) (postductal)

Hypoplasia of aortic arch

AHA: 1Q, '99, 11; 4Q, '88, 8

747.11 Interruption of aortic arch

☑5th **747.2 Other anomalies of aorta**

747.20 Anomaly of aorta, unspecified

747.21 Anomalies of aortic arch

Anomalous origin, right subclavian artery
Dextraposition of aorta
Double aortic arch
Kommerell's diverticulum
Overriding aorta
Persistent:
convolutions, aortic arch
right aortic arch
Vascular ring

EXCLUDES   hypoplasia of aortic arch (747.10)

AHA: 1Q, '03, 15

747.22 Atresia and stenosis of aorta

Absence   }
Aplasia   }
Hypoplasia } of aorta
Stricture }

Supra (valvular)-aortic stenosis

EXCLUDES   congenital aortic (valvular) stenosis or stricture, so stated (746.3)
hypoplasia of aorta in hypoplastic left heart syndrome (746.7)

747.29 Other

Aneurysm of sinus of Valsalva
Congenital:
aneurysm }
dilation   } of aorta

747.3 Anomalies of pulmonary artery

Agenesis   }
Anomaly   }
Atresia   }
Coarctation } of pulmonary artery
Hypoplasia }
Stenosis   }

Pulmonary arteriovenous aneurysm

AHA: 1Q, '94, 15; 4Q, '88, 8

☑5th **747.4 Anomalies of great veins**

747.40 Anomaly of great veins, unspecified

Anomaly NOS of:
pulmonary veins
vena cava

747.41 Total anomalous pulmonary venous connection

Total anomalous pulmonary venous return [TAPVR]:
subdiaphragmatic
supradiaphragmatic

747.42 Partial anomalous pulmonary venous connection

Partial anomalous pulmonary venous return

747.49 Other anomalies of great veins

Absence   }
Congenital } of vena cava (inferior)
stenosis   } (superior)

Persistent:
left posterior cardinal vein
left superior vena cava
Scimitar syndrome
Transposition of pulmonary veins NOS

747.5 Absence or hypoplasia of umbilical artery

Single umbilical artery

☑4th ☑5th Additional Digit Required   Unspecified Code   Other Specified Code   Manifestation Code   ►◄ Revised Text   ● New Code   ▲ Revised Code Title

2005 ICD•9•CM   Volume 1 — 219

Congenital Anomalies

747.6–748.69

✓5ᵗʰ 747.6 Other anomalies of peripheral vascular system

Absence
Anomaly   } of artery or vein, not elsewhere
Atresia   classified

Arteriovenous aneurysm   Congenital:
   (peripheral)   phlebectasia
Arteriovenous malformation   stricture, artery
   of the peripheral   varix
   vascular system   Multiple renal arteries
Congenital:
   aneurysm (peripheral)

   EXCLUDES   *anomalies of:*
                  cerebral vessels (747.81)
                  pulmonary artery (747.3)
                  congenital retinal aneurysm (743.58)
                  hemangioma (228.00-228.09)
                  lymphangioma (228.1)

747.60 Anomaly of the peripheral vascular system, unspecified site

747.61 Gastrointestinal vessel anomaly
     AHA: 3Q '96, 10

747.62 Renal vessel anomaly

747.63 Upper limb vessel anomaly

747.64 Lower limb vessel anomaly

747.69 Anomalies of other specified sites of peripheral vascular system

✓5ᵗʰ 747.8 Other specified anomalies of circulatory system

747.81 Anomalies of cerebrovascular system
Arteriovenous malformation of brain
Cerebral arteriovenous aneurysm, congenital
Congenital anomalies of cerebral vessels

    EXCLUDES   *ruptured cerebral (arterio-venous) aneurysm (430)*

747.82 Spinal vessel anomaly
Arteriovenous malformation of spinal vessel
    AHA: 3Q, '95, 5

747.83 Persistent fetal circulation   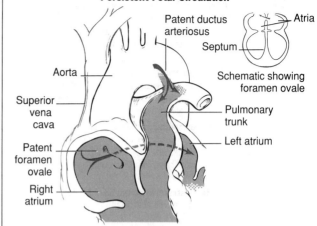 N
Persistent pulmonary hypertension
Primary pulmonary hypertension of newborn
    AHA: 4Q, '02, 62

    DEF: A return to fetal-type circulation due to constriction of pulmonary arterioles and opening of the ductus arteriosus and foramen ovale, right-to-left shunting occurs, oxygenation of the blood does not occur, and the lungs remain constricted after birth; PFC is seen in term or post-term infants causes include asphyxia, meconium aspiration syndrome, acidosis, sepsis, and developmental immaturity.

747.89 Other
Aneurysm, congenital, specified site not elsewhere classified

    EXCLUDES   *congenital aneurysm:*
               coronary (746.85)
               peripheral (747.6)
               pulmonary (747.3)
               retinal (743.58)

    AHA: 4Q, '02, 63

747.9 Unspecified anomaly of circulatory system

✓4ᵗʰ 748 Congenital anomalies of respiratory system
    EXCLUDES   *congenital defect of diaphragm (756.6)*

748.0 Choanal atresia
Atresia   } of nares (anterior)
Congenital stenosis }   (posterior)

    DEF: Occluded posterior nares (choana), bony or membranous due to failure of embryonic bucconasal membrane to rupture.

Persistent Fetal Circulation

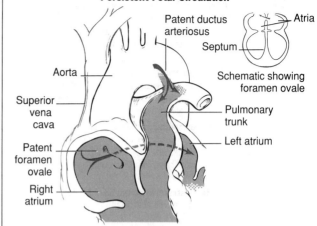

Schematic showing foramen ovale

748.1 Other anomalies of nose
Absent nose   Congenital:
Accessory nose   notching of tip of nose
Cleft nose   perforation of wall of
Congenital: nasal sinus
   deformity of nose   Deformity of wall of nasal
                    sinus

    EXCLUDES   *congenital deviation of nasal septum (754.0)*

748.2 Web of larynx
Web of larynx: Web of larynx:
   NOS   subglottic
   glottic

    DEF: Malformed larynx; marked by thin, translucent, or thick, fibrotic spread between vocal folds; affects speech.

748.3 Other anomalies of larynx, trachea, and bronchus
Absence or agenesis of: Congenital:
   bronchus   dilation, trachea
   larynx   stenosis:
   trachea   larynx
Anomaly(of):   trachea
   cricoid cartilage   tracheocele
   epiglottis   Diverticulum:
   thyroid cartilage   bronchus
   tracheal cartilage   trachea
Atresia (of):   Fissure of epiglottis
   epiglottis   Laryngocele
   glottis   Posterior cleft of cricoid
   larynx   cartilage (congenital)
   trachea   Rudimentary tracheal
Cleft thyroid, cartilage,   bronchus
   congenital   Stridor, laryngeal,
                    congenital

    AHA: 1Q, '99, 14

748.4 Congenital cystic lung
Disease, lung: Honeycomb lung, congenital
   cystic, congenital
   polycystic, congenital

    EXCLUDES   *acquired or unspecified cystic lung (518.89)*

    DEF: Enlarged air spaces of lung parenchyma.

748.5 Agenesis, hypoplasia, and dysplasia of lung
Absence of lung (fissures) (lobe)
Aplasia of lung
Hypoplasia of lung (lobe)
Sequestration of lung

✓5ᵗʰ 748.6 Other anomalies of lung

748.60 Anomaly of lung, unspecified

748.61 Congenital bronchiectasis

748.69 Other
Accessory lung (lobe)
Azygos lobe (fissure), lung

N Newborn Age: 0   P Pediatric Age: 0-17   M Maternity Age: 12-55   A Adult Age: 15-124   MSP Medicare Secondary Payer

Congenital Anomalies

Cleft Lip and Palate

Unilateral cleft lip | No cleft palate

Cleft lip with cleft alveolar ridge | No cleft palate

Unilateral cleft lip and cleft palate — Alveolar ridge — Cleft palate

Prolabium

Bilateral cleft lip and cleft palate

Isolated cleft palate

748.8 **Other specified anomalies of respiratory system**

Abnormal communication between pericardial and pleural sacs
Anomaly, pleural folds
Atresia of nasopharynx
Congenital cyst of mediastinum

748.9 **Unspecified anomaly of respiratory system**

Anomaly of respiratory system NOS

√4ᵗʰ **749 Cleft palate and cleft lip**

√5ᵗʰ **749.0** **Cleft palate**

749.00 **Cleft palate, unspecified**

749.01 **Unilateral, complete**

749.02 **Unilateral, incomplete**

Cleft uvula

749.03 **Bilateral, complete**

749.04 **Bilateral, incomplete**

√5ᵗʰ **749.1** **Cleft lip**

Cheiloschisis   Harelip
Congenital fissure of lip   Labium leporinum

749.10 **Cleft lip, unspecified**

749.11 **Unilateral, complete**

749.12 **Unilateral, incomplete**

749.13 **Bilateral, complete**

749.14 **Bilateral, incomplete**

√5ᵗʰ **749.2** **Cleft palate with cleft lip**

Cheilopalatoschisis

749.20 **Cleft palate with cleft lip, unspecified**

749.21 **Unilateral, complete**

749.22 **Unilateral, incomplete**

749.23 **Bilateral, complete**

AHA: 1Q, '96, 14

749.24 **Bilateral, incomplete**

749.25 **Other combinations**

√4ᵗʰ **750 Other congenital anomalies of upper alimentary tract**

EXCLUDES *dentofacial anomalies (524.0-524.9)*

750.0 **Tongue tie**

Ankyloglossia

DEF: Restricted tongue movement due to lingual frenum extending toward tip of tongue. Tongue may be fused to mouth floor affecting speech.

√5ᵗʰ **750.1** **Other anomalies of tongue**

750.10 **Anomaly of tongue, unspecified**

750.11 **Aglossia**

DEF: Absence of tongue.

750.12 **Congenital adhesions of tongue**

750.13 **Fissure of tongue**

Bifid tongue   Double tongue

750.15 **Macroglossia**

Congenital hypertrophy of tongue

750.16 **Microglossia**

Hypoplasia of tongue

750.19 **Other**

√5ᵗʰ **750.2** **Other specified anomalies of mouth and pharynx**

750.21 **Absence of salivary gland**

750.22 **Accessory salivary gland**

750.23 **Atresia, salivary duct**

Imperforate salivary duct

750.24 **Congenital fistula of salivary gland**

750.25 **Congenital fistula of lip**

Congenital (mucus) lip pits

750.26 **Other specified anomalies of mouth**

Absence of uvula

750.27 **Diverticulum of pharynx**

Pharyngeal pouch

750.29 **Other specified anomalies of pharynx**

Imperforate pharynx

750.3 **Tracheoesophageal fistula, esophageal atresia and stenosis**

Absent esophagus
Atresia of esophagus
Congenital:
  esophageal ring
  stenosis of esophagus
  stricture of esophagus

Congenital fistula:
  esophagobronchial
  esophagotracheal
Imperforate esophagus
Webbed esophagus

750.4 **Other specified anomalies of esophagus**

Dilatation, congenital
Displacement, congenital
Diverticulum } (of) esophagus
Duplication
Giant

Esophageal pouch

EXCLUDES *congenital hiatus hernia (750.6)*

AHA: J-F, '85, 3

750.5 **Congenital hypertrophic pyloric stenosis**

Congenital or infantile:
  constriction
  hypertrophy
  spasm } of pylorus
  stenosis
  stricture

DEF: Obstructed pylorus due to overgrowth of pyloric muscle.

750.6 **Congenital hiatus hernia**

Displacement of cardia through esophageal hiatus

EXCLUDES *congenital diaphragmatic hernia (756.6)*

750.7 **Other specified anomalies of stomach**

Congenital:
  cardiospasm
  hourglass stomach
Displacement of stomach
Diverticulum of stomach, congenital
Duplication of stomach
Megalogastria
Microgastria
Transposition of stomach

750.8 **Other specified anomalies of upper alimentary tract**

748.8–750.8

√4ᵗʰ
√5ᵗʰ Additional Digit Required   Unspecified Code   Other Specified Code   Manifestation Code   ▶◀ Revised Text   ● New Code   ▲ Revised Code Title

Congenital Anomalies

750.9–751.8

750.9   Unspecified anomaly of upper alimentary tract

Congenital:

anomaly NOS
deformity NOS } of upper alimentary tract [any part, except tongue]

✓4ᵗʰ **751   Other congenital anomalies of digestive system**

751.0   Meckel's diverticulum

Meckel's diverticulum (displaced) (hypertrophic)
Persistent:

omphalomesenteric duct
vitelline duct

AHA: ▶1Q, '04, 10◀

DEF: Malformed sacs or appendages of ileum of small intestine; can cause strangulation, volvulus and intussusception.

751.1   Atresia and stenosis of small intestine [P]

Atresia of: Atresia of:
duodenum   intestine NOS
ileum
Congenital:

absence
obstruction } of small intestine or
stenosis   intestine NOS
stricture

Imperforate jejunum

751.2   Atresia and stenosis of large intestine, rectum, and anal canal [P]

Absence:

anus (congenital)
appendix, congenital
large intestine, congenital
rectum

Atresia of:

anus
colon
rectum

Congenital or infantile:

obstruction of large intestine
occlusion of anus
stricture of anus

Imperforate:

anus
rectum

Stricture of rectum, congenital

AHA: 2Q, '98, 16

751.3   Hirschsprung's disease and other congenital functional disorders of colon

Aganglionosis
Congenital dilation of colon
Congenital megacolon
Macrocolon

DEF: Hirschsprung's disease: enlarged or dilated colon (megacolon), with absence of ganglion cells in the narrowed wall distally; causes inability to defecate.

751.4   Anomalies of intestinal fixation

Congenital adhesions: Rotation of cecum or colon:
omental, anomalous   failure of
peritoneal   incomplete
Jackson's membrane   insufficient
Malrotation of colon   Universal mesentery

751.5   Other anomalies of intestine

Congenital diverticulum, colon
Dolichocolon
Duplication of:

anus
appendix
cecum
intestine

Ectopic anus
Megaloappendix
Megaloduodenum
Microcolon
Persistent cloaca
Transposition of:

appendix
colon
intestine

AHA: 3Q, '02, 11; 3Q, '01, 8

✓5ᵗʰ **751.6   Anomalies of gallbladder, bile ducts, and liver**

751.60   Unspecified anomaly of gallbladder, bile ducts, and liver

751.61   Biliary atresia [P]

Congenital:

absence
hypoplasia } of bile duct (common)
obstruction   or passage
stricture

AHA: S-O, '87, 8

751.62   Congenital cystic disease of liver

Congenital polycystic disease of liver
Fibrocystic disease of liver

751.69   Other anomalies of gallbladder, bile ducts, and liver

Absence of:

gallbladder, congenital
liver (lobe)

Accessory:

hepatic ducts
liver

Congenital:

choledochal cyst
hepatomegaly

Duplication of:

biliary duct
cystic duct
gallbladder
liver

Floating:

gallbladder
liver

Intrahepatic gallbladder

AHA: S-O, '87, 8

751.7   Anomalies of pancreas

Absence
Accessory
Agenesis } (of) pancreas
Annular
Hypoplasia

Ectopic pancreatic tissue
Pancreatic heterotopia

EXCLUDES   diabetes mellitus:
congenital (250.0-250.9)
neonatal (775.1)
fibrocystic disease of pancreas (277.00-277.09)

751.8   Other specified anomalies of digestive system

Absence (complete) (partial) of alimentary tract NOS

Duplication
Malposition, congenital } of digestive organs NOS

EXCLUDES   congenital diaphragmatic hernia (756.6)
congenital hiatus hernia (750.6)

[N] Newborn Age: 0   [P] Pediatric Age: 0-17   [M] Maternity Age: 12-55   [A] Adult Age: 15-124   [MSP] Medicare Secondary Payer

751.9   **Unspecified anomaly of digestive system**

Congenital:

anomaly NOS

deformity NOS } of digestive system NOS

✓4th **752 Congenital anomalies of genital organs**

EXCLUDES   *syndromes associated with anomalies in the number and form of chromosomes (758.0-758.9)*

testicular feminization syndrome (257.8)

752.0   **Anomalies of ovaries**   ♀

Absence, congenital

Accessory

Ectopic } (of) ovary

Streak

✓5th **752.1**   **Anomalies of fallopian tubes and broad ligaments**

752.10   **Unspecified anomaly of fallopian tubes and broad ligaments**   ♀

752.11   **Embryonic cyst of fallopian tubes and broad ligaments**   ♀

Cyst: Cyst:

epoophoron   Gartner's duct

fimbrial   parovarian

AHA: S-O, '85, 13

752.19   **Other**   ♀

Absence

Accessory } (of) fallopian tube or broad ligament

Atresia

752.2   **Doubling of uterus**   ♀

Didelphic uterus

Doubling of uterus [any degree] (associated with doubling of cervix and vagina)

752.3   **Other anomalies of uterus**   ♀

Absence, congenital

Agenesis

Aplasia } (of) uterus

Bicornuate

Uterus unicornis

Uterus with only one functioning horn

✓5th **752.4**   **Anomalies of cervix, vagina, and external female genitalia**

752.40   **Unspecified anomaly of cervix, vagina, and external female genitalia**   ♀

752.41   **Embryonic cyst of cervix, vagina, and external female genitalia**   ♀

Cyst of:

canal of Nuck, congenital

vagina, embryonal

vulva, congenital

DEF: Embryonic fluid-filled cysts, of cervix, vagina or external female genitalia.

752.42   **Imperforate hymen**   ♀

DEF: Complete closure of membranous fold around external opening of vagina.

752.49   **Other anomalies of cervix, vagina, and external female genitalia**   ♀

Absence } of cervix, clitoris,

Agenesis   vagina, or vulva

Congenital stenosis or stricture of:

cervical canal

vagina

EXCLUDES   *double vagina associated with total duplication (752.2)*

✓5th **752.5**   **Undescended and retractile testicle**

AHA: 4Q, '96, 33

752.51   **Undescended testis**   ♂

Cryptorchism

Ectopic testis

752.52   **Retractile testis**   ♂

Hypospadias and Epispadias

Labels (left, ventral view): Glans penis; Glandular hypospadias; Penile hypospadias; Scrotal hypospadias; Scrotum; Penile raphe; Scrotal raphe

Labels (right, dorsal view): Normal external urethral orifice; Glans penis; Foreskin (retracted); Epispadias

Hypospadias (ventral view)   **Epispadias (dorsal view)**

✓5th **752.6**   **Hypospadias and epispadias and other penile anomalies**

AHA: 4Q, '96, 34, 35

752.61   **Hypospadias**   ♂

AHA: 3Q, '97, 6

DEF: Abnormal opening of urethra on the ventral surface of the penis or perineum; also a rare defect of vagina.

AHA: ►4Q, '03, 67-68◄

752.62   **Epispadias**   ♂

Anaspadias

DEF: Epispadias: urethra opening on dorsal surface of penis; in females appears as a slit in the upper wall of urethra.

752.63   **Congenital chordee**   ♂

DEF: Ventral bowing of penis due to fibrous band along corpus spongiosum; occurs with hypospadias.

752.64   **Micropenis**   ♂

752.65   **Hidden penis**   ♂

752.69   **Other penile anomalies**   ♂

752.7   **Indeterminate sex and pseudohermaphroditism**

Gynandrism   Pseudohermaphroditism

Hermaphroditism   (male) (female)

Ovotestis   Pure gonadal dysgenesis

EXCLUDES   *pseudohermaphroditism:*

female, with adrenocortical disorder (255.2)

male, with gonadal disorder (257.8)

with specified chromosomal anomaly (758.0-758.9)

testicular feminization syndrome (257.8)

DEF: Pseudohermaphroditism: presence of gonads of one sex and external genitalia of other sex.

✓5th **752.8**   **Other specified anomalies of genital organs**

EXCLUDES   *congenital hydrocele (778.6)*

penile anomalies (752.61-752.69)

phimosis or paraphimosis (605)

752.81   **Scrotal transposition**   ♂

AHA: ►4Q, '03, 67-68◄

752.89   **Other specified anomalies of genital organs**

Absence of: Fusion of testes

prostate   Hypoplasia of testis

spermatic cord   Monorchism

vas deferens   Polyorchism

Anorchism

Aplasia (congenital) of:

prostate

round ligament

testicle

Atresia of:

ejaculatory duct

vas deferens

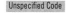 Additional Digit Required   Unspecified Code   Other Specified Code   Manifestation Code   ►◄ Revised Text   ● New Code   ▲ Revised Code Title

2005 ICD•9•CM   **February 2004 • Volume 1 — 223**

Congenital Anomalies

752.9–754.41

752.9 Unspecified anomaly of genital organs
Congenital:
anomaly NOS } of genital organ, not
deformity NOS }   elsewhere classified

√4th **753 Congenital anomalies of urinary system**

753.0 Renal agenesis and dysgenesis
Atrophy of kidney:
congenital
infantile
Congenital absence of kidney(s)
Hypoplasia of kidney(s)

√5th **753.1 Cystic kidney disease**
> EXCLUDES   *acquired cyst of kidney (593.2)*

AHA: 4Q, '90, 3

753.10 Cystic kidney disease, unspecified

753.11 Congenital single renal cyst

753.12 Polycystic kidney, unspecified type

753.13 Polycystic kidney, autosomal dominant
> DEF: Slow progressive disease characterized by bilateral cysts causing increased kidney size and impaired function.

753.14 Polycystic kidney, autosomal recessive
> DEF: Rare disease characterized by multiple cysts involving kidneys and liver, producing renal and hepatic failure in childhood or adolescence.

753.15 Renal dysplasia

753.16 Medullary cystic kidney
Nephronopthisis
> DEF: Diffuse kidney disease results in uremia onset prior to age 20.

753.17 Medullary sponge kidney
> DEF: Dilated collecting tubules; usually asymptomatic but calcinosis in tubules may cause renal insufficiency.

753.19 Other specified cystic kidney disease
Multicystic kidney

√5th **753.2 Obstructive defects of renal pelvis and ureter**
AHA: 4Q, '96, 35

753.20 Unspecified obstructive defect of renal pelvis and ureter

753.21 Congenital obstruction of ureteropelvic junction
> DEF: Stricture at junction of ureter and renal pelvis.

753.22 Congenital obstruction of ureterovesical junction
Adynamic ureter
Congenital hydroureter
> DEF: Stricture at junction of ureter and bladder.

753.23 Congenital ureterocele

753.29 Other

753.3 Other specified anomalies of kidney
Accessory kidney   Fusion of kidneys
Congenital: Giant kidney
   calculus of kidney   Horseshoe kidney
   displaced kidney   Hyperplasia of kidney
Discoid kidney   Lobulation of kidney
Double kidney with   Malrotation of kidney
   double pelvis   Trifid kidney (pelvis)
Ectopic kidney

753.4 Other specified anomalies of ureter
Absent ureter   Double ureter
Accessory ureter   Ectopic ureter
Deviation of ureter   Implantation, anomalous
Displaced ureteric orifice   of ureter

753.5 Exstrophy of urinary bladder
Ectopia vesicae
Extroversion of bladder
> DEF: Absence of lower abdominal and anterior bladder walls with posterior bladder wall protrusion.

753.6 Atresia and stenosis of urethra and bladder neck
Congenital obstruction:
bladder neck
urethra
Congenital stricture of:
urethra (valvular)
urinary meatus
vesicourethral orifice
Imperforate urinary meatus
Impervious urethra
Urethral valve formation

753.7 Anomalies of urachus
Cyst
Fistula } (of) urachussinus
Patent

Persistent umbilical sinus

753.8 Other specified anomalies of bladder and urethra
Absence, congenital of: Congenital urethrorectal
   bladder   fistula
   urethra   Congenital prolapse of:
Accessory: bladder (mucosa)
   bladder   urethra
   urethra   Double:
Congenital: urethra
   diverticulum of bladder   urinary meatus
   hernia of bladder

753.9 Unspecified anomaly of urinary system
Congenital:
anomaly NOS } of urinary system [any part,
deformity NOS }   except urachus]

√4th **754 Certain congenital musculoskeletal deformities**
> INCLUDES   nonteratogenic deformities which are considered to be due to intrauterine malposition and pressure

754.0 Of skull, face, and jaw
Asymmetry of face   Dolichocephaly
Compression facies   Plagiocephaly
Depressions in skull   Potter's facies
Deviation of nasal   Squashed or bent nose,
   septum, congenital   congenital
> EXCLUDES   *dentofacial anomalies (524.0-524.9)*
> *syphilitic saddle nose (090.5)*

754.1 Of sternocleidomastoid muscle
Congenital sternomastoid torticollis
Congenital wryneck
Contracture of sternocleidomastoid (muscle)
Sternomastoid tumor

754.2 Of spine
Congenital postural:
lordosis
scoliosis

√5th **754.3 Congenital dislocation of hip**

754.30 Congenital dislocation of hip, unilateral
Congenital dislocation of hip NOS

754.31 Congenital dislocation of hip, bilateral

754.32 Congenital subluxation of hip, unilateral
Congenital flexion deformity, hip or thigh
Predislocation status of hip at birth
Preluxation of hip, congenital

754.33 Congenital subluxation of hip, bilateral

754.35 Congenital dislocation of one hip with subluxation of other hip

√5th **754.4 Congenital genu recurvatum and bowing of long bones of leg**

754.40 Genu recurvatum
> DEF: Backward curving of knee joint.

754.41 Congenital dislocation of knee (with genu recurvatum)
> DEF: Elevated, outward rotation of heel; also called clubfoot.

N Newborn Age: 0   P Pediatric Age: 0-17   M Maternity Age: 12-55   A Adult Age: 15-124   MSP Medicare Secondary Payer

Congenital Anomalies

754.42–755.29

754.42 Congenital bowing of femur

754.43 Congenital bowing of tibia and fibula

754.44 Congenital bowing of unspecified long bones of leg

√5ᵗʰ **754.5 Varus deformities of feet**

> EXCLUDES   acquired (736.71, 736.75, 736.79)

754.50 Talipes varus
> Congenital varus deformity of foot, unspecified
> Pes varus
> DEF: Inverted foot marked by outer sole resting on ground.

754.51 Talipes equinovarus
> Equinovarus (congenital)

754.52 Metatarsus primus varus
> DEF: Malformed first metatarsal bone, with bone angled toward body.

754.53 Metatarsus varus

754.59 Other
> Talipes calcaneovarus

√5ᵗʰ **754.6 Valgus deformities of feet**

> EXCLUDES   valgus deformity of foot (acquired) (736.79)

754.60 Talipes valgus
> Congenital valgus deformity of foot, unspecified

754.61 Congenital pes planus
> Congenital rocker bottom flat foot
> Flat foot, congenital
> > EXCLUDES   pes planus (acquired) (734)

754.62 Talipes calcaneovalgus

754.69 Other
> Talipes: Talipes:
>   equinovalgus   planovalgus

√5ᵗʰ **754.7 Other deformities of feet**

> EXCLUDES   acquired (736.70-736.79)

754.70 Talipes, unspecified
> Congenital deformity of foot NOS

754.71 Talipes cavus
> Cavus foot (congenital)

754.79 Other
> Asymmetric talipes   Talipes:
> Talipes: equinus
>   calcaneus

√5ᵗʰ **754.8 Other specified nonteratogenic anomalies**

754.81 Pectus excavatum
> Congenital funnel chest

754.82 Pectus carinatum
> Congenital pigeon chest [breast]

754.89 Other
> Club hand (congenital)
> Congenital:
>   deformity of chest wall
>   dislocation of elbow
> Generalized flexion contractures of lower limb joints, congenital
> Spade-like hand (congenital)

√4ᵗʰ **755 Other congenital anomalies of limbs**

> EXCLUDES   those deformities classifiable to 754.0-754.8

√5ᵗʰ **755.0 Polydactyly**

755.00 Polydactyly, unspecified digits
> Supernumerary digits

755.01 Of fingers
> Accessory fingers

755.02 Of toes
> Accessory toes

√5ᵗʰ **755.1 Syndactyly**
> Symphalangy   Webbing of digits

755.10 Of multiple and unspecified sites

755.11 Of fingers without fusion of bone

755.12 Of fingers with fusion of bone

755.13 Of toes without fusion of bone

755.14 Of toes with fusion of bone

√5ᵗʰ **755.2 Reduction deformities of upper limb**

755.20 Unspecified reduction deformity of upper limb
> Ectromelia NOS ⎫
> Hemimelia NOS ⎬ of upper limb
>   ⎭
> Shortening of arm, congenital

755.21 Transverse deficiency of upper limb
> Amelia of upper limb
> Congenital absence of:
>   fingers, all (complete or partial)
>   forearm, including hand and fingers
>   upper limb, complete
> Congenital amputation of upper limb
> Transverse hemimelia of upper limb

755.22 Longitudinal deficiency of upper limb, not elsewhere classified
> Phocomelia NOS of upper limb
> Rudimentary arm

755.23 Longitudinal deficiency, combined, involving humerus, radius, and ulna (complete or incomplete)
> Congenital absence of arm and forearm (complete or incomplete) with or without metacarpal deficiency and/or phalangeal deficiency, incomplete
> Phocomelia, complete, of upper limb

755.24 Longitudinal deficiency, humeral, complete or partial (with or without distal deficiencies, incomplete)
> Congenital absence of humerus (with or without absence of some [but not all] distal elements)
> Proximal phocomelia of upper limb

755.25 Longitudinal deficiency, radioulnar, complete or partial (with or without distal deficiencies, incomplete)
> Congenital absence of radius and ulna (with or without absence of some [but not all] distal elements)
> Distal phocomelia of upper limb

755.26 Longitudinal deficiency, radial, complete or partial (with or without distal deficiencies, incomplete)
> Agenesis of radius
> Congenital absence of radius (with or without absence of some [but not all] distal elements)

755.27 Longitudinal deficiency, ulnar, complete or partial (with or without distal deficiencies, incomplete)
> Agenesis of ulna
> Congenital absence of ulna (with or without absence of some [but not all] distal elements)

755.28 Longitudinal deficiency, carpals or metacarpals, complete or partial (with or without incomplete phalangeal deficiency)

755.29 Longitudinal deficiency, phalanges, complete or partial
> Absence of finger, congenital
> Aphalangia of upper limb, terminal, complete or partial
> > EXCLUDES   terminal deficiency of all five digits (755.21)
> > transverse deficiency of phalanges (755.21)

√4ᵗʰ √5ᵗʰ Additional Digit Required   Unspecified Code   Other Specified Code   Manifestation Code   ▶◀ Revised Text   ● New Code   ▲ Revised Code Title

Congenital Anomalies

755.3–755.67

√5ᵗʰ **755.3 Reduction deformities of lower limb**

755.30 Unspecified reduction deformity of lower limb

Ectromelia NOS }
Hemimelia NOS } of lower limb

Shortening of leg, congenital

755.31 Transverse deficiency of lower limb
Amelia of lower limb
Congenital absence of:
  foot
  leg, including foot and toes
  lower limb, complete
  toes, all, complete
Transverse hemimelia of lower limb

755.32 Longitudinal deficiency of lower limb, not elsewhere classified
Phocomelia NOS of lower limb

755.33 Longitudinal deficiency, combined, involving femur, tibia, and fibula (complete or incomplete)
Congenital absence of thigh and (lower) leg (complete or incomplete) with or without metacarpal deficiency and/or phalangeal deficiency, incomplete
Phocomelia, complete, of lower limb

755.34 Longitudinal deficiency, femoral, complete or partial (with or without distal deficiencies, incomplete)
Congenital absence of femur (with or without absence of some [but not all] distal elements)
Proximal phocomelia of lower limb

755.35 Longitudinal deficiency, tibiofibular, complete or partial (with or without distal deficiencies, incomplete)
Congenital absence of tibia and fibula (with or without absence of some [but not all] distal elements)
Distal phocomelia of lower limb

755.36 Longitudinal deficiency, tibia, complete or partial (with or without distal deficiencies, incomplete)
Agenesis of tibia
Congenital absence of tibia (with or without absence of some [but not all] distal elements)

755.37 Longitudinal deficiency, fibular, complete or partial (with or without distal deficiencies, incomplete)
Agenesis of fibula
Congenital absence of fibula (with or without absence of some [but not all] distal elements)

755.38 Longitudinal deficiency, tarsals or metatarsals, complete or partial (with or without incomplete phalangeal deficiency)

755.39 Longitudinal deficiency, phalanges, complete or partial
Absence of toe, congenital
Aphalangia of lower limb, terminal, complete or partial
EXCLUDES   terminal deficiency of all five digits (755.31)
            transverse deficiency of phalanges (755.31)

755.4 Reduction deformities, unspecified limb
Absence, congenital (complete or partial) of limb NOS
Amelia }
Ectromelia }
Hemimelia } of unspecified limb
Phocomelia }

√5ᵗʰ **755.5 Other anomalies of upper limb, including shoulder girdle**

755.50 Unspecified anomaly of upper limb

755.51 Congenital deformity of clavicle

755.52 Congenital elevation of scapula
Sprengel's deformity

755.53 Radioulnar synostosis

755.54 Madelung's deformity
DEF: Distal ulnar overgrowth or radial shortening; also called carpus curvus.

755.55 Acrocephalosyndactyly
Apert's syndrome
DEF: Premature cranial suture fusion (craniostenosis); marked by cone-shaped or pointed (acrocephaly) head and webbing of the fingers (syndactyly); it is very similar to craniofacial dysostosis.

755.56 Accessory carpal bones

755.57 Macrodactylia (fingers)
DEF: Abnormally large fingers, toes.

755.58 Cleft hand, congenital
Lobster-claw hand
DEF: Extended separation between fingers into metacarpus; also may refer to large fingers and absent middle fingers of hand.

755.59 Other
Cleidocranial dysostosis
Cubitus:
  valgus, congenital
  varus, congenital
EXCLUDES   club hand (congenital) (754.89)
            congenital dislocation of elbow (754.89)

√5ᵗʰ **755.6 Other anomalies of lower limb, including pelvic girdle**

755.60 Unspecified anomaly of lower limb

755.61 Coxa valga, congenital
DEF: Abnormally wide angle between the neck and shaft of the femur.

755.62 Coxa vara, congenital
DEF: Diminished angle between neck and shaft of femur.

755.63 Other congenital deformity of hip (joint)
Congenital anteversion of femur (neck)
EXCLUDES   congenital dislocation of hip (754.30-754.35)
AHA: 1Q, '94, 15; S-O, '84, 15

755.64 Congenital deformity of knee (joint)
Congenital:
  absence of patella
  genu valgum [knock-knee]
  genu varum [bowleg]
Rudimentary patella

755.65 Macrodactylia of toes
DEF: Abnormally large toes.

755.66 Other anomalies of toes
Congenital: Congenital:
  hallux valgus   hammer toe
  hallux varus

755.67 Anomalies of foot, not elsewhere classified
Astragaloscaphoid synostosis
Calcaneonavicular bar
Coalition of calcaneus
Talonavicular synostosis
Tarsal coalitions

N Newborn Age: 0   P Pediatric Age: 0-17   M Maternity Age: 12-55   A Adult Age: 15-124   MSP Medicare Secondary Payer

755.69 Other
Congenital:
  angulation of tibia
  deformity (of):
    ankle (joint)
    sacroiliac (joint)
  fusion of sacroiliac joint

755.8 Other specified anomalies of unspecified limb

755.9 Unspecified anomaly of unspecified limb
Congenital:
  anomaly NOS ⎫
  deformity NOS ⎭ of unspecified limb

> **EXCLUDES** reduction deformity of unspecified limb (755.4)

√4ᵗʰ 756 Other congenital musculoskeletal anomalies

> **EXCLUDES** those deformities classifiable to 754.0-754.8

756.0 Anomalies of skull and face bones

Absence of skull bones　Imperfect fusion of skull
Acrocephaly　　　　　Oxycephaly
Congenital deformity　Platybasia
  of forehead　　　　Premature closure of
Craniosynostosis　　　　cranial sutures
Crouzon's disease　　　Tower skull
Hypertelorism　　　　Trigonocephaly

> **EXCLUDES** acrocephalosyndactyly [Apert's syndrome] (755.55)
> dentofacial anomalies (524.0-524.9)
> skull defects associated with brain anomalies, such as:
>   anencephalus (740.0)
>   encephalocele (742.0)
>   hydrocephalus (742.3)
>   microcephalus (742.1)

AHA: 3Q, '98, 9; 3Q, '96, 15

√5ᵗʰ 756.1 Anomalies of spine

756.10 Anomaly of spine, unspecified

756.11 Spondylolysis, lumbosacral region
Prespondylolisthesis (lumbosacral)
DEF: Bilateral or unilateral defect through the pars interarticularis of a vertebra causes spondylolisthesis.

756.12 Spondylolisthesis
DEF: Downward slipping of lumbar vertebra over next vertebra; usually related to pelvic deformity.

756.13 Absence of vertebra, congenital

756.14 Hemivertebra
DEF: Incomplete development of one side of a vertebra.

756.15 Fusion of spine [vertebra], congenital

756.16 Klippel-Feil syndrome
DEF: Short, wide neck; limits range of motion due to abnormal number of cervical vertebra or fused hemivertebrae.

756.17 Spina bifida occulta
> **EXCLUDES** spina bifida (aperta) (741.0-741.9)

DEF: Spina bifida marked by a bony spinal canal defect without a protrusion of the cord or meninges; it is diagnosed by radiography and has no symptoms.

756.19 Other
Platyspondylia
Supernumerary vertebra

756.2 Cervical rib
Supernumerary rib in the cervical region
DEF: Costa cervicalis: extra rib attached to cervical vertebra.

756.3 Other anomalies of ribs and sternum
Congenital absence of: Congenital:
  rib　　　　　　fissure of sternum
  sternum　　　　fusion of ribs
　　　　　　　　Sternum bifidum

> **EXCLUDES** nonteratogenic deformity of chest wall (754.81-754.89)

756.4 Chondrodystrophy
Achondroplasia　　　　　　Enchondromatosis
Chondrodystrophia (fetalis) Ollier's disease
Dyschondroplasia

> **EXCLUDES** lipochondrodystrophy [Hurler's syndrome] (277.5)
> Morquio's disease (277.5)

AHA: 2Q, '02, 16; S-O, '87, 10

DEF: Abnormal development of cartilage.

√5ᵗʰ 756.5 Osteodystrophies

756.50 Osteodystrophy, unspecified

756.51 Osteogenesis imperfecta
Fragilitas ossium
Osteopsathyrosis
DEF: A collagen disorder commonly characterized by brittle, osteoporotic, easily fractured bones, hypermobility of joints, blue sclerae, and a tendency to hemorrhage.

756.52 Osteopetrosis
DEF: Abnormally dense bone, optic atrophy, hepatosplenomegaly, deafness; sclerosing depletes bone marrow and nerve foramina of skull; often fatal.

756.53 Osteopoikilosis
DEF: Multiple sclerotic foci on ends of long bones, stippling in round, flat bones; identified by x-ray.

756.54 Polyostotic fibrous dysplasia of bone
DEF: Fibrous tissue displaces bone results in segmented ragged-edge café-au-lait spots; occurs in girls of early puberty.

756.55 Chondroectodermal dysplasia
Ellis-van Creveld syndrome
DEF: Inadequate enchondral bone formation; impaired development of hair and teeth, polydactyly, and cardiac septum defects.

756.56 Multiple epiphyseal dysplasia

756.59 Other
Albright (-McCune)-Sternberg syndrome

756.6 Anomalies of diaphragm
Absence of diaphragm　　Congenital hernia:
Congenital hernia:　　　　foramen of Morgagni
  diaphragmatic　　　　Eventration of diaphragm

> **EXCLUDES** congenital hiatus hernia (750.6)

√5ᵗʰ 756.7 Anomalies of abdominal wall

756.70 Anomaly of abdominal wall, unspecified

756.71 Prune belly syndrome
Eagle-Barrett syndrome
Prolapse of bladder mucosa
AHA: 4Q, '97, 44

DEF: Prune belly syndrome: absence of lower rectus abdominis muscle and lower and medial oblique muscles; results in dilated bladder and ureters, dysplastic kidneys and hydronephrosis; more common in male infants with undescended testicles.

√4ᵗʰ
√5ᵗʰ
Additional Digit Required　　Unspecified Code　　　Other Specified Code　　Manifestation Code　　►◄ Revised Text　　● New Code　　▲ Revised Code Title

2005 ICD•9•CM　　　　　　　　　　　　　　　　　　　　　　　　　　　　　**Volume 1 — 227**

Congenital Anomalies

756.79–758.7

756.79 Other congenital anomalies of abdominal wall

Exomphalos   Omphalocele

Gastroschisis

> EXCLUDES   umbilical hernia (551-553 with .1)

DEF: Exomphalos: umbilical hernia prominent navel.

DEF: Gastroschisis: fissure of abdominal wall, results in protruding small or large intestine.

DEF: Omphalocele: hernia of umbilicus due to impaired abdominal wall; results in membrane-covered intestine protruding through peritoneum and amnion.

√5th **756.8 Other specified anomalies of muscle, tendon, fascia, and connective tissue**

756.81 Absence of muscle and tendon

Absence of muscle (pectoral)

756.82 Accessory muscle

756.83 Ehlers-Danlos syndrome

DEF: Danlos syndrome: connective tissue disorder causes hyperextended skin and joints; results in fragile blood vessels with bleeding, poor wound healing and subcutaneous pseudotumors.

756.89 Other

Amyotrophia congenita

Congenital shortening of tendon

AHA: 3Q, '99, 16

756.9 Other and unspecified anomalies of musculoskeletal system

Congenital:

anomaly NOS   } of musculoskeletal system,
deformity NOS }   not elsewhere classified

√4th **757 Congenital anomalies of the integument**

> INCLUDES   anomalies of skin, subcutaneous tissue, hair, nails, and breast

> EXCLUDES   hemangioma (228.00-228.09)
> pigmented nevus (216.0-216.9)

757.0 Hereditary edema of legs

Congenital lymphedema   Milroy's disease

Hereditary trophedema

757.1 Ichthyosis congenita

Congenital ichthyosis

Harlequin fetus

Ichthyosiform erythroderma

DEF: Overproduction of skin cells causes scaling of skin; may result in stillborn fetus or death soon after birth.

757.2 Dermatoglyphic anomalies

Abnormal palmar creases

DEF: Abnormal skin-line patterns of fingers, palms, toes and soles; initial finding of possible chromosomal abnormalities.

√5th **757.3 Other specified anomalies of skin**

757.31 Congenital ectodermal dysplasia

DEF: Tissues and structures originate in embryonic ectoderm; includes anhidrotic and hidrotic ectodermal dysplasia and EEC syndrome.

757.32 Vascular hamartomas

Birthmarks   Strawberry nevus

Port-wine stain

DEF: Benign tumor of blood vessels; due to malformed angioblastic tissues.

757.33 Congenital pigmentary anomalies of skin

Congenital poikiloderma

Urticaria pigmentosa

Xeroderma pigmentosum

> EXCLUDES   albinism (270.2)

757.39 Other

Accessory skin tags, congenital

Congenital scar

Epidermolysis bullosa

Keratoderma (congenital)

> EXCLUDES   pilonidal cyst (685.0-685.1)

757.4 Specified anomalies of hair

Congenital:	Congenital:
alopecia	hypertrichosis
atrichosis	monilethrix
beaded hair	Persistent lanugo

757.5 Specified anomalies of nails

Anonychia	Congenital:
Congenital:	leukonychia
clubnail	onychauxis
koilonychia	pachyonychia

757.6 Specified anomalies of breast

Absent

Accessory   } breast or nipple

Supernumerary

Hypoplasia of breast

> EXCLUDES   absence of pectoral muscle (756.81)

757.8 Other specified anomalies of the integument

757.9 Unspecified anomaly of the integument

Congenital:

anomaly NOS   } of integument
deformity NOS }

√4th **758 Chromosomal anomalies**

> INCLUDES   syndromes associated with anomalies in the number and form of chromosomes

▶Use additional codes for conditions associated with the chromosomal anomalies◀

758.0 Down's syndrome

Mongolism	Trisomy:
Translocation Down's	21 or 22
syndrome	G

758.1 Patau's syndrome

Trisomy:	Trisomy:
13	D_1

DEF: Trisomy of 13th chromosome; characteristic failure to thrive, severe mental impairment, seizures, abnormal eyes, low-set ears and sloped forehead.

758.2 Edwards' syndrome

Trisomy:	Trisomy:
18	E_3

DEF: Trisomy of 18th chromosome; characteristic mental and physical impairments; mainly affects females.

√5th **758.3 Autosomal deletion syndromes**

● **758.31 Cri-du-chat syndrome**

Deletion 5p

DEF: Hereditary congenital syndrome caused by a microdeletion of short arm of chromosome 5; characterized by catlike cry in newborn, microencephaly, severe mental deficiency, and hypertelorism.

● **758.32 Velo-cardio-facial syndrome**

Deletion 22q11.2

● **758.33 Other microdeletions**

Miller-Dieker syndrome

Smith-Magenis syndrome

● **758.39 Other autosomal deletions**

758.4 Balanced autosomal translocation in normal individual

758.5 Other conditions due to autosomal anomalies

Accessory autosomes NEC

758.6 Gonadal dysgenesis

Ovarian dysgenesis   XO syndrome

Turner's syndrome

> EXCLUDES   pure gonadal dysgenesis (752.7)

DEF: Impaired embryonic development of seminiferous tubes; results in small testes, azoospermia, infertility and enlarged mammary glands.

758.7 Klinefelter's syndrome   ♂

XXY syndrome

√5ᵗʰ **758.8** **Other conditions due to chromosome anomalies**

     758.81 **Other conditions due to sex chromosome anomalies**

     758.89 **Other**

758.9 **Conditions due to anomaly of unspecified chromosome**

√4ᵗʰ **759** **Other and unspecified congenital anomalies**

759.0 **Anomalies of spleen**

     Aberrant
     Absent } spleen
     Accessory

     Congenital splenomegaly
     Ectopic spleen
     Lobulation of spleen

759.1 **Anomalies of adrenal gland**

     Aberrant
     Absent } adrenal gland
     Accessory

     EXCLUDES *adrenogenital disorders (255.2)*
     congenital disorders of steroid metabolism (255.2)

759.2 **Anomalies of other endocrine glands**

     Absent parathyroid gland
     Accessory thyroid gland
     Persistent thyroglossal or thyrolingual duct
     Thyroglossal (duct) cyst

     EXCLUDES *congenital:*
     goiter (246.1)
     hypothyroidism (243)

759.3 **Situs inversus**

     Situs inversus or transversus:
     abdominalis
     thoracis
     Transposition of viscera:
     abdominal
     thoracic

     EXCLUDES *dextrocardia without mention of complete transposition (746.87)*

     DEF: Laterally transposed thoracic and abdominal viscera.

759.4 **Conjoined twins**

     Craniopagus   Thoracopagus
     Dicephalus   Xiphopagus
     Pygopagus

759.5 **Tuberous sclerosis**

     Bourneville's disease   Epiloia
     DEF: Hamartomas of brain, retina and viscera, impaired mental ability, seizures and adenoma sebaceum.

759.6 **Other hamartoses, not elsewhere classified**

     Syndrome: Syndrome:
     Peutz-Jeghers   von Hippel-Lindau
     Sturge-Weber (-Dimitri)

     EXCLUDES *neurofibromatosis (237.7)*

     AHA: 3Q, '92, 12

     DEF: Peutz-Jeghers: hereditary syndrome characterized by hamartomas of small intestine.

     DEF: Sturge-Weber: congenital syndrome characterized by unilateral port-wine stain over trigeminal nerve, underlying meninges and cerebral cortex.

     DEF: von Hipple-Lindau: hereditary syndrome of congenital angiomatosis of the retina and cerebellum.

759.7 **Multiple congenital anomalies, so described**

     Congenital:
     anomaly, multiple NOS
     deformity, multiple NOS

√5ᵗʰ **759.8** **Other specified anomalies**

     AHA: S-O, '87, 9; S-O, '85, 11

     759.81 **Prader-Willi syndrome**

     759.82 **Marfan syndrome**
       AHA: 3Q, '93, 11

     759.83 **Fragile X syndrome**
       AHA: 4Q, '94, 41

     759.89 **Other**
       Congenital malformation syndromes affecting multiple systems, not elsewhere classified
       Laurence-Moon-Biedl syndrome
       AHA: 1Q, '01, 3; 3Q, '99, 17, 18; 3Q, '98, 8

759.9 **Congenital anomaly, unspecified**

√4ᵗʰ √5ᵗʰ Additional Digit Required   Unspecified Code   Other Specified Code   Manifestation Code   ▶◀ Revised Text   ● New Code   ▲ Revised Code Title

2005 ICD•9•CM   Volume 1 — 229

15. CERTAIN CONDITIONS ORIGINATING IN THE PERINATAL PERIOD (760-779)

INCLUDES　conditions which have their origin in the perinatal period even though death or morbidity occurs later

Use additional code(s) to further specify condition

MATERNAL CAUSES OF PERINATAL MORBIDITY AND MORTALITY (760-763)

AHA: 2Q, '89, 14; 3Q, '90, 5

✓4ᵗʰ **760　Fetus or newborn affected by maternal conditions which may be unrelated to present pregnancy**

INCLUDES　the listed maternal conditions only when specified as a cause of mortality or morbidity of the fetus or newborn

EXCLUDES　*maternal endocrine and metabolic disorders affecting fetus or newborn (775.0-775.9)*

AHA: 1Q, '94, 8; 2Q, '92, 12; N-D, '84, 11

760.0　Maternal hypertensive disorders
Fetus or newborn affected by maternal conditions classifiable to 642

760.1　Maternal renal and urinary tract diseases
Fetus or newborn affected by maternal conditions classifiable to 580-599

760.2　Maternal infections
Fetus or newborn affected by maternal infectious disease classifiable to 001-136 and 487, but fetus or newborn not manifesting that disease

EXCLUDES　*congenital infectious diseases (771.0-771.8)*

maternal genital tract and other localized infections (760.8)

760.3　Other chronic maternal circulatory and respiratory diseases
Fetus or newborn affected by chronic maternal conditions classifiable to 390-459, 490-519, 745-748

760.4　Maternal nutritional disorders
Fetus or newborn affected by:
maternal disorders classifiable to 260-269
maternal malnutrition NOS

EXCLUDES　*fetal malnutrition (764.10-764.29)*

760.5　Maternal injury
Fetus or newborn affected by maternal conditions classifiable to 800-995

760.6　Surgical operation on mother

EXCLUDES　*cesarean section for present delivery (763.4)*

damage to placenta from amniocentesis, cesarean section, or surgical induction (762.1)

previous surgery to uterus or pelvic organs (763.89)

▲　✓5ᵗʰ **760.7　Noxious influences affecting fetus or newborn via placenta or breast milk**
Fetus or newborn affected by noxious substance transmitted via placenta or breast milk

EXCLUDES　*anesthetic and analgesic drugs administered during labor and delivery (763.5)*

drug withdrawal syndrome in newborn (779.5)

AHA: 3Q, '91, 21

760.70　Unspecified noxious substance
Fetus or newborn affected by:
Drug NEC

760.71　Alcohol
Fetal alcohol syndrome

760.72　Narcotics

760.73　Hallucinogenic agents

760.74　Anti-infectives
Antibiotics

760.75　Cocaine
AHA: 3Q, '94, 6; 2Q, '92, 12; 4Q, '91, 26

760.76　Diethylstilbestrol [DES]
AHA: 4Q, '94, 45

760.79　Other
Fetus or newborn affected by:
immune sera ⎫ transmitted via
medicinal agents ⎬ placenta
NEC ⎪ or breast
toxic substance NEC ⎭ milk

760.8　Other specified maternal conditions affecting fetus or newborn
Maternal genital tract and other localized infection affecting fetus or newborn, but fetus or newborn not manifesting that disease

EXCLUDES　*maternal urinary tract infection affecting fetus or newborn (760.1)*

760.9　Unspecified maternal condition affecting fetus or newborn

✓4ᵗʰ **761　Fetus or newborn affected by maternal complications of pregnancy**

INCLUDES　the listed maternal conditions only when specified as a cause of mortality or morbidity of the fetus or newborn

761.0　Incompetent cervix
DEF: Inadequate functioning of uterine cervix.

761.1　Premature rupture of membranes

761.2　Oligohydramnios
EXCLUDES　*that due to premature rupture of membranes (761.1)*
DEF: Deficient amniotic fluid.

761.3　Polyhydramnios
Hydramnios (acute) (chronic)
DEF: Excess amniotic fluid.

761.4　Ectopic pregnancy
Pregnancy:
abdominal
intraperitoneal
tubal

761.5　Multiple pregnancy
Triplet (pregnancy)　Twin (pregnancy)

761.6　Maternal death

761.7　Malpresentation before labor
Breech presentation ⎫
External version ⎪
Oblique lie ⎬ before labor
Transverse lie ⎪
Unstable lie ⎭

761.8　Other specified maternal complications of pregnancy affecting fetus or newborn
Spontaneous abortion, fetus

761.9　Unspecified maternal complication of pregnancy affecting fetus or newborn

✓4ᵗʰ **762　Fetus or newborn affected by complications of placenta, cord, and membranes**

INCLUDES　the listed maternal conditions only when specified as a cause of mortality or morbidity in the fetus or newborn

AHA: 1Q, '94, 8

762.0　Placenta previa　　　N
DEF: Placenta developed in lower segment of uterus; causes hemorrhaging in last trimester.

✓4ᵗʰ
✓5ᵗʰ Additional Digit Required　　Unspecified Code　　Other Specified Code　　Manifestation Code　　▶◀ Revised Text　　● New Code　　▲ Revised Code Title

Conditions in the Perinatal Period

762.1–764.2

762.1 Other forms of placental separation and hemorrhage N
Abruptio placentae
Antepartum hemorrhage
Damage to placenta from amniocentesis, cesarean section, or surgical induction
Maternal blood loss
Premature separation of placenta
Rupture of marginal sinus

762.2 Other and unspecified morphological and functional abnormalities of placenta N
Placental: Placental:
dysfunction   insufficiency
infarction

762.3 Placental transfusion syndromes N
Placental and cord abnormality resulting in twin-to-twin or other transplacental transfusion
Use additional code to indicate resultant condition in fetus or newborn:
fetal blood loss (772.0)
polycythemia neonatorum (776.4)

762.4 Prolapsed cord N
Cord presentation

762.5 Other compression of umbilical cord N
Cord around neck   Knot in cord
Entanglement of cord   Torsion of cord
AHA: ▶2Q, '03, 9◀

762.6 Other and unspecified conditions of umbilical cord N
Short cord
Thrombosis
Varices } of umbilical cord
Velamentous insertion

Vasa previa
EXCLUDES   infection of umbilical cord (771.4)
single umbilical artery (747.5)

762.7 Chorioamnionitis N
Amnionitis   Placentitis
Membranitis
DEF: Inflamed fetal membrane.

762.8 Other specified abnormalities of chorion and amnion N

762.9 Unspecified abnormality of chorion and amnion N

✓4th **763 Fetus or newborn affected by other complications of labor and delivery**
INCLUDES   the listed conditions only when specified as a cause of mortality or morbidity in the fetus or newborn
AHA: 1Q, '94, 8

763.0 Breech delivery and extraction N

763.1 Other malpresentation, malposition, and disproportion during labor and delivery N
Fetus or newborn affected by:
abnormality of bony pelvis
contracted pelvis
persistent occipitoposterior position
shoulder presentation
transverse lie
conditions classifiable to 652, 653, and 660

763.2 Forceps delivery N
Fetus or newborn affected by forceps extraction

763.3 Delivery by vacuum extractor N

763.4 Cesarean delivery N
EXCLUDES   placental separation or hemorrhage from cesarean section (762.1)

763.5 Maternal anesthesia and analgesia N
Reactions and intoxications from maternal opiates and tranquilizers during labor and delivery
EXCLUDES   drug withdrawal syndrome in newborn (779.5)

763.6 Precipitate delivery N
Rapid second stage

763.7 Abnormal uterine contractions N
Fetus or newborn affected by:
contraction ring
hypertonic labor
hypotonic uterine dysfunction
uterine inertia or dysfunction
conditions classifiable to 661, except 661.3

✓5th **763.8 Other specified complications of labor and delivery affecting fetus or newborn**
AHA: 4Q, '98, 46

     763.81 Abnormality in fetal heart rate or rhythm before the onset of labor N

     763.82 Abnormality in fetal heart rate or rhythm during labor N
     AHA: 4Q, '98, 46

     763.83 Abnormality in fetal heart rate or rhythm, unspecified as to time of onset N

     763.89 Other specified complications of labor and delivery affecting fetus or newborn N
Fetus or newborn affected by:
abnormality of maternal soft tissues
destructive operation on live fetus to facilitate delivery
induction of labor (medical)
previous surgery to uterus or pelvic organs
other conditions classifiable to 650-669
other procedures used in labor and delivery

763.9 Unspecified complication of labor and delivery affecting fetus or newborn N

OTHER CONDITIONS ORIGINATING IN THE PERINATAL PERIOD (764-779)

The following fifth-digit subclassification is for use with category 764 and codes 765.0 and 765.1 to denote birthweight:
0   unspecified [weight]
1   less than 500 grams
2   500-749 grams
3   750-999 grams
4   1,000-1,249 grams
5   1,250-1,499 grams
6   1,500-1,749 grams
7   1,750-1,999 grams
8   2,000-2,499 grams
9   2,500 grams and over

✓4th **764 Slow fetal growth and fetal malnutrition**
AHA: 4Q, '02, 63; 1Q,'94, 8; 2Q, '91, 19; 2Q, '89, 15

✓5th **764.0 "Light-for-dates" without mention of fetal malnutrition** N
Infants underweight for gestational age
"Small-for-dates"

✓5th **764.1 "Light-for-dates" with signs of fetal malnutrition** N
Infants "light-for-dates" classifiable to 764.0, who in addition show signs of fetal malnutrition, such as dry peeling skin and loss of subcutaneous tissue

✓5th **764.2 Fetal malnutrition without mention of "light-for-dates"** N
Infants, not underweight for gestational age, showing signs of fetal malnutrition, such as dry peeling skin and loss of subcutaneous tissue
Intrauterine malnutrition

√5ᵗʰ 764.9 Fetal growth retardation, unspecified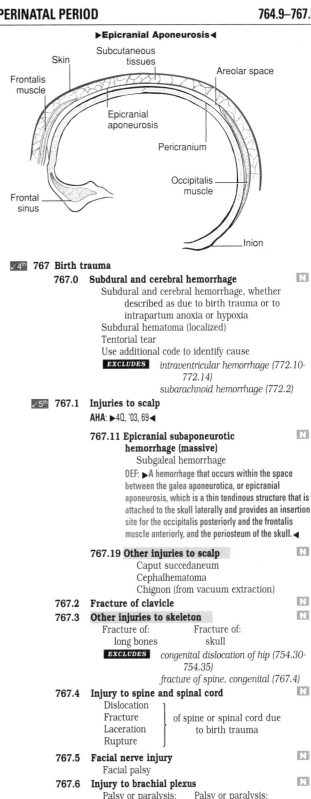
Intrauterine growth retardation
AHA: For code 764.97: 1Q, '97, 6

√4ᵗʰ 765 Disorders relating to short gestation and low birthweight
INCLUDES the listed conditions, without further specification, as causes of mortality, morbidity, or additional care, in fetus or newborn
AHA: 1Q, '97, 6; 1Q, '94, 8; 2Q, '91, 19; 2Q, '89, 15

√5ᵗʰ 765.0 Extreme immaturity
Note: Usually implies a birthweight of less than 1000 grams.
Use additional code for weeks of gestation (765.20-765.29)
AHA: For code 765.03: 4Q, '01, 51
AHA: 4Q, '02, 63

√5ᵗʰ 765.1 Other preterm infants
Note: Usually implies a birthweight of 1000-2499 grams.
Prematurity NOS
Prematurity or small size, not classifiable to 765.0 or as "light-for-dates" in 764
Use additional code for weeks of gestation (765.20-765.29)
AHA: 4Q, '02, 63
AHA: For code 765.10: 1Q, '94, 14
AHA: For code 765.17: 1Q, '97, 6
AHA: For code 765.18: 4Q, '02, 64

√5ᵗʰ 765.2 Weeks of gestation
AHA: 4Q, '02, 63

765.20 Unspecified weeks of gestation
765.21 Less than 24 completed weeks of gestation
765.22 24 completed weeks of gestation
765.23 25-26 completed weeks of gestation
765.24 27-28 completed weeks of gestation
765.25 29-30 completed weeks of gestation
765.26 31-32 completed weeks of gestation
765.27 33-34 completed weeks of gestation
765.28 35-36 completed weeks of gestation
AHA: 4Q, '02, 64
765.29 37 or more completed weeks of gestation

√4ᵗʰ 766 Disorders relating to long gestation and high birthweight
INCLUDES the listed conditions, without further specification, as causes of mortality, morbidity, or additional care, in fetus or newborn

766.0 Exceptionally large baby
Note: Usually implies a birthweight of 4500 grams or more.

766.1 Other "heavy-for-dates" infants
Other fetus or infant "heavy-" or "large-for-dates" regardless of period of gestation

√5ᵗʰ 766.2 Late infant, not "heavy-for-dates"
AHA: ►4Q, '03, 69◄

766.21 Post-term infant
Infant with gestation period over 40 completed weeks to 42 completed weeks

766.22 Prolonged gestation of infant
Infant with gestation period over 42 completed weeks
Postmaturity NOS

►**Epicranial Aponeurosis**◄

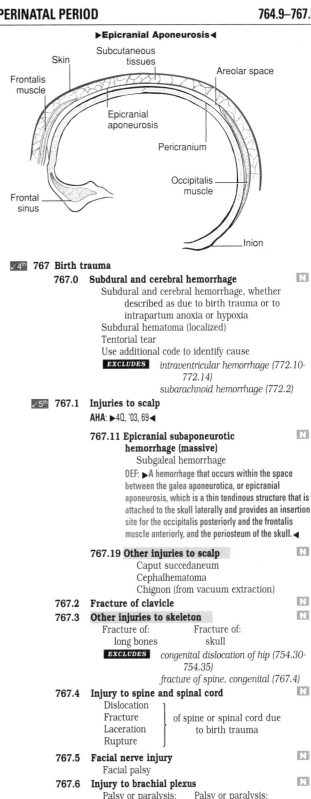

√4ᵗʰ 767 Birth trauma
767.0 Subdural and cerebral hemorrhage
Subdural and cerebral hemorrhage, whether described as due to birth trauma or to intrapartum anoxia or hypoxia
Subdural hematoma (localized)
Tentorial tear
Use additional code to identify cause
EXCLUDES intraventricular hemorrhage (772.10-772.14)
subarachnoid hemorrhage (772.2)

√5ᵗʰ 767.1 Injuries to scalp
AHA: ►4Q, '03, 69◄

767.11 Epicranial subaponeurotic hemorrhage (massive)
Subgaleal hemorrhage
DEF: ►A hemorrhage that occurs within the space between the galea aponeurotica, or epicranial aponeurosis, which is a thin tendinous structure that is attached to the skull laterally and provides an insertion site for the occipitalis posteriorly and the frontalis muscle anteriorly, and the periosteum of the skull.◄

767.19 Other injuries to scalp
Caput succedaneum
Cephalhematoma
Chignon (from vacuum extraction)

767.2 Fracture of clavicle
767.3 Other injuries to skeleton
Fracture of: Fracture of:
  long bones   skull
EXCLUDES congenital dislocation of hip (754.30-754.35)
fracture of spine, congenital (767.4)

767.4 Injury to spine and spinal cord
Dislocation
Fracture   } of spine or spinal cord due
Laceration   } to birth trauma
Rupture

767.5 Facial nerve injury
Facial palsy

767.6 Injury to brachial plexus
Palsy or paralysis: Palsy or paralysis:
  brachial   Klumpke (-Déjérine)
  Erb (-Duchenne)

767.7 Other cranial and peripheral nerve injuries
Phrenic nerve paralysis

767.8 Other specified birth trauma
Eye damage   Rupture of:
Hematoma of: liver
  liver (subcapsular)   spleen
  testes   Scalpel wound
  vulva   Traumatic glaucoma
EXCLUDES hemorrhage classifiable to 772.0-772.9

√4ᵗʰ √5ᵗʰ Additional Digit Required   Unspecified Code   Other Specified Code   Manifestation Code   ►◄ Revised Text   ● New Code   ▲ Revised Code Title

2005 ICD•9•CM   **February 2004 • Volume 1 — 233**

Conditions in the Perinatal Period

764.9–767.8

Conditions in the Perinatal Period

767.9–771.2

767.9 Birth trauma, unspecified [N]
Birth injury NOS

☑4ᵗʰ **768 Intrauterine hypoxia and birth asphyxia**
Use only when associated with newborn morbidity classifiable elsewhere

AHA: 4Q, '92, 20

DEF: Oxygen intake insufficiency due to interrupted placental circulation or premature separation of placenta.

768.0 Fetal death from asphyxia or anoxia before onset of labor or at unspecified time [N]

768.1 Fetal death from asphyxia or anoxia during labor [N]

768.2 Fetal distress before onset of labor, in liveborn infant [N]
Fetal metabolic acidemia before onset of labor, in liveborn infant

768.3 Fetal distress first noted during labor, in liveborn infant [N]
Fetal metabolic acidemia first noted during labor, in liveborn infant

768.4 Fetal distress, unspecified as to time of onset, in liveborn infant [N]
Fetal metabolic acidemia unspecified as to time of onset, in liveborn infant

AHA: N-D, '86, 10

768.5 Severe birth asphyxia [N]
Birth asphyxia with neurologic involvement

AHA: N-D, '86, 3

768.6 Mild or moderate birth asphyxia [N]
Other specified birth asphyxia (without mention of neurologic involvement)

AHA: N-D, '86, 3

768.9 Unspecified birth asphyxia in liveborn infant [N]
Anoxia ⎫
Asphyxia ⎬ NOS, in liveborn infant
Hypoxia ⎭

769 Respiratory distress syndrome [N]
Cardiorespiratory distress syndrome of newborn
Hyaline membrane disease (pulmonary)
Idiopathic respiratory distress syndrome [IRDS or RDS] of newborn
Pulmonary hypoperfusion syndrome
EXCLUDES transient tachypnea of newborn (770.6)

AHA: 1Q, '89, 10; N-D, '86, 6

DEF: Severe chest contractions upon air intake and expiratory grunting; infant appears blue due to oxygen deficiency and has rapid respiratory rate; formerly called hyaline membrane disease.

☑4ᵗʰ **770 Other respiratory conditions of fetus and newborn**

770.0 Congenital pneumonia [N]
Infective pneumonia acquired prenatally
EXCLUDES pneumonia from infection acquired after birth (480.0-486)

770.1 Meconium aspiration syndrome [N]
Aspiration of contents of birth canal NOS
Meconium aspiration below vocal cords
Pneumonitis:
fetal aspiration
meconium

DEF: Aspiration of meconium by the newborn infant prior to delivery. Presence of meconium in the trachea or chest x-ray indicating patchy infiltrates in conjunction with chest hyperextension establishes this diagnosis.

770.2 Interstitial emphysema and related conditions [N]
Pneumomediastinum ⎫
Pneumopericardium ⎬ originating in the
Pneumothorax ⎭ perinatal period

770.3 Pulmonary hemorrhage [N]
Hemorrhage:
alveolar (lung) ⎫
intra-alveolar (lung) ⎬ originating in the
massive pulmonary ⎭ perinatal period

770.4 Primary atelectasis [N]
Pulmonary immaturity NOS

DEF: Alveoli fail to expand causing insufficient air intake by newborn.

770.5 Other and unspecified atelectasis [N]
Atelectasis:
NOS ⎫
partial ⎬ originating in the
secondary ⎭ perinatal period
Pulmonary collapse

770.6 Transitory tachypnea of newborn [N]
Idiopathic tachypnea of newborn
Wet lung syndrome
EXCLUDES respiratory distress syndrome (769)

AHA: 4Q, '95, 4; 1Q, '94, 12; 3Q, '93, 7; 1Q, '89, 10; N-D, '86, 6

DEF: Quick, shallow breathing of newborn; short-term problem.

770.7 Chronic respiratory disease arising in the perinatal period [N]
Bronchopulmonary dysplasia
Interstitial pulmonary fibrosis of prematurity
Wilson-Mikity syndrome

AHA: 2Q, '91, 19; N-D, '86, 11

☑5ᵗʰ **770.8 Other respiratory problems after birth** [N]
AHA: 4Q, '02, 65; 2Q, '98, 10; 2Q, '96, 10

770.81 Primary apnea of newborn [N]
Apneic spells of newborn NOS
Essential apnea of newborn
Sleep apnea of newborn

DEF: Cessation of breathing when a neonate makes no respiratory effort for 15 seconds, resulting in cyanosis and bradycardia.

770.82 Other apnea of newborn [N]
Obstructive apnea of newborn

770.83 Cyanotic attacks of newborn [N]

770.84 Respiratory failure of newborn [N]
EXCLUDES respiratory distress syndrome (769)

770.89 Other respiratory problems after birth [N]

770.9 Unspecified respiratory condition of fetus and newborn [N]

☑4ᵗʰ **771 Infections specific to the perinatal period**
INCLUDES infections acquired before or during birth or via the umbilicus
EXCLUDES congenital pneumonia (770.0)
congenital syphilis (090.0-090.9)
maternal infectious disease as a cause of mortality or morbidity in fetus or newborn, but fetus or newborn not manifesting the disease (760.2)
ophthalmia neonatorum due to gonococcus (098.40)
other infections not specifically classified to this category

AHA: N-D, '85, 4

771.0 Congenital rubella [N]
Congenital rubella pneumonitis

771.1 Congenital cytomegalovirus infection [N]
Congenital cytomegalic inclusion disease

771.2 Other congenital infections [N]
Congenital: Congenital:
herpes simplex   toxoplasmosis
listeriosis   tuberculosis
malaria

[N] Newborn Age: 0   [P] Pediatric Age: 0-17   [M] Maternity Age: 12-55   [A] Adult Age: 15-124   [MSP] Medicare Secondary Payer

771.3 Tetanus neonatorum N
Tetanus omphalitis
EXCLUDES *hypocalcemic tetany (775.4)*
DEF: Severe infection of central nervous system; due to exotoxin of tetanus bacillus from navel infection prompted by nonsterile technique during umbilical ligation.

771.4 Omphalitis of the newborn N
Infection:
navel cord
umbilical stump
EXCLUDES *tetanus omphalitis (771.3)*
DEF: Inflamed umbilicus.

771.5 Neonatal infective mastitis N
EXCLUDES *noninfective neonatal mastitis (778.7)*

771.6 Neonatal conjunctivitis and dacryocystitis N
Ophthalmia neonatorum NOS
EXCLUDES *ophthalmia neonatorum due to gonococcus (098.40)*

771.7 Neonatal Candida infection N
Neonatal moniliasis
Thrush in newborn

√5th **771.8 Other infection specific to the perinatal period**
Use additional code to identify organism
▶(041.00-041.9)◀
AHA: 4Q, '02, 66

771.81 Septicemia [sepsis] of newborn N
771.82 Urinary tract infection of newborn N
771.83 Bacteremia of newborn N
771.89 Other infections specific to the perinatal period N
Intra-amniotic infection of fetus NOS
Infection of newborn NOS

√4th **772 Fetal and neonatal hemorrhage**
EXCLUDES *hematological disorders of fetus and newborn (776.0-776.9)*

772.0 Fetal blood loss N
Fetal blood loss from:
cut end of co-twin's cord
placenta
ruptured cord
vasa previa
Fetal exsanguination
Fetal hemorrhage into:
co-twin
mother's circulation

√5th **772.1 Intraventricular hemorrhage**
Intraventricular hemorrhage from any perinatal cause
AHA: 4Q, '01, 49; 3Q, '92, 8; 4Q, '88, 8

772.10 Unspecified grade N
772.11 Grade I N
Bleeding into germinal matrix
772.12 Grade II N
Bleeding into ventricle
772.13 Grade III N
Bleeding with enlargement of ventricle
AHA: 4Q, '01, 51
772.14 Grade IV N
Bleeding into cerebral cortex

772.2 Subarachnoid hemorrhage N
Subarachnoid hemorrhage from any perinatal cause
EXCLUDES *subdural and cerebral hemorrhage (767.0)*

772.3 Umbilical hemorrhage after birth N
Slipped umbilical ligature

772.4 Gastrointestinal hemorrhage N
EXCLUDES *swallowed maternal blood (777.3)*

772.5 Adrenal hemorrhage N

772.6 Cutaneous hemorrhage N
Bruising
Ecchymoses
Petechiae
Superficial hematoma
} in fetus or newborn

772.8 Other specified hemorrhage of fetus or newborn N
EXCLUDES *hemorrhagic disease of newborn (776.0)*
pulmonary hemorrhage (770.3)

772.9 Unspecified hemorrhage of newborn N

√4th **773 Hemolytic disease of fetus or newborn, due to isoimmunization**
DEF: Hemolytic anemia of fetus or newborn due to maternal antibody formation against fetal erythrocytes; infant blood contains nonmaternal antigen.

773.0 Hemolytic disease due to Rh isoimmunization N
Anemia
Erythroblastosis (fetalis)
Hemolytic disease (fetus) (newborn)
Jaundice
} due to RH: antibodies isoimmunization maternal/fetal incompatibility
Rh hemolytic disease
Rh isoimmunization

773.1 Hemolytic disease due to ABO isoimmunization N
ABO hemolytic disease
ABO isoimmunization
Anemia
Erythroblastosis (fetalis)
Hemolytic disease (fetus) (newborn)
Jaundice
} due to ABO: antibodies isoimmunization maternal/fetal incompatibility
AHA: 3Q, '92, 8
DEF: Incompatible Rh fetal-maternal blood grouping; prematurely destroys red blood cells; detected by Coombs test.

773.2 Hemolytic disease due to other and unspecified isoimmunization N
Eythroblastosis (fetalis) (neonatorum) NOS
Hemolytic disease (fetus) (newborn) NOS
Jaundice or anemia due to other and unspecified blood-group incompatibility
AHA: 1Q, '94, 13

773.3 Hydrops fetalis due to isoimmunization N
Use additional code to identify type of isoimmunization (773.0-773.2)
DEF: Massive edema of entire body and severe anemia; may result in fetal death or stillbirth.

773.4 Kernicterus due to isoimmunization N
Use additional code to identify type of isoimmunization (773.0-773.2)
DEF: Complication of erythroblastosis fetalis associated with severe neural symptoms, high blood bilirubin levels and nerve cell destruction; results in bilirubin-pigmented gray matter of central nervous system.

773.5 Late anemia due to isoimmunization N

√4th **774 Other perinatal jaundice**
774.0 Perinatal jaundice from hereditary hemolytic anemias N
Code first underlying disease (282.0-282.9)

Conditions in the Perinatal Period

774.1 Perinatal jaundice from other excessive hemolysis N
Fetal or neonatal jaundice from:
bruising
drugs or toxins transmitted from mother
infection
polycythemia
swallowed maternal blood
Use additional code to identify cause
EXCLUDES jaundice due to isoimmunization (773.0-773.2)

774.2 Neonatal jaundice associated with preterm delivery N
Hyperbilirubinemia of prematurity
Jaundice due to delayed conjugation associated with preterm delivery
AHA: 3Q, '91, 21

√5th **774.3 Neonatal jaundice due to delayed conjugation from other causes**
774.30 Neonatal jaundice due to delayed conjugation, cause unspecified N
DEF: Jaundice of newborn with abnormal bilirubin metabolism; causes excess accumulated unconjugated bilirubin in blood.

774.31 Neonatal jaundice due to delayed conjugation in diseases classified elsewhere N
Code first underlying diseases as:
congenital hypothyroidism (243)
Crigler-Najjar syndrome (277.4)
Gilbert's syndrome (277.4)

774.39 Other N
Jaundice due to delayed conjugation from causes, such as:
breast milk inhibitors
delayed development of conjugating system

774.4 Perinatal jaundice due to hepatocellular damage N
Fetal or neonatal hepatitis
Giant cell hepatitis
Inspissated bile syndrome

774.5 Perinatal jaundice from other causes N
Code first underlying cause as:
congenital obstruction of bile duct (751.61)
galactosemia (271.1)
Mucoviscidosis (277.00-277.09)

774.6 Unspecified fetal and neonatal jaundice N
Icterus neonatorum
Neonatal hyperbilirubinemia (transient)
Physiologic jaundice NOS in newborn
EXCLUDES that in preterm infants (774.2)
AHA: 1Q, '94, 13; 2Q, '89, 15

774.7 Kernicterus not due to isoimmunization N
Bilirubin encephalopathy
Kernicterus of newborn NOS
EXCLUDES kernicterus due to isoimmunization (773.4)

√4th **775 Endocrine and metabolic disturbances specific to the fetus and newborn**
INCLUDES transitory endocrine and metabolic disturbances caused by the infant's response to maternal endocrine and metabolic factors, its removal from them, or its adjustment to extrauterine existence

775.0 Syndrome of "infant of a diabetic mother" N
Maternal diabetes mellitus affecting fetus or newborn (with hypoglycemia)
AHA: ▶1Q, '04, 7-8;◀ 3Q, '91, 5

775.1 Neonatal diabetes mellitus N
Diabetes mellitus syndrome in newborn infant
AHA: 3Q, '91, 6

775.2 Neonatal myasthenia gravis N
775.3 Neonatal thyrotoxicosis N
Neonatal hyperthyroidism (transient)

775.4 Hypocalcemia and hypomagnesemia of newborn N
Cow's milk hypocalcemia
Hypocalcemic tetany, neonatal
Neonatal hypoparathyroidism
Phosphate-loading hypocalcemia

775.5 Other transitory neonatal electrolyte disturbances N
Dehydration, neonatal

775.6 Neonatal hypoglycemia N
EXCLUDES infant of mother with diabetes mellitus (775.0)
AHA: 1Q, '94, 8

775.7 Late metabolic acidosis of newborn N
775.8 Other transitory neonatal endocrine and metabolic disturbances N
Amino-acid metabolic disorders described as transitory

775.9 Unspecified endocrine and metabolic disturbances specific to the fetus and newborn N

√4th **776 Hematological disorders of fetus and newborn**
INCLUDES disorders specific to the fetus or newborn

776.0 Hemorrhagic disease of newborn N
Hemorrhagic diathesis of newborn
Vitamin K deficiency of newborn
EXCLUDES fetal or neonatal hemorrhage (772.0-772.9)

776.1 Transient neonatal thrombocytopenia N
Neonatal thrombocytopenia due to:
exchange transfusion
idiopathic maternal thrombocytopenia
isoimmunization
DEF: Temporary decrease in blood platelets of newborn.

776.2 Disseminated intravascular coagulation in newborn N
DEF: Disseminated intravascular coagulation of newborn: clotting disorder due to excess thromboplastic agents in blood as a result of disease or trauma; causes blood clotting within vessels and reduces available elements necessary for blood coagulation.

776.3 Other transient neonatal disorders of coagulation N
Transient coagulation defect, newborn

776.4 Polycythemia neonatorum N
Plethora of newborn Polycythemia due to:
Polycythemia due to: maternal-fetal transfusion
donor twin transfusion
DEF: Abnormal increase of total red blood cells of newborn.

776.5 Congenital anemia N
Anemia following fetal blood loss
EXCLUDES anemia due to isoimmunization (773.0-773.2, 773.5)
hereditary hemolytic anemias (282.0-282.9)

776.6 Anemia of prematurity N
776.7 Transient neonatal neutropenia N
Isoimmune neutropenia
Maternal transfer neutropenia
EXCLUDES congenital neutropenia (nontransient) (288.0)
DEF: Decreased neutrophilic leukocytes in blood of newborn.

776.8 Other specified transient hematological disorders N
776.9 Unspecified hematological disorder specific to fetus or newborn N

N Newborn Age: 0   P Pediatric Age: 0-17   M Maternity Age: 12-55   A Adult Age: 15-124   MSP Medicare Secondary Payer

✓4ᵗʰ **777 Perinatal disorders of digestive system**

> INCLUDES   disorders specific to the fetus and newborn
>
> EXCLUDES   *intestinal obstruction classifiable to 560.0-560.9*

777.1 Meconium obstruction   N
> Congenital fecaliths
> Delayed passage of meconium
> Meconium ileus NOS
> Meconium plug syndrome
>> EXCLUDES   *meconium ileus in cystic fibrosis (277.01)*
>
> DEF: Meconium blocked digestive tract of newborn.

777.2 Intestinal obstruction due to inspissated milk   N

777.3 Hematemesis and melena due to swallowed maternal blood   N
> Swallowed blood syndrome in newborn
>> EXCLUDES   *that not due to swallowed maternal blood (772.4)*

777.4 Transitory ileus of newborn   N
>> EXCLUDES   *Hirschsprung's disease (751.3)*

777.5 Necrotizing enterocolitis in fetus or newborn   N
> Pseudomembranous enterocolitis in newborn
>
> DEF: Acute inflammation of small intestine due to pseudomembranous plaque over ulceration; may be due to aggressive antibiotic therapy.

777.6 Perinatal intestinal perforation   N
> Meconium peritonitis

777.8 Other specified perinatal disorders of digestive system   N

777.9 Unspecified perinatal disorder of digestive system   N

✓4ᵗʰ **778 Conditions involving the integument and temperature regulation of fetus and newborn**

778.0 Hydrops fetalis not due to isoimmunization   N
> Idiopathic hydrops
>> EXCLUDES   *hydrops fetalis due to isoimmunization (773.3)*
>
> DEF: Edema of entire body, unrelated to immune response.

778.1 Sclerema neonatorum   N
> Subcutaneous fat necrosis
>
> DEF: Diffuse, rapidly progressing white, waxy, nonpitting hardening of tissue, usually of legs and feet, life-threatening; found in preterm or debilitated infants; unknown etiology.

778.2 Cold injury syndrome of newborn   N

778.3 Other hypothermia of newborn   N

778.4 Other disturbances of temperature regulation of newborn   N
> Dehydration fever in newborn
> Environmentally-induced pyrexia
> Hyperthermia in newborn
> Transitory fever of newborn

778.5 Other and unspecified edema of newborn   N
> Edema neonatorum

778.6 Congenital hydrocele   N
> Congenital hydrocele of tunica vaginalis

778.7 Breast engorgement in newborn   N
> Noninfective mastitis of newborn
>> EXCLUDES   *infective mastitis of newborn (771.5)*

778.8 Other specified conditions involving the integument of fetus and newborn   N
> Urticaria neonatorum
>> EXCLUDES   *impetigo neonatorum (684)*
>> *pemphigus neonatorum (684)*

778.9 Unspecified condition involving the integument and temperature regulation of fetus and newborn   N

✓4ᵗʰ **779 Other and ill-defined conditions originating in the perinatal period**

779.0 Convulsions in newborn   N
> Fits ⎫
> Seizures ⎭ in newborn
>
> AHA: N-D, '94, 11

779.1 Other and unspecified cerebral irritability in newborn   N

779.2 Cerebral depression, coma, and other abnormal cerebral signs   N
> CNS dysfunction in newborn NOS

779.3 Feeding problems in newborn   N
> Regurgitation of food ⎫
> Slow feeding ⎬ in newborn
> Vomiting ⎭
>
> AHA: 2Q, '89, 15

779.4 Drug reactions and intoxications specific to newborn   N
> Gray syndrome from chloramphenicol administration in newborn
>> EXCLUDES   *fetal alcohol syndrome (760.71)*
>> *reactions and intoxications from maternal opiates and tranquilizers (763.5)*

779.5 Drug withdrawal syndrome in newborn   N
> Drug withdrawal syndrome in infant of dependent mother
>> EXCLUDES   *fetal alcohol syndrome (760.71)*
>
> AHA: 3Q, '94, 6

779.6 Termination of pregnancy (fetus)   N
> Fetal death due to:
> induced abortion
> termination of pregnancy
>> EXCLUDES   *spontaneous abortion (fetus) (761.8)*

779.7 Periventricular leukomalacia
> AHA: 4Q, '01, 50, 51
>
> DEF: Necrosis of white matter adjacent to lateral ventricles with the formation of cysts; cause of PVL has not been firmly established, but thought to be related to inadequate blood flow in certain areas of the brain.

✓5ᵗʰ **779.8 Other specified conditions originating in the perinatal period**
> AHA: 4Q, '02, 67; 1Q, '94, 15

779.81 Neonatal bradycardia   N
>> EXCLUDES   *abnormality in fetal heart rate or rhythm complicating labor and delivery (763.81-763.83)*
>> *bradycardia due to birth asphyxia (768.5-768.9)*

779.82 Neonatal tachycardia   N
>> EXCLUDES   *abnormality in fetal heart rate or rhythm complicating labor and delivery (763.81-763.83)*

779.83 Delayed separation of umbilical cord   N
> AHA: ▶4Q, '03, 71◀

779.89 Other specified conditions originating in the perinatal period   N

779.9 Unspecified condition originating in the perinatal period   N
> Congenital debility NOS
> Stillbirth NEC

✓4ᵗʰ / ✓5ᵗʰ Additional Digit Required   Unspecified Code   Other Specified Code   Manifestation Code   ▶◀ Revised Text   ● New Code   ▲ Revised Code Title

16. SYMPTOMS, SIGNS, AND ILL-DEFINED CONDITIONS (780-799)

This section includes symptoms, signs, abnormal results of laboratory or other investigative procedures, and ill-defined conditions regarding which no diagnosis classifiable elsewhere is recorded.

Signs and symptoms that point rather definitely to a given diagnosis are assigned to some category in the preceding part of the classification. In general, categories 780-796 include the more ill-defined conditions and symptoms that point with perhaps equal suspicion to two or more diseases or to two or more systems of the body, and without the necessary study of the case to make a final diagnosis. Practically all categories in this group could be designated as "not otherwise specified," or as "unknown etiology," or as "transient." The Alphabetic Index should be consulted to determine which symptoms and signs are to be allocated here and which to more specific sections of the classification; the residual subcategories numbered .9 are provided for other relevant symptoms which cannot be allocated elsewhere in the classification.

The conditions and signs or symptoms included in categories 780-796 consist of: (a) cases for which no more specific diagnosis can be made even after all facts bearing on the case have been investigated; (b) signs or symptoms existing at the time of initial encounter that proved to be transient and whose causes could not be determined; (c) provisional diagnoses in a patient who failed to return for further investigation or care; (d) cases referred elsewhere for investigation or treatment before the diagnosis was made; (e) cases in which a more precise diagnosis was not available for any other reason; (f) certain symptoms which represent important problems in medical care and which it might be desired to classify in addition to a known cause.

SYMPTOMS (780-789)
AHA: 1Q, '91, 12; 2Q, '90, 3; 2Q, '90, 5; 2Q, '90, 15; M-A, '85, 3

780 General symptoms

780.0 Alteration of consciousness
EXCLUDES coma:
diabetic (250.2-250.3)
hepatic (572.2)
originating in the perinatal period (779.2)
AHA: 4Q, '92, 20

780.01 Coma
AHA: 3Q, '96, 16
DEF: State of unconsciousness from which the patient cannot be awakened.

780.02 Transient alteration of awareness
DEF: Temporary, recurring spells of reduced consciousness.

780.03 Persistent vegetative state
DEF: Persistent wakefulness without consciousness due to nonfunctioning cerebral cortex.

780.09 Other
Drowsiness   Stupor
Semicoma   Unconsciousness
Somnolence

780.1 Hallucinations
Hallucinations: Hallucinations:
NOS   olfactory
auditory   tactile
gustatory
EXCLUDES those associated with mental disorders, as functional psychoses (295.0-298.9)
organic brain syndromes (290.0-294.9, 310.0-310.9)
visual hallucinations (368.16)
DEF: Perception of external stimulus in absence of stimulus; inability to distinguish between real and imagined.

780.2 Syncope and collapse
Blackout   (Near) (Pre) syncope
Fainting   Vasovagal attack
EXCLUDES carotid sinus syncope (337.0)
heat syncope (992.1)
neurocirculatory asthenia (306.2)
orthostatic hypotension (458.0)
shock NOS (785.50)
AHA: 1Q, '02, 6; 3Q, '00, 12; 3Q, '95, 14; N-D, '85, 12
DEF: Sudden unconsciousness due to reduced blood flow to brain.

780.3 Convulsions
EXCLUDES convulsions:
epileptic (345.10-345.91)
in newborn (779.0)
AHA: 2Q, '97, 8; 1Q, '97, 12; 3Q, '94, 9; 1Q, '93, 24; 4Q, '92, 23; N-D, '87, 12
DEF: Sudden, involuntary contractions of the muscles.

780.31 Febrile convulsions
Febrile seizure
AHA: 4Q, '97, 45

780.39 Other convulsions
Convulsive disorder NOS
Fit NOS
Seizure NOS
AHA: 1Q, '03, 7; 2Q, '99, 17; 4Q, '98, 39

780.4 Dizziness and giddiness
Light-headedness
Vertigo NOS
EXCLUDES Ménière's disease and other specified vertiginous syndromes (386.0-386.9)
AHA: ▶2Q, '03, 11;◄ 3Q, '00, 12; 2Q, '97, 9; 2Q, '91, 17
DEF: Whirling sensations in head with feeling of falling.

780.5 Sleep disturbances
EXCLUDES that of nonorganic origin (307.40-307.49)

780.50 Sleep disturbance, unspecified
780.51 Insomnia with sleep apnea
DEF: Transient cessation of breathing disturbing sleep.

780.52 Other insomnia
Insomnia NOS
DEF: Inability to maintain adequate sleep cycle.

780.53 Hypersomnia with sleep apnea
AHA: 1Q, '93, 28; N-D, '85, 4
DEF: Autonomic response inhibited during sleep; causes insufficient oxygen intake, acidosis and pulmonary hypertension.

780.54 Other hypersomnia
Hypersomnia NOS
DEF: Prolonged sleep cycle.

780.55 Disruptions of 24-hour sleep-wake cycle
Inversion of sleep rhythm
Irregular sleep-wake rhythm NOS
Non-24-hour sleep-wake rhythm

Additional Digit Required   Unspecified Code   Other Specified Code   Manifestation Code   ▶◀ Revised Text   ● New Code   ▲ Revised Code Title

Symptoms, Signs, and Ill-Defined Conditions

780.56–781.5

780.56 Dysfunctions associated with sleep stages or arousal from sleep

780.57 Other and unspecified sleep apnea

AHA: 1Q, '01, 6 ; 1Q, '97, 5; 1Q, '93, 28

● **780.58 Sleep related movement disorder**
Periodic limb movement disorder
EXCLUDES   restless leg syndrome (333.99)

780.59 Other

780.6 Fever

Chills with fever   Hyperpyrexia NOS
Fever NOS   Pyrexia
Fever of unknown origin   Pyrexia of unknown
    (FUO)   origin

EXCLUDES   pyrexia of unknown origin (during):
        in newborn (778.4)
        labor (659.2)
        the puerperium (672)

AHA: 3Q, '00, 13; 4Q, '99, 26; 2Q, '91, 8

DEF: Elevated body temperature; no known cause.

✓5ᵗʰ **780.7 Malaise and fatigue**

EXCLUDES   debility, unspecified (799.3)
        fatigue (during):
           combat (308.0-308.9)
           heat (992.6)
           pregnancy (646.8)
        neurasthenia (300.5)
        senile asthenia (797)

AHA: 4Q, '88, 12; M-A, '87, 8

DEF: Indefinite feeling of debility or lack of good health.

780.71 Chronic fatigue syndrome

AHA: 4Q, '98, 48

DEF: Persistent fatigue, symptoms include weak muscles, sore throat, lymphadenitis, headache, depression and mild fever; no known cause; also called chronic mononucleosis, benign myalgic encephalomyelitis, Iceland disease and neurosthenia.

780.79 Other malaise and fatigue
Asthenia NOS
Lethargy
Postviral (asthenic) syndrome
Tiredness

AHA: 1Q, '00, 6; 4Q, '99, 26

DEF: Asthenia: any weakness, lack of strength or loss of energy, especially neuromuscular.

DEF: Lethargy: listlessness, drowsiness, stupor and apathy.

DEF: Postviral (asthenic) syndrome: listlessness, drowsiness, stupor and apathy; follows acute viral infection.

DEF: Tiredness: general exhaustion or fatigue.

▲ **780.8 Generalized hyperhidrosis**
Diaphoresis
Excessive sweating
▶Secondary hyperhidrosis◀
EXCLUDES   ▶focal (localized) (primary) (secondary)
        hyperhidrosis (705.21-705.22)
        Frey's syndrome (705.22)◀

DEF: Excessive sweating, appears as droplets on skin; generalized.

✓5ᵗʰ **780.9 Other general symptoms**
EXCLUDES   hypothermia:
        NOS (accidental) (991.6)
        due to anesthesia (995.89)
        of newborn (778.2-778.3)
        memory disturbance as part of a
           pattern of mental disorder

AHA: 4Q, '02, 67; 4Q, '99, 10; 3Q, '93, 11; N-D, '85, 12

780.91 Fussy infant (baby)   P

780.92 Excessive crying of infant (baby)   P

780.93 Memory loss
Amnesia (retrograde)
Memory loss NOS
EXCLUDES   mild memory disturbance due
        to organic brain damage
        (310.1)
        transient global amnesia
        (437.7)

AHA: 4Q, '03, 71

780.94 Early satiety

AHA: 4Q, '03, 72

DEF: The premature feeling of being full; mechanism of satiety is mutlifactorial.

780.99 Other general symptoms
Chill(s) NOS
Generalized pain
Hypothermia, not associated with low
    environmental temperature

AHA: 4Q, '03, 103

✓4ᵗʰ **781 Symptoms involving nervous and musculoskeletal systems**
EXCLUDES   depression NOS (311)
        disorders specifically relating to:
           back (724.0-724.9)
           hearing (388.0-389.9)
           joint (718.0-719.9)
           limb (729.0-729.9)
           neck (723.0-723.9)
           vision (368.0-369.9)
        pain in limb (729.5)

781.0 Abnormal involuntary movements
Abnormal head movements   Spasms NOS
Fasciculation   Tremor NOS
EXCLUDES   abnormal reflex (796.1)
        chorea NOS (333.5)
        infantile spasms (345.60-345.61)
        spastic paralysis (342.1, 343.0-344.9)
        specified movement disorders
           classifiable to 333 (333.0-333.9)
        that of nonorganic origin (307.2-307.3)

781.1 Disturbances of sensation of smell and taste
Anosmia   Parosmia
Parageusia

DEF: Anosmia: loss of sense of smell due to organic factors, including loss of olfactory nerve conductivity, cerebral disease, nasal fossae formation and peripheral olfactory nerve diseases; can also be psychological disorder.

DEF: Parageusia: distorted sense of taste, or bad taste in mouth.

DEF: Parosmia: distorted sense of smell.

781.2 Abnormality of gait
Gait: Gait:
   ataxic   spastic
   paralytic   staggering
EXCLUDES   ataxia:
        NOS (781.3)
        locomotor (progressive) (094.0)
        difficulty in walking (719.7)

DEF: Abnormal, asymmetric gait.

781.3 Lack of coordination
Ataxia NOS   Muscular incoordination
EXCLUDES   ataxic gait (781.2)
        cerebellar ataxia (334.0-334.9)
        difficulty in walking (719.7)
        vertigo NOS (780.4)

AHA: 3Q, '97, 12

781.4 Transient paralysis of limb
Monoplegia, transient NOS
EXCLUDES   paralysis (342.0-344.9)

781.5 Clubbing of fingers
DEF: Enlarged soft tissue of distal fingers.

N Newborn Age: 0   P Pediatric Age: 0-17   M Maternity Age: 12-55   A Adult Age: 15-124   MSP Medicare Secondary Payer

781.6　Meningismus
　　Dupré's syndrome　　　Meningism
　　AHA: 3Q, '00, 13; J-F, '87, 7

DEF: Condition with signs and symptoms that resemble meningeal irritation; it is associated with febrile illness and dehydration with no evidence of infection.

781.7　Tetany
　　Carpopedal spasm
　　　EXCLUDES　　*tetanus neonatorum (771.3)*
　　　　　　　　　tetany:
　　　　　　　　　　hysterical (300.11)
　　　　　　　　　　newborn (hypocalcemic) (775.4)
　　　　　　　　　　parathyroid (252.1)
　　　　　　　　　　psychogenic (306.0)

DEF: Nerve and muscle hyperexcitability; symptoms include muscle spasms, twitching, cramps, laryngospasm with inspiratory stridor, hyperreflexia and choreiform movements.

781.8　Neurologic neglect syndrome
　　Asomatognosia　　　　Left-sided neglect
　　Hemi-akinesia　　　　Sensory extinction
　　Hemi-inattention　　　Sensory neglect
　　Hemispatial neglect　　Visuospatial neglect
　　AHA: 4Q, '94, 37

√5ᵗʰ **781.9　Other symptoms involving nervous and musculoskeletal systems**
　　AHA: 4Q, '00, 45

　　781.91　Loss of height
　　　　　EXCLUDES　　*osteoporosis (733.00-733.09)*

　　781.92　Abnormal posture

　　781.93　Ocular torticollis
　　　　　AHA: 4Q, '02, 68

DEF: Abnormal head posture as a result of a contracted state of cervical muscles to correct a visual disturbance; either double vision or a visual field defect.

　　781.94　Facial weakness
　　　　Facial droop
　　　　　EXCLUDES　　*facial weakness due to late effect of cerebrovascular accident (438.83)*
　　　　AHA: ▶4Q, '03, 72◀

　　781.99　Other symptoms involving nervous and musculoskeletal systems

√4ᵗʰ **782　Symptoms involving skin and other integumentary tissue**
　　　EXCLUDES　　*symptoms relating to breast (611.71-611.79)*

782.0　Disturbance of skin sensation
　　Anesthesia of skin　　Hypoesthesia
　　Burning or prickling　Numbness
　　　sensation　　　　　Paresthesia
　　Hyperesthesia　　　　Tingling

782.1　Rash and other nonspecific skin eruption
　　Exanthem
　　　EXCLUDES　　*vesicular eruption (709.8)*

782.2　Localized superficial swelling, mass, or lump
　　Subcutaneous nodules
　　　EXCLUDES　　*localized adiposity (278.1)*

782.3　Edema
　　Anasarca　　　　Localized edema NOS
　　Dropsy
　　　EXCLUDES　　*ascites (789.5)*
　　　　　　　　　edema of:
　　　　　　　　　　newborn NOS (778.5)
　　　　　　　　　　pregnancy (642.0-642.9, 646.1)
　　　　　　　　　fluid retention (276.6)
　　　　　　　　　hydrops fetalis (773.3, 778.0)
　　　　　　　　　hydrothorax (511.8)
　　　　　　　　　nutritional edema (260, 262)

AHA: 2Q, '00, 18
DEF: Edema: excess fluid in intercellular body tissue.
DEF: Anasarca: massive edema in all body tissues.
DEF: Dropsy: serous fluid accumulated in body cavity or cellular tissue.
DEF: Localized edema: edema in specific body areas.

782.4　Jaundice, unspecified, not of newborn
　　Cholemia NOS　　　Icterus NOS
　　　EXCLUDES　　*jaundice in newborn (774.0-774.7)*
　　　　　　　　　due to isoimmunization (773.0-773.2, 773.4)

DEF: Bilirubin deposits of skin, causing yellow cast.

782.5　Cyanosis
　　　EXCLUDES　　*newborn (770.83)*

DEF: Deficient oxygen of blood; causes blue cast to skin.

√5ᵗʰ **782.6　Pallor and flushing**
　　782.61　Pallor
　　782.62　Flushing
　　　　Excessive blushing

782.7　Spontaneous ecchymoses
　　Petechiae
　　　EXCLUDES　　*ecchymosis in fetus or newborn (772.6)*
　　　　　　　　　purpura (287.0-287.9)

DEF: Hemorrhagic spots of skin; resemble freckles.

782.8　Changes in skin texture
　　Induration　⎫
　　Thickening　⎬ of skin

782.9　Other symptoms involving skin and integumentary tissues

√4ᵗʰ **783　Symptoms concerning nutrition, metabolism, and development**

783.0　Anorexia
　　Loss of appetite
　　　EXCLUDES　　*anorexia nervosa (307.1)*
　　　　　　　　　loss of appetite of nonorganic origin (307.59)

783.1　Abnormal weight gain
　　　EXCLUDES　　*excessive weight gain in pregnancy (646.1)*
　　　　　　　　　obesity (278.00)
　　　　　　　　　　morbid (278.01)

√5ᵗʰ **783.2　Abnormal loss of weight and underweight**
　　AHA: 4Q, '00, 45

　　783.21　Loss of weight
　　783.22　Underweight

783.3　Feeding difficulties and mismanagement
　　Feeding problem (elderly) (infant)
　　　EXCLUDES　　*feeding disturbance or problems:*
　　　　　　　　　in newborn (779.3)
　　　　　　　　　of nonorganic origin (307.50-307.59)
　　AHA: 3Q, '97, 12

√5ᵗʰ **783.4　Lack of expected normal physiological development in childhood**
　　　EXCLUDES　　*delay in sexual development and puberty (259.0)*
　　　　　　　　　gonadal dysgenesis (758.6)
　　　　　　　　　pituitary dwarfism (253.3)
　　　　　　　　　slow fetal growth and fetal malnutrition (764.00-764.99)
　　　　　　　　　specific delays in mental development (315.0-315.9)
　　AHA: 4Q, '00, 45; 3Q, '97, 4

　　783.40　Lack of normal physiological development, unspecified
　　　　Inadequate development
　　　　Lack of development

　　783.41　Failure to thrive　　　　　　　P
　　　　Failure to gain weight
　　　　AHA: 1Q, '03, 12

DEF: Organic failure to thrive: acute or chronic illness that interferes with nutritional intake, absorption, metabolism excretion and energy requirements. Nonorganic FTT is symptom of neglect or abuse.

√4ᵗʰ / √5ᵗʰ　Additional Digit Required　　Unspecified Code　　Other Specified Code　　Manifestation Code　　▶◀ Revised Text　　● New Code　　▲ Revised Code Title

2005 ICD•9•CM　　　　　　　　　　　　　　　　　　　　　　　　**February 2004 • Volume 1 — 241**

783.42 Delayed milestones   P
Late talker   Late walker

783.43 Short stature
Growth failure   Lack of growth
Growth retardation   Physical retardation
DEF: Constitutional short stature: stature inconsistent with chronological age. Genetic short stature is when skeletal maturation matches chronological age.

783.5 Polydipsia
Excessive thirst

783.6 Polyphagia
Excessive eating   Hyperalimentation NOS
EXCLUDES   disorders of eating of nonorganic origin (307.50-307.59)

783.7 Adult failure to thrive   A

783.9 Other symptoms concerning nutrition, metabolism, and development
Hypometabolism
EXCLUDES   abnormal basal metabolic rate (794.7)
dehydration (276.5)
other disorders of fluid, electrolyte, and acid-base balance (276.0-276.9)

✓4th **784 Symptoms involving head and neck**
EXCLUDES   encephalopathy NOS (348.30)
specific symptoms involving neck classifiable to 723 (723.0-723.9)

784.0 Headache
Facial pain   Pain in head NOS
EXCLUDES   atypical face pain (350.2)
migraine (346.0-346.9)
tension headache (307.81)
AHA: 3Q, '00, 13; 1Q, '90, 4; 3Q, '92, 14

784.1 Throat pain
EXCLUDES   dysphagia (787.2)
neck pain (723.1)
sore throat (462)
chronic (472.1)

784.2 Swelling, mass, or lump in head and neck
Space-occupying lesion, intracranial NOS
AHA: 1Q, '03, 8

784.3 Aphasia
EXCLUDES   developmental aphasia (315.31)
AHA: 4Q. '98, 87; 3Q, '97, 12
DEF: Inability to communicate through speech, written word, or sign language.

✓5th **784.4 Voice disturbance**

784.40 Voice disturbance, unspecified

784.41 Aphonia
Loss of voice

784.49 Other
Change in voice   Hypernasality
Dysphonia   Hyponasality
Hoarseness

784.5 Other speech disturbance
Dysarthria   Slurred speech
Dysphasia
EXCLUDES   stammering and stuttering (307.0)
that of nonorganic origin (307.0, 307.9)

✓5th **784.6 Other symbolic dysfunction**
EXCLUDES   developmental learning delays (315.0-315.9)

784.60 Symbolic dysfunction, unspecified

784.61 Alexia and dyslexia
Alexia (with agraphia)
DEF: Alexia: inability to understand written word due to central brain lesion.
DEF: Dyslexia: ability to recognize letters but inability to read, spell, and write words; genetic.

784.69 Other
Acalculia   Agraphia NOS
Agnosia   Apraxia

784.7 Epistaxis
Hemorrhage from nose   Nosebleed

784.8 Hemorrhage from throat
EXCLUDES   hemoptysis (786.3)

784.9 Other symptoms involving head and neck
Choking sensation   Mouth breathing
Halitosis   Sneezing

✓4th **785 Symptoms involving cardiovascular system**
EXCLUDES   heart failure NOS (428.9)

785.0 Tachycardia, unspecified
Rapid heart beat
EXCLUDES   neonatal tachycardia (779.82)
paroxysmal tachycardia (427.0-427.2)
AHA: 2Q, '03, 11
DEF: Excessively rapid heart rate.

785.1 Palpitations
Awareness of heart beat
EXCLUDES   specified dysrhythmias (427.0-427.9)
DEF: Shock syndrome: associated with myocardial infarction, cardiac tamponade and massive pulmonary embolism; symptoms include mental torpor, reduced blood pressure, tachycardia, pallor and cold, clammy skin.

785.2 Undiagnosed cardiac murmurs
Heart murmurs NOS
AHA: 4Q, '92, 16

785.3 Other abnormal heart sounds
Cardiac dullness, increased or decreased
Friction fremitus, cardiac
Precordial friction

785.4 Gangrene
Gangrene:
NOS
spreading cutaneous
Gangrenous cellulitis
Phagedena
Code first any associated underlying condition
EXCLUDES   gangrene of certain sites — see Alphabetic Index
gangrene with atherosclerosis of the extremities (440.24)
gas gangrene (040.0)
AHA: ▶1Q, '04, 14;◀ 3Q, '91, 12; 3Q, '90, 15; M-A, '86, 12
DEF: Gangrene: necrosis of skin tissue due to bacterial infection, diabetes, embolus and vascular supply loss.
DEF: Gangrenous cellulitis: group A streptococcal infection; begins with severe cellulitis, spreads to superficial and deep fascia; produces gangrene of underlying tissues.

✓5th **785.5 Shock without mention of trauma**

785.50 Shock, unspecified
Failure of peripheral circulation
AHA: 2Q, '96, 10

785.51 Cardiogenic shock
DEF: Peripheral circulatory failure due to heart insufficiencies.

785.52 Septic shock
Shock:
▶endotoxic
gram-negative◀
▶Code first:
systemic inflammatory response syndrome due to infectious process with organ dysfunction (995.92)
systemic inflammatory response syndrome due to non-infectious process with organ dysfunction (995.94)◀
AHA: 4Q, '03, 73, 79

| N Newborn Age: 0 | P Pediatric Age: 0-17 | M Maternity Age: 12-55 | A Adult Age: 15-124 | MSP Medicare Secondary Payer |

242 — Volume 1 • October 2004

2005 ICD•9•CM

785.59 Other
Shock:
hypovolemic

EXCLUDES shock (due to):
anesthetic (995.4)
anaphylactic (995.0)
due to serum (999.4)
electric (994.8)
following abortion (639.5)
lightning (994.0)
obstetrical (669.1)
postoperative (998.0)
traumatic (958.4)

AHA: 2Q, '00, 3

785.6 Enlargement of lymph nodes
Lymphadenopathy   "Swollen glands"

EXCLUDES lymphadenitis (chronic) (289.1-289.3)
acute (683)

785.9 Other symptoms involving cardiovascular system
Bruit (arterial)   Weak pulse

✓4ᵗʰ 786 Symptoms involving respiratory system and other chest symptoms

✓5ᵗʰ 786.0 Dyspnea and respiratory abnormalities

786.00 Respiratory abnormality, unspecified

786.01 Hyperventilation

EXCLUDES hyperventilation, psychogenic (306.1)

DEF: Rapid breathing causes carbon dioxide loss from blood.

786.02 Orthopnea
DEF: Difficulty breathing except in upright position.

786.03 Apnea

EXCLUDES apnea of newborn (770.81, 770.82)
sleep apnea (780.51, 780.53, 780.57)

AHA: 4Q, '98, 50

DEF: Cessation of breathing.

786.04 Cheyne-Stokes respiration
AHA: 4Q, '98, 50

DEF: Rhythmic increase of depth and frequency of breathing with apnea; occurs in frontal lobe and diencephalic dysfunction.

786.05 Shortness of breath
AHA: 4Q, '99, 25; 1Q, '99, 6; 4Q, '98, 50

DEF: Inability to take in sufficient oxygen.

786.06 Tachypnea

EXCLUDES transitory tachypnea of newborn (770.6)

AHA: 4Q, '98, 50

DEF: Abnormal rapid respiratory rate; called hyperventilation.

786.07 Wheezing

EXCLUDES asthma (493.00-493.92)

AHA: 4Q, '98, 50

DEF: Stenosis of respiratory passageway; causes whistling sound; due to asthma, coryza, croup, emphysema, hay fever, edema, and pleural effusion.

786.09 Other

EXCLUDES respiratory distress:
following trauma and surgery (518.5)
newborn (770.89)
syndrome (newborn) (769)
adult (518.5)
respiratory failure (518.81, 518.83-518.84)
newborn (770.84)

AHA: 2Q, '98, 10; 1Q, '97, 7; 1Q, '90, 9

786.1 Stridor

EXCLUDES congenital laryngeal stridor (748.3)

DEF: Obstructed airway causes harsh sound.

786.2 Cough

EXCLUDES cough:
psychogenic (306.1)
smokers' (491.0)
with hemorrhage (786.3)

AHA: 4Q, '99, 26

786.3 Hemoptysis
Cough with hemorrhage
Pulmonary hemorrhage NOS

EXCLUDES pulmonary hemorrhage of newborn (770.3)

AHA: 4Q, '90, 26

DEF: Coughing up blood or blood-stained sputum.

786.4 Abnormal sputum
Abnormal:
amount
color   (of) sputum
odor
Excessive

✓5ᵗʰ 786.5 Chest pain

786.50 Chest pain, unspecified
AHA: 1Q, '03, 6; 1Q, '02, 4; 4Q, '99, 25

786.51 Precordial pain
DEF: Chest pain over heart and lower thorax.

786.52 Painful respiration
Pain: Pleurodynia
anterior chest wall
pleuritic

EXCLUDES epidemic pleurodynia (074.1)

AHA: N-D, '84, 17

786.59 Other
Discomfort
Pressure   } in chest
Tightness

EXCLUDES pain in breast (611.71)

AHA: 1Q, '02, 6

786.6 Swelling, mass, or lump in chest

EXCLUDES lump in breast (611.72)

786.7 Abnormal chest sounds
Abnormal percussion, chest   Rales
Friction sounds, chest   Tympany, chest

EXCLUDES wheezing (786.07)

786.8 Hiccough

EXCLUDES psychogenic hiccough (306.1)

786.9 Other symptoms involving respiratory system and chest
Breath-holding spell

✓4ᵗʰ 787 Symptoms involving digestive system

EXCLUDES constipation (564.00-564.09)
pylorospasm (537.81)
congenital (750.5)

✓5ᵗʰ 787.0 Nausea and vomiting
Emesis

EXCLUDES hematemesis NOS (578.0)
vomiting:
bilious, following gastrointestinal surgery (564.3)
cyclical (536.2)
psychogenic (306.4)
excessive, in pregnancy (643.0-643.9)
habit (536.2)
of newborn (779.3)
psychogenic NOS (307.54)

AHA: M-A, '85, 11

✓4ᵗʰ ✓5ᵗʰ **Additional Digit Required**   **Unspecified Code**   **Other Specified Code**   **Manifestation Code**   ►◄ Revised Text   ● New Code   ▲ Revised Code Title

2005 ICD•9•CM   **Volume 1 — 243**

Symptoms, Signs, and Ill-Defined Conditions

787.01 Nausea with vomiting
AHA: 1Q, '03, 5

787.02 Nausea alone
AHA: 3Q, '00, 12; 2Q, '97, 9

787.03 Vomiting alone

787.1 Heartburn
Pyrosis   Waterbrash
EXCLUDES   dyspepsia or indigestion (536.8)
AHA: 2Q, '01, 6

787.2 Dysphagia
Difficulty in swallowing
AHA: 4Q, '03, 103, 109; 2Q, '01, 4

787.3 Flatulence, eructation, and gas pain
Abdominal distention (gaseous)
Bloating
Tympanites (abdominal) (intestinal)
EXCLUDES   aerophagy (306.4)
DEF: Flatulence: excess air or gas in intestine or stomach.
DEF: Eructation: belching, expelling gas through mouth.
DEF: Gas pain: gaseous pressure affecting gastrointestinal system.

787.4 Visible peristalsis
Hyperperistalsis
DEF: Increase in involuntary movements of intestines.

787.5 Abnormal bowel sounds
Absent bowel sounds
Hyperactive bowel sounds

787.6 Incontinence of feces
Encopresis NOS
Incontinence of sphincter ani
EXCLUDES   that of nonorganic origin (307.7)
AHA: 1Q, '97, 9

787.7 Abnormal feces
Bulky stools
EXCLUDES   abnormal stool content (792.1)
melena:
NOS (578.1)
newborn (772.4, 777.3)

√5th 787.9 Other symptoms involving digestive system
EXCLUDES   gastrointestinal hemorrhage (578.0-578.9)
intestinal obstruction (560.0-560.9)
specific functional digestive disorders:
esophagus (530.0-530.9)
stomach and duodenum (536.0-536.9)
those not elsewhere classified (564.00-564.9)

787.91 Diarrhea
Diarrhea NOS
AHA: 4Q, '95, 54

787.99 Other
Change in bowel habits
Tenesmus (rectal)
DEF: Tenesmus: painful, ineffective straining at the rectum with limited passage of fecal matter.

√4th 788 Symptoms involving urinary system
EXCLUDES   hematuria (599.7)
nonspecific findings on examination of the urine (791.0-791.9)
small kidney of unknown cause (589.0-589.9)
uremia NOS (586)

788.0 Renal colic
Colic (recurrent) of: Colic (recurrent) of:
kidney   ureter
DEF: Kidney pain.

788.1 Dysuria
Painful urination   Strangury

√5th 788.2 Retention of urine
DEF: Inability to void.

788.20 Retention of urine, unspecified
AHA: 3Q, '03, 12-13; 1Q, '03, 6; 3Q, '96, 10

788.21 Incomplete bladder emptying

788.29 Other specified retention of urine

▲ √5th 788.3 Urinary incontinence
Code, if applicable, any causal condition first, such as:
congenital ureterocele (753.23)
genital prolapse ▶(618.00-618.9)◀
EXCLUDES   that of nonorganic origin (307.6)
AHA: 4Q, '92, 22

788.30 Urinary incontinence, unspecified
Enuresis NOS

788.31 Urge incontinence
AHA: 1Q, '00, 19
DEF: Inability to control urination, upon urge to urinate.

788.32 Stress incontinence, male   ♂
EXCLUDES   stress incontinence, female (625.6)
DEF: Inability to control urination associated with weak sphincter in males.

788.33 Mixed incontinence, (male) (female)
Urge and stress
DEF: Urge, stress incontinence: involuntary discharge of urine due to anatomic displacement.

788.34 Incontinence without sensory awareness
DEF: Involuntary discharge of urine without sensory warning.

788.35 Post-void dribbling
DEF: Involuntary discharge of residual urine after voiding.

788.36 Nocturnal enuresis
DEF: Involuntary discharge of urine during the night.

788.37 Continuous leakage
DEF: Continuous, involuntary urine seepage.

788.38 Overflow incontinence

788.39 Other urinary incontinence

√5th 788.4 Frequency of urination and polyuria

788.41 Urinary frequency
Frequency of micturition

788.42 Polyuria
DEF: Excessive urination.

788.43 Nocturia
DEF: Urination affecting sleep patterns.

788.5 Oliguria and anuria
Deficient secretion of urine
Suppression of urinary secretion
EXCLUDES   that complicating:
abortion (634-638 with .3, 639.3)
ectopic or molar pregnancy (639.3)
pregnancy, childbirth, or the puerperium (642.0-642.9, 646.2)
DEF: Oliguria: diminished urinary secretion related to fluid intake.
DEF: Anuria: lack of urinary secretion due to renal failure or obstructed urinary tract.

√5th 788.6 Other abnormality of urination

788.61 Splitting of urinary stream
Intermittent urinary stream

788.62 Slowing of urinary stream
Weak stream

788.63 Urgency of urination
EXCLUDES   urge incontinence (788.31, 788.33)
AHA: 4Q, '03, 74

788.69 Other

N Newborn Age: 0   P Pediatric Age: 0-17   M Maternity Age: 12-55   A Adult Age: 15-124   MSP Medicare Secondary Payer

788.7   **Urethral discharge**
Penile discharge   Urethrorrhea

788.8   **Extravasation of urine**
DEF: Leaking or infiltration of urine into tissues.

788.9   **Other symptoms involving urinary system**
Extrarenal uremia   Vesical:
Vesical: tenesmus
pain
AHA: 4Q, '88, 1

√4ᵗʰ **789 Other symptoms involving abdomen and pelvis**
EXCLUDES   *symptoms referable to genital organs:*
female (625.0-625.9)
male (607.0-608.9)
psychogenic (302.70-302.79)

The following fifth-digit subclassification is to be used for codes 789.0, 789.3, 789.4, 789.6:
0   **unspecified site**
1   **right upper quadrant**
2   **left upper quadrant**
3   **right lower quadrant**
4   **left lower quadrant**
5   **periumbilic**
6   **epigastric**
7   **generalized**
9   **other specified site**
     Multiple sites

√5ᵗʰ **789.0**   **Abdominal pain**
Colic: Cramps, abdominal
NOS
infantile
EXCLUDES   *renal colic (788.0)*
AHA: 1Q, '95, 3; **For code 789.06:** 1Q, '02, 5

789.1   **Hepatomegaly**
Enlargement of liver

789.2   **Splenomegaly**
Enlargement of spleen

√5ᵗʰ **789.3**   **Abdominal or pelvic swelling, mass, or lump**
Diffuse or generalized swelling or mass:
abdominal NOS   umbilical
EXCLUDES   *abdominal distention (gaseous) (787.3)*
ascites (789.5)

√5ᵗʰ **789.4**   **Abdominal rigidity**

789.5   **Ascites**
Fluid in peritoneal cavity
AHA: 4Q, '89, 11
DEF: Serous fluid effusion and accumulation in abdominal cavity.

√5ᵗʰ **789.6**   **Abdominal tenderness**
Rebound tenderness

789.9   **Other symptoms involving abdomen and pelvis**
Umbilical: Umbilical:
bleeding   discharge

NONSPECIFIC ABNORMAL FINDINGS (790-796)
AHA: 2Q, '90, 16

√4ᵗʰ **790 Nonspecific findings on examination of blood**
EXCLUDES   *abnormality of:*
platelets (287.0-287.9)
thrombocytes (287.0-287.9)
white blood cells (288.0-288.9)

√5ᵗʰ **790.0**   **Abnormality of red blood cells**
EXCLUDES   *anemia:*
congenital (776.5)
newborn, due to isoimmunization
(773.0-773.2, 773.5)
of premature infant (776.6)
other specified types (280.0-285.9)
hemoglobin disorders (282.5-282.7)
polycythemia:
familial (289.6)
neonatorum (776.4)
secondary (289.0)
vera (238.4)
AHA: 4Q, '00, 46

790.01   **Precipitous drop in hematocrit**
Drop in hematocrit

790.09   **Other abnormality of red blood cells**
Abnormal red cell morphology NOS
Abnormal red cell volume NOS
Anisocytosis
Poikilocytosis

790.1   **Elevated sedimentation rate**

√5ᵗʰ **790.2**   **Abnormal glucose**
EXCLUDES   *diabetes mellitus (250.00-250.93)*
dysmetabolic syndrome X (277.7)
gestational diabetes (648.8)
glycosuria (791.5)
hypoglycemia (251.2)
that complicating pregnancy, childbirth,
or puerperium (648.8)
AHA: ►4Q, '03, 74;◄ 3Q, '91, 5

790.21   **Impaired fasting glucose**
Elevated fasting glucose

790.22   **Impaired glucose tolerance test (oral)**
Elevated glucose tolerance test

790.29   **Other abnormal glucose**
Abnormal glucose NOS
Abnormal non-fasting glucose
Pre-diabetes NOS

790.3   **Excessive blood level of alcohol**
Elevated blood-alcohol
AHA: S-O, '86, 3

790.4   **Nonspecific elevation of levels of transaminase or lactic acid dehydrogenase [LDH]**

790.5   **Other nonspecific abnormal serum enzyme levels**
Abnormal serum level of:
acid phosphatase
alkaline phosphatase
amylase
lipase
EXCLUDES   *deficiency of circulating enzymes*
(277.6)

790.6   **Other abnormal blood chemistry**
Abnormal blood level of: Abnormal blood level of:
cobalt   magnesium
copper   mineral
iron   zinc
lithium
EXCLUDES   *abnormality of electrolyte or acid-base*
balance (276.0-276.9)
hypoglycemia NOS (251.2)
specific finding indicating abnormality of:
amino-acid transport and
metabolism (270.0-270.9)
carbohydrate transport and
metabolism (271.0-271.9)
lipid metabolism (272.0-272.9)
uremia NOS (586)
AHA: 4Q, '88, 1

790.7   **Bacteremia**
EXCLUDES   *bacteremia of newborn (771.83)*
septicemia (038)
Use additional code to identify organism (041)
AHA: 2Q, '03, 7; 4Q, '93, 29; 3Q, '88, 12
DEF: Laboratory finding of bacteria in the blood in the absence of two or more signs of sepsis; transient in nature, progresses to septicemia with severe infectious process.

790.8   **Viremia, unspecified**
AHA: 4Q, '88, 10
DEF: Presence of a virus in the blood stream.

√5ᵗʰ **790.9**   **Other nonspecific findings on examination of blood**
AHA: 4Q, '93, 29

790.91   **Abnormal arterial blood gases**

√4ᵗʰ √5ᵗʰ Additional Digit Required   Unspecified Code   Other Specified Code   Manifestation Code   ►◄ Revised Text   ● New Code   ▲ Revised Code Title

2005 ICD•9•CM   **February 2004 • Volume 1 — 245**

Symptoms, Signs, and Ill-Defined Conditions

790.92–794.09

790.92 Abnormal coagulation profile
Abnormal or prolonged:
bleeding time
coagulation time
partial thromboplastin time [PTT]
prothrombintime [PT]
EXCLUDES   coagulation (hemorrhagic)
disorders (286.0-286.9)

790.93 Elevated prostate specific antigen, (PSA) A ♂

790.94 Euthyroid sick syndrome
AHA: 4Q, '97, 45
DEF: Transient alteration of thyroid hormone metabolism due to nonthyroid illness or stress.

790.95 Elevated C-reactive protein (CRP)

790.99 Other
AHA: 2Q, '03, 14

✓4th **791 Nonspecific findings on examination of urine**
EXCLUDES   hematuria NOS (599.7)
specific findings indicating abnormality of:
amino-acid transport and metabolism (270.0-270.9)
carbohydrate transport and metabolism (271.0-271.9)

791.0 Proteinuria
Albuminuria
Bence-Jones proteinuria
EXCLUDES   postural proteinuria (593.6)
that arising during pregnancy or the puerperium (642.0-642.9, 646.2)
AHA: 3Q, '91, 8
DEF: Excess protein in urine.

791.1 Chyluria
EXCLUDES   filarial (125.0-125.9)
DEF: Excess chyle in urine.

791.2 Hemoglobinuria
DEF: Free hemoglobin in blood due to rapid hemolysis of red blood cells.

791.3 Myoglobinuria
DEF: Myoglobin (oxygen-transporting pigment) in urine.

791.4 Biliuria
DEF: Bile pigments in urine.

791.5 Glycosuria
EXCLUDES   renal glycosuria (271.4)
DEF: Sugar in urine.

791.6 Acetonuria
Ketonuria
DEF: Excess acetone in urine.

791.7 Other cells and casts in urine

791.9 Other nonspecific findings on examination of urine
Crystalluria   Elevated urine levels of:
Elevated urine levels of: vanillylmandelic
17-ketosteroids   acid [VMA]
catecholamines   Melanuria
indolacetic acid

✓4th **792 Nonspecific abnormal findings in other body substances**
EXCLUDES   that in chromosomal analysis (795.2)

792.0 Cerebrospinal fluid

792.1 Stool contents
Abnormal stool color   Occult stool
Fat in stool   Pus in stool
Mucus in stool
EXCLUDES   blood in stool [melena] (578.1)
newborn (772.4, 777.3)
AHA: 2Q, '92, 9

792.2 Semen   ♂
Abnormal spermatozoa
EXCLUDES   azoospermia (606.0)
oligospermia (606.1)

792.3 Amniotic fluid   M ♀
AHA: N-D, '86, 4
DEF: Nonspecific abnormal findings in amniotic fluid.

792.4 Saliva
EXCLUDES   that in chromosomal analysis (795.2)

792.5 Cloudy (hemodialysis) (peritoneal) dialysis effluent

792.9 Other nonspecific abnormal findings in body substances
Peritoneal fluid   Synovial fluid
Pleural fluid   Vaginal fluids

✓4th **793 Nonspecific abnormal findings on radiological and other examination of body structure**
INCLUDES   nonspecific abnormal findings of:
thermography
ultrasound examination [echogram]
x-ray examination
EXCLUDES   abnormal results of function studies and radioisotope scans (794.0-794.9)

793.0 Skull and head
EXCLUDES   nonspecific abnormal echoencephalogram (794.01)

793.1 Lung field
Coin lesion
Shadow   } (of) lung
DEF: Coin lesion of lung: coin-shaped, solitary pulmonary nodule.

793.2 Other intrathoracic organ
Abnormal: Abnormal:
echocardiogram   ultrasound cardiogram
heart shadow   Mediastinal shift

793.3 Biliary tract
Nonvisualization of gallbladder

793.4 Gastrointestinal tract

793.5 Genitourinary organs
Filling defect: Filling defect:
bladder   ureter
kidney
AHA: 4Q, '00, 46

793.6 Abdominal area, including retroperitoneum

793.7 Musculoskeletal system

✓5th **793.8 Breast**
AHA: 4Q, '01, 51

793.80 Abnormal mammogram, unspecified

793.81 Mammographic microcalcification
DEF: Calcium and cellular debris deposits in the breast that can't be felt but are detected on a mammogram; can be a sign of cancer, benign conditions, or changes in the breast tissue as a result of inflammation, injury, or obstructed duct.

793.89 Other abnormal findings on radiological examination of breast

793.9 Other
Abnormal:
placental finding by x-ray or ultrasound method
radiological findings in skin and subcutaneous tissue
EXCLUDES   abnormal finding by radioisotope localization of placenta (794.9)

✓4th **794 Nonspecific abnormal results of function studies**
INCLUDES   radioisotope:
scans
uptake studies
scintiphotography

✓5th **794.0 Brain and central nervous system**

794.00 Abnormal function study, unspecified

794.01 Abnormal echoencephalogram

794.02 Abnormal electroencephalogram [EEG]

794.09 Other
Abnormal brain scan

N Newborn Age: 0   P Pediatric Age: 0-17   M Maternity Age: 12-55   A Adult Age: 15-124   MSP Medicare Secondary Payer

✓5ᵗʰ **794.1 Peripheral nervous system and special senses**

794.10 Abnormal response to nerve stimulation, unspecified

794.11 Abnormal retinal function studies
Abnormal electroretinogram [ERG]

794.12 Abnormal electro-oculogram [EOG]

794.13 Abnormal visually evoked potential

794.14 Abnormal oculomotor studies

794.15 Abnormal auditory function studies
AHA: ▶1Q, '04, 15-16◀

794.16 Abnormal vestibular function studies

794.17 Abnormal electromyogram [EMG]
EXCLUDES *that of eye (794.14)*

794.19 Other

794.2 Pulmonary
Abnormal lung scan   Reduced:
Reduced: vital capacity
ventilatory capacity

✓5ᵗʰ **794.3 Cardiovascular**

794.30 Abnormal function study, unspecified

794.31 Abnormal electrocardiogram [ECG] [EKG]

794.39 Other
Abnormal: Abnormal:
ballistocardiogram   vectorcardiogram
phonocardiogram

794.4 Kidney
Abnormal renal function test

794.5 Thyroid
Abnormal thyroid: Abnormal thyroid:
scan   uptake

794.6 Other endocrine function study

794.7 Basal metabolism
Abnormal basal metabolic rate [BMR]

794.8 Liver
Abnormal liver scan

794.9 Other
Bladder   Placenta
Pancreas   Spleen

▲ ✓4ᵗʰ **795 Other and nonspecific abnormal cytological, histological, immunological and DNA test findings**
EXCLUDES *nonspecific abnormalities of red blood cells (790.01-790.09)*

▲ ✓5ᵗʰ **795.0 Abnormal Papanicolaou smear of cervix and cervical HPV**
▶Abnormal thin preparation smear of cervix
Abnormal cervical cytology◀
EXCLUDES *carcinoma in-situ of cervix (233.1)*
cervical intraepithelial neoplasia I (CIN I) ▶(622.11)◀
cervical intraepithelial neoplasia II (CIN II) ▶(622.12)◀
cervical intraepithelial neoplasia III (CIN III) (233.1)
▶dyplasia (histologically confirmed) of cervix (uteri) NOS (622.10)◀
▶mild dysplasia (histologically confirmed) (622.11)
moderate dysplasia (histologically confirmed) (622.12)
severe dysplasia (histologically confirmed) (233.1)◀
AHA: 4Q, '02, 69

▲ **795.00 Abnormal glandular Papanicolaou smear of cervix** ♀
▶Atypical endocervical cells NOS
Atypical endometrial cells NOS
Atypical glandular cells NOS◀

▲ **795.01 Papanicolaou smear of cervix with atypical squamous cells of undetermined significance (ASC-US)** ♀

▲ **795.02 Papanicolaou smear of cervix with atypical squamous cells cannot exclude high grade squamous intraepithelial lesion (ASC-H)** ♀

● **795.03 Papanicolaou smear of cervix with low grade squamous intraepithelial lesion (LGSIL)** ♀

● **795.04 Papanicolaou smear of cervix with high grade squamous intraepithelial lesion (HGSIL)** ♀
Cytologic evidence of carcinoma

● **795.05 Cervical high risk human papillomavirus (HPV) DNA test positive** ♀

● **795.08 Unsatisfactory smear** ♀
Inadequate sample

▲ **795.09 Other abnormal Papanicolaou smear of cervix and cervical HPV** ♀
▶Papanicolaou smear of cervix with low risk human papillomavirus (HPV) DNA test positive
Use additional code for associated human papillomavirus (079.4)◀
EXCLUDES ▶ *encounter for Papanicolaou cervical smear to confirm findings of recent normal smear following initial abnormal smear (V72.32)◀*

795.1 Nonspecific abnormal Papanicolaou smear of other site

795.2 Nonspecific abnormal findings on chromosomal analysis
Abnormal karyotype

✓5ᵗʰ **795.3 Nonspecific positive culture findings**
Positive culture findings in:
nose   throat
sputum   wound
EXCLUDES *that of:*
blood (790.7-790.8)
urine (791.9)

795.31 Nonspecific positive findings for anthrax
Positive findings by nasal swab
AHA: 4Q, '02, 70

795.39 Other nonspecific positive culture findings

795.4 Other nonspecific abnormal histological findings

795.5 Nonspecific reaction to tuberculin skin test without active tuberculosis
Abnormal result of Mantoux test
PPD positive
Tuberculin (skin test):
positive
reactor

795.6 False positive serological test for syphilis
False positive Wassermann reaction

✓5ᵗʰ **795.7 Other nonspecific immunological findings**
EXCLUDES *isoimmunization, in pregnancy (656.1-656.2)*
affecting fetus or newborn (773.0-773.2)
AHA: 2Q, '93, 6

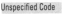
✓4ᵗʰ / ✓5ᵗʰ Additional Digit Required   Unspecified Code   Other Specified Code   Manifestation Code   ▶◀ Revised Text   ● New Code   ▲ Revised Code Title

2005 ICD•9•CM   October 2004 • Volume 1 — 247

Symptoms, Signs, and Ill-Defined Conditions

794.1–795.7

Symptoms, Signs, and Ill-Defined Conditions

795.71–799.9

795.71 Nonspecific serologic evidence of human immunodeficiency virus [HIV]
Inclusive human immunodeficiency [HIV] test (adult) (infant)
Note: This code is ONLY to be used when a test finding is reported as nonspecific. Asymptomatic positive findings are coded to V08. If any HIV infection symptom or condition is present, see code 042. Negative findings are not coded.

EXCLUDES acquired immunodeficiency syndrome [AIDS] (042)
asymptomatic human immunodeficiency virus, [HIV] infection status (V08)
HIV infection, symptomatic (042)
human immunodeficiency virus [HIV] disease (042)
positive (status) NOS (V08)

AHA: 1Q, '93, 21; 1Q, '93, 22; 2Q, '92, 11; J-A, '87, 24

795.79 Other and unspecified nonspecific immunological findings
Raised antibody titer
Raised level of immunoglobulins

✓4th **796 Other nonspecific abnormal findings**

796.0 Nonspecific abnormal toxicological findings
Abnormal levels of heavy metals or drugs in blood, urine, or other tissue
EXCLUDES excessive blood level of alcohol (790.3)
AHA: 1Q, '97, 16

796.1 Abnormal reflex

796.2 Elevated blood pressure reading without diagnosis of hypertension
Note: This category is to be used to record an episode of elevated blood pressure in a patient in whom no formal diagnosis of hypertension has been made, or as an incidental finding.
AHA: 2Q, '03, 11; 3Q, '90, 4; J-A, '84, 12

796.3 Nonspecific low blood pressure reading

796.4 Other abnormal clinical findings
AHA: 1Q, '97, 16

796.5 Abnormal finding on antenatal screening   M ♀
AHA: 4Q, '97, 46

796.6 Abnormal findings on neonatal screening
EXCLUDES nonspecific serologic evidence of human immunodeficiency virus [HIV] (795.71)

796.9 Other

ILL-DEFINED AND UNKNOWN CAUSES OF MORBIDITY AND MORTALITY (797-799)

797 Senility without mention of psychosis
Old age   Senile:
Senescence   debility
Senile asthenia   exhaustion
EXCLUDES senile psychoses (290.0-290.9)

✓4th **798 Sudden death, cause unknown**

798.0 Sudden infant death syndrome   P
Cot death   Sudden death of nonspecific
Crib death   cause in infancy
DEF: Sudden Infant Death Syndrome (SIDS): death of infant under age one due to nonspecific cause.

798.1 Instantaneous death

798.2 Death occurring in less than 24 hours from onset of symptoms, not otherwise explained
Death known not to be violent or instantaneous, for which no cause could be discovered
Died without sign of disease

798.9 Unattended death
Death in circumstances where the body of the deceased was found and no cause could be discovered
Found dead

✓4th **799 Other ill-defined and unknown causes of morbidity and mortality**
DEF: Weakened organ functions due to complex chronic medical conditions.

799.0 Asphyxia
EXCLUDES asphyxia (due to):
carbon monoxide (986)
inhalation of food or foreign body (932-934.9)
newborn (768.0-768.9)
traumatic (994.7)
DEF: Lack of oxygen.

799.1 Respiratory arrest
Cardiorespiratory failure
EXCLUDES cardiac arrest (427.5)
failure of peripheral circulation (785.50)
respiratory distress:
NOS (786.09)
acute (518.82)
following trauma and surgery (518.5)
newborn (770.89)
syndrome (newborn) (769)
adult (following trauma and surgery) (518.5)
other (518.82)
respiratory failure (518.81, 518.83-518.84)
newborn (770.84)
respiratory insufficiency (786.09)
acute (518.82)

799.2 Nervousness
"Nerves"

799.3 Debility, unspecified
EXCLUDES asthenia (780.79)
nervous debility (300.5)
neurasthenia (300.5)
senile asthenia (797)

799.4 Cachexia
Wasting disease
EXCLUDES nutritional marasmus (261)
AHA: 3Q, '90, 17

✓5th **799.8 Other ill-defined conditions**

799.81 Decreased libido   A
Decreased sexual desire
EXCLUDES psychosexual dysfunction with inhibited sexual desire (302.71)
AHA: 4Q, '03, 75

799.89 Other ill-defined conditions
DEF: General ill health and poor nutrition.

799.9 Other unknown and unspecified cause
Undiagnosed disease, not specified as to site or system involved
Unknown cause of morbidity or mortality
AHA: 1Q, '98,.4; 1Q, '90, 20

N Newborn Age: 0   P Pediatric Age: 0-17   M Maternity Age: 12-55   A Adult Age: 15-124   MSP Medicare Secondary Payer

17. INJURY AND POISONING (800-999)

Use E code(s) to identify the cause and intent of the injury or poisoning (E800-E999)

Note:

1. The principle of multiple coding of injuries should be followed wherever possible. Combination categories for multiple injuries are provided for use when there is insufficient detail as to the nature of the individual conditions, or for primary tabulation purposes when it is more convenient to record a single code; otherwise, the component injuries should be coded separately.

   Where multiple sites of injury are specified in the titles, the word "with" indicates involvement of both sites, and the word "and" indicates involvement of either or both sites. The word "finger" thumb.

2. Categories for "late effect" of injuries are to be found at 905-909.

FRACTURES (800-829)

EXCLUDES	malunion (733.81)
	nonunion (733.82)
	pathological or spontaneous fracture (733.10-733.19)
	stress fractures (733.93-733.95)

The terms "condyle," "coronoid process," "ramus," and "symphysis" indicate the portion of the bone fractured, not the name of the bone involved.

The descriptions "closed" and "open" used in the fourth-digit subdivisions include the following terms:

closed (with or without delayed healing):

comminuted	impacted
depressed	linear
elevated	simple
fissured	slipped epiphysis
fracture NOS	spiral
greenstick	

open (with or without delayed healing):

compound	puncture
infected	with foreign body
missile	

A fracture not indicated as closed or open should be classified as closed.

AHA: 4Q, '90, 26; 3Q, '90, 5; 3Q, '90, 13; 2Q, '90, 7; 2Q, '89, 15, S-O, '85, 3

FRACTURE OF SKULL (800-804)

The following fifth-digit subclassification is for use with the appropriate codes in categories 800, 801, 803, and 804:

0　unspecified state of consciousness
1　with no loss of consciousness
2　with brief [less than one hour] loss of consciousness
3　with moderate [1-24 hours] loss of consciousness
4　with prolonged [more than 24 hours] loss of consciousness and return to pre-existing conscious level
5　with prolonged [more than 24 hours] loss of consciousness, without return to pre-existing conscious level

　　Use fifth-digit 5 to designate when a patient is unconscious and dies before regaining consciousness, regardless of the duration of the loss of consciousness

6　with loss of consciousness of unspecified duration

9　with concussion, unspecified

✓4ᵗʰ **800 Fracture of vault of skull**

INCLUDES	frontal bone
	parietal bone

AHA: 4Q, '96, 36

DEF: Fracture of bone that forms skull dome and protects brain.

Fractures

✓5ᵗʰ **800.0** Closed without mention of intracranial injury ⬛MSP
✓5ᵗʰ **800.1** Closed with cerebral laceration and contusion ⬛MSP
✓5ᵗʰ **800.2** Closed with subarachnoid, subdural, and extradural hemorrhage ⬛MSP
✓5ᵗʰ **800.3** Closed with other and unspecified intracranial hemorrhage ⬛MSP
✓5ᵗʰ **800.4** Closed with intracranial injury of other and unspecified nature ⬛MSP
✓5ᵗʰ **800.5** Open without mention of intracranial injury ⬛MSP
✓5ᵗʰ **800.6** Open with cerebral laceration and contusion ⬛MSP
✓5ᵗʰ **800.7** Open with subarachnoid, subdural, and extradural hemorrhage ⬛MSP
✓5ᵗʰ **800.8** Open with other and unspecified intracranial hemorrhage ⬛MSP
✓5ᵗʰ **800.9** Open with intracranial injury of other and unspecified nature ⬛MSP

✓4ᵗʰ **801 Fracture of base of skull**

INCLUDES	fossa:
	anterior
	middle
	posterior
	occiput bone
	orbital roof
	sinus:
	ethmoid
	frontal
	sphenoid bone
	temporal bone

AHA: 4Q, '96, 36

DEF: Fracture of bone that forms skull floor.

✓5ᵗʰ **801.0** Closed without mention of intracranial injury ⬛MSP
✓5ᵗʰ **801.1** Closed with cerebral laceration and contusion ⬛MSP
✓5ᵗʰ **801.2** Closed with subarachnoid, subdural, and extradural hemorrhage ⬛MSP
　　AHA: 4Q, '96, 36
✓5ᵗʰ **801.3** Closed with other and unspecified intracranial hemorrhage ⬛MSP
✓5ᵗʰ **801.4** Closed with intracranial injury of other and unspecified nature ⬛MSP
✓5ᵗʰ **801.5** Open without mention of intracranial injury ⬛MSP
✓5ᵗʰ **801.6** Open with cerebral laceration and contusion ⬛MSP
✓5ᵗʰ **801.7** Open with subarachnoid, subdural, and extradural hemorrhage ⬛MSP
✓5ᵗʰ **801.8** Open with other and unspecified intracranial hemorrhage ⬛MSP
✓5ᵗʰ **801.9** Open with intracranial injury of other and unspecified nature ⬛MSP

✓4ᵗʰ **802 Fracture of face bones**
　　AHA: 4Q, '96, 36

　　802.0 Nasal bones, closed ⬛MSP

✓4ᵗʰ / ✓5ᵗʰ Additional Digit Required　　Unspecified Code　　Other Specified Code　　Manifestation Code　　▶◀ Revised Text　　● New Code　　▲ Revised Code Title

2005 ICD•9•CM　　　　　　　　　　　　　　　　　　　　　　　　　　　　Volume 1 — 249

Injury and Poisoning

802.1–805

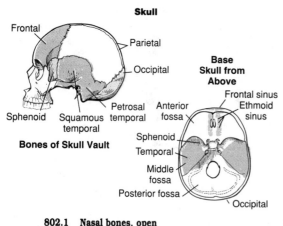

Skull

Frontal
Parietal
Occipital
Sphenoid
Squamous temporal
Petrosal temporal

Bones of Skull Vault

Base Skull from Above

Anterior fossa
Frontal sinus
Ethmoid sinus
Sphenoid
Temporal
Middle fossa
Posterior fossa
Occipital

Facial Fractures

Frontal bone
Nasal bone
LeFort Fracture Types
Orbital floor
Zygomatic bone (malar) and arch
Subcondylar
Body
Angle
Maxilla
Symphysis
Parasymphysis

Type III
Type II
Type I

Common Fracture Sites of Mandible

802.1	Nasal bones, open MSP
✓5th 802.2	Mandible, closed
	Inferior maxilla Lower jaw (bone)
802.20	Unspecified site MSP
802.21	Condylar process MSP
802.22	Subcondylar MSP
802.23	Coronoid process MSP
802.24	Ramus, unspecified MSP
802.25	Angle of jaw MSP
802.26	Symphysis of body MSP
802.27	Alveolar border of body MSP
802.28	Body, other and unspecified MSP
802.29	Multiple sites MSP
✓5th 802.3	Mandible, open
802.30	Unspecified site MSP
802.31	Condylar process MSP
802.32	Subcondylar MSP
802.33	Coronoid process MSP
802.34	Ramus, unspecified MSP
802.35	Angle of jaw MSP
802.36	Symphysis of body MSP
802.37	Alveolar border of body MSP
802.38	Body, other and unspecified MSP
802.39	Multiple sites MSP
802.4	Malar and maxillary bones, closed MSP
	Superior maxilla Zygoma
	Upper jaw (bone) Zygomatic arch
802.5	Malar and maxillary bones, open MSP
802.6	Orbital floor (blow-out), closed MSP
802.7	Orbital floor (blow-out), open MSP
802.8	Other facial bones, closed MSP

      Alveolus   Palate
      Orbit:
         NOS
         part other than roof or floor

    EXCLUDES   orbital:
          floor (802.6)
          roof (801.0-801.9)

802.9	Other facial bones, open MSP
✓4th 803	Other and unqualified skull fractures

    INCLUDES   skull NOS
              skull multiple NOS

    AHA: 4Q, '96, 36

§ ✓5th 803.0	Closed without mention of intracranial injury MSP
§ ✓5th 803.1	Closed with cerebral laceration and contusion MSP
§ ✓5th 803.2	Closed with subarachnoid, subdural, and extradural hemorrhage MSP
§ ✓5th 803.3	Closed with other and unspecified intracranial hemorrhage MSP

§ ✓5th 803.4	Closed with intracranial injury of other and unspecified nature MSP
§ ✓5th 803.5	Open without mention of intracranial injury MSP
§ ✓5th 803.6	Open with cerebral laceration and contusion MSP
§ ✓5th 803.7	Open with subarachnoid, subdural, and extradural hemorrhage MSP
§ ✓5th 803.8	Open with other and unspecified intracranial hemorrhage MSP
§ ✓5th 803.9	Open with intracranial injury of other and unspecified nature MSP
✓4th 804	Multiple fractures involving skull or face with other bones

    AHA: 4Q, '96, 36

§ ✓5th 804.0	Closed without mention of intracranial injury MSP
§ ✓5th 804.1	Closed with cerebral laceration and contusion MSP
§ ✓5th 804.2	Closed with subarachnoid, subdural, and extradural hemorrhage MSP
§ ✓5th 804.3	Closed with other and unspecified intracranial hemorrhage MSP
§ ✓5th 804.4	Closed with intracranial injury of other and unspecified nature MSP
§ ✓5th 804.5	Open without mention of intracranial injury MSP
§ ✓5th 804.6	Open with cerebral laceration and contusion MSP
§ ✓5th 804.7	Open with subarachnoid, subdural, and extradural hemorrage MSP
§ ✓5th 804.8	Open with other and unspecified intracranial hemorrhage MSP
§ ✓5th 804.9	Open with intracranial injury of other and unspecified nature MSP

FRACTURE OF NECK AND TRUNK (805-809)

✓4th 805	Fracture of vertebral column without mention of spinal cord injury

    INCLUDES   neural arch
              spine
              spinous process
              transverse process
              vertebra

The following fifth-digit subclassification is for use with codes 805.0-805.1:

   0   cervical vertebra, unspecified level
   1   first cervical vertebra
   2   second cervical vertebra
   3   third cervical vertebra
   4   fourth cervical vertebra
   5   fifth cervical vertebra
   6   sixth cervical vertebra
   7   seventh cervical vertebra
   8   multiple cervical vertebrae

§ Requires fifth-digit. See beginning of section 800–804 for codes and definitions.

√5th **805.0 Cervical, closed** `MSP`
       Atlas   Axis

√5th **805.1 Cervical, open** `MSP`

805.2 Dorsal [thoracic], closed `MSP`

805.3 Dorsal [thoracic], open `MSP`

805.4 Lumbar, closed `MSP`
       AHA: 4Q, '99, 12

805.5 Lumbar, open `MSP`

805.6 Sacrum and coccyx, closed `MSP`

805.7 Sacrum and coccyx, open `MSP`

805.8 Unspecified, closed `MSP`

805.9 Unspecified, open `MSP`

√4th **806 Fracture of vertebral column with spinal cord injury**
     `INCLUDES` any condition classifiable to 805 with:
           complete or incomplete transverse lesion (of cord)
           hematomyelia
           injury to:
               cauda equina
               nerve
           paralysis
           paraplegia
           quadriplegia
           spinal concussion

√5th **806.0 Cervical, closed**

     806.00 C_1-C_4 level with unspecified spinal cord injury `MSP`
          Cervical region NOS with spinal cord injury NOS

     806.01 C_1-C_4 level with complete lesion of cord `MSP`

     806.02 C_1-C_4 level with anterior cord syndrome `MSP`

     806.03 C_1-C_4 level with central cord syndrome `MSP`

     806.04 C_1-C_4 level with other specified spinal cord injury `MSP`
          C_1-C_4 level with:
              incomplete spinal cord lesion NOS
              posterior cord syndrome

     806.05 C_5-C_7 level with unspecified spinal cord injury `MSP`

     806.06 C_5-C_7 level with complete lesion of cord `MSP`

     806.07 C_5-C_7 level with anterior cord syndrome `MSP`

     806.08 C_5-C_7 level with central cord syndrome `MSP`

     806.09 C_5-C_7 level with other specified spinal cord injury `MSP`
          C_5-C_7 level with:
              incomplete spinal cord lesion NOS
              posterior cord syndrome

√5th **806.1 Cervical, open**

     806.10 C_1-C_4 level with unspecified spinal cord injury `MSP`

     806.11 C_1-C_4 level with complete lesion of cord `MSP`

     806.12 C_1-C_4 level with anterior cord syndrome `MSP`

     806.13 C_1-C_4 level with central cord syndrome `MSP`

     806.14 C_1-C_4 level with other specified spinal cord injury `MSP`
          C_1-C_4 level with:
              incomplete spinal cord lesion NOS
              posterior cord syndrome

Vertebral Column

     806.15 C_5-C_7 level with unspecified spinal cord injury `MSP`

     806.16 C_5-C_7 level with complete lesion of cord `MSP`

     806.17 C_5-C_7 level with anterior cord syndrome `MSP`

     806.18 C_5-C_7 level with central cord syndrome `MSP`

     806.19 C_5-C_7 level with other specified spinal cord injury `MSP`
          C_5-C_7 level with:
              incomplete spinal cord lesion NOS
              posterior cord syndrome

√5th **806.2 Dorsal [thoracic], closed**

     806.20 T_1-T_6 level with unspecified spinal cord injury `MSP`
          Thoracic region NOS with spinal cord injury NOS

     806.21 T_1-T_6 level with complete lesion of cord `MSP`

     806.22 T_1-T_6 level with anterior cord syndrome `MSP`

     806.23 T_1-T_6 level with central cord syndrome `MSP`

     806.24 T_1-T_6 level with other specified spinal cord injury `MSP`
          T_1-T_6 level with:
              incomplete spinal cord lesion NOS
              posterior cord syndrome

     806.25 T_7-T_{12} level with unspecified spinal cord injury `MSP`

     806.26 T_7-T_{12} level with complete lesion of cord `MSP`

     806.27 T_7-T_{12} level with anterior cord syndrome `MSP`

     806.28 T_7-T_{12} level with central cord syndrome `MSP`

√4th   Additional Digit Required   `Unspecified Code`   `Other Specified Code`   `Manifestation Code`   ►◄ Revised Text   ● New Code   ▲ Revised Code Title
√5th

Injury and Poisoning

806.29–810.1

806.29 T_7-T_{12} level with other specified spinal cord injury   `MSP`
     T_7-T_{12} level with:
         incomplete spinal cord lesion NOS
         posterior cord syndrome

✓5th **806.3** Dorsal [thoracic], open

     806.30 T_1-T_6 level with unspecified spinal cord injury   `MSP`

     806.31 T_1-T_6 level with complete lesion of cord   `MSP`

     806.32 T_1-T_6 level with anterior cord syndrome   `MSP`

     806.33 T_1-T_6 level with central cord syndrome   `MSP`

     806.34 T_1-T_6 level with other specified spinal cord injury   `MSP`
         T_1-T_6 level with:
            incomplete spinal cord lesion NOS
            posterior cord syndrome

     806.35 T_7-T_{12} level with unspecified spinal cord injury   `MSP`

     806.36 T_7-T_{12} level with complete lesion of cord   `MSP`

     806.37 T_7-T_{12} level with anterior cord syndrome   `MSP`

     806.38 T_7-T_{12} level with central cord syndrome   `MSP`

     806.39 T_7-T_{12} level with other specified spinal cord injury   `MSP`
         T_7-T_{12} level with:
            incomplete spinal cord lesion NOS
            posterior cord syndrome

806.4 Lumbar, closed   `MSP`
     AHA: 4Q, '99, 11, 13

806.5 Lumbar, open   `MSP`

✓5th **806.6** Sacrum and coccyx, closed

     806.60 With unspecified spinal cord injury   `MSP`

     806.61 With complete cauda equina lesion   `MSP`

     806.62 With other cauda equina injury   `MSP`

     806.69 With other spinal cord injury   `MSP`

✓5th **806.7** Sacrum and coccyx, open

     806.70 With unspecified spinal cord injury   `MSP`

     806.71 With complete cauda equina lesion   `MSP`

     806.72 With other cauda equina injury   `MSP`

     806.79 With other spinal cord injury   `MSP`

806.8 Unspecified, closed   `MSP`

806.9 Unspecified, open   `MSP`

✓4th **807** Fracture of rib(s), sternum, larynx, and trachea

     The following fifth-digit subclassification is for use with codes 807.0-807.1:

         0   rib(s), unspecified
         1   one rib
         2   two ribs
         3   three ribs
         4   four ribs
         5   five ribs
         6   six ribs
         7   seven ribs
         8   eight or more ribs
         9   multiple ribs, unspecified

✓5th **807.0** Rib(s), closed   `MSP`

✓5th **807.1** Rib(s), open   `MSP`

807.2 Sternum, closed   `MSP`
     DEF: Break in flat bone (breast bone) in anterior thorax.

807.3 Sternum, open   `MSP`
     DEF: Break, with open wound, in flat bone in mid anterior thorax.

807.4 Flail chest   `MSP`

807.5 Larynx and trachea, closed   `MSP`
     Hyoid bone   Trachea
     Thyroid cartilage

807.6 Larynx and trachea, open   `MSP`

✓4th **808** Fracture of pelvis

     808.0 Acetabulum, closed

     808.1 Acetabulum, open

     808.2 Pubis, closed

     808.3 Pubis, open

     ✓5th **808.4** Other specified part, closed

         808.41 Ilium

         808.42 Ischium

         808.43 Multiple pelvic fractures with disruption of pelvic circle

         808.49 Other
            Innominate bone   Pelvic rim

     ✓5th **808.5** Other specified part, open

         808.51 Ilium

         808.52 Ischium

         808.53 Multiple pelvic fractures with disruption of pelvic circle

         808.59 Other

     808.8 Unspecified, closed

     808.9 Unspecified, open

✓4th **809** Ill-defined fractures of bones of trunk

     `INCLUDES`   bones of trunk with other bones except those of skull and face
                   multiple bones of trunk

     `EXCLUDES`   *multiple fractures of:*
            pelvic bones alone (808.0-808.9)
            ribs alone (807.0-807.1, 807.4)
            ribs or sternum with limb bones (819.0-
                 819.1, 828.0-828.1)
            skull or face with other bones (804.0-804.9)

     809.0 Fracture of bones of trunk, closed

     809.1 Fracture of bones of trunk, open

FRACTURE OF UPPER LIMB (810-819)

✓4th **810** Fracture of clavicle

     `INCLUDES`   collar bone
                   interligamentous part of clavicle

     The following fifth-digit subclassification is for use with category 810:

         0   unspecified part
            Clavicle NOS
         1   sternal end of clavicle
         2   shaft of clavicle
         3   acromial end of clavicle

     ✓5th **810.0** Closed   `MSP`

     ✓5th **810.1** Open   `MSP`

Pelvis and Pelvic Fractures

Fractures Disrupting Pelvic Circle — Pelvic circle — Stable — Unstable (two-place fracture)

Iliac crest — Ilium — L5 — Pelvic Bones — Sacrum — Coccyx — Pubis — Anterior superior iliac spine — Ischial spine — Acetabulum — Femur — Ischial tuberosity — Pubic symphysis

Acetabular Fractures — Posterior pillar — Transverse

`N` Newborn Age: 0   `P` Pediatric Age: 0-17   `M` Maternity Age: 12-55   `A` Adult Age: 15-124   `MSP` Medicare Secondary Payer

252 — Volume 1   2005 ICD•9•CM

Injury and Poisoning

☑4ᵗʰ **811 Fracture of scapula**

　INCLUDES　shoulder blade

The following fifth-digit subclassification is for use with category 811:

0 unspecified part
1 acromial process
　　Acromion (process)
2 coracoid process
3 glenoid cavity and neck of scapula
9 other

☑5ᵗʰ **811.0 Closed**　　　　　MSP
☑5ᵗʰ **811.1 Open**　　　　　MSP

☑4ᵗʰ **812 Fracture of humerus**

☑5ᵗʰ **812.0 Upper end, closed**

　812.00 Upper end, unspecified part
　　　Proximal end　　Shoulder
　812.01 Surgical neck
　　　Neck of humerus NOS
　812.02 Anatomical neck
　812.03 Greater tuberosity
　812.09 Other
　　　Head　　　　Upper epiphysis

☑5ᵗʰ **812.1 Upper end, open**

　812.10 Upper end, unspecified part
　812.11 Surgical neck
　812.12 Anatomical neck
　812.13 Greater tuberosity
　812.19 Other

☑5ᵗʰ **812.2 Shaft or unspecified part, closed**

　812.20 Unspecified part of humerus
　　　Humerus NOS　　Upper arm NOS
　812.21 Shaft of humerus
　　　AHA: 3Q, '99, 14

☑5ᵗʰ **812.3 Shaft or unspecified part, open**

　812.30 Unspecified part of humerus
　812.31 Shaft of humerus

☑5ᵗʰ **812.4 Lower end, closed**

　　Distal end of humerus
　　Elbow
　812.40 Lower end, unspecified part
　812.41 Supracondylar fracture of humerus
　812.42 Lateral condyle
　　　External condyle
　812.43 Medial condyle
　　　Internal epicondyle
　812.44 Condyle(s), unspecified
　　　Articular process NOS
　　　Lower epiphysis NOS
　812.49 Other
　　　Multiple fractures of lower end
　　　Trochlea

Right Clavicle and Scapula, Anterior View

Right Humerus, Anterior View

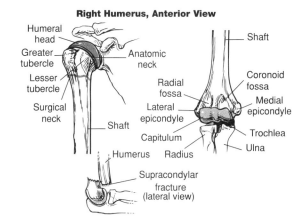

☑5ᵗʰ **812.5 Lower end, open**

　812.50 Lower end, unspecified part
　812.51 Supracondylar fracture of humerus
　812.52 Lateral condyle
　812.53 Medial condyle
　812.54 Condyle(s), unspecified
　812.59 Other

☑4ᵗʰ **813 Fracture of radius and ulna**

☑5ᵗʰ **813.0 Upper end, closed**

　　Proximal end
　813.00 Upper end of forearm, unspecified
　813.01 Olecranon process of ulna
　813.02 Coronoid process of ulna
　813.03 Monteggia's fracture
　　　DEF: Fracture near the head of the ulnar shaft, causing
　　　dislocation of the radial head.
　813.04 Other and unspecified fractures of
　　　　proximal end of ulna (alone)
　　　Multiple fractures of ulna, upper end
　813.05 Head of radius
　813.06 Neck of radius
　813.07 Other and unspecified fractures of
　　　　proximal end of radius (alone)
　　　Multiple fractures of radius, upper end
　813.08 Radius with ulna, upper end [any part]

☑5ᵗʰ **813.1 Upper end, open**

　813.10 Upper end of forearm, unspecified
　813.11 Olecranon process of ulna
　813.12 Coronoid process of ulna
　813.13 Monteggia's fracture
　813.14 Other and unspecified fractures of
　　　　proximal end of ulna (alone)
　813.15 Head of radius
　813.16 Neck of radius
　813.17 Other and unspecified fractures of
　　　　proximal end of radius (alone)
　813.18 Radius with ulna, upper end [any part]

☑5ᵗʰ **813.2 Shaft, closed**

　813.20 Shaft, unspecified
　813.21 Radius (alone)
　813.22 Ulna (alone)
　813.23 Radius with ulna

☑5ᵗʰ **813.3 Shaft, open**

　813.30 Shaft, unspecified
　813.31 Radius (alone)
　813.32 Ulna (alone)
　813.33 Radius with ulna

☑5ᵗʰ **813.4 Lower end, closed**

　　Distal end
　813.40 Lower end of forearm, unspecified

☑4ᵗʰ / ☑5ᵗʰ Additional Digit Required　　Unspecified Code　　Other Specified Code　　Manifestation Code　　▶◀ Revised Text　　● New Code　　▲ Revised Code Title

2005 ICD•9•CM　　　　　**Volume 1 — 253**

811–813.40

Right Radius and Ulna, Anterior View

813.41 Colles' fracture
Smith's fracture
DEF: Break of lower end of radius; associated with backward movement of the radius lower section.

813.42 Other fractures of distal end of radius (alone)
Dupuytren's fracture, radius
Radius, lower end
DEF: Dupuytren's fracture: fracture and dislocation of the forearm; the fracture is of the radius above the wrist, and the dislocation is of the ulna at the lower end.

813.43 Distal end of ulna (alone)
Ulna: Ulna:
head   lower epiphysis
lower end   styloid process

813.44 Radius with ulna, lower end

813.45 Torus fracture of radius
AHA: 4Q, '02, 70

√5th **813.5 Lower end, open**
813.50 Lower end of forearm, unspecified
813.51 Colles' fracture
813.52 Other fractures of distal end of radius (alone)
813.53 Distal end of ulna (alone)
813.54 Radius with ulna, lower end

√5th **813.8 Unspecified part, closed**
813.80 Forearm, unspecified
813.81 Radius (alone)
AHA: 2Q, '98, 19
813.82 Ulna (alone)
813.83 Radius with ulna

√5th **813.9 Unspecified part, open**
813.90 Forearm, unspecified
813.91 Radius (alone)
813.92 Ulna (alone)
813.93 Radius with ulna

√4th **814 Fracture of carpal bone(s)**
The following fifth-digit subclassification is for use with category 814:
0 carpal bone, unspecified
Wrist NOS
1 navicular [scaphoid] of wrist
2 lunate [semilunar] bone of wrist
3 triquetral [cuneiform] bone of wrist
4 pisiform
5 trapezium bone [larger multangular]
6 trapezoid bone [smaller multangular]
7 capitate bone [os magnum]
8 hamate [unciform] bone
9 other

√5th **814.0 Closed**
√5th **814.1 Open**
√4th **815 Fracture of metacarpal bone(s)**
INCLUDES hand [except finger]
metacarpus
The following fifth-digit subclassification is for use with category 815:
0 metacarpal bone(s), site unspecified
1 base of thumb [first] metacarpal
Bennett's fracture
2 base of other metacarpal bone(s)
3 shaft of metacarpal bone(s)
4 neck of metacarpal bone(s)
9 multiple sites of metacarpus

√5th **815.0 Closed**
√5th **815.1 Open**
√4th **816 Fracture of one or more phalanges of hand**
INCLUDES finger(s) thumb
The following fifth-digit subclassification is for use with category 816:
0 phalanx or phalanges, unspecified
1 middle or proximal phalanx or phalanges
2 distal phalanx or phalanges
3 multiple sites

√5th **816.0 Closed**
√5th **816.1 Open**
AHA: For code 816.12: ▶ 4Q, '03, 77 ◀

√4th **817 Multiple fractures of hand bones**
INCLUDES metacarpal bone(s) with phalanx or phalanges of same hand
817.0 Closed
817.1 Open

√4th **818 Ill-defined fractures of upper limb**
INCLUDES arm NOS
multiple bones of same upper limb
EXCLUDES *multiple fractures of:*
metacarpal bone(s) with phalanx or phalanges (817.0-817.1)
phalanges of hand alone (816.0-816.1)
radius with ulna (813.0-813.9)
818.0 Closed
818.1 Open

√4th **819 Multiple fractures involving both upper limbs, and upper limb with rib(s) and sternum**
INCLUDES arm(s) with rib(s) or sternum
both arms [any bones]
819.0 Closed
819.1 Open

Hand Fractures

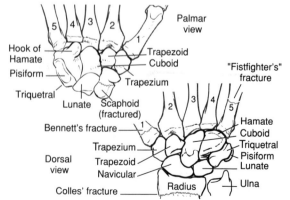

Injury and Poisoning

FRACTURE OF LOWER LIMB (820-829)

✓4th 820 Fracture of neck of femur

✓5th 820.0 Transcervical fracture, closed
    820.00 Intracapsular section, unspecified
    820.01 Epiphysis (separation) (upper)
        Transepiphyseal
    820.02 Midcervical section
        Transcervical NOS
        AHA: 3Q, '03, 12

    820.03 Base of neck
        Cervicotrochanteric section
    820.09 Other
        Head of femur   Subcapital

✓5th 820.1 Transcervical fracture, open
    820.10 Intracapsular section, unspecified
    820.11 Epiphysis (separation) (upper)
    820.12 Midcervical section
    820.13 Base of neck
    820.19 Other

✓5th 820.2 Pertrochanteric fracture, closed
    820.20 Trochanteric section, unspecified
        Trochanter: Trochanter:
          NOS   lesser
          greater
    820.21 Intertrochanteric section
    820.22 Subtrochanteric section

✓5th 820.3 Pertrochanteric fracture, open
    820.30 Trochanteric section, unspecified
    820.31 Intertrochanteric section
    820.32 Subtrochanteric section

    820.8 Unspecified part of neck of femur, closed
        Hip NOS   Neck of femur NOS
    820.9 Unspecified part of neck of femur, open

✓4th 821 Fracture of other and unspecified parts of femur

✓5th 821.0 Shaft or unspecified part, closed
    821.00 Unspecified part of femur
        Thigh   Upper leg
        EXCLUDES   hip NOS (820.8)
    821.01 Shaft
        AHA: 1Q, '99, 5

✓5th 821.1 Shaft or unspecified part, open
    821.10 Unspecified part of femur
    821.11 Shaft

✓5th 821.2 Lower end, closed
        Distal end
    821.20 Lower end, unspecified part
    821.21 Condyle, femoral
    821.22 Epiphysis, lower (separation)
    821.23 Supracondylar fracture of femur
        Multiple fractures of lower end
    821.29 Other
        Multiple fractures of lower end

✓5th 821.3 Lower end, open
    821.30 Lower end, unspecified part
    821.31 Condyle, femoral
    821.32 Epiphysis, lower (separation)
    821.33 Supracondylar fracture of femur
    821.39 Other

✓4th 822 Fracture of patella
    822.0 Closed
    822.1 Open

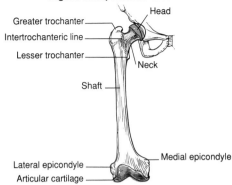
Right Femur, Anterior View

Head
Greater trochanter
Intertrochanteric line
Lesser trochanter
Neck
Shaft
Lateral epicondyle
Medial epicondyle
Articular cartilage

✓4th 823 Fracture of tibia and fibula
    EXCLUDES   *Dupuytren's fracture (824.4-824.5)*
        ankle (824.4-824.5)
        radius (813.42, 813.52)
        Pott's fracture (824.4-824.5)
        that involving ankle (824.0-824.9)

    The following fifth-digit subclassification is for use with category 823:
        0 tibia alone
        1 fibula alone
        2 fibula with tibia

✓5th 823.0 Upper end, closed
        Head   Tibia:
        Proximal end   condyles
                       tuberosity
✓5th 823.1 Upper end, open
✓5th 823.2 Shaft, closed
✓5th 823.3 Shaft, open
✓5th 823.4 Torus fracture
    DEF: A bone deformity in children, occurring commonly in the radius or ulna, in which the bone bends and buckles but does not fracture.
    AHA: 4Q, '02, 70

✓5th 823.8 Unspecified part, closed
    Lower leg NOS
    AHA: For code **823.82:** 1Q, '97, 8

✓5th 823.9 Unspecified part, open

✓4th 824 Fracture of ankle
    824.0 Medial malleolus, closed
        Tibia involving: Tibia involving:
        ankle   malleolus
        AHA: ▶1Q, '04, 9◄

    824.1 Medial malleolus, open
    824.2 Lateral malleolus, closed
        Fibula involving: Fibula involving:
        ankle   malleolus
        AHA: 2Q, '02, 3

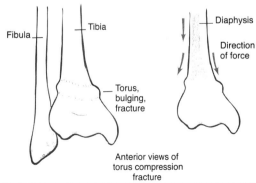
Torus Fracture

Fibula
Tibia
Diaphysis
Direction of force
Torus, bulging, fracture
Anterior views of torus compression fracture

✓4th
✓5th Additional Digit Required   Unspecified Code   Other Specified Code   Manifestation Code   ▶◄ Revised Text   ● New Code   ▲ Revised Code Title

2005 ICD•9•CM   **October 2004 • Volume 1 — 255**

820–824.2

Injury and Poisoning

824.3–830.1

Right Tibia and Fibula, Anterior View

Right Foot, Dorsal

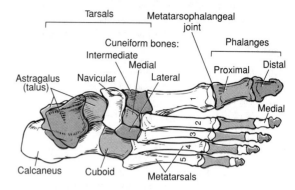

824.3   Lateral malleolus, open

824.4   Bimalleolar, closed

Dupuytren's fracture, fibula   Pott's fracture

DEF: Bimalleolar, closed: Breaking of both nodules (malleoli) on either side of ankle joint, without an open wound.

DEF: Dupuytren's fracture (Pott's fracture): The breaking of the farthest end of the lower leg bone (fibula), with injury to the farthest end joint of the other lower leg bone (tibia).

824.5   Bimalleolar, open

824.6   Trimalleolar, closed

Lateral and medial malleolus with anterior or posterior lip of tibia

824.7   Trimalleolar, open

824.8   Unspecified, closed

Ankle NOS

AHA: 3Q, '00, 12

824.9   Unspecified, open

√4ᵗʰ **825   Fracture of one or more tarsal and metatarsal bones**

825.0   Fracture of calcaneus, closed

Heel bone   Os calcis

825.1   Fracture of calcaneus, open

√5ᵗʰ **825.2   Fracture of other tarsal and metatarsal bones, closed**

825.20   Unspecified bone(s) of foot [except toes]

Instep

825.21   Astragalus

Talus

825.22   Navicular [scaphoid], foot

825.23   Cuboid

825.24   Cuneiform, foot

825.25   Metatarsal bone(s)

825.29   Other

Tarsal with metatarsal bone(s) only

EXCLUDES   calcaneus (825.0)

√5ᵗʰ **825.3   Fracture of other tarsal and metatarsal bones, open**

825.30   Unspecified bone(s) of foot [except toes]

825.31   Astragalus

825.32   Navicular [scaphoid], foot

825.33   Cuboid

825.34   Cuneiform, foot

825.35   Metatarsal bone(s)

825.39   Other

√4ᵗʰ **826   Fracture of one or more phalanges of foot**

INCLUDES   toe(s)

826.0   Closed

826.1   Open

√4ᵗʰ **827   Other, multiple, and ill-defined fractures of lower limb**

INCLUDES   leg NOS

multiple bones of same lower limb

EXCLUDES   multiple fractures of:

ankle bones alone (824.4-824.9)

phalanges of foot alone (826.0-826.1)

tarsal with metatarsal bones (825.29, 825.39)

tibia with fibula (823.0-823.9 with fifth-digit 2)

827.0   Closed

827.1   Open

√4ᵗʰ **828   Multiple fractures involving both lower limbs, lower with upper limb, and lower limb(s) with rib(s) and sternum**

INCLUDES   arm(s) with leg(s) [any bones]

both legs [any bones]

leg(s) with rib(s) or sternum

828.0   Closed   **MSP**

828.1   Open   **MSP**

√4ᵗʰ **829   Fracture of unspecified bones**

829.0   Unspecified bone, closed

829.1   Unspecified bone, open

DISLOCATION (830-839)

INCLUDES   displacement

subluxation

EXCLUDES   congenital dislocation (754.0-755.8)

pathological dislocation (718.2)

recurrent dislocation (718.3)

The descriptions "closed" and "open," used in the fourth-digit subdivisions, include the following terms:

closed: open:

complete   compound

dislocation NOS   infected

partial   with foreign body

simple

uncomplicated

A dislocation not indicated as closed or open should be classified as closed.

AHA: 3Q, '90, 12

√4ᵗʰ **830   Dislocation of jaw**

INCLUDES   jaw (cartilage) (meniscus)

mandible

maxilla (inferior)

temporomandibular (joint)

830.0   Closed dislocation

830.1   Open dislocation

✓4th **831 Dislocation of shoulder**

> **EXCLUDES**   *sternoclavicular joint (839.61, 839.71)*
> *sternum (839.61, 839.71)*

The following fifth-digit subclassification is for use with category 831:

  0 **shoulder, unspecified**
      Humerus NOS
  1 **anterior dislocation of humerus**
  2 **posterior dislocation of humerus**
  3 **inferior dislocation of humerus**
  4 **acromioclavicular (joint)**
      Clavicle
  9 **other**
      Scapula

✓5th **831.0 Closed dislocation**
✓5th **831.1 Open dislocation**

✓4th **832 Dislocation of elbow**

The following fifth-digit subclassification is for use with category 832:

  0 **elbow unspecified**
  1 **anterior dislocation of elbow**
  2 **posterior dislocation of elbow**
  3 **medial dislocation of elbow**
  4 **lateral dislocation of elbow**
  9 **other**

✓5th **832.0 Closed dislocation**
✓5th **832.1 Open dislocation**

✓4th **833 Dislocation of wrist**

The following fifth-digit subclassification is for use with category 833:

  0 **wrist, unspecified part**
      Carpal (bone)
      Radius, distal end
  1 **radioulnar (joint), distal**
  2 **radiocarpal (joint)**
  3 **midcarpal (joint)**
  4 **carpometacarpal (joint)**
  5 **metacarpal (bone), proximal end**
  9 **other**
      Ulna, distal end

✓5th **833.0 Closed dislocation**
✓5th **833.1 Open dislocation**

✓4th **834 Dislocation of finger**

> **INCLUDES**   finger(s)
> phalanx of hand
> thumb

The following fifth-digit subclassification is for use with category 834:

  0 **finger, unspecified part**
  1 **metacarpophalangeal (joint)**
      Metacarpal (bone), distal end
  2 **interphalangeal (joint), hand**

✓5th **834.0 Closed dislocation**
✓5th **834.1 Open dislocation**

✓4th **835 Dislocation of hip**

The following fifth-digit subclassification is for use with category 835:

  0 **dislocation of hip, unspecified**
  1 **posterior dislocation**
  2 **obturator dislocation**
  3 **other anterior dislocation**

✓5th **835.0 Closed dislocation**
✓5th **835.1 Open dislocation**

✓4th **836 Dislocation of knee**

> **EXCLUDES**   *dislocation of knee:*
> *old or pathological (718.2)*
> *recurrent (718.3)*
> *internal derangement of knee joint (717.0-717.5, 717.8-717.9)*
> *old tear of cartilage or meniscus of knee (717.0-717.5, 717.8-717.9)*

836.0 Tear of medial cartilage or meniscus of knee, current

Bucket handle tear:
  NOS   } current injury
  medial meniscus

836.1 Tear of lateral cartilage or meniscus of knee, current

836.2 Other tear of cartilage or meniscus of knee, current

Tear of:
  cartilage   } current injury, not
    (semilunar)   specified as
  meniscus   medial or lateral

836.3 Dislocation of patella, closed

836.4 Dislocation of patella, open

✓5th **836.5 Other dislocation of knee, closed**

  836.50 Dislocation of knee, unspecified
  836.51 Anterior dislocation of tibia, proximal end
      Posterior dislocation of femur, distal end
  836.52 Posterior dislocation of tibia, proximal end
      Anterior dislocation of femur, distal end
  836.53 Medial dislocation of tibia, proximal end
  836.54 Lateral dislocation of tibia, proximal end
  836.59 Other

✓5th **836.6 Other dislocation of knee, open**

  836.60 Dislocation of knee, unspecified
  836.61 Anterior dislocation of tibia, proximal end
  836.62 Posterior dislocation of tibia, proximal end
  836.63 Medial dislocation of tibia, proximal end
  836.64 Lateral dislocation of tibia, proximal end
  836.69 Other

✓4th **837 Dislocation of ankle**

> **INCLUDES**   astragalus
> fibula, distal end
> navicular, foot
> scaphoid, foot
> tibia, distal end

837.0 Closed dislocation

837.1 Open dislocation

✓4th **838 Dislocation of foot**

The following fifth-digit subclassification is for use with category 838:

  0 **foot, unspecified**
  1 **tarsal (bone), joint unspecified**
  2 **midtarsal (joint)**
  3 **tarsometatarsal (joint)**
  4 **metatarsal (bone), joint unspecified**
  5 **metatarsophalangeal (joint)**
  6 **interphalangeal (joint), foot**
  9 **other**
      Phalanx of foot
      Toe(s)

✓5th **838.0 Closed dislocation**
✓5th **838.1 Open dislocation**

✓4th **839 Other, multiple, and ill-defined dislocations**

✓5th **839.0 Cervical vertebra, closed**
    Cervical spine   Neck

  839.00 Cervical vertebra, unspecified   MSP
  839.01 First cervical vertebra   MSP

✓4th
✓5th Additional Digit Required   Unspecified Code   Other Specified Code   Manifestation Code   ▶◀ Revised Text   ● New Code   ▲ Revised Code Title

Injury and Poisoning

839.02–845.09

839.02 Second cervical vertebra `MSP`
839.03 Third cervical vertebra `MSP`
839.04 Fourth cervical vertebra `MSP`
839.05 Fifth cervical vertebra `MSP`
839.06 Sixth cervical vertebra `MSP`
839.07 Seventh cervical vertebra `MSP`
839.08 Multiple cervical vertebrae `MSP`

√5ᵗʰ 839.1 Cervical vertebra, open
839.10 Cervical vertebra, unspecified `MSP`
839.11 First cervical vertebra `MSP`
839.12 Second cervical vertebra `MSP`
839.13 Third cervical vertebra `MSP`
839.14 Fourth cervical vertebra `MSP`
839.15 Fifth cervical vertebra `MSP`
839.16 Sixth cervical vertebra `MSP`
839.17 Seventh cervical vertebra `MSP`
839.18 Multiple cervical vertebrae `MSP`

√5ᵗʰ 839.2 Thoracic and lumbar vertebra, closed
839.20 Lumbar vertebra `MSP`
839.21 Thoracic vertebra `MSP`
     Dorsal [thoracic] vertebra

√5ᵗʰ 839.3 Thoracic and lumbar vertebra, open
839.30 Lumbar vertebra `MSP`
839.31 Thoracic vertebra `MSP`

√5ᵗʰ 839.4 Other vertebra, closed
839.40 Vertebra, unspecified site
     Spine NOS
839.41 Coccyx
839.42 Sacrum
     Sacroiliac (joint)
839.49 Other

√5ᵗʰ 839.5 Other vertebra, open
839.50 Vertebra, unspecified site
839.51 Coccyx
839.52 Sacrum
839.59 Other

√5ᵗʰ 839.6 Other location, closed
839.61 Sternum
     Sternoclavicular joint
839.69 Other
     Pelvis

√5ᵗʰ 839.7 Other location, open
839.71 Sternum `MSP`
839.79 Other `MSP`

839.8 Multiple and ill-defined, closed `MSP`
     Arm
     Back
     Hand
     Multiple locations, except fingers or toes alone
     Other ill-defined locations
     Unspecified location

839.9 Multiple and ill-defined, open `MSP`

SPRAINS AND STRAINS OF JOINTS AND ADJACENT MUSCLES (840-848)

`INCLUDES` avulsion
hemarthrosis
laceration   of:
rupture   joint capsule
sprain   ligament
strain   muscle
tear   tendon

`EXCLUDES` laceration of tendon in open wounds (880-884 and 890-894 with .2)

√4ᵗʰ 840 Sprains and strains of shoulder and upper arm
840.0 Acromioclavicular (joint) (ligament)
840.1 Coracoclavicular (ligament)

840.2 Coracohumeral (ligament)
840.3 Infraspinatus (muscle) (tendon)
840.4 Rotator cuff (capsule)
     `EXCLUDES` complete rupture of rotator cuff, nontraumatic (727.61)
840.5 Subscapularis (muscle)
840.6 Supraspinatus (muscle) (tendon)
840.7 Superior glenoid labrum lesion
     SLAP lesion
     AHA: 4Q,'01, 52

     DEF: Detachment injury of the superior aspect of the glenoid labrum which is the ring of fibrocartilage attached to the rim of the glenoid cavity of the scapula.
840.8 Other specified sites of shoulder and upper arm
840.9 Unspecified site of shoulder and upper arm
     Arm NOS
     Shoulder NOS

√4ᵗʰ 841 Sprains and strains of elbow and forearm
841.0 Radial collateral ligament
841.1 Ulnar collateral ligament
841.2 Radiohumeral (joint)
841.3 Ulnohumeral (joint)
841.8 Other specified sites of elbow and forearm
841.9 Unspecified site of elbow and forearm
     Elbow NOS

√4ᵗʰ 842 Sprains and strains of wrist and hand
√5ᵗʰ 842.0 Wrist
842.00 Unspecified site
842.01 Carpal (joint)
842.02 Radiocarpal (joint) (ligament)
842.09 Other
     Radioulnar joint, distal
√5ᵗʰ 842.1 Hand
842.10 Unspecified site
842.11 Carpometacarpal (joint)
842.12 Metacarpophalangeal (joint)
842.13 Interphalangeal (joint)
842.19 Other
     Midcarpal (joint)

√4ᵗʰ 843 Sprains and strains of hip and thigh
843.0 Iliofemoral (ligament)
843.1 Ischiocapsular (ligament)
843.8 Other specified sites of hip and thigh
843.9 Unspecified site of hip and thigh
     Hip NOS
     Thigh NOS

√4ᵗʰ 844 Sprains and strains of knee and leg
844.0 Lateral collateral ligament of knee
844.1 Medial collateral ligament of knee
844.2 Cruciate ligament of knee
844.3 Tibiofibular (joint) (ligament), superior
844.8 Other specified sites of knee and leg
844.9 Unspecified site of knee and leg
     Knee NOS   Leg NOS

√4ᵗʰ 845 Sprains and strains of ankle and foot
√5ᵗʰ 845.0 Ankle
845.00 Unspecified site
     AHA: 2Q, '02, 3
845.01 Deltoid (ligament), ankle
     Internal collateral (ligament), ankle
845.02 Calcaneofibular (ligament)
845.03 Tibiofibular (ligament), distal
     AHA: ►1Q, '04, 9◄
845.09 Other
     Achilles tendon

`N` Newborn Age: 0   `P` Pediatric Age: 0-17   `M` Maternity Age: 12-55   `A` Adult Age: 15-124   `MSP` Medicare Secondary Payer

☑5ᵗʰ **845.1 Foot**

    845.10 Unspecified site

    845.11 Tarsometatarsal (joint) (ligament)

    845.12 Metatarsophalangeal (joint)

    845.13 Interphalangeal (joint), toe

    845.19 Other

☑4ᵗʰ **846 Sprains and strains of sacroiliac region**

    846.0 Lumbosacral (joint) (ligament)

    846.1 Sacroiliac ligament

    846.2 Sacrospinatus (ligament)

    846.3 Sacrotuberous (ligament)

    846.8 Other specified sites of sacroiliac region

    846.9 Unspecified site of sacroiliac region

☑4ᵗʰ **847 Sprains and strains of other and unspecified parts of back**

    EXCLUDES   lumbosacral (846.0)

    847.0 Neck   MSP

        Anterior longitudinal (ligament), cervical

        Atlanto-axial (joints)

        Atlanto-occipital (joints)

        Whiplash injury

        EXCLUDES   neck injury NOS (959.0)

                 thyroid region (848.2)

    847.1 Thoracic

    847.2 Lumbar

    847.3 Sacrum

        Sacrococcygeal (ligament)

    847.4 Coccyx

    847.9 Unspecified site of back

        Back NOS

☑4ᵗʰ **848 Other and ill-defined sprains and strains**

    848.0 Septal cartilage of nose

    848.1 Jaw

        Temporomandibular (joint) (ligament)

    848.2 Thyroid region

        Cricoarytenoid (joint) (ligament)

        Cricothyroid (joint) (ligament)

        Thyroid cartilage

    848.3 Ribs

        Chondrocostal (joint)

        Costal cartilage } without mention of injury to sternum

☑5ᵗʰ   **848.4 Sternum**

    848.40 Unspecified site

    848.41 Sternoclavicular (joint) (ligament)

    848.42 Chondrosternal (joint)

    848.49 Other

        Xiphoid cartilage

    848.5 Pelvis

        Symphysis pubis

        EXCLUDES   that in childbirth (665.6)

    848.8 Other specified sites of sprains and strains

    848.9 Unspecified site of sprain and strain

INTRACRANIAL INJURY, EXCLUDING THOSE WITH SKULL FRACTURE (850-854)

    EXCLUDES   *intracranial injury with skull fracture (800-801 and 803-804, except .0 and .5)*

        open wound of head without intracranial injury (870.0-873.9)

        skull fracture alone (800-801 and 803-804 with .0, .5)

The description "with open intracranial wound," used in the fourth-digit subdivisions, those specified as open or with mention of infection or foreign body.

The following fifth-digit subclassification is for use with categories 851-854:

  0 unspecified state of consciousness

  1 with no loss of consciousness

  2 with brief [less than one hour] loss of consciousness

  3 with moderate [1-24 hours] loss of consciousness

  4 with prolonged [more than 24 hours] loss of consciousness and return to pre-existing conscious level

  5 with prolonged [more than 24 hours] loss of consciousness, without return to pre-existing conscious level

    Use fifth-digit 5 to designate when a patient is unconscious and dies before regaining consciousness, regardless of the duration of the loss of consciousness

  6 with loss of consciousness of unspecified duration

  9 with concussion, unspecified

AHA: 1Q, '93, 22

☑4ᵗʰ **850 Concussion**

    INCLUDES   commotio cerebri

    EXCLUDES   *concussion with:*

        cerebral laceration or contusion (851.0-851.9)

        cerebral hemorrhage (852-853)

        head injury NOS (959.01)

    AHA: 2Q, '96, 6; 4Q, '90, 24

    850.0 With no loss of consciousness   MSP

        Concussion with mental confusion or disorientation, without loss of consciousness

☑5ᵗʰ   850.1 With brief loss of consciousness

        Loss of consciousness for less than one hour

        AHA: ▶4Q, '03, 76;◀ 1Q, '99, 10; 2Q, '92, 5

        850.11 With loss of consciousness of 30 minutes or less   MSP

        850.12 With loss of consciousness from 31 to 59 minutes   MSP

    850.2 With moderate loss of consciousness   MSP

        Loss of consciousness for 1-24 hours

    850.3 With prolonged loss of consciousness and return to pre-existing conscious level   MSP

        Loss of consciousness for more than 24 hours with complete recovery

    850.4 With prolonged loss of consciousness, without return to pre-existing conscious level   MSP

    850.5 With loss of consciousness of unspecified duration   MSP

    850.9 Concussion, unspecified   MSP

☑4ᵗʰ **851 Cerebral laceration and contusion**

    AHA: 4Q, '96, 36; 1Q, '93, 22; 4Q, '90, 24

☑5ᵗʰ   851.0 Cortex (cerebral) contusion without mention of open intracranial wound   MSP

☑5ᵗʰ   851.1 Cortex (cerebral) contusion with open intracranial wound   MSP

        AHA: 1Q, '92, 9

☑4ᵗʰ ☑5ᵗʰ Additional Digit Required   Unspecified Code   Other Specified Code   Manifestation Code   ▶◀ Revised Text   ● New Code   ▲ Revised Code Title

Injury and Poisoning

851.2–861.0

§ ✓5ᵗʰ **851.2** Cortex (cerebral) laceration without mention of open intracranial wound   MSP

§ ✓5ᵗʰ **851.3** Cortex (cerebral) laceration with open intracranial wound   MSP

§ ✓5ᵗʰ **851.4** Cerebellar or brain stem contusion without mention of open intracranial wound   MSP

§ ✓5ᵗʰ **851.5** Cerebellar or brain stem contusion with open intracranial wound   MSP

§ ✓5ᵗʰ **851.6** Cerebellar or brain stem laceration without mention of open intracranial wound   MSP

§ ✓5ᵗʰ **851.7** Cerebellar or brain stem laceration with open intracranial wound   MSP

§ ✓5ᵗʰ **851.8** Other and unspecified cerebral laceration and contusion, without mention of open intracranial wound   MSP
    Brain (membrane) NOS
    AHA: 4Q, '96, 37

§ ✓5ᵗʰ **851.9** Other and unspecified cerebral laceration and contusion, with open intracranial wound   MSP

✓4ᵗʰ **852** Subarachnoid, subdural, and extradural hemorrhage, following injury
    EXCLUDES   cerebral contusion or laceration (with hemorrhage) (851.0-851.9)
    DEF: Bleeding from lining of brain; due to injury.

§ ✓5ᵗʰ **852.0** Subarachnoid hemorrhage following injury without mention of open intracranial wound   MSP
    Middle meningeal hemorrhage following injury

§ ✓5ᵗʰ **852.1** Subarachnoid hemorrhage following injury with open intracranial wound   MSP

§ ✓5ᵗʰ **852.2** Subdural hemorrhage following injury without mention of open intracranialwound   MSP
    AHA: 4Q, '96, 43

§ ✓5ᵗʰ **852.3** Subdural hemorrhage following injury with open intracranial wound   MSP

Brain

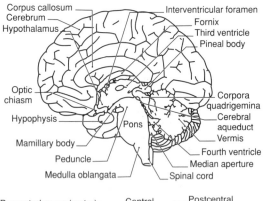

Corpus callosum — Cerebrum — Hypothalamus — / Interventricular foramen / Fornix / Third ventricle / Pineal body

Optic chiasm — / Corpora quadrigemina / Cerebral aqueduct / Vermis

Hypophysis — Pons / Fourth ventricle / Median aperture

Mamillary body — Peduncle — Medulla oblangata — / Spinal cord

Precentral gyrus (motor) — / Central sulcus / Postcentral gyrus (sensory)

Anterior horn of lateral ventricle — Intraventricular foramen — / Body and posterior horn of lateral ventricle

Third ventricle — Lateral sulcus —

Inferior horn of lateral ventricle — Cerebral aqueduct — Lateral aperture — / Fourth ventricle / Median aperture

§ ✓5ᵗʰ **852.4** Extradural hemorrhage following injury without mention of open intracranial wound   MSP
    Epidural hematoma following injury

§ ✓5ᵗʰ **852.5** Extradural hemorrhage following injury with open intracranial wound   MSP

✓4ᵗʰ **853** Other and unspecified intracranial hemorrhage following injury

§ ✓5ᵗʰ **853.0** Without mention of open intracranial wound   MSP
    Cerebral compression due to injury
    Intracranial hematoma following injury
    Traumatic cerebral hemorrhage
    AHA: 3Q, '90, 14

§ ✓5ᵗʰ **853.1** With open intracranial wound   MSP

✓4ᵗʰ **854** Intracranial injury of other and unspecified nature
    INCLUDES   brain injury NOS
    cavernous sinus
    intracranial injury
    EXCLUDES   any condition classifiable to 850-853
    head injury NOS (959.01)
    AHA: 1Q, '99, 10; 2Q, '92, 6

§ ✓5ᵗʰ **854.0** Without mention of open intracranial wound   MSP

§ ✓5ᵗʰ **854.1** With open intracranial wound   MSP

INTERNAL INJURY OF THORAX, ABDOMEN, AND PELVIS (860-869)

INCLUDES   blast injuries
blunt trauma
bruise
concussion injuries (except cerebral)
crushing
hematoma   } of internal organs
laceration
puncture
tear
traumatic rupture

EXCLUDES   concussion NOS (850.0-850.9)
flail chest (807.4)
foreign body entering through orifice (930.0-939.9)
injury to blood vessels (901.0-902.9)

The description "with open wound," used in the fourth-digit subdivisions, those with mention of infection or foreign body.

✓4ᵗʰ **860** Traumatic pneumothorax and hemothorax
    AHA: 2Q, '93, 4

    DEF: Traumatic pneumothorax: air or gas leaking into pleural space of lung due to trauma.

    DEF: Traumatic hemothorax: blood buildup in pleural space of lung due to trauma.

860.0 Pneumothorax without mention of open wound into thorax   MSP

860.1 Pneumothorax with open wound into thorax   MSP

860.2 Hemothorax without mention of open wound into thorax   MSP

860.3 Hemothorax with open wound into thorax   MSP

860.4 Pneumohemothorax without mention of open wound into thorax   MSP

860.5 Pneumohemothorax with open wound into thorax   MSP

✓4ᵗʰ **861** Injury to heart and lung
    EXCLUDES   injury to blood vessels of thorax (901.0-901.9)

✓5ᵗʰ **861.0** Heart, without mention of open wound into thorax
    AHA: 1Q, '92, 9

§ Requires fifth-digit. See beginning of section 850–854 for codes and definitions.

N Newborn Age: 0   P Pediatric Age: 0-17   M Maternity Age: 12-55   A Adult Age: 15-124   MSP Medicare Secondary Payer

861.00 Unspecified injury `MSP`

861.01 Contusion `MSP`
   Cardiac contusion
   Myocardial contusion
   DEF: Bruising within the pericardium with no mention of open wound.

861.02 Laceration without penetration of heart chambers `MSP`
   DEF: Tearing injury of heart tissue, without penetration of chambers; no open wound.

861.03 Laceration with penetration of heart chambers `MSP`

√5ᵗʰ 861.1 Heart, with open wound into thorax
   861.10 Unspecified injury `MSP`
   861.11 Contusion `MSP`
   861.12 Laceration without penetration of heart chambers `MSP`
   861.13 Laceration with penetration of heart chambers `MSP`

√5ᵗʰ 861.2 Lung, without mention of open wound into thorax
   861.20 Unspecified injury `MSP`
   861.21 Contusion `MSP`
      DEF: Bruising of lung without mention of open wound.
   861.22 Laceration `MSP`

√5ᵗʰ 861.3 Lung, with open wound into thorax
   861.30 Unspecified injury `MSP`
   861.31 Contusion `MSP`
   861.32 Laceration `MSP`

√4ᵗʰ 862 Injury to other and unspecified intrathoracic organs
   EXCLUDES *injury to blood vessels of thorax (901.0-901.9)*

862.0 Diaphragm, without mention of open wound into cavity

862.1 Diaphragm, with open wound into cavity

√5ᵗʰ 862.2 Other specified intrathoracic organs, without mention of open wound into cavity
   862.21 Bronchus
   862.22 Esophagus
   862.29 Other
      Pleura   Thymus gland

√5ᵗʰ 862.3 Other specified intrathoracic organs, with open wound into cavity
   862.31 Bronchus
   862.32 Esophagus
   862.39 Other

862.8 Multiple and unspecified intrathoracic organs, without mention of open wound into cavity `MSP`
   Crushed chest
   Multiple intrathoracic organs

862.9 Multiple and unspecified intrathoracic organs, with open wound into cavity

√4ᵗʰ 863 Injury to gastrointestinal tract
   EXCLUDES *anal sphincter laceration during delivery (664.2)*
   bile duct (868.0-868.1 with fifth-digit 2)
   gallbladder (868.0-868.1 with fifth-digit 2)

863.0 Stomach, without mention of open wound into cavity `MSP`

863.1 Stomach, with open wound into cavity `MSP`

√5ᵗʰ 863.2 Small intestine, without mention of open wound into cavity
   863.20 Small intestine, unspecified site `MSP`
   863.21 Duodenum `MSP`
   863.29 Other `MSP`

√5ᵗʰ 863.3 Small intestine, with open wound into cavity
   863.30 Small intestine, unspecified site `MSP`
   863.31 Duodenum `MSP`
   863.39 Other `MSP`

√5ᵗʰ 863.4 Colon or rectum, without mention of open wound into cavity
   863.40 Colon, unspecified site `MSP`
   863.41 Ascending [right] colon `MSP`
   863.42 Transverse colon `MSP`
   863.43 Descending [left] colon `MSP`
   863.44 Sigmoid colon `MSP`
   863.45 Rectum `MSP`
   863.46 Multiple sites in colon and rectum `MSP`
   863.49 Other `MSP`

√5ᵗʰ 863.5 Colon or rectum, with open wound into cavity
   863.50 Colon, unspecified site `MSP`
   863.51 Ascending [right] colon `MSP`
   863.52 Transverse colon `MSP`
   863.53 Descending [left] colon `MSP`
   863.54 Sigmoid colon `MSP`
   863.55 Rectum `MSP`
   863.56 Multiple sites in colon and rectum `MSP`
   863.59 Other `MSP`

√5ᵗʰ 863.8 Other and unspecified gastrointestinal sites, without mention of open wound into cavity `MSP`
   863.80 Gastrointestinal tract, unspecified site `MSP`
   863.81 Pancreas, head `MSP`
   863.82 Pancreas, body `MSP`
   863.83 Pancreas, tail `MSP`
   863.84 Pancreas, multiple and unspecified sites `MSP`
   863.85 Appendix `MSP`
   863.89 Other `MSP`
      Intestine NOS

√5ᵗʰ 863.9 Other and unspecified gastrointestinal sites, with open wound into cavity
   863.90 Gastrointestinal tract, unspecified site `MSP`
   863.91 Pancreas, head `MSP`
   863.92 Pancreas, body `MSP`
   863.93 Pancreas, tail `MSP`
   863.94 Pancreas, multiple and unspecified sites `MSP`
   863.95 Appendix `MSP`
   863.99 Other `MSP`

√4ᵗʰ 864 Injury to liver

The following fifth-digit subclassification is for use with category 864:
   0 unspecified injury
   1 hematoma and contusion
   2 laceration, minor
      Laceration involving capsule only, or without significant involvement of hepatic parenchyma [i.e., less than 1 cm deep]
   3 laceration, moderate
      Laceration involving parenchyma but without major disruption of parenchyma [i.e., less than 10 cm long and less than 3 cm deep]
   4 laceration, major
      Laceration with significant disruption of hepatic parenchyma [i.e., 10 cm long and 3 cm deep]
      Multiple moderate lacerations, with or without hematoma
      Stellate lacerations of liver
   5 laceration, unspecified
   9 other

√5ᵗʰ 864.0 Without mention of open wound into cavity `MSP`
√5ᵗʰ 864.1 With open wound into cavity `MSP`

√4ᵗʰ / √5ᵗʰ Additional Digit Required   Unspecified Code   Other Specified Code   Manifestation Code   ►◄ Revised Text   ● New Code   ▲ Revised Code Title

Injury and Poisoning

865–872.01

√4th **865 Injury to spleen**

The following fifth-digit subclassification is for use with category 865:

0 unspecified injury
1 hematoma without rupture of capsule
2 capsular tears, without major disruption of parenchyma
3 laceration extending into parenchyma
4 massive parenchymal disruption
9 other

√5th **865.0 Without mention of open wound into cavity** `MSP`

√5th **865.1 With open wound into cavity** `MSP`

√4th **866 Injury to kidney**

The following fifth-digit subclassification is for use with category 866:

0 unspecified injury
1 hematoma without rupture of capsule
2 laceration
3 complete disruption of kidney parenchyma

√5th **866.0 Without mention of open wound into cavity** `MSP`

√5th **866.1 With open wound into cavity** `MSP`

√4th **867 Injury to pelvic organs**

> `EXCLUDES` *injury during delivery (664.0-665.9)*

867.0 Bladder and urethra, without mention of open `MSP`
wound into cavity
> AHA: N-D, '85, 15

867.1 Bladder and urethra, with open wound into `MSP`
cavity

867.2 Ureter, without mention of open wound into `MSP`
cavity

867.3 Ureter, with open wound into cavity `MSP`

867.4 Uterus, without mention of open wound ♀ `MSP`
into cavity

867.5 Uterus, with open wound into cavity ♀ `MSP`

867.6 Other specified pelvic organs, without `MSP`
mention of open wound into cavity
> Fallopian tube   Seminal vesicle
> Ovary   Vas deferens
> Prostate

867.7 Other specified pelvic organs, with open `MSP`
wound into cavity

867.8 Unspecified pelvic organ, without mention `MSP`
of open wound into cavity

867.9 Unspecified pelvic organ, with open wound `MSP`
into cavity

√4th **868 Injury to other intra-abdominal organs**

The following fifth-digit subclassification is for use with category 868:

0 unspecified intra-abdominal organ
1 adrenal gland
2 bile duct and gallbladder
3 peritoneum
4 retroperitoneum
9 other and multiple intra-abdominal organs

√5th **868.0 Without mention of open wound into cavity** `MSP`

√5th **868.1 With open wound into cavity** `MSP`

√4th **869 Internal injury to unspecified or ill-defined organs**
> `INCLUDES` internal injury NOS
> multiple internal injury NOS

869.0 Without mention of open wound into cavity `MSP`

869.1 With open wound into cavity `MSP`
> AHA: 2Q, '89, 15

OPEN WOUND (870-897)

> `INCLUDES` animal bite
> avulsion
> cut
> laceration
> puncture wound
> traumatic amputation

> `EXCLUDES` *burn (940.0-949.5)*
> *crushing (925-929.9)*
> *puncture of internal organs (860.0-869.1)*
> *superficial injury (910.0-919.9)*
> *that incidental to:*
>   *dislocation (830.0-839.9)*
>   *fracture (800.0-829.1)*
>   *internal injury (860.0-869.1)*
>   *intracranial injury (851.0-854.1)*

The description "complicated" used in the fourth-digit subdivisions includes those with mention of delayed healing, delayed treatment, foreign body, or infection.

Use additional code to identify infection

AHA: 4Q, '01, 52

OPEN WOUND OF HEAD, NECK, AND TRUNK (870-879)

√4th **870 Open wound of ocular adnexa**

870.0 Laceration of skin of eyelid and periocular area

870.1 Laceration of eyelid, full-thickness, not involving lacrimal passages

870.2 Laceration of eyelid involving lacrimal passages

870.3 Penetrating wound of orbit, without mention of foreign body

870.4 Penetrating wound of orbit with foreign body
> `EXCLUDES` *retained (old) foreign body in orbit (376.6)*

870.8 Other specified open wounds of ocular adnexa

870.9 Unspecified open wound of ocular adnexa

√4th **871 Open wound of eyeball**
> `EXCLUDES` *2nd cranial nerve [optic] injury (950.0-950.9)*
> *3rd cranial nerve [oculomotor] injury (951.0)*

871.0 Ocular laceration without prolapse of intraocular tissue
> AHA: 3Q, '96, 7

> DEF: Tear in ocular tissue without displacing structures.

871.1 Ocular laceration with prolapse or exposure of intraocular tissue

871.2 Rupture of eye with partial loss of intraocular tissue
> DEF: Forcible tearing of eyeball, with tissue loss.

871.3 Avulsion of eye
> Traumatic enucleation
> DEF: Traumatic extraction of eyeball from socket.

871.4 Unspecified laceration of eye

871.5 Penetration of eyeball with magnetic foreign body
> `EXCLUDES` *retained (old) magnetic foreign body in globe (360.50-360.59)*

871.6 Penetration of eyeball with (nonmagnetic) foreign body
> `EXCLUDES` *retained (old) (nonmagnetic) foreign body in globe (360.60-360.69)*

871.7 Unspecified ocular penetration

871.9 Unspecified open wound of eyeball

√4th **872 Open wound of ear**

√5th **872.0 External ear, without mention of complication**

872.00 External ear, unspecified site

872.01 Auricle, ear
> Pinna
> DEF: Open wound of fleshy, outer ear.

`N` Newborn Age: 0   `P` Pediatric Age: 0-17   `M` Maternity Age: 12-55   `A` Adult Age: 15-124   `MSP` Medicare Secondary Payer

872.02　**Auditory canal**
　　DEF: Open wound of passage from external ear to eardrum.

√5ᵗʰ　872.1　**External ear, complicated**
　872.10　External ear, unspecified site
　872.11　**Auricle, ear**
　872.12　**Auditory canal**

√5ᵗʰ　872.6　**Other specified parts of ear, without mention of complication**
　872.61　**Ear drum**
　　　Drumhead　　　Tympanic membrane
　872.62　**Ossicles**
　872.63　**Eustachian tube**
　　DEF: Open wound of channel between nasopharynx and tympanic cavity.
　872.64　**Cochlea**
　　DEF: Open wound of snail shell shaped tube of inner ear.
　872.69　Other and multiple sites

√5ᵗʰ　872.7　**Other specified parts of ear, complicated**
　872.71　**Ear drum**
　872.72　**Ossicles**
　872.73　**Eustachian tube**
　872.74　**Cochlea**
　872.79　Other and multiple sites

872.8　**Ear, part unspecified, without mention of complication**
　　Ear NOS

872.9　Ear, part unspecified, complicated

√4ᵗʰ　873　**Other open wound of head**
　873.0　**Scalp, without mention of complication**
　873.1　**Scalp, complicated**

√5ᵗʰ　873.2　**Nose, without mention of complication**
　873.20　Nose, unspecified site
　873.21　**Nasal septum**
　　DEF: Open wound between nasal passages.
　873.22　**Nasal cavity**
　　DEF: Open wound of nostrils.
　873.23　**Nasal sinus**
　　DEF: Open wound of mucous-lined respiratory cavities.
　873.29　**Multiple sites**

√5ᵗʰ　873.3　**Nose, complicated**
　873.30　Nose, unspecified site
　873.31　**Nasal septum**
　873.32　**Nasal cavity**
　873.33　**Nasal sinus**
　873.39　**Multiple sites**

√5ᵗʰ　873.4　**Face, without mention of complication**
　873.40　Face, unspecified site
　873.41　**Cheek**
　873.42　**Forehead**
　　　Eyebrow
　　AHA: 4Q, '96, 43
　873.43　**Lip**
　873.44　**Jaw**
　873.49　Other and multiple sites

√5ᵗʰ　873.5　**Face, complicated**
　873.50　Face, unspecified site
　873.51　**Cheek**
　873.52　**Forehead**
　873.53　**Lip**
　873.54　**Jaw**
　873.59　Other and multiple sites

√5ᵗʰ　873.6　**Internal structures of mouth, without mention of complication**
　873.60　Mouth, unspecified site
　873.61　**Buccal mucosa**
　　DEF: Open wound of inside of cheek.
　873.62　**Gum (alveolar process)**
　873.63　**Tooth (broken)**
　　AHA: ▶1Q, '04, 17◀
　873.64　**Tongue and floor of mouth**
　873.65　**Palate**
　　DEF: Open wound of roof of mouth.
　873.69　Other and multiple sites

√5ᵗʰ　873.7　**Internal structures of mouth, complicated**
　873.70　Mouth, unspecified site
　873.71　**Buccal mucosa**
　873.72　**Gum (alveolar process)**
　873.73　**Tooth (broken)**
　　AHA: ▶1Q, '04, 17◀
　873.74　**Tongue and floor of mouth**
　873.75　**Palate**
　873.79　Other and multiple sites

873.8　Other and unspecified open wound of head without mention of complication
　　Head NOS

873.9　Other and unspecified open wound of head, complicated

√4ᵗʰ　874　**Open wound of neck**

√5ᵗʰ　874.0　**Larynx and trachea, without mention of complication**
　874.00　**Larynx with trachea**
　874.01　**Larynx**
　874.02　**Trachea**

√5ᵗʰ　874.1　**Larynx and trachea, complicated**
　874.10　**Larynx with trachea**
　874.11　**Larynx**
　874.12　**Trachea**

874.2　**Thyroid gland, without mention of complication**
874.3　**Thyroid gland, complicated**
874.4　**Pharynx, without mention of complication**
　　Cervical esophagus
874.5　**Pharynx, complicated**
874.8　Other and unspecified parts, without mention of complication
　　Nape of neck　　　Throat NOS
　　Supraclavicular region
874.9　Other and unspecified parts, complicated

√4ᵗʰ　875　**Open wound of chest (wall)**
　　EXCLUDES　open wound into thoracic cavity (860.0-862.9)
　　　traumatic pneumothorax and hemothorax (860.1, 860.3, 860.5)
　　AHA: 3Q, '93, 17
　875.0　**Without mention of complication**
　875.1　**Complicated**

√4ᵗʰ　876　**Open wound of back**
　　INCLUDES　loin
　　　lumbar region
　　EXCLUDES　open wound into thoracic cavity (860.0-862.9)
　　　traumatic pneumothorax and hemothorax (860.1, 860.3, 860.5)
　876.0　**Without mention of complication**
　876.1　**Complicated**

√4ᵗʰ　877　**Open wound of buttock**
　　INCLUDES　sacroiliac region
　877.0　**Without mention of complication**
　877.1　**Complicated**

√4ᵗʰ / √5ᵗʰ　Additional Digit Required　　　Unspecified Code　　　Other Specified Code　　　Manifestation Code　　　▶◀ Revised Text　　　● New Code　　　▲ Revised Code Title

Injury and Poisoning

878–893.0

√4ᵗʰ **878 Open wound of genital organs (external), including traumatic amputation**

> **EXCLUDES**   *injury during delivery (664.0-665.9)*
> *internal genital organs (867.0-867.9)*

878.0   **Penis, without mention of complication**   ♂

878.1   **Penis, complicated**   ♂

878.2   **Scrotum and testes, without mention of complication**   ♂

878.3   **Scrotum and testes, complicated**   ♂

878.4   **Vulva, without mention of complication**   ♀
     Labium (majus) (minus)

878.5   **Vulva, complicated**   ♀

878.6   **Vagina, without mention of complication**   ♀

878.7   **Vagina, complicated**   ♀

878.8   **Other and unspecified parts, without mention of complication**

878.9   **Other and unspecified parts, complicated**

√4ᵗʰ **879 Open wound of other and unspecified sites, except limbs**

879.0   **Breast, without mention of complication**

879.1   **Breast, complicated**

879.2   **Abdominal wall, anterior, without mention of complication**
     Abdominal wall NOS   Pubic region
     Epigastric region   Umbilical region
     Hypogastric region
     AHA: 2Q, '91, 22

879.3   **Abdominal wall, anterior, complicated**

879.4   **Abdominal wall, lateral, without mention of complication**
     Flank   Iliac (region)
     Groin   Inguinal region
     Hypochondrium

879.5   **Abdominal wall, lateral, complicated**

879.6   **Other and unspecified parts of trunk, without mention of complication**
     Pelvic region   Trunk NOS
     Perineum

879.7   **Other and unspecified parts of trunk, complicated**

879.8   **Open wound(s) (multiple) of unspecified site(s) without mention of complication**
     Multiple open wounds NOS   Open wound NOS

879.9   **Open wound(s) (multiple) of unspecified site(s), complicated**

OPEN WOUND OF UPPER LIMB (880-887)

AHA: N-D, '85, 5

√4ᵗʰ **880 Open wound of shoulder and upper arm**

The following fifth-digit subclassification is for use with category 880:
     0   shoulder region
     1   scapular region
     2   axillary region
     3   upper arm
     9   multiple sites

√5ᵗʰ 880.0   **Without mention of complication**

√5ᵗʰ 880.1   **Complicated**

√5ᵗʰ 880.2   **With tendon involvement**

√4ᵗʰ **881 Open wound of elbow, forearm, and wrist**

The following fifth-digit subclassification is for use with category 881:
     0   forearm
     1   elbow
     2   wrist

√5ᵗʰ 881.0   **Without mention of complication**

√5ᵗʰ 881.1   **Complicated**

√5ᵗʰ 881.2   **With tendon involvement**

√4ᵗʰ **882 Open wound of hand except finger(s) alone**

882.0   **Without mention of complication**

882.1   **Complicated**

882.2   **With tendon involvement**

√4ᵗʰ **883 Open wound of finger(s)**

> **INCLUDES**   fingernail
> thumb (nail)

883.0   **Without mention of complication**

883.1   **Complicated**

883.2   **With tendon involvement**

√4ᵗʰ **884 Multiple and unspecified open wound of upper limb**

> **INCLUDES**   arm NOS
> multiple sites of one upper limb
> upper limb NOS

884.0   **Without mention of complication**

884.1   **Complicated**

884.2   **With tendon involvement**

√4ᵗʰ **885 Traumatic amputation of thumb (complete) (partial)**

> **INCLUDES**   thumb(s) (with finger(s) of either hand)

885.0   **Without mention of complication**
     AHA: 1Q, '03, 7

885.1   **Complicated**

√4ᵗʰ **886 Traumatic amputation of other finger(s) (complete) (partial)**

> **INCLUDES**   finger(s) of one or both hands, without mention of thumb(s)

886.0   **Without mention of complication**

886.1   **Complicated**

√4ᵗʰ **887 Traumatic amputation of arm and hand (complete) (partial)**

887.0   **Unilateral, below elbow, without mention of complication**   **MSP**

887.1   **Unilateral, below elbow, complicated**   **MSP**

887.2   **Unilateral, at or above elbow, without mention of complication**   **MSP**

887.3   **Unilateral, at or above elbow, complicated**   **MSP**

887.4   **Unilateral, level not specified, without mention of complication**   **MSP**

887.5   **Unilateral, level not specified, complicated**   **MSP**

887.6   **Bilateral [any level], without mention of complication**   **MSP**
     One hand and other arm

887.7   **Bilateral [any level], complicated**   **MSP**

OPEN WOUND OF LOWER LIMB (890-897)

AHA: N-D, '85, 5

√4ᵗʰ **890 Open wound of hip and thigh**

890.0   **Without mention of complication**

890.1   **Complicated**

890.2   **With tendon involvement**

√4ᵗʰ **891 Open wound of knee, leg [except thigh], and ankle**

> **INCLUDES**   leg NOS
> multiple sites of leg, except thigh
> **EXCLUDES**   *that of thigh (890.0-890.2)*
> *with multiple sites of lower limb (894.0-894.2)*

891.0   **Without mention of complication**

891.1   **Complicated**

891.2   **With tendon involvement**

√4ᵗʰ **892 Open wound of foot except toe(s) alone**

> **INCLUDES**   heel

892.0   **Without mention of complication**

892.1   **Complicated**

892.2   **With tendon involvement**

√4ᵗʰ **893 Open wound of toe(s)**

> **INCLUDES**   toenail

893.0   **Without mention of complication**

893.1 Complicated
893.2 With tendon involvement
✓4th **894** Multiple and unspecified open wound of lower limb
INCLUDES lower limb NOS
multiple sites of one lower limb, with thigh
894.0 Without mention of complication
894.1 Complicated
894.2 With tendon involvement
✓4th **895** Traumatic amputation of toe(s) (complete) (partial)
INCLUDES toe(s) of one or both feet
895.0 Without mention of complication
895.1 Complicated
✓4th **896** Traumatic amputation of foot (complete) (partial)
896.0 Unilateral, without mention of complication MSP
896.1 Unilateral, complicated MSP
896.2 Bilateral, without mention of complication MSP
EXCLUDES one foot and other leg (897.6-897.7)
896.3 Bilateral, complicated MSP
✓4th **897** Traumatic amputation of leg(s) (complete) (partial)
897.0 Unilateral, below knee, without mention of complication MSP
897.1 Unilateral, below knee, complicated MSP
897.2 Unilateral, at or above knee, without mention of complication MSP
897.3 Unilateral, at or above knee, complicated MSP
897.4 Unilateral, level not specified, without mention of complication MSP
897.5 Unilateral, level not specified, complicated MSP
897.6 Bilateral [any level], without mention of complication MSP
One foot and other leg
897.7 Bilateral [any level], complicated MSP
AHA: 3Q, '90, 5

INJURY TO BLOOD VESSELS (900-904)

INCLUDES arterial hematoma
avulsion
cut
laceration
rupture
traumatic aneurysm
or fistula
(arteriovenous)
} of blood vessel,
secondary
to other
injuries e.g.,
fracture or
open wound

EXCLUDES accidental puncture or laceration during medical
procedure (998.2)
intracranial hemorrhage following injury (851.0-
854.1)

AHA: 3Q, '90, 5

✓4th **900** Injury to blood vessels of head and neck
✓5th **900.0** Carotid artery
900.00 Carotid artery, unspecified MSP
900.01 Common carotid artery MSP
900.02 External carotid artery MSP
900.03 Internal carotid artery MSP
900.1 Internal jugular vein MSP
✓5th **900.8** Other specified blood vessels of head and neck
900.81 External jugular vein MSP
Jugular vein NOS
900.82 Multiple blood vessels of head and neck MSP
900.89 Other MSP
900.9 Unspecified blood vessel of head and neck MSP
✓4th **901** Injury to blood vessels of thorax
EXCLUDES traumatic hemothorax (860.2-860.5)
901.0 Thoracic aorta
901.1 Innominate and subclavian arteries

901.2 Superior vena cava
901.3 Innominate and subclavian veins
✓5th **901.4** Pulmonary blood vessels
901.40 Pulmonary vessel(s), unspecified
901.41 Pulmonary artery
901.42 Pulmonary vein
✓5th **901.8** Other specified blood vessels of thorax
901.81 Intercostal artery or vein
901.82 Internal mammary artery or vein
901.83 Multiple blood vessels of thorax
901.89 Other
Azygos vein
Hemiazygos vein
901.9 Unspecified blood vessel of thorax
✓4th **902** Injury to blood vessels of abdomen and pelvis
902.0 Abdominal aorta
✓5th **902.1** Inferior vena cava
902.10 Inferior vena cava, unspecified
902.11 Hepatic veins
902.19 Other
✓5th **902.2** Celiac and mesenteric arteries
902.20 Celiac and mesenteric arteries, unspecified
902.21 Gastric artery
902.22 Hepatic artery
902.23 Splenic artery
902.24 Other specified branches of celiac axis
902.25 Superior mesenteric artery (trunk)
902.26 Primary branches of superior mesenteric artery
Ileocolic artery
902.27 Inferior mesenteric artery
902.29 Other
✓5th **902.3** Portal and splenic veins
902.31 Superior mesenteric vein and primary subdivisions
Ileocolic vein
902.32 Inferior mesenteric vein
902.33 Portal vein
902.34 Splenic vein
902.39 Other
Cystic vein   Gastric vein
✓5th **902.4** Renal blood vessels
902.40 Renal vessel(s), unspecified
902.41 Renal artery
902.42 Renal vein
902.49 Other
Suprarenal arteries
✓5th **902.5** Iliac blood vessels
902.50 Iliac vessel(s), unspecified
902.51 Hypogastric artery
902.52 Hypogastric vein
902.53 Iliac artery
902.54 Iliac vein
902.55 Uterine artery ♀
902.56 Uterine vein ♀
902.59 Other
✓5th **902.8** Other specified blood vessels of abdomen and pelvis
902.81 Ovarian artery ♀
902.82 Ovarian vein ♀
902.87 Multiple blood vessels of abdomen and pelvis
902.89 Other
902.9 Unspecified blood vessel of abdomen and pelvis

✓4th ✓5th Additional Digit Required | Unspecified Code | Other Specified Code | Manifestation Code | ►◄ Revised Text | ● New Code | ▲ Revised Code Title

2005 ICD•9•CM | **Volume 1 — 265**

Injury and Poisoning

903–908.0

✓4ᵗʰ **903 Injury to blood vessels of upper extremity**

    ✓5ᵗʰ **903.0 Axillary blood vessels**

        903.00 Axillary vessel(s), unspecified

        903.01 Axillary artery

        903.02 Axillary vein

    903.1 Brachial blood vessels

    903.2 Radial blood vessels

    903.3 Ulnar blood vessels

    903.4 Palmar artery

    903.5 Digital blood vessels

    903.8 Other specified blood vessels of upper extremity

        Multiple blood vessels of upper extremity

    903.9 Unspecified blood vessel of upper extremity

✓4ᵗʰ **904 Injury to blood vessels of lower extremity and unspecified sites**

    904.0 Common femoral artery

        Femoral artery above profunda origin

    904.1 Superficial femoral artery

    904.2 Femoral veins

    904.3 Saphenous veins

        Saphenous vein (greater) (lesser)

    ✓5ᵗʰ **904.4 Popliteal blood vessels**

        904.40 Popliteal vessel(s), unspecified

        904.41 Popliteal artery

        904.42 Popliteal vein

    ✓5ᵗʰ **904.5 Tibial blood vessels**

        904.50 Tibial vessel(s), unspecified

        904.51 Anterior tibial artery

        904.52 Anterior tibial vein

        904.53 Posterior tibial artery

        904.54 Posterior tibial vein

    904.6 Deep plantar blood vessels

    904.7 Other specified blood vessels of lower extremity

        Multiple blood vessels of lower extremity

    904.8 Unspecified blood vessel of lower extremity

    904.9 Unspecified site

        Injury to blood vessel NOS

LATE EFFECTS OF INJURIES, POISONINGS, TOXIC EFFECTS, AND OTHER EXTERNAL CAUSES (905-909)

    Note: These categories are to be used to indicate conditions classifiable to 800-999 as the cause of late effects, which are themselves classified elsewhere. The "late effects" include those specified as such, or as sequelae, which may occur at any time after the acute injury.

✓4ᵗʰ **905 Late effects of musculoskeletal and connective tissue injuries**

    AHA: 1Q, '95, 10; 2Q, '94, 3

    905.0 Late effect of fracture of skull and face bones

        Late effect of injury classifiable to 800-804

        AHA: 3Q, '97, 12

    905.1 Late effect of fracture of spine and trunk without mention of spinal cord lesion

        Late effect of injury classifiable to 805, 807-809

    905.2 Late effect of fracture of upper extremities

        Late effect of injury classifiable to 810-819

    905.3 Late effect of fracture of neck of femur

        Late effect of injury classifiable to 820

    905.4 Late effect of fracture of lower extremities

        Late effect of injury classifiable to 821-827

    905.5 Late effect of fracture of multiple and unspecified bones

        Late effect of injury classifiable to 828-829

    905.6 Late effect of dislocation

        Late effect of injury classifiable to 830-839

    905.7 Late effect of sprain and strain without mention of tendon injury

        Late effect of injury classifiable to 840-848, except tendon injury

    905.8 Late effect of tendon injury

        Late effect of tendon injury due to:

            open wound [injury classifiable to 880-884 with .2, 890-894 with .2]

            sprain and strain [injury classifiable to 840-848]

        AHA: 2Q, '89, 13; 2Q, '89, 15

    905.9 Late effect of traumatic amputation

        Late effect of injury classifiable to 885-887, 895-897

        EXCLUDES   *late amputation stump complication (997.60-997.69)*

✓4ᵗʰ **906 Late effects of injuries to skin and subcutaneous tissues**

    906.0 Late effect of open wound of head, neck, and trunk

        Late effect of injury classifiable to 870-879

    906.1 Late effect of open wound of extremities without mention of tendon injury

        Late effect of injury classifiable to 880-884, 890-894 except .2

    906.2 Late effect of superficial injury

        Late effect of injury classifiable to 910-919

    906.3 Late effect of contusion

        Late effect of injury classifiable to 920-924

    906.4 Late effect of crushing

        Late effect of injury classifiable to 925-929

    906.5 Late effect of burn of eye, face, head, and neck

        Late effect of injury classifiable to 940-941

    906.6 Late effect of burn of wrist and hand

        Late effect of injury classifiable to 944

        AHA: 4Q, '94, 22

    906.7 Late effect of burn of other extremities

        Late effect of injury classifiable to 943 or 945

        AHA: 4Q, '94, 22

    906.8 Late effect of burns of other specified sites

        Late effect of injury classifiable to 942, 946-947

        AHA: 4Q, '94, 22

    906.9 Late effect of burn of unspecified site

        Late effect of injury classifiable to 948-949

        AHA: 4Q, '94, 22

✓4ᵗʰ **907 Late effects of injuries to the nervous system**

    907.0 Late effect of intracranial injury without mention of skull fracture

        Late effect of injury classifiable to 850-854

        AHA: ▶4Q, '03, 103;◄ 3Q, '90, 14

    907.1 Late effect of injury to cranial nerve

        Late effect of injury classifiable to 950-951

    907.2 Late effect of spinal cord injury

        Late effect of injury classifiable to 806, 952

        AHA: ▶4Q, '03, 103;◄ 4Q, '98, 38

    907.3 Late effect of injury to nerve root(s), spinal plexus(es), and other nerves of trunk

        Late effect of injury classifiable to 953-954

    907.4 Late effect of injury to peripheral nerve of shoulder girdle and upper limb

        Late effect of injury classifiable to 955

    907.5 Late effect of injury to peripheral nerve of pelvic girdle and lower limb

        Late effect of injury classifiable to 956

    907.9 Late effect of injury to other and unspecified nerve

        Late effect of injury classifiable to 957

✓4ᵗʰ **908 Late effects of other and unspecified injuries**

    908.0 Late effect of internal injury to chest

        Late effect of injury classifiable to 860-862

Ⓝ Newborn Age: 0   Ⓟ Pediatric Age: 0-17   Ⓜ Maternity Age: 12-55   Ⓐ Adult Age: 15-124   MSP Medicare Secondary Payer

908.1 Late effect of internal injury to intra-abdominal organs
Late effect of injury classifiable to 863-866, 868

908.2 Late effect of internal injury to other internal organs
Late effect of injury classifiable to 867 or 869

908.3 Late effect of injury to blood vessel of head, neck, and extremities
Late effect of injury classifiable to 900, 903-904

908.4 Late effect of injury to blood vessel of thorax, abdomen, and pelvis
Late effect of injury classifiable to 901-902

908.5 Late effect of foreign body in orifice
Late effect of injury classifiable to 930-939

908.6 Late effect of certain complications of trauma
Late effect of complications classifiable to 958

908.9 Late effect of unspecified injury
Late effect of injury classifiable to 959
AHA: 3Q, '00, 4

√4ᵗʰ **909 Late effects of other and unspecified external causes**

909.0 Late effect of poisoning due to drug, medicinal or biological substance
Late effect of conditions classifiable to 960-979
EXCLUDES *late effect of adverse effect of drug, medicinal or biological substance (909.5)*
AHA: ▶4Q, '03, 103◀

909.1 Late effect of toxic effects of nonmedical substances
Late effect of conditions classifiable to 980-989

909.2 Late effect of radiation
Late effect of conditions classifiable to 990

909.3 Late effect of complications of surgical and medical care
Late effect of conditions classifiable to 996-999
AHA: 1Q, '93, 29

909.4 Late effect of certain other external causes
Late effect of conditions classifiable to 991-994

909.5 Late effect of adverse effect of drug, medical or biological substance
EXCLUDES *late effect of poisoning due to drug, medical or biological substance (909.0)*
AHA: 4Q, '94, 48

909.9 Late effect of other and unspecified external causes

SUPERFICIAL INJURY (910-919)

EXCLUDES *burn (blisters) (940.0-949.5)*
contusion (920-924.9)
foreign body:
granuloma (728.82)
inadvertently left in operative wound (998.4)
residual in soft tissue (729.6)
insect bite, venomous (989.5)
open wound with incidental foreign body (870.0-897.7)
AHA: 2Q, '89, 15

√4ᵗʰ **910 Superficial injury of face, neck, and scalp except eye**
INCLUDES   cheek
ear
gum
lip
nose
throat
EXCLUDES *eye and adnexa (918.0-918.9)*

910.0 Abrasion or friction burn without mention of infection

910.1 Abrasion or friction burn, infected

910.2 Blister without mention of infection

910.3 Blister, infected

910.4 Insect bite, nonvenomous, without mention of infection

910.5 Insect bite, nonvenomous, infected

910.6 Superficial foreign body (splinter) without major open wound and without mention of infection

910.7 Superficial foreign body (splinter) without major open wound, infected

910.8 Other and unspecified superficial injury of face, neck, and scalp without mention of infection

910.9 Other and unspecified superficial injury of face, neck, and scalp, infected

√4ᵗʰ **911 Superficial injury of trunk**
INCLUDES   abdominal wall
anus
back
breast
buttock
mchest wall
flank
groin
interscapular region
labium (majus) (minus)
penis
perineum
scrotum
testis
vagina
vulva
EXCLUDES *hip (916.0-916.9)*
scapular region (912.0-912.9)

911.0 Abrasion or friction burn without mention of infection
AHA: 3Q, '01, 10

911.1 Abrasion or friction burn, infected

911.2 Blister without mention of infection

911.3 Blister, infected

911.4 Insect bite, nonvenomous, without mention of infection

911.5 Insect bite, nonvenomous, infected

911.6 Superficial foreign body (splinter) without major open wound and without mention of infection

911.7 Superficial foreign body (splinter) without major open wound, infected

911.8 Other and unspecified superficial injury of trunk, without mention of infection

911.9 Other and unspecified superficial injury of trunk, infected

√4ᵗʰ **912 Superficial injury of shoulder and upper arm**
INCLUDES   axilla
scapular region

912.0 Abrasion or friction burn without mention of infection

912.1 Abrasion or friction burn, infected

912.2 Blister without mention of infection

912.3 Blister, infected

912.4 Insect bite, nonvenomous, without mention of infection

912.5 Insect bite, nonvenomous, infected

912.6 Superficial foreign body (splinter) without major open wound and without mention of infection

912.7 Superficial foreign body (splinter) without major open wound, infected

912.8 Other and unspecified superficial injury of shoulder and upper arm without mention of infection

912.9 Other and unspecified superficial injury of shoulder and upper arm, infected

√4ᵗʰ √5ᵗʰ Additional Digit Required   Unspecified Code   Other Specified Code   Manifestation Code   ▶◀ Revised Text   ● New Code   ▲ Revised Code Title

✓4ᵗʰ **913 Superficial injury of elbow, forearm, and wrist**

913.0 Abrasion or friction burn without mention of infection

913.1 Abrasion or friction burn, infected

913.2 Blister without mention of infection

913.3 Blister, infected

913.4 Insect bite, nonvenomous, without mention of infection

913.5 Insect bite, nonvenomous, infected

913.6 Superficial foreign body (splinter) without major open wound and without mention of infection

913.7 Superficial foreign body (splinter) without major open wound, infected

913.8 Other and unspecified superficial injury of elbow, forearm, and wrist without mention of infection

913.9 Other and unspecified superficial injury of elbow, forearm, and wrist, infected

✓4ᵗʰ **914 Superficial injury of hand(s) except finger(s) alone**

914.0 Abrasion or friction burn without mention of infection

914.1 Abrasion or friction burn, infected

914.2 Blister without mention of infection

914.3 Blister, infected

914.4 Insect bite, nonvenomous, without mention of infection

914.5 Insect bite, nonvenomous, infected

914.6 Superficial foreign body (splinter) without major open wound and without mention of infection

914.7 Superficial foreign body (splinter) without major open wound, infected

914.8 Other and unspecified superficial injury of hand without mention of infection

914.9 Other and unspecified superficial injury of hand, infected

✓4ᵗʰ **915 Superficial injury of finger(s)**

INCLUDES   fingernail
thumb (nail)

915.0 Abrasion or friction burn without mention of infection

915.1 Abrasion or friction burn, infected

915.2 Blister without mention of infection

915.3 Blister, infected

915.4 Insect bite, nonvenomous, without mention of infection

915.5 Insect bite, nonvenomous, infected

915.6 Superficial foreign body (splinter) without major open wound and without mention of infection

915.7 Superficial foreign body (splinter) without major open wound, infected

915.8 Other and unspecified superficial injury of fingers without mention of infection

AHA: 3Q, '01, 10

915.9 Other and unspecified superficial injury of fingers, infected

✓4ᵗʰ **916 Superficial injury of hip, thigh, leg, and ankle**

916.0 Abrasion or friction burn without mention of infection

916.1 Abrasion or friction burn, infected

916.2 Blister without mention of infection

916.3 Blister, infected

916.4 Insect bite, nonvenomous, without mention of infection

916.5 Insect bite, nonvenomous, infected

916.6 Superficial foreign body (splinter) without major open wound and without mention of infection

916.7 Superficial foreign body (splinter) without major open wound, infected

916.8 Other and unspecified superficial injury of hip, thigh, leg, and ankle without mention of infection

916.9 Other and unspecified superficial injury of hip, thigh, leg, and ankle, infected

✓4ᵗʰ **917 Superficial injury of foot and toe(s)**

INCLUDES   heel
toenail

917.0 Abrasion or friction burn without mention of infection

917.1 Abrasion or friction burn, infected

917.2 Blister without mention of infection

917.3 Blister, infected

917.4 Insect bite, nonvenomous, without mention of infection

917.5 Insect bite, nonvenomous, infected

917.6 Superficial foreign body (splinter) without major open wound and without mention of infection

917.7 Superficial foreign body (splinter) without major open wound, infected

917.8 Other and unspecified superficial injury of foot and toes without mention of infection

AHA: 1Q, '03, 13

917.9 Other and unspecified superficial injury of foot and toes, infected

AHA: 1Q, '03, 13

✓4ᵗʰ **918 Superficial injury of eye and adnexa**

EXCLUDES   burn (940.0-940.9)
foreign body on external eye (930.0-930.9)

918.0 **Eyelids and periocular area**

Abrasion   Superficial foreign body
Insect bite   (splinter)

918.1 **Cornea**

Corneal abrasion   Superficial laceration
EXCLUDES   corneal injury due to contact lens (371.82)

918.2 **Conjunctiva**

918.9 **Other and unspecified superficial injuries of eye**

Eye (ball) NOS

✓4ᵗʰ **919 Superficial injury of other, multiple, and unspecified sites**

EXCLUDES   multiple sites classifiable to the same three-digit category (910.0-918.9)

919.0 Abrasion or friction burn without mention of infection

919.1 Abrasion or friction burn, infected

919.2 Blister without mention of infection

919.3 Blister, infected

919.4 Insect bite, nonvenomous, without mention of infection

919.5 Insect bite, nonvenomous, infected

919.6 Superficial foreign body (splinter) without major open wound and without mention of infection

919.7 Superficial foreign body (splinter) without major open wound, infected

919.8 Other and unspecified superficial injury without mention of infection

919.9 Other and unspecified superficial injury, infected

CONTUSION WITH INTACT SKIN SURFACE (920-924)

INCLUDES   bruise   } without fracture or open
               hematoma }   wound

EXCLUDES   concussion (850.0-850.9)
               hemarthrosis (840.0-848.9)
               internal organs (860.0-869.1)
               that incidental to:
                   crushing injury (925-929.9)
                   dislocation (830.0-839.9)
                   fracture (800.0-829.1)
                   internal injury (860.0-869.1)
                   intracranial injury (850.0-854.1)
                   nerve injury (950.0-957.9)
                   open wound (870.0-897.7)

920 Contusion of face, scalp, and neck except eye(s)
   Cheek   Mandibular joint area
   Ear (auricle)   Nose
   Gum   Throat
   Lip

✓4th **921 Contusion of eye and adnexa**
   921.0 Black eye, not otherwise specified
   921.1 Contusion of eyelids and periocular area
   921.2 Contusion of orbital tissues
   921.3 Contusion of eyeball
      AHA: J-A, '85, 16

   921.9 Unspecified contusion of eye
      Injury of eye NOS

✓4th **922 Contusion of trunk**
   922.0 Breast
   922.1 Chest wall
   922.2 Abdominal wall
      Flank   Groin
   ✓5th **922.3 Back**
      AHA: 4Q, '96, 39

      922.31 Back
         EXCLUDES interscapular region (922.33)
      922.32 Buttock
         AHA: 3Q, '99, 14

      922.33 Interscapular region
   922.4 Genital organs
      Labium (majus) (minus)   Vulva
      Penis   Vagina
      Perineum   Testis
      Scrotum
   922.8 Multiple sites of trunk
   922.9 Unspecified part
      Trunk NOS

✓4th **923 Contusion of upper limb**
   ✓5th **923.0 Shoulder and upper arm**
      923.00 Shoulder region
      923.01 Scapular region
      923.02 Axillary region
      923.03 Upper arm
      923.09 Multiple sites
   ✓5th **923.1 Elbow and forearm**
      923.10 Forearm
      923.11 Elbow
   ✓5th **923.2 Wrist and hand(s), except finger(s) alone**
      923.20 Hand(s)
      923.21 Wrist
   923.3 Finger
      Fingernail   Thumb (nail)
   923.8 Multiple sites of upper limb
   923.9 Unspecified part of upper limb
      Arm NOS

✓4th **924 Contusion of lower limb and of other and unspecified sites**
   ✓5th **924.0 Hip and thigh**
      924.00 Thigh
      924.01 Hip
   ✓5th **924.1 Knee and lower leg**
      924.10 Lower leg
      924.11 Knee
   ✓5th **924.2 Ankle and foot, excluding toe(s)**
      924.20 Foot
         Heel
      924.21 Ankle
   924.3 Toe
      Toenail
   924.4 Multiple sites of lower limb
   924.5 Unspecified part of lower limb
      Leg NOS
   924.8 Multiple sites, not elsewhere classified
      AHA: 1Q, '03, 7

   924.9 Unspecified site

CRUSHING INJURY (925-929)
   Use additional code to identify any associated injuries,
         such as:
      fractures (800-829)
      internal injuries (860.0-869.1)
      intracranial injuries (850.0-854.1)
   AHA: ▶4Q, '03, 77;◄ 2Q, '93, 7

✓4th **925 Crushing injury of face, scalp, and neck**
      Cheek   Pharynx
      Ear   Throat
      Larynx
   925.1 Crushing injury of face and scalp   **MSP**
      Cheek   Ear
   925.2 Crushing injury of neck   **MSP**
      Larynx   Throat
      Pharynx

✓4th **926 Crushing injury of trunk**
   926.0 External genitalia
      Labium (majus) (minus) Testis
      Penis   Vulva
      Scrotum
   ✓5th **926.1 Other specified sites**
      926.11 Back
      926.12 Buttock
      926.19 Other
         Breast
   926.8 Multiple sites of trunk   **MSP**
   926.9 Unspecified site
      Trunk NOS

✓4th **927 Crushing injury of upper limb**
   ✓5th **927.0 Shoulder and upper arm**
      927.00 Shoulder region
      927.01 Scapular region
      927.02 Axillary region
      927.03 Upper arm
      927.09 Multiple sites
   ✓5th **927.1 Elbow and forearm**
      927.10 Forearm
      927.11 Elbow
   ✓5th **927.2 Wrist and hand(s), except finger(s) alone**
      927.20 Hand(s)
      927.21 Wrist
   927.3 Finger(s)
      AHA: ▶4Q, '03, 77◄

   927.8 Multiple sites of upper limb
   927.9 Unspecified site
      Arm NOS

✓4th / ✓5th Additional Digit Required   Unspecified Code   Other Specified Code   Manifestation Code   ▶◄ Revised Text   ● New Code   ▲ Revised Code Title

Injury and Poisoning

928–941.0

✓4ᵗʰ **928 Crushing injury of lower limb**

  ✓5ᵗʰ **928.0 Hip and thigh**
     928.00 Thigh
     928.01 Hip

  ✓5ᵗʰ **928.1 Knee and lower leg**
     928.10 Lower leg
     928.11 Knee

  ✓5ᵗʰ **928.2 Ankle and foot, excluding toe(s) alone**
     928.20 Foot
       Heel
     928.21 Ankle

  928.3 Toe(s)

  928.8 Multiple sites of lower limb

  928.9 Unspecified site
    Leg NOS

✓4ᵗʰ **929 Crushing injury of multiple and unspecified sites**

  929.0 Multiple sites, not elsewhere classified   MSP

  929.9 Unspecified site   MSP

EFFECTS OF FOREIGN BODY ENTERING THROUGH ORIFICE (930-939)

EXCLUDES *foreign body:*
granuloma (728.82)
inadvertently left in operative wound (998.4, 998.7)
in open wound (800-839, 851-897)
residual in soft tissues (729.6)
superficial without major open wound (910-919 with .6 or .7)

✓4ᵗʰ **930 Foreign body on external eye**

  EXCLUDES *foreign body in penetrating wound of:*
    eyeball (871.5-871.6)
      retained (old) (360.5-360.6)
    ocular adnexa (870.4)
      retained (old) (376.6)

  930.0 Corneal foreign body

  930.1 Foreign body in conjunctival sac

  930.2 Foreign body in lacrimal punctum

  930.8 Other and combined sites

  930.9 Unspecified site
    External eye NOS

931 Foreign body in ear
  Auditory canal   Auricle

932 Foreign body in nose
  Nasal sinus   Nostril

✓4ᵗʰ **933 Foreign body in pharynx and larynx**

  933.0 Pharynx
    Nasopharynx   Throat NOS

  933.1 Larynx
    Asphyxia due to foreign body
    Choking due to:
      food (regurgitated)
      phlegm

✓4ᵗʰ **934 Foreign body in trachea, bronchus, and lung**

  934.0 Trachea

  934.1 Main bronchus
    AHA: 3Q, '02, 18

  934.8 Other specified parts
    Bronchioles   Lung

  934.9 Respiratory tree, unspecified
    Inhalation of liquid or vomitus, lower respiratory tract NOS

✓4ᵗʰ **935 Foreign body in mouth, esophagus, and stomach**

  935.0 Mouth

  935.1 Esophagus
    AHA: 1Q, '88, 13

  935.2 Stomach

936 Foreign body in intestine and colon

937 Foreign body in anus and rectum
  Rectosigmoid (junction)

938 Foreign body in digestive system, unspecified
  Alimentary tract NOS
  Swallowed foreign body

✓4ᵗʰ **939 Foreign body in genitourinary tract**

  939.0 Bladder and urethra

  939.1 Uterus, any part   ♀
    EXCLUDES *intrauterine contraceptive device:*
      complications from (996.32, 996.65)
      presence of (V45.51)

  939.2 Vulva and vagina   ♀

  939.3 Penis   ♂

  939.9 Unspecified site

BURNS (940-949)

INCLUDES burns from:
  electrical heating appliance
  electricity
  flame
  hot object
  lightning
  radiation
  chemical burns (external) (internal)
  scalds

EXCLUDES *friction burns (910-919 with .0, .1)*
  sunburn (692.71, 692.76-692.77)

AHA: 4Q, 94, 22; 2Q, '90, 7; 4Q, '88, 3; M-A, '86, 9

✓4ᵗʰ **940 Burn confined to eye and adnexa**

  940.0 Chemical burn of eyelids and periocular area

  940.1 Other burns of eyelids and periocular area

  940.2 Alkaline chemical burn of cornea and conjunctival sac

  940.3 Acid chemical burn of cornea and conjunctival sac

  940.4 Other burn of cornea and conjunctival sac

  940.5 Burn with resulting rupture and destruction of eyeball

  940.9 Unspecified burn of eye and adnexa

✓4ᵗʰ **941 Burn of face, head, and neck**

  EXCLUDES *mouth (947.0)*

  The following fifth-digit subclassification is for use with category 941:

    0 face and head, unspecified site
    1 ear [any part]
    2 eye (with other parts of face, head, and neck)
    3 lip(s)
    4 chin
    5 nose (septum)
    6 scalp [any part]
      Temple (region)
    7 forehead and cheek
    8 neck
    9 multiple sites [except with eye] of face, head, and neck

  AHA: 4Q, '94, 22; M-A, '86, 9

  ✓5ᵗʰ **941.0 Unspecified degree**

Burns

Degrees of Burns

First (redness)   Second (blistering)   Third (full thickness)   Deep Third (deep necrosis)   Eschar

---

N Newborn Age: 0   P Pediatric Age: 0-17   M Maternity Age: 12-55   A Adult Age: 15-124   MSP Medicare Secondary Payer

Injury and Poisoning

941.1–947.3

Rule of Nines

Rule of Nines
Estimation of Total Body
Surface Burned

Head and neck 9%

Each arm 9%

Posterior trunk 18%

Anterior trunk 18%

Genitalia 1%

Anterior leg 9%

Posterior leg 9%

✓5th **941.1** Erythema [first degree]

✓5th **941.2** Blisters, epidermal loss [second degree]

✓5th **941.3** Full-thickness skin loss [third degree NOS]

✓5th **941.4** Deep necrosis of underlying tissues [deep third degree] without mention of loss of a body part

✓5th **941.5** Deep necrosis of underlying tissues [deep third degree] with loss of a body part

✓4th **942 Burn of trunk**

> **EXCLUDES**   *scapular region (943.0-943.5 with fifth-digit 6)*

The following fifth-digit subclassification is for use with category 942:

  0   trunk, unspecified site
  1   breast
  2   chest wall, excluding breast and nipple
  3   abdominal wall
      Flank   Groin
  4   back [any part]
      Buttock   Interscapular region
  5   genitalia
      Labium (majus) (minus)   Scrotum
      Penis   Testis
      Perineum   Vulva
  9   other and multiple sites of trunk

AHA: 4Q, '94, 22; M-A, '86, 9

✓5th **942.0** Unspecified degree

✓5th **942.1** Erythema [first degree]

✓5th **942.2** Blisters, epidermal loss [second degree]

✓5th **942.3** Full-thickness skin loss [third degree NOS]

✓5th **942.4** Deep necrosis of underlying tissues [deep third degree] without mention of loss of a body part

✓5th **942.5** Deep necrosis of underlying tissues [deep third degree] with loss of a body part

✓4th **943 Burn of upper limb, except wrist and hand**

The following fifth-digit subclassification is for use with category 943:

  0   upper limb, unspecified site
  1   forearm
  2   elbow
  3   upper arm
  4   axilla
  5   shoulder
  6   scapular region
  9   multiple sites of upper limb, except wrist and hand

AHA: 4Q, '94, 22; M-A, '86, 9

✓5th **943.0** Unspecified degree

✓5th **943.1** Erythema [first degree]

✓5th **943.2** Blisters, epidermal loss [second degree]

✓5th **943.3** Full-thickness skin loss [third degree NOS]

✓5th **943.4** Deep necrosis of underlying tissues [deep third degree] without mention of loss of a body part

✓5th **943.5** Deep necrosis of underlying tissues [deep third degree] with loss of a body part

✓4th **944 Burn of wrist(s) and hand(s)**

The following fifth-digit subclassification is for use with category 944:

  0   hand, unspecified site
  1   single digit [finger (nail)] other than thumb
  2   thumb (nail)
  3   two or more digits, not including thumb
  4   two or more digits including thumb
  5   palm
  6   back of hand
  7   wrist
  8   multiple sites of wrist(s) and hand(s)

✓5th **944.0** Unspecified degree

✓5th **944.1** Erythema [first degree]

✓5th **944.2** Blisters, epidermal loss [second degree]

✓5th **944.3** Full-thickness skin loss [third degree NOS]

✓5th **944.4** Deep necrosis of underlying tissues [deep third degree] without mention of loss of a body part

✓5th **944.5** Deep necrosis of underlying tissues [deep third degree] with loss of a body part

✓4th **945 Burn of lower limb(s)**

The following fifth-digit subclassification is for use with category 945:

  0   lower limb [leg], unspecified site
  1   toe(s) (nail)
  2   foot
  3   ankle
  4   lower leg
  5   knee
  6   thigh [any part]
  9   multiple sites of lower limb(s)

AHA: 4Q, '94, 22; M-A, '86, 9

✓5th **945.0** Unspecified degree

✓5th **945.1** Erythema [first degree]

✓5th **945.2** Blisters, epidermal loss [second degree]

✓5th **945.3** Full-thickness skin loss [third degree NOS]

✓5th **945.4** Deep necrosis of underlying tissues [deep third degree] without mention of loss of a body part

✓5th **945.5** Deep necrosis of underlying tissues [deep third degree] with loss of a body part

✓4th **946 Burns of multiple specified sites**

> **INCLUDES**   burns of sites classifiable to more than one three-digit category in 940-945

> **EXCLUDES**   *multiple burns NOS (949.0-949.5)*

AHA: 4Q, '94, 22; M-A, '86, 9

946.0 Unspecified degree

946.1 Erythema [first degree]

946.2 Blisters, epidermal loss [second degree]

946.3 Full-thickness skin loss [third degree NOS]

946.4 Deep necrosis of underlying tissues [deep third degree] without mention of loss of a body part

946.5 Deep necrosis of underlying tissues [deep third degree] with loss of a body part

✓4th **947 Burn of internal organs**

> **INCLUDES**   burns from chemical agents (ingested)

AHA: 4Q, '94, 22; M-A, '86, 9

947.0 Mouth and pharynx
      Gum   Tongue

947.1 Larynx, trachea, and lung

947.2 Esophagus

947.3 Gastrointestinal tract
      Colon   Small intestine
      Rectum   Stomach

✓4th / ✓5th   Additional Digit Required   Unspecified Code   Other Specified Code   Manifestation Code   ▶◀ Revised Text   ● New Code   ▲ Revised Code Title

Injury and Poisoning

947.4–952.03

947.4 **Vagina and uterus** ♀

947.8 Other specified sites

947.9 Unspecified site

√4th 948 **Burns classified according to extent of body surface involved**

Note: This category is to be used when the site of the burn is unspecified, or with categories 940-947 when the site is specified.

EXCLUDES *sunburn (692.71, 692.76-692.77)*

The following fifth-digit subclassification is for use with category 948 to indicate the percent of body surface with third degree burn; valid digits are in [brackets] under each code:

0 less than 10 percent or unspecified
1 10-19%
2 20-29%
3 30-39%
4 40-49%
5 50-59%
6 60-69%
7 70-79%
8 80-89%
9 90% or more of body surface

AHA: 4Q, '94, 22; 4Q, '88, 3; M-A, '86, 9; N-D, '84, 13

√5th 948.0 **Burn [any degree] involving less than 10 percent of**
[0] **body surface**

√5th 948.1 **10-19 percent of body surface**
[0-1]

√5th 948.2 **20-29 percent of body surface**
[0-2]

√5th 948.3 **30-39 percent of body surface**
[0-3]

√5th 948.4 **40-49 percent of body surface**
[0-4]

√5th 948.5 **50-59 percent of body surface**
[0-5]

√5th 948.6 **60-69 percent of body surface**
[0-6]

√5th 948.7 **70-79 percent of body surface**
[0-7]

√5th 948.8 **80-89 percent of body surface**
[0-8]

√5th 948.9 **90 percent or more of body surface**
[0-9]

√4th 949 **Burn, unspecified**

INCLUDES burn NOS multiple burns NOS

EXCLUDES *burn of unspecified site but with statement of the extent of body surface involved (948.0-948.9)*

AHA: 4Q, '94, 22; M-A, '86, 9

949.0 Unspecified degree

949.1 Erythema [first degree]

949.2 Blisters, epidermal loss [second degree]

949.3 Full-thickness skin loss [third degree NOS]

949.4 **Deep necrosis of underlying tissues [deep third degree] without mention of loss of a body part**

949.5 **Deep necrosis of underlying tissues [deep third degree] with loss of a body part**

Spinal Nerve Roots

INJURY TO NERVES AND SPINAL CORD (950-957)

INCLUDES division of nerve
lesion in continuity
traumatic neuroma   } (with open wound)
traumatic transient
paralysis

EXCLUDES *accidental puncture or laceration during medical procedure (998.2)*

√4th 950 **Injury to optic nerve and pathways**

950.0 **Optic nerve injury**
Second cranial nerve

950.1 **Injury to optic chiasm**

950.2 **Injury to optic pathways**

950.3 **Injury to visual cortex**

950.9 Unspecified
Traumatic blindness NOS

√4th 951 **Injury to other cranial nerve(s)**

951.0 **Injury to oculomotor nerve**
Third cranial nerve

951.1 **Injury to trochlear nerve**
Fourth cranial nerve

951.2 **Injury to trigeminal nerve**
Fifth cranial nerve

951.3 **Injury to abducens nerve**
Sixth cranial nerve

951.4 **Injury to facial nerve**
Seventh cranial nerve

951.5 **Injury to acoustic nerve**
Auditory nerve   Traumatic deafness NOS
Eighth cranial nerve

951.6 **Injury to accessory nerve**
Eleventh cranial nerve

951.7 **Injury to hypoglossal nerve**
Twelfth cranial nerve

951.8 Injury to other specified cranial nerves
Glossopharyngeal [9th cranial] nerve
Olfactory [1st cranial] nerve
Pneumogastric [10th cranial] nerve
Traumatic anosmia NOS
Vagus [10th cranial] nerve

951.9 Injury to unspecified cranial nerve

√4th 952 **Spinal cord injury without evidence of spinal bone injury**

√5th 952.0 **Cervical**

952.00 C_1-C_4 level with unspecified spinal cord injury
Spinal cord injury, cervical region NOS

952.01 C_1-C_4 level with complete lesion of spinal cord

952.02 C_1-C_4 level with anterior cord syndrome

952.03 C_1-C_4 level with central cord syndrome

952.04 C_1-C_4 level with other specified spinal cord injury

    Incomplete spinal cord lesion at C_1-C_4 level:
      NOS
      with posterior cord syndrome

952.05 C_5-C_7 level with unspecified spinal cord injury

952.06 C_5-C_7 level with complete lesion of spinal cord

952.07 C_5-C_7 level with anterior cord syndrome

952.08 C_5-C_7 level with central cord syndrome

952.09 C_5-C_7 level with other specified spinal cord injury

    Incomplete spinal cord lesion at C_5-C_7 level:
      NOS
      with posterior cord syndrome

√5th **952.1** Dorsal [thoracic]

952.10 T_1-T_6 level with unspecified spinal cord injury
    Spinal cord injury, thoracic region NOS

952.11 T_1-T_6 level with complete lesion of spinal cord

952.12 T_1-T_6 level with anterior cord syndrome

952.13 T_1-T_6 level with central cord syndrome

952.14 T_1-T_6 level with other specified spinal cord injury

    Incomplete spinal cord lesion at T_1-T_6 level:
      NOS
      with posterior cord syndrome

952.15 T_7-T_{12} level with unspecified spinal cord injury

952.16 T_7-T_{12} level with complete lesion of spinal cord

952.17 T_7-T_{12} level with anterior cord syndrome

952.18 T_7-T_{12} level with central cord syndrome

952.19 T_7-T_{12} level with other specified spinal cord injury

    Incomplete spinal cord lesion at T_7-T_{12} level:
      NOS
      with posterior cord syndrome

952.2 Lumbar

952.3 Sacral

952.4 Cauda equina

952.8 Multiple sites of spinal cord

952.9 Unspecified site of spinal cord

√4th **953** Injury to nerve roots and spinal plexus

953.0 Cervical root

953.1 Dorsal root

953.2 Lumbar root

953.3 Sacral root

953.4 Brachial plexus

953.5 Lumbosacral plexus

953.8 Multiple sites

953.9 Unspecified site

√4th **954** Injury to other nerve(s) of trunk, excluding shoulder and pelvic girdles

954.0 Cervical sympathetic

954.1 Other sympathetic
    Celiac ganglion or plexus   Splanchnic nerve(s)
    Inferior mesenteric plexus   Stellate ganglion

954.8 Other specified nerve(s) of trunk

954.9 Unspecified nerve of trunk

√4th **955** Injury to peripheral nerve(s) of shoulder girdle and upper limb

955.0 Axillary nerve

955.1 Median nerve

955.2 Ulnar nerve

955.3 Radial nerve

955.4 Musculocutaneous nerve

955.5 Cutaneous sensory nerve, upper limb

955.6 Digital nerve

955.7 Other specified nerve(s) of shoulder girdle and upper limb

955.8 Multiple nerves of shoulder girdle and upper limb

955.9 Unspecified nerve of shoulder girdle and upper limb

√4th **956** Injury to peripheral nerve(s) of pelvic girdle and lower limb

956.0 Sciatic nerve

956.1 Femoral nerve

956.2 Posterior tibial nerve

956.3 Peroneal nerve

956.4 Cutaneous sensory nerve, lower limb

956.5 Other specified nerve(s) of pelvic girdle and lower limb

956.8 Multiple nerves of pelvic girdle and lower limb

956.9 Unspecified nerve of pelvic girdle and lower limb

√4th **957** Injury to other and unspecified nerves

957.0 Superficial nerves of head and neck

957.1 Other specified nerve(s)

957.8 Multiple nerves in several parts
    Multiple nerve injury NOS

957.9 Unspecified site
    Nerve injury NOS

CERTAIN TRAUMATIC COMPLICATIONS AND UNSPECIFIED INJURIES (958-959)

√4th **958** Certain early complications of trauma

    EXCLUDES   *adult respiratory distress syndrome (518.5)*
        flail chest (807.4)
        shock lung (518.5)
        that occurring during or following medical procedures (996.0-999.9)

958.0 Air embolism
    Pneumathemia
    EXCLUDES   *that complicating:*
        abortion (634-638 with .6, 639.6)
        ectopic or molar pregnancy (639.6)
        pregnancy, childbirth, or the puerperium (673.0)

    DEF: Arterial obstruction due to introduction of air bubbles into the veins following surgery or trauma.

958.1 Fat embolism
    EXCLUDES   *that complicating:*
        abortion (634-638 with .6, 639.6)
        pregnancy, childbirth, or the puerperium (673.8)

    DEF: Arterial blockage due to the entrance of fat in circulatory system, after fracture of large bones or administration of corticosteroids.

958.2 Secondary and recurrent hemorrhage

958.3 Posttraumatic wound infection, not elsewhere classified
    EXCLUDES   *infected open wounds — code to complicated open wound of site*

    AHA: 4Q, '01, 53; S-O, '85, 10

958.4 Traumatic shock   **MSP**
    Shock (immediate) (delayed) following injury
    EXCLUDES   *shock:*
        anaphylactic (995.0)
          due to serum (999.4)
        anesthetic (995.4)
        electric (994.8)
        following abortion (639.5)
        lightning (994.0)
        nontraumatic NOS (785.50)
        obstetric (669.1)
        postoperative (998.0)

    DEF: Shock, immediate or delayed following injury.

√4th Additional Digit Required   Unspecified Code   Other Specified Code   Manifestation Code   ►◄ Revised Text   ● New Code   ▲ Revised Code Title

2005 ICD•9•CM   Volume 1 — 273

Injury and Poisoning

958.5–961.1

958.5 Traumatic anuria MSP
Crush syndrome
Renal failure following crushing
EXCLUDES *that due to a medical procedure (997.5)*
DEF: Complete suppression of urinary secretion by kidneys due to trauma.

958.6 Volkmann's ischemic contracture
Posttraumatic muscle contracture
DEF: Muscle deterioration due to loss of blood supply from injury or tourniquet; causes muscle contraction and results in inability to extend the muscles fully.

958.7 Traumatic subcutaneous emphysema
EXCLUDES *subcutaneous emphysema resulting from a procedure (998.81)*

958.8 Other early complications of trauma
AHA: 2Q, '92, 13
DEF: Compartmental syndrome is abnormal pressure in confined anatomical space, as in swollen muscle restricted by fascia.

✓4ᵗʰ 959 Injury, other and unspecified
INCLUDES injury NOS
EXCLUDES *injury NOS of:*
blood vessels (900.0-904.9)
eye (921.0-921.9)
internal organs (860.0-869.1)
intracranial sites (854.0-854.1)
nerves (950.0-951.9, 953.0-957.9)
spinal cord (952.0-952.9)

✓5ᵗʰ 959.0 Head, face and neck
959.01 Head injury, unspecified MSP
EXCLUDES *concussion (850.1-850.9)*
with head injury NOS (850.0-850.9)
head injury NOS with loss of consciousness (850.1-850.5)
specified injuries (850.0-854.1)
AHA: 4Q, '97, 46

959.09 Injury of face and neck MSP
Cheek   Mouth
Ear   Nose
Eyebrow   Throat
Lip
AHA: 4Q, '97, 46

✓5ᵗʰ 959.1 Trunk
EXCLUDES *scapular region (959.2)*
AHA: ▶4Q, '03, 78;◀ 1Q, '99, 10
959.11 Other injury of chest wall
959.12 Other injury of abdomen
959.13 Fracture of corpus cavernosum penis ♂
959.14 Other injury of external genitals
959.19 Other injury of other sites of trunk
Injury of trunk NOS

959.2 Shoulder and upper arm
Axilla   Scapular region
959.3 Elbow, forearm, and wrist
AHA: 1Q, '97, 8
959.4 Hand, except finger
959.5 Finger
Fingernail   Thumb (nail)
959.6 Hip and thigh
Upper leg
959.7 Knee, leg, ankle, and foot
959.8 Other specified sites, including multiple
EXCLUDES *multiple sites classifiable to the same four-digit category (959.0-959.7)*
959.9 Unspecified site

POISONING BY DRUGS, MEDICINAL AND BIOLOGICAL SUBSTANCES (960-979)
INCLUDES overdose of these substances
wrong substance given or taken in error
EXCLUDES *adverse effects ["hypersensitivity," "reaction," etc.] of correct substance properly administered. Such cases are to be classified according to the nature of the adverse effect, such as:*
adverse effect NOS (995.2)
allergic lymphadenitis (289.3)
aspirin gastritis (535.4)
blood disorders (280.0-289.9)
dermatitis:
contact (692.0-692.9)
due to ingestion (693.0-693.9)
nephropathy (583.9)
[The drug giving rise to the adverse effect may be identified by use of categories E930-E949.]
drug dependence (304.0-304.9)
drug reaction and poisoning affecting the newborn (760.0-779.9)
nondependent abuse of drugs (305.0-305.9)
pathological drug intoxication (292.2)
Use additional code to specify the effects of the poisoning
AHA: 2Q, '90, 11

✓4ᵗʰ 960 Poisoning by antibiotics
EXCLUDES *antibiotics:*
ear, nose, and throat (976.6)
eye (976.5)
local (976.0)
960.0 Penicillins
Ampicillin   Cloxacillin
Carbenicillin   Penicillin G
960.1 Antifungal antibiotics
Amphotericin B   Nystatin
Griseofulvin   Trichomycin
EXCLUDES *preparations intended for topical use (976.0-976.9)*
960.2 Chloramphenicol group
Chloramphenicol   Thiamphenicol
960.3 Erythromycin and other macrolides
Oleandomycin   Spiramycin
960.4 Tetracycline group
Doxycycline   Oxytetracycline
Minocycline
960.5 Cephalosporin group
Cephalexin   Cephaloridine
Cephaloglycin   Cephalothin
960.6 Antimycobacterial antibiotics
Cycloserine   Rifampin
Kanamycin   Streptomycin
960.7 Antineoplastic antibiotics
Actinomycin such as:
Bleomycin
Cactinomycin
Dactinomycin
Daunorubicin
Mitomycin
960.8 Other specified antibiotics
960.9 Unspecified antibiotic
✓4ᵗʰ 961 Poisoning by other anti-infectives
EXCLUDES *anti-infectives:*
ear, nose, and throat (976.6)
eye (976.5)
local (976.0)
961.0 Sulfonamides
Sulfadiazine   Sulfamethoxazole
Sulfafurazole
961.1 Arsenical anti-infectives

961.2 Heavy metal anti-infectives
Compounds of: Compounds of:
antimony   lead
bismuth   mercury
EXCLUDES *mercurial diuretics (974.0)*

961.3 Quinoline and hydroxyquinoline derivatives
Chiniofon   Diiodohydroxyquin
EXCLUDES *antimalarial drugs (961.4)*

961.4 Antimalarials and drugs acting on other blood protozoa
Chloroquine   Proguanil [chloroguanide]
Cycloguanil   Pyrimethamine
Primaquine   Quinine

961.5 Other antiprotozoal drugs
Emetine

961.6 Anthelmintics
Hexylresorcinol   Thiabendazole
Piperazine

961.7 Antiviral drugs
Methisazone
EXCLUDES *amantadine (966.4)*
cytarabine (963.1)
idoxuridine (976.5)

961.8 Other antimycobacterial drugs
Ethambutol   Para-aminosalicylic acid
Ethionamide   derivatives
Isoniazid   Sulfones

961.9 Other and unspecified anti-infectives
Flucytosine   Nitrofuran derivatives

962 Poisoning by hormones and synthetic substitutes
EXCLUDES *oxytocic hormones (975.0)*

962.0 Adrenal cortical steroids
Cortisone derivatives
Desoxycorticosterone derivatives
Fluorinated corticosteroids

962.1 Androgens and anabolic congeners
Methandriol   Oxymetholone
Nandrolone   Testosterone

962.2 Ovarian hormones and synthetic substitutes
Contraceptives, oral
Estrogens
Estrogens and progestogens, combined
Progestogens

962.3 Insulins and antidiabetic agents
Acetohexamide
Biguanide derivatives, oral
Chlorpropamide
Glucagon
Insulin
Phenformin
Sulfonylurea derivatives, oral
Tolbutamide
AHA: M-A, '85, 8

962.4 Anterior pituitary hormones
Corticotropin   Somatotropin [growth
Gonadotropin   hormone]

962.5 Posterior pituitary hormones
Vasopressin
EXCLUDES *oxytocic hormones (975.0)*

962.6 Parathyroid and parathyroid derivatives

962.7 Thyroid and thyroid derivatives
Dextrothyroxin   Liothyronine
Levothyroxine sodium   Thyroglobulin

962.8 Antithyroid agents
Iodides   Thiourea
Thiouracil

962.9 Other and unspecified hormones and synthetic substitutes

963 Poisoning by primarily systemic agents

963.0 Antiallergic and antiemetic drugs
Antihistamines   Diphenylpyraline
Chlorpheniramine   Thonzylamine
Diphenhydramine   Tripelennamine
EXCLUDES *phenothiazine-based tranquilizers (969.1)*

963.1 Antineoplastic and immunosuppressive drugs
Azathioprine   Cytarabine
Busulfan   Fluorouracil
Chlorambucil   Mercaptopurine
Cyclophosphamide   thio-TEPA
EXCLUDES *antineoplastic antibiotics (960.7)*

963.2 Acidifying agents

963.3 Alkalizing agents

963.4 Enzymes, not elsewhere classified
Penicillinase

963.5 Vitamins, not elsewhere classified
Vitamin A   Vitamin D
EXCLUDES *nicotinic acid (972.2)*
vitamin K (964.3)

963.8 Other specified systemic agents
Heavy metal antagonists

963.9 Unspecified systemic agent

964 Poisoning by agents primarily affecting blood constituents

964.0 Iron and its compounds
Ferric salts
Ferrous sulfate and other ferrous salts

964.1 Liver preparations and other antianemic agents
Folic acid

964.2 Anticoagulants
Coumarin   Phenindione
Heparin   Warfarin sodium
AHA: 1Q, '94, 22

964.3 Vitamin K [phytonadione]

964.4 Fibrinolysis-affecting drugs
Aminocaproic acid   Streptokinase
Streptodornase   Urokinase

964.5 Anticoagulant antagonists and other coagulants
Hexadimethrine   Protamine sulfate

964.6 Gamma globulin

964.7 Natural blood and blood products
Blood plasma   Packed red cells
Human fibrinogen   Whole blood
EXCLUDES *transfusion reactions (999.4-999.8)*

964.8 Other specified agents affecting blood constituents
Macromolecular blood substitutes
Plasma expanders

964.9 Unspecified agent affecting blood constituents

965 Poisoning by analgesics, antipyretics, and antirheumatics
EXCLUDES *drug dependence (304.0-304.9)*
nondependent abuse (305.0-305.9)

965.0 Opiates and related narcotics
965.00 Opium (alkaloids), unspecified
965.01 Heroin
Diacetylmorphine
965.02 Methadone
965.09 Other
Codeine [methylmorphine]
Meperidine [pethidine]
Morphine

965.1 Salicylates
Acetylsalicylic acid [aspirin]
Salicylic acid salts
AHA: N-D, '94, 15

965.4 Aromatic analgesics, not elsewhere classified
Acetanilid   Phenacetin [acetophenetidin]
Paracetamol [acetaminophen]

Injury and Poisoning

965.5–971.0

965.5 Pyrazole derivatives
Aminophenazone [aminopyrine]
Phenylbutazone

√5th **965.6 Antirheumatics [antiphlogistics]**
    EXCLUDES   *salicylates (965.1)*
                   steroids (962.0-962.9)

    AHA: 4Q, '98, 50

    965.61 Propionic acid derivatives
        Fenoprofen
        Flurbiprofen
        Ibuprofen
        Ketoprofen
        Naproxen
        Oxaprozin
        AHA: 4Q, '98, 50

    965.69 Other antirheumatics
        Gold salts
        Indomethacin

965.7 Other non-narcotic analgesics
Pyrabital

965.8 Other specified analgesics and antipyretics
Pentazocine

965.9 Unspecified analgesic and antipyretic

√4th **966 Poisoning by anticonvulsants and anti-Parkinsonism drugs**

966.0 Oxazolidine derivatives
Paramethadione
Trimethadione

966.1 Hydantoin derivatives
Phenytoin

966.2 Succinimides
Ethosuximide
Phensuximide

966.3 Other and unspecified anticonvulsants
Primidone
    EXCLUDES   *barbiturates (967.0)*
                   sulfonamides (961.0)

966.4 Anti-Parkinsonism drugs
Amantadine
Ethopropazine [profenamine]
Levodopa [L-dopa]

√4th **967 Poisoning by sedatives and hypnotics**
    EXCLUDES   *drug dependence (304.0-304.9)*
                   nondependent abuse (305.0-305.9)

967.0 Barbiturates
Amobarbital [amylobarbitone]
Barbital [barbitone]
Butabarbital [butabarbitone]
Pentobarbital [pentobarbitone]
Phenobarbital [phenobarbitone]
Secobarbital [quinalbarbitone]
    EXCLUDES   *thiobarbiturate anesthetics (968.3)*

967.1 Chloral hydrate group

967.2 Paraldehyde

967.3 Bromine compounds
Bromide   Carbromal (derivatives)

967.4 Methaqualone compounds

967.5 Glutethimide group

967.6 Mixed sedatives, not elsewhere classified

967.8 Other sedatives and hypnotics

967.9 Unspecified sedative or hypnotic
Sleeping:
    drug
    pill   } NOS
    tablet

√4th **968 Poisoning by other central nervous system depressants and anesthetics**
    EXCLUDES   *drug dependence (304.0-304.9)*
                   nondependent abuse (305.0-305.9)

968.0 Central nervous system muscle-tone depressants
Chlorphenesin (carbamate)   Methocarbamol
Mephenesin

968.1 Halothane

968.2 Other gaseous anesthetics
Ether
Halogenated hydrocarbon derivatives, except halothane
Nitrous oxide

968.3 Intravenous anesthetics
Ketamine
Methohexital [methohexitone]
Thiobarbiturates, such as thiopental sodium

968.4 Other and unspecified general anesthetics

968.5 Surface [topical] and infiltration anesthetics
Cocaine   Procaine
Lidocaine [lignocaine]   Tetracaine
    AHA: 1Q, '93, 25

968.6 Peripheral nerve- and plexus-blocking anesthetics

968.7 Spinal anesthetics

968.9 Other and unspecified local anesthetics

√4th **969 Poisoning by psychotropic agents**
    EXCLUDES   *drug dependence (304.0-304.9)*
                   nondependent abuse (305.0-305.9)

969.0 Antidepressants
Amitriptyline
Imipramine
Monoamine oxidase [MAO] inhibitors

969.1 Phenothiazine-based tranquilizers
Chlorpromazine   Prochlorperazine
Fluphenazine   Promazine

969.2 Butyrophenone-based tranquilizers
Haloperidol   Trifluperidol
Spiperone

969.3 Other antipsychotics, neuroleptics, and major tranquilizers

969.4 Benzodiazepine-based tranquilizers
Chlordiazepoxide   Lorazepam
Diazepam   Medazepam
Flurazepam   Nitrazepam

969.5 Other tranquilizers
Hydroxyzine   Meprobamate

969.6 Psychodysleptics [hallucinogens]
Cannabis (derivatives)   Mescaline
Lysergide [LSD]   Psilocin
Marihuana (derivatives)   Psilocybin

969.7 Psychostimulants
Amphetamine   Caffeine
    EXCLUDES   *central appetite depressants (977.0)*
    AHA: ▶2Q, '03, 11◀

969.8 Other specified psychotropic agents

969.9 Unspecified psychotropic agent

√4th **970 Poisoning by central nervous system stimulants**

970.0 Analeptics
Lobeline   Nikethamide

970.1 Opiate antagonists
Levallorphan   Naloxone
Nalorphine

970.8 Other specified central nervous system stimulants

970.9 Unspecified central nervous system stimulant

√4th **971 Poisoning by drugs primarily affecting the autonomic nervous system**

971.0 Parasympathomimetics [cholinergics]
Acetylcholine   Pilocarpine
Anticholinesterase:
    organophosphorus
    reversible

971.1 Parasympatholytics [anticholinergics and antimuscarinics] and spasmolytics
- Atropine
- Homatropine
- Hyoscine [scopolamine]
- Quaternary ammonium derivatives

    EXCLUDES *papaverine (972.5)*

971.2 Sympathomimetics [adrenergics]
- Epinephrine [adrenalin]   Levarterenol [noradrenalin]

971.3 Sympatholytics [antiadrenergics]
- Phenoxybenzamine   Tolazolinehydrochloride

971.9 Unspecified drug primarily affecting autonomic nervous system

√4ᵗʰ 972 Poisoning by agents primarily affecting the cardiovascular system

972.0 Cardiac rhythm regulators
- Practolol
- Procainamide
- Propranolol
- Quinidine

    EXCLUDES *lidocaine (968.5)*

972.1 Cardiotonic glycosides and drugs of similar action
- Digitalis glycosides   Strophanthins
- Digoxin

972.2 Antilipemic and antiarteriosclerotic drugs
- Clofibrate
- Nicotinic acid derivatives

972.3 Ganglion-blocking agents
- Pentamethonium bromide

972.4 Coronary vasodilators
- Dipyridamole
- Nitrates [nitroglycerin]
- Nitrites

972.5 Other vasodilators
- Cyclandelate
- Diazoxide
- Papaverine

    EXCLUDES *nicotinic acid (972.2)*

972.6 Other antihypertensive agents
- Clonidine
- Guanethidine
- Rauwolfia alkaloids
- Reserpine

972.7 Antivaricose drugs, including sclerosing agents
- Sodium morrhuate   Zinc salts

972.8 Capillary-active drugs
- Adrenochrome derivatives   Metaraminol

972.9 Other and unspecified agents primarily affecting the cardiovascular system

√4ᵗʰ 973 Poisoning by agents primarily affecting the gastrointestinal system

973.0 Antacids and antigastric secretion drugs
- Aluminum hydroxide   Magnesium trisilicate

    AHA: 1Q, '03, 19

973.1 Irritant cathartics
- Bisacodyl
- Castor oil
- Phenolphthalein

973.2 Emollient cathartics
- Dioctyl sulfosuccinates

973.3 Other cathartics, including intestinal atonia drugs
- Magnesium sulfate

973.4 Digestants
- Pancreatin
- Papain
- Pepsin

973.5 Antidiarrheal drugs
- Kaolin
- Pectin

    EXCLUDES *anti-infectives (960.0-961.9)*

973.6 Emetics

973.8 Other specified agents primarily affecting the gastrointestinal system

973.9 Unspecified agent primarily affecting the gastrointestinal system

√4ᵗʰ 974 Poisoning by water, mineral, and uric acid metabolism drugs

974.0 Mercurial diuretics
- Chlormerodrin
- Mercaptomerin
- Mersalyl

974.1 Purine derivative diuretics
- Theobromine
- Theophylline

    EXCLUDES *aminophylline [theophylline ethylenediamine] (975.7)*
        caffeine (969.7)

974.2 Carbonic acid anhydrase inhibitors
- Acetazolamide

974.3 Saluretics
- Benzothiadiazides   Chlorothiazide group

974.4 Other diuretics
- Ethacrynic acid
- Furosemide

974.5 Electrolytic, caloric, and water-balance agents

974.6 Other mineral salts, not elsewhere classified

974.7 Uric acid metabolism drugs
- Allopurinol
- Colchicine
- Probenecid

√4ᵗʰ 975 Poisoning by agents primarily acting on the smooth and skeletal muscles and respiratory system

975.0 Oxytocic agents
- Ergot alkaloids
- Oxytocin
- Prostaglandins

975.1 Smooth muscle relaxants
- Adiphenine
- Metaproterenol [orciprenaline]

    EXCLUDES *papaverine (972.5)*

975.2 Skeletal muscle relaxants

975.3 Other and unspecified drugs acting on muscles

975.4 Antitussives
- Dextromethorphan   Pipazethate

975.5 Expectorants
- Acetylcysteine
- Guaifenesin
- Terpin hydrate

975.6 Anti-common cold drugs

975.7 Antiasthmatics
- Aminophylline [theophylline ethylenediamine]

975.8 Other and unspecified respiratory drugs

√4ᵗʰ 976 Poisoning by agents primarily affecting skin and mucous membrane, ophthalmological, otorhinolaryngological, and dental drugs

976.0 Local anti-infectives and anti-inflammatory drugs

976.1 Antipruritics

976.2 Local astringents and local detergents

976.3 Emollients, demulcents, and protectants

976.4 Keratolytics, keratoplastics, other hair treatment drugs and preparations

976.5 Eye anti-infectives and other eye drugs
- Idoxuridine

976.6 Anti-infectives and other drugs and preparations for ear, nose, and throat

976.7 Dental drugs topically applied

    EXCLUDES *anti-infectives (976.0)*
        local anesthetics (968.5)

976.8 Other agents primarily affecting skin and mucous membrane
- Spermicides [vaginal contraceptives]

976.9 Unspecified agent primarily affecting skin and mucous membrane

√4ᵗʰ 977 Poisoning by other and unspecified drugs and medicinal substances

977.0 Dietetics
- Central appetite depressants

977.1 Lipotropic drugs

977.2 Antidotes and chelating agents, not elsewhere classified

977.3 Alcohol deterrents

977.4 Pharmaceutical excipients
- Pharmaceutical adjuncts

977.8 Other specified drugs and medicinal substances
- Contrast media used for diagnostic x-ray procedures
- Diagnostic agents and kits

√4ᵗʰ / √5ᵗʰ Additional Digit Required   Unspecified Code   Other Specified Code   Manifestation Code   ▶◀ Revised Text   ● New Code   ▲ Revised Code Title

Injury and Poisoning

977.9–987.9

977.9   Unspecified drug or medicinal substance

✓4ᵗʰ **978**   Poisoning by bacterial vaccines

     978.0   BCG

     978.1   Typhoid and paratyphoid

     978.2   Cholera

     978.3   Plague

     978.4   Tetanus

     978.5   Diphtheria

     978.6   Pertussis vaccine, including combinations with a pertussis component

     978.8   Other and unspecified bacterial vaccines

     978.9   Mixed bacterial vaccines, except combinations with a pertussis component

✓4ᵗʰ **979**   Poisoning by other vaccines and biological substances

       EXCLUDES   *gamma globulin (964.6)*

     979.0   Smallpox vaccine

     979.1   Rabies vaccine

     979.2   Typhus vaccine

     979.3   Yellow fever vaccine

     979.4   Measles vaccine

     979.5   Poliomyelitis vaccine

     979.6   Other and unspecified viral and rickettsial vaccines

         Mumps vaccine

     979.7   Mixed viral-rickettsial and bacterial vaccines, except combinations with a pertussis component

       EXCLUDES   *combinations with a pertussis component (978.6)*

     979.9   Other and unspecified vaccines and biological substances

TOXIC EFFECTS OF SUBSTANCES CHIEFLY NONMEDICINAL AS TO SOURCE (980-989)

       EXCLUDES   *burns from chemical agents (ingested) (947.0-947.9)*

                     localized toxic effects indexed elsewhere (001.0-799.9)

                     respiratory conditions due to external agents (506.0-508.9)

     Use additional code to specify the nature of the toxic effect

✓4ᵗʰ **980**   Toxic effect of alcohol

     980.0   Ethyl alcohol

         Denatured alcohol   Grain alcohol

         Ethanol

         Use additional code to identify any associated:

            acute alcohol intoxication (305.0)

            in alcoholism (303.0)

            drunkenness (simple) (305.0)

            pathological (291.4)

         AHA: 3Q, '96, 16

     980.1   Methyl alcohol

         Methanol   Wood alcohol

     980.2   Isopropyl alcohol

         Dimethyl carbinol   Rubbing alcohol

         Isopropanol

     980.3   Fusel oil

         Alcohol: Alcohol:

           amyl   propyl

           butyl

     980.8   Other specified alcohols

     980.9   Unspecified alcohol

     981   Toxic effect of petroleum products

         Benzine   Petroleum:

         Gasoline   ether

         Kerosene   naphtha

         Paraffin wax   spirit

✓4ᵗʰ **982**   Toxic effect of solvents other than petroleum-based

     982.0   Benzene and homologues

     982.1   Carbon tetrachloride

     982.2   Carbon disulfide

         Carbon bisulfide

     982.3   Other chlorinated hydrocarbon solvents

         Tetrachloroethylene   Trichloroethylene

         EXCLUDES   *chlorinated hydrocarbon preparations other than solvents (989.2)*

     982.4   Nitroglycol

     982.8   Other nonpetroleum-based solvents

         Acetone

✓4ᵗʰ **983**   Toxic effect of corrosive aromatics, acids, and caustic alkalis

     983.0   Corrosive aromatics

         Carbolic acid or phenol   Cresol

     983.1   Acids

         Acid: Acid:

           hydrochloric   sulfuric

           nitric

     983.2   Caustic alkalis

         Lye   Sodium hydroxide

         Potassium hydroxide

     983.9   Caustic, unspecified

✓4ᵗʰ **984**   Toxic effect of lead and its compounds (including fumes)

       INCLUDES   that from all sources except medicinal substances

     984.0   Inorganic lead compounds

         Lead dioxide   Lead salts

     984.1   Organic lead compounds

         Lead acetate   Tetraethyl lead

     984.8   Other lead compounds

     984.9   Unspecified lead compound

✓4ᵗʰ **985**   Toxic effect of other metals

       INCLUDES   that from all sources except medicinal substances

     985.0   Mercury and its compounds

         Minamata disease

     985.1   Arsenic and its compounds

     985.2   Manganese and its compounds

     985.3   Beryllium and its compounds

     985.4   Antimony and its compounds

     985.5   Cadmium and its compounds

     985.6   Chromium

     985.8   Other specified metals

         Brass fumes   Iron compounds

         Copper salts   Nickel compounds

         AHA: 1Q, '88, 5

     985.9   Unspecified metal

     986   Toxic effect of carbon monoxide

         Carbon monoxide from any source

✓4ᵗʰ **987**   Toxic effect of other gases, fumes, or vapors

     987.0   Liquefied petroleum gases

         Butane   Propane

     987.1   Other hydrocarbon gas

     987.2   Nitrogen oxides

         Nitrogen dioxide   Nitrous fumes

     987.3   Sulfur dioxide

     987.4   Freon

         Dichloromonofluoromethane

     987.5   Lacrimogenic gas

         Bromobenzyl cyanide   Ethyliodoacetate

         Chloroacetophenone

     987.6   Chlorine gas

     987.7   Hydrocyanic acid gas

     987.8   Other specified gases, fumes, or vapors

         Phosgene   Polyester fumes

     987.9   Unspecified gas, fume, or vapor

N   Newborn Age: 0   P   Pediatric Age: 0-17   M   Maternity Age: 12-55   A   Adult Age: 15-124   MSP   Medicare Secondary Payer

✓4ᵗʰ **988 Toxic effect of noxious substances eaten as food**

> **EXCLUDES**   *allergic reaction to food, such as:*
> *gastroenteritis (558.3)*
> *rash (692.5, 693.1)*
> *food poisoning (bacterial) (005.0-005.9)*
> *toxic effects of food contaminants, such as:*
> *aflatoxin and other mycotoxin (989.7)*
> *mercury (985.0)*

988.0   **Fish and shellfish**

988.1   **Mushrooms**

988.2   **Berries and other plants**

988.8   **Other specified noxious substances eaten as food**

988.9   **Unspecified noxious substance eaten as food**

✓4ᵗʰ **989 Toxic effect of other substances, chiefly nonmedicinal as to source**

989.0   **Hydrocyanic acid and cyanides**

> Potassium cyanide   Sodium cyanide
> **EXCLUDES**   *gas and fumes (987.7)*

989.1   **Strychnine and salts**

989.2   **Chlorinated hydrocarbons**

> Aldrin   DDT
> Chlordane   Dieldrin
> **EXCLUDES**   *chlorinated hydrocarbon solvents (982.0-982.3)*

989.3   **Organophosphate and carbamate**

> Carbaryl   Parathion
> Dichlorvos   Phorate
> Malathion   Phosdrin

989.4   **Other pesticides, not elsewhere classified**

> Mixtures of insecticides

989.5   **Venom**

> Bites of venomous snakes, lizards, and spiders
> Tick paralysis

989.6   **Soaps and detergents**

989.7   **Aflatoxin and other mycotoxin [food contaminants]**

✓5ᵗʰ 989.8   **Other substances, chiefly nonmedicinal as to source**

> AHA: 4Q, '95, 60

989.81   **Asbestos**

> **EXCLUDES**   *asbestosis (501)*
> *exposure to asbestos (V15.84)*

989.82   **Latex**

989.83   **Silicone**

> **EXCLUDES**   *silicone used in medical devices, implants and grafts (996.00-996.79)*

989.84   **Tobacco**

989.89   **Other**

989.9   **Unspecified substance, chiefly nonmedicinal as to source**

OTHER AND UNSPECIFIED EFFECTS OF EXTERNAL CAUSES (990-995)

990   **Effects of radiation, unspecified**

> Complication of: Radiation sickness
> phototherapy
> radiation therapy
> **EXCLUDES**   *specified adverse effects of radiation. Such conditions are to be classified according to the nature of the adverse effect, as:*
> *burns (940.0-949.5)*
> *dermatitis (692.7-692.8)*
> *leukemia (204.0-208.9)*
> *pneumonia (508.0)*
> *sunburn (692.71, 692.76-692.77)*
> *[The type of radiation giving rise to the adverse effect may be identified by use of the E codes.]*

✓4ᵗʰ **991 Effects of reduced temperature**

991.0   **Frostbite of face**

991.1   **Frostbite of hand**

991.2   **Frostbite of foot**

991.3   **Frostbite of other and unspecified sites**

991.4   **Immersion foot**

> Trench foot
> DEF: Paresthesia, edema, blotchy cyanosis of foot, the skin is soft (macerated), pale and wrinkled, and the sole is swollen with surface ridging and following sustained immersion in water.

991.5   **Chilblains**

> Erythema pernio   Perniosis
> DEF: Red, swollen, itchy skin; follows damp cold exposure; also associated with pruritus and a burning feeling, in hands, feet, ears, and face in children, legs and toes in women, and hands and fingers in men.

991.6   **Hypothermia**

> Hypothermia (accidental)
> **EXCLUDES**   *hypothermia following anesthesia (995.89)*
> *hypothermia not associated with low environmental temperature (780.99)*
> DEF: Reduced body temperature due to low environmental temperatures.

991.8   **Other specified effects of reduced temperature**

991.9   **Unspecified effect of reduced temperature**

> Effects of freezing or excessive cold NOS

✓4ᵗʰ **992 Effects of heat and light**

> **EXCLUDES**   *burns (940.0-949.5)*
> *diseases of sweat glands due to heat (705.0-705.9)*
> *malignant hyperpyrexia following anesthesia (995.86)*
> *sunburn (692.71, 692.76-692.77)*

992.0   **Heat stroke and sunstroke**

> Heat apoplexy   Siriasis
> Heat pyrexia   Thermoplegia
> Ictus solaris
> DEF: Headache, vertigo, cramps and elevated body temperature due to high environmental temperatures.

992.1   **Heat syncope**

> Heat collapse

992.2   **Heat cramps**

992.3   **Heat exhaustion, anhydrotic**

> Heat prostration due to water depletion
> **EXCLUDES**   *that associated with salt depletion (992.4)*

992.4   **Heat exhaustion due to salt depletion**

> Heat prostration due to salt (and water) depletion

992.5   **Heat exhaustion, unspecified**

> Heat prostration NOS

992.6   **Heat fatigue, transient**

992.7   **Heat edema**

> DEF: Fluid retention due to high environmental temperatures.

992.8   **Other specified heat effects**

992.9   **Unspecified**

✓4ᵗʰ **993 Effects of air pressure**

993.0   **Barotrauma, otitic**

> Aero-otitis media   Effects of high altitude on ears
> DEF: Ringing ears, deafness, pain and vertigo due to air pressure changes.

993.1   **Barotrauma, sinus**

> Aerosinusitis
> Effects of high altitude on sinuses

993.2   **Other and unspecified effects of high altitude**

> Alpine sickness   Hypobaropathy
> Andes disease   Mountain sickness
> Anoxia due to high altitude
> AHA: 3Q, '88, 4

✓4ᵗʰ ✓5ᵗʰ Additional Digit Required   Unspecified Code   Other Specified Code   Manifestation Code   ▶◀ Revised Text   ● New Code   ▲ Revised Code Title

2005 ICD•9•CM   **Volume 1 — 279**

Injury and Poisoning

993.3–995.59

993.3 Caisson disease
Bends   Decompression sickness
Compressed-air disease   Divers' palsy or paralysis
DEF: Rapid reduction in air pressure while breathing compressed air; symptoms include skin lesions, joint pains, respiratory and neurological problems.

993.4 Effects of air pressure caused by explosion
993.8 Other specified effects of air pressure
993.9 Unspecified effect of air pressure

✓4ᵗʰ 994 Effects of other external causes
EXCLUDES certain adverse effects not elsewhere classified (995.0-995.8)

994.0 Effects of lightning
Shock from lightning   Struck by lightning NOS
EXCLUDES burns (940.0-949.5)

994.1 Drowning and nonfatal submersion
Bathing cramp   Immersion
AHA: 3Q, '88, 4

994.2 Effects of hunger
Deprivation of food   Starvation

994.3 Effects of thirst
Deprivation of water

994.4 Exhaustion due to exposure
994.5 Exhaustion due to excessive exertion
Overexertion

994.6 Motion sickness
Air sickness   Travel sickness
Seasickness

994.7 Asphyxiation and strangulation
Suffocation (by):   Suffocation (by):
bedclothes   plastic bag
cave-in   pressure
constriction   strangulation
mechanical
EXCLUDES asphyxia from:
carbon monoxide (986)
inhalation of food or foreign body (932-934.9)
other gases, fumes, and vapors (987.0-987.9)

994.8 Electrocution and nonfatal effects of electric current
Shock from electric current
EXCLUDES electric burns (940.0-949.5)

994.9 Other effects of external causes
Effects of:
abnormal gravitational [G] forces or states
weightlessness

✓4ᵗʰ 995 Certain adverse effects not elsewhere classified
EXCLUDES complications of surgical and medical care (996.0-999.9)

995.0 Other anaphylactic shock
Allergic shock   NOS or due to adverse effect of
Anaphylactic   correct medicinal
reaction   substance properly
Anaphylaxis   administered
Use additional E code to identify external cause, such as:
adverse effects of correct medicinal substance properly administered [E930-E949]
EXCLUDES anaphylactic reaction to serum (999.4)
anaphylactic shock due to adverse food reaction (995.60-995.69)
AHA: 4Q, '93, 30
DEF: Immediate sensitivity response after exposure to specific antigen; results in life-threatening respiratory distress; usually followed by vascular collapse, shock, urticaria, angioedema and pruritus.

995.1 Angioneurotic edema
Giant urticaria
EXCLUDES urticaria:
due to serum (999.5)
other specified (698.2, 708.0-708.9, 757.33)
DEF: Circulatory response of deep dermis, subcutaneous or submucosal tissues; causes localized edema and wheals.

995.2 Unspecified adverse effect of drug, medicinal and biological substance
Adverse effect   (due) to correct medicinal
Allergic reaction   substance properly
Hypersensitivity   administered
Idiosyncrasy
Drug: Drug:
hypersensitivity NOS   reaction NOS
EXCLUDES pathological drug intoxication (292.2)
AHA: 2Q, '97, 12; 3Q, '95, 13; 3Q, '92, 16

995.3 Allergy, unspecified
Allergic reaction NOS   Idiosyncrasy NOS
Hypersensitivity NOS
EXCLUDES allergic reaction NOS to correct medicinal substance properly administered (995.2)
specific types of allergic reaction, such as:
allergic diarrhea (558.3)
dermatitis (691.0-693.9)
hayfever (477.0-477.9)

995.4 Shock due to anesthesia
Shock due to anesthesia in which the correct substance was properly administered
EXCLUDES complications of anesthesia in labor or delivery (668.0-668.9)
overdose or wrong substance given (968.0-969.9)
postoperative shock NOS (998.0)
specified adverse effects of anesthesia classified elsewhere, such as:
anoxic brain damage (348.1)
hepatitis (070.0-070.9), etc.
unspecified adverse effect of anesthesia (995.2)

✓5ᵗʰ 995.5 Child maltreatment syndrome
Use additional code(s), if applicable, to identify any associated injuries
Use additional E code to identify:
nature of abuse (E960-E968)
perpetrator (E967.0-E967.9)
AHA: 1Q, '98, 11

995.50 Child abuse, unspecified P
995.51 Child emotional/psychological abuse P
AHA: 4Q, '96, 38, 40
995.52 Child neglect (nutritional) P
AHA: 4Q, '96, 38, 40
995.53 Child sexual abuse P
AHA: 4Q, '96, 39, 40
995.54 Child physical abuse P
Battered baby or child syndrome
EXCLUDES shaken infant syndrome (995.55)
AHA: 3Q, '99, 14; 4Q, '96, 39, 40
995.55 Shaken infant syndrome P
Use additional code(s) to identify any associated injuries
AHA: 4Q, '96, 40, 43
995.59 Other child abuse and neglect P
Multiple forms of abuse

√5ᵗʰ 995.6 Anaphylactic shock due to adverse food reaction
Anaphylactic shock due to nonpoisonous foods
AHA: 4Q, '93, 30

     995.60 **Due to unspecified food**

     995.61 **Due to peanuts**

     995.62 **Due to crustaceans**

     995.63 **Due to fruits and vegetables**

     995.64 **Due to tree nuts and seeds**

     995.65 **Due to fish**

     995.66 **Due to food additives**

     995.67 **Due to milk products**

     995.68 **Due to eggs**

     995.69 **Due to other specified food**

995.7 Other adverse food reactions, not elsewhere classified
Use additional code to identify the type of reaction, such as:
     hives (708.0)
     wheezing (786.07)

> **EXCLUDES**   *anaphylactic shock due to adverse food reaction (995.60-995.69)*
> *asthma (493.0, 493.9)*
> *dermatitis due to food (693.1)*
>   *in contact with the skin (692.5)*
> *gastroenteritis and colitis due to food (558.3)*
> *rhinitis due to food (477.1)*

√5ᵗʰ 995.8 Other specified adverse effects, not elsewhere classified

     995.80 **Adult maltreatment, unspecified**   🅰
Abused person NOS
Use additional code to identify:
     any associated injury
     perpetrator (E967.0-E967.9)
AHA: 4Q, '96, 41, 43

     995.81 **Adult physical abuse**   🅰
Battered:
     person syndrome NEC
     man
     spouse
     woman
Use additional code to identify:
     any association injury
     nature of abuse (E960-E968)
     perpetrator (E967.0-E967.9)
AHA: 4Q, '96, 42, 43

     995.82 **Adult emotional/psychological abuse**   🅰
Use additional E code to identify perpetrator (E967.0-E967.9)

     995.83 **Adult sexual abuse**   🅰
Use additional code to identify:
     any associated injury
     perpetrator (E967.0-E967.9)

     995.84 **Adult neglect (nutritional)**   🅰
Use addition code to identify:
     intent of neglect (E904.0, E968.4)
     perpetrator (E967.0-E967.9)

     995.85 **Other adult abuse and neglect**   🅰
Multiple forms of abuse and neglect
Use additional code to identify:
     any associated injury
     intent of neglect (E904.0, E968.4)
     nature of abuse (E960-E968)
     perpetrator (E967.0-E967.9)

     995.86 **Malignant hyperthermia**
Malignant hyperpyrexia due to anesthesia
AHA: 4Q, '98, 51

     995.89 **Other**
Hypothermia due to anesthesia
AHA: 3Q, '03, 12

√5ᵗʰ 995.9 Systemic inflammatory response syndrome (SIRS)
►Code first underlying systemic infection◄
AHA: 4Q, '02, 71

DEF: Clinical response to infection or trauma that can trigger an acute inflammatory reaction and progresses to coagulation, impaired fibrinolysis, and organ failure; manifested by two or more of the following symptoms: fever, tachycardia, tachypnea, leukocytosis or leukopenia.

     995.90 **Systemic inflammatory response syndrome, unspecified**
SIRS NOS

     995.91 **Systemic inflammatory response syndrome due to infectious process without organ dysfunction**
Sepsis
AHA: 4Q, '03, 79

     995.92 **Systemic inflammatory response syndrome due to infectious process with organ dysfunction**
Severe sepsis
Use additional code to specify organ dysfunction, such as:
     acute renal failure (584.5-584.9)
     acute respiratory failure (518.81)
     critical illness myopathy (359.81)
     critical illness polyneuropathy (357.82)
     encephalopathy (348.31)
     hepatic failure (570)
     septic shock (785.52)
AHA: 4Q, '03, 73, 79

     995.93 **Systemic inflammatory response syndrome due to noninfectious process without organ dysfunction**

     995.94 **Systemic inflammatory response syndrome due to noninfectious process with organ dysfunction**
Use additional code to specify organ dysfunction, such as:
     acute renal failure (584.5-584.9)
     acute respiratory failure (518.81)
     critical illness myopathy (359.81)
     critical illness polyneuropathy (357.82)
     encephalopathy (348.31)
     hepatic failure (570)
     septic shock (785.52)
AHA: 4Q, '03, 79

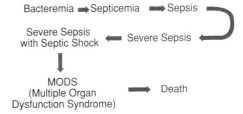

Continuum of Illness Due to Infection

Bacteremia ➡ Septicemia ➡ Sepsis
Severe Sepsis with Septic Shock ⬅ Severe Sepsis ⬅
⬇
MODS (Multiple Organ Dysfunction Syndrome) ➡ Death

Additional Digit Required   Unspecified Code   Other Specified Code   Manifestation Code   ►◄ Revised Text   ● New Code   ▲ Revised Code Title

2005 ICD•9•CM   October 2004 • Volume 1 — 281

Injury and Poisoning

996–996.51

COMPLICATIONS OF SURGICAL AND MEDICAL CARE, NOT ELSEWHERE CLASSIFIED (996-999)

> EXCLUDES *adverse effects of medicinal agents (001.0-799.9, 995.0-995.8)*
> *burns from local applications and irradiation (940.0-949.5)*
> *complications of:*
>   *conditions for which the procedure was performed*
>   *surgical procedures during abortion, labor, and delivery (630-676.9)*
> *poisoning and toxic effects of drugs and chemicals (960.0-989.9)*
> *postoperative conditions in which no complications are present, such as:*
>   *artificial opening status (V44.0-V44.9)*
>   *closure of external stoma (V55.0-V55.9)*
>   *fitting of prosthetic device (V52.0-V52.9)*
> *specified complications classified elsewhere*
>   *anesthetic shock (995.4)*
>   *electrolyte imbalance (276.0-276.9)*
>   *postlaminectomy syndrome (722.80-722.83)*
>   *postmastectomy lymphedema syndrome (457.0)*
>   *postoperative psychosis (293.0-293.9)*
>   *any other condition classified elsewhere in the Alphabetic Index when described as due to a procedure*

√4ʰ **996 Complications peculiar to certain specified procedures**

> INCLUDES *complications, not elsewhere classified, in the use of artificial substitutes [e.g., Dacron, metal, Silastic, Teflon] or natural sources [e.g., bone] involving:*
>   *anastomosis (internal)*
>   *graft (bypass) (patch)*
>   *implant*
>   *internal device:*
>   *catheter*
>   *electronic*
>   *fixation*
>   *prosthetic*
>   *reimplant*
>   *transplant*

> EXCLUDES *accidental puncture or laceration during procedure (998.2)*
> *complications of internal anastomosis of:*
>   *gastrointestinal tract (997.4)*
>   *urinary tract (997.5)*
> *other specified complications classified elsewhere, such as:*
>   *hemolytic anemia (283.1)*
>   *functional cardiac disturbances (429.4)*
>   *serum hepatitis (070.2-070.3)*

AHA: 1Q, '94, 3

√5ʰ **996.0 Mechanical complication of cardiac device, implant, and graft**

Breakdown (mechanical)   Obstruction, mechanical
Displacement   Perforation
Leakage   Protrusion

AHA: 2Q, '93, 9

996.00 Unspecified device, implant, and graft MSP
996.01 Due to cardiac pacemaker (electrode) MSP

AHA: 2Q, '99, 11

996.02 Due to heart valve prosthesis MSP
996.03 Due to coronary bypass graft MSP

> EXCLUDES *atherosclerosis of graft (414.02, 414.03)*
> *embolism [occlusion NOS] [thrombus] of graft (996.72)*

AHA: 2Q, '95, 17; N-D, '86, 5

996.04 Due to automatic implantable cardiac defibrillator
996.09 Other MSP

AHA: 2Q, '93, 9

996.1 Mechanical complication of other vascular device, implant, and graft MSP

femoral-popliteal bypass graft
Mechanical complications involving:
  aortic (bifurcation) graft (replacement)
  arteriovenous:
  dialysis catheter   ⎫
  fistula   ⎬ surgically created
  shunt   ⎭

  balloon (counterpulsation) device, intra-aortic
  carotid artery bypass graft
  umbrella device, vena cava

> EXCLUDES *atherosclerosis of biological graft (440.30-440.32)*
> *embolism [occlusion NOS] [thrombus] of (biological) (synthetic) graft (996.74)*
> *peritoneal dialysis catheter (996.56)*

AHA: 1Q, '02, 13; 1Q, '95, 3

996.2 Mechanical complication of nervous system device, implant, and graft MSP

Mechanical complications involving:
  dorsal column stimulator
  electrodes implanted in brain [brain "pacemaker"]
  peripheral nerve graft
  ventricular (communicating) shunt

AHA: 2Q, '99, 4; S-O, '87, 10

√5ʰ **996.3 Mechanical complication of genitourinary device, implant, and graft**

AHA: 3Q, '01, 13; S-O, '85, 3

996.30 Unspecified device, implant, and graft MSP
996.31 Due to urethral [indwelling] catheter MSP
996.32 Due to intrauterine contraceptive device ♀ MSP
996.39 Other MSP

Cystostomy catheter
Prosthetic reconstruction of vas deferens
Repair (graft) of ureter without mention of resection

> EXCLUDES *complications due to:*
>   *external stoma of urinary tract (997.5)*
>   *internal anastomosis of urinary tract (997.5)*

996.4 Mechanical complication of internal orthopedic device, implant, and graft MSP

Mechanical complications involving:
  external (fixation) device utilizing internal screw(s), pin(s) or other methods of fixation
  grafts of bone, cartilage, muscle, or tendon
  internal (fixation) device such as nail, plate, rod, etc.

> EXCLUDES *complications of external orthopedic device, such as:*
>   *pressure ulcer due to cast ▶(707.00-707.09)◀*

AHA: 2Q, '99, 10; 2Q, '98, 19; 2Q, '96, 11; 3Q, '95, 16; N-D, '85, 11

√5ʰ **996.5 Mechanical complications of other specified prosthetic device, implant, and graft**

Mechanical complications involving:
  prosthetic implant in: prosthetic implant in:
    bile duct   chin
    breast   orbit of eye
  nonabsorbable surgical material NOS
  other graft, implant, and internal device, not elsewhere classified

AHA: 1Q, '98, 11

996.51 Due to corneal graft

996.52 Due to graft of other tissue, not elsewhere classified
Skin graft failure or rejection
> **EXCLUDES** *failure of artificial skin graft (996.55)*
> *failure of decellularized allodermis (996.55)*
> *sloughing of temporary skin allografts or xenografts (pigskin)—omit code*

AHA: 1Q, '96, 10

996.53 Due to ocular lens prosthesis
> **EXCLUDES** *contact lenses—code to condition*

AHA: 1Q, '00, 9

996.54 Due to breast prosthesis
Breast capsule (prosthesis)
Mammary implant

AHA: 2Q, '98, 14; 3Q, '92, 4

996.55 Due to artificial skin graft and decellularized allodermis
Dislodgement   Non-adherence
Displacement   Poor incorporation
Failure   Shearing

AHA: 4Q, '98, 52

996.56 Due to peritoneal dialysis catheter
> **EXCLUDES** *mechanical complication of arteriovenous dialysis catheter (996.1)*

AHA: 4Q, '98, 54

996.57 Due to insulin pump
AHA: 4Q, '03, 81-82

996.59 Due to other implant and internal device, not elsewhere classified
Nonabsorbable surgical material NOS
Prosthetic implant in:
  bile duct
  chin
  orbit of eye

AHA: 2Q, '99, 13; 3Q, '94, 7

√5ᵗʰ **996.6 Infection and inflammatory reaction due to internal prosthetic device, implant, and graft**
Infection (causing obstruction) } due to (presence of) any device, implant, and graft classifiable to 996.0-996.5
Inflammation

Use additional code to identify specified infections
AHA: 2Q, '89, 16; J-F, '87, 14

996.60 Due to unspecified device, implant, and graft

996.61 Due to cardiac device, implant, and graft
Cardiac pacemaker or defibrillator:
  electrode(s), lead(s)
  pulse generator
  subcutaneous pocket
Coronary artery bypass graft
Heart valve prosthesis

996.62 Due to other vascular device, implant, and graft
Arterial graft
Arteriovenous fistula or shunt
Infusion pump
Vascular catheter (arterial) (dialysis) (venous)
AHA: ▶1Q, '04, 5;◀ 4Q, '03, 107, 111; 2Q, '03, 7; 2Q, '94, 13

996.63 Due to nervous system device, implant, and graft
Electrodes implanted in brain
Peripheral nerve graft
Spinal canal catheter
Ventricular (communicating) shunt (catheter)

996.64 Due to indwelling urinary catheter
Use additional code to identify specified infections, such as:
Cystitis (595.0-595.9)
Sepsis (038.0-038.9)

AHA: 3Q, '93, 6

996.65 Due to other genitourinary device, implant, and graft
Intrauterine contraceptive device

AHA: 1Q, '00, 15

996.66 Due to internal joint prosthesis
AHA: 2Q, '91, 18

996.67 Due to other internal orthopedic device, implant, and graft
Bone growth stimulator (electrode)
Internal fixation device (pin) (rod) (screw)

996.68 Due to peritoneal dialysis catheter
Exit-site infection or inflammation

AHA: 4Q, '98, 54

996.69 Due to other internal prosthetic device, implant, and graft
Breast prosthesis
Ocular lens prosthesis
Prosthetic orbital implant

AHA: 4Q, '03, 108; 4Q, '98, 52

√5ᵗʰ **996.7 Other complications of internal (biological) (synthetic) prosthetic device, implant, and graft**
Complication NOS
occlusion NOS
Embolism   } due to (presence of) any device, implant, and graft classifiable to 996.0-996.5
Fibrosis
Hemorrhage
Pain
Stenosis
Thrombus

> **EXCLUDES** *transplant rejection (996.8)*
AHA: 1Q, '89, 9; N-D, '86, 5

996.70 Due to unspecified device, implant, and graft

996.71 Due to heart valve prosthesis

996.72 Due to other cardiac device, implant, and graft
Cardiac pacemaker or defibrillator:
  electrode(s), lead(s)
  subcutaneous pocket
Coronary artery bypass (graft)
> **EXCLUDES** *occlusion due to atherosclerosis (414.02-414.06)*

AHA: 3Q, '01, 20

996.73 Due to renal dialysis device, implant, and graft
AHA: 2Q, '91, 18

996.74 Due to other vascular device, implant, and graft
> **EXCLUDES** *occlusion of biological graft due to atherosclerosis (440.30-440.32)*

AHA: 1Q, '03, 16, 17

996.75 Due to nervous system device, implant, and graft

996.76 Due to genitourinary device, implant, and graft
AHA: 1Q, '00, 15

996.77 Due to internal joint prosthesis

996.78 Due to other internal orthopedic device, implant, and graft
AHA: 2Q, '03, 14

√4ᵗʰ √5ᵗʰ Additional Digit Required   Unspecified Code   Other Specified Code   Manifestation Code   ▶◀ Revised Text   ● New Code   ▲ Revised Code Title

Injury and Poisoning

996.79–997.4

996.79 Due to other internal prosthetic device, implant, and graft
AHA: 1Q, '01, 8; 3Q, '95, 14; 3Q, '92, 4

✓5ᵗʰ **996.8 Complications of transplanted organ**
Transplant failure or rejection
Use additional code to identify nature of complication, such as:
Cytomegalovirus (CMV) infection (078.5)
AHA: 3Q, '01, 12; 3Q, '93, 3, 4; 2Q, '93, 11; 1Q, '93, 24

996.80 Transplanted organ, unspecified

996.81 Kidney
AHA: 3Q, '03, 16; 3Q, '98, 6, 7; 3Q, '94, 8; 2Q, '94, 9; 1Q, '93, 24

996.82 Liver
AHA: 3Q, '03, 17; 3Q, '98, 3, 4

996.83 Heart
AHA: 3Q, '03, 16; 4Q, '02, 53; 3Q, '98, 5

996.84 Lung
AHA: 2Q, '03, 12; 3Q, '98, 5

996.85 Bone marrow
Graft-versus-host disease (acute) (chronic)
AHA: 4Q, '90, 4

996.86 Pancreas

996.87 Intestine

996.89 Other specified transplanted organ
AHA: 3Q, '94, 5

✓5ᵗʰ **996.9 Complications of reattached extremity or body part**

996.90 Unspecified extremity

996.91 Forearm

996.92 Hand

996.93 Finger(s)

996.94 Upper extremity, other and unspecified

996.95 Foot and toe(s)

996.96 Lower extremity, other and unspecified

996.99 Other specified body part

✓4ᵗʰ **997 Complications affecting specified body system, not elsewhere classified**
Use additional code to identify complications
EXCLUDES   the listed conditions when specified as:
causing shock (998.0)
complications of:
anesthesia:
adverse effect (001.0-799.9, 995.0-995.8)
in labor or delivery (668.0-668.9)
poisoning (968.0-969.9)
implanted device or graft (996.0-996.9)
obstetrical procedures (669.0-669.4)
reattached extremity (996.90-996.96)
transplanted organ (996.80-996.89)
AHA: 1Q, '94, 4; 1Q, '93, 26

✓5ᵗʰ **997.0 Nervous system complications**

997.00 Nervous system complication, unspecified

997.01 Central nervous system complication
Anoxic brain damage
Cerebral hypoxia
EXCLUDES   *cerebrovascular hemorrhage or infarction (997.02)*

997.02 Iatrogenic cerebrovascular infarction or hemorrhage
Postoperative stroke
AHA: 4Q, '95, 57

997.09 Other nervous system complications

997.1 Cardiac complications
Cardiac:
arrest
insufficiency   } during or resulting from a
Cardiorespiratory failure   procedure
Heart failure
EXCLUDES   *the listed conditions as long-term effects of cardiac surgery or due to the presence of cardiac prosthetic device (429.4)*
AHA: 2Q, '02, 12

997.2 Peripheral vascular complications
Phlebitis or thrombophlebitis during or resulting from a procedure
EXCLUDES   *the listed conditions due to:*
implant or catheter device (996.62)
infusion, perfusion, or transfusion (999.2)
complications affecting blood vessels (997.71-997.79)
AHA: 1Q, '03, 6; 3Q, '02, 24-26

997.3 Respiratory complications
Mendelson's syndrome   } resulting from a
Pneumonia (aspiration)   procedure
EXCLUDES   *iatrogenic [postoperative] pneumothorax (512.1)*
iatrogenic pulmonary embolism (415.11)
Mendelson's syndrome in labor and delivery (668.0)
specified complications classified elsewhere, such as:
adult respiratory distress syndrome (518.5)
pulmonary edema, postoperative (518.4)
respiratory insufficiency, acute, postoperative (518.5)
shock lung (518.5)
tracheostomy complications (519.00-519.09)
AHA: 1Q, '97, 10; 2Q, '93, 3; 2Q, '93, 9; 4Q, '90, 25

DEF: Mendelson's syndrome: acid pneumonitis due to aspiration of gastric acids, may occur after anesthesia or sedation.

997.4 Digestive system complications
Complications of:
intestinal (internal) anastomosis and bypass, not elsewhere classified, except that involving urinary tract
Hepatic failure
Hepatorenal syndrome   } specified as due to
Intestinal obstruction NOS   a procedure
EXCLUDES   *gastrostomy complications (536.40-536.49)*
specified gastrointestinal complications classified elsewhere, such as:
blind loop syndrome (579.2)
colostomy and enterostomy complications (569.60-569.69)
gastrojejunal ulcer (534.0-534.9)
▶*infection of esophagostomy (530.86)*◄
infection of external stoma (569.61)
▶*mechanical complication of esophagostomy (530.87)*◄
pelvic peritoneal adhesions, female (614.6)
peritoneal adhesions (568.0)
peritoneal adhesions with obstruction (560.81)
postcholecystectomy syndrome (576.0)
postgastric surgery syndromes (564.2)
vomiting following gastrointestinal surgery (564.3)
AHA: 2Q, '01, 4-6; 3Q, '99, 4; 2Q, '99, 14; 3Q, '97, 7; 1Q, '97, 11; 2Q, '95, 7; 1Q, '93, 26; 3Q, '92, 15; 2Q, '89, 15; 1Q, '88, 14

Ⓝ Newborn Age: 0   Ⓟ Pediatric Age: 0-17   Ⓜ Maternity Age: 12-55   Ⓐ Adult Age: 15-124   MSP Medicare Secondary Payer

997.5 Urinary complications
Complications of:
   external stoma of urinary tract
   internal anastomosis and bypass of urinary tract,
     including that involving intestinal tract
Oliguria or anuria ⎫
Renal: ⎬ specified as due to
   failure (acute)   procedure
   insufficiency (acute)
   Tubular necrosis (acute) ⎭

EXCLUDES *specified complications classified*
elsewhere, such as:
postoperative stricture of:
ureter (593.3)
urethra (598.2)

AHA: ▶3Q, '03, 13;◀ 3Q '96, 10, 15; 4Q, '95, 73; 1Q, '92, 13; 2Q, '89,
16; M-A, '87, 10; S-O, '85, 3

√5ᵗʰ **997.6 Amputation stump complication**
EXCLUDES *admission for treatment for a current*
traumatic amputation — code to
complicated traumatic
amputation
phantom limb (syndrome) (353.6)

AHA: 4Q, '95, 82

997.60 Unspecified complication
997.61 Neuroma of amputation stump
DEF: Hyperplasia generated nerve cell mass following
amputation.

997.62 Infection (chronic)
Use additional code to identify organism
AHA: 4Q, '96, 46

997.69 Other

√5ᵗʰ **997.7 Vascular complications of other vessels**
EXCLUDES *peripheral vascular complications (997.2)*

997.71 Vascular complications of mesenteric artery
AHA: 4Q, '01, 53

997.72 Vascular complications of renal artery
997.79 Vascular complications of other
vessels

√5ᵗʰ **997.9 Complications affecting other specified body**
systems, not elsewhere classified
EXCLUDES *specified complications classified*
elsewhere, such as:
broad ligament laceration syndrome
(620.6)
postartificial menopause syndrome
(627.4)
postoperative stricture of vagina
(623.2)

997.91 Hypertension
EXCLUDES *essential hypertension (401.0-*
401.9)

AHA: 4Q, '95, 57

997.99 Other
Vitreous touch syndrome
AHA: 2Q, '94, 12; 1Q, '94, 17

DEF: Vitreous touch syndrome: vitreous protruding
through pupil and attaches to corneal epithelium; causes
aqueous fluid in vitreous body; marked by corneal
edema, loss of lucidity; complication of cataract surgery.

√4ᵗʰ **998 Other complications of procedures, not elsewhere classified**
AHA: 1Q, '94, 4

998.0 Postoperative shock
Collapse NOS   ⎫ during or resulting
Shock (endotoxic)   ⎬ from a surgical
  (hypovolemic) (septic) ⎭ procedure

EXCLUDES *shock:*
anaphylactic due to serum (999.4)
anesthetic (995.4)
electric (994.8)
following abortion (639.5)
obstetric (669.1)
traumatic (958.4)

√5ᵗʰ **998.1 Hemorrhage or hematoma or seroma complicating a**
procedure
EXCLUDES *hemorrhage, hematoma, or seroma:*
complicating cesarean section or
puerperal perineal wound
(674.3)

998.11 Hemorrhage complicating a procedure
AHA: ▶3Q, '03, 13;◀ 1Q, '03, 4; 4Q, '97, 52; 1Q, '97, 10

998.12 Hematoma complicating a procedure
AHA: 1Q, '03, 6; 3Q, '02, 24, 26

998.13 Seroma complicating a procedure
AHA: 4Q, '96, 46; 1Q, '93, 26; 2Q, '92, 15; S-O, '87, 8

998.2 Accidental puncture or laceration during a
procedure
Accidental perforation by catheter or other
   instrument during a procedure on:
  blood vessel
  nerve
  organ
EXCLUDES *iatrogenic [postoperative] pneumothorax*
(512.1)
puncture or laceration caused by
implanted device intentionally left
in operation wound (996.0-996.5)
specified complications classified
elsewhere, such as:
broad ligament laceration syndrome
(620.6)
trauma from instruments during
delivery (664.0-665.9)

AHA: 3Q, '02, 24, 26; 3Q, '94, 6; 3Q, '90, 17; 3Q, '90, 18

√5ᵗʰ **998.3 Disruption of operation wound**
Dehiscence ⎫
Rupture   ⎬ of operation wound

EXCLUDES *disruption of:*
cesarean wound (674.1)
perineal wound, puerperal (674.2)

AHA: 4Q, '02, 73; 1Q, '93, 19

998.31 Disruption of internal operation wound
998.32 Disruption of external operation wound
Disruption of operation wound NOS
AHA: ▶4Q, '03, 104, 106◀

998.4 Foreign body accidentally left during a procedure
Adhesions   ⎫ due to foreign body accidentally left
Obstruction ⎬ in operative wound or body
Perforation ⎭ cavity during a procedure

EXCLUDES *obstruction or perforation caused by*
implanted device intentionally left
in body (996.0-996.5)

AHA: 1Q, '89, 9

√5ᵗʰ **998.5 Postoperative infection**
EXCLUDES *infection due to:*
implanted device (996.60-996.69)
infusion, perfusion, or transfusion
(999.3)
postoperative obstetrical wound
infection (674.3)

√4ᵗʰ
√5ᵗʰ Additional Digit Required   Unspecified Code   Other Specified Code   Manifestation Code   ▶◀ Revised Text   ● New Code   ▲ Revised Code Title

Injury and Poisoning

998.51–999.9

998.51 Infected postoperative seroma
Use additional code to identify organism
AHA: 4Q, '96, 46

998.59 Other postoperative infection

Abscess:
  intra-abdominal
  stitch
  subphrenic   } postoperative
  wound
Septicemia

Use additional code to identify infection
AHA: ▶4Q, '03, 104, 106-107;◀ 3Q, '98, 3; 3Q, '95, 5; 2Q, '95, 7; 3Q, '94, 6; 1Q, '93, 19; J-F, '87, 14

998.6 Persistent postoperative fistula
AHA: J-F, '87, 14

998.7 Acute reaction to foreign substance accidentally left during a procedure
Peritonitis: Peritonitis:
  aseptic   chemical

√5ᵗʰ **998.8 Other specified complications of procedures, not elsewhere classified**
AHA: 4Q, '94, 46; 1Q, '89, 9

998.81 Emphysema (subcutaneous) (surgical) resulting from a procedure

998.82 Cataract fragments in eye following cataract surgery

998.83 Non-healing surgical wound
AHA: 4Q, '96, 47

998.89 Other specified complications
AHA: 3Q, '99, 13; 2Q, '98, 16

998.9 Unspecified complication of procedure, not elsewhere classified
Postoperative complication NOS
EXCLUDES   complication NOS of obstetrical, surgery or procedure (669.4)
AHA: 4Q, '93, 37

√4ᵗʰ **999 Complications of medical care, not elsewhere classified**
INCLUDES   complications, not elsewhere classified, of:
  dialysis (hemodialysis) (peritoneal) (renal)
  extracorporeal circulation
  hyperalimentation therapy
  immunization
  infusion
  inhalation therapy
  injection
  inoculation
  perfusion
  transfusion
  vaccination
  ventilation therapy
EXCLUDES   specified complications classified elsewhere such as:
  complications of implanted device (996.0-996.9)
  contact dermatitis due to drugs (692.3)
  dementia dialysis (294.8)
    transient (293.9)
  dialysis disequilibrium syndrome (276.0-276.9)
  poisoning and toxic effects of drugs and chemicals (960.0-989.9)
  postvaccinal encephalitis (323.5)
  water and electrolyte imbalance (276.0-276.9)

999.0 Generalized vaccinia
DEF: Skin eruption, self-limiting; follows vaccination; due to transient viremia with virus localized in skin.

999.1 Air embolism
Air embolism to any site following infusion, perfusion, or transfusion
EXCLUDES   embolism specified as:
  complicating:
    abortion (634-638 with .6, 639.6)
    ectopic or molar pregnancy (639.6)
    pregnancy, childbirth, or the puerperium (673.0)
  due to implanted device (996.7)
  traumatic (958.0)

999.2 Other vascular complications
Phlebitis   } following infusion,
Thromboembolism   } perfusion, or
Thrombophlebitis   } transfusion
EXCLUDES   the listed conditions when specified as:
  due to implanted device (996.61-996.62. 996.72-996.74)
  postoperative NOS (997.2, 997.71-997.79)
AHA: 2Q, '97, 5

999.3 Other infection
Infection   } following infusion, injection,
Sepsis   } transfusion, or
Septicemia   } vaccination
EXCLUDES   the listed conditions when specified as:
  due to implanted device (996.60-996.69)
  postoperative NOS (998.51-998.59)
AHA: 2Q, '01, 11, 12; 2Q, '97, 5; J-F, '87, 14

999.4 Anaphylactic shock due to serum
EXCLUDES   shock:
  allergic NOS (995.0)
  anaphylactic:
    NOS (995.0)
    due to drugs and chemicals (995.0)
DEF: Life-threatening hypersensitivity to foreign serum; causes respiratory distress, vascular collapse, and shock.

999.5 Other serum reaction
Intoxication by serum   Serum sickness
Protein sickness   Urticaria due to serum
Serum rash
EXCLUDES   serum hepatitis (070.2-070.3)
DEF: Serum sickness: Hypersensitivity to foreign serum; causes fever, hives, swelling, and lymphadenopathy.

999.6 ABO incompatibility reaction
Incompatible blood transfusion
Reaction to blood group incompatibility in infusion or transfusion

999.7 Rh incompatibility reaction
Reactions due to Rh factor in infusion or transfusion

999.8 Other transfusion reaction
Septic shock due to transfusion
Transfusion reaction NOS
EXCLUDES   postoperative shock (998.0)
AHA: 3Q, '00, 9

999.9 Other and unspecified complications of medical care, not elsewhere classified
Complications, not elsewhere classified, of:
  electroshock   }
  inhalation   } therapy
  ultrasound   }
  ventilation   }
Unspecified misadventure of medical care
EXCLUDES   unspecified complication of:
  phototherapy (990)
  radiation therapy (990)
AHA: 1Q, '03, 19; 2Q, '97, 5

N Newborn Age: 0   P Pediatric Age: 0-17   M Maternity Age: 12-55   A Adult Age: 15-124   MSP Medicare Secondary Payer

SUPPLEMENTARY CLASSIFICATION OF FACTORS INFLUENCING HEALTH STATUS AND CONTACT WITH HEALTH SERVICES ▶(V01-V84)◀

This classification is provided to deal with occasions when circumstances other than a disease or injury classifiable to categories 001-999 (the main part of ICD) are recorded as "diagnoses" or "problems." This can arise mainly in three ways:

a) When a person who is not currently sick encounters the health services for some specific purpose, such as to act as a donor of an organ or tissue, to receive prophylactic vaccination, or to discuss a problem which is in itself not a disease or injury. This will be a fairly rare occurrence among hospital inpatients, but will be relatively more common among hospital outpatients and patients of family practitioners, health clinics, etc.

b) When a person with a known disease or injury, whether it is current or resolving, encounters the health care system for a specific treatment of that disease or injury (e.g., dialysis for renal disease; chemotherapy for malignancy; cast change).

c) When some circumstance or problem is present which influences the person's health status but is not in itself a current illness or injury. Such factors may be elicited during population surveys, when the person may or may not be currently sick, or be recorded as an additional factor to be borne in mind when the person is receiving care for some current illness or injury classifiable to categories 001-999.

In the latter circumstances the V code should be used only as a supplementary code and should not be the one selected for use in primary, single cause tabulations. Examples of these circumstances are a personal history of certain diseases, or a person with an artificial heart valve in situ.

AHA: J-F, '87, 8

PERSONS WITH POTENTIAL HEALTH HAZARDS RELATED TO COMMUNICABLE DISEASES (V01-V06)

> **EXCLUDES**   family history of infectious and parasitic diseases (V18.8)
> personal history of infectious and parasitic diseases (V12.0)

✓4ᵗʰ **V01 Contact with or exposure to communicable diseases**

     V01.0 Cholera
         Conditions classifiable to 001

     V01.1 Tuberculosis
         Conditions classifiable to 010-018

     V01.2 Poliomyelitis
         Conditions classifiable to 045

     V01.3 Smallpox
         Conditions classifiable to 050

     V01.4 Rubella
         Conditions classifiable to 056

     V01.5 Rabies
         Conditions classifiable to 071

     V01.6 Venereal diseases
         Conditions classifiable to 090-099

✓5ᵗʰ   **V01.7 Other viral diseases**
         Conditions classifiable to 042-078 and V08, except as above

         AHA: 2Q, '92, 11

         V01.71 Varicella
         V01.79 Other viral diseases

✓5ᵗʰ   **V01.8 Other communicable diseases**
         Conditions classifiable to 001-136, except as above

         AHA: J-A, '87, 24

         V01.81 Anthrax
            AHA: 4Q, '02, 70, 78

         V01.82 Exposure to SARS-associated coronavirus
            AHA: 4Q, '03, 46-47

         V01.83 Escherichia coli (E. coli)
         V01.84 Meningococcus
         V01.89 Other communicable diseases

     V01.9 Unspecified communicable disease

✓4ᵗʰ **V02 Carrier or suspected carrier of infectious diseases**
     AHA: 3Q, '95, 18; 3Q, '94, 4

     V02.0 Cholera
     V02.1 Typhoid
     V02.2 Amebiasis
     V02.3 Other gastrointestinal pathogens
     V02.4 Diphtheria

✓5ᵗʰ   **V02.5 Other specified bacterial diseases**
         V02.51 Group B streptococcus
            AHA: 1Q, '02, 14; 4Q, '98, 56

         V02.52 Other streptococcus
         V02.59 Other specified bacterial disease
            Meningococcal   Staphylococcal

✓5ᵗʰ   **V02.6 Viral hepatitis**
         Hepatitis Australian-antigen [HAA] [SH] carrier
         Serum hepatitis carrier

         V02.60 Viral hepatitis carrier, unspecified
            AHA: 4Q, '97, 47

         V02.61 Hepatitis B carrier
            AHA: 4Q, '97, 47

         V02.62 Hepatitis C carrier
            AHA: 4Q, '97, 47

         V02.69 Other viral hepatitis carrier
            AHA: 4Q, '97, 47

     V02.7 Gonorrhea
     V02.8 Other venereal diseases
     V02.9 Other specified infectious organism
         AHA: 3Q, '95, 18; 1Q, '93, 22; J-A, '87, 24

✓4ᵗʰ **V03 Need for prophylactic vaccination and inoculation against bacterial diseases**

> **EXCLUDES**   vaccination not carried out because of contraindication (V64.0)
> vaccines against combinations of diseases (V06.0-V06.9)

     V03.0 Cholera alone
     V03.1 Typhoid-paratyphoid alone [TAB]
     V03.2 Tuberculosis [BCG]
     V03.3 Plague
     V03.4 Tularemia
     V03.5 Diphtheria alone
     V03.6 Pertussis alone
     V03.7 Tetanus toxoid alone

✓5ᵗʰ   **V03.8 Other specified vaccinations against single bacterial diseases**
         V03.81 Hemophilus influenza, type B [Hib]
         V03.82 Streptococcus pneumoniae [pneumococcus]
         V03.89 Other specified vaccination
            AHA: 2Q, '00, 9

     V03.9 Unspecified single bacterial disease

✓4ᵗʰ **V04 Need for prophylactic vaccination and inoculation against certain viral diseases**

> **EXCLUDES**   vaccines against combinations of diseases (V06.0-V06.9)

     V04.0 Poliomyelitis
     V04.1 Smallpox
     V04.2 Measles alone
     V04.3 Rubella alone
     V04.4 Yellow fever
     V04.5 Rabies
     V04.6 Mumps alone
     V04.7 Common cold

✓4ᵗʰ ✓5ᵗʰ Additional Digit Required   Unspecified Code   Other Specified Code   Manifestation Code   ▶◀ Revised Text   ● New Code   ▲ Revised Code Title

2005 ICD•9•CM   October 2004 • Volume 1 — 287

V Codes

V04.8–V09.91

✓5ᵗʰ **V04.8** **Other viral diseases**
AHA: 4Q, '03, 83

V04.81 Influenza
V04.82 Respiratory syncytial virus (RSV)
V04.89 Other viral diseases

✓4ᵗʰ **V05** **Need for other prophylactic vaccination and inoculation against single diseases**
EXCLUDES vaccines against combinations of diseases (V06.0-V06.9)

V05.0 Arthropod-borne viral encephalitis
V05.1 Other arthropod-borne viral diseases
V05.2 Leishmaniasis
V05.3 Viral hepatitis
V05.4 Varicella
Chickenpox
V05.8 Other specified disease
AHA: 1Q, '01, 4; 3Q, '91, 20

V05.9 Unspecified single disease

✓4ᵗʰ **V06** **Need for prophylactic vaccination and inoculation against combinations of diseases**
Note: Use additional single vaccination codes from categories V03-V05 to identify any vaccinations not included in a combination code.

V06.0 Cholera with typhoid-paratyphoid [cholera+TAB]
V06.1 Diphtheria-tetanus-pertussis, combined [DTP] [DTaP]
AHA: 4Q, '03, 83; 3Q, '98, 13
V06.2 Diphtheria-tetanus-pertussis with typhoid-paratyphoid [DTP+TAB]
V06.3 Diphtheria-tetanus-pertussis with poliomyelitis [DTP+polio]
V06.4 Measles-mumps-rubella [MMR]
V06.5 Tetanus-diphtheria [Td] [DT]
AHA: 4Q, '03, 83
V06.6 Streptococcus pneumoniae [pneumococcus] and influenza
V06.8 Other combinations
EXCLUDES multiple single vaccination codes (V03.0-V05.9)
AHA: 1Q, '94, 19
V06.9 Unspecified combined vaccine

PERSONS WITH NEED FOR ISOLATION, OTHER POTENTIAL HEALTH HAZARDS AND PROPHYLACTIC MEASURES (V07-V09)

✓4ᵗʰ **V07** **Need for isolation and other prophylactic measures**
EXCLUDES prophylactic organ removal (V50.41-V50.49)

V07.0 Isolation
Admission to protect the individual from his surroundings or for isolation of individual after contact with infectious diseases
V07.1 Desensitization to allergens
V07.2 Prophylactic immunotherapy
Administration of:
antivenin
immune sera [gamma globulin]
RhoGAM
tetanus antitoxin
✓5ᵗʰ **V07.3** Other prophylactic chemotherapy
V07.31 Prophylactic fluoride administration
V07.39 Other prophylactic chemotherapy
EXCLUDES maintenance chemotherapy following disease (V58.1)
▲ **V07.4** Hormone replacement therapy (postmenopausal) ♀
V07.8 Other specified prophylactic measure
AHA: 1Q, '92, 11
V07.9 Unspecified prophylactic measure

V08 **Asymptomatic human immunodeficiency virus [HIV] infection status**
HIV positive NOS
Note: This code is ONLY to be used when NO HIV infection symptoms or conditions are present. If any HIV infection symptoms or conditions are present, see code 042.
EXCLUDES AIDS (042)
human immunodeficiency virus [HIV] disease (042)
exposure to HIV ▶(V01.79)◀
nonspecific serologic evidence of HIV (795.71)
symptomatic human immunodeficiency virus [HIV] infection (042)
AHA: 2Q, '99, 8; 3Q, '95, 18

✓4ᵗʰ **V09** **Infection with drug-resistant microorganisms**
Note: This category is intended for use as an additional code for infectious conditions classified elsewhere to indicate the presence of drug-resistance of the infectious organism.
AHA: 3Q, '94, 4; 4Q, '93, 22

V09.0 Infection with microorganisms resistant to penicillins
▶Methicillin-resistant staphylococcus aureus (MRSA)◀
AHA: 4Q, '03, 104, 106
V09.1 Infection with microorganisms resistant to cephalosporins and other B-lactam antibiotics `SDx`
V09.2 Infection with microorganisms resistant to macrolides `SDx`
V09.3 Infection with microorganisms resistant to tetracyclines `SDx`
V09.4 Infection with microorganisms resistant to aminoglycosides `SDx`
✓5ᵗʰ **V09.5** Infection with microorganisms resistant to quinolones and fluoroquinolones
V09.50 Without mention of resistance to multiple quinolones and fluoroquinoles `SDx`
V09.51 With resistance to multiple quinolones and fluoroquinoles `SDx`
V09.6 Infection with microorganisms resistant to sulfonamides `SDx`
✓5ᵗʰ **V09.7** Infection with microorganisms resistant to other specified antimycobacterial agents
EXCLUDES Amikacin (V09.4)
Kanamycin (V09.4)
Streptomycin [SM] (V09.4)
V09.70 Without mention of resistance to multiple antimycobacterial agents `SDx`
V09.71 With resistance to multiple antimycobacterial agents `SDx`
✓5ᵗʰ **V09.8** Infection with microorganisms resistant to other specified drugs
▶Vancomycin (glycopeptide) intermediate staphylococcus aureus (VISA/GISA)
Vancomycin (glycopeptide) resistant enterococcus (VRE)
Vancomycin (glycopeptide) resistant staphylococcus aureus (VRSA/GRSA)◀
V09.80 Without mention of resistance to multiple drugs `SDx`
V09.81 With resistance to multiple drugs `SDx`
✓5ᵗʰ **V09.9** Infection with drug-resistant microorganisms, unspecified
Drug resistance, NOS
V09.90 Without mention of multiple drug resistance `SDx`
V09.91 With multiple drug resistance `SDx`
Multiple drug resistance NOS

PERSONS WITH POTENTIAL HEALTH HAZARDS RELATED TO PERSONAL AND FAMILY HISTORY

EXCLUDES *obstetric patients where the possibility that the fetus might be affected is the reason for observation or management during pregnancy (655.0-655.9)*

AHA: J-F, '87, 1

✓4ᵗʰ **V10 Personal history of malignant neoplasm**
AHA: 4Q, '02, 80; 4Q, '98, 69; 1Q, '95, 4; 3Q, '92, 5; M-J, '85, 10; 2Q, '90, 9

✓5ᵗʰ **V10.0 Gastrointestinal tract**
History of conditions classifiable to 140-159
V10.00 Gastrointestinal tract, unspecified
V10.01 Tongue
V10.02 Other and unspecified oral cavity and pharynx
V10.03 Esophagus
V10.04 Stomach
V10.05 Large intestine
AHA: 3Q, '99, 7; 1Q, '95, 4
V10.06 Rectum, rectosigmoid junction, and anus
V10.07 Liver
V10.09 Other
AHA: ▶4Q, '03, 111◀

✓5ᵗʰ **V10.1 Trachea, bronchus, and lung**
History of conditions classifiable to 162
V10.11 Bronchus and lung
V10.12 Trachea

✓5ᵗʰ **V10.2 Other respiratory and intrathoracic organs**
History of conditions classifiable to 160, 161, 163-165
V10.20 Respiratory organ, unspecified
V10.21 Larynx
AHA: ▶4Q, '03, 108, 110◀
V10.22 Nasal cavities, middle ear, and accessory sinuses
V10.29 Other

V10.3 Breast
History of conditions classifiable to 174 and 175
AHA: ▶2Q, '03, 5;◀4Q, '01, 66; 4Q, '98, 65; 4Q, '97, 50; 1Q, '91, 16; 1Q, '90, 21

✓5ᵗʰ **V10.4 Genital organs**
History of conditions classifiable to 179-187
V10.40 Female genital organ, unspecified   ♀
V10.41 Cervix uteri   ♀
V10.42 Other parts of uterus   ♀
V10.43 Ovary   ♀
V10.44 Other female genital organs   ♀
V10.45 Male genital organ, unspecified   ♂
V10.46 Prostate   ♂
V10.47 Testis   ♂
V10.48 Epididymis   ♂
V10.49 Other male genital organs   ♂

✓5ᵗʰ **V10.5 Urinary organs**
History of conditions classifiable to 188 and 189
V10.50 Urinary organ, unspecified
V10.51 Bladder
V10.52 Kidney
EXCLUDES *renal pelvis (V10.53)*
V10.53 Renal pelvis
AHA: 4Q, '01, 55
V10.59 Other

✓5ᵗʰ **V10.6 Leukemia**
Conditions classifiable to 204-208
EXCLUDES *leukemia in remission (204-208)*
AHA: 2Q, '92, 13; 4Q, '91, 26; 4Q, '90, 3
V10.60 Leukemia, unspecified

V10.61 Lymphoid leukemia
V10.62 Myeloid leukemia
V10.63 Monocytic leukemia
V10.69 Other

✓5ᵗʰ **V10.7 Other lymphatic and hematopoietic neoplasms**
Conditions classifiable to 200-203
EXCLUDES *listed conditions in 200-203 in remission*
AHA: M-J, '85, 18
V10.71 Lymphosarcoma and reticulosarcoma
V10.72 Hodgkin's disease
V10.79 Other

✓5ᵗʰ **V10.8 Personal history of malignant neoplasm of other sites**
History of conditions classifiable to 170-173, 190-195
V10.81 Bone
AHA: ▶2Q, '03, 13◀
V10.82 Malignant melanoma of skin
V10.83 Other malignant neoplasm of skin
V10.84 Eye
V10.85 Brain
AHA: 1Q, '01, 6
V10.86 Other parts of nervous system
EXCLUDES *peripheral sympathetic, and parasympathetic nerves (V10.89)*
V10.87 Thyroid
V10.88 Other endocrine glands and related structures
V10.89 Other

V10.9 Unspecified personal history of malignant neoplasm

✓4ᵗʰ **V11 Personal history of mental disorder**
V11.0 Schizophrenia   SDx
EXCLUDES *that in remission (295.0-295.9 with fifth-digit 5)*
V11.1 Affective disorders   SDx
Personal history of manic-depressive psychosis
EXCLUDES *that in remission (296.0-296.6 with fifth-digit 5, 6)*
V11.2 Neurosis   SDx
V11.3 Alcoholism   SDx
V11.8 Other mental disorders   SDx
V11.9 Unspecified mental disorder   SDx

✓4ᵗʰ **V12 Personal history of certain other diseases**
AHA: 3Q, '92, 11

✓5ᵗʰ **V12.0 Infectious and parasitic diseases**
V12.00 Unspecified infectious and parasitic disease
V12.01 Tuberculosis
V12.02 Poliomyelitis
V12.03 Malaria
V12.09 Other
V12.1 Nutritional deficiency
V12.2 Endocrine, metabolic, and immunity disorders
EXCLUDES *history of allergy (V14.0-V14.9, V15.01-V15.09)*
V12.3 Diseases of blood and blood-forming organs

✓5ᵗʰ **V12.4 Disorders of nervous system and sense organs**
V12.40 Unspecified disorder of nervous system and sense organs
V12.41 Benign neoplasm of the brain
AHA: 4Q, '97, 48
V12.49 Other disorders of nervous system and sense organs
AHA: 4Q, '98, 59

✓4ᵗʰ / ✓5ᵗʰ Additional Digit Required   Unspecified Code   Other Specified Code   Manifestation Code   ▶◀ Revised Text   ● New Code   ▲ Revised Code Title

2005 ICD•9•CM   **February 2004 • Volume 1 — 289**

V Codes

V12.5–V15.82

✓5ᵗʰ **V12.5 Diseases of circulatory system**
    EXCLUDES *old myocardial infarction (412)*
      postmyocardial infarction syndrome (411.0)
    AHA: 4Q, '95, 61

  V12.50 Unspecified circulatory disease
  V12.51 Venous thrombosis and embolism
    Pulmonary embolism
    AHA: 4Q, '03, 108; 1Q, '02, 15

  V12.52 Thrombophlebitis
  V12.59 Other
    AHA: 4Q, '99, 4; 4Q, '98, 88; 4Q, '97, 37

V12.6 Diseases of respiratory system
✓5ᵗʰ **V12.7 Diseases of digestive system**
    AHA: 1Q, '95, 3; 2Q, '89, 16

  V12.70 Unspecified digestive disease
  V12.71 Peptic ulcer disease
  V12.72 Colonic polyps
    AHA: 3Q, '02, 15
  V12.79 Other

✓4ᵗʰ **V13 Personal history of other diseases**
✓5ᵗʰ **V13.0 Disorders of urinary system**
  V13.00 Unspecified urinary disorder
  V13.01 Urinary calculi
  V13.09 Other

V13.1 Trophoblastic disease ♀
    EXCLUDES *supervision during a current pregnancy (V23.1)*

✓5ᵗʰ **V13.2 Other genital system and obstetric disorders**
    EXCLUDES *supervision during a current pregnancy of a woman with poor obstetric history (V23.0-V23.9)*
    habitual aborter (646.3)
    without current pregnancy (629.9)

  V13.21 Personal history of pre-term labor ♀
    EXCLUDES *current pregnancy with history of pre-term labor (V23.41)*
    AHA: 4Q, '02, 78

  V13.29 Other genital system and obstetric disorders ♀

V13.3 Diseases of skin and subcutaneous tissue
V13.4 Arthritis SDx
V13.5 Other musculoskeletal disorders
✓5ᵗʰ **V13.6 Congenital malformations**
    AHA: 4Q, '98, 63

  V13.61 Hypospadias SDx ♂
  V13.69 Other congenital malformations SDx
    AHA: ▶1Q, '04, 16◀

V13.7 Perinatal problems
    EXCLUDES *low birth weight status (V21.30-V21.35)*
V13.8 Other specified diseases
V13.9 Unspecified disease

✓4ᵗʰ **V14 Personal history of allergy to medicinal agents**
V14.0 Penicillin SDx
V14.1 Other antibiotic agent SDx
V14.2 Sulfonamides SDx
V14.3 Other anti-infective agent SDx
V14.4 Anesthetic agent SDx
V14.5 Narcotic agent SDx
V14.6 Analgesic agent SDx
V14.7 Serum or vaccine SDx
V14.8 Other specified medicinal agents SDx
V14.9 Unspecified medicinal agent SDx

✓4ᵗʰ **V15 Other personal history presenting hazards to health**
✓5ᵗʰ **V15.0 Allergy, other than to medicinal agents**
    EXCLUDES *allergy to food substance used as base for medicinal agent (V14.0-V14.9)*
    AHA: 4Q, '00, 42, 49

  V15.01 Allergy to peanuts SDx
  V15.02 Allergy to milk products SDx
    EXCLUDES *lactose intolerance (271.3)*
    AHA: 1Q, '03, 12

  V15.03 Allergy to eggs SDx
  V15.04 Allergy to seafood SDx
    Seafood (octopus) (squid) ink
    Shellfish

  V15.05 Allergy to other foods SDx
    Food additives
    Nuts other than peanuts

  V15.06 Allergy to insects SDx
    Bugs
    Insect bites and stings
    Spiders

  V15.07 Allergy to latex SDx
    Latex sensitivity

  V15.08 Allergy to radiographic dye SDx
    Contrast media used for diagnostic x-ray procedures

  V15.09 Other allergy, other than to medicinal agents SDx

V15.1 Surgery to heart and great vessels SDx
    EXCLUDES *replacement by transplant or other means (V42.1-V42.2, V43.2-V43.4)*
    AHA: ▶1Q, '04, 16◀

V15.2 Surgery to other major organs SDx
    EXCLUDES *replacement by transplant or other means (V42.0-V43.8)*

V15.3 Irradiation SDx
    Previous exposure to therapeutic or other ionizing radiation

✓5ᵗʰ **V15.4 Psychological trauma**
    EXCLUDES *history of condition classifiable to 290-316 (V11.0-V11.9)*

  V15.41 History of physical abuse SDx
    Rape
    AHA: 3Q, '99, 15

  V15.42 History of emotional abuse SDx
    Neglect
    AHA: 3Q, '99, 15

  V15.49 Other SDx
    AHA: 3Q, '99, 15

V15.5 Injury SDx
V15.6 Poisoning SDx
V15.7 Contraception SDx
    EXCLUDES *current contraceptive management (V25.0-V25.4)*
    presence of intrauterine contraceptive device as incidental finding (V45.5)

✓5ᵗʰ **V15.8 Other specified personal history presenting hazards to health**
    AHA: 4Q, '95, 62

  V15.81 Noncompliance with medical treatment SDx
    AHA: 2Q, '03, 7; 2Q, '01, 11; 12, 13; 2Q, '99, 17; 2Q, '97, 11; 1Q, '97, 12; 3Q, '96, 9

  V15.82 History of tobacco use SDx
    EXCLUDES *tobacco dependence (305.1)*

V15.84 Exposure to asbestos `SDx`
V15.85 Exposure to potentially hazardous `SDx`
body fluids
V15.86 Exposure to lead `SDx`
V15.87 History of extracorporeal membrane `SDx`
oxygenation [ECMO]
AHA: 4Q, '03, 84

V15.89 Other `SDx`
AHA: 1Q, '90, 21; N-D, '84, 12

V15.9 Unspecified personal history `SDx`
presenting hazards to health

✓4ᵗʰ V16 Family history of malignant neoplasm
V16.0 Gastrointestinal tract
Family history of condition classifiable to 140-159
AHA: 1Q, '99, 4

V16.1 Trachea, bronchus, and lung
Family history of condition classifiable to 162

V16.2 Other respiratory and intrathoracic organs
Family history of condition classifiable to 160-161,
163-165

V16.3 Breast
Family history of condition classifiable to 174
AHA: 2Q, '03, 4; 2Q, '00, 8; 1Q, '92, 11

✓5ᵗʰ V16.4 Genital organs
Family history of condition classifiable to 179-187
AHA: 4Q, '97, 48

V16.40 Genital organ, unspecified
V16.41 Ovary
V16.42 Prostate
V16.43 Testis
V16.49 Other

✓5ᵗʰ V16.5 Urinary organs
Family history of condition classifiable to 189
V16.51 Kidney
V16.59 Other

V16.6 Leukemia
Family history of condition classifiable to 204-208

V16.7 Other lymphatic and hematopoietic neoplasms
Family history of condition classifiable to 200-203

V16.8 Other specified malignant neoplasm
Family history of other condition classifiable to
140-199

V16.9 Unspecified malignant neoplasm

✓4ᵗʰ V17 Family history of certain chronic disabling diseases
V17.0 Psychiatric condition
EXCLUDES family history of mental retardation
(V18.4)

V17.1 Stroke (cerebrovascular)
V17.2 Other neurological diseases
Epilepsy   Huntington's chorea

V17.3 Ischemic heart disease
V17.4 Other cardiovascular diseases
AHA: ▶1Q, '04, 6◀

V17.5 Asthma
V17.6 Other chronic respiratory conditions
V17.7 Arthritis
V17.8 Other musculoskeletal diseases

✓4ᵗʰ V18 Family history of certain other specific conditions
V18.0 Diabetes mellitus
AHA: ▶1Q, '04, 8◀

V18.1 Other endocrine and metabolic diseases
V18.2 Anemia
V18.3 Other blood disorders
V18.4 Mental retardation
V18.5 Digestive disorders

✓5ᵗʰ V18.6 Kidney diseases
V18.61 Polycystic kidney
V18.69 Other kidney diseases
V18.7 Other genitourinary diseases
V18.8 Infectious and parasitic diseases

✓4ᵗʰ V19 Family history of other conditions
V19.0 Blindness or visual loss
V19.1 Other eye disorders
V19.2 Deafness or hearing loss
V19.3 Other ear disorders
V19.4 Skin conditions
V19.5 Congenital anomalies
V19.6 Allergic disorders
V19.7 Consanguinity
V19.8 Other condition

PERSONS ENCOUNTERING HEALTH SERVICES IN CIRCUMSTANCES RELATED TO REPRODUCTION AND DEVELOPMENT (V20-V29)

✓4ᵗʰ V20 Health supervision of infant or child
V20.0 Foundling `PDx` `P`
V20.1 Other healthy infant or child `PDx`
receiving care
Medical or nursing care supervision of healthy infant
in cases of:
maternal illness, physical or psychiatric
socioeconomic adverse condition at home
too many children at home preventing or
interfering with normal care
AHA: 1Q, '00, 25; 3Q, '89, 14

V20.2 Routine infant or child health check `PDx` `P`
Developmental testing of infant or child
Immunizations appropriate for age
Routine vision and hearing testing
Use additional code(s) to identify:
special screening examination(s) performed
(V73.0-V82.9)
EXCLUDES special screening for developmental
handicaps (V79.3)
AHA: ▶1Q, '04, 15◀

✓4ᵗʰ V21 Constitutional states in development
V21.0 Period of rapid growth in childhood `SDx`
V21.1 Puberty `SDx`
V21.2 Other adolescence `SDx`
✓5ᵗʰ V21.3 Low birth weight status
EXCLUDES history of perinatal problems (V13.7)
AHA: 4Q, '00, 51

V21.30 Low birth weight status, `SDx`
unspecified
V21.31 Low birth weight status, less than `SDx`
500 grams
V21.32 Low birth weight status, 500-999 `SDx`
grams
V21.33 Low birth weight status, 1000-1499 `SDx`
grams
V21.34 Low birth weight status, 1500-1999 `SDx`
grams
V21.35 Low birth weight status, 2000-2500 `SDx`
grams
V21.8 Other specified constitutional `SDx`
states in development
V21.9 Unspecified constitutional state in `SDx`
development

✓4ᵗʰ V22 Normal pregnancy
EXCLUDES pregnancy examination or test, pregnancy
unconfirmed ▶(V72.40)◀

V22.0 Supervision of normal first pregnancy `PDx` ♀
AHA: 3Q, '99, 16

✓4ᵗʰ / ✓5ᵗʰ Additional Digit Required   Unspecified Code   Other Specified Code   Manifestation Code   ▶◀ Revised Text   ● New Code   ▲ Revised Code Title

V Codes

V15.84–V22.0

V22.1 **Supervision of other normal pregnancy** `PDx` ♀
    AHA: 3Q, '99, 16

V22.2 **Pregnant state, incidental** `SDx` ♀
    Pregnant state NOS

✓4ᵗʰ V23 **Supervision of high-risk pregnancy**
    AHA: 1Q, 90, 10

V23.0 **Pregnancy with history of infertility** `M` ♀
V23.1 **Pregnancy with history of trophoblastic** `M` ♀
    disease
    Pregnancy with history of:
      hydatidiform mole
      vesicular mole
    EXCLUDES *that without current pregnancy (V13.1)*

V23.2 **Pregnancy with history of abortion** `M` ♀
    Pregnancy with history of conditions classifiable to
      634-638
    EXCLUDES *habitual aborter:*
        care during pregnancy (646.3)
        that without current pregnancy
         (629.9)

V23.3 **Grand multiparity** `M` ♀
    EXCLUDES *care in relation to labor and delivery*
        (659.4)
        that without current pregnancy (V61.5)

✓5ᵗʰ V23.4 **Pregnancy with other poor obstetric history**
    Pregnancy with history of other conditions
      classifiable to 630-676
    V23.41 **Pregnancy with history of pre-term** `M` ♀
        labor
        AHA: 4Q, '02, 79

    V23.49 **Pregnancy with other poor** `M` ♀
        obstetric history
V23.5 **Pregnancy with other poor reproductive** `M` ♀
    history
    Pregnancy with history of stillbirth or
      neonatal death
V23.7 **Insufficient prenatal care** `M` ♀
    History of little or no prenatal care

✓5ᵗʰ V23.8 **Other high-risk pregnancy**
    AHA: 4Q, '98, 56, 63

    V23.81 **Elderly primigravida** `M` ♀
        First pregnancy in a woman who will be 35
          years of age or older at expected date
          of delivery
        EXCLUDES *elderly primigravida*
           complicating pregnancy
           (659.5)

    V23.82 **Elderly multigravida** `M` ♀
        Second or more pregnancy in a woman who
          will be 35 years of age or older at
          expected date of delivery
        EXCLUDES *elderly multigravida*
           complicating pregnancy
           (659.6)

    V23.83 **Young primigravida** `M` ♀
        First pregnancy in a female less than 16
          years old at expected date of delivery
        EXCLUDES *young primigravida complica-*
           ting pregnancy (659.8)

    V23.84 **Young multigravida** `M` ♀
        Second or more pregnancy in a female less
          than 16 years old at expected date of
          delivery
        EXCLUDES *young multigravida*
           complicating pregnancy
           (659.8)

    V23.89 **Other high-risk pregnancy** `M` ♀
V23.9 **Unspecified high-risk pregnancy** `M` ♀

✓4ᵗʰ V24 **Postpartum care and examination**
    V24.0 **Immediately after delivery** `PDx` `M` ♀
        Care and observation in uncomplicated cases
    V24.1 **Lactating mother** `PDx` ♀
        Supervision of lactation
    V24.2 **Routine postpartum follow-up** `PDx` ♀

✓4ᵗʰ V25 **Encounter for contraceptive management**
    AHA: 4Q, '92, 24

✓5ᵗʰ V25.0 **General counseling and advice**
    V25.01 **Prescription of oral contraceptives** ♀
    V25.02 **Initiation of other contraceptive measures**
        Fitting of diaphragm
        Prescription of foams, creams, or other agents
        AHA: 3Q, '97, 7

    V25.03 **Encounter for emergency contraceptive**
        counseling and prescription
        Encounter for postcoital contraceptive
          counseling and prescription
        AHA: ▶4Q, '03, 84◀

    V25.09 **Other**
        Family planning advice
    V25.1 **Insertion of intrauterine contraceptive device** ♀
    V25.2 **Sterilization**
        Admission for interruption of fallopian tubes or vas
          deferens

    V25.3 **Menstrual extraction** ♀
        Menstrual regulation

✓5ᵗʰ V25.4 **Surveillance of previously prescribed contraceptive**
    methods
        Checking, reinsertion, or removal of contraceptive
          device
        Repeat prescription for contraceptive method
        Routine examination in connection with
          contraceptive maintenance
        EXCLUDES *presence of intrauterine contraceptive*
           device as incidental finding
           (V45.5)

    V25.40 **Contraceptive surveillance, unspecified**
    V25.41 **Contraceptive pill** ♀
    V25.42 **Intrauterine contraceptive device** ♀
        Checking, reinsertion, or removal of
          intrauterine device
    V25.43 **Implantable subdermal contraceptive** ♀
    V25.49 **Other contraceptive method**
        AHA: 3Q, '97, 7

    V25.5 **Insertion of implantable subdermal contraceptive** ♀
    AHA: 3Q, '92, 9

    V25.8 **Other specified contraceptive management**
        Postvasectomy sperm count
        EXCLUDES *sperm count following sterilization*
           reversal (V26.22)
           sperm count for fertility testing (V26.21)
        AHA: 3Q, '96, 9

    V25.9 **Unspecified contraceptive management**

✓4ᵗʰ V26 **Procreative management**
    V26.0 **Tuboplasty or vasoplasty after previous sterilization**
        AHA: 2Q, '95, 10
    V26.1 **Artificial insemination** ♀

✓5ᵗʰ V26.2 **Investigation and testing**
        EXCLUDES *postvasectomy sperm count (V25.8)*
        AHA: 4Q, '00, 56

    V26.21 **Fertility testing**
        Fallopian insufflation
        Sperm count for fertility testing
        EXCLUDES *Genetic counseling and testing*
           (V26.3)

`N` Newborn Age: 0   `P` Pediatric Age: 0-17   `M` Maternity Age: 12-55   `A` Adult Age: 15-124   `MSP` Medicare Secondary Payer

292 — Volume 1 • February 2004   `SDx` Secondary Diagnosis   `PDx` Primary Diagnosis   **2005 ICD•9•CM**

V26.22 Aftercare following sterilization reversal
Fallopian insufflation following sterilization reversal
Sperm count following sterilization reversal

V26.29 Other investigation and testing
AHA: 2Q, '96, 9; N-D, '85, 15

V26.3 Genetic counseling and testing
EXCLUDES   *fertility testing (V26.21)*

     V26.4   General counseling and advice

✓5th **V26.5 Sterilization status**

V26.51 Tubal ligation status   SDx ♀
EXCLUDES   *infertility not due to previous tubal ligation (628.0-628.9)*

V26.52 Vasectomy status   SDx ♂

V26.8 Other specified procreative management

V26.9 Unspecified procreative management

✓4th **V27 Outcome of delivery**
Note: This category is intended for the coding of the outcome of delivery on the mother's record.
AHA: 2Q, '91, 16

V27.0 Single liveborn   M SDx ♀
AHA: 2Q, '03, 9; 2Q, '02, 10; 1Q, '01, 10; 3Q, '00, 5; 4Q, '98, 77; 4Q, '95, 59; 1Q, '92, 9

V27.1 Single stillborn   M SDx ♀
V27.2 Twins, both liveborn   M SDx ♀
V27.3 Twins, one liveborn and one stillborn   M SDx ♀
V27.4 Twins, both stillborn   M SDx ♀
V27.5 Other multiple birth, all liveborn   M SDx ♀
V27.6 Other multiple birth, some liveborn   M SDx ♀
V27.7 Other multiple birth, all stillborn   M SDx ♀
V27.9 Unspecified outcome of delivery   M SDx ♀

Single birth   } outcome to infant
Multiple birth } unspecified

✓4th **V28 Antenatal screening**
EXCLUDES   *abnormal findings on screening — code to findings*
routine prenatal care (V22.0-V23.9)
AHA: ▶1Q, '04, 11◀

V28.0 Screening for chromosomal anomalies by amniocentesis   M ♀

V28.1 Screening for raised alpha-fetoprotein levels in amniotic fluid   M ♀

V28.2 Other screening based on amniocentesis   M ♀

V28.3 Screening for malformation using ultrasonics   ♀

V28.4 Screening for fetal growth retardation using ultrasonics   ♀

V28.5 Screening for isoimmunization   ♀

V28.6 Screening for Streptococcus B   M ♀
AHA: 4Q, '97, 46

V28.8 Other specified antenatal screening   ♀
AHA: 3Q, '99, 16

V28.9 Unspecified antenatal screening   ♀

✓4th **V29 Observation and evaluation of newborns and infants for suspected condition not found**
Note: This category is to be used for newborns, within the neonatal period, (the first 28 days of life) who are suspected of having an abnormal condition resulting from exposure from the mother or the birth process, but without signs or symptoms, and, which after examination and observation, is found not to exist.
AHA: 1Q, '00, 25; 4Q, '94, 47; 1Q, '94, 9; 4Q, '92, 21

V29.0 [1] **Observation for suspected infectious condition**   N PDx
AHA: 1Q, '01, 10

V29.1 [1] **Observation for suspected neurological condition**   N PDx

V29.2 [1] **Observation for suspected respiratory condition**   N PDx

V29.3 [1] **Observation for suspected genetic or metabolic condition**   N PDx
AHA: 4Q, '98, 59, 68

V29.8 [1] **Observation for other specified suspected condition**   N PDx
AHA: 2Q, '03, 15

V29.9 [1] **Observation for unspecified suspected condition**   N PDx
AHA: 1Q, '02, 6

LIVEBORN INFANTS ACCORDING TO TYPE OF BIRTH (V30-V39)

Note: These categories are intended for the coding of liveborn infants who are consuming health care [e.g., crib or bassinet occupancy].

The following fourth-digit subdivisions are for use with categories V30-V39:
   ✓5th   **0 Born in hospital**   N
        1 Born before admission to hospital   N
        2 Born outside hospital and not hospitalized

The following two fifth-digits are for use with the fourth-digit .0, Born in hospital:
        0 delivered without mention of cesarean delivery
        1 delivered by cesarean delivery

AHA: 1Q, '01, 10

✓4th **V30 Single liveborn**   PDx
AHA: 2Q, '03, 9; 4Q, '98, 46, 59; 1Q, '94, 9 ; For code V30.00: ▶ 1Q, '04, 8, 16;◀ 4Q, '03, 68

✓4th **V31 Twin, mate liveborn**   PDx
AHA: 3Q, '92, 10

✓4th **V32 Twin, mate stillborn**   PDx
✓4th **V33 Twin, unspecified**   PDx
✓4th **V34 Other multiple, mates all liveborn**   PDx
✓4th **V35 Other multiple, mates all stillborn**   PDx
✓4th **V36 Other multiple, mates live- and stillborn**   PDx
✓4th **V37 Other multiple, unspecified**   PDx
✓4th **V39 Unspecified**   PDx

PERSONS WITH A CONDITION INFLUENCING THEIR HEALTH STATUS (V40-V49)

Note: These categories are intended for use when these conditions are recorded as "diagnoses" or "problems."

✓4th **V40 Mental and behavioral problems**
V40.0 Problems with learning   SDx
V40.1 Problems with communication [including speech]   SDx
V40.2 Other mental problems   SDx
V40.3 Other behavioral problems   SDx
V40.9 Unspecified mental or behavioral problem   SDx

✓4th **V41 Problems with special senses and other special functions**
V41.0 Problems with sight   SDx
V41.1 Other eye problems   SDx
V41.2 Problems with hearing   SDx
V41.3 Other ear problems   SDx
V41.4 Problems with voice production   SDx
V41.5 Problems with smell and taste   SDx

---

[1] A code from the V30–V39 series may be sequenced before the V29 on the newborn medical record.

✓4th
✓5th Additional Digit Required   Unspecified Code   Other Specified Code   Manifestation Code   ▶◀ Revised Text   ● New Code   ▲ Revised Code Title

V Codes

V41.6–V45.59

V41.6   **Problems with swallowing and mastication** `SDx`

V41.7   **Problems with sexual function** `SDx`

> `EXCLUDES`   *marital problems (V61.10)*
> *psychosexual disorders (302.0-302.9)*

V41.8   **Other problems with special functions** `SDx`

V41.9   **Unspecified problem with special functions** `SDx`

✓4th **V42**   **Organ or tissue replaced by transplant**

> `INCLUDES`   homologous or heterologous (animal) (human) transplant organ status

AHA: 3Q, '98, 3, 4

V42.0   **Kidney** `SDx`
> AHA: 1Q, '03, 10; 3Q, '01, 12

V42.1   **Heart** `SDx`
> AHA: 3Q, '03, 16; 3Q, '01, 13

V42.2   **Heart valve** `SDx`

V42.3   **Skin** `SDx`

V42.4   **Bone** `SDx`

V42.5   **Cornea** `SDx`

V42.6   **Lung** `SDx`

V42.7   **Liver** `SDx`

✓5th **V42.8**   **Other specified organ or tissue**
> AHA: 4Q, '98, 64; 4Q, '97, 49

     V42.81 Bone marrow `SDx`

     V42.82 Peripheral stem cells `SDx`

     V42.83 Pancreas `SDx`
> AHA: 1Q, '03, 10; 2Q, '01, 16

     V42.84 Intestines `SDx`
> AHA: 4Q, '00, 48, 50

     V42.89 Other `SDx`

V42.9   **Unspecified organ or tissue** `SDx`

✓4th **V43**   **Organ or tissue replaced by other means**

> `INCLUDES`   organ or tissue assisted by other means
> replacement of organ by:
>   artificial device
>   mechanical device
>   prosthesis

> `EXCLUDES`   *cardiac pacemaker in situ (V45.01)*
> *fitting and adjustment of prosthetic device*
>   *(V52.0-V52.9)*
> *renal dialysis status (V45.1)*

V43.0   **Eye globe** `SDx`

V43.1   **Lens** `SDx`
> Pseudophakos
> AHA: 4Q, '98, 65

✓5th **V43.2**   **Heart**
> Fully implantable artificial heart
> Heart assist device
> AHA: 4Q, '03, 85

     V43.21 Heart assist device `SDx`

     V43.22 Fully implantable artificial heart

V43.3   **Heart valve** `SDx`
> AHA: 3Q, '02, 13, 14

V43.4   **Blood vessel** `SDx`

V43.5   **Bladder** `SDx`

✓5th **V43.6**   **Joint**

     V43.60 Unspecified joint `SDx`

     V43.61 Shoulder `SDx`

     V43.62 Elbow `SDx`

     V43.63 Wrist `SDx`

     V43.64 Hip `SDx`

     V43.65 Knee `SDx`

     V43.66 Ankle `SDx`

     V43.69 Other `SDx`

V43.7   **Limb** `SDx`

✓5th **V43.8**   **Other organ or tissue**

     V43.81 Larynx `SDx`
> AHA: 4Q, '95, 55

     V43.82 Breast `SDx`
> AHA: 4Q, '95, 55

     V43.83 Artificial skin `SDx`

     V43.89 Other `SDx`

✓4th **V44**   **Artificial opening status**

> `EXCLUDES`   *artificial openings requiring attention or*
> *management (V55.0-V55.9)*

V44.0   **Tracheostomy** `SDx`
> AHA: 4Q, '03, 103, 107, 111; 1Q, '01, 6

V44.1   **Gastrostomy** `SDx`
> AHA: 4Q, '03, 103, 107-108, 110; 1Q, '01, 12; 3Q, '97, 12; 1Q, '93, 26

V44.2   **Ileostomy** `SDx`

V44.3   **Colostomy** `SDx`
> AHA: 4Q, '03, 110

V44.4   **Other artificial opening of gastrointestinal tract** `SDx`

✓5th **V44.5**   **Cystostomy**

     V44.50 Cystostomy, unspecified `SDx`

     V44.51 Cutaneous-vesicostomy `SDx`

     V44.52 Appendico-vesicostomy `SDx`

     V44.59 Other cystostomy `SDx`

V44.6   **Other artificial opening of urinary tract** `SDx`
> Nephrostomy   Urethrostomy
> Ureterostomy

V44.7   **Artificial vagina** `SDx`

V44.8   **Other artificial opening status** `SDx`

V44.9   **Unspecified artificial opening status** `SDx`

✓4th **V45**   **Other postprocedural states**

> `EXCLUDES`   *aftercare management (V51-V58.9)*
> *malfunction or other complication — code to*
>   *condition*

AHA: 4Q, '03, 85

✓5th **V45.0**   **Cardiac device in situ**

> `EXCLUDES`   *artificial heart (V43.22)*
> *heart assist device (V43.21)*

     V45.00 Unspecified cardiac device `SDx`

     V45.01 Cardiac pacemaker `SDx`

     V45.02 Automatic implantable cardiac defibrillator `SDx`

     V45.09 Other specified cardiac device `SDx`
> Carotid sinus pacemaker in situ

V45.1   **Renal dialysis status** `SDx`
> Patient requiring intermittent renal dialysis
> Presence of arterial-venous shunt (for dialysis)

> `EXCLUDES`   *admission for dialysis treatment or*
> *session (V56.0)*

> AHA: ▶1Q, '04, 22-23;◄ 2Q, '03, 7; 2Q, '01, 12, 13

V45.2   **Presence of cerebrospinal fluid drainage device** `SDx`
> Cerebral ventricle (communicating) shunt, valve, or device in situ

> `EXCLUDES`   *malfunction (996.2)*

> AHA: 4Q, '03, 106

V45.3   **Intestinal bypass or anastomosis status** `SDx`

V45.4   **Arthrodesis status** `SDx`
> AHA: N-D, '84, 18

✓5th **V45.5**   **Presence of contraceptive device**

> `EXCLUDES`   *checking, reinsertion, or removal of*
> *device (V25.42)*
> *complication from device (996.32)*
> *insertion of device (V25.1)*

     V45.51 Intrauterine contraceptive device `SDx` ♀

     V45.52 Subdermal contraceptive implant `SDx`

     V45.59 Other `SDx`

`N` Newborn Age: 0   `P` Pediatric Age: 0-17   `M` Maternity Age: 12-55   `A` Adult Age: 15-124   `MSP` Medicare Secondary Payer

V Codes

√5ᵗʰ **V45.6** **States following surgery of eye and adnexa**

Cataract extraction
Filtering bleb   } state following eye surgery
Surgical eyelid adhesion

> **EXCLUDES**   aphakia (379.31)
> artificial eye globe (V43.0)

AHA: 4Q, '98, 65; 4Q, '97, 49

V45.61 Cataract extraction status `SDx`
Use additional code for associated artificial lens status (V43.1)

V45.69 Other states following surgery of `SDx` **eye and adnexa**
AHA: 2Q, '01, 16; 1Q, '98, 10; 4Q, '97, 19

√5ᵗʰ **V45.7** **Acquired absence of organ**
AHA: 4Q, '98, 65; 4Q, '97, 50

V45.71 Acquired absence of breast
AHA: 4Q, '01, 66; 4Q, '97, 50

V45.72 Acquired absence of intestine (large) (small)
V45.73 Acquired absence of kidney
V45.74 Other parts of urinary tract
Bladder
AHA: 4Q, '00, 51

V45.75 Stomach
AHA: 4Q, '00, 51

V45.76 Lung
AHA: 4Q, '00, 51

V45.77 Genital organs
> **EXCLUDES** ► female genital mutilation
> status (629.20-629.23)◄
AHA: 1Q, '03, 13, 14; 4Q, '00, 51

V45.78 Eye
AHA: 4Q, '00, 51

V45.79 Other acquired absence of organ
AHA: 4Q, '00, 51

√5ᵗʰ **V45.8** **Other postprocedural status**

V45.81 Aortocoronary bypass status `SDx`
AHA: 4Q, '03, 105; 3Q, '01, 15; 3Q, '97, 16

V45.82 Percutaneous transluminal coronary `SDx` **angioplasty status**

V45.83 Breast implant removal status `SDx`
AHA: 4Q, '95, 55

V45.84 Dental restoration status `SDx`
Dental crowns status
Dental fillings status
AHA: 4Q, '01, 54

V45.85 Insulin pump status `SDx`
V45.89 Other `SDx`
Presence of neuropacemaker or other electronic device
> **EXCLUDES**   artificial heart valve in situ
> (V43.3)
> vascular prosthesis in situ
> (V43.4)
AHA: 1Q, '95, 11

√4ᵗʰ **V46** **Other dependence on machines**
V46.0 **Aspirator** `SDx`

√5ᵗʰ **V46.1** **Respirator**
Iron lung
AHA: 4Q, '03, 103; 1Q, '01, 12; J-F, '87, 7 3

● **V46.11 Dependence on respirator, status**
● **V46.12 Encounter for respirator dependence during power failure**

V46.2 **Supplemental oxygen** `SDx`
Long-term oxygen therapy
AHA: 4Q, '03, 108; 4Q, '02, 79

V46.8 **Other enabling machines** `SDx`
Hyperbaric chamber
Possum [Patient-Operated-Selector-Mechanism]
> **EXCLUDES**   cardiac pacemaker (V45.0)
> kidney dialysis machine (V45.1)

V46.9 **Unspecified machine dependence** `SDx`

√4ᵗʰ **V47** **Other problems with internal organs**
V47.0 **Deficiencies of internal organs** `SDx`
V47.1 **Mechanical and motor problems with internal** `SDx` **organs**
V47.2 **Other cardiorespiratory problems** `SDx`
Cardiovascular exercise intolerance with pain (with):
  at rest
  less than ordinary activity
  ordinary activity

V47.3 **Other digestive problems** `SDx`
V47.4 **Other urinary problems** `SDx`
V47.5 **Other genital problems** `SDx`
V47.9 **Unspecified** `SDx`

√4ᵗʰ **V48** **Problems with head, neck, and trunk**
V48.0 **Deficiencies of head** `SDx`
> **EXCLUDES**   deficiencies of ears, eyelids, and nose
> (V48.8)

V48.1 **Deficiencies of neck and trunk** `SDx`
V48.2 **Mechanical and motor problems with head** `SDx`
V48.3 **Mechanical and motor problems with neck and trunk**
V48.4 **Sensory problem with head** `SDx`
V48.5 **Sensory problem with neck and trunk** `SDx`
V48.6 **Disfigurements of head** `SDx`
V48.7 **Disfigurements of neck and trunk** `SDx`
V48.8 **Other problems with head, neck, and trunk** `SDx`
V48.9 **Unspecified problem with head, neck, or** `SDx` **trunk**

√4ᵗʰ **V49** **Other conditions influencing health status**
V49.0 **Deficiencies of limbs** `SDx`
V49.1 **Mechanical problems with limbs** `SDx`
V49.2 **Motor problems with limbs** `SDx`
V49.3 **Sensory problems with limbs** `SDx`
V49.4 **Disfigurements of limbs** `SDx`
V49.5 **Other problems of limbs** `SDx`

√5ᵗʰ **V49.6** **Upper limb amputation status**
AHA: 4Q, '98, 42; 4Q, '94, 39

V49.60 Unspecified level `SDx`
V49.61 Thumb `SDx`
V49.62 Other finger(s) `SDx`
V49.63 Hand `SDx`
V49.64 Wrist `SDx`
Disarticulation of wrist
V49.65 Below elbow `SDx`
V49.66 Above elbow `SDx`
Disarticulation of elbow
V49.67 Shoulder `SDx`
Disarticulation of shoulder

√5ᵗʰ **V49.7** **Lower limb amputation status**
AHA: 4Q, '98, 42; 4Q, '94, 39

V49.70 Unspecified level `SDx`
V49.71 Great toe `SDx`
V49.72 Other toe(s) `SDx`
V49.73 Foot `SDx`
V49.74 Ankle `SDx`
Disarticulation of ankle
V49.75 Below knee `SDx`
V49.76 Above knee `SDx`
Disarticulation of knee
V49.77 Hip `SDx`
Disarticulation of hip

V45.61–V49.77

√4ᵗʰ
√5ᵗʰ Additional Digit Required   Unspecified Code   Other Specified Code   Manifestation Code   ►◄ Revised Text   ● New Code   ▲ Revised Code Title

2005 ICD•9•CM   October 2004 • Volume 1 — 295

✓5ᵗʰ **V49.8** **Other specified conditions influencing health status**
AHA: 4Q, '00, 51

V49.81 Asymptomatic postmenopausal
status (age-related) (natural)   A ♂
EXCLUDES   menopausal and
premenopausal
disorders (627.0-627.9)
postsurgical menopause (256.2)
premature menopause (256.31)
symptomatic menopause
(627.0-627.9)
AHA: 4Q, '02, 79; 4Q, '00, 54

V49.82 Dental sealant status   SDx
AHA: 4Q, '01, 54

V49.83 Awaiting organ transplant status

V49.89 Other specified conditions influencing SDx
health status

V49.9 **Unspecified**   SDx

PERSONS ENCOUNTERING HEALTH SERVICES FOR SPECIFIC PROCEDURES AND AFTERCARE (V50-V59)

Note: Categories V51-V58 are intended for use to indicate a
reason for care in patients who may have already been
treated for some disease or injury not now present, or
who are receiving care to consolidate the treatment, to
deal with residual states, or to prevent recurrence.
EXCLUDES   follow-up examination for medical surveillance
following treatment (V67.0-V67.9)

✓4ᵗʰ **V50 Elective surgery for purposes other than remedying health**
states

V50.0 **Hair transplant**

V50.1 **Other plastic surgery for unacceptable**
cosmetic appearance
Breast augmentation or reduction
Face-lift
EXCLUDES   plastic surgery following healed injury
or operation (V51)

V50.2 **Routine or ritual circumcision**   ♂
Circumcision in the absence of significant medical
indication

V50.3 **Ear piercing**

✓5ᵗʰ **V50.4** **Prophylactic organ removal**
EXCLUDES   organ donations (V59.0-V59.9)
therapeutic organ removal — code to
condition
AHA: 4Q, '94, 44

V50.41 Breast

V50.42 Ovary   ♀

V50.49 Other

V50.8 **Other**

V50.9 **Unspecified**

V51 Aftercare involving the use of plastic surgery   SDx
Plastic surgery following healed injury or operation
EXCLUDES   cosmetic plastic surgery (V50.1)
plastic surgery as treatment for current injury —
code to condition
repair of scarred tissue — code to scar

✓4ᵗʰ **V52 Fitting and adjustment of prosthetic device and implant**
INCLUDES   removal of device
EXCLUDES   malfunction or complication of prosthetic device
(996.0-996.7)
status only, without need for care (V43.0-V43.8)
AHA: 4Q, '95, 55 ; 1Q, '90, 7

V52.0 **Artificial arm (complete) (partial)**

V52.1 **Artificial leg (complete) (partial)**

V52.2 **Artificial eye**

V52.3 **Dental prosthetic device**

V52.4 **Breast prosthesis and implant**   ♀
EXCLUDES   admission for implant insertion (V50.1)
AHA: 4Q, '95, 80, 81

V52.8 **Other specified prosthetic device**
AHA: 2Q, '02, 12, 16

V52.9 **Unspecified prosthetic device**

✓4ᵗʰ **V53 Fitting and adjustment of other device**
INCLUDES   removal of device
replacement of device
EXCLUDES   status only, without need for care (V45.0-V45.8)

✓5ᵗʰ **V53.0** **Devices related to nervous system and special**
senses
AHA: 4Q, '98, 66; 4Q, '97, 51

V53.01 Fitting and adjustment of cerebral
ventricular (communicating) shunt
AHA: 4Q, '97, 51

V53.02 Neuropacemaker (brain) (peripheral nerve)
(spinal cord)

V53.09 Fitting and adjustment of other
devices related to nervous system
and special senses
Auditory substitution device
Visual substitution device
AHA: 2Q '99, 4

V53.1 **Spectacles and contact lenses**

V53.2 **Hearing aid**

✓5ᵗʰ **V53.3** **Cardiac device**
Reprogramming
AHA: 3Q, '92, 3; 1Q, '90, 7; M-J, '87, 8 ; N-D, '84, 18

V53.31 Cardiac pacemaker
EXCLUDES   mechanical complication of
cardiac pacemaker
(996.01)
AHA: 1Q, '02, 3

V53.32 Automatic implantable cardiac defibrillator

V53.39 Other cardiac device

V53.4 **Orthodontic devices**

V53.5 **Other intestinal appliance**
EXCLUDES   colostomy (V55.3)
ileostomy (V55.2)
other artificial opening of digestive tract
(V55.4)

V53.6 **Urinary devices**
Urinary catheter
EXCLUDES   cystostomy (V55.5)
nephrostomy (V55.6)
ureterostomy (V55.6)
urethrostomy (V55.6)

V53.7 **Orthopedic devices**
Orthopedic: Orthopedic:
brace   corset
cast   shoes
EXCLUDES   other orthopedic aftercare (V54)

V53.8 **Wheelchair**

✓5ᵗʰ **V53.9** **Other and unspecified device**
AHA: 2Q, '03, 6

V53.90 Unspecified device

V53.91 Fitting and adjustment of insulin pump
Insulin pump titration

V53.99 Other device

✓4ᵗʰ **V54 Other orthopedic aftercare**
EXCLUDES   fitting and adjustment of orthopedic devices
(V53.7)
malfunction of internal orthopedic device (996.4)
other complication of nonmechanical nature
(996.60-996.79)
AHA: 3Q, '95, 3

✓5ᵗʰ **V54.0 Aftercare involving internal fixation device**
> EXCLUDES *malfunction of internal orthopedic device (996.4)*
> *other complication of nonmechanical nature (996.60-996.79)*
> *removal of external fixation device (V54.89)*

AHA: 4Q, '03, 87

V54.01 Encounter for removal of internal fixation device

V54.02 Encounter for lengthening/adjustment of growth rod

V54.09 Other aftercare involving internal fixation device

✓5ᵗʰ **V54.1 Aftercare for healing traumatic fracture**
AHA: 4Q, '02, 80

V54.10 Aftercare for healing traumatic fracture of arm, unspecified

V54.11 Aftercare for healing traumatic fracture of upper arm

V54.12 Aftercare for healing traumatic fracture of lower arm

V54.13 Aftercare for healing traumatic fracture of hip
AHA: 4Q, '03, 103, 105; 2Q, '03, 16

V54.14 Aftercare for healing traumatic fracture of leg, unspecified

V54.15 Aftercare for healing traumatic fracture of upper leg
> EXCLUDES *aftercare for healing traumatic fracture of hip (V54.13)*

V54.16 Aftercare for healing traumatic fracture of lower leg

V54.17 Aftercare for healing traumatic fracture of vertebrae

V54.19 Aftercare for healing traumatic fracture of other bone
AHA: 4Q, '02, 80

✓5ᵗʰ **V54.2 Aftercare for healing pathologic fracture**
AHA: 4Q, '02, 80

V54.20 Aftercare for healing pathologic fracture of arm, unspecified

V54.21 Aftercare for healing pathologic fracture of upper arm

V54.22 Aftercare for healing pathologic fracture of lower arm

V54.23 Aftercare for healing pathologic fracture of hip

V54.24 Aftercare for healing pathologic fracture of leg, unspecified

V54.25 Aftercare for healing pathologic fracture of upper leg
> EXCLUDES *aftercare for healing pathologic fracture of hip (V54.23)*

V54.26 Aftercare for healing pathologic fracture of lower leg

V54.27 Aftercare for healing pathologic fracture of vertebrae
AHA: 4Q, '03, 108

V54.29 Aftercare for healing pathologic fracture of other bone
AHA: 4Q, '02, 80

✓5ᵗʰ **V54.8 Other orthopedic aftercare**
AHA: 3Q, '01, 19; 4Q, '99, 5

V54.81 Aftercare following joint replacement
Use additional code to identify joint replacement site (V43.60-V43.69)
AHA: 4Q, '02, 80

V54.89 Other orthopedic aftercare
Aftercare for healing fracture NOS

V54.9 Unspecified orthopedic aftercare

✓4ᵗʰ **V55 Attention to artificial openings**
> INCLUDES adjustment or repositioning of catheter
> closure
> passage of sounds or bougies
> reforming
> removal or replacement of catheter
> toilet or cleansing
> EXCLUDES *complications of external stoma (519.00-519.09, 569.60-569.69, 997.4, 997.5)*
> *status only, without need for care (V44.0-V44.9)*

V55.0 Tracheostomy

V55.1 Gastrostomy
AHA: 4Q, '99, 9; 3Q, '97, 7, 8; 1Q, '96, 14; 3Q, '95, 13

V55.2 Ileostomy

V55.3 Colostomy
AHA: 3Q, '97, 9

V55.4 Other artificial opening of digestive tract
AHA: 1Q, '03, 10

V55.5 Cystostomy

V55.6 Other artificial opening of urinary tract
Nephrostomy   Urethrostomy
Ureterostomy

V55.7 Artificial vagina

V55.8 Other specified artificial opening

V55.9 Unspecified artificial opening

✓4ᵗʰ **V56 Encounter for dialysis and dialysis catheter care**
Use additional code to identify the associated condition
> EXCLUDES *dialysis preparation — code to condition*

AHA: 4Q, '98, 66; 1Q, '93, 29

V56.0 Extracorporeal dialysis
Dialysis (renal) NOS
> EXCLUDES *dialysis status (V45.1)*

AHA: ▶1Q, '04, 23;◀ 4Q, '00, 40; 3Q, '98, 6; 2Q, '98, 20

V56.1 Fitting and adjustment of extracorporeal dialysis catheter
Removal or replacement of catheter
Toilet or cleansing
Use additional code for any concurrent extracorporeal dialysis (V56.0)
AHA: 2Q, '98, 20

V56.2 Fitting and adjustment of peritoneal dialysis catheter
Use additional code for any concurrent peritoneal dialysis (V56.8)
AHA: 4Q, '98, 55

✓5ᵗʰ **V56.3 Encounter for adequacy testing for dialysis**
AHA: 4Q, '00, 55

V56.31 Encounter for adequacy testing for hemodialysis

V56.32 Encounter for adequacy testing for peritoneal dialysis
Peritoneal equilibration test

V56.8 Other dialysis
Peritoneal dialysis
AHA: 4Q, '98, 55

✓4ᵗʰ **V57 Care involving use of rehabilitation procedures**
Use additional code to identify underlying condition
AHA: 1Q, '02, 19; 3Q, '97, 12; 1Q, '90, 6; S-O, '86, 3

V57.0 Breathing exercises

V57.1 Other physical therapy
Therapeutic and remedial exercises, except breathing
AHA: 4Q, '02, 56; 4Q, '99, 5

✓4ᵗʰ Additional Digit Required | Unspecified Code | Other Specified Code | Manifestation Code | ▶◀ Revised Text | ● New Code | ▲ Revised Code Title
✓5ᵗʰ

V Codes

V57.2–V58.78

☑5ᵗʰ **V57.2 Occupational therapy and vocational rehabilitation**

V57.21 Encounter for occupational therapy
AHA: 4Q, '99, 7

V57.22 Encounter for vocational therapy

V57.3 Speech therapy
AHA: 4Q, '97, 36

V57.4 Orthoptic training

☑5ᵗʰ **V57.8 Other specified rehabilitation procedure**

V57.81 Orthotic training
Gait training in the use of artificial limbs

V57.89 Other
Multiple training or therapy
AHA: 4Q, '03, 105-106, 108; 2Q, '03, 16; 1Q, '02, 16; 3Q, '01, 21; 3Q, '97, 11, 12; S-O, '86, 4

V57.9 Unspecified rehabilitation procedure

☑4ᵗʰ **V58 Encounter for other and unspecified procedures and aftercare**
EXCLUDES   convalescence and palliative care (V66)

V58.0 Radiotherapy PDx
Encounter or admission for radiotherapy
EXCLUDES   encounter for radioactive implant — code to condition
radioactive iodine therapy — code to condition
AHA: 3Q, '92, 5; 2Q, '90, 7; J-F, '87, 13

V58.1 Chemotherapy PDx
Encounter or admission for chemotherapy
EXCLUDES   prophylactic chemotherapy against disease which has never been present (V03.0-V07.9)
AHA: 1Q, '04, 13; 2Q, '03, 16; 3Q, '93, 4; 2Q, '92, 6; 2Q, '91, 17; 2Q, '90, 7; S-O, '84, 5

V58.2 Blood transfusion, without reported diagnosis SDx

V58.3 Attention to surgical dressings and sutures
Change of dressings
Removal of sutures

☑5ᵗʰ **V58.4 Other aftercare following surgery**
EXCLUDES   aftercare following sterilization reversal surgery (V26.22)
attention to artificial openings (V55.0-V55.9)
orthopedic aftercare (V54.0-V54.9)
Note: Codes from this subcategory should be used in conjunction with other aftercare codes to fully identify the reason for the aftercare encounter
AHA: 4Q, '99, 9; N-D, '87, 9

V58.41 Encounter for planned postoperative wound closure
EXCLUDES   disruption of operative wound (998.3)
AHA: 4Q, '99, 15

V58.42 Aftercare following surgery for neoplasm
Conditions classifiable to 140-239
AHA: 4Q, '02, 80

V58.43 Aftercare following surgery for injury and trauma
Conditions classifiable to 800-999
EXCLUDES   aftercare for healing traumatic fracture (V54.10-V54.19)
AHA: 4Q, '02, 80

V58.44 Aftercare following organ transplant
Use additional code to identify the organ transplanted (V42.0-V42.9)

V58.49 Other specified aftercare following surgery
AHA: 1Q, '96, 8, 9

V58.5 Orthodontics SDx
EXCLUDES   fitting and adjustment of orthodontic device (V53.4)

☑5ᵗʰ **V58.6 Long-term (current) drug use**
EXCLUDES   drug abuse (305.00-305.93)
drug dependence (304.00-304.93)
►hormone replacement therapy (postmenopausal) (V07.4)◄
AHA: 4Q, '03, 85; 4Q, '02, 84; 3Q, '02, 15; 4Q, '95, 61

V58.61 Long-term (current) use of anticoagulants SDx
EXCLUDES   ►long-term (current) use of aspirin (V58.66)◄
AHA: 4Q, '03, 108; 3Q, '02, 13-16; 1Q, '02, 15, 16

V58.62 Long-term (current) use of antibiotics SDx
AHA: 4Q, '98, 59

V58.63 Long-term (current) use of antiplatelets/antithrombotics SDx
EXCLUDES   ►long-term (current) use of aspirin (V58.66)◄

V58.64 Long-term (current) use of non-steroidal anti-inflammatories (NSAID) SDx
EXCLUDES   ►long-term (current) use of aspirin (V58.66)◄

V58.65 Long-term (current) use of steroids SDx

V58.66 Long-term (current) use of aspirin

V58.67 Long-term (current) use of insulin

V58.69 Long-term (current) use of other medications SDx
High-risk medications
AHA: 1Q, '03, 11; 2Q, '00, 8; 3Q, '99, 13; 2Q, '99, 17; 1Q, '97, 12; 2Q, '96, 7

☑5ᵗʰ **V58.7 Aftercare following surgery to specified body systems, not elsewhere classified**
Note: Codes from this subcategory should be used in conjunction with other aftercare codes to fully identify the reason for the aftercare encounter
EXCLUDES   ►aftercare following organ transplant (V58.44)
aftercare following surgery for neoplasm (V58.42)◄
AHA: 4Q, '03, 104; 4Q, '02, 80

V58.71 Aftercare following surgery of the sense organs, NEC
Conditions classifiable to 360-379, 380-389

V58.72 Aftercare following surgery of the nervous system, NEC
Conditions classifiable to 320-359
EXCLUDES   aftercare following surgery of the sense organs, NEC (V58.71)

V58.73 Aftercare following surgery of the circulatory system, NEC
Conditions classifiable to 390-459
AHA: 4Q, '03, 105

V58.74 Aftercare following surgery of the respiratory system, NEC
Conditions classifiable to 460-519

V58.75 Aftercare following surgery of the teeth, oral cavity and digestive system, NEC
Conditions classifiable to 520-579

V58.76 Aftercare following surgery of the genitourinary system, NEC
Conditions classifiable to 580-629
EXCLUDES   aftercare following sterilization reversal (V26.22)

V58.77 Aftercare following surgery of the skin and subcutaneous tissue, NEC
Conditions classifiable to 680-709

V58.78 Aftercare following surgery of the musculoskeletal system, NEC
Conditions classifiable to 710-739

Ⓝ Newborn Age: 0   Ⓟ Pediatric Age: 0-17   Ⓜ Maternity Age: 12-55   Ⓐ Adult Age: 15-124   ᴹˢᴾ Medicare Secondary Payer

V Codes

V58.8–V61.6

✓5ᵗʰ V58.8 Other specified procedures and aftercare
AHA: 4Q, '94, 45; 2Q, '94, 8

V58.81 Fitting and adjustment of vascular catheter
Removal or replacement of catheter
Toilet or cleansing
> **EXCLUDES** complication of renal dialysis
> (996.73)
> complication of vascular
> catheter (996.74)
> dialysis preparation — code to
> condition
> encounter for dialysis (V56.0-
> V56.8)
> fitting and adjustment of
> dialysis catheter (V56.1)

V58.82 Fitting and adjustment of nonvascular catheter, NEC
Removal or replacement of catheter
Toilet or cleansing
> **EXCLUDES** fitting and adjustment of
> peritoneal dialysis
> catheter (V56.2)
> fitting and adjustment of
> urinary catheter (V53.6)

V58.83 Encounter for therapeutic drug monitoring
Use additional code for any associated long-term (current) drug use (V58.61-V58.69)
> **EXCLUDES** blood-drug testing for medico-
> legal reasons (V70.4)

AHA: ▶1Q, '04, 13;◀ 4Q, '03, 85; 4Q, '02, 84; 3Q, '02, 13-16

DEF: Drug monitoring: Measurement of the level of a specific drug in the body or measurement of a specific function to assess effectiveness of a drug.

V58.89 Other specified aftercare
AHA: 4Q, '98, 59

V58.9 Unspecified aftercare `SDx`

✓4ᵗʰ V59 Donors
> **EXCLUDES** examination of potential donor (V70.8)
> self-donation of organ or tissue — code to
> condition

AHA: 4Q, '95, 62; 1Q, '90, 10; N-D, '84, 8

✓5ᵗʰ V59.0 Blood
V59.01 Whole blood `PDx`
V59.02 Stem cells `PDx`
V59.09 Other `PDx`
V59.1 Skin `PDx`
V59.2 Bone `PDx`
V59.3 Bone marrow `PDx`
V59.4 Kidney `PDx`
V59.5 Cornea `PDx`
V59.6 Liver `PDx`
V59.8 Other specified organ or tissue `PDx`
AHA: 3Q, '02, 20

V59.9 Unspecified organ or tissue `PDx`

PERSONS ENCOUNTERING HEALTH SERVICES IN OTHER CIRCUMSTANCES (V60-V69)

✓4ᵗʰ V60 Housing, household, and economic circumstances
V60.0 Lack of housing `SDx`
Hobos	Transients
Social migrants	Vagabonds
Tramps	

V60.1 Inadequate housing `SDx`
Lack of heating
Restriction of space
Technical defects in home preventing adequate care

V60.2 Inadequate material resources `SDx`
Economic problem   Poverty NOS

V60.3 Person living alone `SDx`

V60.4 No other household member able to render care `SDx`
Person requiring care (has) (is):
family member too handicapped, ill, or otherwise unsuited to render care
partner temporarily away from home
temporarily away from usual place of abode
> **EXCLUDES** holiday relief care (V60.5)

V60.5 Holiday relief care `SDx`
Provision of health care facilities to a person normally cared for at home, to enable relatives to take a vacation

V60.6 Person living in residential institution `SDx`
Boarding school resident

V60.8 Other specified housing or economic circumstances `SDx`

V60.9 Unspecified housing or economic circumstance `SDx`

✓4ᵗʰ V61 Other family circumstances
> **INCLUDES** when these circumstances or fear of them,
> affecting the person directly involved or
> others, are mentioned as the reason,
> justified or not, for seeking or receiving
> medical advice or care

AHA: 1Q, '90, 9

V61.0 Family disruption
Divorce   Estrangement

✓5ᵗʰ V61.1 Counseling for marital and partner problems
> **EXCLUDES** problems related to:
> psychosexual disorders (302.0-302.9)
> sexual function (V41.7)

V61.10 Counseling for marital and partner problems, unspecified
Marital conflict   Partner conflict

V61.11 Counseling for victim of spousal and partner abuse
> **EXCLUDES** encounter for treatment of
> current injuries due to
> abuse (995.80-995.85)

V61.12 Counseling for perpetrator of spousal and partner abuse

✓5ᵗʰ V61.2 Parent-child problems
V61.20 Counseling for parent-child problem, unspecified
Concern about behavior of child
Parent-child conflict

V61.21 Counseling for victim of child abuse
Child battering   Child neglect
> **EXCLUDES** current injuries due to abuse
> (995.50-995.59)

V61.22 Counseling for perpetrator of parent child abuse
> **EXCLUDES** counseling for non-parental
> abuser (V62.83)

V61.29 Other
Problem concerning adopted or foster child
AHA: 3Q, '99, 16

V61.3 Problems with aged parents or in-laws

✓5ᵗʰ V61.4 Health problems within family
V61.41 Alcoholism in family
V61.49 Other
Care of / Presence of } sick or handicapped person in family or household

V61.5 Multiparity
V61.6 Illegitimacy or illegitimate pregnancy `M` ♀

✓4ᵗʰ / ✓5ᵗʰ Additional Digit Required | Unspecified Code | Other Specified Code | Manifestation Code | ▶◀ Revised Text | ● New Code | ▲ Revised Code Title

V61.7 Other unwanted pregnancy ▢ ♀

V61.8 Other specified family circumstances

Problems with family members NEC

V61.9 Unspecified family circumstance

✓4ᵗʰ V62 Other psychosocial circumstances

INCLUDES those circumstances or fear of them, affecting the person directly involved or others, mentioned as the reason, justified or not, for seeking or receiving medical advice or care

EXCLUDES previous psychological trauma (V15.41-V15.49)

V62.0 Unemployment SDx

EXCLUDES circumstances when main problem is economic inadequacy or poverty (V60.2)

V62.1 Adverse effects of work environment SDx

V62.2 Other occupational circumstances or maladjustment SDx

Career choice problem
Dissatisfaction with employment

V62.3 Educational circumstances SDx

Dissatisfaction with school environment
Educational handicap

V62.4 Social maladjustment SDx

Cultural deprivation
Political, religious, or sex discrimination
Social:
  isolation
  persecution

V62.5 Legal circumstances SDx

Imprisonment   Litigation
Legal investigation   Prosecution

V62.6 Refusal of treatment for reasons of religion or conscience SDx

✓5ᵗʰ V62.8 Other psychological or physical stress, not elsewhere classified

V62.81 Interpersonal problems, not elsewhere classified SDx

V62.82 Bereavement, uncomplicated SDx

EXCLUDES bereavement as adjustment reaction (309.0)

V62.83 Counseling for perpetrator of physical/sexual abuse SDx

EXCLUDES counseling for perpetrator of parental child abuse (V61.22)
counseling for perpetrator of spousal and partner abuse (V61.12)

V62.89 Other SDx

Life circumstance problems
Phase of life problems

V62.9 Unspecified psychosocial circumstance SDx

✓4ᵗʰ V63 Unavailability of other medical facilities for care

AHA: 1Q, '91, 21

V63.0 Residence remote from hospital or other health care facility

V63.1 Medical services in home not available

EXCLUDES no other household member able to render care (V60.4)

AHA: 4Q, '01, 67; 1Q, '01, 12

V63.2 Person awaiting admission to adequate facility elsewhere

V63.8 Other specified reasons for unavailability of medical facilities

Person on waiting list undergoing social agency investigation

V63.9 Unspecified reason for unavailability of medical facilities

✓4ᵗʰ V64 Persons encountering health services for specific procedures, not carried out

V64.0 Vaccination not carried out because of contraindication SDx

V64.1 Surgical or other procedure not carried out because of contraindication SDx

V64.2 Surgical or other procedure not carried out because of patient's decision SDx

AHA: 2Q, '01, 8

V64.3 Procedure not carried out for other reasons SDx

✓5ᵗʰ V64.4 Closed surgical procedure converted to open procedure

AHA: ▶4Q, '03, 87;◀ 4Q, '98, 68; 4Q, '97, 52

V64.41 Laparoscopic surgical procedure converted to open procedure SDx

V64.42 Thoracoscopic surgical procedure converted to open procedure SDx

V64.43 Arthroscopic surgical procedure converted to open procedure SDx

✓4ᵗʰ V65 Other persons seeking consultation

V65.0 Healthy person accompanying sick person

Boarder

✓5ᵗʰ V65.1 Person consulting on behalf of another person

Advice or treatment for nonattending third party

EXCLUDES concern (normal) about sick person in family (V61.41-V61.49)

AHA: ▶4Q, '03, 84◀

V65.11 Pediatric pre-birth visit for expectant mother ▢

V65.19 Other person consulting on behalf of another person

V65.2 Person feigning illness

Malingerer
Peregrinating patient

AHA: 3Q, '99, 20

V65.3 Dietary surveillance and counseling

Dietary surveillance and counseling (in):
  NOS
  colitis
  diabetes mellitus
  food allergies or intolerance
  gastritis
  hypercholesterolemia
  hypoglycemia
  obesity

✓5ᵗʰ V65.4 Other counseling, not elsewhere classified

Health:
  advice
  education
  instruction

EXCLUDES counseling (for):
  contraception (V25.40-V25.49)
  genetic (V26.3)
  on behalf of third party (V65.11-V65.19)
  procreative management (V26.4)

V65.40 Counseling NOS

V65.41 Exercise counseling

V65.42 Counseling on substance use and abuse

V65.43 Counseling on injury prevention

V65.44 Human immunodeficiency virus [HIV] counseling

V65.45 Counseling on other sexually transmitted diseases

V65.46 Encounter for insulin pump training

V65.49 Other specified counseling

AHA: 2Q, '00, 8

V65.5 **Person with feared complaint in whom no diagnosis was made**
Feared condition not demonstrated
Problem was normal state
"Worried well"

V65.8 **Other reasons for seeking consultation**
EXCLUDES   *specified symptoms*
AHA: 3Q, '92, 4

V65.9 **Unspecified reason for consultation**

√4ᵗʰ **V66 Convalescence and palliative care**

V66.0 **Following surgery**   `PDx`
V66.1 **Following radiotherapy**   `PDx`
V66.2 **Following chemotherapy**   `PDx`
V66.3 **Following psychotherapy and other treatment** `PDx`
for mental disorder
V66.4 **Following treatment of fracture**   `PDx`
V66.5 **Following other treatment**   `PDx`
V66.6 **Following combined treatment**   `PDx`
V66.7 **Encounter for palliative care**   `SDx`
End-of-life care
Hospice care
Terminal care
Code first underlying disease
AHA: 4Q, '03, 107; 1Q, '98, 11; 4Q, '96, 47, 48

V66.9 **Unspecified convalescence**   `PDx`
AHA: 4Q, '99, 8

√4ᵗʰ **V67 Follow-up examination**
INCLUDES   surveillance only following completed
treatment
EXCLUDES   *surveillance of contraception (V25.40-V25.49)*
AHA: 2Q, '03, 5; 4Q, '94, 48

√5ᵗʰ **V67.0** **Following surgery**
AHA: 4Q, '00, 56; 4Q, '98, 69; 4Q, '97, 50; 2Q, '95, 8;1Q, '95, 4;
3Q, '92, 11

V67.00 **Following surgery, unspecified**
V67.01 **Follow-up vaginal pap smear**   ♀
Vaginal pap-smear, status-post
hysterectomy for malignant condition
Use additional code to identify:
acquired absence of uterus (V45.77)
personal history of malignant neoplasm
(V10.40-V10.44)
EXCLUDES   *vaginal pap smear status-post*
hysterectomy for non-
malignant condition
(V76.47)

V67.09 **Following other surgery**
EXCLUDES   *sperm count following*
sterilization reversal
(V26.22)
sperm count for fertility testing
(V26.21)
AHA: 3Q, '03, 16; 3Q, '02, 15

V67.1 **Following radiotherapy**
V67.2 **Following chemotherapy**
Cancer chemotherapy follow-up
V67.3 **Following psychotherapy and other**
treatment for mental disorder
V67.4 **Following treatment of healed fracture**
EXCLUDES   *current (healing) fracture aftercare*
(V54.0-V54.9)
AHA: 1Q, '90, 7

√5ᵗʰ **V67.5** **Following other treatment**
V67.51 **Following completed treatment with**
high-risk medications, not elsewhere
classified
EXCLUDES   *long-term (current) drug use*
(V58.61-V58.69)
AHA: 1Q, '99, 5, 6; 4Q, '95, 61 ; 1Q, '90, 18

V67.59 **Other**

V67.6 **Following combined treatment**
V67.9 **Unspecified follow-up examination**

√4ᵗʰ **V68 Encounters for administrative purposes**

V68.0 **Issue of medical certificates**   `PDx`
Issue of medical certificate of:
cause of death
fitness
incapacity
EXCLUDES   *encounter for general medical*
examination (V70.0-V70.9)

V68.1 **Issue of repeat prescriptions**   `PDx`
Issue of repeat prescription for:
appliance
glasses
medications
EXCLUDES   *repeat prescription for contraceptives*
(V25.41-V25.49)

V68.2 **Request for expert evidence**   `PDx`

√5ᵗʰ **V68.8** **Other specified administrative purpose**
V68.81 **Referral of patient without**   `PDx`
examination or treatment
V68.89 **Other**   `PDx`

V68.9 **Unspecified administrative purpose**   `PDx`

√4ᵗʰ **V69 Problems related to lifestyle**
AHA: 4Q, '94, 48

V69.0 **Lack of physical exercise**
V69.1 **Inappropriate diet and eating habits**
EXCLUDES   *anorexia nervosa (307.1)*
bulimia (783.6)
malnutrition and other nutritional
deficiencies (260-269.9)
other and unspecified eating disorders
(307.50-307.59)

V69.2 **High-risk sexual behavior**
V69.3 **Gambling and betting**
EXCLUDES   *pathological gambling (312.31)*
V69.4 **Lack of adequate sleep**
Sleep deprivation
EXCLUDES   *insomnia (780.52)*
V69.8 **Other problems related to lifestyle**
Self-damaging behavior
V69.9 **Problem related to lifestyle, unspecified**

PERSONS WITHOUT REPORTED DIAGNOSIS ENCOUNTERED DURING EXAMINATION AND INVESTIGATION OF INDIVIDUALS AND POPULATIONS ▶(V70-V84)◀

Note: Nonspecific abnormal findings disclosed at the time of
these examinations are classifiable to categories 790-
796.

√4ᵗʰ **V70 General medical examination**
Use additional code(s) to identify any special screening
examination(s) performed (V73.0-V82.9)

V70.0 **Routine general medical examination at a**   `PDx`
health care facility
Health checkup
EXCLUDES   *health checkup of infant or child*
(V20.2)

V70.1 **General psychiatric examination, requested**   `PDx`
by the authority
V70.2 **General psychiatric examination,**   `PDx`
other and unspecified

√4ᵗʰ Additional Digit Required   Unspecified Code   Other Specified Code   Manifestation Code   ▶◀ Revised Text   ● New Code   ▲ Revised Code Title

V Codes

V70.3–V72.41

V70.3 **Other medical examination for administrative purposes** `PDx`

General medical examination for:
   admission to old age home
   adoption
   camp
   driving license
   immigration and naturalization
   insurance certification
   marriage
   prison
   school admission
   sports competition

   EXCLUDES *attendance for issue of medical certificates (V68.0)*
   pre-employment screening (V70.5)

   AHA: 1Q, '90, 6

V70.4 **Examination for medicolegal reasons** `PDx`
   Blood-alcohol tests
   Blood-drug tests
   Paternity testing

   EXCLUDES *examination and observation following:*
   accidents (V71.3, V71.4)
   assault (V71.6)
   rape (V71.5)

V70.5 **Health examination of defined subpopulations** `PDx`
   Armed forces personnel   Prisoners
   Inhabitants of institutions   Prostitutes
   Occupational health   Refugees
     examinations   School children
   Pre-employment screening   Students
   Preschool children

V70.6 **Health examination in population surveys** `PDx`
   EXCLUDES *special screening (V73.0-V82.9)*

V70.7 **Examination of participant in clinical trial**
   Examination of participant or control in clinical research

   AHA: 4Q, '01, 55

V70.8 **Other specified general medical examinations** `PDx`
   Examination of potential donor of organ or tissue

V70.9 **Unspecified general medical examination** `PDx`

√4ᵗʰ **V71** **Observation and evaluation for suspected conditions not found**

   INCLUDES This category is to be used when persons without a diagnosis are suspected of having an abnormal condition, without signs or symptoms, which requires study, but after examination and observation, is found not to exist. This category is also for use for administrative and legal observation status.

   AHA: 4Q, '94, 47; 2Q, '90, 5; M-A, '87, 1

√5ᵗʰ **V71.0** **Observation for suspected mental condition**

   V71.01 **Adult antisocial behavior** `A` `PDx`
     Dyssocial behavior or gang activity in adult without manifest psychiatric disorder

   V71.02 **Childhood or adolescent antisocial behavior** `PDx`
     Dyssocial behavior or gang activity in child or adolescent without manifest psychiatric disorder

   V71.09 **Other suspected mental condition** `PDx`

V71.1 **Observation for suspected malignant neoplasm** `PDx`

V71.2 **Observation for suspected tuberculosis** `PDx`

V71.3 **Observation following accident at work** `PDx`

V71.4 **Observation following other accident** `PDx`
   Examination of individual involved in motor vehicle traffic accident

V71.5 **Observation following alleged rape or seduction** `PDx`
   Examination of victim or culprit

V71.6 **Observation following other inflicted injury** `PDx`
   Examination of victim or culprit

V71.7 **Observation for suspected cardiovascular disease** `PDx`
   AHA: 1Q, '04, 6; 3Q, '90, 10; S-O, '87, 10

√5ᵗʰ **V71.8** **Observation and evaluation for other specified suspected conditions**
   AHA: 4Q, '00, 54 ; 1Q, '90, 19

   V71.81 **Abuse and neglect** `PDx`
     EXCLUDES *adult abuse and neglect (995.80-995.85)*
     child abuse and neglect (995.50-995.59)
     AHA: 4Q, '00, 55

   V71.82 **Observation and evaluation for suspected exposure to anthrax** `PDx`
     AHA: 4Q, '02, 70, 85

   V71.83 **Observation and evaluation for suspected exposure to other biological agent** `PDx`
     AHA: 4Q, '03, 47

   V71.89 **Other specified suspected conditions** `PDx`
     AHA: 2Q, '03, 15

V71.9 **Observation for unspecified suspected condition** `PDx`
   AHA: 1Q, '02, 6

√4ᵗʰ **V72** **Special investigations and examinations**
   INCLUDES routine examination of specific system
   EXCLUDES *general medical examination (V70.0-V70.4)*
   general screening examination of defined population groups (V70.5, V70.6, V70.7)
   routine examination of infant or child (V20.2)
   Use additional code(s) to identify any special screening examination(s) performed (V73.0-V82.9)

V72.0 **Examination of eyes and vision** `PDx`
   AHA: 1Q, '04, 15

V72.1 **Examination of ears and hearing** `PDx`
   AHA: 1Q, '04, 15

V72.2 **Dental examination** `PDx`

√5ᵗʰ **V72.3** **Gynecological examination**
   EXCLUDES *cervical Papanicolaou smear without general gynecological examination (V76.2)*
   routine examination in contraceptive management (V25.40-V25.49)

   V72.31 **Routine gynecological examination** `PDx` ♀
     General gynecological examination with or without Papanicolaou cervical smear
     Pelvic examination (annual) (periodic)
     Use additional code to identify routine vaginal Papanicolaou smear (V76.47)

   V72.32 **Encounter for Papanicolaou cervical smear to confirm findings of recent normal smear following initial abnormal smear** `PDx` ♀

√5ᵗʰ **V72.4** **Pregnancy examination or test**
   EXCLUDES *pregnancy examination with immediate confirmation (V22.0-V22.1)*

   V72.40 **Pregnancy examination or test, pregnancy unconfirmed** `PDx` ♀
     Possible pregnancy, not (yet) confirmed

   V72.41 **Pregnancy examination or test, negative result** `PDx` ♀

`N` Newborn Age: 0   `P` Pediatric Age: 0-17   `M` Maternity Age: 12-55   `A` Adult Age: 15-124   `MSP` Medicare Secondary Payer

302 — Volume 1 • October 2004   `SDx` Secondary Diagnosis   `PDx` Primary Diagnosis   **2005 ICD•9•CM**

V72.5 Radiological examination, not elsewhere classified `SDx`
Routine chest x-ray
`EXCLUDES` examination for suspected tuberculosis (V71.2)
AHA: 1Q, '90, 19

V72.6 Laboratory examination `SDx`
`EXCLUDES` that for suspected disorder (V71.0-V71.9)
AHA: 1Q, '90, 22

V72.7 Diagnostic skin and sensitization tests `PDx`
Allergy tests   Skin tests for hypersensitivity
`EXCLUDES` diagnostic skin tests for bacterial diseases (V74.0-V74.9)

V72.8 Other specified examinations
V72.81 Pre-operative cardiovascular examination `PDx`
V72.82 Pre-operative respiratory examination `PDx`
AHA: 3Q, '96, 14
V72.83 Other specified pre-operative examination `PDx`
AHA: 3Q, '96, 14
V72.84 Pre-operative examination, unspecified `PDx`
V72.85 Other specified examination `PDx`
AHA: 1Q, '04, 12

V72.9 Unspecified examination `PDx`

V73 Special screening examination for viral and chlamydial diseases
AHA: 1Q, '04, 11

V73.0 Poliomyelitis
V73.1 Smallpox
V73.2 Measles
V73.3 Rubella
V73.4 Yellow fever
V73.5 Other arthropod-borne viral diseases
Dengue fever   Viral encephalitis:
Hemorrhagic fever   mosquito-borne
   tick-borne
V73.6 Trachoma
V73.8 Other specified viral and chlamydial diseases
V73.88 Other specified chlamydial diseases
V73.89 Other specified viral diseases
V73.9 Unspecified viral and chlamydial disease
V73.98 Unspecified chlamydial disease
V73.99 Unspecified viral disease

V74 Special screening examination for bacterial and spirochetal diseases
`INCLUDES` diagnostic skin tests for these diseases
AHA: 1Q, '04, 11

V74.0 Cholera
V74.1 Pulmonary tuberculosis
V74.2 Leprosy [Hansen's disease]
V74.3 Diphtheria
V74.4 Bacterial conjunctivitis
V74.5 Venereal disease
V74.6 Yaws
V74.8 Other specified bacterial and spirochetal diseases
Brucellosis   Tetanus
Leptospirosis   Whooping cough
Plague
V74.9 Unspecified bacterial and spirochetal disease

V75 Special screening examination for other infectious diseases
AHA: 1Q, '04, 11

V75.0 Rickettsial diseases
V75.1 Malaria
V75.2 Leishmaniasis
V75.3 Trypanosomiasis
Chagas' disease
Sleeping sickness
V75.4 Mycotic infections
V75.5 Schistosomiasis
V75.6 Filariasis
V75.7 Intestinal helminthiasis
V75.8 Other specified parasitic infections
V75.9 Unspecified infectious disease

V76 Special screening for malignant neoplasms
AHA: 1Q, '04, 11

V76.0 Respiratory organs
V76.1 Breast
AHA: 4Q, '98, 67
V76.10 Breast screening, unspecified
V76.11 Screening mammogram for high-risk patient ♀
AHA: 2Q, '03, 4
V76.12 Other screening mammogram
AHA: 2Q, '03, 3-4
V76.19 Other screening breast examination
V76.2 Cervix ♀
Routine cervical Papanicolaou smear
`EXCLUDES` that as part of a general gynecological examination ▶(V72.31)◀
V76.3 Bladder
V76.4 Other sites
V76.41 Rectum
V76.42 Oral cavity
V76.43 Skin
V76.44 Prostate ♂
V76.45 Testis ♂
V76.46 Ovary ♀
AHA: 4Q, '00, 52
V76.47 Vagina ♀
Vaginal pap smear status-post hysterectomy for non-malignant condition
Use additional code to identify acquired absence of uterus (V45.77)
`EXCLUDES` vaginal pap smear status-post hysterectomy for malignant condition (V67.01)
AHA: 4Q, '00, 52
V76.49 Other sites
AHA: 1Q, '99, 4
V76.5 Intestine
AHA: 4Q, '00, 52
V76.50 Intestine, unspecified
V76.51 Colon
`EXCLUDES` rectum (V76.41)
AHA: 4Q, '01, 56
V76.52 Small intestine
V76.8 Other neoplasm
AHA: 4Q, '00, 52
V76.81 Nervous system
V76.89 Other neoplasm
V76.9 Unspecified

✓4ᵗʰ/✓5ᵗʰ Additional Digit Required   Unspecified Code   Other Specified Code   Manifestation Code   ▶◀ Revised Text   ● New Code   ▲ Revised Code Title

2005 ICD•9•CM   October 2004 • Volume 1 — 303

✓4ᵗʰ **V77 Special screening for endocrine, nutritional, metabolic, and immunity disorders**
AHA: 1Q, '04, 11

V77.0 **Thyroid disorders**
V77.1 **Diabetes mellitus**
V77.2 **Malnutrition**
V77.3 **Phenylketonuria [PKU]**
V77.4 **Galactosemia**
V77.5 **Gout**
V77.6 **Cystic fibrosis**
    Screening for mucoviscidosis
V77.7 **Other inborn errors of metabolism**
V77.8 **Obesity**
✓5ᵗʰ V77.9 **Other and unspecified endocrine, nutritional, metabolic, and immunity disorders**
AHA: 4Q, '00, 53

V77.91 **Screening for lipoid disorders**
    Screening cholesterol level
    Screening for hypercholesterolemia
    Screening for hyperlipidemia
V77.99 **Other and unspecified endocrine, nutritional, metabolic, and immunity disorders**

✓4ᵗʰ **V78 Special screening for disorders of blood and blood-forming organs**
AHA: 1Q, '04, 11

V78.0 **Iron deficiency anemia**
V78.1 **Other and unspecified deficiency anemia**
V78.2 **Sickle cell disease or trait**
V78.3 **Other hemoglobinopathies**
V78.8 **Other disorders of blood and blood-forming organs**
V78.9 **Unspecified disorder of blood and blood-forming organs**

✓4ᵗʰ **V79 Special screening for mental disorders and developmental handicaps**
AHA: 1Q, '04, 11

V79.0 **Depression**
V79.1 **Alcoholism**
V79.2 **Mental retardation**
V79.3 **Developmental handicaps in early childhood**
V79.8 **Other specified mental disorders and developmental handicaps**
V79.9 **Unspecified mental disorder and developmental handicap**

✓4ᵗʰ **V80 Special screening for neurological, eye, and ear diseases**
AHA: 1Q, '04, 11

V80.0 **Neurological conditions**
V80.1 **Glaucoma**
V80.2 **Other eye conditions**
    Screening for:
      cataract
      congenital anomaly of eye
      senile macular lesions
    EXCLUDES *general vision examination (V72.0)*
V80.3 **Ear diseases**
    EXCLUDES *general hearing examination (V72.1)*

✓4ᵗʰ **V81 Special screening for cardiovascular, respiratory, and genitourinary diseases**
AHA: 1Q, '04, 11

V81.0 **Ischemic heart disease**
V81.1 **Hypertension**
V81.2 **Other and unspecified cardiovascular conditions**
V81.3 **Chronic bronchitis and emphysema**

V81.4 **Other and unspecified respiratory conditions**
    EXCLUDES *screening for:*
      lung neoplasm (V76.0)
      pulmonary tuberculosis (V74.1)
V81.5 **Nephropathy**
    Screening for asymptomatic bacteriuria
V81.6 **Other and unspecified genitourinary conditions**

✓4ᵗʰ **V82 Special screening for other conditions**
AHA: 1Q, '04, 11

V82.0 **Skin conditions**
V82.1 **Rheumatoid arthritis**
V82.2 **Other rheumatic disorders**
V82.3 **Congenital dislocation of hip**
V82.4 **Maternal postnatal screening for chromosomal anomalies** ♀
    EXCLUDES *antenatal screening by amniocentesis (V28.0)*
V82.5 **Chemical poisoning and other contamination**
    Screening for:
      heavy metal poisoning
      ingestion of radioactive substance
      poisoning from contaminated water supply
      radiation exposure
V82.6 **Multiphasic screening**
✓5ᵗʰ V82.8 **Other specified conditions**
AHA: 4Q, '00, 53

V82.81 **Osteoporosis**
    Use additional code to identify:
    ►hormone replacement therapy (postmenopausal) status (V07.4)◄
      postmenopausal (age-related) (natural) status (V49.81)
    AHA: 4Q, '00, 54
V82.89 **Other specified conditions**
V82.9 **Unspecified condition**

✓4ᵗʰ **V83 Genetic carrier status**
AHA: 4Q, '02, 79; 4Q, '01, 54

✓5ᵗʰ V83.0 **Hemophilia A carrier**
V83.01 **Asymptomatic hemophilia A carrier**
V83.02 **Symptomatic hemophilia A carrier**
✓5ᵗʰ V83.8 **Other genetic carrier status**
V83.81 **Cystic fibrosis gene carrier**
V83.89 **Other genetic carrier status**

● ✓4ᵗʰ **V84 Genetic susceptibility to disease**
    INCLUDES confirmed abnormal gene
    Use additional code, if applicable, for any associated family history of the disease (V16-V19)

● ✓5ᵗʰ V84.0 **Genetic susceptibility to malignant neoplasm**
    Code first, if applicable, any current malignant neoplasms (140.0-195.8, 200.0-208.9, 230.0-234.9)
    Use additional code, if applicable, for any personal history of malignant neoplasm (V10.0-V10.9)
● V84.01 **Genetic susceptibility to malignant neoplasm of breast**
● V84.02 **Genetic susceptibility to malignant neoplasm of ovary**
● V84.03 **Genetic susceptibility to malignant neoplasm of prostate**
● V84.04 **Genetic susceptibility to malignant neoplasm of endometrium**
● V84.09 **Genetic susceptibility to other malignant neoplasm**
● V84.8 **Genetic susceptibility to other disease**

Ⓝ Newborn Age: 0   Ⓟ Pediatric Age: 0-17   Ⓜ Maternity Age: 12-55   Ⓐ Adult Age: 15-124   MSP Medicare Secondary Payer

SUPPLEMENTARY CLASSIFICATION OF EXTERNAL CAUSES OF INJURY AND POISONING (E800-E999)

This section is provided to permit the classification of environmental events, circumstances, and conditions as the cause of injury, poisoning, and other adverse effects. Where a code from this section is applicable, it is intended that it shall be used in addition to a code from one of the main chapters of ICD-9-CM, indicating the nature of the condition. Certain other conditions which may be stated to be due to external causes are classified in Chapters 1 to 16 of ICD-9-CM. For these, the "E" code classification should be used as an additional code for more detailed analysis.

Machinery accidents [other than those connected with transport] are classifiable to category E919, in which the fourth-digit allows a broad classification of the type of machinery involved. If a more detailed classification of type of machinery is required, it is suggested that the "Classification of Industrial Accidents according to Agency," prepared by the International Labor Office, be used in addition. This is reproduced in Appendix D for optional use.

Categories for "late effects" of accidents and other external causes are to be found at E929, E959, E969, E977, E989, and E999.

DEFINITIONS AND EXAMPLES RELATED TO TRANSPORT ACCIDENTS

(a) A **transport accident** (E800-E848) is any accident involving a device designed primarily for, or being used at the time primarily for, conveying persons or goods from one place to another.

> INCLUDES   accidents involving:
> aircraft and spacecraft (E840-E845)
> watercraft (E830-E838)
> motor vehicle (E810-E825)
> railway (E800-E807)
> other road vehicles (E826-E829)

In classifying accidents which involve more than one kind of transport, the above order of precedence of transport accidents should be used.

Accidents involving agricultural and construction machines, such as tractors, cranes, and bulldozers, are regarded as transport accidents only when these vehicles are under their own power on a highway [otherwise the vehicles are regarded as machinery]. Vehicles which can travel on land or water, such as hovercraft and other amphibious vehicles, are regarded as watercraft when on the water, as motor vehicles when on the highway, and as off-road motor vehicles when on land, but off the highway.

> EXCLUDES   accidents:
> *in sports which involve the use of transport but where the transport vehicle itself was not involved in the accident*
> *involving vehicles which are part of industrial equipment used entirely on industrial premises*
> *occurring during transportation but unrelated to the hazards associated with the means of transportation [e.g., injuries received in a fight on board ship; transport vehicle involved in a cataclysm such as an earthquake]*
> *to persons engaged in the maintenance or repair of transport equipment or vehicle not in motion, unlesss injured by another vehicle in motion*

(b) A **railway accident** is a transport accident involving a railway train or other railway vehicle operated on rails, whether in motion or not.

> EXCLUDES   accidents:
> *in repair shops*
> *in roundhouse or on turntable*
> *on railway premises but not involving a train or other railway vehicle*

(c) A **railway train** or **railway vehicle** is any device with or without cars coupled to it, desiged for traffic on a railway.

> INCLUDES   interurban:
> electric car ⎫ (operated chiefly on its
> streetcar ⎬   own right-of-way,
>   ⎭   not open to other
>   traffic)
>
> railway train, any power [diesel] [electric] [steam]
> funicular
> monorail or two-rail
> subterranean or elevated
> other vehicle designed to run on a railway track

> EXCLUDES   *interurban electric cars [streetcars] specified to be operating on a right-of-way that forms part of the public street or highway [definition (n)]*

(d) A **railway** or **railroad** is a right-of-way designed for traffic on rails, which is used by carriages or wagons transporting passengers or freight, and by other rolling stock, and which is not open to other public vehicular traffic.

(e) A **motor vehicle accident** is a transport accident involving a motor vehicle. It is defined as a motor vehicle traffic accident or as a motor vehicle nontraffic accident according to whether the accident occurs on a public highway or elsewhere.

> EXCLUDES   *injury or damage due to cataclysm*
> *injury or damage while a motor vehicle, not under its own power, is being loaded on, or unloaded from, another conveyance*

(f) A **motor vehicle traffic accident** is any motor vehicle accident occurring on a public highway [i.e., originating, terminating, or involving a vehicle partially on the highway]. A motor vehicle accident is assumed to have occurred on the highway unless another place is specified, except in the case of accidents involving only off-road motor vehicles which are classified as nontraffic accidents unless the contrary is stated.

(g) A **motor vehicle nontraffic accident** is any motor vehicle accident which occurs entirely in any place other than a public highway.

(h) A **public highway [trafficway]** or **street** is the entire width between property lines [or other boundary lines] of every way or place, of which any part is open to the use of the public for purposes of vehicular traffic as a matter of right or custom. A **roadway** is that part of the public highway designed, improved, and ordinarily used, for vehicular travel.

> INCLUDES   approaches (public) to:
> docks
> public building
> station

> EXCLUDES   *driveway (private)*
> *parking lot*
> *ramp*
> *roads in:*
> *airfield*
> *farm*
> *industrial premises*
> *mine*
> *private grounds*
> *quarry*

☑4ᵗʰ Fourth-digit Required   ▶◀ Revised Text   ● New Code   ▲ Revised Code Title

(i) A **motor vehicle** is any mechanically or electrically powered device, not operated on rails, upon which any person or property may be transported or drawn upon a highway. Any object such as a trailer, coaster, sled, or wagon being towed by a motor vehicle is considerd a part of the motor vehicle.

INCLUDES	automobile [any type]
	bus
	construction machinery, farm and industrial machinery, steam roller, tractor, army tank, highway grader, or similar vehicle on wheels or treads, while in transport under own power
	fire engine (motorized)
	motorcycle
	motorized bicycle [moped] or scooter
	trolley bus not operating on rails
	truck
	van

EXCLUDES *devices used solely to move persons or materials within the confines of a building and its premises, such as:*
building elevator
coal car in mine
electric baggage or mail truck used solely within a railroad station
electric truck used solely within an industrial plant
moving overhead crane

(j) A **motorcycle** is a two-wheeled motor vehicle having one or two riding saddles and sometimes having a third wheel for the support of a sidecar. The sidecar is considered part of the motorcycle.

INCLUDES	motorized:
	bicycle [moped]
	scooter
	tricycle

(k) An **off-road motor vehicle** is a motor vehicle of special design, to enable it to negotiate rough or soft terrain or snow. Examples of special design are high construction, special wheels and tires, driven by treads, or support on a cushion of air.

INCLUDES	all terrain vehicle [ATV]
	army tank
	hovercraft, on land or swamp
	snowmobile

(l) A **driver** of a motor vehicle is the occupant of the motor vehicle operating it or intending to operate it. A **motorcyclist** is the driver of a motorcycle. Other authorized occupants of a motor vehicle are **passengers**.

(m) An **other road vehicle** is any device, except a motor vehicle, in, on, or by which any person or property may be transported on a highway.

INCLUDES	animal carrying a person or goods
	animal-drawn vehicles
	animal harnessed to conveyance
	bicycle [pedal cycle]
	streetcar
	tricycle (pedal)

EXCLUDES *pedestrian conveyance [definition (q)]*

(n) A **streetcar** is a device designed and used primarily for transporting persons within a municipality, running on rails, usually subject to normal traffic control signals, and operated principally on a right-of-way that forms part of the traffic way. A trailer being towed by a streetcar is considered a part of the streetcar.

INCLUDES	interurban or intraurban electric or streetcar, when specified to be operating on a street or public highway
	tram (car)
	trolley (car)

(o) A **pedal cycle** is any road transport vehicle operated solely by pedals.

INCLUDES	bicycle
	pedal cycle
	tricycle

EXCLUDES *motorized bicycle [definition (i)]*

(p) A **pedal cyclist** is any person riding on a pedal cycle or in a sidecar attached to such a vehicle.

(q) A **pedestrian conveyance** is any human powered device by which a pedestrian may move other than by walking or by which a walking person may move another pedestrian.

INCLUDES	baby carriage
	coaster wagon
	ice skates
	perambulator
	pushcart
	pushchair
	roller skates
	scooter
	skateboard
	skis
	sled
	wheelchair

(r) A **pedestrian** is any person involved in an accident who was not at the time of the accident riding in or on a motor vehicle, railroad train, streetcar, animal-drawn or other vehicle, or on a bicycle or animal.

INCLUDES	person:
	changing tire of vehicle
	in or operating a pedestrian conveyance
	making adjustment to motor of vehicle
	on foot

(s) A **watercraft** is any device for transporting passengers or goods on the water.

(t) A **small boat** is any watercraft propelled by paddle, oars, or small motor, with a passenger capacity of less than ten.

INCLUDES	boat NOS
	canoe
	coble
	dinghy
	punt
	raft
	rowboat
	rowing shell
	scull
	skiff
	small motorboat

EXCLUDES *barge*
lifeboat (used after abandoning ship)
raft (anchored) being used as a diving platform
yacht

(u) An **aircraft** is any device for transporting passengers or goods in the air.

INCLUDES	airplane [any type]
	balloon
	bomber
	dirigible
	glider (hang)
	military aircraft
	parachute

(v) A **commercial transport aircraft** is any device for collective passenger or freight transportation by air, whether run on commercial lines for profit or by government authorities, with the exception of military craft.

RAILWAY ACCIDENTS (E800-E807)

Note: For definitions of railway accident and related terms see definitions (a) to (d).

EXCLUDES *accidents involving railway train and:*
aircraft (E840.0-E845.9)
motor vehicle (E810.0-E825.9)
watercraft (E830.0-E838.9)

The following fourth-digit subdivisions are for use with categories E800-E807 to identify the injured person:

.0 Railway employee
Any person who by virtue of his employment in connection with a railway, whether by the railway company or not, is at increased risk of involvement in a railway accident, such as:
catering staff of train
driver
guard
porter
postal staff on train
railway fireman
shunter
sleeping car attendant

.1 Passenger on railway
Any authorized person traveling on a train, except a railway employee.

    EXCLUDES *intending passenger waiting at station (.8)*
unauthorized rider on railway vehicle (.8)

.2 Pedestrian
See definition (r)

.3 Pedal cyclist
See definition (p)

.8 Other specified person
Intending passenger or bystander waiting at station
Unauthorized rider on railway vehicle

.9 Unspecified person

√4ᵗʰ E800 Railway accident involving collision with rolling stock
    INCLUDES   collision between railway trains or railway vehicles, any kind
collision NOS on railway
derailment with antecedent collision with rolling stock or NOS

√4ᵗʰ E801 Railway accident involving collision with other object
    INCLUDES   collision of railway train with:
buffers
fallen tree on railway
gates
platform
rock on railway
streetcar
other nonmotor vehicle
other object

    EXCLUDES *collision with:*
aircraft (E840.0-E842.9)
motor vehicle (E810.0-E810.9, E820.0-E822.9)

√4ᵗʰ E802 Railway accident involving derailment without antecedent collision

√4ᵗʰ E803 Railway accident involving explosion, fire, or burning
    EXCLUDES *explosion or fire, with antecedent derailment (E802.0-E802.9)*
explosion or fire, with mention of antecedent collision (E800.0-E801.9)

√4ᵗʰ E804 Fall in, on, or from railway train
    INCLUDES   fall while alighting from or boarding railway train
    EXCLUDES *fall related to collision, derailment, or explosion of railway train (E800.0-E803.9)*

√4ᵗʰ E805 Hit by rolling stock
    INCLUDES   crushed
injured
killed   } by railway train or part
knocked down
run over

    EXCLUDES *pedestrian hit by object set in motion by railway train (E806.0-E806.9)*

√4ᵗʰ E806 Other specified railway accident
    INCLUDES   hit by object falling in railway train
injured by door or window on railway train
nonmotor road vehicle or pedestrian hit by object set in motion by railway train
railway train hit by falling:
earth NOS
rock
tree
other object

    EXCLUDES *railway accident due to cataclysm (E908-E909)*

√4ᵗʰ E807 Railway accident of unspecified nature
    INCLUDES   found dead } on railway right-of-way
injured   } NOS

    railway accident NOS

MOTOR VEHICLE TRAFFIC ACCIDENTS (E810-E819)

Note: For definitions of motor vehicle traffic accident, and related terms, see definitions (e) to (k).

EXCLUDES *accidents involving motor vehicle and aircraft (E840.0-E845.9)*

The following fourth-digit subdivisions are for use with categories E810-E819 to identify the injured person:

.0 Driver of motor vehicle other than motorcycle
See definition (1)

.1 Passenger in motor vehicle other than motorcycle
See definition (1)

.2 Motorcyclist
See definition (1)

.3 Passenger on motorcycle
See definition (1)

.4 Occupant of streetcar

.5 Rider of animal; occupant of animal-drawn vehicle

.6 Pedal cyclist
See definition (p)

.7 Pedestrian
See definition (r)

.8 Other specified person
Occupant of vehicle other than above
Person in railway train involved in accident
Unauthorized rider of motor vehicle

.9 Unspecified person

√4ᵗʰ E810 Motor vehicle traffic accident involving collision with train
    EXCLUDES *motor vehicle collision with object set in motion by railway train (E815.0-E815.9)*
railway train hit by object set in motion by motor vehicle (E818.0-E818.9)

√4ᵗʰ E811 Motor vehicle traffic accident involving re-entrant collision with another motor vehicle
    INCLUDES   collision between motor vehicle which accidentally leaves the roadway then re-enters the same roadway, or the opposite roadway on a divided highway, and another motor vehicle

    EXCLUDES *collision on the same roadway when none of the motor vehicles involved have left and re-entered the highway (E812.0-E812.9)*

√4ᵗʰ Fourth-digit Required   ▶◀ Revised Text   ● New Code   ▲ Revised Code Title

E Codes

E812–E819

§ ✓4ᵗʰ **E812 Other motor vehicle traffic accident involving collision with motor vehicle**

INCLUDES   collision with another motor vehicle parked, stopped, stalled, disabled, or abandoned on the highway
motor vehicle collision NOS

EXCLUDES   *collision with object set in motion by another motor vehicle (E815.0-E815.9)*
re-entrant collision with another motor vehicle (E811.0-E811.9)

§ ✓4ᵗʰ **E813 Motor vehicle traffic accident involving collision with other vehicle**

INCLUDES   collision between motor vehicle, any kind, and:
other road (nonmotor transport) vehicle, such as:
   animal carrying a person
   animal-drawn vehicle
   pedal cycle
   streetcar

EXCLUDES   *collision with:*
object set in motion by nonmotor road vehicle (E815.0-E815.9)
pedestrian (E814.0-E814.9)
nonmotor road vehicle hit by object set in motion by motor vehicle (E818.0-E818.9)

§ ✓4ᵗʰ **E814 Motor vehicle traffic accident involving collision with pedestrian**

INCLUDES   collision between motor vehicle, any kind, and pedestrian
pedestrian dragged, hit, or run over by motor vehicle, any kind

EXCLUDES   *pedestrian hit by object set in motion by motor vehicle (E818.0-E818.9)*

§ ✓4ᵗʰ **E815 Other motor vehicle traffic accident involving collision on the highway**

INCLUDES   collision (due to loss of control) (on highway) between motor vehicle, any kind, and:
   abutment (bridge) (overpass)
   animal (herded) (unattended)
   fallen stone, traffic sign, tree, utility pole
   guard rail or boundary fence
   interhighway divider
   landslide (not moving)
   object set in motion by railway train or road vehicle (motor) (nonmotor)
   object thrown in front of motor vehicle
   other object, fixed, movable, or moving
   safety island
   temporary traffic sign or marker
   wall of cut made for road

EXCLUDES   *collision with:*
any object off the highway (resulting from loss of control) (E816.0-E816.9)
any object which normally would have been off the highway and is not stated to have been on it (E816.0-E816.9)
motor vehicle parked, stopped, stalled, disabled, or abandoned on highway (E812.0-E812.9)
moving landslide (E909)
motor vehicle hit by object:
set in motion by railway train or road vehicle (motor) (nonmotor) (E818.0-E818.9)
thrown into or on vehicle (E818.0-E818.9)

§ ✓4ᵗʰ **E816 Motor vehicle traffic accident due to loss of control, without collision on the highway**

INCLUDES   motor vehicle:
   failing to make curve and:
   going out of control   colliding with
   (due to):   object off
   blowout   the high-
   burst tire   way
   driver falling   overturning
      asleep   stopping
   driver inattention abruptly
   excessive speed   off the
   failure of mech-   highway
      anical part

EXCLUDES   *collision on highway following loss of control (E810.0-E815.9)*
loss of control of motor vehicle following collision on the highway (E810.0-E815.9)

§ ✓4ᵗʰ **E817 Noncollision motor vehicle traffic accident while boarding or alighting**

INCLUDES   fall down stairs of motor
   bus
fall from car in street
injured by moving part while boarding
  of the vehicle   or alighting
trapped by door of
  motor bus

§ ✓4ᵗʰ **E818 Other noncollision motor vehicle traffic accident**

INCLUDES   accidental poisoning from exhaust gas generated by
breakage of any part of
explosion of any part of
fall, jump, or being
  accidentally pushed
  from   motor vehicle
fire starting in   while
hit by object thrown into or in
  on   motion
injured by being thrown
  against some part of, or
  object in
injury from moving part of
object falling in or on
object thrown on

collision of railway train or road vehicle except motor vehicle, with object set in motion by motor vehicle
motor vehicle hit by object set in motion by railway train or road vehicle (motor) (nonmotor)
pedestrian, railway train, or road vehicle (motor) (nonmotor) hit by object set in motion by motor vehicle

EXCLUDES   *collision between motor vehicle and:*
object set in motion by railway train or road vehicle (motor) (nonmotor) (E815.0-E815.9)
object thrown towards the motor vehicle (E815.0-E815.9)
person overcome by carbon monoxide generated by stationary motor vehicle off the roadway with motor running (E868.2)

§ ✓4ᵗʰ **E819 Motor vehicle traffic accident of unspecified nature**

INCLUDES   motor vehicle traffic accident NOS
traffic accident NOS

§ Requires fourth-digit. See beginning of section E810-E819 for codes and definitions.

✓4ᵗʰ Fourth-digit Required   ►◄ Revised Text   ● New Code   ▲ Revised Code Title

MOTOR VEHICLE NONTRAFFIC ACCIDENTS (E820-E825)

Note: For definitions of motor vehicle nontraffic accident and related terms see definition (a) to (k).

INCLUDES   accidents involving motor vehicles being used in recreational or sporting activities off the highway

collision and noncollision motor vehicle accidents occurring entirely off the highway

EXCLUDES   *accidents involving motor vehicle and:*
aircraft (E840.0-E845.9)
watercraft (E830.0-E838.9)
accidents, not on the public highway, involving agricultural and construction machinery but not involving another motor vehicle (E919.0, E919.2, E919.7)

The following fourth-digit subdivisions are for use with categories E820-E825 to identify the injured person:

.0 Driver of motor vehicle other than motorcycle
See definition (l)

.1 Passenger in motor vehicle other than motorcycle
See definition (l)

.2 Motorcyclist
See definition (l)

.3 Passenger on motorcycle
See definition (l)

.4 Occupant of streetcar

.5 Rider of animal; occupant of animal-drawn vehicle

.6 Pedal cyclist
See definition (p)

.7 Pedestrian
See definition (r)

.8 Other specified person
Occupant of vehicle other than above
Person on railway train involved in accident
Unauthorized rider of motor vehicle

.9 Unspecified person

✓4ᵗʰ **E820 Nontraffic accident involving motor-driven snow vehicle**

INCLUDES   breakage of part of | motor-driven
fall from | snow
hit by | vehicle (not
overturning of | on public
run over or dragged by | highway)

collision of motor-driven snow vehicle with:
animal (being ridden) (-drawn vehicle)
another off-road motor vehicle
other motor vehicle, not on public highway
railway train
other object, fixed or movable
injury caused by rough landing of motor-driven snow vehicle (after leaving ground on rough terrain)

EXCLUDES   *accident on the public highway involving motor driven snow vehicle (E810.0-E819.9)*

✓4ᵗʰ **E821 Nontraffic accident involving other off-road motor vehicle**

INCLUDES   breakage of part of | off-road motor
fall from | vehicle,
hit by | except snow
overturning of | vehicle (not
run over or dragged by | on public
thrown against some | highway)
part of or object in |

collision with:
animal (being ridden) (-drawn vehicle)
another off-road motor vehicle, except snow vehicle
other motor vehicle, not on public highway
other object, fixed or movable

EXCLUDES   *accident on public highway involving off-road motor vehicle (E810.0-E819.9)*
collision between motor driven snow vehicle and other off-road motor vehicle (E820.0-E820.9)
hovercraft accident on water (E830.0-E838.9)

✓4ᵗʰ **E822 Other motor vehicle nontraffic accident involving collision with moving object**

INCLUDES   collision, not on public highway, between motor vehicle, except off-road motor vehicle and:
animal
nonmotor vehicle
other motor vehicle, except off-road motor vehicle
pedestrian
railway train
other moving object

EXCLUDES   *collision with:*
motor-driven snow vehicle (E820.0-E820.9)
other off-road motor vehicle (E821.0-E821.9)

✓4ᵗʰ **E823 Other motor vehicle nontraffic accident involving collision with stationary object**

INCLUDES   collision, not on public highway, between motor vehicle, except off-road motor vehicle, and any object, fixed or movable, but not in motion

✓4ᵗʰ **E824 Other motor vehicle nontraffic accident while boarding and alighting**

INCLUDES   fall | while boarding or
injury from moving | alighting from
part of motor | motor vehicle,
vehicle | except off-road
trapped by door of | motor vehicle, not
motor vehicle | on public highway

---

§ ✓4ᵗʰ **E825 Other motor vehicle nontraffic accident of other and unspecified nature**

INCLUDES   accidental poisoning from carbon monoxide generated by

breakage of any part of

explosion of any part of

fall, jump, or being accidentally pushed from   } motor vehicle while in motion, not on public highway

fire starting in

hit by object thrown into, towards, or on

injured by being thrown against some part of, or object in

injury from moving part of

object falling in or on

motor vehicle nontraffic accident NOS

EXCLUDES   *fall from or in stationary motor vehicle (E884.9, E885.9)*

overcome by carbon monoxide or exhaust gas generated by stationary motor vehicle off the roadway with motor running (E868.2)

struck by falling object from or in stationary motor vehicle (E916)

OTHER ROAD VEHICLE ACCIDENTS (E826-E829)

Note: Other road vehicle accidents are transport accidents involving road vehicles other than motor vehicles. For definitions of other road vehicle and related terms see definitions (m) to (o).

INCLUDES   accidents involving other road vehicles being used in recreational or sporting activities

EXCLUDES   *collision of other road vehicle [any] with:*
aircraft (E840.0-E845.9)
motor vehicle (E813.0-E813.9, E820.0-E822.9)
railway train (E801.0-E801.9)

The following fourth-digit subdivisions are for use with categories E826-E829 to identify the injured person.

.0 Pedestrian
See definition (r)

.1 Pedal cyclist
See definition (p)

.2 Rider of animal

.3 Occupant of animal-drawn vehicle

.4 Occupant of streetcar

.8 Other specified person

.9 Unspecified person

✓4ᵗʰ **E826 Pedal cycle accident**

[0-9]   INCLUDES   breakage of any part of pedal cycle
collision between pedal cycle and:
animal (being ridden) (herded) (unattended)
another pedal cycle
any pedestrian
nonmotor road vehicle
other object, fixed, movable, or moving, not set in motion by motor vehicle, railway train, or aircraft
entanglement in wheel of pedal cycle
fall from pedal cycle
hit by object falling or thrown on the pedal cycle
pedal cycle accident NOS
pedal cycle overturned

✓4ᵗʰ **E827 Animal-drawn vehicle accident**

[0,2-4,8,9]   INCLUDES   breakage of any part of vehicle
collision between animal-drawn vehicle and:
animal (being ridden) (herded) (unattended)
nonmotor road vehicle, except pedal cycle
pedestrian, pedestrian conveyance, or pedestrian vehicle
other object, fixed, movable, or moving, not set in motion by motor vehicle, railway train, or aircraft

fall from
knocked down by
overturning of   } animal-drawn vehicle
run over by
thrown from

EXCLUDES   *collision of animal-drawn vehicle with pedal cycle (E826.0-E826.9)*

✓4ᵗʰ **E828 Accident involving animal being ridden**

[0,2,4,8,9]   INCLUDES   collision between animal being ridden and:
another animal
nonmotor road vehicle, except pedal cycle, and animal-drawn vehicle
pedestrian, pedestrian conveyance, or pedestrian vehicle
other object, fixed, movable, or moving, not set in motion by motor vehicle, railway train, or aircraft

fall from
knocked down by   } animal being ridden
thrown from
trampled by

ridden animal stumbled and fell

EXCLUDES   *collision of animal being ridden with:*
animal-drawn vehicle (E827.0-E827.9)
pedal cycle (E826.0-E826.9)

✓4ᵗʰ **E829 Other road vehicle accidents**

[0,4,8,9]   INCLUDES   accident while boarding or alighting from
blow from object in
breakage of any part of
caught in door of-
derailment of   } streetcar nonmotor road vehicle not classifiable to E826-E828
fall in, on, or from
fire in

collision between streetcar or nonmotor road vehicle, except as in E826-E828, and:
animal (not being ridden)
another nonmotor road vehicle not classifiable to E826-E828
pedestrian
other object, fixed, movable, or moving, not set in motion by motor vehicle, railway train, or aircraft
nonmotor road vehicle accident NOS
streetcar accident NOS

EXCLUDES   *collision with:*
animal being ridden (E828.0-E828.9)
animal-drawn vehicle (E827.0-E827.9)
pedal cycle (E826.0-E826.9)

---

§   Requires fourth-digit. Valid digits are in [brackets] under each code. See beginning of section E820-E825 for codes and definitions.

✓4ᵗʰ Fourth-digit Required   ◄► Revised Text   ● New Code   ▲ Revised Code Title

E Codes

E830–E838

WATER TRANSPORT ACCIDENTS (E830-E838)

Note: For definitions of water transport accident and related terms see definitions (a), (s), and (t).

INCLUDES　watercraft accidents in the course of recreational activities

EXCLUDES　*accidents involving both aircraft, including objects set in motion by aircraft, and watercraft (E840.0-E845.9)*

The following fourth-digit subdivisions are for use with categories E830-E838 to identify the injured person:

.0 Occupant of small boat, unpowered

.1 Occupant of small boat, powered

See definition (t)

EXCLUDES　*water skier (.4)*

.2 Occupant of other watercraft — crew

Persons:

engaged in operation of watercraft

providing passenger services [cabin attendants, ship's physician, catering personnel]

working on ship during voyage in other capacity [musician in band, operators of shops and beauty parlors]

.3 Occupant of other watercraft — other than crew

Passenger

Occupant of lifeboat, other than crew, after abandoning ship

.4 Water skier

.5 Swimmer

.6 Dockers, stevedores

Longshoreman employed on the dock in loading and unloading ships

.8 Other specified person

Immigration and custom officials on board ship

Person:

accompanying passenger or member of crew visiting boat

Pilot (guiding ship into port)

.9 Unspecified person

✓4ᵗʰ **E830 Accident to watercraft causing submersion**

INCLUDES　submersion and drowning due to:

boat overturning

boat submerging

falling or jumping from burning ship

falling or jumping from crushed watercraft

ship sinking

other accident to watercraft

✓4ᵗʰ **E831 Accident to watercraft causing other injury**

INCLUDES　any injury, except submersion and drowning, as a result of an accident to watercraft

burned while ship on fire

crushed between ships in collision

crushed by lifeboat after abandoning ship

fall due to collision or other accident to watercraft

hit by falling object due to accident to watercraft

injured in watercraft accident involving collision

struck by boat or part thereof after fall or jump from damaged boat

EXCLUDES　*burns from localized fire or explosion on board ship (E837.0-E837.9)*

✓4ᵗʰ **E832 Other accidental submersion or drowning in water transport accident**

INCLUDES　submersion or drowning as a result of an accident other than accident to the watercraft, such as:

fall:

from gangplank

from ship

overboard

thrown overboard by motion of ship

washed overboard

EXCLUDES　*submersion or drowning of swimmer or diver who voluntarily jumps from boat not involved in an accident (E910.0-E910.9)*

✓4ᵗʰ **E833 Fall on stairs or ladders in water transport**

EXCLUDES　*fall due to accident to watercraft (E831.0-E831.9)*

✓4ᵗʰ **E834 Other fall from one level to another in water transport**

EXCLUDES　*fall due to accident to watercraft (E831.0-E831.9)*

✓4ᵗʰ **E835 Other and unspecified fall in water transport**

EXCLUDES　*fall due to accident to watercraft (E831.0-E831.9)*

✓4ᵗʰ **E836 Machinery accident in water transport**

INCLUDES　injuries in water transport caused by:

deck

engine room

galley

laundry

loading

} machinery

✓4ᵗʰ **E837 Explosion, fire, or burning in watercraft**

INCLUDES　explosion of boiler on steamship

localized fire on ship

EXCLUDES　*burning ship (due to collision or explosion) resulting in:*

submersion or drowning (E830.0-E830.9)

other injury (E831.0-E831.9)

✓4ᵗʰ **E838 Other and unspecified water transport accident**

INCLUDES　accidental poisoning by gases or fumes on ship

atomic power plant malfunction in watercraft

crushed between ship and stationary object [wharf]

crushed between ships without accident to watercraft

crushed by falling object on ship or while loading or unloading

hit by boat while water skiing

struck by boat or part thereof (after fall from boat)

watercraft accident NOS

AIR AND SPACE TRANSPORT ACCIDENTS (E840-E845)

Note: For definition of aircraft and related terms see definitions (u) and (v).

The following fourth-digit subdivisions are for use with categories E840-E845 to identify the injured person. Valid fourth digits are in [brackets] under codes E842-E845.

.0 Occupant of spacecraft

.1 Occupant of military aircraft, any

Crew in military aircraft [air force] [army] [national guard] [navy]

Passenger (civilian) (military) in military aircraft [air force] [army] [national guard] [navy]

Troops in military aircraft [air force] [army] [national guard] [navy]

> **EXCLUDES** *occupants of aircraft operated under jurisdiction of police departments (.5)*
> *parachutist (.7)*

.2 Crew of commercial aircraft (powered) in surface to surface transport

.3 Other occupant of commercial aircraft (powered) in surface to surface transport

Flight personnel:
  not part of crew
  on familiarization flight
Passenger on aircraft (powered) NOS

.4 Occupant of commercial aircraft (powered) in surface to air transport

Occupant [crew] [passenger] of aircraft (powered) engaged in activities, such as:

  aerial spraying (crops) (fire retardants)
  air drops of emergency supplies
  air drops of parachutists, except from military craft
  crop dusting
  lowering of construction material [bridge or telephone pole]
  sky writing

.5 Occupant of other powered aircraft

Occupant [crew][passenger] of aircraft [powered] engaged in activities, such as:

  aerobatic flying
  aircraft racing
  rescue operation
  storm surveillance
  traffic surveillance
  Occupant of private plane NOS

.6 Occupant of unpowered aircraft, except parachutist

Occupant of aircraft classifiable to E842

.7 Parachutist (military) (other)

Person making voluntary descent

> **EXCLUDES** *person making descent after accident to aircraft (.1-.6)*

.8 Ground crew, airline employee

Persons employed at airfields (civil) (military) or launching pads, not occupants of aircraft

.9 Other person

✓4ᵗʰ E840 Accident to powered aircraft at takeoff or landing

INCLUDES	collision of aircraft with any object, fixed, movable, or moving	
	crash	while taking off or landing
	explosion on aircraft	
	fire on aircraft	
	forced landing	

✓4ᵗʰ E841 Accident to powered aircraft, other and unspecified

INCLUDES
aircraft accident NOS
aircraft crash or wreck NOS
any accident to powered aircraft while in transit or when not specified whether in transit, taking off, or landing
collision of aircraft with another aircraft, bird, or any object, while in transit
explosion on aircraft while in transit
fire on aircraft while in transit

✓4ᵗʰ E842 Accident to unpowered aircraft

[6-9]   **INCLUDES**
any accident, except collision with powered aircraft, to:
  balloon
  glider
  hang glider
  kite carrying a person
hit by object falling from unpowered aircraft

✓4ᵗʰ E843 Fall in, on, or from aircraft

[0-9]   **INCLUDES**
accident in boarding or alighting from aircraft, any kind
fall in, on, or from aircraft [any kind], while in transit, taking off, or landing, except when as a result of an accident to aircraft

✓4ᵗʰ E844 Other specified air transport accidents

[0-9]   **INCLUDES**
hit by:
  aircraft
  object falling from aircraft
injury by or from:
  machinery on aircraft
  rotating propeller
  voluntary parachute descent
poisoning by carbon monoxide from aircraft while in transit
} without accident to aircraft
sucked into jet
any accident involving other transport vehicle (motor) (nonmotor) due to being hit by object set in motion by aircraft (powered)

> **EXCLUDES** *air sickness (E903)*
> *effects of:*
> *high altitude (E902.0-E902.1)*
> *pressure change (E902.0-E902.1)*
> *injury in parachute descent due to accident to aircraft (E840.0-E842-9)*

✓4ᵗʰ E845 Accident involving spacecraft

[0,8,9]   **INCLUDES** launching pad accident
EXCLUDES *effects of weightlessness in spacecraft (E928.0)*

VEHICLE ACCIDENTS NOT ELSEWHERE CLASSIFIABLE (E846-E848)

E846 Accidents involving powered vehicles used solely within the buildings and premises of industrial or commercial establishment

Accident to, on, or involving:
    battery powered airport passenger vehicle
    battery powered trucks (baggage) (mail)
    coal car in mine
    logging car
    self propelled truck, industrial
    station baggage truck (powered)
    tram, truck, or tub (powered) in mine or quarry
Collision with:
    pedestrian
    other vehicle or object within premises

Explosion of ⎫
Fall from   ⎬ powered vehicle, industrial
Overturning of ⎪   or commercial
Struck by ⎭

EXCLUDES   accidental poisoning by exhaust gas from vehicle not elsewhere classifiable (E868.2)
          injury by crane, lift (fork), or elevator (E919.2)

E847 Accidents involving cable cars not running on rails

Accident to, on, or involving:
    cable car, not on rails
    ski chair-lift
    ski-lift with gondola
    téléférique
Breakage of cable

Caught or dragged by ⎫
Fall or jump from   ⎬ cable car, not on rails
Object thrown from or in ⎭

E848 Accidents involving other vehicles, not elsewhere classifiable

Accident to, on, or involving:
    ice yacht
    land yacht
    nonmotor, nonroad vehicle NOS

✓4th **E849 Place of occurrence**

The following category is for use to denote the place where the injury or poisoning occurred.

E849.0 Home

Apartment	Private:
Boarding house	garage
Farm house	garden
Home premises	home
House (residential)	walk
Noninstitutional	Swimming pool in private
place of residence	house or garden
Private:	Yard of home
driveway	

EXCLUDES   home under construction but not yet occupied (E849.3)
          institutional place of residence (E849.7)

E849.1 Farm

Farm:
    buildings
    land under cultivation

EXCLUDES   farm house and home premises of farm (E849.0)

E849.2 Mine and quarry

Gravel pit	Tunnel under
Sand pit	construction

E849.3 Industrial place and premises

Building under	Industrial yard
construction	Loading platform (factory)
Dockyard	(store)
Dry dock	Plant, industrial
Factory	Railway yard
building	Shop (place of work)
premises	Warehouse
Garage (place of work)	Workhouse

E849.4 Place for recreation and sport

Amusement park	Public park
Baseball field	Racecourse
Basketball court	Resort NOS
Beach resort	Riding school
Cricket ground	Rifle range
Fives court	Seashore resort
Football field	Skating rink
Golf course	Sports palace
Gymnasium	Stadium
Hockey field	Swimming pool, public
Holiday camp	Tennis court
Ice palace	Vacation resort
Lake resort	
Mountain resort	
Playground, including school playground	

EXCLUDES   that in private house or garden (E849.0)

E849.5 Street and highway

E849.6 Public building

Building (including adjacent grounds) used by the general public or by a particular group of the public, such as:

airport	music hall
bank	nightclub
café	office
casino	office building
church	opera house
cinema	post office
clubhouse	public hall
courthouse	radio broadcasting station
dance hall	restaurant
garage building (for	school (state) (public)
car storage)	(private)
hotel	shop, commercial
market (grocery or	station (bus) (railway)
other	store
commodity)	theater
movie house	

EXCLUDES   home garage (E849.0)
          industrial building or workplace (E849.3)

E849.7 Residential institution

Children's home	Old people's home
Dormitory	Orphanage
Hospital	Prison
Jail	Reform school

E849.8 Other specified places

Beach NOS	Pond or pool (natural)
Canal	Prairie
Caravan site NOS	Public place NOS
Derelict house	Railway line
Desert	Reservoir
Dock	River
Forest	Sea
Harbor	Seashore NOS
Hill	Stream
Lake NOS	Swamp
Mountain	Trailer court
Parking lot	Woods
Parking place	

E849.9 Unspecified place

E Codes

E850–E858.4

ACCIDENTAL POISONING BY DRUGS, MEDICINAL SUBSTANCES, AND BIOLOGICALS (E850-E858)

INCLUDES   accidental overdose of drug, wrong drug given or taken in error, and drug taken inadvertently

accidents in the use of drugs and biologicals in medical and surgical procedures

EXCLUDES   *administration with suicidal or homicidal intent or intent to harm, or in circumstances classifiable to E980-E989 (E950.0-E950.5, E962.0, E980.0-E980.5)*

correct drug properly administered in therapeutic or prophylactic dosage, as the cause of adverse effect (E930.0-E949.9)

See Alphabetic Index for more complete list of specific drugs to be classified under the fourth-digit subdivisions. The American Hospital Formulary numbers can be used to classify new drugs listed by the American Hospital Formulary Service (AHFS). See Appendix C.

✓4th **E850 Accidental poisoning by analgesics, antipyretics, and antirheumatics**

E850.0 Heroin
Diacetylmorphine

E850.1 Methadone

E850.2 Other opiates and related narcotics
Codeine [methylmorphine]   Morphine
Meperidine [pethidine]   Opium (alkaloids)

E850.3 Salicylates
Acetylsalicylic acid [aspirin]
Amino derivatives of salicylic acid
Salicylic acid salts

E850.4 Aromatic analgesics, not elsewhere classified
Acetanilid
Paracetamol [acetaminophen]
Phenacetin [acetophenetidin]

E850.5 Pyrazole derivatives
Aminophenazone [amidopyrine]
Phenylbutazone

E850.6 Antirheumatics [antiphlogistics]
Gold salts   Indomethacin
EXCLUDES   *salicylates (E850.3)*
     steroids (E858.0)

E850.7 Other non-narcotic analgesics
Pyrabital

E850.8 Other specified analgesics and antipyretics
Pentazocine

E850.9 Unspecified analgesic or antipyretic

E851 Accidental poisoning by barbiturates
Amobarbital [amylobarbitone]   Pentobarbital [pentobarbitone]
Barbital [barbitone]   Phenobarbital [phenobarbitone]
Butabarbital [butabarbitone]   Secobarbital [quinalbarbitone]
EXCLUDES   *thiobarbiturates (E855.1)*

✓4th **E852 Accidental poisoning by other sedatives and hypnotics**

E852.0 Chloral hydrate group

E852.1 Paraldehyde

E852.2 Bromine compounds
Bromides   Carbromal (derivatives)

E852.3 Methaqualone compounds

E852.4 Glutethimide group

E852.5 Mixed sedatives, not elsewhere classified

E852.8 Other specified sedatives and hypnotics

E852.9 Unspecified sedative or hypnotic
Sleeping:
   drug
   pill } NOS
   tablet

✓4th **E853 Accidental poisoning by tranquilizers**

E853.0 Phenothiazine-based tranquilizers
Chlorpromazine   Prochlorperazine
Fluphenazine   Promazine

E853.1 Butyrophenone-based tranquilizers
Haloperidol   Trifluperidol
Spiperone

E853.2 Benzodiazepine-based tranquilizers
Chlordiazepoxide   Lorazepam
Diazepam   Medazepam
Flurazepam   Nitrazepam

E853.8 Other specified tranquilizers
Hydroxyzine   Meprobamate

E853.9 Unspecified tranquilizer

✓4th **E854 Accidental poisoning by other psychotropic agents**

E854.0 Antidepressants
Amitriptyline
Imipramine
Monoamine oxidase [MAO] inhibitors

E854.1 Psychodysleptics [hallucinogens]
Cannabis derivatives   Mescaline
Lysergide [LSD]   Psilocin
Marihuana (derivatives)   Psilocybin

E854.2 Psychostimulants
Amphetamine   Caffeine
EXCLUDES   *central appetite depressants (E858.8)*

E854.3 Central nervous system stimulants
Analeptics   Opiate antagonists

E854.8 Other psychotropic agents

✓4th **E855 Accidental poisoning by other drugs acting on central and autonomic nervous system**

E855.0 Anticonvulsant and anti-Parkinsonism drugs
Amantadine
Hydantoin derivatives
Levodopa [L-dopa]
Oxazolidine derivatives [paramethadione] [trimethadione]
Succinimides

E855.1 Other central nervous system depressants
Ether
Gaseous anesthetics
Halogenated hydrocarbon derivatives
Intravenous anesthetics
Thiobarbiturates, such as thiopental sodium

E855.2 Local anesthetics
Cocaine   Procaine
Lidocaine [lignocaine]   Tetracaine

E855.3 Parasympathomimetics [cholinergics]
Acetylcholine   Pilocarpine
Anticholinesterase:
   organophosphorus
   reversible

E855.4 Parasympatholytics [anticholinergics and antimuscarinics] and spasmolytics
Atropine
Homatropine
Hyoscine [scopolamine]
Quaternary ammonium derivatives

E855.5 Sympathomimetics [adrenergics]
Epinephrine [adrenalin]
Levarterenol [noradrenalin]

E855.6 Sympatholytics [antiadrenergics]
Phenoxybenzamine
Tolazoline hydrochloride

E855.8 Other specified drugs acting on central and autonomic nervous systems

E855.9 Unspecified drug acting on central and autonomic nervous systems

E856 Accidental poisoning by antibiotics

E857 Accidental poisoning by other anti-infectives

✓4th **E858 Accidental poisoning by other drugs**

E858.0 Hormones and synthetic substitutes

E858.1 Primarily systemic agents

E858.2 Agents primarily affecting blood constituents

E858.3 Agents primarily affecting cardiovascular system

E858.4 Agents primarily affecting gastrointestinal system

✓4th Fourth-digit Required   ▶◀ Revised Text   ● New Code   ▲ Revised Code Title

E858.5 Water, mineral, and uric acid metabolism drugs

E858.6 Agents primarily acting on the smooth and skeletal muscles and respiratory system

E858.7 Agents primarily affecting skin and mucous membrane, ophthalmological, otorhinolaryngological, and dental drugs

E858.8 Other specified drugs
    Central appetite depressants

E858.9 Unspecified drug

ACCIDENTAL POISONING BY OTHER SOLID AND LIQUID SUBSTANCES, GASES, AND VAPORS (E860-E869)

Note: Categories in this section are intended primarily to indicate the external cause of poisoning states classifiable to 980-989. They may also be used to indicate external causes of localized effects classifiable to 001-799.

✓4ᵗʰ E860 Accidental poisoning by alcohol, not elsewhere classified

E860.0 Alcoholic beverages
    Alcohol in preparations intended for consumption

E860.1 Other and unspecified ethyl alcohol and its products

Denatured alcohol	Grain alcohol NOS
Ethanol NOS	Methylated spirit

E860.2 Methyl alcohol

Methanol	Wood alcohol

E860.3 Isopropyl alcohol

Dimethyl carbinol	Rubbing alcohol subsitute
Isopropanol	Secondary propyl alcohol

E860.4 Fusel oil

Alcohol:	Alcohol:
amyl	propyl
butyl	

E860.8 Other specified alcohols

E860.9 Unspecified alcohol

✓4ᵗʰ E861 Accidental poisoning by cleansing and polishing agents, disinfectants, paints, and varnishes

E861.0 Synthetic detergents and shampoos

E861.1 Soap products

E861.2 Polishes

E861.3 Other cleansing and polishing agents
    Scouring powders

E861.4 Disinfectants
    Household and other disinfectants not ordinarily used on the person
    EXCLUDES *carbolic acid or phenol (E864.0)*

E861.5 Lead paints

E861.6 Other paints and varnishes

Lacquers	Paints, other than lead
Oil colors	White washes

E861.9 Unspecified

✓4ᵗʰ E862 Accidental poisoning by petroleum products, other solvents and their vapors, not elsewhere classified

E862.0 Petroleum solvents

Petroleum:	Petroleum:
ether	naphtha
benzine	

E862.1 Petroleum fuels and cleaners
    Antiknock additives to petroleum fuels
    Gas oils
    Gasoline or petrol
    Kerosene
    EXCLUDES *kerosene insecticides (E863.4)*

E862.2 Lubricating oils

E862.3 Petroleum solids
    Paraffin wax

E862.4 Other specified solvents
    Benzene

E862.9 Unspecified solvent

✓4ᵗʰ E863 Accidental poisoning by agricultural and horticultural chemical and pharmaceutical preparations other than plant foods and fertilizers
    EXCLUDES *plant foods and fertilizers (E866.5)*

E863.0 Insecticides of organochlorine compounds

Benzene hexachloride	Dieldrin
Chlordane	Endrine
DDT	Toxaphene

E863.1 Insecticides of organophosphorus compounds

Demeton	Parathion
Diazinon	Phenylsulphthion
Dichlorvos	Phorate
Malathion	Phosdrin
Methyl parathion	

E863.2 Carbamates

Aldicarb	Propoxur
Carbaryl	

E863.3 Mixtures of insecticides

E863.4 Other and unspecified insecticides
    Kerosene insecticides

E863.5 Herbicides
    2, 4-Dichlorophenoxyacetic acid [2, 4-D]
    2, 4, 5-Trichlorophenoxyacetic acid [2, 4, 5-T]
    Chlorates
    Diquat
    Mixtures of plant foods and fertilizers with herbicides
    Paraquat

E863.6 Fungicides
    Organic mercurials (used in seed dressing)
    Pentachlorophenols

E863.7 Rodenticides

Fluoroacetates	Warfarin
Squill and derivatives	Zinc phosphide
Thallium	

E863.8 Fumigants

Cyanides	Phosphine
Methyl bromide	

E863.9 Other and unspecified

✓4ᵗʰ E864 Accidental poisoning by corrosives and caustics, not elsewhere classified
    EXCLUDES *those as components of disinfectants (E861.4)*

E864.0 Corrosive aromatics
    Carbolic acid or phenol

E864.1 Acids

Acid:	Acid:
hydrochloric	sulfuric
nitric	

E864.2 Caustic alkalis
    Lye

E864.3 Other specified corrosives and caustics

E864.4 Unspecified corrosives and caustics

✓4ᵗʰ E865 Accidental poisoning from poisonous foodstuffs and poisonous plants
    INCLUDES any meat, fish, or shellfish
        plants, berries, and fungi eaten as, or in mistake for, food, or by a child
    EXCLUDES *anaphylactic shock due to adverse food reaction (995.60-995.69)*
        food poisoning (bacterial) (005.0-005.9)
        poisoning and toxic reactions to venomous plants (E905.6-E905.7)

E865.0 Meat

E865.1 Shellfish

E865.2 Other fish

E865.3 Berries and seeds

E865.4 Other specified plants

E865.5 Mushrooms and other fungi

E865.8 Other specified foods

E865.9 Unspecified foodstuff or poisonous plant

✓4ᵗʰ **E866 Accidental poisoning by other and unspecified solid and liquid substances**

> **EXCLUDES**   *these substances as a component of:*
> *medicines (E850.0-E858.9)*
> *paints (E861.5-E861.6)*
> *pesticides (E863.0-E863.9)*
> *petroleum fuels (E862.1)*

E866.0 Lead and its compounds and fumes

E866.1 Mercury and its compounds and fumes

E866.2 Antimony and its compounds and fumes

E866.3 Arsenic and its compounds and fumes

E866.4 Other metals and their compounds and fumes

Beryllium (compounds)   Iron (compounds)
Brass fumes   Manganese (compounds)
Cadmium (compounds)   Nickel (compounds)
Copper salts   Thallium (compounds)

E866.5 Plant foods and fertilizers

> **EXCLUDES**   *mixtures with herbicides (E863.5)*

E866.6 Glues and adhesives

E866.7 Cosmetics

E866.8 Other specified solid or liquid substances

E866.9 Unspecified solid or liquid substance

E867 Accidental poisoning by gas distributed by pipeline

Carbon monoxide from incomplete combustion of piped gas
Coal gas NOS
Liquefied petroleum gas distributed through pipes (pure or mixed with air)
Piped gas (natural) (manufactured)

✓4ᵗʰ **E868 Accidental poisoning by other utility gas and other carbon monoxide**

E868.0 Liquefied petroleum gas distributed in mobile containers

Butane
Liquefied hydrocarbon gas NOS   } or carbon monoxide from incomplete conbustion of these gases
Propane

E868.1 Other and unspecified utility gas

Acetylene
Gas NOS used for lighting, heating, or cooking   } or carbon monoxide from incomplete conbustion of these gases
Water gas

E868.2 Motor vehicle exhaust gas

Exhaust gas from:
    farm tractor, not in transit
    gas engine
    motor pump
    motor vehicle, not in transit
    any type of combustion engine not in watercraft

> **EXCLUDES**   *poisoning by carbon monoxide from:*
> *aircraft while in transit (E844.0-E844.9)*
> *motor vehicle while in transit (E818.0-E818.9)*
> *watercraft whether or not in transit (E838.0-E838.9)*

E868.3 Carbon monoxide from incomplete combustion of other domestic fuels

Carbon monoxide from incomplete combustion of:
    coal
    coke
    kerosene   } in domestic stove or fireplace
    wood

> **EXCLUDES**   *carbon monoxide from smoke and fumes due to conflagration (E890.0-E893.9)*

E868.8 Carbon monoxide from other sources

Carbon monoxide from:
    blast furnace gas
    incomplete combustion of fuels in industrial use
    kiln vapor

E868.9 Unspecified carbon monoxide

✓4ᵗʰ **E869 Accidental poisoning by other gases and vapors**

> **EXCLUDES**   *effects of gases used as anesthetics (E855.1, E938.2)*
> *fumes from heavy metals (E866.0-E866.4)*
> *smoke and fumes due to conflagration or explosion (E890.0-E899)*

E869.0 Nitrogen oxides

E869.1 Sulfur dioxide

E869.2 Freon

E869.3 Lacrimogenic gas [tear gas]

Bromobenzyl cyanide   Ethyliodoacetate
Chloroacetophenone

E869.4 Second-hand tobacco smoke

E869.8 Other specified gases and vapors

Chlorine   Hydrocyanic acid gas

E869.9 Unspecified gases and vapors

MISADVENTURES TO PATIENTS DURING SURGICAL AND MEDICAL CARE (E870-E876)

> **EXCLUDES**   *accidental overdose of drug and wrong drug given in error (E850.0-E858.9)*
> *surgical and medical procedures as the cause of abnormal reaction by the patient, without mention of misadventure at the time of procedure (E878.0-E879.9)*

✓4ᵗʰ **E870 Accidental cut, puncture, perforation, or hemorrhage during medical care**

E870.0 Surgical operation

E870.1 Infusion or transfusion

E870.2 Kidney dialysis or other perfusion

E870.3 Injection or vaccination

E870.4 Endoscopic examination

E870.5 Aspiration of fluid or tissue, puncture, and catheterization

Abdominal paracentesis   Lumbar puncture
Aspirating needle biopsy Thoracentesis
Blood sampling

> **EXCLUDES**   *heart catheterization (E870.6)*

E870.6 Heart catheterization

E870.7 Administration of enema

E870.8 Other specified medical care

E870.9 Unspecified medical care

✓4ᵗʰ **E871 Foreign object left in body during procedure**

E871.0 Surgical operation

E871.1 Infusion or transfusion

E871.2 Kidney dialysis or other perfusion

E871.3 Injection or vaccination

E871.4 Endoscopic examination

E871.5 Aspiration of fluid or tissue, puncture, and catheterization

Abdominal paracentesis Lumbar puncture
Aspiration needle biopsy Thoracentesis
Blood sampling

> **EXCLUDES**   *heart catheterization (E871.6)*

E871.6 Heart catheterization

E871.7 Removal of catheter or packing

E871.8 Other specified procedures

E871.9 Unspecified procedure

✓4ᵗʰ **E872 Failure of sterile precautions during procedure**

E872.0 Surgical operation

E872.1 Infusion or transfusion

E872.2 Kidney dialysis and other perfusion

E872.3 Injection or vaccination

E872.4 Endoscopic examination

E872.5 Aspiration of fluid or tissue, puncture, and catheterization

Abdominal paracentesis   Lumbar puncture
Aspiration needle biopsy Thoracentesis
Blood sampling

> **EXCLUDES**   *heart catheterization (E872.6)*

✓4ᵗʰ Fourth-digit Required   ▶◀ Revised Text   ● New Code   ▲ Revised Code Title

E872.6 **Heart catheterization**

E872.8 **Other specified procedures**

E872.9 **Unspecified procedure**

✓4ᵗʰ **E873 Failure in dosage**

> EXCLUDES *accidental overdose of drug, medicinal or biological substance (E850.0-E858.9)*

E873.0 **Excessive amount of blood or other fluid during transfusion or infusion**

E873.1 **Incorrect dilution of fluid during infusion**

E873.2 **Overdose of radiation in therapy**

E873.3 **Inadvertent exposure of patient to radiation during medical care**

E873.4 **Failure in dosage in electroshock or insulin-shock therapy**

E873.5 **Inappropriate [too hot or too cold] temperature in local application and packing**

E873.6 **Nonadministration of necessary drug or medicinal substance**

E873.8 **Other specified failure in dosage**

E873.9 **Unspecified failure in dosage**

✓4ᵗʰ **E874 Mechanical failure of instrument or apparatus during procedure**

E874.0 **Surgical operation**

E874.1 **Infusion and transfusion**
> Air in system

E874.2 **Kidney dialysis and other perfusion**

E874.3 **Endoscopic examination**

E874.4 **Aspiration of fluid or tissue, puncture, and catheterization**
> Abdominal paracentesis   Lumbar puncture
> Aspiration needle biopsy   Thoracentesis
> Blood sampling
> > EXCLUDES *heart catheterization (E874.5)*

E874.5 **Heart catheterization**

E874.8 **Other specified procedures**

E874.9 **Unspecified procedure**

✓4ᵗʰ **E875 Contaminated or infected blood, other fluid, drug, or biological substance**

> INCLUDES presence of:
> > bacterial pyrogens
> > endotoxin-producing bacteria
> > serum hepatitis-producing agent

E875.0 **Contaminated substance transfused or infused**

E875.1 **Contaminated substance injected or used for vaccination**

E875.2 **Contaminated drug or biological substance administered by other means**

E875.8 **Other**

E875.9 **Unspecified**

✓4ᵗʰ **E876 Other and unspecified misadventures during medical care**

E876.0 **Mismatched blood in transfusion**

E876.1 **Wrong fluid in infusion**

E876.2 **Failure in suture and ligature during surgical operation**

E876.3 **Endotracheal tube wrongly placed during anesthetic procedure**

E876.4 **Failure to introduce or to remove other tube or instrument**
> > EXCLUDES *foreign object left in body during procedure (E871.0-E871.9)*

E876.5 **Performance of inappropriate operation**

E876.8 **Other specified misadventures during medical care**
> Performance of inappropriate treatment NEC

E876.9 **Unspecified misadventure during medical care**

SURGICAL AND MEDICAL PROCEDURES AS THE CAUSE OF ABNORMAL REACTION OF PATIENT OR LATER COMPLICATION, WITHOUT MENTION OF MISADVENTURE AT THE TIME OF PROCEDURE (E878-E879)

> INCLUDES procedures as the cause of abnormal reaction, such as:
> > displacement or malfunction of prosthetic device
> > hepatorenal failure, postoperative
> > malfunction of external stoma
> > postoperative intestinal obstruction
> > rejection of transplanted organ
> EXCLUDES *anesthetic management properly carried out as the cause of adverse effect (E937.0-E938.9)*
> > *infusion and transfusion, without mention of misadventure in the technique of procedure (E930.0-E949.9)*

✓4ᵗʰ **E878 Surgical operation and other surgical procedures as the cause of abnormal reaction of patient, or of later complication, without mention of misadventure at the time of operation**

E878.0 **Surgical operation with transplant of whole organ**
> Transplantation of: Transplantation of:
> > heart   liver
> > kidney

E878.1 **Surgical operation with implant of artificial internal device**
> Cardiac pacemaker   Heart valve prosthesis
> Electrodes implanted in Internal orthopedic
> > brain   device

E878.2 **Surgical operation with anastomosis, bypass, or graft, with natural or artificial tissues used as implant**
> Anastomosis: Graft of blood vessel,
> > arteriovenous   tendon, or skin
> > gastrojejunal
> > EXCLUDES *external stoma (E878.3)*

E878.3 **Surgical operation with formation of external stoma**
> Colostomy   Gastrostomy
> Cystostomy   Ureterostomy
> Duodenostomy

E878.4 **Other restorative surgery**

E878.5 **Amputation of limb(s)**

E878.6 **Removal of other organ (partial) (total)**

E878.8 **Other specified surgical operations and procedures**

E878.9 **Unspecified surgical operations and procedures**

✓4ᵗʰ **E879 Other procedures, without mention of misadventure at the time of procedure, as the cause of abnormal reaction of patient, or of later complication**

E879.0 **Cardiac catheterization**

E879.1 **Kidney dialysis**

E879.2 **Radiological procedure and radiotherapy**
> > EXCLUDES *radio-opaque dyes for diagnostic x-ray procedures (E947.8)*

E879.3 **Shock therapy**
> Electroshock therapy
> Insulin-shock therapy

E879.4 **Aspiration of fluid**
> Lumbar puncture
> Thoracentesis

E879.5 **Insertion of gastric or duodenal sound**

E879.6 **Urinary catheterization**

E879.7 **Blood sampling**

E879.8 **Other specified procedures**
> Blood transfusion

E879.9 **Unspecified procedure**

✓4ᵗʰ Fourth-digit Required   ▶◀ Revised Text   ● New Code   ▲ Revised Code Title

E880–E890.9

ACCIDENTAL FALLS (E880-E888)

EXCLUDES *falls (in or from):*
  burning building (E890.8, E891.8)
  into fire (E890.0-E899)
  into water (with submersion or drowning)
    (E910.0-E910.9)
  machinery (in operation) (E919.0-E919.9)
  on edged, pointed, or sharp object (E920.0-
    E920.9)
  transport vehicle (E800.0-E845.9)
  vehicle not elsewhere classifiable (E846-E848)

☑4ᵗʰ **E880 Fall on or from stairs or steps**

E880.0 Escalator

E880.1 Fall on or from sidewalk curb
  EXCLUDES *fall from moving sidewalk (E885.9)*

E880.9 Other stairs or steps

☑4ᵗʰ **E881 Fall on or from ladders or scaffolding**

E881.0 Fall from ladder

E881.1 Fall from scaffolding

E882 Fall from or out of building or other structure

Fall from: Fall from:
  balcony   turret
  bridge   viaduct
  building   wall
  flagpole   window
  tower   Fall through roof

  EXCLUDES *collapse of a building or structure (E916)*
  fall or jump from burning building (E890.8,
    E891.8)

☑4ᵗʰ **E883 Fall into hole or other opening in surface**

INCLUDES fall into: fall into:
  cavity   shaft
  dock   swimming pool
  hole   tank
  pit   well
  quarry

  EXCLUDES *fall into water NOS (E910.9)*
  that resulting in drowning or submersion
    without mention of injury (E910.0-E910.9)

E883.0 Accident from diving or jumping into water
  [swimming pool]
  Strike or hit:
    against bottom when jumping or diving into water
    wall or board of swimming pool
    water surface

  EXCLUDES *diving with insufficient air supply*
    (E913.2)
  effects of air pressure from diving
    (E902.2)

E883.1 Accidental fall into well

E883.2 Accidental fall into storm drain or manhole

E883.9 Fall into other hole or other opening in surface

☑4ᵗʰ **E884 Other fall from one level to another**

E884.0 Fall from playground equipment
  EXCLUDES *recreational machinery (E919.8)*

E884.1 Fall from cliff

E884.2 Fall from chair

E884.3 Fall from wheelchair

E884.4 Fall from bed

E884.5 Fall from other furniture

E884.6 Fall from commode
  Toilet

E884.9 Other fall from one level to another
  Fall from: Fall from:
    embankment   stationary vehicle
    haystack   tree

☑4ᵗʰ **E885 Fall on same level from slipping, tripping, or stumbling**

E885.0 Fall from (nonmotorized) scooter

E885.1 Fall from roller skates
  In-line skates

E885.2 Fall from skateboard

E885.3 Fall from skis

E885.4 Fall from snowboard

E885.9 Fall from other slipping, tripping, or stumbling
  Fall on moving sidewalk

☑4ᵗʰ **E886 Fall on same level from collision, pushing, or shoving, by or with other person**

  EXCLUDES *crushed or pushed by a crowd or human*
    stampede (E917.1, E917.6)

E886.0 In sports
  Tackles in sports
  EXCLUDES *kicked, stepped on, struck by object, in*
    sports (E917.0, E917.5)

E886.9 Other and unspecified
  Fall from collision of pedestrian (conveyance) with
    another pedestrian (conveyance)

E887 Fracture, cause unspecified

☑4ᵗʰ **E888 Other and unspecified fall**
  Accidental fall NOS   Fall on same level NOS

E888.0 Fall resulting in striking against sharp object
  Use additional external cause code to identify object
    (E920)

E888.1 Fall resulting in striking against other object

E888.8 Other fall

E888.9 Unspecified fall
  Fall NOS

ACCIDENTS CAUSED BY FIRE AND FLAMES (E890-E899)

INCLUDES asphyxia or poisoning due to conflagration or
    ignition
  burning by fire
  secondary fires resulting from explosion

  EXCLUDES *arson (E968.0)*
  fire in or on:
    machinery (in operation) (E919.0-E919.9)
    transport vehicle other than stationary
      vehicle (E800.0-E845.9)
    vehicle not elsewhere classifiable (E846-
      E848)

☑4ᵗʰ **E890 Conflagration in private dwelling**

INCLUDES conflagration in: conflagration in:
  apartment   lodging house
  boarding house   mobile home
  camping place   private garage
  caravan   rooming house
  farmhouse   tenement
  house
  conflagration originating from sources
    classifiable to E893-E898 in the above
    buildings

E890.0 Explosion caused by conflagration

E890.1 Fumes from combustion of polyvinylchloride [PVC] and similar material in conflagration

E890.2 Other smoke and fumes from conflagration

  Carbon monoxide }
  Fumes NOS   from conflagration in
  Smoke NOS   } private building

E890.3 Burning caused by conflagration

E890.8 Other accident resulting from conflagration

  Collapse of   }
  Fall from   burning private
  Hit by object falling from } building
  Jump from   }

E890.9 Unspecified accident resulting from conflagration in private dwelling

---

☑4ᵗʰ Fourth-digit Required   ▶◀ Revised Text   ● New Code   ▲ Revised Code Title

√4ᵗʰ **E891 Conflagration in other and unspecified building or structure**

Conflagration in:	Conflagration in:
barn	farm outbuildings
church	hospital
convalescent and other	hotel
residential home	school
dormitory of educational	store
institution	theater
factory	

Conflagration originating from sources classifiable to E893-E898, in the above buildings

E891.0 Explosion caused by conflagration

E891.1 Fumes from combustion of polyvinylchloride [PVC] and similar material in conflagration

E891.2 Other smoke and fumes from conflagration

Carbon monoxide ⎫ from conflagration in
Fumes NOS ⎬ building or
Smoke NOS ⎭ structure

E891.3 Burning caused by conflagration

E891.8 Other accident resulting from conflagration

Collapse of ⎫
Fall from ⎬ burning building or
Hit by object falling from ⎬ structure
Jump from ⎭

E891.9 Unspecified accident resulting from conflagration of other and unspecified building or structure

E892 Conflagration not in building or structure

Fire (uncontrolled) (in) (of):	Fire (uncontrolled) (in) (of):
forest	prairie
grass	transport vehicle [any],
hay	except while in
lumber	transit
mine	tunnel

√4ᵗʰ **E893 Accident caused by ignition of clothing**

EXCLUDES   *ignition of clothing:*
        from highly inflammable material (E894)
        with conflagration (E890.0-E892)

E893.0 From controlled fire in private dwelling

Ignition of clothing from:
normal fire (charcoal) (coal) ⎫
(electric) (gas) (wood) in: ⎬ in private
brazier ⎬ dwelling
fireplace ⎬ (as listed
furnace ⎬ in E890)
stove ⎭

E893.1 From controlled fire in other building or structure

Ignition of clothing from:
normal fire (charcoal) ⎫
(coal) (electric) ⎬
(gas) (wood) in: ⎬ in other building or
brazier ⎬ structure (as
fireplace ⎬ listed in E81)
furnace ⎬
stove ⎭

E893.2 From controlled fire not in building or structure

Ignition of clothing from:
bonfire (controlled)
brazier fire (controlled), not in building or
    structure
trash fire (controlled)

EXCLUDES   *conflagration not in building (E892)*
        trash fire out of control (E892)

E893.8 From other specified sources

Ignition of clothing from:	Ignition of clothing from:
blowlamp	cigarette
blowtorch	lighter
burning bedspread	matches
candle	pipe
cigar	welding torch

E893.9 Unspecified source

Ignition of clothing (from controlled fire NOS) (in building NOS) NOS

E894 Ignition of highly inflammable material

Ignition of:
benzine ⎫
gasoline ⎬
fat ⎬
kerosene ⎬ (with ignition of clothing)
paraffin ⎬
petrol ⎭

EXCLUDES   *ignition of highly inflammable material with:*
        conflagration (E890.0-E892)
        explosion (E923.0-E923.9)

E895 Accident caused by controlled fire in private dwelling

Burning by (flame of) normal fire
(charcoal) (coal) (electric) ⎫
(gas) (wood) in: ⎬
brazier ⎬ in private dwelling (as
fireplace ⎬ listed in E890)
furnace ⎬
stove ⎭

EXCLUDES   *burning by hot objects not producing fire or*
        flames (E924.0-E924.9)
        ignition of clothing from these sources (E893.0)
        poisoning by carbon monoxide from incomplete
        combustion of fuel (E867-E868.9)
        that with conflagration (E890.0-E890.9)

E896 Accident caused by controlled fire in other and unspecified building or structure

Burning by (flame of) normal fire (charcoal) (coal) (electric)
(gas) (wood) in:
brazier ⎫
fireplace ⎬ in other building or structure (as
furnace ⎬ listed in E891)
stove ⎭

EXCLUDES   *burning by hot objects not producing fire or*
        flames (E924.0-E924.9)
        ignition of clothing from these sources (E893.1)
        poisoning by carbon monoxide from incomplete
        combustion of fuel (E867-E868.9)
        that with conflagration (E891.0-E891.9)

E897 Accident caused by controlled fire not in building or structure

Burns from flame of:
bonfire ⎫
brazier fire, not in building or structure ⎬ controlled
trash fire ⎭

EXCLUDES   *ignition of clothing from these sources (E893.2)*
        trash fire out of control (E892)
        that with conflagration (E892)

√4ᵗʰ **E898 Accident caused by other specified fire and flames**

EXCLUDES   *conflagration (E890.0-E892)*
        that with ignition of:
        clothing (E893.0-E893.9)
        highly inflammable material (E894)

E898.0 Burning bedclothes

Bed set on fire NOS

E898.1 Other

Burning by:	Burning by:
blowlamp	lamp
blowtorch	lighter
candle	matches
cigar	pipe
cigarette	welding torch
fire in room NOS	

E899 Accident caused by unspecified fire

Burning NOS

ACCIDENTS DUE TO NATURAL AND ENVIRONMENTAL FACTORS (E900-E909)

√4ᵗʰ **E900 Excessive heat**

E900.0 Due to weather conditions

Excessive heat as the external cause of:
ictus solaris   sunstroke
siriasis

E900.1 Of man-made origin

Heat (in):   Heat (in):
    boiler room   generated in transport
    drying room   vehicle
    factory   kitchen
    furnace room

E900.9 Of unspecified origin

✓4ᵗʰ E901 Excessive cold

E901.0 Due to weather conditions

Excessive cold as the cause of:
    chilblains NOS
    immersion foot

E901.1 Of man-made origin

Contact with or inhalation of:
    dry ice
    liquid air
    liquid hydrogen
    liquid nitrogen
Prolonged exposure in:
    deep freeze unit
    refrigerator

E901.8 Other specified origin

E901.9 Of unspecified origin

✓4ᵗʰ E902 High and low air pressure and changes in air pressure

E902.0 Residence or prolonged visit at high altitude

Residence or prolonged visit at high altitude as the
    cause of:
    Acosta syndrome
    Alpine sickness
    altitude sickness
    Andes disease
    anoxia, hypoxia
    barotitis, barodontalgia, barosinusitis, otitic
       barotrauma
    hypobarism, hypobaropathy
    mountain sickness
    range disease

E902.1 In aircraft

Sudden change in air pressure in aircraft during
    ascent or descent as the cause of:
    aeroneurosis
    aviators' disease

E902.2 Due to diving

High air pressure from
    rapid descent in water   }   as the cause of:
Reduction in atmospheric   caisson disease
    pressure while   divers' disease
    surfacing from deep   divers' palsy or
    water diving   paralysis

E902.8 Due to other specified causes

Reduction in atmospheric pressure whilesurfacing
    from underground

E902.9 Unspecified cause

E903 Travel and motion

✓4ᵗʰ E904 Hunger, thirst, exposure, and neglect

> **EXCLUDES**   *any condition resulting from homicidal intent*
>   *(E968.0-E968.9)*
>   *hunger, thirst, and exposure resulting from*
>   *accidents connected with transport*
>   *(E800.0-E848)*

E904.0 Abandonment or neglect of infants and helpless persons

Exposure to weather }   resulting from
    conditions   abandonment
Hunger or thirst   or neglect

Desertion of newborn
Inattention at or after birth
Lack of care (helpless person) (infant)

> **EXCLUDES**   *criminal [purposeful] neglect (E968.4)*

E904.1 Lack of food

Lack of food as the cause of:
    inanition
    insufficient nourishment
    starvation

> **EXCLUDES**   *hunger resulting from abandonment or*
>   *neglect (E904.0)*

E904.2 Lack of water

Lack of water as the cause of:
    dehydration   inanition

> **EXCLUDES**   *dehydration due to acute fluid loss*
>   *(276.5)*

E904.3 Exposure (to weather conditions), not elsewhere classifiable

Exposure NOS   Struck by hailstones
Humidity

> **EXCLUDES**   *struck by lightning (E907)*

E904.9 Privation, unqualified

Destitution

✓4ᵗʰ E905 Venomous animals and plants as the cause of poisoning and toxic reactions

> **INCLUDES**   chemical released by animal
>   insects
>   release of venom through fangs, hairs, spines,
>   tentacles, and other venom apparatus

> **EXCLUDES**   *eating of poisonous animals or plants (E865.0-*
>   *E865.9)*

E905.0 Venomous snakes and lizards

Cobra   Mamba
Copperhead snake   Rattlesnake
Coral snake   Sea snake
Fer de lance   Snake (venomous)
Gila monster   Viper
Krait   Water moccasin

> **EXCLUDES**   *bites of snakes and lizards known to*
>   *be nonvenomous (E906.2)*

E905.1 Venomous spiders

Black widow spider   Tarantula (venomous)
Brown spider

E905.2 Scorpion

E905.3 Hornets, wasps, and bees

Yellow jacket

E905.4 Centipede and venomous millipede (tropical)

E905.5 Other venomous arthropods

Sting of: Sting of:
    ant   caterpillar

E905.6 Venomous marine animals and plants

Puncture by sea   Sting of:
    urchin spine   sea anemone
Sting of: sea cucumber
    coral   other marine animal
    jelly fish   or plant
    nematocysts

> **EXCLUDES**   *bites and other injuries caused by*
>   *nonvenomous marine animal*
>   *(E906.2-E906.8)*
>   *bite of sea snake (venomous) (E905.0)*

E905.7 Poisoning and toxic reactions caused by other plants

Injection of poisons or toxins into or through skin by
    plant thorns, spines, or other mechanisms

> **EXCLUDES**   *puncture wound NOS by plant thorns*
>   *or spines (E920.8)*

E905.8 Other specified

E905.9 Unspecified

Sting NOS   Venomous bite NOS

✓4ᵗʰ E906 Other injury caused by animals

> **EXCLUDES**   *poisoning and toxic reactions caused by*
>   *venomous animals and insects (E905.0-*
>   *E905.9)*
>   *road vehicle accident involving animals (E827.0-*
>   *E828.9)*
>   *tripping or falling over an animal (E885.9)*

✓4ᵗʰ Fourth-digit Required   ▶◀ Revised Text   ● New Code   ▲ Revised Code Title

E906.0 Dog bite

E906.1 Rat bite

E906.2 Bite of nonvenomous snakes and lizards

E906.3 Bite of other animal except arthropod
   Cats   Rodents, except rats
   Moray eel   Shark

E906.4 Bite of nonvenomous arthropod
   Insect bite NOS

E906.5 Bite by unspecified animal
   Animal bite NOS

E906.8 Other specified injury caused by animal
   Butted by animal
   Fallen on by horse or other animal, not being ridden
   Gored by animal
   Implantation of quills of porcupine
   Pecked by bird
   Run over by animal, not being ridden
   Stepped on by animal, not being ridden
   EXCLUDES *injury by animal being ridden (E828.0-*
                 E828.9)

E906.9 Unspecified injury caused by animal

E907 Lightning
   EXCLUDES *injury from:*
                 fall of tree or other object caused by lightning
                 (E916)
                 fire caused by lightning (E890.0-E892)

✓4ᵗʰ E908 Cataclysmic storms, and floods resulting from storms
   EXCLUDES *collapse of dam or man-made structure causing*
                 flood (E909.3)

E908.0 Hurricane
   Storm surge
   "Tidal wave" caused by storm action
   Typhoon

E908.1 Tornado
   Cyclone
   Twisters

E908.2 Floods
   Torrential rainfall
   Flash flood
   EXCLUDES *collapse of dam or man-made structure*
                 causing flood (E909.3)

E908.3 Blizzard (snow) (ice)

E908.4 Dust storm

E908.8 Other cataclysmic storms

E908.9 Unspecified cataclysmic storms, and floods
         resulting from storms
   Storm NOS

✓4ᵗʰ E909 Cataclysmic earth surface movements and eruptions

E909.0 Earthquakes

E909.1 Volcanic eruptions
   Burns from lava
   Ash inhalation

E909.2 Avalanche, landslide, or mudslide

E909.3 Collapse of dam or man-made structure

E909.4 Tidalwave caused by earthquake
   Tidalwave NOS
   Tsunami
   EXCLUDES *tidalwave caused by tropical storm*
                 (E908.0)

E909.8 Other cataclysmic earth surface movements and
         eruptions

E909.9 Unspecified cataclysmic earth surface movements
         and eruptions

ACCIDENTS CAUSED BY SUBMERSION, SUFFOCATION, AND FOREIGN BODIES (E910-E915)

✓4ᵗʰ E910 Accidental drowning and submersion
   INCLUDES immersion
                 swimmers' cramp
   EXCLUDES *diving accident (NOS) (resulting in injury except*
                 drowning) (E883.0)
                 diving with insufficient air supply (E913.2)
                 drowning and submersion due to:
                 cataclysm (E908-E909)
                 machinery accident (E919.0-E919.9)
                 transport accident (E800.0-E845.9)
                 effect of high and low air pressure (E902.2)
                 injury from striking against objects while in
                 running water (E917.2)

E910.0 While water-skiing
   Fall from water skis with submersion or drowning
   EXCLUDES *accident to water-skier involving a*
                 watercraft and resulting in
                 submersion or other injury
                 (E830.4, E831.4)

E910.1 While engaged in other sport or recreational
         activity with diving equipment
   Scuba diving NOS   Underwater spear
   Skin diving NOS   fishing NOS

E910.2 While engaged in other sport or recreational
         activity without diving equipment
   Fishing or hunting, except from boat or with diving
         equipment
   Ice skating
   Playing in water
   Surfboarding
   Swimming NOS
   Voluntarily jumping from boat, not involved in
         accident, for swim NOS
   Wading in water
   EXCLUDES *jumping into water to rescue another*
                 person (E910.3)

E910.3 While swimming or diving for purposes other than
         recreation or sport
   Marine salvage
   Pearl diving
   Placement of fishing nets
   Rescue (attempt) of   (with diving
         another person   equipment)
   Underwater construction
         or repairs

E910.4 In bathtub

E910.8 Other accidental drowning or submersion
   Drowning in: Drowning in:
      quenching tank   swimming pool

E910.9 Unspecified accidental drowning or submersion
   Accidental fall into water NOS
   Drowning NOS

E911 Inhalation and ingestion of food causing obstruction of
      respiratory tract or suffocation
   Aspiration and inhalation of food [any] (into respiratory tract)
         NOS
   Asphyxia by
   Choked on   food [including bone, seed in
   Suffocation by   food, regurgitated food]

   Compression of trachea
   Interruption of respiration   by food lodged in
   Obstruction of respiration   esophagus

   Obstruction of pharynx by food (bolus)
   EXCLUDES *injury, except asphyxia and obstruction of*
                 respiratory passage, caused by food
                 (E915)
                 obstruction of esophagus by food without
                 mention of asphyxia or obstruction of
                 respiratory passage (E915)

✓4ᵗʰ Fourth-digit Required   ►◄ Revised Text   ● New Code   ▲ Revised Code Title

E912 Inhalation and ingestion of other object causing obstruction of respiratory tract or suffocation

Aspiration and inhalation of foreign body except food (into respiratory tract) NOS

Foreign object [bean] [marble] in nose

Obstruction of pharynx by foreign body

Compression

Interruption of respiration ⎱ by foreign body in
Obstruction of respiration ⎰ esophagus

> EXCLUDES   *injury, except asphyxia and obstruction of respiratory passage, caused by foreign body (E915)*
> *obstruction of esophagus by foreign body without mention of asphyxia or obstruction in respiratory passage (E915)*

✓4ᵗʰ E913 Accidental mechanical suffocation

> EXCLUDES   *mechanical suffocation from or by:*
> *accidental inhalation or ingestion of:*
> *food (E911)*
> *foreign object (E912)*
> *cataclysm (E908-E909)*
> *explosion (E921.0-E921.9, E923.0-E923.9)*
> *machinery accident (E919.0-E919.9)*

E913.0 In bed or cradle

> EXCLUDES   *suffocation by plastic bag (E913.1)*

E913.1 By plastic bag

E913.2 Due to lack of air (in closed place)

Accidentally closed up in refrigerator or other airtight enclosed space

Diving with insufficient air supply

> EXCLUDES   *suffocation by plastic bag (E913.1)*

E913.3 By falling earth or other substance

Cave-in NOS

> EXCLUDES   *cave-in caused by cataclysmic earth surface movements and eruptions (E909)*
> *struck by cave-in without asphyxiation or suffocation (E916)*

E913.8 Other specified means

Accidental hanging, except in bed or cradle

E913.9 Unspecified means

Asphyxia, mechanical NOS   Suffocation NOS

Strangulation NOS

E914 Foreign body accidentally entering eye and adnexa

> EXCLUDES   *corrosive liquid (E924.1)*

E915 Foreign body accidentally entering other orifice

> EXCLUDES   *aspiration and inhalation of foreign body, any, (into respiratory tract) NOS (E911-E912)*

OTHER ACCIDENTS (E916-E928)

E916 Struck accidentally by falling object

Collapse of building, except on fire

Falling:

rock

snowslide NOS

stone

tree

Object falling from:

machine, not in operation

stationary vehicle

Code first:

collapse of building on fire (E890.0-E891.9)

falling object in:

cataclysm (E908-E909)

machinery accidents (E919.0-E919.9)

transport accidents (E800.0-E845.9)

vehicle accidents not elsewhere classifiable (E846-E848)

object set in motion by:

explosion (E921.0-E921.9, E923.0-E923.9)

firearm (E922.0-E922.9)

projected object (E917.0-E917.9)

✓4ᵗʰ E917 Striking against or struck accidentally by objects or persons

> INCLUDES
> bumping into or against
> colliding with
> kicking against
> stepping on
> struck by
> ⎱ object (moving) (projected) (stationary)
> pedestrian conveyance
> person

> EXCLUDES   *fall from:*
> *collision with another person, except when caused by a crowd (E886.0-E886.9)*
> *stumbling over object (E885.9)*
> *fall resulting in striking against object (E888.0, E888.1)*
> *injury caused by:*
> *assault (E960.0-E960.1, E967.0-E967.9)*
> *cutting or piercing instrument (E920.0-E920.9)*
> *explosion (E921.0-E921.9, E923.0-E923.9)*
> *firearm (E922.0-E922.9)*
> *machinery (E919.0-E919.9)*
> *transport vehicle (E800.0-E845.9)*
> *vehicle not elsewhere classifiable (E846-E848)*

E917.0 In sports without subsequent fall

Kicked or stepped on during game (football) (rugby)

Struck by hit or thrown ball

Struck by hockey stick or puck

E917.1 Caused by a crowd, by collective fear or panic without subsequent fall

Crushed

Pushed ⎱ by crowd or human stampede

Stepped on ⎰

E917.2 In running water without subsequent fall

> EXCLUDES   *drowning or submersion (E910.0-E910.9)*
> *that in sports (E917.0, E917.5)*

E917.3 Furniture without subsequent fall

> EXCLUDES   *fall from furniture (E884.2, E884.4-E884.5)*

E917.4 Other stationary object without subsequent fall

Bath tub

Fence

Lamp-post

E917.5 Object in sports with subsequent fall

Knocked down while boxing

E917.6 Caused by a crowd, by collective fear or panic with subsequent fall

E917.7 Furniture with subsequent fall

> EXCLUDES   *fall from furniture (E884.2, E884.4-E884.5)*

E917.8 Other stationary object with subsequent fall

Bath tub

Fence

Lamp-post

E917.9 Other striking against with or without subsequent fall

E918 Caught accidentally in or between objects

Caught, crushed, jammed, or pinched in or between moving or stationary objects, such as:

escalator

folding object

hand tools, appliances, or implements

sliding door and door frame

under packing crate

washing machine wringer

> EXCLUDES   *injury caused by:*
> *cutting or piercing instrument (E920.0-E920.9)*
> *machinery (E919.0-E919.9)*
> *transport vehicle (E800.0-E845.9)*
> *vehicle not elsewhere classifiable (E846-E848)*
> *struck accidentally by:*
> *falling object (E916)*
> *object (moving) (projected) (E917.0-E917.9)*

✓4ᵗʰ Fourth-digit Required   ►◄ Revised Text   ● New Code   ▲ Revised Code Title

✓4ᵗʰ E919 Accidents caused by machinery

INCLUDES

burned by	
caught in (moving parts of)	
collapse of	
crushed by	
cut or pierced by	
drowning or submersion caused by	
explosion of, on, in	machinery
fall from or into moving part of	(accident)
fire starting in or on	
mechanical suffocation caused by	
object falling from, on, in motion by	
overturning of	
pinned under	
run over by	
struck by	
thrown from	

caught between machinery and other object
machinery accident NOS

EXCLUDES   *accidents involving machinery, not in operation (E884.9, E916-E918)*
injury caused by:
    electric current in connection with machinery (E925.0-E925.9)
    escalator (E880.0, E918)
    explosion of pressure vessel in connection with machinery (E921.0-E921.9)
    moving sidewalk (E885.9)
    powered hand tools, appliances, and implements (E916-E918, E920.0-E921.9, E923.0-E926.9)
    transport vehicle accidents involving machinery (E800.0-E848)
    poisoning by carbon monoxide generated by machine (E868.8)

E919.0 Agricultural machines

Animal-powered agricultural machine	Farm tractor
	Harvester
Combine	Hay mower or rake
Derrick, hay	Reaper
Farm machinery NOS	Thresher

EXCLUDES   *that in transport under own power on the highway (E810.0-E819.9)*
that being towed by another vehicle on the highway (E810.0-E819.9, E827.0-E827.9, E829.0-E829.9)
that involved in accident classifiable to E820-E829 (E820.0-E829.9)

E919.1 Mining and earth-drilling machinery

Bore or drill (land) (seabed)	Shaft lift
Shaft hoist	Under-cutter

EXCLUDES   *coal car, tram, truck, and tub in mine (E846)*

E919.2 Lifting machines and appliances

Chain hoist	
Crane	
Derrick	except in
Elevator (building) (grain)	agricultural
Forklift truck	or mining
Lift	operations
Pulley block	
Winch	

EXCLUDES   *that being towed by another vehicle on the highway (E810.0-E819.9, E827.0-E827.9, E829.0-829.9)*
that in transport under own power on the highway (E810.0-E819.9)
that involved in accident classifiable to E820-E829 (E820.0-E829.9)

E919.3 Metalworking machines

	Metal:
Abrasive wheel	drilling machine
Forging machine	milling machine
Lathe	power press
Mechanical shears	rolling-mill
	sawing machine

E919.4 Woodworking and forming machines

Band saw	Overhead plane
Bench saw	Powered saw
Circular saw	Radial saw
Molding machine	Sander

EXCLUDES   *hand saw (E920.1)*

E919.5 Prime movers, except electrical motors

Gas turbine
Internal combustion engine
Steam engine
Water driven turbine

EXCLUDES   *that being towed by other vehicle on the highway (E810.0-E819.9, E827.0-E827.9, E829.0-E829.9)*
that in transport under own power on the highway (E810.0-E819.9)

E919.6 Transmission machinery

Transmission:	Transmission:
belt	pinion
cable	pulley
chain	shaft
gear	

E919.7 Earth moving, scraping, and other excavating machines

Bulldozer	Steam shovel
Road scraper	

EXCLUDES   *that being towed by other vehicle on the highway (E810.0-E819.9, E827.0-E827.9, E829.0-E829.9)*
that in transport under own power on the highway (E810.0-E819.9)

E919.8 Other specified machinery

Machines for manufacture of:
    clothing
    foodstuffs and beverages
    paper
Printing machine
Recreational machinery
Spinning, weaving, and textile machines

E919.9 Unspecified machinery

✓4ᵗʰ E920 Accidents caused by cutting and piercing instruments or objects

INCLUDES

	object:
accidental injury (by)	edged
	pointed
	sharp

E920.0 Powered lawn mower

E920.1 Other powered hand tools

Any powered hand tool [compressed air] [electric] [explosive cartridge] [hydraulic power], such as:
    drill
    hand saw
    hedge clipper
    rivet gun
    snow blower
    staple gun

EXCLUDES   *band saw (E919.4)*
bench saw (E919.4)

E920.2 Powered household appliances and implements

	Electric:
Blender	fan
Electric:	knife
beater or mixer	sewing machine
can opener	Garbage disposal appliance

E920.3 Knives, swords, and daggers

E920.4 Other hand tools and implements

Axe	Paper cutter
Can opener NOS	Pitchfork
Chisel	Rake
Fork	Scissors
Hand saw	Screwdriver
Hoe	Sewing machine, not powered
Ice pick	Shovel
Needle (sewing)	

E920.5 Hypodermic needle

Contaminated needle

Needle stick

E920.8 Other specified cutting and piercing instruments or objects

Arrow	Nail
Broken glass	Plant thorn
Dart	Splinter
Edge of stiff paper	Tin can lid
Lathe turnings	

> EXCLUDES   *animal spines or quills (E906.8)*
> *flying glass due to explosion (E921.0-E923.9)*

E920.9 Unspecified cutting and piercing instrument or object

✓4ᵗʰ E921 Accident caused by explosion of pressure vessel

> INCLUDES   accidental explosion of pressure vessels, whether or not part of machinery
>
> EXCLUDES   *explosion of pressure vessel on transport vehicle (E800.0-E845.9)*

E921.0 Boilers

E921.1 Gas cylinders

Air tank

Pressure gas tank

E921.8 Other specified pressure vessels

Aerosol can	Pressure cooker
Automobile tire	

E921.9 Unspecified pressure vessel

✓4ᵗʰ E922 Accident caused by firearm, and air gun missile

E922.0 Handgun

Pistol	Revolver

> EXCLUDES   *Verey pistol (E922.8)*

E922.1 Shotgun (automatic)

E922.2 Hunting rifle

E922.3 Military firearms

Army rifle	Machine gun

E922.4 Air gun

BB gun

Pellet gun

E922.5 Paintball gun

E922.8 Other specified firearm missile

Verey pistol [flare]

E922.9 Unspecified firearm missile

Gunshot wound NOS

Shot NOS

✓4ᵗʰ E923 Accident caused by explosive material

> INCLUDES   flash burns and other injuries resulting from explosion of explosive material
> ignition of highly explosive material with explosion
>
> EXCLUDES   *explosion:*
> *in or on machinery (E919.0-E919.9)*
> *on any transport vehicle, except stationary motor vehicle (E800.0-E848)*
> *with conflagration (E890.0, E891.0, E892)*
> *secondary fires resulting from explosion (E890.0-E899)*

E923.0 Fireworks

E923.1 Blasting materials

Blasting cap

Detonator

Dynamite

Explosive [any] used in blasting operations

E923.2 Explosive gases

Acetylene	Fire damp
Butane	Gasoline fumes
Coal gas	Methane
Explosion in mine NOS	Propane

E923.8 Other explosive materials

Bomb	Torpedo
Explosive missile	Explosion in munitions:
Grenade	dump
Mine	factory
Shell	

E923.9 Unspecified explosive material

Explosion NOS

✓4ᵗʰ E924 Accident caused by hot substance or object, caustic or corrosive material, and steam

> EXCLUDES   *burning NOS (E899)*
> *chemical burn resulting from swallowing a corrosive substance (E860.0-E864.4)*
> *fire caused by these substances and objects (E890.0-E894)*
> *radiation burns (E926.0-E926.9)*
> *therapeutic misadventures (E870.0-E876.9)*

E924.0 Hot liquids and vapors, including steam

Burning or scalding by:
- boiling water
- hot or boiling liquids not primarily caustic or corrosive
- liquid metal
- steam
- other hot vapor

> EXCLUDES   *hot (boiling) tap water (E924.2)*

E924.1 Caustic and corrosive substances

Burning by:	Burning by:
acid [any kind]	corrosive substance
ammonia	lye
caustic oven cleaner	vitriol
or other substance	

E924.2 Hot (boiling) tap water

E924.8 Other

Burning by:
- heat from electric heating appliance
- hot object NOS
- light bulb
- steam pipe

E924.9 Unspecified

✓4ᵗʰ E925 Accident caused by electric current

> INCLUDES   electric current from exposed wire, faulty appliance, high voltage cable, live rail, or open electric socket as the cause of:
> - burn
> - cardiac fibrillation
> - convulsion
> - electric shock
> - electrocution
> - puncture wound
> - respiratory paralysis
>
> EXCLUDES   *burn by heat from electrical appliance (E924.8)*
> *lightning (E907)*

E925.0 Domestic wiring and appliances

E925.1 Electric power generating plants, distribution stations, transmission lines

Broken power line

E925.2 Industrial wiring, appliances, and electrical machinery

Conductors	Electrical equipment and
Control apparatus	machinery
	Transformers

E925.8 Other electric current

Wiring and appliances in or on:
- farm [not farmhouse]
- outdoors
- public building
- residential institutions
- schools

▨4ᵗʰ Fourth-digit Required   ▶◀ Revised Text   ● New Code   ▲ Revised Code Title

E925.9 **Unspecified electric current**
  Burns or other injury from electric current NOS
  Electric shock NOS
  Electrocution NOS

✓4ᵗʰ **E926 Exposure to radiation**
  EXCLUDES *abnormal reaction to or complication of*
      treatment without mention of
      misadventure (E879.2)
    atomic power plant malfunction in water
      transport (E838.0-E838.9)
    misadventure to patient in surgical and medical
      procedures (E873.2-E873.3)
    use of radiation in war operations (E996-
      E997.9)

  E926.0 **Radiofrequency radiation**
    Overexposure to: from:
      microwave   high-powered radio and
        radiation   television
      radar radiation   transmitters
      radiofrequency   industrial
      radiofrequency   radiofrequency
        radiation   induction heaters
        [any]   radar installations

  E926.1 **Infrared heaters and lamps**
    Exposure to infrared radiation from heaters and
      lamps as the cause of:
      blistering
      burning
      charring
      inflammatory change
    EXCLUDES *physical contact with heater or lamp*
        (E924.8)

  E926.2 **Visible and ultraviolet light sources**
    Arc lamps   Oxygas welding torch
    Black light sources   Sun rays
    Electrical welding arc Tanning bed
    EXCLUDES *excessive heat from these sources*
        (E900.1-E900.9)

  E926.3 **X-rays and other electromagnetic ionizing radiation**
    Gamma rays   X-rays (hard) (soft)

  E926.4 **Lasers**

  E926.5 **Radioactive isotopes**
    Radiobiologicals   Radiopharmaceuticals

  E926.8 **Other specified radiation**
    Artificially accelerated beams of ionized particles
      generated by:
      betatrons
      synchrotrons

  E926.9 **Unspecified radiation**
    Radiation NOS

E927 Overexertion and strenuous movements
  Excessive physical exercise Strenuous movements in:
  Overexertion (from):   recreational activities
    lifting   other activities
    pulling
    pushing

✓4ᵗʰ **E928 Other and unspecified environmental and accidental causes**
  E928.0 **Prolonged stay in weightless environment**
    Weightlessness in spacecraft (simulator)

  E928.1 **Exposure to noise**
    Noise (pollution)   Supersonic waves
    Sound waves

  E928.2 **Vibration**

  E928.3 **Human bite**

  E928.4 **External constriction caused by hair**

  E928.5 **External constriction caused by other object**

  E928.8 **Other**

E928.9 **Unspecified accident**
  Accident NOS
  Blow NOS   stated as accidentally
  Casualty (not due to war)   inflicted
  Decapitation

  Knocked down
  Killed   stated as accidentally
  Injury [any part of body,   inflicted, but
    or unspecified]   not otherwise
  Mangled   specified
  Wound
  EXCLUDES *fracture, cause unspecified (E887)*
      injuries undetermined whether
        accidentally or purposely inflicted
        (E980.0-E989)

LATE EFFECTS OF ACCIDENTAL INJURY (E929)

Note: This category is to be used to indicate accidental injury
  as the cause of death or disability from late effects,
  which are themselves classifiable elsewhere. The "late
  effects" include conditions reported as such, or as
  sequelae which may occur at any time after the
  attempted suicide or self-inflicted injury.

✓4ᵗʰ **E929 Late effects of accidental injury**
  EXCLUDES *late effects of:*
      surgical and medical procedures (E870.0-
        E879.9)
      therapeutic use of drugs and medicines
        (E930.0-E949.9)

  E929.0 **Late effects of motor vehicle accident**
    Late effects of accidents classifiable to E810-E825

  E929.1 **Late effects of other transport accident**
    Late effects of accidents classifiable to E800-E807,
      E826-E838, E840-E848

  E929.2 **Late effects of accidental poisoning**
    Late effects of accidents classifiable to E850-E858,
      E860-E869

  E929.3 **Late effects of accidental fall**
    Late effects of accidents classifiable to E880-E888

  E929.4 **Late effects of accident caused by fire**
    Late effects of accidents classifiable to E890-E899

  E929.5 **Late effects of accident due to natural and
    environmental factors**
    Late effects of accidents classifiable to E900-E909

  E929.8 **Late effects of other accidents**
    Late effects of accidents classifiable to E910-E928.8

  E929.9 **Late effects of unspecified accident**
    Late effects of accidents classifiable to E928.9

DRUGS, MEDICINAL AND BIOLOGICAL SUBSTANCES CAUSING ADVERSE EFFECTS IN THERAPEUTIC USE (E930-E949)

  INCLUDES correct drug properly administered in
      therapeutic or prophylactic dosage, as
      the cause of any adverse effect including
      allergic or hypersensitivity reactions
  EXCLUDES *accidental overdose of drug and wrong drug*
      given or taken in error (E850.0-E858.9)
    accidents in the technique of administration of
      drug or biological substance, such as
      accidental puncture during injection, or
      contamination of drug (E870.0-E876.9)
    administration with suicidal or homicidal intent
      or intent to harm, or in circumstances
      classifiable to E980-E989 (E950.0-E950.5,
      E962.0, E980.0-E980.5)

  See Alphabetic Index for more complete list of specific
  drugs to be classified under the fourth-digit subdivisions.
  The American Hospital Formulary numbers can be used to
  classify new drugs listed by the American Hospital
  Formulary Service (AHFS). See Appendix C.

✓4ᵗʰ **E930 Antibiotics**
  EXCLUDES *that used as eye, ear, nose, and throat [ENT],*
      and local anti-infectives (E946.0-E946.9)

✓4ᵗʰ Fourth-digit Required   ▶◀ Revised Text   ● New Code   ▲ Revised Code Title

E Codes

E930.0–E934.4

E930.0 Penicillins
Natural
Synthetic
Semisynthetic, such as:
  ampicillin
Semisynthetic, such as:
  cloxacillin
  nafcillin
  oxacillin

E930.1 Antifungal antibiotics
Amphotericin B
Griseofulvin
Hachimycin [trichomycin]
Nystatin

E930.2 Chloramphenicol group
Chloramphenicol
Thiamphenicol

E930.3 Erythromycin and other macrolides
Oleandomycin
Spiramycin

E930.4 Tetracycline group
Doxycycline
Minocycline
Oxytetracycline

E930.5 Cephalosporin group
Cephalexin
Cephaloglycin
Cephaloridine
Cephalothin

E930.6 Antimycobacterial antibiotics
Cycloserine
Kanamycin
Rifampin
Streptomycin

E930.7 Antineoplastic antibiotics
Actinomycins, such as:
  Bleomycin
  Cactinomycin
  Dactinomycin
Actinomycins, such as:
  Daunorubicin
  Mitomycin
EXCLUDES *other antineoplastic drugs (E933.1)*

E930.8 Other specified antibiotics
E930.9 Unspecified antibiotic
✓4th **E931 Other anti-infectives**
EXCLUDES *ENT, and local anti-infectives (E946.0-E946.9)*

E931.0 Sulfonamides
Sulfadiazine
Sulfafurazole
Sulfamethoxazole

E931.1 Arsenical anti-infectives
E931.2 Heavy metal anti-infectives
Compounds of:
  antimony
  bismuth
Compounds of:
  lead
  mercury
EXCLUDES *mercurial diuretics (E944.0)*

E931.3 Quinoline and hydroxyquinoline derivatives
Chiniofon
Diiodohydroxyquin
EXCLUDES *antimalarial drugs (E931.4)*

E931.4 Antimalarials and drugs acting on other blood protozoa
Chloroquine phosphate
Cycloguanil
Primaquine
Proguanil [chloroguanide]
Pyrimethamine
Quinine (sulphate)

E931.5 Other antiprotozoal drugs
Emetine

E931.6 Anthelmintics
Hexylresorcinol
Male fern oleoresin
Piperazine
Thiabendazole

E931.7 Antiviral drugs
Methisazone
EXCLUDES *amantadine (E936.4)*
cytarabine (E933.1)
idoxuridine (E946.5)

E931.8 Other antimycobacterial drugs
Ethambutol
Ethionamide
Isoniazid
Para-aminosalicylic
  acid derivatives
Sulfones

E931.9 Other and unspecified anti-infectives
Flucytosine
Nitrofuranderivatives

✓4th **E932 Hormones and synthetic substitutes**
E932.0 Adrenal cortical steroids
Cortisone derivatives
Desoxycorticosterone derivatives
Fluorinated corticosteroid

E932.1 Androgens and anabolic congeners
Nandrolone phenpropionate
Oxymetholone
Testosterone and preparations

E932.2 Ovarian hormones and synthetic substitutes
Contraceptives, oral
Estrogens
Estrogens and progestogens combined
Progestogens

E932.3 Insulins and antidiabetic agents
Acetohexamide
Biguanide derivatives, oral
Chlorpropamide
Glucagon
Insulin
Phenformin
Sulfonylurea
  derivatives,
  oral
Tolbutamide
EXCLUDES *adverse effect of insulin administered for shock therapy (E879.3)*

E932.4 Anterior pituitary hormones
Corticotropin
Gonadotropin
Somatotropin [growth hormone]

E932.5 Posterior pituitary hormones
Vasopressin
EXCLUDES *oxytocic agents (E945.0)*

E932.6 Parathyroid and parathyroid derivatives
E932.7 Thyroid and thyroid derivatives
Dextrothyroxine
Levothyroxine sodium
Liothyronine
Thyroglobulin

E932.8 Antithyroid agents
Iodides
Thiouracil
Thiourea

E932.9 Other and unspecified hormones and synthetic substitutes
✓4th **E933 Primarily systemic agents**
E933.0 Antiallergic and antiemetic drugs
Antihistamines
Chlorpheniramine
Diphenhydramine
Diphenylpyraline
Thonzylamine
Tripelennamine
EXCLUDES *phenothiazine-based tranquilizers (E939.1)*

E933.1 Antineoplastic and immunosuppressive drugs
Azathioprine
Busulfan
Chlorambucil
Cyclophosphamide
Cytarabine
Fluorouracil
Mechlorethamine hydrochloride
Mercaptopurine
Triethylenethiophosphoramide [thio-TEPA]
EXCLUDES *antineoplastic antibiotics (E930.7)*

E933.2 Acidifying agents
E933.3 Alkalizing agents
E933.4 Enzymes, not elsewhere classified
Penicillinase

E933.5 Vitamins, not elsewhere classified
Vitamin A
Vitamin D
EXCLUDES *nicotinic acid (E942.2)*
vitamin K (E934.3)

E933.8 Other systemic agents, not elsewhere classified
Heavy metal antagonists

E933.9 Unspecified systemic agent
✓4th **E934 Agents primarily affecting blood constituents**
E934.0 Iron and its compounds
Ferric salts
Ferrous sulphate and other ferrous salts

E934.1 Liver preparations and other antianemic agents
Folic acid

E934.2 Anticoagulants
Coumarin
Heparin
Phenindione
Prothrombin synthesis
  inhibitor
Warfarin sodium

E934.3 Vitamin K [phytonadione]
E934.4 Fibrinolysis-affecting drugs
Aminocaproic acid
Streptodornase
Streptokinase
Urokinase

✓4th Fourth-digit Required   ►◄ Revised Text   ● New Code   ▲ Revised Code Title

E934.5 Anticoagulant antagonists and other coagulants
Hexadimethrine bromide
Protamine sulfate

E934.6 Gamma globulin

E934.7 Natural blood and blood products
Blood plasma   Packed red cells
Human fibrinogen   Whole blood

E934.8 Other agents affecting blood constituents
Macromolecular blood substitutes

E934.9 Unspecified agent affecting blood constituents

✓4ᵗʰ **E935 Analgesics, antipyretics, and antirheumatics**

E935.0 Heroin
Diacetylmorphine

E935.1 Methadone

E935.2 Other opiates and related narcotics
Codeine [methylmorphine]   Morphine
Meperidine [pethidine]   Opium (alkaloids)

E935.3 Salicylates
Acetylsalicylic acid [aspirin]
Amino derivatives of salicylic acid
Salicylic acid salts

E935.4 Aromatic analgesics, not elsewhere classified
Acetanilid
Paracetamol [acetaminophen]
Phenacetin [acetophenetidin]

E935.5 Pyrazole derivatives
Aminophenazone [aminopyrine]
Phenylbutazone

E935.6 Antirheumatics [antiphlogistics]
Gold salts   Indomethacin
EXCLUDES   *salicylates (E935.3)*
             steroids (E932.0)

E935.7 Other non-narcotic analgesics
Pyrabital

E935.8 Other specified analgesics and antipyretics
Pentazocine

E935.9 Unspecified analgesic and antipyretic

✓4ᵗʰ **E936 Anticonvulsants and anti-Parkinsonism drugs**

E936.0 Oxazolidine derivatives
Paramethadione
Trimethadione

E936.1 Hydantoin derivatives
Phenytoin

E936.2 Succinimides
Ethosuximide
Phensuximide

E936.3 Other and unspecified anticonvulsants
Beclamide
Primidone

E936.4 Anti-Parkinsonism drugs
Amantadine
Ethopropazine [profenamine]
Levodopa [L-dopa]

✓4ᵗʰ **E937 Sedatives and hypnotics**

E937.0 Barbiturates
Amobarbital [amylobarbitone]
Barbital [barbitone]
Butabarbital [butabarbitone]
Pentobarbital [pentobarbitone]
Phenobarbital [phenobarbitone]
Secobarbital [quinalbarbitone]
EXCLUDES   *thiobarbiturates (E938.3)*

E937.1 Chloral hydrate group

E937.2 Paraldehyde

E937.3 Bromine compounds
Bromide
Carbromal (derivatives)

E937.4 Methaqualone compounds

E937.5 Glutethimide group

E937.6 Mixed sedatives, not elsewhere classified

E937.8 Other sedatives and hypnotics

E937.9 Unspecified
Sleeping:
drug
pill   } NOS
tablet

✓4ᵗʰ **E938 Other central nervous system depressants and anesthetics**

E938.0 Central nervous system muscle-tone depressants
Chlorphenesin (carbamate)
Mephenesin
Methocarbamol

E938.1 Halothane

E938.2 Other gaseous anesthetics
Ether
Halogenated hydrocarbon derivatives, except
     halothane
Nitrous oxide

E938.3 Intravenous anesthetics
Ketamine
Methohexital [methohexitone]
Thiobarbiturates, such as thiopental sodium

E938.4 Other and unspecified general anesthetics

E938.5 Surface and infiltration anesthetics
Cocaine   Procaine
Lidocaine [lignocaine]   Tetracaine

E938.6 Peripheral nerve- and plexus-blocking anesthetics

E938.7 Spinal anesthetics

E938.9 Other and unspecified local anesthetics

✓4ᵗʰ **E939 Psychotropic agents**

E939.0 Antidepressants
Amitriptyline
Imipramine
Monoamine oxidase [MAO] inhibitors

E939.1 Phenothiazine-based tranquilizers
Chlorpromazine   Prochlorperazine
Fluphenazine   Promazine
Phenothiazine

E939.2 Butyrophenone-based tranquilizers
Haloperidol   Trifluperidol
Spiperone

E939.3 Other antipsychotics, neuroleptics, and major tranquilizers

E939.4 Benzodiazepine-based tranquilizers
Chlordiazepoxide   Lorazepam
Diazepam   Medazepam
Flurazepam   Nitrazepam

E939.5 Other tranquilizers
Hydroxyzine   Meprobamate

E939.6 Psychodysleptics [hallucinogens]
Cannabis (derivatives)   Mescaline
Lysergide [LSD]   Psilocin
Marihuana (derivatives)   Psilocybin

E939.7 Psychostimulants
Amphetamine   Caffeine
EXCLUDES   *central appetite depressants (E947.0)*

E939.8 Other psychotropic agents

E939.9 Unspecified psychotropic agent

✓4ᵗʰ **E940 Central nervous system stimulants**

E940.0 Analeptics
Lobeline   Nikethamide

E940.1 Opiate antagonists
Levallorphan   Naloxone
Nalorphine

E940.8 Other specified central nervous system stimulants

E940.9 Unspecified central nervous system stimulant

✓4ᵗʰ **E941 Drugs primarily affecting the autonomic nervous system**

E941.0 Parasympathomimetics [cholinergics]
Acetylcholine
Anticholinesterase:
     organophosphorus
     reversible
Pilocarpine

✓4ᵗʰ Fourth-digit Required   ▶◀ Revised Text   ● New Code   ▲ Revised Code Title

E941.1 Parasympatholytics [anticholinergics and antimuscarinics] and spasmolytics

Atropine	Hyoscine [scopolamine]
Homatropine	Quaternary ammonium derivatives

     EXCLUDES   papaverine (E942.5)

E941.2 Sympathomimetics [adrenergics]

     Epinephrine [adrenalin]   Levarterenol [noradrenalin]

E941.3 Sympatholytics [antiadrenergics]

     Phenoxybenzamine
     Tolazolinehydrochloride

E941.9 Unspecified drug primarily affecting the autonomic nervous system

✓4th **E942 Agents primarily affecting the cardiovascular system**

E942.0 Cardiac rhythm regulators

Practolol	Propranolol
Procainamide	Quinidine

E942.1 Cardiotonic glycosides and drugs of similar action

Digitalis glycosides	Strophanthins
Digoxin	

E942.2 Antilipemic and antiarteriosclerotic drugs

Cholestyramine	Nicotinic acid derivatives
Clofibrate	Sitosterols

     EXCLUDES   dextrothyroxine (E932.7)

E942.3 Ganglion-blocking agents

     Pentamethonium bromide

E942.4 Coronary vasodilators

Dipyridamole	Nitrites
Nitrates [nitroglycerin]	Prenylamine

E942.5 Other vasodilators

Cyclandelate	Hydralazine
Diazoxide	Papaverine

E942.6 Other antihypertensive agents

Clonidine	Rauwolfia alkaloids
Guanethidine	Reserpine

E942.7 Antivaricose drugs, including sclerosing agents

     Monoethanolamine   Zinc salts

E942.8 Capillary-active drugs

     Adrenochrome derivatives
     Bioflavonoids
     Metaraminol

E942.9 Other and unspecified agents primarily affecting the cardiovascular system

✓4th **E943 Agents primarily affecting gastrointestinal system**

E943.0 Antacids and antigastric secretion drugs

     Aluminum hydroxide
     Magnesium trisilicate

E943.1 Irritant cathartics

Bisacodyl	Phenolphthalein
Castor oil	

E943.2 Emollient cathartics

     Sodium dioctyl sulfosuccinate

E943.3 Other cathartics, including intestinal atonia drugs

     Magnesium sulfate

E943.4 Digestants

Pancreatin	Pepsin
Papain	

E943.5 Antidiarrheal drugs

     Bismuth subcarbonatePectin
     Kaolin

     EXCLUDES   anti-infectives (E930.0-E931.9)

E943.6 Emetics

E943.8 Other specified agents primarily affecting the gastrointestinal system

E943.9 Unspecified agent primarily affecting the gastrointestinal system

✓4th **E944 Water, mineral, and uric acid metabolism drugs**

E944.0 Mercurial diuretics

Chlormerodrin	Mercurophylline
Mercaptomerin	Mersalyl

E944.1 Purine derivative diuretics

     Theobromine   Theophylline

     EXCLUDES   aminophylline [theophylline ethylenediamine] (E945.7)

E944.2 Carbonic acid anhydrase inhibitors

     Acetazolamide

E944.3 Saluretics

     Benzothiadiazides   Chlorothiazide group

E944.4 Other diuretics

     Ethacrynic acid   Furosemide

E944.5 Electrolytic, caloric, and water-balance agents

E944.6 Other mineral salts, not elsewhere classified

E944.7 Uric acid metabolism drugs

Cinchophen and congeners	Phenoquin
Colchicine	Probenecid

✓4th **E945 Agents primarily acting on the smooth and skeletal muscles and respiratory system**

E945.0 Oxytocic agents

     Ergot alkaloids
     Prostaglandins

E945.1 Smooth muscle relaxants

     Adiphenine
     Metaproterenol [orciprenaline]

     EXCLUDES   papaverine (E942.5)

E945.2 Skeletal muscle relaxants

     Alcuronium chloride
     Suxamethonium chloride

E945.3 Other and unspecified drugs acting on muscles

E945.4 Antitussives

     Dextromethorphan   Pipazethate hydrochloride

E945.5 Expectorants

Acetylcysteine	Ipecacuanha
Cocillana	Terpin hydrate
Guaifenesin [glyceryl guaiacolate]	

E945.6 Anti-common cold drugs

E945.7 Antiasthmatics

     Aminophylline [theophylline ethylenediamine]

E945.8 Other and unspecified respiratory drugs

✓4th **E946 Agents primarily affecting skin and mucous membrane, ophthalmological, otorhinolaryngological, and dental drugs**

E946.0 Local anti-infectives and anti-inflammatory drugs

E946.1 Antipruritics

E946.2 Local astringents and local detergents

E946.3 Emollients, demulcents, and protectants

E946.4 Keratolytics, kerstoplastics, other hair treatment drugs and preparations

E946.5 Eye anti-infectives and other eye drugs

     Idoxuridine

E946.6 Anti-infectives and other drugs and preparations for ear, nose, and throat

E946.7 Dental drugs topically applied

E946.8 Other agents primarily affecting skin and mucous membrane

     Spermicides

E946.9 Unspecified agent primarily affecting skin and mucous membrane

✓4th **E947 Other and unspecified drugs and medicinal substances**

E947.0 Dietetics

E947.1 Lipotropic drugs

E947.2 Antidotes and chelating agents, not elsewhere classified

E947.3 Alcohol deterrents

E947.4 Pharmaceutical excipients

E947.8 Other drugs and medicinal substances

     Contrast media used for diagnostic x-ray procedures
     Diagnostic agents and kits

E947.9 Unspecified drug or medicinal substance

✓4th **E948 Bacterial vaccines**

E948.0 BCG vaccine

✓4th Fourth-digit Required   ▶◀ Revised Text   ● New Code   ▲ Revised Code Title

E948.1 Typhoid and paratyphoid

E948.2 Cholera

E948.3 Plague

E948.4 Tetanus

E948.5 Diphtheria

E948.6 Pertussis vaccine, including combinations with a pertussis component

E948.8 Other and unspecified bacterial vaccines

E948.9 Mixed bacterial vaccines, except combinations with a pertussis component

√4th E949 Other vaccines and biological substances
> EXCLUDES   *gamma globulin (E934.6)*

E949.0 Smallpox vaccine

E949.1 Rabies vaccine

E949.2 Typhus vaccine

E949.3 Yellow fever vaccine

E949.4 Measles vaccine

E949.5 Poliomyelitis vaccine

E949.6 Other and unspecified viral and rickettsial vaccines
> Mumps vaccine

E949.7 Mixed viral-rickettsial and bacterial vaccines, except combinations with a pertussis component
> EXCLUDES   *combinations with a pertussis component (E948.6)*

E949.9 Other and unspecified vaccines and biological substances

SUICIDE AND SELF-INFLICTED INJURY (E950-E959)
> INCLUDES   injuries in suicide and attempted suicide
> self-inflicted injuries specified as intentional

√4th E950 Suicide and self-inflicted poisoning by solid or liquid substances

E950.0 Analgesics, antipyretics, and antirheumatics

E950.1 Barbiturates

E950.2 Other sedatives and hypnotics

E950.3 Tranquilizers and other psychotropic agents

E950.4 Other specified drugs and medicinal substances

E950.5 Unspecified drug or medicinal substance

E950.6 Agricultural and horticultural chemical and pharmaceutical preparations other than plant foods and fertilizers

E950.7 Corrosive and caustic substances
> Suicide and self-inflicted poisoning by substances
> classifiable to E864

E950.8 Arsenic and its compounds

E950.9 Other and unspecified solid and liquid substances

√4th E951 Suicide and self-inflicted poisoning by gases in domestic use

E951.0 Gas distributed by pipeline

E951.1 Liquefied petroleum gas distributed in mobile containers

E951.8 Other utility gas

√4th E952 Suicide and self-inflicted poisoning by other gases and vapors

E952.0 Motor vehicle exhaust gas

E952.1 Other carbon monoxide

E952.8 Other specified gases and vapors

E952.9 Unspecified gases and vapors

√4th E953 Suicide and self-inflicted injury by hanging, strangulation, and suffocation

E953.0 Hanging

E953.1 Suffocation by plastic bag

E953.8 Other specified means

E953.9 Unspecified means

E954 Suicide and self-inflicted injury by submersion [drowning]

√4th E955 Suicide and self-inflicted injury by firearms, air guns and explosives

E955.0 Handgun

E955.1 Shotgun

E955.2 Hunting rifle

E955.3 Military firearms

E955.4 Other and unspecified firearm
> Gunshot NOS   Shot NOS

E955.5 Explosives

E955.6 Air gun
> BB gun   Pellet gun

E955.7 Paintball gun

E955.9 Unspecified

E956 Suicide and self-inflicted injury by cutting and piercing instrument

√4th E957 Suicide and self-inflicted injuries by jumping from high place

E957.0 Residential premises

E957.1 Other man-made structures

E957.2 Natural sites

E957.9 Unspecified

√4th E958 Suicide and self-inflicted injury by other and unspecified means

E958.0 Jumping or lying before moving object

E958.1 Burns, fire

E958.2 Scald

E958.3 Extremes of cold

E958.4 Electrocution

E958.5 Crashing of motor vehicle

E958.6 Crashing of aircraft

E958.7 Caustic substances, except poisoning
> EXCLUDES   *poisoning by caustic substance
> (E950.7)*

E958.8 Other specified means

E958.9 Unspecified means

E959 Late effects of self-inflicted injury
> Note: This category is to be used to indicate circumstances
> classifiable to E950-E958 as the cause of death or
> disability from late effects, which are themselves
> classifiable elsewhere. The "late effects" include
> conditions reported as such, or as sequelae which may
> occur at any time after the attempted suicide or self-
> inflicted injury.

HOMICIDE AND INJURY PURPOSELY INFLICTED BY OTHER PERSONS (E960-E969)
> INCLUDES   injuries inflicted by another person with intent
> to injure or kill, by any means
> EXCLUDES   *injuries due to:*
> *legal intervention (E970-E978)*
> *operations of war (E990-E999)*
> *terrorism (E979)*

√4th E960 Fight, brawl, rape

E960.0 Unarmed fight or brawl
> Beatings NOS
> Brawl or fight with hands, fists, feet
> Injured or killed in fight NOS
> EXCLUDES   *homicidal:*
> *injury by weapons (E965.0-E966,*
> *E969)*
> *strangulation (E963)*
> *submersion (E964)*

E960.1 Rape

E961 Assault by corrosive or caustic substance, except poisoning
> Injury or death purposely caused by corrosive or caustic
> substance, such as:
> acid [any]
> corrosive substance
> vitriol
> EXCLUDES   *burns from hot liquid (E968.3)*
> *chemical burns from swallowing a corrosive*
> *substance (E962.0-E962.9)*

√4th Fourth-digit Required   ▶◀ Revised Text   ● New Code   ▲ Revised Code Title

E Codes

E962-E978

✓4th **E962 Assault by poisoning**

    E962.0 Drugs and medicinal substances
        Homicidal poisoning by any drug or medicinal substance

    E962.1 Other solid and liquid substances

    E962.2 Other gases and vapors

    E962.9 Unspecified poisoning

E963 Assault by hanging and strangulation

Homicidal (attempt):   Homicidal (attempt):
garrotting or ligature   strangulation
hanging   suffocation

E964 Assault by submersion [drowning]

✓4th **E965 Assault by firearms and explosives**

    E965.0 Handgun
      Pistol   Revolver

    E965.1 Shotgun

    E965.2 Hunting rifle

    E965.3 Military firearms

    E965.4 Other and unspecified firearm

    E965.5 Antipersonnel bomb

    E965.6 Gasoline bomb

    E965.7 Letter bomb

    E965.8 Other specified explosive
      Bomb NOS (placed in):   Dynamite
        car
        house

    E965.9 Unspecified explosive

E966 Assault by cutting and piercing instrument
    Assassination (attempt), homicide (attempt) by any instrument classifiable under E920

Homicidal:
  cut
  puncture } any part of body
  stab
  Stabbed

✓4th **E967 Perpetrator of child and adult abuse**
    Note: Selection of the correct perpetrator code is based on the relationship between the perpetrator and the victim

    E967.0 By father, stepfather, or boyfriend
      Male partner of child's parent or guardian

    E967.1 By other specified person

    E967.2 By mother, stepmother, or girlfriend
      Female partner of child's parent or guardian

    E967.3 By spouse or partner
      Abuse of spouse or partner by ex-spouse or ex-partner

    E967.4 By child

    E967.5 By sibling

    E967.6 By grandparent

    E967.7 By other relative

    E967.8 By non-related caregiver

    E967.9 By unspecified person

✓4th **E968 Assault by other and unspecified means**

    E968.0 Fire
      Arson
      Homicidal burns NOS
      EXCLUDES burns from hot liquid (E968.3)

    E968.1 Pushing from a high place

    E968.2 Striking by blunt or thrown object

    E968.3 Hot liquid
      Homicidal burns by scalding

    E968.4 Criminal neglect
      Abandonment of child, infant, or other helpless person with intent to injure or kill

    E968.5 Transport vehicle
      Being struck by other vehicle or run down with intent to injure
      Pushed in front of, thrown from, or dragged by moving vehicle with intent to injure

    E968.6 Air gun
      BB gun
      Pellet gun

    E968.7 Human bite

    E968.8 Other specified means

    E968.9 Unspecified means
      Assassination (attempt) NOS
      Homicidal (attempt):
        injury NOS
        wound NOS
      Manslaughter (nonaccidental)
      Murder (attempt) NOS
      Violence, non-accidental

E969 Late effects of injury purposely inflicted by other person
    Note: This category is to be used to indicate circumstances classifiable to E960-E968 as the cause of death or disability from late effects, which are themselves classifiable elsewhere. The "late effects" include conditions reported as such, or as sequelae which may occur at any time after injury purposely inflicted by another person.

LEGAL INTERVENTION (E970-E978)

INCLUDES injuries inflicted by the police or other law-enforcing agents, including military on duty, in the course of arresting or attempting to arrest lawbreakers, suppressing disturbances, maintaining order, and other legal action
legal execution

EXCLUDES injuries caused by civil insurrections (E990.0-E999)

E970 Injury due to legal intervention by firearms
  Gunshot wound   Injury by:
  Injury by: rifle pellet or
    machine gun   rubber bullet
    revolver   shot NOS

E971 Injury due to legal intervention by explosives
  Injury by: Injury by:
    dynamite   grenade
    explosive shell   mortar bomb

E972 Injury due to legal intervention by gas
  Asphyxiation by gas   Poisoning by gas
  Injury by tear gas

E973 Injury due to legal intervention by blunt object
  Hit, struck by: Hit, struck by:
    baton (nightstick)   stave
    blunt object

E974 Injury due to legal intervention by cutting and piercing instrument
  Cut   Injured by bayonet
  Incised wound   Stab wound

E975 Injury due to legal intervention by other specified means
  Blow   Manhandling

E976 Injury due to legal intervention by unspecified means

E977 Late effects of injuries due to legal intervention
    Note: This category is to be used to indicate circumstances classifiable to E970-E976 as the cause of death or disability from late effects, which are themselves classifiable elsewhere. The "late effects" include conditions reported as such, or as sequelae, which may occur at any time after the injury due to legal intervention.

E978 Legal execution
    All executions performed at the behest of the judiciary or ruling authority [whether permanent or temporary] as:
  asphyxiation by gas
  beheading, decapitation (by guillotine)
  capital punishment
  electrocution
  hanging
  poisoning
  shooting
  other specified means

TERRORISM (E979)

✓4ᵗʰ E979 Terrorism

> Injuries resulting from the unlawful use of force or violence against persons or property to intimidate or coerce a Government, the civilian population, or any segment thereof, in furtherance of political or social objective

E979.0 Terrorism involving explosion of marine weapons
> Depth-charge
> Marine mine
> Mine NOS, at sea or in harbour
> Sea-based artillery shell
> Torpedo
> Underwater blast

E979.1 Terrorism involving destruction of aircraft
> Aircraft used as a weapon
> Aircraft:
>> burned
>> exploded
>> shot down
> Crushed by falling aircraft

E979.2 Terrorism involving other explosions and fragments
> Antipersonnel bomb (fragments)
> Blast NOS
> Explosion (of):
>> artillery shell
>> breech-block
>> cannon block
>> mortar bomb
>> munitions being used in terrorism
>> NOS
> Fragments from:
>> artillery shell
>> bomb
>> grenade
>> guided missile
>> land-mine
>> rocket
>> shell
>> shrapnel
> Mine NOS

E979.3 Terrorism involving fires, conflagration and hot substances
> Burning building or structure:
>> collapse of
>> fall from
>> hit by falling object in
>> jump from
> Conflagration NOS
> Fire (causing):
>> Asphyxia
>> Burns
>> NOS
>> Other injury
> Melting of fittings and furniture in burning
> Petrol bomb
> Smouldering building or structure

E979.4 Terrorism involving firearms
> Bullet:
>> carbine
>> machine gun
>> pistol
>> rifle
>> rubber (rifle)
> Pellets (shotgun)

E979.5 Terrorism involving nuclear weapons
> Blast effects
> Exposure to ionizing radiation from nuclear weapon
> Fireball effects
> Heat from nuclear weapon
> Other direct and secondary effects of nuclear weapons

E979.6 Terrorism involving biological weapons
> Anthrax
> Cholera
> Smallpox

E979.7 Terrorism involving chemical weapons
> Gases, fumes, chemicals
> Hydrogen cyanide
> Phosgene
> Sarin

E979.8 Terrorism involving other means
> Drowning and submersion
> Lasers
> Piercing or stabbing instruments
> Terrorism NOS

E979.9 Terrorism, secondary effects
> Note: This code is for use to identify conditions occurring subsequent to a terrorist attack not those that are due to the initial terrorist act
>
> **EXCLUDES**   *late effect of terrorist attack (E999.1)*

INJURY UNDETERMINED WHETHER ACCIDENTALLY OR PURPOSELY INFLICTED (E980-E989)

> Note: Categories E980-E989 are for use when it is unspecified or it cannot be determined whether the injuries are accidental (unintentional), suicide (attempted), or assault.

✓4ᵗʰ E980 Poisoning by solid or liquid substances, undetermined whether accidentally or purposely inflicted
> **E980.0 Analgesics, antipyretics, and antirheumatics**
> **E980.1 Barbiturates**
> **E980.2 Other sedatives and hypnotics**
> **E980.3 Tranquilizers and other psychotropic agents**
> **E980.4 Other specified drugs and medicinal substances**
> **E980.5 Unspecified drug or medicinal substance**
> **E980.6 Corrosive and caustic substances**
>> Poisoning, undetermined whether accidental or purposeful, by substances classifiable to E864
> **E980.7 Agricultural and horticultural chemical and pharmaceutical preparations other than plant foods and fertilizers**
> **E980.8 Arsenic and its compounds**
> **E980.9 Other and unspecified solid and liquid substances**

✓4ᵗʰ E981 Poisoning by gases in domestic use, undetermined whether accidentally or purposely inflicted
> **E981.0 Gas distributed by pipeline**
> **E981.1 Liquefied petroleum gas distributed in mobile containers**
> **E981.8 Other utility gas**

✓4ᵗʰ E982 Poisoning by other gases, undetermined whether accidentally or purposely inflicted
> **E982.0 Motor vehicle exhaust gas**
> **E982.1 Other carbon monoxide**
> **E982.8 Other specified gases and vapors**
> **E982.9 Unspecified gases and vapors**

✓4ᵗʰ E983 Hanging, strangulation, or suffocation, undetermined whether accidentally or purposely inflicted
> **E983.0 Hanging**
> **E983.1 Suffocation by plastic bag**
> **E983.8 Other specified means**
> **E983.9 Unspecified means**

E984 Submersion [drowning], undetermined whether accidentally or purposely inflicted

✓4ᵗʰ E985 Injury by firearms, air guns and explosives, undetermined whether accidentally or purposely inflicted
> **E985.0 Handgun**
> **E985.1 Shotgun**
> **E985.2 Hunting rifle**
> **E985.3 Military firearms**
> **E985.4 Other and unspecified firearm**
> **E985.5 Explosives**
> **E985.6 Air gun**
>> BB gun   Pellet gun
> **E985.7 Paintball gun**

✓4ᵗʰ Fourth-digit Required   ◄► Revised Text   ● New Code   ▲ Revised Code Title

E986 Injury by cutting and piercing instruments, undetermined whether accidentally or purposely inflicted

✓4ᵗʰ **E987 Falling from high place, undetermined whether accidentally or purposely inflicted**

    E987.0 Residential premises

    E987.1 Other man-made structures

    E987.2 Natural sites

    E987.9 Unspecified site

✓4ᵗʰ **E988 Injury by other and unspecified means, undetermined whether accidentally or purposely inflicted**

    E988.0 Jumping or lying before moving object

    E988.1 Burns, fire

    E988.2 Scald

    E988.3 Extremes of cold

    E988.4 Electrocution

    E988.5 Crashing of motor vehicle

    E988.6 Crashing of aircraft

    E988.7 Caustic substances, except poisoning

    E988.8 Other specified means

    E988.9 Unspecified means

E989 Late effects of injury, undetermined whether accidentally or purposely inflicted

Note: This category is to be used to indicate circumstances classifiable to E980-E988 as the cause of death or disability from late effects, which are themselves classifiable elsewhere. The "late effects" include conditions reported as such, or as sequelae, which may occur at any time after injury, undetermined whether accidentally or purposely inflicted.

INJURY RESULTING FROM OPERATIONS OF WAR (E990-E999)

INCLUDES injuries to military personnel and civilians caused by war and civil insurrections and occurring during the time of war and insurrection

EXCLUDES *accidents during training of military personnel manufacture of war material and transport, unless attributable to enemy action*

✓4ᵗʰ **E990 Injury due to war operations by fires and conflagrations**

INCLUDES asphyxia, burns, or other injury originating from fire caused by a fire-producing device or indirectly by any conventional weapon

    E990.0 From gasoline bomb

    E990.9 From other and unspecified source

✓4ᵗʰ **E991 Injury due to war operations by bullets and fragments**

    E991.0 Rubber bullets (rifle)

    E991.1 Pellets (rifle)

    E991.2 Other bullets

      Bullet [any, except rubber bullets and pellets]
        carbine
        machine gun
        pistol
        rifle
        shotgun

    E991.3 Antipersonnel bomb (fragments)

    E991.9 Other and unspecified fragments

Fragments from:	Fragments from:
artillery shell	land mine
bombs, except anti-personnel	rockets
grenade	shell
guided missile	Shrapnel

E992 Injury due to war operations by explosion of marine weapons

Depth charge	Sea-based artillery shell
Marine mines	Torpedo
Mine NOS, at sea or in harbor	Underwater blast

E993 Injury due to war operations by other explosion

Accidental explosion of munitions being used in war	Explosion of: artillery shell breech block
Accidental explosion of own weapons	cannon block mortar bomb
Air blast NOS	Injury by weapon burst
Blast NOS	
Explosion NOS	

E994 Injury due to war operations by destruction of aircraft

Airplane: burned exploded	Airplane: shot down Crushed by falling airplane

E995 Injury due to war operations by other and unspecified forms of conventional warfare

Battle wounds
Bayonet injury
Drowned in war operations

E996 Injury due to war operations by nuclear weapons

Blast effects
Exposure to ionizing radiation from nuclear weapons
Fireball effects
Heat
Other direct and secondary effects of nuclear weapons

✓4ᵗʰ **E997 Injury due to war operations by other forms of unconventional warfare**

    E997.0 Lasers

    E997.1 Biological warfare

    E997.2 Gases, fumes, and chemicals

    E997.8 Other specified forms of unconventional warfare

    E997.9 Unspecified form of unconventional warfare

E998 Injury due to war operations but occurring after cessation of hostilities

Injuries due to operations of war but occurring after cessation of hostilities by any means classifiable under E990-E997

Injuries by explosion of bombs or mines placed in the course of operations of war, if the explosion occurred after cessation of hostilities

✓4ᵗʰ **E999 Late effect of injury due to war operations and terrorism**

Note: This category is to be used to indicate circumstances classifiable to E979, E990-E998 as the cause of death or disability from late effects, which are themselves classifiable elsewhere. The "late effects" include conditions reported as such, or as sequelae, which may occur at any time after the injury, resulting from operations of war or terrorism

    E999.0 Late effect of injury due to war operations

    E999.1 Late effect of injury due to terrorism

Official ICD-9-CM Government Appendixes

MORPHOLOGY OF NEOPLASMS

The World Health Organization has published an adaptation of the International Classification of Diseases for oncology (ICD-O). It contains a coded nomenclature for the morphology of neoplasms, which is reproduced here for those who wish to use it in conjunction with Chapter 2 of the International Classification of Diseases, 9th Revision, Clinical Modification.

The morphology code numbers consist of five digits; the first four identify the histological type of the neoplasm and the fifth indicates its behavior. The one-digit behavior code is as follows:

/0   Benign
/1   Uncertain whether benign or malignant
       Borderline malignancy
/2   Carcinoma in situ
       Intraepithelial
       Noninfiltrating
       Noninvasive
/3   Malignant, primary site
/6   Malignant, metastatic site
       Secondary site
/9   Malignant, uncertain whether primary or metastatic site

In the nomenclature below, the morphology code numbers include the behavior code appropriate to the histological type of neoplasm, but this behavior code should be changed if other reported information makes this necessary. For example, "chordoma (M9370/3)" is assumed to be malignant; the term "benign chordoma" should be coded M9370/0. Similarly, "superficial spreading adenocarcinoma (M8143/3)" described as "noninvasive" should be coded M8143/2 and "melanoma (M8720/3)" described as "secondary" should be coded M8720/6.

The following table shows the correspondence between the morphology code and the different sections of Chapter 2:

Morphology Code Histology/Behavior		ICD-9-CM Chapter 2	
Any	0	210-229	Benign neoplasms
M8000- M8004	1	239	Neoplasms of unspecified nature
M8010+	1	235-238	Neoplasms of uncertain behavior
Any	2	230-234	Carcinoma in situ
Any	3	140-195 200-208	Malignant neoplasms, stated or presumed to be primary
Any	6	196-198	Malignant neoplasms, stated or presumed to be secondary

The ICD-O behavior digit /9 is inapplicable in an ICD context, since all malignant neoplasms are presumed to be primary (/3) or secondary (/6) according to other information on the medical record.

Only the first-listed term of the full ICD-O morphology nomenclature appears against each code number in the list below. The ICD-9-CM Alphabetical Index (Volume 2), however, includes all the ICD-O synonyms as well as a number of other morphological names still likely to be encountered on medical records but omitted from ICD-O as outdated or otherwise undesirable.

A coding difficulty sometimes arises where a morphological diagnosis contains two qualifying adjectives that have different code numbers. An example is "transitional cell epidermoid carcinoma." "Transitional cell carcinoma NOS" is M8120/3 and "epidermoid carcinoma NOS" is M8070/3. In such circumstances, the higher number (M8120/3 in this example) should be used, as it is usually more specific.

CODED NOMENCLATURE FOR MORPHOLOGY OF NEOPLASMS

M800   **Neoplasms NOS**
   M8000/0   *Neoplasm, benign*
   M8000/1   *Neoplasm, uncertain whether benign or malignant*
   M8000/3   *Neoplasm, malignant*
   M8000/6   *Neoplasm, metastatic*
   M8000/9   *Neoplasm, malignant, uncertain whether primary or metastatic*
   M8001/0   *Tumor cells, benign*
   M8001/1   *Tumor cells, uncertain whether benign or malignant*
   M8001/3   *Tumor cells, malignant*
   M8002/3   *Malignant tumor, small cell type*
   M8003/3   *Malignant tumor, giant cell type*
   M8004/3   *Malignant tumor, fusiform cell type*
M801-M804   **Epithelial neoplasms NOS**
   M8010/0   *Epithelial tumor, benign*
   M8010/2   *Carcinoma in situ NOS*
   M8010/3   *Carcinoma NOS*
   M8010/6   *Carcinoma, metastatic NOS*
   M8010/9   *Carcinomatosis*
   M8011/0   *Epithelioma, benign*
   M8011/3   *Epithelioma, malignant*
   M8012/3   *Large cell carcinoma NOS*
   M8020/3   *Carcinoma, undifferentiated type NOS*
   M8021/3   *Carcinoma, anaplastic type NOS*
   M8022/3   *Pleomorphic carcinoma*
   M8030/3   *Giant cell and spindle cell carcinoma*
   M8031/3   *Giant cell carcinoma*
   M8032/3   *Spindle cell carcinoma*
   M8033/3   *Pseudosarcomatous carcinoma*
   M8034/3   *Polygonal cell carcinoma*
   M8035/3   *Spheroidal cell carcinoma*
   M8040/1   *Tumorlet*
   M8041/3   *Small cell carcinoma NOS*
   M8042/3   *Oat cell carcinoma*
   M8043/3   *Small cell carcinoma, fusiform cell type*
M805-M808   **Papillary and squamous cell neoplasms**
   M8050/0   *Papilloma NOS (except Papilloma of urinary bladder M8120/1)*
   M8050/2   *Papillary carcinoma in situ*
   M8050/3   *Papillary carcinoma NOS*
   M8051/0   *Verrucous papilloma*
   M8051/3   *Verrucous carcinoma NOS*
   M8052/0   *Squamous cell papilloma*
   M8052/3   *Papillary squamous cell carcinoma*
   M8053/0   *Inverted papilloma*

   M8060/0   *Papillomatosis NOS*
   M8070/2   *Squamous cell carcinoma in situ NOS*
   M8070/3   *Squamous cell carcinoma NOS*
   M8070/6   *Squamous cell carcinoma, metastatic NOS*
   M8071/3   *Squamous cell carcinoma, keratinizing type NOS*
   M8072/3   *Squamous cell carcinoma, large cell, nonkeratinizing type*
   M8073/3   *Squamous cell carcinoma, small cell, nonkeratinizing type*
   M8074/3   *Squamous cell carcinoma, spindle cell type*
   M8075/3   *Adenoid squamous cell carcinoma*
   M8076/2   *Squamous cell carcinoma in situ with questionable stromal invasion*
   M8076/3   *Squamous cell carcinoma, microinvasive*
   M8080/2   *Queyrat's erythroplasia*
   M8081/2   *Bowen's disease*
   M8082/3   *Lymphoepithelial carcinoma*
M809-M811   **Basal cell neoplasms**
   M8090/1   *Basal cell tumor*
   M8090/3   *Basal cell carcinoma NOS*
   M8091/3   *Multicentric basal cell carcinoma*
   M8092/3   *Basal cell carcinoma, morphea type*
   M8093/3   *Basal cell carcinoma, fibroepithelial type*
   M8094/3   *Basosquamous carcinoma*
   M8095/3   *Metatypical carcinoma*
   M8096/0   *Intraepidermal epithelioma of Jadassohn*
   M8100/0   *Trichoepithelioma*
   M8101/0   *Trichofolliculoma*
   M8102/0   *Tricholemmoma*
   M8110/0   *Pilomatrixoma*
M812-M813   **Transitional cell papillomas and carcinomas**
   M8120/0   *Transitional cell papilloma NOS*
   M8120/1   *Urothelial papilloma*
   M8120/2   *Transitional cell carcinoma in situ*
   M8120/3   *Transitional cell carcinoma NOS*
   M8121/0   *Schneiderian papilloma*
   M8121/1   *Transitional cell papilloma, inverted type*
   M8121/3   *Schneiderian carcinoma*
   M8122/3   *Transitional cell carcinoma, spindle cell type*
   M8123/3   *Basaloid carcinoma*
   M8124/3   *Cloacogenic carcinoma*
   M8130/3   *Papillary transitional cell carcinoma*
M814-M838   **Adenomas and adenocarcinomas**
   M8140/0   *Adenoma NOS*
   M8140/1   *Bronchial adenoma NOS*
   M8140/2   *Adenocarcinoma in situ*
   M8140/3   *Adenocarcinoma NOS*
   M8140/6   *Adenocarcinoma, metastatic NOS*
   M8141/3   *Scirrhous adenocarcinoma*
   M8142/3   *Linitis plastica*
   M8143/3   *Superficial spreading adenocarcinoma*
   M8144/3   *Adenocarcinoma, intestinal type*
   M8145/3   *Carcinoma, diffuse type*
   M8146/0   *Monomorphic adenoma*
   M8147/0   *Basal cell adenoma*
   M8150/0   *Islet cell adenoma*
   M8150/3   *Islet cell carcinoma*
   M8151/0   *Insulinoma NOS*
   M8151/3   *Insulinoma, malignant*
   M8152/0   *Glucagonoma NOS*
   M8152/3   *Glucagonoma, malignant*

Appendix A: Morphology of Neoplasms

M8153/1   Gastrinoma NOS
M8153/3   Gastrinoma, malignant
M8154/3   Mixed islet cell and exocrine
          adenocarcinoma
M8160/0   Bile duct adenoma
M8160/3   Cholangiocarcinoma
M8161/0   Bile duct cystadenoma
M8161/3   Bile duct cystadenocarcinoma
M8170/0   Liver cell adenoma
M8170/3   Hepatocellular carcinoma NOS
M8180/0   Hepatocholangioma, benign
M8180/3   Combined hepatocellular carcinoma
          and cholangiocarcinoma
M8190/0   Trabecular adenoma
M8190/3   Trabecular adenocarcinoma
M8191/0   Embryonal adenoma
M8200/0   Eccrine dermal cylindroma
M8200/3   Adenoid cystic carcinoma
M8201/3   Cribriform carcinoma
M8210/0   Adenomatous polyp NOS
M8210/3   Adenocarcinoma in adenomatous
          polyp
M8211/0   Tubular adenoma NOS
M8211/3   Tubular adenocarcinoma
M8220/0   Adenomatous polyposis coli
M8220/3   Adenocarcinoma in adenomatous
          polyposis coli
M8221/0   Multiple adenomatous polyps
M8230/3   Solid carcinoma NOS
M8231/3   Carcinoma simplex
M8240/1   Carcinoid tumor NOS
M8240/3   Carcinoid tumor, malignant
M8241/1   Carcinoid tumor, argentaffin NOS
M8241/3   Carcinoid tumor, argentaffin,
          malignant
M8242/1   Carcinoid tumor, nonargentaffin
          NOS
M8242/3   Carcinoid tumor, nonargentaffin,
          malignant
M8243/3   Mucocarcinoid tumor, malignant
M8244/3   Composite carcinoid
M8250/1   Pulmonary adenomatosis
M8250/3   Bronchiolo-alveolar adenocarcinoma
M8251/0   Alveolar adenoma
M8251/3   Alveolar adenocarcinoma
M8260/0   Papillary adenoma NOS
M8260/3   Papillary adenocarcinoma NOS
M8261/1   Villous adenoma NOS
M8261/3   Adenocarcinoma in villous adenoma
M8262/3   Villous adenocarcinoma
M8263/0   Tubulovillous adenoma
M8270/0   Chromophobe adenoma
M8270/3   Chromophobe carcinoma
M8280/0   Acidophil adenoma
M8280/3   Acidophil carcinoma
M8281/0   Mixed acidophil-basophil adenoma
M8281/3   Mixed acidophil-basophil carcinoma
M8290/0   Oxyphilic adenoma
M8290/3   Oxyphilic adenocarcinoma
M8300/0   Basophil adenoma
M8300/3   Basophil carcinoma
M8310/0   Clear cell adenoma
M8310/3   Clear cell adenocarcinoma NOS
M8311/1   Hypernephroid tumor
M8312/3   Renal cell carcinoma
M8313/0   Clear cell adenofibroma
M8320/3   Granular cell carcinoma
M8321/0   Chief cell adenoma
M8322/0   Water-clear cell adenoma
M8322/3   Water-clear cell adenocarcinoma
M8323/0   Mixed cell adenoma
M8323/3   Mixed cell adenocarcinoma
M8324/0   Lipoadenoma
M8330/0   Follicular adenoma
M8330/3   Follicular adenocarcinoma NOS
M8331/3   Follicular adenocarcinoma, well
          differentiated type

M8332/3   Follicular adenocarcinoma,
          trabecular type
M8333/3   Microfollicular adenoma
M8334/0   Macrofollicular adenoma
M8340/3   Papillary and follicular
          adenocarcinoma
M8350/3   Nonencapsulated sclerosing
          carcinoma
M8360/1   Multiple endocrine adenomas
M8361/1   Juxtaglomerular tumor
M8370/0   Adrenal cortical adenoma NOS
M8370/3   Adrenal cortical carcinoma
M8371/0   Adrenal cortical adenoma, compact
          cell type
M8372/0   Adrenal cortical adenoma, heavily
          pigmented variant
M8373/0   Adrenal cortical adenoma, clear cell
          type
M8374/0   Adrenal cortical adenoma,
          glomerulosa cell type
M8375/0   Adrenal cortical adenoma, mixed
          cell type
M8380/0   Endometrioid adenoma NOS
M8380/1   Endometrioid adenoma, borderline
          malignancy
M8380/3   Endometrioid carcinoma
M8381/0   Endometrioid adenofibroma NOS
M8381/1   Endometrioid adenofibroma,
          borderline malignancy
M8381/3   Endometrioid adenofibroma,
          malignant

**M839-M842   Adnexal and skin appendage
            neoplasms**
M8390/0   Skin appendage adenoma
M8390/3   Skin appendage carcinoma
M8400/0   Sweat gland adenoma
M8400/1   Sweat gland tumor NOS
M8400/3   Sweat gland adenocarcinoma
M8401/0   Apocrine adenoma
M8401/3   Apocrine adenocarcinoma
M8402/0   Eccrine acrospiroma
M8403/0   Eccrine spiradenoma
M8404/0   Hidrocystoma
M8405/0   Papillary hydradenoma
M8406/0   Papillary syringadenoma
M8407/0   Syringoma NOS
M8410/0   Sebaceous adenoma
M8410/3   Sebaceous adenocarcinoma
M8420/0   Ceruminous adenoma
M8420/3   Ceruminous adenocarcinoma

M843   Mucoepidermoid neoplasms
M8430/1   Mucoepidermoid tumor
M8430/3   Mucoepidermoid carcinoma

**M844-M849   Cystic, mucinous, and serous
            neoplasms**
M8440/0   Cystadenoma NOS
M8440/3   Cystadenocarcinoma NOS
M8441/0   Serous cystadenoma NOS
M8441/1   Serous cystadenoma, borderline
          malignancy
M8441/3   Serous cystadenocarcinoma NOS
M8450/0   Papillary cystadenoma NOS
M8450/1   Papillary cystadenoma, borderline
          malignancy
M8450/3   Papillary cystadenocarcinoma NOS
M8460/0   Papillary serous cystadenoma NOS
M8460/1   Papillary serous cystadenoma,
          borderline malignancy
M8460/3   Papillary serous
          cystadenocarcinoma
M8461/0   Serous surface papilloma NOS
M8461/1   Serous surface papilloma,
          borderline malignancy
M8461/3   Serous surface papillary carcinoma
M8470/0   Mucinous cystadenoma NOS
M8470/1   Mucinous cystadenoma, borderline
          malignancy

M8470/3   Mucinous cystadenocarcinoma NOS
M8471/0   Papillary mucinous cystadenoma
          NOS
M8471/1   Papillary mucinous cystadenoma,
          borderline malignancy
M8471/3   Papillary mucinous
          cystadenocarcinoma
M8480/0   Mucinous adenoma
M8480/3   Mucinous adenocarcinoma
M8480/6   Pseudomyxoma peritonei
M8481/3   Mucin-producing adenocarcinoma
M8490/3   Signet ring cell carcinoma
M8490/6   Metastatic signet ring cell
          carcinoma

**M850-M854   Ductal, lobular, and medullary
            neoplasms**
M8500/2   Intraductal carcinoma,
          noninfiltrating NOS
M8500/3   Infiltrating duct carcinoma
M8501/2   Comedocarcinoma, noninfiltrating
M8501/3   Comedocarcinoma NOS
M8502/3   Juvenile carcinoma of the breast
M8503/0   Intraductal papilloma
M8503/2   Noninfiltrating intraductal papillary
          adenocarcinoma
M8504/0   Intracystic papillary adenoma
M8504/2   Noninfiltrating intracystic carcinoma
M8505/0   Intraductal papillomatosis NOS
M8506/0   Subareolar duct papillomatosis
M8510/3   Medullary carcinoma NOS
M8511/3   Medullary carcinoma with amyloid
          stroma
M8512/3   Medullary carcinoma with lymphoid
          stroma
M8520/2   Lobular carcinoma in situ
M8520/3   Lobular carcinoma NOS
M8521/3   Infiltrating ductular carcinoma
M8530/3   Inflammatory carcinoma
M8540/3   Paget's disease, mammary
M8541/3   Paget's disease and infiltrating
          duct carcinoma of breast
M8542/3   Paget's disease, extramammary
          (except Paget's disease of bone)

M855   Acinar cell neoplasms
M8550/0   Acinar cell adenoma
M8550/1   Acinar cell tumor
M8550/3   Acinar cell carcinoma

M856-M858   Complex epithelial neoplasms
M8560/3   Adenosquamous carcinoma
M8561/0   Adenolymphoma
M8570/3   Adenocarcinoma with squamous
          metaplasia
M8571/3   Adenocarcinoma with cartilaginous
          and osseous metaplasia
M8572/3   Adenocarcinoma with spindle cell
          metaplasia
M8573/3   Adenocarcinoma with apocrine
          metaplasia
M8580/0   Thymoma, benign
M8580/3   Thymoma, malignant

M859-M867   Specialized gonadal neoplasms
M8590/1   Sex cord-stromal tumor
M8600/0   Thecoma NOS
M8600/3   Theca cell carcinoma
M8610/0   Luteoma NOS
M8620/0   Granulosa cell tumor NOS
M8620/3   Granulosa cell tumor, malignant
M8621/1   Granulosa cell-theca cell tumor
M8630/0   Androblastoma, benign
M8630/1   Androblastoma NOS
M8630/3   Androblastoma, malignant
M8631/0   Sertoli-Leydig cell tumor
M8632/1   Gynandroblastoma
M8640/0   Tubular androblastoma NOS
M8640/3   Sertoli cell carcinoma
M8641/0   Tubular androblastoma with lipid
          storage

M8650/0	Leydig cell tumor, benign
M8650/1	Leydig cell tumor NOS
M8650/3	Leydig cell tumor, malignant
M8660/0	Hilar cell tumor
M8670/0	Lipid cell tumor of ovary
M8671/0	Adrenal rest tumor

M868-M871 Paragangliomas and glomus tumors

M8680/1	Paraganglioma NOS
M8680/3	Paraganglioma, malignant
M8681/1	Sympathetic paraganglioma
M8682/1	Parasympathetic paraganglioma
M8690/1	Glomus jugulare tumor
M8691/1	Aortic body tumor
M8692/1	Carotid body tumor
M8693/1	Extra-adrenal paraganglioma NOS
M8693/3	Extra-adrenal paraganglioma, malignant
M8700/0	Pheochromocytoma NOS
M8700/3	Pheochromocytoma, malignant
M8710/3	Glomangiosarcoma
M8711/0	Glomus tumor
M8712/0	Glomangioma

M872-M879 Nevi and melanomas

M8720/0	Pigmented nevus NOS
M8720/3	Malignant melanoma NOS
M8721/3	Nodular melanoma
M8722/0	Balloon cell nevus
M8722/3	Balloon cell melanoma
M8723/0	Halo nevus
M8724/0	Fibrous papule of the nose
M8725/0	Neuronevus
M8726/0	Magnocellular nevus
M8730/0	Nonpigmented nevus
M8730/3	Amelanotic melanoma
M8740/0	Junctional nevus
M8740/3	Malignant melanoma in junctional nevus
M8741/2	Precancerous melanosis NOS
M8741/3	Malignant melanoma in precancerous melanosis
M8742/2	Hutchinson's melanotic freckle
M8742/3	Malignant melanoma in Hutchinson's melanotic freckle
M8743/3	Superficial spreading melanoma
M8750/0	Intradermal nevus
M8760/0	Compound nevus
M8761/1	Giant pigmented nevus
M8761/3	Malignant melanoma in giant pigmented nevus
M8770/0	Epithelioid and spindle cell nevus
M8771/3	Epithelioid cell melanoma
M8772/3	Spindle cell melanoma NOS
M8773/3	Spindle cell melanoma, type A
M8774/3	Spindle cell melanoma, type B
M8775/3	Mixed epithelioid and spindle cell melanoma
M8780/0	Blue nevus NOS
M8780/3	Blue nevus, malignant
M8790/0	Cellular blue nevus

M880 Soft tissue tumors and sarcomas NOS

M8800/0	Soft tissue tumor, benign
M8800/3	Sarcoma NOS
M8800/9	Sarcomatosis NOS
M8801/3	Spindle cell sarcoma
M8802/3	Giant cell sarcoma (except of bone M9250/3)
M8803/3	Small cell sarcoma
M8804/3	Epithelioid cell sarcoma

M881-M883 Fibromatous neoplasms

M8810/0	Fibroma NOS
M8810/3	Fibrosarcoma NOS
M8811/0	Fibromyxoma
M8811/3	Fibromyxosarcoma
M8812/0	Periosteal fibroma
M8812/3	Periosteal fibrosarcoma

M8813/0	Fascial fibroma
M8813/3	Fascial fibrosarcoma
M8814/3	Infantile fibrosarcoma
M8820/0	Elastofibroma
M8821/1	Aggressive fibromatosis
M8822/1	Abdominal fibromatosis
M8823/1	Desmoplastic fibroma
M8830/0	Fibrous histiocytoma NOS
M8830/1	Atypical fibrous histiocytoma
M8830/3	Fibrous histiocytoma, malignant
M8831/0	Fibroxanthoma NOS
M8831/1	Atypical fibroxanthoma
M8831/3	Fibroxanthoma, malignant
M8832/0	Dermatofibroma NOS
M8832/1	Dermatofibroma protuberans
M8832/2	Dermatofibrosarcoma NOS

M884 Myxomatous neoplasms

M8840/0	Myxoma NOS
M8840/3	Myxosarcoma

M885-M888 Lipomatous neoplasms

M8850/0	Lipoma NOS
M8850/3	Liposarcoma NOS
M8851/0	Fibrolipoma
M8851/3	Liposarcoma, well differentiated type
M8852/0	Fibromyxolipoma
M8852/3	Myxoid liposarcoma
M8853/3	Round cell liposarcoma
M8854/3	Pleomorphic liposarcoma
M8855/3	Mixed type liposarcoma
M8856/0	Intramuscular lipoma
M8857/0	Spindle cell lipoma
M8860/0	Angiomyolipoma
M8860/3	Angiomyoliposarcoma
M8861/0	Angiolipoma NOS
M8861/1	Angiolipoma, infiltrating
M8870/0	Myelolipoma
M8880/0	Hibernoma
M8881/0	Lipoblastomatosis

M889-M892 Myomatous neoplasms

M8890/0	Leiomyoma NOS
M8890/1	Intravascular leiomyomatosis
M8890/3	Leiomyosarcoma NOS
M8891/1	Epithelioid leiomyoma
M8891/3	Epithelioid leiomyosarcoma
M8892/1	Cellular leiomyoma
M8893/0	Bizarre leiomyoma
M8894/0	Angiomyoma
M8894/3	Angiomyosarcoma
M8895/0	Myoma
M8895/3	Myosarcoma
M8900/0	Rhabdomyoma NOS
M8900/3	Rhabdomyosarcoma NOS
M8901/3	Pleomorphic rhabdomyosarcoma
M8902/3	Mixed type rhabdomyosarcoma
M8903/0	Fetal rhabdomyoma
M8904/0	Adult rhabdomyoma
M8910/3	Embryonal rhabdomyosarcoma
M8920/3	Alveolar rhabdomyosarcoma

M893-M899 Complex mixed and stromal neoplasms

M8930/3	Endometrial stromal sarcoma
M8931/1	Endolymphatic stromal myosis
M8932/0	Adenomyoma
M8940/0	Pleomorphic adenoma
M8940/3	Mixed tumor, malignant NOS
M8950/3	Mullerian mixed tumor
M8951/3	Mesodermal mixed tumor
M8960/1	Mesoblastic nephroma
M8960/3	Nephroblastoma NOS
M8961/3	Epithelial nephroblastoma
M8962/3	Mesenchymal nephroblastoma
M8970/3	Hepatoblastoma
M8980/3	Carcinosarcoma NOS
M8981/3	Carcinosarcoma, embryonal type
M8982/0	Myoepithelioma
M8990/0	Mesenchymoma, benign

M8990/1	Mesenchymoma NOS
M8990/3	Mesenchymoma, malignant
M8991/3	Embryonal sarcoma

M900-M903 Fibroepithelial neoplasms

M9000/0	Brenner tumor NOS
M9000/1	Brenner tumor, borderline malignancy
M9000/3	Brenner tumor, malignant
M9010/0	Fibroadenoma NOS
M9011/0	Intracanalicular fibroadenoma NOS
M9012/0	Pericanalicular fibroadenoma
M9013/0	Adenofibroma NOS
M9014/0	Serous adenofibroma
M9015/0	Mucinous adenofibroma
M9020/0	Cellular intracanalicular fibroadenoma
M9020/1	Cystosarcoma phyllodes NOS
M9020/3	Cystosarcoma phyllodes, malignant
M9030/0	Juvenile fibroadenoma

M904 Synovial neoplasms

M9040/0	Synovioma, benign
M9040/3	Synovial sarcoma NOS
M9041/3	Synovial sarcoma, spindle cell type
M9042/3	Synovial sarcoma, epithelioid cell type
M9043/3	Synovial sarcoma, biphasic type
M9044/3	Clear cell sarcoma of tendons and aponeuroses

M905 Mesothelial neoplasms

M9050/0	Mesothelioma, benign
M9050/3	Mesothelioma, malignant
M9051/0	Fibrous mesothelioma, benign
M9051/3	Fibrous mesothelioma, malignant
M9052/0	Epithelioid mesothelioma, benign
M9052/3	Epithelioid mesothelioma, malignant
M9053/0	Mesothelioma, biphasic type, benign
M9053/3	Mesothelioma, biphasic type, malignant
M9054/0	Adenomatoid tumor NOS

M906-M909 Germ cell neoplasms

M9060/3	Dysgerminoma
M9061/3	Seminoma NOS
M9062/3	Seminoma, anaplastic type
M9063/3	Spermatocytic seminoma
M9064/3	Germinoma
M9070/3	Embryonal carcinoma NOS
M9071/3	Endodermal sinus tumor
M9072/3	Polyembryoma
M9073/1	Gonadoblastoma
M9080/0	Teratoma, benign
M9080/1	Teratoma NOS
M9080/3	Teratoma, malignant NOS
M9081/3	Teratocarcinoma
M9082/3	Malignant teratoma, undifferentiated type
M9083/3	Malignant teratoma, intermediate type
M9084/0	Dermoid cyst
M9084/3	Dermoid cyst with malignant transformation
M9090/0	Struma ovarii NOS
M9090/3	Struma ovarii, malignant
M9091/1	Strumal carcinoid

M910 Trophoblastic neoplasms

M9100/0	Hydatidiform mole NOS
M9100/1	Invasive hydatidiform mole
M9100/3	Choriocarcinoma
M9101/3	Choriocarcinoma combined with teratoma
M9102/3	Malignant teratoma, trophoblastic

M911 Mesonephromas

M9110/0	Mesonephroma, benign
M9110/1	Mesonephric tumor
M9110/3	Mesonephroma, malignant
M9111/1	Endosalpingioma

Appendix A: Morphology of Neoplasms

M912-M916 Blood vessel tumors
M9120/0 Hemangioma NOS
M9120/3 Hemangiosarcoma
M9121/0 Cavernous hemangioma
M9122/0 Venous hemangioma
M9123/0 Racemose hemangioma
M9124/3 Kupffer cell sarcoma
M9130/0 Hemangioendothelioma, benign
M9130/1 Hemangioendothelioma NOS
M9130/3 Hemangioendothelioma, malignant
M9131/0 Capillary hemangioma
M9132/0 Intramuscular hemangioma
M9140/3 Kaposi's sarcoma
M9141/0 Angiokeratoma
M9142/0 Verrucous keratotic hemangioma
M9150/0 Hemangiopericytoma, benign
M9150/1 Hemangiopericytoma NOS
M9150/3 Hemangiopericytoma, malignant
M9160/0 Angiofibroma NOS
M9161/1 Hemangioblastoma

M917 Lymphatic vessel tumors
M9170/0 Lymphangioma NOS
M9170/3 Lymphangiosarcoma
M9171/0 Capillary lymphangioma
M9172/0 Cavernous lymphangioma
M9173/0 Cystic lymphangioma
M9174/0 Lymphangiomyoma
M9174/1 Lymphangiomyomatosis
M9175/0 Hemolymphangioma

M918-M920 Osteomas and osteosarcomas
M9180/0 Osteoma NOS
M9180/3 Osteosarcoma NOS
M9181/3 Chondroblastic osteosarcoma
M9182/3 Fibroblastic osteosarcoma
M9183/3 Telangiectatic osteosarcoma
M9184/3 Osteosarcoma in Paget's disease of bone
M9190/3 Juxtacortical osteosarcoma
M9191/0 Osteoid osteoma NOS
M9200/0 Osteoblastoma

M921-M924 Chondromatous neoplasms
M9210/0 Osteochondroma
M9210/1 Osteochondromatosis NOS
M9220/0 Chondroma NOS
M9220/1 Chondromatosis NOS
M9220/3 Chondrosarcoma NOS
M9221/0 Juxtacortical chondroma
M9221/3 Juxtacortical chondrosarcoma
M9230/0 Chondroblastoma NOS
M9230/3 Chondroblastoma, malignant
M9240/3 Mesenchymal chondrosarcoma
M9241/0 Chondromyxoid fibroma

M925 Giant cell tumors
M9250/1 Giant cell tumor of bone NOS
M9250/3 Giant cell tumor of bone, malignant
M9251/1 Giant cell tumor of soft parts NOS
M9251/3 Malignant giant cell tumor of soft parts

M926 Miscellaneous bone tumors
M9260/3 Ewing's sarcoma
M9261/3 Adamantinoma of long bones
M9262/0 Ossifying fibroma

M927-M934 Odontogenic tumors
M9270/0 Odontogenic tumor, benign
M9270/1 Odontogenic tumor NOS
M9270/3 Odontogenic tumor, malignant
M9271/0 Dentinoma
M9272/0 Cementoma NOS
M9273/0 Cementoblastoma, benign
M9274/0 Cementifying fibroma
M9275/0 Gigantiform cementoma
M9280/0 Odontoma NOS
M9281/0 Compound odontoma
M9282/0 Complex odontoma
M9290/0 Ameloblastic fibro-odontoma
M9290/3 Ameloblastic odontosarcoma
M9300/0 Adenomatoid odontogenic tumor

M9301/0 Calcifying odontogenic cyst
M9310/0 Ameloblastoma NOS
M9310/3 Ameloblastoma, malignant
M9311/0 Odontoameloblastoma
M9312/0 Squamous odontogenic tumor
M9320/0 Odontogenic myxoma
M9321/0 Odontogenic fibroma NOS
M9330/0 Ameloblastic fibroma
M9330/3 Ameloblastic fibrosarcoma
M9340/0 Calcifying epithelial odontogenic tumor

M935-M937 Miscellaneous tumors
M9350/1 Craniopharyngioma
M9360/1 Pinealoma
M9361/1 Pineocytoma
M9362/3 Pineoblastoma
M9363/0 Melanotic neuroectodermal tumor
M9370/3 Chordoma

M938-M948 Gliomas
M9380/3 Glioma, malignant
M9381/3 Gliomatosis cerebri
M9382/3 Mixed glioma
M9383/1 Subependymal glioma
M9384/1 Subependymal giant cell astrocytoma
M9390/0 Choroid plexus papilloma NOS
M9390/3 Choroid plexus papilloma, malignant
M9391/3 Ependymoma NOS
M9392/3 Ependymoma, anaplastic type
M9393/1 Papillary ependymoma
M9394/1 Myxopapillary ependymoma
M9400/3 Astrocytoma NOS
M9401/3 Astrocytoma, anaplastic type
M9410/3 Protoplasmic astrocytoma
M9411/3 Gemistocytic astrocytoma
M9420/3 Fibrillary astrocytoma
M9421/3 Pilocytic astrocytoma
M9422/3 Spongioblastoma NOS
M9423/3 Spongioblastoma polare
M9430/3 Astroblastoma
M9440/3 Glioblastoma NOS
M9441/3 Giant cell glioblastoma
M9442/3 Glioblastoma with sarcomatous component
M9443/3 Primitive polar spongioblastoma
M9450/3 Oligodendroglioma NOS
M9451/3 Oligodendroglioma, anaplastic type
M9460/3 Oligodendroblastoma
M9470/3 Medulloblastoma NOS
M9471/3 Desmoplastic medulloblastoma
M9472/3 Medullomyoblastoma
M9480/3 Cerebellar sarcoma NOS
M9481/3 Monstrocellular sarcoma

M949-M952 Neuroepitheliomatous neoplasms
M9490/0 Ganglioneuroma
M9490/3 Ganglioneuroblastoma
M9491/0 Ganglioneuromatosis
M9500/3 Neuroblastoma NOS
M9501/3 Medulloepithelioma NOS
M9502/3 Teratoid medulloepithelioma
M9503/3 Neuroepithelioma NOS
M9504/3 Spongioneuroblastoma
M9505/1 Ganglioglioma
M9506/0 Neurocytoma
M9507/0 Pacinian tumor
M9510/3 Retinoblastoma NOS
M9511/3 Retinoblastoma, differentiated type
M9512/3 Retinoblastoma, undifferentiated type
M9520/3 Olfactory neurogenic tumor
M9521/3 Esthesioneurocytoma
M9522/3 Esthesioneuroblastoma
M9523/3 Esthesioneuroepithelioma

M953 Meningiomas
M9530/0 Meningioma NOS
M9530/1 Meningiomatosis NOS

M9530/3 Meningioma, malignant
M9531/0 Meningotheliomatous meningioma
M9532/0 Fibrous meningioma
M9533/0 Psammomatous meningioma
M9534/0 Angiomatous meningioma
M9535/0 Hemangioblastic meningioma
M9536/0 Hemangiopericytic meningioma
M9537/0 Transitional meningioma
M9538/1 Papillary meningioma
M9539/3 Meningeal sarcomatosis

M954-M957 Nerve sheath tumor
M9540/0 Neurofibroma NOS
M9540/1 Neurofibromatosis NOS
M9540/3 Neurofibrosarcoma
M9541/0 Melanotic neurofibroma
M9550/0 Plexiform neurofibroma
M9560/0 Neurilemmoma NOS
M9560/1 Neurinomatosis
M9560/3 Neurilemmoma, malignant
M9570/0 Neuroma NOS

M958 Granular cell tumors and alveolar soft part sarcoma
M9580/0 Granular cell tumor NOS
M9580/3 Granular cell tumor, malignant
M9581/3 Alveolar soft part sarcoma

M959-M963 Lymphomas, NOS or diffuse
M9590/0 Lymphomatous tumor, benign
M9590/3 Malignant lymphoma NOS
M9591/3 Malignant lymphoma, non Hodgkin's type
M9600/3 Malignant lymphoma, undifferentiated cell type NOS
M9601/3 Malignant lymphoma, stem cell type
M9602/3 Malignant lymphoma, convoluted cell type NOS
M9610/3 Lymphosarcoma NOS
M9611/3 Malignant lymphoma, lymphoplasmacytoid type
M9612/3 Malignant lymphoma, immunoblastic type
M9613/3 Malignant lymphoma, mixed lymphocytic-histiocytic NOS
M9614/3 Malignant lymphoma, centroblastic-centrocytic, diffuse
M9615/3 Malignant lymphoma, follicular center cell NOS
M9620/3 Malignant lymphoma, lymphocytic, well differentiated NOS
M9621/3 Malignant lymphoma, lymphocytic, intermediate differentiation NOS
M9622/3 Malignant lymphoma, centrocytic
M9623/3 Malignant lymphoma, follicular center cell, cleaved NOS
M9630/3 Malignant lymphoma, lymphocytic, poorly differentiated NOS
M9631/3 Prolymphocytic lymphosarcoma
M9632/3 Malignant lymphoma, centroblastic type NOS
M9633/3 Malignant lymphoma, follicular center cell, noncleaved NOS

M964 Reticulosarcomas
M9640/3 Reticulosarcoma NOS
M9641/3 Reticulosarcoma, pleomorphic cell type
M9642/3 Reticulosarcoma, nodular

M965-M966 Hodgkin's disease
M9650/3 Hodgkin's disease NOS
M9651/3 Hodgkin's disease, lymphocytic predominance
M9652/3 Hodgkin's disease, mixed cellularity
M9653/3 Hodgkin's disease, lymphocytic depletion NOS
M9654/3 Hodgkin's disease, lymphocytic depletion, diffuse fibrosis
M9655/3 Hodgkin's disease, lymphocytic depletion, reticular type

M9656/3	Hodgkin's disease, nodular sclerosis NOS	
M9657/3	Hodgkin's disease, nodular sclerosis, cellular phase	
M9660/3	Hodgkin's paragranuloma	
M9661/3	Hodgkin's granuloma	
M9662/3	Hodgkin's sarcoma	

M969 **Lymphomas, nodular or follicular**

M9690/3	Malignant lymphoma, nodular NOS
M9691/3	Malignant lymphoma, mixed lymphocytic-histiocytic, nodular
M9692/3	Malignant lymphoma, centroblastic-centrocytic, follicular
M9693/3	Malignant lymphoma, lymphocytic, well differentiated, nodular
M9694/3	Malignant lymphoma, lymphocytic, intermediate differentiation, nodular
M9695/3	Malignant lymphoma, follicular center cell, cleaved, follicular
M9696/3	Malignant lymphoma, lymphocytic, poorly differentiated, nodular
M9697/3	Malignant lymphoma, centroblastic type, follicular
M9698/3	Malignant lymphoma, follicular center cell, noncleaved, follicular

M970 **Mycosis fungoides**

M9700/3	Mycosis fungoides
M9701/3	Sezary's disease

M971-M972 **Miscellaneous reticuloendothelial neoplasms**

M9710/3	Microglioma
M9720/3	Malignant histiocytosis
M9721/3	Histiocytic medullary reticulosis
M9722/3	Letterer-Siwe's disease

M973 **Plasma cell tumors**

M9730/3	Plasma cell myeloma
M9731/0	Plasma cell tumor, benign
M9731/1	Plasmacytoma NOS
M9731/3	Plasma cell tumor, malignant

M974 **Mast cell tumors**

M9740/1	Mastocytoma NOS
M9740/3	Mast cell sarcoma
M9741/3	Malignant mastocytosis

M975 **Burkitt's tumor**

M9750/3	Burkitt's tumor

M980-M994 **Leukemias**

M980 **Leukemias NOS**

M9800/3	Leukemia NOS
M9801/3	Acute leukemia NOS
M9802/3	Subacute leukemia NOS
M9803/3	Chronic leukemia NOS
M9804/3	Aleukemic leukemia NOS

M981 **Compound leukemias**

M9810/3	Compound leukemia

M982 **Lymphoid leukemias**

M9820/3	Lymphoid leukemia NOS
M9821/3	Acute lymphoid leukemia
M9822/3	Subacute lymphoid leukemia
M9823/3	Chronic lymphoid leukemia
M9824/3	Aleukemic lymphoid leukemia
M9825/3	Prolymphocytic leukemia

M983 **Plasma cell leukemias**

M9830/3	Plasma cell leukemia

M984 **Erythroleukemias**

M9840/3	Erythroleukemia
M9841/3	Acute erythremia
M9842/3	Chronic erythremia

M985 **Lymphosarcoma cell leukemias**

M9850/3	Lymphosarcoma cell leukemia

M986 **Myeloid leukemias**

M9860/3	Myeloid leukemia NOS
M9861/3	Acute myeloid leukemia
M9862/3	Subacute myeloid leukemia
M9863/3	Chronic myeloid leukemia
M9864/3	Aleukemic myeloid leukemia
M9865/3	Neutrophilic leukemia
M9866/3	Acute promyelocytic leukemia

M987 **Basophilic leukemias**

M9870/3	Basophilic leukemia

M988 **Eosinophilic leukemias**

M9880/3	Eosinophilic leukemia

M989 **Monocytic leukemias**

M9890/3	Monocytic leukemia NOS
M9891/3	Acute monocytic leukemia
M9892/3	Subacute monocytic leukemia
M9893/3	Chronic monocytic leukemia
M9894/3	Aleukemic monocytic leukemia

M990-M994 **Miscellaneous leukemias**

M9900/3	Mast cell leukemia
M9910/3	Megakaryocytic leukemia
M9920/3	Megakaryocytic myelosis
M9930/3	Myeloid sarcoma
M9940/3	Hairy cell leukemia

M995-M997 **Miscellaneous myeloproliferative and lymphoproliferative disorders**

M9950/1	Polycythemia vera
M9951/1	Acute panmyelosis
M9960/1	Chronic myeloproliferative disease
M9961/1	Myelosclerosis with myeloid metaplasia
M9962/1	Idiopathic thrombocythemia
M9970/1	Chronic lymphoproliferative disease

CLASSIFICATION OF DRUGS BY AMERICAN HOSPITAL FORMULARY SERVICE LIST NUMBER AND THEIR ICD-9-CM EQUIVALENTS

The coding of adverse effects of drugs is keyed to the continually revised Hospital Formulary of the American Hospital Formulary Service (AHFS) published under the direction of the American Society of Hospital Pharmacists.

The following section gives the ICD-9-CM diagnosis code for each AHFS list.

AHFS* List		ICD-9-CM Diagnosis Code
4:00	ANTIHISTAMINE DRUGS	963.0
8:00	ANTI-INFECTIVE AGENTS	
8:04	Amebacides	961.5
	hydroxyquinoline derivatives	961.3
	arsenical anti-infectives	961.1
8:08	Anthelmintics	961.6
	quinoline derivatives	961.3
8:12.04	Antifungal Antibiotics	960.1
	nonantibiotics	961.9
8:12.06	Cephalosporins	960.5
8:12.08	Chloramphenicol	960.2
8:12.12	The Erythromycins	960.3
8:12.16	The Penicillins	960.0
8:12.20	The Streptomycins	960.6
8:12.24	The Tetracyclines	960.4
8:12.28	Other Antibiotics	960.8
	antimycobacterial antibiotics	960.6
	macrolides	960.3
8:16	Antituberculars	961.8
	antibiotics	960.6
8:18	Antivirals	961.7
8:20	Plasmodicides (antimalarials)	961.4
8:24	Sulfonamides	961.0
8:26	The Sulfones	961.8
8:28	Treponemicides	961.2
8:32	Trichomonacides	961.5
	hydroxyquinoline derivatives	961.3
	nitrofuran derivatives	961.9
8:36	Urinary Germicides	961.9
	quinoline derivatives	961.3
8:40	Other Anti-Infectives	961.9
10:00	ANTINEOPLASTIC AGENTS	963.1
	antibiotics	960.7
	progestogens	962.2
12:00	AUTONOMIC DRUGS	
12:04	Parasympathomimetic (Cholinergic) Agents	971.0
12:08	Parasympatholytic (Cholinergic Blocking) Agents	971.1
12:12	Sympathomimetic (Adrenergic) Agents	971.2
12:16	Sympatholytic (Adrenergic Blocking) Agents	971.3
12:20	Skeletal Muscle Relaxants	975.2
	central nervous system muscle-tone depressants	968.0
16:00	BLOOD DERIVATIVES	964.7
20:00	BLOOD FORMATION AND COAGULATION	
20:04	Antianemia Drugs	964.1
20:04.04	Iron Preparations	964.0
20:04.08	Liver and Stomach Preparations	964.1
20:12.04	Anticoagulants	964.2
20:12.08	Antiheparin Agents	964.5
20:12.12	Coagulants	964.5
20:12.16	Hemostatics	964.5
	capillary-active drugs	972.8
	fibrinolysis-affecting agents	964.4
	natural products	964.7
24:00	CARDIOVASCULAR DRUGS	
24:04	Cardiac Drugs	972.9
	cardiotonic agents	972.1
	rhythm regulators	972.0
24:06	Antilipemic Agents	972.2
	thyroid derivatives	962.7
24:08	Hypotensive Agents	972.6
	adrenergic blocking agents	971.3
	ganglion-blocking agents	972.3
	vasodilators	972.5
24:12	Vasodilating Agents	972.5
	coronary	972.4

AHFS* List		ICD-9-CM Diagnosis Code
	nicotinic acid derivatives	972.2
24:16	Sclerosing Agents	972.7
28:00	CENTRAL NERVOUS SYSTEM DRUGS	
28:04	General Anesthetics	968.4
	gaseous anesthetics	968.2
	halothane	968.1
	intravenous anesthetics	968.3
28:08	Analgesics and Antipyretics	965.9
	antirheumatics	965.61-965.69
	aromatic analgesics	965.4
	non-narcotics NEC	965.7
	opium alkaloids	965.00
	heroin	965.01
	methadone	965.02
	specified type NEC	965.09
	pyrazole derivatives	965.5
	salicylates	965.1
	specified type NEC	965.8
28:10	Narcotic Antagonists	970.1
28:12	Anticonvulsants	966.3
	barbiturates	967.0
	benzodiazepine-based tranquilizers	969.4
	bromides	967.3
	hydantoin derivatives	966.1
	oxazolidine derivative	966.0
	succinimides	966.2
28:16.04	Antidepressants	969.0
28:16.08	Tranquilizers	969.5
	benzodiazepine-based	969.4
	butyrophenone-based	969.2
	major NEC	969.3
	phenothiazine-based	969.1
28:16.12	Other Psychotherapeutic Agents	969.8
28:20	Respiratory and Cerebral Stimulants	970.9
	analeptics	970.0
	anorexigenic agents	977.0
	psychostimulants	969.7
	specified type NEC	970.8
28:24	Sedatives and Hypnotics	967.9
	barbiturates	967.0
	benzodiazepine-based tranquilizers	969.4
	chloral hydrate group	967.1
	glutethamide group	967.5
	intravenous anesthetics	968.3
	methaqualone	967.4
	paraldehyde	967.2
	phenothiazine-based tranquilizers	969.1
	specified type NEC	967.8
	thiobarbiturates	968.3
	tranquilizer NEC	969.5
36:00	DIAGNOSTIC AGENTS	977.8
40:00	ELECTROLYTE, CALORIC, AND WATER BALANCE AGENTS NEC	974.5
40:04	Acidifying Agents	963.2
40:08	Alkalinizing Agents	963.3
40:10	Ammonia Detoxicants	974.5
40:12	Replacement Solutions NEC	974.5
	plasma volume expanders	964.8
40:16	Sodium-Removing Resins	974.5
40:18	Potassium-Removing Resins	974.5
40:20	Caloric Agents	974.5
40:24	Salt and Sugar Substitutes	974.5
40:28	Diuretics NEC	974.4
	carbonic acid anhydrase inhibitors	974.2
	mercurials	974.0
	purine derivatives	974.1
	saluretics	974.3
40:36	Irrigating Solutions	974.5
40:40	Uricosuric Agents	974.7
44:00	ENZYMES NEC	963.4
	fibrinolysis-affecting agents	964.4
	gastric agents	973.4

Appendix C: Classification of Drugs by AHFS List

AHFS* List	ICD-9-CM Diagnosis Code
48:00 EXPECTORANTS AND COUGH PREPARATIONS	
antihistamine agents	963.0
antitussives	975.4
codeine derivatives	965.09
expectorants	975.5
narcotic agents NEC	965.09
52:00 EYE, EAR, NOSE, AND THROAT PREPARATIONS	
52:04 Anti-Infectives	
ENT	976.6
ophthalmic	976.5
52:04.04 Antibiotics	
ENT	976.6
ophthalmic	976.5
52:04.06 Antivirals	
ENT	976.6
ophthalmic	976.5
52:04.08 Sulfonamides	
ENT	976.6
ophthalmic	976.5
52:04.12 Miscellaneous Anti-Infectives	
ENT	976.6
ophthalmic	976.5
52:08 Anti-Inflammatory Agents	
ENT	976.6
ophthalmic	976.5
52:10 Carbonic Anhydrase Inhibitors	974.2
52:12 Contact Lens Solutions	976.5
52:16 Local Anesthetics	968.5
52:20 Miotics	971.0
52:24 Mydriatics	
adrenergics	971.2
anticholinergics	971.1
antimuscarinics	971.1
parasympatholytics	971.1
spasmolytics	971.1
sympathomimetics	971.2
52:28 Mouth Washes and Gargles	976.6
52:32 Vasoconstrictors	971.2
52:36 Unclassified Agents	
ENT	976.6
ophthalmic	976.5
56:00 GASTROINTESTINAL DRUGS	
56:04 Antacids and Absorbents	973.0
56:08 Anti-Diarrhea Agents	973.5
56:10 Antiflatulents	973.8
56:12 Cathartics NEC	973.3
emollients	973.2
irritants	973.1
56:16 Digestants	973.4
56:20 Emetics and Antiemetics	
antiemetics	963.0
emetics	973.6
56:24 Lipotropic Agents	977.1
60:00 GOLD COMPOUNDS	965.69
64:00 HEAVY METAL ANTAGONISTS	963.8
68:00 HORMONES AND SYNTHETIC SUBSTITUTES	
68:04 Adrenals	962.0
68:08 Androgens	962.1
68:12 Contraceptives	962.2
68:16 Estrogens	962.2
68:18 Gonadotropins	962.4
68:20 Insulins and Antidiabetic Agents	962.3
68:20.08 Insulins	962.3
68:24 Parathyroid	962.6
68:28 Pituitary	
anterior	962.4
posterior	962.5
68:32 Progestogens	962.2
68:34 Other Corpus Luteum Hormones	962.2
68:36 Thyroid and Antithyroid	
antithyroid	962.8
thyroid	962.7

AHFS* List	ICD-9-CM Diagnosis Code
72:00 LOCAL ANESTHETICS NEC	968.9
topical (surface) agents	968.5
infiltrating agents (intradermal)	
(subcutaneous) (submucosal)	968.5
nerve blocking agents (peripheral)	
(plexus) (regional)	968.6
spinal	968.7
76:00 OXYTOCICS	975.0
78:00 RADIOACTIVE AGENTS	990
80:00 SERUMS, TOXOIDS, AND VACCINES	
80:04 Serums	979.9
immune globulin (gamma) (human)	964.6
80:08 Toxoids NEC	978.8
diphtheria	978.5
and tetanus	978.9
with pertussis component	978.6
tetanus	978.4
and diphtheria	978.9
with pertussis component	978.6
80:12 Vaccines NEC	979.9
bacterial NEC	978.8
with	
other bacterial component	978.9
pertussis component	978.6
viral and rickettsial component	979.7
rickettsial NEC	979.6
with	
bacterial component	979.7
pertussis component	978.6
viral component	979.7
viral NEC	979.6
with	
bacterial component	979.7
pertussis component	978.6
rickettsial component	979.7
84:00 SKIN AND MUCOUS MEMBRANE PREPARATIONS	
84:04 Anti-Infectives	976.0
84:04.04 Antibiotics	976.0
84:04.08 Fungicides	976.0
84:04.12 Scabicides and Pediculicides	976.0
84:04.16 Miscellaneous Local Anti-Infectives	976.0
84:06 Anti-Inflammatory Agents	976.0
84:08 Antipruritics and Local Anesthetics	
antipruritics	976.1
local anesthetics	968.5
84:12 Astringents	976.2
84:16 Cell Stimulants and Proliferants	976.8
84:20 Detergents	976.2
84:24 Emollients, Demulcents, and Protectants	976.3
84:28 Keratolytic Agents	976.4
84:32 Keratoplastic Agents	976.4
84:36 Miscellaneous Agents	976.8
86:00 SPASMOLYTIC AGENTS	975.1
antiasthmatics	975.7
papaverine	972.5
theophyllin	974.1
88:00 VITAMINS	
88:04 Vitamin A	963.5
88:08 Vitamin B Complex	963.5
hematopoietic vitamin	964.1
nicotinic acid derivatives	972.2
88:12 Vitamin C	963.5
88:16 Vitamin D	963.5
88:20 Vitamin E	963.5
88:24 Vitamin K Activity	964.3
88:28 Multivitamin Preparations	963.5
92:00 UNCLASSIFIED THERAPEUTIC AGENTS	977.8

* American Hospital Formulary Service

CLASSIFICATION OF INDUSTRIAL ACCIDENTS ACCORDING TO AGENCY

Annex B to the Resolution concerning Statistics of Employment Injuries adopted by the Tenth International Conference of Labor Statisticians on 12 October 1962

1 MACHINES

11 Prime-Movers, except Electrical Motors
111 *Steam engines*
112 *Internal combustion engines*
119 *Others*
12 Transmission Machinery
121 *Transmission shafts*
122 *Transmission belts, cables, pulleys, pinions, chains, gears*
129 *Others*
13 Metalworking Machines
131 *Power presses*
132 *Lathes*
133 *Milling machines*
134 *Abrasive wheels*
135 *Mechanical shears*
136 *Forging machines*
137 *Rolling-mills*
139 *Others*
14 Wood and Assimilated Machines
141 *Circular saws*
142 *Other saws*
143 *Molding machines*
144 *Overhand planes*
149 *Others*
15 Agricultural Machines
151 *Reapers (including combine reapers)*
152 *Threshers*
159 *Others*
16 Mining Machinery
161 *Under-cutters*
169 *Others*
19 Other Machines Not Elsewhere Classified
191 *Earth-moving machines, excavating and scraping machines, except means of transport*
192 *Spinning, weaving and other textile machines*
193 *Machines for the manufacture of foodstuffs and beverages*
194 *Machines for the manufacture of paper*
195 *Printing machines*
199 *Others*

2 MEANS OF TRANSPORT AND LIFTING EQUIPMENT

21 Lifting Machines and Appliances
211 *Cranes*
212 *Lifts and elevators*
213 *Winches*
214 *Pulley blocks*
219 *Others*
22 Means of Rail Transport
221 *Inter-urban railways*
222 *Rail transport in mines, tunnels, quarries, industrial establishments, docks, etc.*
229 *Others*
23 Other Wheeled Means of Transport, Excluding Rail Transport
231 *Tractors*
232 *Lorries*
233 *Trucks*
234 *Motor vehicles, not elsewhere classified*
235 *Animal-drawn vehicles*
236 *Hand-drawn vehicles*
239 *Others*
24 Means of Air Transport
25 Means of Water Transport
251 *Motorized means of water transport*
252 *Non-motorized means of water transport*
26 Other Means of Transport
261 *Cable-cars*
262 *Mechanical conveyors, except cable-cars*
269 *Others*

3 OTHER EQUIPMENT

31 Pressure Vessels
311 *Boilers*
312 *Pressurized containers*
313 *Pressurized piping and accessories*
314 *Gas cylinders*
315 *Caissons, diving equipment*
319 *Others*
32 Furnaces, Ovens, Kilns
321 *Blast furnaces*
322 *Refining furnaces*
323 *Other furnaces*
324 *Kilns*
325 *Ovens*
33 Refrigerating Plants
34 Electrical Installations, Including Electric Motors, but Excluding Electric Hand Tools
341 *Rotating machines*
342 *Conductors*
343 *Transformers*
344 *Control apparatus*
349 *Others*
35 Electric Hand Tools
36 Tools, Implements, and Appliances, Except Electric Hand Tools
361 *Power-driven hand tools, except electric hand tools*
362 *Hand tools, not power-driven*
369 *Others*
37 Ladders, Mobile Ramps
38 Scaffolding
39 Other Equipment, Not Elsewhere Classified

4 MATERIALS, SUBSTANCES AND RADIATIONS

41 Explosives
42 Dusts, Gases, Liquids and Chemicals, Excluding Explosives
421 *Dusts*
422 *Gases, vapors, fumes*
423 *Liquids, not elsewhere classified*
424 *Chemicals, not elsewhere classified*
43 Flying Fragments
44 Radiations
441 *Ionizing radiations*
449 *Others*
49 Other Materials and Substances Not Elsewhere Classified

5 WORKING ENVIRONMENT

51 Outdoor
511 *Weather*
512 *Traffic and working surfaces*
513 *Water*
519 *Others*
52 Indoor
521 *Floors*
522 *Confined quarters*
523 *Stairs*
524 *Other traffic and working surfaces*
525 *Floor openings and wall openings*
526 *Environmental factors (lighting, ventilation, temperature, noise, etc.)*
529 *Others*
53 Underground
531 *Roofs and faces of mine roads and tunnels, etc.*
532 *Floors of mine roads and tunnels, etc.*
533 *Working-faces of mines, tunnels, etc.*
534 *Mine shafts*
535 *Fire*
536 *Water*
539 *Others*

6 OTHER AGENCIES, NOT ELSEWHERE CLASSIFIED

61 Animals
611 *Live animals*
612 *Animal products*
69 Other Agencies, Not Elsewhere Classified

7 AGENCIES NOT CLASSIFIED FOR LACK OF SUFFICIENT DATA

LIST OF THREE-DIGIT CATEGORIES

1. INFECTIOUS AND PARASITIC DISEASES

Intestinal infectious diseases (001-009)
001 Cholera
002 Typhoid and paratyphoid fevers
003 Other salmonella infections
004 Shigellosis
005 Other food poisoning (bacterial)
006 Amebiasis
007 Other protozoal intestinal diseases
008 Intestinal infections due to other organisms
009 Ill-defined intestinal infections

Tuberculosis (010-018)
010 Primary tuberculous infection
011 Pulmonary tuberculosis
012 Other respiratory tuberculosis
013 Tuberculosis of meninges and central nervous system
014 Tuberculosis of intestines, peritoneum, and mesenteric glands
015 Tuberculosis of bones and joints
016 Tuberculosis of genitourinary system
017 Tuberculosis of other organs
018 Miliary tuberculosis

Zoonotic bacterial diseases (020-027)
020 Plague
021 Tularemia
022 Anthrax
023 Brucellosis
024 Glanders
025 Melioidosis
026 Rat-bite fever
027 Other zoonotic bacterial diseases

Other bacterial diseases (030-042)
030 Leprosy
031 Diseases due to other mycobacteria
032 Diphtheria
033 Whooping cough
034 Streptococcal sore throat and scarlatina
035 Erysipelas
036 Meningococcal infection
037 Tetanus
038 Septicemia
039 Actinomycotic infections
040 Other bacterial diseases
041 Bacterial infection in conditions classified elsewhere and of unspecified site

Human immunodeficiency virus (042)
042 Human immunodeficiency virus [HIV] disease

Poliomyelitis and other non-arthropod-borne viral diseases of central nervous system (045-049)
045 Acute poliomyelitis
046 Slow virus infection of central nervous system
047 Meningitis due to enterovirus
048 Other enterovirus diseases of central nervous system
049 Other non-arthropod-borne viral diseases of central nervous system

Viral diseases accompanied by exanthem (050-057)
050 Smallpox
051 Cowpox and paravaccinia
052 Chickenpox
053 Herpes zoster
054 Herpes simplex
055 Measles
056 Rubella
057 Other viral exanthemata

Arthropod-borne viral diseases (060-066)
060 Yellow fever
061 Dengue
062 Mosquito-borne viral encephalitis
063 Tick-borne viral encephalitis
064 Viral encephalitis transmitted by other and unspecified arthropods
065 Arthropod-borne hemorrhagic fever
066 Other arthropod-borne viral diseases

Other diseases due to viruses and Chlamydiae (070-079)
070 Viral hepatitis
071 Rabies
072 Mumps
073 Ornithosis
074 Specific diseases due to Coxsackievirus
075 Infectious mononucleosis
076 Trachoma
077 Other diseases of conjunctiva due to viruses and Chlamydiae
078 Other diseases due to viruses and Chlamydiae
079 Viral infection in conditions classified elsewhere and of unspecified site

Rickettsioses and other arthropod-borne diseases (080-088)
080 Louse-borne [epidemic] typhus
081 Other typhus
082 Tick-borne rickettsioses
083 Other rickettsioses
084 Malaria
085 Leishmaniasis
086 Trypanosomiasis
087 Relapsing fever
088 Other arthropod-borne diseases

Syphilis and other venereal diseases (090-099)
090 Congenital syphilis
091 Early syphilis, symptomatic
092 Early syphilis, latent
093 Cardiovascular syphilis
094 Neurosyphilis
095 Other forms of late syphilis, with symptoms
096 Late syphilis, latent
097 Other and unspecified syphilis
098 Gonococcal infections
099 Other venereal diseases

Other spirochetal diseases (100-104)
100 Leptospirosis
101 Vincent's angina
102 Yaws
103 Pinta
104 Other spirochetal infection

Mycoses (110-118)
110 Dermatophytosis
111 Dermatomycosis, other and unspecified
112 Candidiasis
114 Coccidioidomycosis
115 Histoplasmosis
116 Blastomycotic infection
117 Other mycoses
118 Opportunistic mycoses

Helminthiases (120-129)
120 Schistosomiasis [bilharziasis]
121 Other trematode infections
122 Echinococcosis
123 Other cestode infection
124 Trichinosis
125 Filarial infection and dracontiasis
126 Ancylostomiasis and necatoriasis
127 Other intestinal helminthiases
128 Other and unspecified helminthiases
129 Intestinal parasitism, unspecified

Other infectious and parasitic diseases (130-136)
130 Toxoplasmosis
131 Trichomoniasis
132 Pediculosis and phthirus infestation
133 Acariasis
134 Other infestation
135 Sarcoidosis
136 Other and unspecified infectious and parasitic diseases

Late effects of infectious and parasitic diseases (137-139)
137 Late effects of tuberculosis
138 Late effects of acute poliomyelitis
139 Late effects of other infectious and parasitic diseases

2. NEOPLASMS

Malignant neoplasm of lip, oral cavity, and pharynx (140-149)
140 Malignant neoplasm of lip
141 Malignant neoplasm of tongue
142 Malignant neoplasm of major salivary glands
143 Malignant neoplasm of gum
144 Malignant neoplasm of floor of mouth
145 Malignant neoplasm of other and unspecified parts of mouth
146 Malignant neoplasm of oropharynx
147 Malignant neoplasm of nasopharynx
148 Malignant neoplasm of hypopharynx
149 Malignant neoplasm of other and ill-defined sites within the lip, oral cavity, and pharynx

Malignant neoplasm of digestive organs and peritoneum (150-159)
150 Malignant neoplasm of esophagus
151 Malignant neoplasm of stomach
152 Malignant neoplasm of small intestine, including duodenum
153 Malignant neoplasm of colon
154 Malignant neoplasm of rectum, rectosigmoid junction, and anus
155 Malignant neoplasm of liver and intrahepatic bile ducts
156 Malignant neoplasm of gallbladder and extrahepatic bile ducts
157 Malignant neoplasm of pancreas
158 Malignant neoplasm of retroperitoneum and peritoneum
159 Malignant neoplasm of other and ill-defined sites within the digestive organs and peritoneum

Malignant neoplasm of respiratory and intrathoracic organs (160-165)
160 Malignant neoplasm of nasal cavities, middle ear, and accessory sinuses
161 Malignant neoplasm of larynx
162 Malignant neoplasm of trachea, bronchus, and lung
163 Malignant neoplasm of pleura
164 Malignant neoplasm of thymus, heart, and mediastinum
165 Malignant neoplasm of other and ill-defined sites within the respiratory system and intrathoracic organs

Malignant neoplasm of bone, connective tissue, skin, and breast (170-176)
170 Malignant neoplasm of bone and articular cartilage
171 Malignant neoplasm of connective and other soft tissue
172 Malignant melanoma of skin
173 Other malignant neoplasm of skin
174 Malignant neoplasm of female breast
175 Malignant neoplasm of male breast
176 Kaposi's sarcoma

Malignant neoplasm of genitourinary organs (179-189)
179 Malignant neoplasm of uterus, part unspecified
180 Malignant neoplasm of cervix uteri
181 Malignant neoplasm of placenta
182 Malignant neoplasm of body of uterus
183 Malignant neoplasm of ovary and other uterine adnexa
184 Malignant neoplasm of other and unspecified female genital organs
185 Malignant neoplasm of prostate

186 Malignant neoplasm of testis
187 Malignant neoplasm of penis and other male genital organs
188 Malignant neoplasm of bladder
189 Malignant neoplasm of kidney and other unspecified urinary organs

Malignant neoplasm of other and unspecified sites (190-199)
190 Malignant neoplasm of eye
191 Malignant neoplasm of brain
192 Malignant neoplasm of other and unspecified parts of nervous system
193 Malignant neoplasm of thyroid gland
194 Malignant neoplasm of other endocrine glands and related structures
195 Malignant neoplasm of other and ill-defined sites
196 Secondary and unspecified malignant neoplasm of lymph nodes
197 Secondary malignant neoplasm of respiratory and digestive systems
198 Secondary malignant neoplasm of other specified sites
199 Malignant neoplasm without specification of site

Malignant neoplasm of lymphatic and hematopoietic tissue (200-208)
200 Lymphosarcoma and reticulosarcoma
201 Hodgkin's disease
202 Other malignant neoplasm of lymphoid and histiocytic tissue
203 Multiple myeloma and immunoproliferative neoplasms
204 Lymphoid leukemia
205 Myeloid leukemia
206 Monocytic leukemia
207 Other specified leukemia
208 Leukemia of unspecified cell type

Benign neoplasms (210-229)
210 Benign neoplasm of lip, oral cavity, and pharynx
211 Benign neoplasm of other parts of digestive system
212 Benign neoplasm of respiratory and intrathoracic organs
213 Benign neoplasm of bone and articular cartilage
214 Lipoma
215 Other benign neoplasm of connective and other soft tissue
216 Benign neoplasm of skin
217 Benign neoplasm of breast
218 Uterine leiomyoma
219 Other benign neoplasm of uterus
220 Benign neoplasm of ovary
221 Benign neoplasm of other female genital organs
222 Benign neoplasm of male genital organs
223 Benign neoplasm of kidney and other urinary organs
224 Benign neoplasm of eye
225 Benign neoplasm of brain and other parts of nervous system
226 Benign neoplasm of thyroid gland
227 Benign neoplasm of other endocrine glands and related structures
228 Hemangioma and lymphangioma, any site
229 Benign neoplasm of other and unspecified sites

Carcinoma in situ (230-234)
230 Carcinoma in situ of digestive organs
231 Carcinoma in situ of respiratory system
232 Carcinoma in situ of skin
233 Carcinoma in situ of breast and genitourinary system
234 Carcinoma in situ of other and unspecified sites

Neoplasms of uncertain behavior (235-238)
235 Neoplasm of uncertain behavior of digestive and respiratory systems
236 Neoplasm of uncertain behavior of genitourinary organs
237 Neoplasm of uncertain behavior of endocrine glands and nervous system
238 Neoplasm of uncertain behavior of other and unspecified sites and tissues

Neoplasms of unspecified nature (239)
239 Neoplasm of unspecified nature

3. ENDOCRINE, NUTRITIONAL AND METABOLIC DISEASES, AND IMMUNITY DISORDERS

Disorders of thyroid gland (240-246)
240 Simple and unspecified goiter
241 Nontoxic nodular goiter
242 Thyrotoxicosis with or without goiter
243 Congenital hypothyroidism
244 Acquired hypothyroidism
245 Thyroiditis
246 Other disorders of thyroid

Diseases of other endocrine glands (250-259)
250 Diabetes mellitus
251 Other disorders of pancreatic internal secretion
252 Disorders of parathyroid gland
253 Disorders of the pituitary gland and its hypothalamic control
254 Diseases of thymus gland
255 Disorders of adrenal glands
256 Ovarian dysfunction
257 Testicular dysfunction
258 Polyglandular dysfunction and related disorders
259 Other endocrine disorders

Nutritional deficiencies (260-269)
260 Kwashiorkor
261 Nutritional marasmus
262 Other severe protein-calorie malnutrition
263 Other and unspecified protein-calorie malnutrition
264 Vitamin A deficiency
265 Thiamine and niacin deficiency states
266 Deficiency of B-complex components
267 Ascorbic acid deficiency
268 Vitamin D deficiency
269 Other nutritional deficiencies

Other metabolic disorders and immunity disorders (270-279)
270 Disorders of amino-acid transport and metabolism
271 Disorders of carbohydrate transport and metabolism
272 Disorders of lipoid metabolism
273 Disorders of plasma protein metabolism
274 Gout
275 Disorders of mineral metabolism
276 Disorders of fluid, electrolyte, and acid-base balance
277 Other and unspecified disorders of metabolism
278 Obesity and other hyperalimentation
279 Disorders involving the immune mechanism

4. DISEASES OF BLOOD AND BLOOD-FORMING ORGANS (280-289)
280 Iron deficiency anemias
281 Other deficiency anemias
282 Hereditary hemolytic anemias
283 Acquired hemolytic anemias
284 Aplastic anemia
285 Other and unspecified anemias
286 Coagulation defects
287 Purpura and other hemorrhagic conditions
288 Diseases of white blood cells
289 Other diseases of blood and blood-forming organs

5. MENTAL DISORDERS

Organic psychotic conditions (290-294)
290 Senile and presenile organic psychotic conditions
291 Alcoholic psychoses
292 Drug psychoses
293 Transient organic psychotic conditions
294 Other organic psychotic conditions (chronic)

Other psychoses (295-299)
295 Schizophrenic psychoses
296 Affective psychoses
297 Paranoid states
298 Other nonorganic psychoses
299 Psychoses with origin specific to childhood

Neurotic disorders, personality disorders, and other nonpsychotic mental disorders (300-316)
300 Neurotic disorders
301 Personality disorders
302 Sexual deviations and disorders
303 Alcohol dependence syndrome
304 Drug dependence
305 Nondependent abuse of drugs
306 Physiological malfunction arising from mental factors
307 Special symptoms or syndromes, not elsewhere classified
308 Acute reaction to stress
309 Adjustment reaction
310 Specific nonpsychotic mental disorders following organic brain damage
311 Depressive disorder, not elsewhere classified
312 Disturbance of conduct, not elsewhere classified
313 Disturbance of emotions specific to childhood and adolescence
314 Hyperkinetic syndrome of childhood
315 Specific delays in development
316 Psychic factors associated with diseases classified elsewhere

Mental retardation (317-319)
317 Mild mental retardation
318 Other specified mental retardation
319 Unspecified mental retardation

6. DISEASES OF THE NERVOUS SYSTEM AND SENSE ORGANS

Inflammatory diseases of the central nervous system (320-326)
320 Bacterial meningitis
321 Meningitis due to other organisms
322 Meningitis of unspecified cause
323 Encephalitis, myelitis, and encephalomyelitis
324 Intracranial and intraspinal abscess
325 Phlebitis and thrombophlebitis of intracranial venous sinuses
326 Late effects of intracranial abscess or pyogenic infection

Hereditary and degenerative diseases of the central nervous system (330-337)
330 Cerebral degenerations usually manifest in childhood
331 Other cerebral degenerations
332 Parkinson's disease
333 Other extrapyramidal diseases and abnormal movement disorders
334 Spinocerebellar disease
335 Anterior horn cell disease
336 Other diseases of spinal cord
337 Disorders of the autonomic nervous system

Other disorders of the central nervous system (340-349)
340 Multiple sclerosis
341 Other demyelinating diseases of central nervous system
342 Hemiplegia and hemiparesis

343 Infantile cerebral palsy
344 Other paralytic syndromes
345 Epilepsy
346 Migraine
347 Cataplexy and narcolepsy
348 Other conditions of brain
349 Other and unspecified disorders of the nervous system

Disorders of the peripheral nervous system (350-359)
350 Trigeminal nerve disorders
351 Facial nerve disorders
352 Disorders of other cranial nerves
353 Nerve root and plexus disorders
354 Mononeuritis of upper limb and mononeuritis multiplex
355 Mononeuritis of lower limb
356 Hereditary and idiopathic peripheral neuropathy
357 Inflammatory and toxic neuropathy
358 Myoneural disorders
359 Muscular dystrophies and other myopathies

Disorders of the eye and adnexa (360-379)
360 Disorders of the globe
361 Retinal detachments and defects
362 Other retinal disorders
363 Chorioretinal inflammations and scars and other disorders of choroid
364 Disorders of iris and ciliary body
365 Glaucoma
366 Cataract
367 Disorders of refraction and accommodation
368 Visual disturbances
369 Blindness and low vision
370 Keratitis
371 Corneal opacity and other disorders of cornea
372 Disorders of conjunctiva
373 Inflammation of eyelids
374 Other disorders of eyelids
375 Disorders of lacrimal system
376 Disorders of the orbit
377 Disorders of optic nerve and visual pathways
378 Strabismus and other disorders of binocular eye movements
379 Other disorders of eye

Diseases of the ear and mastoid process (380-389)
380 Disorders of external ear
381 Nonsuppurative otitis media and Eustachian tube disorders
382 Suppurative and unspecified otitis media
383 Mastoiditis and related conditions
384 Other disorders of tympanic membrane
385 Other disorders of middle ear and mastoid
386 Vertiginous syndromes and other disorders of vestibular system
387 Otosclerosis
388 Other disorders of ear
389 Hearing loss

7. DISEASES OF THE CIRCULATORY SYSTEM

Acute rheumatic fever (390-392)
390 Rheumatic fever without mention of heart involvement
391 Rheumatic fever with heart involvement
392 Rheumatic chorea

Chronic rheumatic heart disease (393-398)
393 Chronic rheumatic pericarditis
394 Diseases of mitral valve
395 Diseases of aortic valve
396 Diseases of mitral and aortic valves
397 Diseases of other endocardial structures
398 Other rheumatic heart disease

Hypertensive disease (401-405)
401 Essential hypertension
402 Hypertensive heart disease
403 Hypertensive renal disease
404 Hypertensive heart and renal disease
405 Secondary hypertension

Ischemic heart disease (410-414)
410 Acute myocardial infarction
411 Other acute and subacute form of ischemic heart disease
412 Old myocardial infarction
413 Angina pectoris
414 Other forms of chronic ischemic heart disease

Diseases of pulmonary circulation (415-417)
415 Acute pulmonary heart disease
416 Chronic pulmonary heart disease
417 Other diseases of pulmonary circulation

Other forms of heart disease (420-429)
420 Acute pericarditis
421 Acute and subacute endocarditis
422 Acute myocarditis
423 Other diseases of pericardium
424 Other diseases of endocardium
425 Cardiomyopathy
426 Conduction disorders
427 Cardiac dysrhythmias
428 Heart failure
429 Ill-defined descriptions and complications of heart disease

Cerebrovascular disease (430-438)
430 Subarachnoid hemorrhage
431 Intracerebral hemorrhage
432 Other and unspecified intracranial hemorrhage
433 Occlusion and stenosis of precerebral arteries
434 Occlusion of cerebral arteries
435 Transient cerebral ischemia
436 Acute but ill-defined cerebrovascular disease
437 Other and ill-defined cerebrovascular disease
438 Late effects of cerebrovascular disease

Diseases of arteries, arterioles, and capillaries (440-448)
440 Atherosclerosis
441 Aortic aneurysm and dissection
442 Other aneurysm
443 Other peripheral vascular disease
444 Arterial embolism and thrombosis
445 Atheroembolism
446 Polyarteritis nodosa and allied conditions
447 Other disorders of arteries and arterioles
448 Diseases of capillaries

Diseases of veins and lymphatics, and other diseases of circulatory system (451-459)
451 Phlebitis and thrombophlebitis
452 Portal vein thrombosis
453 Other venous embolism and thrombosis
454 Varicose veins of lower extremities
455 Hemorrhoids
456 Varicose veins of other sites
457 Noninfective disorders of lymphatic channels
458 Hypotension
459 Other disorders of circulatory system

8. DISEASES OF THE RESPIRATORY SYSTEM

Acute respiratory infections (460-466)
460 Acute nasopharyngitis [common cold]
461 Acute sinusitis
462 Acute pharyngitis
463 Acute tonsillitis
464 Acute laryngitis and tracheitis
465 Acute upper respiratory infections of multiple or unspecified sites
466 Acute bronchitis and bronchiolitis

Other diseases of upper respiratory tract (470-478)
470 Deviated nasal septum
471 Nasal polyps
472 Chronic pharyngitis and nasopharyngitis
473 Chronic sinusitis
474 Chronic disease of tonsils and adenoids
475 Peritonsillar abscess
476 Chronic laryngitis and laryngotracheitis
477 Allergic rhinitis
478 Other diseases of upper respiratory tract

Pneumonia and influenza (480-487)
480 Viral pneumonia
481 Pneumococcal pneumonia [Streptococcus pneumoniae pneumonia]
482 Other bacterial pneumonia
483 Pneumonia due to other specified organism
484 Pneumonia in infectious diseases classified elsewhere
485 Bronchopneumonia, organism unspecified
486 Pneumonia, organism unspecified
487 Influenza

Chronic obstructive pulmonary disease and allied conditions (490-496)
490 Bronchitis, not specified as acute or chronic
491 Chronic bronchitis
492 Emphysema
493 Asthma
494 Bronchiectasis
495 Extrinsic allergic alveolitis
496 Chronic airways obstruction, not elsewhere classified

Pneumoconioses and other lung diseases due to external agents (500-508)
500 Coal workers' pneumoconiosis
501 Asbestosis
502 Pneumoconiosis due to other silica or silicates
503 Pneumoconiosis due to other inorganic dust
504 Pneumopathy due to inhalation of other dust
505 Pneumoconiosis, unspecified
506 Respiratory conditions due to chemical fumes and vapors
507 Pneumonitis due to solids and liquids
508 Respiratory conditions due to other and unspecified external agents

Other diseases of respiratory system (510-519)
510 Empyema
511 Pleurisy
512 Pneumothorax
513 Abscess of lung and mediastinum
514 Pulmonary congestion and hypostasis
515 Postinflammatory pulmonary fibrosis
516 Other alveolar and parietoalveolar pneumopathy
517 Lung involvement in conditions classified elsewhere
518 Other diseases of lung
519 Other diseases of respiratory system

9. DISEASES OF THE DIGESTIVE SYSTEM

Diseases of oral cavity, salivary glands, and jaws (520-529)
520 Disorders of tooth development and eruption
521 Diseases of hard tissues of teeth
522 Diseases of pulp and periapical tissues
523 Gingival and periodontal diseases
524 Dentofacial anomalies, including malocclusion
525 Other diseases and conditions of the teeth and supporting structures
526 Diseases of the jaws
527 Diseases of the salivary glands
528 Diseases of the oral soft tissues, excluding lesions specific for gingiva and tongue
529 Diseases and other conditions of the tongue

Diseases of esophagus, stomach, and duodenum (530-537)
530 Diseases of esophagus
531 Gastric ulcer
532 Duodenal ulcer
533 Peptic ulcer, site unspecified
534 Gastrojejunal ulcer
535 Gastritis and duodenitis
536 Disorders of function of stomach
537 Other disorders of stomach and duodenum

Appendicitis (540-543)
540 Acute appendicitis
541 Appendicitis, unqualified
542 Other appendicitis
543 Other diseases of appendix

Hernia of abdominal cavity (550-553)
550 Inguinal hernia
551 Other hernia of abdominal cavity, with gangrene
552 Other hernia of abdominal cavity, with obstruction, but without mention of gangrene
553 Other hernia of abdominal cavity without mention of obstruction or gangrene

Noninfective enteritis and colitis (555-558)
555 Regional enteritis
556 Ulcerative colitis
557 Vascular insufficiency of intestine
558 Other noninfective gastroenteritis and colitis

Other diseases of intestines and peritoneum (560-569)
560 Intestinal obstruction without mention of hernia
562 Diverticula of intestine
564 Functional digestive disorders, not elsewhere classified
565 Anal fissure and fistula
566 Abscess of anal and rectal regions
567 Peritonitis
568 Other disorders of peritoneum
569 Other disorders of intestine

Other diseases of digestive system (570-579)
570 Acute and subacute necrosis of liver
571 Chronic liver disease and cirrhosis
572 Liver abscess and sequelae of chronic liver disease
573 Other disorders of liver
574 Cholelithiasis
575 Other disorders of gallbladder
576 Other disorders of biliary tract
577 Diseases of pancreas
578 Gastrointestinal hemorrhage
579 Intestinal malabsorption

10. DISEASES OF THE GENITOURINARY SYSTEM

Nephritis, nephrotic syndrome, and nephrosis (580-589)
580 Acute glomerulonephritis
581 Nephrotic syndrome
582 Chronic glomerulonephritis
583 Nephritis and nephropathy, not specified as acute or chronic
584 Acute renal failure
585 Chronic renal failure
586 Renal failure, unspecified
587 Renal sclerosis, unspecified
588 Disorders resulting from impaired renal function
589 Small kidney of unknown cause

Other diseases of urinary system (590-599)
590 Infections of kidney
591 Hydronephrosis
592 Calculus of kidney and ureter
593 Other disorders of kidney and ureter
594 Calculus of lower urinary tract
595 Cystitis
596 Other disorders of bladder
597 Urethritis, not sexually transmitted, and urethral syndrome
598 Urethral stricture
599 Other disorders of urethra and urinary tract

Diseases of male genital organs (600-608)
600 Hyperplasia of prostate
601 Inflammatory diseases of prostate
602 Other disorders of prostate
603 Hydrocele
604 Orchitis and epididymitis
605 Redundant prepuce and phimosis
606 Infertility, male
607 Disorders of penis
608 Other disorders of male genital organs

Disorders of breast (610-611)
610 Benign mammary dysplasias
611 Other disorders of breast

Inflammatory disease of female pelvic organs (614-616)
614 Inflammatory disease of ovary, fallopian tube, pelvic cellular tissue, and peritoneum
615 Inflammatory diseases of uterus, except cervix
616 Inflammatory disease of cervix, vagina, and vulva

Other disorders of female genital tract (617-629)
617 Endometriosis
618 Genital prolapse
619 Fistula involving female genital tract
620 Noninflammatory disorders of ovary, fallopian tube, and broad ligament
621 Disorders of uterus, not elsewhere classified
622 Noninflammatory disorders of cervix
623 Noninflammatory disorders of vagina
624 Noninflammatory disorders of vulva and perineum
625 Pain and other symptoms associated with female genital organs
626 Disorders of menstruation and other abnormal bleeding from female genital tract
627 Menopausal and postmenopausal disorders
628 Infertility, female
629 Other disorders of female genital organs

11. COMPLICATIONS OF PREGNANCY, CHILDBIRTH AND THE PUERPERIUM

Ectopic and molar pregnancy and other pregnancy with abortive outcome (630-639)
630 Hydatidiform mole
631 Other abnormal product of conception
632 Missed abortion
633 Ectopic pregnancy
634 Spontaneous abortion
635 Legally induced abortion
636 Illegally induced abortion
637 Unspecified abortion
638 Failed attempted abortion
639 Complications following abortion and ectopic and molar pregnancies

Complications mainly related to pregnancy (640-648)
640 Hemorrhage in early pregnancy
641 Antepartum hemorrhage, abruptio placentae, and placenta previa
642 Hypertension complicating pregnancy, childbirth, and the puerperium
643 Excessive vomiting in pregnancy
644 Early or threatened labor
645 Prolonged pregnancy
646 Other complications of pregnancy, not elsewhere classified
647 Infective and parasitic conditions in the mother classifiable elsewhere but complicating pregnancy, childbirth, and the puerperium
648 Other current conditions in the mother classifiable elsewhere but complicating pregnancy, childbirth, and the puerperium

Normal delivery, and other indications for care in pregnancy, labor, and delivery (650-659)
650 Normal delivery
651 Multiple gestation
652 Malposition and malpresentation of fetus
653 Disproportion
654 Abnormality of organs and soft tissues of pelvis
655 Known or suspected fetal abnormality affecting management of mother
656 Other fetal and placental problems affecting management of mother
657 Polyhydramnios
658 Other problems associated with amniotic cavity and membranes
659 Other indications for care or intervention related to labor and delivery and not elsewhere classified

Complications occurring mainly in the course of labor and delivery (660-669)
660 Obstructed labor
661 Abnormality of forces of labor
662 Long labor
663 Umbilical cord complications
664 Trauma to perineum and vulva during delivery
665 Other obstetrical trauma
666 Postpartum hemorrhage
667 Retained placenta or membranes, without hemorrhage
668 Complications of the administration of anesthetic or other sedation in labor and delivery
669 Other complications of labor and delivery, not elsewhere classified

Complications of the puerperium (670-677)
670 Major puerperal infection
671 Venous complications in pregnancy and the puerperium
672 Pyrexia of unknown origin during the puerperium
673 Obstetrical pulmonary embolism
674 Other and unspecified complications of the puerperium, not elsewhere classified
675 Infections of the breast and nipple associated with childbirth
676 Other disorders of the breast associated with childbirth, and disorders of lactation
677 Late effect of complication of pregnancy, childbirth, and the puerperium

12. DISEASES OF THE SKIN AND SUBCUTANEOUS TISSUE

Infections of skin and subcutaneous tissue (680-686)
680 Carbuncle and furuncle
681 Cellulitis and abscess of finger and toe
682 Other cellulitis and abscess
683 Acute lymphadenitis
684 Impetigo
685 Pilonidal cyst
686 Other local infections of skin and subcutaneous tissue

Other inflammatory conditions of skin and subcutaneous tissue (690-698)
690 Erythematosquamous dermatosis
691 Atopic dermatitis and related conditions
692 Contact dermatitis and other eczema
693 Dermatitis due to substances taken internally
694 Bullous dermatoses
695 Erythematous conditions
696 Psoriasis and similar disorders
697 Lichen
698 Pruritus and related conditions

Other diseases of skin and subcutaneous tissue (700-709)

700 Corns and callosities
701 Other hypertrophic and atrophic conditions of skin
702 Other dermatoses
703 Diseases of nail
704 Diseases of hair and hair follicles
705 Disorders of sweat glands
706 Diseases of sebaceous glands
707 Chronic ulcer of skin
708 Urticaria
709 Other disorders of skin and subcutaneous tissue

13. DISEASES OF THE MUSCULOSKELETAL SYSTEM AND CONNECTIVE TISSUE

Arthropathies and related disorders (710-719)

710 Diffuse diseases of connective tissue
711 Arthropathy associated with infections
712 Crystal arthropathies
713 Arthropathy associated with other disorders classified elsewhere
714 Rheumatoid arthritis and other inflammatory polyarthropathies
715 Osteoarthrosis and allied disorders
716 Other and unspecified arthropathies
717 Internal derangement of knee
718 Other derangement of joint
719 Other and unspecified disorder of joint

Dorsopathies (720-724)

720 Ankylosing spondylitis and other inflammatory spondylopathies
721 Spondylosis and allied disorders
722 Intervertebral disc disorders
723 Other disorders of cervical region
724 Other and unspecified disorders of back

Rheumatism, excluding the back (725-729)

725 Polymyalgia rheumatica
726 Peripheral enthesopathies and allied syndromes
727 Other disorders of synovium, tendon, and bursa
728 Disorders of muscle, ligament, and fascia
729 Other disorders of soft tissues

Osteopathies, chondropathies, and acquired musculoskeletal deformities (730-739)

730 Osteomyelitis, periostitis, and other infections involving bone
731 Osteitis deformans and osteopathies associated with other disorders classified elsewhere
732 Osteochondropathies
733 Other disorders of bone and cartilage
734 Flat foot
735 Acquired deformities of toe
736 Other acquired deformities of limbs
737 Curvature of spine
738 Other acquired deformity
739 Nonallopathic lesions, not elsewhere classified

14. CONGENITAL ANOMALIES

740 Anencephalus and similar anomalies
741 Spina bifida
742 Other congenital anomalies of nervous system
743 Congenital anomalies of eye
744 Congenital anomalies of ear, face, and neck
745 Bulbus cordis anomalies and anomalies of cardiac septal closure
746 Other congenital anomalies of heart
747 Other congenital anomalies of circulatory system
748 Congenital anomalies of respiratory system
749 Cleft palate and cleft lip
750 Other congenital anomalies of upper alimentary tract
751 Other congenital anomalies of digestive system
752 Congenital anomalies of genital organs
753 Congenital anomalies of urinary system
754 Certain congenital musculoskeletal deformities
755 Other congenital anomalies of limbs
756 Other congenital musculoskeletal anomalies
757 Congenital anomalies of the integument
758 Chromosomal anomalies
759 Other and unspecified congenital anomalies

15. CERTAIN CONDITIONS ORIGINATING IN THE PERINATAL PERIOD

Maternal causes of perinatal morbidity and mortality (760-763)

760 Fetus or newborn affected by maternal conditions which may be unrelated to present pregnancy
761 Fetus or newborn affected by maternal complications of pregnancy
762 Fetus or newborn affected by complications of placenta, cord, and membranes
763 Fetus or newborn affected by other complications of labor and delivery

Other conditions originating in the perinatal period (764-779)

764 Slow fetal growth and fetal malnutrition
765 Disorders relating to short gestation and unspecified low birthweight
766 Disorders relating to long gestation and high birthweight
767 Birth trauma
768 Intrauterine hypoxia and birth asphyxia
769 Respiratory distress syndrome
770 Other respiratory conditions of fetus and newborn
771 Infections specific to the perinatal period
772 Fetal and neonatal hemorrhage
773 Hemolytic disease of fetus or newborn, due to isoimmunization
774 Other perinatal jaundice
775 Endocrine and metabolic disturbances specific to the fetus and newborn
776 Hematological disorders of fetus and newborn
777 Perinatal disorders of digestive system
778 Conditions involving the integument and temperature regulation of fetus and newborn
779 Other and ill-defined conditions originating in the perinatal period

16. SYMPTOMS, SIGNS, AND ILL-DEFINED CONDITIONS

Symptoms (780-789)

780 General symptoms
781 Symptoms involving nervous and musculoskeletal systems
782 Symptoms involving skin and other integumentary tissue
783 Symptoms concerning nutrition, metabolism, and development
784 Symptoms involving head and neck
785 Symptoms involving cardiovascular system
786 Symptoms involving respiratory system and other chest symptoms
787 Symptoms involving digestive system
788 Symptoms involving urinary system
789 Other symptoms involving abdomen and pelvis

Nonspecific abnormal findings (790-796)

790 Nonspecific findings on examination of blood
791 Nonspecific findings on examination of urine
792 Nonspecific abnormal findings in other body substances
793 Nonspecific abnormal findings on radiological and other examination of body structure
794 Nonspecific abnormal results of function studies
795 Nonspecific abnormal histological and immunological findings
796 Other nonspecific abnormal findings

Ill-defined and unknown causes of morbidity and mortality (797-799)

797 Senility without mention of psychosis
798 Sudden death, cause unknown
799 Other ill-defined and unknown causes of morbidity and mortality

17. INJURY AND POISONING

Fracture of skull (800-804)

800 Fracture of vault of skull
801 Fracture of base of skull
802 Fracture of face bones
803 Other and unqualified skull fractures
804 Multiple fractures involving skull or face with other bones

Fracture of spine and trunk (805-809)

805 Fracture of vertebral column without mention of spinal cord lesion
806 Fracture of vertebral column with spinal cord lesion
807 Fracture of rib(s), sternum, larynx, and trachea
808 Fracture of pelvis
809 Ill-defined fractures of bones of trunk

Fracture of upper limb (810-819)

810 Fracture of clavicle
811 Fracture of scapula
812 Fracture of humerus
813 Fracture of radius and ulna
814 Fracture of carpal bone(s)
815 Fracture of metacarpal bone(s)
816 Fracture of one or more phalanges of hand
817 Multiple fractures of hand bones
818 Ill-defined fractures of upper limb
819 Multiple fractures involving both upper limbs, and upper limb with rib(s) and sternum

Fracture of lower limb (820-829)

820 Fracture of neck of femur
821 Fracture of other and unspecified parts of femur
822 Fracture of patella
823 Fracture of tibia and fibula
824 Fracture of ankle
825 Fracture of one or more tarsal and metatarsal bones
826 Fracture of one or more phalanges of foot
827 Other, multiple, and ill-defined fractures of lower limb
828 Multiple fractures involving both lower limbs, lower with upper limb, and lower limb(s) with rib(s) and sternum
829 Fracture of unspecified bones

Dislocation (830-839)

830 Dislocation of jaw
831 Dislocation of shoulder
832 Dislocation of elbow
833 Dislocation of wrist
834 Dislocation of finger
835 Dislocation of hip
836 Dislocation of knee
837 Dislocation of ankle
838 Dislocation of foot
839 Other, multiple, and ill-defined dislocations

Sprains and strains of joints and adjacent muscles (840-848)

840 Sprains and strains of shoulder and upper arm
841 Sprains and strains of elbow and forearm
842 Sprains and strains of wrist and hand
843 Sprains and strains of hip and thigh
844 Sprains and strains of knee and leg
845 Sprains and strains of ankle and foot
846 Sprains and strains of sacroiliac region
847 Sprains and strains of other and unspecified parts of back

848 Other and ill-defined sprains and strains

Intracranial injury, excluding those with skull fracture (850-854)
850 Concussion
851 Cerebral laceration and contusion
852 Subarachnoid, subdural, and extradural hemorrhage, following injury
853 Other and unspecified intracranial hemorrhage following injury
854 Intracranial injury of other and unspecified nature

Internal injury of chest, abdomen, and pelvis (860-869)
860 Traumatic pneumothorax and hemothorax
861 Injury to heart and lung
862 Injury to other and unspecified intrathoracic organs
863 Injury to gastrointestinal tract
864 Injury to liver
865 Injury to spleen
866 Injury to kidney
867 Injury to pelvic organs
868 Injury to other intra-abdominal organs
869 Internal injury to unspecified or ill-defined organs

Open wound of head, neck, and trunk (870-879)
870 Open wound of ocular adnexa
871 Open wound of eyeball
872 Open wound of ear
873 Other open wound of head
874 Open wound of neck
875 Open wound of chest (wall)
876 Open wound of back
877 Open wound of buttock
878 Open wound of genital organs (external), including traumatic amputation
879 Open wound of other and unspecified sites, except limbs

Open wound of upper limb (880-887)
880 Open wound of shoulder and upper arm
881 Open wound of elbow, forearm, and wrist
882 Open wound of hand except finger(s) alone
883 Open wound of finger(s)
884 Multiple and unspecified open wound of upper limb
885 Traumatic amputation of thumb (complete) (partial)
886 Traumatic amputation of other finger(s) (complete) (partial)
887 Traumatic amputation of arm and hand (complete) (partial)

Open wound of lower limb (890-897)
890 Open wound of hip and thigh
891 Open wound of knee, leg [except thigh], and ankle
892 Open wound of foot except toe(s) alone
893 Open wound of toe(s)
894 Multiple and unspecified open wound of lower limb
895 Traumatic amputation of toe(s) (complete) (partial)
896 Traumatic amputation of foot (complete) (partial)
897 Traumatic amputation of leg(s) (complete) (partial)

Injury to blood vessels (900-904)
900 Injury to blood vessels of head and neck
901 Injury to blood vessels of thorax
902 Injury to blood vessels of abdomen and pelvis
903 Injury to blood vessels of upper extremity
904 Injury to blood vessels of lower extremity and unspecified sites

Late effects of injuries, poisonings, toxic effects, and other external causes (905-909)
905 Late effects of musculoskeletal and connective tissue injuries
906 Late effects of injuries to skin and subcutaneous tissues
907 Late effects of injuries to the nervous system
908 Late effects of other and unspecified injuries
909 Late effects of other and unspecified external causes

Superficial injury (910-919)
910 Superficial injury of face, neck, and scalp except eye
911 Superficial injury of trunk
912 Superficial injury of shoulder and upper arm
913 Superficial injury of elbow, forearm, and wrist
914 Superficial injury of hand(s) except finger(s) alone
915 Superficial injury of finger(s)
916 Superficial injury of hip, thigh, leg, and ankle
917 Superficial injury of foot and toe(s)
918 Superficial injury of eye and adnexa
919 Superficial injury of other, multiple, and unspecified sites

Contusion with intact skin surface (920-924)
920 Contusion of face, scalp, and neck except eye(s)
921 Contusion of eye and adnexa
922 Contusion of trunk
923 Contusion of upper limb
924 Contusion of lower limb and of other and unspecified sites

Crushing injury (925-929)
925 Crushing injury of face, scalp, and neck
926 Crushing injury of trunk
927 Crushing injury of upper limb
928 Crushing injury of lower limb
929 Crushing injury of multiple and unspecified sites

Effects of foreign body entering through orifice (930-939)
930 Foreign body on external eye
931 Foreign body in ear
932 Foreign body in nose
933 Foreign body in pharynx and larynx
934 Foreign body in trachea, bronchus, and lung
935 Foreign body in mouth, esophagus, and stomach
936 Foreign body in intestine and colon
937 Foreign body in anus and rectum
938 Foreign body in digestive system, unspecified
939 Foreign body in genitourinary tract

Burns (940-949)
940 Burn confined to eye and adnexa
941 Burn of face, head, and neck
942 Burn of trunk
943 Burn of upper limb, except wrist and hand
944 Burn of wrist(s) and hand(s)
945 Burn of lower limb(s)
946 Burns of multiple specified sites
947 Burn of internal organs
948 Burns classified according to extent of body surface involved
949 Burn, unspecified

Injury to nerves and spinal cord (950-957)
950 Injury to optic nerve and pathways
951 Injury to other cranial nerve(s)
952 Spinal cord injury without evidence of spinal bone injury
953 Injury to nerve roots and spinal plexus
954 Injury to other nerve(s) of trunk excluding shoulder and pelvic girdles
955 Injury to peripheral nerve(s) of shoulder girdle and upper limb
956 Injury to peripheral nerve(s) of pelvic girdle and lower limb
957 Injury to other and unspecified nerves

Certain traumatic complications and unspecified injuries (958-959)
958 Certain early complications of trauma
959 Injury, other and unspecified

Poisoning by drugs, medicinals and biological substances (960-979)
960 Poisoning by antibiotics
961 Poisoning by other anti-infectives
962 Poisoning by hormones and synthetic substitutes
963 Poisoning by primarily systemic agents
964 Poisoning by agents primarily affecting blood constituents
965 Poisoning by analgesics, antipyretics, and antirheumatics
966 Poisoning by anticonvulsants and anti-Parkinsonism drugs
967 Poisoning by sedatives and hypnotics
968 Poisoning by other central nervous system depressants and anesthetics
969 Poisoning by psychotropic agents
970 Poisoning by central nervous system stimulants
971 Poisoning by drugs primarily affecting the autonomic nervous system
972 Poisoning by agents primarily affecting the cardiovascular system
973 Poisoning by agents primarily affecting the gastrointestinal system
974 Poisoning by water, mineral, and uric acid metabolism drugs
975 Poisoning by agents primarily acting on the smooth and skeletal muscles and respiratory system
976 Poisoning by agents primarily affecting skin and mucous membrane, ophthalmological, otorhinolaryngological, and dental drugs
977 Poisoning by other and unspecified drugs and medicinals
978 Poisoning by bacterial vaccines
979 Poisoning by other vaccines and biological substances

Toxic effects of substances chiefly nonmedicinal as to source (980-989)
980 Toxic effect of alcohol
981 Toxic effect of petroleum products
982 Toxic effect of solvents other than petroleum-based
983 Toxic effect of corrosive aromatics, acids, and caustic alkalis
984 Toxic effect of lead and its compounds (including fumes)
985 Toxic effect of other metals
986 Toxic effect of carbon monoxide
987 Toxic effect of other gases, fumes, or vapors
988 Toxic effect of noxious substances eaten as food
989 Toxic effect of other substances, chiefly nonmedicinal as to source

Other and unspecified effects of external causes (990-995)
990 Effects of radiation, unspecified
991 Effects of reduced temperature
992 Effects of heat and light
993 Effects of air pressure
994 Effects of other external causes
995 Certain adverse effects, not elsewhere classified

Complications of surgical and medical care, not elsewhere classified (996-999)
996 Complications peculiar to certain specified procedures
997 Complications affecting specified body systems, not elsewhere classified
998 Other complications of procedures, not elsewhere classified
999 Complications of medical care, not elsewhere classified

SUPPLEMENTARY CLASSIFICATION OF FACTORS INFLUENCING HEALTH STATUS AND CONTACT WITH HEALTH SERVICES

Persons with potential health hazards related to communicable diseases (V01-V09)

V01 Contact with or exposure to communicable diseases
V02 Carrier or suspected carrier of infectious diseases
V03 Need for prophylactic vaccination and inoculation against bacterial diseases
V04 Need for prophylactic vaccination and inoculation against certain viral diseases
V05 Need for other prophylactic vaccination and inoculation against single diseases
V06 Need for prophylactic vaccination and inoculation against combinations of diseases
V07 Need for isolation and other prophylactic measures
V08 Asymptomatic human immunodeficiency virus [HIV] infection status
V09 Infection with drug-resistant microorganisms

Persons with potential health hazards related to personal and family history (V10-V19)

V10 Personal history of malignant neoplasm
V11 Personal history of mental disorder
V12 Personal history of certain other diseases
V13 Personal history of other diseases
V14 Personal history of allergy to medicinal agents
V15 Other personal history presenting hazards to health
V16 Family history of malignant neoplasm
V17 Family history of certain chronic disabling diseases
V18 Family history of certain other specific conditions
V19 Family history of other conditions

Persons encountering health services in circumstances related to reproduction and development (V20-V29)

V20 Health supervision of infant or child
V21 Constitutional states in development
V22 Normal pregnancy
V23 Supervision of high-risk pregnancy
V24 Postpartum care and examination
V25 Encounter for contraceptive management
V26 Procreative management
V27 Outcome of delivery
V28 Antenatal screening
V29 Observation and evaluation of newborns and infants for suspected condition not found

Liveborn infants according to type of birth (V30-V39)

V30 Single liveborn
V31 Twin, mate liveborn
V32 Twin, mate stillborn
V33 Twin, unspecified
V34 Other multiple, mates all liveborn
V35 Other multiple, mates all stillborn
V36 Other multiple, mates live- and stillborn
V37 Other multiple, unspecified
V39 Unspecified

Persons with a condition influencing their health status (V40-V49)

V40 Mental and behavioral problems
V41 Problems with special senses and other special functions
V42 Organ or tissue replaced by transplant
V43 Organ or tissue replaced by other means
V44 Artificial opening status
V45 Other postprocedural states
V46 Other dependence on machines
V47 Other problems with internal organs
V48 Problems with head, neck, and trunk
V49 Problems with limbs and other problems

Persons encountering health services for specific procedures and aftercare (V50-V59)

V50 Elective surgery for purposes other than remedying health states
V51 Aftercare involving the use of plastic surgery
V52 Fitting and adjustment of prosthetic device
V53 Fitting and adjustment of other device
V54 Other orthopedic aftercare
V55 Attention to artificial openings
V56 Encounter for dialysis and dialysis catheter care
V57 Care involving use of rehabilitation procedures
V58 Encounter for other and unspecified procedures and aftercare
V59 Donors

Persons encountering health services in other circumstances (V60-V69)

V60 Housing, household, and economic circumstances
V61 Other family circumstances
V62 Other psychosocial circumstances
V63 Unavailability of other medical facilities for care
V64 Persons encountering health services for specific procedures, not carried out
V65 Other persons seeking consultation
V66 Convalescence and palliative care
V67 Follow-up examination
V68 Encounters for administrative purposes
V69 Problems related to lifestyle

Persons without reported diagnosis encountered during examination and investigation of individuals and populations (V70-V84)

V70 General medical examination
V71 Observation and evaluation for suspected conditions not found
V72 Special investigations and examinations
V73 Special screening examination for viral and chlamydial diseases
V74 Special screening examination for bacterial and spirochetal diseases
V75 Special screening examination for other infectious diseases
V76 Special screening for malignant neoplasms
V77 Special screening for endocrine, nutritional, metabolic, and immunity disorders
V78 Special screening for disorders of blood and blood-forming organs
V79 Special screening for mental disorders and developmental handicaps
V80 Special screening for neurological, eye, and ear diseases
V81 Special screening for cardiovascular, respiratory, and genitourinary diseases
V82 Special screening for other conditions
V83 Genetic carrier status
V84 Genetic susceptibility to disease

SUPPLEMENTARY CLASSIFICATION OF EXTERNAL CAUSES OF INJURY AND POISONING

Railway accidents (E800-E807)

E800 Railway accident involving collision with rolling stock
E801 Railway accident involving collision with other object
E802 Railway accident involving derailment without antecedent collision
E803 Railway accident involving explosion, fire, or burning
E804 Fall in, on, or from railway train
E805 Hit by rolling stock
E806 Other specified railway accident
E807 Railway accident of unspecified nature

Motor vehicle traffic accidents (E810-E819)

E810 Motor vehicle traffic accident involving collision with train
E811 Motor vehicle traffic accident involving re-entrant collision with another motor vehicle
E812 Other motor vehicle traffic accident involving collision with another motor vehicle
E813 Motor vehicle traffic accident involving collision with other vehicle
E814 Motor vehicle traffic accident involving collision with pedestrian
E815 Other motor vehicle traffic accident involving collision on the highway
E816 Motor vehicle traffic accident due to loss of control, without collision on the highway
E817 Noncollision motor vehicle traffic accident while boarding or alighting
E818 Other noncollision motor vehicle traffic accident
E819 Motor vehicle traffic accident of unspecified nature

Motor vehicle nontraffic accidents (E820-E825)

E820 Nontraffic accident involving motor-driven snow vehicle
E821 Nontraffic accident involving other off-road motor vehicle
E822 Other motor vehicle nontraffic accident involving collision with moving object
E823 Other motor vehicle nontraffic accident involving collision with stationary object
E824 Other motor vehicle nontraffic accident while boarding and alighting
E825 Other motor vehicle nontraffic accident of other and unspecified nature

Other road vehicle accidents (E826-E829)

E826 Pedal cycle accident
E827 Animal-drawn vehicle accident
E828 Accident involving animal being ridden
E829 Other road vehicle accidents

Water transport accidents (E830-E838)

E830 Accident to watercraft causing submersion
E831 Accident to watercraft causing other injury
E832 Other accidental submersion or drowning in water transport accident
E833 Fall on stairs or ladders in water transport
E834 Other fall from one level to another in water transport
E835 Other and unspecified fall in water transport
E836 Machinery accident in water transport
E837 Explosion, fire, or burning in watercraft
E838 Other and unspecified water transport accident

Air and space transport accidents (E840-E845)

E840 Accident to powered aircraft at takeoff or landing
E841 Accident to powered aircraft, other and unspecified
E842 Accident to unpowered aircraft
E843 Fall in, on, or from aircraft
E844 Other specified air transport accidents
E845 Accident involving spacecraft

Vehicle accidents, not elsewhere classifiable (E846-E849)

E846 Accidents involving powered vehicles used solely within the buildings and premises of an industrial or commercial establishment
E847 Accidents involving cable cars not running on rails
E848 Accidents involving other vehicles, not elsewhere classifiable
E849 Place of occurrence

Accidental poisoning by drugs, medicinal substances, and biologicals (E850-E858)

E850 Accidental poisoning by analgesics, antipyretics, and antirheumatics
E851 Accidental poisoning by barbiturates
E852 Accidental poisoning by other sedatives and hypnotics
E853 Accidental poisoning by tranquilizers

E854 Accidental poisoning by other psychotropic agents
E855 Accidental poisoning by other drugs acting on central and autonomic nervous systems
E856 Accidental poisoning by antibiotics
E857 Accidental poisoning by anti-infectives
E858 Accidental poisoning by other drugs

Accidental poisoning by other solid and liquid substances, gases, and vapors (E860-E869)
E860 Accidental poisoning by alcohol, not elsewhere classified
E861 Accidental poisoning by cleansing and polishing agents, disinfectants, paints, and varnishes
E862 Accidental poisoning by petroleum products, other solvents and their vapors, not elsewhere classified
E863 Accidental poisoning by agricultural and horticultural chemical and pharmaceutical preparations other than plant foods and fertilizers
E864 Accidental poisoning by corrosives and caustics, not elsewhere classified
E865 Accidental poisoning from poisonous foodstuffs and poisonous plants
E866 Accidental poisoning by other and unspecified solid and liquid substances
E867 Accidental poisoning by gas distributed by pipeline
E868 Accidental poisoning by other utility gas and other carbon monoxide
E869 Accidental poisoning by other gases and vapors

Misadventures to patients during surgical and medical care (E870-E876)
E870 Accidental cut, puncture, perforation, or hemorrhage during medical care
E871 Foreign object left in body during procedure
E872 Failure of sterile precautions during procedure
E873 Failure in dosage
E874 Mechanical failure of instrument or apparatus during procedure
E875 Contaminated or infected blood, other fluid, drug, or biological substance
E876 Other and unspecified misadventures during medical care

Surgical and medical procedures as the cause of abnormal reaction of patient or later complication, without mention of misadventure at the time of procedure (E878-E879)
E878 Surgical operation and other surgical procedures as the cause of abnormal reaction of patient, or of later complication, without mention of misadventure at the time of operation
E879 Other procedures, without mention of misadventure at the time of procedure, as the cause of abnormal reaction of patient, or of later complication

Accidental falls (E880-E888)
E880 Fall on or from stairs or steps
E881 Fall on or from ladders or scaffolding
E882 Fall from or out of building or other structure
E883 Fall into hole or other opening in surface
E884 Other fall from one level to another
E885 Fall on same level from slipping, tripping, or stumbling
E886 Fall on same level from collision, pushing, or shoving, by or with other person
E887 Fracture, cause unspecified
E888 Other and unspecified fall

Accidents caused by fire and flames (E890-E899)
E890 Conflagration in private dwelling
E891 Conflagration in other and unspecified building or structure

E892 Conflagration not in building or structure
E893 Accident caused by ignition of clothing
E894 Ignition of highly inflammable material
E895 Accident caused by controlled fire in private dwelling
E896 Accident caused by controlled fire in other and unspecified building or structure
E897 Accident caused by controlled fire not in building or structure
E898 Accident caused by other specified fire and flames
E899 Accident caused by unspecified fire

Accidents due to natural and environmental factors (E900-E909)
E900 Excessive heat
E901 Excessive cold
E902 High and low air pressure and changes in air pressure
E903 Travel and motion
E904 Hunger, thirst, exposure, and neglect
E905 Venomous animals and plants as the cause of poisoning and toxic reactions
E906 Other injury caused by animals
E907 Lightning
E908 Cataclysmic storms, and floods resulting from storms
E909 Cataclysmic earth surface movements and eruptions

Accidents caused by submersion, suffocation, and foreign bodies (E910-E915)
E910 Accidental drowning and submersion
E911 Inhalation and ingestion of food causing obstruction of respiratory tract or suffocation
E912 Inhalation and ingestion of other object causing obstruction of respiratory tract or suffocation
E913 Accidental mechanical suffocation
E914 Foreign body accidentally entering eye and adnexa
E915 Foreign body accidentally entering other orifice

Other accidents (E916-E928)
E916 Struck accidentally by falling object
E917 Striking against or struck accidentally by objects or persons
E918 Caught accidentally in or between objects
E919 Accidents caused by machinery
E920 Accidents caused by cutting and piercing instruments or objects
E921 Accident caused by explosion of pressure vessel
E922 Accident caused by firearm missile
E923 Accident caused by explosive material
E924 Accident caused by hot substance or object, caustic or corrosive material, and steam
E925 Accident caused by electric current
E926 Exposure to radiation
E927 Overexertion and strenuous movements
E928 Other and unspecified environmental and accidental causes

Late effects of accidental injury (E929)
E929 Late effects of accidental injury

Drugs, medicinal and biological substances causing adverse effects in therapeutic use (E930-E949)
E930 Antibiotics
E931 Other anti-infectives
E932 Hormones and synthetic substitutes
E933 Primarily systemic agents
E934 Agents primarily affecting blood constituents
E935 Analgesics, antipyretics, and antirheumatics
E936 Anticonvulsants and anti-Parkinsonism drugs
E937 Sedatives and hypnotics

E938 Other central nervous system depressants and anesthetics
E939 Psychotropic agents
E940 Central nervous system stimulants
E941 Drugs primarily affecting the autonomic nervous system
E942 Agents primarily affecting the cardiovascular system
E943 Agents primarily affecting gastrointestinal system
E944 Water, mineral, and uric acid metabolism drugs
E945 Agents primarily acting on the smooth and skeletal muscles and respiratory system
E946 Agents primarily affecting skin and mucous membrane, ophthalmological, otorhinolaryngological, and dental drugs
E947 Other and unspecified drugs and medicinal substances
E948 Bacterial vaccines
E949 Other vaccines and biological substances

Suicide and self-inflicted injury (E950-E959)
E950 Suicide and self-inflicted poisoning by solid or liquid substances
E951 Suicide and self-inflicted poisoning by gases in domestic use
E952 Suicide and self-inflicted poisoning by other gases and vapors
E953 Suicide and self-inflicted injury by hanging, strangulation, and suffocation
E954 Suicide and self-inflicted injury by submersion [drowning]
E955 Suicide and self-inflicted injury by firearms and explosives
E956 Suicide and self-inflicted injury by cutting and piercing instruments
E957 Suicide and self-inflicted injuries by jumping from high place
E958 Suicide and self-inflicted injury by other and unspecified means
E959 Late effects of self-inflicted injury

Homicide and injury purposely inflicted by other persons (E960-E969)
E960 Fight, brawl, and rape
E961 Assault by corrosive or caustic substance, except poisoning
E962 Assault by poisoning
E963 Assault by hanging and strangulation
E964 Assault by submersion [drowning]
E965 Assault by firearms and explosives
E966 Assault by cutting and piercing instrument
E967 Child and adult battering and other maltreatment
E968 Assault by other and unspecified means
E969 Late effects of injury purposely inflicted by other person

Legal intervention (E970-E978)
E970 Injury due to legal intervention by firearms
E971 Injury due to legal intervention by explosives
E972 Injury due to legal intervention by gas
E973 Injury due to legal intervention by blunt object
E974 Injury due to legal intervention by cutting and piercing instruments
E975 Injury due to legal intervention by other specified means
E976 Injury due to legal intervention by unspecified means
E977 Late effects of injuries due to legal intervention
E978 Legal execution

Terrorism (E979)
E979 Terrorism

Injury undetermined whether accidentally or purposely inflicted (E980-E989)
E980 Poisoning by solid or liquid substances, undetermined whether accidentally or purposely inflicted

E981 Poisoning by gases in domestic use, undetermined whether accidentally or purposely inflicted

E982 Poisoning by other gases, undetermined whether accidentally or purposely inflicted

E983 Hanging, strangulation, or suffocation, undetermined whether accidentally or purposely inflicted

E984 Submersion [drowning], undetermined whether accidentally or purposely inflicted

E985 Injury by firearms and explosives, undetermined whether accidentally or purposely inflicted

E986 Injury by cutting and piercing instruments, undetermined whether accidentally or purposely inflicted

E987 Falling from high place, undetermined whether accidentally or purposely inflicted

E988 Injury by other and unspecified means, undetermined whether accidentally or purposely inflicted

E989 Late effects of injury, undetermined whether accidentally or purposely inflicted

Injury resulting from operations of war (E990-E999)

E990 Injury due to war operations by fires and conflagrations

E991 Injury due to war operations by bullets and fragments

E992 Injury due to war operations by explosion of marine weapons

E993 Injury due to war operations by other explosion

E994 Injury due to war operations by destruction of aircraft

E995 Injury due to war operations by other and unspecified forms of conventional warfare

E996 Injury due to war operations by nuclear weapons

E997 Injury due to war operations by other forms of unconventional warfare

E998 Injury due to war operations but occurring after cessation of hostilities

E999 Late effects of injury due to war operations

Valid Three-digit ICD-9-CM Codes

Three-digit ICD-9-CM codes are used to identify a condition or disease only when a fourth or fifth digit is not available. The following are the only ICD-9-CM codes that are valid without further specificity.

024 Glanders

025 Melioidosis

035 Erysipelas

037 Tetanus

042 Human immunodeficiency virus (HIV) infection

048 Other enterovirus diseases of central nervous system

061 Dengue

064 Viral encephalitis transmitted by other and unspecified arthropods

071 Rabies

075 Infectious mononucleosis

080 Louse-borne [epidemic] typhus

096 Late syphilis, latent

101 Vincent's angina

118 Opportunistic mycoses

124 Trichinosis

129 Intestinal parasitism, unspecified

135 Sarcoidosis

138 Late effects of acute poliomyelitis

179 Malignant neoplasm of uterus, part unspecified

181 Malignant neoplasm of placenta

185 Malignant neoplasm of prostate

193 Malignant neoplasm of thyroid gland

217 Benign neoplasm of breast

220 Benign neoplasm of ovary

226 Benign neoplasm of thyroid gland

243 Congenital hypothyroidism

260 Kwashiorkor

261 Nutritional marasmus

262 Other severe protein-calorie malnutrition

267 Ascorbic acid deficiency

311 Depressive disorder, not elsewhere classified

316 Psychic factors associated with diseases classified elsewhere

317 Mild mental retardation

319 Unspecified mental retardation

325 Phlebitis and thrombophlebitis of intracranial venous sinuses

326 Late effects of intracranial abscess or pyogenic infection

340 Multiple sclerosis

390 Rheumatic fever without mention of heart involvement

393 Chronic rheumatic pericarditis

412 Old myocardial infarction

430 Subarachnoid hemorrhage

431 Intracerebral hemorrhage

436 Acute, but ill-defined, cerebrovascular disease

452 Portal vein thrombosis

460 Acute nasopharyngitis [common cold]

462 Acute pharyngitis

463 Acute tonsillitis

470 Deviated nasal septum

475 Peritonsillar abscess

481 Pneumococcal pneumonia

485 Bronchopneumonia, organism unspecified

486 Pneumonia, organism unspecified

490 Bronchitis, not specified as acute or chronic

496 Chronic airway obstruction, not elsewhere classified

500 Coal workers' pneumoconiosis

501 Asbestosis

502 Pneumoconiosis due to other silica or silicates

503 Pneumoconiosis due to other inorganic dust

504 Pneumoconopathy due to inhalation of other dust

505 Pneumoconiosis, unspecified

514 Pulmonary congestion and hypostasis

515 Postinflammatory pulmonary fibrosis

541 Appendicitis, unqualified

542 Other appendicitis

566 Abscess of anal and rectal regions

570 Acute and subacute necrosis of liver

585 Chronic renal failure

586 Renal failure, unspecified

587 Renal sclerosis, unspecified

591 Hydronephrosis

605 Redundant prepuce and phimosis

630 Hydatidiform mole

631 Other abnormal product of conception

632 Missed abortion

650 Delivery in a completely normal case

677 Late effect of complication of pregnancy, childbirth, and the puerperium

683 Acute lymphadenitis

684 Impetigo

700 Corns and callosities

725 Polymyalgia rheumatica

734 Flat foot

769 Respiratory distress syndrome

797 Senility without mention of psychosis

920 Contusion of face, scalp, and neck except eye(s)

931 Foreign body in ear

932 Foreign body in nose

936 Foreign body in intestine and colon

937 Foreign body in anus and rectum

938 Foreign body in digestive system, unspecified

981 Toxic effect of petroleum products

986 Toxic effect of carbon monoxide

990 Effects of radiation, unspecified

V08 Asymptomatic human immunodeficiency virus [HIV] infection status

V51 Aftercare involving the use of plastic surgery

Abortion

	Spontaneous Abortion (accidental) (early) (late) (miscarriage) (recurrent)				Legally Induced Abortion (elective) (legal) (therapeutic)			
	Incomplete (part of the products of conception are retained)	Complete (all of the products of conception are expelled)	Unspecified	Complication following abortion (separate epidosde of care)	Incomplete (part of the products of conception are retained)	Complete (all of the products of conception are expelled)	Unspecified	Complication following abortion (separate epidosde of care)
Without complication	634.91	634.92	634.90		635.91	635.92	635.90	
With complication of:								
Afibrinogenemia	634.11	634.12	634.10	639.1	635.11	635.12	635.10	639.1
Atrophy, acute yellow	634.71	634.72	634.70	639.8	635.71	635.72	635.70	639.8
Cardiac arrest	634.71	634.72	634.70	639.8	635.71	635.72	635.70	639.8
Cardiac failure	634.71	634.72	634.70	639.8	635.71	635.72	635.70	639.8
Cerebral anoxia	634.71	634.72	634.70	639.8	635.71	635.72	635.70	639.8
Circulatory collapse	634.51	634.52	634.50	639.5	635.51	635.52	635.50	639.5
Defibrination syndrome	634.11	634.12	634.10	639.1	635.11	635.12	635.10	639.1
Electrolyte imbalance	634.41	634.42	634.40	639.4	635.41	635.42	635.40	639.4
Embolism (any type)	634.61	634.62	634.60	639.6	635.61	635.62	635.60	639.6
Endometritis	634.01	634.02	634.00	639.0	635.01	635.02	635.00	639.0
Genital tract infection	634.01	634.02	634.00	639.0	635.01	635.02	635.00	639.0
Hemorrhage, delayed or excessive	634.11	634.12	634.10	639.1	635.11	635.12	635.10	639.1
Intravascular hemolysis	634.11	634.12	634.10	639.1	635.11	635.12	635.10	639.1
Laceration of:								
bladder	634.21	634.22	634.20	639.2	635.21	635.22	635.20	639.2
bowel	634.21	634.22	634.20	639.2	635.21	635.22	635.20	639.2
broad ligament	634.21	634.22	634.20	639.2	635.21	635.22	635.20	639.2
cervix	634.21	634.22	634.20	639.2	635.21	635.22	635.20	639.2
periurethral tissue	634.21	634.22	634.20	639.2	635.21	635.22	635.20	639.2
uterus	634.21	634.22	634.20	639.2	635.21	635.22	635.20	639.2
vagina	634.21	634.22	634.20	639.2	635.21	635.22	635.20	639.2
Metabolic disorder	634.41	634.42	634.40	639.4	635.41	635.42	635.40	639.4
Necrosis of liver	634.71	634.72	634.70	639.8	635.71	635.72	635.70	639.8
Oliguria	634.31	634.32	634.30	639.3	635.31	635.32	635.30	639.3
Other specified complication	634.71	634.72	634.70	639.8	635.71	635.72	635.70	639.8
Parametritis	634.01	634.02	634.00	639.0	635.01	635.02	635.00	639.0
Pelvic infection	634.01	634.02	634.00	639.0	635.01	635.02	635.00	639.0
Pelvic peritonitis	634.01	634.02	634.00	639.0	635.01	635.02	635.00	639.0
Perforation — *See Abortion, by type, laceration*								
Renal failure (acute)	634.31	634.32	634.30	639.3	635.31	635.32	635.30	639.3
Renal shutdown	634.31	634.32	634.30	639.3	635.31	635.32	635.30	639.3
Renal tubular necrosis	634.31	634.32	634.30	639.3	635.31	635.32	635.30	639.3
Salpingitis	634.01	634.02	634.00	639.0	635.01	635.02	635.00	639.0
Salpingo-oophoritis	634.01	634.02	634.00	639.0	635.01	635.02	635.00	639.0
Sepsis NOS	634.01	634.02	634.00	639.0	635.01	635.02	635.00	639.0
Septicemia NOS	634.01	634.02	634.00	639.0	635.01	635.02	635.00	639.0
Shock (postoperative)(septic)	634.51	634.52	634.50	639.5	635.51	635.52	635.50	639.5
Tear — *See Abortion, by type, laceration*								
Unspecified complications	634.81	634.82	634.80	639.9	635.81	635.82	635.80	639.9
Uremia	634.31	634.32	634.30	639.3	635.31	635.32	635.30	639.3
Urinary tract infection	634.71	634.72	634.70	639.8	635.71	635.72	635.70	639.8
UTI (urinary tract infection)	634.71	634.72	634.70	639.8	635.71	635.72	635.70	639.8

Abortion

	Illegally Induced Abortion (criminal) (homicidal) (self-induced)				Unspecified Abortion — Retained products of conception following abortion, not classifiable elsewhere or not otherwise specified			
	Incomplete (part of the products of conception are retained)	Complete (all of the products of conception are expelled)	Unspecified	Complication following abortion (separate epidosde of care)	Incomplete (part of the products of conception are retained)	Complete (all of the products of conception are expelled)	Unspecified	Complication following abortion (separate epidosde of care)
Without complication	636.91	636.92	636.90		637.91	637.92	637.90	
With complication of:								
Afibrinogenemia	636.11	636.12	636.10	639.1	637.11	637.12	637.10	639.1
Atrophy, acute yellow	636.71	636.72	636.70	639.8	637.71	637.72	637.70	639.8
Cardiac arrest	636.71	636.72	636.70	639.8	637.71	637.72	637.70	639.8
Cardiac failure	636.71	636.72	636.70	639.8	637.71	637.72	637.70	639.8
Cerebral anoxia	636.71	636.72	636.70	639.8	637.71	637.72	637.70	639.8
Circulatory collapse	636.51	636.52	636.50	639.5	637.51	637.52	637.50	639.5
Defibrination syndrome	636.11	636.12	636.10	639.1	637.11	637.12	637.10	639.1
Electrolyte imbalance	636.41	636.42	636.40	639.4	637.41	637.42	637.40	639.4
Embolism (any type)	636.61	636.62	636.60	639.6	637.61	637.62	637.60	639.6
Endometritis	636.01	636.02	636.00	639.0	637.01	637.02	637.00	639.0
Genital tract infection	636.01	636.02	636.00	639.0	637.01	637.02	637.00	639.0
Hemorrhage, delayed or excessive	636.11	636.12	636.10	639.1	637.11	637.12	637.10	639.1
Intravascular hemolysis	636.11	636.12	636.10	639.1	637.11	637.12	637.10	639.1
Laceration of:								
bladder	636.21	636.22	636.20	639.2	637.21	637.22	637.20	639.2
bowel	636.21	636.22	636.20	639.2	637.21	637.22	637.20	639.2
broad ligament	636.21	636.22	636.20	639.2	637.21	637.22	637.20	639.2
cervix	636.21	636.22	636.20	639.2	637.21	637.22	637.20	639.2
periurethral tissue	636.21	636.22	636.20	639.2	637.21	637.22	637.20	639.2
uterus	636.21	636.22	636.20	639.2	637.21	637.22	637.20	639.2
vagina	636.21	636.22	636.20	639.2	637.21	637.22	637.20	639.2
Metabolic disorder	636.41	636.42	636.40	639.4	637.41	637.42	637.40	639.4
Necrosis of liver	636.71	636.72	636.70	639.8	637.71	637.72	637.70	639.8
Oliguria	636.31	636.32	636.30	639.3	637.31	637.32	637.30	639.3
Other specified complication	636.71	636.72	636.70	639.8	637.71	637.72	637.70	639.8
Parametritis	636.01	636.02	636.00	639.0	637.01	637.02	637.00	639.0
Pelvic infection	636.01	636.02	636.00	639.0	637.01	637.02	637.00	639.0
Pelvic peritonitis	636.01	636.02	636.00	639.0	637.01	637.02	637.00	639.0
Perforation — See Abortion, by type, laceration								
Renal failure (acute)	636.31	636.32	636.30	639.3	637.31	637.32	637.30	639.3
Renal shutdown	636.31	636.32	636.30	639.3	637.31	637.32	637.30	639.3
Renal tubular necrosis	636.31	636.32	636.30	639.3	637.31	637.32	637.30	639.3
Salpingitis	636.01	636.02	636.00	639.0	637.01	637.02	637.00	639.0
Salpingo-oophoritis	636.01	636.02	636.00	639.0	637.01	637.02	637.00	639.0
Sepsis NOS	636.01	636.02	636.00	639.0	637.01	637.02	637.00	639.0
Septicemia NOS	636.01	636.02	636.00	639.0	637.01	637.02	637.00	639.0
Shock (postoperative) (septic)	636.51	636.52	636.50	639.5	637.51	637.52	637.50	639.5
Specified complication NEC	636.71	636.72	636.70	639.8				
Tear — See Abortion, by type, laceration								
Unspecified complications	636.81	636.82	636.80	639.9	637.81	637.82	637.80	639.9
Uremia	636.31	636.32	636.30	639.3	637.31	637.32	637.30	639.3
Urinary tract infection	636.71	636.72	636.70	639.8	637.71	637.72	637.70	639.8
UTI (urinary tract infection)	636.71	636.72	636.70	639.8	637.71	637.72	637.70	639.8

Abortion Table

Abortion

Abortion	Failed Attempted Abortion Hydatidiform Mole Missed Abortion Other Abnormal Product of Conception			
	Failed Attempted Abortion	**Hydatidiform Mole**	**Missed Abortion (all products of conception retained)**	**Other abnormal product of conception (blighted ovum, fleshy mole, stone mole, carneous mole, mole NOS)**
Without complication	638.9	630	632	631
With complication of:				
Afibrinogenemia	638.1	639.1	639.1	639.1
Atrophy, acute yellow	638.7	639.8	639.8	639.8
Cardiac arrest	638.7	639.8	639.8	639.8
Cardiac failure	638.7	639.8	639.8	639.8
Cerebral anoxia	638.7	639.8	639.8	639.8
Circulatory collapse	638.5	639.5	639.5	639.5
Defibrination syndrome	638.1	639.1	639.1	639.1
Electrolyte imbalance	638.4	639.4	639.4	639.4
Embolism (any type)	638.6	639.6	639.6	639.6
Endometritis	638.0	639.0	639.0	639.0
Genital tract infection	638.0	639.0	639.0	639.0
Hemorrhage, delayed or excessive	638.1	639.1	639.1	639.1
Intravascular hemolysis	638.1	639.1	639.1	639.1
Laceration of:				
bladder	638.2	639.2	639.2	639.2
bowel	638.2	639.2	639.2	639.2
broad ligament	638.2	639.2	639.2	639.2
cervix	638.2	639.2	639.2	639.2
periurethral tissue	638.2	639.2	639.2	639.2
uterus	638.2	639.2	639.2	639.2
vagina	638.2	639.2	639.2	639.2
Metabolic disorder	638.4	639.4	639.4	639.4
Necrosis of liver	638.7	639.8	639.8	639.8
Oliguria	638.3	639.3	639.3	639.3
Other specified complications	638.7	639.8	639.8	639.8
Parametritis	638.0	639.0	639.0	639.0
Pelvic infection	638.0	639.0	639.0	639.0
Pelvic peritonitis	638.0	639.0	639.0	639.0
Perforation — *See Abortion, by type, laceration*				
Renal failure (acute)	638.3	639.3	639.3	639.3
Renal shutdown	638.3	639.3	639.3	639.3
Renal tubular necrosis	638.3	639.3	639.3	639.3
Salpingitis	638.0	639.0	639.0	639.0
Salpingo-oophoritis	638.0	639.0	639.0	639.0
Sepsis NOS	638.0	639.0	639.0	639.0
Septicemia NOS	638.0	639.0	639.0	639.0
Shock (postoperative) (septic)	638.5	639.5	639.5	639.5
Tear — *See Abortion, by type, laceration*				
Unspecified complications	638.8	639.9	639.9	639.9
Urinary tract infection	638.7	639.8	639.8	639.8
UTI (urinary tract infection)	638.7	639.8	639.8	639.8

Abortion Table

Resources

Burn (acid) (cathode ray) (caustic) (chemical) (electric heating appliance) (electricity) (fire) (flame) (hot liquid or object) (irradiation) (lime) (radiation) (steam) (thermal) (x-ray)	Unspecified Degree	First Degree [erythema]	Second Degree [blisters, epidermal loss]	Third Degree NOS [full-thickness skin loss]	Deep Third Degree [without mention of loss of body part]	Deep Third Degree [with loss of a body part]
Abdomen, abdominal (wall) (muscle)	942.03	942.13	942.23	942.33	942.43	942.53
with trunk	942.09	942.19	942.29	942.39	942.49	942.59
Ankle	945.03	945.13	945.23	945.33	945.43	945.53
with lower limb	945.09	945.19	945.29	945.39	945.49	945.59
Anus	942.09	942.19	942.29	942.39	942.49	942.59
Arm(s)	943.00	943.10	943.20	943.30	943.40	943.50
lower	943.01	943.11	943.21	943.31	943.41	943.51
multiple sites, except hand(s) or wrist(s)	943.09	943.19	943.29	943.39	943.49	943.59
upper	943.03	943.13	943.23	943.33	943.43	943.53
Auditory canal (external)	941.01	941.11	941.21	941.31	941.41	941.51
with face or head	941.09	941.19	941.29	941.39	941.49	941.59
Auricle (ear)	941.01	941.11	941.21	941.31	941.41	941.51
with face or head	941.09	941.19	941.29	941.39	941.49	941.59
Axilla	943.04	943.14	943.24	943.34	943.44	943.54
with upper limb, except hand(s) or wrist(s)	943.09	943.19	943.29	943.39	943.49	943.59
Back	942.04	942.14	942.24	942.34	942.44	942.54
with trunk	942.09	942.19	942.29	942.39	942.49	942.59
Biceps						
brachii	943.03	943.13	943.23	943.33	943.43	943.53
femoris	945.06	945.16	945.26	945.36	945.46	945.56
Breast(s)	942.01	942.11	942.21	942.31	942.41	942.51
with trunk	942.09	942.19	942.29	942.39	942.49	942.59
Brow	941.07	941.17	941.27	941.37	941.47	941.57
Buttock(s)	942.04	942.14	942.24	942.34	942.44	942.54
Cheek (cutaneous)	941.07	941.17	941.27	941.37	941.47	941.57
with face or head	941.09	941.19	941.29	941.39	941.49	941.59
Chest wall (anterior)	942.02	942.12	942.22	942.32	942.42	942.52
with trunk	942.09	942.19	942.29	942.39	942.49	942.59
Chin	941.04	941.14	941.24	941.34	941.44	941.54
with face or head	941.09	941.19	941.29	941.39	941.49	941.59
Clitoris	942.05	942.15	942.25	942.35	942.45	942.55
Ear (drum) (external)	941.01	941.11	941.21	941.31	941.41	941.51
with face or head	941.09	941.19	941.29	941.39	941.49	941.59
Elbow	943.02	943.12	943.22	943.32	943.42	943.52
with hand(s) and wrist(s)	946.0	946.1	946.2	946.3	946.4	946.5
with upper limb, except hand(s) or wrist(s)	943.09	943.19	943.29	943.39	943.49	943.59
Entire body	946.0	946.1	946.2	946.3	946.4	946.5
Epididymis	942.05	942.15	942.25	942.35	942.45	942.55
Epigastric region	942.03	942.13	942.23	942.33	942.43	942.53
Extremity						
leg	945.00	945.10	945.20	945.30	945.40	945.50
lower	945.04	945.14	945.24	945.34	945.44	945.54
multiple sites	945.09	945.19	945.29	945.39	945.49	945.59
upper	945.06	945.16	945.26	945.36	945.46	945.56
arm	943.00	943.10	943.20	943.30	943.40	943.50
lower	943.01	943.11	943.21	943.31	943.41	943.51
multiple sites	943.09	943.19	943.29	943.39	943.49	943.59
upper	943.03	943.13	943.23	943.33	943.43	943.53
Eye(s), only — see Eye, eyeball, burn						
with						
face, head or neck	941.02	941.12	941.22	941.32	941.42	941.52
other sites	946.0	946.1	946.2	946.3	946.4	946.5
Face	941.00	941.10	941.20	941.30	941.40	941.50
multiple sites	941.09	941.19	941.29	941.39	941.49	941.59
with eye(s)	941.02	941.12	941.22	941.32	941.42	941.52
Finger (nail) (subungual)	944.01	944.11	944.21	944.31	944.41	944.41
with						
hand(s)	944.08	944.18	944.28	944.38	944.48	944.58
other sites	946.0	946.1	946.2	946.3	946.4	946.5
thumb	944.04	944.14	944.24	944.34	944.44	944.54
multiple digits	944.03	944.13	944.23	944.33	944.43	944.53
with thumb	944.04	944.14	944.24	944.34	944.44	944.54
Foot	945.02	945.12	945.22	945.32	945.42	945.52
with lower limb	945.09	945.19	945.29	945.39	945.49	945.59

Burn (acid) (cathode ray) (caustic) (chemical) (electric heating appliance) (electricity) (fire) (flame) (hot liquid or object) (irradiation) (lime) (radiation) (steam) (thermal) (x-ray)

	Unspecified Degree	First Degree [erythema]	Second Degree [blisters, epidermal loss]	Third Degree NOS [full-thickness skin loss]	Deep Third Degree [without mention of loss of body part]	Deep Third Degree [with loss of a body part]
Forearm(s)	943.01	943.11	943.21	943.31	943.41	943.51
with upper limb, except hand(s) or wrist(s)	943.09	943.19	943.29	943.39	943.49	943.59
Forehead	941.07	941.17	941.27	941.37	941.47	941.57
with face or head	941.09	941.19	941.29	941.39	941.49	941.59
Genitourinary organ(s)						
external	942.05	942.15	942.25	942.35	942.45	942.55
internal—see specific organ or site, burn						
Groin	942.03	942.13	942.23	942.33	942.43	942.53
Hand(s) (and wrist)	944.00	944.10	944.20	944.30	944.40	944.50
back (doral surface)	944.06	944.16	944.26	944.36	944.46	944.56
multiple sites	944.08	944.18	944.28	944.38	944.48	944.58
Head (and face)	941.00	941.10	941.20	941.30	941.40	941.50
multiple sites	941.09	941.19	941.29	941.39	941.49	941.59
Heel	945.02	945.12	945.22	945.32	945.42	945.52
Hip	942.09	942.19	942.29	942.39	942.49	942.59
Internal organ(s) — see specific organ or site, burn						
Knee	945.05	945.15	945.25	945.35	945.45	945.55
with lower limb	945.09	945.19	945.29	945.39	945.49	945.59
Labium (majus) (minus)	942.05	942.15	942.25	942.35	942.45	942.55
Leg	945.00	945.10	945.20	945.30	945.40	945.50
lower	945.04	945.14	945.24	945.34	945.44	945.54
multiple sites	945.09	945.19	945.29	945.39	945.49	945.59
upper	945.06	945.16	945.26	945.36	945.46	945.56
Lip(s)	941.03	941.13	941.23	941.33	941.43	941.53
with face or head	941.09	941.19	941.29	941.39	941.49	941.59
Lumbar region	942.04	942.14	942.24	942.34	942.44	942.54
Malar region	941.07	941.17	941.27	941.37	941.47	941.57
Mastoid region	941.06	941.16	941.26	941.36	941.46	941.56
Membrane, tympanic	941.01	941.11	941.21	941.31	941.41	941.51
Multiple, specified sites, classifiable to more than one category in 940–945	946.0	946.1	946.2	946.3	946.4	946.5
Nasal (septum)	941.05	941.15	941.25	941.35	941.45	941.55
Neck	941.08	941.18	941.28	941.38	941.48	941.58
with face or head	941.09	941.19	941.29	941.39	941.49	941.59
Nose	941.05	941.15	941.25	941.35	941.45	941.55
with face or head	941.09	941.19	941.29	941.39	941.49	941.59
Palm(s)	944.05	944.15	944.25	944.35	944.45	944.55
with hand(s) or wrist(s)	944.08	944.18	944.28	944.38	944.48	944.58
Penis	942.05	942.15	942.25	942.35	942.45	942.55
Perineum	942.05	942.15	942.25	942.35	942.45	942.55
Pubic region	942.05	942.15	942.25	942.35	942.45	942.55
Sacral region	942.04	942.14	942.24	942.34	942.44	942.54
Scalp	941.06	941.16	941.26	941.36	941.46	941.56
with face or head	941.09	941.19	941.29	941.39	941.49	941.59
Scapular region	943.06	943.16	943.26	943.36	943.46	943.56
with upper limb, except hand(s) or wrist(s)	943.09	943.19	943.29	943.39	943.49	943.59
Scrotum	942.05	942.15	942.25	942.35	942.45	942.55
Shoulder(s)	943.05	943.15	943.25	943.35	943.45	943.55
with						
hand(s) and wrist(s)	946.0	946.1	946.2	946.3	946.4	946.5
upper limb, except hand(s) or wrist(s)	943.09	943.19	943.29	943.39	943.49	943.59
Skin, unspecified site	949.0	949.1	949.2	949.3	949.4	949.5
Skull	941.00	941.10	941.20	941.30	941.40	941.50
Submental region	941.04	941.14	941.24	941.34	941.44	941.54
Supraclavicular fossa	941.08	941.18	941.28	941.38	941.48	941.58
Temple	941.06	941.16	941.26	941.36	941.46	941.56
Testicle	942.05	942.15	942.25	942.35	942.45	942.55
Thigh	945.06	945.16	945.26	945.36	945.46	945.56
with lower limb	945.09	945.19	945.29	945.39	945.49	945.59
Thumb(s) (nail)	944.02	944.12	944.22	944.32	944.42	944.52
with finger(s)	944.04	944.14	944.24	944.34	944.44	944.54
with hand(s) or wrist(s)	944.08	944.18	944.28	944.38	944.48	944.58
Toe (nail)	945.01	945.11	945.21	945.31	945.41	945.51
with lower limb	945.09	945.19	945.29	945.39	945.49	945.59

Burn Table

Burn

Burn	Unspecified Degree	First Degree [erythema]	Second Degree [blisters, epidermal loss]	Third Degree NOS [full-thickness skin loss]	Deep Third Degree [without mention of loss of body part]	Deep Third Degree [with loss of a body part]
Trunk	942.00	942.10	942.20	942.30	942.40	942.50
multiple sites	942.09	942.19	942.29	942.39	942.49	942.59
specified site, NEC	942.09	942.19	942.29	942.39	942.49	942.59
Tunica vaginalis	942.05	942.15	942.25	942.35	942.45	942.55
Unspecified site	949.0	949.1	949.2	949.3	949.4	949.5
Vulva	942.05	942.15	942.25	942.35	942.45	942.55
Wrist(s)	944.07	944.17	944.27	944.37	944.47	944.57
with hand(s)	944.08	944.18	944.28	944.38	944.48	944.58

Complications due to (presence of)

Complications due to (presence of)	Mechanical	Infection/inflammatory reaction	Other
aortocoronary bypass graft	996.03	996.61	996.72
arteriovenous			
fistula	996.1	996.62	996.74
shunt		996.62	996.74
artificial heart		996.61	
artificial skin graft	996.55	996.69	996.79
bile duct	996.59	996.69	996.79
blood vessel graft		996.62	996.74
bone growth stimulator	996.4	996.67	996.78
bone marrow transplant	996.85	996.85	996.85
breast implant	996.54	996.69	996.79
bypass graft			
aortocoronary	996.03	996.61	996.72
blood vessel		996.62	996.74
carotid artery		996.62	996.74
coronary artery	996.03	996.61	996.72
femoral-popliteal		996.62	996.74
cardiac			
defibrillator	996.04	996.61	996.72
pulse generator	996.04	996.61	
subcutaneous pocket		996.61	996.72
pacemaker		996.61	996.72
pulse generator		996.61	
subcutaneous pocket		996.61	996.72
valve prosthesis	996.02	996.61	996.71
carotid artery bypass graft		996.62	996.74
catheter			
cystostomy	996.39	996.65	996.76
dialysis		996.62	996.73
peritoneal	996.56	996.68	996.73
spinal	996.2	996.63	996.75
urinary, indwelling	996.31	996.64	996.76
vascular		996.62	996.74
chin implant	996.59	996.69	996.79
contraceptive device (intrauterine)	996.32	996.65	996.76
corneal graft	996.51	996.69	996.79
coronary artery bypass graft	996.03	996.61	996.72
decellularized alodermis	996.55	996.69	996.79
dialysis catheter		996.62	996.73
peritoneal	996.56	996.68	996.73
dorsal column stimulator	996.2	996.63	996.75
electrodes			
brain	996.2	996.63	996.75
heart	996.01	996.61	996.72
esophagostomy	530.87	530.86	
external fixation device	996.4	996.67	996.78
genitourinary device	996.39	996.65	996.76
unspecified	996.30	996.65	996.70
graft			
artificial skin	996.52	996.69	996.79
blood vessel		996.62	996.74
bone	996.4	996.67	996.78
cartilage	996.4	996.67	996.78

Complications due to (presence of)	Mechanical	Infection/inflammatory reaction	Other
graft — *continued*			
carotid artery		996.62	996.74
corneal	996.51	996.69	996.79
coronary artery	996.03	996.61	996.72
femoral-popliteal		996.62	996.74
muscle	996.4	996.67	996.78
peripheral nerve	996.2	996.62	996.75
skin	996.52	996.69	996.79
tendon	996.4	996.67	996.78
ureter	996.39	996.65	996.76
heart assist device		996.61	
heart transplant	996.83	996.83	996.83
infusion pump		996.62	996.74
insulin pump	996.57	996.69	
internal fixation device			
nail	996.4	996.67	996.78
plate	996.4	996.67	996.78
rod	996.4	996.67	996.78
screw	996.4	996.67	996.78
intraaortic balloon		996.62	996.74
joint prosthesis, internal	996.4	996.66	996.77
liver transplant	996.82	996.82	996.82
lung transplant	996.84	996.84	996.84
mammary implant	996.54	996.69	996.79
nervous system device	996.2	996.63	996.75
nonabsorbable surgical material NOS	996.59	996.69	996.79
other vascular device		996.62	996.70
pancreas transplant	996.86	996.86	996.86
prosthetic implant			
bile duct	996.59	996.69	996.79
breast	996.54	996.69	996.79
chin	996.59	996.69	996.79
ocular lens	996.53	996.69	996.79
orbit of eye	996.59	996.69	996.79
vas deferens	996.39	996.65	996.76
shunt			
arteriovenous		996.62	996.74
ventricular	996.2	996.63	996.75
transplanted organ			
bone marrow	996.85	996.85	996.85
heart	996.83	996.83	996.83
liver	996.82	996.82	996.82
lung	996.84	996.84	996.84
other specified organ	996.89	996.89	996.89
pancreas	996.86	996.86	996.86
unspecified organ	996.80	996.80	996.80
umbrella device, vena cava		996.62	996.74
unspecified cardiac device		996.60	996.70
vascular catheter		996.62	996.74
ventricular shunt	996.2	996.63	996.75

Complications Table

Diabetes (brittle) (congenital) (familial) (mellitus) (severe) (slight)	TYPE I		TYPE II or unspecified type — The codes found in these columns are for use even if the patient requires insulin.			Additional Code Required
	Controlled or not stated as uncontrolled	Uncontrolled	Controlled or not stated as uncontrolled	Uncontrolled	Other metabolic disorders or conditions	List these codes after the diabetes code
Without complication or manifestation	250.01	250.03	250.00	250.02		
With complication or manifestation						
coma (ketoacidosis)	250.31	250.33	250.30	250.32		
hyperosmolar (nonketotic)	250.21	250.23	250.20	250.22		
complication NOS	250.91	250.93	250.90	250.92		
specified NEC	250.81	250.83	250.80	250.82		
gangrene	250.71	250.73	250.70	250.72		785.4
hyperosmolarity	250.21	250.23	250.20	250.22		
ketosis, ketoacidosis	250.11	250.13	250.10	250.12		
osteomyelitis	250.81	250.83	250.80	250.82		731.8
specified manifestations NEC	250.81	250.83	250.80	250.82		
Abnormal glucose NOS					790.29	
NOS					790.29	
non-fasting					790.29	
fasting					790.21	
tolerance test					790.22	
Abnormal glucose tolerance test (GTT), elevated glucose tolerance test					790.22	
Acetonemia	250.11	250.13	250.10	250.12		
Acidosis	250.11	250.13	250.10	250.12		
Amyotrophy	250.61	250.63	250.60	250.62		358.1
Aneurysm, micro, retina	250.51	250.53	250.50	250.52		362.01
Angiopathia, angiopathy (peripheral)	250.71	250.73	250.70	250.72		443.81
retinalis (juvenilis)	250.51	250.53	250.50	250.52		362.01
Arthritis, arthropathy	250.61	250.63	250.60	250.62		713.5
Charcôt's	250.61	250.63	250.60	250.62		713.5
neuropathic (Charcôt's)	250.61	250.63	250.60	250.62		713.5
Asymptomatic elevated (abnormal glucose)					790.29	
Ataxia, ataxy, ataxic, locomotor (progressive)	250.61	250.63	250.60	250.62		337.1
Autonomic neuropathy (peripheral)	250.61	250.63	250.60	250.62		337.1
Bone change	250.81	250.83	250.80	250.82		731.8
Bronze, bronzed					275.0	
Cataract diabetic	250.51	250.53	250.50	250.52		366.41
senile (non diabetic)	250.01	250.03	250.00	250.02		366.17
snowflake	250.51	250.53	250.50	250.52		366.41
Charcôt's joint (disease)	250.61	250.63	250.60	250.62		713.5
Chemical					790.29	
Coma (with ketoacidosis)	250.31	250.33	250.30	250.32		
hyperglycemic	250.31	250.33	250.30	250.32		
hyperosmolar (nonketotic)	250.21	250.23	250.20	250.22		
hypoglycemic	250.31	250.33	250.30	250.32		
nondiabetic					251.0	
insulin	250.31	250.33	250.30	250.32		
nondiabetic					251.0	
Kussmaul's	250.31	250.33	250.30	250.32		
prediabetic	250.21	250.23	250.20	250.22		
Complication NOS	250.91	250.93	250.90	250.92		
specified NEC	250.81	250.83	250.80	250.82		
Dermopathy	250.81	250.83	250.80	250.82		709.8
Dietary supervision					V65.3	
Dwarfism-obesity syndrome					258.1	
Ebstein's disease	250.41	250.43	250.40	250.42		581.81
Edema (macula) (retina)	250.51	250.53	250.50	250.52		362.01
Family History					V18.0	
Gangrene	250.71	250.73	250.70	250.72		785.4
Gastroparalysis	250.61	250.63	250.60	250.62		536.3, 337.1
Gastroparesis	250.61	250.63	250.60	250.62		536.3, 337.1

Diabetes Table

Diabetes (brittle) (congenital) (familial) (mellitus) (severe) (slight)	TYPE I		TYPE II or unspecified type The codes found in these columns are for use even if the patient requires insulin.			Additional Code Required
	Controlled or not stated as uncontrolled	Uncontrolled	Controlled or not stated as uncontrolled	Uncontrolled	Other metabolic disorders or conditions	List these codes after the diabetes code
Gestational diabetes						
unspecified. episode. of care delivered w/o antepartum condition					648.80	
					648.81	
with antepartum condition					648.82	
antepartum					648.83	
postpartum					648.84	
Glaucoma	250.51	250.53	250.50	250.52		365.44
Glomerulohyalinosis — diabetic syndrome	250.41	250.43	250.40	250.42		581.81
Glomerulonephritis, chronic	250.41	250.43	250.40	250.42		583.81
with nephrotic syndrome	250.41	250.43	250.40	250.42		581.81
Glomerulosclerosis (intercapillary)	250.41	250.43	250.40	250.42		581.81
Glucose Intolerance					790.22	
Glycogenosis, secondary	250.81	250.83	250.80	250.82		259.8
Hanot-Chauffard (-Troisier) syndrome (bronze diabetes)					275.0	
Hemochromatosis					275.0	
Hirschfeld's disease	250.01	250.01	250.00	250.02		
Hyperglycemia						
with coma	250.31	250.33	250.30	250.32		
diabetic	250.11	250.13	250.10	250.12		
neonatal (transient)					775.1	
nondiabetic					790.6	
postpancreatectomy					251.3	
Hyperosmolar coma	250.21	250.23	250.20	250.22		
Hyperosmolarity	250.21	250.23	250.20	250.22		
Hypertension nephrosis syndrome	250.41	250.43	250.40	250.42		581.81
Hypoglycemia (diabetic) without coma	250.81	250.83	250.80	250.82		
with coma	250.31	250.33	250.30	250.32		
neonatal, transient					775.0	
nondiabetic						
with coma					251.0	
without coma					251.1	
NOS (spontaneous)					251.2	
Hypoglycemic shock	250.81	250.83	250.80	250.82		
Hypoinsulinemia, postsurgical					251.3	
Impaired fasting glucose					790.21	
Impotence	250.61	250.63	250.60	250.62		607.84
Insipidus					253.5	
nephrogenic					588.1	
pituitary					253.5	
vasopressin-resistant					588.1	
Insulin overdose					962.3	
Intercapillary glomerulosclerosis	250.41	250.43	250.40	250.42		581.81
Iridis rubeosis	250.51	250.53	250.50	250.53		364.42
Iritis	250.51	250.53	250.50	250.52		364.42
Ketosis, ketoacidosis	250.11	250.13	250.10	250.12		
Kimmelstiel (-Wilson) disease or syndrome (intercapillary glomerulosclerosis)	250.41	250.43	250.40	250.42		581.81
Kussmaul's coma	250.31	250.33	250.30	250.32		
Lancereaux's (diabetes mellitus with marked emaciation)	250.81	250.83	250.80	250.82		261
Latent (chemical)					790.29	
Lipoidosis	250.81	250.83	250.80	250.82		272.7
Macular edema	250.51	250.53	250.50	250.52		362.01
Microaneurysms, retinal	250.51	250.53	250.50	250.52		362.01
Microangiopathy (peripheral)	250.71	250.73	250.70	250.72		443.81
retinal	250.50	250.53	250.50	250.52		362.01
Mononeuropathy, mononeuritis, unspecified site	250.61	250.63	250.60	250.62		355.9
lower limb, unspecified	250.61	250.63	250.60	250.62		355.8
upper limb, unspecified	250.61	250.63	250.60	250.62		354.9

Diabetes (brittle) (congenital) (familial) (mellitus) (severe) (slight)	TYPE I		TYPE II or unspecified type The codes found in these columns are for use even if the patient requires insulin.			Additional Code Required
	Controlled or not stated as uncontrolled	Uncontrolled	Controlled or not stated as uncontrolled	Uncontrolled	Other metabolic disorders or conditions	List these codes after the diabetes code
Myasthenic syndrome, myasthenia	250.61	250.63	250.60	250.62		358.1
Myelopathy	250.61	250.63	250.60	250.62		336.3
Necrobiosis lipoidica	250.81	250.83	250.80	250.82		709.3
Neonatal, transient hyperglycemia					775.1	
hypoglycemia					775.0	
Nephritis, chronic	250.41	250.43	250.40	250.42		583.81
with nephrotic syndrome	250.41	250.43	250.40	250.42		581.81
Nephropathy	250.41	250.43	250.40	250.42		583.81
Nephrosis (Ebsteins) (syndrome)	250.41	250.43	250.40	250.42		581.81
Neuralgia	250.61	250.63	250.60	250.62		357.2
Neuritis	250.61	250.63	250.60	250.62		357.2
Neurogenic arthropathy	250.61	250.63	250.60	250.62		713.5
Neuropathic arthritis	250.61	250.63	250.60	250.62	713.5	
Neuropathy	250.61	250.63	250.60	250.62		357.2
peripheral	250.61	250.63	250.60	250.62		337.1
Neurophthisis	250.61	250.63	250.60	250.62		357.2
Nonclinical					790.29	
Ophthalmoplegia	250.51	250.53	250.50	250.52		378.86
Oppenheim-Urbach disease or syndrome	250.81	250.83	250.80	250.82		709.3
Osteomyelitis	250.81	250.83	250.80	250.82		731.8
Peripheral angiopathy	250.71	250.73	250.70	250.72		443.81
Peripheral autonomic neuropathy	250.61	250.63	250.60	250.62		337.1
Peripheral vascular disease (occlusive)	250.71	250.73	250.70	250.72		443.81
Phosphate					275.3	
Pierre Mauriac's syndrome (diabetes-dwarfism-obesity)					258.1	
Polyneuropathy, polyneuritis	250.61	250.63	250.60	250.62		357.2
Postpancreatectomy					251.3	
Postsurgical (hypoinsulinemia)					251.3	
Prediabetes					790.29	
Pseudotabes	250.61	250.63	250.60	250.62		337.1
Renal failure, chronic	250.41	250.43	250.40	250.42		585
Renal glycosuria (true)					271.4	
Retinal						
edema	250.51	250.53	250.50	250.52		362.01
hemorrhage	250.51	250.53	250.50	250.52		362.01
microaneurysms	250.51	250.53	250.50	250.52		362.01
Retinitis	250.51	250.53	250.50	250.52		362.01
Retinopathy	250.51	250.53	250.50	250.52		362.01
background (simple)	250.51	250.53	250.50	250.52		362.01
proliferative	250.51	250.53	250.50	250.52		362.02
Rubeosis iridis	250.51	250.53	250.50	250.52		364.42
Secondary						
postsurgical					251.3	
steroid induced					251.8	E932.0
Skin						
dermopathy	250.81	250.83	250.80	250.82		709.8
necrobiosis lipoidica diabeticorum	250.81	250.83	250.80	250.82		709.3
Screening					V77.1	
Steroid induced						
correct substance properly administered					251.8	E932.0
overdose or wrong substance given or taken					962.0	
Stress					790.29	
Subclinical					790.29	
Subliminal					790.29	
Sugar	250.01	250.03	250.00	250.02		
Syndrome						
diabetes-dwarfism-obesity (juvenile)					258.1	

Diabetes Table

Diabetes (brittle) (congenital) (familial) (mellitus) (severe) (slight)	TYPE I		TYPE II or unspecified type. The codes found in these columns are for use even if the patient requires insulin.			Additional Code Required
	Controlled or not stated as uncontrolled	Uncontrolled	Controlled or not stated as uncontrolled	Uncontrolled	Other metabolic disorders or conditions	List these codes after the diabetes code
Syndrome – *continued*						
diabetes mellitus in newborn infant					775.1	
diabetes-nephrosis	250.41	250.43	250.40	250.42		581.81
diabetic amyotrophy	250.61	250.63	250.60	250.62		358.1
Hanot-Chauffard (-Troisier) (bronze diabetes)					275.0	
nephrotic	250.41	250.43	250.40	250.42		581.81
Oppenheim-Urbach (necrobiosis lipoidica diabeticorum)	250.81	250.83	250.80	250.82		709.3
Pierre Mauriac's (diabetes-dwarfism-obesity)					258.1	
renal glomerulohyalinosis-diabetic	250.41	250.43	250.40	250.42		581.81
Syndrome						
Troisier-Hanot-Chauffard (bronze diabetes)					275.0	
Urbach-Oppenheim (necrobiosis lipoidica diabeticorum)	250.81	250.83	250.80	250.82		709.3
Troisier-Hanot-Chauffard syndrome (bronze diabetes)					275.0	
Ulcer (skin), unspecified site	250.81	250.83	250.80	250.82		707.9
lower extremity, unspecified	250.81	250.83	250.80	250.82		707.19
lower extremity, ankle	250.81	250.83	250.80	250.82		707.13
lower extremity, calf	250.81	250.83	250.80	250.82		707.12
lower extremity, heel and midfoot	250.81	250.83	250.80	250.82		707.14
lower extremity, thigh	250.81	250.83	250.80	250.82		707.11
lower extremity, toes	250.81	250.83	250.80	250.82		707.15
specified site NEC	250.81	250.83	250.80	250.82		707.8
unspecified complication	250.91	250.93	250.90	250.92		
Urbach-Oppenheim disease or syndrome (necrobiosis lipoidica diabeticorum)	250.81	250.83	250.80	250.82		709.3
Willis' disease	250.01	250.03	250.00	250.02		
Xanthoma diabeticorum, xanthomatosis	250.81	250.83	250.80	250.82		272.2

Diabetes Table

Site of Hernia	Without Obstruction	With Obstruction	Gangrene (with or without obstruction)
Abdomen (wall)	553.20	552.20	551.20
recurrent	553.21	552.21	551.21
Abdominal, specified site NEC	553.8	552.8	551.8
Appendix	553.8	552.8	551.8
Bilateral — *see* Hernia, by site			
Bladder (sphincter)			
congenital (female) (male)	756.71		
female			
lateral	618.02		
midline	618.01		
male	596.8		
Brain (acquired) (stem)	348.4		
congenital	742.0		
Broad ligament	553.8		
Bubonocele — *see* Hernia, inguinal			
Cecocele — *see also* Hernia, by site	553.9	552.9	551.9
Cerebral (acquired)	348.4		
congenital (endaural)	742.0		
Ciliary body (acquired)	364.8		
traumatic	871.1		
Colic	553.9	552.9	551.9
Colon	553.9	552.9	551.9
Colostomy	569.69		
Cooper's	553.8	552.8	551.8
Crural — *see* Hernia, femoral			
Diaphragm(atic)	553.3	552.3	551.3
congenital (gross defect)	756.6		
traumatic	862.0		
with open wound	862.1		
Direct — *see* Hernia, inguinal			
Disc, intervertebral — *see* Displacement, intervertebral disc			
Diverticulum (intestine)	553.9	552.9	551.9
Double — *see* Hernia, inguinal			
Duodenojejunal	553.8	552.8	551.8
Encysted — *see* Hernia, inguinal			
En glissade — *see* Hernia, inguinal			
Enterocele (*see also* Hernia, by site)	553.9	552.9	551.9
Epigastrocele	553.29	552.29	551.21
recurrent	553.21	552.21	551.21
Enterostomy	569.69		
Epigastric	553.29	552.29	551.29
recurrent	553.21	552.21	551.21
Epigastrocele	553.29	552.29	551.29
recurrent	553.21	552.21	551.21
Epiplocele	553.9	552.9	551.9
Epiplosarcomphalocele	553.1	552.1	551.1
Esophageal (hiatal)	553.3	552.3	551.3
congenital	750.6		
Eventration (chest to colon)	553.3	552.3	551.3
congenital (gross defect)	756.6		
External — *see* Hernia, inguinal			
Fallopian tube	620.4		
Fascia	728.89		
Fat (pad)	729.30		
eye, eyelid	374.34		
knee	729.31		
orbit	374.34		
retro-orbital	374.34		
retropatellar	729.31		
specified site NEC	729.39		
Female			
complete	618.3		
cystocele			
lateral	618.02		
midline	618.01		
with prolapse	618.4		
incomplete	618.2		
fallopian tube	620.4		
ovary, oviduct	620.4		
rectovaginal	618.6		
uterus	621.8		
vaginal	618.6		

Hernia Table

Site of Hernia	Without Obstruction	With Obstruction	Gangrene (with or without obstruction)
Female – *continued*			
vesical			
congenital	756.71		
lateral	618.02		
midline	618.01		
Femoral (unilateral)	553.00	552.00	551.00
bilateral	553.02	552.02	551.02
recurrent	553.03	552.03	551.03
recurrent (unilateral)	553.01	552.01	551.01
Foramen			
Bochdale (acquired)	553.3	552.3	551.3
congenital	756.6		
magnum	348.4		
Morgagni (an) (acquired)	553.3	552.3	551.3
congenital	756.6		
Furnicular (umbilical)	553.1	552.1	551.1
spermatic cord—see Hernia, inguinal			
Gastric mucosa	537.89		
Gastrointestinal tract	553.9	552.9	551.9
Gluteal — *see* Hernia, femoral			
Gruber's	553.8	552.8	551.8
Hesselbach's	553.8	552.8	551.8
Hiatal (esophageal) (sliding)	553.3	552.3	551.3
Holthouse's — *see* Hernia, inguinal			
Incarcerated — *see* Hernia, by site, with obstruction			
Incisional	553.21	552.21	551.21
lumbar	553.8	552.8	551.8
Indirect — *see* Hernia, inguinal			
Infantile — *see* Hernia, inguinal			
Infrapatellar fat pad	729.31		
Inguinal (unilateral) (direct) (double) ((encysted) (external) (furnicular) (indirect) (infantile) (internal) (interstial) (oblique) (scrotal) (sliding)	550.90	550.10	550.00
bilateral	550.92	550.12	550.02
recurrent	550.93	550.13	550.03
recurrent (unilateral)	550.91	550.11	550.01
Internal	553.8	552.8	551.8
Interstitial	553.9	552.9	551.9
Intervertebral cartilage — *see* Displacement, intervertebral disc			
Intestine(al)	553.9	552.9	551.9
Intra-abdominal	553.9	552.9	551.9
Intraparietal	553.9	552.9	551.9
Iris (acquired)	364.8		
traumatic	871.1		
Irreducible — *see* Hernia, by site, with obstruction			
Ischiatic	553.8	552.8	551.8
Lens (acquired)	379.32		
traumatic	871.1		
Linea alba	553.29	552.29	551.29
recurrent	553.21	552.21	551.21
Linea semilunaris	553.29	552.29	551.29
Littre's	553.9	552.9	551.9
Lumbar	553.8	552.8	551.8
intervetebral disc	722.10		
Lung (acquired)	518.89		
congenital	748.69		
Male			
chylocele	608.84		
cystocele	596.8		
scrotal - *see* Hernia, inguinal			
spermatocele	608.1		
congenital	752.8		
testis	550.90	550.10	550.00
bilateral	550.92	550.12	550.02
recurrent	550.93	550.13	550.03
recurrent (unilateral)	550.91	550.11	550.01
vesical	596.8		
congenital	756.71		
Mediastinum	519.3		
Merocele — *see* Hernia, femoral			
Mesenteric (internal)	553.8	552.8	551.8
Mesocolon	553.8	552.8	551.8

Site of Hernia	Without Obstruction	With Obstruction	Gangrene (with or without obstruction)
Muscle (sheath)	728.89		
Nucleus polpous — *see* Displacement, intervertebral disc			
Oblique — *see* Hernia, inguinal			
Obstructive — *see* Hernia, by site with obstruction			
Orbturator	553.8	552.8	551.8
Omental	553.8	552.8	551.8
Omentocele	553.8	552.8	551.8
Orbital fat pad	374.37		
Ovary, oviduct	620.4		
Paracolostomy	569.69		
Paraduodenal	553.8	552.8	551.8
Paraesophageal	553.8	552.8	551.8
congenital	750.6		
Parahiatal	553.8	552.8	551.8
Paraumbilical	553.1	552.1	551.1
Parietal	553.9	552.9	551.9
Perineal	553.8	552.8	551.8
Peritoneal sac, lesser	553.8	552.8	551.8
Petit's	553.8	552.8	551.8
intervertebral disc	722.10		
Popliteal fat pad	729.31		
Postoperative	553.21	552.21	551.21
Prevesical	596.8		
Properitoneal	553.8	552.8	551.8
Pudendal	553.8	552.8	551.8
Rectovaginal	618.6		
Retroperitoneal	553.8	552.8	551.8
Richter's	553.9	552.9	551.9
Rieux's, Reix's	553.8	552.8	551.8
Saint's, triad — *see* Hernia, Diaphragm			
Sarcopiplocele	553.9	552.9	551.9
Sarcoepiplomphalocele	553.9	552.9	551.9
Sciatic	553.8	552.8	551.8
Scrotum, scrotal — *see* Hernia, inguinal			
Sliding			
hiatal	553.3	552.3	551.3
congenital	750.6		
inguinal — *see* Hernia, inguinal			
Spermatocele	608.1		
congenital	752.8		
Spigelian	553.29	552.29	551.29
Spinal — *see* Spina Bifida			
Strangulated — *see* Hernia, by site, wth obstruction			
Supraumbilicus	553.29	552.29	551.29
recurrent	553.21	552.21	551.21
Tendon	727.9		
Testis (nontraumatic)	550.90	550.10	550.00
bilateral	550.92	550.12	550.02
recurrent	550.93	550.13	550.03
recurrent (unilateral)	550.91	550.11	550.01
Thoracic stomach	553.8	552.8	551.8
Treitz's	553.8	552.8	551.8
Triad, Saint's — *see* Hernia, diaphragm			
Umbilical, umbilicus	553.1	552.1	551.1
Unspecified site NEC	553.9	552.9	551.9
Ureter	593.89	593.4	
Uterus	621.8		
Vaginal	618.6		
Velpeau's — *see* Hernia, femoral			
Ventral	553.20	552.20	551.20
incisional	553.21	552.21	551.21
recurrent	553.21	552.21	551.21
Vertebral cartilage — *see* Displacement, intervertebral disc			
Vesical			
congenital (female) (male)	756.71		
female			
lateral	618.02		
midline	618.01		
male	596.8		
Vitreous (acquired)	379.21		
traumatic	871.1		

Hernia Table

Ectopic Pregnancy	Abdominal pregnancy (Intraperitoneal pregnancy)	Tubal pregnancy (Fallopian pregnancy, rupture of fallopian tube due to pregnancy, tubal abortion)	Ovarian pregnancy	Other ectopic pregnancy (Includes the following pregnancy(s): cervical, cornual mural mesometric intraligamentous)	Unspecified ectopic pregnancy
Without complication					
with intrauterine pregnancy	633.01	633.11	633.21	633.81	633.91
without intrauterine pregnancy	633.00	633.10	633.20	633.80	633.90
With complication of:*					
Afibrinogenemia	639.1	639.1	639.1	639.1	639.1
Atrophy, acute yellow	639.8	639.8	639.8	639.8	639.8
Cardiac arrest	639.8	639.8	639.8	639.8	639.8
Cardiac failure	639.8	639.8	639.8	639.8	639.8
Cerebral anoxia	639.8	639.8	639.8	639.8	639.8
Circulatory collapse	639.5	639.5	639.5	639.5	639.5
Defibrination syndrome	639.1	639.1	639.1	639.1	639.1
Electrolyte imbalance	639.4	639.4	639.4	639.4	639.4
Embolism (Any type)	639.6	639.6	639.6	639.6	639.6
Endometritis	639.0	639.0	639.0	639.0	639.0
Genital tract infection	639.0	639.0	639.0	639.0	639.0
Hemorrhage, delayed or excessive	639.1	639.1	639.1	639.1	639.1
Intravascular hemolysis	639.1	639.1	639.1	639.1	639.1
Laceration of:					
bladder	639.2	639.2	639.2	639.2	639.2
bowel	639.2	639.2	639.2	639.2	639.2
broad ligament	639.2	639.2	639.2	639.2	639.2
cervix	639.2	639.2	639.2	639.2	639.2
periurethral tissue	639.2	639.2	639.2	639.2	639.2
uterus	639.2	639.2	639.2	639.2	639.2
vagina	639.2	639.2	639.2	639.2	639.2
Metabolic disorder	639.4	639.4	639.4	639.4	639.4
Necrosis of liver	639.8	639.8	639.8	639.8	639.8
Oliguria	639.3	639.3	639.3	639.3	639.3
Other specified complication	639.8	639.8	639.8	639.8	639.8
Parametritis	639.0	639.0	639.0	639.0	639.0
Pelvic infection	639.0	639.0	639.0	639.0	639.0
Pelvic peritonitis	639.0	639.0	639.0	639.0	639.0
Perforation — *see* Abortion, by type, laceration:					
Renal failure (acute)	639.3	639.3	639.3	639.3	639.3
Renal shutdown	639.3	639.3	639.3	639.3	639.3
Renal tubular necrosis	639.3	639.3	639.3	639.3	639.3
Salpingitis	639.0	639.0	639.0	639.0	639.0
Salpingo-oophoritis	639.0	639.0	639.0	639.0	639.0
Sepsis NOS	639.0	639.0	639.0	639.0	639.0
Septicemia NOS	639.0	639.0	639.0	639.0	639.0
Shock (postoperative)(septic)	639.5	639.5	639.5	639.5	639.5
Tear — *see* Abortion, by type, laceration:					
Unspecified complications	639.9	639.9	639.9	639.9	639.9
Urinary tract infection	639.8	639.8	639.8	639.8	639.8
UTI	639.8	639.8	639.8	639.8	639.8

Ectopic Pregnancy Table

Normal Pregnancy

Pregnancy/Delivery, current (Normal) (Single) (Uterine) (without Sickness)	Code	Special Notes
Normal delivery	650	This code is always a primary diagnosis.
Normal pregnancy		
with other condition not affecting the pregnancy	V22.2	V22.2 should be used in place of any other pregnancy codes and listed second on the claim form. The condition, which does not affect the pregnancy, must be listed first.
First pregnancy	V22.0	Codes V22.0 and V22.1 should never be used in conjunction with any codes from cataegories 640-648 and 651-676.
Second or other normal pregnancy	V22.1	Meaning 2nd, 3rd, 4th etc. pregnancy
Postpartum care and examination		
immediately after delivery	V24.0	Normal uncomplicated cases
lactating mother	V24.1	Supervision of lactating mother
routine postpartum follow-up	V24.2	Care within 6 weeks after delivery
Previous (not effecting current pregnancy)		These codes may be used in conjunction with chapter 11 codes. A thorough review of any pertinent excludes notes (found in the tabular list) is necessary to be certain that these V codes are being used properly.
abortion	V23.2	
difficult delivery	V23.49	
forceps delivery	V23.49	
hemorrhage, antepartum or postpartum	V23.49	
hydatidiform mole	V23.1	
infertility	V23.0	
malignancy NEC	V23.89	
neonatal death	V23.5	
nonobstetrical conditions	V23.89	
premature delivery	V23.41	
pre-term labor	V23.41	
specified NEC	V23.89	
stillbirth	V23.5	
trophoblastic disease	V23.1	
unspecified condition	V23.9	
vesicular mole	V23.1	
Screening, prenatal (for)		If the abnormal finding is known—code the screening and the findings as additional codes
by		
amniocentesis		
chromosomal anomalies	V28.0	N/A
raised alpha-fetoprotein levels (amniotic fluid)	V28.1	N/A
specified, NEC	V28.2	N/A
ultrasound		
fetal growth retardation	V28.4	N/A
malformation	V28.3	N/A
isoimmunization	V28.5	N/A
other specified screening	V28.8	N/A
Streptococcus B	V28.6	N/A
unspecified, screening	V28.9	N/A
Supervision (of) (for)		These codes may be used in conjunction with chapter 11 codes. A thorough review of any pertinent excludes notes (found in the tabular list) is necessary to be certain that these V codes are being used properly.
high-risk	V23.9	
insufficient prenatal care	V23.7	
specified problem NEC	V23.89	
multigravida		Second or more pregnancy
elderly	V23.82	35 years of age or older at expected date of delivery
young	V23.84	Younger than 16 years of age at expected date of delivery
multiparity	V23.3	
normal NEC	V22.1	
first pregnancy	V22.0	
poor		
obstetric history	V23.49	
reproductive history	V23.5	
primigravida		First pregnancy
elderly	V23.81	35 years of age or older at expected date of delivery
young	V23.83	Younger than 16 years of age at expected date of delivery
Unconfirmed	V72.4	
Unwanted NEC	V61.7	

Antepartum Pregnancy Condition or Complication; affecting management of mother	Antepartum condition or complication	Delivered, with or without mention of antepartum condition	Unspecified episode of care	Assign additional code to describe the...	Affecting fetus (coded on the newborn chart only)
Ablatio placentae	641.23	641.21	641.20	N/A	762.1
Abnormal NEC	646.93	646.91	646.90	condition	761.9
amnion	658.93	658.91	658.90	N/A	762.9
cervix	654.63	654.61	654.60	N/A	763.89
causing obstructed labor	660.23	660.21	660.20	cause	763.1
chorion	658.93	658.91	658.90	N/A	762.9
cord (umbilical)	663.93	663.91	663.90	N/A	762.6
fetal chromosomes (suspected)	655.13	655.11	655.10	N/A	758.89
fetal					
heart rate	659.73	659.71	659.70	N/A	763.83
before onset of labor	659.73	659.71	659.70	N/A	763.81
during labor	659.73	659.71	659.70	N/A	763.82
heart rhythm	659.73	659.71	659.70	N/A	763.8
before onset of labor	659.73	659.71	659.70	N/A	763.81
during labor	659.73	659.71	659.70	N/A	763.82
fetus,fetal (suspected) NEC	655.93	655.91	655.90	N/A	779.9
acid-base balance	656.83	656.81	656.80	N/A	768.4
causing disproportion	653.73	653.71	653.70	N/A	763.1
causing obstructed labor	660.13	660.11	660.10	cause	763.1
fetal					
heart rate	659.73	659.71	659.70	N/A	763.83
before onset of labor	659.73	659.71	659.70	N/A	763.81
during labor	659.73	659.71	659.70	N/A	763.82
heart rhythm	659.73	659.71	659.70	N/A	763.83
before onset of labor	659.73	659.71	659.70	N/A	763.81
during labor	659.73	659.71	659.70	N/A	763.82
membranes	658.83	658.81	658.80	N/A	762.9
specified NEC	655.83	655.81	655.80	N/A	779.8
findings, nonspecific	796.5	N/A	N/A	N/A	
(a code from 640-648 should be used first when the management of the mother is affected by the abnormal findings)					
glucose tolerance test	648.83	648.81	648.80	condition	775.0
labor (forces of) NEC	661.93	661.91	661.90	condition	763.7
pelvic organs or tissues NEC	654.93	654.91	654.90	N/A	763.89
causing obstructed labor	660.23	660.21	660.20	cause	763.1
pelvis (bony)	653.03	653.01	653.00	N/A	763.1
causing obstructed labor	660.13	660.11	660.10	cause	763.1
perineum or vulva	654.83	654.81	654.80	N/A	763.89
causing obstructed labor	660.23	660.21	660.20	cause	763.1
placenta, placental (vessel)	656.73	656.71	656.70	N/A	762.2
with hemorrhage	641.83	641.81	641.80	N/A	762.1
position					
cervix	654.43	654.41	654.40	N/A	763.89
causing obstructed labor	660.23	660.21	660.20	cause	763.1
fetus	652.93	652.91	652.90	N/A	763.1
causing obstructed labor	660.03	660.01	660.00	cause	763.1
placenta (low implantation) (previa)	641.03	641.01	641.00	N/A	762.0
with hemorrhage	641.13	641.11	641.10	N/A	762.1
uterus	654.43	654.41	654.40	N/A	763.89
causing obstructed labor	660.23	660.21	660.20	cause	763.1
product(s) of conception NEC	631	N/A	N/A	N/A	
quality of milk	676.83	676.81	676.80	N/A	
shape of uterus	654.43	654.41	654.40	N/A	763.89
causing obstructed labor	660.23	660.21	660.20	cause	763.1
size of fetus	653.53	653.51	653.50	N/A	763.1
causing obstructed labor	660.13	660.11	660.10	cause	763.1
umbilical cord NEC	663.83	663.81	663.80	N/A	762.6
uterus (congenital)	654.03	654.01	654.00	N/A	763.89
causing obstructed labor	660.23	660.21	660.20	cause	763.1
vagina	654.73	654.71	654.70	N/A	763.89
causing obstructed labor	660.23	660.21	660.20	cause	763.1
vulva (acquired) (congenital)	654.83	654.81	654.80	N/A	763.89
causing obstructed labor	660.23	660.21	660.20	cause	763.1
weight gain	646.13	646.11	646.10	condition	761.8
with hypertension (mild) (pre-eclamptic)	642.43	642.41	642.40	N/A	760.0

Antepartum Pregnancy Condition or Complication; affecting management of mother	Antepartum condition or complication	Delivered, with or without mention of antepartum condition	Unspecified episode of care	Assign additional code to describe the...	Affecting fetus (coded on the newborn chart only)
Abnormal NEC – *continued*					
with					
convulsions	642.63	642.61	642.60	N/A	760.0
pre-existing hypertension	642.73	642.71	642.70	N/A	760.0
with severe hypertension	642.53	642.51	642.50	N/A	760.0
Aborter, habitual or recurrent	646.33	646.31	646.30	condition	761.8
Abruption of placenta	641.23	641.21	641.20	N/A	762.1
Abscess					
areola (acute) (chronic)	675.13	675.11	675.10	N/A	
Bartholin's gland	646.63	646.61	646.60	condition	760.8
bladder	646.63	646.61	646.60	condition	760.1
breast (acute) (chronic)	675.13	675.11	675.10		
kidney	646.63	646.61	646.60	condition	760.1
labium (majus) (minus)	646.63	646.61	646.60	condition	760.8
milk	675.13	675.11	675.10	N/A	
nipple	675.03	675.01	675.00	N/A	
subareolar	675.13	675.11	675.10	N/A	
urethra	646.63	646.61	646.60	condition	760.1
vulva	646.63	646.61	646.60	condition	760.8
Absorption (of) (through placenta)					
suspected damage to fetus					
chemical	655.53	655.51	655.50	N/A	760.70
drug	655.53	655.51	655.50	N/A	760.70
Acidosis (fetal) (intrauterine)	656.83	656.81	656.80	N/A	768.4
Addiction					
alcoholic	648.43	648.41	648.40	condition	760.71
suspected fetal damage	655.43	655.41	655.40	N/A	760.71
Adhesion(s), adhesive					
amnion to fetus	658.83	658.81	658.80	N/A	762.89
uterus to abdominal wall	654.43	654.41	654.40	N/A	763.89
causing obstructed labor	660.23	660.21	660.20	cause	763.1
Advanced maternal age (multigravida)	659.63	659.61	659.60	N/A	761.8
primigravida	659.53	659.51	659.50	N/A	761.8
Aerocele	673.03	673.01	673.00	N/A	
AFP (screening for raised levels in amniotic fluid)	V28.1	N/A	N/A	N/A	
Agalactia	676.43	676.41	676.40	N/A	
Air embolism	673.03	673.01	673.00	N/A	
Age					
elderly (35 years of age or older at expected date of delivery)					
multigravida (second or more pregnancy)	659.63	659.61	659.60	N/A	
primigravida (first pregnancy)	659.53	659.51	659.50	N/A	
young (less than 16 years old at expected date of delivery)	659.83	659.81	659.80		
Albuminuria (gravidarum)	646.23	646.21	646.20	condition	760.1
with hypertension (and edema)					760.1
mild	642.43	642.41	642.40	N/A	760.0
severe	642.53	642.51	642.50	N/A	760.0
gestational	646.23	646.21	646.20	condition	760.1
pre-eclamptic (mild)	642.23	642.21	642.20	N/A	760.0
severe	642.53	642.51	642.50	N/A	760.0
Alcohol, alcoholic					
addiction (maternal)	648.43	648.41	648.40	condition	760.71
with suspected fetal damage	655.43	655.41	655.40	N/A	760.71
Alphafetoprotein (screening for raised levels in amniotic fluid)	V28.1	N/A	N/A	N/A	
Amnion (nodosum)	658.83	658.81	658.80	N/A	762.9
Amnionitis	658.43	658.41	658.40	N/A	762.7
Amniotic fluid embolism	673.13	673.11	673.10	N/A	
Amputation of cervix	654.63	654.61	654.60	N/A	763.89
causing obstructed labor	660.23	660.21	660.20	cause	763.1
Android pelvis					
with disproportion (fetopelvic)	653.33	653.31	653.30	N/A	763.1
causing obstructed labor	660.13	660.11	660.10	cause	763.1

Antepartum Pregnancy Table

Antepartum Pregnancy Condition or Complication; affecting management of mother	Antepartum condition or complication	Delivered, with or without mention of antepartum condition	Unspecified episode of care	Assign additional code to describe the...	Affecting fetus (coded on the newborn chart only)
Anemia	648.23	648.21	648.20	condition	760.8
aplastic	648.23	648.21	648.20	condition	760.8
iron (Fe) deficiency	648.23	648.21	648.20	condition	760.8
macrocytic	648.23	648.21	648.20	condition	760.8
megaloblastic	648.23	648.21	648.20	condition	760.8
pernicious	648.23	648.21	648.20	condition	760.8
postpartum	648.23	648.21	648.20	condition	
Anencephalus, anencephaly (fetal)	655.03	655.01	655.00	N/A	
Anesthesia, anesthetic					
complications NEC	668.83	668.81	668.80	condition	
cardiac	668.13	668.11	668.10	condition	763.5
central nervous system	668.23	668.21	668.20	condition	763.5
pulmonary	668.03	668.01	668.00	condition	763.5
death (from) during delivery	668.93	668.91	668.90	condition	761.6
Anomaly, anomalous (congenital)					
cardiovascular system	648.53	648.51	648.50	condition	
cervix	654.63	654.61	654.60	N/A	763.89
causing obstructed labor	660.23	660.21	660.20	cause	763.1
pelvis (bony)	653.03	653.01	653.00	N/A	763.1
causing obstructed labor	660.13	660.11	660.10	cause	763.1
uterus	654.03	654.01	654.00	N/A	763.89
causing obstructed labor	660.23	660.21	660.20	cause	763.1
Anoxia cerebral					
complicating delivery (cesarean) (instrumental)	669.43	669.41	669.40	N/A	
due to obstetric anesthesia or sedation	668.23	668.21	668.20	complication	
Anteversion					
uterus, uterine (cervix)	654.43	654.41	654.40	N/A	763.89
causing obstructed labor	660.23	660.21	660.20	cause	763.1
Anthropoid pelvis					
with disproportion (fetopelvic)	653.23	653.21	653.20	N/A	763.1
causing obstructed labor	660.13	660.11	660.10	cause	763.1
Antibodies (incompatibility)					
ABO	656.23	656.21	656.20	N/A	773.2
anti-C	656.13	656.11	656.10	N/A	773.0
anti-D, cord blood	656.13	656.11	656.10	N/A	773.0
anti-E	656.13	656.11	656.10	N/A	773.0
blood group (ABO)	656.23	656.21	656.20	N/A	773.1
Rh (blood group) (factor)	656.13	656.11	656.10	N/A	773.0
Apoplexia, apoplexy, apoplectic					
placenta	641.23	641.21	641.20	N/A	762.1
uteroplacental	641.23	641.21	641.20	N/A	762.1
Arrest, arrested					
active phase of labor	661.13	661.11	661.10	N/A	763.7
any plane in pelvis complicating delivery	660.13	660.11	660.10	cause	763.1
cardiac					
anesthesia, complicating delivery (cesarean) (instrumental)	668.13 668.13 669.43	668.11 669.41	668.10 669.40	N/A N/A	
deep transverse	660.33	660.31	660.30	cause	763.1
development or growth of fetus	656.53	656.51	656.50	N/A	764.90
transverse (deep)	660.33	660.31	660.30	cause	763.1
Ascites					
fetal, causing fetopelvic disproportion	653.73	653.71	653.70	N/A	763.1
causing obstructed labor	660.13	660.11	660.10	cause	763.1
Aspiration					
acid-pulmonary (syndrome)	668.03	668.01	668.00	complication	
pneumonitis	668.03	668.01	668.00	complication	
Assimilation, pelvis					
with disproportion	653.23	653.21	653.20	N/A	763.1
causing obstructed labor	660.13	660.11	660.10	cause	763.1
Asymmetry					
pelvis with disproportion	653.03	653.01	653.00	N/A	763.1
causing obstructed labor	660.13	660.11	660.10	cause	763.1
Atresia, atretic					
cervix	654.63	654.61	654.60	N/A	763.89
causing obstructed labor	660.23	660.21	660.20	cause	763.1

Antepartum Pregnancy Table

Antepartum Pregnancy Condition or Complication; affecting management of mother	Antepartum condition or complication	Delivered, with or without mention of antepartum condition	Unspecified episode of care	Assign additional code to describe the...	Affecting fetus (coded on the newborn chart only)
Atrophy, atrophic					
breast	676.33	676.31	676.30		
liver (acute) (subacute) (yellow)	646.73	646.71	646.70	complication	
Avulsion (traumatic)					
symphyseal cartilage (inner)	N/A	665.61	665.60	N/A	
Bacilluria, asymptomatic	646.53	646.51	646.50	complication	
Bacteremia					
during labor	659.33	659.31	659.30	N/A	
during pregnancy	647.83	647.81	647.80	condition	
Bacteriuria, asymptomatic	646.53	646.51	646.50	complication	760.1
Band(s), amniotic	658.83	658.81	658.80	N/A	762.8
Bandl's ring (contraction)	661.43	661.41	661.40	N/A	763.7
Bicornis or Bicornuate uterus	654.03	654.01	654.00	N/A	763.89
causing obstructed labor	660.23	660.21	660.20	cause	763.1
Bleeding	641.93	641.91	641.90	N/A	
accidental	641.23	641.21	641.20	N/A	762.1
before 22 completed weeks gestation NEC	640.93	640.91	640.90	N/A	
cerebrovascular	674.03	674.01	674.00	N/A	
due to					
afibrinogenemia or other coagulation defect	641.33	641.31	641.30	N/A	
fibroids	641.83	641.81	641.80	N/A	762.1
marginal sinus (rupture)	641.23	641.21	641.20	N/A	762.1
premature separation, placenta	641.23	641.21	641.20	N/A	762.1
trauma	641.83	641.81	641.80	N/A	
early (before 22 completed weeks gestation)	640.93	640.91	640.90	N/A	
threatened abortion	640.03	640.01	640.00	N/A	
unavoidable	641.13	641.11	641.10	N/A	
Bone disorders	648.73	648.71	648.70	condition	
Borderline pelvis	653.13	653.11	653.10	N/A	763.1
with obstruction during labor	660.13	660.11	660.10	cause	763.1
Braxton Hicks contractions	644.13	N/A	644.10	N/A	
Breech presentation (buttocks) (complete) (frank)	652.23	652.21	652.20	N/A	761.7
with successful version	652.13	652.11	652.10	N/A	763.1
before labor	652.23	652.21	652.20	N/A	761.7
during labor	652.23	652.21	652.20	N/A	763.0
Brow presentation					
complicating delivery	652.43	652.41	652.40		763.1
Bruise					
umbilical cord	663.63	663.61	663.60	N/A	762.6
Caked breast	676.23	676.21	676.20	N/A	
Cardiomyopathy	674.53	674.51	674.50		
Cardiovascular disease	648.63	648.61	648.60	condition	
congenital	648.53	648.51	648.50	condition	
Cellulitis, breast	675.13	675.11	675.10	N/A	
Cephalopelvic disproportion NOS	653.43	653.41	653.40	N/A	763.1
with obstruction during labor	660.13	660.11	660.10	cause	763.1
Cerebrovascular disorders	674.03	674.01	674.00	condition	
Cervicitis	646.63	646.61	646.60	condition	760.8
Cervix					
adhesions	654.63	654.61	654.60	N/A	
anaplasia	654.63	654.61	654.60	N/A	
atypism	654.63	654.61	654.60	N/A	
bands	654.63	654.61	654.60	N/A	
with obstruction during labor	660.23	660.21	660.20	cause	763.1
cervicitis	654.63	654.61	654.60	N/A	
cicatrix	654.63	654.61	654.60	N/A	
cyst	654.63	654.61	654.60	N/A	
dysplasia	654.63	654.61	654.60	N/A	
ectropion	654.63	654.61	654.60	N/A	
endocervicitis	654.63	654.61	654.60	N/A	
erosion	654.63	654.61	654.60	N/A	
hypertrophic elongation	654.63	654.61	654.60	N/A	
incompetence	654.63	654.51	654.50	N/A	761.0
leukoplakia	654.63	654.61	654.60	N/A	
Nabothian (gland) cyst or follicle	654.63	654.61	654.60	N/A	
old laceration	654.63	654.61	654.60	N/A	

Antepartum Pregnancy Table

Antepartum Pregnancy Condition or Complication; affecting management of mother	Antepartum condition or complication	Delivered, with or without mention of antepartum condition	Unspecified episode of care	Assign additional code to describe the...	Affecting fetus (coded on the newborn chart only)
Cervix – *continued*					
polyp	654.63	654.61	654.60	N/A	
stricture and stenosis	654.63	654.61	654.60	N/A	
ulcer	654.63	654.61	654.60	N/A	
Cesarean delivery, section NEC	669.73	669.71	669.70	N/A	763.4
post mortem	669.73	669.71	669.70	N/A	761.6
previous	654.23	654.21	654.20	N/A	
causing obstructed labor	660.23	660.21	660.20	cause	763.1
Chiari-Frommel syndrome	676.63	676.61	676.60	N/A	
Chloasma (gravidarum)	646.83	646.81	646.80	condition	
Chorioamnionitis	658.43	658.41	658.40	N/A	762.7
Cicatrix					
cervix	654.63	654.61	654.60	N/A	
causing obstructed labor	660.23	660.21	660.20	cause	763.1
vagina	654.73	654.71	654.70	N/A	
causing obstructed labor	660.23	660.21	660.20	cause	763.1
Collapse (during or after labor and delivery)					
circulatory (peripheral)	669.13	669.11	669.10	N/A	779.8
lung	668.03	668.01	668.00	N/A	
vascular (peripheral)	669.13	669.11	669.10	N/A	
Colporrhexis	N/A	665.41	665.40	N/A	
Complications NEC	646.93	646.91	646.90	condition	761.9
delivery	669.93	669.91	669.90	N/A	
procedure (instrumental) (manual) (surgical)	669.43	669.41	669.40	N/A	
specified type NEC	669.83	669.81	669.80	N/A	
umbilical cord	663.93	663.91	663.90	N/A	762.6
specified type NEC	663.83	663.81	663.80	N/A	762.6
labor and delivery	669.93	669.91	669.90	N/A	
anesthesia (sedation)	668.93	668.91	668.90	N/A	763.5
cardiac	668.13	668.11	668.10	N/A	
central nervous system	668.23	668.21	668.20	N/A	
pulmonary	668.03	668.01	668.00	N/A	
specified type NEC	668.83	668.81	668.80	N/A	
specified condition NEC	669.83	669.81	669.80	N/A	
intrauterine contraceptive device (IUD)	655.83	655.81	655.80	N/A	
Compound presentation					
complicating delivery	652.83	652.81	652.80	N/A	763.1
causing obstructed labor	660.03	660.01	660.00	cause	763.1
Compression, umbilical cord					
complicating delivery	663.23	663.21	663.20	N/A	762.5
cord around neck	663.13	663.11	663.10	N/A	762.5
cord prolapsed	663.03	663.01	663.00	N/A	762.4
Conjoined twins, causing disproportion (fetopelvic)	653.73	653.71	653.70	N/A	763.1
with obstruction during labor	660.13	660.11	660.10	cause	763.1
Constriction					
ring (uterus)	661.43	661.41	661.40	N/A	763.7
Contractions					
before 37 weeks	644.03	N/A	644.00	N/A	
Braxton Hicks	644.13	N/A	644.10	N/A	
Hicks'	644.13	N/A	644.10	N/A	
hourglass uterus	661.43	661.41	661.40	N/A	763.7
pelvis, complicating delivery	653.13	653.11	653.10	N/A	763.1
causing obstructed labor	660.13	660.11	660.10	cause	763.1
generally contracted	653.13	653.11	653.10	N/A	763.1
causing obstructed labor	660.13	660.11	660.10	cause	763.1
inlet	653.23	653.21	653.20	N/A	763.1
causing obstructed labor	660.13	660.11	660.10	cause	763.1
midpelvic	653.83	653.81	653.80	N/A	763.1
causing obstructed labor	660.13	660.11	660.10	cause	763.1
midplane	653.83	653.81	653.80	N/A	763.1
causing obstructed labor	660.13	660.11	660.10	cause	763.1
outlet	653.33	653.31	653.30	N/A	763.1
causing obstructed labor	660.13	660.11	660.10	cause	763.1
ring (Bandl's)	661.43	661.41	661.40	N/A	763.7
uterus					
abnormal	661.93	661.91	661.90	N/A	763.7
clonic, hourglass or tetanic	661.43	661.41	661.40	N/A	763.7

Antepartum Pregnancy Condition or Complication; affecting management of mother	Antepartum condition or complication	Delivered, with or without mention of antepartum condition	Unspecified episode of care	Assign additional code to describe the...	Affecting fetus (coded on the newborn chart only)
Contractions – *continued*					
dyscoordinate	661.43	661.41	661.40	N/A	763.7
hourglass	661.43	661.41	661.40	N/A	763.7
incoordinate	661.43	661.41	661.40	N/A	763.7
inefficient or poor	661.23	661.21	661.20	N/A	763.7
irregular	661.23	661.21	661.20	N/A	763.7
tetanic	661.43	661.41	661.40	N/A	763.7
Convulsions (eclamptic) (uremic)	642.63	642.61	642.60	N/A	760.0
with pre-existing hypertension	642.73	642.71	642.70	N/A	760.0
Cord, complicating delivery				N/A	
around neck (tightly) (with compression)	663.13	663.11	663.10	N/A	762.5
without compression	663.33	663.31	663.30	N/A	762.6
prolapse, complicating delivery	663.03	663.01	663.00	N/A	762.4
Cornual — *see* Ectopic pregnancy					761.4
CPD	653.43	653.41	653.40	N/A	763.1
causing obstructed labor	660.13	660.11	660.10	cause	763.1
Cracked nipple	676.13	676.11	676.10	N/A	
Cretin, pelvis (with disproportion) (fetopelvic)	653.13	653.11	653.10	N/A	763.1
causing obstructed labor	660.13	660.11	660.10	cause	763.1
Cross birth (of fetus) complicating delivery	652.33	652.31	652.30	N/A	763.1
with successful version	652.13	652.11	652.10	N/A	763.1
causing obstructed labor	660.03	660.01	660.00	cause	763.1
Cyst					
amnion, amniotic	658.83	658.81	658.80	N/A	763.89
chorion	658.83	658.81	658.80	N/A	763.89
ovary	654.43	654.41	654.40	N/A	763.89
causing obstructed labor	660.23	660.21	660.20	cause	763.1
pelvic	654.43	654.41	654.40	N/A	763.89
causing obstructed labor	660.23	660.21	660.20	cause	763.1
Cystitis	646.63	646.61	646.60	condition	760.1
Cystocele	654.43	654.41	654.40	N/A	763.89
causing obstructed labor	660.23	660.21	660.20	cause	763.1
Damage					
coccyx, complicating delivery	N/A	665.61	665.60	N/A	763.89
pelvic (during delivery)					
joint or ligament	N/A	665.61	665.60	N/A	763.89
organ	N/A	665.51	665.50	N/A	763.89
Dates vs uterine size discrepancy	646.83	646.81	646.80		
Dead, fetus					
retained in utero (after 22 completed weeks' gestation)	656.43	656.41	656.40	N/A	779.9
before 22 weeks — *see* Abortion, missed					
syndrome	641.33	641.31	641.30	N/A	779.9
Death					
fetal NEC	646.93	646.91	646.90	condition	779.9
early before 22 weeks gestation — *see* Abortion, missed					
near term	656.43	656.41	656.40	N/A	779.9
maternal, NEC	646.93	646.91	646.90	condition	761.6
during delivery	668.93	668.91	668.90	N/A	
sudden, during delivery	669.93	669.91	669.90	N/A	761.6
under anesthesia NEC	668.93	668.91	668.90	N/A	761.6
Deciduitis	646.63	646.61	646.60	N/A	760.8
Decreased fetal movements	655.73	655.71	655.70	N/A	
Defect, defective					
coagulation (factor)	641.33	641.31	641.30	N/A	762.1
causing hemorrhage of pregnancy or delivery	641.33	641.31	641.30	N/A	762.1
Deficiency, deficient					
coagulation (factor)	641.33	641.31	641.30	N/A	762.1
causing hemorrhage of pregnancy or delivery	641.33	641.31	641.30	N/A	762.1
Deformity					
fetal					
with fetopelvic disproportion	653.73	653.71	653.70	N/A	763.1

Antepartum Pregnancy Table

Antepartum Pregnancy Condition or Complication; affecting management of mother	Antepartum condition or complication	Delivered, with or without mention of antepartum condition	Unspecified episode of care	Assign additional code to describe the...	Affecting fetus (coded on the newborn chart only)
Deformity – *continued*					
causing obstructed labor	660.13	660.11	660.10	N/A	763.1
known or suspected	655.93	655.91	655.90	N/A	763.89
pelvic, pelvis					
with disproportion (fetopelvic)	653.03	653.01	653.00	N/A	763.1
causing obstructed labor	660.13	660.11	660.10	cause	763.1
soft part, organs or tissues NEC	654.93	654.91	654.90	cause	763.89
causing obstructed labor	660.23	660.21	660.20	cause	763.1
Delay, delayed					
any plane in pelvis, complicating delivery	660.13	660.11	660.10	cause	763.1
birth or delivery NEC	662.13	662.11	662.10	N/A	763.89
second twin, triplet, or multiple mate	662.33	662.31	662.30	N/A	763.89
Dependence, maternal					
alcohol, with suspected fetal damage	655.43	655.41	655.40	N/A	779.5
drug	648.33	648.31	648.30	condition	779.5
suspected damage to fetus	655.53	655.51	655.50	N/A	779.5
Depression	648.43	648.41	648.40	condition	
Dermatitis, gestationis	646.83	646.81	646.80	condition	
Detachment					
cervix, annular	N/A	665.31	665.30	N/A	763.89
Development					
incomplete (fetus or newborn)	656.53	656.51	656.50	N/A	763.89
Diabetes					
condition present before pregnancy	648.03	648.01	648.00	condition	775.0
gestational (chemical) (latent)	648.83	648.81	648.80	condition	775.0
Diastasis, recti (abdomen) complicating delivery	665.83	665.81	665.80	N/A	763.89
Difficult delivery NEC	669.93	669.91	669.90	N/A	763.89
Dilatation					
bladder (sphincter)	654.43	654.41	654.40	N/A	763.89
causing obstructed labor	660.23	660.21	660.20	cause	763.1
cervix, complicating delivery	654.63	654.61	654.60	N/A	763.89
incomplete, poor, slow	661.03	661.01	661.00	N/A	763.7
Discrepancy of uterine size to dates	646.83	646.81	646.80	N/A	
Disease, diseased NEC	646.93	646.91	646.90	condition	
breast NEC	676.33	676.31	676.30	N/A	
cerebrovascular, NEC	674.03	674.01	674.00	N/A	
Frommel's	676.63	676.61	676.60	N/A	
heart					
placenta	656.73	656.71	656.70	N/A	762.2
renal NEC	646.23	646.21	646.20	condition	760.1
Valsuani's (progressive pernicious anemia, puerperal)	648.23	648.21	648.20	condition	
venereal NEC	647.23	647.21	647.20	condition	
virus NEC	647.63	647.61	647.60	condition	
with fetal damage	655.33	655.31	655.30	N/A	763.89
Disorders					
breast	676.33	676.31	676.30	N/A	
genital tract or organ	646.63	646.61	646.60	condition	760.8
lactation	676.93	676.91	676.90	N/A	
liver	646.73	646.71	646.70	condition	760.8
mental	648.43	648.41	648.40	condition	
metabolism NEC (in labor and delivery)	669.03	669.01	669.00	N/A	763.89
Displacement, uterus NEC	654.43	654.41	654.40	N/A	763.89
causing obstructed labor	660.23	660.21	660.20	cause	763.1
Disproportion	653.93	653.91	653.90	N/A	763.1
caused by					
conjoined twins	653.73	653.71	653.70	N/A	763.1
contraction, pelvis (general)	653.13	653.11	653.10	N/A	763.1
inlet	653.23	653.21	653.20	N/A	763.1
midpelvic	653.83	653.81	653.80	N/A	763.1
midplane	653.83	653.81	653.80	N/A	763.1
outlet	653.33	653.31	653.30	N/A	763.1

Antepartum Pregnancy Condition or Complication; affecting management of mother	Antepartum condition or complication	Delivered, with or without mention of antepartum condition	Unspecified episode of care	Assign additional code to describe the...	Affecting fetus (coded on the newborn chart only)
Disproportion – *continued*					
fetal NEC	653.53	653.51	653.50	N/A	763.1
ascites	653.73	653.71	653.70	N/A	763.1
hydrocephalus	653.63	653.61	653.60	N/A	763.1
hydrops	653.73	653.71	653.70	N/A	763.1
meningomyelocele	653.73	653.71	653.70	N/A	763.1
sacral teratoma	653.73	653.71	653.70	N/A	763.1
tumor	653.73	653.71	653.70	N/A	763.1
hydrocephalic fetus	653.63	653.61	653.60	N/A	763.1
pelvis, pelvic, abnormality (bony) NEC	653.03	653.01	653.00	N/A	763.1
unusually large fetus	653.53	653.51	653.50	N/A	763.1
causing obstructed labor	660.13	660.11	660.10	cause	763.1
cephalopelvic, normally formed fetus	653.43	653.41	653.40	N/A	763.1
fetopelvic, normally formed fetus	653.43	653.41	653.40	N/A	763.1
causing obstructed labor	660.13	660.11	660.10	cause	763.1
mixed maternal and fetal origin, normally, formed fetus	653.43	653.41	653.40	N/A	763.1
pelvis, pelvic (bony) NEC	653.13	653.11	653.10	N/A	763.1
causing obstructed labor	660.13	660.11	660.10	cause	763.1
specified type NEC	653.83	653.81	653.80	N/A	763.1
Distortion					
lumbar spine				N/A	
with disproportion (fetopelvic)	653.03	653.01	653.00	N/A	763.1
causing obstructed labor	660.13	660.11	660.10	cause	763.1
maternal	669.03	669.01	669.00	N/A	
Distress (fetal)	656.83	656.81	656.80	N/A	763.89
Double uterus	654.03	654.01	654.00	N/A	763.89
causing obstructed labor	660.23	660.21	660.20	cause	763.1
Dropsy, amnion	657.03	657.01	657.00	N/A	761.3
Drug dependence	648.33	648.31	648.30	condition	
Dyscrasia, blood					
with antepartum hemorrhage	641.33	641.31	641.30	N/A	762.1
Dysfunction					
thyroid	648.13	648.11	648.10	condition	
uterus, complicating delivery	661.93	661.91	661.90	N/A	763.7
hypertonic	661.43	661.41	661.40	N/A	763.7
hypotonic, primary	661.03	661.01	661.00	N/A	763.7
secondary	661.13	661.11	661.10	N/A	763.7
Dysplasia of cervix	654.63	654.61	654.60	N/A	763.89
causing obstructed labor	660.23	660.21	660.20	cause	763.1
Dystocia	660.93	660.91	660.90	cause	763.1
cervical	661.03	661.01	661.00	N/A	763.7
contraction ring	661.43	661.41	661.40	N/A	763.7
fetal	660.93	660.91	660.90	cause	763.1
abnormal size	653.53	653.51	653.50	N/A	763.1
causing obstructed labor	660.13	660.11	660.10	cause	763.1
deformity	653.73	653.71	653.70	N/A	763.1
causing obstructed labor	660.13	660.11	660.10	cause	763.1
maternal	660.93	660.91	660.90	N/A	763.1
positional	660.03	660.01	660.00	cause	763.1
shoulder (girdle)	660.43	660.41	660.40	cause	763.1
uterine NEC	661.43	661.41	661.40	N/A	763.7
Early onset of delivery (spontaneous)	N/A	644.21	644.20	N/A	
Preterm neonate birthweight					
Extreme immaturity (**code also weeks of gestation, codes 765.20-765.29**)					
unspecified (weight)					765.00
< 500 gms					765.11
500-749 gms					765.02
750-999 gms					765.03
1,000-1,249 gms					765.04
1,250-1,499 gms					765.05
1,500-1,749 gms					765.06
1,750-1,999 gms					765.07
2,000-2,499 gms					765.08
≥ 2,500 gms					765.09

Antepartum Pregnancy Table

Antepartum Pregnancy Table

Antepartum Pregnancy Condition or Complication; affecting management of mother	Antepartum condition or complication	Delivered, with or without mention of antepartum condition	Unspecified episode of care	Assign additional code to describe the...	Affecting fetus (coded on the newborn chart only)
Early onset of delivery (spontaneous) – *continued*					
Other preterm (**code also weeks of gestation, codes 765.20-765.29**)					
unspecified (weight)					765.10
< 500 gms					765.11
500-749 gms					765.12
750-999 gms					765.13
1,000-1,249 gms					765.14
1,250-1,499 gms					765.15
1,500-1,749 gms					765.16
1,750-1,999 gms					765.17
2,000-2,499 gms					765.18
≥ 2,500 gms					765.19
Preterm neonate weeks of gestation (**code in addition to birthweight, subcategory codes 765.0 and 765.1**)					
unspecified weeks of gestation					765.20
< 24 completed weeks of gestation					765.21
24 completed weeks of gestation					765.22
25-26 completed weeks of gestation					765.23
27-28 completed weeks of gestation					765.24
29-30 completed weeks of gestation					765.25
31-32 completed weeks of gestation					765.26
33-34 completed weeks of gestation					765.27
35-36 completed weeks of gestation					765.28
≥ 37 completed weeks of gestation					765.29
Eclampsia, eclamptic (coma) (convulsions) (delirium)	642.63	642.61	642.60	N/A	760.0
with pre-existing hypertension	642.73	642.71	642.70	N/A	760.0
Edema	646.13	646.11	646.10	condition	
with hypertension — *see* Pregnancy, toxemia					
Effect, adverse					
anesthetic (in labor and delivery) NEC	668.93	668.91	668.90	N/A	763.5
radiation (suspected damage to fetus)	655.63	655.61	655.60	N/A	condition
Effusion, amniotic fluid	658.13	658.11	658.10	N/A	761.1
delayed delivery following	658.23	658.21	658.20	N/A	761.1
Electrolyte imbalance with hyperemesis gravidarum (before 22 completed weeks' gestation)	643.13	643.11	643.10	N/A	761.8
Embolism					
air (pulmonary)	673.03	673.01	673.00	N/A	
amniotic fluid	673.13	673.11	673.10	N/A	
blood clot	673.23	673.21	673.20	N/A	
brain	674.03	674.01	674.00	N/A	
cerebral	674.03	674.01	674.00	N/A	
fat (cerebral) (pulmonary) (systemic)	673.83	673.81	673.80	N/A	
intracranial (venous sinus) (nonpyogenic)	671.53	671.51	671.50	N/A	
pulmonary NEC	673.23	673.21	673.20	N/A	
pyemic	673.33	673.31	673.30	N/A	
septic	673.33	673.31	673.30	N/A	
Emesis (gravidarum) — *see* Pregnancy, vomiting					
Endometritis	646.63	646.61	646.60	condition	760.8
decidual	646.63	646.61	646.60	condition	760.8
Engorgement, breast	676.23	676.21	676.20	N/A	

Antepartum Pregnancy Condition or Complication; affecting management of mother	Antepartum condition or complication	Delivered, with or without mention of antepartum condition	Unspecified episode of care	Assign additional code to describe the...	Affecting fetus (coded on the newborn chart only)
Entanglement, umbilical cord(s)	663.33	663.31	663.30	N/A	762.5
with compression	663.23	663.21	663.20	N/A	762.5
around neck with compression	663.13	663.11	663.10	N/A	762.5
twins in monoamniotic sac	663.23	663.21	663.20	N/A	762.5
Excessive					
large (fetus)	656.63	656.61	656.60	N/A	766.0
with obstructed labor	660.13	660.11	660.10	cause	763.1
causing disproportion	653.53	653.51	653.50	N/A	763.1
causing obstructed labor	660.13	660.11	660.10	cause	763.1
milk secretion	676.63	676.61	676.60	N/A	
weight gain	646.13	646.11	646.10	condition	
Exhaustion (complicating delivery)	669.83	669.81	669.80	N/A	763.89
Extraction					
breech NEC	N/A	669.61	669.60	N/A	763.0
manual NEC	669.83	669.81	669.80	N/A	763.89
Face presentation	652.43	652.41	652.40	N/A	763.1
causing obstructed labor	660.03	660.01	660.00	cause	763.1
Failure, failed					
cervical dilation in labor	661.03	661.01	661.00		763.7
descent of head (at term)	652.53	652.51	652.50	N/A	763.1
in labor	660.03	660.01	660.00	cause	763.1
engagement of head NEC	652.53	652.51	652.50	N/A	763.1
in labor	660.03	660.01	660.00	cause	763.1
fetal head to enter pelvic brim	652.53	652.51	652.50	N/A	763.1
in labor	660.03	660.01	660.00	cause	763.1
forceps NEC	660.73	660.71	660.70	cause	763.1
heart, complicating					
delivery (cesarean) (instrumental)	669.43	669.41	669.40	N/A	
obstetric anesthesia or sedation	668.13	668.11	668.10	N/A	
induction (of labor)	659.13	659.11	659.10	N/A	763.89
by oxytocic drugs (Pitocin)	659.13	659.11	659.10	N/A	763.89
instrumental	659.03	659.01	659.00	N/A	763.89
mechanical	659.03	659.01	659.00	N/A	763.89
medical	659.13	659.11	659.10	N/A	763.89
surgical	659.03	659.01	659.00	N/A	763.89
lactation	676.43	676.41	676.40	N/A	
to progress	661.23	661.21	661.20	N/A	763.89
trial of labor NOS	660.63	660.61	660.60	cause	763.1
vacuum extraction delivery NOS	660.73	660.71	660.70	cause	763.1
ventouse NOS	660.73	660.71	660.70	cause	763.1
False labor (pains)	644.13	N/A	644.10	N/A	
Fatigue	646.83	646.81	646.80	condition	
Fatty metamorphosis of liver	646.73	646.71	646.70	condition	760.8
Fetal					
acidosis	656.33	656.31	656.30	N/A	763.89
bradycardia	659.73	659.71	659.70	N/A	763.83
before onset of labor	659.73	659.71	659.70	N/A	763.81
during labor	659.73	659.71	659.70	N/A	763.82
decreased movements	655.73	655.71	655.70	N/A	763.89
demise (near term)	656.43	656.41	656.40	N/A	cause
early (before 22 weeks completed gestation)	632	N/A	N/A	N/A	761.8
deformity	653.73	653.71	653.70	N/A	763.1
causing obstructed labor	660.13	660.11	660.10	cause	763.1
distress	656.33	656.31	656.30	N/A	
heart rate, abnormal	659.73	659.71	659.70	N/A	763.83
before onset of labor	659.73	659.71	659.70	N/A	763.81
during labor	659.73	659.71	659.70	N/A	763.82
heart rhythm, abnormal	659.73	659.71	659.70	N/A	763.83
before onset of labor	659.73	659.71	659.70	N/A	763.81
during labor	659.73	659.71	659.70	N/A	763.82
movements, decreased	655.73	655.71	655.70	N/A	
Fetomaternal hemorrhage	656.03	656.01	656.00	N/A	772.0
Fibrinolysis	641.33	641.31	641.30	N/A	762.1
Fibroid tumor(s)	654.13	654.11	654.10	N/A	763.89
causing obstructed labor	660.23	660.21	660.20	cause	763.1
Fibromyoma (uterus)	654.13	654.11	654.10	N/A	763.89
causing obstructed labor	660.23	660.21	660.20	cause	763.1

Antepartum Pregnancy Condition or Complication; affecting management of mother	Antepartum condition or complication	Delivered, with or without mention of antepartum condition	Unspecified episode of care	Assign additional code to describe the...	Affecting fetus (coded on the newborn chart only)
Fibrosis, fibrotic					
amnion	658.83	658.81	658.80	N/A	
chorion	658.83	658.81	658.80	N/A	
perineum	654.83	654.81	654.80	N/A	763.8
causing obstructed labor	660.23	660.21	660.20	cause	763.1
Fissure, nipple	676.13	676.11	676.10	N/A	
Fistula					
breast	675.13	675.11	675.10	N/A	
mammary gland	675.13	675.11	675.10	N/A	
Flat, pelvis					
with disproportion (fetopelvic)	653.23	653.21	653.20	N/A	763.1
causing obstructed labor	660.13	660.11	660.10	cause	763.1
Footling presentation	652.83	652.81	652.80	N/A	
with successful version	652.13	652.11	652.10	N/A	
Forced birth or delivery NEC	N/A	669.81	669.80	N/A	763.89
Forceps delivery NEC	N/A	669.51	669.50	N/A	763.2
Fractured coccyx complicating delivery	N/A	665.61	665.60	N/A	
Frommel's disease	676.63	676.61	676.60	N/A	
Frommel-Chiari syndrome	676.63	676.61	676.60	N/A	
Funnel pelvis with disproportion (fetopelvic)	653.33	653.31	653.30	N/A	763.1
causing obstructed labor	660.13	660.11	660.10	cause	763.1
Fusion, hymeno-urethral					
causing obstructed labor	660.13	660.11	660.10	cause	763.1
Galactocele (breast)	676.83	676.81	676.80	N/A	
Galactorrhea	676.63	676.61	676.60	N/A	
Goiter	648.13	648.11	648.10	condition	
Gonococcal infection	647.13	647.11	647.10	condition	760.2
Gonorrhea	647.13	647.11	647.10	condition	760.2
Grand multiparity, affecting labor and delivery	659.43	659.41	659.40	N/A	
Growth fetal (poor)	656.53	656.51	656.50	N/A	764.90
Heart (fetal)					
abnormal					
rate	659.73	659.71	659.70	N/A	763.83
before onset of labor	659.73	659.71	659.70	N/A	763.81
during labor	659.73	659.71	659.70	N/A	763.82
rhythm	659.73	659.71	659.70	N/A	763.83
before onset of labor	659.73	659.71	659.70	N/A	763.81
during labor	659.73	659.71	659.70	N/A	763.82
HELLP (Hemolysis, Elevated Liver function and Low Platelets)	642.53	642.51	642.50	N/A	
Hematoma					
amnion	658.83	658.81	658.80	N/A	
broad ligament	N/A	665.71	665.70	N/A	
complicating delivery (perineum) (vulva)	N/A	664.51	664.50	N/A	
pelvic	N/A	665.71	665.70	N/A	
vagina	N/A	665.71	665.70	N/A	
pelvis, complicating delivery	N/A	665.71	665.70	N/A	
perineal wound complicating delivery	N/A	664.51	664.50	N/A	
umbilical cord	663.63	663.61	663.60	N/A	762.6
vagina	N/A	665.71	665.70	N/A	
vulva, complicating delivery	N/A	664.51	664.50	N/A	767.8
Hemolysis, intravascular	641.33	641.31	641.30	N/A	762.1
Hemolysis, elevated liver function, low platelets syndrome (HELLP)	642.53	642.51	642.50	N/A	
Hemorrhage					
accidental	641.23	641.21	641.20	N/A	762.1
before 22 completed weeks gestation NEC	640.93	640.91	640.90	N/A	
brain	674.03	674.01	674.00	N/A	
cerebrovascular	674.03	674.01	674.00	N/A	
complicating delivery	641.93	641.91	641.90	N/A	762.1
associated with					
afibrinogenemia	641.33	641.31	641.30	N/A	763.89
coagulation defect	641.33	641.31	641.30	N/A	763.89
hyperfibrinolysis	641.33	641.31	641.30	N/A	763.89

Antepartum Pregnancy Condition or Complication; affecting management of mother	Antepartum condition or complication	Delivered, with or without mention of antepartum condition	Unspecified episode of care	Assign additional code to describe the...	Affecting fetus (coded on the newborn chart only)
Hemorrhage –*continued*					
hypofibrinogenemia	641.33	641.31	641.30	N/A	763.89
concealed	641.93	641.91	641.90	N/A	762.1
due to					
afibrinogenemia or other coagulation defect	641.33	641.31	641.30	condition	763.89
fibroids	641.83	641.81	641.80	N/A	763.89
low-lying placenta	641.13	641.11	641.10	N/A	762.0
marginal sinus (rupture)	641.23	641.21	641.20	N/A	762.1
placenta previa	641.13	641.11	641.10	N/A	762.0
premature separation, placenta	641.23	641.21	641.20	N/A	762.1
trauma	641.83	641.81	641.80	N/A	763.89
umbilicus, umbilical cord	663.83	663.81	663.80	N/A	772.0
due to					
afibrinogenemia or other coagulation defect	641.33	641.31	641.30	condition	762.1
fibroids	641.83	641.81	641.80	N/A	762.1
low-lying placenta	641.13	641.11	641.10	N/A	762.1
marginal sinus (rupture)	641.23	641.21	641.20	N/A	762.1
placenta previa	641.13	641.11	641.10	N/A	762.0
premature separation, placenta	641.23	641.21	641.20	N/A	762.1
threatened abortion	640.03	640.01	640.00	N/A	762.1
trauma	641.83	641.81	641.80	N/A	762.1
early (before 22 completed weeks gestation)	640.93	640.91	640.90	N/A	762.1
fetomaternal	656.03	656.01	656.00	N/A	772.0
funis (complicating delivery)	663.83	663.81	663.80	N/A	772.0
intracranial	674.03	674.01	674.00	N/A	
marginal sinus	641.23	641.21	641.20	N/A	762.1
placenta NEC	641.93	641.91	641.90	N/A	762.1
from surgical or instrumental damage	641.83	641.81	641.80	N/A	762.1
previa	641.13	641.11	641.10	N/A	762.0
retroplacental	641.23	641.21	641.20	N/A	762.1
subarachnoid	674.03	674.01	674.00	N/A	
subdural	674.03	674.01	674.00	N/A	
threatened abortion	640.03	640.01	640.00	N/A	
umbilicus, umbilical cord (complicating delivery)	663.83	663.81	663.80	N/A	772.0
unavoidable	641.13	641.11	641.10	N/A	762.0
vasa previa	663.53	663.51	663.50	N/A	772.0
Hemorrhoids	671.83	671.81	671.80	N/A	
Hepatitis	646.73	646.71	646.70	condition	
viral	647.63	647.61	647.60	condition	
Herniation of uterus	654.43	654.41	654.40	N/A	
causing obstructed labor	660.23	660.21	660.20	cause	763.1
Herpes, herpetic	647.63	647.61	647.60	condition	
gestationis	646.83	646.81	646.80	condition	
High head at term	652.43	652.41	652.40	N/A	763.1
HIV	647.63	647.61	647.60	042	
asymptomatic	647.63	647.61	647.60	V08	
Hourglass uterus	661.43	661.41	661.40	N/A	763.7
Hydatidiform mole	630	N/A	N/A	N/A	
previous pregnancy, affecting management of current pregnancy	V23.1	V23.1	V23.1	N/A	
Hydramnios	657.03	657.01	657.00	N/A	761.3
Hydroa gestationis	646.83	646.81	646.80	condition	
Hydrocephalic fetus	655.03	655.01	655.00	N/A	763.1
causing disproportion	653.63	653.61	653.60	N/A	763.1
with obstructed labor	660.13	660.11	660.10	cause	763.1
Hydrops amnii	657.03	657.01	657.00	N/A	
Hydrorrhea	658.13	658.11	658.10	N/A	
Hyperemesis					
before 22 completed weeks of gestation	643.03	643.01	643.00	N/A	761.8
with					
carbohydrate depletion	643.13	643.11	643.10	N/A	761.8
dehydration	643.13	643.11	643.10	N/A	761.8
electrolyte imbalance	643.13	643.11	643.10	N/A	761.8

Antepartum Pregnancy Table

Antepartum Pregnancy Condition or Complication; affecting management of mother	Antepartum condition or complication	Delivered, with or without mention of antepartum condition	Unspecified episode of care	Assign additional code to describe the...	Affecting fetus (coded on the newborn chart only)
Hyperemesis – *continued*					
metabolic disturbance	643.13	643.11	643.10	N/A	761.8
mild	643.03	643.01	643.00	N/A	761.8
severe with metabolic disturbance	643.13	643.11	643.10	N/A	761.8
late (starting 23rd week of gestation)	643.23	643.21	643.20	N/A	761.8
Hypersecretion of milk	676.63	676.61	676.60	N/A	
Hypertension	642.93	642.91	642.90	N/A	760.0
with					
albuminuria (and edema) (mild)	642.43	642.41	642.40	N/A	760.0
severe	642.53	642.51	642.50	N/A	760.0
edema (mild)	642.43	642.41	642.40	N/A	760.0
severe	642.53	642.51	642.50	N/A	760.0
heart disease	642.23	642.21	642.20	N/A	760.0
and renal disease	642.23	642.21	642.20	N/A	760.0
pre-eclampsia or eclampsia	642.73	642.71	642.70	N/A	760.0
renal disease	642.23	642.21	642.20	N/A	760.0
and heart disease	642.23	642.21	642.20	N/A	760.0
benign	642.03	642.01	642.00	N/A	760.0
chronic	642.03	642.01	642.00	N/A	760.0
pre-existing	642.03	642.01	642.00	N/A	760.0
chronic	642.03	642.01	642.00	N/A	760.0
essential	642.03	642.01	642.00	N/A	760.0
with pre-eclampsia or eclampsia	642.73	642.71	642.70	N/A	760.0
gestational	642.33	642.31	642.30	N/A	
malignant	642.23	642.21	642.20	N/A	760.0
chronic	642.23	642.21	642.20	N/A	760.0
with pre-eclampsia or eclampsia	642.73	642.71	642.70	N/A	760.0
pre-existing	642.23	642.21	642.20	N/A	760.0
pre-existing	642.03	642.01	642.00	N/A	
secondary to renal disease	642.13	642.11	642.10	N/A	760.0
with pre-eclampsia or eclampsia	642.73	642.71	642.70	N/A	760.0
transient	642.33	642.31	642.30	N/A	
Hypertensive					
heart and renal disease	642.23	642.21	642.20	N/A	760.0
heart disease	642.23	642.21	642.20	N/A	760.0
renal disease	642.23	642.21	642.20	N/A	760.0
Hyperthyroidism	648.13	648.11	648.10	condition	
Hypertonicity	648.13	648.11	648.10	condition	763.7
Hypertrophy					
breast	676.33	676.31	676.30	N/A	
Hypotension (following labor and delivery)	669.23	669.21	669.20	N/A	
Hypothyroidism	648.13	648.11	648.10	condition	
Hysteralgia	646.83	646.81	646.80	condition	
Icterus gravis	646.73	646.71	646.70	condition	760.8
Illegitimate	V61.6	V61.6	V61.6	N/A	
Imbalance					
electrolyte with hyperemesis gravidarum (before 22 completed weeks' gestation)	643.13	643.11	643.10	N/A	
Immunization					
ABO	656.23	656.21	656.20	N/A	773.1
Rh factor	656.13	656.11	656.10	N/A	773.0
Immunodeficiency to Rh factor	656.13	656.11	656.10	N/A	773.0
Impacted shoulder	660.43	660.41	660.40	cause	763.1
Inadequate development of fetus	656.53	656.51	656.50	N/A	764.90
Incarceration, uterus	654.33	654.31	654.30	N/A	763.1
causing obstructed labor	660.23	660.21	660.20	cause	763.1
Incompatibility, blood groups (ABO)					
ABO	656.23	656.21	656.20	N/A	773.1
Blood (group) (Duffy) (E) (K(ell)) (Kidd) (Lewis) (M) (N) (P) (S) NEC	656.23	656.21	656.20	N/A	773.2
Rh(esus) (blood group) (factor)	656.13	656.11	656.10	N/A	773.0

Antepartum Pregnancy Condition or Complication; affecting management of mother	Antepartum condition or complication	Delivered, with or without mention of antepartum condition	Unspecified episode of care	Assign additional code to describe the...	Affecting fetus (coded on the newborn chart only)
Incompetent cervix (os)	654.53	654.51	654.50	N/A	761.0
causing obstructed labor	660.23	660.21	660.20	cause	763.1
Incoordinate uterus (action) (contractions)	661.43	661.41	661.40	N/A	763.7
In double uterus	654.03	654.01	654.00	N/A	
causing obstructed labor	660.23	660.21	660.20	cause	763.1
Induced					
failed by method of					
drugs	659.13	659.11	659.10	N/A	
mechanical	659.03	659.01	659.00	N/A	
successful — assign code to indicate the reason for the induction					763.89
Indurated breast	676.33	676.31	676.30	N/A	
Inertia, uterus NEC					
primary	661.03	661.01	661.00	N/A	763.7
secondary	661.13	661.11	661.10	N/A	763.7
Infantile					
genitalia, genitals	654.43	654.41	654.40	N/A	763.89
causing obstructed labor	660.23	660.21	660.20	cause	763.1
pelvis	653.13	653.11	653.10	N/A	763.1
causing obstructed labor	660.13	660.11	660.10	cause	763.1
Infarct, infarction					
amnion	658.83	658.81	658.80	N/A	
brain (stem)	674.03	674.01	674.00	N/A	
chorion	658.83	658.81	658.80	N/A	
lung — see Pregnancy, embolism					
placenta	656.73	656.71	656.70	N/A	762.2
Infection	647.93	647.91	647.90	condition	760.2
amniotic fluid	658.43	658.41	658.40	condition	762.7
bladder	646.63	646.61	646.60	condition	
breast (mammary gland)	675.23	675.21	675.20	N/A	
with nipple	675.93	675.91	675.90	N/A	
specified type NEC	675.83	675.81	675.80	N/A	
nonpurulent	675.23	675.21	675.20	N/A	
purulent	675.13	675.11	675.10	N/A	
chorionic plate	658.83	658.81	658.80	N/A	
genital organs	646.63	646.61	646.60	condition	760.8
minor or localized	646.63	646.61	646.60	condition	760.8
intrauterine, complicating delivery	646.63	646.61	646.60	condition	
kidney	646.63	646.61	646.60	condition	760.1
nipple	675.03	675.01	675.00	N/A	
with breast	675.93	675.91	675.90	N/A	
specified type NEC	675.83	675.81	675.80	N/A	
perineal wound minor	646.63	646.61	646.60	condition	760.1
urinary (tract)	646.63	646.61	646.60	condition	760.1
asymptomatic	646.53	646.51	646.50	condition	760.1
UTI	646.63	646.61	646.60	condition	760.1
asymptomatic	646.53	646.51	646.50	condition	760.1
Infective and parasitic diseases NEC	647.83	647.81	647.80	complication	
Infestation	647.93	647.91	647.90	condition	760.8
Inflammation					
areola	675.03	675.01	675.00	N/A	
bladder	646.63	646.61	646.60	condition	760.8
breast (mammary gland)	675.23	675.21	675.20	N/A	
fetal membranes (acute)	658.43	658.41	658.40	N/A	762.7
genital organ	646.63	646.61	646.60	condition	760.8
urinary tract NEC	646.63	646.61	646.60	condition	760.8
Inhalation of stomach contents or secretions in labor and delivery	668.03	668.01	668.00	N/A	
Injury	648.93	648.91	648.90	condition	
birth canal NEC	665.93	665.91	665.90	N/A	763.89
coccyx, complicating delivery	N/A	665.61	665.60	N/A	
genital organs, obstetrical trauma NEC	665.93	665.91	665.90	N/A	763.89
instrumental, obstetrical NEC	665.93	665.91	665.90	N/A	763.89
bladder	N/A	665.51	665.50	N/A	763.89

Antepartum Pregnancy Condition or Complication; affecting management of mother	Antepartum condition or complication	Delivered, with or without mention of antepartum condition	Unspecified episode of care	Assign additional code to describe the...	Affecting fetus (coded on the newborn chart only)
Injury – *continued*					
cervix	N/A	665.31	665.30	N/A	763.89
high vaginal	N/A	665.41	665.40	N/A	763.89
perineal NEC	N/A	664.91	664.90	N/A	763.89
urethra	N/A	665.51	665.50	N/A	763.89
uterus	N/A	665.51	665.50	N/A	763.89
obstetrical NEC	665.93	665.91	665.90	N/A	763.89
pelvic, complicating delivery					
floor N/A	664.11	664.10	N/A	763.89	
joint or ligament	N/A	665.61	665.60	N/A	763.89
organs	N/A	665.51	665.50	N/A	763.89
periurethral tissue, complicating delivery	N/A	665.51	665.50	N/A	763.89
symphysis pubis, complicating delivery	N/A	665.61	665.60	N/A	763.89
Insertion of umbilical cord, lateral or velamentous	663.53	663.51	663.50	N/A	762.6
Insufficient					
prenatal care	V23.7	N/A	N/A	N/A	
weight gain	646.83	646.81	646.80	condition	
Interstitial — *see also* Ectopic pregnancy table	633.8	N/A	N/A	N/A	761.4
Intraligamentous — *see also* Ectopic pregnancy	633.8	N/A	N/A	N/A	761.4
Intramural — *see also* Ectopic pregnancy	633.8	N/A	N/A	N/A	761.4
Intraperitoneal — *see also* Ectopic pregnancy	633.0	N/A	N/A	N/A	761.4
Intoxication					
chemical via placenta or breast milk, suspected	655.53	655.51	655.50	N/A	760.70
drug					
obstetric anesthetic or sedation	668.93	668.91	668.90	N/A	763.5
via placenta or breast milk, suspected	655.53	655.51	655.50	N/A	760.70
septic					
during labor	659.33	659.31	659.30	N/A	
Intrauterine fetal death					
early (before 22 completed weeks of gestation)	632	N/A	N/A	N/A	
near term NEC	656.43	656.41	656.40	N/A	
Isoimmunization (ABO)	656.23	656.21	656.20	N/A	
Rh(esus)	656.13	656.11	656.10	N/A	
Isthmian (with rupture) — *see also* Ectopic Pregnancy	633.1	N/A	N/A	N/A	761.4
Inversion					
nipple	676.33	676.31	676.30		
Ischemia, cerebral	674.03	674.01	674.00	N/A	
Joint disorders	648.73	648.71	648.70	condition	
Knot, umbilical cord (true)	663.23	663.21	663.20	N/A	762.5
Labor					
abnormal NEC	661.93	661.91	661.90	N/A	763.7
arrested active phase	661.13	661.11	661.10	N/A	763.7
desultory	661.23	661.21	661.20	N/A	763.7
dyscoordinate	661.43	661.41	661.40	N/A	763.7
early onset (22-36 weeks gestation)	N/A3	644.21	644.20	N/A	763.7
failed				763.7	
induction	659.13	659.11	659.10	N/A	763.89
mechanical	659.03	659.01	659.00	N/A	763.89
medical (drug)	659.13	659.11	659.10	N/A	763.89
surgical	659.03	659.01	659.00	N/A	763.89
trial (vaginal delivery)	660.63	660.61	660.60	cause	763.1
false	644.13	N/A	644.10	N/A	
hypertonic	661.43	661.41	661.40	N/A	763.7
hypotonic, primary	661.03	661.01	661.00	N/A	763.7
secondary	661.13	661.11	661.10	N/A	763.7
incoordinate	661.43	661.41	661.40	N/A	763.7
irregular	661.23	661.21	661.20	N/A	763.7
long	662.13	662.11	662.10	N/A	763.89
first stage	662.03	662.01	662.00	N/A	763.89

Antepartum Pregnancy Condition or Complication; affecting management of mother	Antepartum condition or complication	Delivered, with or without mention of antepartum condition	Unspecified episode of care	Assign additional code to describe the...	Affecting fetus (coded on the newborn chart only)
Labor – *continued*					
second stage	662.23	662.21	662.20	N/A	763.89
missed (at or near term)	656.43	656.41	656.40	N/A	
obstructed NEC	660.93	660.91	660.90	cause	763.1
specified cause NEC	660.83	660.81	660.80	cause	763.1
pains, spurious	644.13	N/A	644.10	N/A	
precipitate	661.33	661.31	661.30	N/A	763.6
premature	N/A3	644.21	644.20	N/A	
threatened	644.03	N/A	644.00	N/A	
prolonged or protracted	662.13	662.11	662.10	N/A	763.89
first stage	662.03	662.01	662.00	N/A	763.89
second stage	662.23	662.21	662.20	N/A	763.89
threatened NEC	644.13	N/A	644.10	N/A	
undelivered	644.13	N/A	644.10	N/A	
Laceration (obstetrical trauma)					
anus (complicating delivery)	N/A	664.21	664.20	N/A	
with laceration of anal or rectal mucosa	N/A	664.31	664.30	N/A	
bladder	N/A	665.51	665.50	N/A	
bowel	N/A	665.51	665.50	N/A	
broad ligament	N/A	665.61	665.60	N/A	
central, complicating delivery	N/A	664.41	664.40	N/A	
cervix (uteri)	N/A	665.31	665.30	N/A	
fourchette, complicating delivery	N/A	664.01	664.00	N/A	
labia, complicating delivery	N/A	664.01	664.00	N/A	
pelvic (complicating delivery)					
floor (muscles)	N/A	664.11	664.10	N/A	
organ NEC (obstetrical trauma)	N/A	665.51	665.50	N/A	763.89
perineum, complicating delivery	N/A	664.41	664.40	N/A	
first degree	N/A	664.01	664.00	N/A	
second degree	N/A	664.11	664.10	N/A	
third degree	N/A	664.21	664.20	N/A	
fourth degree	N/A	664.31	664.30	N/A	
central	N/A	664.41	664.40	N/A	
involving					
anal sphincter	N/A	664.21	664.20	N/A	
fourchette	N/A	664.01	664.00	N/A	
hymen	N/A	664.01	664.00	N/A	
labia	N/A	664.01	664.00	N/A	
pelvic floor	N/A	664.11	664.10	N/A	
perineal muscles	N/A	664.11	664.10	N/A	
rectovaginal with septum	N/A	664.21	664.20	N/A	
with anal mucosa	N/A	664.31	664.30	N/A	
skin	N/A	664.01	664.00	N/A	
sphincter (anal)	N/A	664.21	664.20	N/A	
with anal mucosa	N/A	664.31	664.30	N/A	
vagina	N/A	664.01	664.00	N/A	
vaginal muscles	N/A	664.11	664.10	N/A	
vulva	N/A	664.01	664.00	N/A	
peritoneum (obstetrical trauma)	N/A	665.51	665.50	N/A	
periurethral tissue (obstetrical trauma)	N/A	665.51	665.50	N/A	
rectovaginal septum	N/A	665.41	665.40	N/A	
with perineum	N/A	664.21	664.20	N/A	
involving anal or rectal mucosa	N/A	664.31	664.30	N/A	
urethra (obstetrical trauma)	N/A	665.51	665.50	N/A	
uterus (obstetrical trauma NEC)	N/A	665.11	665.10	N/A	
vagina (complicating delivery)	N/A	665.41	665.40	N/A	
with perineal involvement	N/A	664.01	664.00	N/A	
first degree	N/A	664.01	664.00	N/A	
second degree	N/A	664.11	664.10	N/A	
third degree	N/A	664.21	664.20	N/A	
fourth degree	N/A	664.31	664.30	N/A	
high	N/A	664.41	664.40	N/A	
muscles	N/A	664.11	664.10	N/A	
sulcus	N/A	665.41	665.40	N/A	
wall	N/A	665.41	665.40	N/A	
vulva (complicating delivery)	N/A	664.01	664.00	N/A	

Antepartum Pregnancy Condition or Complication; affecting management of mother	Antepartum condition or complication	Delivered, with or without mention of antepartum condition	Unspecified episode of care	Assign additional code to describe the...	Affecting fetus (coded on the newborn chart only)
Lactation, lactating (breast)					
defective	676.43	676.41	676.40	N/A	
disorder	676.93	676.91	676.90	N/A	
specified type NEC	676.83	676.81	676.80	N/A	
examination and/or care of mother	V24.1	V24.1	V24.1	N/A	
excessive	676.63	676.61	676.60	N/A	
failed	676.43	676.41	676.40	N/A	
mastitis NEC	675.23	675.21	675.20	N/A	
suppressed	676.53	676.51	676.50	N/A	
Large					
fetus causing disproportion	653.53	653.51	653.50	N/A	763.1
with obstructed labor	660.13	660.11	660.10	cause	763.1
for-dates (fetus)	656.63	656.61	656.60	N/A	766.1
exceptionally (weight of 4500 grams or more)	656.63	656.61	656.60	N/A	766.0
Late effect(s) (of)					
childbirth complication(s)	677	677	677	condition	
complication(s) of					
childbirth	677	677	677	condition	
delivery	677	677	677	condition	
postpartum	677	677	677	condition	
pregnancy	677	677	677	condition	
puerperium	677	677	677	condition	
Lateroversion, uterus	654.43	654.41	654.40	N/A	763.89
causing obstructed labor	660.23	660.21	660.20	cause	763.1
Leakage					
amniotic fluid	658.13	658.11	658.10	N/A	761.1
with delayed delivery	658.23	658.21	658.20	N/A	761.1
blood (microscopic), fetal, into maternal circulation	656.03	656.01	656.00	N/A	
Lesion, vascular of umbilical cord	663.63	663.61	663.60	N/A	762.6
Light-for-dates	656.53	656.51	656.50	N/A	764.00
with signs of fetal malnutrition	656.53	656.51	656.50	N/A	764.10
Listeriosis, suspected fetal damage	655.43	655.41	655.40	N/A	771.2
Lithopedion	656.83	656.81	656.80	N/A	
Locked twins	660.53	660.51	660.50	cause	763.1
Lymphadenitis, breast	675.23	675.21	675.20	N/A	
breast	675.23	675.21	675.20	N/A	
Malaria	647.43	647.41	647.40	condition	
Male type pelvis with disproportion (fetopelvic)	653.23	653.21	653.20	N/A	763.1
causing obstructed labor	660.13	660.11	660.10	cause	763.1
Malformation					
pelvic organs or tissues	654.93	654.91	654.90	N/A	763.89
causing obstructed labor	660.23	660.21	660.20	cause	763.1
placenta	656.73	656.71	656.70	N/A	
umbilical cord (complicating delivery)	663.93	663.91	663.90	N/A	762.6
uterus (congenital)	654.03	654.01	654.00	N/A	
causing obstructed labor	660.23	660.21	660.20	cause	763.1
Malnutrition	648.93	648.91	648.90	condition	
Fetal malnutrition					
Without mention of "light-for dates"					
unspecified (weight)					764.20
< 500 gms					764.21
500-749 gms					764.22
750-999 gms					764.23
1,000-1,249 gms					764.24
1,250-1,499 gms					764.25
1,500-1,749 gms					764.26
1,750-1,999 gms					764.27
2,000-2,499 gms					764.28
≥ 2,500 gms					764.29
With mention of "light-for dates"					
unspecified (weight)					764.10
< 500 gms					764.11
500-749 gms					764.12

Antepartum Pregnancy Condition or Complication; affecting management of mother	Antepartum condition or complication	Delivered, with or without mention of antepartum condition	Unspecified episode of care	Assign additional code to describe the...	Affecting fetus (coded on the newborn chart only)
Malnutrition — *continued*					
750-999 gms					764.13
1,000-1,249 gms					764.14
1,250-1,499 gms					764.15
1,500-1,749 gms					764.16
1,750-1,999 gms					764.17
2,000-2,499 gms					764.18
≥ 2,500 gms					764.19
Malposition					
fetal NEC	652.93	652.91	652.90	N/A	763.1
with successful version	652.13	652.11	652.10	N/A	763.1
before labor	652.93	652.91	652.90	N/A	763.1
in multiple gestation	652.63	652.61	652.60	N/A	763.1
with locking	660.53	660.51	660.50	cause	763.1
causing obstructed labor	660.03	660.01	660.00	cause	763.1
pelvic organs or tissues	654.43	654.41	654.40	N/A	763.89
causing obstructed labor	660.23	660.21	660.20	cause	763.1
specified type NEC	652.83	652.81	652.80	N/A	763.1
causing obstructed labor	660.03	660.01	660.00	cause	763.1
uterus or cervix	654.43	654.41	654.40	N/A	763.89
causing obstructed labor	660.23	660.21	660.20	cause	763.1
Malpresentation					
fetal	652.93	652.91	652.90	N/A	763.1
with successful version	652.13	652.11	652.10	N/A	763.1
in multiple gestation	652.63	652.61	652.60	N/A	763.1
specified type NEC	652.83	652.81	652.80	N/A	763.1
causing obstructed labor	660.03	660.01	660.00	cause	763.1
uterus or cervix	654.43	654.41	654.40	N/A	
causing obstructed labor	660.03	660.01	660.00	cause	763.1
Mammillitis, puerperal	675.23	675.21	675.20	N/A	
Mammitis, puerperal	675.23	675.21	675.20	N/A	
Marginal sinus hemorrhage or rupture	641.23	641.21	641.20	N/A	762.1
Mastitis					
lactational	675.23	675.21	675.20	N/A	
puerperal, (interstitial) (nonpurulent) (parenchymatous)	675.23	675.21	675.20	N/A	
purulent	675.13	675.11	675.10	N/A	
stagnation	675.23	675.21	675.20	N/A	
puerperalis	675.23	675.21	675.20	N/A	
retromammary	675.13	675.11	675.10	N/A	
submammary	675.13	675.11	675.10	N/A	
Maternal obesity syndrome	646.13	646.11	646.10	condition	
Meconium in liquor (staining)	656.83	656.81	656.80	N/A	
Membranitis, fetal	658.43	658.41	658.40	N/A	762.7
Mendelson's syndrome	668.03	668.01	668.00	N/A	
Menstruation during pregnancy	640.83	640.81	640.80	N/A	
Mental disorders	648.43	648.41	648.40	condition	
Mentum presentation	652.43	652.41	652.40	N/A	763.1
causing obstructed labor	660.03	660.01	660.00	cause	763.1
Metaplasia squamous cell amnion	658.83	658.81	658.80	N/A	763.89
Milk					
excess secretion	676.63	676.61	676.60	N/A	
Milk leg (deep vessels)	671.33	671.31	671.30	N/A	
Missed					
delivery (at or near term)	656.43	656.41	656.40	N/A	763.89
labor (at or near term)	656.43	656.41	656.40	N/A	763.89
Morning sickness	643.03	643.01	643.00	N/A	
Multiparity (grand)	659.43	659.41	659.40	N/A	763.8
Myelomeningocele fetal, causing fetopelvic disproportion	653.73	653.71	653.70	N/A	763.1
causing obstructed labor	660.13	660.11	660.10	cause	763.1
Myoma uterus (cervix) (corpus)	654.13	654.11	654.10	N/A	763.89
causing obstructed labor	660.23	660.21	660.20	cause	763.1
Nägele's pelvis with disproportion (fetopelvic)	653.03	653.01	653.00	N/A	763.1
causing obstructed labor	660.13	660.11	660.10	cause	763.1
Necrosis					
genital organ or tract	646.63	646.61	646.60	condition	760.8
kidney, cortical (acute)	646.23	646.21	646.20	condition	760.1

Antepartum Pregnancy Condition or Complication; affecting management of mother	Antepartum condition or complication	Delivered, with or without mention of antepartum condition	Unspecified episode of care	Assign additional code to describe the...	Affecting fetus (coded on the newborn chart only)
Necrosis – *continued*					
tubular	646.23	646.21	646.20	condition	760.1
liver	646.73	646.71	646.70	condition	760.8
placenta	656.73	656.71	656.70	N/A	762.2
renal, cortical	646.23	646.21	646.20	condition	760.1
Nephritis, nephrosis	646.23	646.21	646.20	condition	760.1
with hypertension	642.13	642.11	642.10	N/A	760.0
Nephropathy NEC	646.23	646.21	646.20	condition	
Neuritis (peripheral)	646.43	646.41	646.40	condition	
Nonengagement of head NEC	652.53	652.51	652.50	N/A	763.1
in labor	660.03	660.01	660.00	cause	763.1
Noxious substances transmitted through placenta or breast milk, suspected	655.53	655.51	655.50	N/A	760.70
Nuchal hitch (arm)	652.83	652.81	652.80	N/A	763.1
causing obstructed labor	660.03	660.01	660.00	cause	763.1
Nutritional deficiency	648.93	648.91	648.90	condition	
Obesity	646.13	646.11	646.10	complication	
Oblique lie or presentation	652.33	652.31	652.30	N/A	763.1
with successful version	652.13	652.11	652.10	N/A	763.1
causing obstructed labor	660.03	660.01	660.00	cause	763.1
Obstetrical trauma NEC (complicating delivery)	665.93	665.91	665.90	N/A	763.89
Obstruction, obstructed, obstructive					
labor	660.93	660.91	660.90	cause	763.1
borderline pelvis	660.13	660.11	660.10	cause	763.1
by					
bony pelvis	660.13	660.11	660.10	cause	763.1
deep transverse arrest	660.33	660.31	660.30	cause	763.1
impacted shoulder	660.43	660.41	660.40	cause	763.1
locked twins	660.53	660.51	660.50	cause	763.1
malposition (fetus)	660.03	660.01	660.00	cause	763.1
head during labor	660.33	660.31	660.30	cause	763.1
persistent occipitoposterior position	660.33	660.31	660.30	cause	763.1
soft tissue, pelvic	660.23	660.21	660.20	cause	763.1
Occlusion, precerebral artery NEC	674.03	674.01	674.00	condition	
Oligohydramnios NEC	658.03	658.01	658.00	N/A	761.2
due to premature rupture of membranes	658.13	658.11	658.10	N/A	761.2
Oliguria	646.23	646.21	646.20	condition	
with hypertension — *see* Pregnancy, toxemia					
Oophoritis	646.63	646.61	646.60	condition	
Oversize fetus (weight of 4500 grams or more)	656.63	656.61	656.60	N/A	766.0
causing disproportion	653.53	653.51	653.50	N/A	763.1
with obstructed labor	660.13	660.11	660.10	cause	763.1
Pain(s)	646.83	646.81	646.80	condition	
false labor	644.13	N/A	644.10	N/A	
Papyraceous fetus	646.03	646.01	646.00	condition	779.8
Paralysis, bladder	N/A	665.51	665.50	N/A	
Patent cervix	654.53	654.51	654.50	N/A	761.0
causing obstructed labor	660.23	660.21	660.20	cause	763.1
Pendulous	654.43	654.41	654.40	N/A	763.89
causing obstructed labor	660.23	660.21	660.20	cause	763.1
complication of delivery	N/A	665.11	665.10	N/A	763.89
Perforation					
bladder	N/A	665.51	665.50	N/A	
bowel	N/A	665.51	665.50	N/A	
broad ligament	N/A	665.61	665.60	N/A	
cervix	N/A	665.31	665.30	N/A	
instrumental (complicating delivery)	665.93	665.91	665.90	N/A	
pelvic (floor)	N/A	664.11	664.10	N/A	
organ	N/A	665.51	665.50	N/A	763.89
urethral	N/A	665.51	665.50	N/A	763.89
uterus	N/A	665.51	665.50	N/A	763.89
Persistence					
hymen (tag)	654.83	654.81	654.80	N/A	

Antepartum Pregnancy Condition or Complication; affecting management of mother	Antepartum condition or complication	Delivered, with or without mention of antepartum condition	Unspecified episode of care	Assign additional code to describe the...	Affecting fetus (coded on the newborn chart only)
Persistence – *continued*					
causing obstructed labor	660.23	660.21	660.20	cause	763.1
occiput (anterior or posterior)	660.33	660.31	660.30	cause	763.1
Phlebitis	671.93	671.91	671.90	N/A	760.3
deep	671.33	671.31	671.30	N/A	760.3
intracranial	671.53	671.51	671.50	N/A	
lower extremities	671.23	671.21	671.20	N/A	760.3
specified site NEC	671.53	671.51	671.50	N/A	
superficial	671.23	671.21	671.20	N/A	760.3
Phlegmasia	671.33	671.31	671.30	N/A	760.3
PID	646.63	646.61	646.60	condition	
Pithecoid pelvis (fetopelvic)	653.23	653.21	653.20	N/A	763.1
obstructed labor	660.13	660.11	660.10	cause	763.1
Placenta, placental					
abnormal	656.73	656.71	656.70	N/A	762.2
with hemorrhage	641.83	641.81	641.80	N/A	762.1
abruptio or ablatio	641.23	641.21	641.20	N/A	762.1
absorption (suspected) of					
chemical	655.53	655.51	655.50	N/A	760.79
drug (NEC)	655.53	655.51	655.50	N/A	760.79
accessory lobe	656.73	656.71	656.70	N/A	762.2
with hemorrhage	641.83	641.81	641.80	N/A	762.1
apoplexy	641.23	641.21	641.20	N/A	762.1
battledore	656.73	656.71	656.70	N/A	762.2
with hemorrhage	641.83	641.81	641.80	N/A	762.1
bilobate	656.73	656.71	656.70	N/A	762.2
with hemorrhage	641.83	641.81	641.80	N/A	762.1
bipartita	656.73	656.71	656.70	N/A	762.2
with hemorrhage	641.83	641.81	641.80	N/A	762.1
centralis	641.03	641.01	641.00	N/A	762.0
with hemorrhage	641.13	641.11	641.10	N/A	762.1
circumvallata	656.73	656.71	656.70	N/A	762.2
with hemorrhage	641.83	641.81	641.80	N/A	762.1
cyst (amniotic)	656.73	656.71	656.70	N/A	762.2
with hemorrhage	641.83	641.81	641.80	N/A	762.1
deficiency	656.53	656.51	656.50	N/A	762.2
degeneration	656.53	656.51	656.50	N/A	762.2
detachment	641.23	641.21	641.20	N/A	762.1
dimidiata	656.73	656.71	656.70	N/A	762.2
with hemorrhage	641.83	641.81	641.80	N/A	762.1
disease	656.73	656.71	656.70	N/A	762.2
with hemorrhage	641.83	641.81	641.80	N/A	762.1
duplex	656.73	656.71	656.70	N/A	762.2
with hemorrhage	641.83	641.81	641.80	N/A	762.1
dysfunction	656.53	656.51	656.50	N/A	762.2
fenestrata	656.73	656.71	656.70	N/A	762.2
with hemorrhage	641.83	641.81	641.80	N/A	762.1
fibrosis	656.73	656.71	656.70	N/A	762.2
with hemorrhage	641.83	641.81	641.80	N/A	762.1
hematoma	656.73	656.71	656.70	N/A	762.2
with hemorrhage	641.83	641.81	641.80	N/A	762.1
hemorrhage	641.23	641.21	641.20	N/A	762.1
hormone disturbance	656.73	656.71	656.70	N/A	762.2
with hemorrhage	641.83	641.81	641.80	N/A	762.1
hyperplasia	656.73	656.71	656.70	N/A	762.2
with hemorrhage	641.83	641.81	641.80	N/A	762.1
infarct	656.73	656.71	656.70	N/A	762.2
with hemorrhage	641.83	641.81	641.80	N/A	762.1
insertion, vicious	641.03	641.01	641.00	N/A	762.0
with hemorrhage	641.13	641.11	641.10	N/A	762.1
insufficiency	656.53	656.51	656.50	N/A	762.2
lateral	641.03	641.01	641.00	N/A	762.0
with hemorrhage	641.13	641.11	641.10	N/A	762.1
low implantation	641.03	641.01	641.00	N/A	762.0
with hemorrhage	641.13	641.11	641.10	N/A	762.1
low lying	641.03	641.01	641.00	N/A	762.0
with hemorrhage	641.13	641.11	641.10	N/A	762.1
malformation	656.73	656.71	656.70	N/A	762.2
with hemorrhage	641.83	641.81	641.80	N/A	762.1
malposition	641.03	641.01	641.00	N/A	762.2

Antepartum Pregnancy Table

Antepartum Pregnancy Condition or Complication; affecting management of mother	Antepartum condition or complication	Delivered, with or without mention of antepartum condition	Unspecified episode of care	Assign additional code to describe the...	Affecting fetus (coded on the newborn chart only)
Placenta — *continued*					
with hemorrhage	641.13	641.11	641.10	N/A	762.1
marginalis, marginata	641.03	641.01	641.00	N/A	762.0
with hemorrhage	641.13	641.11	641.10	N/A	762.1
marginal sinus (hemorrhage)	641.23	641.21	641.20	N/A	762.1
membranacea	656.73	656.71	656.70	N/A	762.2
with hemorrhage	641.83	641.81	641.80	N/A	762.1
multiload	656.73	656.71	656.70	N/A	762.2
with hemorrhage	641.83	641.81	641.80	N/A	762.1
necrosis	656.73	656.71	656.70	N/A	762.2
with hemorrhage	641.83	641.81	641.80	N/A	762.1
previa	641.03	641.01	641.00	N/A	762.0
with hemorrhage	641.13	641.11	641.10	N/A	762.1
separation (premature) (undelivered)	641.23	641.21	641.20	N/A	762.1
septuplex	656.73	656.71	656.70	N/A	762.2
with hemorrhage	641.83	641.81	641.80	N/A	762.1
small	656.53	656.51	656.50	N/A	762.2
softening	656.73	656.71	656.70	N/A	762.2
with hemorrhage	641.83	641.81	641.80	N/A	762.1
spuria	656.73	656.71	656.70	N/A	762.2
with hemorrhage	641.83	641.81	641.80	N/A	762.1
succenturiata	656.73	656.71	656.70	N/A	762.2
with hemorrhage	641.83	641.81	641.80	N/A	762.1
syphilitic	647.03	647.01	647.00	condition	760.2
manifest syphilis in the infant or fetus	647.03	647.01	647.00	condition	090.0
transfusion syndromes (fetus)	N/A	N/A	N/A	N/A	762.3
transmission of chemical substance (suspected, affecting pregnancy)	655.53	655.51	655.50	N/A	760.70
trilobate	656.73	656.71	656.70	N/A	762.2
with hemorrhage	641.83	641.81	641.80	N/A	762.1
triplex	656.73	656.71	656.70	N/A	762.2
with hemorrhage	641.83	641.81	641.80	N/A	762.1
varicose vessel	656.73	656.71	656.70	N/A	762.2
with hemorrhage	641.83	641.81	641.80	N/A	762.1
vicious insertion	641.03	641.01	641.00	N/A	
with hemorrhage	641.13	641.11	641.10	N/A	762.0
Placentitis	658.43	658.41	658.40	N/A	762.7
Platypelloid pelvis (disproportion)	653.23	653.21	653.20	N/A	763.1
obstructed labor	660.13	660.11	660.10	cause	763.1
Pneumonitis					
aspiration	668.03	668.01	668.00	condition	
postanesthetic	668.03	668.01	668.00	condition	
postoperative	668.03	668.01	668.00	N/A	
Polygalactia	676.63	676.61	676.60	N/A	
Polyhydramnios	657.03	657.01	657.00	N/A	761.3
Polyp					
cervix	654.63	654.61	654.60	N/A	763.89
obstructed labor	660.23	660.21	660.20	cause	763.1
uterus	654.13	654.11	654.10	N/A	763.89
obstructed labor	660.23	660.21	660.20	cause	763.1
Poor					
contractions labor	661.23	661.21	661.20	N/A	763.7
fetal growth, affecting management	656.53	656.51	656.50	N/A	
Fetal growth retardation unspecified (weight)					764.90
< 500 gms					764.91
500-749 gms					764.92
750-999 gms					764.93
1,000-1,249 gms					764.94
1,250-1,499 gms					764.95
1,500-1,749 gms					764.96
1,750-1,999 gms					764.97
2,000-2,499 gms					764.98
≥ 2,500 gms					764.99
obstetrical history	V23.4	N/A	N/A	N/A	
Position (see also Presentation, fetal)	652.93	652.91	652.90	N/A	763.1
causing obstructed labor	660.03	660.01	660.00	cause	763.1

Antepartum Pregnancy Condition or Complication; affecting management of mother	Antepartum condition or complication	Delivered, with or without mention of antepartum condition	Unspecified episode of care	Assign additional code to describe the...	Affecting fetus (coded on the newborn chart only)
Post-term (over 40 to 42 completed weeks)	645.13	645.11	645.10	N/A	766.21
Prediabetes	648.83	648.81	648.80	condition	
Prolonged (over 42 completed weeks)	645.23	645.21	645.20	N/A	766.22
Pre-eclampsia (mild)	642.43	642.41	642.40	N/A	760.0
with convulsions	642.63	642.61	642.60	N/A	760.0
severe	642.53	642.51	642.50	N/A	760.0
superimposed on pre-existing hypertensive disease	642.73	642.71	642.70	N/A	760.0
Pre-existing condition (prior to pregnancy) affecting current pregnancy					
abnormal glucose tolerance	648.83	648.81	648.80	condition	
anemia	648.23	648.21	648.20	condition	
bone and joint (lower limb)	648.73	648.71	648.70	condition	
cardiovascular	648.63	648.61	648.60	condition	
congenital	648.53	648.51	648.50	condition	
cerebrovascular	674.03	674.01	674.00	N/A	
diabetic	648.03	648.01	648.00	condition	
drug dependence	648.33	648.31	648.30	condition	
genital organ or tract	646.63	646.61	646.60	condition	
gonorrheal	647.13	647.11	647.10	condition	
hypertensive	642.23	642.21	642.20	N/A	
renal	642.13	642.11	642.10	N/A	
infectious	647.93	647.91	647.90	condition	
specified type NEC	647.83	647.81	647.80	condition	
liver	646.73	646.71	646.70	condition	
malarial	647.43	647.41	647.40	condition	
nutritional deficiency	648.93	648.91	648.90	condition	
parasitic NEC	647.83	647.81	647.80	condition	
renal	646.23	646.21	646.20	condition	
hypertensive	642.13	642.11	642.10	N/A	
rubella	647.53	647.51	647.50	condition	
specified condition NEC	648.93	648.91	648.90	condition	
syphilitic	647.03	647.01	647.00	condition	
thyroid	648.13	648.11	648.10	condition	
tuberculous	647.33	647.31	647.30	condition	
urinary	646.63	646.61	646.60	condition	
venereal	647.23	647.21	647.20	condition	
viral NEC	647.63	647.61	647.60	condition	
Premature					
labor	N/A	644.21	644.20	N/A	
threatened	644.03	N/A	644.00	N/A	
rupture of membranes or amnion	658.13	658.11	658.10	N/A	761.1
with delayed delivery	658.23	658.21	658.20	N/A	
Presentation, fetal					
abnormal	652.93	652.91	652.90	N/A	763.1
with successful version	652.13	652.11	652.10	N/A	761.7
causing obstructed labor	660.03	660.01	660.00	cause	763.1
in multiple gestation (one or more)	652.63	652.61	652.60	N/A	763.1
causing obstructed labor	660.03	660.01	660.00	cause	763.1
specified NEC	652.83	652.81	652.80	N/A	763.1
causing obstructed labor	660.03	660.01	660.00	cause	763.1
arm	652.73	652.71	652.70	N/A	763.1
causing obstructed labor	660.03	660.01	660.00	cause	763.1
breech	652.23	652.21	652.20	N/A	761.7
with successful version	652.13	652.11	652.10	N/A	761.7
causing obstructed labor	660.03	660.01	660.00	cause	763.0
brow	652.43	652.41	652.40	N/A	763.1
causing obstructed labor	660.03	660.01	660.00	cause	763.1
cord	663.03	663.01	663.00	N/A	762.5
extended head	652.43	652.41	652.40	N/A	763.1
causing obstructed labor	660.03	660.01	660.00	cause	763.1
face	652.43	652.41	652.40	N/A	763.1
causing obstructed labor	660.03	660.01	660.00	cause	763.1

Antepartum Pregnancy Table

Antepartum Pregnancy Condition or Complication; affecting management of mother	Antepartum condition or complication	Delivered, with or without mention of antepartum condition	Unspecified episode of care	Assign additional code to describe the...	Affecting fetus (coded on the newborn chart only)
Presentation, fetal — *continued*					
to pubes	652.83	652.81	652.80	N/A	763.1
causing obstructed labor	660.33	660.31	660.30	cause	763.1
hand, leg, or foot NEC	652.83	652.81	652.80	N/A	763.1
causing obstructed labor	660.03	660.01	660.00	cause	763.1
mentum	652.43	652.41	652.40	N/A	763.1
causing obstructed labor	660.03	660.01	660.00	cause	763.1
multiple gestation (one fetus or more)	652.63	652.61	652.60	N/A	763.1
causing obstructed labor	660.03	660.01	660.00	cause	763.1
oblique	652.33	652.31	652.30	N/A	763.1
with successful version	652.13	652.11	652.10	N/A	763.1
causing obstructed labor	660.03	660.01	660.00	cause	763.1
shoulder	652.83	652.81	652.80	N/A	763.1
causing obstructed labor	660.03	660.01	660.00	cause	763.1
transverse	652.33	652.31	652.30	N/A	763.1
with successful version	652.13	652.11	652.10	N/A	763.1
causing obstructed labor	660.03	660.01	660.00	cause	763.1
umbilical cord	663.03	663.01	663.00	N/A	
unstable	652.03	652.01	652.00	N/A	763.1
causing obstructed labor	660.03	660.01	660.00	cause	763.1
Previous					
abortion	V23.2	N/A	N/A	N/A	
infertility	V23.0	N/A	N/A	N/A	
nonobstetric condition	V23.89	N/A	N/A	N/A	
poor obstetrical history	V23.49	N/A	N/A	N/A	
premature delivery	V23.41	N/A	N/A	N/A	
trophoblastic disease	V23.1	N/A	N/A	N/A	
Primigravida, elderly	659.53	659.51	659.50	N/A	763.89
Primipara, old	659.53	659.51	659.50	N/A	763.89
Problem (with)					
fetus NOS	656.93	656.91	656.90	N/A	779.9
specified type NEC	656.83	656.81	656.80	N/A	779.8
placenta NOS	656.93	656.91	656.90	N/A	762.2
specified type NEC	656.83	656.81	656.80	N/A	762.2
Prolapse, prolapsed					
arm or hand, complicating delivery	652.73	652.71	652.70	N/A	763.1
causing obstructed labor	660.03	660.01	660.00	cause	763.1
cervix, anterior lip (obstructing labor)	660.23	660.21	660.20	cause	763.1
fetal extremity, complicating delivery	652.83	652.81	652.80	N/A	763.1
causing obstructed labor	660.03	660.01	660.00	cause	763.1
leg, complicating delivery	652.83	652.81	652.80	N/A	763.1
causing obstructed labor	660.03	660.01	660.00	cause	763.1
umbilical cord, complicating delivery	663.03	663.01	663.00	N/A	762.4
uterus	654.43	654.41	654.40	N/A	763.1
causing obstructed labor	660.23	660.21	660.20	cause	763.1
Prolonged					
labor	662.13	662.11	662.10	N/A	763.89
first stage	662.03	662.01	662.00	N/A	763.89
second stage	662.23	662.21	662.20	N/A	763.89
pregnancy over 40 completed weeks to 42 completed weeks	645.13	645.12	645.10	N/A	766.21
pregnancy over 42 completed weeks	645.23	645.21	645.20	N/A	766.22
rupture of membranes (24 hours or more prior to onset of labor)	658.23	658.21	658.20	N/A	761.8
uterine contractions in labor	661.43	661.41	661.40	N/A	763.7
PROM	658.13	658.11	658.10	N/A	761.1
with delayed delivery	658.23	658.21	658.20	N/A	761.8
Prominence, ischial spine or sacral promontory					
with disproportion (fetopelvic)	653.33	653.31	653.30	N/A	763.1
causing obstructed labor	660.13	660.11	660.10	cause	763.1
Proteinuria (gestational)	646.23	646.21	646.20	condition	
with toxemia (mild) (pre-eclamptic)	642.43	642.41	642.40	N/A	760.0

Antepartum Pregnancy Condition or Complication; affecting management of mother	Antepartum condition or complication	Delivered, with or without mention of antepartum condition	Unspecified episode of care	Assign additional code to describe the...	Affecting fetus (coded on the newborn chart only)
Proteinuria (gestational) — *continued*					
convulsions	642.63	642.61	642.60	N/A	760.0
pre-existing hypertension	642.73	642.71	642.70	N/A	760.0
severe	642.53	642.51	642.50	N/A	760.0
Pruritus, pruritic	646.83	646.81	646.80	condition	
Psychosis or psychoneurosis	648.43	648.41	648.40	condition	
Ptyalism	646.83	646.81	646.80	condition	
Pyelitis	646.63	646.61	646.60	condition	760.1
Pyrexia (of unknown origin) (PUO), during labor	659.23	659.21	659.20	N/A	
Quadruplet NEC	651.23	651.21	651.20	N/A	761.5
with fetal loss and retention of one or more fetus(es)	651.53	651.51	651.50	N/A	
Quintuplet NEC	651.83	651.81	651.80	N/A	761.5
with fetal loss and retention of one or more fetus(es)	651.63	651.61	651.60	N/A	
Rachitic with disproportion (fetopelvic)	653.23	653.21	653.20	N/A	763.1
causing obstructed labor	660.13	660.11	660.10	cause	763.1
Rapid second stage (delivery)	661.33	661.31	661.30	N/A	763.6
Reaction obstetric anesthetic or analgesic NEC	668.93	668.91	668.90	N/A	763.5
Rectocele	654.43	654.41	654.40	N/A	763.1
causing obstructed labor	660.23	660.21	660.20	cause	763.1
Renal					
disease or failure NEC	646.23	646.21	646.20	condition	
with secondary hypertension	642.13	642.11	642.10	N/A	
hypertensive	642.23	642.21	642.20	N/A	
Repair of pelvic floor, previous	654.43	654.41	654.40	N/A	763.89
causing obstructed labor	660.23	660.21	660.20	cause	763.1
Retardation fetal growth (intrauterine)	656.53	656.51	656.50	N/A	764.90
Retention, retained					
dead					
fetus (after 22 completed weeks' gestation)	656.43	656.41	656.40	N/A	cause
early fetal death (before 22 completed weeks' gestation)	632	N/A	N/A	N/A	
ovum	631	N/A	N/A	N/A	
Retinitis	646.83	646.81	646.80	condition	
Retraction					
nipple	676.03	676.01	676.00	N/A	
ring, uterus (Bandl's) (pathological)	661.43	661.41	661.40	N/A	763.7
Retroversion, uterus	654.33	654.31	654.30	N/A	763.89
causing obstructed labor	660.23	660.21	660.20	cause	763.1
Rh immunization, incompatibility, or sensitization	656.13	656.11	656.10	N/A	773.0
Rigid, rigidity					
cervix	654.63	654.61	654.60	N/A	763.89
causing obstructed labor	660.23	660.21	660.20	cause	763.1
pelvic floor	654.43	654.41	654.40	N/A	763.89
causing obstructed labor	660.23	660.21	660.20	cause	763.1
perineum or vulva	654.83	654.81	654.80	N/A	763.89
causing obstructed labor	660.23	660.21	660.20	cause	763.1
vagina	654.73	654.71	654.70	N/A	763.89
causing obstructed labor	660.23	660.21	660.20	cause	763.1
Ring(s), complicating delivery					
Bandl's	661.43	661.41	661.40	N/A	763.7
contraction	661.43	661.41	661.40	N/A	763.7
retraction, uterus, pathological	661.43	661.41	661.40	N/A	763.7
Robert's pelvis with disproportion (fetopelvic)	653.03	653.01	653.00	N/A	763.1
causing obstructed labor	660.13	660.11	660.10	cause	763.1
Rubella (German measles)	647.53	647.51	647.50	condition	760.2
with suspected fetal damage	655.33	655.31	655.30	N/A	771.0
Rupture					
abdominal viscera (obstetrical trauma)	N/A	665.51	665.50	N/A	

Antepartum Pregnancy Table

Antepartum Pregnancy Condition or Complication; affecting management of mother	Antepartum condition or complication	Delivered, with or without mention of antepartum condition	Unspecified episode of care	Assign additional code to describe the...	Affecting fetus (coded on the newborn chart only)
Rupture – *continued*					
amnion (premature)	658.13	658.11	658.10	N/A	763.89
with delayed delivery	658.23	658.21	658.20	N/A	763.89
bladder (sphincter), obstetrical trauma	N/A	665.51	665.50	N/A	
cervix (uteri), obstetrical trauma	N/A	665.31	665.30	N/A	
marginal sinus (hemorrhage)	641.23	641.21	641.20	N/A	762.1
membranes (premature)	658.13	658.11	658.10	N/A	761.1
with delayed delivery	658.23	658.21	658.20	N/A	761.1
artificial with delayed delivery following	658.33	658.31	658.30	N/A	761.1
pelvic floor, complicating delivery	N/A	664.11	664.10	N/A	
perineum during delivery	N/A	664.41	664.40	N/A	
umbilical cord	663.83	663.81	663.80	N/A	772.0
urethra (obstetrical trauma)	N/A	665.51	665.50	N/A	
uterus					
before onset of labor	665.03	665.01	665.00	N/A	763.89
during labor	N/A	665.11	665.10	N/A	763.89
vulva, complicating delivery	N/A	664.01	664.00	N/A	
Sacculation, complicating delivery	654.43	654.41	654.40	N/A	763.1
causing obstructed labor	660.23	660.21	660.20	cause	763.1
Salivation (excessive)	646.83	646.81	646.80	condition	
Salpingitis	646.63	646.61	646.60	condition	760.8
Salpingo-oophoritis	646.63	646.61	646.60	condition	760.8
Scar, scarring					
cervix	654.63	654.61	654.60	N/A	763.89
causing obstructed labor	660.23	660.21	660.20	cause	763.1
uterus NEC	654.93	654.91	654.90	N/A	763.89
from previous cesarean delivery	654.23	654.21	654.20	N/A	763.89
causing obstructed labor	660.23	660.21	660.20	cause	763.1
Scoliotic pelvis with disproportion (fetopelvic)	653.03	653.01	653.00	N/A	763.1
causing obstructed labor	660.13	660.11	660.10	cause	763.1
Screening, prenatal (for)					
If the abnormal finding is known — code the findings					
by					
amniocentesis					
chromosomal anomalies	V28.0	N/A	N/A		
raised alpha-fetoprotein levels (amniotic fluid)	V28.1	N/A	N/A		
specified, NEC	V28.2	N/A	N/A		
ultrasound					
fetal growth retardation	V28.4	N/A	N/A		
malformation	V28.3	N/A	N/A		
isoimmunization	V28.5	N/A	N/A		
other specified screening	V28.8	N/A	N/A		
Streptococcus B	V28.6	N/A	N/A		
unspecified, screening	V28.9	N/A	N/A		
Separation (obstetrical trauma)					
pubic bone	N/A	665.61	665.60	N/A	
symphysis pubis	N/A	665.61	665.60	N/A	
Sepsis, complicating labor	659.33	659.31	659.30	N/A	
Septicemia	647.83	647.81	647.80	condition	
Septum, vagina	654.73	654.71	654.70	N/A	763.89
causing obstructed labor	660.23	660.21	660.20	cause	763.1
Sextuplet NEC	651.83	651.81	651.80	N/A	761.5
with fetal loss and retention of one or more fetus(es)	651.63	651.61	651.60	N/A	
Shirodkar suture	654.53	654.51	654.50	N/A	
causing obstructed labor	660.23	660.21	660.20	cause	763.1
Shock					
complicating labor and delivery	669.13	669.11	669.10	N/A	
following labor and deliver	669.13	669.11	669.10	N/A	
Short, shortening, shortness of umbilical cord	663.43	663.41	663.40	N/A	762.6
Sinus, marginal, rupture or bleeding	641.23	641.21	641.20	N/A	762.1
Slow fetal growth	656.53	656.51	656.50	N/A	764.90

Antepartum Pregnancy Condition or Complication; affecting management of mother	Antepartum condition or complication	Delivered, with or without mention of antepartum condition	Unspecified episode of care	Assign additional code to describe the...	Affecting fetus (coded on the newborn chart only)
Small					
for-dates fetus	656.53	656.51	656.50	N/A	764.00
pelvis					
with disproportion (fetopelvic)	653.13	653.11	653.10	N/A	763.1
causing obstructed labor	660.13	660.11	660.10	cause	763.1
Spasms					
cervix, complicating delivery	661.43	661.41	661.40	N/A	763.7
uterus	646.83	646.81	646.80	condition	
complicating delivery	661.43	661.41	661.40	N/A	763.7
complicating labor	661.43	661.41	661.40	N/A	763.7
Specified condition NEC	646.83	646.81	646.80	condition	
Spina bifida (aperta), suspected fetal	655.03	655.01	655.00	N/A	
Spondylolisthesis with disproportion (fetopelvic)	653.33	653.31	653.30	N/A	763.1
causing obstructed labor	660.13	660.11	660.10	cause	763.1
Spondylolysis with disproportion (fetopelvic)	653.33	653.31	653.30	N/A	763.1
causing obstructed labor	660.13	660.11	660.10	cause	763.1
Spondylosis with disproportion (fetopelvic)	653.33	653.31	653.30	N/A	763.1
causing obstructed labor	660.13	660.11	660.10	cause	763.1
Spotting	641.93	641.91	641.90	N/A	
Spurious labor pains	644.13	N/A	644.10	N/A	
Stenosis (cicatricial)					
cervix, cervical (canal)	654.63	654.61	654.60	N/A	763.89
causing obstructed labor	660.23	660.21	660.20	cause	763.1
vagina	654.73	654.71	654.70	N/A	763.89
causing obstructed labor	660.23	660.21	660.20	cause	763.1
Stricture, cervix (canal)	654.63	654.61	654.60	N/A	763.89
causing obstructed labor	660.23	660.21	660.20	cause	763.1
Sudden death					
during childbirth	669.93	669.91	669.90	N/A	
Superfecundation NEC	651.93	651.91	651.90	N/A	
with fetal loss and retention of one or more fetus(es)	651.63	651.61	651.60	N/A	
Superfetation NEC	651.93	651.91	651.90	N/A	
with fetal loss and retention of one or more fetus(es)	651.63	651.61	651.60	N/A	
Supervision (of) (for)					
high-risk	V23.9	N/A	N/A	N/A	
insufficient prenatal care	V23.7	N/A	N/A	N/A	
specified problem NEC	V23.89	N/A	N/A	N/A	
multiparity	V23.3	N/A	N/A	N/A	
normal NEC	V22.1	N/A	N/A	N/A	
first pregnancy	V22.0	N/A	N/A	N/A	
poor	N/A	N/A	N/A		
obstetric history	V23.49	N/A	N/A	N/A	
reproductive history	V23.5	N/A	N/A	N/A	
Suppression of lactation	676.53	676.51	676.50	N/A	
Suppuration, suppurative of breast or mammary gland	675.13	675.11	675.10	N/A	
Surgery, previous					
cervix	654.63	654.61	654.60	N/A	763.89
causing obstructed labor	660.23	660.21	660.20	cause	763.1
pelvic soft tissues NEC	654.93	654.91	654.90	N/A	763.89
causing obstructed labor	660.23	660.21	660.20	cause N/A	763.1
perineum or vulva	654.83	654.81	654.80	N/A	
uterus NEC	654.93	654.91	654.90	N/A	763.89
causing obstructed labor	660.23	660.21	660.20	cause	763.1
from previous cesarean delivery	654.23	654.21	654.20	N/A	
causing obstructed labor	660.23	660.21	660.20	cause	763.1
vagina	654.73	654.71	654.70	N/A	
causing obstructed labor	660.23	660.21	660.20	cause	763.1
Suspended uterus	654.43	654.41	654.40	N/A	763.89
causing obstructed labor	660.23	660.21	660.20	cause	763.1
Suture, Shirodkar (with or without cervical incompetence)	654.53	654.51	654.50	N/A	
causing obstructed labor	660.23	660.21	660.20	cause	763.1

Antepartum Pregnancy Table

Antepartum Pregnancy Condition or Complication; affecting management of mother	Antepartum condition or complication	Delivered, with or without mention of antepartum condition	Unspecified episode of care	Assign additional code to describe the...	Affecting fetus (coded on the newborn chart only)
Syncope complicating delivery	669.23	669.21	669.20	N/A	
Syndrome					
acid pulmonary aspiration (Mendelson's)	668.03	668.01	668.00	N/A	
Chiari-Frommel	676.63	676.61	676.60	N/A	
dead fetus	641.33	641.31	641.30	N/A	
dystocia, dystrophia	654.93	654.91	654.90	N/A	
causing obstructed labor	660.23	660.21	660.20	cause	763.1
Frommel-Chiari	676.63	676.61	676.60	N/A	
H.E.L.L.P (Hemolysis, Elevated Liver function and Low Platelets)	642.53	642.51	642.50	N/A	
hypotension, maternal	669.23	669.21	669.20	N/A	
maternal hypotension	669.23	669.21	669.20	N/A	
Mendelson's (during labor) (obstetric)	668.03	668.01	668.00	N/A	
vanishing twin	651.33	N/A	N/A	N/A	
Syphilis	647.03	647.01	647.00	condition	760.2
Tear, torn					
anus, anal (sphincter), complicating delivery	N/A	664.21	664.20	N/A	763.89
with mucosa	N/A	664.31	664.30	N/A	763.89
bladder, obstetrical trauma	N/A	665.51	665.50	N/A	763.89
bowel, obstetrical trauma	N/A	665.51	665.50	N/A	763.89
broad ligament, obstetrical trauma	N/A	665.51	665.50	N/A	763.89
cervix, obstetrical trauma	N/A	665.31	665.30	N/A	763.89
pelvic					
floor, complicating delivery	N/A	664.11	664.10	N/A	763.89
organ NEC, obstetrical trauma	N/A	665.51	665.50	N/A	763.89
perineum, obstetrical trauma	N/A	665.51	665.50	N/A	763.89
periurethral, obstetrical trauma	N/A	665.51	665.50	N/A	763.89
umbilical cord, complicating delivery	663.83	663.81	663.80	N/A	772.0
urethra, obstetrical trauma	N/A	665.51	665.50	N/A	
vulva, complicating delivery	N/A	664.01	664.00	N/A	763.89
Teratoma, fetal sacral, causing fetopelvic disproportion	653.73	653.71	653.70	N/A	763.1
causing obstructed labor	660.23	660.21	660.20	cause	763.1
Thelitis	675.03	675.01	675.00	N/A	
Threatened				N/A	
abortion or miscarriage	640.03	640.01	640.00	N/A	762.1
labor	644.13	N/A	644.10	N/A	761.8
before 22 completed weeks gestation	640.03	640.01	640.00	N/A	762.1
premature delivery	N/A	644.21	644.20	N/A	761.8
premature labor	644.03	N/A	644.00	N/A	761.8
Thrombophlebitis	671.23	671.21	671.20	N/A	760.3
cerebral (sinus) (vein), nonpyogenic	671.53	671.51	671.50	N/A	760.3
deep	671.33	671.31	671.30	N/A	760.3
intracranial venous sinus, nonpyogenic	671.53	671.51	671.50	N/A	760.3
specified site NEC	671.53	671.51	671.50	N/A	760.3
superficial	671.23	671.21	671.20	N/A	760.3
deep	671.33	671.31	671.30	N/A	760.3
Thrombosis	671.93	671.91	671.90	N/A	
brain (artery) (stem)	674.03	674.01	674.00	N/A	
intracranial, venous sinus (nonpyogenic origin)	671.53	671.51	671.50	N/A	
deep	671.33	671.31	671.30	N/A	760.3
spinal cord	671.53	671.51	671.50	N/A	
superficial	671.23	671.21	671.20	N/A	
umbilical cord (vessels)	663.63	663.61	663.60	N/A	762.6
venous (superficial)	671.23	671.21	671.20	N/A	
deep	671.33	671.31	671.30	N/A	760.3
Thyroid dysfunction	648.13	648.11	648.10	condition	
Thyroiditis	648.13	648.11	648.10	condition	
Thyrotoxicosis	648.13	648.11	648.10	condition	
Tipping pelvis with disproportion (fetopelvic)	653.03	653.01	653.00	N/A	763.1
causing obstructed labor	660.13	660.11	660.10	cause	763.1

Antepartum Pregnancy Condition or Complication; affecting management of mother	Antepartum condition or complication	Delivered, with or without mention of antepartum condition	Unspecified episode of care	Assign additional code to describe the...	Affecting fetus (coded on the newborn chart only)
Torsion of uterus	654.43	654.41	654.40	N/A	
causing obstructed labor	660.23	660.21	660.20	cause	763.1
Toxemia (mild) (pre-eclamptic)	642.43	642.41	642.40	N/A	760.0
with				760.0	
convulsions	642.63	642.61	642.60	N/A	760.0
pre-existing hypertension	642.73	642.71	642.70	N/A	760.0
eclamptic	642.63	642.61	642.60	N/A	760.0
with pre-existing hypertension	642.73	642.71	642.70	N/A	760.0
maternal					
with suspected damage to fetus affecting management of pregnancy	655.43	655.41	655.40	N/A	760.2
manifest to toxoplasmosis in fetus or newborn	655.43	655.41	655.40	N/A	771.2
severe	642.53	642.51	642.50	N/A	760.0
Transmission of chemical substances through the placenta, suspected	655.53	655.51	655.50	N/A	760.70
Transverse					
arrest (deep), in labor	660.33	660.31	660.30	cause	763.1
lie or presentation	652.33	652.31	652.30	N/A	761.7
with successful version	652.13	652.11	652.10		763.1
causing obstructed labor	660.03	660.01	660.00	cause	763.1
Trauma	648.93	648.91	648.90	condition	
causing hemorrhage	641.83	641.81	641.80	N/A	760.5
during delivery NEC	665.93	665.91	665.90	N/A	760.5
obstetrical	665.93	665.91	665.90	N/A	760.5
previous pregnancy (major), affecting management of current pregnancy, childbirth or puerperium	V23.89	V23.89	V23.89	N/A	
Triplet NEC	651.13	651.11	651.10	N/A	761.5
with fetal loss and retention of one or more fetus(es)	651.43	651.41	651.40	N/A	761.5
Trophoblastic disease	630	N/A	N/A	N/A	
previous pregnancy, affecting management of current pregnancy	V23.1	V23.1	V23.1	N/A	
Tubal (with rupture)	633.1	N/A	N/A	N/A	761.4
Tuberculosis	647.33	647.31	647.30	condition	760.2
Tumor					
cervix	654.63	654.61	654.60	N/A	763.89
causing obstructed labor	660.23	660.21	660.20	cause	763.1
fetal, causing disproportion	653.73	653.71	653.70	N/A	763.1
causing obstructed labor	660.13	660.11	660.10	cause	763.1
ovary	654.43	654.41	654.40	N/A	763.89
causing obstructed labor	660.23	660.21	660.20	cause	763.1
pelvic	654.93	654.91	654.90	N/A	763.89
causing obstructed labor	660.23	660.21	660.20	cause	763.1
pelvic organs or tissue NEC	654.43	654.41	654.40	N/A	763.89
causing obstructed labor	660.23	660.21	660.20	cause	763.1
uterus	654.13	654.11	654.10	N/A	763.89
causing obstructed labor	660.23	660.21	660.20	cause	763.1
vagina	654.73	654.71	654.70	N/A	763.89
causing obstructed labor	660.23	660.21	660.20	cause	763.1
vulva	654.83	654.81	654.80	N/A	763.89
causing obstructed labor	660.23	660.21	660.20	cause	763.1
Twin NEC	651.03	651.01	651.00	N/A	761.5
with fetal loss and retention of one or more fetus(es)	651.33	651.31	651.30	N/A	761.5
Unstable lie	652.03	652.01	652.00	N/A	761.7
causing obstructed labor	660.03	660.01	660.00	cause	763.1
Unwanted NEC	V61.7	N/A	N/A	N/A	
Uremia (renal disease or failure) NEC	646.23	646.21	646.20	condition	760.1
with secondary hypertension	642.13	642.11	642.10	N/A	760.0
hypertensive	642.23	642.21	642.20	N/A	760.0
Urethritis	646.63	646.61	646.60	condition	760.1
Uterine size vs. dates discrepancy	646.83	646.81	646.80		
UTI	646.63	646.61	646.60	condition	760.1

Antepartum Pregnancy Table

Antepartum Pregnancy Condition or Complication; affecting management of mother	Antepartum condition or complication	Delivered, with or without mention of antepartum condition	Unspecified episode of care	Assign additional code to describe the...	Affecting fetus (coded on the newborn chart only)
Vaginitis or vulvitis	646.63	646.61	646.60	condition	760.8
Valsuani's disease (progressive pernicious anemia, puerperal)	648.23	648.21	648.20	condition	
Vanishing twin	651.33	N/A	N/A	N/A	
Varicose					
placental vessels	656.73	656.71	656.70	N/A	
veins (legs)	671.03	671.01	671.00	N/A	
perineum	671.13	671.11	671.10	N/A	
vulva	671.13	671.11	671.10	N/A	
Varicosity, labia or vulva	671.13	671.11	671.10	N/A	
Varix (lower extremity)	671.03	671.01	671.00	N/A	
perineum	671.13	671.11	671.10	N/A	
Vulva	671.13	671.11	671.10		N/A
Vasa previa	663.53	663.51	663.50	N/A	762.6
hemorrhage	663.53	663.51	663.50	N/A	772.0
Venereal disease NEC	647.23	647.21	647.20	disease	
Ventouse delivery NEC	N/A	669.51	669.50	N/A	763.3
Version					
before labor	652.13	652.11	652.10	N/A	761.7
causing obstructed labor	660.03	660.01	660.00	cause	763.1
cephalic (correcting previous malposition)	652.13	652.11	652.10	N/A	763.1
causing obstructed labor	660.03	660.01	660.00	cause	763.1
Viral disease NEC	647.63	647.61	647.60	disease	
Vomiting (incoercible) (pernicious) (persistent) (uncontrollable) (vicious	643.93	643.91	643.90	N/A	761.8
due to					
organic disease or other cause	643.83	643.81	643.80	N/A	761.8
specific cause NEC	643.83	643.81	643.80	N/A	761.8
early (mild) (before 22 completed weeks gestation)	643.03	643.01	643.00	N/A	761.8
with				761.8	
carbohydrate depletion	643.13	643.11	643.10	N/A	761.8
dehydration	643.13	643.11	643.10	N/A	761.8
electrolyte imbalance	643.13	643.11	643.10	N/A	761.8
late (after 22 completed weeks gestation)	643.23	643.21	643.20	N/A	761.8
severe (with metabolic disturbance)	643.13	643.11	643.10	N/A	761.8
Vulvitis	646.63	646.61	646.60	condition	760.8
Weight gain	646.13	646.11	646.10	condition	
insufficient	646.83	646.81	646.80	condition	
Young maternal age	659.83	659.81	659.80	N/A	

Postpartum Pregnancy Condition or Complication; affecting management of mother	Postpartum condition or complication	Delivered with mention of postpartum complication	Unspecified episode of care	Assign additional code to describe the...	Affecting newborn (coded on the newborn chart only)
Abnormal NEC					
cervix	654.64	654.62	654.60	N/A	763.89
glucose tolerance test	648.84	648.82	648.80	condition	775.0
pelvic organs or tissues NEC	654.94	654.92	654.90	N/A	763.89
perineum or vulva	654.84	654.82	654.80	N/A	763.89
Abnormal NEC					
position					
cervix	654.44	654.42	654.40	N/A	763.89
uterus	654.44	654.42	654.40	N/A	763.89
quality of milk	676.84	676.82	676.80	N/A	
shape of uterus	654.44	654.42	654.40	N/A	763.89
uterus (congenital)	654.04	654.02	654.00	N/A	763.89
vagina	654.74	654.72	654.70	N/A	763.89
vulva (acquired) (congenital)	654.84	654.82	654.80	N/A	763.89
weight gain	646.14	646.12	646.10	condition	761.8
with hypertension (mild) (pre-eclamptic)	642.44	642.42	642.40	N/A	760.0
with					
convulsions	642.64	642.62	642.60	N/A	760.0

Postpartum Pregnancy Condition or Complication; affecting management of mother	Postpartum condition or complication	Delivered with mention of postpartum complication	Unspecified episode of care	Assign additional code to describe the...	Affecting newborn (coded on the newborn chart only)
Abnormal NEC – *continued*					
pre-existing hypertension	642.74	642.72	642.70	N/A	760.0
with severe hypertension	642.54	642.52	642.50	N/A	760.0
Abscess					
areola (acute) (chronic)	675.14	675.12	675.10	N/A	
Bartholin's gland	646.64	646.62	646.60	condition	760.8
bladder	646.64	646.62	646.60	condition	760.1
breast (acute) (chronic)	675.14	675.12	675.10		
genital organ or tract NEC (postpartum)	670.04	670.02	670.00		
kidney	646.64	646.62	646.60	condition	760.1
labium (majus) (minus)	646.64	646.62	646.60	condition	760.8
milk	675.14	675.12	675.10	N/A	
nipple	675.04	675.02	675.00	N/A	
peritoneum, peritoneal (perforated) (ruptured) postpartum	670.04	670.02	670.00	N/A	
subareolar postpartum	675.14	675.12	675.10	N/A	
urethra	646.64	646.62	646.60	condition	760.1
vulva	646.64	646.62	646.60	condition	760.8
Accreta placenta	667.04	667.02	667.00	N/A	
with hemorrhage	666.04	666.02	666.00	N/A	
Addiction					
alcoholic	648.44	648.42	648.40	condition	760.71
Adherent placenta	667.04	667.02	667.00	N/A	
with hemorrhage	666.04	666.02	666.00	N/A	
Adhesion(s), adhesive					
cervicovaginal (postpartum)	674.84	674.82	674.80	N/A	
uterus to abdominal wall	654.44	654.42	654.40	N/A	763.89
Aerocele	673.04	673.02	673.00	N/A	
Afibrinogenemia (postpartum)	666.34	666.32	666.30	N/A	
AFP (screening for raised levels in amniotic fluid)	V28.1	N/A	N/A	N/A	
Agalactia	676.44	676.42	676.40	N/A	
Air embolism	673.04	673.02	673.00	N/A	
Albuminuria (gravidarum)	646.24	646.22	646.20	condition	760.1
with hypertension (and edema)					760.1
mild	642.44	642.42	642.40	N/A	760.0
severe	642.54	642.52	642.50	N/A	760.0
gestational	646.24	646.22	646.20	condition	760.1
pre-eclamptic (mild)	642.24	642.22	642.20	N/A	760.0
severe	642.54	642.52	642.50	N/A	760.0
Alcohol, alcoholic					
addiction (maternal)	648.44	648.42	648.40	condition	760.71
Alphafetoprotein (screening for raised levels in amniotic fluid)	V28.1	N/A	N/A	N/A	
Amniotic fluid embolism	673.14	673.12	673.10	N/A	
Amputation of cervix	654.64	654.62	654.60	N/A	763.8
Anemia	648.24	648.22	648.20	condition	760.8
aplastic	648.24	648.22	648.20	condition	760.8
iron (Fe) deficiency	648.24	648.22	648.20	condition	760.8
macrocytic	648.24	648.22	648.20	condition	760.8
megaloblastic	648.24	648.22	648.20	condition	760.8
pernicious	648.24	648.22	648.20	condition	760.8
postpartum	648.24	648.22	648.20	condition	
Anesthesia, anesthetic					
complications NEC	668.84	668.82	668.80	condition	763.5
cardiac	668.14	668.12	668.10	condition	763.5
central nervous system	668.24	668.22	668.20	condition	763.5
pulmonary	668.04	668.02	668.00	condition	763.5
death (from) during delivery	668.94	668.92	668.90	condition	761.6
Anomaly, anomalous (congenital)					
cardiovascular system	648.54	648.52	648.50	condition	
cervix	654.64	654.62	654.60	N/A	763.89
uterus	654.04	654.02	654.00	N/A	763.89
Anoxia cerebral					
complicating delivery (cesarean) (instrumental)	669.44	669.42	669.40	N/A	
due to obstetric anesthesia or sedation	668.24	668.22	668.20	complication	

Postpartum Pregnancy Condition or Complication; affecting management of mother	Postpartum condition or complication	Delivered with mention of postpartum complication	Unspecified episode of care	Assign additional code to describe the...	Affecting newborn (coded on the newborn chart only)
Anteversion					
uterus, uterine (cervix)	654.44	654.42	654.40	N/A	763.89
Anuria, postpartum	669.34	669.32	669.30	N/A	
Arrest, arrested					
cardiac					
anesthesia, complicating	668.14	668.12	668.10	N/A	
delivery (cesarean) (instrumental)	669.44	669.42	669.40	N/A	
Aspiration					
acid-pulmonary (syndrome)	668.04	668.02	668.00	complication	
pneumonitis	668.04	668.02	668.00	complication	
Atresia, atretic					
cervix	654.64	654.62	654.60	N/A	763.89
Atrophy, atrophic					
breast, postpartum	676.34	676.32	676.30		
postpartum	674.84	674.82	674.80	N/A	
Atonia, atony, atonic	666.14	666.12	666.10		
Avulsion (traumatic)					
symphyseal cartilage (inner)	665.64	N/A	665.60	N/A	
Bacilluria, asymptomatic	646.54	646.52	646.50	complication	760.1
Bacteremia	647.84	647.82	647.80	condition	
Bacteriuria, asymptomatic	646.54	646.52	646.50	complication	760.1
Bicornis or Bicornuate uterus	654.04	654.02	654.00	N/A	763.89
Bleeding				N/A	
atonic, following delivery	666.14	666.12	666.10	N/A	
cerebrovascular	674.04	674.02	674.00	N/A	
due to					
subinvolution, postpartum	666.24	666.22	666.20	N/A	
Blood, dyscrasia (postpartum)	666.34	666.32	666.30	N/A	
Bone disorders	648.74	648.72	648.70	condition	
Breakdown, perineum	674.24	674.22	674.20	N/A	
Breastfeeding difficulties	676.84	676.82	676.80		
Caked breast (postpartum)	676.24	676.22	676.20	N/A	
Cardiomyopathy	674.54	674.52	674.50	N/A	
Cardiovascular disease	648.64	648.62	648.60	condition	
congenital	648.54	648.52	648.50	condition	
Cellulitis (postpartum)					
breast	675.14	675.12	675.10	N/A	
pelvis	670.04	670.02	670.00	N/A	
Cerebrovascular disorders	674.04	674.02	674.00	condition	
Cervicitis	646.64	646.62	646.60	condition	760.8
Cervix					
adhesions	654.64	654.62	654.60	N/A	
anaplasia	654.64	654.62	654.60	N/A	
atypism	654.64	654.62	654.60	N/A	
bands	654.64	654.62	654.60	N/A	
cervicitis	654.64	654.62	654.60	N/A	
cicatrix	654.64	654.62	654.60	N/A	
cyst	654.64	654.62	654.60	N/A	
dysplasia	654.64	654.62	654.60	N/A	
ectropion	654.64	654.62	654.60	N/A	
endocervicitis	654.64	654.62	654.60	N/A	
erosion	654.64	654.62	654.60	N/A	
hypertrophic elongation	654.64	654.62	654.60	N/A	
incompetence	654.54	654.52	654.50	N/A	761.0
leukoplakia	654.64	654.62	654.60	N/A	
Nabothian (gland) cyst or follicle	654.64	654.62	654.60	N/A	
old laceration	654.64	654.62	654.60	N/A	
polyp	654.64	654.62	654.60	N/A	
stricture and stenosis	654.64	654.62	654.60	N/A	
ulcer	654.64	654.62	654.60	N/A	
Chiari-Frommel syndrome	676.64	676.62	676.60	N/A	
Childbed fever	670.04	670.02	670.00	N/A	
Chloasma (gravidarum)	646.84	646.82	646.80	condition	
Cicatrix					
cervix	654.64	654.62	654.60	N/A	
vagina	654.74	654.72	654.70	N/A	
Circulating anticoagulants	666.34	666.32	666.30	N/A	

Postpartum Pregnancy Condition or Complication; affecting management of mother	Postpartum condition or complication	Delivered with mention of postpartum complication	Unspecified episode of care	Assign additional code to describe the...	Affecting newborn (coded on the newborn chart only)
Collapse (during or after labor and delivery)					
circulatory (peripheral)	669.14	669.12	669.10	N/A	779.8
lung	668.04	668.02	668.00	N/A	
vascular (peripheral)	669.14	669.12	669.10	N/A	
Colporrhexis	665.44	N/A	665.40	N/A	
Complications NEC					
cesarean section wound	674.34	674.32	674.30	N/A	
delivery	669.94	669.92	669.90	N/A	
procedure (instrumental) (manual) (surgical)	669.44	669.42	669.40	N/A	
specified type NEC	669.84	669.82	669.80	N/A	
labor and delivery	669.94	669.92	669.90	N/A	
anesthesia (sedation)	668.94	668.92	668.90	N/A	763.5
cardiac	668.14	668.12	668.10	N/A	
central nervous system	668.24	668.22	668.20	N/A	
pulmonary	668.04	668.02	668.00	N/A	
specified type NEC	668.84	668.82	668.80	N/A	
specified condition NEC	669.84	669.82	669.80	N/A	
perineal repair	674.34	674.32	674.30	N/A	
disruption	674.24	674.22	674.20	N/A	
postpartum NEC	674.94	674.92	674.90	N/A	
surgical wound	674.34	674.32	674.30	N/A	
Convulsions (eclamptic) (uremic)	642.64	642.62	642.60	N/A	760.0
with pre-existing hypertension	642.74	642.72	642.70	N/A	760.0
Cracked nipple (postpartum)	676.14	676.12	676.10	N/A	
Cyst					
ovary	654.44	654.42	654.40	N/A	763.89
pelvic	654.44	654.42	654.40	N/A	763.89
Cystitis	646.64	646.62	646.60	condition	760.1
Cystocele	654.44	654.42	654.40	N/A	763.89
Damage					
coccyx, complicating delivery	665.64	N/A	665.60	N/A	763.89
pelvic (during delivery)					
joint or ligament	665.64	N/A	665.60	N/A	763.89
organ	665.54	N/A	665.50	N/A	763.89
Death, maternal, NEC					
during delivery	668.94	668.92	668.90	N/A	761.6
postpartum (cause not stated) (sudden)	674.94	674.92	674.90	N/A	
sudden, during delivery	669.94	669.92	669.90	N/A	761.6
under anesthesia NEC	668.94	668.92	668.90	N/A	761.6
Deciduitis	646.64	646.62	646.60	N/A	760.8
postpartum	670.04	670.02	670.00	N/A	
Defect, defective coagulation (factor)					
postpartum	666.34	666.32	666.30	N/A	
Deficiency, deficient coagulation (factor)					
postpartum	666.34	666.32	666.30	N/A	
Deformity					
pelvic, pelvis					
soft part, organs or tissues NEC	654.94	654.92	654.90	cause	763.89
Dehiscence (postpartum)					
cesarean wound	674.14	674.12	674.10	N/A	
episiotomy	674.24	674.22	674.20	N/A	
perineal wound	674.24	674.22	674.20	N/A	
uterine wound	674.14	674.12	674.10	N/A	
Dependence, maternal					
drug	648.34	648.32	648.30	condition	779.5
Depression, postpartum	648.44	648.42	648.40	condition	
Dermatitis, gestationis	646.84	646.82	646.80	condition	
Detachment					
cervix, annular	665.34	N/A	665.30	N/A	763.89
Diabetes					
condition present before pregnancy	648.04	648.02	648.00	condition	775.0
gestational (chemical) (latent)	648.84	648.82	648.80	condition	775.0
Diastasis, recti (abdomen) complicating delivery	665.84	665.82	665.80	N/A	763.89

Postpartum Pregnancy Table

Postpartum Pregnancy Table

Postpartum Pregnancy Condition or Complication; affecting management of mother	Postpartum condition or complication	Delivered with mention of postpartum complication	Unspecified episode of care	Assign additional code to describe the...	Affecting newborn (coded on the newborn chart only)
Difficult delivery NEC	669.94	669.92	669.90	N/A	763.89
Difficulty with breast feeding	676.84	676.82	676.80		
Dilatation					
bladder (sphincter)	654.44	654.42	654.40	N/A	763.89
Disease, NEC (postpartum)	674.94	674.92	674.90	N/A	
breast NEC	676.34	676.32	676.30	N/A	
cerebrovascular, NEC	674.04	674.02	674.00	N/A	
Frommel's	676.64	676.62	676.60	N/A	
heart	648.64	648.62	648.60	condition	760.8
postpartum	674.84	674.82	674.80	N/A	
renal NEC	646.24	646.22	646.20	condition	760.1
Valsuani's (progressive pernicious anemia, puerperal)	648.24	648.22	648.20	condition	
venereal NEC	647.24	647.22	647.20	condition	
virus NEC	647.64	647.62	647.60	condition	
Disorders					
breast, postpartum	676.34	676.32	676.30	N/A	
genital tract or organ	646.64	646.62	646.60	condition	760.89
lactation	676.94	676.92	676.90	N/A	
mental	648.44	648.42	648.40	condition	
metabolism NEC (in labor and delivery)	669.04	669.02	669.00	N/A	763.8
Displacement, uterus NEC	654.44	654.42	654.40	N/A	763.8
Disruption, wound					
cesarean operation	674.14	674.12	674.10	N/A	
episiotomy	674.24	674.22	674.20	N/A	
perineal (obstetric)	674.24	674.22	674.20	N/A	
uterine	674.14	674.12	674.10	N/A	
Distortion					
maternal	669.04	669.02	669.00	N/A	
Double uterus	654.04	654.02	654.00	N/A	763.89
Drug dependence	648.34	648.32	648.30	condition	
Dyscrasia, blood					
postpartum	666.34	666.32	666.30	N/A	
Dysfunction					
thyroid	648.14	648.12	648.10	condition	
Dysplasia of cervix	654.64	654.62	654.60	N/A	763.89
Eclampsia, eclamptic (coma) (convulsions) (delirium)	642.64	642.62	642.60	N/A	760.0
with pre-existing hypertension	642.74	642.72	642.70	N/A	760.0
Edema	646.14	646.12	646.10	condition	
with hypertension — see Pregnancy, toxemia					
cervix (postpartum)	674.84	674.82	674.80	N/A	
Effect, adverse					
anesthetic (in labor and delivery) NEC	668.94	668.92	668.90	N/A	763.5
Embolism					
air (pulmonary)	673.04	673.02	673.00	N/A	
amniotic fluid	673.14	673.12	673.10	N/A	
blood clot	673.24	673.22	673.20	N/A	
brain (postpartum)	674.04	674.02	674.00	N/A	
cerebral (postpartum)	674.04	674.02	674.00	N/A	
fat (cerebral) (pulmonary) (systemic)	673.84	673.82	673.80	N/A	
heart	674.84	674.82	674.80	N/A	
intracranial (venous sinus) (nonpyogenic)	671.54	671.52	671.50	N/A	
pulmonary NEC	673.24	673.22	673.20	N/A	
pyemic	673.34	673.32	673.30	N/A	
septic	673.34	673.32	673.30	N/A	
specified NEC	674.84	674.82	674.80	N/A	
Emesis (gravidarum) — see Pregnancy, vomiting					
Endometritis	646.64	646.62	646.60	condition	760.8
decidual	646.64	646.62	646.60	condition	760.8
postpartum	670.04	670.02	670.00	N/A	
Engorgement, breast (postpartum)	676.24	676.22	676.20	N/A	

Postpartum Pregnancy Condition or Complication; affecting management of mother	Postpartum condition or complication	Delivered with mention of postpartum complication	Unspecified episode of care	Assign additional code to describe the...	Affecting newborn (coded on the newborn chart only)
Erysipelas (postpartum, childbirth)	670.04	670.02	670.00	N/A	
Eversion, uterus					
complicating delivery	665.24	665.22	665.20	N/A	763.89
postpartum	674.84	674.82	674.80	N/A	
Excessive					
milk secretion	676.64	676.62	676.60	N/A	
weight gain	646.14	646.12	646.10	condition	
Exhaustion (complicating delivery)	669.84	669.82	669.80	N/A	763.89
Extraction					
manual NEC	669.84	669.82	669.80	N/A	763.89
Extroversion, uterus (complicating delivery)	665.24	665.22	665.20	N/A	763.89
Failure, failed					
heart, complicating					
delivery (cesarean) (instrumental)	669.44	669.42	669.40	N/A	
obstetric anesthesia or sedation	668.14	668.12	668.10	N/A	
lactation	676.44	676.42	676.40	N/A	
renal following labor and delivery (acute)	669.34	669.32	669.30	N/A	
Fatigue	646.84	646.82	646.80	condition	
Febris puerperalis	672.04	672.02	672.00	N/A	
Fever	672.04	672.02	672.00	N/A	
childbed	670.04	670.02	670.00	N/A	
milk	672.04	672.02	672.00	N/A	
sepsis	670.04	670.02	670.00	N/A	
Fibrinolysis postpartum	666.34	666.32	666.30	N/A	
Fibroid tumor(s)	654.14	654.12	654.10	N/A	763.89
Fibromyoma (uterus)	654.14	654.12	654.10	N/A	763.89
Fibrosis, fibrotic					
perineum	654.84	654.82	654.80	N/A	763.89
Fissure, nipple (postpartum)	676.14	676.12	676.10	N/A	
Fistula (postpartum)					
breast	675.14	675.12	675.10	N/A	
mammary gland	675.14	675.12	675.10	N/A	
Forced birth or delivery NEC	669.84	669.82	669.80	N/A	763.89
Fractured coccyx complicating delivery	665.64	N/A	665.60	N/A	
Frommel's disease	676.64	676.62	676.60	N/A	
Frommel-Chiari syndrome	676.64	676.62	676.60	N/A	
Galactocele (breast), postpartum	676.84	676.82	676.80	N/A	
Galactorrhea	676.64	676.62	676.60	N/A	
Gangrene					
gas (bacillus) postpartum, childbirth	670.04	670.02	670.00	N/A	
Goiter	648.14	648.12	648.10	condition	
Gonococcal infection	647.14	647.12	647.10	condition	760.2
Gonorrhea	647.14	647.12	647.10	condition	760.2
HELLP (Hemolysis, Elevated Liver function and Low Platelets)	642.54	642.52	642.50	N/A	
Hematoma					
broad ligament	665.74	665.72	665.70	N/A	
cesarean section wound	674.34	674.32	674.30	N/A	
complicating delivery (perineum) (vulva)	664.54	N/A	664.50	N/A	
pelvic	665.74	665.72	665.70	N/A	
vagina	665.74	665.72	665.70	N/A	
episiotomy	674.34	674.32	674.30	N/A	
obstetrical surgical wound	674.34	674.32	674.30	N/A	
pelvis, complicating delivery	665.74	665.72	665.70	N/A	
perineal wound	674.34	674.32	674.30	N/A	
complicating delivery	664.54	N/A	664.50	N/A	
vagina	665.74	665.72	665.70	N/A	
vulva, complicating delivery	664.54	N/A	664.50	N/A	767.8
Hemolysis, liver dysfunction, low platelets syndrome (HELLP)	642.53	642.51	642.50		
Hemorrhage					
brain (postpartum, childbirth)	674.04	674.02	674.00	N/A	

Postpartum Pregnancy Table

Postpartum Pregnancy Condition or Complication; affecting management of mother	Postpartum condition or complication	Delivered with mention of postpartum complication	Unspecified episode of care	Assign additional code to describe the...	Affecting newborn (coded on the newborn chart only)
Hemorrhage – *continued*					
cerebrovascular	674.04	674.02	674.00	N/A	
cesarean section wound	674.34	674.32	674.30	N/A	
retained					
placenta	666.04	666.02	666.00	N/A	
secundines	666.24	666.22	666.20	N/A	
delayed, postpartum	666.24	666.22	666.20	N/A	
due to					
episiotomy	674.34	674.32	674.30	N/A	
intracranial, postpartum, childbirth	674.04	674.02	674.00	N/A	
obstetrical surgical wound	674.34	674.32	674.30	N/A	
perineal wound	674.34	674.32	674.30	N/A	
postpartum (atonic) (following delivery of placenta)	666.14	666.12	666.10	N/A	
delayed or secondary (after 24 hours)	666.24	666.22	666.20	N/A	
retained placenta	666.04	666.02	666.00	N/A	
third stage	666.04	666.02	666.00	N/A	
subarachnoid, postpartum, childbirth	674.04	674.02	674.00	N/A	
subdural, postpartum, childbirth	674.04	674.02	674.00	N/A	
third stage	666.04	666.02	666.00	N/A	
Hemorrhoids	671.84	671.82	671.80	N/A	
Hepatitis, viral	647.64	647.62	647.60	condition	
Herniation of uterus	654.44	654.42	654.40	N/A	
Herpes, herpetic	647.64	647.62	647.60	condition	
gestationis	646.84	646.82	646.80	condition	
Hydroa gestationis	646.84	646.82	646.80	condition	
Hypersecretion of milk	676.64	676.62	676.60	N/A	
Hypertension	642.94	642.92	642.90	N/A	760.0
with					
albuminuria (and edema) (mild)	642.44	642.42	642.40	N/A	760.0
severe	642.54	642.52	642.50	N/A	760.0
edema (mild)	642.44	642.42	642.40	N/A	760.0
severe	642.54	642.52	642.50	N/A	760.0
heart disease	642.24	642.22	642.20	N/A	760.0
and renal disease	642.24	642.22	642.20	N/A	760.0
pre-eclampsia or eclampsia	642.74	642.72	642.70	N/A	760.0
renal disease	642.24	642.22	642.20	N/A	760.0
and heart disease	642.24	642.22	642.20	N/A	760.0
benign	642.04	642.02	642.00	N/A	760.0
chronic	642.04	642.02	642.00	N/A	760.0
pre-existing	642.04	642.02	642.00	N/A	760.0
chronic	642.04	642.02	642.00	N/A	760.0
essential	642.04	642.02	642.00	N/A	760.0
with pre-eclampsia or eclampsia	642.74	642.72	642.70	N/A	760.0
gestational	642.34	642.32	642.30	N/A	
malignant	642.24	642.22	642.20	N/A	760.0
chronic	642.24	642.22	642.20	N/A	760.0
with pre-eclampsia or eclampsia	642.74	642.72	642.70	N/A	760.0
pre-existing	642.24	642.22	642.20	N/A	760.0
pre-existing	642.04	642.02	642.00	N/A	
secondary to renal disease	642.14	642.12	642.10	N/A	760.0
with pre-eclampsia or eclampsia	642.74	642.72	642.70	N/A	760.0
transient	642.34	642.32	642.30	N/A	
Hypertensive					
heart and renal disease	642.24	642.22	642.20	N/A	760.0
heart disease	642.24	642.22	642.20	N/A	760.0
renal disease	642.24	642.22	642.20	N/A	760.0
Hyperthyroidism	648.14	648.12	648.10	condition	
Hypotonic uterus	666.14	666.12	666.10		
Hypertonicity	648.14	648.12	648.10	condition	763.7
Hypertrophy					
breast (postpartum)	676.34	676.32	676.30	N/A	
uterus (postpartum)	674.84	674.82	674.80	N/A	

Postpartum Pregnancy Condition or Complication; affecting management of mother	Postpartum condition or complication	Delivered with mention of postpartum complication	Unspecified episode of care	Assign additional code to describe the...	Affecting newborn (coded on the newborn chart only)
Hypotension (following labor and delivery)	669.24	669.22	669.20	N/A	
Hypothyroidism	648.14	648.12	648.10	condition	
Hysteralgia	646.84	646.82	646.80	condition	
Incarceration, uterus	654.34	654.32	654.30	N/A	763.1
Incompetent cervix (os)	654.54	654.52	654.50	N/A	761.0
Increased anticoagulants (postpartum)	666.34	666.32	666.30	N/A	
In double uterus	654.04	654.02	654.00	N/A	763.89
Indurated breast (postpartum)	676.34	676.32	676.30	N/A	
Inertia of uterus	666.14	666.12	666.10		
Infantile					
genitalia, genitals	654.44	654.42	654.40	N/A	763.89
Infarct, infarction					
brain (stem), postpartum, childbirth	674.04	674.02	674.00	N/A	
Infection	647.94	647.92	647.90	condition	760.2
bladder	646.64	646.62	646.60	condition	
breast (mammary gland), postpartum	675.24	675.22	675.20	N/A	
with nipple	675.94	675.92	675.90	N/A	
specified type NEC	675.84	675.82	675.80	N/A	
nonpurulent	675.24	675.22	675.20	N/A	
purulent	675.14	675.12	675.10	N/A	
cesarean section wound	674.34	674.32	674.30	N/A	
episiotomy	674.34	674.32	674.30	N/A	
genital organs	646.64	646.62	646.60	condition	760.8
postpartum, childbirth	670.04	670.02	670.00	N/A	760.8
major	670.04	670.02	670.00	N/A	760.8
minor or localized	646.64	646.62	646.60	condition	760.8
intrauterine, complicating delivery	646.64	646.62	646.60	condition	
kidney	646.64	646.62	646.60	condition	760.1
nipple	675.04	675.02	675.00	N/A	
with breast	675.94	675.92	675.90	N/A	
specified type NEC	675.84	675.82	675.80	N/A	
perineal wound (obstetrical)	674.34	674.32	674.30	N/A	
postpartum (major)	670.04	670.02	670.00	N/A	
minor	646.64	646.62	646.60	condition	
urinary (tract)	646.64	646.62	646.60	condition	760.1
asymptomatic	646.54	646.52	646.50	condition	760.1
UTI	646.64	646.62	646.60	condition	760.1
asymptomatic	646.54	646.52	646.50	condition	760.1
Infective and parasitic diseases NEC	647.84	647.82	647.80	complication	
Infestation	647.94	647.92	647.90	condition	760.8
Inflammation					
areola, postpartum	675.04	675.02	675.00	N/A	
bladder	646.64	646.62	646.60	condition	760.8
breast (mammary gland), postpartum	675.24	675.22	675.20	N/A	
genital organ	646.64	646.62	646.60	condition	760.8
urinary tract NEC	646.64	646.62	646.60	condition	760.8
Inhalation of stomach contents or secretions in labor and delivery	668.04	668.02	668.00	N/A	
Injury	648.94	648.92	648.90	condition	
birth canal NEC	665.94	665.92	665.90	N/A	763.89
coccyx, complicating delivery	665.64	N/A	665.60	N/A	
genital organs, obstetrical trauma NEC	665.94	665.92	665.90	N/A	763.89
instrumental, obstetrical NEC	665.94	665.92	665.90	N/A	763.89
bladder	665.54	N/A	665.50	N/A	763.89
cervix	665.34	N/A	665.30	N/A	763.89
high vaginal	665.44	N/A	665.40	N/A	763.89
perineal NEC	664.94	N/A	664.90	N/A	763.89
urethra	665.54	N/A	665.50	N/A	763.89
uterus	665.54	N/A	665.50	N/A	763.89
obstetrical NEC	665.94	665.92	665.90	N/A	763.89
pelvic, complicating delivery					
floor	664.14	N/A	664.10	N/A	763.89
joint or ligament	665.64	N/A	665.60	N/A	763.89

Postpartum Pregnancy Table

Postpartum Pregnancy Condition or Complication; affecting management of mother	Postpartum condition or complication	Delivered with mention of postpartum complication	Unspecified episode of care	Assign additional code to describe the...	Affecting newborn (coded on the newborn chart only)
Injury – *continued*					
organs	665.54	N/A	665.50	N/A	763.89
periurethral tissue, complicating delivery	665.54	N/A	665.50	N/A	763.89
symphysis pubis, complicating delivery	665.64	N/A	665.60	N/A	763.89
Insufficient					
prenatal care	V23.7	N/A	N/A	N/A	
weight gain	646.84	646.82	646.80	condition	
Newborn "light-for-dates"					
Without mention of fetal malnutrition					
unspecified (weight)					764.00
< 500 gms					764.01
500-749 gms					764.02
750-999 gms					764.03
1,000-1,249 gms					764.04
1,250-1,499 gms					764.05
1,500-1,749 gms					764.06
1,750-1,999 gms					764.07
2,000-2,499 gms					764.08
≥ 2,500 gms					764.09
Intoxication					
drug					
obstetric anesthetic or sedation	668.94	668.92	668.90	N/A	763.5
septic, postpartum, childbirth	670.04	670.02	670.00	N/A	
Inversion					
nipple, postpartum	676.34	676.32	676.30		
uterus, complicating delivery	665.24	665.22	665.20		763.89
Ischemia, cerebral (postpartum, childbirth)	674.04	674.02	674.00	N/A	
Joint disorders	648.74	648.72	648.70	condition	
Laceration (obstetrical trauma)					
anus	664.24	N/A	664.20	N/A	
with laceration of anal or rectal mucosa	664.34	N/A	664.30	N/A	
bladder	665.54	N/A	665.50	N/A	
bowel	665.54	N/A	665.50	N/A	
broad ligament	665.64	N/A	665.60	N/A	
central	664.44	N/A	664.40	N/A	
cervix (uteri)	665.34	N/A	665.30	N/A	
fourchette	664.04	N/A	664.00	N/A	
labia	664.04	N/A	664.00	N/A	
pelvic					
floor (muscles)	664.14	N/A	664.10	N/A	
organ NEC	665.54	N/A	665.50	N/A	
perineum	664.44	N/A	664.40	N/A	
first degree	664.04	N/A	664.00	N/A	
second degree	664.14	N/A	664.10	N/A	
third degree	664.24	N/A	664.20	N/A	
fourth degree	664.34	N/A	664.30	N/A	
central	664.44	N/A	664.40	N/A	
involving					
anal sphincter	664.24	N/A	664.20	N/A	
fourchette	664.04	N/A	664.00	N/A	
hymen	664.04	N/A	664.00	N/A	
labia	664.04	N/A	664.00	N/A	
pelvic floor	664.14	N/A	664.10	N/A	
perineal muscles	664.14	N/A	664.10	N/A	
rectovaginal with septum	664.24	N/A	664.20	N/A	
with anal mucosa	664.34	N/A	664.30	N/A	
skin	664.04	N/A	664.00	N/A	
sphincter (anal)	664.24	N/A	664.20	N/A	
with anal mucosa	664.34	N/A	664.30	N/A	
vagina	664.04	N/A	664.00	N/A	
vaginal muscles	664.14	N/A	664.10	N/A	
vulva	664.04	N/A	664.00	N/A	
secondary	674.24	674.22	674.20	N/A	
peritoneum (obstetrical trauma)	665.54	N/A	665.50	N/A	

Postpartum Pregnancy Condition or Complication; affecting management of mother	Postpartum condition or complication	Delivered with mention of postpartum complication	Unspecified episode of care	Assign additional code to describe the...	Affecting newborn (coded on the newborn chart only)
Laceration (obstetrical trauma – *continued*					
periurethral tissue (obstetrical trauma)	665.54	N/A	665.50	N/A	
rectovaginal septum	665.44	N/A	665.40	N/A	
with perineum	664.24	N/A	664.20	N/A	
involving anal or rectal mucosa	664.34	N/A	664.30	N/A	
urethra (obstetrical trauma)	665.54	N/A	665.50	N/A	
vagina (complicating delivery)	665.44	N/A	665.40	N/A	
with perineal involvement	664.04	N/A	664.00	N/A	
first degree	664.04	N/A	664.00	N/A	
second degree	664.14	N/A	664.10	N/A	
third degree	664.24	N/A	664.20	N/A	
fourth degree	664.34	N/A	664.30	N/A	
high	664.44	N/A	664.40	N/A	
muscles	664.14	N/A	664.10	N/A	
sulcus	665.44	N/A	665.40	N/A	
wall	665.44	N/A	665.40	N/A	
vulva (complicating delivery)	664.04	N/A	664.00	N/A	
Lactation, lactating (breast) (postpartum)					
defective	676.44	676.42	676.40	N/A	
disorder	676.94	676.92	676.90	N/A	
specified type NEC	676.84	676.82	676.80	N/A	
examination and/or care of mother	V24.1	V24.1	V24.1	N/A	
excessive	676.64	676.62	676.60	N/A	
failed	676.44	676.42	676.40	N/A	
mastitis NEC	675.24	675.22	675.20	N/A	
suppressed	676.54	676.52	676.50	N/A	
Late effect(s) (of)					
childbirth complication(s)	677	677	677	condition	
complication(s) of					
childbirth	677	677	677	condition	
delivery	677	677	677	condition	
postpartum	677	677	677	condition	
pregnancy	677	677	677	condition	
puerperium	677	677	677	condition	
Lateroversion, uterus	654.44	654.42	654.40	N/A	763.89
Lymphadenitis, breast postpartum	675.24	675.22	675.20	N/A	
Lymphangitis (postpartum)	670.04	670.02	670.00	N/A	
breast	675.24	675.22	675.20	N/A	
Malaria	647.44	647.42	647.40	condition	
Malformation					
pelvic organs or tissues	654.94	654.92	654.90	N/A	763.89
uterus (congenital)	654.04	654.02	654.00	N/A	
Malnutrition	648.94	648.92	648.90	condition	
Malposition					
pelvic organs or tissues	654.44	654.42	654.40	N/A	763.89
uterus or cervix	654.44	654.42	654.40	N/A	763.89
Malpresentation					
uterus or cervix	654.44	654.42	654.40	N/A	
Mammillitis, puerperal, postpartum	675.24	675.22	675.20	N/A	
Mammitis, puerperal, postpartum	675.24	675.22	675.20	N/A	
Mastitis					
lactational	675.24	675.22	675.20	N/A	
puerperal, postpartum, (interstitial) (nonpurulent) (parenchymatous)	675.24	675.22	675.20	N/A	
purulent	675.14	675.12	675.10	N/A	
stagnation	675.24	675.22	675.20	N/A	
puerperalis	675.24	675.22	675.20	N/A	
retromammary (puerperal, postpartum	675.14	675.12	675.10	N/A	
submammary (puerperal, postpartum	675.14	675.12	675.10	N/A	
Maternal obesity syndrome	646.14	646.12	646.10	condition	

Postpartum Pregnancy Table

Postpartum Pregnancy Condition or Complication; affecting management of mother	Postpartum condition or complication	Delivered with mention of postpartum complication	Unspecified episode of care	Assign additional code to describe the...	Affecting newborn (coded on the newborn chart only)
Membrane, retained (complicating delivery) (with hemorrhage)	666.24	666.22	666.20	N/A	
without hemorrhage	667.14	667.12	667.10	N/A	
Mendelson's syndrome	668.04	668.02	668.00	N/A	
Mental disorders	648.44	648.42	648.40	condition	
Metritis (puerperal, postpartum, childbirth)	670.04	670.02	670.00	N/A	
Metrorrhagia, postpartum	666.24	666.22	666.20	N/A	
Milk					
excess secretion	676.64	676.62	676.60	N/A	
fever	672.04	672.02	672.00	N/A	
retention	672.04	672.02	672.00	N/A	
Milk leg (deep vessels)	671.44	671.42	671.40	N/A	
Myocardiopathy (postpartum)	674.84	674.82	674.80	N/A	
Myoma uterus (cervix) (corpus)	654.14	654.12	654.10	N/A	763.89
Myxedema (postpartum)	674.84	674.82	674.80	N/A	
Necrosis					
genital organ or tract	646.64	646.62	646.60	condition	760.8
kidney, cortical (acute)	646.24	646.22	646.20	condition	760.1
following labor and delivery	669.34	669.32	669.30	N/A	
tubular	646.24	646.22	646.20	condition	760.1
following labor and delivery	669.34	669.32	669.30	N/A	
liver, puerperal, postpartum	674.84	674.82	674.80	N/A	
renal, cortical	646.24	646.22	646.20	condition	760.1
Nephritis, nephrosis	646.24	646.22	646.20	condition	760.1
with hypertension	642.14	642.12	642.10	N/A	760.0
Nephropathy NEC	646.24	646.22	646.20	condition	
Neuritis (peripheral)	646.44	646.42	646.40	condition	
puerperal, postpartum	646.44	646.42	646.40	condition	
Nutritional deficiency	648.94	648.92	648.90	condition	
Obesity	646.14	646.12	646.10	complication	
Obstetrical trauma NEC (complicating delivery)	665.94	665.92	665.90	N/A	763.89
Occlusion, precerebral artery NEC (puerperal, postpartum, childbirth)	674.04	674.02	674.00	condition	
Oliguria	646.24	646.22	646.20	condition	
with hypertension — see Pregnancy, toxemia					
following labor and delivery (postpartum)	669.34	669.32	669.30	N/A	
Oophoritis	646.64	646.62	646.60	condition	
Pain(s),	646.84	646.82	646.80	condition	
Paralysis, bladder	665.54	N/A	665.50	N/A	
Parametritis	670.04	670.02	670.00	N/A	
Patent cervix	654.54	654.52	654.50	N/A	761.0
Pelvic Inflammatory Disease	646.64	646.62	646.60	condition	
Pendulous abdomen	654.44	654.42	654.40	N/A	763.89
Perforation					
bladder	665.54	N/A	665.50	N/A	
bowel	665.54	N/A	665.50	N/A	
broad ligament	665.64	N/A	665.60	N/A	
cervix	665.34	N/A	665.30	N/A	
instrumental (complicating delivery)	665.94	665.92	665.90	N/A	
pelvic (floor)	664.14	N/A	664.10	N/A	
organ	665.54	N/A	665.50	N/A	763.89
urethral	665.54	N/A	665.50	N/A	763.89
uterus	665.54	N/A	665.50	N/A	763.89
Peritonitis	670.04	670.02	670.00	N/A	
Persistence					
hymen (tag)	654.84	654.82	654.80	N/A	
Phlebitis	671.94	671.92	671.90	N/A	760.3
deep, postpartum	671.44	671.42	671.40	N/A	
intracranial	671.54	671.52	671.50	N/A	
lower extremities	671.24	671.22	671.20	N/A	760.3
specified site NEC	671.54	671.52	671.50	N/A	
superficial	671.24	671.22	671.20	N/A	760.3
Phlegmasia	671.44	671.42	671.40	N/A	

Postpartum Pregnancy Condition or Complication; affecting management of mother	Postpartum condition or complication	Delivered with mention of postpartum complication	Unspecified episode of care	Assign additional code to describe the...	Affecting newborn (coded on the newborn chart only)
PID	646.64	646.62	646.60	condition	
Placenta, placental					
accreta	667.04	667.02	667.00	N/A	
with hemorrhage	666.04	666.02	666.00	N/A	
adherent	667.04	667.02	667.00	N/A	
with hemorrhage	666.04	666.02	666.00	N/A	
increta	667.04	667.02	667.00	N/A	
with hemorrhage	666.04	666.02	666.00	N/A	
percreta	667.04	667.02	667.00	N/A	
with hemorrhage	666.04	666.02	666.00	N/A	
polyp	674.44	674.42	674.40	N/A	
retention (without hemorrhage)	667.04	667.02	667.00	N/A	
fragments (delayed hemorrhage)	666.24	666.22	666.20	N/A	
without hemorrhage	667.14	667.12	667.10	N/A	
hemorrhage	666.04	666.02	666.00	N/A	
postpartum	666.24	666.22	666.20	N/A	
syphilitic	647.04	647.02	647.00	condition	760.2
manifest syphilis in the infant or fetus	647.04	647.02	647.00	condition	090.0
trapped	667.04	667.02	667.00	N/A	
with hemorrhage	666.04	666.02	666.00	N/A	
Pneumonitis					
aspiration	668.04	668.02	668.00	condition	
postanesthetic	668.04	668.02	668.00	condition	
postoperative	668.04	668.02	668.00	N/A	
Polygalactia	676.64	676.62	676.60	N/A	
Polyp					
cervix	654.64	654.62	654.60	N/A	763.89
placenta	674.44	674.42	674.40	N/A	
uterus	654.14	654.12	654.10	N/A	763.89
Postpartum					
abscess					
areola (acute) (chronic)	675.14	675.12	675.10	N/A	
Bartholin's gland	646.64	646.62	646.60	condition	
breast (acute) (chronic) (mammary)	675.14	675.12	675.10	N/A	
cervix (uteri)	670.04	670.02	670.00	N/A	
fallopian tube	670.04	670.02	670.00	N/A	
genital organ or tract NEC	670.04	670.02	670.00	N/A	
kidney	646.64	646.62	646.60	condition	
labium (majus) (minus)	646.64	646.62	646.60	condition	
mesosalpinx	670.04	670.02	670.00	N/A	
milk	675.14	675.12	675.10	N/A	
nabothian	646.64	646.62	646.60	condition	
nipple	675.04	675.02	675.00	N/A	
ovary	670.04	670.02	670.00	N/A	
oviduct	670.04	670.02	670.00	N/A	
para-uterine	670.04	670.02	670.00	N/A	
pelvic	670.04	670.02	670.00	N/A	
perimetric	670.04	670.02	670.00	N/A	
peritoneum, peritoneal (perforated) (ruptured)	670.04	670.02	670.00	N/A	
periuterine	670.04	670.02	670.00	N/A	
retro-uterine	670.04	670.02	670.00	N/A	
subareolar	675.14	675.12	675.10	N/A	
suprapelvic	670.04	670.02	670.00	N/A	
tubal (ruptured)	670.04	670.02	670.00	N/A	
tubo-ovarian	670.04	670.02	670.00	N/A	
urethra	646.64	646.62	646.60	condition	
urinary tract NEC	646.64	646.62	646.60	condition	
uterine, uterus	670.04	670.02	670.00	N/A	
vagina (wall)	646.64	646.62	646.60	condition	
vaginorectal	646.64	646.62	646.60	condition	
vulva	646.64	646.62	646.60	condition	
vulvovaginal gland	646.64	646.62	646.60	condition	
accident	674.94	674.92	674.90	N/A	
adnexitis	670.04	670.02	670.00	N/A	
afibrinogenemia, or other coagulation defect	666.34	666.32	666.30	N/A	

Postpartum Pregnancy Condition or Complication; affecting management of mother	Postpartum condition or complication	Delivered with mention of postpartum complication	Unspecified episode of care	Assign additional code to describe the...	Affecting newborn (coded on the newborn chart only)
Postpartum – *continued*					
albuminuria (acute) (subacute)	646.24	646.22	646.20	condition	
pre-eclamptic	642.44	642.42	642.40	N/A	
anemia (conditions classifiable to 280-285)	648.24	648.22	648.20	condition	
anuria	669.34	669.32	669.30	N/A	
apoplexy	674.04	674.02	674.00	N/A	
asymptomatic bacteriuria	646.54	646.52	646.50	condition	
blood dyscrasia	666.34	666.32	666.30	N/A	
breast atrophy	676.34	676.32	676.30	N/A	
caked breast	676.24	676.22	676.20	N/A	
cardiomyopathy	674.54	674.52	674.50	N/A	
cerebrovascular disorder (conditions classifiable to 430-434, 436-437)	674.04	674.02	674.00	condition	
complications NOS	674.94	674.92	674.90	N/A	
specified type NEC	674.84	674.82	674.80	N/A	
cracked nipple	676.14	676.12	676.10	N/A	
deciduitis (acute)	670.04	670.02	670.00	N/A	
disease	674.94	674.92	674.90	N/A	
beast NEC	676.34	676.32	676.30	N/A	
cerebrovascular (acute)	674.04	674.02	674.00	condition	
pelvic inflammatory	670.04	670.02	670.00	N/A	
PID	670.04	670.02	670.00	N/A	
tubo-ovarian	670.04	670.02	670.00	N/A	
disorder					
lactation	676.94	676.92	676.90	N/A	
specified type NEC	676.84	676.82	676.80	N/A	
disruption					
cesarean wound	674.14	674.12	674.10	N/A	
episiotomy wound	674.24	674.22	674.20	N/A	
perineal laceration wound	674.24	674.22	674.20	N/A	
embolism (pulmonary)	673.24	673.22	673.20	N/A	
air	673.04	673.02	673.00	N/A	
amniotic fluid	673.14	673.12	673.10	N/A	
blood clot	673.24	673.22	673.20	N/A	
brain or cerebral	674.04	674.02	674.00	N/A	
cardiac	674.84	674.82	674.80	N/A	
fat	673.84	673.82	673.80	N/A	
intracranial sinus (venous)	671.54	671.52	671.50	N/A	
pyemic	673.34	673.32	673.30	N/A	
septic	673.34	673.32	673.30	N/A	
spinal cord	671.54	671.52	671.50	N/A	
endometritis (conditions classifiable to 615.0-615.9)	670.04	670.02	670.00	N/A	
engorgement, breasts	676.24	676.22	676.20	N/A	
erysipelas	670.04	670.02	670.00	N/A	
failure					
lactation	676.44	676.42	676.40	N/A	
renal, acute	669.34	669.32	669.30	N/A	
fever					
meaning sepsis	670.04	670.02	670.00	N/A	
meaning pyrexia (of unknown origin)	672.04	672.02	672.00	N/A	
fissure, nipple	676.14	676.12	676.10	N/A	
fistula					
breast (mammary gland)	675.14	675.12	675.10	N/A	
nipple	675.04	675.02	675.00	N/A	
galactophoritis	675.24	675.22	675.20	N/A	
galactorrhea	676.64	676.62	676.60	N/A	
gangrene (gas) (uterus)	670.04	670.02	670.00	N/A	
hematoma, subdural	674.04	674.02	674.00	N/A	
hematosalpinx, infectional	670.04	670.02	670.00	N/A	
hemiplegia, cerebral	674.04	674.02	674.00	N/A	
hemorrhage	666.14	666.12	666.10	N/A	
brain	674.04	674.02	674.00	N/A	
bulbar	674.04	674.02	674.00	N/A	
cerebellar	674.04	674.02	674.00	N/A	
cerebral	674.04	674.02	674.00	N/A	

Postpartum Pregnancy Condition or Complication; affecting management of mother	Postpartum condition or complication	Delivered with mention of postpartum complication	Unspecified episode of care	Assign additional code to describe the...	Affecting newborn (coded on the newborn chart only)
Postpartum – *continued*					
delayed (after 24 hours) (uterine)	666.24	666.22	666.20	N/A	
extradural	674.04	674.02	674.00	N/A	
internal capsule	674.04	674.02	674.00	N/A	
intracranial	674.04	674.02	674.00	N/A	
intrapontine	674.04	674.02	674.00	N/A	
meningeal	674.04	674.02	674.00	N/A	
pontine	674.04	674.02	674.00	N/A	
subarachnoid	674.04	674.02	674.00	N/A	
subcortical	674.04	674.02	674.00	N/A	
subdural	674.04	674.02	674.00	N/A	
uterine, delayed	666.24	666.22	666.20	N/A	
ventricular	674.04	674.02	674.00	N/A	
hemorrhoids	671.84	671.82	671.80	N/A	
hepatorenal syndrome	674.84	674.82	674.80	N/A	
hypertrophy (breast) (mammary gland)	676.34	676.32	676.30	N/A	
induration breast (fibrous)	676.34	676.32	676.30	N/A	
infection					
Bartholin's gland	646.64	646.62	646.60	condition	
breast (acute) (chronic) (mammary)	675.24	675.22	675.20	N/A	
with nipple	675.94	675.92	675.90	N/A	
specified type NEC	675.84	675.82	675.80	N/A	
cervix (uteri)	646.64	646.62	646.60	condition	
endocervix	646.64	646.62	646.60	condition	
fallopian tube	670.04	670.02	670.00	N/A	
generalized	670.04	670.02	670.00	N/A	
genital tract (major)	670.04	670.02	670.00	N/A	
minor or localized	646.64	646.62	646.60	condition	
kidney	646.64	646.62	646.60	condition	
mammary gland	675.24	675.22	675.20	N/A	
with nipple	675.94	675.92	675.90	N/A	
specified type NEC	675.84	675.82	675.80	N/A	
nipple	675.04	675.02	675.00	N/A	
with breast	675.94	675.92	675.90	N/A	
specified type NEC	675.84	675.82	675.80	N/A	
ovary	670.04	670.02	670.00	N/A	
pelvic	670.04	670.02	670.00	N/A	
peritoneum,	670.04	670.02	670.00	N/A	
renal	646.64	646.62	646.60	condition	
tubo-ovarian	670.04	670.02	670.00	N/A	
urinary tract NEC	646.64	646.62	646.60	condition	
asymptomatic	646.54	646.52	646.50	condition	
uterine, uterus	670.04	670.02	670.00	N/A	
vagina	646.64	646.62	646.60	condition	
inflammation — *see also* Postpartum, infection					
areola (acute) (chronic)	675.14	675.12	675.10	N/A	
Bartholin's gland	646.64	646.62	646.60	condition	
breast	675.24	675.22	675.20	N/A	
cervix (uteri)	646.64	646.62	646.60	condition	
fallopian tube	670.04	670.02	670.00	N/A	
genital organ or tract NEC	670.04	670.02	670.00	N/A	
localized	646.64	646.62	646.60	condition	
mammary gland	675.24	675.22	675.20	N/A	
nipple	675.04	675.02	675.00	N/A	
ovary	670.04	670.02	670.00	N/A	
oviduct	670.04	670.02	670.00	N/A	
pelvis	670.04	670.02	670.00	N/A	
periuterine	670.04	670.02	670.00	N/A	
tubal	670.04	670.02	670.00	N/A	
vagina	646.64	646.62	646.60	condition	
inversion, nipple	676.34	676.32	676.30	N/A	
ischemia, cerebral	674.04	674.02	674.00	N/A	
lymphangitis	670.04	670.02	670.00	N/A	
breast	675.24	675.22	675.20	N/A	
mammillitis	675.04	675.02	675.00	N/A	
mastitis	675.24	675.22	675.20	N/A	

Postpartum Pregnancy Table

Postpartum Pregnancy Table

Postpartum Pregnancy Condition or Complication; affecting management of mother	Postpartum condition or complication	Delivered with mention of postpartum complication	Unspecified episode of care	Assign additional code to describe the...	Affecting newborn (coded on the newborn chart only)
Postpartum – *continued*					
purulent	675.14	675.12	675.10	N/A	
retromammary	675.14	675.12	675.10	N/A	
submammary	675.14	675.12	675.10	N/A	
metritis (septic) (suppurative)	670.04	670.02	670.00	N/A	
metroperitonitis	670.04	670.02	670.00	N/A	
metrorrhagia	666.24	666.22	666.20	N/A	
metrosalpingitis	670.04	670.02	670.00	N/A	
metrovaginitis	670.04	670.02	670.00	N/A	
milk leg	671.44	671.42	671.40	N/A	
monoplegia, cerebral	674.04	674.02	674.00	N/A	
necrosis				N/A	
kidney, tubular	669.34	669.32	669.30	N/A	
liver (acute) (subacute) (conditions classifiable to 570)	674.84	674.82	674.80	N/A	
ovary	670.04	670.02	670.00	N/A	
renal cortex	669.34	669.32	669.30	N/A	
occlusion, precerebral artery	674.04	674.02	674.00	N/A	
oliguria	669.34	669.32	669.30	N/A	
oophoritis	670.04	670.02	670.00	N/A	
ovaritis	670.04	670.02	670.00	N/A	
paralysis				N/A	
bladder (sphincter)	665.54	N/A	665.50	N/A	
cerebral	674.04	674.02	674.00	N/A	
paralytic stroke	674.04	674.02	674.00	N/A	
parametritis	670.04	670.02	670.00	N/A	
paravaginitis	646.64	646.62	646.60	condition	
pelviperitonitis	670.04	670.02	670.00	N/A	
perimetritis	670.04	670.02	670.00	N/A	
perimetrosalpingitis	670.04	670.02	670.00	N/A	
perinephritis	646.64	646.62	646.60	condition	
perioophoritis	670.04	670.02	670.00	N/A	
perisalpingitis	670.04	670.02	670.00	N/A	
peritoneal infection	670.04	670.02	670.00	N/A	
peritonitis (pelvic)	670.04	670.02	670.00	N/A	
perivaginitis	646.64	646.62	646.60	condition	
phlebitis	671.94	671.92	671.90	N/A	
deep	671.44	671.42	671.40	N/A	
intracranial sinus (venous)	671.54	671.52	671.50	N/A	
pelvic	671.44	671.42	671.40	N/A	
specified site NEC	671.54	671.52	671.50	N/A	
superficial	671.24	671.22	671.20	N/A	
phlegmasia alba dolens	671.44	671.42	671.40	N/A	
placental polyp	674.44	674.42	674.40	N/A	
prediabetes	648.84	648.82	648.80	condition	
pyelitis	646.64	646.62	646.60	condition	
pyelocystitis	646.64	646.62	646.60	condition	
pyelohydronephrosis	646.64	646.62	646.60	condition	
pyelonephritis	646.64	646.62	646.60	condition	
pyelonephrosis	646.64	646.62	646.60	condition	
pyemia	670.04	670.02	670.00	N/A	
pyocystitis	646.64	646.62	646.60	condition	
pyohemia	670.04	670.02	670.00	N/A	
pyometra	670.04	670.02	670.00	N/A	
pyonephritis	646.64	646.62	646.60	condition	
pyonephrosis	646.64	646.62	646.60	condition	
pyo-oophoritis	670.04	670.02	670.00	N/A	
pyosalpingitis	670.04	670.02	670.00	N/A	
pyosalpinx	670.04	670.02	670.00	N/A	
pyrexia (of unknown origin)	672.04	672.02	672.00	N/A	
renal					
disease NEC	646.24	646.22	646.20	condition	
failure, acute	669.34	669.32	669.30	N/A	
retention					
decidua (fragments) (with delayed hemorrhage)	666.24	666.22	666.20	N/A	
without hemorrhage	667.14	667.12	667.10	N/A	
placenta (fragments) (with delayed hemorrhage)	666.24	666.22	666.20	N/A	

Postpartum Pregnancy Condition or Complication; affecting management of mother	Postpartum condition or complication	Delivered with mention of postpartum complication	Unspecified episode of care	Assign additional code to describe the...	Affecting newborn (coded on the newborn chart only)
Postpartum – *continued*					
without hemorrhage	667.14	667.12	667.10	N/A	
secundines (fragments) (with delayed hemorrhage)	666.24	666.22	666.20	N/A	
without hemorrhage	667.14	667.12	667.10	N/A	
retracted nipple	676.04	676.02	676.00	N/A	
salpingitis	670.04	670.02	670.00	N/A	
salpingo-oophoritis	670.04	670.02	670.00	N/A	
salpingo-ovaritis	670.04	670.02	670.00	N/A	
salpingoperitonitis	670.04	670.02	670.00	N/A	
sapremia	670.04	670.02	670.00	N/A	
secondary perineal tear	674.24	674.22	674.20	N/A	
sepsis (pelvic)	670.04	670.02	670.00	N/A	
septicemia	670.04	670.02	670.00	N/A	771.81
subinvolution (uterus)	674.84	674.82	674.80	N/A	
sudden death (cause unknown)	674.94	674.92	674.90	N/A	
tetanus	670.04	670.02	670.00	N/A	
thelitis	675.04	675.02	675.00	N/A	
thrombocytopenia	666.34	666.32	666.30	N/A	
thrombophlebitis (superficial)	671.24	671.22	671.20	N/A	
deep	671.44	671.42	671.40	N/A	
pelvic	671.44	671.42	671.40	N/A	
specified site NEC	671.54	671.52	671.50	N/A	
uremia	669.34	669.32	669.30	N/A	
vaginitis (conditions classifiable to 616.1)	646.64	646.62	646.60	condition	
varicose veins (legs)	671.04	671.02	671.00	N/A	
vulva or perineum	671.14	671.12	671.10	N/A	
vulvitis (conditions classifiable to 616.1)	646.64	646.62	646.60	condition	
vulvovaginitis (conditions classifiable to 616.1)	646.64	646.62	646.60	condition	
white leg	671.44	671.42	671.40	N/A	
Prediabetes	648.84	648.82	648.80	condition	
Pre-eclampsia (mild)	642.44	642.42	642.40	N/A	760.0
with convulsions	642.64	642.62	642.60	N/A	760.0
severe	642.54	642.52	642.50	N/A	760.0
superimposed on pre-existing hypertensive disease	642.74	642.72	642.70	N/A	760.0
Pre-existing condition (prior to pregnancy) affecting current pregnancy					
abnormal glucose tolerance	648.84	648.82	648.80	condition	
anemia	648.24	648.22	648.20	condition	
bone and joint (lower limb)	648.74	648.72	648.70	condition	
cardiovascular	648.64	648.62	648.60	condition	
congenital	648.54	648.52	648.50	condition	
cerebrovascular	674.04	674.02	674.00	N/A	
diabetic	648.04	648.02	648.00	condition	
drug dependence	648.34	648.32	648.30	condition	
genital organ or tract	646.64	646.62	646.60	condition	
gonorrheal	647.14	647.12	647.10	condition	
hypertensive	642.24	642.22	642.20	N/A	
renal	642.14	642.12	642.10	N/A	
infectious	647.94	647.92	647.90	condition	
specified type NEC	647.84	647.82	647.80	condition	
malarial	647.44	647.42	647.40	condition	
nutritional deficiency	648.94	648.92	648.90	condition	
parasitic NEC	647.84	647.82	647.80	condition	
renal	646.24	646.22	646.20	condition	
hypertensive	642.14	642.12	642.10	N/A	
rubella	647.54	647.52	647.50	condition	
specified condition NEC	648.94	648.92	648.90	condition	
syphilitic	647.04	647.02	647.00	condition	
thyroid	648.14	648.12	648.10	condition	
tuberculous	647.34	647.32	647.30	condition	
urinary	646.64	646.62	646.60	condition	
venereal	647.24	647.22	647.20	condition	
viral NEC	647.64	647.62	647.60	condition	
Proteinuria (gestational)	646.24	646.22	646.20	condition	
with toxemia (mild) (pre-eclamptic)	642.44	642.42	642.40	N/A	760.0

Postpartum Pregnancy Table

Postpartum Pregnancy Condition or Complication; affecting management of mother	Postpartum condition or complication	Delivered with mention of postpartum complication	Unspecified episode of care	Assign additional code to describe the...	Affecting newborn (coded on the newborn chart only)
Proteinuria – *continued*					
with toxemia					
with convulsion	642.64	642.62	642.60	N/A	760.0
with pre-existing hypertension	642.74	642.72	642.70	N/A	760.0
severe	642.54	642.52	642.50	N/A	760.0
Pruritus, pruritic	646.84	646.82	646.80	condition	
Psychosis or psychoneurosis	648.44	648.42	648.40	condition	
Ptyalism	646.84	646.82	646.80	condition	
Pyelitis	646.64	646.62	646.60	condition	760.1
Pyrexia (of unknown origin) (PUO)					
postpartum	672.04	672.02	672.00	N/A	
Reaction obstetric anesthetic or analgesic NEC	668.94	668.92	668.90	N/A	763.5
Rectocele	654.44	654.42	654.40	N/A	763.1
Renal					
disease or failure NEC	646.24	646.22	646.20	condition	
with secondary hypertension	642.14	642.12	642.10	N/A	
hypertensive	642.24	642.22	642.20	N/A	
shutdown following labor and delivery	669.34	669.32	669.30	N/A	
Repair of pelvic floor, previous	654.44	654.42	654.40	N/A	763.89
Retention, retained					
decidua (following delivery) (fragments)	667.14	667.12	667.10	N/A	
with hemorrhage	666.24	666.22	666.20	N/A	
membranes (following delivery)	667.14	667.12	667.10	N/A	
with hemorrhage	666.24	666.22	666.20	N/A	
milk (postpartum)	676.24	676.22	676.20	N/A	
placenta (total) (without hemorrhage)	667.04	667.02	667.00	N/A	
with hemorrhage	666.04	666.02	666.00	N/A	
portions or fragments	667.14	667.12	667.10	N/A	
with hemorrhage	666.24	666.22	666.20	N/A	
secundines (following delivery)	667.14	667.12	667.10	N/A	
with hemorrhage	666.24	666.22	666.20	N/A	
complicating puerperium (delayed hemorrhage)	666.24	666.22	666.20	N/A	
Retinitis	646.84	646.82	646.80	condition	
Retraction					
nipple (postpartum)	676.04	676.02	676.00	N/A	
Retroversion, uterus	654.34	654.32	654.30	N/A	763.89
Rigid, rigidity					
cervix	654.64	654.62	654.60	N/A	763.89
pelvic floor	654.44	654.42	654.40	N/A	763.89
perineum or vulva	654.84	654.82	654.80	N/A	763.89
vagina	654.74	654.72	654.70	N/A	763.89
Rubella (German measles)	647.54	647.52	647.50	condition	760.2
Rupture					
abdominal viscera	665.54	N/A	665.50	N/A	
bladder (sphincter)	665.54	N/A	665.50	N/A	
cervix (uteri)	665.34	N/A	665.30	N/A	
pelvic floor	664.14	N/A	664.10	N/A	
perineum	664.44	N/A	664.40	N/A	
urethra	665.54	N/A	665.50	N/A	
vulva	664.04	N/A	664.00	N/A	
Sacculation	654.44	654.42	654.40	N/A	763.1
Salivation (excessive)	646.84	646.82	646.80	condition	
Salpingitis	646.64	646.62	646.60	condition	760.8
postpartum	670.04	670.02	670.00	N/A	
Salpingo-oophoritis	646.64	646.62	646.60	condition	760.8
postpartum	670.04	670.02	670.00	N/A	
Scar, scarring					
cervix	654.64	654.62	654.60	N/A	763.89
uterus NEC	654.94	654.92	654.90	N/A	763.89
Separation (obstetrical trauma)					
pubic bone	665.64	N/A	665.60	N/A	
symphysis pubis	665.64	N/A	665.60	N/A	
Sepsis, postpartum	670.04	670.02	670.00	N/A	
Septicemia	647.84	647.82	647.80	condition	771.81
postpartum	670.04	670.02	670.00	N/A	
Septum, vagina	654.74	654.72	654.70	N/A	763.89

Postpartum Pregnancy Condition or Complication; affecting management of mother	Postpartum condition or complication	Delivered with mention of postpartum complication	Unspecified episode of care	Assign additional code to describe the...	Affecting newborn (coded on the newborn chart only)
Shirodkar suture	654.54	654.52	654.50	N/A	
Shock					
complicating labor and delivery	669.14	669.12	669.10	N/A	
following labor and deliver	669.14	669.12	669.10	N/A	
Spasms					
uterus	646.84	646.82	646.80	condition	
Specified condition NEC	646.84	646.82	646.80	condition	
Stenosis (cicatricial)					
cervix, cervical (canal)	654.64	654.62	654.60	N/A	763.89
vagina	654.74	654.72	654.70	N/A	763.89
Stricture, cervix (canal)	654.64	654.62	654.60	N/A	763.89
Subinvolution of uterus (postpartum)	674.84	674.82	674.80	N/A	
Sudden death					
during childbirth	669.94	669.92	669.90	N/A	
postpartum	674.94	674.92	674.90	N/A	
Suppression of lactation	676.54	676.52	676.50	N/A	
Suppuration, suppurative of breast or mammary gland (postpartum)	675.14	675.12	675.10	N/A	
Surgery, previous					
cervix	654.64	654.62	654.60	N/A	763.89
pelvic soft tissues NEC	654.94	654.92	654.90	N/A	763.89
perineum or vulva	654.84	654.82	654.80	N/A	
uterus NEC	654.94	654.92	654.90	N/A	763.89
vagina	654.74	654.72	654.70	N/A	
Suspended uterus	654.44	654.42	654.40	N/A	763.89
Suture, Shirodkar (with or without cervical incompetence)	654.54	654.52	654.50	N/A	
Syncope complicating delivery	669.24	669.22	669.20	N/A	
Syndrome					
acid pulmonary aspiration (Mendelson's)	668.04	668.02	668.00	N/A	
Chiari-Frommel	676.64	676.62	676.60	N/A	
dystocia, dystrophia	654.94	654.92	654.90	N/A	
Frommel-Chiari	676.64	676.62	676.60	N/A	
H.E.L.L.P (Hemolysis, Elevated Liver function and Low Platelets)	642.54	642.52	642.50	N/A	
hepatorenal following delivery	674.84	674.82	674.80	N/A	
hypotension, maternal	669.24	669.22	669.20	N/A	
maternal hypotension	669.24	669.22	669.20	N/A	
Mendelson's (during labor) (obstetric)	668.04	668.02	668.00	N/A	
Syphilis	647.04	647.02	647.00	condition	760.2
Tear, torn					
anus, anal (sphincter),	664.24	N/A	664.20	N/A	763.89
with mucosa	664.34	N/A	664.30	N/A	763.89
bladder	665.54	N/A	665.50	N/A	763.89
bowel	665.54	N/A	665.50	N/A	763.89
broad ligament	665.54	N/A	665.50	N/A	763.89
cervix	665.34	N/A	665.30	N/A	763.89
pelvic					
floor	664.14	N/A	664.10	N/A	763.89
organ NEC	665.54	N/A	665.50	N/A	763.89
perineum	665.54	N/A	665.50	N/A	763.89
periurethral	665.54	N/A	665.50	N/A	763.89
urethra	665.54	N/A	665.50	N/A	
vulva	664.04	N/A	664.00	N/A	763.89
Tetanus, tetanic (puerperal, postpartum, childbirth)	670.04	670.02	670.00	N/A	
Thelitis (puerperal, postpartum)	675.04	675.02	675.00	N/A	
Thrombocytopenia (postpartum)	666.34	666.32	666.30	N/A	
Thrombophlebitis	671.24	671.22	671.20	N/A	760.3
cerebral (sinus) (vein), nonpyogenic	671.54	671.52	671.50	N/A	760.3
intracranial venous sinus, nonpyogenic	671.54	671.52	671.50	N/A	760.3
pelvic, postpartum	671.44	671.42	671.40	N/A	
specified site NEC	671.54	671.52	671.50	N/A	760.3
superficial	671.24	671.22	671.20	N/A	760.3

Postpartum Pregnancy Table

Postpartum Pregnancy Table

Postpartum Pregnancy Condition or Complication; affecting management of mother	Postpartum condition or complication	Delivered with mention of postpartum complication	Unspecified episode of care	Assign additional code to describe the...	Affecting newborn (coded on the newborn chart only)
Thrombosis	671.94	671.92	671.90	N/A	
brain (artery) (stem)	674.04	674.02	674.00	N/A	
intracranial, venous sinus (nonpyogenic origin)	671.54	671.52	671.50	N/A	
postpartum	671.94	671.92	671.90	N/A	
brain (artery) (stem)	674.04	674.02	674.00	N/A	
venous	671.54	671.52	671.50	N/A	760.3
cardiac	674.84	674.82	674.80	N/A	
cerebral (artery)	674.04	674.02	674.00	N/A	
venous	671.54	671.52	671.50	N/A	760.3
deep (vein)	671.44	671.42	671.40	N/A	
intracranial sinus (nonpyogenic) (venous)	671.54	671.52	671.50	N/A	760.3
pelvic	671.44	671.42	671.40	N/A	
pulmonary (artery)	673.24	673.22	673.20	N/A	
specified site NEC	671.54	671.52	671.50	N/A	
superficial	671.24	671.22	671.20	N/A	
spinal cord	671.54	671.52	671.50	N/A	
superficial	671.24	671.22	671.20	N/A	
venous (superficial)	671.24	671.22	671.20	N/A	
Thyroid dysfunction	648.14	648.12	648.10	condition	
Thyroiditis	648.14	648.12	648.10	condition	
Thyrotoxicosis	648.14	648.12	648.10	condition	
Torsion of uterus	654.44	654.42	654.40	N/A	
Toxemia (mild) (pre-eclamptic)	642.44	642.42	642.40	N/A	760.0
with				760.0	
convulsions	642.64	642.62	642.60	N/A	760.0
pre-existing hypertension	642.74	642.72	642.70	N/A	760.0
eclamptic	642.64	642.62	642.60	N/A	760.0
with pre-existing hypertension	642.74	642.72	642.70	N/A	760.0
severe	642.54	642.52	642.50	N/A	760.0
Trapped placenta (without hemorrhage)	666.04	666.02	666.00	N/A	
with hemorrhage	667.04	667.02	667.00	N/A	
Trauma	648.94	648.92	648.90	condition	
during delivery NEC	665.94	665.92	665.90	N/A	760.5
obstetrical	665.94	665.92	665.90	N/A	760.5
previous pregnancy (major), affecting childbirth or postpartum management	V23.89	V23.89	V23.89	N/A	
Tuberculosis	647.34	647.32	647.30	condition	760.2
Tumor					
cervix	654.64	654.62	654.60	N/A	763.89
ovary	654.44	654.42	654.40	N/A	763.89
pelvic	654.94	654.92	654.90	N/A	763.89
pelvic organs or tissue NEC	654.44	654.42	654.40	N/A	763.89
uterus	654.14	654.12	654.10	N/A	763.89
vagina	654.74	654.72	654.70	N/A	763.89
vulva	654.84	654.82	654.80	N/A	763.89
Uremia (renal disease or failure) NEC	646.24	646.22	646.20	condition	760.1
with secondary hypertension	642.14	642.12	642.10	N/A	760.0
complicating labor and delivery	669.34	669.32	669.30	N/A	
hypertensive	642.24	642.22	642.20	N/A	760.0
Urethritis	646.64	646.62	646.60	condition	760.1
Urinary Tract Infection	646.64	646.62	646.60	condition	760.1
UTI	646.64	646.62	646.60	condition	760.1
Vaginitis or vulvitis	646.64	646.62	646.60	condition	760.8
Valsuani's disease (progressive pernicious anemia, puerperal)	648.24	648.22	648.20	condition	
Varicose					
veins (legs)	671.04	671.02	671.00	N/A	
perineum	671.14	671.12	671.10	N/A	
vulva	671.14	671.12	671.10	N/A	
Varicosity, labia or vulva	671.14	671.12	671.10	N/A	
Varix (lower extremity)	671.04	671.02	671.00	N/A	
perineum	671.14	671.12	671.10	N/A	
vulva	671.14	671.12	671.10	N/A	
Venereal disease NEC	647.24	647.22	647.20	disease	
Viral disease NEC	647.64	647.62	647.60	disease	
Vulvitis	646.64	646.62	646.60	condition	760.8
Weight gain	646.14	646.12	646.10	condition	
insufficient	646.84	646.82	646.80	condition	
White leg, postpartum, childbirth	671.44	671.42	671.40	N/A	